Companion to Clinical Neurology
Second Edition

Companion to
Clinical Neurology

SECOND EDITION

WILLIAM PRYSE-PHILLIPS

MD, FRCP (Lond.), FRCP (C), DPM

Professor of Medicine (Neurology)
Memorial University
St. John's, Newfoundland, Canada

OXFORD

UNIVERSITY PRESS

2003

OXFORD
UNIVERSITY PRESS

Oxford   New York
Auckland   Bangkok   Buenos Aires   Cape Town   Chennai
Dar es Salaam   Delhi   Hong Kong   Istanbul   Karachi   Kolkata
Kuala Lumpur   Madrid   Melbourne   Mexico City   Mumbai
Nairobi   São Paulo   Shanghai   Taipei   Tokyo   Toronto

Library of Congress Cataloging-in-Publication Data
Pryse-Phillips, William.
Companion to clinical neurology /
William Pryse-Phillips.—2nd ed.
p. ; cm.   Includes bibliographical references.
ISBN 0-19-515938-1
1. Neurology—Dictionaries. I. Title.
[DNLM: 1. Neurology—Dictionary—English.
2. Nervous System Diseases—Dictionary—English.
Wl 13 P973c 2003]   RC334 .P79 2003   616.8'03—dc21   2002029294

2 4 6 8 9 7 5 3 1

Printed in the United States of America
on acid-free paper

Preface to the Second Edition

The kind comments of those who wrote reviews of the first edition of my *Companion* delighted me. I am particularly pleased that what was written originally for my own use as a practicing clinical neurologist was also found appropriate by so many of my colleagues and I was further honored when Japanese colleagues called for an edition in their own language.

The format of the book has not changed in this second edition. I have continued to list certain items twice if either of their two names seems likely to be the word or phrase that requires authentication, and have selected from some thousands of journal articles scanned only those definitions, criteria, or comments that were most meaningful to me. I have made comments that may not amuse the General Staff, but they come from where the action is: in the trenches.

Advances in neurology are occurring at least as fast as in any other area of medicine and I recognize that in the year between the delivery of my manuscript and its publication, new information will have been presented that will make some of my definitions passé. I ask the reader's forbearance. I also must restate the comment I made in preparing the first edition of my *Companion*: "I have aimed [only] for reasonable completeness," suitable for almost all (but of course not quite all) the situations that the clinical neurologist is likely to meet in which an authoritative definition is required. The decisions on what to include and to exclude were mine, based on my experience and my enthusiasms, so this is a very personal compilation, stemming from my insights (and sometimes probably the lack of them) into the neurology of today that rides upon yesterday's shoulders. I offer it with the hope that it will inform and occasionally divert my colleagues and that it will benefit their patients.

St. John's, Newfoundland   W.P-P.
Canada

Preface to the First Edition

A confused and equivocal terminology is the fruitful parent of confused and equivocal thinking.

—*Sir Francis Walshe, 1947*

One of the most difficult tasks for the beginning neurologist is that of understanding the jargon of the subject. It has been estimated that over 20,000 new words are learned or at least interpreted by a mature physician; a high percentage of them must be used in neurology. Not only derivations from Latin and Greek, but also eponymous disorders, names of chemicals, acronyms, neologisms, and pet-names spill repeatedly from neurologists' lips. Because they are not all widely known they often cloud meaning and impair communication although their original intent was to define, to categorize, or to distinguish concepts, clinical experience, or scientific truths.

Who were all these people whose names are attached to syndromes or diseases or tests? How do dysphagia and dysphasia differ? Why isn't Bell's phenomenon the same as Bell's palsy and why doesn't it involve the long thoracic nerve of Bell? Is there common ground in the definition of criteria for this or that condition? Such questions are naive to a neurologist, but need an answer when asked by students or by physicians who are not so trained, or by professional workers in allied disciplines.

Companion to Clinical Neurology is a personal endeavour to provide answers to questions like these. I have tried to incorporate within it some science, some art, some history, some practical experience. It is also a hive in which nest numerous bees formerly resident in my bonnet and which needed more *Lebensraum*. It is designed for the bedside and, I hope, for a reasonably low shelf in a room where a physician does his or her work. At least one reference is included for most of the entries delineating diseases, usually representing that publication on the subject which brought the material first to attention or one to which the interested reader may turn in order to receive more precise directions along the road to further knowledge; but in some instances it is to that paper on the subject which I enjoyed reading most.

The *Companion* is designed as a guide wherein the menu of neurological practice is laid out and from which suggestions for further reading may be obtained. I have assembled what I believe to be the best published definitions of neurological phenomena, and where none is available, have provided a brief description of my own. This is not a treatise on differential diagnosis; only, when a word or a phrase is encountered which is not fully understood. I trust that it will have been given a definition here, and in certain cases, some background to reinforce memorization.

My selection of items or names for inclusion has been on the basis of what problems I think a neurologist might expect to meet over the years of clinical practice. The major entry is in each case that name which I believe to be the one most commonly used, and therefore the most recognizable. Bracketed thereafter are synonyms also in recent use. Where words other than major entries are printed in boldface, this indicates that the item is itself a separate entry; italics indicate foreign words, emphasis, journals, or variants not entered elsewhere. Where two or more authors have given their names to a condition, the reference given is to that paper first appearing, or occasionally to that which corrected the errors of the first with such dexterity that the alternate eponym is preferable—as with Jakob and Creutzfeldt. However, where usage of the two (or three or, God help us, more) names has led to numerous variations depending on the order in which those names are placed, only that combination which seemed to me to be the most familiar has been included. The same restriction applies to the seemingly endless permutations of derived Latinisms, only a few of which appear. To save the bother of incessant turning of pages, brief summaries of some conditions are also included under their alternative names.

In this *Companion* I have aimed for reasonable completeness, but realize that neurology is too large a subject for one head to contain. Among the readers of this book there will be many with special knowledge which could lead to improvements upon some of the definitions that I have attempted here; their kind offers of contributions would be accepted with delight and acknowledged with gratitude.

W.P-P.

Foreword to the First Edition

In these days of publish-or-perish, novelty seldom rises above the flat sea of new reviews and books that simply confirm what's already well known. Dr. Pryse-Phillips, however, has chosen a new tack and, in the process, brought us an astonishingly large, clinically oriented compendium of things neurological. In form, *Companion to Clinical Neurology* takes its place alongside such source references as the renowned and informative *Oxford Companions*. Its contents describe at varying length but with great clarity the phenomenological world of clinical neurology from its hesitant beginning over a century ago to its current vigorous strength. Ranging between brief, identifying sentences defining minor neurological facts to longer descriptions about diseases and their classifications, Pryse-Phillips depicts or explains neurology's bygone leaders as well as its symptoms, signs, syndromes, diseases, eponyms, operative procedures, and diagnostic tests. In the breadth of its topics the book has a gently nostalgic, British-Continental flavor of a more relaxed scientific day. Nevertheless, it by no means ignores American sources or recent contributions, including genetic classifications.

Certain features stand out. The *Companion* gives special attention to the clinical expressions and electrophysiological mechanisms of the epilepsies. The text also interestingly and informatively reflects Pryse-Phillips' longstanding interest in neurology's cognitive and behavioral aspects. But these are just a few of its extraordinary riches. Did you, the reader, know that although Munchausen's syndrome was named by Ascher in 1951, the disorder's content had been described by Meige in his graduation thesis (Paris) in 1893? Or that the condition has three synonyms and three subsets? I didn't. Would you be surprised to find that ataxia has been defined in 41 different forms, or that it is included in 40 different identified syndromes? I was. These historic pearls and many others await the reader's eye, whether to entertain as nightly pre-sleep browsing or to act as a sourcebook from which to identify past foundations of tomorrow's neuroscience.

Companion to Clinical Neurology provides a remarkably thorough, pithy view of the world of clinical neurology and its close co-disciplines. With well over 15,000 entries and 5,000 references, it successfully reflects the prodigious (and nowadays rare) scholarship of its author. Within these pages the novitiate will discover the past richness of clinical neurology, and experienced neurologists will find informative explanations about all kinds of common and arcane aspects of their discipline's heritage.

In short, *Companion to Clinical Neurology* provides the best compact source I know in which one can quickly refresh one's memory about a fact well known or dig out a hitherto unknown item about the most philosophically and biologically interesting of all the medical specialties.

Fred Plum, M.D.

Acknowledgments

During the years that I wrote the first edition of this book, many people gave me help and advice. In particular I was fortunate in being able to access the private collection of medical biographies compiled by (the late) Mr. Austin Seckersen, formerly of the Bodleian Library at the University of Oxford. His generosity greatly speeded the completion of the work. The initial writing was done during a sabbatical year from Memorial University. I thank Lord Walton, then Warden of Green College, and Professor John Newsom-Davis of the University of Oxford for providing me with a visiting scholarship at Green College and with membership of the Department of Neurology.

Substantial assistance in the writing of the first edition was provided by Drs. Milton Alter, Peter Dunne, Roger Duvoisin, Joseph Foley, Anita Harding, Andrew Kertesz, Wayne Massey, David Neary, Charles Poser, R. Mark Sadler, Patrick Sweeney, P.K. Thomas, and James Woodrow. Mr. Theo Dunnett of the Bodleian Library provided skilled help without limit in the location and selection of sources, particularly in the production of the illustrations in this second edition.

The writing of this second edition was done during another sabbatical year from Memorial University and I thank Dr. Ian Bowmer, Dean of Medicine, for providing this essential opportunity. Huge assistance was lent by Dr. Heather Arnold, Dr. Bijal Mehta, and Dr. Scott Sloka in scrutinising the neurological papers published in English since the first edition, while they were studying medicine at Memorial. Many corrections and additions were suggested by Dr. Homer J. Moore, of San Diego, CA, to whom I offer my hearty thanks.

Items substantially contributed by others acknowledged here are followed by their initials in the text.

This compilation required the reproduction of items from some hundreds of individual sources, for which today fees are commonly required. I thank the American Academy of Sleep Medicine, the American Medical Association, the American Psychiatric Association, Blackwell Science, the British Medical Association, the Canadian Journal of Neurological Sciences, Elsevier Science, the United States Government, John Wiley and Sons Inc., and the World Health Organization in particular for waiving such fees; without their gracious support of an academic endeavor such as this, the book would have been impossible to produce.

The material from the American Association of Electrodiagnostic Medicine's Glossary of Terms in Electrodiagnostic Medicine © 2001 is used freely by kind permission of the AAEM (Nomenclature Committee: Lawrence H. Phillips II, M.D., Chair, Andrew J. Haig, M.D., William Litchy, M.D., Chair; Mark Hallett, M.D., Raymond G. Auger, M.D., Charles K. Jablecki, M.D., Ernest M. Baran, M.D., M.S.B.M.E., Dale J. Lange, M.D., Francis J. Bonner Jr., M.D., Janice M. Massey, M.D., M.E. Brandstater, M.B.B.S., Ph.D., FRCP, Lawrence R. Robinson, M.D., Daniel Dumitru, M.D., Ph.D., Margaret A. Turk, M.D., Bjorn Falck, M.D., Ph.D., Jacqueline J. Wertsch, M.D., Andrew J. Gitter, M.D., and Asa J. Wilbourn, M.D.). Again, I offer my sincere thanks.

The lines from "voices to voices, lip to lip" are reprinted as an *envoi* from *Complete Poems*, 1904–1962, by E. E. Cummings, edited by George J. Firmage, by permission of Liveright Publishing Corporation. Copyright © 1926, 1954, 1991 by the Trustees for the E. E. Cummings Trust. Copyright © 1985 by George James Firmage.

In some instances an original reference was not available to me; I acknowledge again with pleasure (and with admiration) the work of Dr. Michael Baraitser and Dr. Robin Winter and their colleagues that led to the publication of the Neurogenetic Database; this and the encyclopedic works of Dr. Victor McKusick and (through his superb website) Dr. Alan Pestronk provided me with data on and analyses of a number of disorders that I would have missed otherwise.

I am especially grateful to my new editor, Fiona Stevens, Nancy Wolitzer, Jerri Hurlbutt, and the Oxford University Press for their confidence in me and in my book and for their labors in making it as good as it could be.

And I thank my family, Gwyneth, Amy, and Sam for their continual support, and for understanding the realities of an academic life.

Companion to Clinical Neurology

AAA syndromes   See **Allgrove syndrome.**

A band   Dark, anisotropic thick filaments in muscle which with the I bands make up a myofibril. Upon them is a dark transverse M line surrounded by a lighter H-zone.

A pattern deviation   A nonparalytic form of horizontal strabismus or **tropia** in which the visual axes are directed to closer objects (**esotropia**) as the subject looks up or separate (**exotropia**) as the subject looks down. Thus the horizontal deviation of the visual axes varies with the vertical position of the eyes.[3330] See also **V pattern deviation**, which is the reverse of this.

A test   (Random Letter Test) A simple test of **vigilance** in which the examiner reads out a random series of letters, and the patient is required to tap on the table with a pencil whenever a specific letter such as *A* is spoken.

A wave   A compound muscle action potential that follows the **M wave,** evoked consistently from a muscle by submaximal electric stimuli and frequently abolished by supramaximal stimuli. Its amplitude is similar to that of an F wave, but the latency is more constant. The A wave usually occurs before the F wave, but may occur afterwards. It is thought to be due to extra discharges in the nerve, ephapses, or axonal branching. This term is preferred over *axon reflex, axon wave*, or *axon response*. Compare with the **F wave.**[10] (From the 2001 Report of the Nomenclature Committee of the American Association of Electromyography and Electrodiagnosis. Used by permission, copyright © 2001, AAEM.)

A₁, A₂ electrodes   The conventional terms in electroencephalography for recording electrodes placed respectively on the left and right ears.

A_c electrode   The conventional term in electroencephalography for a recording electrode placed on the contralateral ear with respect to any other electrode.

Aase-Smith syndrome   A congenital dysmorphic syndrome characterized by cardiac and skeletal abnormalities, adrenal tumors, **holoprosencephaly**, **Dandy-Walker malformation,** and hydrocephalus.[16]

AB variant   A form of gangliosidosis characterized by deficiency of GM₂ activator factor, leading to the accumulation of GM₂ ganglioside. See **GM₂ gangliosidosis.**

Abadie, Charles A.   (1842–1932) French ophthalmologist who practiced in Paris. He described alcohol injection of the Gasserian ganglion for **trigeminal neuralgia** as well as the **Abadie sign** (Dalrymple sign), retraction of the upper lid as a result of contraction of the levator palpebrae muscles in hyperthyroidism.[17]

Abadie, Jean-Louis-Irenée-Jean   (1873–1946) French neurologist and psychiatrist who graduated with a the-

sis on the internal capsule and who became professor of nervous and mental diseases in Bordeaux. He described the **Abadie sign** in 1905; his other publications dealt with such topics as hysterical polyuria, epilepsy, tabes, and diabetes insipidus.

Abadie sign   Loss of deep pain sensation, shown by insensibility to hard pressure upon the Achilles' tendon in patients with **tabes dorsalis;** it was said to have been the third most common sign in that condition. See also **Biernacki sign** and **Pitres sign,** each of which are also typically positive in tabes.

abasia   An inability to maintain an upright posture, as described with **astasia** by **Blocq** in patients with hysterical disorders.[606]

abasic gait apraxia   A syndrome resulting from small hemorrhages into the posterior internal capsule and/or putamen bilaterally, manifesting clinically as an inability to maintain the upright stance or to walk, although the muscle actions underlying these activities are unaffected when the subject makes the same movements while lying down.[5114]

ABC syndrome   (angry backfiring C nocioceptor syndrome) A fanciful term for what is likely to be the **complex regional pain syndrome.**

Abdallat neurocutaneous syndrome   A congenital dysmorphic syndrome characterized by patchy depigmentation of skin and hair, spasticity, and sensorimotor peripheral neuropathy.[337]

abdominal epilepsy   The occurrence of abdominal pain or vomiting as the sole or major manifestation of a partial seizure in children.[1503]

This nonconvulsive seizure disorder occurs principally in children and is characterized by brief attacks of borborygmi, vomiting, pallor or flushing of the face, perspiration, and severe colicky periumbilical pain, frequently associated with altered consciousness and brief and simple automatisms. Coexisting EEG abnormalities include bilateral spike-and-wave, polyspike-and-wave, low-voltage fast, and 10-Hz fast activity.[56]

abdominal migraine   Recurrent attacks of abdominal pain, vomiting, pallor, and sometimes fever in school-age children who have a family history of migraine and who, in many cases, later go on to develop more typical migrainous features.[359] The pain is usually a diffuse burning or aching in periumbilical or epigastric regions, and may have been preceded by well-recognized prodromal symptoms of migraine.

abdominal neuroblastoma   See **neuroblastoma.**

abdominal pain–nerve entrapment syndrome   Unilateral segmental pain felt in the abdominal wall and due to entrapment of cutaneous nerves as they pass through its muscular layer, usually at the outer border of the rectus sheath. The origin of the pain is localized to a point below the examining finger, and it is worsened by tensing the abdominal muscles, as with trunk flexion in the supine position.

abdominal paradox   Inward movement of the abdominal wall during inspiration, as seen in some cases of neuromuscular disease leading to ventilatory failure.

abdominal (muscle) reflex   Contraction of the rectus abdominis and other muscles of the abdominal wall in response to a tap on the muscle itself or at the upper or lower end of the rectus abdominis. The reflex is not always found in the normal subject, but may be increased in patients with pyramidal lesions above T6.

Numerous sites for the elicitation of the reflex have been described, including the rectus abdominis lateral to the umbilicus, the nipple, the symphysis pubis, the anterior superior iliac spine, the costal margin, or the thoracic wall. Another method described is to insert the finger into the umbilicus and to tap it.[3324]

abdominal (skin) reflex   Contraction of the muscles of the abdominal wall such that the umbilicus is drawn slightly towards the site of a gentle scratch of the overlying skin in any of the four quadrants. It was first described by Rosenbach in 1876.[3324]

This represents a spinal polysynaptic reflex that is normally present, but it may be absent in pyramidal lesions at sites above T6, and in multiple sclerosis, because of diminished excitability of the spinal reflex center.[3182] It is seldom present after pregnancies, in the very obese, and in those who have had numerous abdominal operations. When the cord lesion is at T10, the reflex will only be present over the upper half of the abdomen. Further localization of a spinal cord lesion according to the presence of the reflex in upper, middle, and lower abdominal regions is of more theoretical than practical value.

abdominal reflex dissociation   Augmentation of the **abdominal muscle reflex** with disappearance of the **abdominal skin reflex;** a sign of an upper motor neuron lesion above T6.[3324]

abducens   (Lat, to lead away from) The sixth cranial nerve, described by Eustachius in 1564, and so called because it supplies the lateral rectus muscle which draws the eye to the side, away from the midline.

abduction   The movement by which part of the body is drawn away from the sagittal line or a digit is drawn aside from the medial line of the hand. See also (ocular) **duction.**

abduction nystagmus   (ataxic nystagmus, internuclear ophthalmoplegia) A form of dissociated nystagmus in which the abnormal movement is seen in the abducting eye either exclusively or else far more obviously than in the other eye, which may fail to adduct normally. See **internuclear ophthalmoplegia.**

abductor digiti quinti sign   Slight abduction of the fifth finger on one side when patients with mild hemiparesis extend the arms out in front of them. When this is seen bilaterally, however, the sign has no significance.[128]

The phenomenon was noted by **Wartenberg,** but he ascribed it to cerebellar disease. The **Souques sign,** in which all the fingers are separated, is similar, as is the **pinky finger sign.**

abductor laryngeal paralysis   A dominantly inherited congenital syndrome manifesting as hoarse voice and dysphagia.[337]

Abercrombie, John   (1781–1844) Scottish physician who published the first book devoted to the neuropathology of both the central and the peripheral nervous systems, in which he classified three types of apoplexy (1828). He was also the first to describe **subdural empyema.**

Aberfeld syndrome   A recessively inherited syndrome of myotonia, dwarfism, multiple joint contractures, facial dysmorphism, blepharophimosis, poor muscle development, and bone disease, resembling **Morquio-Brailsford disease.**[24]

aberrant regeneration   The inappropriate redirection of fibers sprouting from a site of injury. This has been described most typically in compression of the third cranial nerve by an intracavernous meningioma. In this situation retraction of the upper eyelid on downward gaze or adduction of the eye, restricted upward movement of the globe, and impairment of the pupillary light response are found.[623]

abetalipoproteinemia   (Bassen-Kornzweig syndrome) A recessively inherited, progressive ataxic syndrome of early childhood, due to a deficiency of apoprotein B, which is an important factor in transporting lipids from the intestine to the plasma. The responsible gene is located on chromosome 2 at 2p24. The accompanying neuropathy is probably due to vitamin E deficiency.

Clinically, the disease resembles **Friedreich ataxia,** with cerebellar signs, ptosis, ophthalmoplegia, and sensorimotor neuropathy, but in addition pigmentary retinopathy and steatorrhea are found, low-density lipoproteins are absent from the plasma, triglyceride and cholesterol levels and chylomicron counts are low, and acanthocytes are found in fresh smears.[2439] See also **cerebellar ataxias** (*variants*).

abiotrophic dementia   See **Creutzfeldt-Jakob disease.**

abiotrophy   (Gr, lack of + organism + turn) Derived by Sir William **Gowers,** this term signifies the cessation of growth of an organ. It is used to label a process whereby the previously normal metabolism of certain cell lines ceases, frequently as an age-related process. The word was first used by Gowers in his discussion of the spinocerebellar degenerations.

Diseases labeled abiotrophic include Huntington chorea, adult-onset acid maltase deficiency, Parkinson disease, amyotrophic lateral sclerosis, and many more, but as the infective, genetic, or other etiologies of neurological diseases are progressively discovered, the blanket term seems to have less and less usefulness. Probably the last condition to warrant the name of abiotrophy will be such age-related changes as cortical cell loss producing memory impairment.

able autism See **Asperger syndrome.**

ablepharon Absence of the eyelids. In the most severe form, the skin of the forehead and the skin of the face are fused but the condition may be incomplete or unilateral. Autosomal recessive inheritance has been shown in many cases.

abluminal Outside the lumen of a vessel, such as a blood vessel.

abnormal illness behavior See **hysteria.**

abnormal involuntary movement scale A five-point scale for the evaluation of abnormal involuntary movements affecting the face and mouth, the extremities, and the trunk, with an added global judgement of severity.

The assessment is based upon a formal examination in which subjects remove their shoes and socks and sit with their legs apart, their feet flat on the floor and their hands on their knees or hanging unsupported. Opening of the mouth; protrusion of the tongue; tapping the thumb with each finger as fast as possible; standing; extending both arms in front; walking; and alternate flexion and extension of the arms are then observed and the abnormalities rated between 0 (none, normal) and 4 (severe). The muscles of facial expression, lips and perioral regions, jaw, tongue, upper and lower limbs, and trunk are examined separately, and a global assessment is made of the severity of any abnormal movements and of the incapacity which they induce.[4541]

abnormal swallowing syndrome Brief awakenings from normal sleep as a result of aspiration of normal secretions that have not been swallowed efficiently, leading to choking and coughing[2323] (see also **sleep disorders**[234]).

abortive disseminated encephalitis (Redlich encephalitis) See **encephalitis lethargica.**

abscess, cerebral A circumscribed collection of pus. The first accurate account of the phenomenon was that of Hermann Lebert (1813–1878), a French physician, in 1856, although Sauveur Morand (1697–1773), a French surgeon, is credited with a successful drainage procedure for temporosphenoidal abscess in 1752.[4979] MacEwen performed the first modern procedure.[3548] An historical review was published by Garfield.[2029] See also **epidural abscess**, **spinal subdural abscess.**

absence epilepsy (petit mal epilepsy, centrencephalic epilepsy, minor motor seizures, myoclonic-astatic seizures, myokinetic epilepsy, typical absence attacks, pyknolepsy) A seizure disorder in which the seizures consist typically of frequent brief (2–15 seconds) alterations in consciousness without motor accompaniments apart from fluttering of the eyelids, automatisms, or association with myoclonic or atonic seizures (*complex absences*). In all cases there is an immediate return to normal activity and mentation at the end of the attack. In *simple absence attacks*, there is only impairment of consciousness, although simple and limited motor activity such as eyelid fluttering may occur. A hereditary tendency is notable in some families.[3515]

The following diagnostic criteria of the ILAE have been reviewed:[679]

1. A form of epilepsy with onset before puberty (childhood AE), or before age 17 years (juvenile AE)
2. Occurring in previously mentally and neurologically normal children
3. Absences are the initial type of seizures
4. Very frequent absence seizures of any kind occur, except myoclonic absences
5. Absence seizures are associated on the EEG with bilateral, symmetric, and synchronous discharge of regular 3/second spike-and-wave complexes on a normal background activity. Less regular spike–wave activity is possible, when compatible with a diagnosis of typical absences.

Typical and atypical forms are recognized. In the *typical form*, the clinical manifestations are as above, and the EEG shows generalized, synchronous, symmetrical 2.5-Hz (or more) spike-and-wave or multiple spike-and-wave activity. In the *atypical form* (see **atypical absences**), such activity is at <2.5 Hz or is >2.5 Hz but with irregular frequency or asymmetrical voltage; clinically the duration is greater, and abnormal interictal records, multiple seizure types including myoclonus and loss of postural tone, mental retardation, and developmental delay are all more common while automatisms are less so. Substantial overlap occurs between the two varieties.

In further *variant forms*, myoclonic jerks, versive movements, or atonic periods are associated, in which case the tendency for the typical or complex absence attacks to cease at puberty is not manifest. Generalized tonic-clonic seizures may also occur in patients with typical absence attacks,[2631] as may myoclonus.

The term was first employed to describe temporary mental confusion by Louis-Florentin Calmeil (1798–1895), a French physician, in his graduate thesis on epilepsy.

absence seizures Generalized nonconvulsive epileptic seizures expressed mainly by disturbances of consciousness with little if any motor activity. Typical absence seizures are characterized by symmetrical and synchronous 3-Hz spike–wave complexes; atypical absences are associated with other EEG patterns including spike–wave complexes at slower rates, small-amplitude fast activity, or rhythmic, high-voltage 10-Hz activity.[1694]

absence status (petit mal status, spike–wave stupor, non-convulsive status, minor status) An epileptic syndrome characterized by clouding of consciousness, apathy, or stupor with fluctuating confusion, interspersed with atonic or myoclonic head nods, fluttering of the eyelids, or slight erratic myoclonus of the face or segments of the limbs, lasting from hours to days. These behavioral changes are accompanied by generalized continuous or near-continuous EEG abnormalities, usually comprising complexes of spikes and slow waves occurring at 3 Hz (2.5–6 Hz) and representing a change from the usual interictal EEG pattern. Incoordination resembling that of cerebellar ataxia may also occur. The condition is usually found in subjects with preexisting generalized epileptic syndromes, such as the **Lennox-Gastaut syndrome.** See also **twilight states, status epilepticus, complex partial status.**

In a *variant form*, similar features appear in adults without any preexisting seizure disorder, who show rhythmic irregular spike–wave discharges on the EEG.[5542]

absent muscles The congenital absence of certain muscles such as the pectoralis, serratus anterior, latissimus dorsi, trapezius, supraspinatus, or thenar muscles.

The more usual occurrence of deficiency in the right rather than the left pectoralis is unexplained. See **Souques syndrome.**

absolute refractory period That interval following depolarization of a nerve or muscle during which it cannot be excited by further stimuli.

abstraction ability The ability to discern the meaning or significance of ideas. The ability to think in nonrepresentative rather than in concrete terms, to form concepts, use categories, generalize from a single instance, apply procedural rules, and distinguish the properties of a part from the mass of the whole.

Abul Quasim Arabian physician of the tenth century, whose writings contained the first known account of **experiential hallucinations** in epilepsy.

abulia (Gr, without + will) A state in which the patient manifests lack of initiative and spontaneity, with preserved consciousness. An apathetic blunting of feeling, drive, mentation, and behavior such that all actions are performed slowly after a delay.

Clinically, it is a sign of lesions such as a tumor affecting the under side of the frontal lobes, bilateral lacunar strokes, or **normal pressure hydrocephalus.**[3852]

Academy of Neurological and Orthopedic Medicine and Surgery A professional society. Address: 522 Rossmore Drive, Las Vegas, NV 89110. Tel: 702-452-9538.

acalculia Difficulties in calculating, with or without problems in the identification and naming of printed figures, but usually accompanied by inability to copy (**acopia**). The condition was described and named by Henschen in 1919. Lesions of the dominant frontal or parieto-occipital lobes are responsible. Hécaen[2505] defined three forms:

Aphasic acalculia Impaired comprehension and writing of numbers due to a lesion of the dominant hemisphere.

Visuospatial acalculia Defective alignment of numbers and of arithmetic grammar, yet normal comprehension of the numbers themselves.

Anarithmic acalculia An inability to comprehend numeration and the principles of mathematics, often accompanied by other evidence of dominant hemisphere lesions. See also **anarithmia.**

acanthamoebocytosis Infection with *Acanthamoeba polyphaga*, usually acquired from swimming in infected pools. The neurological complications include meningoencephalitis.

acanthocytes (Gr, thorn + cells) Red cells with a spiky outline, seen only in fresh blood smear preparations.

acanthocytosis The presence of **acanthocytes** (spiky red cells) in the blood; a finding in **abetalipoproteinemia, familial hypobetalipoproteinemia, amyotrophic chorea with acanthocytosis, HARP syndrome, Hallervorden-Spatz disease, mitochondrial cytopathies, Wolman disease,** and the **McLeod phenotype.**[2435,5350] See **neuroacanthocytosis.**

acatalasemia A **peroxisomal disorder** without neurological features.

acataposis (Gr, not + to swallow) Dysphagia.

acceleration injury An injury resulting from sudden movement of the head and neck in relation to the rest of the body. The older term, *whiplash*, though more evocative to a jury, has now been superseded.

acceleration injury syndrome An alleged posttraumatic syndrome of persistent neck pain, headache, dizziness and disequilibration, impaired concentration, irritability, and emotional lability following such an injury, usually caused by a motor vehicle accident. The underlying pathology, if any, is not determined.

accelerator nerves The sympathetic nerves to the heart.

accessory nerve The eleventh cranial nerve, so named by Thomas **Willis** in his *Cerebri Anatome* (1664) because he realized that it receives additional fibers from the C2–3 spinal roots.

accessory nerve palsy A focal motor neuropathy causing weakness and wasting of the sternomastoid and/or trapezius muscles.

The most common cause is surgical trauma at the time of lymph node biopsy; blunt trauma is etiologically less common.[523]

accident neurosis See **disability neurosis.**

accommodation   1. In neuronal physiology, a rise in the threshold transmembrane depolarization required to initiate a spike, when depolarization is slow or a subthreshold depolarization is maintained. In the older literature, the observation that the final intensity of current applied in a slowly rising fashion to stimulate a nerve was greater than the intensity of a pulse of current required to stimulate the same nerve. The latter may largely be an artifact of the nerve sheath and bears little relation to true accommodation as measured intracellularly. (From the 2001 Report of the Nomenclature Committee of the American Association of Electromyography and Electrodiagnosis.[10] Used by permission, copyright © 2001, AAEM.)

2. In the older literature, *accommodation* was used to describe the observation that the final intensity of current applied in a slowly rising fashion to stimulate a nerve was greater than the intensity of a pulse of current required to stimulate the same nerve. The latter may largely be an artifact of the nerve sheath and bears little relation to true accommodation as measured intracellularly.

3. (ocular) The process whereby the lens changes its shape to refract more, and the pupil constricts as the eyes converge, in order to improve the focusing of objects at a short range. Retinal blur is diminished and, as in the case of cameras, the smaller aperture improves the depth of focus. The power of accommodation decreases with age because of decreased power of the ciliary muscle and decreased elasticity of the lens. The phenomenon was first described by Thomas Young (1773–1829), an English physician, at the age of 20.

accommodation curve   See **strength–duration curve.**

accommodative effort syndrome   Blurring of images with persisting near fixation, due to impaired ocular divergence with a normal near point for accommodation and convergence, and with an **esophoria** during near vision, which is relieved by plus lenses.[4605]

accommodative insufficiency   Impairment of accommodation for near vision, as a result of congenital or of acquired causes, the latter including disorders both of the eye and of the central and peripheral nervous systems and muscles.

acephalgic migraine   (migraine equivalent) The occurrence of a migraine aura without the succeeding headache, more commonly seen in patients of advanced age. Symptoms of cortical or brainstem dysfunction occur, with gradual onset, and are less than an hour in duration. In childhood, occipital seizures may cause the same symptoms. See also **migraine without aura.** A familial form has been described.[5125]

aceruloplasminemia   A recessively inherited syndrome affecting iron metabolism manifesting cerebellar ataxia, early dementia, involuntary movements, reti-nal dystrophy, and diabetes, and with absence of ceruloplasmin in the plasma.[3457]

acervuli   See **psammoma bodies.**

acesis   (from Gr, to heal) A cure.

acetylcholine   Acetyl trimethyl-β-acetyl-ethylammonium hydroxide, a transmitter substance liberated from terminals of the vagus nerve (Otto Loewi, 1921), from parasympathetic synapses, and from motor nerve endings (Sir Henry Dale, 1933, 1936).

acetylcholine deficiency   A variant syndrome of childhood **myasthenia gravis,** in which a deficiency of acetylcholine at the nerve terminals is due to a defect in resynthesis at that site.[2469]

acetylcholine receptor deficiency   A recessively inherited myasthenia-like syndrome characterized by a marked deficiency of acetylcholine receptors and presenting clinically as bulbar, limb, and ocular muscle weakness from infancy and electrically marked by small, miniature end-plate potentials.[1202]

acetylcholinesterase deficiency   A rare variant syndrome of infantile **myasthenia gravis** in which the acetylcholine is not hydrolyzed after its release at the end plate, leading to prolonged depolarization and repetitive potentials following a single stimulus.[1668]

The clinical features resemble those of other forms of myasthenia, with weakness and fatigability of the bulbar, extraocular, and spinal musculature, but EMG studies reveal repetitive muscle action potentials in response to single nerve stimulation as well as the usual decrementing response to repetitive stimuli.

achalasia   Failure of relaxation of any kind of hollow tube, as in the case of degeneration of Auerbach's plexus in the esophagus, which leads to impaired esophageal contractions presenting clinically as dysphagia or vomiting. The condition usually occurs in infancy.[3904]

achalasia and microcephaly   A congenital syndrome characterized by this disorder of esophageal motility, with accompanying microcephaly and mental and developmental delay.[337]

Achard-Foix-Mouzon syndrome   Reduction of the number of lumbar or sacrococcygeal vertebrae, usually associated with a **conus medullaris syndrome** and sometimes causing leg weakness as well.[30]

achee   See **akee.**

Achilles reflex   (triceps surae reflex) The ankle jerk.

Achilles tendon   The gastrocnemius tendon inserting into the calcaneum, so named because of the association with Achilles' heel.

The fable underlying the nomenclature is that the mother of this Greek hero held him by the heel when dipping him into the river Styx, a procedure conferring invulnerability to all those parts touched by the water.

The heel was not protected and it was a wound to this region delivered by his enemy Paris that killed him. In these days of flourishing neuromythology, it is unwise to scoff at this kind of story.

Achillodynia (Albert disease, Swediaur disease) Pain in the heel due to Achilles tendonitis. It was first described in 1893 by Edward Albert (1841–1900), an Austrian surgeon.[4979]

achondroplasia A craniofacial dysplasia in which the formation of enchondral bone is also deficient. The condition is dominantly inherited in 20% of cases. The major clinical features are facial dysmorphism, dwarfism, tripod hands, and lumbar lordosis. See also **Jeune syndrome** and **Ellis-van Creveld syndrome,** which are similar.

The condition was described by Parrot in 1878 and in greater detail by Pierre **Marie** in 1880.

ACHOO See **photic sneeze reflex.**

Achor-Smith syndrome A syndrome of acute skeletal muscle degeneration with profound weakness in the setting of prolonged nutritional deficiency with features of pernicious anemia, sprue, and pellagra, complicated by acute diarrhea resulting in hypokalemia and severe renal insufficiency.

achromasia (Gr, lack of + color) The impaired uptake of chemical stains by cells undergoing chromatolysis.

achromatic Having or producing no color; a term applied to those lenses which cause no color dispersion.

achromatopsia (Gr, lack of + color + eyesight) (color blindness, cortical or central achromatopsia) An acquired disorder of color perception involving all or part of the visual field, with preservation of vision for form. The retinal color receptors are not affected. The condition is frequently associated with visual agnosia and with a field defect. It is caused by focal damage to the visual association cortex or its subjacent white matter.[1260] See also **dyschromatopsia, cone dystrophy.**

In a *variant form*, the same problem is inherited as a sex-linked deficit.

acid albumen turbidity test A screening test for the detection of mucopolysaccharides in blood or urine.

acid maltase (D-1,4- and D-1,6-glucosidase) A lysosomal enzyme which hydrolyzes glycogen, maltose, and other oligosaccharides to yield free glucose.

acid maltase deficiency See **glycogen storage diseases.**

acid phosphatase deficiency A recessively inherited syndrome of intermittent vomiting, hypotonia, lethargy, opisthotonus, and death in early infancy due to deficiency of lysosomal acid phosphatase.[4057]

acidemia See **organic acidemia.**

Ackerman's angle A measurement at the skull base, considered characteristic in encephalocele and hydrocephalus but not now in use. It was described in 1882 by Konrad Ackerman (1825–1896), a German pathologist who was a professor at Rostock.

acne fulminans with inflammatory myopathy A syndrome characterized by the sudden onset of severe ulcerative acne of the chest, back, and face, associated with fever and leukocytosis and accompanied by pain in the pelvic girdle muscles with wasting, myalgia, and arthralgia but with normal serum creatine kinase levels.[4169]

acopia Difficulty in making a copy on paper from a printed or written text, regardless of whether reading is affected or not.

acoria (aplestia) Inability to attain satiety after eating.

Acosta disease See **acute mountain sickness.**

acoustic EMG (AMG; acoustic myography) A record of the sounds emitted by muscles during their contraction as a result of mechanical vibrations set up within the muscle. The mean frequency of the sounds increases in parallel with the contractile force derived. The technique is used in monitoring fatigue and force of contraction, and in the control of prosthetic devices.[10,375]

acoustic myography See **acoustic EMG.**

acoustic neuroma A benign tumor of the vestibular portion of the eighth cranial nerve, and actually a schwannoma. It was first described by **Cushing** in 1917[1229] and accounts for 5%–10% of all intracranial tumors.

Clinically, hearing loss, tinnitus, and dysequilibrium lead to headache, incoordination and imbalance, involvement of adjacent cranial nerves, and eventually symptoms of increased intracranial pressure and bulbar symptoms. The use of **computerized axial tomography, magnetic resonance imaging,** and **brainstem auditory evoked responses** in the diagnosis of the condition has been reviewed.[2467]

Acoustic Neuroma Association A charitable organization in this field. Address: 600 Peachtree Parkway, Suite 108, Cumming, GA 30041. E-mail: anausa@aol.com. Web site: http://www.anausa.org.

Acoustic Neuroma Association of Canada A charitable organization. Address: PO Box 369, Edmonton, Alberta, Canada T5J 2J6. Tel: (403) 428-3384. Web site: http://www.anac.ca.

acoustic reflex Contraction of the stapedius muscles bilaterally in response to a loud sound, recorded by measuring the acoustic impedance in the ear. The quietest sound producing such a contraction is known as the *acoustic threshold*; it is elevated in lesions of the cochlear nerve, but also with seventh cranial nerve or middle ear disease.

acoustic startle reflex   Violent muscle jerks following an unexpected sound stimulus, as in **stiff person syndrome** and **hyperekplexia.**

acoustic threshold   See **acoustic reflex.**

acousticomotor seizures   See **startle epilepsy.**

acousticopalpebral reflex   See **palpebral reflex.**

acquired central alveolar hypoventilation   A syndrome of hypoventilation occurring during sleep, typically related to bilateral posterolateral medullary lesions, which are most often vascular occlusions.[1423]

acquired epileptic aphasia   See **Landau-Kleffner syndrome.**

acquired fixation nystagmus   See **acquired nystagmus, fixation nystagmus.**

acquired hepatocerebral encephalopathy   (portosystemic shunt encephalopathy, non-Wilsonian hepatocerebral degeneration) A cerebral degenerative disease complicating chronic liver failure and producing a syndrome of drowsiness, impaired memory, ataxia, dysarthria, asterixis, choreoathetosis, and progressive dementia. The pathological hallmarks of the disorder are the presence of plump (Alzheimer type II) astrocytes in the striatum, cortex, and dentate nucleus and of spongy changes in the third cerebral cortical layer in laminar distribution.

The condition was described by Victor and Adams in 1965, although F. Morel had noted a similar condition in 1939.[3971]

A *variant condition* is *early childhood hepatocerebral degeneration*, in which progressive liver disease (the Huttenlocher variant of **Alpers disease**) and brain disease are manifest by recurrent partial, secondarily generalized seizures followed by mental and motor regression. The liver disease is exacerbated by valproic acid administration.[549]

In another *variant form*, the clinical appearances are those of **Wilson disease** but the metabolic disorder affecting copper is distinct.[2146] See also **non-Wilsonian extrapyramidal disease.**

acquired horizontal jerk nystagmus   The most common form of acquired nystagmus, subdivided between **vestibular** and **gaze-evoked** or **gaze-paretic** forms.

acquired immunodeficiency syndrome (AIDS)   Infection with the human immunodeficiency virus (HIV), a lentivirus that causes systemic and neurological disease, the latter by primary infection, malignancy, or through opportunistic infection. The various neurological syndromes produced have been classified:[3728,5662]

Chart A–1. Neurological Complications of Acquired Immunodeficiency Syndrome

Opportunistic Infection

CNS toxoplasmosis
Cryptococcal meningitis
Progressive multifocal leukoencephalopathy
Herpesvirus infections

Malignancy

Primary CNS lymphoma
Systemic lymphoma

Primary Infection

AIDS-related dementia (see HIV encephalopathy)
HIV encephalopathy
HIV myelopathy
Acute atypical meningitis
Acute sensory neuropathy
AIDS radiculopathy

See also **HIV-associated** conditions.

acquired inflammatory demyelinating polyneuropathies   Inflammatory demyelinating diseases of the peripheral nerves and nerve roots, often with extensive secondary axonal degeneration and resulting from immunological disturbances. Acute (**acute inflammatory demyelinating polyneuropathy**), chronic (**chronic inflammatory demyelinating polyneuropathy**), and dysproteinemic or paraneoplastic (**gammopathic neuropathy**) forms are described.[77]

acquired mutism   A condition of complete absence of speech that is not associated with other aphasic symptomatology or alteration of consciousness. See **mutism, cerebellar mutism.**

acquired myotonia   See **idiopathic neuromyotonia.**

acquired pendular nystagmus   A rare form of horizontal, vertical, or rotatory nystagmus in which the phases are similar in duration in each direction, as a result of which there is no "jerk" component. It leads to complaints of burred vision with oscillopsia and is often associated with a head tremor. The usual causes are cerebellar or brainstem disease, most likely due to vascular or demyelinating pathologies.[2278] It is also a feature of the syndrome of oculopalatal myoclonus.[272]

acquired slow-channel syndrome   See **myasthenia gravis.**

acquired verbal–auditory agnosia with convulsive disorder   See **Landau-Kleffner syndrome.**

acrocallosal syndrome   (Nelson syndrome, Schinzel syndrome) A dysmorphic syndrome characterized by unusual facial appearance, mental retardation, absent corpus callosum, duplication of the halluces, and mental retardation.[4097] Macrocephaly and clinodactyly are also common, and hyperreflexia with hypotonia is usual.[4970]

acrocephalopolysyndactyly   The combination of cranial vault abnormality with polysyndactyly. At least four forms are differentiated:[335]

Type I (**Noack syndrome, Pfeiffer syndrome**) A (dominantly inherited?) syndrome of acrocephaly, large toes with syndactyly, and brachydactyly of the toes and sometimes of the fingers.

Type II (**Carpenter syndrome**) The combination of acrocephaly, polysyndactyly, short stature, obesity, mental retardation (usually), and congenital cardiac defects.[4731]

Type III The combination of acrocephaly, syndactyly of fingers and toes, and other skeletal abnormalities.[4882]

Type IV A congenital dysmorphic syndrome characterized by acrocephalopolysyndactyly, and craniosynostosis.[335]

Hootnick-Holmes syndrome is a further *variant form* characterized by webbed fingers, polysyndactyly and craniostenosis.[2641]

See also **acrocephalosyndactyly, Apert syndrome.**

acrocephalosyndactyly Dominantly inherited syndromes characterized by the occurrence of both tower skull and fusion of digits. The distinction between some of the syndromes that follow may be artificial.[335]

Type I See **Apert syndrome.**

Type II Probably the same as **Apert syndrome.**

Type III (**Saethre-Chozen syndrome**) A congenital dysmorphic syndrome characterized also by low frontal hairline, ptosis, facial asymmetry, and soft tissue syndactyly of the hands.[544]

Type IV (**Waardenburg syndrome**) A rare congenital dysmorphic syndrome characterized by genital, digital, and cardiac anomalies, acrocephaly, and craniosynostosis.[5522]

Type V (**Pfeiffer syndrome**) A rare congenital dysmorphic syndrome characterized by acrocephaly, hypertelorism with normal intelligence, and soft tissue syndactyly of the hands.[3661] See **Pfeiffer syndrome.**

Other *variants* without CNS findings are recorded.[335] See also **Carpenter syndrome.**

acrocephaly (Gr, pointed + head) A developmental defect in skull shape such that the anteroposterior diameter is reduced, the occiput is flattened, and the forehead is high, as with fusion of both of the coronal or of all the cranial sutures. See also **Crouzon syndrome.**

acrodermatitis chronica atrophicans (Hopf syndrome) A chronically progressive dermatological disease of young adults, probably of spirochetal origin and tickborne, leading to widespread livid blue-red discoloration of the skin and later dermal atrophy.[2644] It is often complicated by an asymmetric sensory polyneuropathy.[4169]

acrodermatitis enteropathica See **subacute myelo-opticoneuropathy.**

acrodynia (Gr, the extremities + pain) 1. See **Pink disease.** 2. The distal limb pain felt in nutritional neuropathies and in ergotism. The term is now seldom used.

acrodysostosis A congenital dysmorphic syndrome characterized by short stature, psychomotor retardation, brachycephaly, thick calvarium, and hydrocephalus.[5188]

acrodystrophic neuropathy A sensory neuropathy causing painless plantar ulcers or trophic changes, often with destruction of the bones, hands, and feet.

In this group are the **hereditary sensory and autonomic neuropathies** and some acquired neuropathies such as those due to **leprosy, diabetes,** and alcoholism.[4878]

acrofacial dysostosis See **orofaciodigital syndrome 2.**

acrofacial syndrome See **fetal hydantoin syndrome.**

acromegalic myopathy A syndrome of mild proximal muscle weakness with elevated levels of serum creatine kinase and associated with hypertrophy of both type 1 and type 2 muscle fibers in patchy distribution,[3685] sometimes seen in this condition of excess growth hormone production.

In a *variant form*, muscle hypertrophy is the only abnormality.

acromegalic neuropathy An uncommon, severe, debilitating, progressive peripheral neuropathy complicating hypothyroidism, with marked enlargement of the peripheral nerves and characterized by endoneurial hypertrophy and axonal degeneration.[5351] Features of the **carpal tunnel syndrome** may be the earliest presentation.

acromial reflex Flexion of the elbow in response to a tap on the coracoid or the acromion, present in upper motor neuron lesions affecting that limb[4723] and probably resulting from transmitted vibrations rather than from direct stretch of any tendon.

acromicria A skeletal deformity appearing in many congenital syndromes, characterized by smallness of the extremities.

acro-osteolysis with osteoporosis See **osteopetrosis.**

acroparesthesia Tingling sensations in the distal parts of the limbs, the classic complaint of people with **carpal tunnel syndrome,** but also voiced by some with sensory polyneuropathies.

acroparesthesia syndrome See **carpal tunnel syndrome.**

acropathy Disfiguring damage sustained by the most distal parts of the body—the digits, ears, and nose, for example. This is seen in many mutilating sensory neuropathies[5534] such as **hereditary sensory and autonomic neuropathies** and **leprosy,** as well as with cord lesions interrupting pain pathways, such as **syringomyelia.**

acrus The term of Hippocrates for the state of the body when it is at the height of its well-being.

acrylamide An industrial polymer used to form slurries, which is toxic to axons since it impairs the process of fast (bidirectional) axonal transport, leading to **dying-back neuropathies.**

Acta Neurochiurgica A neurosurgical journal. Web site: http://link.springer.de/link/service/journals/00701/about.htm.

Acta Neurologica Belgica   (*Acta Neurol. Belg.*) A neurological journal. Address: Association des Sociétés Scientifiques Medicales Belgiques, 43 rue des Champs Elyssées, B-1050 Brussels, Belgium. Web site: http://www.ulb.ac.be/medecine/loce/Acta_Medica_Belgica/journal/Acta_Neurologica_Belgica.htm

Acta Neurologica Scandinavica (*Acta Neurol. Scand.*) A neurological journal published by Blackwell/Munksgaard. Web site: www/blackwellmunksgaard.com/actaneurologica.

Acta Neuropathologica   A neuropathological journal. Web site: http://link.springer.de/link/service/journals/00401/index.htm.

actin   A structural protein in vertebrate muscles.

action myoclonus   (intention myoclonus) Brief, sudden, arrhythmic, fine, or coarse myoclonic jerks followed by a period of inhibition, excited by willed movements and startle, affecting variable muscle groups but usually those activated voluntarily and leading to fragmentation of contraction. It is the characteristic finding in the **Lance-Adams syndrome.**[3240] See also **myoclonus.**

action myoclonus–renal failure syndrome   A recessively inherited syndrome characterized by severe progressive action myoclonus, finger tremor, ataxia, dysarthria, seizures, and renal failure requiring transplantation by the third decade, but without mental involvement.[166]

action myotonia   Delayed muscle relaxation following voluntary contraction of the muscle.

action potential (AP)   The brief regenerative electric potential that propagates along a single axon or muscle fiber membrane. An all-or-none phenomenon; whenever the stimulus is at or above threshold, the action potential generated has a constant size and configuration. See also **compound action potential, motor unit action potential.** (From the 2001 Report of the Nomenclature Committee of the American Association of Electromyography and Electrodiagnosis.[10] Used by permission, copyright © 2001, AAEM.)

action tremor   1. Physiological tremor accentuated by muscle contraction, as seen both in normal subjects and in those with **Parkinson disease.** 2. Any tremor or voluntary contraction of muscles, including postural, kinetic, and isometric tremors.[1422] See also **cerebellar tremors.**

activated protein C resistance factor   (Leiden) A dominantly inherited disorder resulting in an increased liability to stroke and due to a mutation at 1q23.

activation   1. In physiology, a general term for the initiation of a process. 2. The process of motor unit action potential firing. The force of muscle contraction is determined by the number of motor units and their firing rate. (From the 2001 Report of the Nomenclature Committee of the American Association of Elec-

tromyography and Electrodiagnosis.[10] Used by permission, copyright © 2001, AAEM.)

activation procedure   A technique used to detect defects of neuromuscular transmission during repetitive nerve stimulation testing. Most commonly a sustained voluntary contraction is performed to elicit facilitation or postactivation depression. (From the 2001 Report of the Nomenclature Committee of the American Association of Electromyography and Electrodiagnosis.[10] Used by permission, copyright © 2001, AAEM.)

activator mutant   A form of **gangliosidosis** with two *variants*:

> *Infantile (AB variant)* A disorder presenting similarly to Tay-Sachs disease (**GM₂ gangliosidosis**) with the infantile onset of myoclonus, seizures, hypotonia, and, later, spasticity, dementia, and death. A cherry-red retinal spot is present.[4906]
>
> *Adult (AB variant)* A syndrome of adult-onset normal-pressure hydrocephalus, seizures, and dementia with increased hexosaminidase A and B activity.[335]

active continence   The maintenance of bladder outlet closure at rest through increased reflex activity in the pudendal nerve, which causes increased activity in the striated muscle around the urethra and thus increases the resistance to fluid flow.

active electrode   (exploring electrode, input terminal 1, grid 1, G1) The recording electrode close to the source of the activity to be recorded. In EEG, the first of two inputs to a differential amplifier. [RMS] See also **recording electrode.**

active sleep   A sleep stage in newborn children, similar to **REM sleep.**

activities of daily living   (ADL) The range of those behaviors which are normally required for personal self-maintenance and independent life within a community. These activities are usually divided between two categories. *Physical ADL* represents the most basic personal care tasks, such as feeding, excretion (bowels, bladder), toileting, dressing, cleanliness (grooming, bathing), and motility (transfers, wheelchair, walking, stairs). *Instrumental ADL* embodies more complex activities, including handling of personal finances, preparing meals, shopping, using the telephone, traveling and housework.

Items included within extended ADL include the following:[349]

Getting About	Household Activities	Other Activities
Carrying a hot drink	Washing up	Gardening
Working outside	Washing clothes	Managing money
Crossing roads	Housework	Going out socially
Getting in/out of a car	Shopping	Employment/work
Using public transport	Making hot drinks/snack	Hobbies/leisure
Driving a car	Reading	
	Telephoning	
	Writing	

Scores on ADL scales correlate well with scores on psychometric test batteries.[2] See also **Katz Activities of Daily Living scale, Physical Self-Maintenance scale, Instrumental Activities of Daily Living scale, Functional Assessment Staging.**

acuity   A term expressing the efficiency of a sensory pathway. It is most often employed in the realm of vision, normal acuity being the ability to resolve an image at a distance similar to that required by a normal population. Thus a visual acuity of 20/40 implies that the subject is only capable of resolving images 20 feet away while the normal population can do so when it is 40 feet away. Auditory acuity is also measureable, but measurements of tactile acuity are complex and unresolved.

acupressure   (Gr, needle + to press) Formerly a method of arresting hemorrhage; currently the term used for a system of pain relief by digital or other pressure on certain sites on a patient's body known only to practitioners of the mystery.

acupuncture   An Oriental system of treatment of disease by the insertion and subsequent rotation of long needles through the tautened skin, the insertions being made along certain charted meridians. Acupuncture was introduced into England in 1683 by a Dr. Rhyne but was not accepted again until espoused by Berlioz in 1816.

acusia   (acousis) The faculty of hearing.

acute   Sudden, urgent, short-term, or fast-appearing.

acute abstinence encephalopathy   An acute confusional state occurring on withdrawal from a cerebral depressant agent which had been chronically ingested. **Delirium tremens** is an example.

acute acquired postconvulsive hemiplegia   See **HHE syndrome.**

acute active multiple sclerosis   That form of **multiple sclerosis** characterized by extensive areas of confluent demyelination within the brainstem or spinal cord and leading to death within months of the clinical onset of the disease.

acute alcoholic myopathy   An acute syndrome of muscle pain, tenderness, swelling, weakness, and wasting of proximal muscles with myoglobinuria and consequent renal failure,[1626,1627] following another bout of excessive ingestion of alcohol by chronic alcoholics.

Pathologically the condition is marked by myofibrillar degeneration, especially of type 1 fibers. See also **alcoholic myopathy, acute hypokalemic myopathy of alcoholism.**

acute amnestic syndromes   See **Wernicke-Korsakoff syndrome.**

acute anterior poliomyelitis   See **poliomyelitis.**

acute areflexic paralysis   A syndrome occurring in malnourished patients who become acutely hypophosphatemic as a result of being fed with nutrients which do not contain phosphate.

Clinically, initial paresthesias lead to acute muscular weakness affecting the ocular and bulbar as well as the truncal and limb muscles; areflexia; sensory neuropathy; and ageusia. Central signs include somnolence or coma, confusional states, seizures, and pyramidal signs. The serum phosphorus level is always below 1 mg/dl and the signs remit when the levels are raised.[5164]

acute ascending polyneuropathy   See **acute inflammatory demyelinating polyneuropathy.**

acute ataxia   See **acute cerebellar ataxia.**

acute atrophic paralysis   A defunct name for **poliomyelitis.**

acute atypical meningitis   A manifestation of the initial direct infection of the meninges or brain with HIV and presenting a self-limited syndrome of meningitis, headache, long tract signs, and cranial nerve deficits.[2615]

acute autonomic neuropathy   An uncommon syndrome, usually affecting healthy young people. Presentation is often dramatic with gastrointestinal involvement heralding widespread dysautonomia. Acute autonomic neuropathy can be primarily cholinergic without orthostatic hypotension (26%) or pandysautonomic (74%), involving sympathetic adrenergic functions. Onset has been temporally related to viral syndromes in 20% of cases, with autonomic deficits usually evolving over 1 to 3 weeks. Gastroparesis (69%) and syncope (12%) are frequent presenting complaints. Spinal fluid protein levels are often (75%) elevated in pandysautonomic subtypes. Prolonged and incomplete recovery is the rule (60%), with persistent gastroparesis and orthostatic hypotension.

Other specific diseases that occasionally mimic acute autonomic neuropathy include botulism, porphyria, amyloidosis, and paracarcinomatous neuropathies. Acute autonomic neuropathy shares several clinical features with and is likely to be a variant of **acute inflammatory demyelinating polyneuropathy,** suggesting an immune-mediated pathogenesis.[2468] See also **autonomic neuropathy.**

acute axonal motor neuropathy   See **Chinese paralytic syndrome.**

acute axonal motor neuropathy with anti-GM$_1$ antibodies and _Campylobacter_ infection   See **immune-mediated neuropathies.**

acute benign hydrocephalus   (Marie-See syndrome) **Idiopathic intracranial hypertension** occurring in children as a result of the excessive ingestion of vitamin A.

acute brachial neuropathy   See **neuralgic amyotrophy.**

acute brachial plexitis   See **neuralgic amyotrophy.**

acute brachial plexopathy   See **neuralgic amyotrophy.**

acute brain swelling   See **parainfectious noninflammatory encephalomyelitis, cerebral edema.**

acute central cervical spinal cord injury   Acute hyperextension injury to the cervical spine producing hemorrhagic necrosis of the central cord. See **central cord syndrome**. The resulting clinical syndrome is of weakness (greater in the arms than in the legs), variable impairment of sensation below the level of the lesion, and urinary incontinence.[4984] See also **hematomyelia, Minor disease.**

acute cerebellar ataxia   1. (Zappert syndrome, acute cerebellitis) An acute reversible cerebellitis following viral infections such as varicella or after immunization and presenting with truncal, gait, and limb ataxia and **opsoclonus**.[2172] The prognosis for full recovery is good.[1119] 2. (Westphal-Leyden syndrome) An acute ataxic syndrome described in an adult by Leyden in 1891 and having both cerebral (cerebellar) and peripheral (sensory) forms.[3391] The condition was thought not to be a toxic manifestation and may have represented a postinfectious or demyelinating disorder. It is not clearly distinguished from Zappert syndrome.

acute cerebellar degeneration   A pan-cerebellar syndrome manifesting as ataxia and dysarthria in which there are no antibodies to Yo antigen or Purkinje cells and unassociated with underlying carcinoma or other structural disease.[4768]

acute cerebellitis   See **acute cerebellar ataxia.**

acute cerebral schistosomiasis   An acute encephalitis or encephalomyelitis presenting with personality change, angioneurotic edema, and pyramidal signs but progressing to coma with seizures. Marked peripheral eosinophilia is detected. The condition may be a form of allergic encephalopathy.[6030] See also **chronic cerebral schistosomiasis.**

acute compartment syndrome of the thigh   A potentially devastating disorder due to damage to neural and vascular structures as the result of acute swelling of the thigh muscles as a result of severe (or sometimes not severe) trauma.[5023,5761]

Compartment syndromes occur wherever muscles are overlain by fascial coverings. The **anterior tibial syndrome** is the best known, but other sites include the supraspinatus, anconeus and forearm muscles, the abdomen, and the posterior thigh and foot.

acute confusional migraine (dysphrenic migraine)   An agitated and confused state lasting minutes to hours and occurring occasionally in children (and even less commonly in adults) with a personal or family history of migraine. The confusional episode is not itself accompanied by headache, however.[2039]

acute corticosteroid myopathy   An acute necrotizing myopathy associated with the use of corticosteroids with or without neuromuscular junction blocking agents, occasionally seen in patients in intensive care. See **acute quadriplegic myopathy.**

acute delayed measles encephalitis   A chronic progressive encephalopathy occurring 3 months after an attack of measles and characterized by high antimeasles antibody levels, the presence of intranuclear inclusions in glial and neuronal nuclei, destruction of the ependyma, hydrocephalus, and, clinically, intractable **epilepsia partialis continua** and coma.[3533] See also **subacute sclerosing panencephalitis.**

acute dialysis encephalopathy   See **dialysis encephalopathy.**

acute dialysis neuropathy   An asymmetrical sensorimotor neuropathy (an acute **multiple mononeuropathy**) considered to be caused by ischemia due to vasoconstriction, occurring in patients with chronic renal failure undergoing dialysis.[3863]

acute disseminated encephalomyelitis   (ADEM, post- or parainfectious encephalomyelitis) An acute monophasic postinfectious or postvaccinial autoallergic, inflammatory, and demyelinating encephalopathy with major effects on the white matter of the cerebral hemispheres, cerebellum, optic nerves, and spinal cord. It is characterized pathologically by the presence of perivascular mononuclear cell infiltration in the brain and spinal cord, edema of the white matter, and variable perivenous and confluent demyelination with relative preservation of axons.

The name was applied by C.F. **Westphal** in 1872, but the condition was only defined pathologically by Hurst in 1941.[2713]

Clinically it is manifested by the acute onset of fever, meningismus, nausea and vomiting, seizures, and altered consciousness, with developing evidence of widespread CNS damage such as reduced consciousness, bilateral optic neuritis and other cranial nerve palsies, visual field defects, aphasia, hemiparesis, seizures, and cerebellar ataxia, all developing days or weeks after a viral or streptococcal infection or other immunologic challenge.[84] MRI studies reveal multifocal areas of increased signal intensity on T2-weighted sequences, enhancing with contrast, in both white and gray matter. In most cases, recovery occurs with steroid therapy, but a third of patients later develop **multiple sclerosis.**[5029]

When acute and fulminating with multiple intracerebral hemorrhages, the condition is known as *acute hemorrhagic leukoencephalitis* or Strumpell-Leichtenstern syndrome.[5389]

See also **brainstem encephalitis, Miller Fisher**

syndrome, multiphasic disseminated encephalomyelitis.

acute disseminated perivenous encephalomyelitis See acute disseminated encephalomyelitis.

acute dystonia of thalamic origin A lacunar syndrome.[1853]

acute encephalopathy of infancy (fatal infantile mitochondrial disease) A fatal mitochondrial disease with complex IV or cytochrome-*c* oxidase deficiency, presenting in neonates with hypotonia, vomiting, weakness, ptosis, and areflexia with renal tubular acidosis and sometimes cardiomyopathy and lactic acidosis.[335,1455]

acute flexion-extension injury See whiplash; acceleration injury syndrome.

acute fulminant myoglobinuric polymyositis A form of polymyositis distinguished from other forms by its extreme severity and by the presence of picornavirus-like particles in the muscles.[1987]

acute hemiconcern A transient behavioral syndrome rarely following stroke involving the territory of the right anterior parietal artery, in which patients with profound left hemisensory loss persistently examine and manipulate the left side of their bodies with their intact right arm.[627]

acute hemiplegia of childhood Hemiplegia occurring in early childhood, due to occlusive vascular disease or from unknown causes, as opposed to those cases in which trauma, heart disease, infection, sickle-cell disease or other pathologies can be incriminated.[5255] See also moyamoya disease.

acute hemorrhagic leukoencephalitis (acute necrotizing hemorrhagic encephalopathy, Strumpell-Leichtenstern syndrome) A form of autoallergic encephalitis following a viral illness in young adults, representing the most severe form of acute disseminated encephalomyelitis, in which there is inflammation within and around vessels with petechial hemorrhages, maximal in white matter. All of these features, except the petechiae, resemble those of experimental allergic encephalomyelitis.

The condition is usually acute and fatal, but patients with slow progression and even with recovery have been described.[2675] It was first described by Hurst in 1941 from Australia.

acute hypokalemic myopathy of alcoholism An acute myopathy without muscle pain, tenderness, or swelling, associated with severe hypokalemia within the context of alcoholism.[4842]

acute illness myopathy See Hopkins syndrome, critical care myopathy.

acute infantile hemiplegia The abrupt occurrence of a brain infarct (usually thrombotic in nature) in a previously healthy infant or child who lacks any predisposing condition. Coma, seizures, and fever often re-

sult from the localized defect. The causes of the condition have been reviewed by Golden.[2164]

acute infantile spinal muscular atrophy type 1 See hereditary motor neuropathy.

acute infectious torticollis An epidemic syndrome reported only in China, characterized by the occurrence of nonspecific prodromal symptoms suggesting viral infection, followed by painful spasm of the neck muscles with head tilt, torticollis, tongue stiffness, and spasm of other muscles including the oculomotor, lingual, and oral muscles, and distant dystonia.[4100]

acute inflammatory demyelinating polyneuropathy (acute ascending polyneuropathy, Landry-Guillain-Barré [-Strohl] syndrome, acute postinfective polyradiculoneuropathy, acute plexitis, etc; Jablonski[2764] lists 21 synonyms) Forms of peripheral neuropathy of uncertain cause but with an immune-mediated pathology, characterized by lymphocytic infiltration of the peripheral nerves and by destruction of myelin. The basis of the condition is the occurrence of aberrant immune responses directed against components of peripheral nerve, likely following cytomegalovirus, Epstein-Barr virus, HIV, or vaccinia virus infection.

Clinically this presents typically as an acute or subacute polyneuropathy with progressive motor weakness, areflexia, minor sensory changes, and almost invariably some autonomic instability.[2316,3258] The face is often involved, the eyes rarely so (except in the Miller Fisher variant). Antecedent events are often detected, these events typically including virus infections, surgery, trauma, malignancy, injection of sera and vaccines, or the presence of lymphoma or other malignancies, although in many cases there are no known preceding events. Symptoms reach their nadir in less than 3 weeks, but 80% of patients improve to some degree by 6 weeks.

The CSF protein is frequently raised but the cell count is not (albuminocytologic dissociation). The disease presents one of the classic "catch-22" dilemmas: those who respond best to plasmapheresis are also those whose signs have progressed rapidly over the first week, but the best response is obtained when this treatment is given in the first 7 days.

Descriptive clinical[228] and electrodiagnostic[83] criteria have been defined (but criticized by Poser[4505]) and some are reproduced in Chart A–2. Organizations devoted to this condition include the following: American Autoimmune Related Diseases Association 22100 Gratiot Avenue Eastpointe, East Detroit, MI 48201-2227. Tel: 586-776-3900; 800-598-4668. E-mail:aarda@aol.com. Web site: http://www.aarda.org; and the Guillain-Barre Syndrome Foundation International P.O. Box 262 Wynnewood, PA 19096. E-mail: gbint@netcom.com. Tel: 610-667-0131. Web site: http://www.webmast.com/gbs.

The condition was first reported by Wardrop and Ollivier in 1834–1837 and then by Jean-Baptiste-Octave Landry (1826–1865), a French physician, who correctly concluded in 1859 that it is a disease of the peripheral nerves. Guillain and Barré added the CSF findings ("Dissociation Albumino-Cytologique" or Sicard-Foix syndrome) in 1891.

Antibodies to GM_1, GD_{1a}, LM_1, sulfatide, and other glycolipids are variously detectable.[5990]

Chart A–2. Diagnostic Criteria for Guillain-Barre Syndrome (Acute Infectious Polyneuropathy)

I. *Features required for diagnosis*
  A. Progressive motor weakness of more than one limb. The degree ranges from minimal weakness of the legs, with or without mild areflexia, to total paralysis of the muscles of all four extremities and the trunk, bulbar and facial paralysis, and external ophthalmoplegia.
  B. Areflexia (loss of tendon jerks). Universal areflexia is the rule, although distal areflexia with definite hyporeflexia of the biceps and knee jerks will suffice if other features are consistent.
II. *Features strongly suggestive of the diagnosis*
  A. Clinical features (ranked in order of importance)
    1. Progression. Symptoms and signs of motor weakness develop rapidly but cease to progress by 4 weeks into the illness. Approximately 50% will reach the nadir by 2 weeks, 80% by 3 weeks, and more than 90% by 4 weeks.
    2. Relative symmetry. Symmetry is seldom absolute, but usually, if one limb is affected, the opposite is as well.
    3. Mild sensory symptoms or signs
    4. Cranial nerve involvement. Facial weakness occurs in approximately 50% and is frequently bilateral. Other cranial nerves may be involved, particularly those innervating the tongue and muscles of deglutition, and sometimes the extraocular motor nerves. On occasion (less than 50%) the neuropathy may begin in the nerves to the extraocular muscles or other cranial nerves.
    5. Recovery. It usually begins 2 to 4 weeks after progression stops. Recovery may be delayed for months. Most patients recover functionally.
    6. Autonomic dysfunction. Tachycardia and other arrhythmias, postural hypotension, hypertension, and vasomotor symptoms, when present, support the diagnosis. These findings may fluctuate. Care must be exercised to exclude other bases for these symptoms, such as pulmonary embolism.
    7. Absence of fever at the onset of neuritic symptoms
    8. Absence of manifestations of systemic illness or constitutional symptoms or both, either preceding or coinciding with onset of neuropathy
  Variants (not ranked). The presence of one of these need not rule out the diagnosis if other features are strongly supportive, but the presence of two of them makes the diagnosis unlikely.
    1. Fever at onset of neuritic symptoms
    2. Severe sensory loss with pain
    3. Progression beyond 4 weeks. Occasionally, a patient's disease will continue to progress for much longer than 4 weeks or the patient will have a minor relapse.
    4. Cessation of progression without recovery or with major permanent residual deficit remaining
    5. Sphincter function. Usually the sphincters are not

affected, but transient bladder paralysis may occur during the evolution of symptoms.
    6. CNS involvement. Ordinarily, Guillain-Barre syndrome is thought of as a disease of the peripheral nervous system. Evidence of CNS involvement is controversial. In occasional patients, such findings as severe ataxia interpretable as cerebellar in origin, dysarthria, extensor plantar responses, and ill-defined sensory levels are demonstrable, and these need not exclude the diagnosis if other features are typical.
  B. CSF features strongly supportive of the diagnosis
    1. CSF protein. After the first week of symptoms, CSF protein is elevated or has been shown to rise on serial lumbar punctures.
    2. CSF cells. Counts of 10 or fewer mononuclear leukocytes/mm^3 in CSF
  Variants include the following:
    1. No CSF protein rise in the period of 1 to 10 weeks after the onset of symptoms (rare)
    2. Counts of 10 to 50 mononuclear leukocytes/mm^3 in CSF (common in patients seropositive for HIV, however)
  C. Electrodiagnostic features strongly supportive of the diagnosis (see below). Approximately 80% will have evidence of nerve conduction slowing or block at some point during the illness. Conduction velocity is usually less than 60% of normal, but the process is patchy and not all nerves are affected. Distal latencies may be increased to as much as three times the normal amount. Use of F-wave responses often gives good indication of slowing over proximal portions of nerve trunks and roots. Up to 20% of patients will have normal conduction studies. Conduction studies may not become abnormal until several weeks into the illness.
III. *Features casting doubt on the diagnosis*
  A. Marked, persistent asymmetry of weakness
  B. Persistent bladder or bowel dysfunction
  C. Bladder or bowel dysfunction at onset
  D. More than 50 mononuclear leukocytes/mm^3 in CSF
  E. Presence of polymorphonuclear leukocytes in CSF
  F. Sharp sensory level
IV. *Features that rule out the diagnosis*
  A. Current history of hexacarbon abuse (volatile solvents; n-hexane and methyl n-butyl ketone). This includes huffing of paint lacquer vapors or addictive glue sniffing.
  B. Abnormal porphyrin metabolism indicating a diagnosis of acute intermittent porphyria. This would manifest as increased excretion of porphobilinogen and δ-aminolevulinic acid in the urine.
  C. A history or finding of recent diphtheritic infection, either faucial or wound, with or without myocarditis
  D. Features clinically consistent with lead neuropathy (upper limb weakness with prominent wrist drop; may be asymmetrical) and evidence of lead intoxication
  E. Occurrence of a purely sensory syndrome
  F. A definite diagnosis of a condition such as poliomyelitis, botulism, hysterical paralysis, or toxic neuropathy (e.g., from nitrofurantoin, dapsone, or organophosphorus compounds), which occasionally may be confused with Guillain-Barré syndrome

Criteria established by an ad hoc committee of the NINCDS, Dr. A.K. Asbury, Chairman, and reproduced by kind permission.[228]

Proposed electrodiagnostic criteria for demyelination of peripheral nerve are included but a more recent classification[2361] is as follows.

Chart A–2A. Criteria for Electrophysiological Classification

1. Normal (All the following are found in all nerves tested)
   DML ≤100% ULN
   F wave present with latency ≤100% ULN
   MCV ≥100% LLN
   dCMAP ≥100% LLN
   pCMAP ≥100% LLN
   pCMAP/dCMAP ratio >0.5
2. Primary demyelinating
   (At least one of the following in each of at least two nerves, or at least two of the following in one nerve if all others inexcitable and dCMAP ≥10% LLN)
   MCV <90% LLN (85% if dCMAP <50% LLN)
   DML >110% ULN (120% if dCMAP <100% LLN)
   pCMAP/dCMAP ratio <0.5 and dCMAP ≥20% LLN
   F-response latency >120% ULN
3. Primary axonal
   None of the above features of demyelination in any nerve (except one demyelinating feature allowed in one nerve if dCMAP <10% LLN, and dCMAP <80% LLN in at least two nerves)
4. lnexcitable
   dCMAP absent in all nerves (or present in only one nerve with dCMAP <10% LLN)
5. Equivocal
   Does not exactly fit criteria for any other group

dCMAP, compound muscle action potential amplitude after distal stimulation; DML, distal motor latency; LLN, lower limit of normal; MCV, motor conduction velocity; pCMAP, compound muscle action potential amplitude after proximal stimulation; ULN, upper limit of normal. (Modified from Ho et al.[2592a])

About 5% of patients with this condition will show evidence of axonal damage.[228,229] See also **demyelination.**

Simpler clinical criteria for the typical syndrome (and variants) have been suggested by Ropper et al.[4772] and are reproduced here by kind permission of the authors and of F.A. Davis Co., Ltd.

Clinical Features

1. Weakness that is approximately symmetric in all the limbs
2. Paresthesias in the feet and hands
3. Areflexia or hyporeflexia in all limbs by 1 week
4. Progression of the above three features over several days to 1 month

Laboratory Abnormalities That Confirm the Diagnosis

5. Elevated CSF protein concentration (>45 mg/dl) within 3 weeks from onset
6. Abnormalities of F waves (absence, dispersion, impersistence) in at least two limbs, or motor nerve conduction block, or slowing (motor nerve conduction velocity below 80% of normal)

Variants of the usual clinical syndrome include **Ataxia, areflexia, and facial diplegia**

Acute motor axonal neuropathy (AMAN) (an acute axonal form with a poor prognosis for recovery, often due to *Campylobacter infection*)[1756]

Acute motor and sensory neuropathy (AMASN) see **acute motor axonal neuropathy.**

Acute pandysautonomia

Acute sensory neuronopathy

Miller Fisher syndrome

Polyneuritis cranialis

A *pharyngeal-cervical-brachial variant* has the following diagnostic criteria, suggested by Ropper et al.[4772] and reproduced here by kind permission of the authors and of F.A. Davis Co., Ltd.

Clinical Features

1. Paresthesias in the feet and hands
2. No weakness or respiratory failure
3. Areflexia or hyporeflexia in all limbs by 1 week
4. Distally diminished sensation involving mainly vibration and joint position
5. Proximal progression of numbness and sensory loss on the limbs over several days to 1 month
6. Improvement in paresthesias and sensory loss by 2 to 4 months from onset

Laboratory Abnormalities That Confirm the Diagnosis

7. Elevated CSF protein concentration (>45 mg/dl) within 3 weeks of onset
8. Severe sensory nerve conduction abnormalities
9. Minimal motor conduction and late response abnormalities

Anti-GD_{1a} and anti-GT_{1a} antibodies have been detected in some cases of this condition.

A *pure motor variant* has the following diagnostic criteria, suggested by Ropper et al.[4772] and reproduced here by kind permission of the authors and of F.A. Davis Co, Ltd.

Clinical Features

1. Progressive, relatively symmetric weakness in all limbs
2. No paresthesias or sensory loss
3. Areflexia or hyporeflexia in all limbs by 1 week
4. Progression of weakness over 1 day to 3 weeks

Laboratory Abnormalities That Confirm the Diagnosis

5. Elevated CSF protein concentration (>45 mg/dl) within 3 weeks of onset
6. Abnormalities of F waves in at least two limbs or motor nerve conduction block, or slowing
7. Normal sensory nerve potentials

A *paraparetic variant* has the following diagnostic criteria, suggested by Ropper et al.[4772] and reproduced here by kind permission of the authors and of F.A. Davis Co, Ltd.

Clinical Features

1. Progressive leg weakness over 1–3 weeks
2. Areflexia or hyporeflexia in the legs by 1 week of illness
3. Normal (or virtually normal) power and reflexes in the arms and cranial nerve innervated muscles
4. Minimal or no paresthesias or sensory loss

Laboratory Abnormalities That Confirm the Diagnosis

5. Variable, usually slight, elevation of CSF protein concentration
6. Abnormal motor nerve conduction and late responses in the legs

Facial diplegia which presents with ataxia and are-flexia but with minimal limb weakness or sensory deficit.[986]

Acute ophthalmoparesis without ataxia is a rare form presenting with relatively symmetric ophthalmoparesis progressing over 4 weeks, unaccompanied by ataxia or limb weakness. The condition usually follows an infectious illness. The CSF shows albuminocytological dissociation and anti-GQ1b IgG antibodies are detectable in the serum.[4199]

Acute small fiber sensory neuropathy 1. A pure sensory variant presenting with acute numbness and burning dysesthesias in a symmetric glove-and-stocking distribution in the limbs, with normal muscle strength, areflexia, and electrophysiological evidence of demyelinating neuropathy. The CSF protein levels may be raised. The condition increases for up to a month and then slowly remits. (Oh S. et al. Neurology 2001;56:82–6) 2. A similar syndrome in which however there is evidence only of thin sensory fiber involvement, the electrodiagnostic studies being normal and the muscle stretch reflexes retained. (Seneviratne U and Gunasekera S. J. Neurol. Neurosurg. Psychiatr. 2002;72:540–2)

acute intermittent porphyria   A dominantly inherited disorder characterized by deficiency of hydroxymethylbilane synthase (porphobilinogen deaminase) and manifesting episodes of acute abdominal pain, vomiting, and porphyrinuria, sometimes with acute distal motor axonopathy. Exacerbations are triggered in most instances by exposure to environmental triggers (barbiturates, dilantin, griseofulvin, sulfonamides, estrogens; alcohol; infections; or starvation).[4756] The responsible gene maps to 11q23.2–qter.

Neurological features complicate a third of attacks and include the acute or subacute occurrence of proximal motor neuropathy affecting the arms more than the legs (often asymmetrically) as well as the face and autonomic system in the setting of other features of the disease, including abdominal pain, vomiting, tachycardia, hypertension, and often seizures. Delirium, psychosis, and neurotic behavior patterns are mental features described, as in the case of King George III of England. Sensory loss may be detected in the **bathing suit area.** The ankle jerks are preserved but all other muscle stretch reflexes are diminished.

Widespread central, peripheral, and autonomic system lesions have been found.[5402]

acute intrinsic myelopathy   (acute transverse myelitis, acute necrotic myelopathy) An acutely developing spinal cord lesion, involving both sides of the cord at one or more adjacent levels, ascending or static, occurring at any age without prior neurological features and due to neither compression nor surgery. The condition may remain at one level or may ascend through new levels of the cord. Onset in less than 3 weeks of symmetrical motor and sensory dysfunction referable to a distinct spinal cord level, with sphincter dysfunction, are typical features.

Typically this occurs as a postinfectious autoimmune demyelinating condition, but ischemic infarction, bleeding from arteriovenous malformations, demyelinating disease, viral infections, and paraneoplastic syndromes are other causes.[5946] See also **acute necrotic myelopathy, acute toxic myelopathy.**

acute lethal catatonia   Muscle rigidity with an increase in creatine kinase levels without involuntary movements or autonomic signs in subjects exposed to neuroleptic drugs.

The condition represents a rare variant of the **neuroleptic malignant syndrome,** from which it cannot be distinguished clinically.[40]

acute midbrain syndrome   See **diencephalic autonomic seizures.**

acute motor axonal neuropathy (AMAN)   An axonal form of acute inflammatory polyneuropathy characterized clinically by rapid onset of weakness, an early nadir, distal weakness initially, relative sparing of cranial nerves, and occurrence mainly in summer. Many cases are associated with *C. jejuni* infection and the presence of IgG anti-GM$_1$ antibodies, some of which may be cross-reactive with lipopolysaccharides. AMAN may also occur following infusion of parenteral gangliosides, composed primarily of GM$_1$. These disorders have been further subdivided on the basis of electrophysiology and pathology into acute motor axonal neuropathy (AMAN) and *acute motor-sensory axonal neuropathy* (AMSAN).

Pathologic findings in AMAN and AMSAN include axonal degeneration of the affected nerves and the presence of periaxonal macrophages (in motor roots in AMAN and in motor and sensory roots in AMSAN). The cause is unknown. *Campylobacter* infections, present in many patients with AMAN and in other forms of Guillain-Barré syndrome, may play a role in triggering such a process possibly by "molecular mimicry."[1756,3767]

acute mountain sickness   (Acosta syndrome) A clinical syndrome comprising headache, insomnia, anorexia, nausea, dizziness, dyspnea, peripheral edema, vomiting, and incoordination, occurring between 6 and 24 hours after attainment of high elevations, peaking on the second or third day and resolving after about a week.

While it is usually self-limiting, the syndrome can progress to pulmonary and cerebral edema. It is hypothesized that the pathogenesis is increased cerebral blood flow and early cerebral edema in all cases as a result of hypoxia, which itself is due to improper or too-rapid acclimatization.[2359] See also **altitude insomnia.**

acute myelitis   See **acute intrinsic myelopathy.**

acute necrotic myelopathy (myelomalacia) A form of **acute intrinsic myelopathy** presenting with flaccid paralysis and total sensory loss ascending over a few days from the legs to the thoracic regions or higher with loss of sphincter control and without recovery.

Pathologically, the condition is characterized by extensive necrosis of the white matter, more than of the gray matter, of a large part of the cord, without vascular disease or neoplasia but sometimes with evidence of inflammation.[5946] Changes in the CSF are inconstant but may include an abnormally high protein content, either with few cells or with pleocytosis.

The condition is thought to be a form of **acute disseminated encephalomyelitis** or of **Devic disease** but a similar syndrome may be associated with carcinoma or tuberculosis or with some toxic or infectious agent, or it may represent a postinfectious phenomenon.[4509] See also **subacute necrotic myelopathy.**

acute (necrotic) myopathy A myopathy complicating infection with influenza A or B virus, Coxsackie virus B5, echovirus 9, adenovirus 21, Epstein-Barr virus, or herpes simplex virus and presenting with lymphadenopathy, proximal myopathic weakness, muscle pain and cramp, and myoglobinuria due to rhabdomyolysis. Biopsy shows phagocytosis and fiber necrosis.

A similar myopathy may complicate carcinoma or alcoholism.

See also **acute fulminant myoglobinuric polymyositis, acute quadriplegic myopathy, myoglobinuria, Hopkins syndrome.**

acute necrotizing encephalopathy of childhood A syndrome of coma, seizures, vomiting, hyperpyrexia and hepatomegaly reported in Japanese children following acute respiratory infections. The presence of diarrhea and of raised CSF protein and the absence of hyperammonemia or hypoglycemia are considered to differentiate the condition from **Reye syndrome.**[3923]

acute necrotizing hemorrhagic encephalopathy See **acute hemorrhagic leukoencephalitis.**

acute necrotizing myopathy of intensive care. See **quadriplegic myopathy.**

acute non-suppurative encephalitis See **parainfectious noninflammatory encephalomyelts.**

acute ocular oscillations See **opsoclonus.**

acute onset lethargia and prolonged abulia A syndrome resulting from infarction of the genu of the left internal capsule. See **strategic-infarct dementia, capsular genu syndrome, multi-infarct dementia.**

acute ophthalmoparesis without ataxia See **acute inflammatory demyelinating neuropathy** (*variants*).

acute painful ophthalmoplegia A syndrome closely resembling **superior orbital fissure syndrome** but with frequent involvement of the optic nerve, reported from the Far East.[5502]

acute pandysautonomia See **autonomic neuropathy (1).**

acute peripheral vestibulopathy (vestibular neuronitis, labyrinthitis, neurolabyrinthitis) A clinical syndrome of vertigo and vomiting, falls, past-pointing towards the affected side, horizontal or rotatory direction-fixed spontaneous nystagmus towards the affected side, unilateral canal paresis, and normal hearing. While it is usually supposed to have a viral origin affecting the eighth nerve and/or the labyrinth, pontine lesions can produce an identical syndrome.[5559]

acute persistent akathisia A variety of chronic **akathisia** in which the abnormal movements appear shortly after institution of therapy with a neuroleptic agent, and which persist.[843]

acute phase shift of sleep See **rapid time zone change syndrome.**

acute plexitis See **acute inflammatory demyelinating polyneuropathy.**

acute polioclastic encephalitis A form of encephalitis in which the gray matter of the cerebral cortex bears the brunt of the damage caused by the inflammatory process.

acute polymyopathy A rapidly progressive syndrome of proximal weakness, muscle pain, tenderness, and swelling with elevated creatinine kinase levels. It is considered to be due to deficiency of essential fatty acids during prolonged total peripheral nutrition.[5355] See also **acute (necrotic) myopathy, polymyositis.**

acute polyneuropathy with edema Beriberi in modern form.[1295]

acute polyradiculitis See **acute inflammatory demyelinating polyneuropathy.**

acute postasthmatic amyotrophy See **Hopkins syndrome.**

acute posterior multifocal placoid pigment epitheliopathy A syndrome characterized by sudden, usually binocular, blurring of vision, in which multifocal yellowish-white lesions are seen in the pigment epithelium of the retina. The disease, considered to be a manifestation of diffuse cerebral vasculitis, is usually self-limiting and visual function returns eventually.[2045]

acute postinfectious encephalomyelitis See **acute disseminated encephalomyelitis.**

acute postinfective polyradiculoneuropathy See **acute inflammatory demyelinating polyneuropathy.**

acute quadriplegic myopathy (acute necrotizing myopathy of intensive care, thick filament myopathy, floppy person syndrome) A syndrome of severe, rapid-onset, diffuse myopathic weakness complicating urgent steroid therapy, as in the course of treatment of acute asthmatic attacks, with or without the addition of non-depolarizing blocking agents.[2582, 6134] Typically, the clinical picture is of flaccid quadriparesis with ventilatory muscle involvement, marked wasting, and hyporeflexia. EMG findings are a mix of neuropathic, myopathic, and end-plate abnormalities. Muscle biopsy reveals severe atrophy of most muscle fibers, with disorganization and necrosis of myofibrils and selective loss of thick (myosin) filaments.[2582] See also **Hopkins syndrome, acute (necrotic) myopathy, critical illness polyneuropathy.**

acute rhabdomyolysis An uncommon acute, necrotic myopathy occurring during various viral infections and causing muscle destruction with myoglobinuria. Clinically, muscle pain, tenderness, weakness, and myoglobinuria occur, sometimes complicated by renal failure. See **acute (necrotic) myopathy.**

A similar but more limited syndrome occurs in association with heavy, unaccustomed exercise. See **squat-jump myoglobinuria, rhabdomyolysis.**

acute sensory (ataxic) neuronopathy An acutely developing, monophasic, purely sensory neuropathy involving mainly large-fiber modalities in the limbs and trunk with sensory ataxia and areflexia, and in which the underlying lesions are thought to be of the dorsal root and gasserian ganglion cells. The condition is probably immune mediated, or due to vascular causes in the absence of underlying carcinoma. The autonomic system may also be involved; occasionally, muscle stretch reflexes are preserved.[4217]

The syndrome has also been recorded following exposure to adriamycin, pyridoxine, mercury, and antibiotics and following infections with herpes zoster. The prognosis for recovery is poor.[5337]

acute serous encephalitis (Brown-Symmers disease) A rapidly progressive encephalopathy characterized by irritability, anorexia, vomiting, and evidence of raised intracranial pressure with bulbar signs in the form of respiratory irregularity. Ptosis, nystagmus, papilledema, convulsions, contraction of the angle of the mouth, muscle twitching, rigidity of the neck, hemiplegia, and coma lead to death in untreated children within 2 days.[789] See **parainfectious noninflammatory encephalomyelitis, acute disseminated encephalomyelitis.**

acute severe combined demyelination The concurrence of Guillain-Barré syndrome and acute disseminated encephalomyelitis in acute and fulminant form, presenting with acute onset of coma and flaccid, areflexic quadriparesis, elevated CSF protein levels and delayed F waves, and with MRI evidence of extensive multifocal demyelination. Prompt clinical response followed by recovery may be achieved by treatment with corticosteroids.[160]

acute sinus headache This definition and the following diagnostic criteria are suggested by the Headache Classification Committee of the International Headache Society and are reproduced by kind permission.[1051]

  A. Purulent discharge in the nasal passage, either spontaneous or by suction

  B. Pathological findings in one or more of the following tests:
      X-ray examination, CT, or MRI
      Nasal endoscopy

  C. Simultaneous onset of headache and sinusitis

  D. Headache location: in acute frontal sinusitis, headache is located directly over the sinus and may radiate to the vertex or behind the eyes; in acute maxillary sinusitis, headache is located over the antral area and may radiate to the upper teeth or to the forehead; in acute ethmoiditis, headache is located between and behind the eyes and may radiate to the temporal area; in acute sphenoiditis, headache is located in the occipital area, the vertex, the frontal region, or behind the eyes.

  E. Headache disappears after treatment of acute sinusitis.

In this context it should be noted that the condition of chronic sinus headache probably does not exist, most cases having features allowing the diagnosis of **migraine.**

acute small fiber sensory neuropathy See **acute inflammatory polyneuropathy.**

acute superior hemorrhagic polioencephalitis The term of **Gayet** for what is now known as **Wernicke-Korsakoff syndrome.**

acute suppurative myositis (pyomyositis) Direct bacterial (or syphilitic) infection of muscle, with staphylococci, clostridia, streptococci, and anaerobes being the organisms most commonly isolated.

Clinically, the findings are of localized pain, tenderness, and swelling with systemic evidence of infection. The condition is uncommon in temperate regions, especially since paraldehyde is now seldom administered intramuscularly.

acute symptomatic seizures See **situation-related seizures.**

acute syphilitic meningitis A benign meningitic illness occurring in the secondary stage of syphilis but without fever, but often complicated by hydrocephalus or cranial nerve involvement. The CSF almost always shows abnormality. The illness usually occurs at the same time as the rash and within 2 years of infection. Cerebrovascular syphilitic syndromes follow within years at most.

acute thalamic esotropia Adduction of one eye, which remains immobile while the other eye responds normally to vestibulo-ocular stimulation, in the presence of altered consciousness, long tract signs, and impaired upward gaze. The condition results from lesions of the contralateral posterior thalamus.[2178]

acute thyrotoxic encephalomyelopathy (Waldenstrom syndrome) An acute complication of hyperthyroidism, usually seen in the elderly, who present with sixth, seventh, and bulbar cranial nerve palsies, an hallucinatory psychosis with lethargy and apathy or excitement, and a variety of signs of cortical dysfunction. Eventually, they slip into a coma.[5805] See also **thyrotoxic crises.**

acute thyrotoxic myopathy   Rapidly progressive bulbar weakness complicating a thyroid storm (acute hyperthyroidism); a condition of uncertain nature, with myasthenia, periodic paralysis, and encephalopathy also having been suggested as the underlying cause.

acute toxic encephalopathy   See **parainfectious noninflammatory encephalomyelitis.**

acute toxic myelopathy   An **acute intrinsic myelopathy** occasionally associated with intravenous illicit drug usage, spinal angiography, aortic angiography, intrathecal penicillin or chemotherapautic injections, or spinal anesthesia. See also **lathyrism.**

acute transverse myelitis   See **acute intrinsic myelopathy.**

acute vertical myoclonus   Vertical, pendular, large-amplitude oscillations of the eyes, occurring in some patients with recent brainstem strokes.[3330]

acute viral encephalitis   Infection of the substance of the brain by a virus (such as herpes simplex, Epstein-Barr, mumps, influenza, Coxsackie, or echo), leading to disease which may be mild and transient or fulminant and lethal.

Clinically, headache, hemiparesis, fever, nausea, drowsiness, coma, neck stiffness, papilledema, seizures, and various other neurological signs are the most common findings. The CSF may be under increased pressure; it contains mononuclear cells (and typically red cells in herpes encephalitis) but the protein level may be normal. EEG abnormalities usually include generalized or focal slowing, or bursts of spike-and-wave activity.[3003]

acute Werdnig-Hoffman disease   See **hereditary motor neuropathy.**

acyl coenzyme A dehydrogenase deficiency   Recessively inherited mitochondrial diseases of childhood, characterized by disorders of the short-, medium-, or long-chain forms of the enzyme. Medium-chain acyl coenzyme A dehydrogenase deficiency is perhaps the most common disorder of fatty acid oxidation.

Clinical features variously include vomiting, coma, muscle weakness (lipid myopathy with cardiomyopathy), and mental retardation. Hepatomegaly, nonketotic hypoglycemia, myoglobinuria resulting from rhabdomyolysis, and dicarboxylic aciduria are usual laboratory features of these conditions.[5315]

Multiple acyl coenzyme A dehydrogenase deficiency is listed under **glutaric aciduria type 2.**

adacrya   (Gr, without + to weep) Inability to form tears.

adamantinoma   (Gr, hard mineral substance) See **craniopharyngioma.**

Adamkiewicz, Albert   (1850–1921) Polish professor of pathology at Kraków. The artery of Adamkiewicz is a branch of the abdominal aorta, representing the major segmental arterial supply of the spinal cord at that level, which it approaches close to or at L1, usually from the left side. Adamkiewicz also described the demilunes found beneath the neurilemma of medullated nerves.

Adams, Robert   (1771–1875) Dublin physician.

Adams syndrome   (tachycardia and hypertension) A congenital syndrome characterized by microphthalmia, cataract, ECG abnormality, aminoaciduria, renal stones, hypertension, and seizures.[337]

Adams-Stokes-Morgagni syndrome   (Stokes-Adams syndrome) Syncope of cardiac origin, the usual cause being complete atrioventricular block, with bradycardia usually at a rate below 40/min.[36]

Morgagni's original (1761) note in his *De Sedibus et Causis Morborum* (Letter the Ninth, which treats of epilepsy) clearly describes seizures with cessation of the heart beat, but Adams's report was more precise in detail. Stokes published his observations in 1846.

adaptation   1. A decline in the response to a repetitive stimulus. 2. A decline in the frequency of the spike discharge as typically recorded from sensory axons in response to a maintained stimulus.[10] 3. (neuro-ophthalmology) Diminished responsiveness of central mechanisms in response to a persistent abnormality disturbing function. Adaptation modifies the direct effects of a neurological lesion; thus the nystagmus in **internuclear ophthalmoplegia** reflects the excessive innervation of the weak medial rectus with spillover to the abducting eye. Saccadic dysmetria and macrosaccadic oscillations occur in **myasthenia gravis** and with cerebellar lesions as adaptive changes to weakness, but become maladaptive when strength returns temporarily in the Tensilon test.

adaptation rate   The rate at which a sensory receptor reduces its afferent discharge in response to a persisting adequate stimulus.

adaptive behavior   The capacity of an individual to function with respect to the physical and the human environment. See also **Vineland Adaptive Behavior Scale, Woodcock-Johnson Scales of Independent Behavior, Minnesota Child Development Inventory, Adaptive Behavior Scale.**

Adaptive Behavior Scale   A questionnaire used in the assessment of levels of functioning and maladaptive behavior in retarded people or those with acquired brain damage.[4136]

Addenbrooke's Cognitive Evaluation   A short instrument for early detection of dementia, expanding the **MMSE.** It consists of six components evaluating orientation (10 points), attention (8), memory (35), verbal fluency (14), language (28), and visuospatial ability (5). The orientation and attention components are as in the MMSE. The memory component evaluates episodic memory (recall of three items from the MMSE plus a "name and address learning and delayed recall" test) and semantic memory. The language component requires naming of 12 line drawings, repetition of words and sentences, reading regular and irregular words, and comprehension and writing tasks. The visuospatial test requires copying of overlapping pentagons (from the MMSE) and of a wire cube and drawing a clock face. Verbal fluency examines letter fluency for words beginning with the letter *P* and category fluency for animals. Scores for each of the six domains can be calculated separately; their sum gives a composite score out of 100. The MMSE score can also be calculated.

The instrument can be reviewed as an appendix on the *Neurology* Web site, www.neurology.org.[3697]

Addison disease   The systemic disorder stemming from a deficiency of corticosteroid hormones as a result of adrenal disease. Neurological complications include a mild myopathy, and a syndrome of idiopathic intracranial hypertension, with or without cerebral edema and encephalopathy.

Addison, Thomas   (1793–1860) English physician who trained in Edinburgh but spent almost all of his professional life as Physician to Guy's Hospital in London, where he showed particular interest in the skin and described pernicious anemia, adrenal failure, xanthomas, vitiligo (Addison-Gull disease), and morphoea.

adducted thumbs syndrome   See **Christian syndrome, craniosynostosis.**

adduction   (from Lat, to lead towards) The movement by which a body part is drawn towards the sagittal line or a finger moves towards the center line of the hand. See also (ocular) **duction.**

adduction lag   A reduction in the amplitude and velocity of the (adducting) fast phase of jerk nystagmus induced in the eye on the same side as a lesion of the median longitudinal fasciculus (**internuclear ophthalmoplegia**).[5232]

adductor reflex   Adduction of the abducted leg in response to a tap on the medial epicondyle of the femur and, in cases of pyramidal disease, from many other sites on the pelvis, leg, and spine (*spinal adductor reflex*). It is a marker for lower motor neuron lesions at L2 and, like other muscle stretch reflexes, is increased in pyramidal tract disease.

adductor reflex of the foot   (Hirschberg sign) Stroking the inner border of the foot from the hallux back towards the heel leads to adduction, inversion, and plantar flexion of the foot because of contraction of the tibialis posterior in patients with pyramidal tract disease.

adductor spread of knee jerk   See **developmental reflexes.**

Adelaide craniosynostosis   A rare, dominantly inherited syndrome linked to chromosome 4p. See also **craniosynostosis.**

adenoma sebaceum   (Bourneville disease) A papular skin lesion in **tuberous sclerosis,** first described in 1826 by Pierre Rayer (1793–1867), a French dermatologist, although Pringle had already noted the facial lesions.

adenylate deaminase deficiency   See **muscle adenylate deaminase deficiency.**

adermonervia   (Gr, lack of + skin + nerves) Loss of skin sensation.

adhalin   (from Arabic, muscle) A 50-kd dystrophin-associated glycoprotein (α-sarcoglycan), a component of the sarcoglycan complex of the muscle cell membrane. The disorders consequent upon deficiency of the protein were first detected in North Africa, hence the derivation of the term.

adhalinopathies   (α-sarcoglycanopathies) Unusual, heterogeneous forms of muscular dystrophy characterized by deficiency of adhalin and presenting clinically as severe childhood autosomal recessive muscular dystrophy (SCARMD) resembling **Duchenne dystrophy** in its clinical features and course but without involvement of the cardiac, facial, ocular, or pharyngeal muscles. This form has been mapped to chromosome 17q21 and is due to a primary defect of adhalin. In another form presenting as a milder limb girdle muscular dystrophy, the absence of adhalin is secondary to a separate defect on chromosome 13q12 or 4q12.[1725] See also **quadriceps myopathy, severe childhood autosomal recessive muscular dystrophy.**

Primary adhalinopathy may be a common cause of autosomal recessive muscular dystrophy of variable severity.[4437]

adhesive arachnoiditis   (chronic idiopathic adhesive arachnoiditis) Chronic inflammation of the arachnoid membrane, usually in lumbar regions, constricting the spinal cord, the nerve roots, and the blood vessels and leading to a slowly progressive ascending myelopathy or to multiple painful radiculopathies.

This condition was a complication of myelography when using oily contrast media or the injection of any foreign substance into the subarachnoid space, and also was a complication of syphilis and chronic granulomatous diseases, but such causes are now rare. When the condition is detected, commonly no cause is found. See **spinal arachnoiditis.**

adhesive capsulitis of the shoulder   See **Duplay syndrome.**

adiadochokinesis   See **dysdiadochokinesis.**

adiaphoresis   (Gr, lack of + to throw off by perspiration) Lack of sweating.

Adie pupil   (tonic pupil, pupillotonic pseudotabes, Markus syndrome, pseudo-Argyll Robertson pupil, myotonic pupillary reaction, Saenger syndrome, Kehrer-Adie syndrome, iridoplegia interna, pseudotonic pupillotonia) The condition in which one enlarged pupil (seldom both) reacts extremely slowly, if at all, to light but does constrict on prolonged accommodation and then remains persistently constricted after the stimulus is removed. It is usually seen in young women.

The lesion causing the partial denervation of the pupillary sphincter is in the ciliary ganglion; it is diagnosed definitively by the hypersensitivity of the pupil to 0.125% **pilocarpine** or 2.5% **methacholine** and is a benign condition which nevertheless disturbs the naive who look into a mirror and notice a single dilated pupil. Scheie had previously introduced the methacholine test; Adie concluded that the lesion was in the postganglionic parasympathetic fibers, as the pupils showed denervation hypersensitivity to that substance.

This pupillary phenomenon was reported by Piltz in 1899 and by at least three other authors before Holmes and Adie[41, 2623] each reported it in 1931. The pupillary changes are often combined with reduction or loss of the muscle stretch reflexes in the legs (**Holmes-Adie syndrome**), as reported by both authors,[43, 4420] and occasionally by anhidrosis or by generalized weakness.

Adie, William John   (1887–1935) An Australian neurologist who trained in Edinburgh and in Europe before being appointed to the staff of the **National Hospital,** Queen Square, and the Charing Cross Hospital. During World War I he was mentioned in despatches for gallantry and for devising a temporary gas mask, consisting of clothing soaked in urine.[1829]

He wrote on a variety of subjects, such as **narcolepsy** (in his M.D. thesis), **myotonic dystrophy,** pituitary tumors, and **multiple sclerosis,** but is best remembered for his 1931 description[41] of the pupillary anomaly that bears his name, although he gave credit to colleagues for describing it in 1902. However, the first report was probably that of James Ware[5047] in a paper read to the Royal Society in 1812, and others thereafter had briefly noted the phenomenon as well.

Adie-Critchley syndrome   Forced grasping and groping in cases of tumor of the contralateral frontal lobe, described by these authors in 1927.[42]

Adie-Holmes syndrome   See **Adie pupil, Holmes-Adie syndrome.**

adiposis dolorosa   See **Dercum disease.**

adiposogenital syndrome   Arrest or delay in sexual development, with obesity, and due to destruction of the tuberal nuclei of the hypothalamus. The cause of most cases is not determined, but a craniopharyngioma is present in some cases.

adipsia   A decreased sensation of thirst, usually due to damage to the osmoreceptors of the anterior hypothalamus, such that in the presence of a high plasma osmolality. There is an inappropriate lack of thirst and water losses are not replenished by drinking.

The hypothalamic lesion may also cause a reduction in antidiuretic hormone secretion, so that the problem of thirst is complicated by excessive water loss.[170]

adjustment sleep disorder   Sleep disturbances temporally related to acute stress, conflict, or environmental change causing emotional arousal. The complaints of insomnia or excessive sleepiness are related in time to an identifiable stressor and remit if the stress is removed, or if adaptation to it improves. Polysomnography reveals an increased sleep latency, reduced sleep efficiency, or increased number and duration of awakenings; a prolonged total sleep time; or reduced mean sleep latency on the **minimum sleep latency test.**[234]

adolescent familial cramps   A relatively benign X-linked recessively or dominantly inherited myopathic syndrome of adolescence, characterized by cramps following exercise, elevated serum creatine kinase levels, normal production of lactate by muscle under ischemic conditions, and minimal weakness or wasting.[2424] See **cramps.**

adolescent stretch syncope   The occurrence of syncope when the subject stretches the truck with the neck hyperextended, resulting from compression of the craniocervical arteries.[5398]

ADR syndrome   (ataxia, deafness, mental retardation) See **cerebellar ataxias, Richards Rundle syndrome.**

adrenal hypoplasia with mental retardation and muscular dystrophy   See **Renier syndrome.**

adrenergic receptors   (adrenoceptors) Sites of the action of noradrenaline in the CNS. There are three types of receptor: α_1 (found in the cerebral cortex and thalamus), α_2, and β.

adrenocorticotrophic hormone   A peptide secreted by the hypothalamus, affecting functions within the CNS to do with task discrimination, approach-avoidance behavior, and memory.

adrenoleukodystrophy   (Siemerling-Creutzfeldt disease, sudanophilic leukodystrophy, melanodermic leukodystrophy, adrenoleukomyeloneuropathy, adrenomyelodystrophy; OMIM 300100) A group of progressive, X-linked recessive, peroxisomal degenerative disorders of myelin (leukodystrophies), the responsible gene mapping to Xq28. They are characterized by a deficiency of lignoceroyl coenzyme A synthetase.

The diagnosis is established by finding abnormal levels of very long–chain (C_{26}) fatty acids (VLCFAs) in the plasma, cultured fibroblasts and brain,[4012, 4013] for which a single peroxisomal deficiency is responsible. The abnormal VLCFA levels are considered responsible for interference with myelin formation, shown by the presence of severe myelinoclastic diffuse sclerosis not sparing the U fibers, especially in parieto-occipital regions. Axonal loss also occurs. Raised CSF protein levels, abnormal EEGs and nucleide scans, and the biochemical consequences of primary adrenal failure are also found.

The condition was first reported by Creutzfeldt in 1923, although Schilder had published reports of patients with various other white matter diseases (some accompanying adrenal insufficiency) in 1911. The status of **Schilder disease** as a separate entity is uncertain; it may not exist.

In the classical *X-linked juvenile variety* of adrenoleukodystrophy, the onset of symptoms is in childhood or youth, with progressive gait disturbance due to myelopathy, often with neuropathy and hypoadrenalism, sometimes with extrapyramidal or cerebellar signs, demyelinating sensorimotor peripheral neuropathy, and unmyelinated fiber loss.[2281]

In younger children with the X-linked form, progressive encephalopathy with cortical blindness, dementia, deafness, optic atrophy, and seizures are described; the same features may appear only later in life in males and are sometimes manifested in female carriers. Isolated myelopathy and isolated hypoadrenalism are other rare phenotypes.

At least six different phenotypes are recognized:

Childhood cerebral adrenoleukodystrophy A variant characterized by rapidly progressive cerebral demyelination

Adolescent cerebral adrenoleukodystrophy A phenotype similar to the childhood form but with slightly later age of onset

Adult cerebral adrenoleukodystrophy (OMIM 169500) A rare, dominantly inherited variant sometimes presenting with psychosis

Adrenomyeloneuropathy An X-linked metabolic defect in which deficiency of peroxisomal oxidation of VLCFAs leads to accumulation of these acids, especially hexocosanoate (C26:0), with a high C26/C22 ratio in plasma and fibroblasts. The gene locus has been mapped at Xq28. The condition is a clinically and genetically distinct variant of childhood adrenoleukodystrophy.[2281] It presents as a syndrome of adrenal insufficiency beginning in youth or early adult life, with the later development of progressive spastic paraparesis in the third decade, hypogonadism, and distal, axonal, dying-back, symmetrical polyneuropathy with autonomic involvement (causing impotence and sphincter disturbances) beginning in early adult life. Cerebellar dysfunction, dementia, and hemiparesis are also described.

X-linked Addison disease without neurological involvement

Asymptomatic forms[5727]

The current classification of the following three conditions is uncertain.

Naidu variant A disorder characterized by neonatal seizures, hypotonia, hepatomegaly, hypsarrhythmia, and developmental delay, with elevated VLCFA levels but normal liver peroxisomes[4062]

Infantile sudanophilic leukodystrophy A disorder resembling typical adrenoleukodystrophy beginning in infancy and is characterized by severe seizures and psychomotor retardation.[566] It resembles (and may be the same as) **Zellweger syndrome,** another peroxisomal disorder.

Neonatal adrenoleukodystrophy (recessive type) A congenital **peroxisomal disorder** in which multiple peroxisomal functions are deficient, inherited in a recessive manner, and characterized by frontal bossing, cataract, optic atrophy, pigmentary retinal degeneration, enlarged liver, adrenal hypoplasia, dementia, seizures, nystagmus, cerebral atrophy, diffusely increased skin pigmentation, and hyperpipecolic acidemia.[2993, 2994] Clinically, the features are almost identical to those of **Zellweger syndrome,** differing only in the milder involvement and longer survival of the affected infant (death ensuing at ages up to 10 years).[4773]

See also **female adrenoleukodystrophy, Pelizaeus-Merzbacher disease.**

adrenoleukomyeloneuropathy See **adrenoleukodystrophy.**

adrenomyelodystrophy See **adrenoleukodystrophy.**

adrenomyeloneuropathy See **adrenoleukodystrophy.**

Adrian, Edgar Douglas, Lord (1889–1977) English physiologist who was educated at Cambridge, where his neurophysiological studies included important research leading to the elucidation of the **all-or-nothing response.** He trained in neurology at the **National Hospital** and served in military hospitals during the World War I, returning thereafter to Cambridge, where he devoted the rest of his life to studies of the electrical reactions of muscle and nerve, the physiology of the retinal receptors, the all-or-nothing response,[48] receptor adaptation to stimuli (1926), the EEG, and the general principles of neural transmission, introducing many new investigative techniques, including coaxial needles for electromyography. For these studies he shared the Nobel Prize in 1932 with C.S. **Sherrington.** He was the first scientist to acknowledge and understand the significance of Hans **Berger's** EEG work, which had been ridiculed as artefact by others, and on which he elaborated.

He was made professor of physiology at Cambridge in 1937 and later became Master of Trinity College, after that vice-chancellor and then chancellor of the university. He was president of the Royal Society from 1951 to 1955, and was raised to the peerage on relinquishing that position.

Adson, Alfred Washington (1887–1951) American surgeon at the Mayo Clinic, Rochester, MN.

Adson syndrome (Naffziger syndrome) See **thoracic outlet syndrome.**

Adson test   A maneuver for the diagnosis of vasogenic thoracic outlet syndrome. The subject leans forward with the neck extended and turned to one or the other side, and then inhales deeply. Elevation of the rib cage puts further pressure on the subclavian artery and thus reduces the radial pulse on the side to which the head is turned. However, the same phenomenon occurs in many asymptomatic people, so the value of the test is unproven. Even the existence of the syndrome is disputed.[50] The performance of a Valsalva maneuver during hyperextension of the neck is an alternative method of doing this test.

adult acid maltase deficiency   See **glycogen storage disease.**

adult amaurotic idiocy   See **Martha-Alma disease.**

adult amylopectinosis   See **glycogen storage diseases.**

adult cretinism   (Gull syndrome) See **myxedema.**[2330]

adult myoclonic epilepsy   A syndrome of idiopathic generalized epilepsy in which myoclonic seizures beginning in adult life accompany absence or generalized tonic-clonic seizures. The family history is usually positive for seizures. The clinical examination and imaging studies are normal. The EEG shows generalized epileptiform abnormalities.[2119]

adult occult hydrocephalus   See **normal pressure hydrocephalus.**

adult polyglucosan body disease   A rare neurological disorder of unknown cause characterized by diffuse central and peripheral nervous system dysfunction, manifesting clinically as progressive upper and lower motor neurone involvement of the limbs, disturbances of the sphincters, sensory loss, and cognitive impairment. Pathologically, the condition is distinguished by the widespread accumulation of polyglucosan bodies throughout the nervous system.

The condition is considered to be inherited as an autosomal recessive trait in which abnormalities of branching enzyme activity in white cells are implicated,[3475, 4733] but it is likely to be heterogeneous.

adult polysaccharidosis   A rare syndrome characterized by the intracellular accumulation of abnormal polysaccharides resembling amylopectin in the form of cytoplasmic spheroids similar to those of **Lafora body disease** but presenting in adult life.

Clinically, the condition starts with paraparesis, progressing to quadriparesis, sensory loss in the legs, dementia, and death.[4409]

adult proximal spinal muscular atrophy   See **hereditary motor neuropathy** (*variants*).

adult spinal muscular atrophy   See **hereditary motor neuropathy, type 4.**

adult-onset dementia with argyrophilic grains   A progressive dementing disorder with clinical features indistinguishable from **Alzheimer disease** but in which no tangles are found in the cerebral cortex and with argyrophilic grains staining positive with Alz-50 monoclonal antibody.[2759]

adult-onset cerebellar ataxia and sensory deafness (of Schimke) See **cerebellar ataxias** (*variants*).

adult-onset foot dystonia   A rare form of localized **dystonia**, sometimes occurring as a presenting feature of Parkinson disease.[3117]

adult-onset leukodystrophies   See **18q syndrome, adrenoleukodystrophy, Alexander disease, Canavan disease, Cockayne syndrome, Krabbe disease, metachromatic leukodystrophy, multiple sulfatase deficiency, Pelizaeus-Merzbacher disease, childhood ataxia with CNS hypomyelination, sudanophilic leukodystrophies.**

Although most of these conditions more commonly start in childhood, all can occasionally appear first in adult life.[395]

advanced sleep phase syndrome   (phase lead, phase advance, evening somnolence and early morning wakefulness) A syndrome of persistent and consistent expedition in the times of sleep onset and of waking compared to the times that were formerly normal for that patient, leading to complaints of excessive evening sleepiness and of early waking. Sleep architecture is normal.[4268] In this disorder the major sleep episode is advanced in relation to the desired clock-time, resulting in symptoms of compelling evening sleepiness and an awakening that is earlier than desired. The following diagnostic criteria have been suggested:[234]

A. Inability to stay awake until the desired bedtime or inability to remain asleep until the desired time of awakening.

B. There is a phase advance of the major sleep episode in relation to the desired time for sleep.

C. Symptoms are present for at least 3 months.

D. When not required to remain awake until the desired (later) bedtime, patients will

  1. Have a habitual sleep period that is of normal quality and duration, with sleep onset earlier than desired;

  2. Awaken spontaneously earlier than desired;

  3. Maintain stable entrainment to a 24-hour sleep-wake pattern.

E. Does not meet criteria for any other disorder causing inability to maintain sleep or excessive sleepiness.

Adapted from *The International Classification of Sleep Disorders Diagnostic and Coding Manual.* Rochester, MN: American Sleep Disorders Association, © 1990. Reproduced by kind permission of the American Academy of Sleep Medicine.

Advances in Applied Neurological Sciences   (*Adv. Appl. Neurol. Sci.*) A neurological journal. Address: Springer-Verlag New York, Inc., 175 Fifth Avenue, New York, NY 10010.

Advances in Neurogerontology   (*Adv. Neurogerontol.*) A neurological subspecialty journal. Address: Praeger

Publishers, 1 Madison Avenue, New York, NY 10010–3603.

Advances in Neurology   (*Adv. Neurol.*) A neurological review book series. Address: Raven Press, 1185 Avenue of the Americas, Department 1B, New York, NY 10036.

Advances in Neuropsychology and Behavioral Neurology   (*Adv. Neuropsychol. Behav. Neurol.*) A neurological journal. Address: Guilford Publications, Inc., Journals Department, 72 Spring Street, New York, NY 10012.

adversive seizure   A variety of partial complex epilepsy in which there is tonic or clonic deviation of the head and eyes to one side with or without jerking of the arm on that side and the adoption of a raised, flexed posture of that arm.

Though formerly regarded as indicating that the origin of the seizure is in the frontal lobe on the side from which the head turns away, the localizing value of the sign is now questioned.

adynamesthesia   (Gr, lack of + power + feeling) Lack of appreciation of the force applied in a motor act, described with lesions in the contralateral prerolandic cortex.[4745]

adynamia   (Gr, lack of + power). Weakness.

adynamia episodica hereditaria, adynamia-hyperkalemia   (Gamstorp syndrome) See **familial periodic paralysis.**[2014]

adynamia periodica hereditaria   A dominantly inherited disorder of the muscle membrane with secondary effects on potassium metabolism in which attacks of muscle weakness with areflexia and percussion myotonia occur from childhood onwards, precipitated by rest after exercise, hunger, and cold. See **familial periodic paralysis** (*hyperkalemic form*).

aerocele   See **pneumo(cephalo)cele.**

aerotitis syndrome   Middle ear petechiae and inflammation following barotrauma and leading to complaints of fullness or pain in the ear, mild conduction deafness, and vertigo.[1563]

aesthesiometer   An instrument for measuring the sense of touch on the skin.

aesthesioneuroblastoma   (olfactory neuroblastoma) See **neuroblastoma**.

afebrile occasional seizures   Simple or complex motor seizures occurring as a symptom of underlying brain disease and not recurring after the underlying cause is no longer operating.

The list of causes includes intracranial infections or other encephalopathies, metabolic diseases, and head trauma.[56]

affect   (feeling-tone) The range, depth, and appropriateness of a subject's emotional responsiveness.

affective-psychic seizure   (dreamy state, psychic variant, automatism, vertige épileptique, psychomotor seizure) A form of simple partial seizure (thus without alteration of consciousness) characterized by alterations in mood or cognitive function as a result of the epileptic discharge. The seizures resemble those of complex partial type inasmuch as they may also be components of such attacks, and they have similar pathologies.

afferent   (Lat, carrying toward) Applied to neural impulses running into the CNS from the periphery, or to impulses running toward any identified structure.

Affiliated National Dystonia Association   A charitable organization comprising **the Dystonia Medical Research Foundation** and the **National Spasmodic Dysphonia Association. WE MOVE** also participates. The association awards research grants to discover the cause and cure of dystonia. It also sponsors symposia for the medical profession and for patients, and publishes educational materials and a newsletter and builds chapters and patient support groups.

Address: c/o Dystonia Foundation, One E. Wacker Dr., Ste. 2900, Chicago, IL 60601-2001. Tel: 312-755-0198.

affricate   A consonant which is produced by first blocking the airflow, as for a stop, and then slowly releasing it, causing turbulence as in a fricative sound—for example, /c/ as in cheese.[3505]

African trypanosomiasis   See **sleeping sickness.**

afterdischarge   1. The continuation of action potentials in a neuron, axon, or muscle fiber following the termination of an applied stimulus. 2. The continuation of firing of muscle action potentials after cessation of voluntary activation, for example, in myotonia. (From the 2001 Report of the Nomenclature Committee of the American Association of Electromyography and Electrodiagnosis.[10] Used by permission, copyright © 2001, AAEM.) 3. An EEG seizure pattern following repetitive electrical stimulation of a discrete area of the brain via cortical or intracerebral electrodes. 4. A burst of rhythmic activity following a transient such as an evoked potential or a spike. (Adapted from the 1974 Report of the Committee on Terminology, IFCN,[989] © 1974. With permission from Elsevier Science.)

afterimage   The persistence of a visual image after extinction of the original stimulus as a result of retinal changes during exposure to it. The perception may be similar to that of a photographic negative.

afternoon ectropion   Weakness of the periocular muscles increasing during the day and leading thus to ectropion in the evening in patients with **myasthenia gravis.**[5824]

after-nystagmus   Transient **nystagmus** occurring after a period of rotation of the body (as in a **Barany**

chair) has ceased, as a result of the continued movement of endolymph.

afterpotential   The membrane potential between the end of the spike and the time when the membrane potential is restored to its resting value. The membrane during this period may be depolarized or hyperpolarized at different times. (From the 2001 Report of the Nomenclature Committee of the American Association of Electromyography and Electrodiagnosis.[10] Reproduced by permission of the Association.

age   Years of life, the groupings being arbitrarily defined in 1879 as embryonic (9 months), infancy to 3 years, childhood to 12 years, adolescence to 25 years, maturity to 50 years, and decline thereafter. Boyhood and girlhood are defined as the period from the second dentition to puberty.[4512]

age-associated memory impairment   (age-associated cognitive decline, benign senescent forgetfulness) A state of minor cognitive impairment in the form of disturbances of memory function in people aged over 50 years.[1193] The following diagnostic criteria have been suggested (From Crook TH, Larrabee GJ. Age-associated memory impairment: Diagnostic Criteria and treatment strategies. Psychopharm Bull. 1988;2: 509–14, by permission of MediaWorks.[1191, 3747])

I. *Inclusion*
   A. Patient aged over 50 years
   B. Complaints of gradually progressive memory loss reflected in everyday circumstances
   C. Memory test performance at least 1 standard deviation below the mean established for young adults on a standardized test of recent memory (e.g., **Benton Visual Retention Test,** Logical Memory Scale, or Associate Learning subtests of the **Wechsler Memory Scale**)
   D. Evidence of adequate intellectual function as determined by a scaled score of at least 9 on the Vocabulary subtest of the **Wechsler Adult Intelligence Scale**
   E. Absence of dementia, as suggested by a score of 24 or higher on the **Mini-Mental State Examination**
II. *Exclusion*
   A. Evidence of delirium, confusion, or alteration in consciousness or of any general medical or neurological disorder which could cause cognitive deterioration
   B. History of any infective or inflammatory brain disease
   C. Evidence of significant cerebrovascular pathology; repeated head injury; or depression, mania, or any other major psychiatric disorder
   D. Current diagnosis or history of substance abuse or use of psychotropic drug in the previous month

Whether this condition blends over time into a true dementing illness remains to be seen; now, as at the time of publication of the first edition of this book, the author prognosticates that it will eventually be shown to do so.

agenesis   The failure of the formation of a body part during embryological development. In the case of the corpus callosum, agenesis may occur alone or in association with other cerebral malformations or as part of a number of other syndromes such as alobar **holoproscencephaly,** and it may also be a marker for certain inherited metabolic diseases.[3120, 3838]

Agenesis of the cerebellar vermis may be asymptomatic or may be associated with impaired motor coordination.

agenesis of the cerebellar vermis   See **Joubert syndrome.**

agenesis of the cerebellum   An uncommon malformation characterized by improper development of the dentate nuclei, vermis, and cerebellar peduncles.[3091] Unilateral maldevelopment of the cerebellum is more common.

agenesis of the corpus callosum   (callosal agenesis) A dysmorphic developmental syndrome presenting clinically with brachycephaly, hypertelorism, and hyperhidrosis in childhood with abnormality in consciousness, flushing, poor temperature control, and mental and developmental delay.[444] **Microcephaly** and **heterotopias** may be associated. Both recessive and X-linked kinships have been described.

The anatomical defect was described first by Reil in 1812. The same anomaly complicates a number of other congenital degenerative syndromes.[335]

Variants include the following:

Agenesis of the corpus callosum, X-linked A congenital syndrome comprising megacolon, adducted thumbs, and mental and developmental delay in addition to the dysmorphogenesis.[2924]

Agenesis of the corpus callosum with hypothermia A syndrome that has been reported in childhood and adult life. Some cases show spongy white matter disease.[4452]

Agenesis of the corpus callosum with anterior horn cell disease (Charlevoix County disease) A dysmorphic condition described in Quebec in which the agenesis is complicated by lower motor neuron lesions causing flaccid quadriparesis, areflexia, sensory neuropathy, and mental retardation.[163]

See also **acrocallosal syndrome.**

agenesis of the septum pellucidum with porencephaly   A congenital dysmorphic syndrome characterized by heterotopias within the cerebrum; microcephaly, hydranencephaly, or porencephaly; polymicrogyria; and absence of the septum pellucidum.

Clinically, it manifests with mental and developmental delay, pyramidal signs, and dystonia.[337]

ageotropic nystagmus   (apogeotropic nystagmus) See **vestibular nystagmus.**

age-related cognitive decline   See **age-associated memory impairment.**

ageusia   (Gr, lack of + the sensation of taste). Loss of taste sensation, usually resulting from lesions of the chorda tympani, and less commonly as a result of disorders of the brainstem or of the temporal lobes.

aggressive myoclonic epilepsies   A syndrome characterized by myoclonic jerks which are fragmental and usually erratic. See **progressive myoclonic epilepsy.**

agnathia-holoprosencephaly A congenital dysmorphic syndrome characterized by an absent or small mandible and holoprosencephaly.[337]

agnosia Impairment of the ability to recognize stimuli which were formerly recognized, in the absence of disturbances of perception, intellect, or language and due to acquired lesions of the cerebral cortex. In Teuber's words, perceptions are stripped of meaning; vision, hearing, and tactile sensations may also be affected.

The term was coined by Sigmund Freud in 1891, but others, using the terms *visual perceptive centers, asymbolia,* and *imperceptions,* had clearly recognized the existence of the condition.[3857] The causal lesions are usually in the posterior part of the parietal lobe, but can be in the callosum or deeper white matter where they act to disconnect the speech area from the primary sensory cortex. This indicates that, as Geschwind had originally proposed, most agnosias are modality-specific naming defects with a marked confabulatory response and represent disconnection syndromes.

Visual agnosia is "a disorder of higher behaviour confined to the visual realm in which an alert, attentive, intelligent and non-aphasic patient with normal visual perception gives evidence of not knowing the meaning of [or of not recognizing visual] stimuli."[1260]

Prosopagnosia (from Gr, a face + to know) is a form of visual agnosia characterized by the inability to recognize previously known faces or other complex visual stimuli and to learn new ones. Generic recognition may remain (a face) but specific recognition (Uncle Fred) is lost, indicating a failure of visually triggered episodic memory. Bilateral lesions of the central visual system are responsible.

Visual object agnosia is often associated with prosopagnosia and with failures of generic recognition. The lesions are bilateral and extensive, affecting the ventral and mesial occipitotemporal visual cortex. Object agnosia without prosopagnosia is sometimes seen with a unilateral lesion of the left occipitotemporal region.

See also **apperceptive agnosia, associative agnosia.**

agnosopsia The ability to discriminate in the absence of awareness of what is being discriminated. See **Riddoch syndrome.**

agonist 1. (prime mover, protagonist) A muscle, the major action of which is to produce a particular movement in question. See **prime mover, antagonist**. 2. A chemical substance that binds to a receptor, exciting it.

agoraphobia (Gr, an assembly or marketplace + fear) Pathological fear of open spaces; the term was introduced by **Westphal** in 1871.[5933]

agrammatic aphasia See **Broca aphasia.**

agrammatism (telegraphic speech, nonfluent aphasia) An aphasic disorder that impairs syntax rather than vocabulary and that leads to effortful, dysprosodic speech, often with associated dysarthria and improper sentence construction. It results from an inability to organize words so that sentences follow grammatical rules, and from the improper use or nonuse of grammatical morphemes (e.g., conjunctions, prepositions, and bound inflectional affixes such as *-ed, -ment,* or *-ing*).[2190]

The substantive content of speech uttered is high but the supporting grammar distortion makes the speech sound like pidgin English or a telegram. The causal lesion is in the Sylvian cortex. This term was first used by **Pick** in 1913.

agranular cortex The motor strip, containing pyramidal rather than granular cells.

agraphesthesia Lack of the ability to perceive figures drawn on the skin, as with lesions of the contralateral parietal lobe, subcortical structures, spinal cord, and the peripheral nerves.

This is a sensitive and consistent indicator of defective perception of cutaneous sensory space but it is not of value in localizing the cause of sensory disturbance to the parietal lobe. The faculty had been identified by Hall and Donaldson in 1885 but the word was only introduced 40 years later.[451] See also **tactile agnosia.**

agraphia (Gr, lack of + writing) Difficulty experienced in self-expression by means of writing.[1179] The term is generally restricted to that inability to write due to a cerebral lesion but which is not traceable to a gross motor handicap. The first modern descriptions were those of Jean Pitres (1848–1928) in 1884, and of **Déjèrine.**[1339]

Various classifications exist:

Anterior agraphia Writing is characterized by large, crude, and scrawled letters, written usually with the left hand in dextrals who have suffered an anterior lesion of the dominant hemisphere.

Posterior agraphia Writing is characterized by well-formed letters composed into sentences but with omissions, misspellings, and incorrect word order, seen in dextrals who have suffered a posterior lesion of the dominant hemisphere.

Visuospatial agraphia Writing is characterized by inappropriate placement of normal words and letters on the page, as seen in patients who have suffered a nondominant hemisphere lesion.

An alternative descriptive classification[399] recognizes the following:

Aphasic agraphia The agraphia accompanies Broca, Wernicke, conduction, or transcortical sensory dysphasia.

Agraphia with alexia (parietal agraphia) This disorder occurs with dominant parietal lobe lesions and leads to the poor formation of letters and to spelling errors.

Pure agraphia Writing is characterized by poor spelling, although the words are well formed; neither alexia nor aphasia is present.

Apraxic agraphia This dominant parietal lobe syndrome is characterized by difficulty forming letters and words when writing spontaneously or to dictation, often accompanied by errors in copying and in oral spelling.

Spatial agraphia Writing is distorted by abnormal placement of the letters on the page, often explicable by visual neglect, since a nondominant parietal lobe lesion is the usual cause.

To these forms the following may yet be added:

Deep agraphia A disorder characterized by lexicalizations and semantic errors. [AK]

Surface agraphia A disorder in which irregular spelling is regularized. [AK]

Phonological agraphia A disorder in which there is specific impairment of the conversion from phoneme to grapheme and in which dictated nonwords cannot be transcribed. [AK]

agraphia with alexia   See **agraphia.**

agrypnia   (Gr, lack of + sleep) Total and prolonged absence of sleep. A condition characterized by total insomnia without tiredness.[1831]

It has been described in *agrypnia with fibrillary chorea of Morvan*[4005] as a syndrome of unknown cause characterized by complete absence of sleep and of sleepiness, evening hallucinations, generalized fasciculations and paresthesias, and abnormal movements as in Morvan disease. Some relief of the agrypnia has been obtained by oral 5-hydroxytryptophan ingestion. The cause is unknown; both viral infection and mercury poisoning have been incriminated.

Aguecheek disease   A literary allusion to the Shakespearean character, Sir Andrew Aguecheek in *Twelfth Night* (1602), whose former intellect appears to have been commendable: "[he] . . . plays o'the viol de Gamboys, and speaks three or four languages word for word without the book and hath all the good gifts of Nature" (Act I, Scene 3), but, having been drunk nightly, lost important mental powers: " . . . for many do call me a fool" (Act II, Scene 5). Moreover, his drinking companion Sir Toby Belch considered that " . . . if you were to find so much blood in [Andrew's] liver as would clog the foot of a flea, I'll eat the rest of the anatomy."

Shakespeare gave Sir Andrew himself some insight: "Methinks I have no more wit than a Christian or an ordinary man has; but I am a great eater of beef, and I believe that does harm to my wit." Summerskill[5412] has neatly suggested that this was the first account of **chronic portosystemic encephalopathy.**

Aguilar syndrome   A congenital dysmorphic syndrome characterized by conjunctival telangiectasias, immunoglobulin deficiency, seizures, and mental and developmental delay.[54] See **ataxia–telangiectasia-like syndrome.**

agyria   Absence of gyri in the cerebral cortex. See **lissencephaly.**

ai   An old Gascon word for tenosynovitis.

Aicardi syndrome   The association of **infantile spasms, agenesis of the corpus callosum,** and chori-

oretinal lacunae. Other features of note are myoclonus, psychomotor deterioration, optic hypoplasia, chorioretinopathy, vertebral, and other dysplastic bony anomalies including microcephaly, asynchronous burst–suppression EEG patterns in the two hemispheres, and female gender. The condition was described in 1969.

An unidentified intrauterine insult during the first trimester was considered to be the cause,[527] but the condition may be X-linked dominant (at Xp22) with lethality in affected males.[335]

Aicardi Syndrome Foundation   A charitable organization in this field. Address: 450 Winterwood Drive, Roselle, IL 60172. Tel: 800-374-8518. E-mail: aicardi@aol.com. Web site: http://www.aicardi.com.

Aicardi-Goutières syndrome   (microcephaly with basal ganglion calcification) A congenital leukodystrophy syndrome, autosomal recessive but genetically heterogeneous, and characterized by microcephaly, seizures, basal ganglion calcification, hydrocephalus, and mental and developmental delay.[61]

AIDS   See **HIV disease** Organizations offering information and support in this disease include the *Elizabeth Glaser Pediatric AIDS Foundation* (Address: 2950 31st St. Suite 125, Santa Monica, CA 90405. Tel: 310-314-1459; 888-499-4673. E-mail: info@pedAIDS.org. Web site: http://www.pedAIDS.org); the *American Foundation for AIDS Research* (Address: 120 Wall St. 13th Floor, New York, NY 10005-3902. Tel: 212-806-1600. E-mail: publications@amfar.org. Web site: http://www.amfar.org); the *National Association of People with AIDS* (Address: 1413K Street, NW 7th Floor Washington, DC 20005-3442. Tel: 202-898-0414 ext. 124. E-mail: imbrevelle@napwa.org. Web site: http://www.napwa.org); the *National NeuroAIDS Tissue Consortium* (Address: 1050 Forest Hill Road, Staten Island, NY 10314. E-mail: Joanna@hivbrainbanks.org. Tel: 800-510-1678. Web site: http://www.hivbrainbanks.org); and the *National Institute of Allergy and Infectious Diseases* (NIAID) (Address: National Institutes of Health, 31 Center Drive, Rm. 7A50 MSC 2520 Bethesda, MD 20892-2520. Tel: 301-496-5717. Web site: http://www.niaid.nih.gov).

AIDS radiculopathy   An inflammatory demyelinating polyneuropathy resembling **acute** or **chronic inflammatory demyelinating polyneuropathy,** considered to be immune mediated and to reflect disordered immune regulation in patients infected with the human T-cell lymphotropic virus type III.

A predominantly sensory mixed axonal-demyelinating polyneuropathy is also found in patients with AIDS-related complex, and features of multiple mononeuropathy also occur in some of these patients. Another neuropathy with painful dysesthesias and symmetrical distal sensory loss has also been reported.[1135, 5244] See also **HIV-associated progressive polyneuropathy.**

AIDS-dementia complex   See **HIV encephalopathy.**

AIDS-related dementia   See **HIV encephalopathy.**

ainhum   Spontaneous amputation of the smallest toes without anesthesia; a tropical disease seen in the Black races.

akataphasia   (Gr, negative + to declare) See **Broca aphasia.**

akathisia   (Gr, an inability to stay down) A feeling of restlessness or an irresistible urge to move, of which the patient is painfully aware. The urge is usually expressed as complex, stereotyped, and repetitive movements. The condition is most commonly induced by dopamine receptor–blocking drugs.[2096]

Complex stereotypies, accompanied by restlessness, are also common in patients with akathisia. Both early **acute persistent** and *chronic tardive* forms have been distinguished, the former when the dose of a neuroleptic drug is being increased and the latter at a late stage of therapy, during its reduction. See also **restless legs syndrome, Tourette syndrome.**

The following rating scale has been designed:[4865]

Subjective

(Rate each 0 = absent, 1 = mild, 2 = moderate, 3 = severe)
1. Feeling of restlessness, especially in the legs
2. Inability to keep the legs still.
3. Inability to remain still, standing or sitting.

Objective

(Rate each 0 = absent, 1 = mild, 2 = moderate, 3 = severe)
1. Sitting:
   Semipurposeful/purposeless leg/feet movements
   Semipurposeful hand/arm movements
   Shifting body position in chair
   Inability to remain seated
2. Standing:
   Purposeless/semipurposeful leg/feet movements
   Shifting weight from foot to foot or walking on the spot
   Inability to remain standing in one place (walking/pacing)

Reproduced from Sachev P and Loneragan C. Low dose apomorphine challenge in tardive akathisia. *Neurology* 1993;43:544–7, by permission.

akee   (achee) A West Indian fruit containing hypoglycin, an inhibitor of acyl coenzyme A dehydrogenases. Intoxication leads to a picture resembling **isovaleric acidemia.**[3835]

akinesia   (akinesis) (Gr, lack of + set in motion) Defined by an ad hoc committee of the World Federation of Neurology as a movement disorder "characterized by poverty and slowness of initiation and execution of willed and associated movements, and difficulty in changing one motor pattern to another in the absence of paralysis. This may include an inability to sustain repetitive movements and difficulty in performing repetitive motor acts and may vary in severity from slight (sometimes called hypokinesia) to severe and complete immobility."[6038]

akinesia algera   (Möbius syndrome, atremia) The loss of voluntary motion as a result of pain produced by such motion. In the absence of any detectable physical disease likely to be responsible, the condition is considered to be functional or psychogenic.[5286]

akinesthesia   Loss of directional sensitivity in the skin and joints.

akinetic freezing of gait   A hypokinetic form of fluctuation in parkinsonian patients on long-term levadopa therapy.

akinetic mutism   (**persistent vegetative state**) The term introduced by Cairns[870] for the state in which patients appear awake and maintain a sleep–wake cycle but are unable to communicate in any way (that is, not by speech, by gesture, or by facial expression). The condition is characterized by continuous or prolonged deep NREM hypersomnia or coma with some retention of eye movements but with loss of REM sleep and of arousal mechanisms. The **Glasgow Coma Scale** score will be 4-1-1 or less.

Cairns' original patient had an epidermoid tumor of the third ventricle, but patients with lesions in the region of the thalamus, basal ganglia, anterior cingulate gyrus, or pons, or with obstructive hydrocephalus and those with **Creutzfeldt-Jakob** disease may also enter this state. Those with lesions of the paramedian part of the posterior diencephalon, the anterior thalamic peduncle, or the midbrain are said to have posterior or mesencephalic akinetic mutism and those with bifrontal lesions disconnecting the cingulate cortex, to have the anterior or frontal form.

Since damage to both afferent and efferent pathways and to the rostral reticular activating system has caused the syndrome, it cannot be called homogeneous, although the clinical syndrome shows little variation. See **persistent vegetative state** (the preferred term), also **de-efferented state.**

akinetic rigid syndromes   Degenerative brain diseases producing these features.[6031]

They include **Wilson disease; dopa-responsive dystonia; Juvenile Huntington disease; SCA3/MJD; DRPLA; Pelizaeus-Merzbacher disease; ataxia-telangiectasia; Lesch-Nyhan syndrome; Hallervorden-Spatz disease; familial prion diseases;** autosomal dominant and autosomal recessive juvenile **Parkinson disease; X-linked dystonia parkinsonism** (**Lubag**), and **DDPAC.**

akinetic rigidity   See **arteriosclerotic rigidity.**

akinetic seizures   (centrencephalic myoclonic-astatic petit mal seizures) A syndrome in which seizures manifest by sudden and complete loss of muscle tone or absences are accompanied by severe mental retardation and often by major motor (grand mal) seizures.[2705] See also **Lennox-Gastaut syndrome.**

akinetic syndrome   See **Parkinson disease.**

akinetic-rigid syndrome   Loss of the ability to initiate and execute movements, associated with a loss of postural stability; negative symptoms, as typically seen in basal ganglion syndromes such as Parkinson disease but also as a result of heatstroke, as a toxic effect and in numerous neyrological disorders. The subject was reviewed by Riley and Lang in 1996.[4697]

akinetopsia   See **cerebral akinetopsia.**

akopia   See **acopia.**

Akureyri disease   See **von Economo disease.**

Alajouanine syndrome   Congenital bilateral paralysis of the sixth and seventh cranial nerves, with clubfoot.[67]

Alajouanine, Theophile   (1869–1959) French neurologist who was a pupil of the **Déjèrines** in Paris.

Alajouanine-Foix syndrome   See **subacute necrotic myelopathy.**

alalia   (Gr, lack of + to talk) Speechlessness due to paralysis of the vocal apparatus.

Aland disease   An X-linked disease reported (only) from the Aland Islands, characterized by deafness, seizures, mental retardation, latent nystagmus, and tapetoretinal degeneration.[1911]

alaninuria–microcephaly–dwarfism–diabetes syndrome   See **Stimmler syndrome.**

alarm reaction   The first of the three stages of adaptive reaction to stressful situations defined by Hans **Selye.** It is marked by strong sympathetic activity, sufficient for the fight-or-flight response.

alarm clock headache   The term reflects the regularity of the attacks of head pain in many of these patients. See **cluster headache.**

Albers-Schonberg disease   (osteopetrosis, osteosclerosis fragilis, marble bone disease) A dominantly or recessively inherited syndrome characterized by increased density of the bones throughout the skeleton with unusual brittleness and associated with anemia and macrocephaly. The condition occasionally leads to cranial nerve (e.g., I, II, III, V, VII, VIII) palsies, nystagmus, or hydrocephalus.[3085, 5651]

In the condition was described in 1904 by Heinreich Ernst Albers-Schonberg (1865–1921), a German radiologist and professor at Hamburg University, who devoted his life to the study of X-rays and clinical radiology without being fully aware of their dangers.[78] See also **osteopetrosis.**

In a *variant form*, osteopetrosis is combined with syndactyly.[5651]

Albert disease   See **achillodynia.**

Albert test   A test of visual neglect in which the subject is required to cross out a series of lines ruled on a sheet of paper; the percentage of lines left uncrossed gives a score which in patients with acute stroke is related to cognitive outcome 6 months later.[80] See also **neglect.**

albinism   Hereditary syndromes characterized by deficiency of melanin production in the eyes and/or skin. Most have no neurological complications other than congenital nystagmus.

The Rev. Mr. Spooner, a classicist don and warden of New College Oxford, was albino and it has been suggested that his verbal distortions ("Sir! You have hissed all my mystery lectures; you shall leave Oxford by the town drain") could be accounted for by his nystagmus which jumbled the words that he read; however, his abnormal speech was by all accounts spontaneous as much as read, so this explanation may be insufficient.

albinism with degenerative features   A dominantly inherited syndrome of deaf-mutism with albinism.[5583]

Albright hereditary osteodystrophy   (Fuller Albright syndrome, osteitis fibrosa disseminata, polyostotic fibrous dysplasia) A rare disorder with onset in childhood, characterized by replacement of bone by fibrous tissue, bony cysts, precocious puberty in female patients, areas of brown skin pigmentation, and, in some cases, papilledema and optic atrophy.[86]

Albright syndrome   (pseudohypoparathyroidism and pseudopseudo hypoparathyroidism) A congenital dysmetabolic, dysmorphic **neurocutaneous syndrome** characterized by obesity; short stature; brachydactyly; dental anomalies; precocious puberty in females; hypocalcemia; intracranial, intramuscular, and subcutaneous calcification; skin hyperpigmentation; and mental and developmental delay.[3] Ocular symptoms reported include proptosis, visual field defects, optic atrophy, and papilledema.[86]

albumino-cytologic dissociation   A marked increase in the level of protein in the cerebrospinal fluid without a similarly large increase in the cell count. See **Froin syndrome.**

alcohol   A sedative drug, relaxing inhibitions first and the cause of much social and medical misery as well as of transient emotional relief. King Darius of the Persians had inscribed on his tomb, "I could drink much wine and bear it well" and William Pitt found that he could retire during a lively debate for a couple of bottles of port to refresh and enliven his faculties, but most heavy drinkers (i.e., more than three drinks per day for men or two for women) suffer some medical consequences; some of the neurological problems are listed in the following entries.

alcohol-dependent sleep disorder   A disorder characterized by the assisted initiation of sleep by the sustained ingestion of ethanol, used here for its sedative effect.[234] Other alcoholic patients claim that they persistently wake up too early in the morning.

alcoholic cerebellar degeneration   A uniform syndrome in chronic alcoholics resulting from atrophy, especially of the cerebellar vermis. The clinical features include a broad-based, staggering gait, impaired heel–toe walking, slow leg tremor, and terminal oscillations in the finger–nose test with minimal involvement of the arms and without nystagmus or dysarthria.

The disorder is associated with destruction of all the neurocellular elements of the cerebellar cortex, and with damage to the anterior and superior aspects of the vermis and the olivary nuclei. Cerebral cortical atrophy is also likely to accompany this syndrome.[2574]

alcoholic dementia   Widespread affections of intellectual function, subtle or severe, occurring in chronic alcoholics who have no evidence of Alzheimer disease, of multi-infarct dementia, nor of the **Wernicke-Korsakoff syndrome** (which is the diagnosis usually applied in cases where the onset was not abrupt), and in whom there is a tendency for cortical shrinkage and ventricular dilatation on head CT scans.[3425] The absence of any typical pathology makes the existence of the entity as a primary condition suspect, however.[5759] See also **Marchiafava-Bignami disease, pellagrous encephalopathy, acquired hepatocerebral encephalopathy.**

alcoholic encephalopathy   Alcohol-engendered **pellagra** affecting the brain, leading to central chromatolysis, especially marked in the brainstem pontine nuclei and cerebellar dentate nuclei, and in the nuclei of the third, sixth, seventh, and eighth cranial nerves.[2481]

alcoholic myopathy   A syndrome of acute or chronic weakness due to the toxic effects of alcohol.

The *acute form* (**acute alcoholic myopathy**) is a necrotizing myopathy presenting with muscle pain, tenderness, swelling, and weakness which begins during a period of heavy alcohol intake. Myoglobinuria is commonly detectable, as are other manifestations of acute alcohol toxicity or withdrawal, many of which lead to excessive muscular activity.[1627]

The *chronic form* is a slowly progressive, painless proximal myopathy with retained reflexes, affecting the legs more than the arms. It improves with cessation of alcohol ingestion and improved nutrition.[1627]

A form associated with *hypokalemia* (**acute hypokalemic myopathy of alcoholism**) is also described.[2683]

alcoholic neuropathy   (athrodynia a potu) A painful centripetal sensorimotor axonal neuropathy due to nutritional deficiencies in alcoholics. The condition was first described in 1779 by Lettsom (1744–1815), a physician in the Virgin Islands, and then in 1822 by James Jackson, Sr. (1777–1867).

Clinically, insidiously progressive, distal weakness, paresthesias, and burning pain are the usual symptoms, felt in the legs much more than in the arms; hyperesthesias and hyperpathias are also common complaints. Symmetrical hyporeflexia, distal weakness, and the usual features of sensorimotor and autonomic neuropathy, with trophic changes, are typical signs.

A variant is *acute alcoholic axonal polyneuropathy*, presenting with flaccid tetraplegia and areflexia in subjects with malnutrition related to heavy alcohol consumption.[6016] See also **Wernicke-Korsakoff syndrome, Strachan syndrome, beriberi.**

alcoholic paraplegia   Weakness of the legs associated with excessive alcohol abuse, described first in 1868 by Samuel Wilks (1824–1911), physician to Guy's Hospital, London.[5974]

The condition is likely to represent either a severe motor neuropathy or a proximal myopathy, as described in the preceding entries.

Alcoholics Anonymous   General Services Office Address: Box 459, Grand Central Station, New York, NY 10017. A Web site allowing contact with the whole system is at http://www.aa-uk.org.uk/lists/Alanon.htm

aldolase A deficiency   A congenital dysmorphic syndrome characterized by dwarfism; strabismus; ptosis; dental, dermal, skeletal, and cardiac anomalies; enlarged liver; microcephaly; and mental and developmental delay.[337]

alertness   A phasic, graded state of arousal in which the subject is awake and responsive to environmental stimuli.

Alexander disease   (fibrinoid degeneration of astrocytes, dysmyelinogenic leukodystrophy; OMIM 203450) A rare sporadic leukodystrophy, usually occurring in infants, and characterized by fibrinoid degeneration of astrocytes which contain deposits resembling **Rosenthal fibers,** with widespread demyelination but preservation of neurons. Its biochemical basis is undefined. Linkage to 11q13 has been established.

The major clinical features include psychomotor retardation, growth delay, seizures, spastic quadriparesis, and megalencephaly; death ensues within a few years. The condition was described by W.S. Alexander in 1949.[97]

Variants include: a *localized form* in infants, characterized by spastic dysarthria, dysphagia, and fasciculations,[337] and the *juvenile type*, characterized by self-mutation, seizures, bulbar weakness, nystagmus, ataxia, and pyramidal signs.[668]

Even rarer *adult forms* are characterized by manifest dementia, dysarthria, ataxia, intracranial calcification, cerebral gliosis, and diffuse demyelination.[4857] One report describes familial occurrence, with added palatal myoclonus.[5017]

Alexander Graham Bell Association for the Deaf   A charitable organization. Address: 3417 Volta Pl. NW, Washington, D.C. 20007-778.

Alexander's laws   1. The amplitude of the nystagmus caused by central lesion changes with the direction of gaze, being greater when gaze is directed in the direction of the fast phase.[4728] 2. Nystagmus of vestibular origin is separable into three degrees. In the first, it is present only when gaze is in the direction of the fast phase of the nystagmus; in the second, it is also present in the primary position; and in the third, it is present when gaze is in any direction. Thus, in sum, nystagmus of vestibular origin is of greatest amplitude when the subject looks in the direction of its fast component. This last series of statements was enunciated by Dr. Gustav Alexander, an Austrian otolaryngologist, in 1912.

alexia   (Gr, lack of + lexicon) Inability to comprehend the meaning of written or printed language symbols.[1172] Auditory comprehension is retained and spontaneous speech is normal in the pure form, which is rare.

The condition was separated from other varieties of language impairment in 1885 by Lichtheim. **Déjèrine** described the two major varieties (*with agraphia* and *without agraphia*, see following entries) in 1891–1892, and determined that the left angular gyrus is the center for the interpretation of the visual images which constitute written language.

A third form (*anterior or frontal alexia*; preangular, literal alexia, letter blindness) also exists, in association with **Broca aphasia** due to a lesion in the posterior part of the dominant frontal lobe. It may represent inability to read out loud while internal comprehension is retained (in which case it is not really an alexia at all), or the exposure of a lifelong reading problem, but is most often a feature of the primary lesion.

Its features include **syntactic alexia** and anomia for letters, though there is some success with comprehension of spelled words. Spelling aloud is poor. There is severe agraphia; poor ability to comprehend spelled words and to spell aloud; nonfluent aphasia; poor, clumsy copying with omissions; and accompanying right hemiparesis, motor apraxia, and mild sensory loss.[463, 467]

A fourth form, *deep dyslexia*, is a condition of total alexia and agraphia with an added lack of comprehension of words spelled out, and is due to a lesion of the posterior parts of the cortical language areas. It occurs usually in the context of recovery from total alexia. In this condition, a patient can read only by lexical semantic association, which leads to speech containing a number of synonyms which are spoken in place of the words read. See **deep dyslexia.**

alexia with agraphia   (central alexia; associative, verbal, literal, semantic, subangular, aphasic, total, parietal-temporal, letter, aphasic, or cortical alexia; angular gyrus syndrome; word and letter blindness; word blindness; acquired illiteracy) A symptom complex identified by **Déjèrine** in 1891, comprising impaired reading and naming, especially of letters but also of words (literal and verbal alexia); severe impairment of both spontaneous writing and writing to dictation, with retention of only a slavish ability to copy (agraphia); and an inability to comprehend spelled words and to spell aloud. Fluent aphasia, anomia, right hemisensory deficits with hemianopia, and the features of **Gerstmann syndrome** are occasionally found. The causal lesion is in the dominant parietotemporal region.[1339]

alexia without agraphia   (posterior, occipital, sensory, verbal, agnosic, optic, associative, spleniooccipital, postangular, visual or pure alexia; pure word blindness) A **disconnection syndrome** described by **Déjèrine** (1892) and the first for which clear anatomical evidence was forthcoming. The major feature is an inability to read letters, words, or musical notation, in association with a right hemianopia and difficulties with color naming. Copying, writing spontaneously and to dictation, and the interpretation of pictures and letter naming are preserved, however, and verbal output is fluent and appropriate. Comprehension of spelled words and spelling aloud are retained. A patient with the syndrome was recorded by Johann Schmidt in 1673 as follows: "He could not read written characters, much less combine them in any way. He did not know a single letter nor could he distinguish one from the other. But it is remarkable that, if some name were given to him to be written, he could write it readily, spelling it correctly. However, he could not read what he had written even though it was in his own hand."

The causal lesions are of the left occipital lobe and of the splenium of the corpus callosum, disconnecting the intact right visual cortex (area 18) from the left angular gyrus.[2080]

alexithymia   A trait of personality characterized by difficulty in verbalizing one's perceived emotions.

algesthesis   (Gr, pain + perception) An antique term for any painful condition.

algetic   (Gr, pain) Producing pain.

algodystrophy   (Sudeck atrophy) See **reflex sympathetic dystrophy, causalgia.**

algoneurodystrophy   See **reflex sympathetic dystrophy.**

Alice-in-Wonderland syndrome   (depersonalization syndrome, Lilliputian syndrome) A syndrome of bizarre disturbances of the body image, feelings of levitation, alteration of the sense of the passage of time, depersonalization, **metamorphopsia,** and doubting of personality that may occur in the setting of migraine, epilepsy, parietal lobe disease, hypnagogic states, schizophrenia, delirious states, or ingestion of hallucinogens. In migraine at least, the patient retains insight into the unreality of the experiences. The syndrome is also well described in children.[2665]

The same feelings of detachment, unreal changes in the outside world, fantastic distortions of the sizes and shapes of people and things, and the bewilderment that plagued Alice also affect the victims of this syndrome, as was noted by J.W. Todd in 1955.[5596] The fact that Lewis Carroll suffered from migraine may also have led to the appellation,[3818] and as Alice drank several mysterious vials of liquid before her strange experiences, so also have a number of victims of this syndrome ingested drugs such as LSD and hashish.[5047]

alien hand (limb) syndromes   (la main étrangère; anarchic hand) Failure to recognize ownership of a limb in the absence of visual cues, associated with autonomous activity of that limb, which are perceived by the subject as outside one's control; thus a circumstance in which one of the patient's hands behaves idiosyncratically and automatically in a way which the patient finds foreign, or at least uncooperative. It usually complicates a callosal lesion, and may be accompanied by grasp reflexes, cortical myoclonus, involuntary groping towards (or manipulation of) objects perceived, intermanual conflict, mirror movements, and motor perseveration.[329]

Three forms are recognized. The *callosal form* is characterized by intermanual conflict and the *frontal type* by reflex grasping. The former usually occurs in the nondominant hand and is temporary, while the latter is due to left medial frontal lesions with callosal involvement and is persistent; alien phenomena are seen in the contralateral dominant hand.[4969] A major recent review is that of Fisher.[1864] A *sensory alien hand syndrome* is also described; the right arm carries out involuntary movements of choking and attack on the left side of the body following a stroke in right posterior cerebral artery territory. Multiple disorders of primary sensation, sensory processing, hemispatial attention and visual association, and severe left arm ataxia are also present.[276]

In a *variant form* that may be ictal, the phenomenon occurs paroxysmally. The cortical lesions described were frontomedial or posteroparietal.[3331]

alien tissue lesions   Hamartomatous masses commonly found in the temporal lobes of patients operated on for complex partial seizures.

They are of three main types. *Glial forms* may be astroglial or oligodendroglial; *mixed neuroglial forms* include gangliogliomas and cortical dysplasias, neither of which acts like a tumor. The *vascular lesions* occurring in this context represent angiomatous malformations.[6]

aliquorrhea   A syndrome of low intracranial pressure following lumbar puncture or traumatic meningeal tears, and occasionally seen with subdural hematomas or occurring spontaneously.

The leading clinical symptom is headache occurring in the upright position, which fades quickly when the recumbent position is attained. See also **spontaneous intracranial hypotension.**

allachesthesia   See **alloesthesia.**

allele (allelic) diseases   Diseases with differing manifestations but resulting from a disorder of the same gene. Conditions in which the same genetic abnormality leads to differing clinical manifestations.

Allen reflex   1. (Gonda reflex) A variant of the **Babinski reflex** in which dorsiflexion of the hallux is sought in response to downward stretching and sudden release of the second toe. See also **Stransky reflex.**

2. (Cleckley reflex) A variant of the **Babinski reflex** in which dorsiflexion of the hallux is sought in response to upward flicking and sudden release of the second toe.

Allen diagnostic scale   A scoring system devised to aid in the clinical diagnosis of the pathology underlying acute stroke.[108]

Variable	Clinical Feature	Score
Apoplectic onset with two or more of the following: loss of consciousness, headache within 2 hours, vomiting, or neck stiffness	None or 1	0
	Two or more	21.9
Level of consciousness 24 hours after admission	Alert	0
	Drowsy	7.3
	Coma	14.6
Plantar responses	Both down or one upgoing	0
	Bilaterally upgoing	7.1
Diastolic blood pressure 24 hours after admission	×0.17	7
History of angina, claudication or diabetes	None	0
	1 or more	−3.7
History of hypertension	Not present	0
	Present	−3.7
Previous transient ischemic attack or stroke	None	0
	Any previous event	−6.7
Heart disease	None	0
	Aortic or mitral murmur	−4.3
	Cardiac failure	−4.3
	Cardiomyopathy	−4.3
	Atrial fibrillation	−4/3
	Cardiomegaly on chest X-ray	−4.3
	Myocardial infarct in past 6–12 months	−4.3
Constant heart disease		−12

From Allen CMC. Clinical diagnosis of the acute stroke syndrome. Quart J Med 1983;52:515–23, reprinted with permission.

A score of <4 suggests ischemic stroke and a score of >24 suggests intracranial hemorrhage with fair reliability.[945] See also **Siriraj score, NIH Stroke Scale, Canadian Neurological Scale.**

Allen score   A scale with prognostic value in patients with stroke. The following features are recorded:
Age in years
Loss of consciousness at onset of stroke
Drowsy or comatose 24 hours after onset (or later)

Complete limb paralysis (no movement better than palpable contraction, MRC 1)
Higher cerebral dysfunction (HCD)
  Aphasia and/or
  Parietal deficit:
    Sensory or visual inattention or
    Visuospatial neglect or
    Loss of joint position sense
  Homonymous visual field deficit to confrontation (HHA)

Calculation of score

Constant (start with)	+40
Complete limb paralysis	−12
HCD with HHA and hemiplegia	−11
Drowsy/comatose at 24 hours	−10
Age in years	−(age × 0.4)
Initial loss of consciousness	−9
Uncomplicated hemiparesis	+8

Patients with a score of <0 are likely to die or to have severe impairments if they live. Those with a score >0 will probably survive and will walk again.[109]

Allen-Dent syndrome See **argininosuccinase deficiency, citrullinemia.**

allergic angiitis and granulomatosis (Churg-Strauss syndrome) Vasculitic syndromes characterized by fibrinoid necrosis with eosinophilic and granulomatous tissue reactivity in capillaries, venules, and the small and medium-sized muscular arteries.[5377] See **Churg-Strauss syndrome.** The clinical presentations resemble those of **polyarteritis nodosa.**[2414]

In a *variant form, necrotizing granulomatous angiitis with a predilection for the CNS* (Feisen-Cravioto syndrome), the effects are confined to the brain and spinal cord.

allergic polyneuritis A subacute motor neuropathy following prophylactic immunization against **rabies.**[3301]

allesthesia See **alloesthesia.**

Allgrove syndrome (ALADIN, AAA syndrome; OMIM 231550) A rare recessive or dominantly inherited multisystem degenerative disease of childhood, (chromosome 12q13) characterized by alacrima, achalasia, and sensorimotor polyneuropathy with insensitivity to ACTH largely as a result of cholinergic nerve dysfunction.[113] The condition may be a peroxisomal disorder.

Alliance of Genetic Support Groups A charitable organization. Address: 35 Wisconsin Circle, Ste. 440, Chevy Chase, MD 20815. Tel: 301-652-5553 1-800-336-GENE.

Allison leg jitters See **restless legs syndrome.**

all-median hand The anomalous condition in which all of the intrinsic hand muscles are supplied by the median nerve, which normally supplies only the opponens and abductor pollicis brevis, the lateral two lumbricals, and half of the flexor pollicis brevis.

The clinical significance is slight unless the patient happens to receive an ulnar nerve lesion, in which case the hand continues to function normally, or a median nerve lesion, in which case it does not function at all.[3623]

allo- Greek prefix signifying *other.*

allocheiria (allochiria) Faulty localization of a stimulus, such that subjects touched on the left hand claim that they were touched on the right; a sign of right (nondominant) parietal lobe disease, described by **Bamberger** and by Obersteiner in 1881.

allochiria See **allocheiria.**

allocortex (rhinencephalon) The four-layered, differentiated paleocortex including the hippocampal formation and the pyriform cortex. With the **corticoid areas,** it constitutes the cortical expression of the **limbic system.**

allodynia (Gr, other + pain) (hyperpathia, hyperalgesia) Pain felt following a stimulus that is not usually noxious and does not normally cause pain. This frequently occurs in association with **causalgia** following prior axonal injury, and indicates the presence of hyperexcitable axonal sprouts able to generate electrical impulses ab initio or else to encourage **ephaptic transmission.** Sensitization of peripheral nociceptors and disinhibition or sensitization within parts of the central nervous system are other postulated mechanisms.[2008]

alloesthesia (allesthesia) 1. Displacement of a sensation—usually tactile or visual—away from the true position of the stimulating object. Thus a patient with a right parietal lesion touched on the left hand which is resting on a table may claim that it was actually the table that was touched. 2. Displacement of a perception (in any modality) from the correct to another side or site, seen with lesions of the right parietal lobe or spinal cord. Thus with visual alloesthesia, the percept may be displaced from an intact to a blind half-field.

Obersteiner described the sign first in 1880 in a patient with a spinal cord lesion and others have noted it in patients with hysteria or parietal lobe lesions. It is thought that damage to the crossing fibers causes sensory inputs to be channelled through uncrossed fibers on the opposite side.[2969]

allokinesis 1. Perception of an ordinary nonpruritic stimulus as itchy.[5173] (HJM) 2. The performance of movements requested of the patient by the wrong limb. Thus a paralyzed left arm will not obey a request to touch an object, but the left leg will do so involuntarily.[1858]

allophones Minor variations in a phoneme.

all-or-nothing (none) response (of sensory nerve fibers). A phenomenon described first by Keith Lucas but further analyzed by **Adrian** in 1918 and then more fully 4 years later.[48] Adrian stated the all-or-nothing principle as follows: "In a normal nerve fibre, where the impulse is not conducted with a decrement, the intensity of the impulse at any point depends only on the local condition of the fiber at that point [but neither] on the strength of the stimulus which set the impulse in motion nor on the amount of reduction which the impulse may have suffered in regions of decrement as it passed down the nerve."[48]

allotriogeusia   (Gr, another + taste) Perversion of taste. See **ageusia.**

all-ulnar hand   Anomalous motor innervation of all of the intrinsic hand muscles by the ulnar nerve, the sensory innervation pattern being normal. The anatomical basis is the Riche-Cannieu anastomosis, through which the motor fibers from the median nerve transfer to the ulnar in the palm.[4868]

alogia   Poverty of speech production and content.

alopecia–mental retardation–seizures syndrome   A congenital dysmorphic syndrome in which alopecia, fine, brittle hair, dental caries, seizures, and mental and developmental delay are associated. See **dermotrichic syndrome.**

Alpers, Bernard Jacob   (1900–1981) American neurologist who trained at Harvard and studied as a postgraduate in Madrid with **Rio Hortega**. He was Professor and Chairman of Neurology at Jefferson Medical College, Philadelphia, for 27 years. He described the infantile gray matter degenerative disease named for him in 1931. His comment on differential diagnosis, "based on collective data, clinical problems deal entirely with pertinent possibilities and not with a long list of all possibilities," represents a message which, in the context of Grand Rounds, has still not been widely understood.

Alpers disease   (progressive neuronal degeneration of childhood with liver disease, progressive cerebral poliodystrophy; spongy glioneuronal dystrophy; diffuse cerebral degeneration in infancy; diffuse progressive cerebral cortical atrophy; progressive neuronal degeneration of childhood; Christensen-Krabbé syndrome) A rare, sporadic, or recessively inherited mitochondrial disease of unknown cause in which there is degeneration of the gray matter and glial tissue, and a subacute hepatitis beginning early in life, often after normal infancy.

Clinically, the disease is characterized by progressive mental deterioration, developmental delay, spasticity, myoclonus and generalized convulsions, choreoathetosis, ataxia, optic atrophy with blindness, deafness, and early death from liver failure with abnormal lactate and pyruvate metabolism.[120] The differences between this condition and **Leigh disease** are questionable.

Adolescent onset has also been recorded. See also **familial poliodystrophy.**

alpha coma   (alpha pattern coma) The presence of an EEG pattern predominantly within the alpha frequency band, paradoxically resembling waking EEG patterns but unreactive to touch, sound, or pain and often widely distributed over the head, seen in apparently comatose patients. See **persistent vegetative state** (the preferred term).

This is most commonly seen in hypoxic patients following cardiac arrest, those with localized brainstem lesions at or just caudal to the pontomesencephalic junction, or those with drug intoxication or concussion.[266, 5762]

Outcome may be predicted by the reactivity of the EEG to noxious stimuli. The finding carries a poor prognosis; the few survivors seldom have meaningful recovery.[2925]

alpha rhythm   Regular, rhythmic activity on the EEG at 8–13 Hz occurring during wakefulness over the posterior regions of the head, generally with higher voltage over the occipital area. Its amplitude is variable but is mostly below 50 uV in the adult and it is best seen with the eyes closed and under conditions of physical relaxation and relative mental inactivity. The rhythm is blocked or attenuated by attention (especially visual), mental effort, and drowsiness.

The use of the term must be restricted to those rhythms which fulfil all these criteria. Activities in the alpha band that differ from the alpha rhythm as regards their topography and/or reactivity either have specific appellations (for instance, the mu rhythm) or should be referred to as rhythms of alpha frequency. Cf. rhythm of alpha frequency. (Adapted from the 1974 Report of the Committee on Terminology, IFCN,[989] © 1974. With permission from Elsevier Science.)

alpha variant rhythms   Certain characteristic EEG rhythms which are recorded most prominently over the posterior regions of the head and differ in frequency but resemble in reactivity the alpha rhythm. Cf. fast alpha variant rhythm, slow alpha variant rhythms. (Adapted from the 1974 Report of the Committee on Terminology, IFCN,[989] © 1974. With permission from Elsevier Science). This rhythm tends to have a frequency that is the harmonic of the fundamental EEG rhythm.

alpha-aminoadipic aciduria   A rare diffuse encephalopathy, probably recessively inherited and a possible cause of mental retardation, characterized by this urinary finding.[1833]

alpha-fetoprotein   A protein. The levels of this protein are elevated in the amniotic fluid of fetuses who have neural tube deficits. Acetylcholinesterase levels, however, have more specificity.

alpha-galactosidase   The enzyme deficient in **Fabry disease.**

alpha-glycerophosphate dehydrogenase deficiency   See **glycerol-phosphate dehydrogenase deficiency.**

alpha-ketoadipicaciduria A rare diffuse encephalopathy of infants due to an error in lysine metabolism (failure of conversion of α-ketoadipic acid to glutaryl coenzyme A) and characterized by impairment of mental and physical development, metabolic acidosis, skin rash, hypotonia, and seizures.[5915]

alpha-methyl-aceto-acetyl-coenzyme A β-ketothiolase deficiency A hyperammonemic syndrome causing accumulation of aceto-acetic and other organic acids, and clinically characterized by episodic vomiting, impairment of consciousness, seizures, hyperglycemia, and ketoacidosis.[1302]

alpha-methyl-β-hydroxybutyric aciduria A diffuse encephalopathy due to deficiency in thiolase activity, characterized by mental retardation, metabolic acidosis, and altered consciousness.[1302]

alpine sickness See **altitude insomnia.**

Alport, A. Cecil (1890–1959) American physician.

Alport syndrome (dominant nephritis and hearing loss) A dominantly or incomplete sex-linked recessively inherited disease of childhood, characterized by progressive renal impairment with interstitial foamy cells in the kidneys; neural deafness; abnormalities of the lens, including spherophakia and cataracts; macular degeneration; and optic nerve **Drusen.**[125, 1954]

ALS See **amyotrophic lateral sclerosis.**

ALS and Neuromuscular Research Foundation A charitable organization. Address: California Pacific Medical Center, 3698 California St., Room 545, San Francisco, CA 94118. Tel: 415-923-3604.

ALS Association A charitable organization dedicated to finding the cause and cure of this disease. It provides funding for research grants, conducts scientific symposia and health-care professional education programs, provides patient counseling, and conducts public education programs. Address: 21021 Ventura Blvd., Ste 321, Woodland Hills, CA 91364-2206. Tel: 818-340-7500; fax: 1-800-782-4747.

ALS-Parkinson-dementia syndromes See **amyotrophic lateral sclerosis** (*variants*).

ALS Society of Canada A charitable organization dedicated to providing care and finding the cure for ALS. Web site: http://www.als.ca/.

Alstrom-Hallgren syndrome (recessive retinal degeneration, diabetes, obesity, and hearing loss) A rare recessively transmitted syndrome of infancy or childhood characterized by loss of central vision because of pigmentary retinal degeneration (cone-rod dystrophy), diabetes mellitus, progressive neural deafness, hypogonadism, interstitial nephropathy, and sometimes acanthosis nigricans, mental retardation, or obesity.[127] See also **Bardet-Biedel syndrome, Usher syndrome.**

alternans nystagmus See **periodic nystagmus.**

alternate brachial diplegia See **cruciate paralysis.**

alternate cover test See **cover test.**

laternate fixation The ability of a subject to fixate with either eye with equal facility.

alternate inferior paralysis See **Millard-Gubler syndrome.**

alternate paralysis A condition described in the nineteenth century, in which there is paralysis of movement on one side of the body and of sensation on the other.[4512] A low brainstem lesion could account for this rare occurrence.

alternating abducent hemiplegia See **Raymond syndrome.**

alternating contraction anisocoria A rare consequence of damage to the pathway from the pretectal area to the Edinger-Westphal nucleus. There is increased reactivity of the affected eye to light, but the size of the pupils is equal in darkness.

alternating current nystagmus See **vestibular nystagmus.**

alternating eye deviation sign Consistent deviation of the eyes in parallel away from the side on which the examiner is standing, occurring when the examiner attempts to open the subject's eyes. The condition is considered to be a conversion reaction.[217]

alternating hemiplegia Paresis of cranial nerves on one side of the body and of the trunk and limbs on the other, constituting clear evidence of a lesion of the brainstem. The term was introduced by Gubler. See also the **Weber, Benedikt, Foville, Millard-Gubler, Jackson** and **Villaret syndromes** and the **alternating hypoglossal hemiplegia syndrome.**

alternating hemiplegia of childhood A rare progressive disease with onset before the age of 18 months, characterized by sudden and repeated attacks of hemiplegia lasting hours to days, involving each side alternately, relieved by sleep, associated with other paroxysmal phenomena (tonic attacks, posturing, nystagmus, chorea, or athetosis) or with autonomic disturbances, and with progressive mental and neurological deterioration.[57]

Ocular palsies and fixed motor deficits are additional features described. In infancy, screaming attacks may precede the motor manifestations.[931] See also **periodic syndromes.** The condition may reflect mitochondrial dysfunction.

In *variant forms*, the condition is dominantly inherited,[3871] affects all four limbs, or is a benign syndrome occurring repetitively during sleep.

The syndrome also appears in *infantile hypotonia and paroxysmal dystonia, paroxysmal symptomatic alternating dystonia with hemiparesis*, **migraine coma,** *alter-*

nating diplegia with livedo reticularis, and **pyruvate dehydrogenase deficiency.**[162]

alternating Horner syndrome   The apparent alternation of the side on which there is a **Horner syndrome**. This represents a *variant* in which the miosis, ptosis, and facial flushing in patients with lower cervical cord disease alternate from side to side over days, presumably as a result of a lesion of the ciliospinal centers of Budge.[2001]

Another explanation would be that one side is normal but that on the other, the manifestations of the Horner syndrome alternate with those of a **Pourfour du Petit syndrome.**

alternating hypoglossal hemiplegia syndrome   (anterior bulbar syndrome, Déjèrine syndrome) A vascular medial brainstem syndrome in which damage to the pyramid and twelfth cranial nerve nucleus on one side causes wasting and weakness of the tongue with anesthesia of the soft palate and posterior pharyngeal wall on the same side as the infarct, and a contralateral hemiparesis.

In a *variant form*, (*alternating hypoglossal hemiplegia-hemianesthesia syndrome*), contralateral numbness also occurs, due to involvement of the medial lemniscus. See also **Déjèrine syndromes.**

alternating nystagmus   See **periodic nystagmus.**

alternating oculomotor paralysis   See **Weber syndrome.**

alternating parallel syndrome   The association of spastic hemiparesis, cerebellar ataxia, and trigeminal analgesia on the side of a brainstem lesion, with analgesia of the trunk and limbs on the contralateral side, due to an adjacent or extending lesion affecting the cervical cord.[5599]

alternating sensory loss   Impairment of certain modalities of sensation on different sides of the head and of the trunk and limbs. Thus, in the lateral medullary syndrome, damage to the descending spinal nucleus and tract and to the ascending spinothalamic pathway leads to loss of pain and temperature sensation over the face on the same side and of the trunk and limbs on the other side. See **alternating thermoanalgesia, alternating hemiplegia.**

alternating sequences test   A test of concentration, planning, and resistance to interference, in which the subject is required to write some lines of alternating letters or shapes.[3521]

alternating thermoanalgesia   A subjective diminution of the sense of sharp pain and of temperature on one side of the face and the opposite side of the trunk and limbs. See **alternating sensory loss.**

This combination of signs signifies the presence of a lateral brainstem lesion, as in the **Wallenberg syndrome or the anterior inferior cerebellar artery syndrome.**

alternating windmill nystagmus   See **circular nystagmus.**

alternobaric vertigo   An acute form of vestibular vertigo occurring in pilots during marked change in altitude, usually following straining movements (Valsalva) designed to "clear the ears," and always due to obstruction of the eustachian tubes. Nystagmus and oscillopsia are usual accompaniments.

altitude insomnia   (acute mountain sickness, Acosta disease, Andes disease, Alpine sickness, hypobaropathy) An acute insomnia usually accompanied by headaches, loss of appetite, and fatigue following ascent to high altitudes. Diagnostic criteria include the following:[234]

A. A complaint of insomnia
B. A temporally related ascent to a high altitude (typically above 4000 m)
C. Polysomnographic monitoring that demonstrates
   1. Reduced total sleep duration, decreased sleep efficiency with an increased sleep latency, and increased arousals and awake time
   2. A pattern of periodic breathing during sleep
   3. Oxygen desaturation during sleep
D. Other medical or psychiatric disorders can be present but are not the cause of the primary complaint.
E. The complaint is not caused by other sleep disorders, such as obstructive sleep apnea syndrome, central sleep apnea syndrome, or other causes of insomnia.

Adapted from *The International Classification of Sleep Disorders Diagnostic and Coding Manual.* Rochester, MN: American Sleep Disorders Association, © 1990. Reproduced by kind permission of the American Academy of Sleep Medicine.

altitudinal defects   Visual field defects which do not cross the equator of vision (but may cross the vertical meridian) and which indicate the presence of an acquired lesion of the retina or choroid, or of the more proximal portion of the visual pathway. They also occur with congenital hypoplasia of the optic nerve.

altitudinal hemianopia   Loss of half of the visual field above or below the (horizontal) equator. This is usually evidence of retinal vascular insufficiency or of anterior ischemic optic neuropathy. See also **hemianopia, altitudinal defects.**

altitudinal neglect   Neglect of half of the visual field above or below the equator. This is usually evidence of bilateral parietal lobe lesions.[4597]

alveolar hypoventilation DIMS (disorders of initiating and maintaining sleep) syndrome   A syndrome of insomnia due to the disruption of sleep occasioned by central apnea superimposed upon hypopnea with alveolar hypoventilation, associated with daytime unresponsiveness to chemical regulators of ventilation (see also **sleep disorders** and **Ondine's curse**).

alveolar hypoventilation DOES (disorders of excessive sleep) syndrome   The appearance or worsening during sleep of conditions characterized by impaired ventilation (reduced tidal volume or respiratory rate) but without prolonged apneic spells. See **sleep disorders.**

alveolar sarcoma   A rare malignant primary tumor of muscle occurring in children and young adults, in which muscle cell differentiation can be differentiated microscopically.

Alzheimer, Alois   (1864–1915) German neuropsychiatrist and pathologist, and a professor of psychiatry in Munich and then Breslau. He first described the disease named for him in a lecture given in Tubingen in 1906, publishing this a year later. **Kraepelin,** with whom he was working, recognized the description as definitive and named the disease for Alzheimer in 1910.

Alzheimer also made important contributions in the areas of syphilis, Huntington and Parkinson diseases, and vascular dementias,[5047] although these contributions are less well remembered.

Alzheimer Association   A charitable organization with 217 chapters nationwide. Research, education, chapter formation, advocacy, and patient and family services are its goals. Funding is available for pilot and multiyear research proposals in the basic, clinical, and social sciences with relevance to Alzheimer disease. Address: 919 N. Michigan Ave., Ste. 1000, Chicago, IL 60611-1696. Tel: 312-335-8700. E-mail: info@alz.org. Web site: http://www.alz.org.

Alzheimer disease   The proper term for what was formerly known by the pejorative term *senile dementia* (introduced by **Binswanger** in 1898). At last it has become a respectable subject for research, in part because of the economic threat that it poses to civilization as the population ages and the prevalence increases. Order has been brought to the clinical diagnostic process by the acceptance of diagnostic guidelines (see Charts A–3 and A–4). Progressive memory loss, aphasia, apraxias, and visuospatial abnormalities are the most important features. Criteria for pathological diagnosis have also been defined; cortical atrophy, neuronal loss, "senile" plaques, vacuoles, neurofibrillary tangles (the earliest change observed), and meningeal fibrosis are characteristic; all were described by Alzheimer verbally in 1906 or in subsequent publications in 1907[133] and 1911.[2959] Internet sites of interest include www.alz.org, www.alzforum.org, www.alzheimer.ca, and www.alzheimer's.org.

See also **dementia** and **Pick disease,** from which latter the diagnosis may be difficult.[3827]

Chart A–3. NINCDS Criteria for the Clinical Diagnosis of Alzheimer Disease[4079]

I. *Criteria for the clinical diagnosis of PROBABLE Alzheimer disease*
 A. Dementia, established by clinical examination and documented by the **Mini-Mental State Examination,** the **Blessed Dementia Scale,** or some similar examination, and confirmed by neuropsychological tests
 B. Deficits in two or more areas of cognition
 C. Progressive worsening of memory and other cognitive functions
 D. No disturbance of consciousness
 E. Onset between ages 40 and 90, most often after age 65
 F. Absence of systemic disorders or other brain diseases that in and of themselves could account for the progressive deficits in memory and cognition
II. *Criteria supporting diagnosis of PROBABLE Alzheimer disease*
 A. Progressive deterioration of specific cognitive functions such as language (aphasia), motor skills (apraxia), and perception (agnosia)
 B. Impaired activities of daily living and altered patterns of behavior
 C. Family history of similar disorders, particularly if confirmed neuropathologically
 D. Laboratory results: normal lumbar puncture as evaluated by standard techniques; normal pattern or nonspecific changes in EEG, such as increased slow-wave activity; and evidence of cerebral atrophy on CT scanning with progression documented by serial observation
III. *Features that make the diagnosis of PROBABLE Alzheimer disease uncertain or unlikely*
 A. Sudden, apoplectic onset
 B. Focal neurological findings such as hemiparesis, sensory loss, visual field deficits, and incoordination early in the course of the illness
 C. Seizures or gait disturbances at the onset or very early in the course of the illness
IV. *Clinical diagnosis of POSSIBLE Alzheimer disease*
 A. May be made on the basis of the dementia syndrome, in the absence of other neurological, psychiatric, or systemic disorders sufficient to cause dementia, and in the presence of variations in the onset, presentation, or clinical course
 B. May be made in the presence of a second systemic or brain disorder sufficient to produce dementia, which is not considered to be the cause of the dementia
 C. Should be used in research studies when a single, gradually progressive severe cognitive deficit is identified in the absence of other identifiable cause

Alternative Research Diagnostic Criteria have been formulated, e.g., by Berg.[488] The new American Psychiatric Association DSM-IV criteria follow.

Chart A–4. Alzheimer Disease Diagnostic Criteria

A. The development of multiple cognitive deficits as manifested by both
 1. Memory impairment (inability to learn new information and inability to recall previously learned information) and
 2. Cognitive impairment, manifested by at least one of the following
  a. Aphasia (language disturbance)
  b. Apraxia (inability to carry out motor activities despite intact comprehension and motor function)
  c. Agnosia (failure to recognize or identify objects despite intact sensory function)
  d. Disturbance in executive functioning (i.e., planning, organizing, sequencing, abstracting)

B. The cognitive deficits in Criteria A1 and A2 each cause significant impairment in social or occupational functioning and represent a significant decline from a previous level of functioning

C. The course is characterized by gradual onset and cognitive decline.

D. The cognitive deficits in Criteria A1 and A2 are not due to any of the following
1. Other central nervous system conditions that cause progressive deficits in memory and cognition (e.g., cerebrovascular disease, **Parkinson disease, Huntington disease, subdural hematoma, normal pressure hydrocephalus**).
2. Systemic nonpsychiatric medical conditions that are known to cause dementia (e.g. hypothyroidism, vitamin B12 or folic acid deficiency, niacin deficiency, hypercalcemia, neurosyphilis, HIV infection).
3. Substance-induced conditions.

E. The deficits do not occur exclusively during the course of delirium.

F. The disturbance is not better accounted for by another Axis 1 disorder (e.g., major depressive disorder, schizophrenia).

Adapted slightly and reprinted with kind permission from the Diagnostic and Statistical Manual of Mental Disorders, Fourth Edition, Text Revision. Copyright 2000. American Psychiatric Association Washington, DC, *without fee.*[150]

Variants include the following:

Alzheimer disease with spongy changes and myoclonus A syndrome in which the onset of dementia is between the ages of 20 and 50, with myoclonic seizures. Pathologically, cerebral atrophy, neurofibrillary tangles, senile plaques, and spongy changes are found in the brain.[337]

Familial Alzheimer disease Relatively uncommon dominantly inherited types of the disease.[335] Early-onset forms are associated with the gene presenilin 1 on chromosome 14 (14q24), amyloid precursor protein on chromosome 21 (21q11.2–21q21), or presenilin 2 on chromosome 2. A later-onset form maps to chromosome 19 (19q13). In each case, the clinical picture is much the same as that in patients with the sporadic form.

Visual variant of Alzheimer disease A form characterized by early visual agnosia and abnormal contrast sensitivity without defects of acuity or color vision, slowly progressing over years to a demented state with the pathological features of Alzheimer disease.[3375]

Alzheimer disease with cerebrovascular disease A category of dementia reserved for patients fulfilling the clinical criteria for possible **Alzheimer disease** who also present clinical or brain-imaging evidence of relevant cerebrovascular disease.

Early onset Alzheimer disease A dominantly inherited variant mapping to chromosome 14q 23.

Alzheimer disease with spastic paraparesis See **familial British dementia.**

A *psychotic phenotype* characterized by a rapid decline in cognitive and functional capacities and a tendency toward agressive behavior with a suggestive familial basis.[5448]

Alzheimer Disease and Associated Disorders A

professional subspecialty journal. Web site: http://www.alzheimerjournal.com/.

Alzheimer Disease Assessment Battery A computer-based behavioral assessment package designed to detect deterioration of cognitive functioning in **Alzheimer disease.**[717]

The battery examines intellectual deterioration, pathological memory loss, word-finding disturbance, and spatial disorientation. A selective reminding task is incorporated and word fluency, spatial disorientation, and remote memory are also assessed.

Alzheimer Disease Assessment Scale A 21-item scale designed to assess the severity of cognitive and noncognitive behavioral impairments in a patient with dementia due to **Alzheimer disease.**

The scale includes short neuropsychological tests and items rated by the clinical examiner on the basis of observation of the patient's behavior and after an interview with the caregiver. It is divided into two sections, the first employing short tests of memory, language, and praxis to give a *cognitive subscale*, and the second rating mood, distractibility, vegetative functions, agitation, delusions, hallucinations, and concentration to give a 10-item *noncognitive subscale.*[4779]

Alzheimer Disease Society A charitable organization. Address: 3rd floor, Bank Buildings, Fulham Broadway, London SW6 1EP, United Kingdom.

Alzheimer Foundation An organization devoted to facilitating clinical and basic research in Alzheimer disease. The official journal of the foundation is the *Journal of Geriatric Psychiatry and Neurology.* Address: 8177 South Harvard, M/C-114, Tulsa, OK 74137. A Web site allowing access to many others, is at http://www.alz.org.

Alzheimer Society of Canada A charitable organization. Address: 491. Lawrence Avenue West, Ste. 501, Toronto, Ontario, M5M 1C7 Canada.

Alzheimer type I astrocyte An astrocyte with a large lobulated vesicular nucleus and abundant vacuolated cytoplasm, resulting from aberrant cell division and described in the striatum of patients with **Wilson disease** and with other chronic liver diseases.

Alzheimer type II astrocyte An astrocyte with a large, irregularly shaped and lobulated nucleus encompassed by a narrow rim of poorly staining cytoplasm. It is characteristically found in patients with ammonia toxicity, as in hepatic failure.

Alzheimer's Disease Education and Referral Center (ADEAR) A charitable organization in this field. Address: P.O. Box 8250 Silver Spring, MD 20907-8250. Tel: 301-495-3311, 800-438-4380. E-mail: adear@alzheimers.org. Web site: http://www.alzheimers.org.

akinetic rigidity See **arteriosclerotic rigidity.**

Amalric syndrome (macular dystrophy–deaf-muteness syndrome) A recessively inherited syndrome of congenital partial deafness, and atypical pigmentary retinopathy without impaired night vision.[134] The similarities to **Alport, Cockayne, Lawrence-Moon-Biedel,** and **Hallgren** syndromes are notable.

amaurosis (from Gr, darkness) The term used by Hippocrates for "a becoming dull of sight" and in seventeenth-century England for the condition "when the sight is gone and no fault is to be seen."[5204] It is now used almost exclusively for **transient monocular blindness** of vascular origin.

amaurosis congenita See **Leber disease.**

amaurosis fugax A term signifying **transient monocular blindness** (TMB), the latter being a more precise and contemporary label. It is usually due to platelet-cholesterol emboli but in about 20% of cases is migrainous. Since the etiological diagnosis is almost impossible to make clinically, the precision of studies of the various treatments for amaurosis is questionable.

Wray has discerned four types, differentiated by their underlying pathologies,[6045] and reproduced by kind permission.

Type 1 (transient retinal ischemia–embolic) is characterized by the abrupt loss of all or a portion of the vision in one eye, lasting seconds to minutes, with total recovery. The partial visual impairment may be described as a curtain—ascending, descending, or moving sideways—and producing a uniocular altitudinal or hemianopic defect. Patients may experience a central scotoma, a paracentral scotoma, or an area of segmental visual loss. In addition, they may complain of vertical or horizontal stationary scintillating scotomas, which may be associated with (*a*) vague, irregular, background shadows that rapidly move to the periphery and (*b*) vague, irregular shadows suddenly appearing paracentrally and moving toward the periphery in seconds. Intensely bright, tiny scintillating lights suddenly appear paracentrally and move peripherally (seconds) in a straight horizontal line, leaving behind a faint glowing line for 2 or 3 seconds.

Most commonly, the visual loss is complete, the patient stating that everything is "completely black." Vision recovers in seconds to minutes, with recovery taking longer than loss. *Variants* include graying, dimming, or blurring of vision.

The pathophysiological mechanism is thought to be arterial occlusion due to emboli to the ophthalmic artery or to the retinal artery.

Type 2 (retinal vascular insufficiency–hypoperfusion) is characterized by a less rapid onset of visual loss. In general, it is of longer duration, lasting minutes to hours (thus temporary rather than transient). Many of these patients complain of peculiar visual aberrations such as loss of or excessive contrast vision, dazzle, photographic negative imagery, flickering lights, photopsias, and dyschromatopsias. In addition, many experience a blurring or total loss of vision when they go out into (or come in from) bright light, or upon assuming a sitting or an upright position. The visual loss is often described as a concentric contraction of the visual field ("iris diaphragm effect"), especially when it is bilateral. Rarely, a patient will report blindness after eating. Often, while reading, the subject will complain that the page becomes excessively bright. Complaints of chronic ocular or retro-ocular pain of an insidious and aching nature are also recorded.

In all of these cases there is severe carotid stenosis, either ipsilaterally or bilaterally, marked by low perfusion pressures on ophthalmodynamometric testing.

Type 3 (angiospastic form) is characterized by the sudden onset of total visual loss or progressive contraction of the visual field sparing fixation. These attacks are usually short-lived in terms of minutes, but may be prolonged. Direct observations of the fundus during such attacks have revealed (*a*) narrowing of the retinal arteries and veins, cessation of blood flow, segmentation of the blood columns, and optic disc pallor, and (*b*) narrowing of the retinal veins.

Fluorescein angiography reveals early filling of the optic disc capillaries with late filling (30 seconds) of the retinal arterioles in the former case (*a*), and a delay in filling of the central retinal artery in the latter (*b*). Many of these patients have a known migraine diathesis.

Type 4 (idiopathic forms) is a "wastebasket" category in which the signs and symptoms defy classification. The type of visual disturbance in this group of patients closely resembles that of type 1, except for the duration of the attack, which may be very short (like a transient obscuration of vision) or very long (thus resembling a type 3 attack). In general, the patients suffer from multiple attacks, some occurring as frequently as one or two times per day. No identifiable pathophysiological mechanism can be determined[837] but anticardiolipid antibodies may be tarred with guilt by association.

amaurosis-hemiplegia syndrome (Espildora-Luque syndrome) Blindness in one eye with contralateral hemiparesis, due to reflex spasm of the homolateral middle cerebral artery (as originally described), to separate emboli to that artery, or to occlusion of the internal carotid at the takeoff of the ophthalmic artery.[1459] See **Espildora-Luque syndrome.**

amaurotic familial idiocy (Tay-Sachs disease) The original term for the **gangliosidoses,** applied by Bernard Sachs (1858–1954), an American neurologist. The term is now defunct, having been replaced by the names of the two broad categories of disease which the condition represents, namely the **gangliosidoses** and the **neuronal ceroid lipofuscinoses.**

amaurotic pupil A pupil that does not constrict despite maximal light stimulation of the eye, because of damage to the afferent pathway.

ambient echolalia The use of words suggested by irrelevant local visual or auditory stimuli rather than by the context of the conversation. This occurs as a manifestation of delirious states and some dementias.[1858]

ambiguo-hypoglossal paralysis   See **Tapia syndrome.**

ambiguo-spinothalamic syndrome   See **Avellis syndrome.**

ambiopia   See **diplopia.**

ambulation index   A simple scale of some value in assessing the stage of disease in multiple sclerosis.[2194]

amblyaphia   (Gr, dulled + the sense of touch) Numbness.

amblyopia   (Gr, dulled or blunted + eye) Impairment or loss of vision in a healthy eye which is not due to an error in refraction nor to other disease of the eye itself.

Squint and **anisometria** are the commoner causes, although Hippocrates used the word for dimness of vision in old age, which indicates that the use of the word has been modified substantially.

Amblyopia ex anopsia is diminished vision due to suppression of images from a ("lazy") strabismic eye.

AMC   See **arthrogryposis multiplex congenita.**

amebiasis   Infection with *Naegleria* or with *Entamoeba histolytica*; in each case, a potential cause of meningoencephalitis or of cerebral abscess.[929]

ameloblastoma   See **craniopharyngioma.**

amenorrhea-galactorrhea syndrome   The occurrence of these problems due to the excessive secretion of prolactin by a pituitary basophilic adenoma.

American Academy of Cerebral Developmental Medicine   A professional organization. Address: 2315 Westwood Ave., PO Box 11086, Richmond, VA 23230.

American Academy of Clinical Neurophysiology   A professional organization. Address: 5700 Old Orchard Road, First floor, Skokie, IL 60077-1057. Tel: 708-966-0050.

American Academy of Neurological and Orthopaedic Medicine and Surgery   A professional organization. Address: 320 Ranchero Drive, Ste. 108, Las Vegas, NV 89102.

American Academy of Neurological Surgery   A professional organization. Address: Massachussetts General Hospital, Department of Neurosurgery, Fruit Street, Boston, MA 02114. Tel: 617-726-2000.

American Academy of Neurology (AAN)   A leading professional organization founded in 1948 against the strident opposition of some members of the **American Neurological Association** (ANA), in order to cater to the educational and scientific needs of all neurologists and to be a forum for the younger members of the discipline. Unlike the ANA, the AAN offers ordinary membership to any individual with Board qualifications, and associate and junior membership categories are also available. Fellows are elected from the ranks of those clinical neurologist members who have attended sufficient annual meetings.

Dr A.B. **Baker** was the prime mover in the founding of the academy, in March 1948; he and Drs. Forster, Aird, and **Wartenberg** were the first directors. The house journal is *Neurology.* The early history of the academy was recounted by Brown.[794] Address: 2221 University Ave. SE, Ste. 335, Minneapolis, MN 55414. Tel: 612-623-8115; fax: 612-623-3504. Web site: http://www.aan.com.

American Academy of Pain Management   A professional specialist organization. Web site: http://www.aa-painmanage.org/.

American Academy of Sleep Medicine   (formerly American Sleep Disorders Association) A professional organization. Web site: http://www.aasmnet.org/.

American Association for the Study of Headache   See **American Headache Society.**

American Association of Acoustic Neuroma   A professional organization. P.O. Box 398, Carlisle, PA 17013. Tel: 717-249-4783; fax: 717-249-0353.

American Association of Electrodiagnostic Medicine   (formerly the American Association of Electromyography and Electrodiagnosis) A professional society concerned with education, practice standards, and research into neuromuscular disease, founded in 1953 by Dr. James G. Golseth, an American neurologist. *Muscle and Nerve* is the official publication of the association. Internet address: www.aaem.net. Tel: 507-288-0100.

American Association of Electrodiagnostic Technologists   A professional organization. Address: Box 40, Davey, NE 68336.

American Association of Neurological Surgeons   A professional society. Address: 625 N. Michigan Ave., Ste. 1519, Chicago, IL 60611. Tel: 312-993-0043. Web site: http://www.neurosurgery.org/aans/.

American Association of Neuropathologists   A professional society of neuropathologists seeking to advance research and training. Address: 1300 Morris Park Ave., Bronx, NY. 10461. Tel: 212-430–2495. Web site: http://www.aanp-jnen.com/aanpframes.html.

American Association of Neuroscience   A professional organization. Address: 224 N. Des Plaines, Ste. 601, Chicago, IL 60661. Tel: 312-993-0043.

American Association of Neuroscience Nurses   A professional organization. Web site: http://www.aann.org/.

American Association of Physical Medicine and Rehabilitation   A professional organization. Address: One IBM Plaza, Suite 2500, Chicago, IL 60611-3604. Tel: 312-464-9700. E-mail: info@aapmr.org. Web site: http://www.aapmr.org.

American Autoimmune Related Diseases Association A charitable organization in this field. Address: 22100 Gratiot Ave. Eastpointe, East Detroit, MI 48201-2227. Tel: 586-776-3900; 800-598-4668. E-mail: aarda@aol.com. Web site: http://www.aarda.org.

American Behcet's Disease Association A charitable organization in this field. Address: P.O. Box 15247, Chattanooga, TN 37415. Tel: 800-723-4238. E-mail: mharting@ix.netcom.com. Web site: http://www.behcets.com.

American Board of Clinical Neurophysiology A professional organization. Address: 1111 Lac de Ville Blvd. Rochester, NY, 14618. Tel: 804-627-0713.

American Board of Electrodiagnostic Medicine An independent, autonomous credentialling body establishing and promulgating criteria for certification through a combination of academic training, clinical experience, and examination components selected on the basis of their relationship to knowledge, competence, or achievement in the field of electrodiagnostic medicine. Address: 21 Second St. SW, Rochester, MN 55902. Tel: 507-288-0100.

American Board of Electroencephalography and Neurophysiology A body established to control the process of specialization and to oversee the recognition of those considered to be qualified in electroencephalography and related disciplines. Address: 850 Elm Grove Rd., Elm Grove, WI 53122.

American Board of Neurological Surgery An American regulatory body. Address: School of Medicine, LSU Medical Center, 1542 Tulane Avenue, New Orleans, LA 70112. Tel: 504-568-5036.

American Board of Psychiatry and Neurology A body established in 1934 to control the process of specialization and to oversee the recognition of those considered to be qualified in these disciplines.

American Brain Tumor Association A charitable association in this field. Address: 2720 River Road, Suite 146, Des Plaines, Illinois, 60018. Tel: 708-827-9910; and at 3725 N Talman Avenue, Chicago, IL 60618-4712. Tel. 1-800-886-2282. Web site: http://www.abta.org/.

American Chronic Pain Association A charitable organization providing support and information on this condition. Address: PO Box 850, Rocklin, CA 95677. Tel: 916-632-0922. Web site: http://www.theacpa.org/.

American College of Neuropsychopharmacology A professional association. Address: 134 Wesley Hall, Vanderbilt University, Nashville, TN 37240. Tel: 615-322-7417.

American Council for Headache Education (ACHE) A charitable organization concerned with public education about the nature and management of headache. Address: 19 Mantua Rd., Mt. Royal, NJ 08061. Tel: 856-423-0258. Web site: http://www.achenet.org/.

American Electroencephalographic Society A professional organization for physicians and others with interests in basic systems neurobiology, neuroimaging, and neurobehavior. Address: 1 Regency Dr., PO Box 30, Bloomfield, CT 06002. Tel: 203-243-3977.

American Epilepsy Society A professional society promoting interdisciplinary communication and the exchange of basic and clinical information about epilepsy. Address: 638 Prospect Ave., Hartford, CT 06105. Tel: 203-232-4825. Web site: http://www.aesnet.org/.

American Foundation for the Blind A charitable organization. Address: 15 W. 16th St., New York, NY 10011. Tel: 212-620-2000.

American Headache Society A professional organization for physicians and others interested in the study and management of headache and facial pain, founded in 1959. Its objectives are to promote the exchange of ideas concerning the cause and treatment of headache and related painful disorders, the education of physicians and other health professionals, and the encouragement of scientific research. Address: 19 Mantua Rd., Mount Royal, NJ 08061. Tel: 856-423-0043. Web site: http://ahsnet.org.

American Heart Association A charitable organization providing support and information on vascular disease, including stroke. Address: 7272 Greenville Ave., Dallas, TX 75231. Tel: 214-373-6300. Web site: http://www.americanheart.org.

American Journal of EEG Technology (*Am. J. EEG Technol.*) A subspecialty EEG journal. Address: ASET Executive Office, 204 West 7th St., Carroll, IA 51401.

American Journal of Neuroradiology (*AJNR Am J Neuroradiol*) A neuro-radiological journal. Address: Waverly Press Inc., 428 E. Preston St., Baltimore, MD 21202. Web site: http.www.ajnr.org/.

American Lyme Disease Foundation, Inc. A charitable association in this field. Address: Royal Executive Park. 3. International Dr., Rye Brook, NY 10573. Tel: 914-277-6970.

American Medical Electroencephalographic Association A professional organization. Address: 850 Elm Grove Rd., Elm Grove, WI 53122. Tel: 414-796-1149.

American Narcolepsy Association A charitable organization providing support and information on this condition. Address: PO Box 26230, San Francisco, CA 94126-6230. Tel: 415-788-4793.

American Neurological Association (ANA) A leading professional society devoted to the cultivation of neurological science in its normal and pathological relations, founded by William **Hammond,** J.J. Putnam, and others in 1875. The ANA was the first of the national neurological associations to be formed, the British one coming into existence in 1886, the French one in 1899, and the German one in 1907.

The neurological trauma cases produced by the Civil War led to a great increase in interest in neurology in the latter half of the nineteenth century in the United States and the ANA flourished, with Ramsay **Hunt,** C.L. **Dana,** Bernard **Sachs,** Pearce Bailey, Charles K. Mills, Silas Weir **Mitchell,** George Beard, and James Jewell among its members.

The association's journal was the *Archives of Neurology* until 1975, when it sponsored the ***Annals of Neurology*** under the editorship of Dr. Fred Plum. A retrospective anniversary volume was published in 1975.[1402] Membership today is by election and requires evidence of significant scientific contributions on the part of the candidate. Address: 2221 University Ave. SE, Ste. 350, Minneapolis, MN 55414. Tel: 612-623-2401. Web site: http://www.aneuroa.org.

American Pain Society   A charitable association in this field. Address: 5700 Old Orchard Road, Skokie, IL 60077. Tel: 708-966-5595. Web site: http://www.ampainsoc.org.

American Paralysis Association   A charitable organization concerned with research, care, and treatment of spinal cord injury and other paralyzing or disabling conditions. Address: 500 Morris Ave., Springfield, NJ 07081. Tel: 201-379-2690 or 1-800-225-0292. A related Web site is at http://www.familyvillage.wisc.edu/lib_sci.htm.

American Paraplegia Society   A charitable organization providing support and information on this condition. Address: 75-20 Astoria Blvd., Jackson Heights, NY 11370. Tel: 718-303-3782. Web site: http://www.apssci.org.

American Parkinson Disease Association   A charitable organization that provides an educational, referral, and support program to medical professionals, patients and their families, and the public at large through regional symposia and educational literature and videotapes. The association has 48 information and referral centers, 90 chapters, and more than 350 support groups. It also sponsors research on Parkinson disease by funding advanced centers for research, fellowships, and research grants. Address: 60 Bay St., Ste. 401, Staten Island, NY 10301. Tel: 1-800-223-2732. Web site: http://www.apdaparkinson.com.

American Psychiatric Association *Diagnostic and Statistical Manual*   A compilation, revised periodically, of all psychiatric and many neurological disorders, with diagnostic criteria. The *Diagnostic and Statistical Manual, Fourth Edition* (Text Revision) is the current volume.[150]

American Sleep Apnea Association   A charitable organization in this field. Address: 1424 K St. NW, Suite 302, Washington, DC 20005. Tel: 202-293-3650. E-mail: asaa@sleepapnea.org. Web site: http://www.sleepapnea.org.

American Sleep Disorders Association   (now American Academy of Sleep Medicine) A professional organization made up primarily of physicians and scientists in the multidisciplinary fields of sleep disorders medicine. The association establishes standards for evaluation and treatment of disorders of sleep and alertness, provides educational materials and courses for physicians, promotes research on sleep mechanisms, and represents the sleep discipline to reimbursement agencies, regulatory bodies, and the public. Address: 1610 Fourteenth St. N.W., Ste. 300, Rochester, MN 55901. Tel: 507-287-6006. Web site: http://www.asda.org. See also http://www.sleepapnea.org.

American Sleep Disorders Association Diagnostic Classification of Sleep Disorders   See **sleep disorders.**

American Society for Clinical Evoked Potentials   A professional organization. Address: 41 East Point Rd., White Plains, NY 10601.

American Society for Stereotactic and Functional Neurosurgery   A professional organization. Address: Division of Neurosurgery, 636431 Fannen, University of Texas Medical School, Houston, TX 77030. Tel: 713-792-2121.

American Society of Electroneurodiagnostic Technologists   The national professional organization for EEG/EP/PSG/NCV technologists, physicians, managers, institutions, and students. It provides education, employment services, a newsletter, insurance services, and an annual scientific forum and publishes the *American Journal of EEG Technology*. Address: 204 W. 7th St., Carroll, IA 51401-2317. Tel: 712-792-2978.

American Society of Neuroimaging   A professional scientific organization dedicated to the advancement of all types of neuroimaging through literature and the promotion of scientific and educational programs. Address: 2221 University Ave. SE, Ste. 340, Minneapolis, MN 55414. Tel: 612-623-2404. Web site: http://www.asnweb.org.

American Society of Neuroradiology   A professional association. Address: Rush Presbyterian Medical Center, 1753 West Congress Parkway, Chicago, IL 60612. Tel: 312-942-5000.

American Society of Neurorehabilitation   A professional organization dedicated to improving patient care and fostering and encouraging research, teaching, and training in all areas of neurorehabilitation. Address: 2221 University Ave. SE, Ste. 360, Minneapolis, MN 55414. Tel: 612-623-2405. Web site: http://www.asnr.com.

American Speech Language Hearing Association (ASHA)   A chairtable organization in this field. Address: 10801 Rockville Pike, Rockville, MD 20852-3279. Tel: 301-897-5700; 800-638-8255. E-mail: actioncenter@asha.org. Web site: http://www.asha.org.

American Syringomyelia Alliance Project   A charitable organization providing support and information on this condition. Address: PO Box 1586, Longview, TX 75606-1586. Tel: 903-236-7079; 1-800-ASAP-282. Web site: http://www.asap4sm.com.

American Tinnitus Association   A charitable organization providing support and information on this condition. Address: PO Box 5, Portland, OR 97207. Tel: 503-248-0024, 503-248-9985. Web site: http://www.ata. org.

American Tourette Syndrome Association   A charitable organization providing support and information on this condition. Address: 42–40 Bell Blvd., Bayside, NY 11361-2861. Tel: 718-224-299, 1-800-237-0717. See also the Web site: http://www.nlm.nih.gov/medlineplus/tourettesyndrome.html.

amimia   Loss of the power to copy gestures.

Amin-Amat syndrome   (inverse Marcus Gunn phenomenon, inverse jaw-winking) A rare condition in which the homolateral eye closes as the external pterygoid muscle moves the jaw to the opposite side. It is due to inhibition of the levator palpebrae during the activation of the fifth nerve; in some cases this occurs as a congenital anomaly.[3499]

aminoacidopathies   Inborn errors of metabolism presenting usually in the neonatal period with depression of neurological function and increase or decrease in muscle tone. See **hyperglycinemia, homocystinuria, hypervalinemia, phenylketonuria, maple syrup urine disease.**

aminoaciduria–retardation–dwarfism and muscular dystrophy syndrome   See **Stransky syndrome.**

Ammon, Friedrich Augustus von   (1799–1861) German physician who studied medicine in Leipzig and Göttingen, specialized in ophthalmology in Dresden, and was then Professor of Pathology and Materia Medica at that university.

Ammon's horn   The hippocampus. The god Jupiter was considered capable of assuming the form of a ram, in which guise his name was Ammon. The name refers to the shape of a ram's horn.

Ammon's horn sclerosis   Gliosis of the hippocampus, the most common single lesion found in the temporal lobectomy specimens of patients with **complex partial seizures.** It was first described by Sommer in 1880.

amnemonic   (Gr, lack of + memory) Diseases characterized by loss of memory.

amnesia   (Gr, lack of + memory) Forgetfulness, or inability to learn new material currently perceived unless repeatedly rehearsed. Amnesia exists both for events and for facts. Broca's use of the word in the phrase *ver-*

bal amnesia, meaning "impaired word-finding," is no longer current. See also **hysterical amnesia, post-traumatic amnesia, primary amnesia, retrograde amnesia, opographical amnesia, transient global amnesia.**

Amnesia Association   A charitable organization. Address: 25 Prebend Gardens, London W4 1TN, United Kingdom.

amnesic aphasia   Originally, a fluent aphasia; see **anomic aphasia.**

amnesic automatisms   An occasional feature of the narcolepsy complex, in which the subject acts automatically (but usually appropriately) without subsequent recall. See also **transient global amnesia.**

amnesic stroke   Persistent or transient amnesic syndromes resulting from infarction in the territory of the posterior cerebral arteries, usually accompanied by visual field deficits. Rarely, unilateral (usually left-sided) infarctions in the territories of the posterior cerebral, anterior choroidal, or thalamic penetrating arteries affecting the hippocampus or thalamus may cause a similar pure amnesic state.[4276]

amnestic   A term for diseases causing loss of memory.

amnestic aphasia   A form of aphasia in which there is a failure to recall the names of people or of other nouns in conversation when they are presented visually or verbally.

amnestic color anomia   An inability to recall the names of colors but with retention of the ability to distinguish them.

amnestic disorder   A disorder of memory due to bilateral lesions of the hippocampal–limbic circuit. The American Psychiatric Association suggests the following *diagnostic guidelines*:[150]

A. The development of memory disorder as manifested by the inability to learn new information or the inability to recall previously learned information.

B. The memory disturbance causes significant impairment in social or occupational functioning and represents a significant decline from a previous level of functioning.

C. The memory disturbance does not occur exclusively during the course of a delirium or a dementia.

D. There is evidence from the history, physical examination, or laboratory findings that the disturbance is a direct physiological consequence of a general medical condition (including physical trauma).

Adapted slightly from the Diagnostic and Statistical Manual of Mental Disorders. Fourth Edition (text revision). Copyright 2000. American Psychiatric Association Washington, DC. Reprinted by kind permission.

An amnestic syndrome with anterograde, retrograde, and post-event amnesia and relative preservation of recognition memory[1980] can also occur after basal forebrain infarction.

amnestic-confabulatory syndrome   See **Korsakoff syndrome.**

amniotic bands A congenital dysmorphic syndrome caused by compression of the fetus by fibrous bands of amniotic origin in utero.

The clinical results of this include omphalocele, constriction rings of the arms, legs, or digits, and syndactyly. **Craniosynostosis, hydrocephalus, holoproscencephaly, encephalocele,** and **cranial meningocele** have all been described in association.[2682]

amoeboid movements Variable distortions of a dilated pupil, considered to reflect excessive activity in the ciliary ganglion or of the long ciliary nerve.[5824]

amok A self-limited syndrome of spontaneous, wild, and murderous agitation, the word coming from Malaya, where this behavior is described with greater frequency than elsewhere, mainly in young men. Whether the cause is toxic or psychological is not determined.

amorphin A structural protein in the Z lines of muscle.

amorphosynthesis 1. A *variant term for* **constructional apraxia** as a result of parietal lobe dysfunction. 2. Inability to comprehend or be aware of parts or functions of the body. Tactile extinction would be a minor form of this condition, hemi-asomatagnosia a maximal form.[1399] See also **Anton-Babinski syndrome.**

amphigory Fluent, grammatical, but nonsensical or irrelevant speech in demented patients who do not have dysphasia.[1848] Central and medial temporal lobe lesions are usually responsible.

amphiphilic drug myopathy Forms of myopathy associated with the ingestion of large, cationic amphiphilic molecules (i.e., with both hydrophilic and hydrophobic sites). Such agents include imipramine, amiodarone, chloroquine, colchicine, etc.[3188]

amphoamphoterodiplopia (Gr, both + both + two + double sight) Diplopia which is both uni- and binocular. The length of the word is inversely proportional to the importance of the condition.

amplitude With reference to an action potential, the maximum voltage difference between two points, usually baseline to peak or peak to peak. By convention, the amplitude of potentials that have an initial negative deflection from the baseline, such as the compound muscle action potential and the antidromic sensory nerve action potential are measured from baseline to the most negative peak. In contrast, the amplitude of a compound sensory nerve action potential, motor unit potential, fibrillation potential, positive sharp wave, fasciculation potential, and most other action potentials is measured from the most positive peak to the most negative peak. (From the 2001 Report of the Nomenclature Committee of the American Association of Electromyography and Electrodiagnosis.[10] Used by permission, copyright © 2001, AAEM.)

amplitude decay The percent change in the amplitude of the M wave or the compound sensory nerve action potential between two different stimulation points along the nerve. Decay = 100* (amplitude$_{distal}$ − amplitude$_{proximal}$/amplitude$_{distal}$). Useful in the evaluation of conduction block. Abnormal decay without increased temporal dispersion may indicate a conduction block.

Ampole syndrome A congenital dysmorphic syndrome characterized by short stature, strabismus, double ureters, arachnodactyly, skeletal deformities, dry skin, seizures, and mental and developmental delay.[337]

amputation illusion A sensation that may occur after spinal cord injury in which the subject feels that an anesthetic part is no longer present at all.[5154]

amputation neuroma A swelling at the distal end of the proximal segment of a cut nerve, composed of bundles of randomly oriented axons (**neurites**), Schwann cells, and connective tissue.

Amsterdam dwarfism See **De Lange syndrome.**

Amsterdam Short-term Memory (ASTM) Test A test of memory and concentration, reported to be of value in detecting malingering in subjects after whiplash injury, leading to the suggestion that the cognitive complaints of non-malingering post-whiplash patients are likely to result from chronic pain, chronic fatigue, or depression.[4974]

amusement park stroke Stroke usually due to dissection of a vertebral artery, as a result of hyperextension of the neck during a roller-coaster ride. Headache and subdural hematoma are other complications of this leisure activity.[844]

amusia (Gr, lack of + to do with the Muses—in this case, those concerned with melodies) Inability to discern the elements of music such as rhythm, pitch, melody, modulation, intonation, and accentuation of musical sounds. Like aphasia, this has both expressive and receptive forms, both of which seem to be unusually common among people who otherwise appear healthy and many of whom today are in the forefront of composition.

The faculty of musical expression is probably dependent on the normal function of the anterior parts of the right or left temporal and posterior inferior frontal convolutions. On the sensory side, *tone deafness* and *note blindness* were the other terms suggested by Knoblauch (1888) for those disorders of communication involving music which correspond to aphasia in the realm of language. The **Luria-Nebraska** Test Battery examines some such functions.

Numerous other disorders have also been identified in the musical field,[3857] including motor and sensory amusia, *paramusia, musical agraphia, amnestic amusia, musical alexia, instrumental apraxia,* and **amimia.**

amyelotrophy (Gr, lack of + marrow + nourishment) Atrophy of the spinal cord.

amygdala (Gr, almond) A nucleus, part of the limbic system, situated deep in the inferomesial aspect of the temporal lobe at the tail of the caudate. Its major roles are in motivation, affect, and emotional display.

amygdalar sclerosis Severe neuronal loss and sclerosis in the amygdala without accompanying hippocampal pathology, associated with seizures and described in subjects who have had temporal lobe surgery for that indication.[3883]

amygdalo-hippocampal seizures (mesiobasal limbic or rhinencephalic seizures) Hippocampal seizures are the most common form; the symptoms are those described under **temporal lobe syndromes** except that auditory symptoms may not occur. The interictal scalp EEG may be normal, or may show interictal uni- or bilateral temporal sharp or slow waves, which may be synchronous or asynchronous. The intracranial interictal EEG may show mesial anterior temporal spikes or sharp waves.

Clinically, the seizures are characterized by rising epigastric discomfort, nausea, marked autonomic signs, and other symptoms including borborygmi, belching, pallor, fullness of the face, flushing of the face, arrest of respiration, pupillary dilatation, fear, panic, and olfactory-gustatory hallucinations,[1114] and the seizures tend to increase during REM sleep.

amyloid (β-amyloid protein) (from Lat, starch) An insoluble fibrous membrane protein, part of the β-amyloid precursor protein, which exhibits green birefringence in polarized light after staining with Congo Red. It is encoded by a gene on chromosome 21. The β-protein form is found in the CNS in neurofibrillary tangles, in plaques, and in the walls of cerebral vessels, typically in **congophilic angiopathy, Alzheimer disease,** and **Down syndrome.** The prion protein form is found in scrapie and in **Jakob-Creutzfeldt** disease.

Primary amyloidosis is that form associated with the AL amyloid protein, an immunoglobulin light-chain fragment produced by plasma cells. The same amyloid protein is also found with **multiple myeloma,** Waldenstrom **macroglobulinemia,** and **agammaglobulinemia.** The main findings are cardiac and renal, but painful sensorimotor and autonomic peripheral axonal neuropathy and amyloid myopathy are neurological complications, mainly in elderly men. Genetic forms are also recognized; see **familial amyloid neuropathy** and below.

In *secondary amyloidosis* (as with various chronic diseases, Hodgkin disease, and familial Mediterranean fever) the protein is of the AA type, derived from a plasma protein precursor in patients with chronic inflammatory disease or with malignancy such as renal cell carcinoma and Hodgkin disease. Yet other forms of amyloid protein are expressed in dialysis patients and those with different mitotic lesions or **Alzheimer disease.**

In a *variant* form, *AA amyloidosis* may be associated with autonomic neuropathy, vestibulocochlear dysfunction, and lattice corneal dystrophy.[5659]

amyloid angiopathy See **congophilic angiopathy.**

amyloid myopathy An occasional manifestation of primary systemic amyloidosis in which there is infiltration of muscles with amyloid material, forming nodules and compressing muscle fibers and leading to atrophy or pseudohypertrophy, weakness, hardness or muscles, macroglossia, and hoarseness. The EMG findings are of chronic myositis.[2078, 2841]

amyloid neuropathy Forms of neuropathy characterized by the deposition of amyloid (fragments of an immunoglobulin light chain) within tissues in cases of sporadic **amyloidosis.** *Primary amyloid neuropathy* presents with sensorimotor polyneuropathy, **carpal tunnel syndrome,** and **autonomic neuropathy,** complicating renal and cardiac failure.[35] *Secondary amyloidosis* leads only to entrapment neuropathies. See also **familial amyloid neuropathy.**

amyloid-associated muscle pseudohypertrophy General hypertrophy of muscles attributed to the deposition of extracellular amyloid within skeletal muscles, producing proximal limb stiffness, aching, and weakness.[4702]

amyloidoma Large deposits of amyloid material within the parenchyma of the nervous system, where they may give rise to clinical features resembling those of a tumor.[1086]

amyloidopathies Neurodegenerative disorders characterized by the production/deposition of normal or abnormal amyloid material within cells of the nervous system. **Alzheimer disease,** some forms of **systemic amyloidosis,** and **familial British** (or Danish) dementia are examples.

amyloidosis Deposition of **amyloid** within tissues, as occurs in familial, primary, or secondary amyloidosis. See **familial amyloid neuropathy, myeloma, gammopathic neuropathy.**

amylo-transglucosidase deficiency See **glycogen storage diseases.**

amylo-1,6-glucosidase debrancher deficiency See **glycogen storage diseases.**

amyoplasia congenita See **arthrogryposis multiplex congenita.**

amyostatic syndrome (Gr, lack of + muscle + standing still) An old term for tremor in **Parkinson disease.**

amyosthenia   (Gr, lack of + muscle + force) Weakness.

amyotonia congenita   (Oppenheim disease) A sporadic congenital disorder characterized by muscular weakness and hypotonia at birth without local muscle wasting, mainly peripherally, and with no tendency to spread to muscles previously unaffected. The usual course is for progressive improvement, even with a return of muscle stretch reflexes.

Despite these guidelines to the clinical features, so many exceptions to the original rules governing the diagnosis have been recorded that it is more likely that this is not a disease *sui generis* but represents either a nonprogressive myopathy or a form of **hereditary motor neuropathy**.[5669]

The term replaced Oppenheim's *myatonia congenita* because the latter was too similar to **myotonia congenita,** but was itself later replaced at the suggestion of Walton by **benign congenital hypotonia**[7 7] and then by the vernacular **floppy baby syndrome.**

See also **benign congenital hypotonia, Oppenheim disease, hereditary motor neuropathy type 1.**

amyotrophic cervical myelopathy   A sporadic syndrome of asymmetric muscular atrophy of the distal upper limbs seen predominantly in young males and reported mainly from Japan.[5602]

amyotrophic choreoacanthocytosis   (amyotrophic choreoathetosis) A rare, dominantly or recessively inherited disease with adult onset, characterized by orofacial dyskinesias, chorea, lip or tongue biting, and neurogenic muscular atrophy accompanied by atrophy of the caudate nuclei and acanthocytosis but without abnormalities in plasma lipoproteins.[2290, 5071] See also **neuroacanthocytosis.**

Criteria for the diagnosis have been suggested;[3376] these include extrapyramidal movement disorders, generalized muscle weakness, acanthocytosis (1%–50%), normal intelligence, and, in some cases, ataxia, epilepsy, or schizophrenia.

amyotrophic choreoathetosis   See **amyotrophic chorea-acanthocytosis.**

amyotrophic dystonic paraplegia   A syndrome of slowly progressive dystonia, spasticity, weakness, and muscle wasting, dominantly inherited with variable expression. The dystonia affects the bulbar, trunk, and limb muscles and is accompanied over time by spastic paraparesis and later by neurogenic muscle atrophy.[2121]

amyotrophic lateral sclerosis   (ALS; Charcot syndrome; Aran syndrome; motor neurone disease; progressive muscular atrophy; Aran-Duchenne disease; progressive bulbar palsy; progressive muscular atrophy; primary lateral sclerosis; Mills disease; Lou Gehrig disease) A sporadic, fatal, degenerative disease of unknown cause occurring in adult life, in which pure involvement of the cranial and spinal upper and lower motor neuron systems is manifested by rapid, inexorably progressive, and ultimately generalized muscle weakness and wasting and by pyramidal signs.

Clinically, older adults are affected with any combination of upper and lower motor signs such as weakness, wasting, fasciculations, and hyperreflexia, witnessing damage to the bulbar and spinal motor nuclei and pyramidal tracts, although the ocular muscles are spared. The course is usually fatal within 5 years of onset. Stages of involvement based on single-fiber EMG data (early reinnervation; well-compensated reinnervation; early decompensation–late reinnervation; and late decompensation–reinnervation failure) have been defined.[5443]

This group includes sporadic cases with atypical features: e.g., ophthalmoplegia; nystagmus; sporadic multisystem disorders with amyotrophy, cerebellar disorder, and ophthalmoplegia; **monomelic;** and other restricted forms. See also **motor neuronal disorders.**

Pathologically, there is loss of the large motor neurons in the cerebral cortex, brainstem and spinal cord, leading to a combination of upper and lower motor neuron lesions. Subclinical involvement of other neuronal systems also occurs.[5483]

This invariably fatal disease is survived only by medical students and impressionable neurologists who notice the extent of their (normal) fasciculations for the first time. Although it is subsumed under the category of **abiotrophy,** studies of the Chamorro and other Guamian peoples indicate that toxicity from ingestion of the cycad root may be the cause of the **ALS–Parkinson–dementia complex** prevalent there, and by extension it is supposed that toxic causes may in fact be important in ALS as well.

The stem condition was identified by Duchenne[1536] and the main forms recorded by Aran in the following year,[204] by Cruveilhier in 1852, and by Charcot[973] in 1881, who also introduced the term *amyotrophic lateral sclerosis.* Marie reviewed the validity of the syndrome in 1897[3615] and Poser reviewed the diagnostic criteria for the disease.[4502] A recent review is that of Rowland and Shneider.[4830] Chart A–5 lists the stages of involvement of individual muscles in ALS.

Charitable organizations in this field include: The *Family Caregiver Alliance* (Address: 690 Market St., Suite 600, San Francisco, CA 94104. Tel: 415-434-3388; 800-445-8106. E-mail: info@caregiver.org. Web site: http://www.caregiver.org); the **ALS Association;** the **ALS Society of Canada;** the *Forbes Norris ALS Research Center* (Address: California Pacific Medical Center, 2324 Sacramento St., San Francisco, CA 94115. Tel: 415-923-3604); and the *Les Turner ALS Foundation* (Address: 8142 North Lawndale Ave. Skokie, IL 60076. Tel: 888-ALS-1107; 847-679-3311. Web site: info@ lesturnerals.org).

Chart A–5. Stage of Involvement of Individual Muscles in Amyotrophic Lateral Sclerosis

Stage	Strength	Wasting	Fiber Density	Jitter
1	Normal	None	Normal/ slightly increased <2.5	None/ slightly increased
2	Normal	None	Increased >2.5	Increased
3	Weak and easily fatiguable	Often present	Markedly increased	Markedly increased
4	Very weak	Prominent	Slightly increased, may be unrecordable	Prominent if recordable

Criteria for the diagnosis of ALS were defined at a workshop held under the auspices of the World Federation of Neurology in 1989[6037] and have since been further revised (Subcommittee on Motor Neuron Diseases of World Federation of Neurology Research Group on Neuromuscular Diseases, El Escorial. Criteria for the diagnosis of amyotrophic lateral sclerosis. © 1997–2002 World Federation of Neurology.) Web site: http://www.wfnals.org/Articles/elescorial1988.htm

Chart A–6. Revised Criteria for the Diagnosis of Amyotrophic Lateral Sclerosis

Requirements for the Diagnosis of Amyotrophic Lateral Sclerosis

The diagnosis of amyotrophic lateral sclerosis (ALS) requires
A. The presence of
   1. Evidence of lower motor neuron (LMN) degeneration by clinical, electrophysiological, or neuropathologic examination,
   2. Evidence of upper motor neuron (UMN) degeneration by clinical examination, and
   3. Progressive spread of symptoms or signs within a region or to other regions, as determined by history or examination,
together with
B. The absence of
   1. Electrophysiological and pathological evidence of other disease processes that might explain the signs of LMN and/or UMN degeneration, and
   2. Neuroimaging evidence of other disease processes that might explain the observed clinical and electrophysiological signs.

Clinical Studies in the Diagnosis of Amyotrophic Lateral Sclerosis

A careful history, physical, and neurological examination must be conducted to search for clinical evidence of UMN and LMN signs in four regions (brainstem or cervical, thoracic, or lumbosacral spinal cord) of the CNS. Ancillary tests should be reasonably applied, as clinically indicated, to exclude other disease processes. These should include electrodiagnostic, neurophysiological, neuroimaging, and clinical laboratory studies. Clinical evidence of LMN and UMN degeneration is required for the diagnosis of ALS.

The clinical diagnosis of ALS, without pathological confirmation, may be categorized into various levels of certainty by clinical assessment alone, depending on the presence of UMN and LMN signs together in the same topographical anatomic region in the brainstem (bulbar cranial motor neurons), or cervical, thoracic, or lumbosacral spinal cord (anterior horn motor neurons). The terms *clinically definite ALS* and *clinically probable ALS* are used to describe these categories of clinical diagnostic certainty on clinical criteria alone, as follows:

Clinically definite ALS There is clinical evidence alone of the presence of UMN, as well as LMN signs, in three regions.

Clinically probable ALS There is clinical evidence alone of UMN and LMN signs in at least two regions with some UMN signs necessarily rostral to (above) the LMN signs. The terms *clinically probable ALS–Laboratory-supported* and *clinically possible ALS* are used to describe these categories of clinical certainty on clinical and criteria or only clinical criteria.

Clinically probable–laboratory-supported ALS Clinical signs of UMN and LMN dysfunction are in only one region, or when UMN signs alone are present in one region, and LMN signs defined by EMG criteria are present in at least two limbs, with proper application of neuroimaging and clinical laboratory protocols to exclude other causes.

Clinically possible ALS Clinical signs of UMN and LMN dysfunction are found together in only one region or UMN signs are found alone in two or more regions, or LMN signs are found rostral to UMN signs and the diagnosis of clinically probable–laboratory-supported ALS cannot be proven by evidence on clinical grounds in conjunction with electrodiagnostic, neurophysiologic, neuroimaging, or clinical laboratory studies. Other diagnoses must have been excluded to accept a diagnosis of clinically possible ALS.

(Clinically suspected ALS is a pure LMN syndrome, in which the diagnosis of ALS cannot be regarded as sufficiently certain to include the patient in a research study. Hence, this category was deleted from the revised El Escorial Criteria for the Diagnosis of ALS.)

Clinical Types and Patterns of Amyotrophic Lateral Sclerosis

1. *Sporadic ALS* ALS occurs alone or is present incidentally with other preexisting disease processes.
2. *Genetically determined (familial, hereditary) ALS* ALS, present in one or more generations, is associated with different modes of inheritance and defined pathogenic mutations such as superoxide dismutase-1 (SOD-1) mutations or hexosaminidase A/B deficiency. ALS may occur as a genetically determined disease, and in some cases, the pathogenic mutation has been determined, e.g., mutations of the SOD-1 gene. When there is a family history of such a defined pathogenic mutation, the diagnosis may be upgraded to *clinically definite familial–laboratory-supported ALS* or ALS presenting with progressive upper and/or lower motor neuron signs in at least a single region (in the absence of another cause for the abnormal neurological signs). However, in genetically determined cases where the gene has not been identified (even if linkage is established), the criteria for the diagnosis of sporadic ALS apply.
3. *ALS plus syndromes* ALS is present in association with clinical features of other neurological diseases that develop in addition to the phenotype of ALS or develop in parallel with the ALS, e.g., extrapyramidal features or dementia.

4. *ALS with laboratory abnormalities of uncertain significance* ALS is present in association with laboratory-defined abnormalities that are of uncertain significance to the pathogenesis of ALS.

5. *ALS-mimic syndromes* These syndromes occur as a consequence of other, non-ALS pathogenic processes, and do not represent other forms of ALS. ALS-mimic syndromes include the post-poliomyelitis syndrome; multifocal motor neuropathy with or without conduction block; endocrinopathies, especially hyperparathyroid or hyperthyroid states; lead intoxication; infections; and paraneoplastic syndromes.

Electrophysiological Studies in the Diagnosis of Amyotrophic Lateral Sclerosis

Patients in whom the diagnosis of ALS is considered on clinical grounds should have electrophysiological studies performed to confirm LMN dysfunction in clinically affected regions, detect electrophysiological evidence of LMN dysfunction in clinically uninvolved regions, and exclude other pathophysiological processes. These electrophysiological studies should be performed by qualified physicians according to established standards. It is essential to interpret the electrophysiological results in conjunction with the clinical and other ancillary findings. The El Escorial criteria for electrophysiological studies are given below.

Electrophysiological features required to identify definite primary LMN degeneration include all of the following:

Reduced interference pattern with firing rates higher than 10 Hz

Large motor unit potential (MUP; large amplitude, long duration)

Fibrillation potentials

Electrophyiological features that support the identification of probable primary LMN degeneration include one or both of the following:

Reduced recruitment or large MUP and fibrillation potentials and unstable MUP

Reduced motor unit estimates and increased macro-EMG MUP

Electrophysiological features that support the identification of possible primary LMN degeneration include one or more of the following:

Reduced recruitment, large MUP, fibrillation potentials, or unstable MUP alone

Polyphasic MUP or increased single fiber density alone

Low-amplitude MUP if the disease has lasted more than 5 years, or if there is associated atrophy

Low-amplitude compound motor action potential (CMAP)

CMAP change between proximal and distal sites of stimulation that is uniform along the length of the nerve

Up to 30% decrement in motor conduction velocity–established normal values if a low-amplitude CMAP is above 10% of normal is present

Up to 50% decrement in motor conduction velocity–established normal values if the CMAP is less than 10% of normal

Up to 20% decrement of the CMAP on 2-Hz repetitive stimulation

Up to 10% decrement in sensory nerve conduction velocity and action potential amplitude from established normal values

Complex repetitive discharges

Presence [originally published as "absence"] of fasciculations

These criteria, however, have been persuasively criticized by Wilbourn. (Wilbourn AJ. Clinical neurophysiology in the diagnosis of amyotrophic lateral sclerosis J. Neurol. Sci. 1998;160 (Suppl. 1):S25–S29.)

Neuroimaging Studies in the Diagnosis of Amytrophic Lateral Sclerosis

Neuroimaging studies should be selected in order to exclude other conditions which may cause UMN and/or LMN signs that may simulate sporadic ALS. There are no neuroimaging tests which provide positive support for the diagnosis of ALS, although there are neuroimaging methods (e.g., nuclear magnetic resonance [NMR] spectroscopy) that may in the future support the diagnosis of UMN involvement. Rarely, brain T2-weighted MRI may show increased signal in the corticospinal tracts.

Clinical Laboratory Studies in the Diagnosis of Amyotrophic Lateral Sclerosis

The diagnostic process employed to confirm the diagnosis of sporadic ALS when the diagnosis is uncertain includes repeated clinical examinations to document progression, repeated electrophysiological and/or neuroimaging examinations to exclude structural disorders, and laboratory examinations to exclude other disorders or support the diagnosis of ALS plus syndromes, ALS-mimic syndromes, or ALS with laboratory abnormalities of uncertain significance.

Neuropathological Studies in the Diagnosis of Amyotrophic Lateral Sclerosis

The diagnosis of sporadic ALS may be supported or excluded by muscle and/or biopsy studies in the living patient. The diagnosis of sporadic ALS may be proven or excluded by autopsy examination.

Alternative Diagnostic Criteria for Amyotrophic Lateral Sclerosis[4802]

The diagnosis of ALS requires the presence of each of the following:

LMN signs in at least two limbs

UMN signs in at least one region (bulbar, cervical, or lumbosacral)

Progression of the disease, defined as increasingly symptomatic impairment by history. This may involve the same or new regions.

The diagnosis of ALS requires the absence of each of the following:

Sensory signs (except those attributable to aging)

Neurogenic sphincter abnormalities

Clinically evident CNS disease apart from ALS, with a natural history of progression (e.g., Parkinson disease, dementia)

Clinically evident peripheral nervous system disease with a natural history of progression (e.g., diabetic polyneuropathy, hereditary polyneuropathy)

Amytrophic lateral sclerosis variants comprise clinical syndromes in which the predominant presentation is that seen in sporadic ALS, but that includes one or more additional features. These features are outlined below.

I. *Forms with documented genetic transmission*

   A. *Familial ALS* (Hirano-Lewy body disease) In uncommon instances the condition is a familial trait, usually compatible with an autosomal dominant mode of transmission.[4035] The responsible gene maps to chromosome 21.q22.1–q22.2. Recessive transmission of the pure syndrome has also been described. In most cases, pyramidal and posterior column signs are present; in some, dementia and/or extrapyramidal signs (parkinsonism) are found as well.[129,2581,5469]

Familial ALS and Related Disorders: Known Inheritance Patterns[5383]

Inheritance Pattern	Chromosomal Linkage	Unique Features
Autosomal Dominant		
ALS 1	21q22.1	Cu/Zn superoxide dismutase mutations
ALS X	Xpll–q12	Adult onset
ALS 3		Adult onset; absence of linkage to Cu/Zn superoxide dismutase
ALS 4	9q34	Juvenile onset, complete penetrance; very slow progression; distal limb amyotrophy with pyramidal signs
ALS 6	9q21–22	Frontotemporal dementia associated
ALS with bulbar onset		Japanese family; juvenile onset with prominent early-onset bulbar dysfunction; slow progression; dementia
NFH	22q12.1–q22	Mutations in KSP repeats (not observed in familial ALS; only found in sporadic ALS)
Autosomal Recessive		
ALS 2	2q33–q35	Spastic pseudobulbar syndrome with spastic paraplegia; childhood onset; slow progression
ALS 5	15q15.1–q21.1	Not pseudobulbar; distal amyotrophy; minor spasticity; long-term survival
Brown-Vialetto-Van Laere syndrome		Progressive bulbar paralysis; childhood onset; progressive deafness; pyramidal signs
X-linked		
Kennedy syndrome	Xq12	Progressive muscle atrophy; gynecomastia; reduced fertility; androgen receptor gene mutation (trinucleotide [CAG] repeat)
Miscellaneous		
Hexosaminidase A, B	15q23–q24	Late-onset GM_2 gangliosidosis

Disinhibition-dementia-parkinsonism-amyotrophy syndrome Chr 17   Allelic with frontotemporal dementia and parkinsonism

   B. *Adult polyglycosan body disease*

   C. *Amyotrophic lateral sclerosis with autosomal dominant familial* **Parkinsonism**[5307]

   D. *Motor neuron disease with presenile dementia* This variant is characterized by the onset in mature adult life of dementia (**Pick disease**), ophthalmoplegias, and cerebral atrophy, along with the usual features of ALS.[674]

   E. *Familial juvenile motor neuron disease* (juvenile bulbar palsy) A slowly progressive variant characterized by the onset in childhood of bulbar and spinal muscle atrophy with pyramidal signs.[2403] See **Fazio-Londe disease.** The gene maps to 2q 33–35. In another form of juvenile ALS, dementia is associated.

   F. *Progressive muscular atrophy with microcephaly and mental retardation*[5293]

   G. *Corticospinal tract deficit and axonal motor polyneuropathy,* in which weakness, intermittent dysphagia, weight loss, atrophy, and fasciculations of the distal muscles, pseudobulbar dysarthria, hyperactive reflexes, and upgoing plantar responses are found without sensory loss in patients with hyperparathyroidism.[1869]

   H. *Autosomal dominant juvenile amyotrophic lateral sclerosis* A form of chronic motor neuron disease characterized by combined upper and (mainly distal) lower motor neuron symptoms and signs with onset prior to age 25 years, linked to the chromosome 9q34 region (ALS4).[4566]

   I. *Juvenile spinal muscular atrophy of the distal upper extremity* A syndrome in which the features of ALS are accompanied by minipolymyoclonus of the fingers and worsening of symptoms with cold. It has been described in young male Japanese and is caused by a structural abnormality of the cervical cord.

   J. **X-linked bulbospinal muscular atrophy** (Kennedy disease), **adult GM_2 gangliosidosis, Machado-Joseph disease, multiple system atrophy,** and **hexosaminidase A deficiency** are phenotypically similar.

II. *Forms with unusual age at presentation or unusual course*

   A. *Sporadic juvenile ALS.* A variant in which neuronal inclusions derived from the Nissl substance are formed, and with neurofibrillary degeneration in the motor cortex.[3804]

   B. *Progressive muscular atrophy with malignant course* A form that is fatal within 1 year, but that is not clearly different from autosomal dominant ALS.

   C. *Slow motor neuron disease* A variant in which survival extends well beyond 5 years, and in which the etiology may differ from that of the more usual forms.

   D. *Subacute reversible motor neuron disease* A syndrome of weakness and wasting with fasciculations and some upper motor neurone signs occurring in adults with spontaneous resolution of the signs over a year, in the absence of any other demonstrable pathology.[5663]

   E. *Brachial amyotrophic diplegia* A sporadic form in which weakness and muscle atrophy without pyramidal signs affects only only the upper limbs and is slowly progressive over years. A "man-in-the-barrel" syndrome results.[2954]

III. *Geographic location (Western Pacific, Guam, Kii, etc.)*

    A. *ALS-Parkinson-dementia syndrome of Guam* (**Lytico-Bodig**, Hirano parkinsonism/dementia, Western Pacific ALS) A disease of the Chamorro race of the Western Pacific island of Guam in the Mariana Island group, first described by Hirano and others in 1961, at which time it accounted for 10% of adult deaths. The condition also occurs in clusters in Japan and Western New Guinea. Insidious but severe progressive dementia, parkinsonism, and motor neuron involvement occur in any combination in adult patients, especially males; all show the reptilian stare, akinesia, and stooped posture of typical Parkinson disease, but tremor is slight or absent and rigidity is often absent too. Ophthalmoplegia, cerebellar and pyramidal signs, and evidence of dementia may be found, but typical signs of ALS are found in only about one-third of the cases. Death occurs within 3–5 years of the onset of symptoms.[2580]

Intensive study of the Chamorros has shown this to be a toxic disease as a result of eating flour made of the seeds of the False Sago palm *Cycas circinalis,* which contains an excitatory nonprotein amino acid neurotoxin;[5272] the disease is manifested in those who are genetically susceptible.

A similar condition is recognized among the Japanese people on the Kii peninsula and among the Akai and Ayau people of Western New Guinea.

    B. **Madras type** A form characterized by bulbar palsy, hearing loss, and minipolymyoclonus of the fingers, recorded in southern India. The pattern of inheritance is uncertain.

IV. *Forms with concurrent dementia*

    A. Amyotrophic lateral sclerosis phenotypes with the pathological features of **Martha-Alma (Hallervorden-Spatz) disease**[674] or with *aphasic dementia*[936] have been described.

    B. *Amyotrophic lateral sclerosis–Parkinson–dementia syndrome* The association of these three entities occurs as a sporadic or familial disease, most commonly seen in Guam (see III-A, above) but also in Europeans, in whom it may be inherited as a recessive trait.[2580] The pathological features of typical ALS are occasionally accompanied by mild dementia, language disturbance, or parkinsonism, but this is more common in subjects with the familial form of the disease.[4982]

V. *Forms with extrapyramidal signs (may be recessively inherited)*

    A. **Amyotrophic dystonic paraplegia**

VI. *Forms with objective sensory, autonomic or cerebellar abnormalities*

    A. *Amyotrophic lateral sclerosis with posterior column involvement* A variant which is dominantly inherited with clinical and pathological features of degeneration of upper and lower motor neurons and with posterior column demyelination.[1681]

    B. *Spinal muscular atrophy with ALS, spinocerebellar ataxia, and deafness*

    C. *Motor neuron disease (ALS) with sensory involvement* A variant characterized by the onset in mature adult life of loss of pain and temperature sensation along with the usual features of ALS

    D. **Progressive muscular atrophy with ALS** An entity of uncertain validity, presenting as a combination of **hereditary motor and sensory neuropathy** and pyramidal features

    E. *Spastic paraplegia with amyotrophy of hands*

    F. *Focal motor neuron disease* See **monomelic spinal muscular atrophy.**

    G. *Amytrophic lateral sclerosis with ophthalmoplegia* A rare variant in which there is extensive neuronal loss and gliosis in the nuclei of the third, fourth, and sixth cranial nerves[2473]

    H. Forms with associated evidence of degeneration of the posterior columns or other tracts in the spinal cord, of **tics,** or of **Luyso-pallidal-nigral atrophy**

VII. *Forms with involvement of other body systems or with other identified disease*

    A. *Amyotrophic lateral sclerosis with hyperparathyroidism* A syndrome of corticospinal tract deficit and axonal motor polyneuropathy. In this syndrome weakness, intermittent dysphagia, weight loss, atrophy and fasciculations of the distal muscles, pseudobulbar dysarthria, hyperactive reflexes, and up-going plantar responses are found without sensory loss in patients with hyperparathyroidism.[1869]

    B. *Paraneoplastic ALS* Here the typical findings of ALS are associated with underlying bronchial carcinoma, and remit when the tumor is resected.[3906] Carcinomatous motor neuron disease is only possibly a specific syndrome but amyotrophy may be seen in paraneoplastic encephalomyelopathy and may improve after removal of the tumor.

    C. *Amyotrophic lateral sclerosis with plasma cell dyscrasia and monoclonal paraproteinemia,* such as Waldenstrom macroglobulinemia, multiple myeloma, or chronic lymphatic leukemia. Both monoclonal and polyclonal gammopathies involving either IgM or IgG have been detected.[3779] See **gammopathic neuropathy.**

    D. Amytrophic lateral sclerosis associated with adrenocorticotrophic hormone deficiency.[2727]

ALS-like syndromes resemble but are not ALS and include spondylotic myelopathy, vascular, lymphoma, non-tumor endocrine abnormalities, hyperthyroidism, hyperparathyroidism, prior irradiation of the spinal cord, acute infection, postinfectious, monoclonal gammopathy, dysimmune states such as multifocal motor neuropathy with conduction block, exogenous toxins such as lead,[881] and genetic/acquired enzyme defects such as hexosaminidase A deficiency in younger patients. (Adapted from the Scottish MND Register.[5039])

Amyotrophic Lateral Sclerosis and Other Motor Neuron Disorders The official publication of the **World Federation of Neurology Research Group on Motor Neuron Disease**, published by Martin Dunitz. Web site: http://www.tandf.co.uk/journals/alphalist.html.

Amyotrophic Lateral Sclerosis Association See **ALS Association.**

Amyotrophic Lateral Sclerosis score A standardized method of assessment of motor functions in patients with ALS, which are rated as 3 (normal), 2 (impaired), 1 (trace), or 0.

Items assessed include holding up the head, chewing food, swallowing, speaking, turning in bed, sitting up, emptying the bowel and bladder, breathing and coughing. Subjects are also scored on writing their name, fastening buttons or zippers, feeding themselves, gripping objects, lifting themselves, lifting a book or a tray, lifting a fork or a pencil, changing arm position, climbing one flight of stairs, walking one block, walking across a room, walking with assistance, standing up, and changing position. Stretch reflexes in the arms and legs, the jaw jerk, and the plantar responses bilaterally are also assessed, as are fasciculations and wasting in the face, tongue, arms, shoulders, legs, and hips. Emotional lability, fatigability, and leg rigidity are other factors examined. The theoretical maximum score is 100.[4164]

Amyotrophic Lateral Sclerosis Society of Canada   A charitable organization. Address: 90 Adelaide St. E., Ste. B-101, Toronto, Ontario, Canada M5C 2R4. Tel: 416-362-0269.

amyotrophic syphilitic myelopathy   See **Erb syphilitic amyotrophy.**

amyotrophy   (from Lat, lack of + muscle + growth) Muscle atrophy. The word is used in the context of acute shoulder girdle pain and weakness (**neuralgic amyotrophy**), **syphilitic amyotrophy, diabetic amyotrophy,** and various genetically determined malformations; but as it is descriptive rather than definitive, its employment is properly limited. There is a convention, however, that it is used when the seat of the pathology is in the anterior horn cells.

The word is an unfortunate neologism; while lack of muscle growth is indeed present in patients with amyotrophy, the word *atrophy* is better known to us, and *myoatrophy* would have been a better construction. But since *amyotrophy* has been around for twice as long as has this author, he will not tilt at windmills.

anabolic GM₃ gangliosidosis   See **hematosidosis.**

anaerobic threshold   The level of muscular activity at which respiratory rate, plasma lactate levels, and other signs of anaerobic metabolic activity first appear.

anal reflex   The *superficial* anal reflex is a (polysynaptic) reflex contraction of the anal sphincter in response to stimulation of the perianal skin, mediated by the somatic fibers at S4–5, described by Rossimolo in 1891. It is lost in tabes dorsalis and with local lesions at these levels.

The *deep (internal)* reflex consists of the contraction of the internal anal sphincter muscle in response to muscle stretch, as by the gloved finger introduced, and is mediated by sympathetic fibers from L1–L2.

anal triangle   An anatomical region, the two sides of which are formed by the gluteus maximus and the base

by the superficial transverse perineal muscles. The anus, along with the surrounding external anal sphincter, is in the middle. The entire area is covered by the levator ani.

analgagnosia   Unawareness of the unpleasant qualities of painful stimuli, as shown by the subject's lack of reactivity to them.

analgesia   (Gr, lack of + pain) 1. Insensibility to pain, or lack of pain sensation, without effects on consciousness. 2. Reduction or loss of sensitivity to a stimulus which would normally be painful. This meaning, however, is often included in the nonspecific term **anesthesia.**

analgesia panaris   See **hereditary sensory neuropathy type 2.**

analgesic rebound headache   (analgesic headache; rebound headache; medication induced headache; ergotamine headache) A headache syndrome with clinical characteristics of both **migraine** and **tension-type headaches,** occurring in chronic migraine or tension-type headache sufferers who have taken to consuming acetylsalicylic acid, acetaminophen, nonsteroidal anti-inflammatory agents, benzodiazepines, ergot compounds, caffeine, narcotics, barbiturates, or combinations of these agents in increasing doses and on a regular basis, usually daily.[4595] A headache with characteristics of **hemicrania continua** has also been reported as a *variant.*

The mechanism is unknown, but the morning accentuation of the symptom would support chemical dependence such that the headaches are triggered by falling analgesic levels. This perpetuates and worsens instead of alleviating the headaches. See **rebound headache.**

analphalipoproteinemia   See **Tangier disease.**

anamnesia   (Gr, anew + memory) Recollection of phenomena prior to a given period in the disease.

anamnestic   Recalling to memory. Thus as *anamnesis*, the history of the disease.

anamnestic color blindness   Difficulty in finding the correct word for a colored object, errors being made in which the patient may perseverate. This is probably a combination of a mild disorder of visual perception and minimal dysphasia.

anapeiratic   (Gr, to do again, to repeat exercises) The term applied by **Hammond** to those pareses brought on by excessive use of a body part. See **occupational cramps.**

anaplastic meningioma   See **meningioma.**

anarchic hand   See **alien hand.**

anarithmia   Inability to comprehend numeration and the principles of mathematics, as presumably is the case in **Gerstmann syndrome.** See also **acalculia.**

anarithmic acalculia   See **acalculia.**

anarthria   Complete inability to articulate speech sounds, due to local causes or to lesions of the medulla, pons, or bulbar cranial nerves. The original Greek derivation actually indicates a defect or absence of the limbs.

anastic aphasia   See **anomia.**

anastomosis   (Gr, to bring to a mouth) The communication of the branches of vessels with one another, as if one mouth (or open end of a vessel) were joined to another.

anaudia   (Gr, negative + speech) See **aphonia.** The term has also been employed for **catalepsy.**

ancient change   The presence of large, pleomorphic, scattered, hyperchromatic nuclei within **Schwannomas,** and particularly in long-standing acoustic neuromas.[6]

Ander disease   See **Dercum disease.**

Andermann syndrome   1. See **Landau-Kleffner syndrome.** 2. (**agenesis of the corpus callosum**) A congenital dysmorphic syndrome characterized by hypertelorism, strabismus, ptosis, nystagmus, facial and generalized weakness, scoliosis, pes cavus, callosal agenesis, and mental and developmental delay.[3277]

Andersen brown forehead ring   (linea fusca) A brown pigmentation on the forehead, found in some patients with chronic CNS diseases, especially postencephalitic parkinsonism and syphilis. The cause is unknown.[3865]

Andersen disease   (glycogen storage disease type IV; D-1,4 glucan 6-glucosyltransferase brancher enzyme deficiency). The major features are hepatic cirrhosis, splenomegaly, hypotonia with muscle atrophy (especially in the legs), and delay in acquisition of motor skills.[169] See **glycogen storage diseases.**

Andersen, Dorothy   (1901–1963) American pediatrician and pathologist.

Andersen syndrome   (Klein-Lisak syndrome) A rare entity comprising potassium-ensitive periodic paralysis without myotonia, ventricular arrhythmias leading potentially to syncope or sudden death, and dysmorphisms (clinodactyly, syndactyly, hypoplastic mandible, hypertelorism, low-set ears). A prolonged QTc interval is detected in many cases. Tubular aggregates may be found on muscle biopsy. A dominant *variant* has been reported.[5500]

Anderson, W.   (1842–1900) English surgeon and anatomist at St. Thomas' Hospital, where he was also a dermatologist.

Anderson-Fabry disease   A rare X-linked lysosomal storage disorder due to deficiency of α-galactosidase A, which results in the deposition of neutral glycosphingolipids (mainly trihexosyl ceramide) in endothelial and smooth muscle cells.

The clinical features include a skin rash (**angiokeratoma**); pain and paresthesias in the extremities; abnormalities of cutaneous thermal sensation; episodic painful crises, sometimes precipitated by exercise or other stress; acroparesthesias; and a tendency toward acute ischemic hemorrhagic brain lesions. Death is due to renal failure and cerebrovascular accidents.[172,588,1728]

Andes disease   See **altitude insomnia.**

Andrade neuropathy   (**familial amyloid neuropathy,** Portuguese neuropathy) A dominantly inherited acropathic sensorimotor and autonomic neuropathy with adult onset, complicating primary amyloidosis, in which gastrointestinal complaints (cyclic diarrhea and constipation) are common.[174]

André-Thomas   (1867–1961) French neurologist, born in Paris, where he trained in Medicine, serving under **Raymond,** Bouchard, and **Déjèrine.** After graduation he worked as chef de laboratoire for Déjèrine, remaining at the **Salpetrière** until 1917, but was not accepted onto the staff. From 1911 until his death he was attached to the Hôpital Saint-Joseph. He assumed the hyphen between his Christian name and surname in order to distinguish himself from André Thomas, the contemporary physiologist.

His contributions to neurology extend over about 70 years, the greater part concerned with clinical and anatomical studies of the cerebellum and spinal cord, psychotherapy, and neurophysiology. He commenced his studies of the development of the newborn at the age of 78; these culminated in his landmark book, *The Neurological Examination of the Infant* (1954, in collaboration).

André-Thomas sign   (Springlike phenomenon) This is essentially the same as **rebound.**[4723]

anemic headache   A frontal or generalized headache, once considered to be associated with increased blood flow in patients with severe anemia.

anencephaly   (Gr, lack of + brain) (acrania, exencephaly, craniorachischisis) A lethal defect due to failure of the cephalad part of the neural tube to form, resulting in the complete absence of development of the cerebral hemispheres[1351] and of the vault of the skull. This developmental aberration is commonly accompanied by failure of closure of the neural tube, presenting as **myelocele** or **meningomyelocele.**

It is suggested that anencephalics are capable of performing certain of those intellectual functions commonly considered to require the presence of cerebral cortex, but they seldom live long enough for evidence of this to be detected.

anerethisia   (Gr, lack of + to excite) Lack of incentive or motivation.

anergy   (Gr, lack of + energy) (anergia, anenergia) Lack of strength, vigor, or energy.

anesthesia   (Gr, lack of + sensation) Lack of feeling, though not necessarily of pain. The term was suggested by Oliver Wendell Holmes (1804–1894), the American physician and author, in a letter to Dr. William Morton, an American dentist who pioneered the use of pain-relieving agents in his practice. Holmes used the diphthong.

anesthesia dolorosa   1. Painful anesthesia or dysesthesia, often related to surgical trauma of the trigeminal ganglion, evoked most frequently after rhizotomy or thermocoagulation has been performed for treatment of idiopathic trigeminal neuralgia.

Anaesthesia dolorosa may also follow upon trauma to the trigeminal complex and, rarely, after vascular lesions of the central trigeminal pathways. This definition and the following diagnostic criteria are suggested by the Headache Classification Committee of the International Headache Society and are reproduced by kind permission.
   A. Pain or dysesthesia is limited to the distribution of one or more divisions of the trigeminal nerve.
   B. Sensation to pinprick is diminished over the affected area.
   C. Symptoms follow a lesion of the trigeminal nerve or its central projections.[1051]
   2. Painful insensitivity of a body part, occurring as a result of incomplete nerve injury, usually traumatic or postherpetic.

anesthetic leprosy   (Danielsson-Boeck disease) A form of **leprosy** in which hyperesthesia gives way to anesthesia with mutilation.[1274] See **leprosy.**

aneurysm   (Gr, a widening) An expansion of the diameter of a blood vessel, usually an artery, due to disease of its wall. Various forms occur:

Berry ("saccular") aneurysms (naturalistic, not eponymic) are focal "blowouts" at points where arteries bifurcate, at which sites there is attenuation of the medial muscular and of the elastic layers of the arterial wall. They are found on the vessels of the anterior circulation in 85% of cases; in 25% of cases, more than one aneurysm is present.

Cirsoid (Gr, enlargement of a vein + likeness) or racemose (Lat; clusters) aneurysms are irregular dilatations of arteries, causing to many sinuous bulges.

Dissecting aneurysms are those occurring in both intracranial and extracranial arteries in which there is a tear in the media, the blood under pressure rupturing and splitting the media before tracking back into the true lumen of the vessel at a higher level.

Fusiform aneurysms (dolichoectasia, atherosclerotic aneurysm) are dilatations of the whole circumference over a length of the vessel, mainly caused by atheroma. They are found most commonly in the vertebrobasilar and internal carotid arteries in elderly people, and pro-duce symptoms mainly by compression of adjacent structures.[1818]

Mycotic aneurysms are focal dilatations of cerebral arteries resulting from inflammation of the walls of the vessels, tending distally and usually occurring as a complication of bacteremia.

aneurysm of the great vein of Galen   Aneurysmal dilatation of this vein as a result of the shunting of excessive amounts of arterial blood into it, seen in infants with developmental cerebrovascular anomalies such as **arteriovenous malformations.**

In early infancy, the usual presentation is with high-output cardiac failure, accompanied by a cranial bruit,[5193] while in later months the aneurysm may act as a mass lesion causing aqueductal compression and resulting hydrocephalus; seizures and dilated scalp veins are other features of note. When the presentation is not until later childhood, seizures, the effects of intracranial bleeding, and both brainstem and cerebellar findings are commonly noted, but usually no bruit is audible.

anfracta cerebri   The cerebral fissures.

anfractuosity   (Lat, a turning or bending around) Applied to the sulci between the cerebral convolutions.

Angelman syndrome   (happy puppet syndrome; OMIM 105830) A congenital neurobehavioral disorder characterized by brachycephaly, microcephaly, and a horizontal depression in the occipital bone; cerebral atrophy and primary optic atrophy; multifocal seizures with **hypsarrhythmia;** ataxic, jerky (puppet-like) limb movements (hence the alternative name); prognathism; unusually protrusive tongue; easily provoked and prolonged paroxysms of laughter but no speech; hypopigmentation; and mental and developmental delay.[182] A microdeletion at chromosome 15q11–q13 is present, almost always of maternal inheritance.

See also **Prader-Willi syndrome,** in which the same deletion is of paternal inheritance.

Angelucci syndrome   (allergic conjunctivitis syndrome) A syndrome of recurrent conjunctivitis, often associated with dermal and mucosal pruritic lesions and occasionally with signs of proximal myopathy.[183] The cause is unknown.

angiectasia   (Gr, a blood vessel + dilation) Pathological widening of the blood vessels, usually applied to dilatation of the capillaries (telangiectasis).

angioblastic meningioma   See **meningioma.**

angiodysgenetic myelomalacia   See **subacute necrotic myelopathy** (Foix-Alajouanine syndrome).

angioendotheliomatosis   Invasion of cerebral and other blood vessels by anaplastic malignant cells.

angiographically occult CNS vascular malformation   Slow-flow vascular lesions within the brain which appear avascular on angiography. They include venous angioma, telangiectasis, thrombosed arteriovenous angioma, and cavernous angioma.

angiography   A series of techniques for visualizing the anatomy and pathology of the arterial system by means of the injection of radio-opaque dyes with X-ray imaging; ultrasound (**Doppler studies;** or **magnetic resonance imaging**).

The first of these was introduced by the Portuguese surgeon Egaz Moniz in 1936, providing the first opportunity for physicians to obtain even an indirect representation of the intracranial structures. A history of angiography has been written by Gurdjian.[2336]

angioid streaks   (Knapp syndrome) Brown or gray lines visible on the retinae. They represent defects in Brusch's membrane or other retinal degenerative changes, and resemble blood vessels except that they are not usually directed radially.

Angioid streaks are typically seen in **pseudoxanthoma elasticum** but also occur in other diseases of the retinal vessels[3094] and are occasionally found in normal subjects.

angiokeratoma   Warty growths in the skin with telangiectasia, the skin lesion clustered in the swimming trunk area, characteristic of **Anderson-Fabry disease** and in Mibelli disease, described first in 1877 by Dr. E.W. Cottle (d. 1919), an English physician.[4979]

angiokeratoma corporis diffusum (universale) (Fabry disease) See **Anderson-Fabry disease.**

angiolipoma   A rare benign tumor composed of adipose tissue and abnormal vascular elements, usually in the posterior epidural space of the spinal canal and sometimes infiltrating local bone.[1919]

angioma   A common vascular malformation (rather than a true neoplasm), comprising four types:

  Arteriovenous malformations
  Capillary telangiectases
  Cavernous angiomas (cavernomas) Compact aggregations of sinusoidal blood vessels with minimal or no neural tissue between the vessels, most common within the brainstem and in Sylvian regions and sometimes multiple. Calcification may occur. Clinically, bleeding is uncommon, but seizures may occur.
  Venous angiomas (developmental venous anomalies) Common malformations consisting of loose collections of venous channels with intervening neural tissue, situated anywhere in the nervous system and often multiple. They are seldom symptomatic.

angioma capillare et venosum calcificans   See **Sturge-Weber syndrome.**

angiomatosis meningo-oculofacialis   See **Sturge-Weber syndrome.**

angiomatosis retinae (cystica)   See **von Hippel–Lindau disease.**

angiomatosis retino-cerebellaris   See **von Hippel–Lindau disease.**

angiomatous malformation   See **arteriovenous malformation.**

angiomatous meningioma   See **meningioma.**

angioparalytic hemicrania   See **hemiplegic migraine.**

angiopathia retinae juvenalis   See **Eales disease.**

angiopathic myopathy   An ischemic myopathy complicating polyarteritis nodosa or giant-cell arteritis.[3301]

angiopathic neuropathy   Typically, a **multiple mononeuropathy** causing pain, weakness, and sensory loss in the distribution of a number of nerves as a result of numerous nerve microinfarcts in small-vessel occlusive diseases, causing both axonal damage and demyelination. Diabetes and polyarteritis are the more common causes.[1572]

angiophrasia   The repetitive insertion of a meaningless sound into otherwise normal speech, as in "hemming and hawing."

angiosarcoma   A vascular sarcoma.

angiosclerotic paroxysmal myasthenia   (Determan) See **Charcot.**

angiostrongyliasis   An infestation by *Angiostrongylus cantonensis*, acquired through the ingestion of inadequately cooked snails, prawns or frogs, or the vegetable matter upon which they have resided. Both sensory radiculopathies and CNS infestation are complications.

Anglade, Dominique   (b. 1867) French neurologist who first demonstrated the value of Victoria Blue as a staining technique for neuroglia, according to Lasègue.[3285]

angle tumors   Conventionally synonymous with cerebellopontine angle tumors. The typical syndrome was first described in accurate detail by **Cushing,**[1229] who noted that there had been reports as far back as 1830 but based his account on a personal series of 30 such cases. Tinnitus; deafness; vertigo; suboccipital discomfort; frank cerebellar signs; involvement of the fifth, sixth, seventh, and bulbar cranial nerves; features of raised intracranial pressure; and "cerebellar crises" (extreme suboccipital pain with neck retraction and reduction in consciousness, angor animi, bradycardia and apnea, indicating intermittent increases in intracranial pressure) occurred, generally in that order.

angular gyrus syndrome   The clinical effects of damage to the heteromodal cortex adjacent to Wernicke area, including any combination of anomia, alexia, acalculia, constructional deficits, dysgraphia, defects in finger identification, and left/right naming difficulties. See also **Gerstmann syndromes, alexia.**

anhedonia   A term used mainly in psychiatry, signifying the inability to experience pleasure and loss of the power of enjoyment. By extension, it represents a telling symptom of depressed affect.

anhidrosis (Gr, lack of + sweat) Absence of sweating; a local phenomenon with damage to specific sympathetic cholinergic pathways, or a generalized problem as a result of degenerative or chemically induced sympathetic failure.

The condition may occur congenitally as a recessively inherited trait in which there is a failure of differentiation of sweat glands.[3569] See also **Riley-Day syndrome, multiple system atrophy, familial amyloid neuropathy.**

anhidrotic ectodermal dysplasia (Christ-Siemens-Touraine syndrome) An X-linked recessive syndrome comprising anhidrosis, hypotrichosis, saddle nose, dental anomalies, periorbital pigmentation, and sometimes mental delay.[5690]

anhydromyelia (Gr, lack of + water + marrow) Deficiency of CSF.

anima (derivative of Lat; soul or spirit) The soul or vital life-force, applied also to the intellectual principle of humans.

aniridia A dominantly inherited congenital malformation characterized by absence of the iris, usually bilaterally, associated with photophobia, amblyopia, nystagmus, and sometimes ataxia.[5105] Other anomalies are also described in a few of the patients.

In a *variant form* (*aniridia, mental retardation, genital abnormalities*), these features and nystagmus, cataract, and glaucoma are found in association with abnormalities of chromosome 11p13.[4137] See also **Gillespie syndrome.**

aniseikonia Perception of one object viewed by the two eyes as having two different sizes or shapes.

anismus Constipation due to functional obstruction of the pelvic outlet by paradoxical contraction of the striated sphincter muscles during defecation straining. This may represent a focal dystonia.[3693]

anisocoria (Gr, negative + equal + pupil) Inequality of the diameter of the pupils of 0.4 mm or more, suggesting the presence of a lesion of the sympathetic pathway to the eye on one side or of the parasympathetic pathway on the other if any disease is present at all.

In this form, *simple, essential, or central anisocoria*, the pupils react to light and accommodation, the difference in their size is maintained under different conditions of illumination, and pharmacological responses are normal. The condition is regarded as a normal variant.

anisometropia (Gr, negative + equal + measure + eye) A difference in the refraction of the two eyes; or a difference in the anteroposterior diameter of the two eyes. In each case, it is a common cause of **amblyopia.**

anisomorphic gliosis The irregular orientation of the glial fibers in severely damaged neural tissues.

anisosthenic (Gr, negative + the same + strength) Inequality in the force of contraction of different muscles.

ankyloblepharon The presence of a variable degree of fusion of the lid margins, a malformation that may be dominantly or recessively inherited.

ankylosis (from Gr, the bend of the arm) A stiffening of a joint by disease.

Annals of Neurology The journal of the American Neurological Association (Web site: http://www.aneuroa.org/) and of the Child Neurology Society (Web site: http://www.childneurologysociety.org/), publishing articles on all aspects of the human nervous system, both normal and abnormal is published by John Wiley & Sons Inc. *Wiley InterScience.* Web site: http://www3.interscience.wiley.com/cgi-bin/jtoc?ID=76507645.

annectant gyri The convolutions passing from the parietal to the occipital lobes.[2240]

Annual Review of Neuroscience (*Annu. Rev. Neurosci.*) A neurological/neuroscience review book series. Address: Annual Reviews Inc., 4139 El Camino Way, Palo Alto, CA 94303-0897. Web site: http://neuro.annualreviews.org/.

anodal block A local block of nerve conduction caused by membrane hyperpolarization under a stimulating anode. Does not occur in routine clinical studies, since it is possible for the anode to routinely result in nerve depolarization if sufficient current intensities are used. (From the 2001 Report of the Nomenclature Committee of the American Association of Electromyography and Electrodiagnosis.[10] Used by permission, copyright © 2001, AAEM.)

anode The positive terminal of an electric current source. cf. **cathode.**

anodyne (Gr, lack of + pain) An analgesic medicine; until the earliest part of this century the word was applied to drugs such as opium, chloroform, and hemp, only the last of which is easily obtainable today.

anomalous reflex A reflex with no known survival value, e.g., vomiting with vertigo.

anomia (from Lat, deprivative + a name) The inability to generate and utter names; a facility impaired in all forms of aphasia but also in many cerebral diseases not causing aphasia. Four forms are distinguished:[468]

> *Word-production anomia* The patient knows the required name but is unable to produce it correctly without some form of cuing, because of difficulty in initiating articulation, or in evoking the word, or as a result of **paraphasia.**
> *Word-selection anomia* A pure word-finding problem in which the patient can recognize and describe the function of the object presented, but cannot evoke its name.
> *Semantic anomia* A failure of both the comprehension and the use of the name of an object; a situation in which the word has lost its semantic meaning for the patient.

Disconnection anomia Inability to evoke the name of an object presented in one modality while the word is recalled when it is presented in another (*modality-specific anomia*); a naming failure in a single category only, such as color (*category specific anomia*); and inability to name an object recognized after placement in the left hand, as after callosal section (*callosal anomia*).

See also **progressive pure anomia.**

anomic aphasia   The most common form of aphasia, characterized by fluency, retention of repetition, and fair or good comprehension but poor naming ability. The anomia is a defect of naming, not of recognition. Semantic errors and the use of circumlocutions and general words ("thing", "whatsit", "you know") for specific nouns are characteristic. The lesion is of the low angular gyrus and posterior middle temporal gyrus but the phenomenon is also a socially pervasive form of communication (?) in modern teenagers.

anophthalmia   (Gr, lack or + eye) A rare, usually recessively inherited **craniofacial malformation** characterized by a lack of traces even of ocular development as the result of failure of formation of the primary optic vesicle.[2738] See also the syndromes of **Goldenhar, Wildervanck, Franceschetti, and Hallermann and Streiff.**

Another *variant* is *anophthalmia with intracranial germinoma*, a congenital syndrome in which the anophthalmia is complicated by polyuria, hypopituitarism, hydrocephalus, cerebral teratoma, and mental and developmental delay.[337]

anopsia   (Gr, lack of + vision) Loss of sight.

anorexia hysterica   See **anorexia nervosa.**

anorexia nervosa   (Gr, lack of + appetite) (apepsia hysterica; anorexia hysterica) An eating disorder (psychogenic food refusal) characterized by an exaggerated fear of obesity, a desire for thinness, and a distorted body image.

The condition was first described by Richard Morton in 1689, but there is some evidence that Mary, Queen of Scots had suffered from this disorder in the previous century. The name was coined by Sir William **Gull** in 1874 but is not fully accurate, as many patients retain a feeling of hunger at least until well into the illness.[886, 2030]

The *American Psychiatric Association DSM IV Criteria for the Diagnosis of Anorexia Nervosa* (available at http://www.psychologynet.org/dsm.html) are as follows:[150]

Early signs may include withdrawal from family and friends, increased sensitivity to criticism, sudden increased interest in physical activity, anxiety, or depressive symptoms.

Refusal to maintain body weight at or above a minimally normal weight for age and height (e.g., weight loss leading to maintenance of body weight less than 85% of that expected; or failure to make expected weight gain during period of growth, leading to body weight less than 85% of that expected).

Intense fear of gaining weight or becoming fat, even though underweight.

Disturbance in the way in which one's body weight or shape is experienced, undue influence of body weight or shape on self-evaluation, or denial of the seriousness of the current low body weight.

In postmenarcheal females, amenorrhea, i.e., the absence of at least three consecutive menstrual cycles. (A woman is considered to have amenorrhea if her periods occur only following hormone, e.g., estrogen, administration.)

Restricting type: During the current episode of anorexia nervosa, the person has not regularly engaged in binge-eating or purging behavior (i.e., self-induced vomiting or the misuse of laxatives, diuretics, or enemas).

Binge-eating/purging type: During the current episode of anorexia nervosa, the person has regularly engaged in binge-eating or purging behavior (i.e., self-induced vomiting or the misuse of laxatives, diuretics, or enemas).

anorgasmia   Inability to experience orgasm, due to psychological reasons, medications, local genital causes, or lesions of the anterolateral spinal cord or of the nervi erigentes.[503]

anosmia   (Gr, lack of + smell) Loss of the sense of smell. When unilateral, it suggests the presence of local nasal disease or of a mass lesion such as a meningioma, glioma, or abscess in the anterior cranial fossa; when bilateral, its localizing value is diluted and either local nasal or intracranial disorders may be responsible. The condition may be inherited as an autosomal dominant trait.[5185] See also **Kallmann syndrome.**

anosognosia   (denial syndrome) A term introduced by Josef **Babinski** for the unawareness or denial of physical deficits.[287] This is seen most often with lesions of the right parietal lobe, in which case the unawareness is of the deficits on the left side of the body. This may actually lead to denial of ownership of a (paretic) limb, usually the left, in patients with infarct of the right supramarginal cortex or the thalamocortical radiations projecting to it. In a minor key, the phenomenon consists merely of unconcern about an admitted deficit. Denial of numerous other kinds of deficit such as those of memory, sight, praxis, or speech also occurs. See also **simultagnosia.**

anosognosic graphopmimia   See hypergraphia.

anoxic myelopathy   The occurrence of symmetrical gray matter lesions in the spinal cords of patients who had suffered systemic anoxic episodes or circulatory arrest. These changes, though generalized, are most marked in lumbosacral regions.[278]

anoxic seizures   A heterogeneous group of paroxysmal events that include some degree of abrogation of consciousness and various motor and sensory phenomena occurring as a result of cortical anoxia and representing a type of **nonepileptic seizure.**

ansa   (Lat, a handle). A curved structure.

ansa hypoglossi   A looped branch running between the twelfth cranial nerve and the cervical plexus.

ansa lenticularis   A fiber tract carrying impulses from the globus pallidus to the thalamus.

ansa subclavia   The left recurrent laryngeal nerve.

antagonist   1. A muscle, the main action of which opposes the function of another (**agonist**) muscle. See also **synergist**. 2. A chemical substance that binds to a receptor and inhibits its activity.

antagonistic anterior tibial reflex   (Piotrowski reflex) Plantar flexion at the ankle in response to a tap on the tibialis anterior muscle belly. The reflex is sometimes elicited in patients with pyramidal lesions. See **Piotrowski sign.**

antagonistic reflexes   Occasional variant forms of the usual deep reflexes, modified in certain conditions by the underlying pathology and by the method of elicitation.[5858]

antalgic   (Gr, against + pain) Analgesic.

antalgic gait   Limping as a result of pain felt (from any cause, such as arthropathy) during walking.

antebrachium   (Lat, before + arm) The forearm.

antecollis   (Lat, before + neck) A focal dystonia characterized by sustained involuntary contractions of the neck muscles, which result in abnormal flexion of the head on the neck. See **cervical dystonia.**

anterior   (rostral) In front.

anterior agraphia   See **agraphia.**

anterior alexia   See **alexia.**

anterior apraxia   See **apraxia.**

anterior bulbar syndrome   Anterior spinal artery occlusion causing ischemic infarction of the pyramid, the twelfth cranial nerve, and possibly the medial lemniscus, thus producing a homolateral hypoglossal paralysis and contralateral hemiparesis (and hemianesthesia). It was first described by Déjèrine.[2764] See also **alternating hypoglossal hemiplegia syndrome, Déjèrine syndromes.**

anterior cavernous syndrome   A syndrome of painful ophthalmoplegia with **Horner syndrome** and trigeminal anesthesia due to a lesion in this situation. It was first described in detail by **Jefferson**[2764] and later by Foix in 1925. See **Tolosa-Hunt syndrome.**

anterior cerebral artery syndromes   Occlusion of the main trunk proximal to Heubner's artery leading to severe contralateral hemiplegia with sensory loss over the leg, urinary incontinence, emotional and intellectual changes, and left-sided apraxia with a right-side occlusion, or transcortical aphasia if it is on the left. Sensory neglect and micrographia have also been described in this circumstance.

Occlusion distal to Heubner's artery leads to hemiplegia with crural predominance, indefinite sensory impairment, left-sided ideomotor apraxia, forced grasping and groping in the left arm, dysphasia with a left-sided occlusion, and emotional and intellectual changes. Main stem occlusions distal to this point lead to crural paresis and mental changes only.

Occlusion of Heubner's artery alone leads to hemiparesis affecting the arm more than the face or leg, and occlusions of other arterial branches cause varying degrees of crural weakness only.[1166]

anterior choroidal artery   A branch of the internal carotid artery supplying part of the posterior limb of the internal capsule, the lateral geniculate body, the globus pallidus, part of the optic radiation, and the middle third of the crus cerebri. Occlusion leads to a constant clinical picture. See **anterior choroidal artery syndrome.**

anterior choroidal artery syndrome   (von Monakow syndrome) The occurrence of contralateral hemiplegia, hemianesthesia, and homonymous hemianopia without cognitive deficit, due to occlusion or hemorrhage of the artery with infarction of the posterior limb of the internal capsule or the medial globus pallidus, the ventral posterolateral thalamus, and the lateral geniculate body.[5327]

Left-sided spatial neglect and minor speech disturbances may also occur according to the side of the infarction.[1326] Despite the eponymous attribution, Foix and Chavanay gave a complete description in 1925.[1898]

anterior cingulate gyrus epilepsy   A variety of frontal focal cortical epilepsy involving the pericallosal gyrus. It has variable clinical manifestations including head turning, head dropping, apparent absences, and psychotic behavior and there is no typical EEG pattern[4911]

anterior cingulate syndrome   Apathy, akinesia, drowsiness, and mutism, said to be fatal in weeks. The causative lesion is more likely to be of the thalamus with secondary expansion effects on the corpus callosum, since surgical removal of the anterior cingulate gyri causes no such signs.

anterior cornual syndrome   (Schantz syndrome) Damage to the anterior horn cells in a segment of the spinal cord, resulting from any one of the various possible pathologies.

anterior crural syndrome   See **anterior tibial syndrome.**

anterior encephalocele   The congenital appearance of a frontal cranial meningocele. See **dysraphism.**

anterior ethmoidal nerve syndrome   Bilateral recurrent nasal pain or severe headache with neck stiffness lasting a day or more at a time.[846] The nature of this condition requires further study.

anterior frontopolar region seizures A form of epilepsy. Anterior frontopolar seizure patterns include forced thinking or initial loss of contact and adversive movements of head and eyes, with possible evolution including contraversive movements and axial clonic jerks and falls and autonomic signs. (From the revised ILAE Classification,[1114] reproduced by kind permission.)

anterior horn cell disease with cerebellar hypoplasia in infants See **hereditary motor neuropathy** (*variants*).

anterior horn cell disease with pontocerebellar hypoplasia See **hereditary motor neuropathy** (*variants*).

anterior inferior cerebellar artery syndrome The constellation of signs following infarction of the territory supplied by this artery.

The signs include vertigo and nystagmus; tinnitus and homolateral deafness; gait and homolateral limb ataxia; homolateral facial palsy; **alternating thermoanalgesia** (homolateral face, contralateral trunk and limb involvement); and homolateral **Horner syndrome.**

anterior internuclear ophthalmoplegia See **internuclear ophthalmoplegia.** It not certain that Lutz and Lhermitte's differentiation between the so-called anterior and posterior forms of the syndrome is appropriate.

anterior interosseous nerve syndrome (Kiloh-Nevin syndrome) Weakness and wasting of flexor pollicis longus, of that part of the flexor digitorum profundus innervated by the median nerve, and of pronator quadratus as a result of proximal compression of the anterior interosseous branch of the median nerve between the two heads of pronator teres, usually by a fibrous band or as a result of local trauma.[4190]

The flexor carpi radialis and flexor digitorum sublimis are spared, being supplied by the main trunk of the median nerve. The pronator teres is seldom affected. See also **pinch sign.**

anterior ischemic optic neuropathy Infarction of the laminar and retrolaminar parts of the optic nerve due to small-vessel disease of the choroidal or posterior ciliary branches of the ophthalmic arteries. The condition is most commonly associated with hypertension or **giant cell arteritis** (when it is frequently bilateral), other collagen-vascular diseases, **drusen,** diabetes, and such vascular disorders as hypotension resulting from blood loss; nevertheless, over a quarter of the patients have no detectable underlying disease.

Clinically, the major features are abrupt painless visual field loss, with an **altitudinal defect** and pallor and swelling of all or only a sector of the optic nerve head, later leading to **optic atrophy.** Peripapillary hemorrhages are commonly seen in the acute stages.[624]

anterior midline structure syndrome See **Zeman-King syndrome.**

anterior opercular syndrome (Foix-Chavanay-Marie syndrome, facio-linguo-pharyngo-masticatory diplegia) Loss of voluntary control of facial, pharyngeal, lingual, masticatory, and sometimes ocular muscle activity due to bilateral anterior perisylvian lesions involving the primary motor cortex within the frontal and parietal opercula. Bilateral opercular polymicrogyria or infarction is the usual causes.[3601]

Clinically, the *acquired form* of the condition is characterized by acute onset, inability to perform voluntary movements with the bulbar muscles, decreased gag reflex, and absence of **emotionalism.** In the *developmental form*, inability to protrude or wiggle the tongue, seizures, mild mental retardation, and brisk reflexes with normal Babinski responses are typical features.[1897] Bilateral infarcts or herpes encephalitis is usually responsible. See also **bilateral central macrogyria, epilepsy, pseudobulbar palsy and mental retardation.**

anterior slow alpha of drowsiness An EEG pattern recorded in drowsiness from midline frontocentral regions; also distinct from true alpha activity by virtue of being slightly slower.[786]

anterior spinal artery syndrome (Beck syndrome) Infarction of the anterior portion of the spinal cord due to occlusion of the anterior spinal artery, leading abruptly to pain, pyramidal and spinothalamic deficits, and loss of sphincter control below the level of the lesion and to pain, hyperalgesia, and evidence of a lower motor neuron lesion at its site. The senses of vibration and of joint position are spared.

Such infarcts are most usual in thoracic regions, the clinical picture varying with the level of cord involvement. Aortic dissection, syphilis, and aortic surgery are the most common causes of the condition, which was first described by Preobrashenski in 1904,[4519] although a fuller account was later provided by Beck.[414]

anterior spinal hernia Thoracic myelopathy due to anterior spinal artery segmental branch ischemia in a cord chronically trapped in a congenital anterior meningocele.[5939]

anterior-superior cerebellar artery syndrome The clinical picture resulting from infarcts in the territory of this artery.[4492] The typical clinical presentation includes dysarthria, unsteadiness and/or vertigo, homolateral limb ataxia, and dysmetria with axial lateropulsion, but it may also mimic the lacunar **dysarthria clumsy hand syndrome.** Coma at onset (or delayed) and tetraplegia are also described. Cardiogenic embolism is the commonest single cause.

anterior tarsal tunnel syndrome Entrapment of the terminal parts of the mixed deep peroneal nerve below the inferior extensor retinaculum, presenting clinically with numbness and tingling over the first web space of the foot and frequently with a **Tinel sign** over the sensory branch of the deep peroneal nerve on the anterior aspect of the ankle.[4498]

anterior tibial sign   Involuntary extension of the hallux with forcible flexion of the hip; seen in pyramidal lesions.[4723]

anterior tibial syndrome   (anterior crural syndrome; march syndrome) Pain in the anterior tibial compartment with weakness of the muscles and sensory loss in the distribution of the anterior tibial nerve, due to swelling of the muscles with a resultant increase in local pressure below the fascial covering of the compartment, and with subsequent ischemic necrosis of all the soft tissues within it.[4026]

The condition was first described by Karl Beck, and later by **Vogt** in 1943.

anterocollis   A form of sporadic focal **dystonia.**

anterograde   Forward.

anterograde amnesia   1. (anterograde memory deficits) Loss of the capacity for learning new material. This term corresponds to memory difficulties as they are usually understood. See also **retrograde amnesia.** 2. Loss of recall for events following a neurological deficit.

anthropology   The study of the characteristics of past and present human populations. Subdivisions of anthropology include the sociocultural, archaeological, biological, and linguistic branches.

anthropomorphism   The ascription of human characteristics to animals.

anti-   (Lat, against) A prefix signifying "in opposition to."

antiamphiphysin antibodies   Antibodies detected rarely in patients with breast cancer who manifest paraneoplastic encephalomyelitis or stiff-person syndromes.[1253]

anti-basal ganglion antibodies   Markers of the presence of a postinfectious autoimmune inflammatory disorder, usually following a streptococcal infection. The syndromes include **Sydenham chorea, PANDAs,** and **acute disseminated encephalomyelitis.**

anti-CAR antibodies   Antibodies detected in some patients with small cell lung cancer who manifest photoreceptor degeneration.[1253] (*cancer-associated retinopathy*)

anticardiolipin antibodies   Circulating immunoglobulin A, G, and M antibodies associated with a tendency toward arterial or venous thrombosis and thrombocytopenia, in part as a result of inhibition of prostacycline release from the endothelial walls.

Associations with ischemic (multiple) cerebral infarction, **Sneddon syndrome, chorea,** seizures, **optic neuritis, acute inflammatory demyelinating polyneuropathy,** and **migraine** have been shown.[550]

anticholinergic syndrome   The association of fever, flushing, dilated pupils and drowsiness, delirium, or coma, sometimes with extrapyramidal signs, as a result of a toxic reaction to anticholinergic drugs.[1775]

anticipatory nystagmus   Predictive, slow eye movements that occur prior to ramp or step target movements of the eyes, interspersed with saccades in the opposite direction.[1368] See **induced nystagmus.**

anticipatory postural reflexes   Alterations of the position of the trunk and limbs prior to the performance of a movement of the whole body. An example is the truncal and leg flexion that precedes the rising from a chair.[4180]

anticonvulsant   A drug that inhibits epileptic seizures. As many such agents have other effects (such as inhibition of activity in pain pathways), use of the term is only appropriate in the context of epilepsy.

anti-CV$_2$ antibodies   Antibodies detected in some patients with small-cell lung cancer who manifest encephalomyelitis or cerebellar degeneration syndromes.[1253]

antidepressant   A drug that elevates depressed mood. As many such agents have other effects (such as the prophylaxis of migraine), use of the term is only appropriate in the context of depression.

antidromic   Propagation of a nerve impulse in the direction opposite to physiologic conduction—e.g., conduction along motor nerve fibers away from the muscle and conduction along sensory fibers away from the spinal cord. Cf. **orthodromic.** (From the 2001 Report of the Nomenclature Committee of the American Association of Electromyography and Electrodiagnosis.[10] Used by permission, copyright © 2001, AAEM.)

anti-GM$_1$ antibodies   Antibodies directed at ganglioside epitopes, capable of inducing conduction block and associated with the clinical conditions **multifocal neuropathy with conduction block,** a motor variant of **chronic inflammatory demyelinating ganglioradiculopathy, amyotrophic lateral sclerosis** (seldom), and other motor neuropathies.

anti-GQ$_{1b}$ antibody syndrome   The common autoimmune mechanism in **Miller Fisher syndrome, acute inflammatory demyelinating polyneuropathy, Bickerstaff brain stem encephalitis,** and **acute ophthalmoparesis without ataxia.**[4199]

anti-Hu antibodies   Antibodies directed at neuronal nuclei in the CNS and peripheral nervous system, characteristically found in paraneoplastic encephalomyelitis affecting the cerebellum and limbic system and with sensory and autonomic neuropathies. Small-cell lung cancer and neuroblastoma are the more common underlying tumors.[1252, 3942]

anti-Jo-1 antibodies   Antibodies present in some syndromes characterized by muscle weakness and pain, the Raynaud phenomenon, interstitial lung disease, arthritis, and skin rashes.[4025]

anti-Ma antibodies Antibodies detected to Ma1 and Ma2 proteins in patients with various cancers who manifest paraneoplastic limbic, cerebellar, and brainstem syndromes.[1253]

anti-MAG-associated neuropathy See **immune-mediated neuropathies.**

anti-MysB antibodies Antibodies detected rarely in patients with small-cell lung cancer who manifest a myasthenic syndrome.[1253]

anti-neuronal antibodies Autoantibodies occasionally identified in the serum of patients with a paraneoplastic disorder of the nervous system. The *antinucleoprotein antibody* (Hu) is mainly associated with small-cell carcinoma of the lung, while the *anti-Purkinje* antibody is usually found in patients with breast or ovarian cancer.[3943] Anti-Ro/SS-A and anti-La/SSB antibodies occur in some patients with **Sjogren syndrome.** Anti-Yo antibodies are found in paraneoplastic cerebellar degeneration. Other neuronal antigens include myelin-associated glycoprotein, GM_1, GQ_{1b} and other gangliosides, and sulfatide and chondroitin sulfate.[4555]

antiphospholipid antibodies A family of immunoglobulin antibodies to phospholipids, including the lupus anticoagulant and anticardiolipin antibodies (IgG, IgM, and IgA isotypes). They are most commonly found in women, in people aged less than 50 years, and in those with cerebral, optic, and other ischemic syndromes, headaches, thrombotic events, biologically false-positive reactions to syphilis, or thrombocytopenia. They also occur in 1%–2% of the general population and in up to 50% of patients with **systemic lupus erythematosus.**

These antibodies may be considered markers of stroke risk, but their precise relationship to the event is uncertain.[3378]

antiphospholipid antibody syndrome A thrombophilic disorder defined by the presence in the blood of the lupus anticoagulant or anticardiolipin antibodies, usually in high titer, and clinically by recurrent fetal losses, recurrent arterial or venous thromboses, or thrombocytopenia.[3378]

Patients who are antiphospholipid antibody positive and who present with recurrent fetal loss, venous or arterial occlusion, or thrombocytopenia but without clinical evidence of systemic lupus erythematosus are said to have the primary syndrome. The cerebral syndromes may involve the small or the larger arteries, presenting a **stroke,** transient ischemic attack, or **multi-infarct dementia.**[742] Occasional neurological presentations include transverse myelitis, chorea, and a syndrome resembling **acute inflammatory demyelinating polyneuropathy.** See also **Sneddon syndrome.**[2562]

anti-Ri antibodies Antibodies detected rarely in patients with breast cancer who manifest opsoclonuis, nystagmus, dysarthria, and ataxia.[1252, 3942]

antisaccades Deviations of the eyes from a central fixation point not *towards* a new visual stimulus but *away from* it. Failure to make such movements in the test situation is evidence of frontal lobe dysfunction.[3066]

anti-Ta antibodies Antibodies detected rarely in some patients with testicular cancer who manifest a paraneoplastic syndrome of limbic and brainstem encephalitis.[1253]

antithrombin III deficiency A dominantly inherited disorder of hemaglobin predisposing patients to stroke and due to a mutation in the antithrombin III gene at 1q23–25.

anti-Tr antibodies Antibodies detected rarely in patients with Hodgkin lymphoma who manifest a paraneoplastic syndrome of cerebellar degeneration.[1253]

anti-VGCC antibodies Antibodies detected in some patients with small-cell lung cancer who manifest a paraneoplastic myasthenic (Lambert-Eaton) syndrome.[1253]

anti-Yo antibodies Antibodies detected rarely in patients with breast or ovarian cancer who manifest a paraneoplastic subacute cerebellar syndrome with nystagmus and dysarthria.[1252, 3942]

Anton, Gabriel (1858–1933) Austrian neurologist who worked with **Meynert** before holding appointments successively in Innsbruck, Graz, and Halle (where he succeeded **Wernicke** in 1905). In 1899 he described a loss of awareness of focal cerebral somatosensory defects in patients suffering from visual agnosia or word deafness (*anosognosia* in **Babinski**'s terminology).

Anton syndrome Anosognosia for blindness, with denial of that blindness. Such usage actually extends the definition of the syndrome described by Anton in 1899.

Although overtly unable to see, often because of bilateral occipital lobe ischemic damage, the patients deny that this is so and may resort to confabulation about things "seen."[188 4625] **Allocheiria** is another inconstant accompaniment.

Anton-Babinski syndrome Anosognosia, usually for a left hemiparesis, because this is classically a result of a right parietal lesion. The patient is commonly unaware of the paralysis or, if aware, remains indifferent.

The names of Redlich and Bonvicini are also sometimes attached to this condition, but their reports were up to 20 years later than those of Anton and Babinski.

Antonini type A areas Regions within **Schwannomas** characterized by sheaths of spindle cells with long nuclei and fine intercellular cytoplasmic processes.[6]

Antonini type B areas Regions within **Schwannomas** characterized by populations of cells with small round nuclei and fine cytoplasmic processes intermixed with mast cells.[6]

anxietas tibiarum   See **restless legs syndrome.**

Anyane Yeboa syndrome (clefting–corneal opacity–retardation) A congenital dysmorphic syndrome characterized by short stature, cloudy corneae, cleft upper lip and palate, urinary system anomalies, hydrocephalus, and mental and developmental delay.[337]

aortic arch arteritis   See **aortic arch disease.**

aortic arch disease (Takayasu disease; pulseless disease; aortic arch arteritis) An obliterative panarteritis affecting the major branches of the arch of the aorta, usually in young women, and leading to cerebral and systemic ischemic symptoms and loss of pulses at the appropriate sites. Evidence of the formation of a collateral circulation, cardiac enlargement, systemic hypertension in the legs, and an elevated erythrocyte sedimentation rate are also characteristic.[5473]

The condition was described by Broadbent in 1875 (as "subclavian stenosis") and by Takayasu in 1908. Sixteen synonyms are listed by Jablonski.[2764, 2765]

In a *variant* of the syndrome (*aortic arch syndrome*), similar features occur, mainly in young males in the Far East, in the absence of such arteritic pathology and without evidence of fibromuscular hyperplasia or atheroma. There is, however, intense collagen proliferation at the origins of the great vessels leaving the aorta.[1246]

APACHE score A severity-of-disease classification system deriving a point score based upon the initial values of 12 routine physiological measurements, age, and previous health status. Increasing scores are closely correlated with the risk of subsequent hospital death.[3096]

apallic syndrome The original term of Kretschmer[3159] for the **persistent vegetative state.**

apathetic thyrotoxicosis A variant form of acute hyperthyroidism in the elderly, characterized by lethargy, depression, abdominal pain, nausea, and vomiting.

apathy (Gr, without + feeling) A state characterized by a reduction in spontaneous action and speech, with delayed, short, slow, or absent responses to stimuli and a flat affect.[912]

Apathy, abulia from frontal lobe disorders, psychomotor retardation in depression, and bradykinesia with "bradyphrenia" from extrapyramidal disorders can be difficult to tell apart clinically.[3383] Apathy does not correlate well with depression but does correlate with lowered cognitive function. See also **athymhormia.**

ape hand (simian hand) Generalized atrophy and weakness of the intrinsic muscles of the hand, leading to a decline of the position of the thumb into the plane of the palm, as in severe motor neuropathies with predominant effects on the median nerve.[574]

Apelt-Gerkin-Lenz syndrome See **cleft lip–palate and tetraphocomelia.**

apepsia hysterica   See **anorexia nervosa.**

aperiodic 1. EEG waves or complexes occurring in a sequence but at an irregular rate. 2. EEG waves or complexes occurring intermittently at irregular intervals. (Adapted from the 1974 Report of the Committee on Terminology, IFCN,[989] © 1974. With permission from Elsevier Science.)

aperiodic alternating nystagmus See **periodic alternating nystagmus.**

Apert, Eugene (1868–1940) French pediatrician practicing in Paris, with a major interest in developmental abnormalities.

Apert syndrome (type 1 acrocephalosyndactyly; Apert-Park-Powers syndrome; syndrome of Lobstein, van der Hoeve, Spurway, Henzschell, von Ammon, Looser, or Eddowes) A rare, sporadic (rarely autosomal dominant) craniofacial malformation stemming from abnormal bony fusion (craniostenosis) affecting the skull (**acrocephaly, turricephaly, brachycephaly**), facial bones, hands, and feet (**syndactyly**). In some cases, the inability of the skull to expand leads to increased intracranial pressure as the brain grows, leading to ophthalmoplegia, optic atrophy with visual failure, and mental retardation. Shallow orbits are responsible for the slight exophthalmos. Agenesis of the corpus callosum or of limbic structures, blue sclerae, deafness, bilateral fourth cranial nerve palsy and bony fragility are also reported.[192] Linkage to chromosome 10q has been achieved.

It was first described by Oribasius (325–403 A.D.) and may have been recognized by Homer, whose hero Thersites was described as if being so afflicted. It was reviewed and fully described in 1906 by Apert after a preceding description by Troquart in 1886.

The skull shape of Louis-Philippe of France ("tête en poire") may have been due to such brachycephaly. The conditions of acrocephaly and acrocephalosyndactyly have been reviewed by Ferriman[1801] and by Baraitser.[335] See also **Crouzon syndrome, acrocephalosyndactyly.**

Apert-Park-Powers syndrome See **Apert syndrome.**

Apgar scores A practical, semiquantitative method of evaluation of the newborn infant, the observations being made 1 minute after birth and sometimes repeated at 10 minutes.

In the scale, up to 2 points may be given each for respiratory effort, reflex irritability, muscle tone, heart rate, and color.[193] The scale has predictive value in terms of future motor and mental development.

Score	Heart Rate	Respiratory Effort	Reflex Irritability	Muscle Tone	Color
2	100–140	Normal cry	Normal	Good	Pink
1	100	Irregular and shallow	Depressed	Fair	Fair
0	>60	Apnea	Absent	Flaccid	Cyanotic

aphagia algera   The loss of the ability to eat as a result of pain produced by eating, leading to emaciation. In the absence of any detectable physical disease likely to be responsible, the condition is considered to be functional or psychogenic.[5286] See also **akinesia algera.**

aphakia   (Gr, negative + a lentil) The condition of absence of the lens of the eye.

aphasia   (Gr, lack of + speech) (dysphasia) A disturbance of word choice and/or grammar or of comprehension in communicating through language, due to brain disease; a disturbance in communication using language, not primarily due to motor or sensory deficits. Or, in the terms of Sir Henry **Head,** a disorder of symbolic formulation and expression.

The first modern report of motor aphasia was by **Broca,** who demonstrated a case (of "aphemie") in 1861 associated with a lesion of the left second and third frontal convolutions. Broca later correctly narrowed the site of the lesion to the posterior part of the left inferior frontal convolution, although Pierre **Marie** sectioned that patient's brain in 1906 and found that the lesion was much more extensive.[3616]

The condition had been described by Hippocrates and by Schmidt in 1679 and was recognized by Carl von Linne (Linnaeus) in 1745. In 1683 Peter Rommeliu (1643–1708) described what he called a "rare form of aphonia." His lucid description, the embodiment of the modern aphasia examination, identifies the syndrome as Broca aphasia. Alexia, paraphasia, unawareness of defects, amnesic aphasia, jargon aphasia, and agraphia had also been mentioned variously by others before the nineteenth century.[3857] In 1825, Bouillard noted that the faculty for forming words could be lost even though the muscles of articulation were intact, and in 1836, Marc Dax stated that the site of speech memories was the left hemisphere. **Trousseau** suggested the use of the word *aphasia* rather than *aphemie* in 1864. A survey of the earliest accounts of aphasia from those of Hippocrates on was provided by Benton and Joynt, who noted that most of the forms of aphasia had been described piecemeal before Broca's contribution.[475] The early history has also been reviewed.[4690]

Bedside screening tests have been devised; see **Frenchay Aphasia Screening Test, Sheffield Screening Test for Acquired Language Disorders.**

The sensory type of aphasia was first described as such by **Wernicke** in 1874, although others had written of the deficits before him. The most important summations of knowledge have been those of Henry **Head,** whose two-volume work, *Aphasia and Kindred Disorders of Speech*, was published in 1926,[2496] and more recently that of Critchley.[2581]

See also **Broca aphasia, Wernicke aphasia, conduction aphasia, transcortical aphasia, global aphasia, nonoptic aphasia.**

Aphasia, Apraxia, Agnosia   A subspecialty neurological journal. Address: Biolinguistics, P.O. Box 11356, Chicago, IL 60611.

aphasia batteries   Standardized schemes for the diagnosis and assessment of aphasic disorders, for use informally at the bedside or in the neuropsychology laboratory.

Batteries in common clinical use include the **Western Aphasia Battery,**[3018] the **Aphasia Language Performance Scales, the Boston Diagnostic Aphasia Examination,**[2191] the Eisenson Examination for Aphasia,[1621] the **Minnesota Test for the Differential Diagnosis of Aphasia,** and the **Porch Index** of Communicative Ability.[4491]

Screening tests include the **Aphasia Screening Test,** and the **Token Test.** The use of these (and other) tools is reviewed by Lezak.[3392]

Aphasia Language Performance Scale   A formalized, portable interview technique for assessing a patient's skills in listening, talking, reading, and writing.

Aphasia quotient   The relationship of fluency, information, comprehension, repetition, and naming scores on the **Western Aphasia Battery** to the hypothetical normal score of 100, as a measure of the severity of language impairment.[3024]

Aphasia Screening Test   A popular instrument for the assessment, classification, and grading of language dysfunction and some nonlanguage communications skills.[2399] The test is included within the **Halstead-Reitan Test Battery.**

The following truncated version is suggested as a tool for distinguishing between right and left hemisphere damage:[2521]

1. Copy a square, a Greek cross, and a triangle without lifting the pencil from the paper.
2. Name each copied figure.
3. Spell each name.
4. Repeat "He shouted the warning" and then explain and write it down.

Patients with left hemisphere lesions may be able to copy the designs but not to write, but those with right hemisphere lesions will be able to write but may not manage to reproduce the designs.[3392] The test differentiates between patients with right and with left hemisphere lesions, but should not be relied upon to do more than that.

aphasia-agnosia-apraxia syndrome   (Pick syndrome, Bianchi syndrome) The combination of dementia, apperceptive blindness, and loss of reflex gaze.[4625] See **posterior cortical dementia.**

aphasic acalculia   See **acalculia.**

aphasic agraphia   See **agraphia.**

aphasic perseveration therapy   A method of reducing aphasic errors by encouraging speech free from that

perseveration which is considered to be an integral component of aphasic symptoms.[2528]

aphasiology A study of the phenomena of central disorders of language.[1178]

Aphasiology A specialist professional journal published by Taylor and Francis Psychology Press. Web site: http://www.tandf.co.uk/journals/pp/02687038.html.

aphemia 1. (pure word dumbness; cortical dumbness; cortical anarthria; simple aphasia; subcortical motor aphasia; ataxic aphasia; severe apraxia of speech) A nonfluent aphasia characterized by a disturbance of oral verbal output, in which spoken language is poorly articulated, slow and effortful, and repetition is impaired. Comprehension, word choice, grammar, syntax, and writing are not affected.

The syndrome commonly evolves from an initial state of right hemiparesis and mutism. The underlying lesion interrupts the path from Broca's area to the motor area.[462]

The word was originally selected by **Broca** to indicate loss of articulate speech due to a cerebral lesion, the motor and sensory functions remaining unaffected, but it was rejected by **Trousseau** in 1864 because a literal translation from modern Greek is *infamy*, which seems inappropriate.

Bastian thought that, in aphasia, the area for kinesthetic images for words was destroyed and thinking thus disturbed; in aphemia, he considered the lesion to be of the motor paths linking this area with the muscles of articulation, so that intellectual functions remained. The lesion is now considered to be restricted within Broca's area or in the subjacent cortex.[3937] See also **aphasia, foreign accent syndrome, diplegia with dissociation, oral-buccal apraxia.**

2. Selective loss of volitional (as opposed to emotional) movements, as in the case of the facial muscles in the **anterior operculum syndrome.**[4959]

apheresis (Gr, to take away) (plasmapheresis) The term used for the separation of the constituents of blood by centrifugation, after which the protein fractions containing the antibodies responsible for the pathology can be removed and the remainder of the blood, with added albumin, replaced.

aphonia (Gr, negative + the voice) 1. The inability to produce vocal sounds or phonate. 2. Loss of the power of intonation, although articulation is preserved (obsolete).

aphonia clericorum Loss of speech due to laryngitis, from excessive use of the voice.

aphrasia (Gr, negative + to speak) Broca's term for **aphasia.**

aphthongia (Gr, negative + a clear sound) A peculiar affection described by Fleury, allied to stuttering, in which an attempt to speak brings on spasm of the tongue and of the muscles attached to the hyoid bone[2240] and representing dysarthria due to orofacial dystonia with spasm of the hypoglossus. The condition has certain similarities to **writer's cramp.**

aplestia (acoria) Inability to attain satiety after eating.

apnea (Gr, negative + to breathe) Cessation of the ventilatory airflow for at least 10 seconds.

apnea index The number of periods of apnea occurring in the course of 1 hour of sleep, recorded by **polysomnography.** The normal value is 5 or less.

apnea test A necessary test in **brain death** protocols. The comatose patient is ventilated with pure oxygen (or oxygen with CO_2) for 10 minutes, after which ventilation is terminated but a passive flow of oxygen is maintained for 10 minutes. Spontaneous ventilatory efforts stimulated by a rise in $PaCO_2$ over 60 mmHg indicate retention of some brainstem function.

apneic spells Cessation of airflow at the nose and mouth lasting longer than 10 seconds. See **sleep apnea.**

apneic threshold The partial pressure of arterial CO_2 below which respiratory motor output is so inhibited that the normal breathing rhythm is significantly disrupted; a pathophysiological mechanism involved in sleep apnea.[1383]

apneusis See **apneustic breathing.**

apneustic breathing (Gr, lack of + to breathe) A respiratory pattern in which the usual pause taken at the end of expiration is replaced by one at the end of inspiration. Pauses at the end of inspiration lasting 2 or 3 seconds may alternate with pauses at the end of expiration and reflect damage to the respiratory control mechanisms in the mid- or caudal pons. Apneustic breathing is therefore a late sign of rostrocaudal deterioration. In comatose patients, this pattern of respiration has serious significance because the probable cause is a lesion low in the pons.

apneustic center A site in the caudal pons adjacent to the trigeminal motor nucleus, damage to which may lead to apneustic breathing.

apoceruloplasmin deficiency A recessively inherited syndrome characterized by adult-onset blepharospasm with facial dystonia, high-density basal ganglion lesions on CT scans, low serum copper and ceruloplasmin levels (but no **Kayser-Fleischer rings**), low serum apoceruloplasmin and intestinal copper absorption, but increased liver uptake of copper.[3920]

apo-E A plasma glycoprotein involved in lipid metaboism, with three variants (apo-E2, E3, and E4) The E4 allele is associated with decreased longevity, raised plasma cholesterol, and **Alzheimer disease.**

apogeotropic nystagmus See **vestibular nystagmus.**

apomorphine test The assessment of motor functions such as tapping and walking before and repetitively after a subcutaneous injection of apomorphine, a dopamine receptor. Doses are increased from 1 up to 10 mg until either a positive response occurs or intolerance develops. The test is considered to predict responsiveness to L-dopa administration in parkinsonian syndromes and may differentiate idiopathic Lewy body Parkinson disease from **parkinsonism-plus** syndromes such as multisystem atrophy and cerebellar atrophy.[1319]

aponeurotic ptosis   Drooping of the upper lid in association with lengthening or disease of the aponeurosis. The muscle function is normal but the upper lid is seen to be thinned above the tarsal plate.[1320]

apoplexy   (Gr, a violent striking down) A sudden, sometimes catastrophic event such as a stroke, or hemorrhage into an organ, usually the brain. In Hippocratic writings, the word was also used for paralysis of part of the body occurring as a result of a stroke.[1046] The term was also used by Areteus and Galen and can be found in Chaucer; the meaning was a paralysis of *all* the body with loss of sensation, motion, and understanding, while for partial paralyses the term *palsy* was used. Johann **Wepfer** (1620–1695) demonstrated in 1658 that hemorrhage into the brain was the cause[4979] and Marshall **Hall** agreed. **Abercrombie** differentiated three forms, corresponding to subarachnoid hemorrhage, left middle cerebral artery occlusion, and intracerebral bleeding. The term *pontine apoplexy* was used from 1845 for primary intrapontine hemorrhage and *cerebellar apoplexy*, similarly.

The word is also used today for acute events affecting the labyrinth or the pituitary. The former is typically due to occlusion of the artery of the internal auditory meatus, the latter a life-threatening condition in which pituitary infarction leads to the acute onset of ophthalmoplegia with bilateral amaurosis, drowsiness, or coma; subarachnoid hemorrhage, CSF pleocytosis, and increased protein are also usually associated.

apoptosis   A gene-directed process of programmed cell death characterized by raised levels of cytosolic calcium in the dying cells, triggering digesting endonuclease activity without inflammatory changes. The process is normal in the embryo and in healthy adult tissues, leading in the latter case to the disposal of neutrophils and the elimination of self-reactive T-cell clones.[104,4660] Prevention of apoptosis is a therapeutic option in ischemic and traumatic brain disease.[9]

apparent/real nystagmus   See **stepping-around nystagmus.**

apperception   Sensation accompanied by comprehension of what is perceived.

apperceptive agnosia   An inability to recognize objects in the absence of a primary visual sensory deficit seen in patients with lesions of the right hemisphere. Lissauer considered that visual perception began with a stage of conscious awareness of a sensory impression

(apperception) followed by a stage in which associating semantic ideas added meaning.[3429]

appetite   An emotion requiring the satisfaction of a perceived need.

approach–avoidance equilibrium   A state of immobility in which a stimulus to act is balanced by a countervailing disincentive.

apractagnosia   (minor hemisphere syndrome) Unawareness of the significance of painful sensations, disturbances of the body schema, denial of contralateral hemiparesis, lack of spontaneous movement of the contralateral side, dressing apraxia, **asymbolia for pain,** and loss of visuospatial functions and orientation due to lesions of the minor (effectively, the right) hemisphere.[2506] The term is not specific, since it encompasses too many separate symptoms, and is thus seldom employed now. See also **anosognosia, constructional apraxia.**

apractagnosia for spatial orientation   See **visuospatial agnosia.**

apraxia   1. An inability to use body parts successfully. 2. An inability to carry out learned skilled, purposeful movements to command or in imitation, despite intact motor and sensory systems, good comprehension, normal volition and cognition, and full cooperation. The subject thus cannot produce the correct movement in response to a verbal command, nor imitate correctly a movement performed by the examiner, nor perform a movement correctly in response to a scene or object, nor handle an object correctly. 3. The loss of those mental faculties required to guide or execute purposeful movements, not explained by elementary motor or sensory deficits, impairment of perception or comprehension, or severe mental deterioration.

The first definition (of Nathan) is appropriate when apraxias occur as a result of a lesion of the motor system, as in the case of apraxic dysarthria in the **anterior operculum syndrome.** Geschwind suggested[2080] that apraxias result from disconnections of the posterior speech area from the association areas lying anterior to the primary motor cortex, and from disconnections of the visual association areas from these "motor association areas." Sparing of whole-body movements is not uncommon in such cases, perhaps because of preservation of the **Bundle of Turck.**

The recognition of apraxia and its first classification were the work of Hugo Karl Liepmann (1863–1925), a German neurologist, in 1900. He described three varieties,[3409] but further subgroups are defined today:

1. *Ideomotor apraxia* (motor apraxia) The inability to perform a motor act on command which can be performed spontaneously, so that the implementation of the gesture in a precise motor program is disrupted. In right-handed subjects, it is associated with lesions of the left hemisphere and thus is a common finding in patients with aphasia. Further subcategories include *sympathetic dys-*

praxia; the failure of a patient with Broca's aphasia to perform actions to command with the left hand; *parietal apraxia* resulting from damage to the arcuate fasciculus; *callosal apraxia*, an inability of the patient to perform an action with one hand while he can do so with the other, as in cases of anterior lesions of the corpus callosum; and *anterior* or *frontal apraxia*, in which the subject fails in the performance of tasks requiring bimanual interaction, because of a lesion of the left supplementary motor area.[748]

2. *Ideational apraxia* (conceptual apraxia) This connotes the inability to perform the coordinated sequence of actions that constitute a goal-directed activity despite the patient's ability to perform the individual components in isolation; or the inability to select and use objects as a result of disruption of the normal integration of systems subserving the functional knowledge of actions and those involved in object knowledge.[3332]

3. *Limb-kinetic apraxia* Limb apraxia has been divided between forms because of a failure of a conceptual system (ideational apraxia, above) and impairment of the production of the movement—ideomotor or limb-kinetic apraxia—which is an entity of doubtful validity, the clumsiness that forms the basis for the condition probably being due to paresis.

Specific forms of apraxia (slightly modified here) have been defined by Koski et al. (2002)[3138]

Buccofacial apraxia Impairment in performing mouth or face actions on verbal command or imitation (see also **orofacial apraxia**)

Conceptual apraxia A form in which the concept of the action is lost, characterized by an impaired ability to use tools and to understand meaningful gestures

Constructional apraxia Inability to assemble component parts into a coherent whole

Ideational apraxia Impairment in the sequential use of multiple objects. Traditionally, the term is also used to refer to impairment in the concept of an action. The term *conceptual apraxia* (see above) was coined to distinguish between these two dissociable impairments.

Ideomotor apraxia Impairment in the performance of skilled movements on verbal command or in imitation. It is most commonly characterized by spatial or temporal errors in movement execution.

Limb apraxia The term used to refer to ideomotor apraxia of the limbs. It frequently includes impaired performance of actions that also depend on the hands and fingers.

Limb-kinetic apraxia Slowness and stiffness of movements with a loss of fine and precise movements

Optical apraxia Impairment in performing saccadic eye movements on command

Orofacial apraxia Impairment in performing mouth or face actions on verbal command or imitation (see also *buccofacial apraxia*, above)

Speech apraxia Selective impairment in ability to produce speech sounds

Tactile apraxia Impairment of hand movements for the use of and interaction with an object, in the presence of preserved intransitive movements

Unimodal apraxia Any form of apraxia that is specific to actions demonstrated in a single modality, e.g., visual but not auditory

Reprinted from Koski L, Lacoboni MN, Mazziotta JC. Deconstructing stroke: understanding disorders of intentional movement after stroke. *Curr Opin Neurol Neurosurg.* 2002;**15:**–71, by kind permission.

See also the following entries and **Bruns gait apraxia, lid apraxia, apraxia of eyelid opening, dressing apraxia, Luria-Nebraska battery.**

apraxia for dressing   See **dressing apraxia.**

apraxia of eyelid opening   (blepharocolysis, eyelid apraxia, focal eyelid dystonia, eyelid freezing, involuntary levatoro inhibition) A supranuclear disorder manifested by an inability of the alert subject to open the closed lids at will, in the absence of **ptosis** from any cause, of failed language comprehension, and of **blepharospasm.**

The responsible lesion may be in the right hemisphere, in both, or in the basal ganglia; and is due to inhibition of normal tonic activity in the levator muscle.[2875, 2981] It may be an accompaniment of such basal ganglion syndromes as **Parkinson** or **Wilson disease.**[1426]

apraxia of gait   See **apraxic gait, Bruns gait apraxia.**

apraxia of gaze   A supranuclear disorder characterized by a transient, atonic inability to move the eyes in the direction desired, or to scan a picture for features surrounding the central point, in the absence of evidence of a lower motor neurone lesion of the third, fourth, or sixth cranial nerves.

The condition is a feature of **progressive supranuclear palsy** and of various pyramidal syndromes of hemispheric origin; and may occur in the **Balint syndrome.**

apraxia of lid closure   (compulsive lid opening) The inability of awake patients to initiate or sustain lid closure voluntarily in the presence of intact reflex lid closure, due to bilateral hemispheric damage.[2975]

apraxia of speech   Impairment of purposive speech with word-finding errors and paraphasias, while emotional or automatic speech is unaffected; as occurs with inferior frontal lesions in the dominant hemisphere.[1285]

apraxic agraphia   An agraphic syndrome characterized by a selective disturbance of writing in the absence of any abnormality in letter or name selection, so that in the pure variety, spelling and reading are intact and there are no other disturbances of language function.[399] The causal lesion may be frontal, parietal, or thalamic.

apraxic dysarthria   Inability to make purposeful speech sounds in the absence of **dysphasia,** as occurs in the **anterior operculum syndrome.**[3601]

apraxic gait   (apractic gait, magnetic gait, **Bruns gait apraxia**) Inability to initiate the process of forward motion by alternating steps, although the power and coordination of the legs are normal in the lying and sitting positions. The maintenance of the feet on the floor, removed only with great effort, has led to the alternative name *magnetic gait*.

aproscencephaly with Rieger-type eye anomalies   A congenital syndrome characterized by anterior chamber abnormalities, adrenal hypoplasia, and aproscencephaly.[337]

aprosodia (aprosody)   Lack of **prosody** in speech, which thus loses the inflections that add meaning and emotional content so that patients talk as though the language used were foreign to them.

Prosody is an affective component of language, as is emotional gesturing, and is organized within the right hemisphere in a manner similar to left hemispheric language functions so that motor, sensory, global, transcortical, and conduction forms of aprosodia may be differentiated.[4801]

In *motor aprosodia* the lesion affects the right frontal and anterior parietal opercula and produces speech that is flat, devoid of emotional tone, and unaccompanied by gestures. Repetition of affective prosody is impaired but its comprehension and the interpretation of emotional gesturing remain.

In *sensory aprosodia* emotional prosody in speech and active gesturing are normal but their visual and auditory comprehension is impaired, as is their repetition. The lesion is of the right posterior temporal and parietal opercula.

In *global aprosodia* due to a large right perisylvian lesion, affect can neither be displayed nor comprehended. A left hemiparesis is also likely to be present.

Transcortical aprosodias resemble the motor, sensory, and global forms, except that repetition is preserved.

Impairment of both the production and comprehension of language components such as stress, pauses, cadences, accent, melody, and intonation that allow the translation of internal states is termed *affective aprosodia*.[912]

aqueduct of Sylvius   (cerebral aqueduct) The narrow passage between the third and fourth ventricles described by Franciscus de la Boe (**Sylvius**) in about 1650.

aqueduct syndrome   See **syndrome of the mesencephalic gray matter.** See also **Sylvian aqueduct syndrome.**

aqueductal forking   A developmental error in which representation of the aqueduct for part of its course is by two distinct channels in the sagittal plane, separated from each other by normal nervous tissue.[1512]

aqueductal stenosis   Narrowing of the aqueduct of Sylvius in the absence of branching of the channel, gliosis, inflammation, or tumor; a cause of **noncommunicating hydrocephalus.**[1512]

Acquired causes or congenital narrowing, forking, or gliosis of the aqueduct or the presence of a septum may be responsible.

arachnoid   (Gr, resembling a spider's web) The word was used by Herophilus and later by Galen for any thin membrane. In neurology it refers to the gossamer thin (but watertight) middle layer of the three meninges enclosing, with the pia mater, the CSF. Its anatomy was described in 1800 by Bichat.[5204]

arachnoid cysts   (leptomeningeal cysts) Benign, nongenetic, slowly growing cysts composed of a thickened and fibrotic arachnoid membrane, usually situated over the lateral aspects of the hemispheres or within the spinal canal and containing CSF. They are considered to represent maldevelopment of the cerebral meninges.

They are most common in the region of the Sylvian fissure and have been blamed for cognitive impairment, seizures, developmental delay, headache, hydrocephalus, focal signs, and raised intracranial pressure, but are most often asymptomatic. See also **porencephalic cyst.**[5930]

arachnoid diverticula   (spinal arachnoid cyst; leptomeningeal cyst; intradural meningeal cyst; circumscribed serous spinal meningitis; localized adhesive spinal arachnoiditis; meningeal hydrops). Small diverticula in free communication with the subarachnoid space, arising from the septum posticum of Schwalbe (a sagittal membrane dividing the posterior spinal subarachnoid space) and occasionally causing pain, percussion tenderness, and myelopathic signs in erect adult subjects.[3039]

Aran disease   See **amyotrophic lateral sclerosis.**

Aran, Francois-Amilcar   (1817–1861) French physician who was born in Bordeaux but who trained and worked in Paris. He was mainly interested in cardiology but described progressive muscular atrophy (**amyotrophic lateral sclerosis**) in 1850, a year after **Duchenne** (whose work he acknowledged) but 3 years before Cruveilhier, whose name is also sometimes attached to the syndrome.

Aran-Duchenne disease   See **amyotrophic lateral sclerosis.**

arbovirus encephalitis   Direct viral infections of the brain due to RNA viruses of the togavirus, bunyaviruses, or reoviruses class. Most are zoonoses of birds or lower vertebrates and are transmitted through an arthropod vector, such as mosquitoes or ticks. The *togavirus* diseases include Eastern, Western, Venezuelan, and Semlicki forest encephalitis. St. Louis, Japanese, Murray Valley, West Nile, Ilheus, Russian, Spring, Summer, and Central European encephalitis, and Louping ill and Powassan encephalitis are also produced by *flaviviruses* of the togavirus group. *Bunyavirus*-caused encephalitides are those of the California encephalitis group. *Reoviruses* include Colorado tickborn encephalitis and Bhanja.[6030]

arcade of Fröhse   A fibrous tunnel at the origin of the supinator muscle, under which runs the posterior interosseous nerve as it enters the forearm. This is thus a place where that nerve may be entrapped.

arceau rhythm   See **mu rhythm.**

archenteric cyst   See **neurenteric cyst.**

Archimedes spiral   Fine motor coordination may be assessed by getting the subject to draw a two-dimensional spiral figure from the center outwards. Tremor, athetosis, and other involuntary movement disorders and also pyramidal lesions may disturb the smooth execution of the drawing.

architectonics   The microscopical study of the appearances of cells and fibers in the cerebral cortex, leading to the definition of morphologically distinct areas. The major work was done by **Korbimian Brodmann, von Economo,** and the **Vogts.**

Archives de Neurologie   A neurological journal founded by **Charcot** in 1880 and edited by him until his death in 1893.

Archives of Neurology   (*Arch. Neurol.*) An American neurological journal founded in 1959 with Harold **Wolff** as the first chief editor. It was sponsored by the American Neurological Association and published by the American Medical Association, taking over from the *Archives of Neurology and Psychiatry.* Address: American Medical Association; 535 N. Dearborn St., Chicago, IL 60610. Web site: http://archneur.ama-assn.org.

The American Neurological Association later adopted the newly formed *Annals of Neurology* as its official organ.

Archives of Neurology and Psychiatry   A professional journal founded in 1918 with Weisenburg as editor, to provide a vehicle for neurological papers that were not then finding adequate space in the *Journal of Nervous and Mental Diseases.*

arctic hysteria   (Myriatchit) See **Latah.**

arcuate fasciculus   (Lat, bowed + a bundle) A cerebral fiber pathway originating in the cortex of the supratemporal plane, arching posteriorly around the Sylvian fissure and running in the superior longitudinal fasciculus across the insula, to the lower frontal region. This and the local auditory cortex, insula and supramarginal gyrus are the structures damaged in patients with **conduction aphasia,** in which the faculty of word repetition is especially affected.[1265]

arcuate scotoma   A visual field defect described first by **Bjerrum.**[591] It has a curved shape, skirting the central fixation spot, and is due to segmental (compressive) lesions of the optic nerve fibers running from the temporal retina both above and below the maculopapillar bundle.

area postrema   A region in the floor of the fourth ventricle where the blood–brain barrier is deficient.

areflexia without pupillary changes   A benign and nonprogressive anomaly of unknown cause.[5702] See also **Holmes-Adie syndrome.**

areflexic syncope(syndrome)   See **paralytic postural syncope.**

Aretaeus of Cappadocia   (A.D. 81–138) Physician who described complex partial seizures (following a depressed skull fracture) and gave a full account of the different forms of **aura.** Noting the contralateral signs, he postulated decussation of the motor pathways in the brain. He also introduced the terms *paraplegia* (localized loss of touch and movement), *paresis* (loss of motor power only), and *apoplexy* (a generalized loss of movement, sensation, and understanding).

arginase deficiency   (argininemia) A very rare recessively inherited hyperammonemic syndrome presenting as a diffuse encephalopathy in infancy or childhood, with added features of microcephaly, developmental delay, seizures, spasticity, ataxia, chorea, athetosis, opisthotonos, persistent vomiting, and intolerance of protein feeds.[5248] Argininemia, arginemia, and aminoaciduria are characteristic findings.[2439]

argininemia   See **arginase deficiency.**

argininosuccinase deficiency   (Allen-Dent syndrome; citrullinemia) A rare, usually recessively inherited hyperammonemic disorder presenting in childhood with toe-walking, vomiting, lethargy, and failure to thrive, usually followed in 6–12 months by progressive developmental delay, seizures, abnormal involuntary movements, ataxia, parapaaresis, friability of the hair, attention-deficit/hyperactivity disorder, hepatomegaly, and persistent vomiting. A few patients with nearly normal development have been reported.[105] Plasma citrulline levels are markedly raised.

argininosuccinic aciduria   A rare, recessive hyperammonemic syndrome due to deficiency of arginosuccinate lysase. The abnormal gene is located on chromosome 7 (7cen–q11.2).

The condition presents clinically with lethargy, seizures, and coma in newborn children who have sparse, brittle, and coarse hair. Failure to thrive, seizures, hepatosplenomegaly, jaundice, and mental retardation are the usual presenting features in infancy, and seizures, ataxia, and psychomotor retardation, often with episodic vomiting and hypotonia, in childhood. Aminoacidemia, moderate citrullinemia, and hyperammonemia are noted at all ages.[944]

Argyll Robertson, Douglas Moray Cooper Lamb (1837–1909) Scottish ophthalmologist who trained in Edinburgh, St. Andrews, and Berlin. After his studies abroad he returned to Edinburgh and eventually became President of the Royal College of Surgeons of that city. He gave credit to the German neurologist **Remak**

for first showing him the pupillary abnormality that now bears his own name.

Argyll Robertson pupils   Pupils that are small, irregular, unequal, and effectively not reactive to light, though reactive to accommodation.

Described in 1869, the lesion is of the pathways between the pretectal region of the midbrain and the Edinger-Westphal nucleus. Syphilis is the classic etiology, but other mesencephalic lesions and diabetes may also be responsible. The inequality and irregularity of the spastic pupils are not explained by the known neurological defects;[4719] possibly syphilitic iritis producing local scarring is the immediate cause.[212]

argyrophilic brain disease   A dementing disease in which silver-staining fibrils are detected throughout the cortex rather than the usual plaques and tangles of **Alzheimer disease,** which this condition otherwise resembles closely.[2759]

arhinencephaly   A congenital malformation in which the olfactory pathway is absent. It is neither a morphological nor a single etiological entity, since numerous associated malformations of the eyes, pyramidal pathways, cerebellum and dentato-olivary complex, craniofacial dysmorphisms, and cardiac, renal, and endocrine disorders are variously described in association.[3108] See also **olfactory dysgenesis, holoproscencephaly.**

Arieti-Gray syndrome   See **Sturge-Weber syndrome.**

arm recoil   The arms of the supine infant are first flexed maximally and then extended; in the normal mature infant the arms return to the fully flexed position.

arm-diaphragm synkinesis   Arm movements occurring in time with respiratory movements, as a result of aberrant regeneration of phrenic nerve fibers following brachial plexus or cervical root lesions.[5449]

arm-dropping test   See **Bekhterev signs,** No. 9.

Armendares syndrome   An X-linked recessive or autosomal recessive syndrome characterized by microcephaly with cranial asymmetry, craniosynostosis, small face, microcephaly, high-arched palate, ptosis, pigmentary retinopathy, short stature, delayed skeletal maturation, short fifth fingers, and simian creases of the hand.[216] See also **craniosynostosis.**

Arnold, Friedrich   (1803–1890) German anatomist who in 1838 made precise differentiation between the frontal, parietal, occipital, and temporosphenoidal lobes. He also described the frontopontine tract, the arcuate nuclei, the otic ganglion, and the auricular branch of the vagus nerve and its canal.

Arnold, Julius   (1835–1915) Heidelberg physician (the son of Friedrich) who described **superior laryn-**

geal neuralgia[2764] and the **Chiari malformation** (3 years after Chiari).

Arnold syndrome   See **superior laryngeal neuralgia.**

Arnold-Chiari malformation   See **Chiari malformation.**

Arnold's nerve cough   Coughing with stabbing pain felt in the suboccipital region, thought to be due to irritation of the auricular branch of the vagus nerve.[72]

aromatic L-amino acid decarboxylase deficiency   A rare recessively inherited inborn error of metabolism in which absence of this enzyme prevents the synthesis of normal amounts of catecholamines and of serotonin.

Clinically, the disorder is characterized by oculogyric crises and extreme axial hypotonia, with hypokinesia and athetosis. Ptosis, sweating, lability of blood pressure and temperature, and nasal congestion witness the catecholamine deficiency. Abnormal sleep, feeding difficulties, and esophageal reflux are other features. A response to monoamine oxidase A inhibitors and to dopamine agonists is reported.[2721]

arousal   1. An abrupt change from a deeper to a lighter stage of non-rapid eye movement sleep or from rapid eye movement sleep to the awake state.[249] 2. A period of at least 1.5 seconds in which there is increased EMG activity in association with a return of desynchronization of the EEG during sleep.

arousal disorders   Parasomnias occurring in the first third of nocturnal sleep during stages 3 or 4 of NREM sleep, when the subject is unrousable. A spectrum of behaviors is identified, increasing in severity from face rubbing, chewing, and mumbling through sleeptalking, sitting up in bed, sleepwalking, thrashing about in bed, night terrors, and panic attacks. See **parasomnias, confusional arousals, sleepwalking, sleep terrors.**

array   A regular arrangement of electrodes over the scalp or brain or within the brain substance.

arrhythmic activity   A sequence of waves of inconstant period. cf. rhythm.

arrhythmokinesis   Disturbances in rapid alternating ballistic movements in patients with cerebellar dysfunction.[5927]

Arroyo sign   Sluggishness of the pupillary light reaction in hypoadrenalism.[4723]

arterial gas embolism   Air embolism occurring typically when a diver ascends (decompresses) without exhaling, as a result of which the air in the respiratory passages expands and causes alveolar rupture, the air entering the systemic circulation.

Pain, respiratory distress, and cerebral and brainstem signs are the usual sequelae.[2275]

arterial stationary wave   An angiographic appearance resembling ringed constrictions, described in the distal part of the internal carotid artery in Tolosa-Hunt syndrome (**superior orbital fissure syndrome**).

arteriography   The depiction of the lumen of the larger arteries by X-rays, the artery having been injected with a radio-opaque medium. The technique was introduced by Egas Moniz (1874–1955).[1611]

arteriosclerotic parkinsonism   See **frontal gait disorder, isolated gait ignition failure.**

arteriosclerotic rigidity   (akinetic rigidity, hypertonia of opposition, paratonia) The expression employed by Macdonald Critchley for increased muscular resistance to passive stretch, made worse by instructions given to the patient to relax. It thus resembles **paratonia.**

arteriovenous fistula   Any connection between an artery and a vein allowing arterial blood to flow into the venous system directly without interposed capillaries. See **spinal dural arteriovenous fistula.**

arteriovenous malformation   (AVM) (tumor circoidius; racemose aneurysm; racemose angioma; angiomatous malformation) An uncommon congenital vascular malformation (**angioma**) in which gliotic neural tissue is present between the vascular elements. It is due to an arrest in development that results in the formation of direct artery-to-vein communications of any size from cryptic to tumorous, without an intervening capillary bed. The condition may be familial.

The lesion evolves during life with increased blood flow and attenuation of distended venous channels, leading to clinical manifestations usually after the second decade. Hemorrhage, ischemia resulting from steal of arterial blood, irritation of the underlying brain, and local brain atrophy may be responsible for the clinical manifestations, which include intracerebral or subarachnoid bleeding, seizures, focal signs, headache, bruits, and even cardiac failure in patients with large-volume shunts through the malformation.[3158, 4414, 5330]

See also **angioma, cerebral blood vessel hamartoma, aneurysm of the vein of Galen, capillary telangiectasia, cavernous angioma, venous malformations.** A grading system for all forms of AVM has been suggested.[5275]

A *variant* is *spinal avm, epidermal nevus*, and *rhabdomyosarcoma.*[5009]

arteriovenous malformations with cavernous hemangiomas   A dominantly inherited syndrome of **cerebral blood vessel hamartoma** in which both of these abnormalities occur, without skin or retinal lesions.[3179]

arteritis   Inflammatory disease of the arterial walls. See **giant-cell arteritis.**

artery of migraine   The posterior cerebral artery,[1857] so called because of the close association between migraine and visual disturbances.

artery of Percheron   A perforating artery branching from the precommunal part of the posterior cerebral artery and supplying the upper paramedian midbrain and thalamus.

arthrogryposis   (Gr, joint + to become bent) Congenital ankylosis of more than one joint. A condition of fixation of joints due to contractures in local tissues, occurring either in isolation or in association with neural or muscular diseases in childhood (**arthrogryposis multiplex congenita**).

Arthrogryposis Association   A charitable organization. Address: 106 Herkheimer St., Northville, NY 11710.

arthrogryposis multiplex congenita   (AMC) (multiple congenital articular rigidities; amyoplasia congenita; Guerin-Stern disease; myodystrophia fetalis deformans) A group of uncommon disorders of infants and children characterized by multiple fibrotic joint contractures appearing at or just after birth, leading to immobility of the limbs with fixation in certain postures due to contracture of the muscles.[2306] The spine and temporomandibular joints, however, are never affected.

Most cases are sporadic, and are neither neural nor myopathic in origin; presumably this form is not heritable and represents an intrauterine or developmental disorder of joints. However, AMC may be associated with either neuropathic or myopathic disease[328, 1507] and may be inherited either as a dominant or as a recessive characteristic. The syndrome was first described by Otto in 1841.

Congenital cerebral maldevelopments such as micropolygyria, heterotopias, dilated ventricles, absent corticospinal tracts, anterior horn cell degeneration, and facial nerve nuclear degeneration may accompany the joint disorder.[2640] Absence of abdominal muscles, myelocele, club feet, dislocation of hips and knees, congenital heart disease and hernias are also described in association.

Variant forms include the following:
1. Arthrogryposis is *dominantly inherited* but neither atrophy nor weakness are apparent.[1240]
2. The anterior horn cells of the spinal cord are affected, and there is liver disease with pigment overload and renal dysfunction. Death ensues within weeks or months.[4125]
3. Multiple articular rigidities and nodular protuberances of the anterior vertebral columns are present with an almost total absence of myelin and Schwann cells.[4398]
4. *Dominantly inherited lower motor neuron disorder with arthrogryposis* is a nonprogressive, congenital disorder restricted to the lower part of the body, with atrophy of spinal motor neurons and absence of muscle spindles.[3165] Expression of the gene is variable.[1887]
5. The *myopathic type* is characterized by the occurrence of arthrogryposis with a primary myopathic disorder, such as **congenital muscular dystrophy.**
6. *AMC* associated with pulmonary hypoplasia
7. Distal X-linked *AMC* also manifesting anterior horn cell disease

8. AMC accompanying a congenital neuropathy[2640]
See also **Kuskowim disease.**

arthrokinetic-induced nystagmus (Stransky nystagmus; somatosensory nystagmus) That form of nystagmus induced in darkness by passive movement of the arm. The fast phase beats away from the arm that is moved.

articulated labials Those consonants (*B, P, M, W*) which depend for their utterance on intact lip function. See also **modified labials, dentolabials.**

articulation The distinct utterance of vocal speech sounds.

artifact (artefact) 1. Any potential difference due to an extracerebral source recorded in EEG tracings. 2. Any modification of the EEG caused by extracerebral factors such as alterations of the media surrounding the brain, instrumental distortion, or malfunction and operational errors. (Adapted from the 1974 Report of the Committee on Terminology, IFCN,[989] © 1974. With permission from Elsevier Science.) 3. Any symptom or physical sign that is unrelated to the pathology that induced the present consultation. 4. A voltage change generated by a biologic or nonbiologic source other than the ones of interest. The stimulus artifact (or shock artifact) represents cutaneous spread of stimulating current to the recording electrode and the delay in return to baseline, which is dependent on the ability of filters to respond to high voltage. Stimulus artifacts may precede or overlap the activity of interest.

Movement artifact refers to a change in the recorded activity caused by movement of the recording electrodes. (From the 2001 Report of the Nomenclature Committee of the American Association of Electromyography and Electrodiagnosis.[10] Used by permission, copyright © 2001, AAEM.)

artistic agnosia Inability to comprehend the nuances of an artistic production. An uncommon sign of right hemisphere disease.

arylsulfatase A family of enzymes coded on chromosome 22 responsible for cleaving the sulfatase ester from the galactose portion of the sulfatide molecule. Sulfatase A is deficient in metachromatic leukodystrophy. The B and C forms are also missing in the condition of multiple sulfatase deficiency.

ascending neuritis An inflammatory reaction in the peripheral nerves capable of progressing proximally and thereby leading to dysfunction of the CNS as hypothesized by **Charcot.** In the absence of supportive evidence, the hypothesis generates intestinal rather than cerebral sympathy.

Aschner cardiac phenomenon See **oculocardiac reflex.**

Aschner sign See **oculocardiac reflex.**

asemasia (Gr, lack of + to show by signs) Loss of the power of communication by language or by signs.

aseptic meningitis (lymphocytic choriomeningitis) 1. A disease with acute onset characterized by meningeal signs, pleocytosis in the CSF (mainly mononuclear cells), and sterile CSF culture. 2. A benign lymphocytic meningitis due to an RNA virus, usually transmitted by mice, in which the cellular response is monocytic (lymphocytic) rather than granulocytic.

Clinically, a typical meningitis illness follows a prodromal febrile, influenza-like illness after 4–7 days, and lasts for up to 4 weeks, with minor residua such as arthralgias and drowsiness being common over the next few months. In the acute stage, the CSF shows monocytic pleocytosis but glucose levels are normal and cultures are negative.

A **chronic benign lymphocytic** form of meningitis also occurs.[2647]

The term was first applied in 1920 by James Bourne Ayer (b. 1882), a Boston neurologist.[2995]

Ashworth scale A validated scale for assessing the severity of spasticity, when such an assessment is important:

0. No increase in muscle tone
1. Slight increase in tone, giving a catch when the affected part is moved in flexion or extension, followed by minimal resistance throughout the remainder of the range of movement
2. More marked increase in tone through most of the range of movement, but the affected parts are easily moved
3. Considerable increase in tone, making passive movement difficult
4. Affected part rigid in flexion or extension[639]

See also **spasm score.**

asimultagnosia (extinction, sensory competition) Difficulty in perceiving the whole of the visual field at one time, or in appreciating the occurrence of simultaneously presented tactile or auditory stimuli on each side of the body.

Those affected with the visual form see their field piecemeal and identify objects in parts of it only, thus failing to enumerate the number of objects (crosses, letters, etc.) written on a card, although those that they *do* perceive, they perceive normally. The condition is a feature of **Balint syndrome.**

asomatognosia 1. Lack of awareness of the deep sensations (joint position sense, deep pain, muscle sense) from part of the body, usually due to posterior column or peripheral nerve (thick-fiber) disease. 2. Inability to recognize a paretic limb as one's own. See also **anosognosia.**

asomnia Pathologically persistent wakefulness. See **agrypnia.**

aspartate A dicarboxylic acid excitatory neurotransmitter.

aspartylglycosaminuria   A rare, recessively inherited lysosomal storage disease producing diffuse encephalopathy and presenting as intellectual retardation from infancy, accompanied by skin photosensitivity; short neck and short stature; brachycephaly; facial dysmorphism; joint laxity; macroglossia; behavioral disturbances; pyramidal, retinal, and corneal abnormalities; glycoasparginuria; and aminoaciduria.

The biopsy of almost any tissue shows the presence of vacuoles in the cytoplasm. The responsible gene has been located at 4q24–qter.[4482]

Asperger syndrome   (able autism) A minor form of autism in which there are few if any problems with language and learning, though many in the realm of social interaction. Expressively, subjects lack empathy and appear self-centered and are only comfortable in predictable situations. They may not use appropriate loudness levels, may make socially unacceptable statements about the appearance of others (see **verbal dysdecorum**), or yawn widely as one talks to them, and may miss the nonliteral meaning of language and/or the suprasegmental intent of language communicated through prosodic rhythm and melody as opposed to the words said, as well as the nonverbal message. Many also demonstrate a kind of rigidity in thought and behavior, which presents as obsessional behavior. See the Web site http://www.ummed.edu/pub/o/ozbayrak/asperger.html.

Asperger Syndrome Coalition of the U.S.   A charitable organization in this field. Address: PO Box 351268, Jacksonville, FL 32235-1268. E-mail: info@asc-us.org. Tel: 866-427-7747. Web site: http://www.asc-us.org.

aspergillosis   Infection with *Aspergillus fumigatus*, seldom affecting the nervous system, but occasionally causing cerebral abscess, basal meningitis, or septic infarction of the brain.

associated movements   1. Tonic or postural reflex reactions (i.e., variations in muscle tone or attitude), typically appearing in hemiparetic limbs and characterized by long latency, constant form, and slow development and decline. Their adequate stimulus is tonically maintained, voluntary contraction of some other part of the skeletal musculature.[5829] 2. An involuntary association between the movements of paralyzed limbs and other parts of the body; thus a paralyzed arm may be adducted strongly during a yawn.[5564]

associated nystagmus   See **induced nystagmus.**

Association Canadienne de l'Ataxie de Friedreich   A Canadian charitable organization. Address: 5620 rue C.A. Jobin, Montreal, PQ, H1P 1H8 Canada. Tel: 514-321-8684.

association cortex   1. Those parts of the cerebral cortex not recognized as having specific motor or sensory functions, although lesions of these regions lead to deficits in attention, sensation, language, and other higher cerebral functions.[1541] 2. Homotypical six-layered isocortex, some of which is modality-specific (*unimodal*) and some, *heteromodal* (polymodal, multimodal, supramodal, polysensory or high-order association cortex) in its response to differing kinds of stimulation.

The unimodal areas act as obligatory relays for the intracortical transfer of sensory information from the primary reception areas to other parts of the cortex. The heteromodal areas allow intermodal association and have close relationships with limbic and paralimbic function. Lesions here give rise to complex, multimodality disorders such as **Gerstmann syndrome,** confusional states, or **Balint syndrome.**[3851]

Association for Alzheimer's Disease and Related Disorders   A charitable organization. Address: 70 East Lake Street, Chicago, IL 60601. Tel: 312-853-3060. Web site: http://www.alzhi.org.

Association for Brain Tumor Research   A national charitable organization providing free written information about brain tumors and treatment options, including facts about medical specialists, facilities, and support groups. The organization also funds medical research. Address: 208 South LaSalle Street, Ste 1426, Chicago, IL 60604. Tel: 312-782-4311. Web site: http://www.abta.org.

Association for Children and Adults with Learning Disabilities   A charitable organization. Address: 4156 Library Road, Pittsburgh, PA 15234. Tel: 412-881-2253.

Association for Neuro-Metabolic Disorders   A charitable organization in this field. Address: c/o Cheryl Volk, 5223 Brookfield Lane, Sylvania, OH 43560. Tel: 419-885-1497. E-mail: VOLK4OLKS@aol.com.

Association for Persons with Severe Handicaps   A charitable organization. Address: 7010 Roosevelt Way NE, Seattle, WA 98115. Tel: 206-361-8870.

Association for Research in Nervous and Mental Disease   A professional organization. Address: 1. Gustave Levy Place, PO Box 1052, New York, NY 10029.

Association Française contre les Myopathies   A charitable organization. Address: 13 Place de Rungis, 75013 Paris, France. Tel: 1-4565-1300.

Association of British Neurologists   A professional society. Address: Ormond House, 27 Boswell Street, London WC1N 3JZ, UK. Web site: http://www.the-abn.org.

Association of Professional Sleep Disorders   A grouping of the three major U.S. societies involved with clinical and research studies on sleep. Address: 604 Second St. SW, Rochester, MN 55902. Tel: 507-287-6006.

Association of Rehabilitation Nurses   A professional organization. Address: 2506 Gross Point Rd., Evanston, IL 60201. Tel: 708-966-3433.

Association of Sleep Disorders Centers   A professional organization of centers conducting research and clinical investiation of sleep disorders, with activities in education, quality control, and cooperative research. Address: PO Box YY, East Setauket, NY 11733. Tel: 516-473-8964. Web site: http://www.asda.org/professional.htm.

associative agnosia   One of the two forms of agnosia differentiated by Lissauer (1891), the other being **apperceptive agnosia** (in which the perceptual mechanism is thought to be disturbed). Associative agnosia is a true defect of recognition, due to an impairment of the normal processing mechanisms of the associative cortex by which perceived stimuli are matched with previously encoded information to allow recognition. As a result, the perception is normal but it is stripped of its meaning; thus there is a loss of the ability to identify objects seen,[977] so that while an object seen may be drawn accurately, the subject nevertheless does not recognize what it is.

associative visual agnosia without alexia   A rare syndrome in which the subject is unable to appreciate the meaning of visually presented, nonverbal but meaningful stimuli, while perception of such stimuli through other channels is retained. A right hemianopia is usually present.

The condition represents the effect of both an interhemispheric visual–verbal disconnection and a specific categorization defect for visual, nonverbal, meaningful stimuli.[83]

astasia trepidante   (astasia trepidans) A peculiar fear of walking, occurring rarely in elderly people in whom no specific abnormalities can be found to explain their apprehension. Occasionally, they may be so fearful of walking that they will not take a step at all and "freeze"; when encouraged to step out, they may clutch onto things or drop to their knees. In many cases, **normal pressure hydrocephalus** is considered to be the cause, and in some cases it is.

The **Petren gait** is a dilute version of the same condition.

astasia-abasia   The inability to maintain an upright posture, despite normal function of the legs in bed; usually a manifestation of hysteria. The opposite condition (legs paralyzed in bed but able to sustain gait) is also recognized.[606] The words mean "inability to stand and walk." It may be better to use the term *hysterical dysbasia* for the difficulty with gait and the term *stasibasiphobia* for the fear of standing or walking. In hysterical dysbasia there is often marked swaying from side to side, with superfluous movements; the patient may fall far to the side or to the front or back when walking but is usually able to regain balance without falling to the floor. If a fall does occur, it is in a theatrical manner but usually without injury. It can frequently be demonstrated in hysterical dysbasia that, although unable to

walk forwards, the patient may be able to walk backwards or to one side or even to run without difficulty.

Charcot, in describing this as "a special variety of motor feebleness of the legs from want of coordination in relation to position in rest and progression," indicated that he regarded the condition as an ability to move the legs in the recumbent but not in the upright position. See also **Blocq syndrome, frontal disequilibrium, subcortical disequilibrium.**

astatesthesia   Inability to recognize the position of a limb in space.

astereognosis   A failure of judgement regarding the spatial characteristics of a tactile stimulus, due to a lesion of the contralateral parietal cortex.

asterixis   (negative myoclonus) Brief, irregular, and jerky movements resulting from the temporary loss of muscle stimulation during which muscle tone is lost from an extended limb. This leads to momentary dropping of all or part of it (lapses in posture),[6093] or to a tremor when the interruptions in innervation last <200 msec.

When bilateral, asterixis is the result of metabolic or toxic diseases, such as renal or hepatic failure; when unilateral, lesions of the opposite hemisphere or of the midbrain or brainstem on either side are responsible.[4640] Truncal asterixis is also described.

asteroid hyalitis   Deposition of calcium compounds in the vitreous humor as a result of trauma or in the elderly.

asthenia   (Gr, lack of + strength) 1. A languid, fragile, and vulnerable constitutional tendency, leaving the subject prone to complaints but without diagnosable disease. 2. Generalized weakness or disinclination to attempt muscular activity. 3. Early subjective fatigue preventing the continuation of motor activity without clinical or laboratory-demonstrated weakness.[2381] See also **fatigue.**

asthenia crurum dolorosa (paresthetica)   See **Ekbom syndrome.**

asthenia of upward gaze   Progressive ptosis with descent of the globe after the maintenance of upward gaze for a minute or so; a sign of end-plate fatigue in **myasthenia gravis.**

asthenic bulbar paralysis   See **myasthenia gravis.**

asthenic ophthalmoplegia   Ocular **myasthenia gravis.**

asthenopia   (Gr, lack of + strength + eye) (accomodative asthenopia) Frontal headache, fatigue, and failure of continued accomodation (leading to complaints of blurred or indistinct vision) and of concentration, occurring in some subjects after prolonged close work. 2. A similar phenomenon occurs during the later stages of recovery from cortical blindness.

asthmatic amyotrophy   See **Hopkins syndrome.**

astigmatism   (Gr, lack of + a point) A defect of the refractive media of the eye in which parallel rays of light arising from a single source are not brought to a common point on the retina, usually due to differences in the curvature of the cornea at different places.[2331]

astonagaza   See **dancing mania.**

astroblastoma   See **astrocytoma.**

astrocyte   (Gr, star + cell) A glial cell in the CNS. *Gemistocytic* astrocytes (goose-fat cells), plump reactive astrocytes found abundantly in areas of demyelination, and *protoplasmic* astrocytes (now type 1), found largely in gray matter, were the two forms differentiated by Ramon y **Cajal** in 1881. *Fibrous* astrocytes (spider cells) are abundant in white matter and in the optic nerve.

astrocytoma   A slowly growing primary neuroectodermal tumor of the cerebrum, cerebellum, or spinal cord composed of astrocytic cells with fine fibrillary processes and indistinct cell borders in well-differentiated types and lacking both collagen and reticulin fibers. Glial fibrillary acidic protein is present in most astrocytoma cells.

On the basis of their distribution, histology, and predominant cell type, the following forms are recognized:

Fibrillary (diffuse) The commonest (90%) form of astrocytoma, occurring particularly in the cerebral hemispheres of adults or in the pons in children. The tumor is graded[4707] between astrocytoma, malignant (anaplastic) astrocytoma, and glioblastoma multiforme (in which malignant change is seen in discrete areas of previously well-differentiated astrocytomas arising in the cerebral hemispheres of adults).[6]

Pilocytic Relatively slowly growing fibrillary astrocytic tumors occurring particularly in the cerebellum, hypothalamus, optic nerve and chiasm, and the brainstem in children. The tumors are characterized by the elongation of some of their constituent cells lying in parallel rows and by the presence of **Rosenthal fibers.**

Less common forms include the following:

Subependymal giant-cell astrocytomas Calcified astrocytomas found in the thalamus and periventricular regions in some patients with **tuberous sclerosis**

Protoplasmic astrocytomas Tumors containing stellate cells with fine processes and minimal neuroglial fibers

Gemistocytic astrocytomas Tumors containing plump cells with eosinophilic cytoplasm displacing the nucleus peripherally

Pleomorphic xanthoastrocytomas More malignant tumors with exceptionally large cells, occasionally found in the superficial cortex of the hemispheres in young people

Astroblastomas Poorly differentiated astrocytomas with pleomorphism, mitoses, and perivascular rosette formation

These histological differences do not correlate well with prognosis, however, and an alternative method of classification defines the astrocytoma as a mildly hypercellular tumor with pleomorphism but without vascular proliferation nor necrosis; the anaplastic astrocytoma as a tumor with vascular proliferation, moderate pleomorphism and hypercellularity; and the glioblastoma multiforme as the same with added necrosis.[838]

In yet another system, nuclear atypia, mitoses, endothelial proliferation, and necrosis are used as the criteria for grading.[1304]

In a *variant* familial syndrome, cutaneous malignant melanomas are associated.[2961]

astrocytosis   See **gliosis.**

astroglia   Astrocytes of all kinds.

astroglial neoplasms   An encompassing term for all tumors arising from astrocytes.

astrogliosis   Proliferation of astrocytes (mainly type 1) in response to local injury. See **gliosis.**

asymbolia (e)   (Gr, lack of + a sign) Loss of the power of forming or comprehending a symbol of thought, in any medium. The term was suggested by Finkelberg as more encompassing than **aphasia.**[4512]

asymbolia for pain   Unawareness of the unpleasant qualities of painful sensations, first described by Schilder and Stengel in 1938. A patient can distinguish between sensations, e.g., sharp from dull, but shows no response to either pain or threatening gestures while such a response is seen to verbal threats.

The syndrome is strongly associated with lesions of the dominant parietal lobe and may be accompanied by the features of **Gerstmann syndrome.**

asymmetric cortical degenerative syndromes   Dementing disorders with features suggesting only localized cortical involvement, at least in the early stages.[935] See **primary progressive aphasia, frontal lobe dementia, parietal degeneration.**

asymmetric crying facies   (cardiofacial syndrome) Unilateral weakness of the depressor muscles of the lower lip, which only appears in infants when they cry. The sign itself is of small import, except that it may be a marker for other congenital anomalies, usually cardiac.[2219]

Although this is usually considered to represent damage to fibers of the VII cranial nerve, the facts that the weakness is only of the lower quadrant and appears only with emotional movements, and that any other deficits are on the same side of the body as the facial weakness suggest that the original lesion is cerebral.

asymmetric limb weakness with motor conduction block   An acquired syndrome of slowly progressive, asymmetric, multifocal limb weakness with regions of profound, circumscribed motor conduction block in proximal or intermediate limb regions, sparing the extremities, the cranial nerves, and sensory fibers.[3155] See **multifocal motor neuropathy with conduction block.**

asymmetry   1. The unequal amplitude, form, or frequency of EEG activity over homologous areas on opposite sides of the head. 2. The unequal development of EEG waves about the baseline.

asymptomatic carotid bruit   The presence of an audible bruit over a carotid artery in the absence of a history of neurological deficit. The finding suggests that the subject has generalized arteriosclerosis and has a 1% annual risk of stroke (but is at considerably greater risk of myocardial infarction). Detection of such a bruit was once regarded as an indication for carotid endarterectomy rather than cardiac evaluation (a decision analogous to repairing the stable door after the horse has been sold), but conservative management is now more widely advocated unless the carotid stenosis is extreme.[6074]

asymptomatic neurosyphilis   A mild spirochetal meningitis without clinical effect but due to active treponemal invasion, commonly within months of infection and accompanied by an inflammatory reaction and positive reagin tests in the CSF. Untreated, progression to a symptomatic form of neurosyphilis is likely.

asymptomatic polysomographic finding   Features that are recorded during polysomnography but are not the basis of any subjective complaints.[249]

asynchrony   The nonsimultaneous occurrence of EEG activities over regions on the same side or on opposite sides of the head.

asynergia   (asynergy) 1. A disturbance in the normal cooperation of agonists and antagonists, as is supposed to occur with disease of the cerebellum. 2. The inability to perform the various components of a movement at the right time and in the appropriate order or place. See **dyssynergia.**

asynkinesia   A consistent pattern of impairment in the ability to perform two tasks simultaneously with the two hands (e.g., drawing a triangle while squeezing a bulb). The deficit is described in **Parkinson disease.**[802]

atavism   Some strange recurrence to a primitive past; with more resemblance to remote ancestors than to parents (OED). A number of pathological states, e.g., **Down syndrome** and recidivism, were ascribed to atavism until genetic research determined the nature of the former and sociology demonstrated that the latter was explicable without reference to genetics at all. However, as Medawar points out, reappearance of a recessive trait in remote descendants as a manifestation of a recessive gene could be regarded as atavism too.

atavistic speech   See **Worster-Drought-Allen syndrome.**

ataxia   (Gr, without + order; disarranged) (ataxy) A term of Hippocrates, still in general use to characterize incoordination or awkwardness in the performance of a motor task. This may be due to lesions of the motor (including cerebellar) or sensory pathways or to local factors such as arthritis.

When due to impairment of cerebellar function, it is known as *cerebellar ataxia* and when due to loss of proprioceptive information, as *sensory, special sensory,* or *posterior column ataxia.*

In *frontal ataxia* the disorder of movements results from a lesion of the contralateral frontocorticopontine pathway; *parietal ataxia* is better regarded as a form of **apraxia.** *Truncal ataxia* is that form in which sitting and standing stance are mainly affected, due to a lesion of the (midline) archicerebellum. *Gait ataxia* is wide based and staggering; it is due to lesions of the paleocerebellum (vermis and anterior lobe).

See also **cerebellar disease, posterior column ataxia, retinitis pigmentosa.** For quantitation of ataxia, see **Nobile-Orazio Ataxia Scale** and the Web site http://www.ataxia.org.

ataxia and adult-onset dementia   An X-linked syndrome of early-onset ataxia, tremor, and pyramidal signs and slowly progressive dementia with onset in adult life. Optic atrophy and extrapyramidal findings are not part of this syndrome.[1746]

ataxia and albinism   See **cerebellar ataxias** (*variants*).

ataxia and cirrhosis   See **cerebellar ataxias** (*variants*).

ataxia and hypergonadotrophic hypogonadism (of Skre)   See **cerebellar ataxias** (*variants*).

ataxia and other neurological deficits with hyperuricemia   See **cerebellar ataxias** (*variants*).

ataxia, aniridia, and mental retardation   See **cerebellar ataxias** (*variants*).

ataxia, areflexia, and facial diplegia   A variant of **acute inflammatory demyelinating polyneuropathy** in which the seventh cranial nerves are affected bilaterally, the CSF protein is elevated, and ataxia and areflexia are typically found in the virtual absence of limb weakness or significant sensory disturbances. The prognosis for recovery is excellent.[986]

ataxia, areflexia, and ophthalmoplegia   A variant presentation of **acute inflammatory demyelinating polyneuropathy.** See **Miller Fisher syndrome.**

ataxia, cataracts, hemiballismus, and dementia   See **cerebellar ataxias** (*variants*).

ataxia, deaf-mutism, and muscular wasting 1, early onset   See **cerebellar ataxias** (*variants*).

ataxia, deaf-mutism, and muscular wasting 2, late onset   See **cerebellar ataxias** (*variants*).

ataxia, deafness, and leukodystrophy   A progressive familial disorder of early onset with unknown cause.[3365]

ataxia hereditaria   See **Friedreich ataxia.**

ataxia, ichthyosis, and hepatosplenomegaly (of Harper)   See **cerebellar ataxias** (*variants*).

ataxia, juvenile cataract, myopathy, and mental retardation   See **cerebellar ataxias** (*variants*).

ataxia muscularis   see **Thomsen disease.**

ataxia oligophrenia myocardial sclerosis, sensory deafness   See **cerebellar ataxias** (*variants*).

ataxia, photomyoclonus, skeletal deformities   See **cerebellar ataxias** (*variants*).

ataxia, sensory deafness, and optic atrophy   See **cerebellar ataxias** (*variants*).

Ataxia Telangiectasia Children's Project   A charitable organization in this field. Address: 668 South Military Trail, Deerfield Beach, FL 33442-3023. Tel: 954-481-6611; 800-543-5728. E-mail: Info@atcp.org. Web site: http://www.atcp.org.

Ataxia Telangiectasia Medical Research Foundation A charitable organization in this field. Address: 5241 Round Meadow Rd., Hidden Hills, CA 91302 Tel: 818-704-8146. E-mail: becca4435@aol.com.

Ataxia Telangiectasia Project   A charitable organization in this field. Address: 3002 Enfield Rd., Austin, TX 78703. Tel: 512-472-3417. E-mail: A-TProject@austin.rr.com. Web site: http://www.atproject.org.

ataxia-telangiectasia   (Louis-Bar syndrome) A rare, recessively inherited syndrome of neurological deterioration and failure of DNA repair in which there are breaks on chromosome 11 at 11q22–q23. The condition is named for Mme. Louis-Bar, who gave the first complete description.[3480]

The main clinical features are the onset in infancy of progressive cerebellar ataxia (mainly truncal) with dysarthria; telangiectasia of the bulbar conjunctiva and malar areas of the face; progeric changes in the skin and hair; chorea and athetosis; apraxia of eye movements with impaired pursuit, gaze-holding, and convergence; mental retardation; demyelinating sensorimotor neuropathy with hyporeflexia; predisposition to malignancies; recurrent sinopulmonary infections; and hypersensitivity to ionizing radiation.

Increased serum α-fetoprotein, deficiency of immunoglobulins, absent or hypoplastic thymus and T-cell deficiency with impairment of the synthesis of antibodies, and degeneration of the cerebellar cortex, dentate nucleus, inferior olives, and cranial nerve nuclei are other notable characteristics.[1550, 3549, 3751] See also the Web site: http://www.ninds.nih.gov/health_and_medical/disorders/a-t.htm.

Variants include the following:

1. *Ataxia without telangiectasia* An inherited ataxic syndrome with onset in infancy or childhood and also characterized by dysarthria, immunoglobulin deficiency, dementia, dystonia, ophthalmoplegia, athetosis, and neurogenic muscle atrophy.[337]
2. A syndrome of ataxia, choreoathetosis, and horizontal and vertical ocular motor apraxia.[60]

ataxia with downbeat nystagmus   See **cerebellar ataxias** (*variants*).

ataxia with hypogonadism and retinopathy   See **cerebellar ataxias** (*variants*).

ataxia with motor neuron disease   See **cerebellar ataxias** (*variants*).

ataxia with paroxysmal dystonia   See **cerebellar ataxias** (*variants*).

ataxia with sensory neuropathy   A syndrome characterized by the onset in childhood of speech defect/dysarthria, cerebellar signs, and demyelinating sensorimotor neuropathy.

Developmental deformities of the cerebellum, pons, and basal ganglia are also found.[337]

ataxia without telangiectasia   See **ataxia-telangiectasia.**

ataxia-analgia hysterica   (Briquet ataxia) Inability to maintain the upright posture with anesthesia of the skin; a psychogenic disorder described by **Briquet** in 1859.

ataxia-ocular motor apraxia   See **cerebellar ataxias** (*variants*).

ataxia-plus   See **Machado-Joseph disease.**

ataxia–telangiectasia-like   syndrome   (epilepsy-telangiectasia syndrome) A recessively inherited dysmorphic syndrome characterized by conjunctival telangiectasias, brachydactyly, seizures, and mental retardation.

ataxic aphasia   The term of **Lichtheim** for the disconnection syndrome in which the pathway from Broca's area to the motor areas is interrupted, producing nonfluent speech with poor repetition but with preservation of both writing and comprehension. See **Broca aphasia, aphemia.**

ataxic cerebral palsy   See **congenital cerebellar hypoplasia.**

ataxic conjugate movements   See **opsoclonus.**

ataxic diplegia   A congenital syndrome characterized by T-cell deficiency, absence, or hypoplasia of the thymus, spasticity, and ataxia.[337]

ataxic gait   An irregular, lurching, wide-based gait, the steps taken irregularly and of unequal length; falls to the side are common because of impairment of righting reflexes. This form of gait disturbance is accentuated when the subject attempts to walk on a narrow base, as with heel–toe walking.

ataxic hemiparesis   (dysarthria–clumsy hand syndrome, homolateral ataxia and crural paresis) A **lacunar syndrome** in which weakness and cerebellar ataxia occur on the same side of the body, the leg being most affected.

The lesion is in the posterior limb of the internal capsule or in the basis pontis on the side opposite the signs in most cases.[1866, 2191]

ataxic neuropathy   Any form of neuropathy in which the thick fibers subserving proprioception are particularly affected. See **sensory ataxia, chronic sensory gangliopathies.**

ataxic nystagmus   (abduction nystagmus, internuclear ophthalmoplegia). A form of dissociated nystagmus seen in the abducting eye either exclusively or far more than in the other eye, which may fail to adduct normally. See **abduction nystagmus, internuclear ophthalmoplegia, saccadic pulses.**

ataxic paramyotonia   (Gr, beside + a muscle + a stretching) (paramyotonia) An acquired nervous disease characterized by tonic spasms in certain muscle groups associated with ataxia and both sensory and motor deficits, described by **Gowers.**

ataxic syndromes   Inherited or acquired conditions characterized by the appearance of limb or truncal ataxia, nystagmus, and other signs of cerebellar and other neurological impairment at varying stages of life. The biochemical causes of the several conditions are not completely known and the group may be regarded as a set of variants of the forms of inherited **cerebellar ataxias** listed elsewhere, to which group some of these possibly belong.

ataxic tremor   See **cerebellar tremors.**

ataxic tropical neuropathy   A diffuse affection of the CNS producing optic atrophy and sensory ataxia as a result of chronic cyanide poisoning from the excessive consumption of cassava root, seen in Central and West African countries. See **Nigerian neuropathy.**[2362]

ataxy   See **ataxia, cerebellar ataxia.**

atelencephaly   A congenital dysmorphic syndrome characterized by microcephaly, hydranencephaly or porencephaly, hydrocephalus, and cerebral atrophy.[337]

ateliosis   (from Gr, incompleteness + a state) Dwarfism with incomplete development of all body organs (as in the Lorain-Levi syndrome); a term introduced by Gilford in 1902 but which has not been much employed.

atelo-   (Gr, imperfect development of) Prefix connoting maldevelopment, thus *ateloencephalia, atelomyelia,* and *atelostomia* indicate imperfect development of the brain, the spine, or the mouth, respectively.

atherothrombotic brain infarction   Cerebral infarction due to occlusion of a supplying vessel that is the site of atherosclerosis.

Diagnostic criteria include the following:

1. The rapid onset and persistence for over 24 hours of focal neurological symptoms or signs such as uni- or binocular visual loss; dysphasia or dysarthria; symptoms of bulbar paresis; uni- or bilateral paresis; uni- or bilateral sensory impairment; disturbance in the level of consciousness, *and*
2. Stenosis or obstruction of a carotid or vertebral artery or a major branch thereof shown by some form of angiography; *or* abnormal uptake of tracer elements consistent with infarction on radionucleide brain scan or SPECT scan; *or* focal abnormality consistent with infarction on CT or MRI scan.

athetoid cerebral palsy   See **athetoid syndrome.**

athetoid syndrome   (double athetosis, infantile partial striatal sclerosis, little disease with involuntary movements, distal dystonia) A nonprogressive but evolving form of **cerebral palsy** caused by damage to the basal ganglia of the full-term brain, and characterized by impairment of postural reflexes, arrhythmic involuntary movements, and dysarthria, with sparing of sensation, ocular movements, and often intelligence.

Affected children thus cannot sit, cannot move at will, and cannot talk, but yet take everything in.[1900] Intranatal asphyxia or neonatal jaundice are the usual etiologies and marbling of the basal ganglia (**état marbré**) is the typical pathology.

A *variant* is BD MCA (athetoid cerebral palsy), a congenital dysmorphic syndrome characterized by microphthalmia, colobomas of the iris, blue sclera, breast and skeletal anomalies, microcephaly, pyramidal and extrapyramidal signs, and mental and developmental delay.[337]

athétose double   (Fr, bilateral athetosis) A severe form of cerebral palsy manifesting with bilateral athetosis and profound mental delay, described by Paul Oulmont.[7]

athetosis   (Gr, lack of + a fixed place; thus, without a fixed position) (Hammond disease) An involuntary movement disorder characterized by irregular, forceful, slow, writhing movements generally of the extremities, very often with finger movements and with co-contraction of agonists and antagonists. Primary and secondary causes are recognized.[2408, 6038]

Both negative and positive phenomena have been described as costituting the clinical features. The *negative phenomena* include impairment of postural reactions, dysarthria, and early paresis of upward gaze. The *positive phenomena* comprise athetotic involuntary movements (a release of anticipatory postural reactions) and the athetoid "dance on hot bricks," dysphagia, and snorting, which witness athetosis of the bulbar muscles.

In certain syndromes in which athetosis is the dominant feature, other phenomena such as **intention tremors** and signs witnessing the release of brainstem and other primitive reflexes (an overactive bite reflex and **Moro response,** extension spasms, asymmetrical **tonic neck reflexes,** eye-avoiding and face-avoiding reactions) also may emerge.[1900]

The condition was described and named by William **Hammond** in 1871[2408] but had previously been known (as *morbus sacer*). Hammond was incorrect in maintaining that the movements persist in sleep, as they do not. Sir Victor **Horsley** showed in 1909 that excision of the precentral cortex relieved or abolished the movements.[2659]

In 1911 the Vogts defined *double athetosis* (bilateral athetosis) as a pure striatal syndrome, the clinical correlate of the **état marbré,** which they also distinguished. See also **athetoid syndrome, spinal pseudoathetosis.**

athrodynia à potu   See **alcoholic neuropathy.**

athymhormia   Loss of self-psychic activation, or a lack of motivation, with apathy, aspontaneity, and loss of motor and affective drive but without suffering or cognitive impairment. The cause is usually bilateral infarcts in the region of the centrum semiovale.[912]

Atkin oculo-cerebro-acral syndrome   An X-linked congenital dysmorphic syndrome characterized by seizures, skeletal, ocular, cardiac, and renal malformations, delayed closure of fontanelles, and cerebellar atrophy with the Dandy-Walker malformation with macrocephaly and mental and developmental delay.[255]

atlantoaxial dislocation   Abnormal congenital or acquired mobility between **atlas** and **axis** as a result of absence or nonfusion of the odontoid peg, or of abnormal laxity of the ligament binding the odontoid to the anterior arch of the atlas.[5282]

Such forward displacement of the atlas may occur as a result of trauma or as a congenital anomaly (as in **Down syndrome**). The narrowing of the spinal canal may lead to chronic compressive or ischemic myelopathy affecting the posterior columns and pyramidal tracts most severely and leading to extensive degeneration of anterior horn cells throughout the cervical cord.

Clinically, affected people complain of neck pain, stiffness, and both static and progressive symptoms which mainly indicate damage to the upper motor neuron in the spinal cord, with less evidence of lower motor neuron or posterior column involvement. Cranial nerve palsies are not a feature. The dislocation may be congenital in Asian people.[5795]

Three forms are defined:
1. Occipitalization of the atlas with fusion of the second and third cervical vertebrae, posterior dislocation of the odontoid, and cord compression as a result of maldevelopment of the transverse ligament
2. Maldevelopment of the odontoid process only
3. Dislocation of the odontoid only during flexion of the neck

atlanto-dens interval   The separation of the first and second cervical vertebrae, normally less than 5 mm. A greater separation suggests the presence of atlantoaxial dislocation.

atlas   The first cervical vertebra, carrying the weight of the head. It is named for the Greek mythological figure who was changed by Perseus into stone—the Atlas mountain that was so lofty that it was considered to hold up the sky. A variation of the myth, more relevant to the function of the vertebra under discussion, has Atlas supporting variously the pillars of heaven or the earth upon his shoulders (hence the name for a book of maps), which led Vesalius to name the vertebra so.

atonia-astasia   See **Foerster atonic diplegia.**[2764]

atonic absences   Atypical absences accompanied by loss of postural tone. See **atonic seizures.**

atonic cerebral diplegia   A congenital "cerebral palsy" syndrome comprising flaccid weakness with marked delay in the attainment of motor milestones, severe mental defect, and absent or rudimentary speech. Microcephaly, seizures, and congenital heart disease may also be associated.[1518]

atonic seizures   (atonic absences) Epileptic syndromes characterized by the sudden loss of motor power and leading to sudden falls or slumping of all or part of the body and accompanied on EEG by slow spike–waves, 3-Hz spike–waves, polyspike and waves, or fast recruiting rhythms, and on EMG by suppression of normal tonic activity in the involved muscles.[56]

atonic-sclerotic muscular dystrophy   See **congenital muscular dystrophy.**

atremia   See **akinesia algera.**

atrophia myotonica   See **myotonic dystrophy.**

atrophy   (Gr, Negative + to nourish) Emaciation or wasting, usually of muscles, and most often accompanied by loss of strength.

Progressive muscular atrophy is a term for **amyotrophic lateral sclerosis.**

attack (of multiple sclerosis)   The occurrence of a symptom or symptoms of neurological dysfunction in the setting of multiple sclerosis, with or without objective confirmation, and lasting more than 24 hours.[4504]

attention   The complex capacity for focusing upon one of a number of competing sensory stimuli or for maintaining readiness to record specific stimuli, without being distracted by others that are extraneous.

Orientation, exploration, concentration, motivation and vigilance are prerequisites for, or aspects of, this capacity, while attention itself is the major prerequisite for intellectual, reflective and meaningful motor activity. The faculty is particularly likely to be disturbed when a lesion affects the frontal lobe.[3851] Useful tests include the Trailmaking test and tests of cancellation, reversal of digits, and serial-seven subtractions.

The processes underlying attention include *Tonic Attention*, which requires mechanisms regulating the span or efficiency of vigilance, and *Selective Attention*, which determines its object.

attention-deficit/hyperactivity disorder   (ADHD) A condition predominantly seen in childhood in which the patient manifests stimulus-oriented behavior, distractibility, shortened attention span, lack of tolerance of frustration, and lack of fear.[1548]

Lack of investment of organization and maintenance of attention and effort in completing tasks; inability to inhibit impulsive responses; lack of modulation of arousal levels to meet the demands of the situation; and unusually strong inclination to seek immediate gratification are considered the primary deficits.[3, 1504] The cause is unknown.

Diagnostic criteria for attention deficit hyperactivity disorder have been defined, as follows:[150]

A. Either 1 or 2 are present:
1. Six or more of the following symptoms of inattention have persisted for at least 6 months to a degree that is maladaptive and inconsistent with developmental level:
   a. Often fails to give close attention to details or makes careless mistakes in schoolwork, work, or other activities
   b. Often has difficulty sustaining attention in tasks or play activities
   c. Often does not seem to Iisten when spoken to directly
   d. Often does not follow through on instructions and fails to finish schoolwork, chores, or duties in the workplace (not due to oppositional behavior or failure to understand instructions)
   e. Often has difficulty organizing tasks and activities
   f. Often avoids, dislikes, or is reluctant to engage in tasks that require sustained mental effort (such as schoolwork or homework)
   g. Often loses things necessary for tasks or activities (toys, school assignments, pencils, books, or tools)
   h. Is often easily distracted by extraneous stimuli
   i. Is often forgetful in daily activities
2. Six or more of the following symptoms of *hyperactivity–impulsivity* have persisted for at least 6 months to a degree that is maladaptive and inconsistent with developmental level:

Hyperactivity
   a. Often fidgets with hands or feel or squirms in seat
   b. Often leaves seat in classroom or in other situations in which remaining seated is expected
   c. Often runs about or climbs excessively in situations in which it is inappropriate (in adolescents or adults, may be limited to subjective feelings of restlessness)
   d. Often has difficulty playing or engaging in leisure activities quietly
   e. Is often "on the go" or often acts as if "driven by a motor"
   f. Often talks excessively

Impulsivity
   g. Often blurts out answers before questions have been completed
   h. Often has difficulty awaiting turn
   i. Often interrupts or intrudes on others (such as butting Into conversations or games)

B. Some hyperactive, impulsive, or inattentive symptoms that caused impairment were present before age 7 years.
C. Some impairment from the symptoms is present in two or more settings (such as in school or work and at home).
D. There must be clear evidence of clinically significant impairment in social, academic, or occupational functioning.
E. The symptoms do not occur exclusively during the course of a pervasive developmental disorder, schizophrenia, or another psychotic disorder and are not better accounted for by another mental disorder (such as a mood, anxiety, dissociative, or personality disorder).

Diagnosis
   ADHD, predominantly inattentive type: Meets inattention criteria only (section A1) for the last 6 months
   ADHD, predominantly hyperactive–impulsive type: Meets hyperactive–impulsive criteria only (section A2) for the last 6 months
   ADHD, combined type: Meets criteria in sections A1 and A2 for the last 6 months

Adapted slightly and reprinted by kind permission of the American Psychiatric Association Washington, DC, without fee from the *Diagnostic and Statistical Manual of Mental Disorders, Fourth Edition, Text Revision. Copyright 2000.*

attenuation   1. Reduction in amplitude of EEG activity. This may occur transiently in response to physiological or other stimuli, such as electrical stimulation of the brain, or can result from pathological conditions. Cf. **blocking.** 2. Reduction of sensitivity of an EEG channel, i.e., decrease in output pen deflection by operation of the sensitivity or filter controls. It is customarily expressed as relative reduction of sensitivity at certain stated frequencies. (Adapted from the 1974 Report of the Committee on Terminology, IFCN[989] © 1974. With permission from Elsevier Science.) 3. Decrease in any neurological phenomenon induced by some extrinsic factor.

attitude en chien de fusil   The French term for that posture of rigid trunk extension and maximal flexion of the hips and knees (resembling that of a gundog keeping down) adopted by patients with severe meningeal irritation.

atypical absences   Absence seizures unassociated with the typical 3-Hz spike–wave pattern and marked clinically by a brief period of immobility with staring, decreased responsiveness, and, on the EEG, bursts of diffuse and often asymmetrically slow spike–waves at rates of up to 2.5 Hz or the various EEG patterns associated with tonic seizures.[56] The attacks have slower onset and termination and tend to occur more often and for longer than typical absence attacks. In some cases, motor activity is retained during the seizure.[1137]

atypical Alzheimer disease   See **congophilic angiopathy.**

atypical bobbing   See **reverse ocular bobbing.**

atypical cluster headache   A dubious entity, in which otherwise typical cluster headaches are accompanied by interparoxysmal changes in the EEG and by episodes of retrobulbar neuritis.

atypical facial pain   A facial pain syndrome without overt cause and usually associated with psychiatric disturbances, particularly depression. It occurs mainly in women after the age of 40 and is described as boring or burning and persistent, ill localized, and sometimes affecting both sides of the face.

The syndrome (*facial pain not fulfilling criteria in groups 11 and 12*) has been defined by the International

Headache Society Classification Committee[1051] as follows (amended and reproduced by kind permission): persistent facial pain that does not have the characteristics of the cranial neuralgias (classified elsewhere) and which is not associated with physical signs or a demonstrable organic cause.

A. The pain is present daily and persists for most or all of the day.

B. It is confined at onset to a limited area on one side of the face but may spread to the upper or lower jaws or to a wider area of the face or neck. It is deep and poorly localized.

C. The pain is not associated with sensory loss or other physical signs.

D. Laboratory investigations including X-ray of face and jaws do not demonstrate any relevant abnormality.

Atypical trigeminal neuralgia exhibits both episodic, lancinating unilateral facial pains with shock-free intervals and variable-intensity but constant unilateral facial pain, thus combining features of both classical trigeminal neuralgia and trigeminal neuropathy.

atypical myopathy with myofibrillar aggregates See **myofibrillar myopathy.**

atypical neurologic disease syndrome Assorted symptom complexes experienced initially by women after the surgical insertion of bags containing silicone in submammary regions, but more recently following other traumatic life events, such as participation in military conflict, and characterized by multiple apparent rheumatological or neurological complaints without accompanying clinical or laboratory abnormalities. Fatigue, myalgias, memory problems, blurred vision, numbness, impaired balance, etc. are the usual presentations. See also **silicone encephalopathy.**

A learned judgment delivered in an Alabama (U.S.) court appears to have taken responsibility for defining medical criteria for nonmedical (or at least nonorganic) disorders; these are reproduced here with some editing but without critical comment, in order to save this author from having to invoke the First Amendment.

1. A diagnosis of atypical neurological disease syndrome (ANDS) shall be based on the clinical findings and laboratory tests set forth below. The clinical and laboratory presentation of these neurologic syndromes will have an atypical presentation from the natural disease and will also have additional neuromuscular, rheumatic, or nonspecific autoimmune signs and symptoms.

2. Eligibility for ANDS requires both:
   Satisfying the requirements for one of the four neurologic disease types set forth in paragraph 5 below, and
   Any three additional (nonduplicative) neuromuscular, rheumatic, or nonspecific symptoms or findings set forth in the definition for atypical connective tissue disease (ACTD).

3. An individual will fit into this category if her primary symptoms are characteristic of a neurologic disease as diagnosed by a Board-certified neurologist or by a physician Board certified in internal medicine.

4. If the individual's qualified medical doctor determines that a symptom is clearly and specifically caused by a source other than breast implants, that symptom will not be utilized in the diagnosis of ANDS unless the Claims Office determines that other submissions indicate that the symptom should be utilized. A symptom that may be caused only in part by a source other than breast implants is not excluded from such utilization.

5. Neurological disease types:

Polyneuropathies. This disease category requires a diagnosis of polyneuropathy that is confirmed by one or more of the following:

• Objectively demonstrated loss of sensation to pinprick, vibration, touch, or position
• Proximal or distal muscle weakness
• Tingling and/or burning pain in the extremities
• Signs of dysesthesia
• Loss of tendon reflex
• Plus one or more of the following laboratory findings:
• Abnormal levels of anti-mag or anti-sulfatide or anti-GM_1 antibodies
• Abnormal sural nerve biopsy
• Abnormal electrodiagnostic testing (EMG or nerve conduction studies, etc.)

Multiple sclerosis-like syndrome. This disease category requires definite evidence of CNS disease, with a history and physical findings compatible with multiple sclerosis or multiple sclerosis–like syndrome, involving one or more of the following signs and symptoms:

• Weakness in the pyramidal distribution
• Evidence of optic neuritis documented by an ophthalmologist
• Increased deep tendon reflexes
• Absent superficial abdominal reflexes
• Ataxia or dysdiadochokinesia as the sign of cerebellar involvement
• Neurologically induced tremors
• Internuclear ophthalmoplegia and/or bladder or speech involvement secondary to CNS disease

Plus one or more of the following:

• Abnormal brain MRI with foci of increased signal abnormality suggestive of demyelinating lesions
• Delayed visual-evoked responses or abnormal-evoked potentials
• Abnormal CSF with oligoclonal bands

Amyotrophic lateral sclerosis-like syndrome. This disease category requires documented evidence of progressive upper and widespread lower motor neuron involvement, plus one or more of the following:

• Neurologic autoantibodies such as anti-mag, anti-sulfatide, and anti-GM_1
• Abnormal sural nerve biopsy
• Chronic inflammation on muscle or nerve biopsies
• Abnormal EMG
• Documentation on neurologic examination of both upper and lower motor neuron disease and/or bulbar involvement

Disease of neuromuscular junction. This disease category requires a diagnosis of myasthenia gravis or myasthenia gravis–like syndrome or disorders of the neuromuscular junction made by a Board-certified neurologist and confirmed by abnormal EMG showing typical findings of decrement on repetitive stimulation testing and/or elevated acetylcholine receptor antibodies.

atypical ocular bobbing See **reverse ocular bobbing.**

atypical parkinsonism Syndromes resembling **Parkinson disease** in which there occur early involvement of speech, gait, or balance; relative paucity of tremor; symmetrical involvement; increased axial rather than limb tone; and poor response to levadopa treatment. MRI scans may show increased T2 signal intensities in the putamen and caudate, perhaps reflecting the accumulation of iron in those sites. Two major groups are defined: **progressive supranuclear palsy** and **multiple system degeneration,** the latter encompassing **striatonigral degeneration, Shy-Drager syndrome,** and **olivopontocerebellar atrophy. See also corticobasal degeneration.**

atypical partial benign epilepsy of childhood An epileptic syndrome in which the onset is between 2 and 6 years of age in children with previously normal development and examination. They display at least two different seizure types, including partial nocturnal seizures, generalized atonic clonic seizures, brief absences, massive myoclonic jerks, and atonic seizures occurring in clusters lasting up to a month and separated by free intervals of several months' duration. The EEG shows intense diffuse slow spike–wave activity during slow-wave sleep in these periods. Focal spikes and central regions are recorded in the awake state. Atonic seizures and mental deterioration do not occur and the disease appears to remit before the age of 9 years.[56]

atypical rapid spike–wave activity See **irregular generalized spike–wave activity.**

atypical repetitive spike-and-slow-waves A term referring to paroxysms consisting of a sequence of spike-and-slow-wave complexes which occur bilaterally and synchronously but do not meet one or more of the criteria of 3-Hz spike-and-slow-waves. (Adapted from the 1974 Report of the Committee on Terminology, IFCN,[989] © 1974. With permission from Elsevier Science.)

atypical sensory syndrome A pattern of sensory loss involving all sensations, but only in isolated parts of the body, and occurring with variously sited infarcts of a parietal lobe.[383] See also **parietal stroke.**

atypical teratoma See **dysgerminoma, germinoma.**

atz See **wolfing reflex.**

audiogenic epilepsy See **musciogenic epilepsy.**

audiokinetic nystagmus A form of jerk nystagmus induced in darkness by a loud noise, the source of which rotates around the subject.

audiometry Techniques for the quantitative measurement of auditory acuity. See also **Bekesy audiometry.**

audiospinal reaction Brief (startle-like) muscle contraction of the trunk and limbs in response to an unexpected, loud auditory stimulus. The response can be quantitated by examining the facilitation of the **H reflex** that it induces.[1373]

auditory affective agnosia Impairment in the comprehension of affective speech, as opposed to propositional speech; this may occur in subjects with right hemisphere dysfunction and a neglect syndrome.[2518]

auditory agnosia A disorder of recognition of sounds in a subject with normal hearing, alertness, and intelligence. Both *verbal* (inability to interpret spoken language) and *nonverbal types* (inability to interpret nonverbal sounds) occur[2518] the former is due to bilateral lesions of the auditory cortex, the latter to a similar lesion on the right side. See also **cortical deafness.**

auditory evoked potential Electric waveforms of biologic origin elicited in response to sound stimuli, classified by their latency as short-latency brainstem auditory evoked potential (BAEP) with a latency of up to 10 msec, middle-latency with a latency of 10 to 50 msec, and long-latency with a latency of over 50 msec. See **brainstem auditory evoked potential.** (From the 2001 Report of the Nomenclature Committee of the American Association of Electromyography and Electrodiagnosis.[10] Used by permission, copyright © 2001, AAEM.)

auditory imperception (word deafness) Failure of patients to comprehend the meaning of what they hear although they know well that the sounds represent speech.[828, 4694] See **word deafness.**

auditory neuropathy An acquired or hereditary condition still under study, characterized by hearing deficits (especially for speech), normal cochlear function; and abnormal brainstem auditory evoked potentials.[5323]

auditory receptive dysphasia See **Wernicke aphasia.**

Auditory Verbal Learning Test A memory test, requiring the subject to learn 15 nouns in five trials, recalling them 20 minutes later, after which a recognition test is given.[5715]

auditory vertigo Illusory physiological sensations of movement of the self (with audiokinetic nystagmus) induced by moving sound fields.[727]

auditory-oculogyric reflex Immediate turning of the head and eyes in the direction of an unexpected, sudden, and loud noise. This cochlear reflex was once invoked as a test for hysterical deafness.[4723]

auditory-palpebral reflex (cochleopalpebral reflex) Immediate blinking in response to a sudden, loud, and unexpected sound.[4723] See **palpebral reflex.**

Auerbach, Leopold (1828–1897) German anatomist and neuropathologist, of Breslau.

Auerbach's plexus (myenteric plexus) The autonomic plexus between the circular and the longitudinal coats of the intestinal wall described by Auerbach in 1862.[2995]

augmentation An increase in the amplitude of recorded electrical activity.

Aujesky, Aladar (1869–1933) Hungarian pathologist, working in Budapest, who described the "scratching pest."

aura (Gr, a soft breath of wind) 1. The events comprising that part of an epileptic seizure which a subject can recall afterwards. The classical form, known to Aretaeus of Cappadocia and to Galen, was the **epigastric aura** ". . . as if a blast of cold air ascended from the lowest parts toward the heart and head."[5204] 2. Reversible neurological symptoms that may precede, accompany, or follow the pain phase of a migraine.

aural vertigo See **Ménière syndrome.**

auricular myoclonus Repetitive, intermittent, or constant clonic movements of the antitragicus muscle at rates of up to 70 Hz, suppressed only by strong contraction of the limbs, as a result of excessive irritability of the facial nerve of unknown cause.[3059]

auriculotemporal neuralgia See **superior laryngeal neuralgia.**

auriculotemporal syndrome (gustatory sweating, chorda tympani syndrome) Flushing and sweating of one side of the face during mastication, particularly when eating highly spiced foods, as a result of abnormal regeneration of the terminal axons of parasympathetic fibers following damage to the auriculotemporal nerve, a branch of the mandibular.[1953] See **Frey syndrome.**

auscultatory percussion A technique designed to detect intracranial mass lesions. The examiner percusses the frontal bone in the midline while listening with a stethoscope applied successively to different parts of the scalp; reduction in perceived sound intensity is claimed to indicate the presence of an intracranial mass between the site of tapping and the area of reduced sound transmission.[2298]

Austin disease See **multiple sulfatase deficiency.**

Austin fluff test A screening test for the detection of metachromatic lipids.[267]

Austin variant See **metachromatic leukodystrophy.**

Australian X disease See **Murray Valley encephalitis.**

Austregesilo, Antonio (1876–1956?) Brazilian neurologist and psychiatrist, who was professor of clinical medicine and then of neurology in Rio de Janeiro. He described epidemic neuromyelitis following an epidemic in 1931 and wrote particularly on tropical neurology, extrapyramidal disorders, and Schilder disease, and in addition the elicitation of the Babinski response

by stimulation of the thigh, recognizing this as being due to spread of the receptive area for the reflex.

autism The term of Bleuler for that form of psychosis in which the individual is "divorced from reality." The word is used now, after Kanner, for a long-life, static developmental disorder with a genetic basis, comprising a spectrum of biological or organic childhood psychoses (infantile autism or autistic disorder) which may be postencephalitic (*autism with polioencephalopathy*), schizophrenic, or, probably very commonly, due to central agnosias. Lesions that are bilateral, cortical, and subcortical and that affect the mesolimbic structures are considered most likely to be responsible.

Clinical manifestations include profound impairment in social relationships, severe developmental disturbances of verbal and nonverbal communication, ritualistic and compulsive behavior, and disturbances of motility and of attention. Perseveration, concreteness of thought, affective blunting, and lack of insight into the thinking of others are usual features. Seizures and cognitive disturbances may also be present,[1359, 1372] as may any of a range of defined neurological conditions such as chromosomal abnormalities, **Rett syndrome, phenylketonuria,** etc.[58] See also **Asperger syndrome**

The DSM-IV TR criteria for diagnosis of 299.00 *Autistic Disorder* are as follows:[150]

A. A total of six (or more) items from (1), (2), and (3), with two from (1), and at least one each from (2) and (3):

1. Qualitative impairment in social interaction, manifest by at least two of the following:

Marked impairment in the use of multiple nonverbal behaviors, such as eye-to-eye gaze, facial expression, body postures, and gestures, to regulate social interaction

Failure to develop peer relationships appropriate to developmental level

Lack of spontaneous seeking to share enjoyment, interests, or achievements with other people (e.g., by lack of showing, bringing, or pointing out objects of interest)

Lack of social or emotional reciprocity

2. Qualitative impairment in communication, as manifest by at least one of the following:

Delay in, or total lack of, the development of spoken language (not accompanied by an attempt to compensate through alternative modes of communication such as gesture or mime)

In individuals with adequate speech, marked impairment in the ability to initiate or sustain a conversation with others

Stereotyped and repetitive use of language, or idiosyncratic language

Lack of varied, spontaneous make-believe, or social imitative play appropriate to developmental level

3. Restrictive repetitive and stereotypic patterns of behavior, interests, and activities, as manifested by at least one of the following:

Encompassing preoccupation with one or more stereotyped and restricted patterns of interest that is abnormal either in intensity or focus

Apparently inflexible adherence to specific nonfunctional routines or rituals

Stereotyped and repetitive motor mannerisms (e.g., hand or finger flapping or twisting, or complex whole-body movements)

Persistent preoccupation with parts of objects

B. Delays or abnormal functioning in at least one of the following areas, with onset prior to age 3 years:

1. Social interaction
2. Language as used in social communication
3. Symbolic or imaginative play

C. The disturbance is not better accounted for by Rett's disorder or childhood disintegrative disorder.

The other pervasive developmental disorders include Asperger's disorder, Rett syndrome, childhood disintegrative disorder, pervasive developmental disorder–not otherwise specified (PDD-NOS), or atypical autism.

(Reprinted from the Diagnostic and Statistical Manual of Mental Disorders, Fourth Edition, Text Revision V, without fee, by kind permission of the American Psychiatric Association, Washington, DC. Copyright 2000.)

A practice guideline for screening and diagnosis has been developed by the American Academy of Neurology.[1814]

Autism Network International (ANI) A charitable organization in this field. Address: P.O. Box 35448, Syracuse, NY 13235-5448. E-mail: jisincla@mailbox. syr.edu. Web site: http://www.ani.ac.

Autism Society of America A charitable organization in this field. Address: 7910 Woodmont Ave., Suite 300, Bethesda, MD 20814-3067. Tel: 301-657-0881; 800-328-8476. E-mail: info@autism-society.org. Web site: http://www.autism-society.org.

Autism Society of Canada 129 Yorkville Ave., Ste 202, Toronto, Ontario, M5R 1C4 Canada. Tel: 416-922-0302; fax: 416-922-1032. Web site: http://autismsocietycanada.ca.

autism with polioencephalopathy See **autism.**

autochthonous Proceeding from within the self, as opposed to being triggered by external stimuli. The term is usually used in the descriptions of forms of delusional activity.

autoecholalia See **palilalia.**

autolysis Enzymatic autodigestion of cells in which there is initially clumping of the chromatin, swelling of mitochondria, and dispersion of ribosomes. The process is typified by the changes occurring in the brain when it remains warm and unfixed after death.

automatic behavior syndrome The frequent occurrence of complex automatisms lasting seconds to hours and involving activities not requiring great learned skill, during a state of altered consciousness due to repetitive microsleeps, a state that is facilitated by performing repetitive or boring tasks such as long drives inducing drowsiness. There is amnesia for events occurring during the episode, which occurs in patients with **narcolepsy** and other causes of **excessive daytime sleepiness.**[2321]

automatic bladder Reflex contraction of the bladder wall with relaxation of its sphincter, in response to increased distension pressure, occurring when the bladder has lost its upper motor neuron or lower motor neuron innervation. As a result, normal cortical inhibition is impossible and the bladder discharges, usually with low volumes of urine contained therein, as a result of its own inherent response to stretch of the detrusor. Such automatic expulsion of the contents of the bladder occurs some 25 days after complete division of the spinal cord, when the bladder contents reach a certain amount. At this time, the sphincter relaxes and urine is passed involuntarily.

Automatic micturition may be facilitated by any afferent stimulus passing into the lower part of the cord, especially if it evokes a flexor spasm, or by deep breathing. Generalized sweating due to activity of the nervous system below the level of the lesion may accompany the bladder contraction.

In a different form in which there is a lower motor neuron lesion as a result of damage to the cauda equina or conus medullaris, contractions occur initially but later distension or infection leads to damage to the stretch receptors in the bladder wall, and overdistension occurs with dribbling incontinence. In a third form, following complete division of the spinal cord above L5, the reflex is intact but detrusor contraction occurs in response to stretch without inhibition from higher levels.[2499]

automatic decomposition EMG (ADEMG) A computerized method for extracting individual motor unit action potentials from an interference pattern. (From the 2001 Report of the Nomenclature Committee of the American Association of Electromyography and Electrodiagnosis.[10] Used by permission, copyright © 2001, AAEM.)

automatic language Overlearned sequences of speech (such as numbers or the alphabet) and emotional speech such as expletives.

automatism 1. More-or-less coordinated and adapted involuntary activity that would be purposeful if the subject were aware of it, occurring during a state of clouding of consciousness, either in the course of or after an epileptic seizure and usually followed by amnesia for the event.[1073, 2776] 2. Behavioral sequences that unfold without voluntary control and usually with loss or impairment of awareness, as components of **complex partial,** prolonged absence, or other types of seizures, or postictally. In a few cases consciousness is retained during the performance of the automatic movement.[3813] See also **affective-psychic seizures.**

autonomic (Gr, self + law, hence self-governing or automatic) The term **autonomic nervous system** was suggested by **Langley** for the sympathetic and parasympathetic systems in about 1898.

autonomic diencephalic epilepsy   Unusual seizures, manifestations of which include apnea, stridor, laryngospasm, chest pain, and cardiac arrhythmias. See **Penfield syndrome.**

Autonomic Disorders Association   A charitable organization. Address: Sarah Matheson Trust, Pickering Unit, St. Mary's Hospital, Praed Street, London W2 1 NY, UK. Tel: 0171-886-1520. Web site: http://www. edinburgh.gov.uk/HEBS/UKHealthAdviceGroups/ ukhealthadvicegroupsautonomicdisordersassociation-saramathesontrustAdasmt.html.

autonomic dysfunction syndrome   See **diencephalic autonomic seizures.**

autonomic dysreflexia   (autonomic hyperreflexia) The occurrence of paroxysmal hypertensive episodes, headache, sweating, and bradycardia in response to nonspecific stimuli such as bladder distension or pain below the level of a spinal cord lesion and due to disconnection of spinal sympathetic centers from supraspinal control. See **Head-Riddoch syndrome.**

autonomic function tests   Measurements of end-organ responsiveness to the activation of neural reflex arcs, reflecting autonomic function. The noninvasive tests in more general use[4610] include the following:

Sympathetic Division

1. One drop of 4%–10% cocaine dilates the pupil if the postganglionic sympathetic activity is intact but will not have this effect if there is a lesion of the sympathetic pathway at any site. Cocaine blocks the reuptake of adrenaline from the synaptic cleft.

2. One drop of 0.1% (1 in 1000) adrenaline has no effect on a normal pupil but causes dilatation when there is postganglionic failure due to denervation supersensitivity.

3. One drop of 1% hydroxyamphetamine (Paredrine) dilates the normal pupil by releasing noradrenaline from the nerve ending into the synaptic cleft; absence of dilation signifies a lesion of the third neurone. Dilation lag occurs when the active dilation of the pupil is because of lack of sympathetic activity.

4. Postural hypotension. A fall in blood pressure of more than 30 mmHg systolic and more than 20 mmHg diastolic on standing for 2 minutes is abnormal; but if the heart rate increases, this may be evidence of reduced blood volume. The arm must be extended horizontally during the test. Orthostatic stress tests may accentuate abnormalities; have the patient do 12 squats (or take sublingual glyceryl trinitrite) and then repeat the blood pressure recording.

5. Isometric exercise (sustained handgrip) should increase systolic and diastolic blood pressures by 15 mmHg; heart rate and cardiac output also increase.[1723]

6. **Cold pressor test.** The hand is immersed in ice water for 1 minute, as a result of which the blood pressure should rise by 20/15 mmHg.

7. **Thermoregulatory sweat test.** The naked patient is heated by more than 1°C, and that area of the skin painted with alizarin-red which has changed color is measured. This test assesses the postganglionic sympathetic (cholinergic) activity.[3486] Quinizarin[1453,2342] was formerly used.

8. Supine noradrenaline and vanillylmandelic acid levels provide information about net postganglionic adrenergic activity. With preganglionic lesions, supine noradrenaline levels are normal but there will be no response to standing.

9. **Psychogalvanic response.** This test assesses a polysynaptic, postganglionic somatosympathetic reflex pathway, skin voltage changing in response to emotion, an electrical shock, or an inspiratory gasp.[3487]

10. **Quantitative sudomotor axon reflex test** (Q-SART). A 10% solution of acetylcholine is iontophoresed into the skin of the proximal foot and medial forearm for 10 mA-minutes. This will produce sweating within 1–2 minutes in preganglionic but not in postganglionic sympathetic disorders.

11. Intradermal acetylcholine injection leads normally to a sweating response. This test and the preceding test assess postganglionic sympathetic sudomotor function.[147, 1697]

12. Silastic imprint. Pilocarpine iontophoresis over skin covered with silastic, which is marked by each sweat droplet.[3007]

13. Skin vasomotor reflexes. In this test, the skin blood flow is measured by a laser Doppler flowmeter in the toe or finger pads. The stimulus employed may be an inspiratory gasp, contralateral cold stimulation, the response to standing, or the Valsalva maneuver.[3485]

14. **Venoarteriolar reflex.** A local axon reflex, relying on postganglionic sympathetic C-fiber activity which normally increases total peripheral resistance. Reflex arteriolar constriction should reduce the blood flow by half in response to a rise in venous transmural pressure of more than 25 mmHg, as by lowering the leg 40 cm.

15. Baroreflex activity. The alteration in heart rate with sudden or sustained changes in blood pressure is assessed.[3486]

Parasympathetic Division

1. One drop of 2.5% methacholine or 0.125% pilocarpine has no effect on a normal pupil but constricts one with pre- or postganglionic parasympathetic denervation (supersensitivity again).

2. **Sinus arrhythmia.** Beat-to-beat variation during respiration depends on cardiac parasympathetic activity. Normally, the heart beats faster (so the R-R interval shortens) towards the end of inspiration, and beats slower (the R-R interval lengthens) towards the end of expiration. With normal vagal activity, the ECG recorded at six respirations per minute should demonstrate differences of 15 beats per minute (bpm) between inspiration and expiration. A change of less than 10 bpm suggests abnormal vagal activity.

3. **E:I ratio.** The mean of the longest R-R interval during expiration divided by the mean of the shortest R-R interval during inspiration should be more than 1.2 in patients aged less than 40 years. The test is a modified way of expressing the beat-to-beat variation in heart rate with simple breathing.

4. **30:15 ratio.** The ratio of the R-R intervals at the 30th and the 15th beats after rising to a standing position from a lying position. A ratio of less than 1.03 is abnormal, and

suggests a lesion of the vagus pathway. The supine-to-erect heart rate normally increases by 11–29 bpm, the maximum usually occurring at the 15th beat and the heart slowing to a stable rate by the 30th beat.

5. Carotid sinus massage should cause bradycardia.

6. Atropine, 1 mg IV, should increase heart rate by 30–40 bpm.

7. **Valsalva ratio.** This is an expression of the maximum heart rate generated by a Valsalva maneuver (blowing against 40 mmHg for 15 seconds) divided by the minimum rate occurring within 30 seconds of the maximum rate. The ratio of the longest to the shortest R-R interval should be 1.45 in young people. This is more accurately measured invasively.

8. The bulbocavernosus reflex and anal sphincter tone can be assessed with specialized instrumentation.

Invasive tests, including measurements of skin blood flow during mental arithmetic or with an inspiratory gasp, hot/cold stimulation, or radiant heating, need a well-tuned autonomic laboratory. The tests currently most favored have been reviewed.[8]

autonomic hyperreflexia syndrome See **Head-Riddoch syndrome.**

autonomic nervous system (vegetative nervous system) A division of the nervous system responsible for the automatic regulation of all the other systems of the body. Its existence was known to Galen, who regarded the sympathetic chain and the ninth, tenth, and eleventh nerve complex as forming the sixth nerve in his classification. He was also aware of the superior cervical ganglion and the rami communicantes.

It was Eustachius (1524–1574) who differentiated the vagus from the sympathetic, but the relative functions of the two systems were not considered until **Pourfour DuPetit** (1644–1741) sectioned the sympathetic chain in a dog and observed the resulting features of Horner syndrome. **Remak** first described unmyelinated nerve fibers in 1838 and believed that they arose from the sympathetic chain. Kolliker, Claude **Bernard,** and **Brown-Séquard** each demonstrated sympathetic vasoconstrictor effects, while E.F. and E.H. Weber slowed the heart by vagal stimulation and introduced the concept of inhibition in the nervous system. Hering and Breuer discovered the pulmonary reflex resulting from inflation of the lung in 1868.

W.H. Gaskell (1874–1914) and John Newport Langley (1852–1925), working in Cambridge, described pre- and postganglionic neurons, noted the antagonistic functions of the sympathetic and parasympathetic systems (respectively exciting and inhibiting glandular and smooth muscle activity), and divided the autonomic system between the cranial (bulbar) and sacral parasympathetic and thoracolumbar sympathetic outflows. It was Langley who suggested the name *autonomic nervous system.*[32]

autonomic neuropathy 1. (acute autonomic neuropathy, acute pandysautonomia) The acute or suba-cute onset of pandysautonomia occurring over several weeks, followed by recovery and usually unaccompanied by evidence of involvement of the central or peripheral nervous systems, preceding infection and other systemic disease. The condition is possibly a *variant form* of **acute inflammatory demyelinating polyneuropathy.**

Clinically, lethargy, tiredness, postural hypotension, blurred vision with pupillary paresis, anhidrosis, dry mouth, abdominal pain, constipation, urinary retention, and impotence are the usual features.[5558] *Pure cholinergic dysautonomia* has also been described.[3776]

Ropper et al.[4772] have defined diagnostic criteria for the *pure autonomic variant* of **acute inflammatory demyelinating polyneuropathy** as follows, reproduced here by kind permission of the authors and of F.A. Davis, Inc.

Clinical Features
Progressive sympathetic and parasympathetic dysfunction over 1–3 weeks
No limb weakness, ophthalmoplegia, or ataxia
Areflexia or hyporeflexia by 1 week
Improvement of some autonomic dysfunction by 2–4 months

Laboratory Abnormalities That Confirm the Diagnosis
Elevated CSF protein concentration
Normal (or virtually normal) motor nerve conduction studies, and abnormal sensory nerve conduction studies

2. Neuropathies affecting the autonomic nervous system as part of a more generalized affection as with diabetes, amyloidosis, porphyria, and the **hereditary sensory and autonomic neuropathies,** etc.[3776]

Autonomic Neuroscience: Basic and Clinical (formerly the *Journal of the Autonomic Nervous System*). The official publication of The International Society for Autonomic Neuroscience. Web site: http://www.isanweb.org.

autonomic storm See **episodic autonomic dysreflexia; diencephalic autonomic seizures.**

Autonomic Symptom Profile A question bank assessing secretomotor function, male sexual dysfunction, urinary, gastrointestinal, pupillomotor, vasomotor and sleep functions, and reflex syncope.[5401]

autonomous bladder 1. (reflex neurogenic bladder) The state of the bladder following loss of all supraspinal inhibitory influences; the volume tolerated is reduced and reflex emptying occurs through a contracted sphincter. 2. (autonomous or paralytic neurogenic bladder) The state of the bladder deprived of lower motor neuron innervation or in the early stages of spinal shock; the bladder is flaccid and dilated, with dribbling incontinence through a lax sphincter and loss of voluntary control of the initiation or termination of voiding.

autophagy The localization of intracellular debris and organelles within membranes of the endoplasmic reticulum.

autoregulation   The ability of the brain to maintain a constant cerebral blood flow despite changes in perfusion pressure by variation in size of precapillary resistance vessels (arterioles). A metabolic mechanism is likely, perhaps based on the release of adenosine or other vasodilator metabolites with incipient hypoxia. With fully relaxed smooth muscle, increases in transmural pressure cause passive widening of the lumen. If the smooth muscle is normally responsive, increased transmural pressure causes constriction and decreased pressure, dilatation. Maximum dilatation occurs below 60 and above 160 mmHg. (Below or above those levels, the perfusion rate follows the perfusion pressure—i.e., autoregulation is lost.)

With severe hypertension, the arterioles dilate maximally and the **blood–brain barrier** breaks down. Substances such as protein cross as a result of increased vesicular transport and endothelial disruption, not by opening of the tight junctions. The result is edema.

autosomal dominant cerebellar ataxia (ADCA, olivopontocerebellar atrophy) A group of spinocerebellar degenerations including what were once known as **Sanger-Brown** and **Marie ataxias** and **olivopontocerebellar, "primary" parenchymatous cerebellar cortical,** and **cerebellopontine atrophies,** with onset in young adult life. In these conditions, cerebellar and corticospinal features coexist variously with optic atrophy, involuntary movements (chorea, dystonia or Parkinsonian features), lower motor neuron lesions, ptosis, myoclonus, bulbar palsy, pigmentary retinal degeneration, and/or ophthalmoplegia; sensory loss is not found.

Harding[2438] classified them as follows:

ADCA I Cerebellar ataxia associated with supranuclear ophthalmoplegia, optic atrophy, dementia, lower motor neurone lesions, and/or extrapyramidal features. Pathologically, there is degeneration of the spinal cord, brainstem nuclei and cerebellar afferent pathways. This class is genetically heterogeneous.

ADCA II Cerebellar ataxia, visual failure due to pigmentary retinal degeneration and sometimes dementia, and both pyramidal and extrapyramidal features

ADCA III A rare pure cerebellar ataxia with onset over the age of 50 years

ADCA IV Cerebellar ataxia with photosensitive myoclonus and deafness

A few rare, dominantly inherited forms remain: one with *periodic ataxic manifestations,* another *associated with essential tremor,* and others still whose various manifestations demonstrate that these disorders are essentially **multiple system degenerations,** potentially involving almost any part of the nervous system.

Variant forms are autosomal or X-linked recessively inherited or occur sporadically.

autosomal dominant cerebellar atrophy with optic atrophy, progressive external ophthalmoplegia, dementia, extrapyramidal signs, and lower motor neuron lesions   See **Joseph disease.**

autosomal dominant chin tremor   See **hereditary quivering of the chin.**

autosomal dominant episodic ataxia   A heterogenous condition characterized by episodic ataxia and clinical response to acetazolamide. In many cases nystagmus is also found. In various kindreds paroxysmal ataxia, paroxysmal choreoathetosis, and myotonia are also described.[2016] See **episodic ataxia.**

autosomal dominant juvenile amyotrophic lateral sclerosis   See **amyotrophic lateral sclerosis.**

autosomal dominant muscular dystrophy with humeropelvic distribution and cardiomyopathy   See **myopathies.**

autosomal dominant myopathy with myofibrillar inclusions   See myofibrillar myopathy.

autosomal dominant nocturnal frontal lobe epilepsy   A dominantly inherited syndrome of brief clusters of nocturnal seizures preceded by an aura, lasting less than a minute, with onset in childhood. Tonic spasms or hyperkinetic motor seizures are the usual phenotypes. Partial awareness may be maintained. Linkage to both 20q (OMIM 600513) and 15q (OMIM 603204) have been established. The latter presents with tonic hyperkinetic movements resembling parasomnias.

A diagnosis of **parasomnia** or of **paroxysmal nocturnal dystonia** is often made if sleep EEGs are not available.[4947]

autosomal dominant partial epilepsy with variable foci   A syndrome with onset in childhood in which heterogeneous complex partial or secondarily generalized seizures occur in members of the same family, by day or night. Interictal EEGs are abnormal in the patients and in some asymptomatic relatives.[4947]

autosomal dominant rolandic epilepsy with speech dyspraxia   A syndrome with onset in early childhood of typical nocturnal rolandic seizures, centrotemporal spikes in the interictal EEG with the addition of speech dyspraxia, and cognitive deterioration becoming severe in subsequent generations as a result of anticipation.[4947]

autosomal dominant torsion dystonia   See **dopa-responsive dystonia.**

autosomal recessive muscular dystrophy   A severe and progressive recessively inherited muscular dystrophy characterized by the onset in childhood of proximal muscle weakness and atrophy affecting the girdle and truncal muscles predominantly. Joint contractures, pseudohypertrophy, scoliosis, cardiomyopathy, calf hypertrophy, and markedly raised serum creatine kinase levels are other features.

The best-recognized form, also known as **adhalinopathy,** is characterized by at least near-complete absence of this muscle membrane protein with normal dystrophin staining. The gene responsible is located on chromosome 17q. The clinical disorders reported range from severe childhood muscular dystrophy resembling **Duchenne dystrophy** (but seldom with cardiomyopathy and with a more benign course) to a late-onset syndrome of mild myopathic muscle weakness.[4437] Another form is due to a mutation of a gene on 13q, which is hardly distinguishable from **Duchenne dystrophy** except for the absence here of mental retardation and the occurrence of the disorder mainly (so far) in Tunisian patients.[447] See also **severe childhood autosomal recessive muscular dystrophy.**

There is marked variability in the intensity of symptoms and severity of the course of the disease between siblings.[2402] See also **limb-girdle muscular dystrophy, myopathies.**

autosomal recessive sensory neuropathy See **hereditary sensory neuropathy.**

autotopagnosia Impairment in the localization and naming of one's own body parts, described by **Pick** in 1908.

Avellis, Georg (1864–1916) German laryngologist.

Avellis syndrome (ambiguo-spinothalamic syndrome) Paralysis of one vocal cord and the same side of the pharynx and soft palate (tenth cranial nerve) with contralateral hemianesthesia, due to a lesion of the medullary tegmentum affecting the vagal nuclei and the spinothalamic tract, or from a lesion at the jugular foramen. Horner syndrome or contralateral spinothalamic tract deficits may be associated.[269]

In the original cases, only the ninth and tenth cranial nerves were affected, and the lesion was most likely at the jugular foramen; but the more generalized effects of a medullary lesion are now regarded as appropriately placed with the condition.

average potential reference (Goldman-Offner reference) An average of the potentials of all or of many EEG electrodes, used as a reference.

averaging A method for extracting time-locked potentials from random background noise by sequentially adding traces and dividing by the total number of traces.

aviation neurology The branch of neurology concerning fitness to fly in an airplane as aircrew or passenger. Guidelines for fitness status were compiled by a committee of the American Medical Association and published in 1979.

Avicenna (980–1036) Persian physician and Islamic philosopher. His book on the laws of medicine was published in Arabic and, when translated into Latin, served as a basic textbook for medicine in Europe until the eithteenth century. In it he described facial palsy, trigeminal neuralgia, and perhaps hemifacial spasm, and introduced the word *epilepsy.*[139]

AVM Support Group A charitable organization. 107 Bella Vista Way, San Francisco, CA 94127. Tel: 415-421-7330

awakening The return to the polysomnographically defined awake state from any non-rapid eye movement stage or from rapid eye movement sleep, characterized by the appearance of alpha and beta waves on the EEG, tonic EMG activity, voluntary eye movements, and eye blinking.[249] See also **arousal.**

awakening grand mal An epileptic syndrome, representing a form of primary generalized epilepsy of adolescence, characterized by the onset, after the age of 8 and usually in the mid-teen years, of primary generalized seizures, occurring mainly in the half hour following awakening but sometimes also during sleep. Seizures are easily provoked by deprivation of sleep and by photic stimulation. See also **juvenile myoclonic epilepsy.**

Axelrod sensory neuropathy with skeletal dysplasia A congenital dysmorphic syndrome characterized by skeletal deformities, absent or sparse tears, seizures, sensory and autonomic neuropathy, and craniorachischisis.[337]

Axenfeld, Karl Theodor Paul Polycarpus (1867–1930) German ophthalmologist.

Axenfeld-Schurenberg syndrome (cyclic oculomotor paralysis) A congenital unilateral third cranial nerve palsy with mydriasis alternating with phases of pupillary constriction and contraction of muscles supplied by the third nerve, and thus leading to elevation of the upper lid and nasal deviation of the eye (although lateral deviation is also described).[275] See also **cyclic oculomotor palsy.**

axial dystonia Dystonia affecting the back and trunk, causing scoliosis, lordosis, tortipelvis, etc.

axial hyperkinesia Rocking at the hips in a to-and-fro movement, often with an element of pelvic thrusting. It is seen in some patients with dystonic states, such as **tardive dyskinesia.**

axial myopia Congenital increase in the anteroposterior diameter of the eye, leading to the appearance of unilateral proptosis of up to 4 mm.[4267]

axial skeletal–neural dysraphic disorders Complex developmental malformations due to original paraxial mesodermal insufficiency affecting the formation of the axial basicranium, and the elevation of the neural folds interfering with their closure. Three fundamental types are recognized, in which the skeletal, neural, and oropharyngeal elements are partially or totally unclosed (e.g. **anencephaly** and **occipital encephalocele**) or are closed but abnormal (e.g., **Chiari malformation**).[3624]

axial tonic seizures Seizures in which stiffening of the posterior neck muscles produces an erect posture of the head. Opening of the eyes and mouth, rigidity of the paraspinal and abdominal muscles, and apnea are other common characteristics.[2055]

axilemma (axolemma, Mauthner's sheath) The axon sheath. Ludwig Mauthner (1840–1894), a Bohemian ophthalmologist, described and so named it in 1882.

axilla (Gr, the point on which a wheel revolves + arm) The armpit.

axillary nerve palsy (circumflex nerve palsy) A mononeuropathy occurring particularly as a result of dislocation of the shoulder, and leading to weakness and wasting of the deltoid and teres minor muscles and to a patch of numbness over the lateral aspect of the shoulder and upper arm.

axis The second cervical vertebra.

axis cylinder (axon, Remak's band) The core and conducting element of the nerve fiber; the long extension of a neuronal cell body containing **microtubules, neurofilaments,** and **smooth endoplasmic reticulum.**

Robert Remak (1815–1865), a German physiologist and neurologist, described and named it in 1838.[4979]

axon The conducting element of the nerve trunk. See **axis cylinder.**

axon reaction See **chromatolysis.**

axon reflex (axon response, axon wave) A late response recorded from nerves after peripheral stimulation and disappearing when the stimulus is supramaximal. It may witness **ephaptic transmission,** and is detected in neuropathies or after nerve injury.[1991] See also **A wave.**

axon reflex test Local vasodilation with the production of a flare normally follows a prick delivered through one drop of 1% histamine solution placed on the skin, indicating that the axons in that region are intact. See also **autonomic function tests.**

axon response A triple response in the skin, consisting of local vasodilatation, formation of a wheal, and further surrounding vasodilatation (the flare) occurring after the intradermal injection of 1% histamine acid phosphate or a strong local tactile stimulus. See also **axon reflex.**

It is present normally and in areas in which denervation has occurred as a result of preganglionic nerve lesions. With postganglionic nerve lesions, the response is not present in anesthetic regions, when it thus represents a hopeful prognostic sign.[659]

axon stains Histological enhancement methods used to demonstrate axons preferentially. These include the Bodian and Bielschowsky methods employing silver salts and a reducing agent. See also **myelin stains.**

axon wave See **axon reflex.**

axonal cross-talk See **ephaptic transmission.**

axonal degenerations Forms of neuropathy in which the basic fault is disruption of neuronal metabolism to the extent that axonal transport mechanisms fail. See also **Wallerian degeneration.**

axonal sheath Three concentric layers of tissue about the axon. From within outwards, these comprise the Schwann cells and two connective tissue membranes, the neurilemma and the endoneurium. In some nerves, a layer of myelin is interposed between the Schwann cell layer and the axon.

axonal transport (axoplasmic transport) The process whereby constituents of the axoplasm pass both centrifugally from and centripetally towards the perikaryon. Two systems exist: the slow transport system is that process whereby the constituents of axoplasm such as **neurofilaments** and **microtubules** are delivered from the cell body down the axon to its terminal at rates of up to 3 mm/day; the fast system is bidirectional and carries substances of high molecular weight (small vesicles, mitochondria, and membrane-bound tubules) at speeds of up to 400 mm/day both towards and away from the cell body.

The existence of such a system was correctly surmised by Descartes, although he was unaware of the electrical properties of nerves.

axonopathy Disease of the axon, as opposed to disease primarily affecting the neuronal cell body (which is called **neuronopathy**). In the dying-back form, there is initial degeneration of the longer fibers with progression of the lesion from distal to proximal.

axonotmesis A lesion of a peripheral nerve producing discontinuity of axons, while the supporting structures of the nerve (Schwann tubes, endoneurium, and perineurium) are more or less preserved. There is nevertheless such disturbance of the nerve fibers that true Wallerian degeneration occurs peripherally.

The condition represents one of the three types of nerve injury described by Seddon,[5048] the others being **neurapraxia** and **neurotmesis.**

axoplasm The circulating cytoplasm contained within the axonal tubes.

axorhizomelic tonic seizures A type of tonic seizure which begins in the same way as axial tonic seizures but which continues with tonic contraction of the proximal part of the contralateral arm, causing abduction and elevation of the semiflexed arm and shoulder.

axotomy, axonotomy See **axonotmesis.**

Azorean disease (Azorean ataxia, Joseph disease). A dominantly inherited syndrome with **cerebellar ataxia.** See **Machado-Joseph disease.**

B

B cells   Type B lymphocytes which are the precursors of immunoglobulin-producing cells.

B waves   Spontaneous oscillations of intracranial pressure of between 10 and 50 mmHg, occurring at 0.5- to 2-minute intervals during sleep and in patients with periodic (**Cheyne-Stokes**) respirations.

Baastrup disease   The presence of lumbar pain due to soft tissue disease affecting the interspinous ligaments and adjacent soft tissues.[280]

Babcock sentence   "One thing that a nation must have to become rich and great is a large, secure supply of wood." The inability to repeat exactly this rather pedestrian economic statement after three presentations was once considered a strong indication of impaired short-term memory, but three-item recall sequences are now more fashionable.

Babes nodules   Collections of microglia in the nervous system, found in in **rabies.**

Babiński, Josef-Francois-Felix   (1857–1932) French neurologist of Polish descent who became chef de clinique under **Charcot,** following Pierre **Marie** and preceding Gilles de la **Tourette.** He did not succeed **Charcot** as professor at the Salpêtrière for internal political reasons, but instead led the neurology service at the Pitié, an adjacent Paris hospital, from 1895. He remained a bachelor, living with his older brother Henri, a gourmet of distinction.

Babiński regarded his work on spinal cord compression to be his best, but today his most lasting legacy is considered to be the sign bearing his name, which he described in 1896 (in 28 lines). He is also remembered for his definition of many cerebellar signs and for the introduction of the terms **dysdiadochokinesis** and **asynergia;** for the platysma, reinforcement, trunk-thigh, and **pronator signs;** and for the **Babinski-Frölich (adiposo-genital) syndrome,** which he described in 1900, a year before Fröhlich. The **Babinski-Nageotte** and **Anton-Babinski** (anosognosia) **syndromes** also bear witness to his astonishing clinical perspicacity. It is also remembered that he pointed out that the hysterical symptoms of many patients at the Salpétrière died with Charcot. He was an early proponent of the use of the reflex hammer.

Babinski attracted many important neurologists from abroad to his service, but his failure to gain appointment at the **Salpétrière** reduced his influence within France, although he was a founder of the Société de Neurologie, edited the *Revue Neurologique,* and was elected to the Parisian Academy of Medicine in 1914. In the end, dispassionately, from abroad, he was properly regarded as the most outstanding of all the pupils of Charcot.[2750] Like Henry **Head,** he died from complications of **Parkinson disease.**

Babinski signs   1. Described by Babinski as "the phenomenon of the toes," the sign consists of the upward (dorsiflexion or extension) movement of the hallux with uncomfortable or painful stimulation of the sole of the foot, while the normal response would be for the toes to move downwards. As he noted in his original[283] or in later papers published between 1896 and 1903, flexion at the hip and knee, ankle dorsiflexion, and fanning of the toes ("signe de l'éventail") may also occur.

The sign is present (upgoing toe) in the presence of a disturbance in the pyramidal system, regardless of its duration, intensity, or extent, and it represents a part of the flexion reflex in humans.

Marshall **Hall, Vulpian,** and **Strumpell** had previously noted this phenomenon and **Remak** had described extension of the hallux on plantar stimulation in transverse myelitis 3 years before, but Babinski investigated the phenomenon in depth, principally in an attempt to distinguish organic from hysterical weakness, and deserves the eponym. Some reports show him using a feather, but his words indicate that he elicited the sign by pricking the skin of the sole.[283]

Numerous other methods of eliciting the sign (**Chaddock, Bing, Oppenheim, Gordon, Thomas, Stransky,** etc.) have also been described, and are complementary but rather less useful.[5729]

2. Diminution or absence of the Achilles reflex in sciatica. Babinski introduced the preferred method of examining the reflex, with the patient kneeling.

3. Fanning of the toes on the side on which there is clinical evidence of a pyramidal lesion, when the supine patient attempts to sit up.

4. Greater contraction of the platysma on the healthy than on the affected side in hemiparesis, tested by getting the patient to open the mouth wide or to try to whistle.

5. (**pronator sign**) Increased pronation of the paretic arm in hemiparetic states, such that when the examiner places the patient's hands in a position of supination, only the hand on the side affected returns to the pronated position.

6. Pupillary changes with aortic aneurysms.[284] See **Horner syndrome.**

7. Paradoxical raising of the eyebrow on the side of hemifacial spasm as a result of contraction of the frontalis muscle as well as the orbicularis oculi.[286]

8. The **plantar push**

Babinski trunk-thigh test   (combined flexion phenomenon) If the recumbent patient with leg weakness is asked to sit up with his arms flexed over his chest, the legs may move as follows:
- Involuntary flexion of the paretic limb occurs in organic hemiplegia; the heel may lift off the examining table.
- Involuntary flexion of both limbs occurs in organic paraplegia.

- Only the normal leg is flexed in hysterical hemiparesis.
- Neither leg is flexed in hysterical paraparesis.

Thus an unusual situation obtains, namely that the retention of some movement denotes the presence of organic disease.

Babinski-Fröhlich syndrome (pituitary tumor without acromegaly but with genital arrest) See **Fröhlich syndrome.**

Babinski-Froment syndrome Post-traumatic paralysis with hypotonia and hyporeflexia but with excessive mechanical excitability. A syndrome of wartime, with an uncertain basis.[288]

Babinski-Nageotte syndrome (medullary tegmental paralysis, combined lateral and medial medullary syndrome) A paramedian pontomedullary lesion causing homolateral **Horner syndrome;** ipsilateral weakness of the soft palate, pharynx, larynx, and tongue; loss of taste of the posterior third of the tongue; cerebellar ataxia with nystagmus; and contralateral hemiparesis and hemianesthesia.[289]

The **Cestan-Chenais syndrome** is almost identical.

Babinski-Weil test The blindfolded patient with a vestibular disorder, when asked to take 10 steps forward and 10 back, deviates to the right while walking forward and to the left going back, or vice versa. This gait pattern has been termed *star walking.*

Babkin reflex (hand–mouth reflex) Opening of the mouth and flexion of the forearm and the neck when the palm of a normal infant is pressed. The reflex is normally present until the fourth month of life.

backaveraging Averaging a signal that occurs in a time epoch preceding a triggering event. It is often used to extract a time-locked EEG signal preceding voluntary or involuntary movement, usually triggered by the onset of the EMG activity of the movement. An example is the **Bereitschaftspotential.** (From the 2001 Report of the Nomenclature Committee of the American Association of Electromyography and Electrodiagnosis.[10] Used by permission, copyright © 2001, AAEM.)

backfiring The discharge of an antidromically activated motor neuron.

background activity 1. Any EEG activity representing the setting in which a given normal or abnormal pattern appears and from which such pattern is distinguished. This is not, however, a synonym for any individual rhythm such as the alpha rhythm. (Adapted from the report of the Committee on Terminology, IFCN,[989] © 1974, with permission from Elsevier Science.) 2. In electromyography, no background activity is normally recorded unless the needle tip is close to a motor end plate. See **end-plate noise.**

back-handing The process of arising from the squatting position with the aid of the hands placed on the floor

beside and behind the feet to give a push upward; a sign of mild pelvic girdle weakness. See also **Gowers signs.**

back-kneeing Locking of the knee in hyperextension, a posture adopted by patients with quadriceps weakness in order to prevent sudden flexion at the joint while walking or standing.

back-up saccades See **catch-up saccades.**

Badal, Jules (1840–1929) French neuro-ophthalmologist, the first holder of a chair in that subject in France (at Bordeaux). He was at first a soldier, being decorated in the field during the Franco-Prussian War, but left the army for medicine. In 1888 he published a description of his patient Valerie, who developed a posteclamptic state of visual disorientation with features of what is now known as **Gerstmann syndrome.** See also **posterior leukoencephalopathy.**

Badal-Gerstmann syndrome See **Gerstmann syndromes.**

BADS syndrome The association of a loss of the **Bell phenomenon** with **corneal anesthesia** and a dry eye in a patient with seventh cranial nerve palsy, leading to traumatic corneal damage.

Baer nystagmus See **reflex sensory nystagmus.**

Baetz-Greenwalt syndrome A congenital dysmorphic syndrome characterized also by microcephaly, holoprosencephaly, or arhinencephaly and by congenital cardiac anomalies.[337]

bag fibers Intrafusal muscle fibers of two types, one reacting to the velocity and acceleration of stretch and the other to the acceleration of the stretching force.

Bailey, Pearce (1902–1976) American neurologist, who trained in medicine at Princeton and Columbia, receiving also a Ph.D. in psychology from the Sorbonne, before training in neurology at Bellevue Hospital in New York. His later clinical post was as professor at Georgetown University. He was the first director of the National Institute of Neurological and Communicative Disorders and Stroke, where he organized an intensive program of research into seizure disorders, multiple sclerosis, muscular disease, perinatal disease, and diseases of the eye and ear, training and assisting the careers of many now-prominent scholar–neurologists.

Bailey was a founder of the World Federation of Neurology and both nationally and internationally was prominent in the organization of associations dedicated to the furtherance of social, research, or clinical goals within the neurological sciences. The Pearce Bailey Medal and Prize of the Epilepsy Foundation of America were created in his honor.

Bailey, Perceval (1892–1973) American neurosurgeon, anatomist, and scholar who trained in medicine at Chicago, and Northwestern Universities and then studied with **Cushing** at Harvard, in Chicago and in

Paris. Returning to Harvard, he embarked upon a study of cerebral tumors, which culminated in his classification of gliomas, completed while working under Cushing, who, in the tradition of nineteenth century European schools, published it himself in 1926. Bailey continued to collaborate with Cushing on tumor classification but returned to the University of Chicago in 1928 where he became head of the Department of Neurology and Neurosurgery. His major work was *Intracranial Tumors of Infancy and Childhood* (1939), published in collaboration. He transferred to the University of Illinois in 1940, where he continued his work until retirement.[7]

Bailey-Cushing tumor   See **medulloblastoma.**

Baillarger, Jules-Gabriel-Francois   (1809–1890) An outstanding figure in French neurology and psychiatry in the nineteenth century. He worked at the Salpétrière from 1840, where he described the cycles of manic-depressive illness and melancholic stupor and wrote extensively on hallucinations, syphilis, and brain anatomy until his retirement in 1870.[297,298]

Jules-Gabriel-Francois Baillarger

Baillarger lines   The bands of fibers visible to the naked eye in sections of the occipital cortex. The striae Gennarii are such laminations. Six layers were descried by Baillarger, a finding later confirmed histologically by **Remak.**

Baillarger sign   Unilateral dilatation of the pupil in tertiary syphilis, for which Baillarger could adduce no good explanation.[297]

Baillarger syndrome   See **Frey syndrome.**

Baillarger-Jackson principle   The ability of aphasic patients to enunciate words involuntarily that they cannot utter at will.[68]

The phenomenon puts one in mind of the words of Dr. Samuel Johnson: "Things too silly to be said may yet be sung."

Baillie, Matthew   (1761–1823) Scottish morbid anatomist who gave the first accounts of cerebral pathology.

Bainbridge, Francis Arthur   (1874–1921) English physiologist who was professor of physiology successively at Durham and at St. Bartholemew's Hospital in London.[1750] His best-remembered work was that showing that cardiac acceleration occurs as a result of inhibition of vagal tone, as by an increase in blood pressure or distension of the right atrium.

Bainbridge reflex   Increased sympathetic activity with tachycardia in response to an increase in venous and in right atrial pressure, due to vagal inhibition.

Bajonet posture   Hyperpronation and hyperflexion of the hands and feet with permanent dorsiflexion of the hallux (**pseudo-Babinski sign**), seen in some basal ganglion disorders such as the later stages of parkinsonism and **pallidal atrophies.**

balance   The maintenance of the upright posture during sitting, standing, and locomotion through the detection and correction of displacement of the line of gravity beyond the base of support.

balanced amplifier   An amplifier that consists of two identical single-ended amplifiers operated as a pair but in opposite phases.

Balci oculocerebral syndrome   A congenital dysmorphic syndrome characterized by cloudy corneae or sclerocornea, microphthalmia, mental and developmental delay, seizures, microcephaly, and spasticity with aminoaciduria.[337]

balderdash syndrome   A colloquial term for **Ganser syndrome.**

Balduzzi reflex   Adduction and inward rotation of the contralateral leg in response to the vibration set up by a tap on the sole of the foot, present in normal subjects but increased in patients with pyramidal tract disease.

The sign was described in 1926 by Ottorino Balduzzi, an Italian neurologist at the University of Rome.[305]

Balint, Rudolf   (1874–1929) Hungarian neurologist, professor at the University of Budapest.

Balint syndrome   1. (Balint-Holmes syndrome, psychic paralysis of visual fixation, cortical paralysis of visual fixation) A rare syndrome resulting from bilateral parietooccipital disease and characterized by inability to direct the eyes to a certain point in the visual field despite the retention of intact eye movements (ocular apraxia, psychic paralysis of gaze); **optic ataxia,** a disorder of visual reaching; inability to read; impaired depth perception and fluctuating visual inattention for any stimulus not exciting the macula (visual disorientation or **simultagnosia.**)[3008]

Balint's patient had left-sided visual inattention but inability to perform directed movements with the right hand (his left handed movements were faultless), suggesting a **disconnection syndrome.** Fragments of receptive aphasia, agraphia, and ideomotor apraxia may coexist.[308,5671]

2. Loss of all voluntary extraocular movements and pupillary paralysis with retention of reflex eye movements, seen in hyperthyroidism.[5047]

Balint-Holmes syndrome   See **Balint syndrome.**

balking   The increasingly angry refusal of demented patients to cooperate in the routine procedures of daily care.

Baller-Gerold syndrome   (craniosynostosis and radial aplasia) A recessively inherited congenital syndrome characterized by craniosynostosis affecting the coronal suture, and by short stature, radial aplasia, and absent fingers.[309]

ballet dancer's foot   A focal occupational dystonia affecting the foot muscles.[5335]

Ballet, Gilbert   (1853–1916) French neurologist and psychiatrist who trained in Limoges and Paris, became chef de clinique to **Charcot,** rising through the ranks to professor of the history of medicine and then of mental diseases in 1908.

Ballet sign   Retention of the pupillary reflexes despite external ophthalmoplegia in **dysthyroid ophthalmopathy.**

Ballet syndrome   External ophthalmoplegia with paresis of the muscles supplied by the fifth, seventh, and twelfth cranial nerves and by the vagus in patients with hyperthyroidism.[310]

ballism   (ballismus) (from Gr, to dance) Extensive, vigorous, fast, poorly patterned, nonadaptive movements of the facial, limb, or truncal muscles. These violent, flinging, involuntary movements are due to lesions of the subthalamic nucleus of Luys, most often following a **lacunar stroke.**

Hemiballism is the term applied when the movements are unilateral, as is more common. *Paraballism* denotes bilateral ballism.

ballismic cerebral palsy   An ill-defined form of cerebral palsy characterized by uni- or bilateral ballism affecting the arms or legs.

ballistic   Not subject to modification after initiation.

ballistic movement overflow myoclonus   A form of **essential myoclonus,** characterized by involuntary movements occurring in 50- to 100-msec bursts of activity in the agonist muscle, accelerating a limb, followed by the same in the antagonist muscles (slowing it down) and then by further brief contraction in the agonist. The phenomenon has been described in patients with **familial essential myoclonus.**

This pattern differs from that occurring in *reticular* and in *cortical loop myoclonus,* in which the duration of the burst is only 10–30 msec.[2387]

ballismus   See **ballism.**

balloon cells   Grossly distended neurons with displacement of the nucleus and Nissl substance to the periphery, as in the **gangliosidoses,** in which the undegraded gangliosides distend neuronal cell bodies.

Balo concentric sclerosis   (encephalitis periaxialis concentrica) A rare subacute, progressive dysmyelinating disease, perhaps a variant of **multiple sclerosis,** described by Balo in Hungary in 1927. Bands of intact myelin alternating with zones of demyelination are found in the white matter, especially of the frontal lobes, varying in size from 1 to 3 cm and arranged in irregular concentric rings, witnessing the patchy destruction of myelin with reformation at the edge of each large plaque and thus explaining the laminated appearance. The axons are intact within these foci.[311]

The clinical features include progressive spastic paralysis and other widely varying evidence of diffuse cerebral disease, with childhood onset.

Balo, Jozsef Matyas   (1895–1979) Hungarian pathologist who trained and worked at the University of Budapest where he became chairman of the department of pathology and, for a period, dean of the medical school. He reported his case of concentric sclerosis in 1926.

Baltic myoclonus   (Nordic myoclonus, Unverricht-Lundborg-Lafora syndrome) A recessively inherited form of **progressive myoclonic epilepsy.** The onset of the myoclonus and tonic-clonic seizures is between 8 and 13 years, while such neurological signs as gradual intellectual failure, dysarthria, ataxia, and intention tremor appear later. Absence and drop attacks sometimes occur. The myoclonus may be precipitated by movement, stress, and sensory stimuli and repetitive morning myoclonus is common. Survival into adult life is usual. The gene locus has been mapped to chromosome 21. The diagnostic feature of Lafora body disease is the PAS-positive inclusion body found in neurons throughout the gray matter of the brain, including the dentate nucleus of the cerebellum, and on biopsy of axillary skin, liver, or skeletal muscle.

The syndrome was first reported by Unverricht in 1891 and appears to occur mainly in the populations of eastern Sweden and Finland, determining the name.[5689] There is suggestive evidence that **dyssynergia cerebellaris myoclonica** is the same condition as this disease. See also **Unverricht-Lundborg-Lafora syndrome** (which differs only in a slightly older onset age and earlier onset of intellectual impairment).

Bamberger disease (palmus) The sudden onset of clonic spasms of the legs, producing a jumping or springing motion. It was sometimes a manifestation of hysteria, sometimes of psychosis. Guttmann (1867), Frey (1875), and Gowers[2240] also wrote on the same condition, which they thought in at least some cases was organic. Bamberger also described **allocheiria.**

The author has seen one possible case but knows of no other report in the last century.[2238] See **saltatory spasm.**

Bamberger, H von (1822–1888) German physician who trained in Prague and Vienna, and later became professor of pathology first at Wurzburg University and then at Vienna. In 1872 he described the findings now regarded as typical of **Pick disease,** as well as the disease entered above.

band A portion of the frequency spectrum of the EEG, including the delta, theta, alpha, and beta bands.

band heterotopia A form of gray matter heterotopia in which there is premature arrest of gray matter migration resulting in a symmetric band of subcortical gray matter, referred to as the "double cortex sign. There may be some associated cortical pachygyria. Clinically, patients manifest an age-related epileptogenic encephalopathy with multiple types of generalized seizures and progressive cognitive decline. Association with the *Lennox-Gastaut syndrome* has been reported.[353] See **diffuse cortical dysplasia.**

band keratopathy Horizontal ribbons of calcium deposition in the cornea and conjunctiva, occurring in hypercalcemic states.

bands of Büngner Chains of multiplying Schwann cells which act as templates for the regenerating axons following **Wallerian degeneration.**

bandwidth (EEG channel) The range of frequencies between which the response of an EEG channel is within stated limits. This is determined by the frequency response of the amplifier–writer combination and the frequency filters used.

The manner in which the EEG channel bandwidth is specified by different manufacturers is not standardized at present. For instance, in a given instrument, a bandwidth of 0.5–50 Hz may indicate that frequencies of 0.5 and 50 Hz are attenuated 30° (3 dB) or another stated percent, with intermediate frequencies being attenuated less. (Adapted from the report of the Committee on Terminology, IFCN[989], © 1974, with permission from Elsevier Science).

Bannayan-Zonana syndrome A congenital dysmorphic syndrome characterized by mental and developmental delay, macrocephaly, unusual frequency of brain tumors such as capillary or cavernous hemangiomas, subcutaneous lipomas, and musculoskeletal maldevelopment.[3872]

Bannwarth syndrome (lymphocytic meningoradiculitis) Subacute or chronic lymphocytic meningitis due to tick-borne infection with *Borrelia burgdorferi* and presenting with severe radicular pain and sensory and motor signs associated with cranial nerve palsies, especially facial paralysis.[331] See **Lyme disease** (of which this is the European version).

Baraitser syndrome A craniofacial malformation syndrome characterized by cleft lip or palate, choroidal **colobomas,** seizures, mental retardation, short broad digits, and renal dysplasia.[338]

Bárány positional vertigo see **benign positional vertigo.**

Robert Bárány

Bárány, Robert (1876–1936) Hungarian otologist born in Vienna who studied medicine, psychiatry, and neurology in Austria and Germany. He was awarded the Nobel prize in 1914 for his work on otovestibular physiology and medicine. Although originally working in Vienna, he was captured by the Russian forces while a physician in the Austro-Hungarian army during the World War I (although he was himself a pacifist) and was interned as a prisoner, being released by the Czar to work in Uppsala at the behest of Prince Carl of Sweden.

His publications on the genesis of vertigo and on caloric testing have not been disputed; he first noted that nystagmus followed aural lavage, and that the direction of the fast component was away from the cooled side, leading him to propose that the caloric response occurred as a result of the movement of fluid in the semicircular canals. His invention of the rotating chair was based upon his reasoning that gravitational forces would have the same effect.

Bárány sign   Complete or partial reduction of the response of the labyrinth to caloric stimulation.

Bárány syndrome   Unilateral posterior headache, periodic ipsilateral deafness, vertigo, tinnitus, and imperfect pointing.[339] See also **Ménière disease.**

Bárány test   1. (*caloric test*) Production of nystagmus by irrigation of the external auditory meatus with hot and with cold water. Hot water irrigation leads to nystagmus with its fast component to the same side; with cold water irrigation the fast component is to the opposite side. Reduction in the amplitude and duration of the nystagmus indicates the presence of labyrinthine disease. The test was introduced by Bárány in 1906.

2. (*pointing test*) The subject points to a stationary object first with the eyes open and then with them closed; deviation of the arm(s) only with the eyes closed suggests a posterior column lesion, while deviation both with the eyes open and with them closed suggests ipsilateral cerebellar or vestibular disease. In such conditions, the deviation of the arm is in the same direction as the slow component of any accompanying nystagmus.

3. (*chair test*) Rotation of a subject who is sitting on a chair wearing opaque lenses and with the head inclined 30° forward (in order to bring the horizontal semicircular canals into the true horizontal plane). With normal labyrinthine function, horizontal nystagmus is produced in the direction opposite to the direction of rotation, and lasts about 10–30 seconds.

Barbeau, André   (1931–1986) Quebec neurologist, professor at the University of Montreal who trained in Chicago and Montreal, and who became a leading figure in Canadian neurology as a result of his dynamic interest in neurogenetic diseases and movement disorders.

barber's chair sign   See **Lhermitte sign.**

Barber syndrome   A congenital dysmorphic syndrome characterized also by skeletal maldevelopment, mental and developmental delay, microcephaly, microphthalmia, ptosis and blepharophimosis, and spina bifida occulta.[337]

Bard sign   Nystagmus due to an organic lesion increases in amplitude with fixation of a moving object, but with congenital nystagmus, this may cause the abnormal movements to cease.

Bardet, Georges   (b. 1885) Parisian physician.

Bardet-Biedl syndrome   A recessively inherited syndrome manifesting obesity, severe pigmentary retinal dystrophy, renal failure, syndactyly, brachydactyly, and (less often) polydactyly.[346,563]

It represents a variant form of **Laurence-Moon-Biedl syndrome,** from which it differs through the absence of spastic paraparesis. However, mental retardation, diabetes, congenital cardiac anomalies, multiple renal cysts, hydronephrosis and hypogenitalism (males), or hypogonadism (females) are other features described.[2265,2456]

baresthesia   The sense of weight or graded pressure.

barkers   See **dancing mania.**

Barlow, Sir Thomas   (1845–1945) London physician, who described **acute disseminated encephalomyelitis** following measles, in 1887.

Barnard-Scholz syndrome   A syndrome of retinal degeneration and ophthalmoplegia of unknown cause; one of the original patients at least had syphilis, another had cerebellar signs.[361]

Reports that the condition resembles **Kjellin syndrome** appear mistaken, as spastic paraplegia was not a feature of the cases reported by Barnard and Scholz.

barognosis   The ability to discriminate between weights using the cutaneous, muscle, tendon, and joint senses. Disturbance of the faculty was investigated by Gordon **Holmes** after 1910, who determined that subjects with unilateral cerebellar disease tend to overestimate weights placed in the ataxic hand. Parietal lesions may also be responsible.

baroreceptor   Specialized detector of pressure change situated in the carotid sinus and aortic arch and relaying information to the nucleus tractus solitarius along the ninth cranial nerve. Increase in blood pressure leads to reflex bradycardia and decrease in both peripheral resistance and myocardial contractility.

baroreflex   Alteration in blood pressure as a result of stimulation of the baroreceptors in the great vessels of the neck, buffering changes in arterial blood pressure in order to avoid excessive fluctuations, thus they mediate the blood pressure response to standing, carotid sinus compression, etc.[2279]

baroreflex failure syndrome   A syndrome of labile or sustained hypertension alternating with hypotension, and tachycardia resulting from lesions of the carotid sinus, its afferent pathways, or the brainstem. Sweating, flushing, headache, and emotional lability are other symptoms recorded.

Tachycardia occurs with such stresses as the ice-water immersion test and bradycardia with sedation; but hypotension resulting from nitroprusside infusion does not cause tachycardia, nor does phenylephrine-induced hypertension lead to bradycardia. Generalized autonomic failure is seldom an accompaniment.[4720]

barotrauma   The effects on the body of alterations in atmospheric pressure, as with deep-water diving or ascent to high altitudes. The sinuses, middle ears, nervous system, and skin are especially affected in the various syndromes.[1418]

Barré, J.A. (1880–1967) French physician who interned with Babinski in Paris and worked with **Guillain** during the First World War. He became professor of neurology in Strasbourg in 1919, working largely on vestibular functions.

Barré sign The patient, lying prone, is unable to keep the lower leg vertical on the side of a pyramidal lesion when the knees are flexed.

Barré syndrome (Barré-Lieou syndrome, posterior cervical sympathetic syndrome) Occipital headache, corneal ulceration with pain in the eyes as well as in the ears, vertigo, tinnitus, vasomotor disorders, and facial spasm, thought to be due to irritation of the sympathetic plexus on the vertebral artery in patients with rheumatism of the cervical spine.

The condition was first described in 1928 in the thesis of Dr. Y.C. Lieou, a student of Barré in Strasbourg. See also **acceleration injury syndrome,**[372] **whiplash, cervical migraine.**

Barré-Lieou syndrome See **Barré syndrome.**

Darrow Neurological Institute A nonprofit neurological research institution. Address: 305 W. Thomas Rd., Phoenix, AZ 85013. Tel: 602-285-3186.

Bartel nystagmus See **induced nystagmus.**

bartender's sign Extension of the shoulder so that the elbow is pulled backwards—a trick used by patients with weakness of the biceps to resist the examiner's attempt to extend the elbow.

The name derives from the pulling movement made by bartenders who draw beer from a barrel in the old-fashioned way without the benefit of compressed air.

Barth syndrome An X-linked dilated cardiomyopathy linked to chromosome Xp28 (allelic with X-linked fatal infantile cardiomyopathy) and due to a mutation in the Tafazzin protein. The clinical features include onset in infancy with mild and non-progressive hypotonia, learning disability and lethal dilated cardiomyopathy.

A variant is *Barth-like syndrome with mtRNA Leu mutations* which may be progressive or self-limiting. See http://www.neuro.wustl.edu/neuromuscular/msys/cardiac.html#barth.

Barthel Index of Activities of Daily Living A 10-item reliable instrument for the assessment by an observer of a patient's actual abilities in self-care and ambulation, of particular use in assessing the degree of dependence in the elderly.[3455,3573] A score of greater than 60 correlates with eventual return to home and of greater than 95 indicates independent self-care. The drawback to the Barthel Index is its lack of inclusion of cognitive and language function. See Chart B–1. A five-item short form (rating transfers, bathing, use of the

toilet, stair climbing, and mobility) has also been validated.[2594]

See also **Functional Impairment Measure, Functional Independence Measure, stroke scales, disability scales, Katz Activities of Daily Living Index, Nottingham 10-point Activities of Daily Living Index, Rivermead Activities of Daily Living Scale.**

Chart B–1. Barthel Index of Activities of Daily Living

Self-care Index

1. Drinking from a cup
2. Eating
3. Dressing upper body
4. Dressing lower body
5. Putting on brace or artificial limb
6. Grooming
7. Washing or bathing
8. Urinary incontinence
9. Bowel incontinence

Mobility Index

10. Getting into and out of chair
11. Getting onto and off toilet
12. Getting into and out of bathtub or shower
13. Walking 50 yards on level surface
14. Walking up/down one flight of stairs
15. Propelling or pushing wheelchair (if not able to walk)

Barthel Index

Feeding

Independent, able to apply any necessary device, feeds in reasonable time	10
Needs help, e.g., for cutting food	5
Totally dependent	0

Bathing

Performs without assistance	5
Cannot perform without assistance	0

Personal toilet (grooming)

Washes face, combs hair, brushes teeth, shaves (manages electric razor plug)	5
Needs assistance	0

Dressing

Independent—ties shoes, fastens fasteners, applies braces	10
Needs help but does at least half of task in reasonable time	5
Totally dependent	0

Bowel control

No accidents—able to use enema or suppository, if needed	10
Occasional accidents or needs help with enema or suppository	5
Frequent accidents	0

Bladder control

No accidents—can use/care for collecting device if used	10
Occasional accidents or needs help with device	5
Incontinent, needs indwelling catheter	0

Toilet transfers

Independent with toilet or bedpan, handles clothes, wipes, flushes, or cleans pan	10
Needs help for balance, handling clothes or toilet paper	5
No use of toilet, bedridden	0

Chair/bed transfers

Independent, including using wheelchair locks, lifting footrests	15
Minimum assistance or supervision	10
Able to sit but needs maximum assistance to transfer	5
Completely bedridden, use of chair impossible	0

Ambulation

Independent for 50 yards (45 meters), may use assisting devices, except for rolling walker	15
With help for 50 yards (45 meters)	10
Independent with wheelchair for 50 yards (45 meters), only if unable to walk	5
Sits on wheelchair but cannot wheel self	0

Stair climbing

Independent—may use assisting devices	10
Needs help or supervision	5
Cannot climb stairs	0

Modifications to this part of the instrument (mainly as regards scoring) have been suggested.

Bartschi-Rochaix syndrome   See **cervical migraine.**

basal cell nevus syndrome   A chromosomal disorder characterized by mental retardation, frontal and biparietal bossing, hyperteleorism, basal cell nevi, and an increased frequency of **medulloblastomas** or **astrocytomas.**[2222]

basal electrode   An electrode placed close to the base of the skull, such as nasopharyngeal and sphenoidal electrodes.

basal ganglia   The term of **Gowers** (1885) for the deep cerebral nuclei concerned with the elaboration of motor activity and including the caudate, putamen and globus pallidus, substantia nigra, subthalamic nucleus, and amygdala. These he referred to as the "dark basement of the brain."

basal ganglion calcification with mental retardation and steatorrhea   A rare syndrome with these features. See also **striatopallidal calcification, bilateral occipital calcification, epilepsy, and celiac disease.**

basal ganglion disorders   A popular inclusive term for those syndromes that manifest, *inter alia,* athetosis, ballism, chorea, dystonia, or parkinsonism.

basal ganglion "epilepsy"   Paroxysmal **dystonias** lasting a few seconds or minutes only. Despite the (old) name, the movements do not represent epilepsy or seizures at all.

basal vein of Rosenthal   A neuroradiological landmark, the basal cerebral vein is a tributary of the internal cerebral vein. It was described by Friedrich Rosenthal (1780–1829) a German anatomist.

basal-frontal syndrome   See **Foster Kennedy syndrome.**

Basedow disease   Exophthalmic goiter, described by Basedow in Germany in 1840, but in England by **Graves** 5 years and by **Parry** 15 years previously.

Basedow, Karl Adolph von   (1799–1854) German physician.

Basedow paraplegia   A subacute areflexic motor polyneuropathy affecting the legs in patients with hyperthyroidism, with sparing of sphincter functions.[1020] The attribution to Basedow was made by Charcot.[1762]

That this entity and **acute inflammatory demyelinating polyneuropathy** are different conditions remains uncertain. Proximal myopathy is another complication with a similar presentation. See **hyperthyroidism.**

baseline   (isoelectric line) 1. (EEG) Strictly, a line obtained when an identical voltage is applied to the two input terminals of an EEG amplifier or when the instrument is in the calibrate position but no calibration signal is applied. 2. Colloquially, an imaginary line corresponding to the approximate mean value of all the EEG activity assessed visually in an EEG derivation over a period of time. (Adapted from the report of the Committee on Terminology, IFCN,[989] © 1974, with permission from Elsevier Science.) 3. A potential recorded from a biologic system while the system is at rest. 4. A flat trace on the recording instrument. (From the 2001 Report of the Nomenclature Committee of the American Association of Electromyography and Electrodiagnosis.[10] Used by permission, copyright © 2001, AAEM.)

basilar   (Gr, arising from the base of a thing) Term denoting its Greek derivation.

basilar artery migraine   See **basilar migraine.**

basilar impression   (basilar invagination) A deformity of the base of the skull, consisting of an elevation into the cranial cavity of a variable part of the bony rim of the foramen magnum, not always associated with an increase in the basal angle of the skull and thus not quite the same as platybasia.[5282] The condition was first described by Ackerman in 1790, but this term was first used by Berg and Retzius in 1855.

The upward movement of the rim of the foramen magnum elevates the floor of the posterior fossa so that the upper cervical spine invaginates the posterior fossa, thus diminishing its volume. The basal angle of the skull (Weckler's angle, normally 132°–145°) is increased to over 150°. The importance of measuring this angle is now lost, since diagnosis is so readily made with MRI scanning.

Invagination is common in conditions marked by softening of the bones, such as Paget disease, osteomalacia, and rickets; is associated with shortness of the neck; and may lead to local pain, raised intracranial pressure, bilateral cerebellar disturbance, interference of the function of the lower cranial nerves, or high spinal cord compression.[4198] See also **platybasia.**

basilar insufficiency   See **vertebrobasilar insufficiency.**

basilar invagination   See **basilar impression.**

basilar migraine   (basilar artery migraine, Bickerstaff migraine, syncopal migraine, vertebrobasilar migraine). Migraine with aura symptoms clearly originating from the brainstem or cerebellum or from both occipital lobes. The headache is preceded by symptoms of dysfunction in the vertebrobasilar territory, including alteration of consciousness in the form of stupor or coma. See also **migraine-coma.**

The following diagnostic criteria are suggested by the Headache Classification Committee of the International Headache Society (from Classification of headache disorders, cranial neuralgias and facial pains; and diagnostic criteria for primary headache disorders. *Cephalalgia* 1988;**8**(Suppl):1–96),[1051] reproduced by kind permission).

  A. Fulfils criteria for **migraine with aura**
  B. Two or more aura symptoms of the following types: visual symptoms in both the temporal and nasal fields of both eyes, dysarthria, vertigo, tinnitus, decreased hearing, double vision, ataxia, bilateral paresthesias, bilateral pareses, decreased level of consciousness. The paresthesias are mainly of the distal limbs.

The condition is characterized by signs compatible with ischemia in the territory of the posterior circulation, presumably on the basis of migrainous vasospasm, occurring typically in adolescent and preadolescent females. The attacks usually last less than 1 hour and usually precede a severe migrainous headache. Common symptoms include bilateral scintillating visual scotomata, ataxia, nausea, and vomiting. Rarer symptoms are nystagmus and decreased hearing. Bickerstaff's description, published in 1961, has not been equalled.[552]

A *variant* is the combination of *basilar migraine, seizures, and severe epileptiform EEG abnormalities.* This is a benign syndrome in adolescents, characterized by the occurrence of rare focal or generalized seizures and rhythmic temporo-occipital spike–wave complexes in association with the clinical features of basilar migraine as detailed above.[878] Whether this is the same condition as **benign occipital epilepsy of childhood** or is a different one is not yet determined.

basket brain   A developmental abnormality characterized by the presence of bilateral fluid-filled cysts in the cerebral hemispheres. The condition represents a milder degree of damage than **hydranencephaly.**

Bassen, F.A.   (b. 1903) Canadian-born internist and hematologist, who practiced at Mount Sinai Hospital in New York.

Bassen-Kornzweig syndrome   See **abetalipoproteinemia.**[381]

Bassoe syndrome   A congenital dysmorphic syndrome characterized by distal myopathic weakness, cataract, ptosis, kyphosis, hypogonadotrophic hypogonadism, gonadal dysgenesis, and osteoporosis.[337]

Bastian aphasia   See **Wernicke aphasia. Bastian** described this disorder 5 years before Wernicke did.

Bastian, Henry Charlton   (1837–1915) English neurologist, professor of medicine at University College Hospital, London, and on the staff of the **National Hospital,** Queen Square. His publications include excellent descriptions of spinal shock, pareses, word deafness, word blindness, and other aphasias,[387] and a successful book, *The Brain as the Organ of Mind* (1880). Nevertheless, he appears to have been outshone by contemporary luminaries of greater incandescence. His dictum "We think in words," the basis of the **phonological system** of speech, will not, however, be eclipsed, although his beliefs in the essential unity of living and nonliving matter and in spontaneous generation have not been popularly accepted.

Henry Charlton Bastian

Bastian's law Transverse lesions of the spinal cord above the lumbar enlargement result in the abolition of the muscle stretch reflexes in the legs.[388] This is true enough in the early stages during the period of spinal shock, but not later on.

Batelle Developmental Inventory A developmental screening test assessing gross and fine motor development, academic, social, and cognitive skills, receptive and expressive language activity, and self-help skills. The inventory is suitable for children up to 8 years of age. It relies upon a questionnaire, observation of the child, and specific testing.

bathing suit area The shoulder and pelvic girdle regions of the trunk, distinguished only because sensory losses may occasionally be found in such areas in, e.g., **acute intermittent porphyria** or **leprosy.** Changes in fashion have made this appellation seriously outdated.

bathmocephaly (from Gr, threshold + head) A developmental malformation characterized by parieto-occipital overdevelopment with marked prominence of the occiput.

bathyesthesia Deep sensibility—awareness of sensations emanating from muscles, tendons, joints, etc., and including the senses of position, movement, and deep pressure, as well as vibration.

Batson's plexus The prevertebral venous plexus, a valveless system extending from the dural venous sinuses and thought to act as a potential path for the distribution of infection or tumor cells.

Batten disease (Batten-Vogt disease, neuronal ceroid lipofuscinosis) A storage disease in which ceroid and lipofuscin are deposited but in which the underlying enzymatic defect is uncertain. See **neuronal ceroid lipofuscinosis.**

Batten Disease Support and Research Association A charitable association in this field. Address: 2660 Parsons Ave., Columbus, OH 43207. Web site: http://www.basva.org/index.htm.

Batten, Frederic Eustace (1865–1918) English neurologist who trained at Cambridge and St. Bartholomew's Hospital and whose clinical career was based at the **National Hospital** and the Hospital for Sick Children, where he concentrated mainly upon the pathology of diseases of the nervous system in children. He described cerebellar diplegia (**ataxic cerebral palsy**) in 1908 and noted that both congenital and acquired causes were relevant, and progressive muscular atrophy a year after the report by Werdnig in Germany. His first work on cerebroretinal degeneration was published in 1903.

Batten-Gibb disease See **myotonic dystrophy.**

Batten-Mayou disease See **neuronal ceroid lipofuscinosis, gangliosidoses.**

Batten-Russell-Collier disease See **diencephalic syndrome.**

Batten-Steinert-Curschmann disease See **myotonic dystrophy.**

Batten-Turner syndrome See **congenital muscular dystrophy.**[5670]

Batten-Vogt disease See **neuronal ceroid lipofuscinosis.**

battered baby syndrome The effect of nonaccidental trauma to infants, resulting in skeletal and soft tissue injury. Neurological lesions include concussion, subdural hematomas, skull fractures, cerebral contusions, and **diffuse axonal injury.**[5787]

Battle sign Bruising and swelling of the skin behind the ear and over the mastoid, as occurs with local skull fractures and with dural sinus thrombosis.[1829]

Battle, W.H. (1855–1936) English surgeon, practicing at St. Thomas' and the Royal Free Hospitals in London.

Bayle, Antoine-Laurent-Jesse (1799–1858) French psychiatrist and pathologist, whose thesis after internship gave the first definitive account of **general paralysis of the insane** (although this condition had been recorded by Esquirol) in which he described the delusions of grandeur, delirium, dementia, paresis, tremor, ataxia, gait disturbance, sensory loss, and deafness, and the chronic adhesive arachnoiditis. Unfortunately, his thesis was received with antagonism by the medical establishment, and Bayle drifted away from neurology to general medicine and bibliography. He summarized the features of general paralysis superbly, as follows:[402]

> The symptoms of chronic arachnoiditis can all be included in the condition of general incomplete paralysis and derangement of the intellectual functions. . . . First, enunciation is noticeably impeded, the gait is unsteady, the disorder of the patient's understanding is manifested by a weakening of his intelligence and a monomaniacal dementia that more or less dominates the sick man, who is often considerably elated.
>
> In the second stage, speech disturbance and partial paralysis of the arms may [remain the same or] become worse. The dementia remains maniacal and general, often accompanied by dominant ideas; the patient may become agitated, a condition varying with his volubility and mobility; this causes him to become restless . . . and occasionally his furor is completely violent and uncontrollable.
>
> Finally, the third period is usually characterized by a state of dementia and a partial paralysis which may be partial or complete. The patient's speech is faltering, tremulous and sometimes unintelligible. The gait is vacillating, staggering or even impossible. . . . Understanding is extremely weakened; he retains only a few ideas that are incoherent and fixed and at this stage he becomes calm and immobile, though at times he may have periods of severe agitation. This stage . . . ends in paralysis and complete idiocy [with] tremors and convulsive movements.

The correctness of his original conclusions that the

mental symptoms and paralysis were the consequence of the changes he recorded in the brain and meninges was only confirmed 2 years after Bayles' death, by **Baillarger.**

Bayle disease   See **general paralysis of the insane.**

Bayle, Francois   (1622–1709) French physician who first noted calcification and plaques in the arterial walls and related these appearances of arterial atherosclerosis to apoplexy.

Bayley scales of infant development   A measure of sensorimotor development in infants up to the age of 30 months.[3]

BBB syndrome   See **Opitz syndrome.**

BD MCA   See **athetoid syndrome.**

Beals syndrome   A dominantly inherited disorder in which the appearance of Marfan syndrome is complicated by the presence of multiple contractures, dysmorphic ears, and congenital cardiac defects.[4580]

(BEAM-D) Scale   See **Behavioral and Emotional Activities Manifested in Dementia Scale.**

Bean syndrome   See **blue rubber bleb nevus syndrome.**

Beard, George Miller   (1839–1883) American physician. After training at Yale and in New York, interrupted by a period in Lincoln's navy, he practiced neuropsychiatry at the New York Hospital and introduced the concept of **neurasthenia,**[406] devoting most of his energy to that dubious entity, which he treated with vigor, electrotherapy, and some success. His book *American Nervousness* (Boston, 1881) inspired many to believe in the organicity of their symptoms.

Beard-Valleix points   See **Valleix points.**

Beare syndrome   A congenital dysmorphic syndrome characterized by short stature, sensorineural deafness, ichthyosis, erythema, abnormal nails, sensorimotor neuropathy, and mental and developmental delay.[337]

Beck Depression Inventory   A self-report questionnaire devised by Dr. Aaron Beck, with 21 groups of statements to do with both psychological and somatic symptoms, designed to determine the level of depression but frequently used as a screening test.[413] In disabled people, the scale may measure distress rather than depression.[5792] See also **Hamilton Rating Scale, Zung Self-Rating Depression Scale.**

Beck, Karl   German neurologist at Heidelberg who described the white rami in 1846.

Beck syndrome   See **anterior spinal artery syndrome.**

Becker muscle dystrophy   An X-linked recessive muscular dystrophy with the gene locus in the Xp21 band (on the short arm of the X chromosome).

Clinically, the disease is allelic with, and resembling, **Duchenne dystrophy** in every clinical feature excepting its later onset; facial sparing; lesser severity of somatic, cardiac, and enzymatic manifestations; slower rate of progression; and resultant longer survival.[418]

Becker myotonia   The autosomal recessive form of **myotonia congenita.**

Becker, P.E.   German geneticist whose work was done mainly at the Universities of Freyburg and Göttingen, where he was professor of human genetics. His publications concentrated upon the myotonic and other muscular dystrophies.[1829]

Beckwith-Wiedemann syndrome   A chromosomal anomaly (duplication of the terminal segment of 11p) characterized clinically by high birth weight and rapid postnatal growth, neonatal leucine-induced hypoglycemia with seizures, macrosomia with macroglossia and muscular hypertrophy, microcephaly, umbilical hernia, and renal hyperplasia. Additional features may include facial nevus flammeus.[1110,5879]

Beemer syndrome   A congenital dysmorphic syndrome characterized by delayed closure of the fontanelles, wide cranial sutures, hydrocephalus, Fallot tetralogy, ambiguous genitalia, and osteopetrosis.[337]

beer potomania   See **beer-drinkers hyponatremia.**

beer-drinkers hyponatremia   (beer-drinkers potomania) A hypo-osmolar state with low-serum sodium and potassium levels, resulting from the intake of large quantities of low-electrolyte fluid. Fatigue, confusion, and seizures are the common clinical results.

The mechanism is considered to be a combination of primary polydipsia and impaired water excretion in subjects with an excessive water load (e.g., 5 liters of beer daily), and with a low intake of solutes and protein. As a result, urea formation is reduced too, so that there is insufficient solute available to allow excretion of the water.[2572]

Beevor, Charles Edward   (1854–1908) British neurologist who trained at University College Hospital and in Europe before joining the staff of the **National Hospital,** Queen Square. There he worked closely with Sir Victor **Horsley** on cerebral localization. Such work established him as one of the leading British neurologists, a reputation further solidified by his complete description of the arterial supply to the brain.[424]

Beevor signs   1. In the supine patient with a cord lesion at T9–T10, attempted flexion of the neck and upper trunk leads to upward movement of the umbilicus, due to weakness of the lower half of the rectus abdominis.

2. Contraction of both agonists and antagonists during attempted muscle contraction in hysterical states, described by Beevor in 1904.

BEHAVE AD   See **Behavioral Pathology in Alzheimer Disease.**

Behavioral and Emotional Activities Manifested in Dementia (BEAM-D) A validated rating scale of behaviors that are directly observable (such as wandering and aggression) and of those signs that must be inferred from the subject's behaviors (such as delusions and hallucinations). It is used mainly to assess the effects of treatment in dementing conditions.[5189]

Behavioral Assesment of Dysexecutive syndrome A validated schedule for assessing executive deficits in schizophrenia and dementing disorders.[5994]

Behavioral Dyscontrol Scale (BDS) A measure of frontal lobe impairment designed to predict the capacity for independent regulation of purposeful behavior. It has been shown to predict functional autonomy and both impulsivity and apathy among geriatric patients. The scale appears to assess a different functional domain than that of the MMSE and similar measures, which rely heavily on the evaluation of orientation and gross cognitive status.[2973,4834]

Behavioral Inattention Test A battery of tests for the assessment of visuospatial neglect, including pointing to objects and reading a menu and a newspaper, sensitive for detecting lesions of both the right and left hemisphere.[5366] The battery employs six conventional tests: line crossing (**Albert test**); letter cancellation; star cancellation; figure and shape copying; line bisection; and representational drawing, and nine behavioral tests: picture scanning; telephone dialing; menu reading; article reading; telling and setting the time (digital clock); coin sorting; address and sentence copying; map navigation; and card sorting.[5995]

Behavioural Neurology A journal publishing mainly on the relationship between disordered human behavior and underlying biological mechanisms. Web site: http://www.iospress.nl/site/html/09534180.html.

Behavioral Pathology in Alzheimer disease (BEHAVE-AD) A 25-item scale designed to chart behavioral symptoms related to Alzheimer disease and to measure treatment outcomes, the ratings made by clinicians who interview the patient and also by a caregiver. Such items as delusional ideation, hallucinations, disturbances in activity, aggression, sleep disturbances, affective symptoms, and anxiety symptoms are examined.[4645]

Behavioral Problem Checklist An instrument designed to assess the range of behavioral problems that dementia patients may exhibit when living at home, and the upset caused to family members or other caregivers. The instrument is an expansion and modification of the memory and behaviorial problems checklist of Zarit and incorporates additional items. The frequency, duration, and reaction to 52 separate activities or normal behaviors are scored.

Behavioral rating scales See **Geriatric Rating Scale; Sandoz Clinical Assessment–Geriatric; Dementia Rating Scale; Vineland Social Maturity Scale; Adaptive Behavior Scale; Glasgow Coma Scale; Galveston Orientation and Amnesia Test; Glasgow Outcome Scale; Rappaport Disability Rating Scale; quality of life.**

behaviorism A psychological paradigm, the theory underlying it being that all overt human behavior is the result of the building up of a series of conditioned reflexes throughout life.

Behavioural Neurology A subspecialty neurological journal. Address: Rapid Communications Oxford Ltd., The Old Malthouse, Paradise Street, Oxford 0X1 1LD, England.

Behçet, Halushi (1889–1948) Turkish dermatologist.

Behçet syndrome (triple symptom complex, oculo-bucco-genital syndrome) A chronic, recurrent, systemic vasculitic syndrome of unknown etiology, thought originally[427] to comprise the triad of recurrent oral and genital aphthous ulcers and hypopyon iritis. Today, a combination of recurrent oral ulceration with any two of the following—recurrent genital ulcerations, eye lesions, skin lesions, and a positive pathergy test—is considered to be the appropriate criterion.[4201]

In some cases, synovitis, cutaneous pustules, erythema nodosum, meningoencephalitis, systemic and pulmonary arterial aneurysms, phlebitis and intestinal ulcers are added features and subclinical involvement of the CNS is also common,[531] occurring in about a third of sufferers who are usually young males. The diverse syndromes include meningo-encephalitis involving the optic nerves, brainstem, spinal cord, and cerebral hemispheres, seizures, benign intracranial hypertension (probably following cerebral venous thrombosis), various focal signs, parkinsonism, and dementia.[4202] Peripheral nerve involvement also occurs, but rarely.

The first description of the disease was that of Hippocrates in his third *Book of Endemic Diseases.* At least 18 synonyms for the condition are recorded.[2764,3033]

Behr, Carl Julius Peter (b. 1876) German ophthalmologist who studied in Freyburg, Kiel, Munich, and Berlin, actually graduating from Kiel University. After holding various positions he became professor of ophthalmology at Hamburg University.

Behr disease 1. (Behr syndrome, complicated hereditary infantile optic atrophy, optic atrophy–ataxia syndrome) A recessively inherited combination of degeneration of the maculae with chorioretinitis, optic atrophy and pigmentary retinopathy, cerebellar and pyramidal signs, peripheral sensory axonal neuropathy, and mental retardation, with onset in early childhood.[428] 2. (central tapetoretinal degeneration) A foveal dystrophy of adults.[429] 3. Calcification in the basal ganglia in hyperparathyroidism.[5553]

Behr pupil   Dilation of the pupil opposite the side of damage to the optic tract. The sign is inconsistent and of no utility.

Behr syndrome   See **Behr disease.**

Békésy audiometry   An audiometric test measuring the increments in volume that are required for a patient to hear continuous rather than interrupted tones at low levels of stimulation. Five categories of abnormality have been differentiated and the test can distinguish between cochlear and retrocochlear lesions.

Bekhterev layer   A plane of the cerebral cortex between the Baillarger lines and the tangential fibers.

Bekhterev nucleus   The superior vestibular nucleus in the brainstem.

Bekhterev nystagmus   (Bekhterev phenomenon, compensatory nystagmus) Reversal of the direction of the eye and head nystagmus and body turning induced by unilateral labyrinthectomy when the second labyrinth is also removed. See **vestibular nystagmus.**

Bekhterev phenomenon   See **Bekhterev nystagmus.**

Bekhterev signs   A number of signs described by Bekhterev, of greater or less clinical utility.

1. The Russian alternative to the **Babinski sign,** described independently but in a language less conducive to international understanding
2. Paradoxical dilation of a pupil with light stimulation in syphilis
3. Plantar flexion of the foot when the dorsum is tapped with a percussion hammer, seen in pyramidal tract disease
4. In pyramidal disease of the cord and in hemiplegia: "where the foot is passively bent in a plantar direction, when released, dorsal flexion of the foot occurs with flexion of the knee and the hip on the opposite side."[4723]
5. (*hypogastric reflex*) Normal contraction of the muscles of the lower part of the abdominal wall when the thigh is scratched
6. Lack of pain when the peroneal nerve is compressed, seen in tertiary neurosyphilis. This is the same as the **Biernacki sign,** but in a different nerve. It also resembles the **Abadie sign.**
7. (*nasal reflex*) Contraction of the facial muscles on the same side when the nose is tickled. This is a normal phenomenon.
8. When the patient with severe sciatic nerve irritation extends the sound leg, the affected leg cannot be extended at all.
9. (*arm dropping test*) When the arms are supported with the shoulders and elbows flexed and the support is suddenly removed, they will fall to the side after a momentary delay in normal subjects, but will "hang" in the air for a second or so in patients with pyramidal disease.
10. Extension and adduction of the thumb in response to a gentle pressure sliding down the border of the radius. This is a sign of pyramidal tract disease.[1349a]

Bekhterev, Vladimir Mikhailovich von   (1857–1927) Russian neuropathologist and psychiatrist at Kazan and later in Leningrad. He trained with Fleschig, **Meynert, Westphal,** and **Charcot** and authored over 500 papers on anatomy, the vestibular system, cortical localization, and psychology. He described spondylitis deformans (Bekhterev-Marie-Strumpell disease) as well as the conditions defined in the following entries. He maintained poor relations with Pavlov, his colleague at Leningrad, who did not consider his work to be of much merit.[1829]

Bekhterev-Brissaud syndrome   Spasmodic laughter and weeping in patients with hemiplegia; probably the first account of **pathological emotionality,** since involvement of the brainstem was suggested by the original papers of Brissaud.[435,758]

Bekhterev-Mendel reflex   Elicitation of the **plantar muscle reflex** by tapping on the dorsum of the foot, thus depressing it, lengthening the arch, and stretching the plantar muscles. This in turn leads to plantar flexion of the toes, with dorsiflexion being the normal response.

Belgian Society of Clinical Neurophysiology   A professional organization. Contact: Professor J.E. Desmedt, Université Libre de Bruxelles, Unité de Récherche sur le cerveau, 115 bd de Waterloo B-1000, Bruxelles, Belgium.

Bell, Luther   Nineteenth-century American psychiatrist and superintendent of an asylum in Somerville, Massachusetts.

Bell mania   Acute delirium.

Bell-Magendie law   The anterior spinal roots are motor, the posterior roots sensory.

The name of Sir Charles **Bell** should not really join that of **Magendie** here, because no such conclusion was drawn by him until after Magendie had published his account.

Bell palsy   (facial palsy, refrigeration palsy, rheumatic palsy) Facial paralysis due to a lesion of the seventh cranial nerve peripheral to the brainstem and commonly in the facial canal, where viral infection (HSV) is considered one likely cause.

Pain in the mastoid region may be the first symptom, after which the face is weak, as shown by inability to wrinkle the forehead or to close the eye on that side, tearing, dysarthria due to drooping of the corner of the mouth, and loss of the nasolabial fold. The sense of taste may be lost over the anterior two-thirds of the tongue. Recovery occurs within 6 months in over 80% of patients.[438]

The alternative name reflects the long-held but unproven belief that cooling of the face may precipitate the palsy, as Bell himself noted in one case. Melotte[3823] indicates that an account of the palsy was given by Richard Powell 8 years before Bell's classic description. Recurrent facial palsy may in some instances be familial when it carries a worse prognosis for recovery.[93]

A *variant form* is *familial recurrent Bell palsy with ocular motor palsies,* a dominantly inherited syndrome with the first episode of facial weakness occurring at any age and of the first episode of oculomotor paresis (with pupillary sparing) occurring in mature adult life. The pathogenesis is unknown.[93]

Bell phenomenon   (palpebro-oculogyric reflex) The normal tendency of the eyes to roll upward when a person tries to close them. In the presence of facial palsy, with resulting paralysis of the orbicularis oculi, this deviation, normally hidden, is visible, since the eye is no longer covered by the eyelid. Bell described it in 1823.[439]

Bell, Sir Charles   (1774–1842) Scottish anatomist, surgeon, and artist who went to London in 1804, returning as professor of surgery at the University of Edinburgh in 1835. Many of his discoveries were enabled in part by his attendance on the wounded after the battles of Corunna and Waterloo. He was a man of great good humor, acknowledged as the leading anatomist of his day. He described facial palsy in 1821, and later reported **myotonia** and pseudohypertrophic muscular dystrophy. He determined that muscles only twitched when the anterior spinal roots were sectioned, but thought that these roots carried both motor and sensory impulses. He was aware that posterior root section produced loss of pain but thought that the pathway for unconscious impressions (position sense) was through the posterior roots to the cerebellum; it was **Magendie** who showed their general sensory function, in 1822, a view that Bell accepted fully.

Bell also noted that the trigeminal nerve has both motor and sensory functions. He identified the long thoracic nerve,[438] and was the first to postulate the existence of a "sixth" sense, that of movement in muscles or joints; this and many other of his anatomical findings were published in his books *The Anatomy of the Body* (1802) or *The Nervous System of the Human Body* (1830).

His engaging personality prompted the text of his epitaph in Hallow Churchyard, Worcestershire:

Sacred to the Memory
of
Sir Charles Bell
who, after Unfolding with
Unrivalled Sagacity, Patience and Success
the Wonderful Structure of our Mortal
Bodies, Esteemed Lightly of his Greatest Discoveries
Except only as they Tended to Impress
Himself and Others with a Deeper Sense
of
The Infinite Wisdom and Ineffable Goodness
of the
Almighty Creator.

belly-dancers' dystonia   Focal dyskinetic movements affecting the abdominal wall musculature, most often as an unwanted effect of metoclopramide. Forward thrusting of the pelvis is another such movement similarly occasioned.[2730]

Bender Gestalt Test   A test of visuospatial praxis in which the subject is required to copy designs shown for a brief period.[447] The results allow comment upon right hemisphere and frontal lobe functions.

Bender, Morris B.   (d. 1983) American neurologist at Mount Sinai Hospital, New York. His major area of interest was neuro-ophthalmology and the higher functions associated with vision. A superb intuitive clinician and teacher, he was rewarded with a personal Chair in Clinical Neurology and was at one time president of the **American Neurological Association.**

Bender-type myopathy   See **congenital myopathy.**

bending reflex   Flexion of the elbow and shoulder when the wrist is forcibly passively flexed; it is present in normal subjects but is markedly increased with bifrontal lesions, especially those affecting the parasagittal, precentral regions. In severe cases, the elbow flexion can be elicited by gentle radial deviation of the patient's wrist (radial bending reflex). The reflexes of **Leri** and of **Mayer** are related.[5083]

bending-over vertigo   The physiological occurrence of vertigo or postural imbalance induced when a subject bends maximally at the waist, caused by the same mechanism as **head-extension vertigo** with the addition of increased intracranial pressure.[727]

bends   See **decompression sickness.**

Benedek klazomania   (Gr, klazo, I howl) Compulsive palilalic shouting in postencephalitic patients, differentiated by Benedek from the encephalitic complications of rage attacks, somnambulism, delirium, chorea, and parkinsonism, the latter having been present in all of his postencephalitic patients.[453]

Benedek, Laszlo   (b. 1887) Hungarian. Professor of Neuropsychiatry at Debrecen University and later at Budapest.

benediction hand   The appearance of the hand when trying to make a fist when there is a high lesion of the median nerve, preventing flexion of the index and middle fingers because of paresis of the flexor digitorum sublimis and of the median half of the flexor digitorum profundus.

Benedikt inferior syndrome   A pontine lesion, usually vascular, causing contralateral hemiplegia, hemiataxia, and sensory change.[4723]

Benedikt, Moritz   (1835–1920) Austrian physician who practiced in Vienna. His interest in cerebral localization led him to embrace phrenology, in the course of which studies he was one of the first physicians to X-ray the skull. His description of the syndrome now known by his name (1889) was brief and somewhat distorted by the facts that his 4-year-old patient also had a left cerebellar and many frontal tuberculomas, a right cingulate gyrus lesion and another in the cerebral peduncle, and syphilis; but his intuitive localization of the lesion responsible to the midbrain was nevertheless correct.[454]

He was also a pioneer in electrotherapy and in the study of the occupational neuroses.

Moritz Benedikt

Benedikt syndrome (tegmental syndrome) The association of a third cranial nerve palsy with ipsilateral cerebellar tremor and contralateral **rubral tremor,** involuntary movements resembling parkinsonian tremor, and hemiparesis, usually as a result of a small infarct or tumor in the region of the red nucleus which damages both this and the adjacent corticospinal fibers in the cerebral peduncle.[456] Benedikt actually described it in a patient with a tuberculoma at that site.

In this syndrome, motor fibers cross to the red nucleus from the contralateral dentate nucleus, and then cross back to influence the performance of motor actions on the other side of the body, while the corticospinal fibers are also uncrossed at this level, resulting in the unusual association of both cerebellar-like and pyramidal findings on the same side.[454]

benign abducens nerve palsy of childhood A rare, self-limiting condition seen in infancy and childhood. The diagnosis is essentially one of exclusion.[1081]

benign acute childhood myositis (myalgia cruris epidemica) An acute infectious syndrome of children causing muscle inflammation, after which myalgia involves the calves and thighs more frequently than other muscles; mild weakness and local tenderness are present and serum creatine kinase levels are markedly increased.[187] Recovery usually occurs within a week.

Influenza A and B, parainfluenza virus, and adenovirus 2 are the commoner causal agents. See also **postinfluenzal myositis.**

benign age and localization-related idiopathic epilepsy See **benign childhood epilepsy with centrotemporal spikes, benign childhood epilepsy with occipital paroxysms.**

benign cerebral vasculitis An inflammatory disorder of the intracranial arteries associated with segmental narrowing seen on angiography. The condition may be asymptomatic or seizures and focal neurological signs may result. The reversibility of the arteriographic findings and the absence of biopsy reports allow speculation that vasospasm (rather than vasculitis) is the cause in at least some cases.[5068]

benign childhood epilepsy with affective symptoms A disputed epileptic syndrome, in which frequent, brief periods of extreme fear occur in young children, without alteration in consciousness but with the usual autonomic symptoms of extreme anxiety. No consistent EEG abnormality is associated.

The condition appears to be self-limiting within a year or two, clearing without residua.[1251,4317]

benign childhood epilepsy with centrotemporal spikes (rolandic seizures, sylvian epilepsy, benign epilepsy, benign sylvian seizures with midtemporal spike foci, benign childhood epilepsy with rolandic paroxysmal discharges, lingual syndrome, centrotemporal epilepsy; OMIM 117100) A common form of `benign age and localization-related idiopathic epilepsy characterized by brief, simple, partial, hemifacial motor seizures, frequently having associated somatosensory symptoms that have a tendency to evolve into generalized tonic-clonic seizures. Both seizure types are often related to sleep. The onset of these attacks is between the ages of 3 and 13 years (peak: 9–10 years), and recovery occurs spontaneously before the age of 16 years. Genetic predisposition is frequent (linked to chromosome 15q14), and there is male predominance.[3464]

The EEG shows blunt, high-voltage centrotemporal spikes, often followed by slow waves that are activated by sleep and tend to spread or shift from side to side. (Adapted from Commission for classification and terminology, ILAE. Proposal for Revised Classifications of Epilepsies and Epileptic syndromes. *Epilepsia* 1989; **30**:389–399.)[1114]

In brief, it is a rare example of a distinct syndrome of epilepsy, occurring mainly during sleep in prepubertal children who are without neurological or intellectual abnormalities. The seizures are usually brief and infrequent, and the whole disorder only occupies a few years of the child's life.[56] The seizures tend to be controllable without great difficulty, and after their termination, the child is left without physical or psychological handicap.[3355]

Despite the usual eponym, given above, the syndrome was actually first described by Martinus Rulando in 1597.[5733]

Variant forms include one in which the condition is dominantly inherited and complicated by speech dyspraxia,[4946] and *malignant rolandic-sylvian epilepsy,* a form characterized by refractory sensorimotor seizures, cognitive disturbances, normal MRI findings, perisylvian spikes on magnetoencephalography, and frontotemporal spikes on the EEG.[4275]

benign childhood epilepsy with frontal or with midline spikes   A syndrome with clinical features resembling those of **benign childhood epilepsy with centrotemporal spikes** in which, however, the spikes are recorded from these differing locations.

benign childhood epilepsy with occipital paroxysms   A form of **benign age and localization-related idiopathic epilepsy** occurring before the age of 13 years and characterized by unequivocal clinical evidence of epileptic seizures (mainly tonic deviation of the eyes and vomiting, often with evolution to generalized tonic-clonic or to simple motor seizures) and with paroxysms maximal in the occipital areas on at least one EEG, and neither clinical nor EEG manifestations of primary generalized epilepsy nor of any other distinctive syndrome; no evidence of neurological or intellectual deficit; and a normal appearance of the CT brain scan.[2053,4316]

benign childhood epilepsy with rolandic paroxysmal discharges   See **benign childhood epilepsy with centrotemporal spikes.**

benign childhood epilepsy with somatosensory-evoked spikes   An epileptic syndrome of children in the first decade, characterized clinically by daytime versive seizures affecting the head and body, not always with alteration in consciousness, and electrically by sharp- and slow-wave complexes recorded in parietal or parasagittal regions, elicited by somatosensory stimulation, such as tapping the limbs. The attacks tend to remit after a year or so.[4317]

benign childhood partial epilepsies   A group of syndromes characterized by the occurrence of partial epileptic seizures in young children, occurring over the space of a few years only, usually at night, and often accompanied by hypersalivation, vomiting, headache, pallor, and sweating. Abundant high-amplitude, focal, sharp- and slow-wave discharges are recorded interictally on the EEG from various cephalic regions, especially during sleep, but all other tests give normal results. Febrile convulsions are common in these children.

The syndromes delineated to date include **benign childhood epilepsy with affective symptoms; benign childhood epilepsy with centrotemporal spikes; Panayiotopoulos syndrome; benign childhood epilepsy with occipital paroxysms; benign childhood epilepsy with somatosensory evoked spikes;** and **benign childhood epilepsy with frontal or with midline spikes.**[4317] See also **Landau-Kleffner syndrome.**

benign congenital hypotonia   A syndrome diagnosed on the basis of a clinical impression that an infant shows more hypotonia than weakness. This is unlikely to be a single entity and some of the conditions are probably not even myopathic. See **benign congenital myopathy.**

benign congenital myopathy   (Oppenheim disease, myotonia, amyotonia congenita, benign congenital hypotonia, minimal change myopathy, floppy infant syndrome) A heterogeneous group of conditions affecting infants in which hypotonia, muscle weakness, and lax (hypermobile) joints but normal muscle biopsy, serum enzymes, and EMG findings are the major features.[1744]

The subjects correctly diagnosed in retrospect are those that recover after the first year of life. Others (obviously not suffering from a benign disease) die of respiratory complications of their weakness[4250,5669,5837] and should be classified as having some other condition.

When combined with hyperexcitability of the CNS, the condition has been known as *Ullrich syndrome.*[2764,5838]

benign congenital myotonia   See **benign hereditary myopathy.**

benign cough headache   Headache precipitated by coughing, yet in the absence of any intracranial disorder. This definition and the following diagnostic criteria are suggested by the Headache Classification Committee of the International Headache Society (from Classification of headache disorders, cranial neuralgias and facial pains; and diagnostic criteria for primary headache disorders. *Cephalalgia* 1988;**8**[Suppl]:1–96[1051]).

A. Is a bilateral headache of sudden onset, lasting less than 1 minute, and precipitated by coughing

B. May be prevented by avoiding coughing

C. May be diagnosed only after structural lesions such as posterior fossa tumor have been excluded by neuroimaging

benign distal cranial arteritis   See **isolated benign cerebral vasculitis.**

benign dystonia   A congenital dystonic syndrome characterized by dystonias without accompanying features.[337]

benign early-onset Parkinson disease   A parkinsonian syndrome characterized by unilateral tremor and rigidity of long duration and minimal progression with onset usually in the fourth decade, sometimes following a severe febrile illness.[5036]

benign encephalomyelitis   See **postinfection fatigue syndrome.**

benign epilepsy of children with rolandic spikes   See **benign childhood epilepsy with centrotemporal spikes.**

benign epilepsy with occipital paroxysms See **benign occipital epilepsy of childhood.**

benign epileptic aphasia One of the benign focal (partial) epilepsies of childhood manifesting with pure intermittent speech disturbances. See **benign occipital epilepsy of childhood, occipital lober epilepsy and intercalated migraine.**

benign epileptiform transients of sleep (small/big/large sharp spikes) The appearance of spike activity between 5 and 135 mV recorded on the EEG uni- or bilaterally over the anterior and middle temporal lobe regions of young people during non–rapid eye movement sleep stages 1 and 2, especially after a period of sleep deprivation; first described by Grey-Walter.

They are considered to have no pathological significance, but their differentiation from similar spikes associated with partial epilepsy of temporal lobe origin may cause confusion.[5943] See also **small sharp spikes.**

benign episodic mydriasis Intermittent unilateral pupillary dilation, of unknown cause.[1602,2388]

benign essential blepharospasm See **blepharospasm.**

Benign Essential Blepharospasm/Meige Research Foundation, Inc . A nonprofit organization dedicated to finding the cause of and cure for blepharospasm, Meige disease, and related disorders. The foundation has support groups nationwide in the United States, promotes awareness and research, distributes educational materials to patients and physicians, and serves as a referral clearing house. Address: PO Box 12468, Beaumont, TX 77726-2468. Tel: 409-832-0788.

benign essential chorea See **hereditary nonprogressive chorea.**

benign essential tremor See **essential tremor.**[1267]

benign exertional headache Headache precipitated by any form of exercise. Subvarieties, such as *weight-lifters headache* and *effort headache in runners*,[3676] are recognized. This definition and the following diagnostic criteria are suggested by the Headache Classification Committee of the International Headache Society (from Classification of headache disorders, cranial neuralgias and facial pains; and diagnostic criteria for primary headache disorders. *Cephalalgia* 1988;**8**[Suppl]: 1–96[1051]).

   A. Is specifically brought on by physical exercise
   B. Is bilateral, throbbing in nature at onset and may develop migrainous features in those patients susceptible to migraine (code for migraine first)
   C. Lasts from 5 minutes to 24 hours
   D. Is prevented by avoiding excessive exertion, particularly in hot weather or at high altitude
   D. Is not associated with any systemic or intracranial disorder

benign familial chorea See **hereditary nonprogressive chorea.**

benign familial infantile convulsions (OMIM 601764) A dominantly inhertited epilepsy syndrome linked to chromosomes 16 and 19q11–13 and characterized by the occurrence of seizures, typically after the age of 4 months, over a short period. The foci are parieto-occipital. Paroxysmal choreoathetosis may be associated at a later age.[507]

benign familial macrocephaly A syndrome with the following diagnostic criteria suggested by De Myer,[1384] adapted here (see Chart B–2).

Chart B–2. Criteria for the Clinical Diagnosis of Benign Familial Macrocephaly

The occipitofrontal diameter is >2 standard deviations above the mean or >98th percentile.
There is no increase in intracranial pressure (as would be shown by bulging fontanelle, palpably split sutures, or persistent vomiting.
Neurological and developmental examinations are normal.
Neurocutaneous stigmata and other somatic anomalies are absent.
There is a family history of megalencephaly.
Follow-up visits establish the normality of the patient's developmental course, and the occipitofrontal circumference curve levels off and, although it remains high, begins to parallel the normal curve.
Radiographic findings demonstrate normal or only slightly enlarged ventricles in one of the family members with an enlarged occipitofrontal circumference, establishing that the condition is megalencephaly, not arrested hydrocephalus or another lesion.
Chemical screening tests for metabolic disorders or lysosomal enzyme deficits are negative in those patients lacking some of the other criteria.

Adapted from De Myer W. Megalencephaly; types, clinical syndromes and management. Pediatr. Neurol. 1986;2:321–327, reproduced by kind permission from Elsevier Science.

benign familial myoclonic epilepsy See **Rabot epilepsy.**

benign familial neonatal convulsions (OMIM 121200) A dominantly inherited epileptic syndrome in which multiple generalized tonic-clonic seizures occur daily, starting on or after the second day of life (but always in the first month), and disappearing spontaneously within weeks, although occasional seizures may occur thereafter[2926] in a variant form. The physical examination findings and the children's subsequent neurodevelopmental progress are normal. The responsible genes have been mapped to chromosome 20q13.3 and 8q24.

Ocular, autonomic, tonic, and respiratory seizure manifestations and automatisms are also recorded.[4760]

benign fasciculation potential A fasciculation potential occurring (in retrospect) in the context of a nonprogressive neuromuscular disorder. Unfortunately, its electrical characteristics do not allow confident distinction from fasciculations occurring in progressive neuromuscular disorders, so the value of the term is questionable.

benign fasciculations and cramps (Denny-Brown and Foley syndrome) The occurrence of fasciculations in healthy people who do not have other features suggesting **amyotrophic lateral sclerosis** or of other lower motor neuron disorders such as weakness or wasting, and neither EMG nor biopsy show evidence of denervation.[1401,4626]

The fasciculations are most commonly in the leg muscles but can affect any region, and tend to recur in the same point of a muscle on any particular occasion. The cramps are usually felt in the calf muscles. The origin of the disorder is not known, but progression to **amyotrophic lateral sclerosis** is seldom seen; only about 6% of subjects aged 45 years and older with fasciculations as their only complaint go on to develop this disorder.

benign focal amyotrophy A sporadic syndrome of nonprogressive asymmetrical uni- or bilateral segmental muscle weakness and atrophy localized to one limb or both homologous limbs markedly, occurring in young males. Sensory loss and CNS involvement do not occur. The electrophysiological, radiological, and muscle histopathological findings suggest chronic focal anterior horn cell disease.[3041] See **monomelic amyotrophy** and **hereditary motor neuropathy,** of which this is likely to be a variant.

benign focal atrophy See **monomelic amyotrophy.**

benign focal epilepsy See **benign childhood epilepsy with centrotemporal spikes.**

benign focal epilepsy with centrotemporal spikes See **benign childhood epilepsy with centrotemporal spikes.**

benign focal epilepsy with occipital lobe spike waves See **occipital lobe epilepsy and intercalated migraine.**

benign hereditary chorea A syndrome characterized by chorea affecting all body parts, clumsy gait, sometimes with dystonia, and with onset in infancy, childhood, or youth.[4563,4732] The condition is mapped to 14q. This is surely no more than a variety of **hereditary nonprogressive chorea.**

benign hereditary myopathy See **benign congenital myopathy.**

benign idiopathic dystonia Dystonia occurring in the first year of life, ceasing by 18 months of age.[5979] See **dystonia.**

benign infantile mitochondrial myopathy (mitochondria-lipid-glycogen disease of muscle) A reversible expression of inherited deficiency in cytochrome-*c* oxidase (complex IV), leading clinically to hypotonia, weakness, macroglossia, and lactic acidosis after birth, which, however, abates over months and leads only to residual mild proximal weakness.[1448]

benign influenzal myopathy A transient painful affection of the legs, with elevated serum creatine kinase levels, seen occasionally in children recovering from acute influenzal infections.[3868]

benign intracranial hypertension One of two acceptable alternative terms for the syndrome of increased intracranial pressure in the absence of a causative mass lesion, documented elsewhere in this book under **idiopathic intracranial hypertension.**

benign intracranial hypertension headache The following diagnostic criteria are suggested by the Headache Classification Committee of the International Headache Society (from Classification of headache disorders, cranial neuralgias and facial pains; and diagnostic criteria for primary headache disorders. *Cephalalgia* 1988;8[Suppl]:1–96[1051]).

A. Patient suffers from benign intracranial hypertension fulfilling the following criteria: increased intracranial pressure (>200 mm H_2O) measured by epidural or intraventricular pressure monitoring or by lumbar puncture; normal neurological examination except for papilledema and possibly sixth cranial nerve palsy; no mass lesion and no ventricular enlargement on neuroimaging; normal or low protein concentration and normal white blood cell count in CSF; no clinical nor neuroimaging suspicion of venous sinus thrombosis.

B. Headache intensity and frequency related to variations of intracranial pressure with a time lag of less than 24 hours.

benign juvenile focal muscular atrophy of upper extremities See **monomelic amyotrophy.**

benign masturbatory cephalalgia An acute **benign exertional headache,** usually experienced in private.[5768] See **headache associated with sexual activity.**

benign monoclonal gammopathy See **paraproteinemic neuropathy.**

benign monomelic amyotrophy See **monomelic amyotrophy.**

benign motor neuron disorder See **cramp fasciculation syndrome.**

benign multiple sclerosis That form of multiple sclerosis which, having been present for more than 10 years with a relapsing and remitting course, has left the patient with little functional disability (rating less than 3 on the **Kurtzke scale**).

benign muscular dystrophy with contractures A variant of **Emery-Dreifuss syndrome** with likely autosomal dominant inheritance, characterized by proximal myopathy, contractures, and rigidity of paraspinal muscles without cardiomyopathy.[295]

A dominant pattern of inheritance is likely, but Y-to-Y transmission is also possible.[295]

benign myalgic encephalomyelitis See **chronic fatigue syndrome.**

benign myoclonic epilepsy in childhood   See **benign myoclonic epilepsy in infancy.**

benign myoclonic epilepsy in infancy (benign neonatal sleep myoclonus, benign myoclonic epilepsy in childhood) A rare syndrome characterized by a partial arousal response manifesting as bilateral, synchronous, and repetitive rhythmic jerking of the limbs with occasional jerks of the trunk, fingers, wrists, elbows, and ankles, occurring without other clinical abnormality during any phase of sleep in some otherwise-normal neonates up to the age of 2 years.[1143] The jerks occur in clusters of four or five at about 1 per second, and involve mainly the limbs, occasionally affecting distal muscle roots most obviously. The onset is usually in the first week of life. The disorder is self-limited and benign, lasting at most a few months,[234] and may be classified as a **parasomnia.** There is often a family history of convulsions or epilepsy. Examination is normal.

They are not accompanied by any other type of seizure, although generalized tonic-clonic seizures may occur during adolescence and are easily controlled by appropriate treatment. The epilepsy may be accompanied by a relative delay of intellectual development and minor personality disorders. EEG recording shows generalized 3-Hz spike–waves occurring in brief bursts during the early stages of sleep. (Adapted by permission from Commission for Classification and Terminology, ILAE. Proposal for revised classifications of epilepsies and epileptic syndromes. *Epilepsia* 1989;**30:** 389–399.[1114])

benign myoclonus of early infancy A clinical syndrome of repetitive jerking movements resembling **West syndrome** but self-limiting by the age of 2 years and lacking the neurological and developmental arrest, the **hypsarrhythmic** EEG pattern, and the fatal prognosis of that condition.[3465] It is considered to be a form of **tic disorder.**

benign myoclonus of infancy   See **myoclonus.**

benign myopathy A dominantly inherited syndrome with onset in childhood after normal infantile motor development, and characterized by weakness of the neck flexors, girdle muscles and limb extensors, and, in some cases, by flexion contracture of the elbows and by hyporeflexia. Muscle biopsy findings are nonspecific but suggest myopathy.[2860]

benign neonatal convulsions (fifth-day fits) Frequently repeated clonic or apneic seizures occurring at about the fifth day of life, without known etiology or concomitant metabolic disturbance. The interictal EEG often shows alternating sharp theta waves. There is no recurrence of seizures and psychomotor development is not affected. (By permission from Commission for Classification and Terminology, ILAE. Proposal for revised classifications of epilepsies and epileptic syndromes. *Epilepsia* 1989;**30:**389–399.[1114])

benign neonatal familial convulsions Rare, dominantly inherited disorders manifesting most commonly on the second and third days of life, with frequently repeated clonic or apneic seizures lasting for a few days or weeks, without specific EEG criteria. The history and investigations reveal no etiologic factors. About 14% of these patients later develop epilepsy, commonly in adult life. (From Commission for Classification and Terminology, ILAE. Proposal for revised classifications of epilepsies and epileptic syndromes. *Epilepsia* 1989;**30:** 389–399 by permission.[1114]) The responsible gene lies at chromosome 20q 13.3.

benign neonatal sleep myoclonus   See **benign myoclonic epilepsy in infancy.**

benign occipital epilepsy of childhood (benign epilepsy with occipital paroxysms, BEOPS) One of the benign focal (partial) epilepsies of childhood, and thus related to **benign childhood epilepsy with centrotemporal spikes** and **benign epileptic aphasia.** Clinically, the condition presents in the middle of the first decade with infrequent and easily controlled seizures comprising positive or negative visual phenomena, without focal neurological or ocular signs or mental disturbance but with striking irregular occipital spike–wave discharges on the EEG.[2053] In a number of cases these are followed by hemisensory, motor or psychomotor seizures, and migraine-like headaches.[2051]

benign occipital spikes The appearance of uniform diphasic or triphasic sharp waves over one or both occipital regions, attenuated by eye opening but activated by sleep. The electrographic finding is most commonly associated with migraine; seizures if they occur at all, usually remit after puberty.[2051]

benign paroxysmal cranial neuralgia (cephalgia fugax) A benign syndrome of unknown cause, characterized by the occurrence of frequent, repetitive (1–20 per day), sharp, neuralgia-like head pains occurring in bouts, with long remissions between them.[4379]

benign paroxysmal positional vertigo   See **benign positional vertigo.**

benign paroxysmal torticollis in infancy A self-limited disorder with onset during the first month of life, recurring at varying intervals until the age of 1–5 years and characterized by periods of torticollic posturing of the head.[1091]

benign paroxysmal vertigo of childhood (paroxysmal torticollis in infancy) Multiple, brief, sporadic episodes of true vertigo occurring in otherwise healthy children aged between 1 and 5 years who stop all activities, appear frightened, refuse to move or stand, and may be nauseated or vomit.

The condition may be a migraine equivalent of childhood or adolescence. It remits spontaneously after some years. The International Headache Society criteria require a normal neurological examination and a normal EEG, since recurrent vertigo can be a symptom of epilepsy (**tornado epilepsy**).[1404] See also **periodic syndromes.**

benign partial epilepsy of childhood   A syndrome of benign seizures occurring only during sleep, involving mainly the mouth and face, disappearing by puberty, and accompanied by marked rolandic spike discharges during rapid eye movement sleep periods but the EEG is normal interictally.[4207] The neurological examination is normal. See **benign childhood epilepsy with centrotemporal spikes,** which is surely the same thing.

benign partial epilepsy of childhood with occipital paroxysms   A syndrome characterized by interictal paroxysms of high-amplitude spike–waves or sharp waves, recurring more or less rhythmically on the occipital and posterotemporal areas of one or both hemispheres, and occurring only when the eyes are closed. Ictally, the initial visual symptoms such as amaurosis, phosphenes, visual illusions, or hallucinations are often followed by a hemiclonic seizure or by automatisms when the occipital discharge spreads to central or temporal regions. A migraine-like headache ensues in a quarter of the cases.

benign partial epilepsy with affective symptoms during the attacks   The ictal symptomatology is mainly constituted by a terror feeling and autonomic signs without evident loss of consciousness. EEG abnormalities are variable and situated in frontal and mid-temporal areas.

benign partial epilepsy with centrotemporal spikes of childhood   The most frequent and the best known of the benign partial epilepsies, characterized by genetic predisposition, male predominance; onset between 3 and 13 years, and recovery before 15–16 years. Seizures are brief hemifacial motor, with frequent associated somatosensory symptoms, and are usually nocturnal, sometimes tending to become generalized in this case. The *EEG* shows blunt, high-voltage centrotemporal spikes, often followed by slow-waves, which are activated by sleep and tend to spread and/or shift from side to side.

benign partial epilepsy with extreme somatosensory evoked potentials   A form of **benign partial epilepsy of childhood,** with affected children having large somatosensory evoked potentials evoked by heel-tapping. Later, spontaneous EEG abnormalities in the parietal area and partial motor seizures with adversion appear.

benign partial epilepsy with occipital sharp waves   See **benign childhood epilepsy with occipital paroxysms.**

benign pontine hypertrophy   Although the condition is neither benign nor truly hypertrophic, the name was once applied to slowly growing pontine gliomas.

benign positional vertigo   (BPPV; benign peripheral/paroxysmal positional vertigo, paroxysmal positional nystagmus) A common syndrome characterized by acute, transient, episodic, rotational vertigo, precipitated (after a few seconds latency) by rapid changes in the position of the head, characteristically declining after seconds or minutes and fatiguing with repeated postural changes. Nausea, vomiting, and peripheral nystagmus are typically associated.[318,3270]

The cause is uncertain but may be the dislocation and random movement of the canaliths (otoconia) that stimulate the hair cells in the posterior (less commonly the horizontal) semicircular canals of the undermost ear. The condition was first described by Barany in 1921.[339] It is frequently relieved by the **Semont** or the **Epley liberatory maneuvers.**

Variants include a disabling form;[2813] a form in which a horizontal semicircular canal is implicated—in this type the nystagmus is direction changing, horizontal, and non-fatiguing; and a form in which the nystagmus is direction changing, probably because of pathology affecting the horizontal semicircular canal.[314]

See also **Dix-Hallpike maneuver, Semont liberatory maneuver, Epley maneuver.**

benign postural myoclonus   A rare syndrome manifesting position-dependent myoclonus, responsive to clonazepam and valproic acid.

benign recurrent vertigo   A benign recurrent episodic syndrome of vertigo, nausea, vomiting, and hyperhidrosis without evidence of vestibulopathy, occurring mainly on waking and seen in women with a personal (or at least a family) history of recurrent headaches at the time of their menstrual periods.[3973]

benign rolandic epilepsy   (benign focal epilepsy linked to 15q) See **benign childhood epilepsy with centrotemporal spikes.**

benign senescent forgetfulness   A nonprogressive, fluctuating amnestic syndrome in elderly people, whose recollection of remote names and dates, but not of events, is impaired on certain occasions, the data bubbling up later.[3150] See **age-associated memory impairment.**

benign sensorimotor epilepsy with parietal spikes   See **extreme somatosensory evoked potential.**

benign sex headache   See **headache associated with sexual activity.**

benign sixth nerve palsy   Isolated, painless, and self-limited paresis of one of the sixth nerves in children, occurring 10–20 days after an upper respiratory infection.[3103]

benign spinal muscular atrophy with calf hypertrophy   See **hereditary motor neuropathy.**

benign sporadic sleep spikes   See **small sharp spikes.**

benign sylvian seizures with midtemporal spike foci
See **benign childhood epilepsy with centrotemporal spikes.**

benign symmetric lipomatosis   See **familial multiple symmetrical lipomatosis with peripheral neuropathy.**

benign torticollis of infancy   Recurrent attacks in which the head tilts, occurring during the first year of life and persisting for a few months to several years. The attacks occur predominantly in the morning and last between 2 and 24 hours. Associated symptoms include irritability, drowsiness, pallor or flushing, and dysequilibrium.[1404] The etiology is not determined.

benign tremulous parkinsonism   A syndrome of isolated tremor without other signs of **Parkinson disease,** occurring in a single limb, in elderly patients, and without progression over the course of years of observation.

benign tumors   Tumors which are slowly growing and noninvasive, and which show no vascular proliferation, few mitoses, and minimal necrosis histologically.

benign X-linked muscular dystrophy   (Waida dystrophy) A variant form of muscular dystrophy characterized by the onset in youth of proximal and distal muscle atrophy and weakness, pseudohypertrophy, and cardiomyopathy.[337] See **Becker muscle dystrophy.**

bent knee pulling   A variation of the **femoral stretch** maneuver in which the examiner passively extends the patient's hip by pulling backward on the foot with the knee flexed, and exerting forward pressure on the buttock, with the patient in the semiprone position. The action stretches the femoral nerve. Pain felt as a result is a useful sign of root irritation at L3.[2768]

bent spine syndrome   (camptocormia; from Gr, bent + tree trunk) A focal axial myopathy seen mainly in elderly people and causing progressive paravertebral muscle weakness, leading to a posture of anterior flexion of the trunk, with bent spine on standing but normal supine posture. Weakness of the neck extensors may lead to dropping of the head. Serum creatine kinase is normal or moderately increased, paraspinal EMG is nonspecific, and biopsy is myopathic. The syndrome may be caused by a late-onset paraspinal muscle dystrophy but is heterogeneous in origin.[5074]

Benton Visual Retention Test   A test of visuospatial praxis and nonverbal memory in which the subject sees, and is required to memorize and later to reproduce, a series of simple but progressively more complex line drawings.

It is said to be useful in distinguishing between the normal elderly and those with **Alzheimer disease.**[472]

Benton-van Allen Test of Facial Discrimination   A pictorial test for visual agnosia.

Berant syndrome   A dominantly inherited congenital syndrome characterized by acrocephaly, elbow joint and radio-ulnar synostosis, and craniosynostosis affecting the sagittal suture.[480]

Berdon syndrome   See **megacystis-microcolon-intestinal hypoperistalsis syndrome.**

Bereitschafts potential   (readiness potential) An EEG potential recorded maximally at the vertex, probably emanating from the supplementary motor area and preceding a self-paced voluntary movement.[1435] It is a component of the movement-related cortical potential. See also **backaveraging.**

Bergara-Wartenberg sign   Loss of those fine vibrations which are palpable when the examiner places his finger on the closed eyelids of a normal patient. The sign is positive in patients with facial palsy.[490]

Berger, E   (1855–1926) Austrian ophthalmologist who studied in Vienna, Berlin, and Paris, where he later set up in practice, becoming Professor of Ophthalmology at the École de Médicine. He was a voluminous writer on many aspects of ophthalmology.

Berger, Johannes (Hans)   (1873–1941) German physiologist who trained at Jena University, where he became professor of psychiatry, succeeding **Binswanger.** He was the first to record cortical electrical potentials in humans (1924), describing the alpha and the beta rhythms.[492] In 1932 he established the association in humans between unilateral spike discharges on the EEG and contralateral clonic jerks. He died by his own hand in 1941. He was an outspoken anti-Nazi and the régime had closed his clinic for that reason, over which he became despondent.

Berger, Oskar   (1844–1885) German neurologist and neuropathologist who studied in Breslau, Berlin, and Vienna, graduating from Berlin University and eventually becoming professor at Breslau where his main interests were hypnotism, neuropathology, neuralgias, and electrotherapy.

Berger paresthesia   Distal paresthesias in young subjects. Berger's paper was published in a Breslau journal in 1879, but no pathology was reported, and it is likely that the condition represents benign nerve compression, as with the **carpal tunnel syndrome.**

Berger rhythm   The alpha rhythm of the EEG.

Berger sign   Irregularity of the pupil, which may be elliptical in the early stages of tertiary syphilis.[491]

Bergeron disease   (electric chorea) A disease of childhood characterized by violent rhythmical spasms ceasing in sleep and with a short and benign course. In this the condition differs from Dubini disease, which was frequently fatal.

The first description was attributed to Dr. E.-J. Bergeron in 1880 by his pupil René Berland in his graduation thesis (University of Paris), but the condition had been previously noted by James Begbie in 1847.[425,5047]

Its nature remains unexplained. See also **Dubini disease.**

Bergeron, Etienne-Jules   (1817–1900) French pediatrician who trained in Paris and worked in the French military and at the Hôpital Trousseau, as well as being prominent in the field of public health.

Bergmann glial cells   A layer of astrocytes within the Purkinje layer of the cerebellar cortex which hypertrophy in those conditions in which the Purkinje cells atrophy. They were described by Gottlieb Bergmann (1781–1861), a German physician.

Bergmeister papilla   An ocular remnant of the anterior hyaloid artery producing a preretinal fibrous veil. Another remnant, placed further anteriorly, is known as a *Mittendorf dot.*

beriberi   (probably derived from a Singhalese word signifying weakness, the repetition adding emphasis). A syndrome of cardiomyopathy and sensorimotor peripheral neuropathy resulting from dietary deficiency of vitamin B_1 (thiamine).

The condition was first described in the East Indies in 1642 by Jacob Bontius, a Dutch physician. In 1889, another Dutch physician, Christiaan Eijkman, demonstrated that the dietary deficiency was due to a lack of the polishings of rice (the husks), which is where the thiamine is. More recently, the name has been used in remote areas to refer to any form of severe neuropathy. It is still seen in Third World countries in starvation areas, in severely dietarily deprived alcoholics, and occasionally in people on severely restricted fad diets.

The chronic, dry, *atrophic form* represents a mainly motor neuropathy and occurs in alcoholics. The *subacute form* is a centripetal symmetrical sensorimotor neuropathy affecting especially those limbs most utilized in the individual's activities of daily living, with the later addition of cardiac failure.

Acute beriberi is a syndrome of chest pain with cardiac failure, and leads rapidly to death.[4460]

Berlin syndrome   A recessively inherited dysmorphic syndrome of physical and mental retardation with generalized mottling of the skin, hyperkeratosis, reduced sweating, and impaired eruption of the teeth.[509]

Berman disease   See **mucolipidosis.**

Berman syndrome   A familial, perhaps recessive disorder characterized by progressive ataxia, deafness, mental retardation, and signs of both upper and lower motor neuron lesions.

The condition resembles the **Richards-Rundle syndrome,** except that it lacks the endocrinopathy and aminoaciduria.[515]

Bernard, Claude   (1813–1878) An outstanding French physician and physiologist who was first apprenticed to an apothecary and embarked upon a career as a playwright (with very modest success) before he became a medical student and a pupil of **Magendie** in Paris, graduating in 1839. He described the ocular changes that are now known as **Horner syndrome** in 1862, 7 years before Horner did,[518] and also discovered the existence of vasomotor nerves.[517]

Bernard was also the first to describe the action of curare in producing neuromuscular blockade, although the muscle remained susceptible to direct stimulation, and he first identified the *milieu intérieur,* gluconeogenesis, the functions of gastric secretions and lipolysis by pancreatic secretions. His book *An Introduction to the Study of Experimental Medicine* (1865) laid the foundations for the scientific study of the human body. Among the honors accorded him was the issuance of a French stamp bearing his portrait and carrying a surcharge to be used for the support of unemployed intellectuals.

Bernard-Horner syndrome   See **Horner syndrome.**

Bernhardt, Martin   (1844–1915) German neurologist who graduated from Berlin University and later worked with Leyden and Westphal. He himself was eventually professor at Berlin. He described **meralgia paresthetica** in 1878 and a form of progressive spinal muscular atrophy in 1893, as well as publishing good descriptions of cerebral tumors, syphilitic apoplexy, and diseases of the spinal cord.

Bernhardt-Roth (Rot) paresthesia   See **meralgia paresthetica.**

Berry aneurysm   See **aneurysm.**

Berry pins   A set of three 8-cm pins with white, green, or red spots of different sizes painted on their globular heads, used for the assessment of the central visual fields by confrontation at the bedside.[522]

Berry spot test   A test for detecting mucopolysaccharides, used in the diagnosis of Hurler syndrome, one of the **mucopolysaccharidoses.**

Bertolotti syndrome   Numbness, pain, and/or hypersensitivity in the distribution of the sciatic nerve associated with sacralization of the fifth lumbar vertebra.[525]

Bertolotti-Garcin syndrome   See **Garcin syndrome.**

Besnier-Boeck-Schaumann disease   See **sarcoidosis.**

Bessman-Baldwin syndrome   A recessively inherited syndrome characterized by blindness due to pigmentary macular degeneration, seizures, and mental and motor retardation. Excessive urinary excretion of carnitine and of various amino acids is another features of the syndrome.[532]

beta band   EEG activity in the frequency band over 13 Hz. Practically, most EEG machines using pen writers appreciably attenuate all frequencies higher than 75 Hz, and the customary use of relatively slow paper speeds further limits the interpreter's ability to resolve visually waves of frequencies over 35 Hz. However, this does not justify limiting unduly the high-frequency response of the EEG channels, for EEG waves include transients such as spikes and sharp waves with components at frequencies above 50 Hz. (Adapted from the report of the Committee on Terminology, IFCN,[989] © 1974, with permission from Elsevier Science.)

beta rhythm In general, any EEG rhythm faster than 13 Hz, but more characteristically used to describe a rhythm from 13 to 35 Hz recorded over the fronto-central regions of the head during wakefulness. The amplitude of such beta rhythm is variable but is mostly below 30 uV. Other beta rhythms are most prominent in other locations or are diffuse. (Adapted from the report of the Committee on Terminology, IFCN,[989] © 1974, with permission from Elsevier Science.)

This rhythm is especially susceptible to enhancement by medications such as benzodiazepines and barbiturates.

beta-enolase deficiency A defect of distal glycolysis that may present as a metabolic myopathy, manifesting myalgias, and exercise intolerance during adult-life.[1111]

See also **phosphoglycerate kinase, phosphoglycerate mutase, lactate dehydrogenase,** and **aldolase A deficiencies.**

beta-galactosidase-neuraminidase deficiency See **galactosialidosis.**

beta-glucuronidase deficiency See **mucopolysaccharidoses.**

beta-hydroxyisovaleric aciduria A syndrome of hereditary motor neuropathy resembling type 1 **hereditary motor neuropathy,** with associated abnormal aminoaciduria, and leading to early death. The condition is considered to be due to a failure of the enzymes in the leucine degradation pathway.[1631]

beta-interferon The first therapy for remitting-relapsing multiple sclerosis shown to be capable of reducing the number of exacerbations of the disease, at least during the first 3 years in which it is taken.

beta-ketothiolase deficiency (short-chain 3-ketothiolase deficiency) An inborn error of metabolism presenting in infancy with intermittent acidosis, hyperammonemia, lethargy, vomiting, feeding difficulty, hyponatremia, hyperkalemia and alteration in consciousness down to coma. Aminoaciduria is not a feature of the syndrome.[1301]

beta-methylcrotonylglycinuria A rare **organic acidemia** presenting in infancy with **infantile spasms,** lethargy, irritability, tachypnea, feeding difficulties, and failure to thrive.[335]

Bethlem myopathy (early-onset benign autosomal dominant limb girdle myopathy with contractures) A dominantly inherited, slowly progressive muscle disease with onset of limb girdle weakness and mild atrophy in infancy or childhood, without facial or cardiac involvement. Contractures of the fingers, elbows, and ankles are common. The first evidence may be reduction in fetal movements in the last trimester, hypotonia in the neonatal period, or weakness and contractures presenting in early childhood, but the onset can also be in late adult life with mild, diffuse proximal rather than distal weakness, occasional respiratory muscle weakness, cramps, and falls. The condition may arrest at any time and it is compatible with a normal life span,[2860] although some disability is usual after the age of 50 years.

Serum creatine kinase levels are normal or slightly elevated, the EMG is myopathic, and muscle biopsy is indicative of non-specific myopathy. The condition has been mapped variously to chromosome 21q22.3 and to 2q37 loci.

Better Hearing Institute A charitable organization. Address: Box 1840, Washington, DC 20013.

Betz cells The largest motor pyramidal cells of the fifth cerebral cortical layer.[536]

Betz, Vladimir Aleksandrovich (1834–1894) Russian professor of anatomy at Kiev University (1868–1889).[1478] He described the giant pyramidal cells in 1874.

Beveridge syndrome A congenital dysmorphic syndrome characterized by macrocephaly, delayed closure of the fontanelles and cranial sutures, skeletal maldevelopments, visceromegaly, rhizomelia of the upper limbs, and patchy depigmentation of the skin.[337]

Bezold-Jarisch reflex Reflex cardiovascular depression with vasodilation and bradycardia (vasovagal syncope) The circulatory response changes from the normal maintenance of arterial pressure, to parasympathetic activation and sympathetic inhibition, causing hypotension. This change is triggered by reduced cardiac venous return leading to mechanical or chemical stimulation in the heart left ventricle, where the afferent limb of the reflex evidently arises, (HJM) as well as through affective mechanisms such as pain or fear. It is probably mediated in part via afferent nerves from the heart, but also by various noncardiac baroreceptors which may become paradoxically active. This response may occur during regional anesthesia, hemorrhage, or supine inferior vena cava compression in pregnancy; these factors are additive when combined. In these circumstances, hypotension may be more severe than that caused by bradycardia alone, because of unappreciated vasodilation.[1249,3056] See also **neurocardiogenic syncope.**

Bianchi syndrome The occurrence of sensory aphasia, apraxia, and alexia occurring in patients with left-sided lesions involving the parietal lobe, with transient hemiplegia and hemianesthesia, and described by Leonardo Bianchi (1848–1927),[545] an Italian psychiatrist. See **aphasia-agnosia-apraxia syndrome.**

bias People who survive a disease for some time (prevalent cases) may differ from new (incident) cases by virtue of a confounding factor that is actually enhancing survival rather than acting as an etiologic factor.[4124]

biceps femoris reflex Contraction of this muscle in response to a tap over its tendon just above the fibular head. This is one of the few reflexes allowing assessment of the L5 reflex arc. See also **external hamstring reflex.**

biceps reflex Contraction of the biceps in response to a tap on its tendon, usually elicited by placing the examiner's index finger over the biceps tendon and tapping the finger, thus both palpating and visualizing the resultant muscle contraction. The reflex is increased in pyramidal disease affecting that limb and diminished with C5,6 lesions.

Bichat, Marie-François-Xavier (1771–1802) Anatomist, histologist, and physician at the Hotel-Dieu in Paris from the unusually early age of 28. Among his many contributions were his descriptions of the arachnoid membrane and of the subarachnoid space.[548]

Bickerstaff brainstem "encephalitis" A syndrome of ophthalmoplegia, ataxia, and normal or decreased muscle stretch reflexes, preceded by a febrile illness and leading to gradual paralysis of cranial nerve function, descending from the oculomotor muscles to the whole brainstem with slow subsequent recovery, during which a parkinsonian picture may develop transiently. During the acute illness, drowsiness or a moribund state may occur, although with supportive care, patients slowly return to normal, without sequelae. Cortical EEG abnormalities and areflexia are also described. As in Miller Fisher syndrome, IgG anti-GQ$_{1b}$ antibodies are frequently present. Deafness, ataxia, and extensor plantar responses have been recorded. MRI scans and brainstem evoked responses have suggested the presence of a brainstem lesion and there is pleocytosis in the CSF.[90,553] The condition tends to occur in small groups in geographically related areas.

The relationship of this condition to the **Miller Fisher syndrome** (a variant of **acute inflammatory demyelinating polyneuropathy**) is likely to be intimate; indeed, they may be identical,[6003] since anti-GQ$_{1b}$ antibodies are not limited by the blood–brain barrier in the sites of their attack. The increased cells in the CSF, normal peripheral nerve conduction studies, and localized abnormality of evoked potentials in typical cases of "brainstem encephalitis" suggest that the condition may well involve the brainstem, with or without peripheral nerve involvement,[6067] but the simultaneous involvement of both sites has been recorded and central and peripheral demyelination can occur together. See also **basilar migraine.**

Bickerstaff, Edwin R. Contemporary English neurologist.

Bickerstaff migraine See **basilar migraine.**

bicuculline A potent epileptogenic agent which acts by blockade of gamma-aminohydroxybutyric acid, the inhibitory neurotransmitter.

Biedel, Arthur (1869–1933) Polish endocrinologist.

Bielschowsky, Alfred (1871–1940) German ophthalmologist practicing in Berlin, who gave the first account of **internuclear ophthalmoplegia**.[560] See also **Roth-Bielschowsky syndrome.**

Bielschowsky head tilt test Patients with diplopia due to a fourth cranial nerve palsy will note that the images fuse if they tilt the head toward the opposite shoulder but separate further when they tilt the head toward the side of the fourth nerve palsy. As an example, with a left fourth nerve palsy, the vertical deviation is more marked when the head is tilted down toward the left shoulder, and less marked when the head is tilted the other way.

Bielschowsky, Max (1869–1940) German neurobiologist, a student under Edinger and Nissl, who graduated from Munich University and worked with Weigl and Edinger before moving to the Neurobiological Institute in Berlin. There his work was mainly on cytoarchitecture (**Vogt** was the director of the institute). He sought asylum from the Nazis in Spain and then in Holland in 1936, but was brought back by threat; he fled to England just before the start of the World War II.

He introduced the technique for the silver staining of neurons which is still the basis of that now used, and investigated the pathology of numerous brain diseases, such as that listed below.[7]

Max Bielschowsky

Bielschowsky bodies   Intraneuronal inclusion bodies restricted to neurons in the external pallidum in cases of choreoathetosis and cerebral palsy.[3461] See also **corpora amylacea, Lafora bodies.**

Bielschowsky-(Dollinger)-Jansky disease   (late infantile amaurotic familial idiocy) A rare, recessively inherited lipid storage disease characterized by seizures in early childhood, mental and motor impairment, cerebellar atrophy, and retinal degeneration (without the **cherry-red spot**), described by Bielschowsky in 1914.[561] See **neuronal ceroid lipidosis.**

Bielschowsky-Lutz-Cogan syndrome   See **internuclear ophthalmoplegia.**

Biemond, Arie   (b. 1902) Dutch neurologist, who trained in Amsterdam, where he later became professor of neurology.

Biemond ataxia   (OMIM 176250) A rare, dominantly inherited spinocerebellar degeneration resembling SCA4 with onset in youth or young adult life, and in which there is loss of posterior root ganglion cells with posterior column demyelination and of cerebellar Purkinje cells. Loss of vibration and postural sense and areflexia are the usual clinical manifestations,[564] although scoliosis may also be associated.[335] The condition has been mapped to the short arm of chromosome 16.

There is uncertainty as to whether this is a specific disorder, even though it is often referred to as a syndrome of pure posterior column ataxia (sensory ataxia). Primary degeneration of the large dorsal root ganglion cells would cause exactly the same symptoms (loss of thick-fiber sensory functions and hypo- or areflexia).[2439] The condition was first described by Mollaret in 1929.

A *variant* is a recessively inherited form with added pigmentary retinopathy.[2569]

See also **familial posterior column ataxia, cerebellar ataxias.**

Biemond syndrome   1. (brachydactyly-ataxia) A congenital, dominantly inherited, dysmorphic syndrome characterized by brachydactyly, abnormal metatarsals, and cerebellar signs.[562]

2. (obesity–polydactyly–iris coloboma) A congenital, recessive, dysmorphic syndrome characterized by obesity, iris coloboma, pigmentary retinal degeneration, hypogonadotrophic hypogonadism, polydactyly, hydrocephalus, and mental and developmental delay.[563] See **hydrocephalus with polydactyly.**

Biernacki sign   Anesthesia in ulnar distribution or absence of pain when the ulnar nerve is pinched, described in tertiary neurosyphilis.[4723]

big blind spot syndrome   The occurrence of an enlarged blind spot in the absence of any optic disk edema, the increased size of the blind spot being due to focal peripapillary retinopathy. Central acuity and color vision are unaffected but a sharply defined scotoma is present, corresponding to the blind spot. The syndrome appears to be evanescent.[1885] See also **multiple evanescent white dot syndrome, papillophlebitis.**

big Broca aphasia   See **Broca aphasia.**

big/large spikes   See **benign epileptiform transients of sleep.**

Bignami, Amico   (1862–1929) Italian pathologist who graduated from the University of Rome, where he became professor of general pathology in 1902. Most of his important communications were made in conjunction with **Marchiafava.**

Bijlsma syndrome   A congenital dysmorphic syndrome characterized by aqueduct stenosis with hydrocephalus and gaze palsies, spasticity, and mental and developmental delay.[337]

Bikele sign   1. Resistance to extension of the elbow when the arm is elevated at the shoulder in patients with **neuralgic amyotrophy,** probably due to traction upon the irritated nerve roots.[5877] 2. Pain felt in the shoulder with contraction of the biceps, when the abducted, externally rotated arm is extended. The sign is described in patients with cerebral tumor[5047] or meningism.

bilateral   (Gr, double + the side) On both sides.

bilateral biparietal atrophy   See **posterior cortical atrophy.**

bilateral central macrogyria   (epilepsy, pseudobulbar palsy and mental retardation, developmental Foix-Chavany-Marie syndrome) A neuronal migration disorder manifesting pseudobulbar palsy, mild pyramidal signs, mild mental retardation, and intractable secondary or multifocal epileptic syndromes (such as **infantile spasms,** generalized tonic-clonic or partial complex seizures, atonic attacks, head-dropping spells). The bilateral cerebral macrogyria is demonstrable on MRI scans.[3205]

bilateral distal vertebral artery occlusion   A rare syndrome with grave prognosis seen in patients with marked vasculopathy and characterized by the slow progression of signs of cerebellar and lateral medullary ischemia due to chronically reduced perfusion in vertebrobasilar territory, with a tendency to sudden death.[897]

bilateral facial agenesis   See **mandibulofacial dysostosis.**

bilateral facial spasm   See **blepharospasm.**

bilateral frontal polymicrogyria   See **polymicrogyria.**

bilateral occipital calcification, epilepsy, and celiac disease   An uncommon epileptic syndrome resembling **Sturge-Weber disease,** and characterized by malabsorption; bilateral cortical and subcortical calcifications, mainly posteriorly but sometimes extending into frontal regions; and partial epilepsy. The latter may consist either of occipital seizures with a benign course and without mental deterioration or neurological signs, or of drug-resistant occipital seizures with mental deterioration. No cutaneous abnormalities are described, there is no lobar atrophy, and MRI scans are normal.[3566]

bilateral paraspasm   See **dystonia.**

bilateral periventricular nodular heterotopia (OMIM 300049) A malformation of neuronal migraition or proloferation in which nodular masses of gray matter line the lateral ventricles and protrude into its lumen. Most cases have been female, who present with various types of seizure but who are otherwise normal. The condition is dominant and mapped to chromosome Xq28.

In a *variant* form in boys, mental retardation and frontonasal malformations also occur.[1481,2310] See also **X-linked lissencephaly, congenital bilateral perisylvian syndrome, subcortical band heterotopia.**

bilateral simultaneous optic neuropathy   See **optic neuropathy.**

bilateral striatal necrosis, dystonia, and optic atrophy   A rare syndrome, probably recessively inherited, characterized by dystonic movements and postures, generalized hypokinesia, subacute visual loss, and bilateral selective striatal necrotic lesions visualized by CT and MRI scans. Cognitive functions are unimpaired.[3364] See also **Leigh disease, infantile bilateral striatal necrosis, Leber optic atrophy.**

bilateral vestibular paresis   Loss of vestibular function following local infection, leading to **sensory ataxia** when the eyes can no longer compensate for the loss of vestibular input. Rotation and caloric stimulation tests do not induce vertigo for the same reason.[1034]

bilirubin encephalopathy   See **kernicterus.**

bimodal extinction   The failure to perceive and report sensory signals from one side in more than one mode, e.g., tactile and visual.

binasal hemianopia   Isolated loss of both of the nasal fields of vision due to bilateral involvement of the uncrossed fibers at the optic chiasm, typically as a result of displacement of these fibers by a local mass lesion or increased intracranial pressure, or because of their compression by masses such as aneurysms of the internal carotid artery or meningiomas, which are often (but not always) bilateral.[4197]

binaural   (Lat, twice + ear) Relating to both ears.

Binet, Alfred   (1856–1911) French psychologist, who, with Theodor Simon, devised the first validated test of intelligence at the request of the French government. The early tests gave a "mental age," and allowed classifications of intellectually impaired people as *idiots* (mental age, 1–2 years), *imbeciles* (3–7 years), and *morons* (8–12 years). Above that age, people were classified as backward, normal, or advanced.

Later, an intelligence quotient was calculated as the mental age divided by the chronological age and expressed as a percentage. The Binet-Simon tests led to refinements such as the Stanford-Binet and Herring-Binet tests, derivatives of which are still in use.

Bing headache (syndrome)   See **cluster headache.**

Bing reflex   1. Watering of the eyes when eating food with a strong taste. 2. A variant method of eliciting the Babinski response, whereby the dorsum of the foot is pricked with a pin.[574]

Bing, Robert Paul   (1878–1956) Swiss neurologist and neuropathologist, who studied under **Horsley,** His, **Edinger, Oppenheim,** and **Déjèrine,** eventually becoming professor of neurology at Basel University. His *Kompendium* (1909) was a manual of localization in clinical neurology based on a superb exposition of clinical neuroanatomy; it was translated into three languages and most recently revised in English by Webb **Haymaker** (1969). The book remains, however, an essential introduction to the subject for aspiring neurologists. It was followed by his *Lehrbuch der Nerven-Krankheiten* (1913), the fifth edition of which was also translated by Haymaker in 1939.

Robert Paul Bing

Bing-Neel syndrome   A syndrome of encephalomyelopathy and polyradiculopathy in association with macroglobulinemia.

Systemic clinical features include fever, emaciation, anorexia, weight loss, and lymphadenopathy; common neurological findings are personality change, delusions, dementia, and variously pyramidal, cerebellar, and unclear sensory findings. The erythrocyte sedimentation rate is elevated, and IgM hyperglobulinemia, resembling **Waldenstrom macroglobulinemia,** is usual.[573]

Dr. Bing is an American and Dr. A.V. Neel a Scandinavian physician.

binocular   (Lat, twice + eyes) Relating to both eyes.

binocular diplopia   See **diplopia.**

Binswanger disease   (Binswanger encephalitis, subacute arteriosclerotic encephalopathy, progressive subcortical arteriosclerotic encephalopathy, encephalitis subcorticalis chronica progressiva, lacunar dementia). An entity characterized by an ischemic periventricular leukoencephalopathy typically sparing the arcuate subcortical U fibers and manifested clinically by subcortical frontal executive dysfunction, parkinsonian gait disturbances, urinary incontinence, mood changes, and pseudobulbar palsy. It is one of the most common forms of vascular dementia in the elderly. Clinically, it may be suspected in middle-aged hypertensive patients with evidence of systemic vascular disease who develop insidious, fluctuating **subcortical dementia** with especial involvement of memory, mood, and cognition; seizures; as well as evidence of pyramidal, extrapyramidal, and cerebellar[457] dysfunction presenting as mild strokes.

This leukoencephalopathy is likely caused by hypoxia-ischemia of distal watershed periventricular territories, the combined effects of arteriolosclerosis and elongation of medullary arterioles, dilatation of the perivascular spaces (état criblé), and decreased brain perfusion from hypotension or low cardiac output. Lacunes may be markers of Binswanger-type lesions in these patients. Increased fibrinogen levels and hyperviscosity may be found.[901,1868]

Binswanger did not provide a full account of the neuropathology of the condition (this was remedied by **Nissl** and by **Alzheimer,** who also named the disease), and his patients were not notably hypertensive. One assumes with slight justification that the condition defined as follows is that which Binswanger actually described. Criteria for the diagnosis of Binswanger disease have been suggested[459] (see Chart B–3).

Binswanger differentiated this condition from syphilis (although in retrospect it is likely that his patient did have syphilis), and his pathological examination showed the presence of arteriolosclerosis, hemorrhages, and infarcts deep in the cerebral hemispheres, extensive white matter atrophy mainly in the periventricular and occipitotemporal distribution and only slight atrophy of the cortex.[577] The pathological features of note are **lacunes,** subcortical white matter demyelination, the **état criblé,** neuronal loss, gliosis, ventricular dilatation, and atheroma of the larger cerebral vessels. CT scans show enlarged ventricles, symmetrical periventricular lucencies, and lacunar and sometimes cortical infarcts.

Olszewski emphasized the presence of the lacunes in 1962 and suggested the term *subcortical arteriosclerotic encephalopathy,* but the eponym presumes less and is preferred for its brevity. The definitive major review is that of Babikian and Ropper.[282]

A familial form of Binswanger disease presenting in younger patients in the absence of vascular risk factors should raise the possibility of cerebral autosomal dominant arteriopathy with subcortical infarcts and leukoencephalopathy (CADASIL).

Binswanger encephalitis   See **Binswanger disease.**

Chart B–3. Criteria for the Diagnosis of Binswanger Disease

1. Dementia must be established by clinical examination and confirmed by neuropsychological tests.
2. One finding from two of the following three groups must be present:
   The presence of a vascular risk factor or evidence of systemic vascular disease (e.g., hypertension, diabetes, a history of myocardial infarction, cardiac arrhythmia, or congestive heart failure),
   Evidence of focal cerebrovascular disease (e.g., a history of stroke, or demonstration of focal pyramidal or sensory signs), or
   Evidence of "subcortical" cerebral dysfunction (e.g., parkinsonian, magnetic, or "senile" gait, parkinsonian or gegenhalten rigidity, or a history of incontinence secondary to a spastic bladder).
3. The radiological criteria require bilateral **leukoaraiosis** on CT or bilateral and multiple or diffuse subcortical high-signal T2-weighted lesions greater than 2×2 mm on MRI scans.

The proposed criteria lose their validity in the presence of
1. Multiple or bilateral cortical lesions on CT or MRI scans, or
2. Severe dementia (e.g, **Mini-Mental State** score of less than 10).

Adapted from Bennett DA, Wilson RS, Gilley DW et al. Clinical diagnosis of Binswanger's disease. J. Neurol. Neurosurg. Psychiatry 1990; **53:***961–965, by kind permission.[459]*

Otto Ludwig Bingswanger

Binswanger, Otto Ludwig   (1852–1929) Swiss physician who qualified in Medicine at Zurich University and who later studied psychiatry under Meynert in Vienna. He became professor of psychiatry at Jena University and directed a military hospital during the World War I. He is best remembered for his paper "The Differentiation of Progressive General Paralysis," published in 1894,[577] in which he suggested a vascular rather than a syphilitic cause for the dementing syndrome now named for him, but he also wrote extensively on epilepsy, hysteria, and delirium. He retired, following a severe attack of "Spanish" influenza (**encephalitis lethargica**) in 1919.

biological clocks Pacemaking mechanisms in the brain controlling circadian rhythms, likely situated within the suprachiasmatic nuclei in the anterior hypothalamus.

biopsy The surgical removal of tissue (such as muscle, nerve or brain) for microscopic or bacteriological study.

biopterin deficiency See **phenylketonuria.**

Biot breathing A pattern of respiration marked by irregular grouping of the breaths that vary in depth and between which there are apneic pauses of different lengths. These occur in patients with dorsolateral medullary lesions and in such diffuse diseases as meningitis and uremia. The pattern is not (as has sometimes been suggested) regular, rapid, or rhythmical.

Dr. C. Biot (b. 1848) was a French physician who published his description in 1876 while an intern in Lyon.[578]

biotin-responsive encephalopathy (OMIM 252260) A recessively inherited, progressive neurological syndrome of early childhood due to deficiency of biotinidase.[6023] It is mapped to 3p25.

Clinically, the disease is phenotypically diverse, and may be characterized by alopecia, skin rash, encephalopathy, ataxia, hypotonia, hearing loss, myoclonus, neonatal seizures, developmental delay, lactic acidosis, and/or aminoaciduria.[4885]

The condition is one cause of the **Ramsay-Hunt syndrome** of seizures, myoclonus, and ataxia. See **multiple carboxylase deficiency.**

biotin-responsive multiple carboxylase deficiency See **holocarboxylase deficiency.**

biphasic action potential An action potential that crosses the baseline only once, producing two phases (one above and the other below the baseline).

biphasic end-plate activity See **end-plate activity.**

biphasic motor reaction The occurrence of a **flexor reflex** followed by extension of the legs in patients with incomplete spinal cord lesions, after any form of stimulation given to sites below the level of the lesion.

biphasic wave See **diphasic wave.**

bipolar With two opposite poles or states. Hence *bipolar depression, bipolar cells* (neurons with two axons), and the following entries.

bipolar derivation A recording from a pair of exploring electrodes. See also **exploring electrode, bipolar montage.**

bipolar montage Multiple bipolar derivations in which no electrode is common to all derivations. In most cases, bipolar derivations are linked, i.e., adjacent derivations from electrodes along the same array have one electrode in common, connected to the input terminal 2 of one amplifier and to the input terminal 1 of the following amplifier. See also **referential montage.** (Adapted from the report of the Committee on Terminology, IFCN,[989] © 1974, with permission from Elsevier Science.)

bipolar needle electrode A recording electrode that measures the voltage between two insulated wires cemented side-by-side in a steel cannula. The bare tips of the electrodes are flush with the level of the cannula which may serve as a ground. (From the 2001 Report of the Nomenclature Committee of the American Association of Electromyography and Electrodiagnosis.[10] Used by permission, copyright © 2001, AAEM.)

bird-like face syndrome See **Seckel bird-headed dwarfism.**

Birnbaum syndrome A syndrome characterized by chronic progressive chorea with cerebellar atrophy, described in 1941.[587]

bisynchronous A tautologous contraction the equally tautologous term "bilaterally synchronous."

bitemporal hemianopia Loss or reduction in efficacy of the visual field on the temporal side in each eye. The first complete analytic description was in 1915 by Cushing and Walker,[1233] who pointed out that the usual cause was a hypophyseal tumor and that the defects were rarely symmetrical.

They divided such visual defects into eight stages according to their severity, among which stage 1 represented a slant in the upper boundary of the temporal field and a corresponding quadrantic defect in the color peripheries; stage 4 represented hemianopsia, often with macular sparing; and stage 8 indicated complete blindness.

The development of the deficit was charted by Traquair, who showed that it characteristically begins in the upper outer quadrant, proceeding clockwise in the right and counterclockwise in the left field, so that the upper nasal quadrant remains intact longest. The central defect behaves in the same way.[5625]

See also **hemianopia, Traquair scotoma.**

bizarre high-frequency discharge See **complex repetitive discharge.**

bizarre repetitive discharge See **complex repetitive discharge.**

bizarre repetitive potential See **complex repetitive discharge.**

Bjerrum, Jamik Peterson (1851–1926) Danish professor of ophthalmology in Copenhagen, who described **arcuate scotomas** in patients with glaucoma in 1890. He also developed the tangent screen, which is still in general use, employing a cloth pinned to the door of his office.[1829]

Bjerrum screen (tangent screen) A dark felt cloth 1 meter square marked with a central point, radii, and concentric rings, set vertically in a darkened room, upon which the subject gazes while a lighted object is brought into the field of vision from the periphery as a test of the peripheral visual fields and the extent of the blind spot.

Björnstadt syndrome See **pili torti.**

black widow spider An arachid, the venom of which induces the rapid release of transmitter from nerve terminals, causing initial muscular contractions followed by paralysis. This may be fatal in young children and the frail elderly.

The spider (so called because the female eats her mate) is recognized by the characteristic red "hourglass" pattern on her belly.

bladder disorders See **automatic bladder, deafferented bladder, hypertonic bladder, incontinence, motor paralytic bladder.**

Blanchet syndrome Unilateral lumbar meningopolyradiculoneuritis associated with inflammation of the lumbar sympathetic chain.[599] Further reports of this syndrome are not available and the nature of the condition is unknown.

blast (Gr, bud) a suffix denoting development.

blepharismus (from Gr, the eyelid) Winking.

blepharoclonus Repetitive blinking, sometimes heralding the later development of **blepharospasm.** See **spasmus nictitans.**

blepharocolysis (Gr, an eyelid + inhibition) A supranuclear movement disorder characterized by a transient atonic inability to initiate eyelid opening in the absence of a definable lesion of the supranuclear or infranuclear oculomotor pathways, described most often in patients with pyramidal or extrapyramidal diseases. The disorder is thus not actually an apraxia at all. See **apraxia of lid opening.**

blepharonasofacial syndrome A dominantly inherited dysmorphic syndrome characterized by stenosis of the lacrimal puncta, syndactyly, pyramidal and cerebellar signs, dystonia, and mental retardation.[4352]

blepharophimosis A dominantly inherited condition characterized by shortness and narrowing of the palpebral fissures, shortening of the upper eyelid (with deficiency of the levator palpebrae superioris also contributing to ptosis), hypoplasia of the orbicularis oculi, and flattening of the root of the nose.[4]

blepharophimosis syndrome A heterogeneous dominantly inherited, congenital, dysmorphic syndrome characterized by blepharophimosis and, variously, ptosis, telecanthus, nystagmus, strabismus, reversible joint contractures, cleft palate, dolichocephaly, arachnodactyly, skeletal and cerebellar dysgeneses, hypotonia, and mandibular hypoplasia.[1877] See also **Marden-Walker syndrome, Schwartz-Jampel syndrome.**

Congenital blepharophimosis is a *variant* characterized by general diminution of the palpebral fissure in all its dimensions but with the eyelids normally differentiated. Associated eye defects include nystagmus, microphthalmos, anophthalmos, ptosis, epicanthus inversus, and hypermetropia. Facial dysmorphisms are also frequently associated. The condition may be dominantly inherited as uncomplicated blepharophimosis, in association with microphthalmos and anophthalmos; with rigidity and dysfunction of the extraocular muscles, or as part of the **Waardenburg syndrome.**

The following criteria for the diagnosis of congenital blepharophimosis have been suggested:[5437]
1. Diminution of the palpebral fissure in the range of 10–15 mm long and 2–4 mm wide on opening of the lids. The measurements remain constant throughout life.
2. The distance between the internal canthi often equals double the length of the palpebral fissure.
3. A flattened nasal bridge is present.
4. The aplasia of the palpebral levators and the tautness of the skin cause stiffness of the lids and obliteration of the tarsal folds.
5. The eyelid descends over the cornea and covers the pupil. For improvement the head is usually tilted back and there is continued overaction of the occipitofrontalis muscle.
6. The eyelids are defectively developed with thin, smooth atrophic skin and rudimentary tarsal plates.
7. The eyelashes are underdeveloped and grow irregularly.
8. There is lateral displacement of the lachrymal puncta and elongation of the lateral.
9. The lack of contact within the bulb and the lids especially nasally results in epiphera.

blepharoplegia (Gr, eyelid + weakness) Ptosis due to paresis of the levator palpebrae.

blepharoptosis (Gr, eyelid + a fall) Drooping of the upper eyelid. See **ptosis.**

blepharoschisis A malformation affecting the eyelids which may be a simple cleft up to complete absence (*ablepharon*).[4] See also **coloboma.**

blepharospasm (facial paraspasm, bilateral facial spasm, benign essential blepharospasm) Symmetrical, repetitive, involuntary, sustained, tight closure of the eyes as a result of involuntary contractions of the orbiculari oculi, in the absence of ocular pathology,[2256,2808] although the R2 component of the **blink reflex** is abnormally prolonged.

The condition represents a focal dystonic syndrome, most common in adult women. The muscular contractions are often increased by bright light and reduced by other voluntary activity, despite which they may be so intractable as to produce functional blindness.[1649,2811] See also **Meige syndrome.**

Rating scales for blepharospasm have been constructed.[1729]

In a *variant form,* patients with **Parkinson disease** or **progressive supranuclear palsy** are unable to initiate or sustain eye opening in the absence of overt spasm of the orbicularis muscles.[1648]

blepharospasm-oromandibular dystonia   See **Brueghel syndrome.**

Blessed-Roth dementia instruments   (Newcastle Dementia Scale, Information-Memory-Concentration Test) A two-part measure designed to quantify the cognitive and behavioral symptoms of dementia, comparing these manifestations with measures of underlying brain neuropathology. Some of the elements have been included in the **CAMDEX**[4814] and the CERAD Instrument.[3997]

The *Blessed Dementia Scale* is a behavioral rating scale evaluating functional and emotional impairment and consisting of 22 items measuring changes in performance of everyday activities, self-care habits, and personality interests and drives. The Blessed Information-Memory-Concentration Test[603] is a well-validated measure of cognitive impairment. Dr G. Blessed is a neuropsychologist in Newcastle, UK. See **Information-Memory-Concentration Test.**

blind headache   A once-popular term for **migraine.**

blind spot   A physiological defect in the visual fields due to the absence of rod and cone receptors on the head of the optic nerve. Its presence was first remarked in 1688 by E. Mariotte (1620–1684), a French physicist, who also described the **red reflex.**

blindisms   (digito-ocular maneuver) The repetitive rubbing of the eyes, an action performed frequently by some people with congenital pigmentary retinal degenerations.

blindsight   The capacity to detect (or at least make saccadic movements in the direction of) visual stimuli presented within the area of a field defect in the absence of acknowledged awareness. This may occur when the blindness results from damage to the striate cortex.[5901]

blink rate   The frequency of involuntary repetitive blinking. In the normal subject this is 24 ± 15 per minute. The rate is decreased in depressive illnesses, **Parkinson disease,** and **progressive supranuclear palsy.**[4851]

blink reflex

1. Clinically, closure of the eyes with sudden visual stimulation or with tactile stimulation of the upper part of the face. The reflex was known to Descartes and to Jean Fernel (1506–1588). See also **palpebral reflex, orbicularis oculi reflex.**
2. In electromyography, **compound muscle action potentials** evoked from orbicularis oculi muscles as a result of brief electric or mechanical stimuli applied to the cutaneous area

innervated by the supraorbital (or less commonly, the infraorbital) branch of the trigeminal nerve. Typically, there is an early compound muscle action potential (R1 wave) ipsilateral to the stimulation site with a latency of about 10 msec and a bilateral late compound muscle action potential (R2 wave) with a latency of approximately 30 msec. Generally, only the R2 wave is associated with a visible contraction of the muscle. The configuration, amplitude, duration, and latency of the two components, along with the sites of recording and stimulation, should be specified. The Rl and R2 waves are oligosynaptic and polysynaptic brainstem reflexes, respectively. Together they are called the *blink reflex.* The afferent arc is provided by the sensory branches of the trigeminal nerve and the efferent arc is provided by facial nerve motor fibers. (From the 2001 Report of the Nomenclature Committee of the American Association of Electromyography and Electrodiagnosis.[10] Used by permission, copyright © 2001, AAEM.)

The reflex is considered abnormal when there is unilateral loss of R1; unilateral delay by 1.4 msec or more; or uni- or bilateral delay above the age-related mean + 2.5 SEM.[2643]

blink response   See **blink reflex.**

blink-saccade synkinesis   The tendency for blink and saccadic movements to occur together. This is both normal and efficient, although normally, either movement may be made alone. Inability to make saccades without blinking has been described as a sign of posterior fossa disease.[6110]

blip syndrome   Irregularly recurrent, momentary sensations in the head suggesting impending loss of consciousness, felt in the relaxed state, by subjects without evidence of neurological disease. It has a benign prognosis.[3239]

See also **exploding head syndrome.**

blips   Torsional eye deviations during and after saccadic eye movements.[2526]

Bliss symbols   A pictographic, ideographic writing system of about 100 symbols developed by Charles K. Bliss that can be decoded in all languages and is intended to function as an auxiliary language for international communication. It has been adapted as a communication medium for prereading, severely communicatively impaired children.

The symbols express both items and ideas, and are laid out on large cards, enabling the subject to point to them successively in order to convey information or requests.[3788] However, newer language systems such as *Rebus* and *Picsyms* have been adopted more widely because many people find them easier to learn.

blitz-nick-salaam krampfe   See **West syndrome.**

Bloch, Bruno   (1878–1933) Swiss physician.

Bloch-Sulzberger syndrome   See **incontinentia pigmenti.**

Block Design Test   A constructional task forming a subtest of the **Wechsler Adult Intelligence Scale,** in which the subject is required to manipulate multiple-patterned blocks in order to match a composite pattern presented on a card, a measure of (right hemisphere) spatial functioning.[5889]

block vertebral anomaly A rare spinal column and cord anomaly with scoliosis, abnormal rib cage, and local myelopathy resulting from a failure of segmentation at the affected level.[4972]

blocking 1. The apparent temporary obliteration of EEG rhythms in response to physiological or other stimuli such as electrical stimulation of the brain. See **attenuation.** 2. A condition of temporary unresponsiveness of the EEG amplifier caused by major overload and manifested initially by extreme flat-topped pen excursion(s) lasting up to a few seconds. See also **clipping.** (Adapted from the report of the Committee on Terminology, IFCN,[989] © 1974, with permission from Elsevier Science.) 3. A brief interruption of a train of thought with a temporary difficulty in logical verbal expression. Although this is a common occurrence in the normal, fatigued person and increases with age, repetitive brief periods of complete inhibition of thought is a symptom of schizophrenia of the first rank, and can occur in depressive illness. 4. A term used in **single fiber electromyography** to describe dropout of one or more components of the potential during sequential firings. If more than one component drops out simultaneously it is described as concomitant blocking. This is usually seen when jitter values exceed 80 to 100 μsec. A sign of abnormal neuromuscular transmission, which may be due to primary neuromuscular transmission disorders, such as myasthenia gravis and other myasthenic syndromes. Also seen as a result of degeneration and reinnervation in neuropathies or myopathies. Concomitant blocking may be generated by a split muscle fiber or failure of conduction at an axon branch serving several muscle fibers. (From the 2001 Report of the Nomenclature Committee of the American Association of Electromyography and Electrodiagnosis.[10] Used by permission, copyright © 2001, AAEM.)

blocking reaction The abrupt inhibition or cessation of a voluntary movement.

Blocq, Paul-Oscar (1860–1896) French neuropsychiatrist, born and trained in Paris, where he worked at the Salpêtrière before his premature death. He published his own textbook in 1894, contributed chapters on chorea and syphilis to Charcot's *Traité de Médicine,* and described the syndrome of **astasia-abasia** in 1888.[606]

Blocq syndrome (astasia-abasia) Hysterical inability to walk or even stand, although all movements are normal in the lying position. Jacoud, Charcot, and Weir Mitchell had touched upon the subject, but Blocq's 1888 monograph was the definitive text.[606] As he put it, the patient "can even jump in some cases or walk on all fours, but has lost the memory of the specialized movements necessary to hold himself upright (astasia) and to walk (abasia)."

All but one of Blocq's patients were under 28 years old. By his description there appears to be some resemblance to Bamberger's saltatory spasms, but Blocq denied this. In fact, both were manifestations of hysteria. However, with vermis lesions (e.g., due to medulloblastoma in children), leg movements may be unimpaired in recumbency even though the gait is very ataxic. [JF]

blood–brain barrier A physicochemical mechanism whereby solutes and materials in suspension in the blood are held back from entering the internal environment of the brain.

The search for the nature of this barrier was initiated by Ehrlich in 1886 as a result of his work on aniline dyes as staining reagents, during which he noticed that the vital acid dyes such as trypan blue stained everything in the body except the brain, which *was,* however, stained by the basic dyes. In 1913, Goldman injected acid dyes into the ventricles and showed that they did then stain the brain tissue, indicating the presence of a selectively permeable barrier between blood and brain, considered to be at the level of the endothelial cell.[5610]

Within the brain, only the area postrema, median eminence, pineal gland, neurohypophysis, pineal crest, and a few other areas are not shielded by this barrier. Clinically, it is highly effective in preventing entry into the CNS of various medications, including some antibiotics. The barrier may, however, be lowered by inflammation, as in meningitis, and by certain other toxins. The barrier is crossed more easily by nonionized, low-molecular-weight, lipid-soluble molecules.

Bloom syndrome A congenital dysmorphic syndrome characterized also by microcephaly, short stature, hirsutism, facial telangiectasias, vitiligo, café-au-lait spots, and photosensitivity of the skin.[5085]

blowout fracture A fracture of the floor of the orbit as a result of blunt trauma to the globe or to the inferior orbital rim. Multiple ocular motor palsies may result, and entrapment of the inferior rectus muscle within the fracture may lead to restriction of upward gaze.[3330]

blue diaper syndrome (Drummond syndrome) A recessively inherited diffuse encephalopathy characterized by hypercalcemia, nephrocalcinosis, and indicanuria. Craniostenosis, mental retardation, and dwarfism are less constant features.

The condition is due to the slow absorption of tryptophan from the bowel, followed by its conversion to indoles, which are absorbed and excreted in the urine to produce the bluish staining.[1519]

blue edema See **Charcot edema.**

blue jeans syndrome Compression of the sciatic nerve by shrinking wet jeans.[3696]

blue rubber bleb nevus syndrome An uncommon congenital neurocutaneous disorder manifesting blue hemangiomas of the skin and vascular malformations of internal organs, sometimes including the brain and its venous sinuses but more commonly the gastrointestinal tract. Seizures may be a complication. It was first described by William Bean in 1958.[4929]

B-mode ultrasonography A technique whereby high-frequency sound waves are transmitted through tissues, the returning echoes providing an image of the area evaluated.

It allows identification of the arterial wall and lumen of vessels to the extent that even minor disease of the internal carotid can be detected, but it does not readily distinguish flowing blood from clot.

bobbing See **ocular bobbing.**

bobble-headed doll syndrome A congenital syndrome characterized by intermittent, arrhythmic, to-and-fro (flexion-extension) bobbing or nodding movements of the head at 2–3 Hz associated with rhythmic flexion and extension of the arms and legs in the presence of severe, slowly progressive hydrocephalus. It is usually caused by a tumor of the third ventricle, but tumors of the corpus callosum, frontal lobe, or basal ganglia may also be responsible.[477,5961]

Generalized obesity, optic atrophy, behavioral problems, emotional lability, sensory deficits, choroid plexus tumors, and arachnoid cysts are other reported features.

Boder-Sedgwick syndrome See **ataxia-telangiectasia.**

Bodian, David (b. 1910) American anatomist.

Bodian stain A method for staining nerve fibers and nerve endings, using colloidal silver, invented by Bodian in 1936.[617]

body clock That mechanism within the brain which regulates cycles of human activity as a pacemaker. It is considered to exist within the suprachiasmatic nucleus.

body image agnosia See **topographical agnosia, finger agnosia.**

body righting reflex See **righting reflexes.**

body schema See **body scheme.**

body scheme (body schema) The term of **Head, Holmes,** and **Brain** for an individual's conception of his body's size, shape and position, the body parts, right and left sides, etc.

The mechanism is directly involved when a person cannot recognize parts of his own body, a phenomenon termed *asomatagnosia.*

Boe, Franciscus de la (1614–1672) Dutch physiologist and professor of the practice of medicine at Leyden; also known as **Sylvius.** He described the lateral (sylvian) fissure in 1637, and named the aqueduct, although he was not the first to describe it. He also made the first differentiation between static, postural, and action tremors.

Bogorad, F.A. (fl. 1928) Russian neurologist.

Bogorad syndrome See **crocodile tears,** the syndrome aptly named by Bogorad in 1928,[625] but previously described by **Oppenheim** in 1913.

bombesin A peptide found in the brain and in the gastrointestinal tract that causes a feeling of satiety.

bonbon sign Movement of the tongue inside the mouth, producing a bulge in the cheek, as though the subject has a candy in her mouth. It is seen in dystonic or choreic states.

Bondin-Barbizet syndrome See **epileptic endocrine syndrome.**

Bonhoeffer, Karl Ludwig (1868–1948) German psychiatrist who studied in Tübingen and Munich. After psychiatric training in France and Germany, he was assistant to **Wernicke** and later succeeded Kraepelin at Heidelberg University before moving on, eventually to Berlin University, as professor of psychiatry. He authored nearly 100 publications on various topics in neurology, psychiatry, pathology, and alcoholism. He died 3 years after his son, a Lutheran pastor, was hanged for outspoken criticism of the Nazi régime.

Bonhoeffer symptom Chorea, which he considered to be caused by a lesion in a region posterior to the optic thalamus, presumably the caudate, in which case he was right.[652]

Bonhoeffer syndrome (exogenous psychosis) See **delirium.**

Bonnet, Amedée (1809–1858) French surgeon who trained in Lyon and Paris and after internship there returned to Lyon University, where he became professor of clinical surgery in due course.

Charles Bonnet

Bonnet, Charles (1720–1793) Swiss lawyer, naturalist and philosopher. A wealthy man, he never practiced law (which he disliked) but rather studied natural history. He wrote on sensation and discernment in plants, and anticipated Darwin's theory of evolution, by implication. His studies of respiratory pores in Lepidoptera led to his election as a fellow of the Royal Society, although he never left Switzerland.[5047] After his sight failed, he turned from biology to philosophy. He described the **Bonnet syndrome** in his grandfather.

Bonnet, Paul French ophthalmologist in Lyon.

Bonnet sign Pain in the back occurring with adduction of the thigh, but not when the flexion is passively performed without the adduction; it is positive in lumbosacral root irritation. The sign was described incidentally, in Bonnet's two-volume book on joint disease (1845).

Bonnet syndrome (syndrome of Charles Bonnet) 1. The occurrence in elderly people with normal mental faculties of recurrent, vivid, dynamic, neutral, or pleasant visual pseudohallucinations. The original description was of this problem and autoscopy occurring in Charles Bonnet's grandfather who had had an operation for cataract 11 years before: "his double, the smoker, appeared regularly each evening the moment he lit his pipe. Immediately after he would describe another decoration or some other vision; and having jested over these fictions of the brain, he would calmly resume his discourse."[654] Strangely, when Charles Bonnet also went blind at the end of his life, he also experienced visual hallucinations.[1258]

The condition is not all that rare if elderly people are asked directly about such experiences, but they seldom volunteer the information. Although originally described in people with eye disease, it may also occur as a cortical dissociation syndrome described by Paul Bonnet.

2. (trigeminosympathetic neuralgia) **Trigeminal neuralgia** with **Horner syndrome** and with vasomotor disturbance in the area supplied by the trigeminal nerve.[655,5047] The condition may be a form of **Raeder syndrome.**

3. (Bonnet-Déchaume-Blanc syndrome, neuroretinoangiomatosis) Unilateral tortuosity of the retinal vessels (cirsoid aneurysms) with vascular malformations of the orbit or midbrain and of the face, described by Paul Bonnet and his colleagues in 1937.[656,657]

Miscellaneous other lesions of the orbits, central or peripheral nervous systems, or skin are also described. See also **Wyburn-Mason syndrome,** which may be the same thing.

Bonnet-Collet syndrome See **Collet-Sicard syndrome.**

Bonnet-Dechaume-Blanc syndrome See **Bonnet syndrome (2).**

Bonnevie, Kristine (1872–1950) Norwegian zoologist.

Bonnevie-Ullrich syndrome A sporadic congenital syndrome characterized by ptosis, ophthalmopareses, cataracts, hyperelastic skin, hypertrichosis, muscular hypotrophy, and lymphangiectatic edema of the extremities. The condition may be a variant of Turner syndrome.[2987]

Bonnier, Paul (1861–1918) French physician.

Bonnier syndrome (Deiter's nucleus syndrome) Vertigo, pallor, tachycardia, somnolence, trigeminal pain, weakness, and marked apprehension; contralateral hemiplegia may be a feature. The syndrome is due to a vascular or neoplastic lesion of Deiter's nucleus.[660]

Bontius, Jacobus (1592–1631) Dutch physician who gave the first account of **beriberi** and of **nutritional amblyopia** in his book *De Medicina Indorum* after working for the Dutch East India Company.

Boorgard angle (foraminobasilar angle) The angle defined by the intersection of the plane of the clivus and the plane of the foramen magnum, normally 126°–136°. The value changes with age and increase is not always associated with genuine basilar invagination, so this measurement is now little employed.[5282]

borderland of epilepsy The term of Sir William **Gowers** for a group of disorders including fainting, vagal and vasovagal attacks, vertigo, migraine, and sleep disorders which by their abrupt onset, repetitive nature, and brief duration resemble seizure disorders.

The clinical characteristics of these conditions, with speculations on their underlying pathophysiology, were published by Gowers in a book of the same name in 1907.[2237]

borderzone infarction Infarctions along the boundaries of recognized vascular territories, most commonly following an episode of profound reduction in global cerebral perfusion.

Bordier-Fränkel sign Upward and outward deviation of the eye on the side of a peripheral facial nerve lesion.[4723]

Börjeson-Forssman-Lehmann syndrome A rare, X-linked recessive dysmorphic syndrome (or at least expressed fully only in males), consisting of severe obesity, genital infantilism, hypogonadism, seizures, mental retardation, hypothyroidism, narrow palpebral fissures, and cromegaloid facial appearance. Short stature, nystagmus, strabismus, ptosis, blepharophimosis, microcephaly, seizures, and hypogonadotrophic hypogonadism are also described.[666,5047]

Borna virus A recently detected virus capable of causing damage to the central nervous system (especially to the hippocampus) without evidence of inflammation.[4840]

Bornholm disease See **epidemic pleurodynia.**

borreliosis (relapsing fever) Infection with *Borrelia recurrentis,* a spirochete transmitted to humans by lice or ticks. The disease is characterized by malaise, high fever, headache, vomiting, and myalgias followed by hepatosplenomegaly with jaundice, bronchitis, a petechial skin rash, and meningoencephalopathy causing confusion, drowsiness up to coma, seizures, and focal neurological signs. The CSF often shows a lymphocytic pleocytosis. Further but milder relapses of the initial illness occur over the next few weeks.[826] Acrodermatitis chronica atrophicans is a late manifestation and is associated with a distal sensory polyneuropathy.[3047] See also **Lyme disease.**

Borries syndrome   Headache, fever, increased cells and protein in the CSF, and focal signs suggesting brain abscess but in fact due to localized nonsuppurative encephalitis.[669]

The condition was described in 1921 by G.V.T. Borries, a Danish physician in Copenhagen.

Bors-Comarr classification   A system for grading the degree of bladder involvement, introduced for the management of patients following spinal shock.[670] See Chart B–4.

Chart B–4. Bors-Comarr Classification of Bladder Disorders

Complete Lesions Above Conus (S2–4); Somatic Upper Motor Neuron Lesion

Balanced (automatic or neurogenic reflex bladder)	Small capacity, increased residual urine; reflex, spontaneous or conditioned initiation; no inhibition; no desire to void
Imbalanced	Initially flaccid-atonic with large capacity, 400 ml or more; later autonomous with capacity 150–250 ml; finally spastic, with capacity <150 ml

Incomplete Lesions above Conus (S2–4); Somatic Upper Motor Neuron Lesion

Balanced (uninhibited neurogenic bladder)	Residual 10–20%, capacity 200–300 ml; desire to micturate present; initiation precipitate; inhibition inadequate
Imbalanced	Residual 10% or more; capacity 200–1000 ml or more

Complete Lesions At or Below Conus (S2–4); Somatic Lower Motor Neuron Lesion

Balanced (autonomous/automatic bladder)	Residual 0–10%, capacity 400 ml or more; desire to micturate absent; initiation with straining; inhibition passive
Imbalanced	Residual 10% or more; capacity 400 ml or more

Incomplete Lesions At or Below Conus (S2–4); Somatic Lower Motor Neuron Lesion

Balanced	Residual 0–10%, capacity 300–400 ml; desire to micturate present; initiation with straining or normal; inhibition active but inadequate;
Imbalanced (tabetic bladder)	Residual 10% or more; capacity 600 ml or more; sensation absent

*The term balanced here refers to coordinated coordination of the forces of expulsion and relaxation. The amount of residual urine is considered to be in proportion to the imbalance between these functions. (From Bors E. Urological aspects of rehabilitation in spinal cord injuries. Copyright 1951. American Medical Association. JAMA 1951;**146**:225–229.[670])*

Boston craniosynostosis   A dominantly inherited form of craniosynostrosis mapped to chromosome 5q

Boston Diagnostic Aphasia Examination   A comprehensive instrument for assessing language, in particular spontaneous speech, naming, repetition, comprehension of oral language, reading, and writing, used for classifying as well as detecting aphasias.[2192]

The examination may be prolonged and requires expertise on the part of the interviewer.

Boston Naming Test   A sensitive test of visual confrontation naming ability, in which the subject is required to name a series of 60 objects presented as line drawings, with standardized verbal or phonemic clues being provided when initial recognition fails.[2921]

A shorter version is also available, for use with demented patients.[3550]

Boston sign   Intermittent descent of the globe on downward gaze, seen in **dysthyroid orbitopathy.**[4723]

Boston Society of Psychiatry and Neurology   One of the oldest medical societies in the United States, it was founded in 1880, largely with the inspiration of Walter Channing, for the informal and social discussion of medical subjects. Its proceeding were reported in the *Boston Medical and Surgical Reporter* (the forerunner of the *New England Journal of Medicine*). Members have continued to present and discuss topics in both psychiatry and neurology at monthly meetings held continuously since its founding.[1686]

bottoms-up dissection   Dissection of the extracranial carotid artery, considered to have been produced by repetitive neck extension during the act of throwing back the head in order to drain the contents of drinking glasses.[5644]

botulinus toxin   A group of seven serologically distinct neuroparalytic toxins produced by *Clostridium botulinum*, all of which block the release of acetylcholine by the nerve terminal and cause slowly reversible effects indistinguishable from typical denervation. The type A toxin is used therapeutically to produce local suppression of muscle contraction in certain **dystonias** and in **hemifacial spasm.** Guidelines for its use were suggested by the American Academy of Neurology in 1990.[13]

The use of the agent in the management of headaches and of the facial evidences of aging is less well substantiated.

botulism   (from Lat, a sausage) Poisoning with the exotoxin of *Clostridium botulinus* (commonly of types

A, B, and E), initially described after poisoning by infected sausages.

The toxin binds to cholinergic nerve terminals, inhibiting acetylcholine release and clinically leading to weakness, especially of the ocular and bulbar muscles, acute autonomic dysfunction (pupillary dilatation occurs in half the cases), and gastrointestinal symptoms. The electrical signs resemble those of the **Lambert-Eaton myasthenic syndrome** but nerve conduction velocities are normal.

Infantile botulism results from botulinal neurotoxin produced in vivo following colonization of the gastrointestinal tract in children aged 1 to 9 months. The disease spectrum varies from "failure to thrive" to "the floppy baby syndrome" (the most common form) and sudden infant death syndrome or "crib death." Typical symptoms in the floppy baby syndrome include lethargy, diminished sucking, constipation, weakness, feeble cry, and diminished spontaneous activity with loss of head control, followed by extensive flaccid paralysis.[998,999]

Adult botulism is usually caused by ingestion of preformed toxin, less often from wound infection. Progressive descending paralysis develops, involving extraocular, bilbar, respiratory, and proximal more than distal limb muscle weakness with autonomic dysfunction.

Bouchard, Charles   (1837–1909?) French neurologist who trained in Lyon and Paris; he studied under **Charcot** at the **Salpétrière** for some of this time and co-authored a number of papers with him, particularly on the relationship of miliary aneurysms to cerebral hemorrhage, the subject of his doctoral thesis. Bouchard rose quickly in the hierarchy and was appointed professor of general pathology at the University of Paris in 1879. After this, however, he distanced himself from Charcot and strove for the advancement of his own students against Charcot's; thus he prevented the appointment of **Babinski** to the position of *professeur agrégé*.[2750]

bouche de Tapir   (Fr, mouth of a tapir) Involuntary protrusion of the upper lip, a sign of bilateral facial weakness as in some cases of facial myopathy, described by Karl **Westphal** in 1886.

Bouillard, Jean-Baptiste   (1796–1881) French physician, professor of medicine at the Charité in Paris. He differentiated between expressive and receptive dysphasias and localized the lesion to the frontal lobes.

boundary infarct   See **watershed infarct.**

Bourdon test   A test of attention in which the subject is required to strike out all the examples of a given letter in a line of printed random letters.

Bourneville, Desiré-Magloire   (1840–1909) French physician who trained under **Charcot** and became pediatric neurologist and psychiatrist at the Bicêtre hospital in Paris where he was in charge of care of the mentally retarded patients. Apart from his description of **tuberous sclerosis,** he also demonstrated the virtual identity of cretinism and myxedema (1880), wrote on multiple sclerosis, hysteria, medical photography, and thermometry, and was a founder both of the French *Archives de Neurologie* in 1880 and of *La Presse Medicale.* Bourneville was an important figure in arranging the publication of Charcot's lectures.

He described tuberous sclerosis in 1880,[682,683] the same year as Hartdegen in Germany reported the condition independently (but von Recklinghausen[1181] had already noted the same features in 1863). Outside medicine, he was elected to the Chambre des Deputés in Paris in 1873, and introduced legislation to improve hospital conditions and medical practice in obstetrics.[7]

Desiré-Magloire Bourneville

Bourneville disease   See **tuberous sclerosis.**

Bourneville-Brissaud disease   See **tuberous sclerosis.**

Bourneville-Pellizzi disease   See **tuberous sclerosis.**

Bourneville-Pringle disease   See **tuberous sclerosis.**

bovine spongiform encephalopathy   ("mad cow disease") A neurological disease transmitted by an unconventional, resistant agent (an aberrant isoform of prion protein), with a latency of some 18 months. This is a "slow virus" disease, equivalent to the disease **scrapie** in cattle.[5914]

The possibility that this condition might be responsible for a future outbreak of Jakob-Creutzfeldt disease has recently caused concern in the United Kingdom.

Bowditch law   Peripheral nerve fibers do not fatigue with repetitive stimulation; a truth enunciated by Henry Pickering Bowditch (1840–1911), an American physiologist, in 1890 (and 6 years previously by Nikolai Wedensky in Russia).[4979]

bowed-head sign   (Gould sign) Forward flexion of the head on the neck in an effort to compensate for an inferior hemianopia.

bowel-bladder functional scale   A sensitive questionnaire developed to assess the nature and severity of sphincter dysfunction, mainly in patients with **multiple sclerosis.**[5668]

Bowen-Conradi syndrome   A lethal, congenital, recessively inherited dysmorphic syndrome characterized also by dolicho- or scaphocephaly, microcephaly, dwarfism, and other musculoskeletal maldevelopments. The condition has been reported to occur among the Hutterite people of North America.[689]

bowing reflex   If an infant with anencephaly is placed in the supine position and the thigh is extended at the hip joints, the head then lifts itself slowly in flexion, and the trunk does the same, so that the infant achieves the sitting position. The reflex is seen only in anencephalic children or in normal premature infants of 7 months gestation.[4370]

bow-leggedness   See **genu varum.**

bowlers' cramp   An occupational dystonic syndrome described in cricketers, whose attempts to put spin on the ball being bowled lead instead to involuntary gripping of it.[4536]

Bowman membrane   The anterior elastic membrane of the cornea.

Bowman, Sir William   (1816–1892) English ophthalmic surgeon and anatomist, professor of anatomy and physiology at King's College, London.[1478]

bowstring sign   (Cram test) A sign of lumbar root irritation elicited by flexing the hip with the knee flexed 30°, the heel resting on the examiner's shoulder; the examiner presses upon the posterior tibial nerve in the popliteal fossa with her thumb and then depresses the knee into extension. Pain felt in the leg or in the low back suggests root irritation.[1154]

bow-tie atrophy   The pattern of retinal atrophy secondary to the presence of a lesion at the junction of the optic tract and chiasm, damaging the fibers from the homolateral temporal and contralateral nasal retinas. Relative superior and inferior temporal atrophy of the homolateral disk and nasal and temporal atrophy of the contralateral disk occurs, the abnormal region being defined by the normal arcuate fibers above and below.[4116]

bow-tie nystagmus   A drug-induced oscillation of the eyes consisting of upbeat nystagmus coupled with alternating horizontal saccades synchronized with the vertical fast phases; thus the movement of the eyes traces the outline of a bow tie (diabolo, butterfly,

etc.).[1368] See also **induced nystagmus, anticipatory nystagmus.**

Box and Block Test   A manipulation task, assessing dexterity in the arms and hands.[2194]

boxing   An organized attempt of two people to inflict head injuries upon one another for the pleasure of the spectators and (if the latter pay to witness the event) for the profit of the promoter.

While acutely inflicted injuries such as concussion are deemed especially praiseworthy, the causation of post-concussion syndrome, intracranial hemorrhage, and cerebral contusion do not detract from the victor's kudos, while chronic traumatic encephalopathy in boxers is only taken into account outside public scrutiny.

The neurological aspects of this "sport" have been reviewed.[2882]

Boyle, Robert   Seventeenth-century English chemist and member of the Royal Society who gave an account of a diurnal variety of **essential tremor,** relieved by drinking a chocolate liqueur.

brachial   (from Lat, arm) Of or pertaining to the arm.

brachial amyotrophic diplegia   A slowly progressive variety of **amyotrophic lateral sclerosis** in which a lower motor neuron syndrome is confined to the arms and shoulder girdle, often for some years.[2954]

brachial neuritis   See **neuralgic amyotrophy.**

brachial neuropathy   Any neuropathic disorder affecting the brachial plexus or its branches peripherally in the arms.[3427]

brachial plexopathy   See **neuralgic amyotrophy, hypertrophic brachial plexus neuropathy.**

brachial plexus neuropathy   See **neuralgic amyotrophy, hypertrophic brachial plexus neuropathy.**

brachial-basilar insufficiency syndrome   See **subclavian steal syndrome.**

brachialgia statica progressiva   Nocturnal arm paresthesiae. See **sensory perineuritis.** The condition is probably actually **carpal tunnel syndrome.**

brachioradialis reflex   (supinator, radial, forearm or styloradial reflex) Contraction of this muscle in response to a sudden stretch caused by a tap on the radius. It is increased as a result of an upper motor neuron lesion sited above C6.

Brachmann–de Lange syndrome   See **de Lange syndrome.**

brachy-   (Gr, short) Prefix denoting its etymological meaning.

brachycephaly   (Gr, short + head) A craniofacial dysmorphism characterized by premature bilateral fusion of the coronal sutures which leads to a relative increase in the transverse compared with the longitudinal diameter of the skull (usually quoted as being above 80% or in a ratio of 4:5).[4]

The appearance is of recession of the supraorbital rim and of the forehead (which bulges out above the root of the nose) while the temporal fossa bulges laterally in compensation. One or both orbits show an elliptic "Harlequin" or "devil-like" appearance. Upward growth of the skull leads to **turricephaly** and if the anterior fontanelle is slow to close, the top of the head has a pointed appearance (**acrocephaly**).

Clinically, cleft palate and syndactyly occur often and raised intracranial pressure, blindness, and mental retardation are sometimes associated.

brachydactyly-ataxia See **Biemond syndrome.**

brachydactyly-spheroplakia See **Weill-Marchesani syndrome.**

brachytherapy The implantation of radioactive materials by catheter directly into a tumor.

Bradborn sign (Thorburn phenomenon) Adoption of a posture of flexion of the wrist and fingers when the arm is adducted at the shoulder and flexed at the elbow, seen in patients with bilateral C7 lesions.

When unilateral, this is also known as the *Jolly sign.*

Bradbury-Eggleston triad Orthostatic hypotension, impotence, and anhidrosis, as components of the **Shy-Drager syndrome** or of **progressive autonomic failure.**

bradycoria Slowing of the pupillary reaction to light or accommodation.

bradykinesia (Gr, slow + movement) Abnormal slowness in the execution of motor tasks, as in depressive illness, hypothyroidism, parkinsonism, and disinclination to undertake the task in hand.

bradykinin A neuropeptide vasodilator.

bradylalia (Gr, slow + babbling) Slowness and monotony in speech with pauses between syllables, as in **parkinsonism** and with **pseudobulbar palsy.**

bradyphrasia Slowness of speech due to slowness of the underlying mental operations.[4512]

bradyphrenia Slowness in thinking, as suggested by delay in responding to questions. See also **abulia.**

Bragard sign Aggravation of back pain induced during straight-leg raising as a result of passive dorsiflexion of the ankle.[374] The **Sicard sign** is the same, except that in this case only the hallux is dorsiflexed.

Braid, James (1795–1860) English surgeon in Manchester who attended a series of popular demonstrations of hypnotism in 1841. He was converted into believing that it was "a simple, speedy and certain method for throwing the nervous system into a new condition, which may be rendered eminently available in the cure of certain disorders," and in 1843 published a book (*Neurypnology*) on the subject, advocating its use for

the treatment of hysterical paralysis, tic douloureux, headache, epilepsy, palpitations, etc.

In this and other publications, however, he did explode the fancies of the Mesmerists and showed that the basis of the state was suggestion. He also introduced the term *hypnotism.*

Braid strabismus Accommodation for close vision of an object held above the line of sight, reputedly useful in the attainment of the hypnotic state.

Braidism Hypnosis or mesmerism.

Braille A system for the reading of words adapted in 1830 by Louis Braille (1809–1852), a blind French teacher of the blind, from a prototype designed by Charles Barbier 10 years before.[705] It uses 63 groups of raised points 2.5 or 3 mm apart to represent each letter or punctuation mark, and can be read fluently by a blind person using one finger (the *reading finger*) of each hand, but less well or not at all when using other fingers. Although complex, the system remains that most often used today, despite the introduction of other systems, such as the English method of Dr. William Moon (1845).

brain What this is all about. The word is a generic term for that part of the CNS within the cranium subserving (as Sherrington regarded it in essence) the management of the muscles but also the regulation of the bodily functions of the animal, its will, and the apparatus required for perception of the internal and external environment.

The word is derived from the Anglo-Saxon word *braegen,* which could have a common root with the Greek **bregma.**

Brain A professional journal of neurology, published continuously since April 1878. Bucknill, Crighton-Brown, Ferrier, and Hughlings-Jackson were the first editors but Dr. A. de Watteville took over the editorship in 1886 with committee assistance until 1900 and Henry **Head** occupied the editor's chair from shortly thereafter.

The publication was adopted by the Neurological Society of London as its organ in 1887, 2 years after its foundation. It is currently published by Oxford University Press, Walton St., Oxford 0X2 6DP, UK. Web site: http://brain.oupjournals.org/.

Brain and Development (*Brain Dev.*) A Japanese pediatric journal of neurodevelopment, founded in 1979. Web site: http:www.elsevier.nl/locate/Braindev.

Brain and Language (*Brain Lang.*) A neurological journal. Address: Academic Press Inc., 1250 6th Avenue, San Diego, CA 92101.

Brain and Mind An electronic (web-based) neuroscience magazine. Web site: http://www.epub.org/br/cm/.

Brain and Nerve (*No To Shinkei*) A neurological journal. Address: Igaku Shoin Ltd., 5-24-3 Hongo Bunkyo-ku, Tokyo 113-91, Japan.

brain attack A term introduced to remind all those who treat stroke lightly that this condition requires and is benefited by emergency management in the same way as is heart attack.

Brain Attack Coalition A professional group dedicated to improving stroke care and comprising the **American Academy of Neurology, American Association of Neurological Surgeons, American College of Emergency Physicians,** American Heart Association Stroke Council, **American Society of Neuroradiology, National Institute of Neurological Disease and Stroke, National Stroke Association.** Web site: www.stroke-site.org.

brain autolysis Enzymatic autodigestion of the brain, following prolonged circulatory stoppage and death.

brain death (cerebral death) Loss of the clinical function of the brain, including the brainstem when the proximate cause is known and demonstrably irreversible. The three cardinal findings upon which the clinical diagnosis is based are coma or unresponsiveness, absence of brainstem reflexes, and apnea. The concept of brain death was created out of advances in therapeutic technology. The criteria for determining brain death in adults and in children suggested by the President's Commission are reproduced in Charts B–5 and B–6. Competing but not necessarily conflicting alternatives have also been published.[5530] See also **persistent vegetative state.**

Chart B–5. Criteria for the Determination of Brain Death

An individual presenting the findings in either section A (cardiopulmonary) or section B (neurological) is dead. In either section a diagnosis of death requires that both *cessation of functions,* as set forth in subsection 1, and *irreversibility,* as set forth in subsection 2, be demonstrated.

A. An individual with irreversible cessation of circulatory and respiratory functions is dead.
 1. Cessation is recognized by an appropriate clinical examination. Clinical examination will disclose absence of responsiveness, heartbeat, and respiratory effort. Medical circumstances may require the use of confirmatory tests, such as an ECG.
 2. Irreversibility is recognized by persistent cessation of functions during an appropriate period of observation and/or trial of therapy.

In clinical situations where death is expected, where the course has been gradual, and where irregular agonal respiration or heartbeat finally ceases, the period of observation following the cessation may be only the few minutes required to complete the examination. Similarly, if resuscitation is not undertaken and ventricular fibrillation and standstill develop in a monitored patient, the required period of observation thereafter may be as short as a few minutes. When a possible death is unobserved, unexpected, or sudden, the examination may need to be more detailed and repeated over a longer period, while appropriate resuscitative effort is maintained as a test of cardiovascular responsiveness. Diagnosis in individuals who are first observed with rigor mortis or putrefaction may require only the observation period necessary to establish that fact.

B. An individual with irreversible cessation of all functions of the entire brain, including the brainstem, is dead. The "functions of the entire brain" that are relevant to the diagnosis are those that are clinically ascertainable. Where indicated, the clinical diagnosis is subject to confirmation by laboratory tests, as described in the following portions of the text. Consultation with a physician experienced in this diagnosis is advisable.
 1. Cessation is recognized when evaluation discloses findings of a and b:
  a. Cerebral functions are absent, and there must be deep coma, that is, cerebral unreceptivity and unresponsivity. Medical circumstances may require the use of confirmatory studies such as an EEG or blood-flow study.
  b. Brainstem functions are absent.

Reliable testing of brainstem reflexes requires a perceptive and experienced physician using adequate stimuli. Pupillary light, corneal, oculocephalic, oculovestibular, oropharyngeal, and respiratory (apnea) reflexes should be tested. When these reflexes cannot be adequately assessed, confirmatory tests are recommended.

Adequate testing for apnea is very important. An accepted method is ventilation with pure oxygen or an oxygen and carbon dioxide mixture for ten minutes before withdrawal of the ventilator, followed by passive flow of oxygen. (This procedure allows Pa_{CO_2} to rise without hazardous hypoxia.) Hypercarbia adequately stimulates respiratory effort within 30 seconds when Pa_{CO_2} is >60 mmHg. A 10-minute period of apnea is usually sufficient to attain this level of hypercarbia. Testing of arterial blood gases can be used to confirm this level. Spontaneous breathing efforts indicate that part of the brainstem is functioning.

Peripheral nervous system activity and spinal cord reflexes may persist after death. True decerebrate or decorticate posturing or seizures are inconsistent with the diagnosis of death.
 2. Irreversibility is recognized when evaluation discloses findings of a and b and c:
  a. The cause of coma is established and is sufficient to account for the loss of brain functions. . . . Most difficulties with the determination of death on the basis of neurological criteria have resulted from inadequate attention to this basic diagnostic prerequisite. In addition to a careful clinical examination and investigation of history, relevant knowledge of causation may be acquired by CT scan, measurement of core temperature, drug screening, EEG, angiography, or other procedures.
  b. The possibility of recovery of any brain functions is excluded, and the most important reversible conditions are sedation, hypothermia, neuromuscular blockade, and shock. In the unusual circumstance where a sufficient cause cannot be established, irreversibility can be reliably inferred only after extensive evaluation for drug intoxication, extended observation, and other testing. A determination that blood flow to the brain is absent can be used to demonstrate a sufficient and irreversible condition.
  c. The cessation of all brain functions persists for an appropriate period of observation and/or trial of therapy.

Even when coma is known to have started at an earlier time, the absence of all brain functions must be established by an experienced physician at the initiation of the observation period. The duration of observation periods is a matter of clinical judgment, and some physicians recommend shorter or longer periods than those given here.

Except for patients with drug intoxication, hypothermia, young age, or shock, medical centers with substantial experience in diagnosing death neurologically report no cases of brain functions returning following a 6-hour cessation, documented by clinical examination and confirmatory EEG. In the absence of confirmatory tests, a period of observation of at least 12 hours is recommended when an irreversible condition is well established. For anoxic brain damage where the extent of damage is more difficult to ascertain, observation for 24 hours is generally desirable. In anoxic injury, the observation period may be reduced if a test shows cessation of cerebral blood flow or if an EEG shows electrocerebral silence in an adult patient without drug intoxication, hypothermia, or shock.

Confirmation of clinical findings by EEG is desirable when objective documentation is needed to substantiate the clinical findings. Electrocerebral silence verifies irreversible loss of cortical function except in patients with drug intoxication or hypothermia. (Important technical details are provided in "Minimal Technical Standards for EEG Recording in Suspected Cerebral Death" [Guidelines in EEG 1980, Atlanta, American Electroencephalographic Society, 1980, section 4, pp 19–24].) When joined with the clinical findings of absent brainstem functions, electrocerebral silence confirms the diagnosis.

Complete cessation of circulation to the normothermic adult brain for more than 10 minutes is incompatible with survival of brain tissue. Documentation of this circulatory failure is therefore evidence of death of the entire brain. Four-vessel intracranial angiography is definitive for diagnosing cessation of circulation to the entire brain (both cerebrum and posterior fossa) but entails substantial practical difficulties and risks. Tests are available that assess circulation only in the cerebral hemispheres, namely radioisotope bolus cerebral angiography and gamma camera imaging with radioisotope cerebral angiography. Without complicating conditions, absent cerebral blood flow as measured by these tests, in conjunction with the clinical determination of cessation of all brain functions for at least 6 hours, is diagnostic of death.

Complicating Conditions

A. *Drug and metabolic intoxication.* Drug intoxication is the most serious problem in the determination of death, especially when multiple drugs are used. Cessation of brain functions caused by the sedative and anesthetic drugs, such as barbiturates, benzodiazepines, meprobamate, methaqualone, and trichloroethylene, may be completely reversible even though they produce clinical cessation of brain functions and electrocerebral silence. In cases where there is any likelihood of sedative presence, toxicology screening for all likely drugs is required. If exogenous intoxication is found, death may not be declared until the intoxicant is metabolized or intracranial circulation is tested and found to have ceased.

Total paralysis may cause unresponsiveness, areflexia, and apnea that closely simulates death. Exposure to drugs such as neuromuscular blocking agents or aminoglyco-

side antibiotics, and diseases such as myasthenia gravis are usually apparent by careful review of the history. Prolonged paralysis after use of succinylcholine chloride and related drugs requires evaluation for pseudocholinesterase deficiency. If there is any question, low-dose atropine stimulation, electromyogram, peripheral nerve stimulation, EEG, tests of intracranial circulation, or extended observation, as indicated, will make the diagnosis clear.

In drug-induced coma, EEG activity may return or persist while the patient remains unresponsive, and therefore the EEG may be an important evaluation along with extended observation. If the EEG shows electrocerebral silence, short-latency auditory or somatosensory-evoked potentials may be used to test brainstem functions, since these potentials are unlikely to be affected by drugs.

Some severe illnesses (e.g., hepatic encephalopathy, hyperosmolar coma, and preterminal uremia) can cause deep coma. Before irreversible cessation of brain functions can be determined, metabolic abnormalities should be considered and, if possible, corrected. Confirmatory tests of circulation or EEG may be necessary.

B. *Hypothermia.* Criteria for reliable recognition of death are not available in the presence of hypothermia (below 32.2°C core temperature). The variables of cerebral circulation in hypothermic patients are not sufficiently well studied to know whether tests of absent or diminished circulation are confirmatory. Hypothermia can mimic brain death by ordinary clinical criteria and can protect against neurological damage due to hypoxia. Further complications arise since hypothermia also usually precedes and follows death. If these complicating factors make it unclear whether an individual is alive, the only available measure to resolve the issue is to restore normothermia. Hypothermia is not a common cause of difficulty in the determination of death.

C. *Children.* The brains of infants and young children have increased resistance to damage and may recover substantial functions even after exhibiting unresponsiveness on neurological examination for longer periods compared with adults. Physicians should be particularly cautious in applying neurological criteria to determine death in children younger than 5 years.

D. *Shock.* Physicians should also be particularly cautious in applying neurological criteria to determine death in patients in shock because the reduction in cerebral circulation can render clinical examination and laboratory tests unreliable.

Reproduced by permission. From President's Commission. Guidelines for the determination of death. JAMA 1981;246:2184–2186. Copyright (1981), American Medical Association.

Chart B–6. Guidelines for the Determination of Brain Death in Children

History

The critical initial assessment is the clinical history and examination. The most important factor is determination of the proximate cause of coma to ensure absence of remediable or reversible conditions. Most difficulties with the determination of death on the basis of neurological criteria have resulted from overlooking this basic fact. Especially important are detection of toxic and metabolic disorders, sedative-hypnotic drugs, paralytic agents, hypothermia, hypotension, and surgically remediable conditions. The physical examination is necessary to determine the failure of brain function.

Physical Examination Criteria

1. Coma and apnea must coexist. The patient must exhibit complete loss of consciousness, vocalization, and volitional activity.
2. Absence of brainstem function as defined by:
   a. Midposition or fully dilated pupils that do not respond to light. Drugs may influence and invalidate pupillary assessment.
   b. Absence of spontaneous eye movements and those induced by oculocephalic and caloric (oculovestibular) testing.
   c. Absence of movement of bulbar musculature including facial and oropharyngeal muscles. The corneal, gag, cough, sucking, and rooting reflexes are absent.
   d. Respiratory movements are absent with the patient off the respirator. Apnea testing using standardized methods can be performed but this is done after other criteria are met.
3. The patient must not be significantly hypothermic or hypotensive for age.
4. Flaccid tone and absence of spontaneous or induced movements, excluding spinal cord events such as reflex withdrawal or spinal myoclonus, should exist.
5. The examination should remain consistent with brain death throughout the observation and testing period.

Observation Periods According to Age

The recommended observation period depends on the age of the patient and the laboratory test utilized.

7 days to 2 months The American Neurological Association Task Force recommends two examinations and EEGs separated by at least 48 hours.

2 months to 1 year The Task Force recommends two examinations and EEGs separated by at least 24 hours. A repeat examination and EEG are not necessary if a concomitant radionuclide angiograpahic (CRAG) study demonstrates no visualization of cerebral arteries.

Over 1 year When an irreversible cause exists, laboratory testing is not required and the Task Force recommends an observation period of at least 12 hours. There are conditions, particularly hypoxic-ischemic encephalopathy, in which it is difficult to assess the extent and reversibility of brain damage. This is particularly true if the first examination is performed soon after the acute event. Therefore, in this situation, the Task Force recommends a more prolonged period of at least 24 hours of observation. The observation period may be reduced if the EEG demonstrates electrocerebral silence or the CRAG does not visualize cerebral arteries.

Laboratory Testing

Electroencephalography Electroencephalography to document electrocerebral silence should, if performed, be done over a 30-minute period using standardized techniques for brain death determinations. In small children it may not be possible to meet the standard requirement for 10-cm electrode separation. The inter-electrode distance should be decreased proportional to the patient's head size. Drug concentrations should be insufficient to suppress EEG activity.

Angiography CRAG confirms cerebral death by demonstrating the lack of visualization of the cerebral circulation. A technically satisfactory CRAG that demonstrates arrest of carotid circulation at the base of the skull and absence of intracranial arterial circulation can be considered confirmatory of brain death, even though there may be some visualization of the intracranial venous sinuses. The value of this study in infants under 2 months is under investigation. Contrast angiography can document lack of effective blood flow to the brain.

From American Neurological Association Task Force. Guidelines for the determination of brain death in children. Ann Neurol 1987;21:616–617, reproduced by permission.

brain distension See **normal pressure hydrocephalus.**

brain electrical activity mapping (BEAM) A computer-controlled method for collecting and displaying spatiotemporal information brain electrical contained in recordings from multiple scalp electrodes, whereby colored topographic maps of regional electrical activity (EEG or evoked potential) are displayed.[1545] The place of this technique vis-à-vis other methods for the diagnostic localisation of cerebral lesions is still undetermined.

brain ferrocalcinosis See **striopallidal calcification.**

brain fever See **chronic fatigue syndrome.**

brain herniation Displacement of brain structures as a result of pressure from an expanding mass lesion elsewhere in the cranium. Examples are a cerebellar pressure cone at the foramen magnum, uncal herniation down through the tentorium, transtentorial herniation of the brainstem, subfalcial herniation of the cinguate gyrus and upward cerebellar herniation through the tentorium. The relevance of these tissue shifts has been questioned, the suggestion being made that the only really important event is midbrain compression as a result of lateral shift at the level of the tentorium.[1863]

Brain Information Service Address: Health Science Room 43–67, University of California at Los Angeles, Los Angeles, CA 90024.

Brain Injury (*Brain Inj.*) A subspecialty neurological journal. Address: Taylor & Francis Ltd., Rankine Road Basingstoke, Hampshire RG24 0PR, UK. Web site: http://www.tandf.co.uk/journals/titles/02699052.html.

Brain Injury Association A charitable association in this field. Address: 1776 Massachusetts Ave., N.W., Ste. 1000, Washington, DC. Tel: 202-296-6443, 800-444-6443. Web site: http://www.blausa.org.

brain mapping A digital technique whereby the EEG tracing from 16–32 electrodes arranged in a grid pattern is analyzed to create an isoelectric display of the electrical field over the head, usually in color. It can be used to study the topography of any feature at a point in time, or to average recurring events, as with evoked potentials. Its usefulness stems from the ease with which such abnormalities may be seen or localized, rather than from its ability to show features invisible to trained electroencephalographers. The technic is not a substitute for neuroimaging in any form.[575]

brain reflex   (quadripedal reflex) The flexed arm of a hemiparetic patient extends when the patient assumes the quadripedal position.[4723]

Brain Research   (*Brain Res.*) A neurological journal. Address: Elsevier Science Publishers B V, P.O. Box 211, 1000 AE Amsterdam, The Netherlands.

Brain Research Bulletin   (*Brain Res. Bull.*) The official journal of the *International Behavioral Neuroscience Society*. Web site: http://www.brb.cf.ac.uk/.

Brain Research Fund Foundation of London   A charitable association in this field. Address: 111 Waterloo St., Ste 600, London, Ontario N6B 2M4, Canada. Tel: 519-642-7755.

brain sand   Gritty particles (**psammoma bodies**) found in certain cerebral tumors, such as meningiomas, but also in many normal people.

brain shift   The movement of parts of the brain across the midline or downward in response to the effects of an intracranial mass lesion.

Such displacements include those of the cingulate gyrus herniating beneath the falx; of the uncus or cerebellar tonsils, which descend through the tentorial aperture or the foramen magnum, respectively; and of the brainstem, which moves across the midline and also downward. In the case of masses within the posterior fossa, upward herniation of the cerebellum may also occur.

brain stones   See **cerebral calculi.**

Brain Tissue Resource Center   An association promoting research through the collection and banking of human postmortem brain tissue. Address: Mailman Research Center, McLean Hospital, 115 Mill St., Belmont, MA 02178.

brain tumor   Benign or malignant neoplasms of the brain. These have been classified by the World Health Organization as in Chart B–7. Most of the entries are cataloged in this book under their individual names. The grading is available at http://neurosurgery.mgh.harvard.edu/newwhobt.htm

Chart B–7. Neuroepithelial Tumors of the Central Nervous System and Other CNS Neoplasms

Neuroepithelial Tumors of the Central Nervous System

1. *Astrocytic tumors* (glial tumors—categories I–V; see Grading of Astrocytic Tumors, below. They may also be subclassified as invasive or noninvasive, although this is not formally part of the WHO system. The noninvasive tumor types are indicated below. Categories in italics are also not recognized by the new WHO classification system, but are in common use.)
   1. Astrocytoma (WHO grade II)
      Variants: protoplasmic, gemistocytic, fibrillary, mixed
   2. Anaplastic (malignant) astrocytoma (WHO grade III)
      Hemispheric, diencephalic, optic, brainstem, and cerebellar sites
   3. Glioblastoma multiforme (WHO grade IV)
      Variants: giant cell glioblastoma, gliosarcoma
   4. Pilocytic astrocytoma (noninvasive, WHO grade I)
      Hemispheric, diencephalic, optic, brain stem, and cerebellar sites
   5. Subependymal giant cell astrocytoma (noninvasive, WHO grade I)
   6. Pleomorphic xanthroastrocytoma (noninvasive, WHO grade I)
2. Oligodendroglial tumors
   1. Oligodendroglioma (WHO grade II)
   2. Anaplastic (malignant) oligodendroglioma (WHO grade III)
3. Ependymal cell tumors
   1. Ependymoma (WHO grade II)
      Variants: cellular, papillary, epithelial, clear cell, and mixed
   2. Anaplastic ependymoma (WHO grade III)
   3. Myxopapillary ependymoma
   4. Subependymoma (WHO grade I)
4. Mixed gliomas
   1. Mixed oligoastrocytoma (WHO grade II)
   2. Anaplastic (malignant) oligodastrocytoma (WHO grade III)
   3. Other (e.g., ependymo-astrocytoma)
5. Neuroepithelial tumors of uncertain origin
   1. Polar spongioblastoma (WHO grade IV)
   2. Astroblastoma (WHO grade IV)
   3. Gliomatosis cerebri (WHO grade IV)
6. Tumors of the choroid plexus
   1. Choroid plexus papilloma
   2. Chodroid plexus carcinoma (anaplastic choroid plexus papilloma)
7. Neuronal and mixed neuronal-glial tumors
   1. Gangliocytoma
   2. Dysplastic gangliocytoma of the cerebellum (Lhermitte-Duclos)
   3. Ganglioglioma
   4. Anaplastic (malignant) ganglioglioma
   5. Desmoplastic infantile ganglioglioma (*desmoplastic infantile astrocytoma*)
   6. Central neurocytoma
   7. Dysembryoplastic neuroepithelial tumor
   8. Olfactory neuroblastoma (esthesioneuroblastoma)
      Variant: olfactory neuroepithelioma
8. Pineal parenchyma tumors
   1. Pineocytoma
   2. Pineoblastoma
   3. Mixed pineocytoma/pineoblastoma
9. Tumors with neuroblastic or glioblastic elements (embryonal tumors)
   1. Medulloepithelioma
   2. Primitive neuroectodermal tumors with multipotent differentiation

i. Medulloblastoma (variants: medullomyoblastoma, melanocytic medulloblastoma, desmoplastic medulloblastoma)
ii. Cerebral primitive neuroectodermal tumor
3. Neuroblastoma
(Variant: ganglioneuroblastoma)
4. Retinoblastoma
5. Ependymoblastoma

Other CNS Neoplasms

1. *Tumors of the sellar region*
   1. Pituitary adenoma
   2. Pituitary carcinoma
   3. Craniopharyngioma
2. *Hematopoietic tumors*
   1. Primary malignant lymphomas
   2. Plasmacytoma
   3. Granulocytic sarcoma and others
3. *Germ cell tumors*
   1. Germinoma
   2. Embryonal carcinoma
   3. Yolk sac tumor (endodermal sinus tumor)
   4. Choriocarcinoma
   5. Teratoma
   6. Mixed germ cell tumors
4. Tumors of the meninges
   1. Meningioma
      Variants: meningothelial, fibrous (fibroblastic), transitional (mixed), psammomatous, angiomatous, microcystic, secretory, clear cell, chordoid, lymphoplasmacyte-rich, and metaplastic subtypes
   2. Atypical meningioma
   3. Anaplastic (malignant) meningioma
5. Non-meningothelial tumors of the meninges
   1. Benign mesenchymal
      Osteocartilaginous tumors, lipoma, fibrous histiocytoma, and others
   2. Malignant mesenchymal
      Chondrosarcoma, hemangiopericytoma, rhabdomyosarcoma, meningeal sarcomatosis, and others
   3. Primary melanocytic lesions
      Diffuse melanosis, melanocytoma, maliganant melanoma, and the variant meningeal melanomatosis
   4. Hemopoietic neoplasms
      Malignant lymphoma, plasmactoma, granulocytic sarcoma)
5. Tumors of uncertain histogenesis
   Hemangioblastoma (capillary hemangioblastoma)
6. Tumors of cranial and spinal nerves
   1. Schwannoma (neurinoma, neurilemoma)
      Cellular, plexiform, and melanotic subtypes
   2. Neurofibroma
      Circumscribed (solitary) neurofibroma, plexiform neurofibroma
   3. Malignant peripheral nerve sheath tumor (malignant schwannoma)
      Epithelioid, divergent mesenchymal or epithelial differentiation, melanotic
7. Local extensions from regional tumors
   1. Paraganglioma (chemodectoma)
   2. Chordoma

3. Chondroma
4. Chondrosarcoma
5. Carcinoma
8. Metastatic tumours
9. Unclassified tumors
10. Cysts and tumor-like lesions
    1. Rathke cleft cyst
    2. Epidermoid
    3. Dermoid
    4. Colloid cyst of the third ventricle
    5. Enterogenous cyst
    6. Neuroglial cyst
    7. Granular cell tumor (choristoma, pituicytoma)
    8. Hypothalamic neuronal hamartoma
    9. Nasal glial heterotopia
    10. Plasma cell granuloma

A number of grading systems are in common use for tumors of astrocytic lineage (i.e., astrocytomas, anaplastic astrocytomas, and glioblastomas). Grades are assigned solely on the basis of microsopic appearance of the tumor. The numerical grade assigned for a given tumor, however, can vary depending on which grading system is used, as illustrated by the following table. Thus, it is important to specify the grading system referred to when a grade is specified. The St. Anne/Mayo grade has proven to correlate better with survival than the previously common Kernohan grading system. It can only be applied to invasive tumors of astrocytic lineage; it is otherwise similar to the WHO grading system.

Grading of Astrocytic Tumors

WHO designation	WHO Grade*	Kernohan Grade*
Pilocytic astrocytoma	I	I
Astrocytoma	II	I, II
Anaplastic (malignant astrocytoma)	III	II, III
Glioblastoma	IV	III, IV

The WHO and Kernohan systems are not criteria based. Thus, a given tumor may not fall under the same designation in all three systems.

Brain Tumor Foundation for Children Inc.   A charitable organization. Address: 2231 Perimeter Park Drive, Ste 9, Atlanta, GA 30341. Tel: 404-458-5564.

Brain, W. Russell   (Lord Brain, 1895–1966) Preeminent English neurologist who trained at Oxford and at the London Hospital before entering neurology as a junior staff member at the Maida Vale Hospital for Nervous Diseases. He was elected to a consultant appointment at both hospitals and practiced from them for all of his professional life. His honors included the presidency of the Royal College of Physicians of London and of the Association of British Neurologists, Fellowship of the Royal Society, a peerage, and honors bestowed by other universities, royal societies and foreign institutions. He was editor of *Brain* from 1954 until his death.

Lord Brain's research contributions were essentially clinical, leading him to define first or to describe best such conditions as the carpal tunnel syndrome, dysthyroid ophthalmopathy, some paraneoplastic syndromes, the dysphasias, and the complications of cervical spondylosis. His textbooks *Diseases of the Nervous*

System and the shorter *Clinical Neurology* were each a model of clarity, selectiveness, and accuracy, and both went into several editions during his lifetime and thereafter. His literary output turned to the poetical and philosophical later in his life (*Some Reflections on Genius and Other Essays* in 1960 and *Tea with Walter de la Mare* in 1957). In addition, he was well placed to guide public and political opinion in matters relating to humanitarian care of the sick and numerous aspects of public health policy, responsibilities which he fulfilled completely. He was acknowledged at his death to be the foremost neurologist in England by virtue of his abilities in every field of endeavor to which he turned his hand or his heart.

Brain Tumor Society   A national voluntary health agency. Address: 124 Watertown St., Suite 3H, Watertown, MA 02472-2500. Tel: 617-924-9997; 800-770-8287. E-mail: info@tbts.org. Web site: http://www.tbts.org.

brainstem attack   See **diencephalic autonomic seizures.**

brainstem auditory evoked potentials   (BAEP) Electric waveforms of biologic origin elicited in response to sound stimuli. These normally consist of a sequence of up to seven waves, designated I to VII, which occur during the first 10 msec after the onset of the stimulus and have positive polarity at the vertex of the head.[146] (From the 2001 Report of the Nomenclature Committee of the American Association of Electromyography and Electrodiagnosis.[10] Used by permission, copyright © 2001, AAEM.)

The generators for waves I–V are the acoustic nerve, cochlear nuclei, superior olivary nuclei, lateral lemniscus and inferior colliculi, respectively. The generators for waves VI and VII are uncertain.

Recording of BAEPs may be of value in the assessment of brainstem function in a variety of disorders, including multiple sclerosis, central pontine myelinolysis, and brain death.[1007]

brainstem encephalitis   See **Bickerstaff brainstem encephalitis.**[90]

brainstem gliomas   Diffuse malignant tumors of the brainstem, usually arising in childhood, adolescence, or early adult life, with death supervening within a year. Diffuse intrinsic pontine, tectal, and cervicomedullary locations are described.[2319] See also **gliomas.**

brainstem hallucinations   Pure visual hallucinations resulting from lesions of the midbrain, pons, or thalamus.[1862] See **peduncular hallucinosis.**

brainstem ptosis   Bilateral ptosis in alert patients without pupillary changes in the setting of brainstem infarctions. The cause is not known.[1847]

brainstem reflexes   Colloquially, the **corneal, gag, oculocephalic, oculovestibular,** and **cough reflexes.**

The **carotid sinus, cardiorespiratory,** and other vegetative reflexes are not usually included under this heading.

braking saccades   Saccades that stop the movement of the quick phase of jerk nystagmus, preceding the ensuing slow drift of the eyes which comprises the next part of the cycle.

Bramwell, Byrom   (1847–1931) Scottish physician, who contributed substantially to the understanding of the principles of localization within the spinal cord[714] and of tumors of the nervous system.

branch atheromatous disease   Narrowing or occlusion of the mouth of a branching artery by an atheromatous process different from lipohyalinosis, considered to be a potential cause of **lacunar syndromes.**[899]

branched-chain ketoaciduria   (maple syrup urine disease) A congenital dysmetabolic syndrome characterized by neonatal seizures and feeding problems, hypotonia alternating with dystonia, and aminoaciduria. The condition progresses to seizures, coma, and death. Classic, intermediate, intermittent and thiamine-responsive types have been differentiated.[335]

Another *variant* is *maple syrup urine disease, variant form,* a congenital syndrome characterized by neonatal feeding problems, seizures and disturbed consciousness, hypotonia, ophthalmoplegia, twelfth cranial nerve palsy, and aminoaciduria.

brancher enzyme deficiency   A rare recessively inherited and fatal form of glycogen storage disease characterized by the accumulation of polysaccharides in the liver, brain, and both cardiac and skeletal muscle.

The condition presents in infancy with hypotonia and weakness and is fatal within 2 years.[3782] See also **glycogen storage diseases.**

branchial muscle hypertrophy   See **branchial myopathy.**

branchial myoclonus   Rhythmical myoclonus-like movements of the palate, pharynx, larynx, tongue, and face (the branchial musculature), occurring as a hereditary disease or as a result of disease affecting the dentatorubroolivary pathways in the brainstem (the **Guillain-Mollaret triangle**).

branchial myopathy   (hypertrophic branchial myopathy, branchial muscle hypertrophy) A rare syndrome of unknown cause, characterized by tender hypertrophy of the temporalis and masseter muscles.[3230,3585]

brass arm   (telegraphist's cramp) A repetitive strain injury. See **occupational cramp.**

brassfounders ague   Sweating, nervousness, and paresthesias, possibly as a result of zinc oxide poisoning.

Brauch-Romberg sign   See **Romberg sign.**

Bravais, Louis   French physician who gave an account of focal (hemiplegic) seizures in his thesis on graduation from the University of Paris in 1827, thus antedating even Richard **Bright.**

brawny induration   (old Fr; slice of flesh + from Lat; to make hard) Discoloration and abnormal firmness developing in soft tissues, as in cellulitis.

breach rhythm   Nonepileptogenic mu-like EEG activity recorded in the vicinity of a skull defect.[3075] See also **wicket rhythm.**

breadcrumbing tremor   An alternative name for the **pill-rolling tremor** of parkinsonism.

breath-holding spells   Forms of **reflex syncope** in children. Episodes of altered consciousness occurring in children under the age of 5 years. Two forms are defined: *cyanotic* spells result from performing a Valsalva maneuver and are characterized by emotional provocation, apnea in expiration, cyanosis, brief stiffening of the body, and loss of consciousness, in that order, before the infant breathes again and regains awareness. See also **sobbing spasms.** *Pallid breath-holding spells* (**reflex anoxic seizures**) are provoked by minor head trauma and are characterized by pallor, accelerated loss of consciousness, and stiffening of the trunk and limbs with myoclonus and downbeating of the eyes, and result from asystole due to vagal cardiac standstill. Crying is seldom a feature.[3466]

breathlessness with effort intolerance   See **chronic fatigue syndrome.**

Breathnach syndrome   (premature aging with telangiectasias) A congenital dysmorphic syndrome characterized by pigmentary retinopathy, chorioretinitis, and intracranial calcification with seizures. Multiple fractures, skin telangiectasia, and angiokeratomas are other manifestations.[337]

Bregeat syndrome   An embryologic malformation comprising angiomatosis of the oculo-orbital vessels, homolateral thalamencephalic angioma of the choroidal plexus, and contralateral cutaneous angioma on the forehead. The condition is thus very similar to the **Wyburn-Mason syndrome.**[733]

bregma   (Gr, to moisten) The fore-part of the head, the anterior fontanelle at the junction of the coronal and sagittal sutures of the skull, which is soft and moist in the newborn. The word was used by Aristotle and Galen to apply to the **vertex,** but **Broca** applied it as we use it now.

bregmocardiac reflex   Bradycardia occurring as a result of compression of the anterior fontanelle in infants.

Bremer, Friedreich Wilhelm   (fl. 1926) German neurologist at Munich University whose major work on dysraphism was published in 1926.[734] He was also the first to show changes in the EEG during different sleep stages and used the **cerveau isolé** preparation (in which the transection is performed behind the third nerve nucleus) in the cat to show that coma can occur with the EEG appearance of non–rapid eye movement sleep; contrasting this with the findings in the **encephale isolé** preparation (in which a cut is made at the level of the cervicomedullary junction), when normal sleep–wake cycles are retained.

Bremer syndrome   See **dysraphism.**

Breughel syndrome   (blepharospasm-oromandibular dystonia, Meige syndrome) A **cranial dystonia** marked by combinations of prolonged involuntary spasmodic contractions of the muscles of the face, mouth, tongue, and jaw, due to a disorder of the basal ganglia in the elderly, the blepharospasm often making the patients functionally blind.

  The condition is named after the contorted facial expressions of the individuals depicted in some of the paintings of Peter Breughel the elder, a Flemish artist (1712–1765)[3639,3814] Unlike those of Breughel, the equally graphic depictions of dystonia by William Blake do not include representations of oromandibular dystonia.

Brickner phenomenon   **Oscillopsia,** originally described in multiple sclerosis.[744]

Brickner, Richard Max   (1896–1959) American neurologist in New York, who studied extensively the effects of temperature on function in **multiple sclerosis.**

Brief Cognitive Rating Scale   (BCRS) An instrument designed to assess the severity of cognitive decline, employed widely in the investigation of pharmacological agents used in the treatment of cognitive dysfunction in elderly people. See Chart B–8. The test excludes measures of mood change but provides scores of concentration, recent and remote memory, orientation, and functioning and self-care. In a modification (BCRS part 2), speech and language capacity, psychomotor function, mood and behavior, praxis, and calculation ability are also assessed.[4646,4649]

Chart B–8. Brief Cognitive Rating Scale

1. Concentration

1. No objective or subjective evidence of deficit in concentration
2. Subjective decrement in concentration ability
3. Minor objective signs of poor concentration (e.g., serial 7's)
4. Definite concentration deficit for background (e.g., marked deficit on serial 7's; frequent deficit in subtraction of serial 4's from 40)
5. Marked concentration deficit (e.g., gives months backwards or problem with serial 2's from 20)
6. Forgets the concentration task. Frequently begins to count forwards when asked to count backwards from 10 by 1's.
7. Marked difficulty counting forward to 10 by 1's

2. Recent memory

1. No objective or subjective evidence of deficit
2. Subjective impairment only (forgetting names more than before)
3. Deficit in recall of specific events evident on detailed questioning. No deficit in the recall of major recent events
4. Cannot recall major events of previous weekend or week. Scanty knowledge (not detailed) of current events, favorite TV shows, etc.
5. Unsure of weather, current president, or current address
6. Occasional knowledge of some recent events. Little or no idea of current address, weather, etc.
7. No knowledge of any recent events

3. Past memory

1. No subjective or objective impairment in present memory
2. Subjective impairment only. Can recall two or more primary school teachers
3. Some gaps in past memory upon detailed questioning. Able to recall at least one childhood teacher and/or one childhood friend
4. Clear-cut deficit. The spouse recalls more of the patient's past than the patient. Cannot recall childhood friends and/or teachers but knows the names of most schools attended. Confuses chronology in reciting personal history
5. Major past events sometimes not recalled (e.g., names of schools attended)
6. Some residual memory of past (e.g., may recall country of birth or former occupation)
7. No memory of the past

4. Orientation

1. No deficit in memory for time, place, or identity of self or others
2. Subjective impairment only. Knows time to nearest hour, location
3. Any mistake in time >2 hours; day of week >1 day; date >3 days
4. Mistakes in month >10 days, or year >1 month
5. Unsure of month and/or year and/or season; unsure of locale
6. No idea of date. Identifies spouse but may not recall name. Knows own name
7. Cannot identify spouse. May be unsure of personal identity.

5. Functioning and self-care

1. No difficulty, either subjectively or objectively
2. Complains of forgetting location of objects. Subjective work difficulties
3. Decreased job functioning evident to co-workers. Difficulty in traveling to new locations
4. Decreased ability to perform complex tasks (e.g., planning dinner for guests, handling finances, marketing, etc.)
5. Needs help in choosing proper clothing
6. Needs help in feeding, toileting, bathing, and/or ambulating
7. Requires constant assistance in all activities of daily life

From Reisberg, 1988.[4649]

Brief Psychiatric Rating Scale   A relatively short observer-rated scale assessing 16 items including depressive symptoms, with the object of assessing changes after treatment.[4281] The scale concentrates on psychopathology, with less emphasis on the manifestations of dementia such as somatic and self-care factors.

A similar scale for the assessment of geriatric patients has also been constructed.[4366]

brief small abundant motor-unit action potentials A pattern of voluntary EMG activity which suggests, but is by no means diagnostic of, primary myopathy.[1675] See **BSAPPs.**

Brief Symptom Inventory   A self-report questionnaire used for individual screening of depressive symptoms.[1415]

Bright, Richard   (1789–1858) English physician and pathologist born in Bristol. After training in Edinburgh, at Guy's Hospital, and in Europe, he practiced in London where he was appointed physician to Guy's Hospital in 1824. He is best remembered for his descriptions of chronic renal disease and of various neurological conditions, collected in the two volumes of his *Reports of Medical Cases* (1827–1831), in which *inter alia* he described the features of certain seizure types, recognizing the sensory march,[745] painful lateralized seizures, secondary generalization of focal seizures, ictal amaurosis, and olfactory auras.

His account of postictal paralysis preceded that of **R.B. Todd.** He described absence attacks as follows: "Often it is the momentary absence of mind, the eye fixed in thought, yet gazing vacantly, no convulsion, no sound, the occupation of the hand ceases while the mind for the moment is annihilated; the cloud passes off, the intellect returns and often unconscious that its operation has been suspended, the patient resumes the occupation in which he was engaged."

He obtained and himself performed autopsies whenever possible, leading both to a superb pathological collection (retained at Guy's) and to contemporary recognition of the value of understanding the pathology of disease. Thus he was able to show that focal epilepsy was as likely to originate from brain disease as was the generalized variety, at a time when **Brown-Séquard,** for example, was advocating amputations for the control of focal seizures.[6088]

He was also a noted geologist; his collection, expanded by the purchase of the fossil section of that amassed by James **Parkinson,** passed eventually to the Institute of Geological Sciences.

Briquet, Paul   (1796–1881) French physician whose two theses were on varicose veins and artificial illumination, respectively, but who also published on tuberculosis, cholera, and hysteria.

Briquet syndrome   1. Aphonia and dyspnea, considered by Briquet (1859) to be due to hysterical paralysis of the diaphragm; this is almost certainly the **hyper-**

ventilation syndrome. 2. Hysteria, specifically hysterical anesthesia of the skin with consequent imprecision of movements ("ataxia"). Briquet regarded this as a "neurosis of the brain" in which unpleasant environmental events acted upon the "affective part" of the brain in a susceptible and predisposed person. His book[750] finally disposed of the old concept that hysteria was in some way associated with wanderings of the uterus. 3. A chronic illness characterized by the occurrence of multiple symptoms affecting multiple organ systems, resulting from **conversion disorder.**

His work and concepts of hysteria have been reviewed.[3577]

Brissaud convolution   The gyrus parietalis transversus.

Brissaud disease   (chorea variabilis) See **Tourette syndrome** (which was in fact what he was describing).[751]

Brissaud, Edouard   (1852–1909) French neuropsychiatrist. As a student he trained under **Charcot,** Millard, and **Lasègue** and after graduation became chef de clinique at the Pitié. He later deputized for Charcot in his absences, filling the Chair at the Salpétrière temporarily after Charcot's death.

He was elected professor of the history of medicine in the Faculté de Médicine in Paris, and later was professor of pathology. With Pierre **Marie** he founded the *Revue Neurologique* in 1893. Brissaud wrote extensively on such subjects as neuroanatomy, hysteria, asthma, acromegaly, parkinsonism, syphilis, involuntary movements, hypnosis, and medical history. He also gave a good account of **tuberous sclerosis,** but after Bourneville. **Horsley** operated on his brain tumor in Paris, but this did not prolong his life.

Edouard Brissaud

Brissaud infantilism   A syndrome of the persistence of infantile characteristics beyond the age of puberty, with retarded growth and delayed mental development. Round, chubby face, underdeveloped genitalia, dwarfism, lack of body hair, and delayed epiphyseal ossification are characteristic. The condition probably represents infantile myxedema.[752]

Brissaud reflex   Contraction of the tensor fascia lata in response to scratching the sole of the foot; seen in pyramidal disease.

Brissaud syndrome   1. See **Brissaud infantilism.** 2. Sinistrosis ("shell-shock"), but the term was used by him to describe the features of traumatic or **compensation neurosis:** "It is a pathological attitude in an injured person who refuses to recognise that he is cured as he genuinely believes that he has not obtained just legal compensation for the injury received. He is basically a claimant who over-estimated his right to be indemnified."[753]

Brissaud-Lereboullet syndrome   (hemicraniosis) Hemifacial and hemicranial hyperostosis associated with underlying meningiomas or sarcomas, raised intracranial pressure, visual disturbances, exophthalmos, and seizures.

The condition probably represents sarcomatous change in a long-standing meningioma.[754]

Brissaud-Marie syndrome   Hysterical glossolabial paralysis in which the deviation of the face and of the tongue are unphysiological with respect to the limb weakness.[755,757,4723]

Brissaud-Meige syndrome   See **hemifacial spasm.**

Brissaud-Sicard syndrome   Facial hemispasm associated with contralateral hemiparesis due to a caudal-ventral pontine lesion, described in 1908.[756]

Bristowe, John Syer   (fl. 1885) English neurologist and Fellow of the Royal Society who described the effects of callosal tumors in *Brain* in 1885.

Bristowe syndrome   (callosal syndrome) The pattern of symptoms associated with tumors of the corpus callosum, comprising negativism, disturbances of memory, concentration, and personality, and hemiparesis.[121] Tumors affecting the anterior part of the corpus callosum may lead to apraxias of the left hand as well.

British Journal of Neurosurgery   A professional specialist journal published for the Society of British Neurosurgeons. Web site: http://www.tandf.co.uk/journals/titles/02688697.html.

British Medical Journal (BMJ)   A general medical journal, also publishing items of neurological interest. Access to the journal is free, on-line: http://bmj.com/.

Brixa-Koppens sign   See **Gowers signs.**

broad A-band disease   A benign congenital myopathy characterized clinically by neonatal hypotonia, with or without congenital blindness due to retinal dystrophy, and delay in speech amd development. Ultrastructural abnormalities include disorganization of myosin thick filaments leading to a loss of A band/I band demarcation and an impression of broadening of the A band. See also **Leber congenital amaurosis.**[4028]

Broadbent apoplexy   Intracerebral hemorrhage which penetrates into the ventricles.[762]

Broadbent law   With a lesion of the upper motor neuron above the facial colliculus in the pons, the hand and arm are most affected, the leg next so, and the lower face and tongue only slightly.

Broadbent, Sir William Henry   (1835–1907) English neurologist and cardiologist who trained in Manchester and London, studying further under Trousseau in Paris after graduation. He practiced largely from St. Mary's Hospital, London, and was elected a fellow of the Royal Society in 1896. He was created a baronet as a result of his services as Physician to Queen Victoria and King Edward VII.

His neurological publications concerned hemiplegia, aphasia, and the preceding two entries.

Broca aphasia   (Broca dysphasia, nonfluent aphasia, agrammatic aphasia). A classic nonfluent dysphasia characterized by awkward slow and effortful articulation, loss of **prosody,** impairment of repetition and naming, and restriction to simple grammatical forms in speech and writing (**agrammatism**) so that spontaneous speech is of a telegraphic type.

Agrammatism leads to the use of single words, words with a high substantive content (nouns and verbs), but few articles, pronouns, prepositions, or conjunctions. The normal syntactic relations are lost. Repetition and confrontation naming are also much affected but there is relative preservation of comprehension. Phonetic disintegration (mainly shown as trouble in initiating speech and in selecting and blending words) and mispronunciation of phonemes (such as *B* for *P*) also occur.

The causative lesion involves the posterior part of inferior frontal gyrus of the dominant hemisphere, the anterior parietal region, the insula, and both banks of the rolandic fissure with deep extension.[763] The condition has been separated into two types:

Persisting Broca aphasia (big or true Broca aphasia) This type usually begins with a global aphasia and right-sided paresis with evolution to a state in which spoken language is comprehended but a nonfluent and agrammatical speech with poor repetition remains, which is due to extensive damage affecting not only the inferior left frontal gyrus but also the surrounding cortex and the underlying white matter and basal ganglia, as above.

Broca area infarction syndrome (little, mild, or acute Broca aphasia) A nonfluent agrammatic output is present at the beginning of the disorder, comprehension is preserved, and the speech disturbance improves to a state of near normality except for some impairment in prosody. Any initial **mutism** is replaced by rapidly abating dyspraxic

and effortful articulation and there is significant permanent disturbance in language function. The lesion responsible is a restricted infarction of the posterior portion of the dominant inferior frontal gyrus.[3937]

Broca dysphasia   See **Broca aphasia.**

Broca, Pierre-Paul   (1824–1880) French anthropologist, anatomist, and professor of clinical surgery at the Bicêtre in Paris; later a politician. He described hemispheric dominance and determined that right-handedness was associated with the representation of speech in the left hemisphere, thus defining the anatomical correlate of nonfluent aphasia (1861).[763] He also described the major features of motor or expressive aphasia in his patient Tan, and was the first to trephine for a cerebral abscess which he had localized correctly by clinical means (the only means available).

He reported in 1865 the cases of eight aphasic ("aphemic") right-handers with left hemisphere lesions and stated that the left inferior frontal convolution was the center for articulate speech.[764,2533] He also described muscular dystrophy before **Duchenne,** rickets, the treatment of cerebral aneurysms, clubfeet, fractures, and the use of hypnotism in surgery.

As an anthropologist he was interested in craniology (naming the inion, bregma, dacryon, lambda, metopion, obelion, and opisthion) and he was involved in the discovery and reports on Neanderthal man. He founded the French school of anthropology.

Pierre-Paul Broca

Broca's area   (Broca's convolution) The motor speech area; the posterior part of the inferior (third) frontal convolution, on the left side in a large majority of people.

Broca's area infarction syndrome   See **Broca aphasia.**

Broca's convolution   See **Broca area.**

Brodmann areas   Fifty-two cortical areas, containing 11 regions distinguished by the structure and disposition of their cellular layers (**cytoarchitectonics**) defined by Brodmann in 1903–1908.[1478]

Brodmann, Korbinian   (1868–1918) German physician who initially trained in psychiatry in Jena, Frankfurt, and Berlin but who later was appointed in succession professor of anatomy in Tübingen, Halle, and Munich, where he pioneered the study of **cytoarchitectonics.**

Brody syndrome   (Lambert-Brody syndrome) A recessive muscle disease of childhood mapped to chromosome 16p12; and due to functional deficiency of Ca^{2+} ATPase in the sarcoplasmic reticulum of fast-twitch skeletal muscle. It is characterized clinically by impaired muscle relaxation after voluntary contraction, with cramps, stiffness and myalgia being induced by exercise and cold. Progression is slow. The EMG shows that the cramps are electrically silent. Muscle biopsy reveals only type II fiber atrophy.[266,481,766] Dominant inheritance has also been reported.

bromide   A halogen, introduced by Locock for the treatment of "hysterical" epilepsy in 1857,[3451] on the bases that epilepsy was (at least in some cases) a manifestation of abnormal sexual tendencies, and that bromides had been found to cause impotence. As a result of Locock's paper, Dr. C.B. Radcliffe and Sir Samuel Wilks both generalized the indications for its use to treatment of organic epilepsy.

bromide partition test   A chemical test performed on CSF samples providing evidence for or against a diagnosis of tuberculous meningitis.[3591]

bronx cheer   A derogatory expression, a compound of eructation and retching. When involuntary, it is classified as a complex vocal tic, a manifestation of **Tourette syndrome;** when voluntary, it is merely an expression of opinion.

Brossard, Jules   (1855–1911) French physician.

Brossard scapulodistal syndrome   A **scapuloperoneal syndrome,** probably recessively inherited.[782]

Brown ataxia   See **Sanger Brown ataxia.**

Brown, Charles Leonard   (b. 1899) American pathologist, practicing in Boston and New York.

Brown, Jason W.   American neurologist in Los Angeles.

Brown, Sanger   (1852–1928) Canadian-born neurologist who trained in medicine at Bellevue. He intro-

duced a new system of classification of patients at the mental hospital where he was first appointed which led to the discharge of a number of them. He achieved prominence in psychiatry, going on to be medical superintendent in other hospitals in the northeastern United States.

In 1886 he studied neurology with Sharpey-Shafer in London and established the role of the occipital lobe in vision. He settled in Chicago in 1890, becoming professor of forensic medicine and hygiene at Rush and of clinical neurology at the University of Illinois.

Sanger Brown

Brown syndrome   (a syndrome of the neural crest) Loss of deep pain sensitivity, retention of superficial pain, autonomic dysfunction, hypoplasia of dental enamel, meningeal thickening and cystic change, hyporeflexia, mild mental retardation, and blond hair, blue-green eyes, and a fair complexion.[795]

The authors suggested that this association of signs indicated that there was a failure of differentiation of the neural crest as the underlying embryonic abnormality.

See **superior oblique tendon syndrome.** The condition was described by Dr. H.W. Brown in 1950.

Brown-Peterson paradigm   A test used for the assessment of short-term memory. It typically consists of the presentation of a set of three items, after which the patient is asked to engage in some distracting activity such as counting backward from a three-digit number for between 2 and 30 seconds. Reproduction of the originally presented material is then requested. Between 10 and 20 trials are usually administered.[4424]

Brown-Séquard, Charles-Edouard (1817–1894) A neurologist of Eurasian and Irish-American parentage who was born in Mauritius but who trained in Paris, first for a literary and later for a medical career. Trousseau was one of his teachers, and after graduation he worked with Baron Larrey. In his thesis on the physiology of the spinal cord, accepted in Paris in 1846; he described the sensory decussation within the cord. Constrained by the Second Empire and short of money, he left France and visited New York and then Mauritius (where he was given a gold medal to commemorate his handling of a cholera epidemic) before settling to practice in Richmond, Virginia in 1855. He felt it proper to withdraw from this city following a tactless remark of his about slavery, and the resulting remarks of others upon his own mixed blood.

He returned to Paris in that year and published his findings on the functions of the adrenal glands. In 1858 he lectured in London, Glasgow, and Dublin, after which he was held in the highest esteem and was elected Fellow of the Royal Society and also Fellow of the Royal College of Physicians in 1860. At this time he was appointed as the first physician to the **National Hospital,** Queen Square, a position that he held until 1863 when he accepted the Chair of Nervous Pathology at Harvard. There he remained until the death of his wife in 1868, when he returned to Paris and accepted the Chair of Experimental Physiology at the Faculté de Médicine. In 1872 he returned to New York and remarried, but he went again to Paris on the death of his second wife 2 years later.

In 1877 he accepted the post of professor of physiology at Geneva, married for the third time, and remained in Geneva for a year before succeeding Claude **Bernard** as professor of experimental medicine at the Collège de France in Paris, a post that he retained until his death.

Although noted for many physiological observations, including that of caloric testing 45 years before **Bárány,** his name is chiefly remembered for his descriptions in 1850 and 1851 of the syndrome resulting from lateral hemisection of the spinal cord, popularly (but probably incorrectly) thought to have been brought to his attention by the activities of the Parisian mafioso who settled their scores with stilettos so thin as to be able to penetrate into the spinal canal[809] and for his demonstration that excision of the adrenal glands was followed by features of Addison disease.

His medical interests exceeded neurology,[5672] and he reported late in life on the effects he experienced from the self-injection of an extract of guinea pig testicles, which he regarded as entirely satisfactory.

Charles-Edouard Brown-Séquard

Brown-Séquard spinal epilepsy Muscle spasms arising because of the presence of an irritative lesion affecting the motor fibers in the spinal cord. Despite the name, the condition is not truly epileptic but rather a form of segmental myoclonus.[574]

Brown-Séquard syndrome Damage to the lateral half of the spinal cord, leading to ipsilateral loss of pyramidal and posterior column function and contralateral spinothalamic loss, with evidence of a root lesion at the site of the cord injury. Direct trauma was once, and extrinsic compressive lesion is now, the most common cause.[809]

Brown-Symmers disease (acute serous encephalitis) See **acute disseminated encephalomyelitis.**[789]

Brown–Vialetto–Van Laere syndrome See **pontobulbar palsy with deafness.**

Bruch membrane The structure supporting the pigmented epithelial layer overlying the rods and cones in the retina.

Bruck–de Lange syndrome A fatal infantile syndrome of psychomotor delay, extrapyramidal rigidity, movement disorder, and local or generalized muscular hypertrophy.[1356] See **De Lange syndrome.**

Brudzinski, Josef (1874–1917) Polish physician who graduated from Moscow and specialized in pediatrics. After a tour of European schools he returned to Warsaw and then was appointed head of a children's hospital in Lodz, transferring to Warsaw again as rector of the university. The sign for which he is best remembered (described below) was described in 1909.[810]

Brudzinski signs 1. *Neck phenomenon* Flexion of the hips and knees (sometimes with extension of the hallux and fanning of the toes) in response to passive neck flexion.

2. *Contralateral leg sign* The involuntary flexion or extension of one leg in response to forceful passive flexion of the other leg at the hip (straight leg raising).[810] In each case it is a sign of meningeal irritation or inflammation. *The reciprocal contralateral leg sign* is seen when one leg is flexed at the hip and knee and the other is extended. When the flexed limb is lowered to the bed, the other leg flexes.

3. (*Cheek sign*) Flexion of the elbows with upward jerking of both arms in response to pressure on the cheeks.[811]

4. (*Symphysis sign*) Flexion of the legs in response to suprapubic pressure.[374]

Most of these signs were described in patients with tuberculous meningitis.[4723,5047]

bruit   (Fr, noise) An abnormal sound generated as a result of the turbulent flow of blood within arteries and heard through a stethoscope.

bruit de pôt fêlé   See **cracked-pot note.**

Brumback syndrome   A congenital dysmorphic syndrome characterized by microcephaly, cerebral atrophy, agenesis of the corpus callosum, and **Brushfield spots** on the iris.

Brunauer syndrome   A dominantly inherited syndrome of mental retardation, defective enamel formation and hyperhidrosis with hyperkeratosis of the palms and soles.[2221]

Bruns ataxia   See **Bruns gait apraxia.**

Bruns gait apraxia   (Bruns ataxia, apractic or magnetic gait) Inability to initiate the process of forward motion by alternating steps, although the power and coordination of the legs is normal in the lying or sitting positions. The maintenance of the feet on the floor, removed only with great effort, has led to the alternative name *magnetic gait.*

This static ataxia in the presence of frontal lobe disorders is due to involvement of the descending efferent frontocerebellar fibres and was originally described in the setting of frontal lobe tumors but is now more commonly seen in frontal ischemic disease. The constellation of abulia, psychomotor retardation, primitive reflexes, and ideomotor apraxia with cerebellar findings is suggestive.[816]

The entity is of uncertain validity, and has been considered to have cerebellar, apraxic, agnosic, and labyrinthine components.[818] See **frontal dysequilibrium.**

Bruns, Ludwig   (1858–1916) German neurologist, who studied at Munich and Göttingen Universities and trained in neurology with Hitzig and later in Paris. After some time in Berlin with **Westphal** and **Oppenheim,** he left to direct the Department of Internal Medicine at Hanover University where he was later appointed professor.

In 1892 he described the gait disorder named for him[816] and wrote on hysteria, callosal tumors, goiter, tetanus, parkinsonism, the optic nerve, birth injuries, and diabetes. He was also the author (in collaboration) of a large and influential *Textbook of Pediatric Neurology.*[818]

Ludwig Bruns

Bruns nystagmus   The combination of small-amplitude, rapid-jerk nystagmus in the primary position, beating away from the side of an extraaxial mass lesion compressing the vestibular nerve and the brainstem, in association with slow, large-amplitude, gaze-evoked, or gaze-paretic nystagmus toward the side of the lesion.[6075]

The syndrome occurs typically with cerebellopontine angle tumors characterized by **gaze paretic nystagmus** evoked by gaze to the side of the tumor and by **vestibular nystagmus** evoked by gaze to the opposite side.

Bruns syndrome   Vertigo, vomiting headache, and visual disturbance during change in head posture; a sign of cerebral tumors, usually in the posterior fossa but also occurring with, for example, bilateral subdural hematomas.[817]

The original description was of a man with cysticercosis, who had no symptoms unless he moved his head quickly.[122]

Brushfield spots   Mottled or speckled, white or light yellow pin-points regularly placed in a ring near the outer margin of the iris, found in 90% of people with **Down syndrome** and in about a quarter of normal subjects when they are known as **Wolfflin nodules.**

Brushfield could not find the spots in patients with brown irides.[819]

Brushfield syndrome   See **Sturge-Weber syndrome.**

Brushfield, Thomas   (1856–1933) English psychiatrist working in mental deficiency.

Brushfield-Wyatt syndrome   Generalized and trigeminal port-wine stains with a calcified angioma in the underlying cerebral hemisphere producing hemianopia and hemiparesis, and mental defect.[820] The similarity to **Sturge-Weber syndrome** is obvious.

The term has also been used for **tuberous sclerosis.**

bruxism   (nocturnal tooth-grinding) A stereotyped movement disorder occurring during partial arousal from sleep (and thus a **parasomnia**), characterized by unconscious tight jaw closure with stereotyped rhythmic grinding of the teeth occurring especially during non–rapid eye movement stage 2 sleep, unassociated with EEG abnormalities.[4923] See also **sleep disorders.**[234] Damage to the teeth and to the temporomandibular joints may result. The condition also occurs during periods of rapid eye movement sleep.

bruxomania   Persistent, conscious tooth-grinding.

BSA(P)Ps   (**B**rief, **S**mall, **A**bundant **P**olyphasic **P**otentials) A recruitment pattern of motor unit action potentials recorded during electromyography, usually during minimal contraction and usually suggesting the presence of primary muscle disease. Although the term is discouraged by the American Association of Electromyography and Electrodiagnosis Nomenclature Subcommittee,[10] the pattern is quite distinctive and the acronym quite satisfactory to most electromyographers.

buccal apraxia   (oral apraxia) Impairment in performing mouth or face actions on verbal command or imitation (see also **orofacial apraxia**) or in performing learned, skilled movements with the facial and bulbar muscles—for example, inability to protrude the tongue to command. With this is associated difficulty in imitating meaningless movements made by the examiner. The responsible lesion is of the opercula or the anterior perisylvian regions.[29,3138] See also **apraxia.**

buccal reflex   (snouting; Toulouse, Vurpas, oral, nasomental reflex) Approximation of the lips when the upper lip is tapped; a sign of pseudobulbar palsy. See also **orbicularis oris reflex.**

For a sign of relatively slight importance, this number of alternative names is peculiar.

Buchem syndrome   See **hyperostosis corticalis generalisata familiaris.**

buckling sign   Involuntary flexion of the extended knee when the hip is flexed during straight-leg raising. This is evidence of irritation of the sciatic spinal nerve roots. See **Brudzinski signs #2;** *contralateral leg sign.*

buckthorn neuropathy   (tullidora) A toxic syndrome characterized by flaccid ascending motor weakness and ataxia, resulting from the ingestion of the berries of *Karwinskia humboldtiana,* a Central American shrub. The pathological changes include both segmental demyelination of the motor nerves and neuronopathy.[3905]

Budge centers   The spinal cord at C7–T6, from which fibers pass out to the sympathetic chain, named the *ciliospinal center* by Budge and Waller; they also identified the *genitospinal center* in the sacral cord.

Budge, Julius Ludwig   (1811–1884) Professor of anatomy and physiology in Bonn and later in Pomerania.[1478]

buffer amplifier   An amplifier generally with a voltage gain of 1, a high-input impedance and a low-output impedance, and used to isolate the input signal from the loading effects of an immediately following circuit. In some EEG machines, each input is connected to a buffer amplifier located in the jack box to reduce cable artifact and interference. (Adapted from the report of the Committee on Terminology, IFCN,[989] © 1974, with permission from Elsevier Science.)

bulbar   (from Gr, a bulb or any rounded structure) Of or pertaining to the medulla oblongata.

bulbar encephalitis   See **Bickerstaff brainstem encephalitis.**

bulbar myoclonus   See **palatal myoclonus.**

bulbar palsy   Lower motor neuron weakness of those muscles supplied by the seventh through twelfth cranial nerves as a result usually of pontomedullary lesions, motor neuropathies, nerve compression at the skull base, or **myasthenia gravis;** and leading thus to weakness of the face and tongue, dysphagia, dysarthria, and dysphonia.

The first description was that of John Bunyan in 1680.

bulbar palsy with deafness   See **Vialetto–van Laere syndrome.**

bulbar palsy with deafness and pigmentary retinopathy   See **hereditary motor neuropathy** (*variants*).

bulbar palsy with olivopontocerebellar atrophy   See **cerebellar ataxias.**

bulbar spinal muscular atrophy of childhood   See **Fazio-Londe disease.**

bulbar spinal muscular atrophy with deafness   See **Vialetto–van Laere syndrome.**

bulbocavernosus reflex   (virile reflex) Sudden contraction of the bulbocavernosus and ischiocavernosus muscles and of the anal sphincter with squeezing or irritation of the glans penis or clitoris. The same reflex can be elicited with electrical stimulation of the dorsal nerve of the penis, with recording by a single-fiber needle in the bulbocavernosus muscle.[5772]

The reflex was described as a normal phenomenon in 1890 by Jacques **Onanoff,** but he noted that it is absent with advancing age and regarded it more useful as evidence of retained virility than of neurological disease, considering that when it was present in impotent or in neurasthenic patients, it signified that the condition did not have an organic basis. Absence of the reflex suggests a neurogenic cause for bladder dysfunction, indicating neural integrity of L5–S5, but mainly of the S2, 3, 4 segments. The response is increased in patients with pyramidal tract lesions.[1700]

bulbomimic reflex (Mondonesi reflex) In metabolic coma, eyeball pressure leads to bilateral facial grimacing; with coma due to a focal brain lesion, the grimace is seen on one side only.

bulbospinal neuronopathy (spinal and bulbar muscular atrophy, Kennedy syndrome) A heterogeneous group of disorders of unknown cause affecting infants or young adults who present with distal weakness, fasciculations, and postural tremor. Twitching of the chin is a typical complaint. Dysarthria and dysphagia follow later. The depression of muscle stretch reflexes and the detection of mild sensory disturbances differentiate the condition from motor neuron disease and from hereditary motor neuropathies.

Inheritance by all modes has been described at some time, and the course of the disease shows extreme variability.

Variant forms include the following:
1. *Kennedy syndrome* (Kennedy-Alter-Sung syndrome) A benign X-linked bulbospinal neuronopathy due to a CAG repeat mapping to Xq21.3–q12, also with onset in adult life, in which gynecomastia, bulbar and facial weakness, fasciculations, hypertrophy and cramping of the calves and postural tremor are the more prominent features.[3006] **Progressive proximal spinal and bulbar atrophy of late onset** is probably the same condition.
2. The juvenile form of X-linked proximal spinal muscular atrophy, with calf enlargement
3. A rare phenotype of **GM$_2$ gangliosidosis**[5554]
4. *Familial bulbospinal neuronopathy with optic atrophy*[A327]

bulbospinal system Pathways that originate in the brainstem, descend to spinal levels, and are concerned in the control of movement and of posture.

bulimia (Gr, a particle + hunger) Morbid hunger; excessive appetite with decreased satiety after eating.

bulimia nervosa (Gr, a particle + hunger) (binge eating) 1. Morbid hunger; excessive appetite with decreased satiety after eating. 2. A chronic but self-limiting eating disorder characterized by an episodic desire to eat large amounts of food, accompanied by a sense of loss of control and often of depression; each episode is followed by purging, starvation, and fasting.

As with **anorexia,** the patients manifest a fear of fatness, a desire for thinness, a distorted body image, and a denial of illness.[4855] The American Psychiatric Association criteria (DSM-IV-TR)[150] amplify this description.

Bull angle The angle between the plane of the hard palate and the plane of the atlas vertebra on a true lat-

eral skull X-ray film. The normal angle is <5°, while patients with basilar impression often have an angle measuring over 13°.[832]

Although a popular measure, it has been criticized because the first reference point is not part of the base of the skull, and is therefore unsuitable when defining the relationship of different parts thereof, such as the rim of the foramen magnum.

bulldog reflex Involuntary clenching of the teeth in response to the sensation of any object placed between them; shown by some patients with frontal lobe tumors.[574]

Bumke, Oswald Conrad Edward (1877–1950) German neurologist and psychiatrist who studied medicine in various German universities, graduating from Kiel University. He rose through the ranks in Freyberg, Halle, Rostock, Breslau, Leipzig, and Munich, succeeding Kraepelin at Munich University. He is best remembered for describing the pupillary sign, but he also published extensively on various psychiatric topics.[5047]

He collaborated with **Foerster** in the production of the *Handbuch der Neurologie* (1935–1937), which became the most influential book (in 17 volumes) on the subject in European neurology. He attended Lenin in his last illness (a stroke).

Bumke (anxiety) pupils Dilatation of the normal pupil in response to a stressful psychic stimulus, with an impaired light response. The sign was described by Bumke in his book *Die Pupillenstörungen* (Jena, 1903), and is said to be absent in schizophrenia.

bundle of Turck A fiber pathway running from the posterior temporal region to the pontine nuclei and from there to the cerebellar vermis. It is probably responsible for the retention of whole-body movements in cases of apraxia.

bungarotoxin (a-BTX) The lethal factor in the venom of the banded krait, which binds so completely and specifically to acetylcholine receptor sites that it supplies a method for their quantification.

Büngner bands Basal laminae which assist in the orientation of sprouting axons.

Bunina bodies Eosinophilic, rounded, or elongated intracytoplasmic inclusion bodies with clear haloes found in the motor neurons of the spinal cord, brainstem, and motor cortex in **amyotrophic lateral sclerosis.**

Burdach column (fasciculus cuneatus) The lateral part of the posterior (dorsal) columns of the spinal cord, named by Burdach in 1819. The medial part (fasciculus gracilis) is named for **Goll.** The Burdach nucleus is the cuneate nucleus. See also **cuneate fasciculus and nucleus.**

Burdach, Karl Friedrich (1776–1847) German physician, anatomist, and physiologist, and professor in these disciplines in Dorpat and then Königsberg. He was a member of the *Naturphilosophen* group, concerned with speculative generalizations on brain functions.

He introduced the terms *biology* and *morphology* to medicine and named the globus pallidus (1819), internal capsule, putamen, lenticular nucleus, red nucleus, cingulum, cuneus, and amygdaloid nucleus and classified the thalamic nuclei, as well as writing widely in other areas of pathology and physiology.[3856] He named the fasciculus cuneatus, and discovered the red nucleus before Stilling. He was also a neuroanatomical historian; in his *Vom Baue und Leben des Gehirns* (1819–1826) he attributed to **Willis** the first description of the corpus striatum, pyramids, olives, and the anterior commissure, and the description of the anatomy of the connections of the cerebellar peduncles, the stria medullaris, and the eleventh cranial nerve.

Burkitt lymphoma   A multicentric tumor composed of poorly differentiated lymphoid cells, common in East Africa and described by Sir Denis Burkitt from Uganda in 1958. Clinically, swellings of the jaw, orbit, and face and ovarian infiltration are the usual features.

Neurological complications include direct or ischemic myelopathy, multiple cranial neuropathies affecting especially the oculomotor and seventh cranial nerves, malignant meningitis, seizures, and delirium.

burn encephalopathy   The acute onset of reduction in the level of consciousness, often with confusion, seizures, or neurological signs, or any of these in combination, in patients (especially children) suffering from severe burns.

The syndrome is not homogeneous. It affects some 5% of children at risk (usually with over 30% of the body surface burned) within a few days of the injury, but is usually reversible. Multiple metabolic problems are considered to be responsible.[3932] The syndrome was first noted by Dupuytren in 1832.

burn neuropathy   Multiple mononeuropathies occurring in severely burned patients, often with associated complications of sepsis. Vascular occlusion of the vasa nervorum, direct thermal injury, and a disseminated neurotoxin are suggested as mechanisms.[3637]

Burnett syndrome   (milk-alkali syndrome) The occurrence of weakness, depression, nausea, headache, and mental confusion in patients with hypercalcemia and alkalosis, due to excessive intake of milk and soluble alkalis.[845]

Burnier, Louis-Rene   (1880–1952) French dermatologist practicing in Paris.

Burnier syndrome   (hypophysial nanism) A syndrome of short stature, optic atrophy, and adiposogenital dystrophy, with or without obesity, due to a pituitary tumor destroying the anterior lobe in childhood.[847]

burning feet syndrome   (Gopalan syndrome, hot feet, happy feet, painful feet, jittery legs) A sensory neuropathy causing aching, burning, numbness, tingling, and aching in the legs with vasodilation of the feet, worse with heat and better with cold. It is generally due to deficiency in B-complex vitamins, as occurs in malnutrition states and uremia,[2201] but a dominantly inherited form has been reported.[5362]

burning hands syndrome   A forme fruste of the **central cord syndrome** in which limited injury has spared many of the fibers usually affected in that condition but has led to reduced input into the spinothalamic tract from the cervical segments.[3633]

burning mouth syndrome   (glossodynia, glossopyrosis, oral dysesthesias) A syndrome of persistent awareness of a painful, burning sensation in the mouth and/or tongue seen mainly in mature adult women.

The causes are multifactorial; ill-fitting dentures, vitamin B deficiency, anxiety, depression, and cancerphobia are all cited as etiological factors.[3233]

Burns syndrome   See **oculoauriculocutaneous syndrome.**

burst   A group of waves that appear and disappear abruptly and are distinguished from background activity by differences in frequency for and/or amplitude. The term does not imply abnormality and is not a synonym for **paroxysm.** (Adapted from the report of the Committee on Terminology, IFCN,[989] © 1974, with permission from Elsevier Science.)

burst lobe   The occurrence of an intracerebral or intracerebellar hematoma in continuity with a subdural hematoma, following cerebral trauma.

burst neurons   Neurons which, with pause neurons, are found in the paramedian pontine reticular formation (PPRF) and which generate the high-frequency burst discharges that act as the command for saccades to occur.

burst suppression   An EEG pattern characterized by bursts of theta and/or delta waves, at times intermixed with faster waves and with intervening periods of relative quiescence.

The term should be used to describe the EEG effects of some anesthetic drugs at certain levels of anesthesia. (Adapted from the report of the Committee on Terminology, IFCN,[989] © 1974, with permission from Elsevier Science.)

The pattern is typically seen in hypoxic brain damage and in prolonged status epilepticus, and it indicates significant compromise of the brain's metabolic integrity, with a poor prognosis.

Burton sign   The blue line in the gums just below their junction with the teeth in chronic lead poisoning, described by Dr. H. Burton (1799–1849), a physician at St. Thomas' Hospital in London.

Buschke Cued Recall Test   A test of memory (using confrontation naming) which coordinates the encoding and retrieval of new information for cued recall with an initial search strategy. The subject is required to name the objects shown in a series of pictures (e.g, "Which one is a piece of clothing?"), is prompted if he fails to name it, and finally is told the answer. Following a distracting task, the subject is required to recall as many of the 12 pictures shown as possible.[852,853]

Buschke-Fuld selective reminding procedure   A test of recent memory in which the subject learns 12 words over a dozen trials, being reminded only of those words that he failed to recall on the preceding trial. After 12 trials, the subject is required to note from a multiple-choice list those words with which he had difficulty.[853] The test is very sensitive to the presence of cognitive change.

Busse-Buschke disease   See **cryptococcal meningitis.**

butterfly area   The nasal and adjacent malar regions of the face.

butterfly glioma   A glioma that has spread from one hemisphere to the other directly through the corpus callosum. These lesions may have started within the corpus callosum and, by infiltrating both frontal lobes, lead either to increasing stupor or to emotional lability, irritability, or delusional states.

butterfly infarct   The pattern of infarction with occlusion of the precommunal part of the posterior cerebral artery, and thus of the penetrating arteries springing from it; and involving the medial part of the midbrain tegmentum and the medial part of the thalamus bilaterally.

Pupillary disorders and disturbances of eye movement result.

Buzzard, E.F.   (1871–1945) English physician, Regius Professor of Medicine at Oxford.

Buzzard reflex   A variant of the knee jerk, in this case obtained as the patient sits with the toes pressing on the floor as a facilitatory maneuver.[4723] See **nociceptive reflex.**

Bywaters syndrome   Traumatic/ischemic myositis with myoglobinemia and myoglobinuria and shock, sometimes leading to renal failure and usually described after extensive crush injuries.[864]

C

C fibers Unmyelinated sensory nerve fibers in the peripheral nervous system, feeding in from receptors that respond to temperature, chemical, and high-threshold mechanical stimulation.

C reflex An abnormal reflex response representing the electrophysiologic correlate of sensory evoked myoclonus. The term *C* was chosen to indicate that the reflex might be mediated in the cerebral cortex. This is sometimes, but not always, true.[10]

This enhanced long-latency EMG response is found in a stimulated muscle (and sometimes in the homologous muscle on the opposite side), particularly in patients with myoclonic disorders, time locked to a peripheral nerve electrical stimulus and equating a myoclonic jerk.

C syndrome (Opitz trigonocephaly syndrome) A recessively inherited craniofacial malformation syndrome characterized by trigonocephaly and microcephaly with ridging in the metopic region due to synostosis of the metopic suture, hypotelorism, Mongoloid slant to the eyes, epicanthic folds, strabismus, short neck, congenital cardiac malformations, and skeletal anomalies including syndactyly.[4247,4256]

C waves (Traub-Hering waves) Low-amplitude fluctuations of the CSF pressure occurring at 4–8/minute, normally present but enhanced in states of raised intracranial pressure. The waves correspond with changes in arterial blood pressure.

cacacusis Frightening echoes of mechanical sounds or of words heard or said, symptomatic of right hemisphere lesions.[4894] See also **palinacousis.**

CACH (childhood ataxia with diffuse CNS hypomyelination; vanishing white matter disease) A heterogeneous leukodystrophic condition of childhood with variable course resulting from maldevelopments of myelin formation, (dys- or hypomyelination) rather than demyelination.[4960,5719] See **fatal infantile leukodystrophy.**

cachectic myopathy (neuromyopathy) A syndrome of proximal atrophy with relative retention of power. Both neuropathic and myopathic causes are suspected, while the underlying problem is considered to be nutritional.

cachexia (Gr; bad + a habit) Severe loss of subcutaneous tissue and muscle bulk, the latter without commensurate weakness; muscle biopsy shows the presence of scattered atrophic fibers. The condition is the result of severe malnutrition, malignancy, or other systemic illness.

Cachexia mercurialis was the term applied to widespread ulceration occurring in syphilitic patients treated with mercury; *cachexia saturnia* is an old term for chronic lead poisoning.

cachodia (Gr, a bad smell) Having a bad smell.

cacogenesis (Gr, bad + origin) A morbid malformation, such as a monster.

cacogeusia (Gr, bad + taste) The perception that all food in the mouth has a foul taste; a symptom of local disease, partial damage to the olfactory nerve, or depressive illness.

cacophonia (Gr, bad + lack of + voice) Hoarseness of the voice.

cacosmia (Gr, bad + smell) Perception of all food as having a foul smell. The causes are similar to those of **cacogeusia.**

CADASIL See **cerebral autosomal dominant arteriopathy with subcortical infarcts and leukoencephalopathy.**

cadiva insania (Lat, falling + senseless) An ancient term for epilepsy.

caducus (Lat, falling) A term indicating falling—hence *caducus morbus,* another ancient term for epilepsy.

Cadwalader, Thomas (1708–1779) American physician who first described lead palsy and lead colic in his *Essay on the West Indian Dry-Gripes,* published in Philadelphia by Benjamin Franklin in 1746.[4723]

caeruleus (ceruleus) (from Lat, dark blue) Blue, azure.

café-au-lait spots Brown skin macules, possessed by many healthy people but a diagnostic requirement for **von Recklinghausen** disease, in which there must be more than six present. Of these, at least one should measure over 5 mm in its longest axis in prepubertal people; after puberty, at least one should measure more than 15 mm.

caffeine withdrawal headache A variety of **rebound headache** for which the following diagnostic criteria are suggested:[1051]

    A. Patient has consumed caffeine daily or at a rate of ≥15 g monthly
    B. Occurs within 24 hours after last caffeine intake
    C. Is relieved within 1 hour by taking 100 mg of caffeine

Caffey-Silverman syndrome See **infantile cortical hyperostosis.**

cage paralysis Vitamin B_{12} deficiency in captive primates fed a fruit diet deficient in that vitamin.

caida de mollera See **fallen fontanelle.**

Cairns, Sir Hugh William Bell (1896–1952) Australian neurosurgeon, born and educated in Adelaide and seeing service in World War I before returning to Australia to graduate in 1917. He was then elected to a Rhodes scholarship at Balliol College, Oxford, and, following that, worked at the London Hospital. After studying with Harvey **Cushing** on a Rockefeller fellowship, he turned to neurosurgery and later joined the staff first of the London Hospital and the **National Hospitals** for Nervous Diseases in Queen Square and Maida Vale and subsequently of the Radcliffe Infirmary as the first Regius Professor of Surgery at the University of Oxford.

During the World War II he established and ran a head injury base hospital in Oxford and organized mobile neurosurgical teams for the front. He designed a crash helmet and leg guard for motor cyclists, which saved many lives and prevented many fractures. His numerous publications include studies of gliomas and subdural hematomas, the use of antibiotics, problems of consciousness, and neuro-ophthalmology.[2824,5014]

Sir Hugh William Bell Cairns

Cairns syndrome 1. **persistent vegetative state** with near-complete loss of all but ocular movements and of emotional response. "Oft-repeated commands may be carried out in a feeble, slow and incomplete manner but usually there are no movements of a voluntary character."[870] Voluntary extraocular movements, chewing, swallowing, and breathing are maintained. There is incontinence and, in some cases, decorticate rigidity. Fluctuations may occur.

The condition is produced by lesions in and around the third ventricle. Cairns considered this state to be due to a disorder of cortical function secondary to a diencephalic lesion.[870] 2. Hydrocephalus due to blockage of the CSF pathways by meningitic exudate.[869]

caisson disease See **decompression sickness.**

Cajal cells Astrocytes.

Cajal, Santiago Ramon y (1852–1934) Spanish neurohistologist and anatomist who trained in Saragossa. He was appointed professor of anatomy at Valencia University at the age of 29 but later transferred to Bologna and then returned to Spain as professor of histology and morbid anatomy in Madrid. His major work, *Histologie du système nerveuse de l'homme and des vertèbres* (Paris, 1909–1911), established him as the father of neurohistology, although some of the credit belongs to Camillo **Golgi,** a modification of whose silver stain Cajal used, and with whom he shared the Nobel prize for 1906. His textbook of general pathology[4578] became a standard source. Cajal also introduced a silver nitrate stain to show the content of the neuronal cytoplasm; this stain was employed by **Alzheimer** to demonstrate neurofibrillary tangles. Among his students or collaborators were **Lorente de No, Lafora,** and Wilder **Penfield.**

Cajal enunciated his neuronal theory in three parts. First, nerve cells are independent elements that do not anastomose (as in a syncytium) but make contact only at specific points. Second, nervous impulses are always transmitted from the cell body out to the axon; and third, the axon conducts *away from* the cell body. His autobiography has recently been published.[4579]

Cajal stain A metallic impregnation method of staining astrocytes, using gold chloride sublimate.

calamus scriptorius (Lat, a quill or reed + of a writer) The inverted triangle, somewhat resembling the point of a pen, on the dorsum of the medulla in the floor of the fourth ventricle; so named by Herophilus, a Greek physician and anatomist in Athens (335–280 B.C.)

calcification of the basal ganglia 1. An asymptomatic condition discovered fortuitously on X-ray studies, CT scans, or MRI scans of the head. 2. Calcium deposition in the basal ganglia as occurs in numerous progressive white matter degenerations, true and pseudohypoparathyroidism, hyperparathyroidism, mitochondrial cytopathies, some infections including HIV infection and toxoplasmosis, tuberous sclerosis, Down syndrome, and systemic lupus erythematosus, as well as following many forms of toxic, radiation, or other damage to neural tissue. See **striatopallidal calcification.**

3. A specific fatal syndrome in infants who present with microcephaly, bilateral spasticity, dystonia, and CSF lymphocytosis.[61] See also **choroidocerebral calcification syndrome.**

calcinosis universalis See **Profichet syndrome.**

calcitonin myopathy A myopathic syndrome characterized by medullary carcinoma of the thyroid, neuromas of the tongue and eyelid, prominence of the lips and stigmata of **Marfan syndrome,** and skin pigmentation.[1220]

calcium ATPase deficiency   A rare disorder of muscle characterized by exertional muscle contractures with rhabdomyolysis and impaired muscle relaxation, due to a deficiency in sarcoplasmic reticulum-ATPase.[4473]

calcium gene-related peptide   A neurotransmitter normally found at cholinergic sites in the motor system but also released in the walls of cranial vessels in migraine attacks, at which sites it has a local inflammatory action.

Calderon syndrome (kinky hair–photosensitivity–mental retardation) A congenital dysmorphic syndrome characterized by sparse, brittle, and kinky hair, absent eyebrows and eyelashes, skin photosensitivity, and mental and developmental delay.[337] See also **Menkes disease.**

calibration   1. The testing and recording of the responses of EEG channels to voltage differences applied to the input terminals of their respective amplifiers. DC (usually) or AC voltages of magnitude comparable to the amplitudes of EEG waves are used. 2. The testing of the accuracy of paper speed regulation by means of a time marker. (Adapted from the report of the Committee on Terminology, IFCN,[989] © 1974, with permission from Elsevier Science.)

California encephalitis   Direct viral infection of brain due to bunyavirus members of the arbovirus group. Clinically, the disease typically affects children in the central and eastern parts of the United States and southern Canada and occurs seasonally, mainly in early fall, presenting with typical features of encephalitis with focal neurological signs and stupor but with a low mortality and few residua.[2864]

California Verbal Learning Test   A recently developed test of aural learning, recall, and recognition memory for a list of words over five trials and allowing assessment of different components of memory as well as of retrieval strategy and other executive functions.[1363]

Call-Fleming syndrome   The occurrence of vasospasm following subarachnoid hemorrhage or hemorrhagic stroke. The clinical presentation is with seizures, and initially fluctuating neurological deficits but permanent neurological disability ensues. (Call GK. et al. *Stroke* 1988;19:1159–70.)

callosal agenesis   Failure of formation of the corpus callosum due to a developmental failure during embryogenesis. See **agenesis of the corpus callosum.**

callosal anomia   See **anomia.**

callosal apraxia   Apraxia of the left hand resulting from infarction of the corpus callosum.[5873] See **apraxia.**

callosal disconnection   The association of tactile anomia, agraphia, and apraxia affecting the left hand,

described in **multiple sclerosis.**[4985] Left-ear suppression on dichotic listening tasks is another feature of the syndrome.

callosal fissure   The space between the dorsum of the corpus callosum and the overlying hemisphere.

callosal syndrome   See **Bristowe syndrome.**

callosotomy   Section of the corpus callosum: a surgical therapy for intractable generalized and akinetic seizure disorders for half a century, now more widely accepted than previously on account of reduced morbidity from the use of microsurgical techniques.[4206]

Calmeil, Louis-Florentin (1798–1895)   French physician who described **general paralysis** in a book in 1826, immediately after **Bayle**'s description of the same condition. He also introduced the term *absence* into medicine.

calmodulin   The main calcium-binding protein in cells. Ca^{2+} ATPase is the main enzyme responsible for its removal. With depletion of high-energy phosphates resulting from ischemia, the Ca^{2+} ATPase system quits and Ca^{2+} levels increase within cells. High Ca^{2+} levels are cytotoxic, and cell death only occurs in the presence of Ca^{2+}.

caloric after-nystagmus   See **vestibular nystagmus.**

caloric nystagmus   Nystagmus of the type seen in peripheral vestibular lesions and induced by warm or cold stimulation of the labyrinths. Cold stimulation leads to nystagmus with its fast component away from the irrigated side, and warm stimulation produces nystagmus in the other direction. See **vestibular nystagmus.**

caloric paresis   A relative decrease in the responsiveness of one side compared with the other on caloric testing. See **canal paresis.**

caloric tests   (caloric irrigation tests) The introduction of hot or cold (44°C or 30°C) water or air into the external auditory meatus to test eighth (vestibular) cranial nerve function through stimulation of the receptors in the semicircular canals. The change in ambient temperature sets up convection currents in the endolymph of the horizontal semicircular canal when the subject lies supine with the head elevated 30° from the horizontal. These induce vertigo and nystagmus (with the fast component away from the canal when irrigated with cold, and toward the canal when irrigated with warm) in the normal subject, the maximal velocity of the slow component being recorded using electronystagmography.

See also **canal paresis, directional preponderance, Barany test.**

calvaria, calvarium   (from Lat, baldness) The vault of the cranium.

calvarial hyperostosis   (Morgagni syndrome) See **hyperostosis frontalis interna.**

CAMDEX (**Cam**bridge **D**iagnostic **Ex**amination) A highly reliable clinical instrument of value in diagnosing dementia, in measuring cognitive impairment, and in assessing behavior and adaptation in everyday life. The measure includes a standardized, structured interview with a relative or other caregiver and incorporates data from other sources, including a patient interview, a cognitive examination, and interviewer observations. Three diagnostic scores (for organicity, multi-infarct dementia, and depression) can be derived. Items of the **Blessed Dementia Scale** are included within the CAMDEX as one of the measures of cognitive decline.[4814] See also the **CERAD** Instrument.[3998]

camel sign   The appearance of a sensory action potential with two peaks when recorded over the median nerve at the wrist with stimulation of the fourth finger.

The mechanism concerns the innervation of the fourth finger by both the ulnar and the median nerves; in **carpal tunnel syndrome** a small-amplitude ulnar sensory nerve action potential can be recorded from over the median nerve, as can the delayed median sensory nerve action potential, the two producing the "double-humped" appearance. The sign was originally noted by Dr. Charles Simpson of Victoria, British Columbia, who also pointed out that the normal response is a potential with a single peak (the dromedary response), the abnormal one having two, like a Bactrian camel.[5175]

Camera syndrome   (neuralgic osteopathy) Lumbosacral inflammatory osteopathy of adults, causing radiculopathic pain, which is worse at night, and weight loss.[524] The similarity to ankylosing spondylitis is great.

CAMFAK syndrome   A recessively inherited syndrome of **CA**taracts, **M**icrocephaly, **F**ailure to thrive, **A**rthrogryposis, and **K**yphoscoliosis, also presenting with decreased myelination in the CNS, cerebral calcifications, pyramidal signs, and peripheral neuropathy.

Whether this condition has its own identity or is merely a severe variant of **Cockayne syndrome** is not yet determined.[5477]

campimetry   The measurement or plotting of the visual fields.

camptocormia   (from Gr, kamptos [curved] + kormos [the trunk]; functional bent back, Souques disease) 1. A bizarre posture of maximal trunk flexion, adopted primarily while walking. In some cases, this is a hysterical condition in which the spine is greatly flexed, even though it remains flexible and in which there is compensatory extension of the head on the neck. It was first described by Sir Benjamin **Brodie** in 1837 and has been known by his name; practically all the cases seen early in the last century were in soldiers during the two World Wars. **Hurst** regarded it as always hysterical in nature.[5267] 2. In the elderly, however, this name is given to an acquired kyphosis increasing during walking, totally reducible in the dorsal horizontal position and

sometimes accompanied by other neurological or systemic disorders.[2576] 3. Severe neck flexion resulting from e.g. motor neuron diseases; myopathies such as **inclusion body myositis, facioscapulohumeral dystrophy** or **nemaline myopathy;** or **Parkinson** disease or its variants.[5684a]

camptodactyly   A dominantly inherited abnormality of the hands characterized by permanent flexion of one of more fingers, usually at the proximal interphalangeal joints.[3256]

In *variant* forms, deafness and muscular hypoplasia are also described. The condition is also a feature of various other congenital malformation syndromes. See also **CAP disease, Pena-Shokeir phenotypes, Tel-Hashomer camptodactyly, camptomelic variant.**

camptomelic dwarfism   See **camptomelic variant.**

camptomelic syndrome   See **camptomelic variant.**

camptomelic variant   (camptomelic syndrome, camptomelic dwarfism) a congenital dysmorphic syndrome characterized by dwarfism, hypertelorism, nasal hemangiomas, micrognathia, cleft palate, platyspondyly, mesomelia of upper and lower limbs and skeletal anomalies of the skull, long bones and spine with delayed closure of the fontanelles, wide cranial sutures, and hydrocephalus.[3634]

Camurati-Engelman syndrome   A genetic craniotubular hyperostotic and osteosclerotic syndrome stemming from active overgrowth of bone, in which sclerosis and hyperostosis of the base of the skull and the long bones appear in the first year, associated with conductive deafness and proximal and distal myopathic weakness. The condition has been reviewed.[3593] See **progressive diaphyseal dysplasia.**

Canadian Association for Narcolepsy   A charitable association. Address: 14 Carluke Crescent, Apt. 207, Willowdale, Ontario, M2L 2H8 Canada. Tel: 416-222-7890.

Canadian Association of Neurological Nurses.   A professional organization. Web site: http://www.cann.ca/.

Canadian Association for Neuroscience   A professional organization founded to promote communication among neuroscientists throughout Canada; to represent the interests of Canadian neuroscientists at national and international levels; to promote research in all disciplines contributing to the understanding of the nervous system; to contribute to the advancement of education in the Neurosciences; and to provide for and assist in the dissemination to the general public of the results of current neuroscience research and its significance in relation to health and disease. Web site: http://www.ucalgary.ca/UofC/Others/CAN/.

Canadian Brain Tissue Bank   A resource organization. Address: Banting Institute, Room 128, 100 College St., Toronto, Ontario, Canada M5G 1L5.

Canadian Brain Tumour Consortium   A charitable organization providing information and support to patients with brain tumors. Web site: http://www.cbtc.ca/.

Canadian Cerebral Palsy Association   A charitable organization. Address: 975 St. Joseph Blvd., Ste 200 Hull, Quebec, J8Z 1W8 Canada. Tel: 819-771-3113.

Canadian Congress of Neurological Sciences   An organization subsuming all Canadian clinical neuroscience societies and publishing the *Canadian Journal of Neurological Sciences.* Address: P.O. Box 5456, Station A, Calgary, AB, T2H 1X8 Canada. Tel: 403-229-9544. Web site: http://www.ccns.org/CSCNpage.htm.

Canadian Down Syndrome Society   A charitable organization. Address: 2837 76th Avenue No., 206, Surrey, BC, V3W 2V3 Canada. Tel: 604-599-6009.

Canadian Epilepsy Consortium   A national investigator network of over 40 academic and community based neurologists who specialize in treating both pediatric and adult patients with epilepsy. Web site: http://www.epilepsyconsortium.ca/.

Canadian Headache Society   A professional society. Address: C/o Dr. Marek Gawel, Sunnybrook Health Science Centre, 2075 Bayview Ave., Toronto, Ontario, Canada M4N 3M5. Tel: 416-323-7506.

Canadian Journal of Neurological Sciences   (Can. J. Neurol. Sci.) The official organ of the Canadian Neurological, Neurosurgical, Child Neurology, and Clinical Neurophysiology Societies (Canadian Congress of Neurological Sciences). Address: P.O. Box 4220, Station C, Calgary, Alberta, Canada T2T 5N1. Web site: http://www.canjneurolsci.org/.

Canadian League Against Epilepsy   The Canadian chapter of the **International League Against Epilepsy.** Membership consists primarily of physicians with a particular interest in epilepsy. Web site: http://www.clae.org/.

Canadian Mental Health Association   A charitable organization. Address: 180 Dundas St. W, Ste 2301, Toronto, Ontario, M5G 1Z8 Canada. Tel: 416-977-5580.

Canadian Movement Disorder Group   A professional organization. Web site: www.cmdg.org/.

Canadian Neurological Coalition   A group formed by the association of a number of Canadian charitable foundations concerned with various neurological disorders for the purposes of advocacy, information sharing, and the support of research. Address: 100 College St., Ste. 126, Toronto, Ontario, Canada M5G 1L5. Tel: 416-596-7043.

Canadian Neurological Scale   A semiquantitative tool for the assessment of neurologic function. It was designed primarily for use in patients following cerebrovascular accident, in whom it has been shown to be both valid and reliable. The scale rates mentation (level of consciousness, orientation, and speech); motor weakness (face and both proximal and distal arm and leg function); and motor re-sponses, comparing the two sides with respect to the face, arms, and legs[1141] (see Chart C–1).

Chart C–1. Canadian Neurological Scale

Level of Consciousness

Alert: Normal consciousness

Drowsy: The patient, when stimulated verbally, remains awake and alert for a short period of time but tends to doze even when examined.

Stuporous: The patient responds to loud verbal stimuli and/or strong touch, and may vocalize but does not become alert or completely wake up.

Comatose: The patient responds to deep pain (i.e., sternal pressure).

1. Only by purposeful movement of limb towards noxious stimuli and/or grimacing and/or moaning (no verbal response)
2. By nonpurposeful movements, flexion of upper limbs (i.e., decortication), or extension of upper limbs (i.e. decerebration)
3. No response to noxious stimuli.

Note: If the patient is alert or drowsy, monitor progress with Section A, but if stuporous or comatose, monitor with Section B (see below).

Mentation

1. Orientation
   A. Oriented: Patient is oriented to both place (i.e., city or hospital) and time (i.e., patient must give at least correct month and year). If early in month (i.e., first 3 days), previous month is acceptable. Speech can be dysarthric (mispronounced or slurred) but intelligible.
   B. Disoriented or nonapplicable: If for any reason patient cannot answer the preceding questions on orientation (i.e., does not know answer, gives wrong answer, answers only partially, cannot express self either by lack of words or unintelligible speech, or finally ignores questions).
2. Speech (language and pronunciation)
   A. Receptive language: The patient is asked:
      a. "Close your eyes."
      b. "Does a stone sink in water?"
      c. "Point to the ceiling." Repeat twice if necessary.
      If the patient obeys three commands, continue to B. Expressive language, but if the patient obeys only two commands or less, score the receptive defect in the Speech Scale, and then proceed directly to motor function testing.
   B. Expressive language: In this section pay special attention not only to the answers but also to word pronunciation, e.g., dysarthria or slurring.
      a. Ask the patient to name a pencil, key, and watch; make sure that the patient can see them. If the patient names only two or less of them, score "expressive defect" on Speech Scale but if three objects are correctly named, proceed to b.
      b. Ask the patient:
      "What do you do with a pencil?"
      "What do you do with a key ?"
      "What do you do with a watch?"
      If three questions are correctly answered, score "normal speech."

Note: (*1*) The above scoring system relates to language only.

Problems with pronunciation of words (dysarthria or slurred speech) are graded directly on the Speech Scale below. (2) The patient should always be scored according to worst speech deficit (i.e., language score or mispronunciation) (3) Do not mimic commands in Section A, Receptive language.

Speech Scale

Normal speech: Answers all commands and questions in Speech section; patient can have slurred speech (dysarthria) but still be intelligible.

Expressive defect: The patient obeys commands in the receptive language section but makes one or more errors in the section on expressive language and/or mispronounces words (slurred speech), so that the speech is totally or partially unintelligible (severe dysarthria).

Receptive defect: The patient obeys only two or less commands in the section on receptive language.

Motor Function

When evaluating strength and range of motion in limbs, always submit both limbs to same testing (i.e., apply same resistance at same position bilaterally).

Section A1. For patients who do not have comprehension problems (i.e., normal speech or expressive defect only)

1. Face
   Ask patient to show teeth or gums.
   No weakness: symmetrical grin, no asymmetry in smile
   Weakness: facial asymmetry; one corner of mouth lower than other, either at rest or while showing teeth

2. Upper limb (proximal)
   The patient should be tested in sitting position if possible. Test: abduction arms (to 90°)
   If the patient is lying in bed, elevate arms to approximately 45° to 90°. The strength in both arms is to be tested simultaneously; resistance must be applied at midpoint between shoulder and elbow at all times.

3. Upper limb (distal)
   The patient is tested in the sitting or the lying position with the arms elevated and is asked to make fists and to extend the wrists. Compare the range of movement in both wrists simultaneously.
   If there is a full range of extension in both wrists, proceed to test strength by applying resistance separately to both fists while stabilizing the patient's arms firmly.

4. Lower limb
   The patient lying in bed for testing should always be scored according to the worst deficit, either a or b. Test:
   a. Hip flexion. Ask patient to flex thighs towards trunk with knees flexed to 90°. Movement in both thighs is tested separately.
   b. Dorsiflexion of foot. Ask patient to point toes and foot upward. Compare both feet simultaneously (i.e., complete and partial movement).
   In both a and b, apply resistance alternately to each thigh and foot after the full movement has been completed to test strength.

Gradation of Motor Deficit

No detectable weakness
Mild weakness: normal range of motion against gravity, but succumbs to resistance by observer either partially or totally

Significant weakness: cannot completely overcome gravity in range of motion (i.e., partial movement)

Total weakness: absence of motion in movement tested or only contraction of muscles without actual movement of limb

Section A2. For patients with comprehension problems (i.e., receptive defect in Speech Scale). Motor function in this section can be monitored in one of two ways:

1. The ability of the patient to maintain a fixed posture in the upper or lower limbs for a few (3–5) seconds. The observer will alternately place the limbs in the desired position.
   a. Upper limbs: place arms outstretched at 90° in front of patient.
   b. Lower limbs: flex thighs with knees flexed at 90°.
   c. Facial power: have the patient mimic your own grin.
   If the patient does not cooperate, then proceed to:

2. Comparison of motor response to a noxious stimuli (i.e., pressure on the nail-bed of the fingers or toes with a pencil. Facial response (grimacing) to pain is tested by applying pressure on sternum.
   a. Face (grimacing)
      Symmetrical
      Asymmetrical (note side)
   b. Upper limbs
      Equal motor response: patient can maintain the fixed posture equally in both upper limbs for a few seconds or withdraws equally on both sides to pain.
      Unequal motor response: patient cannot maintain the fixed posture equally on both sides; weakness is noted on one side or there is an unequal withdrawal to pain. Note the side on which the withdrawal is not as brisk.
   c. Lower limbs
      Equal motor response: patient can maintain the fixed posture equally in both lower limbs for a few seconds or withdraws equally on both sides to pain.
      Unequal motor response: patient cannot maintain the fixed posture equally on both sides; weakness is noted on one side or there is an unequal withdrawal to pain. Note the side where withdrawal is not as brisk.

Symptomatology

1 Presenting Symptoms	2 New Symptoms (recurrence)
Type	Type
Localization	Localization
Duration	Duration
Frequency	Frequency

The above symptoms and any remarks should be noted in the progress notes. The side of the weakness should always be identified and the modalities graded numerically on the score sheet. If the patient is stuporous or comatose, monitor progress with the **Glasgow coma scale.**

Scoring

Mentation

Level of consciousness	Alert	30
	Drowsy	15
Orientation	Oriented	10
	Disoriented or NA	00
Speech	Normal	10
	Expressive deficit	05
	Receptive deficit	00

Motor functions: weakness (no comprehension deficit)

Face	None	05
	Present	00
Arm: proximal	None	15
	Mild	10
	Significant	05
	Total	00
Arm: distal	None	15
	Mild	10
	Significant	05
	Total	00
Leg: proximal	None	15
	Mild	10
	Significant	05
	Total	00
Leg: distal	None	15
	Mild	10
	Significant	05
	Total	00

With comprehension deficit: motor response

Face	Symmetrical	05
	Asymmetrical	00
Arms	Equal	15
	Unequal	00
Legs	Equal	15
	Unequal	00

NA, not applicable. (Adapted with permission from Coté R, Battista RN, Wolfson C, et al. The Canadian Neurolgical Scale: validation and reliability assessment. Neurology 1989;**39**:638–643, © Elsevier Science.)

Canadian Neuropathy Association   A charitable organization that provides support and for people with neuropathies. Address: c/o Garry Cyr, 9273 Snoddon Rd., Pefferlaw, Ontario, L0E-1N0 Canada. Tel: 705-437-3881. Web site: www.canadianneuropathyassociation.org/.

Canadian Paraplegia Association   A charitable organization. Address: 520 Sutherland Drive, Toronto, ON, Canada M4G 3V9.

Canadian Porphyria Foundation Inc.   A charitable organization providing support and information on this condition. Address: PO Box 1206, Neepawa, MB, R0J 1H0 Canada. Tel: 204-476-2800.

Canadian Rett Syndrome Association   A charitable organization providing support and information on this condition. Address: 555 Fairway Rd., Ste 301, Kitchener, Ontario, N2C 1X4 Canada. Tel: 416-494-1954.

Canadian Stroke Consortium   A professional organization promoting and assisting stroke research in Canada. Address: 1131A Leslie Street, Suite 205 Toronto, Ontario M3C 3L8. Web site: http://www.strokeconsortium.ca/.

canal   (Lat, a furrow) Grooves in or passages through bone or other tissues; thus Arnold's canal for the lesser superficial petrosal nerve, Huguier's canal for the chorda tympani, and Jacobson's canal for the tympanic branch of the ninth cranial nerve. The spinal canal was identified by **Etienne.**

canal paresis   Decreased responsiveness of the vestibular apparatus as shown by reduced duration of nystagmus in response to caloric stimulation with water 7°C above or below body temperature. The lesion may lie anywhere between the vestibular nuclei in the brainstem and the semicircular canals, but when due to a central lesion, the nystagmus is not enhanced by preventing visual fixation.[1928] See also **directional preponderance.**

canalolithiasis   A state in which the calcific particles normally present in the semicircular canals move abnormally in response to postural changes of the head, exciting the hair cell receptors of the canals and producing an hallucination of rotation. This is considered especially relevant in the genesis of posterior canal **benign positional vertigo.**

See also **cupolithiasis.**

Canavan leukodystrophy   (Canavan–van Bogaert-Bertrand disease, aspartoacyclase deficiency spongy degeneration of infancy, infantile CNS spongy degeneration, cavitating leukodystrophy; OMIM 271900) A rare, recessively inherited leukodystrophy, considered to be due to asparto-acylase deficiency, in which spongy vacuolation of the brain and spinal cord and demyelination are the pathological hallmarks.[3] It is mapped to 17pter–p13, and experimental gene therapy has been reported.

The *neonatal form* presents with hypotonia and failure to thrive, and is lethal.

The *infantile form* is a recessively inherited syndrome occurring among Eastern European Jewish children, and is characterized pathologically by **lissencephaly,** spongy degeneration and vacuolation of the cerebral white matter, and loss of myelin with little glial reaction. Increased urinary excretion of *N*-acetyl-aspartic acid is a characteristic finding. The main clinical features include the early onset of psychomotor arrest, **megalencephaly,** seizures, and drooping of the head due to particular weakness of the neck muscles. Myoclonus, spasticity, involuntary movements, optic atrophy, blindness, and deafness also occur before the final phase of decerebration, and death occurs before the age of 5 years.[887]

The *juvenile form* begins after the age of 5 years and is characterized by a progressive cerebellar syndrome, optic atrophy, pigmentary retinal degeneration, and dementia.

The condition was first differentiated by Van Bogaert and Bertrand in 1949. Canavan herself had considered the condition to be a form of **Schilder disease.**

A *variant* condition is *cavitating leukodystrophy with autonomic failure,* characterized by the onset in young adult life of ataxia, orthostatic hypotension, neurogenic bladder, spasticity, and constipation in the presence of the same pathological findings.

Canavan, Myrtelle M. (1879–1953) American neuropathologist who trained at the Women's Medical College in Philadelphia and who became pathologist at the Boston State Hospital and later curator of the Warren Anatomical Museum at Harvard. Her paper on a form of spongy degeneration was published in 1931.

Canavan–Van Bogaert–Bertrand disease See **Canavan leukodystrophy.**

cancellation tests Tests of attention, specifically for visual neglect, in which the subject is required to find and circle all instances of a specific letter in a field of printed letters or of a specific design in a printed field of designs.[3851]

cancer-associated retinopathy (CAR syndrome)[3083] See **paraneoplastic syndromes.**

candle drippings The irregular outgrowths of the ependyma into the ventricles, producing small, tumor-like nodules containing excessive numbers of astrocytes, calcium, and groups of bizarre and vacuolated cells of large diameter, as in **tuberous sclerosis.**

Cannon, Walter Bradford (1871–1945) American neurologist and professor of physiology at Harvard, who described stress reactions in the autonomic nervous system and showed that sympathetic nerves liberate a substance ("sympathin") which has an adrenaline-like action, and is indeed adrenaline. He was also a pioneer in the physiology of the gastrointestinal tract, suffering excessive X-ray exposure as a result.

His emergency theory, summarized today by the phrase "fight or flight" in relation to the functions of the sympathetic nervous system, provided the basis for Hans **Selye**'s categorization of the body's reactions to chronic stress.

Walter Bradford Cannon

Cannon's law (law of denervation) Denervated end-organs are supersensitive to their physiological transmitters.

Cantelli sign (Widowitz sign, doll's-eye sign) Dissociated movements of the head and the eyes in diphtheria. When the head is raised, the eyes are lowered, and vice versa.[4723] This is not the same as the abnormalities of **doll's head eye movements** described in comatose patients with brainstem lesions.

Cao syndrome (agenesis of corpus callosum and microcephaly) A congenital dysmorphic syndrome characterized by optic atrophy, pigmented retinas, microcephaly, spasticity, aqueduct stenosis, and callosal agenesis with mental and developmental delay.[337]

CAP congenital myopathy See **CAP disease.**

CAP disease (CAP congenital myopathy) A nonprogressive congenital myopathy associated with **C**amptodactyly, **A**rthropathy, and **P**ericarditis. Neurological features are facial, proximal, and distal atrophy and weakness, short stature, high palate, kyphoscoliosis, pectus excavatum, and seizures.

Pathologically, the condition is distinguished by a lack of ATPase peripherally in many of the myofibrils, a decrease of myosin, and an abnormal sarcomere pattern.[1809]

Capgras, J.M. (1873–1950) French psychiatrist.

Capgras syndrome (Fr, *l'illusion des sosies,* the illusion of doubles) A chronic delusional psychosis occurring in clear consciousness, in which patients make the remarkable complaint that certain people whom they see (usually family members) are only their own doubles; or that they have replaced another person of emotional importance to the patient, such as the spouse.[893,5632]

capillary hemangioma See **nevus flammeus.**

capillary leak syndrome A potentially fatal condition characterized by generalized increased permeability of capillaries and presenting with widespread edema, including cerebral edema, and multiple microinfarctions.[4980]

capillary nevus See **nevus flammeus.**

capillary telangiectasia A small **vascular malformation** composed of multiple irregular clusters of dilated capillaries, usually separated by some neural parenchyma and found in the cerebral cortex, white matter, or brainstem (mainly in the pons).

Occasionally they bleed and lead to destruction of small regions locally, producing seizures or focal deficits such as hearing loss, ataxia, vertigo, diplopia, and limb weakness.[6,4937] They are also found in association with Weber-Rendu-Osler disease but are usually of no clinical significance.[5330]

Cappeto syndrome A disease of unknown cause, possibly immune based and certainly resembling **systemic lupus erythematosus** in its usual occurrence in young women and its clinical features. These include multiple retinal branch occlusions with retinal hemorrhages, field defects, gaze palsies, and encephalopathy with confusion, psychosis, seizures, pyramidal signs, and almost any other neurological signs.[892]

capsaicin   A neurotoxic agent derived from red peppers (paprika) which initially causes pain but later analgesia to chemical and heat stimuli (but not to mechanical touch) by first stimulating and then blocking unmyelinated sensory fibers. It is used topically in the treatment of **postherpetic neuralgia.**[5872]

capsular genu syndrome   A faciolingual stroke syndrome in which the infarct or hemorrhage is limited to the genu of the internal capsule, leading to contralateral facial and lingual hemiparesis with dysarthria but with only mild limb weakness.[631]

When the inferior part of the internal capsule is infarcted, fluctuating alertness, hypokinesia, memory disturbances, and **abulia** are typical clinical features; the whole may resemble **akinetic mutism.** The syndrome is considered to be a result of occlusion of the perforating vessels arising from the internal carotid, anterior cerebral, or anterior choroidal arteries supplying the thalamic peduncles. The condition was first described by **Déjèrine.**[1342]

capsular warning syndrome   (crescendo TIAs) A distinct syndrome of repetitive motor and/or sensory transient ischemic attacks affecting the face, arm, and leg, considered to be related to the region of the internal capsule and frequently succeeded by evidence of capsular infarction, usually lacunar in nature.[51,1492]

The ischemia is most often due to hemodynamic phenomena in diseased single, small penetrating vessels. When cerebral infarction develops it is usually lacunar and involves a single penetrating vessel, although occasionally striatocapsular or anterior choroidal artery territory infarction occurs.

capsulothalamic syndrome   See **thalamic syndrome.**

CAR syndrome   See **paraneoplastic syndromes.**

car toll neuropathy   Compression of the sciatic nerve under the piriformis muscle, in this case by loose change carried in the hip pocket of the driver of the car.[512] See **piriformis syndrome, toilet seat neuropathy, credit card wallet sciatica.**

carbamyl phosphate synthetase deficiency   A rare, congenital **hyperammonemic syndrome** leading to severe leukoencephalopathy with neonatal feeding problems, altered consciousness, cyclic vomiting, seizures, and secondary cerebrovascular disease, usually in infants with mental and developmental delay (but also described in an adult). The condition is due to deficiency of the enzyme essential in the early stages of the urea cycle.[5820] The responsible gene maps to chromosome 2p.

A *variant* is an incomplete form that appears in later childhood.[94]

carbohydrate-deficient glycoprotein syndrome   A group of recessively inherited metabolic disorders. Type 1 presents with early-onset psychomotor retardation and pigmentary retinopathy, usually combined with mild hepatic dysfunction, facial dysmorphisms, subcutaneous lipodystrophy, stroke-like episodes during childhood, and generalized seizures. Thoracic deformities are also described. The prognosis for life is good. Types 2 and 3 are associated with demyelination or hypomyelination and are less well recognized. Patients with type 3 manifest severe psychomotor retardation, tetrapareses, cerebral and optic atrophy, retinal pigmentary degeneration, and cerebellar hypoplasia.[5358] A raised serum level of carbohydrate-deficient transferrin is a marker for the condition.[5358]

carbon dioxide narcosis   A generalized encephalopathy with increased cerebral blood flow and cerebral edema, resulting from chronic ventilatory insufficiency and carbon dioxide retention.

carbon monoxide encephalopathy   A severe encephalopathy resulting from the conversion of oxyhemoglobin to carboxyhemoglobin, a compound that does not liberate oxygen with the same facility as oxyhemoglobin. The resulting histotoxic anoxia leads to reduction in consciousness, in the early stages. In fatal cases, cerebral edema, petechial hemorrhages, degeneration of the globus pallidus, and, eventually, leukoencephalopathy occur.[680]

carbonic anhydrase II deficiency   (marble brain disease) A congenital dysmorphic syndrome characterized by short stature, deafness, optic atrophy with blindness, abnormal dental development, renal tubular acidosis, proximal and distal myopathic weakness, myopathy, intracranial calcifications, multiple fractures, osteosclerosis or osteopetrosis, wide metaphyses, and mental and developmental delay.[337]

carcinoid myopathy   An acquired proximal myopathy with advanced atrophy of type 2 muscle fibers, developing in subjects with carcinoid syndrome of long standing.[5440]

carcinomatous meningitis   (meningeal carcinomatosis) A rare, usually fatal form of intracranial metastatic disease in which the leptomeninges are diffusely invaded by metastatic tumor cells, coating the surface of the brain and spinal cord and infiltrating the **Virchow-Robin spaces.** The most common primary sites are the breast and lung; melanomas can produce a similar picture.

Both clinically and pathologically, the condition resembles meningitis rather than tumor. Headache, visual failure, raised intracranial pressure, multiple cranial nerve palsies, areflexia, meningism, and a variable degree of dementia are the leading clinical features.[1835] See also **cerebral metastases.**[5865]

carcinomatous myopathy A syndrome of mono-myositis multiplex with the chief complaint of pain of sudden onset of a few days' duration as a result of infarction, possibly from nonbacterial thrombotic endocarditis,[2512] or of direct carcinomatous emboli to the proximal muscles.[1500]

Generalized muscle atrophy (**cachexia**) in association with systemic carcinoma and acute myonecrosis complicating distant carcinoma[5692] are further syndromes under this heading.

carcinomatous neuromyopathy Syndromes of proximal and axial weakness, usually neurogenic in origin. They are most often considered to be the result of an autoimmune attack but may also be associated with the treatment for an underlying carcinoma with, e.g., steroids. See **paraneoplastic syndromes.**

carcinomatous sensory neuropathy A **paraneoplastic syndrome** of dorsal root ganglionitis and neuronal degeneration presenting subacutely with isolated sensory loss, usually in association with oatcell carcinoma of the lung. See **paraneoplastic sensory neuropathy.**

cardiac syncope Syncope due to diminished cardiac output as a result of dysrhythmia or outflow obstruction.

cardinal points reflex Deviation of the lip and the tongue to the point where a baby's lip is touched by the examiner's finger. Further movements of the finger up toward the nose or down to the chin lead to extension and to flexion of the neck, respectively.

cardinal positions of gaze The nine classic points to which gaze may be directed. They comprise up-left, up-center, up-right; left, center, and right in the horizontal plane; and down-left, down-center, and down-right.

cardioembolic stroke See **cardiogenic embolism.**

cardiofacial syndrome See **asymmetrical crying facies.**

cardiogenic dementia Impairment in cognitive function occurring in patients with cardiac dysrhythmia and resulting relative hypotension and impairment of cerebral perfusion.[3260]

cardiogenic embolism (cardioembolic stroke) Emboli arising from the heart and proceeding to the cerebral circulation. They are considered to account for cerebral ischemic infarction in 15% of cases of stroke.

The cardiac pathologies responsible and therapeutic methods have been reviewed, and the clinical features suggesting embolism are listed below.[948] Diagnostic criteria have also been suggested[2071,3891] (see Charts C–2 to C–4). A problem in diagnosis is that emboli are often dispatched when the heart rhythm reverts to normal after a period of fibrillation. [JF]

Chart C–2. Clinical Features of Cerebral Embolism

1. Abrupt onset of maximal deficit
2. Presence of a potentially embolic source
3. Multiple brain infarcts involving the cortex or cerebellum in multiple vascular territories
4. Hemorrhagic infarct shown by computed tomography
5. Absence of atherosclerotic arterial disease by angiography
6. Angiographic evidence of vanishing occlusions
7. Evidence of embolism to other organs
8. Cardiac thrombi demonstrated by various imaging techniques

---

Chart C–3. Diagnostic Criteria for Cardiogenic Cerebral Embolism

Definite Cardioembolic Stroke

All of the following features are evident:

1. No antecedent TIAs in the same vascular distribution within 2 weeks of stroke onset
2. Maximal neurologic deficit at stroke onset
3. CT or MRI evidence of lesion ≥2 cm or involving cortex or symptoms suggesting cortical involvement
4. Arterial imaging showing no evidence of significant occlusive disease (≥50% linear stenosis in proximal large vessel supply)

Probable Cardioembolic Stroke

One of the following features is present:

1. At least two of 1, 2, 3, above; no lacunar syndrome is present; *and* arterial imaging is required with no evidence of significant occlusive disease
2. Vertebrobasilar distribution *and* 1, 2, 3, above are all true *and* there is no arterial imaging

Adapted from Miller et al. (1993).[3891]

Chart C–4. Diagnostic Criteria for Cerebral Embolism (2)

Criteria for the Diagnosis of Cardiac-Originating Embolism

Presence of any *one* of the following:

1. Mitral stenosis
2. Prosthetic valve
3. Endocarditis
4. Myocardial infarction within 6 weeks of qualifying stroke
5. Myocardial aneurysm
6. Intracardiac clot or mass
7. Mitral valve prolapse, age under 45, in the absence of a reasonable alternative explanation for the qualifying stroke

Or, the presence of any *two* of the following:

1. Atrial fibrillation (chronic or paroxysmal)
2. Sick sinus syndrome
3. Recent involvement of more than one vascular territory
4. Seizure at onset
5. Hemorrhagic infarct
6. Cerebral artery branch occlusion(s) without overt evidence of extracranial or cavernous sinus carotid disease on arteriography

Adapted from Gent M, Blakeley J, Easton JD, et al. Canadian-American Ticlopidine Study; Thrombo-Embolic Stroke. Stroke 1988;19:1203–10[2071] and reproduced by permission, © Elsevier Science.

cardioinhibitory syncope   Fainting due to extreme bradycardia resulting from excessive vagal stimulation of the heart. The effect is clinically demonstrable by increasing vagal cardiac activity by placing pressure on the eyeball—the *oculocardiac reflex*. See **cardiac syncope.**

cardioskeletal myopathy with intrasarcoplasmic dense granulofilamentous material   See **myofibrillar myopathy.**

cardiovascular autonomic reflex testing   Studies of pulse rate or blood pressure with deep breathing, Valsalva maneuver, or tilting. See **autonomic function tests.**

cardiovocal syndrome   See **Ortner syndrome.**

CARE   Acronym for the **C**omprehensive **A**ssessment and **R**eferral **E**valuation, a long, semistructured interview instrument that covers psychiatric symptoms, physical symptoms, and performance in the activities of daily living, and requests information about nutrition and economic matters. A short form is available.[2338]

The tool has been widely used in the assessment of elderly people who might need referral to health or social services.[2339]

Carney complex   (Swiss syndrome) A dominantly inherited disorder characterized by mesenchymal and peripheral nerve tumors, skin pigmentation, and endocrine overactivity.[1571] See **familial Cushing syndrome.**

carnitine   A small, water-soluble molecule, both synthesized in the liver and ingested, which is stored in skeletal and cardiac muscle, where it plays an important role in the transport of the coenzyme A–fatty acid complex across the mitochondrial membrane, and thus in energy availability. It is also concerned in the buffering of organic acids.

carnitine deficiency   A diffuse disorder, of which two major forms have been defined: muscular and systemic.[1459]

Type 1 lipid storage myopathy (myopathic carnitine deficiency) is a recessively inherited lipid storage vacuolar myopathy leading to fluctuating but progressive proximal muscle weakness and kyphoscoliosis. Lipid excess is confined to muscle and low levels of carnitine are found in type 1 muscle fibers[1211] but not in the serum. In some cases, oral L-carnitine ingestion reverses the signs of the disease,[1660] which has resulted from a deficit in the carnitine acyl-carnitine carrier system.

Type 2 lipid storage myopathy (systemic carnitine deficiency) is a recessively inherited syndrome with onset in infancy or childhood, and leading to episodic attacks of metabolic acidosis and hypoglycemia causing encephalopathy, and to slowly progressive proximal weakness with lipid storage in muscles, cardiomyopathy, and low carnitine levels in liver, heart, and muscle.

The affected infants may present with features resembling **Reye syndrome** with nausea, vomiting, liver failure, encephalopathy, and lipid storage myopathy.[1459,2938]

In a *variant form, dominant lipid myopathy with normal carnitine,* lifelong weakness and fat intolerance are associated with lipid storage in type 1 muscle fibers and with type 2 muscle fiber atrophy.[244]

Low carnitine levels are found secondarily in patients with cirrhosis or schistosomiasis, in those on dialysis, and in those with chronic renal failure not on dialysis, as well as in people receiving total parenteral nutrition or suffering from Fanconi syndrome, **mitochondrial myopathies,** organic acidemias, or muscular dystrophy. The cardiomyopathy of dialysis is due to carnitine deficiency. See also **lipid myopathies.**

carnitine palmityl transferase deficiency   An autosomal or sex-linked recessively inherited lipid storage myopathy due to deficiency of this enzyme, which is normally involved in fatty acid metabolism in muscles.

Clinically, it presents in infancy as a generalized lethal disease with severe cardiomyopathy; or in childhood, youth, or adult life with exercise intolerance, muscle pain and cramp, recurrent myoglobinuria with nephropathy, and chronic myopathic girdle weakness[1451,2688] following prolonged exertion, fasting or cold.[808] Fat intolerance and raised serum triglyceride levels are usually detected.[923] During fasting, serum creatine kinase levels remain low and ketogenesis is normal. Deficiency of the enzyme may be associated with susceptibility to **malignant hyperthermia.**

In *variant forms,* CPT_2 is deficient in skeletal muscle and leukocytes but the CPT^1 level is normal.[4988]

A lipid myopathy is associated with reduced exercise capacity, intolerance to fasting, and reduced concentration of carnitine in muscle and serum, but with normal CPTase activity. The possibility of flavoprotein deficiency is adduced.[924]

Myoglobinuria and weakness occur, progressing even to acute respiratory failure following an infection (*adult* form).[529]

Carnitine deficiency is induced by repeated *hemodialysis.*[394]

Carnitine deficiency accompanies a riboflavine-responsive **lipid myopathy.**[924]

carnosinase deficiency   See **carnosinemia.**

carnosine   A neuropeptide substance.

carnosinemia   (carnosinase deficiency) A congenital, recessively inherited, neurodegenerative syndrome characterized by kyphoscoliosis, aminoaciduria, arachnodactyly, and cerebral atrophy with myoclonic and generalized tonic-clonic seizures, pyramidal and extrapyramidal signs, and severe progressive psychomotor retardation[4416] in the presence of high plasma levels of carnosine.

caroticocavernous fistula (Foix-Jefferson syndrome) Rupture of an aneurysm of the intracavernous internal carotid artery creating an arteriovenous anastomosis, with arterial blood thus flowing into the sinus.

Local pain, an ocular bruit (often audible to the patient), visual loss, and diplopia are the usual symptoms, and retinal congestion and pulsatile exophthalmos with variable lesions of the third, fourth, ophthalmic fifth, and sixth cranial nerves are characteristic signs.[28]

carotid (from Gr, to cast into a deep sleep, to throttle) The arteries of the neck were so called because it was known in ancient times that animals became sleepy when these vessels were compressed, a fact known to professional wrestlers today.

carotid artery syndrome 1. (ocular ischemic syndrome) Transient or permanent painless visual loss, lachrymation, visual field losses due to retinal ischemia, vascular retinopathy, and transient ischemic attacks, due to reduced flow within, or emboli from, the homolateral carotid artery. See **ocular ischemic syndrome.** 2. See **red-eyed shunt syndrome.**

carotid body A chromaffin-containing chemoreceptor situated at the bifurcation of the common carotid artery.

carotid body tumor (ganglion nodosum tumor) A chromaffinoma (chemodectoma) that infiltrates the region of the jugular foramen and leads to complaints of pulsatile tinnitus, hoarseness, and dysarthria due to dysfunction of cranial nerves VII, IX, and X, and local pain. Compression of the carotid sinus may also occur, leading to bradycardia and syncope.

The first pathological account was given in 1891 by Felix Marchand (1846–1928), a German pathologist.

carotid compression test (Matas test) Digital massage of the carotid sinuses, and then compression of the two carotid arteries in turn during electroencephalography, with the patient's head facing forward or turned to the left or right, in an attempt to assess the adequacy of blood flow in the carotid and vertebral systems as judged by the clinical or EEG changes induced.

The method is now seldom employed; hypotension, cardiac asystole, displacement of atheromatous debris, and ischemic stroke are potential hazards, a vague idea of arterial patency being the questionable reward.

carotid hypoplasia See **familial hypoplasia of the carotid arteries.**

carotid sinus A dilatation of the proximal portion of the internal carotid artery, containing baroreceptors that send information on blood pressure via the ninth nerve to the medulla.

carotid sinus hypersensitivity (carotid sinus syncope/syndrome, Charcot-Weiss-Baker syndrome[971]) Syncope, confusion, faintness, or seizures resulting from decreased cerebral perfusion due to extreme bradycardia in response to excessive afferent input from the carotid sinus, usually in older patients with atheroma, in whom it may lead to significant morbidity related to trauma suffered during falls.

The *cardioinhibitory* form is diagnosed when stimulation of the carotid sinuses leads to 3 seconds of cardiac asystole or atrioventricular block; the less common *depressor* type is said to occur when a drop in blood pressure of 50 mmHg results. Slowing of the pulse by 30 bpm or a fall in blood pressure of 30 mmHg characterizes borderline states.[4953] The syndrome was first described in 1933 by Soma Weiss (1898–1942) and James P. Baker, two American physicians.[4979,1266]

carotid sinus reflex Bradycardia resulting from increased pressure within the carotid sinuses; a parasympathetic response on both the afferent and efferent sides.[5606] Either an increase in blood pressure or manipulation of the sinus by pressure from without will normally induce slowing of the heart rate.

The reflex is mediated by the ninth and tenth cranial nerves; it was first described by Torald Sollamn (b. 1874), an American pharmacologist, but his description was amplified by Heinrich Hering (1866–1948), a German physiologist, in 1923. See also **carotid sinus hypersensitivity.**

carotid sinus syncope/syndrome See **carotid sinus hypersensitivity.**

carotid tubercle The mass on the anterior aspect of the transverse processes of the sixth cervical vertebra, in front of which lies the carotid artery.

carotidynia (facial migraine, atypical facial neuralgia, Hilger syndrome) A dull, intermittent, aching pain in the neck and in the lower half of the face, sometimes with a throbbing component, with tenderness of the carotid artery. The condition is thought to arise from the adventitial coat of the common carotid artery, either as a form of migraine or as a result of subclinical carotid artery dissection, but superior laryngeal neuralgia has been suggested as another possible cause[4241] and the nonspecificity of the pathologies causing transient unilateral neck pain has led to a suggestion that the whole condition be expunged from medical nosology.[579]

The condition was initially described in 1927, but more fully by Dr. J.A. Hilger.[2573]

carpal tunnel syndrome A common entity in which affected subjects (who are usually female) complain of paresthesias, numbness, and pain in the hands, especially on waking and following repetitive manual tasks. The cause is compression of the median nerve beneath the transverse carpal ligament at the wrist, the cure surgical decompression.

The original description by Putnam[4548] seems to have been ignored until the syndrome was rediscovered by **Phalen** at the Cleveland Clinic, and by Lord **Brain** in London in 1946. See also **Phalen sign, flick sign.**

Diagnostic guidelines have been suggested by the American Academy of Neurology[12] (see Chart C–5.) The Association also lists differential diagnostic possibilities, confirmatory studies, further diagnostic tests, and treatment.[12]

Familial carpal tunnel syndrome is an occasional *variant*, with its usual onset in adult life.[1278]

Chart C–5. Diagnostic Guidelines for Carpal Tunnel Syndrome

1. History: The likelihood of carpal tunnel syndrome increases with the number of standard symptoms and provocative factors listed below:

   Dull, aching discomfort in the hand, forearm, or upper arm

   Paresthesias in the hand

   Weakness or clumsiness of the hand

   Dry skin, swelling, or color changes in the hand

   Occurrence of any of these symptoms within the median distribution

   Provocative factors are sleep, sustained hand and/or arm positions, and repetitive actions of the hand or wrist. Mitigating factors are changes in hand posture and shaking the hand.

2. Physical examination:

   It may be normal.

   Symptoms are elicited by tapping or direct pressure over the median nerve at the wrist (**Tinel sign**) or with forced extension or flexion of the wrist (**Phalen sign**).

   Sensory loss is in the median nerve distribution.

   Weakness or atrophy of the thenar muscles is present.

   Dry skin is apparent on the digits 1–3.

Adapted from the American Academy of Neurology Quality Standards Committee. Practice Parameters; Carpal Tunnel Syndrome (1993).[143a]

The median-thenar to ulnar-thenar latency difference (TTLD), and the median-thenar to ulnar-hypothenar latency difference (THLD) may be the most sensitive electrodiagnostic tests in this condition. The abnormal cutoffs are TTLD, 0.8 msec; THLD, 1.2 msec.

In *severe carpal tunnel syndrome* the subject has wasting of the thenar eminence as well as the usual signs listed above.

Carpenter syndrome (acrocephalopolysyndactyly) A rare recessively inherited disorder characterized by premature fusion of all the cranial sutures, which leads to **acrocephaly** and **brachycephaly.**

Facial dysmorphism, corneal opacities, mental retardation, obesity, syndactyly, pes cavus, polydactyly, congenital cardiac anomalies, and aminoaciduria are also described.[914] See also **acrocallosal syndrome, acrocephalosyndactyly.**

carphology (Gr, chaff + to collect) Picking at the bedclothes, once thought characteristic of typhoidal delirium but in fact a nonspecific sign both of delirium and dementia.

carpometacarpal reflex (carpophalangeal reflex, von Bechterew reflex) Flexion of the fingers in response to a tap on the back of the wrist when the arm is extended;

a sign with the same significance as the **finger flexion reflex,** of which it is a *variant.*

carpopedal spasm Cupping of the palm of the hand with extension of the fingers and adduction of the thumb as a result of spasm of the intrinsic hand muscles in **tetany.** It is typically due to abnormal calcium control of sodium channels leading to axonal hyperexcitability, as in hypomagnesemia, hypoparathyroidism, and respiratory alkalosis normocalcemic tetany. All forms are worsened by alkalosis resulting from hyperventilation and by ischemia. A dominantly inherited form is described. Electromyographically, there are spontaneous repetitive discharges at up to to 300 Hz arising in peripheral axons.

carpophalangeal reflex See **carpometacarpal reflex.**

carpus (Gr, the wrist). Pertaining to the wrist.

Carraro syndrome A recessively inherited syndrome characterized by the absence of the tibias and by nerve deafness.[919]

Carrión disease See **Oroya fever.**

carus (Gr, heavy sleep) An ancient term for deep sleep or coma and also for loss of sensation and voluntary movement.

Casal, Gaspar (1679–1759) Spanish physician who wrote the first definitive account of the features of **pellagra,** including the pigmentation of the upper chest wall sometimes known as the *Casal necklace.*

Casserio, Giulio See **Gasser,** Johann Lorenz.

Castro-Gago syndrome (microcephaly–albinism–limb defects) A congenital dysmorphic syndrome characterized by generalized depigmentation of the hair and skin, acral defects such as hypoplastic phalanges and absent or hypoplastic hallux, microcephaly, and mental and developmental delay.[337]

cat box effect A familiar name applied by H.H. Jasper to the activation of the cat's EEG through increased activity of the reticular activating system, brought on by the desire of the cat to urinate.

cat cry syndrome See **cri du chat syndrome.**

cat eye syndrome (coloboma–anal atresia syndrome) A chromosomal disorder characterized by colobomas of the iris and choroid, facial dysmorphisms, urogenital anomalies, congenital cardiac defects, and mental and developmental delay. In many cases, trisomy 22 is present.[2911]

CAT scan See **computerized axial tomography.**

cat scratch encephalitis A nonfatal syndrome of encephalopathy (or myelopathy, radiculopathy, or cerebellar ataxia) due to *Bartonella henselae,* distinguished by the normalcy of the CSF. Seizures and a variety of neurological signs occur with meningism. It complicates *cat scratch disease,* a benign and self-limited disorder manifested usually in children by a skin rash, local lymphadenopathy, and fever.[3385,3534,4481]

CAT syndrome   A congenital dysmorphic syndrome characterized also by skeletal anomalies affecting the skull, spine, facial and limb bones and teeth, sparse fine hair, muscle atrophy, metaphyseal dysplasia, ichthyosis, and mental and developmental delay.[337]

cataclysmic migraine   An unusual vascular episode in the territory of the posterior cerebral artery, in which headache, visual symptoms, sensory and motor deficits, and signs of involvement of the third cranial nerve develop suddenly, clearing but leaving permanent neurological sequelae such as a hemianopias. The syndrome is more common in females, especially those below the age of 40.[1855] See **posterior cerebral artery syndrome.**

catalentia   Paracelsus' term for **epilepsy.**

catalepsy   (from Gr, a seizure) Increase in muscle tone, leading to the assumption of fixed postures that can be held for long periods without fatigue or other voluntary movement. It is usually associated with psychiatric disease (including schizophrenia and hysteria) or epilepsy.

The term has also been used in quite the opposite sense for the astatic, falling attacks in **narcolepsy.**

catalepsy of awakening   See **sleep paralysis.**

cataleptic hallucinatory fear syndrome   See **Rosenthal syndrome.**

cataphasia   (Gr, an affirmative proposition) Spontaneous or evoked repetition of the same word or phrase.

cataphora   (Gr, to fall down) An ancient alternative term for deep sleep or coma.

cataplexy   (Gr, to strike down) A rapid eye movement sleep disorder triggered by events that stir the emotions and consisting of the sudden, episodic, reversible, generalized, or localized loss of muscle power and areflexia, without any alteration of consciousness and with abrupt return to normal after a few seconds. It is considered to represent a dissociation of awareness and behavior.

The clinical manifestations range from a sagging of the jaw, with flexion of the neck and knees, up to sudden powerlessness of abrupt onset lasting between seconds and half an hour. If the attack lasts more than a minute, a dreamlike state supervenes.[2321] The sphincters are not affected but other features of the narcoleptic tetrad are often present. The episodes may occur unprovoked or as a reaction to an emotional stimulus, tiredness or a heavy meal. Unilateral cataplexy is also described but is extremely rare.

The term was known to Hippocrates, to whom it denoted any sudden illness, but in its modern form was first applied by Henneberg in 1916. See also **narcolepsy** and the ASDA Diagnostic Classification.[234]

cataptosis   (from Gr, to fall down) The term of Galen for epilepsy, apoplexy, or sudden paralysis.

cataract–sensorineural deafness syndrome   A dominantly inherited syndrome in which the deafness is progressive.[4058]

cataract–spasticity–mental retardation syndrome (Martsolf syndrome) A recessively inherited congenital dysmorphic syndrome characterized by cataract, ataxia, spasticity, and mental and developmental delay.[3662]

cataracts–renal tubular necrosis–encephalopathy See **Crome syndrome.**

catastrophic migraine   (cataclysmic migraine). See **posterior cerebral artery syndrome.**[1857]

catastrophic reaction   A brief emotional outburst, the behavioral response of a brain-injured or demented subject to frustration, sorrow, and anger because of inability to cope in the performance of a task. The reaction is characterized by acute anxiety, agitation and tearfulness, cessation of meaningful or cooperative activity, and sometimes uncontrolled hostility. It is associated especially with nonfluent aphasias and with left opercular lesions, and likely results from disturbances in frontotemporal-limbic-basal ganglion circuitry.[911]

Catastrophic Reaction Scale   An 11-item instrument quantitating the severity of this reaction during the clinical interview.[5321]

catathrenia   A parasomnia characterized by abnormal groaning during expiration in stage II non–rapid eye movement (NREM) or REM sleep.[5757]

catatonia   (from Gr, stretching tight, depressed)[5204] A psychiatric and motor disturbance characterized by the presence of at least one motor sign (catalepsy, posturing, or waxy flexibility) in combination with at least one sign of psychosocial withdrawal or excitement and/or bizarre repetitive movements (mutism, negativism, grimacing, impulsiveness, stereotypes, mannerisms, command automatism, echopraxia/echolalia, or verbigeration).

The condition was first described by **Kahlbaum** in 1868 and is most commonly associated with affective illnesses and schizophrenia but also occurs in a wide range of metabolic, systemic, toxic, and organic cerebral diseases.[1350]

catch-up saccades   (back-up saccades) Brief, small, corrective saccades that augment the velocity of pursuit movements so that they will match that of the moving visual target.

When the velocity of the pursuit movements is too high, *back-up saccades* exert a braking function with the same purpose. See **gain of pursuit eye movements.**

category fluency test   A test of language in which subjects are asked to generate the names of as many different kinds of fruit, vegetables, or animals as they can in 1 minute. See also **letter fluency test.**

category test   (of Halstead) A sensitive test of abstract reasoning, concept formation, and organizational ability in which the subject is required to discern similarities and differences between, and to sort and classify, colored shapes on changing bases of reference.

category-specific anomia   See **anomia.**

category-specific dysphasia   The selective preservation or impairment of specific semantic categories among patients with aphasia; these include specific deficits in comprehension of the names of body parts or of colors or inanimate objects.

cathode   The negative pole of a galvanic battery.

cathodic   (Gr, downward + a way) Proceeding downward, as in the case of the efferent nerve impulse.

cation   An electrically charged body that seeks the negative pole in an electrical field.

Catlin mark   (fenestra parietalia symmetricae, foramina parietalia permagna) A familial anomaly consisting of bilateral defects in the parietal bones, first described by Lancisi in 1707.

Clinically, the subjects are themselves aware of the defects, but headaches and seizures have only loosely been associated.[3068]

catochus   (Gr, from + to detain) An ancient term for **catalepsy** and for **persistent vegetative state.**

Caton, Richard   (1842–1926) Scottish physician, whose physiological researches led to the first (1874) description of the electrical potential changes in the brain while he was a lecturer at Liverpool University, where he later became professor of physiology.[5280] His work was not recognized until **Berger** referred to it in his important paper in 1929.

cattle-trucking   Retinal arteriolar stasis; the breaking-up of the columns of blood in the retinal arterioles, seen after death. The sign is sometimes dignified by the names of Salsbury and Melvin.

Caucasian   A term used first in 1776 by Blumenbach to define the white-skinned races and more recently employed by those who do not know that the word *europoid* is anthropologically more correct.

cauda equina   (Lat, a tail + of a horse) The nerve roots of the lumbar and sacral segments which, on leaving the cord within the dural sac, stream downward with something like the appearance of a horse's tail.

cauda equina syndrome   Weakness, reflex change, pain, and sensory disturbances in the territory of any of the roots forming the cauda equina (L2, 3, 4, 5, and S1), but often sparing the conus medullaris and thus bladder and bowel sphincter function and the motor and sensory functions of S2, 3, and 4 (**sacral sparing**). Compression by an intra- or extradural mass is the most common cause. So-called intermittent claudica-

tion of the cord[2968] is a *variant* due to **lumbar spinal stenosis.**

It must be noted that lesions seldom affect the nervous system in this nicely classified manner, so that the features of both of these syndromes often occur together.[4824] See also **conus medullaris syndrome.**

caudal   Towards the tail; posterior.

caudal dysplasia syndrome   See **caudal regression syndrome.**

caudal regression syndrome   (caudal dysplasia syndrome, sacral agenesis, mermaid syndrome) A congenital developmental disorder characterized by spinal dysraphism, complete or partial absence (aplasia) of the bony structures of the lower spine (sacrum and coccyx), anal anomalies, aplasia of the lumber facets, and usually visceral anomalies, incontinence, and a neurogenic bladder, depending on the extent of involvement of the lumbosacral cord and roots.[1545,4920,5909]

The cause of the syndrome is unknown, but maternal diabetes is a common association, while in other cases autosomal dominant inheritance has been recorded.

caudate   (Lat, equipped with a tail) A nucleus within the basal ganglion complex, its long "tail" curving around in a C-shape.

cauloplegia   (Gr, stem + a stroke) Paralysis of the penis.[4512] Presumably this means impotence.

causalgia   (Gr, burning heat) (reflex dystrophy, shoulder-hand syndrome, mimoausalgia, algodystrophy, neurodynia, traumatic neuralgia, post-traumatic pain syndrome, reflex sympathetic dystrophy, sympathalgia, Sudeck atrophy, minor causalgia, sympathalgia, deafferentation pain; see **complex regional pain syndrome.**) A syndrome of severe, persistent burning pain, felt commonly in the distribution of a nerve at any time following partial damage to that nerve (especially the proximal median, ulnar, or sciatic), but also felt in more distant regions, occurring in patients with nontraumatic nerve lesions or a phantom limb, and accompanied by sudomotor and vasomotor changes and eventually secondary atrophy of skin, joints, muscle, and bone in the affected region.[4996] Abnormal discharges in sympathetic efferents, sensitization of peripheral receptors, or ephaptic tramsmission between sympathetic and nociceptiv afferent fibers have been incriminated in causation; sensitision of spinal cord nociceptive neurons is a likely central mechanism.

Typically, the subject cannot bear anything to touch the affected areas, and heat, movement, and emotion worsen it although local cooling or block of the sympathetic fibers at a proximal level may provide relief. Tremor, dystonias, and chorea occur in a few cases. The syndrome also occurs sometimes with diseases of the CNS such as stroke, myelopathy, cervical osteoarthritis, and multiple sclerosis, with immobility after myocardial infarction, following frostbite and burns, and with phenobarbital ingestion.

Stages have been defined: the acute stage of pain, hyperpathia and allodynia, lasts weeks after injury and is succeeded by the dystrophic stage for about 3 months. The pain then radiates more widely, joints swell, muscles atrophy, and osteopososis can be shown. The atrophic stage is the end-stage of the condition, in which there are irreversible trophic changes in the skin and underlying structures, with joint contractures.

Weir **Mitchell,** as a result of his Civil War experiences, saw this condition frequently and applied the term to this type of severe, persistent and burning pain following nerve injury,[3909] although the first modern account was that of Denmark,[1387] whose patient had been injured in the Peninsular War. The term is probably best reserved for the combination of burning pain and autonomic disturbances occurring in the circumstances he described (nerve injury), the syndrome similar in whole or part (or when arising in other contexts) being termed **reflex sympathetic dystrophy.** See also **deafferentation pain.**

cautious gait   (elderly gait, senile gait) A gait disorder characterized by a normal to mildly widened base, short and slow stride, and *en bloc* turns. There is no hesitancy in initiating gait, and no shuffling nor freezing. Cadence and foot clearance of the support surface are normal. Mild disequilibrium (as judged by the response to a push and the difficulty in balancing on one foot) also occurs.

Most patients with this gait pattern are aware of impaired balance and express the need for caution to avoid falls. Other neurological symptoms and signs are generally mild and do not form a consistent picture. The pattern is associated with musculoskeletal lesions in the peripheral or central nervous systems. (Adapted from Nutt, et al.[4180])

cava septi pellucidi et vergae   (fifth ventricle, ventricle of Arantius, pseudocele) Cavities within the septum pellucidum, developing at the site of fusion of the two cerebral hemispheres as a secondary cleavage with necrobiosis as the fibers of the corpus callosum cross the midline.

The cavities (vergae being the posterior of the two and closing first) are normally present during prenatal life but are obliterated in most people within weeks of birth. Although they may rarely enlarge to obliterate the foramina of Monro, thus producing hydrocephalus, in an overwhelming majority of cases they have no clinical effects at all.[5102] Their presence was first recorded by Julius Caesar Arantius (1530–1589), an Italian physician, in 1571.[4979]

Cavanagh variant   See **hereditary spastic paraparesis.**

cavernoma   See **cavernous angioma.**

cavernous angioma   (hemangioma, cavernoma) Benign vascular malformations consisting of masses of abnormally dilated and undifferentiated sinusoidal vascular channels with no direct arteriovenous communication, lined by a single layer of endothelium and packed together with little or no neural tissue between.[6,3968] They also occur in the skin and liver.

When dominantly inherited, cavernous angiomas are often multiple, occuring mainly in the cerebral hemispheres, less often in the pons and spinal cord. Seizures and the effects of hemorrhage are the usual neurological presentations. They are seldom visualized on arteriograms because of the slow flow of the blood within them, but they are well shown on CT and MRI scans. Clinically, they are characterized by either the lack of symptoms, or by seizures, headaches, or focal neurological signs, which may result from intracerebral hemorrhage. On T2-weighted MRI scans they show as tiny hypodense areas, or as larger areas of mixed signal intensity with a low-intensity rim, due to the deposition of hemosiderin.[4664] A responsible gene (*CCM1*) has been mapped to chromosome 7q11–q22. See also **arteriovenous malformation, angioma.**

cavernous sinus   A plexus of small veins within a split in the dural sac beside the pituitary, through which the internal carotid artery and cranial nerves III, IV, V (ophthalmic division), and VI pass.

cavernous sinus syndrome   Painful dysfunction of cranial nerves III, IV, VI, of the first (and occasionally second) division of the fifth nerve and in some cases of the sympathetic fibers, due to a lesion within the cavernous sinus.

The syndrome was described by Foix in 1922[1894] and by Jefferson in 1938.[2823] See **superior orbital fissure syndrome.**

cavernous sinus syndrome of Raeder   See **superior orbital fissure syndrome.**

cavernous sinus thrombosis   Occlusion of the venous channels comprising the cavernous sinus.[1475] It occurs most commonly secondary to sepsis, in the preantibiotic era, especially mastoiditis, but may occur with marantic conditions such as severe dehydration, and in cachectic states associated with cancer.

Diagnostic criteria were suggested by Eagleton[1592] prior to the introduction of modern investigative procedures, and are listed below:
1. Known site of infection, or septicemia
2. Early destructive signs (full retinal veins, proptosis, exophthalmos, collateral venous circulation)
3. Oculomotor pareses and trigeminal nerve involvement
4. Neighborhood abscesses from the thrombophlebitis situated in the orbit, nasopharynx, occiput, or neck
5. Symptoms of complicating disease (headache, papilledema, meningeal signs)

cavernous sinus–lateral wall syndrome   See **superior orbital fissure syndrome.**

cavernous sinus–nasopharyngeal tumor syndrome   See **Godtfredsen syndrome.**

cavitating sudanophilic leukodystrophy   A group of demyelinating diseases occurring at any time of life and characterized clinically by developmental delay or dementia, tonic or clonic seizures, cerebellar and pyramidal signs, and cavitating changes in the CNS.[191] See **Canavan leukodystrophy.**

cavum   (from Lat, a hollow). A cavity or space.

cavum septi pellucidi   (Lat, a compartment or hole + a fence + transparent) (the "fifth ventricle") A cystic structure within the septum pellucidum, occurring as a developmental variant and declining in prevalence with age.[3560]

This is a common incidental finding in normal subjects, but may also be associated with **holoproscencephaly,** optic nerve hypoplasia, or the following syndrome, and may be acquired as a result of cranial trauma or hydrocephalus,[3884] or itself act as a cause of obstructive hydrocephalus.

cavum vergae   A congenital syndrome characterized by macrocephaly, posteriorly sited cavum septi pellucidi, and mental or developmental delay.[3884]

Cawthorne-Cooksey exercises   A regimen of physical therapy exercises for the eyes and body designed to diminish vertigo due to labyrinthine lesions. See also **Semont liberatory maneuver.**

CDC National Preventation Information Network   A Government-sponsored service in the United States. Address: CDC NPIN, P.O. Box 6003, Rockville, MD 20849-6003. Tel: 1-800-458-5231. See also http://www.natip.org/.

cebocephaly   (from Lat, a monkey + head) A form of frontal median clefting of the face, in which there is orbital hypotelorism with a single blind nostril, the nasal cavity being correctly placed but with no septum nor columella.[335]

-cele   (Gr, a tumor) Suffix denoting tumor.

celiac disease   A malabsorption syndrome manifesting intolerance to dietary gluten. In some 10% of cases, neurological syndromes occur, such as peripheral neuropathy, progressive multifocal leukoencephalopathy, cerebellar ataxia, progressive myoclonic ataxia, dementia, or myopathy.[4394]

cellulalgia   1. Unusually severe pain felt with gentle compression (pinching) of the skin. This is a characteristic feature in patients with **myofascial pain syndromes** and with **cervicogenic headaches** and may represent referred hyperesthesia, although the underlying pathology is quite uncertain. 2. Thickened and tender skin in the territory of one dermatome, the root of which is irritated or compressed.[3578]

Celsus, Aurelius Cornelius   (53 B.C. to 7 A.D.) Roman gentleman and writer on medicine, probably not a doctor, even though occasionally described as physician to Caligula. He compiled Greek medical writings into a book, *De Medicina,* which flourished but was later lost, bursting forth again in 1478 as one of the first books to be made after the invention of printing and remaining a standard medical text for nearly 300 years at a time when "many men would not look at the new moon out of respect for the old." In it, Celsus described anesthetic leprosy, migraine, seizures, apoplexy, paralysis, hydrocephalus, spinal injury, and facial neuralgia. See also **Paracelsus.**

Center for Epidemiological Studies Depression Scale (CES-D) A self-report questionnaire found to be both reliable and valid as a screening tool to identify the presence of depressive symptoms; see Chart C–6. The interview is given by a nurse who shows the depression scale response cards to the patient and asks the patient (for each item) to pick the card "which best describes how you felt or behaved this past week," recording the responses on a form.[4568,5136]

Chart C–6. Center for Epidemiological Studies Depression Scale

Depression scale

0	Rarely or none of the time (<1 day)
1	Some or a little of the time (1–2 days)
2	Occasionally or a moderate amount of time (3–4 days)
3	Most or all of the time (5–7 days)

Statements

1. I was bothered by things that usually don't bother me.
2. I did not feel like eating; my appetite was poor.
3. I felt that I could not shake off the blues even with help from my family or friends.
4. I felt that I was just as good as other people.
5. I had trouble keeping my mind on what I was doing.
6. I felt depressed (blue or down).
7. I felt that everything I did was an effort.
8. I felt hopeful about the future.
9. I thought my life had been a failure.
10. I felt fearful.
11. My sleep was restless.
12. I was happy.
13. I talked less than usual.
14. I felt lonely.
15. People were unfriendly.
16. I enjoyed life.
17. I had crying spells.
18. I felt sad.
19. I felt that people disliked me.
20. I could not get "going."

Adapted from Radloff LS. The CES-D Scale. Appl. Psychol. Meas. 1977;1:385–401[4568] and reproduced by kind permission of Dr. David Weiss.

central alveolar hypoventilation syndrome   A disorder characterized by ventilatory impairment resulting in arterial oxygen desaturation that is worsened by sleep, and occurring in patients with normal mechanical properties of the lung. Diagnostic criteria have been suggested[234] (see Chart C–7).

Chart C–7. Central Alveolar Hypoventilation
Syndrome

A. The patient can have a complaint of either insomnia or excessive sleepiness. The patient is usually unaware of the clinical features observed by others, such as hypoventilation during sleep.
B. Frequent episodes of shallow breathing occur during sleep.
C. Primary lung disease, skeletal malformations, or peripheral neuromuscular disorder affecting ventilation is absent.
D. Polysomnographic monitoring demonstrates:
   1. Episodes of shallow breathing greater than 10 seconds in duration associated with arterial oxygen desaturation, and one or more of the following:
   2. Frequent arousals from sleep associated with the breathing disturbances;
   3. Brady-tachycardia; and
   4. A minimal sleep latency test that demonstrates mean sleep latency of less than 10 minutes.
E. The syndrome can be associated with neurological disorders that affect the CNS control of breathing.
F. Other sleep disorders can be present, e.g., periodic limb moment disorder, central sleep apnea syndrome, or obstructive sleep apnea syndrome.

Adapted from the ASDA Diagnostic Classification Steering Committee. The International Classification of Sleep Disorders Diagnostic and Coding Manual. *Rochester, MN: American Sleep Disorders Association, 1990. Reproduced by kind permission of the American Academy of Sleep Medicine.*

See also congenital central hypoventilation syndrome.

central and peripheral demyelination   A syndrome comprising features of both **multiple sclerosis** and **chronic inflammatory demyelinating polyradiculoneuropathy.**[5552] See **chronic demyelinating neuropathy with multifocal CNS demyelination.**

central anisocoria   Variable inequality of the pupils with normal light reactions at all times and with normal dilation in response to psychosensory or pharmacological stimuli.

A lesion of the brainstem, as in **multiple sclerosis,** has been considered to be causal.[5824]

central anticholinergic syndrome   Signs suggesting atropine poisoning (dry, flushed, and warm skin, dilated pupils, decreased bowel sounds and urinary retention, and confusion) occurring as a result of exposure of the CNS to anticholinergic agents in toxic concentrations. See **anticholinergic syndrome.**

central aphasia   A form of aphasia described by Goldstein, now regarded as an incomplete form of **Wernicke (receptive) aphasia** resembling **conduction aphasia.**

central cervical cord syndrome   See **central cord syndrome.**

central conduction time   The latencies between stimulation of the cortical motor areas and the cervical cord, and the onset of the peripheral response. Either a magnetic stimulator or stimulation using a low-output impedance stimulator is employed.

The technique allows assessment of conduction in the descending motor pathways between the cortex and the cord, and has been found useful in demonstrating lesions of this pathway in, e.g., multiple sclerosis.[3896] See also **central motor conduction.**

central congenital alveolar hypoventilation   See **central alveolar hypoventilation syndrome.**

central cord syndrome   The occurrence of signs of spinothalamic and pyramidal tract dysfunction below, and of areflexia and hyper- or hypoesthesia at the site of a lesion affecting the central regions of the spinal cord. This may follow hyperextension injuries and other causes of ischemia, or may be the manifestation of intrinsic cord tumors, infections, or syringomyelia.[4584]

The *central cervical cord syndrome* leads to complaints of severe pain in the shoulder girdle region and arms, with weakness of the upper more than of the lower limbs, retention of urine, and variable impairment of sensation below the level of the lesion. It results from central cord lesions following severe hyperextension injuries to the cervical spine[2646] or midline cervical disk protrusion.

See also **burning hands syndrome.**

central core disease   (Shy-Magee disease) An uncommon, dominantly inherited or sporadic nonprogressive myopathy in which frozen sections of muscle demonstrate single or multiple regions within type 1 myofibers which lack reactivity for oxidative enzymes, phosphorylase, and glycogen, and which have a smudgy appearance with the modified trichrome stain. Electron microscopy of the **cores** shows lack or absence of mitochondria, reduced glycogen content, and changes in the contractile apparatus. The gene responsible is located at 19q12–q13.1.

The clinical features include onset in infancy, proximal muscle weakness and hypotonia with delayed motor development, and, in adults, mild proximal weakness affecting the pelvic girdle mainly, and the facial muscles in some cases. At any age, flat feet, kyphoscoliosis, pes cavus, congenital dislocation of the hips, joint contractures, poor temperature control, and stiffness of the muscles during exercise are often found. Eye movements are normal. The condition is a cause of "idiopathic" hyperCKemia.

The appearance of the central cores may be a nonspecific marker of a metabolic disorder. The condition was first recognized by Shy and Magee in 1956.[5152] Patients with this condition are at risk of **malignant hyperthermia.**[5142]

Variants include *multicore disease,* a syndrome of nonprogressive weakness in which small, short cores lie transversely across the muscle fiber;[1666] *minicore disease,* in which very small foci of Z-line streaming are seen within the muscle fibers;[1223] and a form with *muscle diphosphatase deficiency* presenting as a nonfamilial congenital nonprogressive myopathy.[2929]

central dazzle   See **central photophobia.**

central deafness   See **word deafness.**

central electromyography   The electrodiagnostic study of reflexes and of the control of movement by the spinal cord and brain, using for example **transcranial magnetic stimulation.** See also **central motor conduction.**

Central European encephalitis   A direct infection of brain by a flavivirus member of the togavirus group of arboviruses, characterized by an illness resembling **Russian spring-summer encephalitis,** except that it is milder and usually resolves without sequelae.[6030]

central facial palsy   Weakness of the lower quadrant of the face due to a lesion of the upper motor neuron pathway from the contralateral hemisphere. When isolated, this may be a **lacunar syndrome.**[2677]

The upper quadrant (the forehead) is largely spared because the neurons innervating the frontalis muscles receive (supranuclear) input from the motor cortex of both hemispheres, but those innervating the muscles of the lower half do not.

See also **volitional facial palsy, emotional facial palsy, lacunes.**

central fatigue   Failure to maintain sustained maximal force because of an unidentified, nonvolitional safety mechanism within the CNS which shuts off the neuromuscular unit when the latter seems to be at risk of damage from excessive contraction.[777] The organic nature of the problem was proved by the slowness of recovery times of motor-evoked potential amplitudes using transcranial magnetic stimulation.[3408]

central glare   See **central photophobia.**

central hematomyelia   Traumatic myelopathy, the clinical features resembling those of **syringomyelia** but in this case resulting from bleeding into the substance of the spinal cord.[3901] See **Minor disease.**

central herniation   1. The lateral and forward shift of the diencephalon and the downward-thrusting of the centrum semiovale through the tentorium cerebelli as a result of raised intracranial pressure, and giving rise to the **central syndrome.** 2. Backward protrusion of a herniating intervertebral disk in the midline.

central midtemporal spikes   (rolandic or sylvian spikes) Uniform diphasic or triphasic sharp waves occurring focally in the central and midtemporal regions in children between the ages of 4 and 13 years of age, unilaterally, bilaterally, or shifting between the two sides. The number of sharp waves is markedly increased by sleep and discharges may be absent during the waking state. The EEG finding is not necessarily associated with clinical seizure activity.[3356]

central motor conduction   The speed of conduction in central motor pathways, estimated by measurement of the latency of response in a muscle with magnetic stimulation of the motor cortex and of the appropriate nerve roots.[2737]

central nervous deficiency syndrome   Garland's term for the syndrome affecting starved prisoners of war who developed failing vision with optic atrophy, nerve deafness, and numbness and paresthesias of the legs, presumably because of nutritional deficiencies.[2033] See also **Strachan syndrome.**

central nervous system   The brain, the second cranial nerve, and the spinal cord.

Central Nervous System and Brain Disorders Network   An alliance of the National Foundation for Brain Research, the National Association for Clinical NeuroServices, and the National Coalition for Research in Neurological Disorders. Web site: http://www.brainnet.org/

central neurofibromatosis   See **neurofibromatosis, Gardner syndrome.**

central neurogenic hyperventilation   Hyperventilation characterized by sustained tachypnea that persists despite an elevated arterial pO_2 and pH and a low arterial pCO_2. It occurs in the absence of a respiratory stimulant and persists during sleep. In most cases it is due to hepatic encephalopathy or brainstem tumors, or is a sign of rostral–caudal deterioration in patients with generalized brain swelling. The mechanism of its occurrence is uncertain.[4463]

central nystagmus   A direction-changing nystagmus caused by a lesion of the CNS (as opposed to disease of the eyes or of the labyrinths), usually in the cerebellum or brainstem. Vertical, horizontal, or torsional forms occur; they may be uni- or bidirectional and are neither fatiguable nor suppressed by fixation. Other signs of CNS dysfunction are commonly present. Any vertigo accompanying it is relatively mild. See **direction-changing nystagmus.**

central oscillopsia   Subjective awareness of movement of visual images resulting from brainstem or temporal lobe disorders affecting the central vestibular apparatus.

central pain   (funicular pain) Deeply felt, amorphous, indefinable, and severe pain arising from lesions (almost all of which are strokes) completely or mainly confined to the CNS, with a latent period between injury and onset and invariably associated with some sensory disturbance.

Such pain is felt in regions distant from, but related to, spinal cord or cerebral lesions. Diffuse paresthesias, **allodynia,** and **hyperpathia** are commonly associated.

The mechanisms are unknown—up- or downregulation of receptors for adrenergic transmitters; sensitization of C nociceptors with low thresholds, capable of prolonged discharges after sensitization;

abnormal hypersensitivity of damaged fibers; the generation of new receptors; alteration in the central pattern of impulse conduction; alterations in inhibitory mechanisms; and activation of secondary polysynaptic pathways are all possibilities but in every case there appears to be some interruption of the spinothalamocortical nociceptive pathways.[502,2733]

See also **thalamic syndrome.**

central paroxysmal positional nystagmus A form of positional nystagmus in any direction, lasting 30 seconds or so, that is non-fatiguing and accopmpanied by other features of brainstem disese.

central photophobia (central glare, **central dazzle**) A subjective complaint of excessive brightness in patients with an homonymous hemianopia, probably in association with a calcarine lesion and interpretable as the visual correlate of paresthesia.[1214,1847] The same symptom may result from digitalis poisoning.

central pontine myelinolysis A condition characterized by a single confluent focal area of myelin destruction in the central pons with relative preservation of axons, in the absence of inflammatory changes.

It has been associated with various metabolic abnormalities such as alcoholism and too rapid correction of profound hyponatremia (faster than 12 mmol/L/day), and may reflect swelling of the interdigitated crossing fibers in the pons; however, lesions are also found in the pontine tegmentum, the mesencephalon, the deep cerebral nuclei, and the subcortical white matter.

Clinically, coma, seizures, and acutely evolving signs of corticospinal, cerebellar, and lower cranial nerve dysfunction are the major features.[4156,4523]

A similar syndrome may complicate foci of demyelination elsewhere than the central pons, and in some cases the condition is due to hypoxia rather than to abnormalities of sodium regulation.

central razzle Excessive discomfort from stimulation by loud sounds because of cortical lesions and thought to be due to loss of a centrifugal inhibitory pathway that may function to sharpen images.[258]

central retinal artery occlusion An ophthalmological emergency occurring mainly in the elderly, in which retinal ischemia and infarction cause acute and severe visual loss, with attenuation of the retinal vessels, retinal pallor and edema, and a **cherry-red spot.**

The usual cause is an arterial embolism, arteritis, or vasospasm; in the case of the first of these, massage of the eye and lowering of intraocular pressure may improve the chances of restoring some sight.[196]

central retinal vein occlusion An acquired disorder causing reduction in vision, swelling of the optic nerve head, dilation of the retinal veins, and hemorrhages in the retinal nerve fiber layer.

The cause is usually not determined, but the condition may be associated with hypertension and other vascular diseases.[2985] One cause may be compression of the vein by a dilated, atheromatous central retinal artery. See also **venous stasis retinopathy.**

central scotoma 1. A defect in the field of vision corresponding to that part of the field subtended by the macula, due to a lesion of the papillomacular fibers. 2. A defect in the field of vision which is surrounded by an intact field. See **scotoma.**

central serous retinopathy (central angiospastic retinopathy) A syndrome of unknown cause occurring in young adult males, characterized by the accumulation of serous fluid at one macula or beneath the retina or the adjacent pigmented epithelium. Clinical features include complaints of metamorphopsia, positive scotomas, and micropsia. The prognosis for recovery is good but in about a quarter of all cases the condition recurs.

central sleep apnea syndrome A disorder characterized by a cessation or decrease of ventilatory effort during rapid eye movement sleep, usually with associated oxygen desaturation and without any accompanying respiratory effort, as a result of an unusually high apneic threshold. The condition may occur as a complication of numerous CNS lesions, hypoxia, and metabolic diseases but is most commonly found in healthy people at high altitudes. Diagnostic criteria have been suggested by the American Sleep Disorders Association[234] (see Chart C–8).

Chart C–8. Central Sleep Apnea Syndrome

A. The patient has a complaint of either insomnia or excessive sleepiness. Occasionally the patient may be unaware of clinical features observed by others.

B. Frequent episodes of shallow or absent breathing during sleep.

C. Associated features include at least one of the following:
    1. Gasps, grunts or choking during sleep,
    2. Frequent body movements, or
    3. Cyanosis during sleep.

D. Polysomnographic monitoring demonstrates:
    1. Central apneic pauses >10 seconds (20 seconds in infancy) in duration, and one or more of the following:
    2. Frequent arousals from sleep associated with the apneas,
    3. Brady-tachycardia, or
    4. Oxygen desaturation in association with the apneic episodes, with or without
    5. A **minimal sleep latency test** that demonstrates mean sleep latency of less than 10 minutes.

E. Other sleep disorders can be present, e.g., periodic limb movement disorder, obstructive sleep apnea syndrome, or **central alveolar hypoventilation syndrome.**

Adapted from the ASDA Diagnostic Classification Steering Committee. The International Classification of Sleep Disorders Diagnostic and Coding Manual. Rochester, MN: American Sleep Disorders Association, 1990. Reproduced by kind permission of the American Academy of Sleep Medicine.

central syndrome Downward displacement of the upper brainstem at the junction with the diencephalon through the tentorial opening, leading to an orderly sequence of events that witness the functional disturbance of progressively more caudal levels of the brainstem.[4466] These include reduction in conscious level and Cheyne-Stokes respirations (*diencephalic stage*); midposition fixed pupils, loss of oculocephalic reflexes, and central neurogenic hyperventilation (*pontine stage*); decorticate posturing, ataxic or no respirations, bradycardia, and hypertension (*medullary stage*); and ultimately death.

central tapetoretinal degeneration   See **Behr disease.**

central tegmental tract   Fibers that descend from the red nucleus and elsewhere in the lower diencephalon and mesencephalon, running to the ipsilateral olive. It was first described by von Bechterew in 1885. Bilateral lesions of the tract appear to induce the phenomenon of **palatal myoclonus.**

central vestibular nystagmus   See **vestibular nystagmus.**

central vestibular vertigo   That form of vertigo caused by lesions of the vestibular nuclei or of the vestibulocerebellum, and characterized by change in direction with gaze to either side. The nystagmus may be pendular and can be purely horizontal, vertical, or rotatory.

central-distal axonopathy   Axonal damage in the peripheral extremities of axons within the CNS, one cause of which is prolonged low-level exposure to acrylamide, an industrial polymer, while the effects of MPTP, clioquinol, and lathyrism and possibly the biochemical deficits underlying **Friedreich ataxia** and **hereditary spastic paraplegia** are others.

The clinical syndromes produced include the subacutely evolving onset and evolution of sensorimotor/autonomic peripheral neuropathy, spasticity, optic atrophy, and cerebellar ataxia.[5549] See also **subacute myelo-opticoneuropathy.**

centrencephalic epilepsy   The term applied to the supposed site of origin of generalized tonic-clonic seizures, based on the fact that bilateral epileptic discharges can be set up in homologous areas of the two hemispheres following stimulation of subcortical structures such as the intralaminar thalamic nuclei of experimental animals.

In 1938 **Penfield** considered that one area in the nervous system functions to integrate the electrical activity of the two hemispheres, probably the rostral brainstem and thalamus, and that this area also constituted the neural substratum of consciousness.

Abnormal discharges in this region would give rise to those seizures that Penfield labeled *centrencephalic.* However, it is notable that lesions of other parts of the brain may also induce seizures with exactly the same clinical and electrographic characteristics. See **absence seizures.**

centrencephalic myoclonic-astatic epilepsy   (infantile myoclonic petit mal, centrencephalic myoclonic-astatic petit mal, true myoclonic epilepsy) Forms of myoclonic-astatic epilepsy for which there is no detectable pathological basis. In such cases there is frequently a positive family history of seizures.[1497] The patient may be mentally normal or retarded, and first exhibits symptoms usually in the second to fifth years of life. Myoclonic and atonic seizures, absences, petit mal status, tonic seizures, etc. are the usual phenotypes. See **akinetic seizures, juvenile myoclonic epilepsy of Janz, centrencephalic epilepsy.**

centrencephalic myoclonic-astatic petit mal   See **centrencephalic myoclonic-astatic epilepsy.**

centrifugal   (Lat, center + fleeing from) Movement of a phenomenon (such as sensory loss in developing peripheral neuropathy) from proximal to distal parts of the body.

centrifugal nerve   A motor nerve.

centripetal   (Lat, center + seeking) Movement of a phenomenon (such as sensory loss in developing peripheral neuropathy) from distal to proximal parts of the body.

centripetal nystagmus   A form of **gaze-evoked nystagmus** that increases with prolonged eccentric gaze, but may reverse in direction if the position of the eyes is maintained longer. It is most commonly seen in ocular **myasthenia gravis**[3318] or in diseases of the cerebellum.

See also **rebound nystagmus,** in which nystagmus in the opposite direction occurs when the eyes are returned from the deviated to the primary position.

centrocecal scotoma   A scotoma that involves the area of the visual field subtended between the macula and the blind spot. It reflects pathology affecting the fibers running to the optic nerve head from the macula and from the retina between the macula and the optic disk.

centronuclear myopathies   (myotubular myopathies) Sporadic or variously inherited **congenital myopathies** with occasional onset in childhood or adult life, characterized by the presence of structures resembling fetal myotubes and central nuclei in the extrafusal muscle fibers with predominance and hypotrophy of type I fibers.[1744,5115] The most common form maps to Xq27–q28, but autosomal dominant and recessive forms are also recorded.

Among these there is a high proportion of histochemical type 2 fibers resembling myotubes (with a peripheral ring of myofibrils and a central area in which myofibrillar components and nuclei are present). Type 1 fiber atrophy and the nonspecific features of myopathy are other common findings.[3985,5294]

Clinically, the appearances vary; facial, extraocular, and limb weakness with equinovarus deformity of the feet and, in adults, a syndrome of moderate limb-girdle weakness have both been associated with these biopsy appearances, although a syndrome of nonprogressive myopathy with weakness of the facial and extraocular muscles and hypotonia is a characteristic presentation. Muscle pain and stiffness after exertion with relief by rest are other common symptoms.

It is possible that **centronuclear** myopathies and **type 1 fiber atrophy with central nuclei** are forms of the same disease.[535]

Variant members of the class include *X-linked recessive centronuclear (myotubular) myopathy* (OMIM 310400), a fatal congenital myopathy presenting with weak fetal movements, fetal distress, respiratory distress in the neonate, proximal myopathic weakness, hypotonia, and atrophy. Tubular aggregates are found in muscle biopsy specimens.[5160] The responsible gene maps to Xq28.[5741]

Centronuclear myopathy with type 1 fiber atrophy and myotubules is a slowly progressive form of centronuclear myopathy with onset in childhood, affecting the muscles of the pelvic girdle and legs, in which the muscle biopsy reveals type 1 fiber atrophy, central nuclei, and fibers resembling myotubes.[535]

Another *variant* is a form in which *type 1 fiber hypotrophy and fingerprint inclusions* are found in muscle biopsy specimens. The clinical syndrome includes slowly progressive muscular weakness and features of Malins syndrome.[4175]

A *dominantly inherited form* presents in youth or adult life with proximal muscle wasting, with the facial, extraocular, and distal muscles sometimes being involved as well. The condition is slowly progressive and can be compatible with a normal life span. Muscle biopsy shows central nuclei with a clear surrounding zone in 60% of the fibers, for both types 1 and 2.[3774]

In other *dominantly or recessively inherited forms* presenting in childhood or adult life, proximal muscle weakness and wasting with sparing of the cranial muscles, with calf muscle hypertrophy[567] or with cardiomyopathy, have been reported.

centrotemporal epilepsy See **benign childhood epilepsy with centrotemporal spikes.**

centrum ovale infarcts Stroke from acute infarction in the centrum ovale which receives its blood supply from the superficial (pial) middle cerebral artery (MCA) system through perforating medullary branches that course toward the lateral ventricles.[632]

centrum semiovale The hemispheric mass of gray and white matter that remains at the top of the brainstem when the cerebrum is removed. It comprises the basal ganglia and internal capsules.

cephalaea An ancient term for a form of headache resembling migraine.

cephalalgia (Gr, the head + pain) Headache.

Cephalalgia The organ of the International Headache Society, devoted to the topic of headache and related pains. Web site: www.cephalalgia.org.

cephalgia fugax See **benign paroxysmal cranial neuralgia.**

cephalic (Gr, pertaining to the head).

cephalic bellows sound A cranial bruit heard best over the anterior fontanelle of children with hydrocephalus and raised intracranial pressure. It was described first in 1833 by Dr. John Dix Fisher (1797–1850), a physician in Massachussetts,[2209] who thought the sound indicated the presence of cerebral pathology, but it was dismissed by Osler as being without pathological significance in 1880.

cephalic index A craniometric sign, the breadth of the head divided by the length and multiplied by 100, the product having no known significance.

cephalic tetanus (Rose tetanus, Rose-Villar syndrome) A form of **tetanus** affecting the facial or oculomotor muscles.

cephalitis An ancient term for inflammation of the brain and its membranes.

cephalocele Herniation of the intracranial contents through a defect in the skull. Such midline craniocerebral cystic defects result from failure in the normal development of the neural tube and consist of **meningoceles,** within which there is no neural tissue, and **encephaloceles** proper, in which some neural tissue is present.[3773] They are classified as *primary* (occipital, parietal, **sincipital,** and basal) and *secondary* (following surgery or trauma or with a craniofacial cleft).[1307]

cephalohematoma (Gr, head + blood + a mass) A blood clot lying beneath the scalp but outside the cranium, seen most often in infants as a complication of a traumatic delivery.

cephalo-oculocutaneous telangiectasia See **Louis-Bar syndrome.**

cephaloponia (Gr, head + pain) An ancient term for a severe or heavy pain in the head.

cephalosyndactyly See **Waardenbeng syndrome.**

CERAD The **C**onsortium to **E**stablish a **R**egistry for **A**lzheimer **D**isease, a research group formed in the United States to standardize examination techniques, facilitate cooperative study, and perform annual assessments on a defined population.[3998] The Web site is acessible through http://www.alz.washington.edu/ceradrt.html.

CERAD Global Deterioration Scale (GDS) A rating instrument for staging the magnitude of cognitive and functional impairment in normal aging, age-associated memory impairment, and primary degenerative dementia, composed of a battery of tests designed to provide brief and accurate assessment of the presenting symptoms. The levels of cognitive functioning are rated from no cognitive decline to very mild, moderate, moderately severe, severe, and very severe decline, and for each of these, full notation of definitions are given.[3998]

CERAD test battery   A selection of tests designed to provide a brief and accurate assessment of the presenting manifestations and cognitive changes in patients with **Alzheimer disease** or other cognitive disorders in the elderly.

Aside from information on demographics, a drug inventory, and history, physical and general neurological examinations are performed and a diagnostic impression recorded. Tests of verbal fluency, the modified Boston Naming Test, the Mini-Mental State Examination, tests of constructional praxis, word lists to recall, and word list recognition tests are also administered.[3997]

ceramidase deficiency   See **Farber disease.**

ceramide lactoside lipidosis   (ceramidosis) See **Farber disease.**

cerebellar abscess   A purulent collection within the cerebellum, usually associated with pyogenic inflammation of the middle ear.

Clinically, headache, vomiting, drowsiness, ataxia of gait and limb movements, nystagmus, meningism, and evidence of increased intracranial pressure are the leading features.

cerebellar ataxia   (ataxy, Zappert syndrome) 1. An inclusive term for all the clinical motor manifestations of cerebellar disease, especially incoordination or awkwardness in the performance of a motor task due to disease of the cerebellum or its connections.

The term thus begs the question; "What are the signs of cerebellar disease?" Although an experienced clinician may have no doubt that certain mild abnormalities of voluntary movements are due to loss of cerebellar coordinating functions, no precise differentiation between these abnormalities and those caused by e.g., proprioceptive disorders or subtle weakness from corticospinal lesions is possible, other than by the exclusion of such alternatives by determining that the other signs of such lesions are not to be found. All of the tests to elicit "cerebellar signs" (discoordination, dysmetria, dysdiadochokinesis, etc.) may in fact be abnormal on the basis of frontal lobe, internal capsule, or other pathway lesions.

2. (*cerebellar ataxias*, spinocerebellar ataxias) Inherited diseases of the cerebellum or of its connections, presenting with typical signs of cerebellar dysfunction and frequently complicated damage to other parts of the nervous system. These are distinguished here from those conditions that have no known hereditary basis, which are classified here.

A recent comprehensive classification of the multi-

tude of the inherited cerebellar ataxias is that of Harding,[2440] who defined five groups, to which the condition of **hereditary spastic paraparesis** may be added conveniently. Chart C–9 is based upon that classification, adapted and with the addition of syndromes taken from the extensive listing by Baraitser[335] and others.

Chart C–9. The Idiopathic Dominantly Inherited Ataxias

ADCA Type I

These are late-onset (usually after 20 years) ataxias with variable added signs. A compilation from various sources[2407,4952,5403] and from Dr. Will Garrett, personal communication, follows.

Spinocerebellar ataxia type 1 (SCA1) Autosomal dominant form with a locus on chromosome 6p22–p23. Clinically, gait disturbance and speech problems are the typical onset symptoms, developing usually in the twenties; ophthalmoplegia, optic atrophy, pyramidal and extrapyramidal signs, peripheral sensorimotor neuropathy, mild dementia, and amyotrophy follow. This is the most frequent single example of the SCAs reported to date.[4260a] A CAG repeat has been incriminated.

SCA2 Autosomal dominant form on 12q23–q24.1.[4083a] Clinically, this resembles SCA1 but the hyporeflexia is more pronounced, saccades are particularly slow, and both myoclonus and cramps are reported.[437] In variant forms, there is also Parkinsonism[2347] or retinal degeneration.[461]

SCA3/Machado-Joseph disease Autosomal dominant form on 14q24.3–q32.1 I. This dominantly inherited syndrome with onset usually in mid-adult life comprises progressive ataxia and supervening pyramidal signs, dysarthria, and vertical gaze pareses associated with cerebellar and brainstem atrophy with perioral fasciculations. Optic atrophy, chorea, parkinsonism, dystonic or rigid dystonias, distal weakness and wasting, and retained reflexes are common additional findings; saccade velocities are not reduced in some kinships. The responsible gene maps to 6p24–p23.[2440,5015] The condition was first described in detail by Menzel in 1891.[3839] See also **Joseph disease.**

SCA4 Located on 16q24.ter or 16q22.1. A form with prominent sensory axonal neuropathy and hyporeflexia but without eye movement disorders.[1881a]

SCA12 Located on 5q31–33. This autosomal dominant syndrome is characterized clinically by action tremor in the head and arms with onset in the fourth decade of hyperreflexia and mild to moderate cerebellar signs such as ataxia, dysmetria, and dysarthria. Parkinsonism and dementia have been recorded later in life.[4221] The syndrome results from an unstable CAG repeat in the gene *PPP 2R2B.*

ADCA Type II: Ataxia with Pigmentary Retinal Degeneration/Progressive Macular Degeneration

Clinically, the cerebellar syndrome is accompanied by progressive visual loss and evidence of anterior horn cell degeneration. It is mapped to 3p12–p21.1[1654]

SCA7 Located on 3p12–13 11. This syndrome, resembling SCA1 with onset usually in childhood, comprises progressive visual failure (maculopathy), ataxia, seizures, and supervening gaze pareses. Pyramidal signs including hyperreflexia, posterior column sensory loss, and dementia are also reported. The syndrome is associated with atrophic changes in the cerebellum, basal ganglia, and spinal cord.[2236,5894] This must be the same condition as that formerly called *ADCA II: with pigmentary retinal degeneration/progressive macular degeneration.*

ADCA Type III: "Pure" Cerebellar Ataxias with Late Onset

(Adult-onset cerebellar ataxia, olivopontocerebellar atrophy, parenchymatous cerebellar cortical atrophy, cerebellopontine atrophy, late cortical cerebellar atrophy, Marie-Foix Alajouanine syndrome, Thomas atrophy) This group of ataxic disorders is of unknown etiology with onset usually after the age of 50 years.[2438] Corticospinal, extrapyramidal, and ocular features are not prominent and sensory loss is absent. The chief pathological change is cerebellar cortical atrophy with loss of the Purkinje cell layer.[179,2605]

SCA5 Located on 11q13 (11 cen). This form presents as a slowly developing cerebellar and pyramidal syndrome in the third decade, with global cerebellar atrophy.[4589a]

SCA6 Located on 19p13. This dominantly inherited form resembles SCA5 but is manifested in older adults and posterior column function is impaired. Life span is normal. Downbeat nystagmus is an added feature but the brainstem is otherwise unaffected. The mutation is allelic with episodic ataxia type 2[1997,2079,5347] and linked to **familial hemiplegic migraine** both clinically and through shared abnormalities of the CACNA1A P/Q type calcium channel α_1 subunit.

SCA8 Located on 13q21. This is a slowly progressive form with cerebellar, pyramidal, and cognitive signs.[2897]

SCA11 Life span is normal. This form is not yet mapped.

Others

SCA9 Located on a chromosomal site not yet determined.

SCA10 Located on 22q13. This pure cerebellar syndrome has seizures as an added feature, and is described from Mexico.[4606] A similar phenotype has been mapped to 22q.13.[3704]

SCA13 Located on 19q. This recessive form manifests in childhood. Psychomotor failure is reported.

SCA14 Located on 19q

SCA 15 (Unknown locus) This pure ataxic syndrome is reported in a single Australian family.[5371]

SCA16 Autosomal dominant form on 8q 22.1–24.1. Head and hand tremors are reported.

SCA17 Not completely characterized.

Dentato-rubro-pallido-luysian atrophy (DRPLA) Located on 12 p

SCA types 1, 2, 3, 6 and 7, 12, and DRPLA stem from mutations consisting of expanded and unstable CAG trinucleotide repeats. SCA8 results from an expansion of a CTG trinucleotide repeat. The types of mutations responsible for SCA4 and 5 and for SCA9 through 11 are unknown.[5403] See also **Ramsay Hunt syndrome; mitochondrial diseases.**

ADCA Type IV

Cerebellar signs with myoclonus and deafness characterize ths group (see Chart C–10) which may not be a distinct entity. See *May-White syndrome* below, and **MERRF.**

Chart C–10. The (Spino)Cerebellar Ataxias

I. *Congenital inherited ataxias*
   A. Congenital ataxia with mental retardation with or without spasticity (includes pontoneocerebellar and granule cell hypoplasia); which are autosomal recessive or dominant, or X-linked. The various syndromes identified include the following:

   Angelman syndrome

   Ataxia with photomyoclonus A dominantly inherited syndrome characterized by extreme sensitivity to light, and with myoclonus, cerebellar ataxia, ataxic gait, pes cavus, kyphosis, and dementia.[1625] The condition may also manifest later in life. This condition and **MERRF** (Myoclonus Epilepsy with Ragged Red Fibers) are probably the same.

   Cerebellar hemisphere hypoplasia (congenital granular cell hypoplasia) A syndrome of ataxia and mental retardation, each of variable severity.[5957]

   Congenital ataxia with choroidal coloboma (**Pfeiffer syndrome**)

   Congenital cerebellar atrophy A dominantly inherited syndrome in which ataxia complicates early mild motor delay.[1994]

   Lhermitte-Duclos disease (*granular cell hypertrophy*)

   Neonatal cerebellar atrophy with retinal dystrophy A fatal syndrome of neonatal ataxia with retinal dystrophy and limitation of joint movement complicated by diarrhea, vomiting, pericardial effusion, and hepatic fibrosis.

   Olivopontocerebellar atrophy with hepatic cirrhosis and retinal dystrophy A congenital inherited ataxic syndrome with cerebellar hemisphere hypoplasia, characterized by pericarditis, neonatal feeding problems, hypotonia, pigmentary retinopathy, abnormal enlarged liver, joint contractures, and mental and developmental delay.[337]

   Paine syndrome

   Pontocerebellar hypoplasia

   Progressive ataxia, retinal degeneration, peripheral neuropathy, myopathy, and mental subnormality A rare congenital syndrome in which the above manifestations are accompanied by hypoparathyroidism, dwarfism, malabsorption and cholelithiasis.[2181]

   NARP syndrome (Neuropathy, Ataxia and Retinitis Pigmentosa).

   B. **Joubert syndrome** (congenital ataxia, recessively inherited, with episodic hyperpnea, abnormal eye movements, and mental retardation)

   C. **Gillespie syndrome** Congenital ataxia with partial aniridia, infantile spasms, choreoathetosis, and mental and developmental delay. The inheritance pattern is undefined.[2118]

   D. *Dysequilibrium syndrome* A rare, congenital, nonprogressive, autosomal recessively inherited ataxic syndrome characterized by ataxia, hypotonia, severe postural disturbance, strabismus, delay in achieving language, and often severe mental and motor retardation.[2368]

II. *Ataxias with known metabolic or other cause*
   A. Intermittent ataxic syndromes
      Hyperammonemias
         Citrullinemia (ornithine transcarbylamase deficiency)

Argininosuccinuria
Arginase deficiency
Hyperornithinemia
Aminoacidurias
Hartnup disease
Pyruvate and lactic acid dysmetabolism
PDH deficiency
B. Progressive ataxic syndromes
Abetalipoproteinemia
Adrenoleukodystrophy
Celiac disease
Cerebrotendinous xanthomatosis
GDH deficiency
Hexosaminidase deficiency (GM$_2$ gangliosidosis)
Hypobetalipoproteinemia
Hypoxanthine-guanine phosphoribotransferase
deficiency
Krabbe leukodystrophy
Metachromatic leukodystrophy
Mitochondrial encephalomyopathies
Neuronal ceroid lipofuscinosis
Sialidosis
Sphingomyelin storage disorders
Vitamin E deficiency
Wilson disease
X-linked ataxia, ichthyosis, and tapetoretinal dys-
trophy (arylsulfatase C deficiency); see **metachro-
matic leukodystrophy**
C. Ataxic disorders associated with defective DNA repair
Ataxia-telangiectasia
Xeroderma pigmentosum
Cockayne syndrome
III. *Early-onset ataxias of unknown cause (onset usually before
20 years)*
Friedreich ataxia Among the spinocerebellar degenera-
tions in this group, this is the form most commonly diagnosed,
but such a statement (while true globally) is inappropriate in
certain parts of the world, where variants may be far more frequent. Next most commonly reported is the syndrome of
early-onset cerebellar ataxia with retained reflexes (next entry). Most of these syndromes are recessively inherited and differ from Friedreich ataxia in the absence (with certain exceptions as below) of optic atrophy, diabetes, cardiac involvement,
and severe skeletal deformity.

Early-onset cerebellar ataxia of unknown cause (Friedreich
ataxia with retained reflexes) This syndrome resembles
Friedreich ataxia but with retention of the muscle stretch
reflexes and with a better prospect of continuing function.[3090]

This group includes ataxic syndromes complicated by myoclonus (see **Ramsay Hunt syndrome**) while occasional
families have also been described in which the ataxia is associated with deafness, tapetoretinal or pigmentary retinal
degeneration, optic atrophy, macular degeneration, dementia, extrapyramidal disorders, peripheral neuropathy, etc., as
follows:

Ataxia with isolated vitamin E deficiency
Hypo- or hypergonadism
Ataxia with hypergonadotrophic hypogonadism (Skre
syndrome) A recessively inherited syndrome of gait
and limb ataxia, also characterized by cataract, primary amenorrhea, streak ovaries, small testes, oph-

thalmoplegias, loss of pain sensation, and mental and
developmental delay.[3710]
Ataxia with hypogonadotrophic hypergodadism (Holmes
syndrome) A recessively inherited syndrome of gait
and limb ataxia, with onset in youth or early adult
life. The condition is also characterized by pigmentary retinopathy, small penis and testes, pes cavus,
dementia, hypotonia, dysarthria, choreoathetosis,
distal weakness and wasting, loss of pain and joint
position senses, short stature, and mental and developmental delay.[2619]
Myoclonus
Ramsay Hunt syndrome This represents more than
one condition, including **mitochondrial encephalomyopathy, sialidosis,** and **Baltic myoclonus.** See
progressive myoclonus epilepsy.
**Childhood ataxia with diffuse central nervous system
demyelination** A progressive neurological disorder,
also classified as a leukodystrophy, characterized clinically by progressive ataxic diplegia with onset before
the age of 5 and with MRI and pathological evidence
of confluent white matter disease.[4960] See **CACH.**
Childhood deafness
Ataxia with sensory deafness and optic atrophy A dominantly inherited ataxic syndrome with onset in
childhood, characterized by sensorineural deafness,
optic atrophy, and neurogenic muscle atrophy.[337]
Congenital deafness
Ataxia with deaf-mutism and muscular wasting 1. (early
onset) A congenital inherited ataxic syndrome characterized by sensorineural deafness, pyramidal signs,
neurogenic muscle atrophy with fasciculations, and
thick-fiber sensory neuropathy.[1714] 2. (late onset) An
inherited ataxic syndrome characterized by sensorineural deafness, endocrinopathy, spasticity, axonal motor neuropathy, and thick-fiber sensory neuropathy.[1714]
Optic atrophy with or without mental retardation
Behr syndrome
Richards-Rundle syndrome
Cataract and mental retardation
Marinesco Sjögren syndrome A recessively inherited
ataxic syndrome with onset in childhood, also characterized by cataract, proximal and distal myopathy, and
mental and developmental delay.[3623]
Pigmentary retinopathy
Ataxia with retinal degeneration A dominantly inherited ataxic syndrome characterized variously by such
additional features as macular degeneration, optic atrophy, pigmentary retinopathy, nerve deafness, peripheral neuropathy, mental retardation, external ophthalmoplegia, pyramidal and extrapyramidal signs,
myoclonus, myocardial sclerosis and skin lesions, and
the presence of abnormal mitochondria.[2440,2804] Kinships in which this syndrome is recessively inherited
are also described.[2440] See also **MERRF.**

Other *variant early-onset ataxias of unknown etiology* include the following:
Ataxia with albinism An inherited ataxic syndrome characterized by dysarthria, motor neuropathy, diffuse depigmentation of skin, and mental and developmental
delay.[337]

Ataxia with deaf-mutism and muscular wasting 1. (early onset) A congenital inherited ataxic syndrome characterized by sensorineural deafness, pyramidal signs, neurogenic muscle atrophy with fasciculations, and thick-fiber sensory neuropathy.[2070] 2. (late onset) An inherited ataxic syndrome with onset in adult life, characterized by sensorineural deafness, endocrinopathy, spasticity, axonal motor neuropathy, and thick-fiber sensory neuropathy.[2070]

Ataxia with ocular motor apraxia An inherited ataxic syndrome with onset in infancy or childhood also characterized by chorea and athetosis.[60] This and **ataxia-telangiectasia** are possibly the same condition.

Ataxia with pallidonigroluysian atrophy and Lewy bodies[3989]

Ataxia with paroxysmal dystonia An inherited ataxic syndrome with onset in infancy or childhood, also characterized by dysarthria, paroxysmal dystonia, and pyramidal signs.[2250]

Ataxia with pupillary paralysis A static inherited ataxic syndrome with onset in early adult life in which these features accompany kyphoscoliosis, sixth nerve palsy, cataract, kyphoscoliosis and pes cavus.[5425]

Benign cerebellatr ataxia with extensive thermoanalgesia A dominantly inherited variant with associated demyelinating neuropathy affecting especially the smaller fibers.[4483]

Early onset ataxia with cardiomyopathy and retained reflexes A variant phenotype of Friedreich ataxia, also mapping to chromosome 9q.[4304]

Familial intermittent ataxia An X-linked recessive, paroxysmal ataxic syndrome with onset in infancy or early childhood, also characterized by dysarthria, apraxias, neurodegenerative regression, and abnormal lactate and pyruvate metabolism.[3444]

Familial spinocerebellar degeneration with corneal dystrophy An inherited ataxic syndrome with congenital or infantile onset, also characterized by cloudy corneas.[337]

Jeune syndrome

Myokymia and periodic ataxia An inherited ataxic syndrome with onset in infancy and also characterized by paroxysmal dystonia and myokymia.[4712]

Progressive visual and hearing loss, progressive spastic paraplegia, cerebellar ataxia, and dementia A syndrome with these findings is inherited either as a dominant or as a recessive trait.

Spino-olivocerebellar degeneration with ophthalmoplegia A recessively inherited ataxic syndrome characterized by colobomas of the optic nerve, dementia, ophthalmoplegia, paraplegia, demyelination, and pancytopenia.[1279]

Wadia-Swami syndrome

X-linked cerebellar ataxias Rare syndromes characterized by various combinations of visual loss, mild spastic paraparesis, mental slowing, myoclonic seizures, extrapyramidal deficits, posterior column demyelination, peripheral motor neuropathy, and pes cavus with onset in infancy.[224,2440]

Other rare *variants* occur (summarized by Baraitser[335]) in which cerebellar ataxia is combined with brachydactyly and nystagmus, erythrokeratodermia, glutathione deficiency, or skin hyperpigmentation.

IV. Late-onset ataxias

This group of dominantly inherited ataxic syndromes has an onset usually after 20 years of age, and is accompanied in most cases by other neurological features such as dementia, optic atrophy, pigmentary retinopathy, or extrapyramidal signs.

Other *variant* forms include the following:

Cerebellar ataxia with myoclonus and deafness (May-White syndrome) A very slowly progressive, dominantly inherited syndrome characterized by the onset in late childhood or adolescence of cerebellar ataxia and impaired vision due to pigmentary retinopathy. Spasticity occurs in some cases, but mental deterioration is not found.[3715]

Idiopathic late-onset cerebellar ataxia A heterogeneous group of familial or sporadic cerebellar syndromes without a known familial basis.[2436]

Adult-onset autosomal recessive ataxia with thalamic lesions described once in a Finnish family.[4589]

Adult-onset cerebellar ataxia and sensory deafness (of Schimke) An inherited ataxic syndrome with onset in adult life, also manifesting sensorineural deafness and high arches of the feet.[337]

Familial periodic ataxia A syndrome characterized by the onset in childhood of attacks of ataxia, dysarthria, vertigo, and nystagmus lasting hours to days. Drowsiness, headache, fever, and vomiting may also occur. A response to acetazolamide has been reported. The signs usually remit completely between attacks.[1490] Similarities to **basilar migraine** are notable.

Ataxia and other neurological deficits with hyperuricemia An inherited ataxic syndrome with onset in youth or adult life, characterized by ophthalmoplegia, facial palsy, sensorineural deafness, dysarthria, cardiomyopathy, nephropathy, and hyperuricemia.[337]

Ataxia with cataracts, hemiballismus, and dementia An inherited ataxic syndrome with onset in adult life, also characterized by cataract, tics, pyramidal and extrapyramidal signs, muscle cramp, and dementia.[337]

Ataxia with downbeat nystagmus A recessively inherited ataxic syndrome with onset in young adult life characterized also by dysarthria, dysphagia, vertical nystagmus, and pyramidal signs.[337]

Ataxia with fasciculations A dominantly inherited condition with onset in young adult life, described (once) in India.[5184]

Ataxia with ichthyosis and hepatosplenomegaly (of Harper) An inherited ataxic syndrome with onset in mature adult life, characterized by dysarthria, enlarged liver and spleen, dementia, ophthalmoplegia, hyperkeratosis, and ichthyosis.[337]

Benign hereditary cerebellar ataxia with extensive thermoanalgesia A dominantly inherited variant in which a length-dependent axonal neuropathy results from the loss of primary sensory afferents subserving pain and temperature sensation.[4483]

Spinocerebellar degeneration with motor system involvement A rare variant with onset in adult life, characterized by ataxia, amyotrophy, and ophthalmoplegia, resembling the spinocerebellar degenerative diseases.[2486] Pyramidal signs and generalized neuropathic muscle atrophy and weakness leading to respiratory difficulties have also been described in this cluster.

Ataxia with vitamin E deficiency[4277]

Ataxia-telangiectasia

Spinopontine degeneration

Ataxia with photomyoclonus and skeletal deformities An inherited ataxic syndrome with onset in adult life and characterized by dysarthria kyphosis, high arches of feet, dementia, and myoclonus.[337]

Autosomal recessive late-onset ataxia A rare, recessively inherited syndrome with onset in adult life, characterized by ataxia, supranuclear ophthalmoplegias, facial impassivity, pseudobulbar and pyramidal signs, peripheral neuropathy, and pure cerebellar cortical atrophy.[2443] Thalamic lesions also may occur.[4589]

Familial cerebellar ataxia with cerebrovascular amyloid An inherited ataxic syndrome with onset in young adult life, characterized by dementia, pyramidal signs, and cerebrovascular disease.[3482]

Familial spastic ataxia A dominantly inherited ataxic syndrome with onset at any age, characterized by spastic-ataxic dysarthria, dementia, vertical nystagmus, optic atrophy, pyramidal signs, and variable sensory neuropathic signs.

Late-onset hereditary ataxia with global thermoanalgesia and absence of fungiform papillae on the tongue An ataxic syndrome, probably dominantly inherited, with these features and sensorineural deafness, canal paresis, ageusia, and numerous signs of autonomic disease, thus resembling **hereditary sensory and autonomic neuropathy** types 2 or 3. The onset in the single Japanese report published was in mid-adult life.[1986]

IVa. *Late-onset recessive ataxias*
These are very rare; no diagnostic criteria are available.

Baraitser[335] summarized the reports of the adult-onset cerebellar ataxias in group IV above (cerebellar ataxia plus) and classified them as follows:

1. Syndromes with added ophthalmological signs and pyramidal or extrapyramidal signs
2. Syndromes with added retinitis pigmentosa
3. Syndromes with added peripheral neuropathy; in which features of **hereditary motor and sensory neuropathy** are found in association with cerebellar ataxia. One such syndrome is *Ziegler syndrome,* in which ataxia, rigidity, fasciculations, parkinsonism, and signs of peripheral neuropathy are found.
4. Late-onset pure cerebellar ataxias without associated features. These comprise two groups of "pure" ataxic syndromes with onset in adult life:
   A. *Recessive inheritance* Those ataxias inherited recessively are rarer than other recessive ataxias. They may be variously associated with downbeat nystagmus, hypogonadism, deafness, pigmentary retinopathy, or optic atrophy.
   B. *Dominant inheritance* These are rare syndromes in which affected family members also show other features apart from the ataxia and which thus are not completely pure.[2436]

Cerebellar ataxia is also a feature of the following syndromes, noted elsewhere:

Ataxia-telangiectasia	Chediak-Higashi syndrome
Flynn-Aird syndrome	Hartnup disease
Ketotic hyperglycinemia	Nonketotic hyperglycinemia
Pyruvate decarboxylase deficiency	Richards Rundle syndrome
Intermittent branched-chain ketoaciduria	

See also **Biemond ataxia, Kuru, hypertrophia musculorum vera, periodic ataxias, idiopathic late-onset cerebellar ataxias, Joseph disease, delayed-onset cerebellar syndrome.**

V. *Episodic ataxias* (periodic ataxias, hereditary paroxysmal cerebellar ataxia)

These are channelopathies, of which two dominantly inherited forms are decribed, one with brief attacks from childhood, precipitated by exercise and startle and complicated by jouint contractures and myokymia, mapping to 12p and due to a mutation of the potassium channel gene *KCNA1*. The other is characterized by attacks lasting hours to days, precipitated by stress, exercise, and fatigue, with a progressive cerebellar syndrome and permanent gaze-evoked nystagmus; it maps to 19p. Both respond to acetazolamide.[2407] See also **pyruvate decarboxylase deficiency, pyruvate dehydrogenase deficiency, maple syrup urine disease, Hartnup disease,** and defects of ammomia metabolism.

VI. *Hereditary spastic parapareses/paraplegias*
This final group again includes both pure and complicated forms. An historical review was provided by Konigsmark and Weiner.[3125] See **hereditary spastic paraparesis.**

Adapted from Harding AE. Clinical features and classification of inherited ataxias. Advances in Neurology, *Chapter 1. New York: Raven Press, 1993, and Baraitser M. The Genetics of Neurological Disorders. Oxford: Oxford University Press, 1990. A further classification, relying upon genetic data, will surely be adopted in time.*

cerebellar ataxia with celiac disease The concurrence of these conditions; the patients do not have specific or diagnostic neurological signs other than the ataxia.[4394]

cerebellar ataxia with crossed third nerve palsy (Claude syndrome) A **lacunar syndrome** presenting with dysarthria, cerebellar ataxia, and facial numbness.[1853,1867]

cerebellar ataxia with hypogonadotrophic hypogonadism See **cerebellar ataxias.**

cerebellar ataxia with myoclonus and deafness See **cerebellar ataxias.**

cerebellar ataxia with retained reflexes See **cerebellar ataxias.**

cerebellar ataxia with retinal degeneration See **cerebellar ataxias.**

cerebellar catalepsy sign Oscillation of the trunk and legs of patients with cerebellar lesions when their legs, flexed at the hips and knees, are passively raised from the bed. The sign was described by **Babiński** in 1902, but has not found favor.[285]

cerebellar cataplexy (cerebellar catatonia) The ability of certain patients with cerebellar disease to hold a static posture of the legs with statuesque immobility while they cannot walk or move the legs through space without gross ataxia. The phenomenon differentiates between sensory ataxias and those of cerebellar origin.[1350] This sign was first described by Babiński in 1902.

cerebellar catatonia See **cerebellar cataplexy.**

cerebellar cognitive affective syndrome Behavioral changes occurring in patients with lesions involving the posterior lobe of the cerebellum and the vermis, characterized by impairment of executive functions such as planning, set-shifting, verbal fluency, abstract reasoning, and working memory; difficulties with spatial cognition including visual–spatial organization and memory; personality change with blunting of affect or disinhibited and inappropriate behavior; and language deficits including agrammatism and dysprosodia. Lesions of the anterior lobe of the cerebellum produce only minor changes in executive and visual–spatial functions.

The constellation of deficits is suggestive of disruption of the cerebellar modulation of neural circuits that link prefrontal, posterior parietal, superior temporal, and limbic cortices with the cerebellum.[4973]

cerebellar cortical degeneration   An autoimmune nonmetastatic **paraneoplastic syndrome** of the CNS manifesting evidence of widespread cerebellar atrophy with loss of Purkinje cells, occurring in patients with carcinoma of the bronchus or ovary or with lymphoma, and in which an immunologic response induced by the tumor causes a secondary immune reaction in specific brain areas because of shared antigens.[711]

cerebellar diaschisis   A reduction in blood flow and oxygen utilization in the cerebellar hemisphere contralateral to a supratentorial infarct,[369,370] due to an interruption of afferent input along the corticopontocerebellar pathway.

cerebellar diplegia   The term applied by Frederick **Batten** in 1903 to what is now known as *ataxic cerebral palsy.*

cerebellar disorders   Syndromes characterized by **ataxia, nystagmus,** alterations in muscle tone, and **gait disorder** resulting from disorders affecting the cerebellum or its connections.

These are classified in this book as **cerebellar ataxias** in which there is a known hereditary basis for the condition; as **ataxic syndromes** in which the ataxia is a major feature but no familial tendency is known; and randomly, where cerebellar signs occur as one feature of other syndromes.

cerebellar hemangioblastoma   A malignant vascular tumor of the cerebellum, commonly occurring in patients with **Von Hippel–Lindau** disease.

cerebellar hemisphere hypoplasia   See **cerebellar ataxias.**

cerebellar imitation synkineses   Similar movements occurring in the hand or foot 200 msec or so after the contralateral one is moved. This may occur in patients with cerebellar degenerative diseases.[2891]

cerebellar migraine   A distinct form of late-onset autosomal dominant **cerebellar ataxia** in which the ataxia occurs during recovery from attacks of hemiplegic migraine, the patients ultimately suffering from persistent ataxia, with cerebellar atrophy shown radiologically.[4665] See also **familial hemiplegic migraine.**

cerebellar mutism   (mutism and subsequent dysarthria) Loss of speech a day or two after an acute cerebellar event such as removal of a chronic mid-cerebellar tumor, or with stroke or encephalitis. Speech returns usually within 6 months, but is marred by severe dysarthria. Consciousness is retained and there are no accompanying deficits on examination of the lower cranial nerves, but in children, neurobehavioral disorders and pyramidal signs may be manifest. The mechanism is not determined but the condition is associated with hydrocephalus at presentation, localization of the tumor adjacent to the IV ventricle, and postsurgical edema of the pontine tegmentum.[1305,5724]

cerebellar outflow tremor   See **rubral or midbrain tremor.**

cerebellar posture   A term introduced by **Batten** in 1903 for that position of the head in which "the occiput is turned to one side and the chin to the other and at the same time flexed to the side to which the occiput was directed." The same posture occurs after labyrinthine extirpation and "is the result of interference with a tonic reflex in which the extensor muscles of the neck, under the influence of impulses from the labyrinths, are maintained in a state of tonus adequate to resist the effect of gravity on the head."[706]

cerebellar seizures   See **diencephalic autonomic seizures.**

cerebellar signs   Postural **hypotonia, pendular reflexes, asthenia** and fatigability, **ataxia, decomposition of movement, asynergy, nystagmus, dysmetria, tremor,** loss of associated movements, drooping of the shoulder, and abnormalities in the rate, regularity, and force of voluntary movements occurring as a result of disease of the cerebellum or of its connections.[2625] See **cerebellar tremors.** In patients with cerebellar tumors, symptoms and signs have been defined as vertigo, deafness, tinnitus, weakness in homolateral conjugate gaze, sixth nerve palsies, skew deviation, horizontal jerk nystagmus, involvment of the fifth and seventh cranial nerves, homolateral limb weakness with asthenia, paresis of homolateral trunk muscles, hypotonia of the homolateral limbs, ataxia with reeling gait, intention tremor, postural deficits, and variable muscle stretch reflex activity.[5357]

cerebellar tonic seizures   See **diencephalic autonomic seizures.**

cerebellar tremors   Various forms of involuntary alternating movement due to disease of the cerebellum or of its connections. Such tremors are proximal, occur with movement, displace the limb at right angles to the intended direction of movement, and increase in amplitude when they approach the target. The frequency is usually <5 Hz.

The various forms of cerebellar tremor have been classified by Sabra and Hallet[4864] (see Chart C–11). See also **titubation.**

Chart C–11. Varieties of Cerebellar Tremor

Action tremor A tremor occurring with postural maintenance or goal-directed movement.

Cerebellar tremor at rest A tremor seen when the body part appears to be completely relaxed, although there is actually some slight background muscular contraction.

Epipaxic postural tremor A tremor occurring just after the performance of a goal-directed movement.

Intention tremor (kinetic cerebellar, ataxia or hyperkinetic tremor) A tremor appearing with goal-directed movements, often worse terminally.

Mild postural cerebellar tremor (postural, simple, static, propaxic postural, or epipaxic postural tremors) A mild tremor occurring early or late during sustained postural maintenance or just before (propaxic) or after (epipaxic) a goal-directed movement.

Propaxic postural tremor A tremor occurring just before the performance of a goal-directed movement.

Severe postural cerebellar tremor (rubral, superior cerebellar peduncle, peduncular, or hyperkinetic tremor) A severe tremor at 2.5–4 Hz occurring with postural maintenance, present at rest, persisting during maintenance of a posture, and worsening with goal-directed movements. It is usually associated with **dysmetria.**

Adapted from Sabra AF, Hallett M. Action tremor witrh alternating activity in antagonist muscles. Neurology 1984;34:151–156, by permission.

cerebello-olivary degeneration A dominantly inherited form of cerebellar ataxia[2619] with abnormal motor and sensory conduction in peripheral nerves. See **Holmes disease.**

cerebellopontine angle tumor Any extraaxial mass situated beside the pontomedullary junction and abutting the internal auditory meatus. Pressure upon the roots of cranial nerves V, VII, and VIII and on the cerebellum are responsible for the usual clinical findings.[320] The most common form is the vestibular schwannoma.

cerebellum (Lat, diminutive of brain) The hindbrain, situated in the posterior fossa and behind the pons. It was considered to be the seat of sexual appetite by Fraser (1880) but was shown to function in the coordination of voluntary movements by **Flourens,** and regarded as the head ganglion of the proprioceptive system by **Sherrington.** The name was first applied by Erasistratus, a Greek physician and anatomist, about 300–250 B.C.

cerebral (from Lat, cerebrum, the brain) Pertaining to the brain.

cerebral abscess An infective lesion of the brain substance. Though commonly bacterial, other organisms may produce focal encephalitis with liquefaction and the formation of a capsule, which are the hallmarks of an abscess. *Toxoplasma, Cryptococcus,* and *Mycobacterium tuberculosis* arc all nonpyogenic causes of abscess, but pyogenic abscesses are more common.

Infection may spread hematologically from a distant site, particularly in patients with congenital heart disease, or it may spread directly from infected cranial structures such as the middle ear or the nasal sinuses. The clinical features are those of increased intracranial pressure, focal deficits, and meningeal inflammation in any combination. The frequency of cerebral abscesses, particularly of those due to toxoplasmosis, is now increasing in the wake of the epidemic of HIV infections.

The first systematic account was published in 1856 by Hermann Lebert (1813–1878).

cerebral acanthocytosis A hereditary syndrome of tics, self-mutilation, dystonia, and personality change associated with the presence of acanthocytes in the fresh peripheral blood smear. See **neuroacanthocytosis.**

cerebral akinetopsia (cerebral motion blindness) A syndrome in which a patient loses specifically the ability to perceive visual motion, as a result of cortical lesions outside the striate area.[6116]

cerebral amyloid angiopathy (congophilic angiopathy, cerebral angiopathy, dyshoric angiopathy) An age-related condition characterized by deposition of amyloid fibrils outside the internal elastic lamina of the small and medium-sized leptomeningeal vessels and the pial and cortical arterioles, with acellular thickening of their walls. The amorphous, eosinophilic amyloid material stains with Congo Red and shows birefringence under polarized light. The peripheral vessels are unaffected.

The condition is progressively more common in older populations; it occurs sporadically, but dominantly inherited forms have been described in Iceland and The Netherlands.[2947] The vessels affected are those running from the leptomeninges to the cerebral cortex, leading to hypoperfusion and multiple small infarcts and hemorrhages into the cortex (lobar hemorrhages) and to demyelination of the underlying white matter. Systemic amyloidosis is not present.

Clinically, the picture is that of multiple or recurrent lobar intracerebral hemorrhages with pyramidal signs, internal and external ophthalmoplegias, and dementia (if there are symptoms at all; the condition has been detected in healthy elderly people and in those with **Alzheimer disease** or dementing illnesses of that type[815]). For further discussion of the dementing syndrome, see **congophilic angiopathy.**

Variants are listed under **familial amyloid neuropathy.**

cerebral aneurysmal arteriopathy Diffuse dilation of the arteries arising from the circle of Willis, due to hypoperfusion and/or septic emboli and seen particularly in children with AIDS.[1534]

cerebral angiomas Arteriovenous communications established through the medium of a mass of abnormal cerebral vessels which take the place of the usual capillary bed. The usual clinical presentation is with focal seizures followed by **Todd paresis** in patients aged less than 30 years at the first presentation, and who develop a slowly progressive hemiparesis or sensory loss on the affected side. In some cases, headache, subarachnoid hemorrhage, or the presence of a bruit suggests the diagnosis.[3553]

cerebral angiopathy   (dyshoric angiopathy) See **cerebral amyloid angiopathy.**

cerebral angiopathy of toxemia   Multisegment narrowing of the cerebral arteries resulting from hypertension-induced vasoconstriction in women with toxemia of pregnancy. The syndrome presents with headache, focal neurological signs, seizures, and decreased consciousness, and there may be lymphocytic pleocytosis in the CSF.

The prognosis is generally favorable.[5641]

cerebral apophysis   The pineal gland.

cerebral apoplexy   Intracerebral hemorrhage.

cerebral atonic-astatic syndrome   See **Forster syndrome.**

cerebral auscultation   See **cephalic bellows sound.**

cerebral autosomal dominant arteriopathy with subcortical infarcts and leukoencephalopathy (CADASIL)   A dominantly inherited, systemic vascular disease and a cause of multiple infarcts in adults, mainly in the white matter, basal ganglia, and leptomeninges. The clinical presentation is usually with multiple episodes of migraine (usually associated with aura) in young adult life, leading later to recurrent subcortical infarcts with pseudobulbar palsy and vascular dementia. Other manifestations appearing within 20 years of onset include gait disturbance, pseudobulbar palsy, mood disturbances, neurosensory hearing loss, urinary incontinence, cognitive impairment, and seizures. The dementia has a subcortical and frontal presentation, with behavioral symptoms, amnesia, disturbed executive functions, bradyphrenia, slowing of information processing, and frontal symptoms without aphasia, apraxia, or agnosia.

The condition is due to a Notch 3 mutation on chromosome 19p13 (or 19p12). Histopathologically, an eosinophilic granular deposit is seen in the media of the small penetrating cerebral arteries causing vascular obliteration and multiple infarcts, mainly in the white matter, basal ganglia, and leptomeninges. Magnetic resonance imaging shows hyperintensities in the periventricular and deep white matter, basal ganglia, and brainstem, but the diagnosis is best made by skin biopsy, which shows granular, electron-dense osmophilic material.[951,1598,4844]

cerebral beriberi   See **Wernicke syndrome.**

cerebral blood flow   The totality of the volume of blood delivered to the brain. This is usually constant at 55 ml/100 g/min if the pCO_2 is constant, depending on local activation. Measurement is with intracarotid or inhaled Xenon[133,] a gamma emitter, using the Kety-Schmidt equation (the amount of a substance entering or leaving the brain in a given time is equal to the difference in its arteriovenous concentration times blood flow; thus the cerebral metabolic rate of oxygen = $PaO_2 - PvO_2 \times$ blood flow).

Two clearance rates are normally measured: fast from gray matter and slow from white matter and scalp.

cerebral calcifications and cerebellar hypoplasia   A congenital syndrome of optic nerve colobomas leading to blindness with hypotonia, myoclonic seizures, microcephaly, quadriplegia, and mental and developmental delay.

Cerebral and cerebellar atrophy with intracranial calcifications and the **Dandy-Walker malformation** are also found.[337]

cerebral calculi   (brain stones) Large, solitary, or multiple, well-circumscribed, bony hard areas of pathological cerebral calcification, within preexisting cerebral tumors, hemorrhage, inflammation, or degenerative pathology. Clinically, if symptomatic, they usually present with recurrent seizures.[5581]

cerebral cortex   (Gr, brain + rind or bark) The outer surface of the brain, composed largely of neuronal cell bodies and glial tissue. The six-layered cortex was first described and illustrated by Berlin in his inaugural thesis of 1858; following this insight, he continued on to become a distinguished ophthalmologist. Three- and four-layered cortex is also found, the former as the olfactory cortex and the latter as the cerebral expression of the limbic system.

cerebral death   See **brain death.**

cerebral diplegia   See **Little disease.** The term applied by Sigmund **Freud** to cerebral palsies with bilateral involvement. The condition had been recognized, however, by Nicholas André in 1741.

cerebral diplopia   (polyopia) A rare symptom of perception of more than one object as a result of a lesion of the occipital lobe. The underlying mechanism is not precisely determined.[452]

cerebral dominance   Specialization of one hemisphere for the performance of a function in humans and animals, influenced by both genetic and nongenetic factors.

Dominance varies according to the modality examined; thus, while almost all right-handers have left hemispheric dominance for speech, so do at least 60% of left-handers. Commonly, the left hemisphere is dominant for language and manual skills, while the right is more involved in certain spatial and musical abilities, attention, and many aspects of emotion.[2083]

Broca in 1863 and **Dax** in 1865 first stated that language functions resided in the left hemisphere in right-handed people.

cerebral dropsy   See **hydrocephalus.**

cerebral dyschromatopsia   Acquired defects in color perception resulting (rarely) from cerebral lesions, usually in the parietal or occipital regions.[4381]

cerebral dysgenesis   Disorders of embryological development of the brain. These have been classified by Cochrane and colleagues[1063a] as follows (see Chart C–12).

Chart C–12. Types of Cerebral Dysgenesis

A. *Dysgenesis presenting because of or associated with ventriculomegaly.*
   1. Hydrocephalus is usually present.
      Dandy-Walker syndrome
      Aqueductal stenosis
      Chiari type 2 malformation
      Lhermitte-Duclos disease
   2. Hydrocephalus may not be present.
      Lobar **holoprosencephaly**
      Agenesis of the corpus callosum associated with a dorsal sac.
   3. Hydrocephalus is not usually present.
      Alobar **holoprosencephaly**
      Megalencephaly
      Periventricular **heterotopias**
B. *Dysgenesis presenting because of craniofacial dysmorphism*
   1. **Encephalocele** (occipital/frontobasal/sphenoidal)
   2. **Amniotic band syndrome**
C. *Dysgenesis presenting because of focal neurological dysfunction*
   1. Hypothalamic hamartomas
   2. Cortical dysplasia
   3. **Chiari malformation**

Adapted from Cochrane DD, Poskitt KJ, Normal MG. Surgical implications of cerebral dysgenesis. Can J Neurol Sci 1991;18:181–195, by kind permission.

cerebral edema   An increase in the volume of the brain as a result of an increase in the water content of the brain itself. Three major forms are recognized:[1875]

Vasogenic edema, which is due to increased capillary permeability, as with tumors, abscess, or purulent meningitis resulting from damage to the vessel walls. The fluid, a protein-containing filtrate, collects mainly in the white matter, increasing the extracellular fluid volume.

Cytotoxic edema, in which cellular swelling affects the neurons and glia in both the gray and white matter, as with hypoxia or hypo-osmolality states. The extracelluar volume is decreased here.

Interstitial edema, in which there is increased brain fluid due to a reduction in absorption of CSF. This occurs initially in the periventricular white matter, as in obstructive hydrocephalus. The extracellular fluid volume is increased.

cerebral embolism   Occlusion of a cerebral blood vessel by a clot of blood or a mass of other material (cholesterol, air, cardiac valve fragments, etc.). This may be symptomless or may lead to clinical evidence of a stroke syndrome.[948] See **cardiogenic embolism.**

cerebral enlargement   See **normal pressure hydrocephalus.**

cerebral equipotentiality   The concept that all parts of the cortex are functionally equivalent. The concept was propounded by Golz in 1812 and grew during the eighteenth century, gaining further strength from **Flourens'** and **Lashley's** demonstrations that intelligent behavior in rats (learning to run mazes after ablation of their cerebral cortex) was determined by the amount of tissue removed rather than by the actual site of its removal. Lashley called this the Law of Mass Action, but he himself modified this later by suggesting that *area* rather that *total* equipotentiality was more likely.

cerebral gigantism   (Sotos syndrome) A dominantly inherited or sporadic congenital dysmorphic syndrome characterized by increased birth weight and body length for the first 5 years or so of life, with the rapid development of acromegalic features, accelerated skeletal maturation, macrocrania, hypertelorism, dolichocephaly or scaphocephaly, renal tumors, seizures, strabismus, and mental and developmental delay. Prognathism, antimongolian slant, high-arched palate, mental retardation, and ataxia are other usual clinical signs.[5262]

cerebral granulomatous angiitis   See **isolated angiitis of the nervous system.**

cerebral hemispheric attention vise   The right hemisphere is considered to activate spacial representational mechanisms in both hemispheres, while the left can only activate its own. Damage to the right hemisphere then causes reduced arousal in both hemispheres, prevents left hemispheric symptoms from compensating for the deficit, and results in left-sided neglect, whereas damage to the left-hand side will still allow the right hemisphere to function in overcoming right-sided neglect.[3054]

cerebral hemorrhage   Bleeding into the brain substance. Most commonly, this occurs as a result of the rupture of small, deep, penetrating arterioles in the basal ganglia, deep cerebral white matter, pons, or cerebellum, typically in hypertensive patients, but trauma, hemostatic disorders, and vascular pathologies such as aneurysms and angiomas are other important, if less common, causes.

A *variant* is *lobar cerebral hemorrhage,* in which the bleeding is into the cortex or the subjacent white matter, usually as a result of local structural disease, trauma, or **cerebral amyloid angiopathy.**

cerebral hydatid disease   The presence of intracerebral cysts as accidental parasites of echinococcus granularis. The condition is usually seen in children who come into close contact with dogs in sheep-rearing areas. The symptoms are mainly of raised intracranial pressure, seizures, and focal signs with the Schroeder tetrad.[6030] Rupture of the cyst, most often due to puncture during surgery when the disease was neither anticipated nor diagnosed preoperatively, produces a chamical meningeal reaction that may be lethal.

Craniovertebral hydatid disease is a *variant* condition in which hydatid cysts are found mainly within the lower thoracic vertebrae or in extraspinal soft tissue masses that infiltrate or compress the spinal cord or, with high cervical lesions, cause cranial nerve pareses.[5003,5004] See also **Schroeder tetrad.**

cerebral hypoperfusion   Reduction in blood supply to the whole brain (or to a defined region of the brain) to such a degree as to induce symptoms.

cerebral hypoxia   A reduction in the supply of oxygen to the brain to such as degree as to induce symptoms. This may reflect either **cerebral hypoperfusion** or a diminution of the arterial p_aO_2.

cerebral infantile paralysis   (Strumpell disease) Poliomyelitis extending from its usual major site of attack in the spinal cord, to cause encephalitis. See **Strumpell disease.**

cerebral infarction   Irreversible ischemic damage to all cell types within a region of the brain, usually following incomplete ischemia.

cerebral ischemia   That condition marked by inadequate blood supply to the brain, either locally or globally and with or without symptoms arising as a result.

cerebral lymphoma   (microglioma) Primary malignant lymphomas of the CNS. Spinal (extradural) lymphomas also occur. See **primary CNS lymphoma, HIV.**

cerebral malaria   A diffuse encephalopathy following infection with *Plasmodium falciparum*, transmitted by the bites of female anopheles mosquitoes. The condition is found in Central Africa, Southeast Asia, South America, India, and Central America, but cerebral complications ensue in only some 2% of cases of *P. falciparum* infection, mainly in infants and those who have had no previous exposure to such infection.

Such complications are due to occlusion of small cerebral vessels by clumps of cells and plasmodia, giving rise to a number of defined syndromes reflecting the numerous vessels that may be occluded. Clinically, chills, rigors, and headache, followed by periods of high fever with delirium, more severe headache, and abdominal pain occur at 48-hour intervals. Neurologically, meningitic, mono- or hemiplegic, cerebellar, myelitic, aphasic, and comatose forms, and others manifesting various focal neurological syndromes resulting from spinal or peripheral nerve involvement, are reported.[1289,6030]

In adults, criteria for the diagnosis have been suggested.[4120,4121]

cerebral metastases   Secondary tumors of the brain or meninges, arising most commonly from the lung, breast, kidney, or thyroid gland. Choriocarcinomas, malignant melanoma, and leukemias are the other more common types of secondary malignancy directly affecting the nervous system.

cerebral microangiopathy   See **idiopathic calcification of the basal ganglia.**

cerebral motion blindness   See **cerebral akinetopsia.**

cerebral nerve   See **cranial nerve.**

cerebral palsy   (Little disease) A symptom complex comprising nonprogressive (but not unchanging) disorders of posture and movement, sometimes with epilepsy, visuomotor, or other learning difficulties or extrapyramidal syndromes, secondary to lesions or anomalies of the brain arising in the early stages of its development or (in a minority of cases) to postneonatal events such as meningoencephalitis, vascular occlusion, or trauma.

The condition is classed as a **static encephalopathy** and is segregated according to the extremities involved—hence mono-, hemi-, di-, and quadriplegic forms. It is supposed to arise as a result of cerebral insults, either congenital or sustained during pregnancy (such as anoxia or infections), or in the perinatal period (such as intracerebral hemorrhage or anoxia), but major risk factors include maternal mental retardation, the presence of congenital malformations outside the CNS, birth weight below 2000 g, and breech presentation (though not breech delivery). Most affected children do not show evidence of severe fetal distress during labor nor of depression of cerebral function in the neonatal period.[835,4095] A discussion of causes and mechanisms has been published.[3174]

Named varieties include the following:
Ataxic cerebral palsy
Ataxic diplegia A combination of **ataxic cerebral palsy** and signs of corticospinal tract dysfunction
Athetoid type A congenital syndrome manifesting cerebellar ataxia, with rigidity, athetosis, and often dystonia. See **athetoid syndrome.**
Dyskinetic cerebral palsy
Hemiparetic cerebral palsy
Hypotonic cerebral palsy
Spastic cerebral palsy (**Little disease**) A congenital syndrome manifesting microcephaly, pyramidal signs (hemiparesis, paraparesis, quadriparesis), spasticity, athetosis, myoclonus, and mental and developmental delay.

An historical review has been published.[2739] See also **Little, W.J.; Gowers, W.; Hammond, W.; Foerster, W.**

Cerebral Palsy Bulletin   See *Developmental Medicine and Child Neurology.*

cerebral peduncle syndrome   (Leyden syndrome) See **Weber syndrome.**

cerebral perfusion pressure   The difference between the mean arterial blood pressure and the intracranial pressure. Cerebral blood flow can usually be maintained by autoregulation until the perfusion pressure falls below 40 mmHg.

cerebral pseudosclerosis   See **Wilson disease.**

cerebral ptosis   Bilateral, often asymmetrical ptosis occurring in association with acute right hemisphere lesions and conjugate deviation of the eyes to the right.[1565,3351]

cerebral radionecrosis   Necrosis of brain tissue as a late complication of prior radiotherapy.

Clinically, the damaged brain tissue acts as an expanding mass lesion, producing increased intracranial pressure, focal deficits, and seizures, or causes a milder syndrome of progressive intellectual deficits with seizures.

cerebral salt-wasting syndrome   Natriuresis despite hyponatremia and contraction of the extracellular volume, occurring in the presence of an intracerebral lesion. See **syndrome of inappropriate ADH secretion.**

cerebral signs, nonspecific   Nonlocalizing but suggestive evidence of organic pathology in the brain. These include **perseveration, drowsiness,** irritability, inversion of sleep rhythms, **amnesia,** and personality changes.

cerebral thrombosis   The occlusion of an artery supplying the brain as a result of disease of the arterial wall in situ, as opposed to embolism from a point in the vascular system closer to the heart. The result is commonly atherothrombotic brain infarction.

cerebral tumors   Benign or malignant tumors of the brain. By popular extension, tumors of the meninges and blood vessels may also be included with them, although properly these are intracranial/intraspinal but not necessarily cerebral. A listing is given in Chart C–13.

Chart C–13. Neuroectodermal Tumors

Astrocytoma
Glioblastoma
Oligodendroglioma
Cerebellar astrocytoma
Medulloblastoma
Brainstem glioma
Ependymoma

Other Tumors

Meningioma
Hemangioma, hemangioblastoma
Secondary tumors
Lymphoproliferative diseases
Chordoma
Neurofibromas
Neurilemmoma
Craniopharyngioma
Pituitary adenoma
Reticulum cell sarcoma (microgliomatosis)

cerebral vasculitis   Inflammatory disease of the arteries supplying the brain. See **giant cell arteritis, isolated benign cerebral vasculitis.**

cerebral venous thrombosis   Thrombotic occlusion of the great venous sinuses or of other cerebral veins; the superior sagittal sinus is that most often affected. Both septic and aseptic forms are recognized; the former are less common than in past years while the latter have occurred, especially in young adults, with a wide range of associated diseases, most of which impact upon coagulation.[270,5730]

Clinical syndromes resulting include the usual features of raised intracranial pressure; headache; reduced conscious level; seizures; and various focal deficits pointing to the hemispheric or posterior fossa lesion, which is usually a venous infarct.[271,686] The causes have been reviewed.[685]

See also **cord sign, empty delta sign.**

cerebral ventricostium   The spontaneous formation of a communication between the cerebral ventricles and the surface of the brain in patients with hydrocephalus.[2915]

cerebration   The use of the brain; thinking (colloquial).

Cerebri Anatome   The anatomical masterpiece of Thomas **Willis,** published in 1664.

cerebritis   Inflammation of the substance of the brain. The term is most commonly employed to denote the earliest stages of pyogenic infection, which progress to abscess formation.

cerebroarthrodigital syndrome   A congenital dysmorphic syndrome characterized by absence of the sacrum, reduction deformity of the arms, absent fingers or oligodactyly, brachydactyly, joint contractures, hypoplasia of muscles, microcephaly, and hydrocephalus.[5302]

cerebrocardiac neurosis   See **depersonalisation.**

cerebrocerebellar lissencephaly   A congenital malformation characterized by **lissencephaly** of the cerebrum, cerebellum, and corpus callosum, with mental and developmental delay.[4157] See **lissencephaly.**

cerebrocostomandibular syndrome   A congenital, recessively inherited dysmorphic syndrome characterized by dwarfism, micrognathia, cleft palate, narrow thorax, tracheal anomalies, and mental and developmental delay.[5161]

cerebrofaciothoracic dysplasia   See **Pascual-Castroviejo syndrome.**

cerebrohepatorenal syndrome   See **Zellweger disease.**

cerebromacular degeneration (cerebromacular dystrophy, Stock-Spielmeyer-Vogt disease) See **gangliosidoses, neuronal ceroid lipofuscinosis.**

cerebromacular dystrophy   See **cerebromacular degenerations.**

cerebromalacia   (Lat, and Gr, brain + softness) Local softening of the brain, usually as the result of ischemia.

cerebromedullary disconnection   See **locked-in syndrome.**

cerebro-ocular dysgenesis   See **Walker-Warburg syndrome.**

cerebro-ocular dysplasia with muscular dystrophy See **congenital muscular dystrophy** (*variants*), **Walker-Warburg syndrome.**

cerebro-oculofacioskeletal syndrome   A recessively inherited congenital dysmorphic syndrome characterized by microphthalmia, cataract, blepharophimosis, micrognathia, rocker-bottom feet, vertical talus bones, camptodactyly, intracranial calcifications, agenesis of the corpus callosum, microcephaly, and mental and developmental delay.[4399] See **Pena-Shokeir syndrome.**

cerebro-oculomuscular syndrome   (COMS) A congenital syndrome characterized by cloudy corneas, microphthalmia, colobomas of the iris, cataract, hypoplasia of the optic nerve or retina, optic atrophy, pigmentary retinopathy, and blindness, with adducted thumbs, joint contractures, macrocephaly, distal myopathic weakness, cerebral atrophy, aqueduct stenosis, hydrocephalus, lissencephaly, the **Dandy-Walker malformation,** and mental and developmental delay.[2514] See **congenital muscular dystrophy, Walker-Warburg syndrome.**

cerebro-osteonephrodysplasia   A congenital dysmorphic syndrome characterized also by dwarfism; large tongue; umbilical hernia; protuberant abdomen; enlarged liver and spleen; skeletal anomalies including clefts of the vertebrae, platyspondyly, brachycephaly, microcephaly, delayed closure of fontanelles, camptodactyly, and rhizomelia of the limbs; nephropathy; seizures; spasticity; fasciculations; cerebral atrophy; hydrocephalus; and mental and developmental delay.[337]

cerebroretinal angiomatosis   See **von Hippel–Lindau disease.**

cerebroretinal arteriovenous aneurysm   See **Wyburn-Mason syndrome.**

cerebroretinal degeneration   See **neuronal ceroid lipofuscinosis.**

cerebroretinal lipofuscinosis   See **neuronal ceroid lipofuscinosis.**

cerebroretinal vasculopathy   (hereditary cerebroretinal vasculopathy) A rare, dominantly inherited disorder presenting with progressive visual loss, dysarthria, intellectual decline, and gait disturbances starting after the age of 30 years and due to the presence of abnormalities of small blood vessels in the retina and brain and of cerebral pseudotumors. Periventricular leukoencephalopathy suggesting small vessel occlusions is evident on MRI scans.[2255]

cerebroside   Phosphate-free nitrogenous lipids containing galactose and found in brain myelin.

cerebroside lipidosis   See **glucosylceramide lipidosis.**

cerebrospinal   Relating both to the brain and the spinal cord.

cerebrospinal block syndrome   See **Zange-Kindler syndrome.**

cerebrospinal fever   Meningococcal meningitis.

cerebrospinal fluid   (CSF) A clear, watery secretion of the choroid plexus and brain. The existence of the CSF was proved by Domenic **Cotugno** (1736–1822), an Italian anatomist, in 1764, but the term was not used until introduced by Magendie in 1827.[5204] The first analyses of the fluid were performed nearly a hundred years later (Corning, 1855), preceding the studies of **Quincke.**

The fluid is formed principally by the choroid plexus within the ventricles but also from brain extracellular fluid, enters the subarachnoid space through the foramina of Luschka and **Magendie,** and circulates (the third circulation of Harvey **Cushing**) down into the spinal canal before rising again and passing diffusely over the hemispheres to its final site of absorption by the pacchionian granulations in the dural venous sinuses, minimal amounts also being absorbed through the arachnoid root sleeves along the cranial and spinal nerve roots. It functions as a protective support for the brain and cord, as a pathway for neurotransmitters, as a metabolic sink, and possibly as a coolant. The methods of secretion and absorption and the normal pressure, cytology, and biochemistry of the fluid have been reviewed.[1236,1875,3527]

cerebrospinal fluid fistula headache   The following diagnostic criteria are suggested by the Headache Classification Committee of the International Headache Society:[1051]

A. Post-traumatic, postoperative, or idiopathic CSF leak demonstrated by measurement of glucose concentration in leaking fluid, or by leakage of spinally injected dye or radioactive tracer

B. Headache characteristics as for **post–lumbar puncture headache**

C. Headache disappears within 14 days after effective treatment of fistula

(Reproduced with permission from Classification of headache disorders, cranial neuralgias and facial pains, and diagnostic criteria for primary headache disorders. *Cephalalgia* 1988;**8**[suppl]:1–96).

cerebrospinal fluid hypovolemia   See **idiopathic intracranial hypotension**

cerebrospinal fluid rhinorrhea   Escape of CSF through the anterior cranial fossa to the nasal cavities. The causes are divided between those which are traumatic and those which are not, the latter group including cases of high- and normal-pressure leaks.[4238]

cerebrotendinous xanthomatosis (cholestanolosis; OMIM 213700) A rare autosomal recessive lipid storage disease characterized by the deposition of cholestanol (a cholesterol metabolite) in the body tissues (replacing cholesterol in the myelin of the central and peripheral nervous systems) and by raised plasma levels of cholestanol; the result of a defect in the activity of sterol 27-hydroxylase, a mitochondrial enzyme responsible for the synthesis of bile acids.[5708] The genetic abnormality maps to 2q33–ter.

Clinically, the disease is manifest in early life with cataracts, xanthomatous swelling of tendons (particularly the Achilles tendons), mild mental slowing, ataxia and eventually cerebellar and pyramidal signs, and a sensorimotor peripheral neuropathy. Seizures, early atheroma, osteoporosis, bone fractures, pes cavus, hypercholestanolemia, and myopathic facies are other features. The condition progresses to a state of spastic, dysarthric helplessness and death, usually before the age of 30 years.[498,2439] The condition was first described by van Bogaert in 1937.

cerebrovascular disease   See **strokes.**

Cerebrovascular Diseases A neurological subspecialty journal. Address: S. Karger AG, P.O. Box 10, Allschwilerstrasse, CH-4009 Basel, Switzerland. Web site: http://www.karger.ch/journals/ced/ced_jh.htm.

cerebrovascular insufficiency The term of **Denny-Brown** denoting episodes of focal reversible ischemia of the brain resulting from failure of the collateral blood supply, as occur during systemic hypotension in people with severe but previously subclinical carotid or vertebrobasilar disease, leading to a reduction in perfusion pressure in defined brain regions.[6119]

Cardiac abnormalities or mere postural change may be responsible for the hypotensive episodes. The clinical effects include brief, repetitive episodes of transient neurological dysfunction (amaurosis, clumsiness, weakness, paresthesias, etc.), frequently with involuntary jerking of the affected limbs, accompanied by slow activity on the EEG.[2057] See also **limb shaking.**

cerebrovascular reserve 1. The capacity of the brain to withstand a limited period of ischemia without undergoing infarction. 2. The capacity of the cerebral circulation to protect the brain from the potentially damaging effects of ischemia by maintaining the delivery of glucose and oxygen despite reductions in local or global perfusion pressure.

cerebrovascular syphilis A form of tertiary syphilis in which arteritis leads to vascular occlusion, usually in the territory of the middle cerebral artery, after a prolonged prodrome of nonspecific headaches, malaise, vertigo, insomnia, etc. The CSF cell count, protein, and serology findings are always abnormal.

cerebrum (Lat, the brain) Originally the whole thing, but the cerebellum was differentiated by Erasistratus in

the third century B.C. The word appeared in English in 1565.[5204]

ceroid An acid-fast, sudanophilic fluorescent substance of unknown chemical composition which is found in human tissues such as liver, muscle, intestine, and nervous system, in association with several disease processes. See **lipofuscin.**

ceroid lipofuscinosis See **neuronal ceroid lipofuscinosis.**

ceroid storage disease A disease resulting from an inborn metabolic error and once known as *Landing-Oppenheim disease,*[3251] but now subdivided according to the causative chemical deficits. See **neuronal ceroid lipofuscinosis.**

ceruleus See **caeruleus.** Lat, sky-blue.

ceruloplasmin deficiency with hemosiderosis A hereditary syndrome of progressive dementia, extrapyramidal disorders, cerebellar ataxia, and diabetes mellitus with low-serum cereloplasmin and raised ferritin levels, reported from Japan.[3990]

cerveau isolé A physiological preparation, with the brain (classically of a cat) being isolated from the remainder of the CNS by a cut at the intercollicular level, just beneath the third nerve nucleus.[735] Interruption of the activity of the ascending reticular activating system leads to permanent sleep, apart from the motor and sensory effects.

cervical (from Lat, the neck). Pertaining to the neck.

cervical acceleration injury See **whiplash.**

cervical band syndrome A form of **thoracic outlet syndrome,** supposed to be produced by pressure upon the lower fibers of the brachial plexus by a fibrous tissue remnant stretching from the transverse processes of the lowest cervical vertebra to the clavicle. The existence of such bands, which are visible only to surgeons and which cannot be imaged, must be very uncommon.

cervical dystonia (spasmodic torticollis, idiopathic cervical dystonia [ICD]) The most common form of adult-onset focal **dystonia** characterized by sustained involuntary contractions of the neck muscles, which result in abnormal movements and postures of the head and neck. Tremor may be associated.[2810] Dystonia in other regions and concomitant head or hand tremor are also present in a minority of cases. When the onset is in adult life the symptoms do not generalize, but segmental spread may occur and pain can increase independent of the dystonia.

Because the movements are not always spasmodic and because torticollis is not the invariable clinical result of the muscle contractions (**laterocollis, retrocollis,** and **antecollis** also occur), the alternative term is now preferred to that used for over a century. The etiology is unknown; painful trauma may be involved in the pathogenesis of the condition but the underlying physiology is speculative. In inherited adult-onset cervical dystonia, linkage to chromosome 18p has been demonstrated.[1300]

cervical migraine   (posterior cervical sympathetic syndrome of Barré, Bartschi-Rochaix syndrome, cervical vertigo syndrome) A syndrome characterized by occipital headache, scotomas, vertigo, tinnitus, vasomotor disorders, paresthesiae, facial spasm, and neck stiffness, ascribed by M.J. Barré[373] to irritation of the sympathetic plexus around the vertebral artery in patients with cervical arthropathy.

Whether this represents **migraine** or **vertebrobasilar insufficiency** or arises as a result of structural pathology in the cervical spine is not determined.[4161] See also **cervicogenic headache.**

cervical nystagmus   (neck torsion nystagmus, vertebrobasilar insufficiency nystagmus) A form of jerk nystagmus with or without other vestibular signs, supposed to result from lesions of the proprioceptive mechanisms in the cervical cord, but which is commonly due either to toxicity or to positional changes.

cervical radiculopathy   Compression or ischemia of the cervical nerve roots as a result of local degenerative or other disease.

The clinical features have been analyzed and comprise pain in the neck, shoulders, arm, or forearm; paresthesias, muscle weakness and atrophy, hyporeflexia, and objective disturbances of sensation in the appropriate dermatomal distributions.[6084] The following diagnostic criteria have been suggested:
1. Symptoms
   A. Pain in the neck, the arm, or both
   B. Paresthesias, dysesthesias, or hypesthesia in nerve root distribution
   C. Muscle weakness
2. Signs
   A. Sensory changes in dermatomal distribution
   B. Weakness, atrophy, or fasciculation in myotomal distribution
   C. Unilaterally diminished muscle stretch reflexes
3. Diagnostic procedures
   A. EMG evidence of acute denervation in cervical paraspinal muscles or in a myotome
   B. Demonstrable abormality on myelography, CT-assisted myelography, or MRI, correlating with the clinical features
   C. Identification of an affected cervical root at operation

The diagnosis of definite radiculopathy can be made in the presence of criteria 3C; 3A; 2A, 2B, and 2C; or 3B and 1A and either 1B or 1C. The diagnosis of probable radiculopathy can be made in the presence of more than one of criteria 1A, 1B, and 1C with any one of criteria 2; or with any one of criteria 1 with 3B; or 1A with any two of criteria 2.

Cervical radiculopathy is deemed *not* present if only one of criteria 1 is present; in the presence of an abnormal imaging test without evidence of a recent radiculopathy; or if the EMG changes suggest chronicity rather than a recent cervical root injury (amended from the criteria of Dr. William J. Litchy, with many thanks).

cervical rib   A benign anomaly, first described by Naffziger[4060] and sometimes detected in patients who complain of neck or arm pain and who are then at risk of operation to remove the rib, which is thought to be causing a **thoracic outlet syndrome.**

cervical spinal muscular atrophy   See **hereditary motor neuropathy, type 1.**

cervical spondylosis   Degenerative changes in the vertebrae and their joints and in the annulus fibrosus of the disks with or without accompanying arthritis of the synovial joints of the cervical spine (cervical osteoarthritis) leading to any combination of degeneration or prolapse of the intervertebral disks, thickening and buckling of the ligamentum flavum, and osteophyte formation.[4375] The local fibrosis, hypertrophy, and distortion lead sometimes to ischemic or compressive effects upon the spinal cord and nerve roots at the affected levels.

The condition was recognized as a cause of paraplegia by Strümpell in 1888, but only in 1926 was it shown (by Eliott) that spondylotic narrowing of the intervertebral foramina could lead to radicular symptoms.[710]

cervical spondylotic myelopathy   Ischemic-compressive disease of the spinal cord resulting from degenerative arthropathy of the cervical spine, in particular affecting the intervertebral disks and the zygapophyseal joints and leading to hypertrophy of the ligamentum flavum. Disc protrusion compounds the clinical deficit.[5487] Clinically, compression leads to conduction block in the cord, especially between C3 and C5, producing pyramidal signs and evidence of root compression. Compression of the vertebral arteries augmenting cord ischemia is another complication.

The condition had attracted little attention until the papers of Brain and Wilkinson demonstrated the ability of such incursions upon the spinal canal to compromise the functions of the cord at this site. The further studies of Yoss et al.[6084] confirmed the clinical and radiological picture, which is composed of the triad of reduced mobility of the neck, long tract signs below (often far below) the level of the lesion(s), and local radiculopathic features.

Thoracic myelopathy is far less common; local tumors or disk herniation are the more common causes.

See also **midcervical central cord syndrome.**

cervical sympathetic irritation syndrome   See **Pourfour du Petit syndrome.**

cervical vertigo   Subjective hallucinations of rotational acceleration thought likely to arise as a result of lesions of the cervical proprioceptive mechanisms. The existence of the phenomenon in humans is, however, controversial.[726]

cervical vertigo syndrome See **cervical migraine.**

cervicobrachial neuralgia Pain felt in the neck and referred to the regions of the arm supplied by the four lower cervical and the first thoracic roots.

cervicocollic reflex A muscle stretch reflex allowing compensatory adjustments to the position of the head in response to neck and truncal movements.

cervicogenic headache Recurrent, persistent, uni- or bilateral, moderate to severe pulsating head pain in any region, referred from a primary nociceptive source in the musculoskeletal tissues innervated by the cranial nerves, but usually associated with disease of the cervical spine.

Consistent reproduction of the pain by neck movement, painful limitation of neck movement, accentuation of pain with sudden head movement, abnormal postures of the head and neck, abnormal mobility of the craniocervical junction, and sensory abnormalities implicating the upper cervical cord or lower medulla are features characteristically associated.[1604] Dizziness, conjunctival injection, phonophobia, photophobia, nausea, and vomiting are also described, which have led to persistent concerns since Liveing's contention in 1873 that the differentiation of this condition from **migraine** is inappropriate.[1603] Although neck structures play a role in the pathophysiology of some headaches, clinical patterns indicating a neck–headache relationship have still not been adequately defined. Further rigorous studies are needed to confirm the validity of cervicogenic headache as an entity.[3349]

Diagnostic criteria have been suggested[5198] (see Chart C–14). However, the validity of the syndrome is not universally accepted. See also **posterior cervical sympathetic syndrome, cervical migraine.**

Chart C–14. Diagnostic Criteria for Cervicogenic Headache

Following is a variant form of the diagnostic criteria proposed by Sjaastad et al. (1990).[5198] and reviewed by Antonaci et al.:[189]

1. Unilateral headache without side shift
2. Symptoms and signs of neck involvement
   a. Pain triggered by neck movement and/or sustained awkward position and/or external pressure over the ipsilateral upper, posterior neck, or occipital region
   b. Ipsilateral neck, shoulder, and arm pain of a rather vague, nonradicular nature
   c. Reduced range of motion in the cervical spine
3. Pain episodes of varying duration or fluctuating, continuous pain
4. Moderate, non-excruciating pain, usually of a non-throbbing nature
5. Pain starting in the neck, eventually spreading to oculofrontotemporal areas, where the maximum pain is often located
6. Anaesthetic blockades of the major occipital nerve and/or

the C2 root or other appropriate blockades on the symptomatic side abolish the pain transiently, provided
   a. Complete anesthesia is obtained or
   b. A whiplash (neck trauma) is sustained a relatively short time prior to the onset
7. Various attack-related phenomena include autonomic symptoms and signs, nausea, vomiting (ipsilateral edema), and flushing mostly in the periocular area; dizziness; photo- and phonophobia; and blurred vision on the eye ipsilateral to the pain.

cervicolinguomasticatory syndrome (Kulenkampff-Tarnow syndrome) Probably an earlier description of **Meige syndrome.** See **tardive dyskinesia.**

cervico-ocular reflex (neck-eye loop) A postural reflex elicited by angular motion of the trunk relative to the fixed head or vice versa, holding still the position of the eyes and head to ensure gaze stability during movement of the trunk.[771]

cervico-oculoacoustic syndrome See **Wildervanck syndrome.**

cervico-osteofacial syndrome See **Wildervanck syndrome.**

CES-D Scale See **Center for Epidemiologic Studies Depression Scale.**

Céstan, Étienne Jacques-Marie-Raymond (1872–1933) French neurologist and psychiatrist who worked at the **Salpétrière** for some years as *chef de clinique* to **Raymond,** before returning to his native Toulouse, where he practiced as professor of mental and nervous diseases or of clinical medicine.

His publications spanned numerous areas of neuropathology and clinical neurology without any one focus.

Céstan syndrome (Céstan-Chenais syndrome) Unilateral paralysis of the soft palate and vocal cords with **Horner syndrome,** ataxia, alternating hemiplegia and hemianesthesia for proprioception, and discriminative touch (medial lemniscus); the spinothalamic fibers, placed laterally, are spared.

The syndrome is due to infarction of the medial part of the medullary tegmentum as a result of vertebral artery occlusion below the origin of the posterior inferior cerebellar artery.[950] It was first described by Dr. Céstan and by Dr. L.J. Chenais (1872–1950), who was also a French physician.

Céstan-Chenais syndrome See **Céstan syndrome.**

Céstan-Lejonne syndrome See **Emery-Dreifuss syndrome.**

cGy The unit of measurement of radiation.

Chaddock, Charles Gilbert (1861–1936) American neurologist and psychiatrist who trained in Michigan and later in Paris under **Babiński** at the Bicêtre. He became professor of neurological diseases at the St. Louis

University School of Medicine. He is remembered for the sign next following and for having translated Kraft-Ebing's work *Psychopathia Sexualis* and some of **Babiński**'s papers into English.[1750]

Chaddock reflex   1. (*external malleolar sign*) A variant method of eliciting the **Babiński reflex** (plantar reflex) by scratching the skin below the lateral malleolus from behind forward, its advantage being the lesser amount of withdrawal excited. There is evidence that this is the only method with greater sensitivity than the original.[953] The same method had been described by Kisaku Yoshimura, a Japanese physician, in 1906, 5 years before Chaddock's description. The reversed Chaddock sign[5494] is the same thing done (obviously) backwards. 2. (*wrist sign*) Flexion of the wrist and abduction of the fingers when the ulnar side of the lower forearm is stimulated; seen in pyramidal tract disease.[4723]

chaeromania   (from Gr, to rejoice + madness) Mania or euphoria, a psychotic state characterized by unwonted cheerfulness.

Chagas disease   An arthropod-borne zoonosis due to infection with *Trypanosoma cruzi,* first described by Chagas in 1907. The clinical features are those of chronic meningitis with evidence of cortical inflammation and demyelination; late in the course of the disease there is evidence of autonomic neuropathy.[5288] See **South American trypanosomiasis.**

chair tests   1. The production of nystagmus in the direction opposite rotation when the subjects revolve on a chair with their head flexed 30° forward (to bring the horizontal semicircular canal truly into a horizontal position) and while wearing **Frenzel glasses.** The test was described by **Bárány.**

The normal response after rotation of the chair to the right is for horizontal jerk nystagmus to the left to persist for 10–30 seconds. See **Bárány test.**

2. *Chair test* If the chair on which the normal subject sits is suddenly tilted backward, the subject will reflexly sit forward. The subject with bilateral labyrinthine lesions or with **Parkinson disease** makes no such reaction.

chalasia   (from Gr, chalasis; to relax or grow languid) 1. A term of Hippocrates for relaxation. 2. Failure of contraction of the cardiac sphincter of the stomach, leading to acid reflux.

chalastic fits   (inhibitory epilepsy) Attacks of general limpness, resembling **cataplexy** but symptomatic of lesions affecting the medial aspects of both frontal lobes.[1708]

Chalfont Seizure Severity Scale   A scale that assesses and scores the components of seizure attacks that cause patients the greatest disturbance. Factors such as the presence of falling, injuries, loss of awareness, and any

warning of seizures; the occurrence of dropping objects, incontinence, automatisms and convulsions; and duration of the seizures and the time taken to regain normal functioning are rated.[1549] See also **National Hospital Seizure Severity Scale,** which is derived from the Chalfont Scale.

Chamberlain line   A line drawn on a true lateral X-ray of the skull from the back of the hard palate to the posterior border of the foramen magnum. The line normally crosses above all parts of the atlas and axis; if basilar impression is present, part of the odontoid process and, in severe cases, other parts of the axis and of the atlas project above this line. However, the same is true in some normal subjects and a better measurement is that of the **Bull angle.**[832]

Chamberlain, W.E.   (b. 1891) American radiologist in Philadelphia.

chameleon tongue   Involuntary withdrawal of the tongue which is being protruded voluntarily; a sign commonly seen in patients with chorea.

champagne-cork papilledema   Severe papilledema such that the optic nerve head bulges forward and extends outward in all directions into the vitreous humor, thus resembling a champagne cork (or a mushroom).

chancre   An indolent, painless skin or mucosal ulcer at the site of a primary infection with *Treponema pallidum,* which can be isolated from it.

channel   The complete system for the detection, amplification, and display of potential differences between a pair of electrodes.

channelopathies   Genetically determined metabolic disturbances of the calcium, chloride, or potassium voltage-gated ion channels in the cell membrane, leading to disparate manifestations. Many of the disorders recognized are listed below, some with notes on the sites of the chrosomal anomaly.

Disorder	Site of Chromosomal Anomaly
Familial periodic paralysis hyperkalemic (sodium)	SCN4A, 17q23–25b
Familial periodic paralysis hypokalemic (calcium or potassium channels)	CACNLA3
Paramyotonia congenita (sodium)	SCN4A 17q 23–25
Myotonia congenita (Thomsen, Becker) (chloride)	CLCN1; 7q
Myotonia fluctuans (sodium)	
Myotonia permanens (sodium)	
Episodic ataxia with myokymia	CACNA1 12p13
Autosomal dominant nocturnal frontal lobe epilepsy	CHRNA4
Malignant hyperthermia (ryanodine)	
Central core disease	
Andersen syndrome (potassium)	
Long Q-T syndrome 1–5	
Startle	
Benign familial neonatal convulsions	29q 13. 8q24?

ADFNLE	20q13
Generalized epilepsy with febrile seizures	19q13
Juvenile myoclonic epilepsy (Janz)	6p
Febrile convulsions	8q
Benign familial infantile convulsions	18q?
Partial epilepsy	10q22
X-linked infantile spasms	Xp 11.4
Unverricht-Lundberg syndrome	21q22
Lafora body disease	6q 24
Cherry-red spot–myoclonus syndrome	6p 21.3
MERRF mt DNA	
Batten disease	16p 12.1
Juvenile **Gaucher disease**	1q 21
Familial hemiplegic migraine (episodic ataxia 2 is closely linked)	CACNL4
Calcium channelopathies	
Familial adult myoclonic epilepsy	8q 24

chanson de parler   See **prosody**.

Chapple syndrome   Unilateral facial weakness with contralateral laryngeal palsy occurring in the newborn. The latter problem is thought to be due to compression of the superior laryngeal nerve by the thyroid cartilage in utero as a consequence of excessive lateral flexion of the neck.[968] The syndrome was described by Dr. Charles Chapple of Philadelphia in 1956.

Charcot artery   The lenticulostriate branch of the middle cerebral artery, known as the "artery of cerebral hemorrhage."

Charcot disease   1. See **amyotrophic lateral sclerosis**.[980] 2. Chorea in the elderly, of which Charcot gave the neat description: "the movements are gesticulatory; they cover a wide area, are irregular, unrhythmical, contradictory, and render the accomplishment of any definite act a difficult matter."[974] The status of the disorder may be in some doubt.

Charcot edema   (blue edema) Non-pitting stasis edema, coldness, and peripheral cyanosis, usually with sensory loss and weakness and occurring as a result of disuse of a limb—a manifestation of hysterical paralyses in many of Charcot's patients but also sometimes seen following injury or stroke.[2313]

Charcot, Jean-Martin   (1825–1893) French neurologist, psychiatrist, and anatomist. After graduation from the University of Paris in 1853 he interned at the Salpêtrière, an asylum in Paris for the mentally ill and for those suffering from various chronic diseases, for 4 years from 1858, seeing there a huge variety of previously unclassified disease. He returned in 1862 as attending physician and over the next 30 years developed it into a school of neurology that became internationally famous. He was elected professor of pathological anatomy in 1872, succeeding Vulpian; 10 years after that, a special chair of nervous diseases was created for him, although his observations did not extend solely to neurology—as witness his accounts of Charcot-Leyden

crystals in the sputum of asthmatics, of intermittent claudication, and of biliary (Charcot) fever.

The starting point for this triumph was his meticulous recording of physical signs in all the 5000 patients housed in the hospital, signs that he later attributed to the specific neurological lesions found when the patients came to autopsy. This was the clinico-anatomic method that became the hallmark of the **Salpêtrière** and later of neurology in general. From 1866, Charcot offered lectures on neurological subjects that quickly became popular as a result of the inclusion of pathophysiology with the clinical demonstrations, his own dominating and self-assured manner, and the theatricality of the presentations. At these sessions (the Tuesday Lectures), symptoms, diagnoses, and pathology were discussed, focusing on a number of patients brought in for demonstration. The extent to which he actually examined (as opposed to observed) the patients is unclear.

Charcot's private practice was large, his hospital practice even larger. Honored in his day, he may be considered in retrospect to be the father of modern neurology. His studies encompassed rheumatism and changes in abdominal organs and lungs in old age, organic disease of the nervous system such as muscular atrophy, poliomyelitis, aneurysms, multiple sclerosis (differentiated for the first time in the Tuesday Lectures of 1868), and motor neuron disease (**amyotrophic lateral sclerosis**), in which he demonstrated the involvement of the anterior roots as well as the lateral columns in 1869, stroke syndromes, Ménière syndrome, tabetic arthropathy and lightning pains, encephalitis, cord compression, cerebral hemorrhage, hysteria and hypnotism, and the psychoneuroses as well as art as applied to the nervous system. It was Charcot who differentiated tics from chorea. His complete works were published in nine volumes. The Tuesday Lectures were translated into English after 1877 by George Sigerson (New Sydenham Society).[2154,5047]

Charcot joint   Painless, often gross deformity and destruction of joints in tabes dorsalis and other conditions (e.g., syringomyelia, hereditary sensory neuropathy) in which the sensation of pain is lost.[970] The absence of proprioceptive sense is also likely to be relevant by denying restraint to the muscular contractions and thus permitting abnormal joint positions to be assumed. [JF] See also **neurogenic arthropathy**.

Charcot sign   Elevation of the eyebrow on the side of a peripheral facial palsy and its depression when the patient attempts to close the eye.

The sign has also been interpreted as consisting of depression of the eyebrows when the eyes are closed, indicating blepharospasm; or their elevation, indicating apraxia of eye closure.

Charcot syndrome   See **amyotrophic lateral sclerosis**.

Charcot triad   The combination of nystagmus, intention tremor, and scanning speech, which Charcot suggested was diagnostic of **multiple sclerosis.**[975] This is no longer considered to be so.

Charcot vertigo   (laryngeal vertigo, laryngeal epilepsy) The occurrence of syncope or vertigo caused by a severe bout of coughing, sometimes with laryngospasm.[976]

That this actually represents epilepsy is unproven, though it has been suggested to be so.[5952] **Cough syncope** is a more likely cause.

Charcot-Bouchard aneurysm   A defect in the muscular coat of an arteriole among the deep penetrating vessels of the brain affected by **lipohyalinosis** in chronically hypertensive people. These are most often in the basal ganglia, thalamus, pons, and cerebellum. The arteriolar wall here consists merely of the intimal layer and some surrounding gliosis. As a result, it is fragile, and in the event of its rupture in association with increased blood pressure, bleeding will not be controllable by the usual mechanism of muscle spasm.

Charcot-Erb paresis   (syphilitic myelitis) See **Erb-Charcot syndrome.**

Charcot-Joffroy syndrome   See **hypertrophic spinal meningitis.**

Charcot-Marie-Tooth Association   A charitable organization that provides education and support to patients with Charcot-Marie-Tooth disease and their families, as well as to the medical/scientific community. The association's program is composed of a quarterly newsletter, regional conferences, a medical referral system, a videotape program, and area support groups. The association also maintains a registry of patients with the disease. Address: 601 Upland Ave., Upland, PA 19015-2496. Tel: 215-499-7486.

Charcot-Marie-Tooth disease   See **hereditary motor and sensory neuropathies.** While Charcot and Marie[981] had priority of publication, they considered the condition to be a myelopathy, an error corrected by Tooth (who noted that **Virchow** had already described the same condition).

Charcot-Marie-Tooth disease with distal spinal muscular atrophy   See **hereditary motor and sensory neuropathy, type 2.**

Charcot-Marie-Tooth disease with progressive ataxia and tremor   See **hereditary motor and sensory neuropathy, type 1.**

Charcot-Marie-Tooth International   A charitable organization. Address: 1 Springbank Dr., St. Catherines, Ontario, L2S 2K1 Canada. Tel: 416-687-3630.

Charcot-Weiss-Baker syndrome   See **carotid sinus hypersensitivity.**

Charcot-Wilbrand syndrome   Visual agnosia with an inability to revisualize images formerly seen, due to an infarct in the territory of the posterior cerebral artery.[978]

Dr. H. Wilbrand (1851–1935) was a German neuro-ophthalmologist, and a professor at Hamburg University.

CHARGE association syndrome   A congenital dysmorphic syndrome characterized by **C**olobomas of iris and retina, congenital **H**eart disease, choanal **A**tresia, mental and developmental **R**etardation, **G**enital hypoplasia and cryptorchid testes, **E**ar deformities, and deafness. Four of these six manifestations are taken as sufficient for the diagnosis.

Facial palsy, cleft palate, hypopituitarism, esophageal and renal deformities, etc., also occur but could not be worked into the acronym.[2376]

Charlevoix-Saguenay spastic ataxic syndrome   A recessive form of slowly progressive complicated hereditary spastic paraplegia with onset in childhood, first reported from Quebec and mapped to chromosome 13q11–12.[4030]

Clinically, the pyramidal syndrome is accompanied by dysarthria, ataxia, and abnormal eye movements; mitral incompetence and a motor neuropathy may be associated.[676] See **hereditary spastic paraplegia;** but the condition could equally well be classified as an early-onset **cerebellar ataxia** with retained reflexes.

Charlie M syndrome   A congenital syndrome characterized by ocular hyperteleorism, facial paralysis, cleft palate, and digital and dental abnormalities.[2213]

Charlin Correa, Carlos   (1885–1945) A Chilean ophthalmologist.

Charlin syndrome   Brief bouts of severe unilateral pain at the root and ala of the nose accompanied by catarrh, uveitis with photophobia, conjunctivitis, and lacrimation.[983] See **ciliary neuralgia.**

The problem has been considered to be a selective neuritis of the maxillary branch of the trigeminal nerve, but may equally well be a form of **cluster headache.**

Chaslin gliosis   (marginal gliosis) A condensation of usually delicate horizontal glial fibers that are normally found in the cortex, immediately beneath the pial surface, thought to be the consequence of convulsions. The gliosis is ubiquitous but most noticeable in the hippocampal gyrus and the surface of Ammon's horn; in severe cases it may extend through the cortex down to the subependymal regions.

Chaslin, Pierre   French pathologist, who first described the appearances of gliosis.[987]

chasma   See **yawning.**

Chassaignac disease   Pain in the limbs caused by trauma in children aged between 2 and 5 years, leading to incomplete paralysis or pseudoparalysis and with prompt and full recovery.[988]

It was described by Charles-Marie-Édouard Chassaignac (1805–1879), who was a French physician.

CHAT classification of stroke   A brief method of classifying the **C**linical, **H**istorical, **A**rterial (anatomical) and **T**arget (pathological) features that relate to the stroke process.[520]

chatterbox syndrome   See **cocktail party syndrome.**

Chavany, J-A. E.   (1892–1959) French neurologist.

Chavany-Brunhes syndrome   The occurrence of headaches and various other (probably psychogenic) complaints in patients who are found to have benign calcification of the falx. The original description[991] suggested a causal association.

check reflex   Involuntary inhibition of a muscular contraction with a degree of restitution. Thus, when a patient's arm is extended horizontally in front of her and downward pressure on the wrist is applied by the examiner, and when that pressure is suddenly released, the arm normally flies upward for a short distance, then stops and descends slightly. The latter movement is known as *rebound* or *recoil*. Failure to inhibit the upward movement and loss of the downward restitution are together considered signs of cerebellar disease on the same side and are due to abnormal slowing of the desired contraction or relaxation of muscles required to maintain the position of the limb when the resistance is removed.

"When a person attempts to execute movement against resistance with a normal limb, and the resistance is suddenly removed, the limb rapidly moves a short distance in the desired direction till abruptly checked, or it may recoil. In a spastic limb, the amount of recoil is excessive; in functional cases there may be neither primary movement, nor recoil. In homolateral cerebellar disease, the range of movement is excessive, generally continued till it is no longer mechanically possible, and there is little or no recoil."[5357]

checkerboard fields   Alternating squares of different colors, conveniently represented upon a television monitor. Repeated reversals of the colors of the squares (e.g., black becomes white, white becomes black) is the most effective stimulus known for the formation of **visual evoked responses.**

Chediak, Moises   (b. 1903) Cuban physician, professor of clinical pathology in Havana.

Chediak-Higashi disease   A rare, congenital, recessively inherited **neurocutaneous syndrome** manifesting partial oculocutaneous albinism in childhood, with photophobia, decreased lacrimation, peripheral neuropathy, enlarged liver, spleen, and lymph glands, and signs of cerebellar and basal ganglion disease with intermittent febrile episodes.

Other neurological signs such as mental and developmental delay, seizures, papilledema, nystagmus, ataxia, and motor neuropathy have also been recorded. The diagnosis is confirmed by the finding of peroxidase-positive panleukocytic granules. Only a few patients live into their adult years, usually because of recurrent infections[609] or the development of lymphomas.

Dr. O. Higashi is a Japanese pediatrician.

Chedoke-McMaster Stroke Assessment Disability Inventory   A two-part scale measuring the physical impairments and disabilities affecting patients after stroke and yielding scores on shoulder pain, postural control, the arm, the hand, the leg, and the foot[2243] (see Chart C–15). See also **stroke scales.**

Chart C–15. Chedoke-McMaster Stroke Assessment Disability Inventory

Gross motor function index

1. Supine to side lying on strong side
2. Supine to side lying on weak side
3. Side lying to long sitting through strong side
4. Side lying to sitting on side of the bed through strong side
5. Side lying to sitting on side of the bed through weak side
6. Standing
7. Transfer to and from bed toward strong side
8. Transfer to and from bed toward weak side
9. Transfer up and down from floor and chair
10. Transfer up and down from floor and standing

Walking index

11. Walking indoors
12. Walking outdoors, over rough ground, ramps, and curbs
13. Walking outdoors several blocks
14. Stairs
15. Age- and sex-appropriate walking distance (in meters) for 2 minutes (2-point bonus)

Scoring key

Independence (no helper)

7. Complete independence (timely, safely)
6. Modified independence (device)

Modified dependence (helper)

5. Supervision
4. Minimal assist (subject = 75%)
3. Moderate assist (subject = 50%)

Complete dependence (helper)

2. Maximal assist (subject = 25%)
1. Total assist (subject = 0%)

*Adapted from Gowland C, Stratford P, Ward M, et al. Measuring physical impairment and disability with the Chedoke-McMaster Stroke Assessment. Stroke 1993;**24**:58–63.[2243] Reproduced by permission.*

cheek sign   See **Brudzinski signs.**

cheilalgia   (Gr, lip + pain) Pain in the lips.

cheiralgia paresthetica   (Gr, the hand + pain) (cheiralgia, Wartenberg disease) Isolated painful neuropathy of the superficial branch of the radial nerve, described by Wartenberg in 1917.

cheirooral migraine   Migraine headaches preceded by an aura comprising paresthesias of the hand and cheek on one side, sometimes combined with aphasia.

cheirooral syndrome   The combination of a sensory defect around the corner of the mouth and on the homolateral palm of the hand or thumb, due to a small lesion in the contralateral parietal cortex, or less often in the contralateral corona radiata, or in the pons (where the medial lemniscus is involved).[3701,4236]

chemical meningitis   A syndrome of meningism associated with the rupture of a dermoid cyst, or resulting from the presence of blood or chemicals in the CSF. The cells in the CSF are largely of mononuclear type. A similar syndrome occurs rarely as a complication of primary cerebral tumors.

chemoaffinity   The hypothesis of Sperry that each developing neuron or group of neurons acquires a distinct chemical label that defines both its functional class and its position within the population of neurons of which it is a part, and to identify and form connections with their target cells, such as receptor organs.

chemodactoma   A benign, highly vascular, locally invasive paraganglioma of non-chromaffin cells, often arising in the glomus jugulare region and characterized by the presence of thin-walled vessels and clear cells with intervening reticulin.[4185] See **glomus jugulare tumor, carotid body tumor.**

chemonucleolysis   An invasive therapeutic procedure involving the injection of digesting enzymes (chymopapain) into an intervertebral disk to cause it to shrink as the nucleus pulposus is digested, thus relieving symptoms of disk protrusion. The effectiveness of the procedure in patients with prolapsed intervertebral disks, neurological signs, and failed conservative therapy is not questioned, but the unwanted effects of the injection include anaphylaxis and transverse myelitis.

chemopallidectomy   The production of destructive lesions in the globus pallidus by stereotaxic procaine or alcohol injection as a therapeutic measure to relieve rigidity and tremor in **Parkinson disease.**

Both the newer operation of ventrolateral thalamotomy and the advent of useful oral medications led to the abandonment of this technique, which was popular in the 1950s; but should such a measure be required at this time to contain severe and resistant tremors, radiofrequency lesions would be used rather than chemicals.

chemoreceptors   Carotid and aortic bodies sensitive to alterations in the tissue tensions of pH, oxygen, and carbon dioxide. Decreased arterial pO_2, increased pCO_2, or decreased pH of the blood leads to hyperpnoea and redistribution of blood to cerebral and coronary beds, but induces vasoconstriction.

Similar bodies in the floor of the medulla are sensitive to changes in the pH of the CSF, a fall leading to hyperpnoea.

Chernogubov syndrome   See **Ehlers-Danlos syndrome.**

cherry-red spot   The appearance of the macula that remains red when surrounded by a pale retina, reflecting the storage of an opaque material in the perifoveal ganglion cells; a characteristic sign in Tay-Sachs disease (classic **GM₂ gangliosidosis**) and in numerous other neuronal storage diseases, in central retinal artery occlusion, and in macular trauma or hemorrhage.

In patients with storage diseases, disappearance of the spot occurs when the retinal ganglion cells atrophy. Fourteen conditions in which the spot is seen have been listed.[3071]

cherry-red spot–myoclonus syndrome   (type I juvenile sialidosis) A lysosomal storage disease in which sialyloligosaccharides are accumulated, manifesting corneal clouding and the retinal spot in childhood with the later appearance of severe, progressive, stimulus-sensitive myoclonus and generalized seizures, hypotonia, hyperreflexia, and dysarthria.[4593] See **sialidosis type I.**

The association of such abnormalities also occurs in Tay-Sachs disease, Niemann-Pick disease, **GM₁** and **GM₂ gangliosidoses, metachromatic leukodystrophy,** and the **glycogenoses.**

cheshire cat sign   1. The inappropriate persistence of a smile on the face of a patient with myotonic dystrophy.[1607] 2. The situations described by Bywaters in which patients exhibit the typical features of a condition although the diagnosis cannot be confirmed by pathological examination, or in which patients have a disease without any clinical evidence of it.[863]

cheval de frise   A device made of a hexagonal beam to which were attached radial wooden stakes or iron spikes, placed atop a wall to repel invaders. The pattern resulting resembles, in the minds of some migraineurs, the visual auras of migraine attacks.[4458]

chewing oscillopsia   See **oscillopsia.**

Cheyne disease   (the English malady) Morbid concern about health matters, considered by George Cheyne to be due to the moisture and variability of the climate in the British isles.[1004]

Cheyne, George   (1671–1743) Scottish physician who studied in Edinburgh and Aberdeen, was elected to the Royal Society within a year of graduation, and entered practice in London. He enjoyed a somewhat intemperate way of life, became ill, renounced his former indulgences, and retired to Bath where his publications advocated temperance and a strict regimen in daily life, suggested methods of treating the gout, and advised on diet. Much of this material must have been written on the basis of personal experience.[5047] He is best remembered for his book *The English Malady.*

Cheyne, John   (1777–1836) Scottish physician, though physician to the Dublin hospitals, and an early neuropathologist, who published accounts of acute hydrocephalus that was probably due to tuberculous meningitis, and of ischemic stroke and subarachnoid hemorrhage, drawn in part from the pathological specimens of his friend Sir Charles **Bell**. Although he presciently blamed stress, alcohol, and tobacco as causes of strokes, he is best remembered for his description of periodic (Cheyne-Stokes) respirations in 1818, 35 years before **Stokes** (who acknowledged this). Neither seems to have been aware that Robert **Whytt** had also remarked upon the phenomenon.

Cheyne-Stokes respiration   The occurrence of a series of inspirations increasing to a maximum and then declining in force and length until a state of apparent apnea is established, when, after a more or less prolonged period, sometimes of apparent death, a low inspiration, followed by one more decided, marks the commencement of a new ascending and then descending series of inspirations. Cheyne described this phenomenon in a patient as follows: "For several days his breathing was irregular; it would cease entirely for a quarter of a minute, then it would become very perceptible, although very low, then by degrees it became heaving and quick, and then it would gradually cease again; this revolution in the state of his breathing occupied about a minute, during which there were about thirty acts of respiration."[1005]

The phenomenon was named for John **Cheyne** and for William Stokes (1804–1878) an Irish physician, Regius Professor of Medicine at Dublin University from 1845.

Hans Chiari

Chiari, Hans   (1851–1916) Austrian pathologist who trained in Vienna and worked there with Heschl before moving to Prague and later to Strasbourg. He described the first three of the malformations bearing his name between 1891 and 1896. Other contributions include his de-

scription of choriocarcinoma, thrombosis of the hepatic vein (Budd-Chiari syndrome), and, in 1906, recognition of the association of carotid artery plaques with thrombi in the intracranial portion of the carotid artery.[3760]

Chiari malformation   (Arnold-Chiari malformation, List syndrome)[3430] Congenital caudal displacement of the brainstem, cerebellum, spinal cord, cervical spine, and posterior fossa, often manifesting only in adult life. A short neck, obstructive hydrocephalus, cerebellar signs, evidence of damage to the lower cranial nerves, and nystagmus are the principal manifestations when the disorder becomes symptomatic, but a syringomyelic syndrome (lumbosacral radiculopathy) may also occur and the condition may be complicated by meningomyelocele.[221]

In *type 1* (adult type, familial occipital dysplasia, Arnold-Chiari-Schwalbe-Gredig-Penfield-Coburn syndrome), there is downward displacement of the pons, medulla, fourth ventricle, and cerebellar tonsils down to or through the foramen magnum, associated with spinal dysraphism and sometimes with hydrocephalus. This usually presents with pyramidal or cerebellar signs, downbeat nystagmus, hydrocephalus, and variable cranial nerve disturbances in adult life. Syringomyelia is also commonly present. The condition may be dominantly inherited.[3969]

In *type 2* (infantile type, Chiari type) the fourth ventricle may descend far down into the cervical spine, and the hypoplastic cerebellar vermis and tonsils and possibly the elongated medulla all herniate down through, and may impact within, the foramen magnum. Meningomyelocele is associated.

This is the most common form and presents in infancy or childhood. Spina bifida of any degree, platybasia, assimilation of the atlas with the occipital bones, **Klippel-Feil syndrome,** hydrocephalus, and other cerebral anomalies (microgyria, tectal anomalies) often coexist.

John Cleland in England had also described this anomaly in 1883; **Arnold** further described one case in 1894.[7]

Type 3 (Chiari-Parker-McConnell-Aring) is characterized by downward displacement of the medulla and cerebellar tonsils with an accompanying occipital encephalocele through which the cerebellum projects.

Type 4 is cerebellar hypoplasia, the same condition as the **Dandy-Walker** cyst.

Despite the usual eponymous title, the first description was actually that of John Cleland (an English anatomist, surgeon and poet) in 1883, but the report of Chiari in 1891 drew more attention.[1009]

chiasma   (Gr, two lines crossing like an *X*) The decussation of the fibers of the optic nerve.

chiasmal apoplexy   An acutely evolving syndrome of retro-orbital or frontal headache with abrupt visual loss due to hemorrhage into the optic chiasm. Young adults are most often affected.

The underlying pathology is most commonly a small intrachiasmatic arteriovenous malformation.[3581]

chiasmal syndrome The clinical effects of compression of the chiasm in the presence of a normally sized sella turcica by, for instance, a pituitary adenoma or a suprasellar meningioma.

The clinical features include complaints of visual deterioration with dimming of vision, diplopia, headache, and vertigo, and on examination a central scotoma, bitemporal field defects, and optic atrophy are found.[1231] See **Cushing syndrome.** See also **hemifield slide, postfixation blindness.**

Child Behaviour Checklist A rating instrument for child behavior, used in the classification of pediatric neurobehavioral disorders.[31]

Child Neurology Society A professional organization of child neurologists. Address: 475 Cleveland Ave. N., Ste. 220, St. Paul, MN 55104-5051. Tel: 651-641-1584.

childhood absence epilepsy (pyknolepsy; OMIM 600131) An uncommon seizure disorder occurring in children of school age (peak manifestation age 6–7 years), with a strong genetic predisposition in otherwise normal children. It appears more frequently in girls than in boys and is characterized by very frequent absences (several to many per day), typically precipitated by hyperventilation. The neurological examination is normal.

The EEG reveals bilateral, synchronous, symmetrical spike–wave complexes, usually at 3 Hz on a normal background activity. During adolescence, generalized tonic-clonic seizures may develop. Otherwise, absences may remit or, more rarely, persist as the only seizure type. (Adapted from Commission for Classification and Terminology, ILAE. Proposal for revised classifications of epilepsies and epileptic syndromes. *Epilepsia* 1989; **30**:389–399.[1114])

Some develop GTC seizures in adolescence or early adulthood.

childhood ataxia with diffuse CNS hypomyelination (**fatal infantile leukodystrophy,** CACH, vanishing white matter disease) A progressive heterogeneous leukodystrophic disorder of unknown etiology with onset in childhood, sometimes following cranial trauma or fever. It is characterized by normal head size, ataxic diplegia, lack of dementia, late optic atrophy, and a diffuse, confluent CNS white matter abnormality on CT and MRI scans shown pathologically to be due to hypomyelination.[4960,5719] The condition has also been reported to occur first in adult life.[395]

childhood dermatomyositis or polymyositis associated with vasculitis (juvenile dermatomyositis) An acquired, progressive, noninfectious, nongranulomatous, proximal, painful inflammatory myopathy of children or youths with a slow, relapsing, or monophasic course. Clinically, a skin rash and calcinosis are both common in association with the weakness. Pathologically, muscle fiber necrosis is rare and limited to lesions resembling infarcts; capillary necrosis at the periphery of muscle fascicles, the presence of undulating tubules in endothelial cells, lymphocytes, pericytes, and pseudosatellite cells, and variable inflammatory infiltrates in connective tissue septa are the major features.[915]

A strong association with HLA class II DQa1*0501 antigen has been shown.

childhood epilepsy with centrotemporal spikes See **benign rolandic epilepsy.**

childhood epilepsy with occipital paroxysms The syndrome is, in general, similar to that of benign childhood epilepsy with centrotemporal spikes. The seizures start with visual symptoms (amaurosis, phosphenes, illusions, or hallucinations) and are often followed by a hemiclonic seizure or automatisms. In 25% of cases, the seizures are immediately followed by migrainous headache. The EEG has paroxysms of high-amplitude spike–waves or sharp waves recurring rhythmically on the occipital and posterior temporal areas of one or both hemispheres, but only when the eyes are closed. During seizures, the occipital discharge may spread to the central or temporal region. At present, no definite statement on prognosis is possible. (Adapted from Commission for Classification and Terminology, ILAE. Proposal for revised classifications of epilepsies and epileptic syndromes. *Epilepsia* 1989;**30**:389–399.[1114]) Other criteria have been suggested as follows:[4316]

1. Unequivocal clinical evidence of epileptic seizures and paroxysms maximal in the occipital areas on at least one EEG, and no clinical nor EEG manifestations of primary generalized epilepsy or of another distinctive epileptic syndrome;
2. No evidence of neurological or intellectual deficit; and
3. Normal appearance of CT brain scan.

childhood muscular dystrophies See **limb-girdle muscular dystrophies** (LGMD 2B), distal myopathy (**Miyoshi myopathy**), which are both deficient in this same gene product; and **Fukuyama** congenital muscular dystrophy.[5654]

childhood myoclonic epilepsies See **myoclonus.**

childhood polymyositis Inflammatory muscle disease occurring before the (arbitrary) age of 16. See **polymyositis.**

A *variant form* is *acquired infantile polymyositis,* which is a variant of **childhood polymyositis** presenting in infancy with hypotonia without CNS involvement and showing a good response to steroid therapy.[5563]

childhood schizophrenia See **Heller disease.**

childhood-onset DIMS Difficulties in the initiation and maintenance of sleep starting before puberty and persisting into adult life, resulting in complaints of insomnia. See also ASDA diagnostic classification, **sleep disorders.**[234]

childhood-onset idiopathic torsion dystonia A syndrome presenting first after the age of 6 years with arm dystonia but without rest tremor, bradykinesia, or rigidity. Any response to levadopa is but slight.[840]

childhood-onset parkinsonism A parkinsonian syndrome presenting first before the age of 12 years, with foot dystonia, rest tremor, bradykinesia, and rigidity. A response to levadopa is notable.[2075]

Children's Brain Tumor Foundation A charitable organization. Address: 35 Alpine Lane, Chappaqua, NY 10514. Tel: 914-238-4917.

Child's Brain See **Pediatric Neurosciences.**

Children's Coma Score A scale designed for use with infants and toddlers aged 0–3 years who have incurred head injury (see Chart C–16).[4572]

Chart C–16. Children's Coma Score

Score response	
Ocular response	
4	Pursuit
3	Extraocular muscles intact and reactive pupils
2	Fixed pupils, *or* extraocular movements impaired
1	Fixed pupils *and* extraocular movements impaired
Verbal response	
3	Cries
2	Spontaneous respirations
1	Apneic
Motor response	
4	Flexes and extends
3	Withdraws from painful stimuli
2	Hypertonic
1	Flaccid

From Raimondi AJ, Hirschauer J. Head injury in the infant and toddler: Coma scoring and outcome scale. Child's Brain 1984;11:12–35. Reproduced by permission.

See also **Glasgow Coma scale.**

Child's Nervous System The official journal of the International, European and Korean Societies for Paediatric Neurosurgery, published by Springer. Web site: http://link.springer.de/link/service/journals/00381/index.htm.

chimera An organism created from the genetic material of two different species. The term is derived from the Greek word signifying a monster.

Chinese paralytic syndrome An acute axonal motor neuropathy occurring in the summer months and causing a rapidly progressive ascending tetraparesis in children or young adults, often with ventilatory failure but without sensory changes, fever, CSF pleocytosis, or systemic illness.

In some cases, anti-GM$_1$ antibodies suggesting recent *Campylobacter* infection are detectable. The prognosis is good if the severe complications are appropriately managed.

The name was applied as a result of the first reports of the disorder that had affected many children in Northern China, but the infection is worldwide.[2102,3767,3768] See also **immune-mediated neuropathies.**

Chinese restaurant syndrome (Kwok's quease, post-sinocibal syndrome, Sin-Cib-Syn) Monosodium glutamate (MSG) poisoning, manifesting as tightness of the masseters, limb paresthesias, burning of the face, limbs, and chest, and precordial discomfort occurring after ingestion of MSG (usually in a restaurant serving Chinese food) but self-limited over a few hours.[3208]

chiralgia See **cheiralgia paresthetica.**

chirismus An old term for spasm of the wrists, hands, or fingers during a convulsion.

chiromegaly Trophic changes leading to proliferation of the soft tissues of the hand, as in some cases of syringomyelia.

chiropodal paralysis Weakness and atrophy of the small muscles of the hands and feet, once thought typical of arsenical polyneuritis but in fact common in almost every form of motor neuropathy.

chloroma (Balfour disease) A rare condition in which hyperplasia of the leukocyte parent cells, usually myeloblasts, results in widespread tumor formation, frequently affecting the orbits and skull. The eponym follows the report of Dr. J.H. Balfour to the Medico-Chiurgical Society in 1834 but the nature of the syndrome is uncertain.

chlorosis (from Gr, greening) Until the early twentieth century, this was considered a disease entity, affecting young women around puberty and manifest by a greenish pallor, oligomenorrhea, and numerous symptoms that would today be regarded as evidence of hypochondriasis. See **chronic fatigue syndrome.**

Chodzko reflex Contraction of several muscles of the arm on one or both sides when the manubrium is percussed,[1015] presumably witnessing hyperirritability of some kind.

Dr. W. Chodkzo was a Polish neurologist.

choked disk See **papilledema.**

cholecystokinin A complex of octapeptide neurotransmitter hormones found in the gut and in the brain with a role in feeding behavior.

cholestanol A biological substance closely resembling cholesterol, deposited in **cholestanolosis.**

cholestanolosis See **cerebrotendinous xanthomatosis.**

cholesteatoma Small tumors usually found on the base of the skull, for instance, at the cerebellopontine angle, and composed of epithelial cells arranged in concentric layers.

cholesterol emboli syndrome (atheromatous embolization) A multisystem disorder caused by peripheral embolization of cholesterol crystals, for example, after angiography, aortic surgery, or other trauma. The findings may occur remotely, even months after the inciting event.

Clinical features include blue toe syndrome, gangrene, livedo reticularis; pain in the legs, feet, toes, abdomen, flank, or back; hematuria; accelerated hypertension; impaired renal function; and (less commonly) spinal cord, penile, splenic, or adrenal infarction.[443]

cholinergic crisis An acute exacerbation of myasthenia-like symptoms of weakness and fatigability (**cholinergic paralysis**), often with evidence of generalized parasympathetic overactivity, as a result of excessive ingestion of anticholinergic drugs, in a patient with **myasthenia gravis.**

The condition mimics, and is hardly differentiated clinically from, **myasthenic crisis.** The use of edrophonium for diagnosis in this situation is dangerous, but a régime comprising discontinuation of anticholinesterase drugs, and ventilatory support and time invariably provides the answer.

cholinergic paralysis Weakness as a result of excessive depolarization of the motor end-plate. Poisoning with anticholinesterase compounds such as nerve gases, depolarizing drugs, or black widow spider venom are typical causes. See also **neuromuscular transmission defects.**

cholosis An extinct term for lameness.

chondrodystrophia calcificans punctata congenita See **Conradi-Hünerman syndrome.**

chondrodytrophic myotonia See **Schwartz-Jampel syndrome.**

chondroectodermal dysplasia See **Ellis–van Creveld syndrome.**

chondromas Benign cartilaginous tumors which occasionally arise from the synchrondroses at the base of the skull or from the vault.[3215]

chopper A device consisting of a mechanical or electronic switch used in some EEG amplifiers for interrupting (chopping) D.C. and low-frequency A.C. signals and converting them into square waves of relatively high frequency. The same device may provide synchronous rectification of these square waves after amplification to reconvert them to the form of the original signal at the output. (Adapted from the report of the Committee on Terminology, IFCN[989], © 1974, with permission from Elsevier Science.)

chopper amplifier A direct current amplifier in which a chopper interrupts D.C. and low-frequency

A.C. signals and converts them into square waves of relatively high frequency. These are magnified by an A.C. amplifier and then reconverted by synchronous rectification to the form of the original signal at the output. (Adapted from the report of the Committee on Terminology, IFCN,[989] © 1974, with permission from Elsevier Science.)

chorda (Lat, the string, as of a musical instrument) A tendon or fiber bundle.

chorda tympani (Gr, bowstring + drum) A branch of the seventh cranial nerve, crossing through the middle ear applied to the eardrum and carrying afferent fibers subserving taste sensation from the anterior two-thirds of the tongue. It was first described by Bartolommeo Eustachius (1524–1574), an Italian anatomist, in 1563.[4979]

chordoma An uncommon tumor arising from the remnants of the primitive notochord, either in the clivus at the base of the cranium or at the level of the sacrum. It was first described and named by Moritz Ribbert (1855–1920), a Swiss pathologist.[4979]

Symptoms occur as a result of local compression of neurological and other structures. Histologically, they are characterized by sheets of **physaliphorous cells** containing periodic acid-Schiff–positive material, bone fragments, keratin, S-100 protein, and epithelial membrane antigen.[6]

chorea (Gr, dancing; Fr, folie musculaire) Excessive spontaneous, irregular, random, brief, abrupt, nonrepetitive, irregular movements with distal predominance, flowing randomly from one body part to another. They result from numerous diseases of the basal ganglia, including the caudate nucleus. The severity of the movements varies from mild motor restlessness and fidgeting to constant, dance-like, or even violent and disabling instability of limbs, posture, and gait.

The names of four saints (Vitus [Guy], Valentine, Modesti, and John) have been associated with chorea over the ages. Power and Sedgwick (1882) identify 39 varieties of chorea; apart from the succeeding entries, these include diaphragmatic or laryngeal chorea (probably hiccoughs), chorea dimitiata (hemichorea), epidemic chorea, chorea magna and chorea germanorum (dancing mania, epidemic or hysterical chorea or tarantulism), chorea nutans (head nodding), chorea festinans and saltatoria (forms in which the subject is compelled to run or jump), and chorea senilis, an inaccurate synonym for **Parkinson disease.**[4512]

For a historical review, see McHenry.[3760] See also the following entries and **dystonic choreoathetosis induced by exercise, familial inverted choreoathetosis** and **kinesigenic choreoathetosis, benign hereditary chorea, benign essential chorea, hereditary progressive chorea without dementia, Huntington disease, Sydenham chorea.**

chorea anglorum   See **Sydenham chorea.**

chorea electrica   (Bergeron disease, electric chorea) See **Dubini disease.**

chorea fibrillaris   See **Morvan chorea.**

chorea gravidarum   Monosymptomatic chorea resembling that of **Sydenham chorea** but occurring during the earlier months of pregnancy.[484]

chorea lascivia   The name applied by Paracelsus to **dancing mania.**

chorea major   Originally dancing mania, now **Huntington chorea,** if employed at all.

chorea minor   (chorea anglorum) See **Sydenham chorea.**

chorea progressive hereditaria   See **Huntington disease.**

chorea St. Viti   See **Sydenham chorea.**

chorea variabilis   A term used both for **Tourette syndrome** and **Brissaud disease.**

chorea with curvilinear bodies   A rare, possibly recessively inherited syndrome characterized by chorea, paroxysmal dystonia, intractable tonic-clonic seizures, pyramidal signs, and mental and developmental delay with onset in childhood. Curvilinear bodies are detected in brain neurons and in peripheral white cells.[1248]

chorea-amyotrophy with chronic hemolytic anemia   A condition resembling **choreoacanthocytosis** except for the substitution of hemolytic anemia for the acanthocytosis.

Clinically, the disorder appears in adult life and manifests facial and vocal tics, tongue-biting, pes cavus, hyporeflexia, neuropathy or myopathy, and increase in serum creatine kinase levels.[5273] See also **Fotopoulos syndrome.**

choreic gait   Unsteady progression with irregular lurches induced by involuntary choreic movements of the legs, giving an impression fancifully described as dance-like.

choreic hand   Flexion of the wrist with overextension of the metocarpophalangeal joints when the arms are extended in front of the body.[6000]

choreiform syndrome   The persistent movements and akathisiac restlessness in school-age boys with the **attention defect hyperactivity syndrome.** The validity of the syndrome is uncertain.[4517]

choreoacanthocytosis   See **neuroacanthocytosis.**

choreoathetosis   While **chorea** and **athetosis** are clinically different and result from lesions in different areas of the basal ganglia, they often coexist; but more often this term reflects the uncertainty of the observer as to which condition is being viewed.

choreoathetosis/spasticity disease   A syndrome with these features mapped to 1p, a region containing a cluster of potassium (K+) channel genes.

choreoathetotic cerebral palsy   See **cerebral palsy.** The original description of athetosis was by **Hammond** in 1867.

choreofacient   An agent that produces limb tremor; the name was formerly applied to heavy metals such as mercury.

choreomania   Epidemic chorea. See **dancing mania.**

choresthesia   (Gr, place + sensation) A term encompassing the somatic sense of space, and thus a synthesis of joint position sense, depth sense, and two-point discrimination.[4661,5212]

choristoma   A benign, microscopic, granular cell tumor of the neurohypophysis, usually found accidentally in elderly people.

choroid   (Gr, chorion + like) A vascular structure; thus the vascular layer of the eye or the secretory villi beneath the ependyma and within the cerebral ventricles.

choroid plexus papilloma   An uncommon, benign, primary neuroectodermal vascular tumor arising from the choroid plexus in the lateral ventricles in children and the fourth ventricles in adults. Benign (well-differentiated) forms are characterized histologically by an uniform columnar epithelium with few mitoses, frequent calcification, and positive staining for carbonic anhydrase C, S-100 protein, **glial acidic fibrillary protein,** and cytokeratins; malignant (poorly differentiated) forms show pleomorphism, irregularity of structure, and local invasiveness and stain only for cytokeratins.[6]

Clinically, they may lead to a syndrome of headache with raised intracranial pressure without localizing signs and with seizures, but they may remain asymptomatic.

choroideremia   An X-linked recessive condition (Xq21.2) causing retinitis pigmentosa, choroidal degeneration, and visual loss.[1160]

choroiditis   Inflammation of the choroid layer of the eye.

choroidocerebral calcification syndrome   A rare syndrome of mental retardation, dense calcification of the lateral ventricular choroid plexus, and increased CSF protein, seen first in infancy.[5183]

Christensen-Krabbe syndrome   See **Alpers disease.**

Christian syndrome   1. (adducted thumbs syndrome, Christian-Andrews-Conneally-Molar syndrome) A congenital, recessively inherited dysmorphic syndrome characterized also by brachydactyly, hirsutism, micrognathia, cleft palate, pectus excavatum, adducted thumbs, club foot, ophthalmoplegia, muscle fasciculations, preaxial polysyndactyly, varus joint contractures, craniosynostosis with microcephaly and hypertelorism, and mental and developmental delay.[1028] See also **craniosynostosis**. 2. An X-linked syndrome characterized by dwarfism, ridging of the metopic sutures, cervical vertebral fusion, thoracic and sacral vertebral deformities, sixth cranial nerve palsy, and imperforate anus.[1027]

Christian-Andrews-Conneally-Molar syndrome (adducted thumbs syndrome) See **Christian syndrome** (1).

chromatic sensitive epilepsy A seizure disorder in boys who convulse while watching cartoons on television. Like many others, they were not known to suffer from epilepsy, although some had a family history of epilepsy. The flickering blue and red background is considered to be the most important precipitating factor.

chromatin-positive Turner syndrome See **Noonan syndrome**.

chromatolysis (axon reaction) Morphologic changes within neuronal cell bodies, including the disruption, dispersal, and eventual disappearance of the granular endoplasmic reticulum (Nissl substance) as a result of damage to its axon. There is loss of stainable material from a damaged neuron.

Two forms are described. In *central chromatolysis,* the loss of basophilic Nissl substance leads to eosinophilic staining of the cytoplasm, initially close to the cell nucleus. When chromatolysis occurs as a response to *axonal injury,* the Nissl substance degenerates, but also the nucleus moves to an eccentric position, the nucleolus enlarges, and swelling of the perikaryon and basophilia within the cytoplasm occurs. The word was introduced by **Marinesco** in 1909.

chromatopsia The perception of colors that invest objects seen or their background.

chromophobe adenoma A benign pituitary tumor, the cells of which take up little stain. The tumor provides evidence of its existence mainly through exerting local pressure on the surrounding structures (optic chiasm, hypothalamus, cavernous sinus), rather than through the effects of its hormonal secretions.

chromosome 4p partial deletion A dysmorphic syndrome characterized also by mental and physical delay, nystagmus, ptosis, and strabismus.[213] See **Wolf-Hirschorn syndrome**.

chromosome 5p deletion See **cri du chat syndrome**.

chromosome 13 trisomy syndrome (Patau syndrome) See **trisomy 13 syndrome**.

chromosome 18 partial deletion 1. (long arm; de Grouchy syndrome) A congenital dysmorphic syndrome manifesting midface dysplasia, short stature, mental and physical delay, nystagmus, seizures, hypotonia, optic atrophy, retinal degeneration, and congen-

ital cardiac anomalies.[3296] 2. (short arm) A congenital dysmorphic syndrome with midface dysplasia, manifesting also mental and physical delay, hypertelorism, epicanthic folds, strabismus, and (later) aphasia. Arhinencephaly or microcephaly are also reported in some cases.[2784]

chromosome 21q deletion A congenital dysmorphic syndrome characterized by microcephaly, hypertonia, antimongoloid slant, mental delay, and pyloric stenosis.[4651]

chromotopia Loss of the perception of colors when there is no loss for white objects. Clinically, it is usually a hemichromatopia, due to a lesion of the contralateral pathways less severe than is required to produce hemianopia.

chronaxie (chronaxy) (Gr, time + value) The time for which a current twice as strong as the galvanic threshold must flow in order to excite the muscle stimulated. The concept was introduced by Louis Lapique (b. 1866), a French physiologist, in 1909. Both the term and the concept are obsolete. See **strength–duration curve**.

chronaxy See **chronaxie**.

chronic (Gr, concerning time) Long continued.

chronic acquired hepatocerebral degeneration A heterogeneous disorder affecting patients with portosystemic collaterals or surgically created shunts. Clinical presentations can be neuropsychiatric (apathy, lethargy, dementia, excessive somnolence) or a movement disorder (dysarthria, ataxia, tremor, choreoathetosis that affects the cranial musculature predominantly but also that of the trunk and extremities; parkinsonism, myoclonus, pyramidal signs, and/or dystonia). Diffuse muscular rigidity, grasp reflexes, tremor at rest, nystagmus, action myoclonus, and persistent asterixis are less common signs. A coarse, rhythmic tremor of the arms in certain sustained postures and diffuse slowing on the EEG complete the typical clinical picture. Elevation of the blood ammonia level or an abnormality of ammonia tolerance are typical findings.

Cortical laminar necrosis and polymicrocavitation in the cortex and basal ganglia are combined with cerebral and cerebellar atrophy. Microscopically, Alzheimer type II astrocytes and cytoplasmic glycogen granules are characteristic. Recent neuroradiological observations in patients with liver failure have shown a specific magnetic resonance imaging appearance with a hyperintense T1 signal in the pallidum, putamen, and, rarely, the mesencephalon.[2862]

chronic AIDS encephalopathy See **HIV-associated cognitive/motor complex**.

chronic akathisia A form of drug-induced akathisia in which the abnormal movements occur either as the neuroleptic dose is being increased early in therapy (**acute persistent akathisia**) or coincide with a reduction of the dose at the end of the course of treatment (**tardive akathisia**).[843]

chronic alcoholic myopathy   See **alcoholic myopathy, Schultze test.**

chronic anterior poliomyelitis   (Cruveilhier atrophy) See **amyotrophic lateral sclerosis.**

chronic asymmetric spinal muscular atrophy   A rare syndrome, more common in males, with its onset in the first four decades of life and manifesting slowly progressive asymmetrical neurogenic muscular atrophy (usually of one arm) without bulbar or pyramidal involvement and with slight depression of the muscle stretch reflexes.[2442]

Patients with this condition probably represent that small proportion of those diagnosed as having **amyotrophic lateral sclerosis** whose survival is prolonged. See also **hereditary motor neuropathy** (*variants*).

chronic atrophic paralysis   An old name for **hereditary motor neuropathy.**

chronic axon loss polyradiculoneuropathy   See **chronic inflammatory demyelinating polyradiculoneuropathy.**

chronic benign lymphocytic meningitis   (chronic lymphocytic meningitis) A benign and chronic syndrome of headache, depression, malaise, and subtle personality change in patients with persistent elevation of CSF cell counts following an episode of meningitis. The etiology is unknown,[2647] but rarely conditions such as Wegener'granulomatosis and multiple sclerosis are found. A subgroup of patients responds to corticosteroids.[982]

chronic brain syndrome   Dementia. The term is inappropriate, evasive, and redundant. See **dementia.**

chronic brain syndrome of infantile hydrocephalus   See **cocktail party syndrome.**

chronic cerebral schistosomiasis   A granulomatous disease resulting from invasion of the brain, usually by *Schistosoma japonicum.* The granulomas may produce focal signs and frequently seizures.[6030]

chronic childhood spinal muscular atrophy   (Werdnig-Hoffman, Oppenheimer, [Wohlfart-]Kugelberg-Welander disease, Krabbe universal muscular hypoplasia, amyotonia congenita, hereditary proximal SMA, infantile muscular atrophy) A recessively (seldom dominantly inherited) syndrome manifesting progressive disorder of anterior horn cells with initial proximal selectivity but without pyramidal tract involvement, which does not itself cause death in less than 18 months. Most cases have their onset before the age of 8 years.[4383] See **hereditary motor neuropathy, types 1, 2, 3.**

chronic chorea   See **trigeminal neuralgia.**

chronic cluster headache   (chronic migrainous neuralgia) Headache in which the attacks occur for more than 1 year without remission or with remissions lasting less than 14 days. (see Chart C–17.)

Chart C–17. Chronic Cluster Headache

A. All letter headings of **cluster headache**
B. Absence of remission phases for 1 year or more with remissions lasting less than 14 days[1051]

Two subvarieties are defined:

Chronic cluster headache unremitting from onset (primary chronic cluster)

A. All letter headings of **chronic cluster headache**
B. Absence of remission periods lasting 14 days or more from onset

Chronic cluster headache evolved from episodic (secondary chronic cluster)

A. All letter headings of **chronic cluster headache**
B. At least one interim remission period lasting 14 days or more within 1 year after onset, followed by unremitting course for at least 1 year

Adapted from the Headache Classification Committee of the International Headache Society. Classification of headache disorders, cranial neuralgias and facial pains; and diagnostic criteria for primary headache disorders. Cephalalgia 1988;8(Suppl):1–96.[1051] *Reproduced by kind permission.*

chronic congenital TORCH encephalopathies   Polio-encephalopathies resulting from intrauterine infection with **T**oxoplasmosis, **O**ther viruses, **R**ubella, **C**ytomegalovirus, or **H**erpesvirus, or with *treponema.*

Developmental delay, myoclonic seizures, retinopathy, hepatosplenomegaly, and hematological disorders are potential consequences common to all these infections.[1822]

chronic congenital toxoplasmosis with late degeneration   A polioencephalopathy characterized by the development of chorioretinitis, intracranial calcification, cerebral cortical atrophy, microcephaly, and various neurological signs in infants after 3 months of age with congenital toxoplasmosis that had formerly been asymptomatic.[1588] See **congenital toxoplasmosis.**

chronic cytomegalovirus disease   An encephalopathy resulting from prenatal or perinatal cytomegalovirus infection, the virus acting like a slow virus infection, and liable to cause mild hydrocephalus progressing to extensive loss of brain substance or polycystic encephalomalacia. The virus can be cultured in the urine or leukocytes, indicating that it is capable of causing both static and progressive encephalopathies. The static encephalopathy usually consists of microcephaly, spasticity, seizures, and retinal abnormalities with hearing loss and mental retardation. In the progressive form, the virus has not been cultured from the brain.[729]

chronic dacryoadenitis   See **orbital pseudotumor syndrome.**

chronic daily headache   A compound headache syndrome characterized by persistence, clinical features reminiscent of both migraine and tension-type headache, and debilitation, all in the absence of evidence of organic disease. It has been subclassified as follows:

Primary chronic daily headache disorders include transformed migraine, chronic tension-type headache, new daily persistent headache, and hemicrania continua.

Secondary causes include post-traumatic headache, cervical spine disorders, and headache associated with vascular disease and nonvascular intracranial disorders. Most patients with chronic daily headache overuse symptomatic medication.[5156] See **chronic tension-type headache, transformed migraine, new daily persistent headache, hemicrania continua** (primary types); **and post-traumatic headache, cervicogenic headache, rebound headache** (secondary types). A classification has been attempted.[5157]

chronic demyelinating neuropathy with multifocal CNS demyelination (central and peripheral demyelination) A syndrome combining the features of chronic demyelinating peripheral neuropathy with slow nerve conduction velocities, peripheral nerve hypertrophy, and elevation of the CSF protein levels. Its onset is insidious and there is continuous progression with evidence of multifocal lesions in the CNS, including optic neuritis, brainstem involvement, and cerebellar and pyramidal signs, with episodic expression.[5552] These findings actually fulfil the diagnostic criteria for clinically definite **multiple sclerosis.**

The findings suggest the coincidence of a chronic inflammatory demyelinating polyneuropathy and multiple sclerosis, which might represent central and peripheral responses to a common antigen at some time past.

chronic encephalitis of Rasmussen   See **Rasmussen encephalitis.**

chronic encephalopathy with hepatic insufficiency See **acquired hepatocerebral degeneration.**

chronic encephalopathy with pulmonary insufficiency   See **chronic pulmonary encephalopathy.**

chronic Epstein-Barr virus infection   1. A syndrome of recurrent fever, upper respiratory tract infections, lymphadenopathy, fatigue, malaise, uveitis, keratitis, conjunctivitis, and corneal edema due to persistent or reactivating EB virus infection.[6027] 2. See **chronic fatigue syndrome.**

chronic factitious disorder with physical symptoms See **Munchausen syndrome.**

chronic familial vascular encephalopathy   See **familial subcortical dementia with arteriosclerotic leukoencephalopathy.**

chronic fatigue syndrome   (Royal Free disease, Iceland disease) A combination of the symptoms of apparent weakness, lack of mental drive, listlessness, and fatigue (easy tiring after exertion) in the absence of demonstrable organic pathology, substantially reducing a patient's daily activities for over 6 months.

Numerous other conditions can be subsumed under this heading with greater or lesser degrees of confidence; effort syndrome, *Da Costa syndrome, benign myalgic encephalomyelitis, chronic Epstein-Barr virus infection, postviral asthenia, postinfection fatigue syndrome, brain fever, breathlessness with effort intolerance, melancholy, the vapors, chlorosis, neurasthenia, repetitive strain injury,* and other named conditions have been considered by many to have no organic cause, while just as many others claim (or once claimed, for there is a fashion to these things) that these are physical rather than mental illnesses.

The presence of the above-mentioned symptoms without appropriate physical signs and a tendency in some instances for the symptoms to spread in communities with epidemic speed are the only notable clinical features. Objective testing of patients with typical fatigue syndromes revealed normal muscle strength in one recent study,[3446] though this is disputed. The demonstration of slowed reaction times, impaired performance on complex attentional amd memory tasks, and slowness in acquiring and processing new information suggest that an organic cause remains to be found.[4017]

Fatigue can be of central or peripheral origin, and particularly in the former case may not yet be susceptible to etiologic diagnosis, thus it may be best to keep an open mind with respect to the possible cause in any one case.[5437] Discussions on the very existence of this contentious syndrome as an organic entity have been emotional.

Criteria for the diagnosis have been suggested[2632] (see Chart C–18). Both of the *major criteria* (the new onset of a persisting or relapsing, debilitating fatigue that is not resolved by rest in bed, with a reduction of daily activity to less than half of the patient's premorbid activity for at least 6 months; and the exclusion of other causes of similar symptoms) and 6 of the *minor criteria* (fever, sore throat, myalgia, muscle weakness, arthralgia, headaches, and neuropsychological symptoms) must be fulfilled for the diagnosis to be made.

Chart C–18. Guidelines for the Diagnosis of Chronic Fatigue Syndrome

Chronic Fatigue Syndrome (CFS)

a. A syndrome characterized by fatigue as the principal symptom
b. Of definite onset and not life-long
c. Fatigue is severe and disabling, and affects physical and mental functioning.
d. Fatigue is present for more than 50% of the time for a minimum of 6 months.

e. Other symptoms also occur, particularly myalgia, and mood and sleep disturbance.

Exclusion criteria include the following:

a. Patients with established medical conditions known to produce chronic fatigue (e.g., severe anemia)

b. Psychiatric disorders, e.g., schizophrenia, manic depressive illness, substance abuse, eating disorder, or proven organic brain disease. Depressive illness, anxiety disorders, and hyperventilation syndrome are not necessarily reasons for exclusion.

Postinfectious Fatigue Syndrome (PIFS)

This is a subtype of CFS in which the condition either follows an infection or is associated with a current infection (benign postinfection myositis).[5024] Whether such associated infection is of etiological significance requires further study. To meet research criteria for PIFS, patients must:

1. Fulfil criteria for CFS as above, and
2. Fulfil the following additional criteria:
   a. There is definite evidence of infection at onset (patient's self-report is not sufficiently reliable).
   b. Corroboration of infection by laboratory evidence.

Adapted from Holmes GP, Kaplan JE, Gantz NM, et al. Chronic fatigue syndrome; a working case definition. Ann Intern Med 1988;108:387-389. Reproduced by permission.

chronic Guillain-Barré syndrome   See **chronic inflammatory demyelinating polyradiculoneuropathy.**

chronic hepatic encephalopathy and parkinsonism   (acquired (non-Wilsonian) chronic hepatocerebral degeneration) A syndrome of variable dementia, with a rather characteristic dysarthria, ataxia, intention tremor, and choreoathetosis that affects the cranial musculature predominantly but also that of the trunk and extremities; a coarse rhythmic tremor of the arms, maximized in certain sustained postures, pyramidal tract signs, and diffuse slowing on the EEG complete the typical clinical picture. Diffuse muscular rigidity, grasp reflexes, tremor at rest, nystagmus, and persistent asterixis are less common signs. Action myoclonus and combined system disease of the spinal cord have been found in isolated instances

The condition may complicate any type of liver disease (postnecrotic, portal, and biliary cirrhosis). All patients have had portal-systemic collaterals or surgically created shunts and have either an elevation of blood ammonia levels or abnormal ammonia tolerance. The major neuropathologic changes consist of a diffuse but patchy cortical laminar or pseudolaminar necrosis and polymicrocavitation at the corticomedullary junctions and in the striatum. In addition, there is a diffuse increase in the size and number of protoplasmic astrocytes, as is so often encountered in other forms of liver failure.

chronic hereditary spinocerebellar degeneration see **cerebellar ataxias.**

chronic hexosaminidase A and B deficiency   See **hexosaminidase deficiency.**

chronic hyperphosphatemia tarda   See **hyperostosis corticalis generalisata.**

chronic idiopathic adhesive arachnoiditis   Smouldering inflammation of the arachnoid membrane, seldom due to a cause that can be determined (although fungi may occasionally be responsible[1312]), leading to constriction and ischemia of the cord and the nerve roots at those levels. See **adhesive arachnoiditis.**

chronic idiopathic anhidrosis   The condition of isolated local failure of sudomotor function in adult life, with other evidence of autonomic failure being absent. Both pre- and postganglionic lesions may be responsible for the anhidrosis, which is not total, but which involves wide areas of the body, not always in contiguous sites.

Clinically, the patients manifest heat intolerance, becoming flushed, dizzy, dyspneic, and weak in high ambient temperatures, in which they do not sweat.[3487]

chronic idiopathic ataxic neuropathy   Sensory ataxia due to a chronic, large-fiber pure sensory neuronopathy, the principal lesion being of the dorsal root ganglia in the absence of cancer, nutritional deficiency, pyridoxine abuse, or previous acute infectious polyneuropathy. Sural nerve biopsy reveals severe destruction of myelinated axons.

The clinical features include paresthesias, profound disturbance of proprioception and kinesthetic sense, absent muscle stretch reflexes, and normal muscle strength.[1242,5171] The EMG and motor conduction speeds are normal but sensory potentials cannot be recorded. See also **chronic inflammatory demyelinating polyradiculoneuropathy, progressive sensory radiculopathy.**

chronic idiopathic axonal polyneuropathy   See **chronic inflammatory demyelinating polyradiculoneuropathy.**

chronic idiopathic headache   See **chronic tension-type headache unassociated with disorder of pericranial muscles.**

chronic immune demyelinating polyneuropathy (CIDP)   See **chronic inflammatory demyelinating polyradiculoneuropathy.**

chronic infantile spinal muscular atrophy   See **hereditary motor neuropathy, type 2.**

chronic inflammatory demyelinating polyradiculoneuropathy   (CIDP, relapsing corticosteroid-dependent polyneuritis, steroid-responsive recurrent polyneuropathy, relapsing hypertrophic neuritis, subacute demyelinating proximal and distal polyneuropathy, chronic axon loss polyradiculoneuropathy, chronic idiopathic axonal polyneuropathy, chronic Guillain-Barré syndrome) A heterogeneous syndrome of acquired, subacute or chronic, symmetrical, slowly progressive or relapsing polyneuropathies with pathological or electrophysiological evidence of demyelination and inflammatory cell infiltration within nerves, occurring mainly in adult males in the absence of detectable underlying causal disease such as carcinoma, paraproteinemia, etc. (CIDP-1). In the presence of such pathologies, the appellation *CIDP-2* has been suggested.

The neuropathy is usually sensorimotor, but pure motor and sensory forms also occur (see **chronic sensory demyelinating neuropathy**). The interval between onset and nadir of this condition is greater than 4 weeks and the average duration from onset to peak deficit is between 3 and 15 years. Sensory and autonomic changes are more common and identifiable antecedent events less common than in the acute form. Clinically there is hypo- or areflexia with often asymmetrical distal > proximal weakness; pain, painful paresthesias or numbness, autonomic signs, and clinically evident nerve hypertrophy may be noted. Mild, symmetric facial, or bulbar weakness occurs occasionally. The course is chronic and progressive in most cases, taking up to 2 years to reach a plateau. About a third of cases have a relapsing course. Two-thirds of patients respond to steroid therapy, most of the remainder to other forms of immunosuppression.[366,3733]

Pathologically, onion bulbs are seen in the peripheral nerves; the CSF protein is high and myelopathy can occur because of cord compression from the enlarged nerve roots.[3869] Electrophysiologic testing reveals conduction block, marked slowing of nerve conduction velocities, temporal dispersion of the CMAP, prolonged distal latencies, and impersistence of F waves. Serum IgM and IgG autoantibodies against tubulin are characteristic. MRI may show hypertrophy of spinal roots and plexus, especially in cases of long duration. Pathologically, the spinal roots and peripheral nerves may show mild inflammation but demyelination and remyelination are more typical. Anti-GM$_1$ ganglioside antibodies are seldom found.

In a minority of cases, periventricular, subcortical, and brainstem white matter lesions indistinguishable from those seen in multiple sclerosis are also seen, supporting the existence of a central–peripheral inflammatory demyelinating syndrome.[3830,4056] See **chronic demyelinating neuropathy with multifocal CNS demyelination.**

Variants include forms with onset in childhood (when the disease may be monophasic with remission) and associations with diabetes and serum M-proteins. In a few cases, a multifocal presentation, perineuritis, sensory manifestations, and arm involvement have been noted. Pathologically, there is patchy loss of myelinated axons with some axonal regeneration.

Multifocal demyelinating CIDP (Lewis-Sumner syndrome), is a slowly progressive, or relapsing–remitting disorder of adult life presenting with asymmetric, mainly distal weakness in the arms more than the legs. Occasionally, a proximal syndrome involving the phrenic or suprascapular nerves occurs. Sensory loss is mainly distal but is rarely severe or disabling. Electrophysiology shows multifocal conduction block and variably slowed nerve conduction velocities with prolonged distal latencies. The CSF is raised but usually <100 mg/dl IgM anti-GM$_1$ antibodies are not present. MRI may show swollen nerves in brachial plexus. Pathologically, there is patchy demyelination and some axonal loss.

Various sets of criteria for the diagnosis[11,366] have been blended by Saperstein et al.[4918]and are presented below (see Chart C–19). Electrodiagnostic criteria for demyelination (from a different source) follow.

Chart C–19. Chronic Inflammatory Demyelinating Polyradiculoneuropathy

1. Clinical

Mandatory Clinical Features

Major: symmetric proximal and distal weakness
Minor: exclusively distal weakness or sensory loss
Hypo- or areflexia (this will usually involve all four limbs)
Duration of 2 months or more

Laboratory Features

Mandatory: CSF protein >45 mg/dl
Supportive: Cell count <10/mm^3
Nerve biopsy shows predominant features of demyelination*
Electrodiagnostic studies (see below)

Requirements for Diagnostic Categories

Definite: Clinical major electrodiagnostic and CSF (biopsy not mandatory)
Probable: Clinical major electrodiagnostic or CSF and biopsy
Possible: Clinical major and I of 3 laboratory features

Unequivocal nerve biopsy evidence of demyelination and remyelination includes demyelination shown by either electron microscopy (>5 fibers) or teased fiber studies (>12% of 50 teased fibers, minimum of four internodes each, demonstrating demyelination/remyelination); subperineurial or endoneurial edema; mononuclear cell infiltration; onion bulb formation; and prominent variation in the degree of demyelination between fascicles.

Exclusion factors would be vasculitis, neurofilamentous swollen axons, amyloid deposits, or intracytoplasmic inclusions in Schwann cells or macrophages indicating adrenoleukodystrophy, metachromatic leukodystrophy, globoid cell leukodystrophy, or other evidence of specific pathology.

Clinical exclusions noted in the 1991 American Academy of Neurology Ad Hoc Committee recommendations[11] were the following:

1. Mutilation of hands or feet, retinitis pigmentosa, ichthyosis, appropriate history of drug or toxic exposure known to cause a similar peripheral neuropathy, or family history of a genetically based peripheral neuropathy
2. Sensory level
3. Unequivocal sphincter disturbance

*From Saperstein D.S., Katz JS, Barohn RJ. Clinical spectrum of chronic acquired demyelinating polyneuropathies. Muscle Nerve 2001;**24**:311–24. © 2001. Reprinted by permission of John Wiley and Sons, Inc.*

2. Physiological Studies[2695]

Neurophysiological Criteria for Diagnosis of CIDP[4198]

Either

1. Partial conduction block or abnormal temporal dispersion of conduction must be present in at least two nerves, and there must be significantly reduced conduction velocity, or significantly prolonged distal motor latency, or absent or significantly prolonged minimum F-wave latency in at least one other nerve; or

2. In the absence of block or dispersion, significantly reduced conduction velocity, or significantly prolonged distal motor latency, or absent or significantly prolonged minimum F-wave latency must be present in at least three nerves; or

3. In the presence of significant neurophysiological abnormalities in only two nerves, unequivocal histological evidence of demyelinating or demyelinated nerve fibers in a nerve biopsy must also be present.

Recording Technique

The following nerves are tested on both sides unless the criteria are fulfilled by studying a smaller number of nerves or points:

Median (wrist, elbow, axilla)
Ulnar (wrist, elbow, axilla, Erb's point)
Peroneal (ankle, below fibular head, above fibular head)
Tibial (ankle, popliteal fossa)
Ten consecutive F waves are recorded from each nerve, and the minimal latency is measured.

Definitions

Partial conduction block <15% change in duration between proximal and distal sites and >20% drop in negative peak area and peak-to-peak amplitude

Abnormal temporal dispersion and possible conduction block >15% change in duration between proximal and distal sites and >20% drop in negative peak area or peak-to-peak amplitude between proximal and distal sites; additional studies such as stimulation across short segments or recording of individual motor units required for confirmation

Significantly reduced conduction velocity <80% of lower limit of normal or, if distal motor compound muscle action potential amplitude <80% of normal, <70% of lower limit of normal

Significantly prolonged distal motor latency >125% of upper limit of normal or, if amplitude <80% of normal, >150% of upper limit of normal

Significantly delayed minimum F-wave latency >120% of upper limit of normal or, if amplitude <80% of normal, >150% of upper limit of normal.

Laboratory Studies

Depending on the results of the laboratory tests, those patients meeting the criteria above will be classified into the groups listed below.

The following studies are suggested: complete blood count, erythrocyte sedimentation rate, creatine kinase, antinuclear antibody, ANA, routine biochemical screen, thyroid function tests, serum and urine immunoglobulin studies (to include either immunofixation electrophoresis or immunoelectrophoresis), and HIV and hepatitis serology. The list of laboratory studies is not comprehensive. For instance, in certain clinical circumstances other studies may be indicated, such as phytanic acid, long-chain fatty acids, porphyrins, urine heavy metals, α-lipoprotein, β-lipoprotein, glucose tolerance test, imaging studies of the CNS, and lymph node or bone marrow biopsy.

Idiopathic CIDP is said to occur when there is no concurrent disease. The presence of such disease (depending on laboratory studies or other clinical features) indicates that the patient has an *acquired demyelinating polyneuropathy*. The conditions thus far described include thyrotoxicosis, HIV infection, monoclonal gammopathy, hereditary motor and sensory neuropathy, chronic active hepatitis, inflammatory bowel disease, systemic lupus erythematosus, monoclonal or biclonal gammopathy (macroglobulinemia, POEMS syndrome, osteosclerotic myeloma), Castleman disease, diabetes, CNS demyelinating disease, and Hodgkin disease.

After Hughes RAC, Bensa S, Willison H, et al. Randomized Controlled Trial of Intravenous Immunoglobulin versus Oral Prednisolone in Chronic Inflammatory Demyelinating Polyneuropathy. Ann. Neurol. 2001;50: 195–201, by permission.

Variant forms include the following:

Chronic demyelinating neuropathy with multifocal CNS demyelination[5552] A central–peripheral inflammatory demyelinating syndrome in which periventricular, subcortical, and brainstem white matter lesions indistinguishable from those seen in multiple sclerosis are found in association with the peripheral neuropathy.[3830]

A *sensory form* with distal pansensory loss and pain, and normal power or minimal distal weakness. Electrophysiology shows evidence of motor and sensory demyelination, conduction block, slow nerve conduction velocity and long distal latency in which the manifestations are more of a sensory than of a motor deficit.[4214]

An adult form in which the pathology suggests mainly axonal involvement.[5685]

Childhood CIDP A variant often following infections or vaccinations and with a monophasic or chronic course, with weakness and disability persisting in some cases. The disease here may be monophasic with remission.

CIDP associated with IgG or IgA M-protein A clinical syndrome similar to typical CIDP with slowly progressive symmetric weakness.

CIDP + diabetes mellitus A condition similar to CIDP, but the subjects are older, gait imbalance is especially marked, and there is evidence of significant axonal loss.

An *infantile form* is an hypertrophic, demyelinating, sensorimotor peripheral neuropathy with muscle weakness and atrophy, accompanied by scoliosis, pes cavus, and raised CSF protein levels.

In a few cases, a multifocal presentation, perineuritis, sensory manifestations, and arm involvement have been noted. See also **monoclonal gammopathy of uncertain significance,** the clinical features of which may be identical with those of CIDP. See also the Web site www.neuro.wustl.edu/neuromuscular/ for detailed current information.

chronic insomnia Prolonged difficulty in sleeping; **primary chronic insomnia, chronic pseudo-insomnia,** insomnia due to other disease, and forms due to another sleep disorder are distinguished.[4337]

chronic juvenile amyotrophic lateral sclerosis   See **hereditary motor system disease, hereditary motor neuropathy, type 3.**

chronic limb-girdle myasthenia gravis   See **myasthenia gravis.**

chronic lymphocytic leukemia   A group of malignancies characterized by the proliferation of small, immunologically mature lymphoid cells in the peripheral blood, most of which are B cell in origin. Neurological complications include *H. Zoster* and other opportunistic infections and, less commonly, direct invasion or hemorrhage in the central nervous system.[692]

chronic lymphocytic meningitis   An insidious progressive cause of headache and cognitive and neurological impairment that is sometimes responsive to corticosteroids. Leptomeningeal biopsy and long-term follow-up seldom identify the underlying cause in these patients.[982] See also **chronic benign lymphocytic meningitis.**

chronic manganese encephalopathy   A syndrome of involuntary movement disorders characterized by widespread cell loss in the caudate and putamen as a result of chronic manganese intoxication.[6061]

chronic meningitis   That form of meningitis in which the clinical and CSF abnormalities persist for longer than 4 weeks.[1644] Tuberculosis, brucellosis, and spirochetal infections are the most common infectious causes; granulomatous diseases and neoplastic meningeal disorders are others.

chronic migrainous neuralgia   See **chronic cluster headache.**

chronic motor axonal neuropathy   A diffuse inflammatory motor polyradiculoneuropathy not associated with the presence of anti-GM_1 antibodies or paraproteinemia.[2226] See also **chronic inflammatory dysimmune polyneuropathy.**

chronic motor tic disorder   A syndrome of stereotyped, unifocal, and unvarying motor or vocal tics (not both), occurring for over a year and usually presenting in adult life. The condition probably falls within the spectrum of **Tourette syndrome.**[2163]

chronic muscle contraction headache   See **chronic tension-type headache associated with disorder of pericranial muscles.**

chronic myelopathy   (progressive myelopathy) An isolated, slowly progressive unifocal myelopathy with predominantly motor findings, considered to be due to a single site of involvement by **multiple sclerosis** in patients in whom **amyotrophic lateral sclerosis, structural lesions,** and **subacute combined degeneration of the cord** have been excluded.[4368]

chronic myopathy   The rare production of a syndrome of muscle weakness and wasting in children as a result of persisting viral infection.[3687]

chronic neurogenic quadriceps amyotrophy   A rare focal wasting disease of the thighs, with childhood onset. See **Furukawa syndrome**[1998] and **hereditary motor neuropathy** (*variants*).

Chronic Pain Outreach   A charitable organization. Address: 822 Wycliff Court, Manassas, VA 22110.

chronic pain syndromes   These are listed variously by name in this book. A taxonomy has been devised by the International Association for the Study of Pain.[2723]

chronic paroxysmal hemicrania   (Sjaastad syndrome) Attacks with largely the same characteristics of pain and associated symptoms and signs as **cluster headache,** but shorter lasting, more frequent, and occurring mostly in females; there is absolute effectiveness of indomethacin. This definition and the diagnostic criteria are suggested by the Headache Classification Committee of the International Headache Society[1051] (see Chart C–20). This type of head pain almost exactly resembles **cluster headache,** the notable differences being the increased frequency (and reduced duration) of the pains, its predilection for women, precipitation often by neck movement, and the near-specific responsiveness to indomethacin.

Chart C–20. Chronic Paroxysmal Hemicrania; Diagnostic Criteria

A. At least 50 attacks fulfilling B–E below
B. Attacks of severe unilateral orbital, supraorbital and/or temporal pain always on the same side lasting 2 to 45 minutes
C. Attack frequency greater than 5 a day for more than half of the time (periods with lower frequency may occur)
D. Pain is associated with at least one of the following signs/symptoms on the pain side: conjunctival injection, lacrimation, nasal congestion, rhinorrhea, ptosis, eyelid edema
E. Absolute effectiveness of indomethacin (150 mg/day or less)
F. At least one of the following:
   History and physical and neurological examinations do not suggest one of the disorders listed in groups 5–11.
   History and/or physical and/or neurological examinations do suggest such disorder, but it is ruled out by appropriate investigations.
   Such disorder is present, but chronic paroxysmal hemicrania does not occur for the first time in close temporal relation to the disorder.

From Headache Classification Committee of the International Headache Society. Classification of headache disorders, cranial neuralgias and facial pains; and diagnostic criteria for primary headache disorders. Cephalalgia 1988;8(Suppl.):1–96. Reprinted by kind permission of Blackwell Science.

chronic paroxysmal hemicrania–tic syndrome   A rare **trigeminal-autonomic cephalalgia** in which these two syndromes occcur together.[6136]

chronic polymyositis   (acquired inflammatory polyneuropathy, late-life muscular dystrophy, menopausal muscular dystrophy) A very slowly progressive form of **idiopathic inflammatory polymyositis** occurring in adult life, affecting the arms and legs, often asymmetrically, without pain, muscle swelling, or associated skin changes.

In a *variant* form, intranuclear and intracytoplasmic aggregates with tubular structures are found on muscle biopsy.[1022]

chronic polyneuropathy of undetermined cause Sensory, motor, or mixed neuropathies usually with onset in mature adult life, symmetrical and present for more than 1 year. They are usually accompanied by mild slowing of motor conduction, an impairment of sensory conduction, and chronic axonal degeneration shown on sural nerve biopsy.

The condition is slowly progressive only and in some two-thirds of patients, prolonged follow-up does not yield any clues as to the underlying etiology. The group has been thought to make up some 13% of an unselected series of patients with peripheral neuropathy referred to a neurological center.[3778]

chronic polyradiculoneuropathy of infancy A fatal syndrome of progressive muscular weakness and wasting with areflexia and elevation of the CSF protein levels occurring in infancy, and characterized pathologically by near-total deficiency of myelin in the cranial and spinal nerve roots.[2949]

chronic portosystemic encephalopathy See **acquired hepatocerebral encephalopathy.**

chronic post-traumatic headache A headache syndrome without special features that is indistinguishable from chronic tension-type headache and migraine without aura. It is associated with reduced regional cerebral blood flow and hemispheric asymmetries, which supports an organic basis.[2350] See also **post-traumatic headache.**

chronic progressive dementia See **Alzheimer disease.**

chronic progressive encephalitis A slow-virus disease of brain possibly associated with preceding infection with the virus of **Russian spring-summer encephalitis,** clinically manifesting as mental, visual, auditory, pyramidal, and cerebellar disorders.

chronic progressive external ophthalmoplegia (CPEO; von Graefe syndrome) Disorders of conjugate gaze, usually without diplopia, but with marked ptosis. The syndrome may be accompanied by any of various other clinical features including dementia, mitochondrial myopathy, and encephalopathy (**Leigh disease**). It is often caused by deletions in mitochondrial DNA and is conveniently classified as an encephalomyeloneuromyopathy, thus ending the tedious disputes of the last 20 years as to whether the disorder is of central or peripheral origin. Clinically, the syndromes are usually dominantly inherited. The ophthalmoplegia (a constant) may be associated with weakness of other muscle groups and/or with evidence of central or peripheral nervous system dysfunction. See **Kearns-Sayre syndrome, mitochondrial diseases, progressive external ophthalmoplegia.**

chronic progressive myelopathy The clinical entity of a slowly progressive spastic paraparesis (spastic gait, leg weakness and hyperreflexia, and variable degrees of sensory loss) without evidence of spinal cord compression, disseminated lesions, or disease of the lower motor neurons. Most of these patients are eventually considered to suffer from **multiple sclerosis.**[4368]

chronic progressive radiation myelopathy See **radiation myelopathy.**

chronic progressive spinobulbar spasticity A syndrome characterized by spasticity, dysphasia, and twelfth cranial nerve abnormalities with onset in adult life.[337]

chronic pseudoinsomnia The complaint of insomnia starting in adult life with daytime sleepiness and malaise, but without demonstrable abnormality of the duration or structure of sleep on investigation in the sleep laboratory.

chronic psychogenic headache See **chronic tension-type headache unassociated with disorder of pericranial muscles.**

chronic pulmonary encephalopathy (chronic encephalopathy with pulmonary insufficiency) A progressive degenerative disease of premature infants with severe respiratory distress. Cerebral cortical and brainstem forms are differentiated, each with a fatal prognosis.[1643,3835]

chronic relapsing plexus neuropathy with persistent conduction block See **multifocal inflammatory CIDP variant, multifocal inflammatory demyelinating neuropathy.**

chronic relapsing polyneuropathy The term applied to those forms of **chronic inflammatory demyelinating polyradiculoneuropathy** in which remissions and recurrences occur.

chronic segmental spinal muscular atrophy of the upper limbs A sporadic or familial disorder characterized by juvenile onset, uni- or bilateral localization of muscle atrophy to the hands and forearms, and a benign course.[2585]

chronic sensory ataxic neuropathy See **chronic sensory demyelinating neuropathy.**

chronic sensory demyelinating neuropathy (chronic sensory ganglionopathy) A form of **chronic inflammatory demyelinating neuropathy** with its pathology localized mainly in the dorsal root ganglion cells, characterized by the subacute or chronic progression of a pure sensory neuropathy (though with electrical evidence that the demyelinating process affects motor as well as sensory fibers), loss of proprioceptive and kinaesthetic sensation, raised CSF protein, and a good response to immunosuppression.[4214] Malignancies, Sjogren syndrome, and paraproteinemic and idiopathic causes are recognized.[2899]

chronic sensory ganglionopathy See **chronic sensory demyelinating neuropathy.**

chronic sensory neuropathy (chronic sensory ganglionopathy) An insidiously progressive large-fiber sensory neuronopathy with ataxia as its most prominent clinical feature.[5171] See **chronic idiopathic ataxic neuropathy.**

chronic spinal meningitis (radicular myelopathy associated with spinal neuronitis, meningitis circumscripta spinalis) A rapidly progressive radicular myelopathy due to extensive spinal meningitis, often occurring as a first expression of tuberculosis in the nervous system.

Syphilis, pyogenic organisms, *Cryptococcus* and chemicals may also be causal in a few cases. The condition was first described by Harley in 1909. See **spinal arachnoiditis.**

chronic spinal muscular atrophy with pallidal degeneration See **hereditary motor neuropathy** (*variants*).

chronic subdural hematoma (pachymeningitis hemorrhagica interna) Subdural hemorrhage present at 2 weeks or more after head trauma which has displaced the brain in an anterior–posterior direction, tearing the veins as they enter the superior longitudinal sinus and leading to blood loss into the subdural space, with the eventual formation of a membrane.

Clinical signs typically include headache, depression of consciousness, and fluctuating focal deficits; increased intracranial pressure and such transient neurological signs as weakness, dysarthria, dysphasia, and visual field deficits are also recorded as presenting signs. The condition is an important cause of reversible dementia.

The latent interval between the trauma and the development of clinical signs may be months or years,[5646] so that patients and their family and friends may be unaware of the occurrence of the preceding head trauma.

chronic tension-type headache (chronic daily headache) Headache present for at least 15 days a month during at least 6 months. The headache is usually pressing/tightening in quality, mild or moderate in severity, bilateral, and does not worsen with routine physical activity. Nausea, photophobia, or phonophobia may occur. This definition and the diagnostic criteria are suggested by the Headache Classification Committee of the International Headache Society (see Chart C–21). The definition is valid but the diverse manifestations of this heterogeneous form of headache may not always comply.

Chart C–21. Chronic Tension-Type Headache: Diagnostic Criteria

A. Average headache frequency ≥15 days/month (180 days/year) for ≥6 months fulfilling criteria B–D, listed below
B. At least two of the following pain characteristics:
  1. Pressing/tightening quality
  2. Mild or moderate severity (may inhibit, but does not prohibit activities)
  3. Bilateral location
  4. No aggravation by walking stairs or similar routine physical activity
C. Both of the following:
  1. No vomiting, and
  2. No more than one of nausea, photophobia, or phonophobia
D. At least one of the following:
  1. History, and physical and neurological examinations do not suggest one of the disorders listed in groups 5–11 of the International Headache Society Classification scheme (see **headache**)
  2. History and/or physical and/or neurological examinations do suggest such disorder, but it is ruled out by appropriate investigations
  3. Such disorder is present, but tension-type headache does not occur for the first time in close temporal relation to the disorder.

From Classification of headache disorders, cranial neuralgias and facial pains; and diagnostic criteria for primary headache disorders. Cephalalgia 1988;8(suppl):1–96.[1051] Reprinted by kind permission of Blackwell Science.

chronic tension-type headache associated with disorder of pericranial muscles (chronic muscle contraction headache) Chronic tension-type headache associated with increased levels of tenderness and/or EMG activity of pericranial muscles. This definition and the following diagnostic criteria are suggested by the Headache Classification Committee of the International Headache Society (from Classification of headache disorders, cranial neuralgias and facial pains; and diagnostic criteria for primary headache disorders. *Cephalalgia* 1988;**8**[suppl]:1–96).
  A. Fulfils criteria for **chronic tension-type headache**
  B. At least one of the following: increased tenderness of pericranial muscles demonstrated by manual palpation or using pressure algometer, or increased EMG activity in pericranial muscles at rest or during physiological tests. In such cases there may be localized areas of cervico-occipital muscle tenderness with particularly painful nodules or trigger points on palpation.

chronic tension-type headache unassociated with disorder of pericranial muscles (chronic idiopathic headache, chronic psychogenic headache) Chronic tension-type headache with normal levels of tenderness and/or EMG activity in pericranial muscles. This definition and the following diagnostic criteria are suggested by the Headache Classification Committee of the International Headache Society (from Classification of headache disorders, cranial neuralgias and facial pains; and diagnostic criteria for primary headache disorders. *Cephalalgia* 1988;**8**[Suppl]:1–96), by kind permission.

A. Fulfils criteria for **chronic tension-type headache**

B. No increased tenderness of pericranial muscles. If peprformed, EMG of pericranial muscles shows normal levels of activity.

chronic tetanus   A rare *variant* occurring in patients partially immune to tetanus, and producing such symptoms as stiffness and muscle spasms, worsened by volitional movements and startle, and lasting months. Electrodiagnostic studies and muscle biopsy study show evidence of motor neuropathy.[4712]

chronic tetany   (sporadic tetany) See **idiopathic neuromyotonia.**

chronic tic disorder   See **Tourette syndrome.**

chronic TORCH encephalopathy with myoclonia   A variant of **chronic congenital TORCH encephalopathies** with this added complication.

chronic traumatic edema   See **reflex sympathetic dystrophy.**

chronic Werdnig-Hoffmann disease   See **hereditary motor neuropathy, type 2.**

chronodispersion   The difference between minimum and maximum latency values in a series of *F* **waves.**

chronotaraxis   A disturbance of temporal orientation, time interval estimation, or chronological order of events for symptoms that is peculiar to circumscribed lesions of the anterior ventral and mediodorsal thalamic nuclei.[5276]

chronotherapy   A form of therapy for sleep disorders in which the times for waking and sleeping are rigidly prescribed.

Churg-Strauss syndrome   (leucocytoclastic angiitis, allergic granulomatosis, eosinophilic granulomatous vasculitis) An autoallergic vasculopathy of unknown cause, not certainly defined as a specific entity as characterized as part of the spectrum of polyarteritis nodosa. Clinically, it is characterized by asthma, fever, hypereosinophilia with widespread necrotizing arteritis, erythema multiforme, allergic rhinitis, and extravascular granulomatosis. Neurological features occur in about 25% of cases and include deficits of cranial nerves II, III, VII, and VIII, myositis, and polyneuropathy or multiple mononeuropathy,[5377] and other focal deficits such as the Balint syndrome and Churg-Strauss syndrome. See also **allergic angiitis** and granulomatosis.

Chvostek, Franz   (1835–1884) Austrian physician who trained in Vienna and worked there for all of his life. He published an account of his sign in 1876. His other contributions were in various fields of internal medicine.

Chvostek sign   Tapping over the facial nerve anterior to the ear leads to twitching of the homolateral facial muscles due to hyperexcitability of the nerve, as in hypocalcemic tetany.

The related **Chvostek phenomenon** consists of hyperexcitabilty of any of the peripheral nerves to percussion, as in cases of tetanus.[1037]

chymopapain   A proteolytic digestive enzyme used for **chemonucleolysis.**

cicatrix   A gliotic scar in the CNS, often leading to the local origination of epileptic discharges and detectable during life by **MRI.**

ciguatera   A widespread ichthyosarcotoxaemia with dramatic and clinically important neurological features. The clinical syndrome results from the ingestion of ciguatera toxin, a substance found in various species of periequatorial reef fish as the result of their ingestion of algae containing the toxin that increases the permeability of membranes to sodium. Captain James Cook suffered from this in 1777, probably as a result of eating a large grouper; the condition is most common in Polynesian and Caribbean waters. The neurotoxin is stored in the viscera of fish that have eaten the dinoflagellate and concentrated it upwards throughout the food chain towards progressively larger species, including humans. Both Pacific (P-CTX-1) and Caribbean (C-CTX-1) ciguatoxins are potent, heat-stable, lipophilic sodium-channel activator toxins that bind to and maintain open the voltage-sensitive sodium channel on the cell membranes of all excitable tissues.

The clinical manifestations include oral and peripheral paresthesias, dysesthesias and allodynia, metallic taste, pruritis, nausea, vomiting, malaise, anorexia, burning joint pain, **cold reversal,** diarrhea, vomiting, skin itching, cramps, and joint and muscle pains. Temperature perception reversal is sometimes described as "pathognomonic" for ciguatera. Cerebellar dysfunction, hyporeflexia, cranial nerve palsies, and (rarely) respiratory paralysis have also been recorded. Autonomic dysfunction leads to hypotension, bradycardia, dilated pupils, and hypersalivation in severe cases.[1025,4382] The differential diagnosis includes organophosphate, botulinus, tetrodotoxin, and neurologic shellfish poisoning. See also **tetrodotoxin, scombroid, paralytic shellfish poisoning, domoic acid.**

ciliary   (from Lat, the eyelid or eyelash). Pertinent to the eyelid.

ciliary arteries   Anterior and posterior, long and short branches of the ophthalmic artery supplying the external ocular muscles, and the conjunctiva, sclera, ciliary apparatus, and choroid.

ciliary body   The ciliary muscle and anterior part of the choroid (corona ciliaris), with specialized functions in secreting the aqueous fluid into the anterior chamber of the eye. It was known to **Herodotus** (ca. 290 B.C.), but the term was applied by **Fallopius** (ca. 1550 A.D.) to the whole of the anterior part of the choroid, the restrictive definition being made by Frederich Henle (1809–1885), a German anatomist.

ciliary ganglion   A ganglion situated immediately behind the eye, in which relay parasympathetic fibers destined for the ciliary body, and sympathetic fibers with a similar destination pass through without synapsing. It was described by Ànders Retzius (1796–1860), a Swedish anatomist (ca. 1840).[4979]

ciliary muscles   Smooth muscles of the ciliary body, the circumferential fibers described in 1858 by Heinrich Muller (1820–1864) and the radial in 1847 by William Bowman (1816–1892).[4979] Together they control the aperture of the pupil and the degree of curvature of the lens.

ciliary neuralgia   Intermittent bouts of severe pain in the cheek, temple, and eye. See **cluster headache, Charlin syndrome.**

ciliary reflex   Touching the eyelashes causes blinking of the homolateral eyelid.[6064]

ciliospinal center of Budge   The site of the cell bodies of the second neuron of the descending sympathetic pathway, situated at the C8–T2 cord levels. Their fibers are pupillodilator neurons.

ciliospinal reflex   Dilation of the pupil homolateral to a painful stimulus such as pinching the neck. The presence of the sign indicates the integrity of the afferent pathway through the cervical nerves and of the efferent sympathetic pathway that traverses the whole of the brainstem.

cilosis   (from Lat, an eyelash) Spasmodic trembling of the eyelid. A form of facial **myokymia.**

cinchona   The extract of the bark of the Peruvian oak, so named after the Countess of Cinchon, wife of the Spanish Governor of Peru, who was cured of a fever (presumably malaria) through its use. The active principle is quinine.

cinchonism   Quinine toxicity, manifest by headache, tinnitus, tremor, pallor, and jaundice.

cinerea   (Lat, ash-colored). Hence tuber cinereum—the "grey root" of the pituitary.

cinesialgia   (Gr, movement + pain) An extinct term for painful muscle cramps or muscle pain during contraction.

cinetic   (from Gr, with reference to motion) Now usually written as *kinetic.*

cingulate   (from Lat, a belt or girdle) Encompassing.

cingulate gyrus   The four-layered paleocortex representing the cortical expression of the **limbic system** and sited above the corpus callosum on the medial aspect of the frontal lobes.

cingulate gyrus syndrome   See **Nielsen syndrome.**

cingulate seizures   A seizure disorder in which the seizure patterns are complex partial with complex motor gestural automatisms at the onset. Autonomic signs are common, as are changes in mood and affect. (Adapted from Commission for Classification and Terminology, ILAE. Proposal for revised classifications of epilepsies and epileptic syndromes. *Epilepsia* 1989;**30:**389–399.[1114])

These complex partial seizures often end with a temper tantrum. They may be provoked by stress, and are often accompanied by frequent absence attacks, autonomic disturbances, and motor signs.[3722]

cingulosynapsis   A form of lobar **holoproscencephaly** in which the hemispheres are well developed but joined by a band of neocortex over the corpus callosum.[3108]

cinonosos   (Gr, to move + disease) An obsolete term for any disease affecting muscular motion.

circadian rhythm   Alternations of sleeping and waking, and of activity, body temperature, and hormonal levels with a cycle of about a day, paced by a "clock" function within the suprachiasmatic nucleus. Two circadian rhythms exist, each with a 25-hour length: the sleep–wake/growth hormone/urinary electrolytes cycle and the rapid eye movement sleep/cortisol/body temperature cycle.

circadian rhythm sleep disorders   Varieties of **dyssomnia** reflecting disturbance of the timing of sleep rather than its nature. They are classified by the **American Sleep Disorders Association** as follows:[234]

1. **Time zone change (jet lag) syndrome**
2. **Shift work sleep disorder**
3. **Irregular sleep–wake pattern**
4. **Delayed sleep phase syndrome**
5. **Advanced sleep phase syndrome**
6. **Non–24-hour sleep–wake disorder**
7. Circadian rhythm sleep disorder not otherwise specified.

See also **sleep disorders.**

circle of Haller   The network of blood vessels surrounding the optic nerves; also the attachments of the mitral and tricuspid valves in the heart.

circle of Willis   The anastomotic ring of arteries (two posterior cerebral, posterior communicating, internal carotid, and anterior cerebral; one anterior communicating and the basilar) which encircles the pituitary stalk anterior and inferior to the base of the brain.

It was first depicted in 1647 by Johann Vesling, but Thomas **Willis** further defined the structures in 1664 and his name is applied to the configuration.

circular nystagmus   (diagonal, elliptic, oblique, alternating windmill, circumduction, gyratory, radiary nystagmus) Types of acquired pendular nystagmus in which the fine, fast, vertical, and horizontal oscillations are in opposite directions. In circular nystagmus, they have similar amplitudes; in elliptical nystagmus, they are different. The resulting ocular movements are as their names suggest. The retinal image and the perceived motion (**oscillopsia**) are in the same direction as the eye movement.[1368]

Such disorders are most commonly due to brainstem disease but are sometimes congenital.

circumduction   An abnormality of gait in which the pelvis is elevated on the side of a hemiparesis when the weight is borne on the other leg, in order that the affected leg (longer now as a result of hip and knee extension and ankle plantar flexion) does not scrape upon the ground.

circumduction nystagmus   See **circular nystagmus.**

circumferential bipolar montage   A montage consisting of derivations from pairs of electrodes along circumferential arrays. (Adapted from the report of the Committee on Terminology, IFCN,[989] © 1974, with permission from Elsevier Science.)

circumlocution   Discursive wordiness, indirectly providing information rather than defining the objects to be communicated. Charles Dickens' Mr. Micawber is a well-drawn example, but he did not appear to suffer from that amnesic aphasia, which is a typical pathology causing this form of speech disturbance.

circumscribed cortical atrophy   See **Pick disease.**

circumscribed serous spinal meningitis   See **arachnoid diverticula.**

circumscript meningitis   See **subdural empyema.**

cirsoid aneurysm of the scalp   A congenital syndrome characterized by paroxysmal vascular headaches and the presence of cirsoid aneurysms.[337] See also **aneurysm.**

cisterna chiasmatica   The subarachnoid space between the optic chiasm and the rostral end of the corpus callosum.

cisterna interpeduncularis   The subarachnoid space between the crura cerebri (cerebral peduncles).

cisterna magna   (Lat, large reservoir) The subarachnoid space behind the transverse fissure of the cerebellum.

cisternal block syndrome   See **Zange-Kindler syndrome.**

cisternal puncture   Insertion of a needle through the atlanto-occipital membrane into the cisterna magna. This is done to collect a CSF sample when it cannot be obtained at the usual lumbar site, or to insert contrast medium above the level of a spinal block. Precise measurement of the depth of the puncture is required, since the next structure to be encountered after the cistern is the medulla oblongata. The procedure was introduced by Obregia in 1908 and further refined by James B. Ayer (b. 1882), an American neurologist, in 1920.

cisternography   An invasive test designed to assess the circulation of the CSF, performed by the injection of a radionuclide such as radioiodinated albumin into the lumbar subarachnoid space, the passage of this marker indicating CSF flow patterns when the spine and later the head are scanned with a gamma camera at intervals over the following 72 hours.

citrullinemia   (Allen-Dent syndrome) A recessively inherited hyperammonemic syndrome of infants due to deficiency of argininosuccinate synthetase, an essential enzyme in the urea cycle. The responsible gene maps to 9q34. Three forms (neonatal/infantile types I and III, and adult type II) are recognized. The genetic defect of the latter is in the "citrin" gene (*SLC25A13*) and the clinical manifestations are mainly those of hepatic encephalopathy with raised plasma levels of citrulline and ammonia.[2728]

Types I and III are characterized by attacks of ataxia, vomiting, irritability, seizures, involuntary movements, seizures, and confusion which occur from early childhood, precipitated by dietary protein and fever in children who are mentally retarded.[3784] High plasma levels of argininosuccinic acid are found.[5722] Although the condition may be lethal because of brain edema, in some cases it is actually asymptomatic.

A variant is reported from Japan, in which the onset is in adult life, presenting with cyclical bizarre, behavior patterns, dysarthria, and motor weakness, with dementia and hepatomegaly following. See also **argininosuccinase deficiency.**

Clarke column   The dorsal or posterior columns of the spinal cord[1478] (nucleus dorsalis), described by **Clarke** in 1851.

Clarke cells   Pigmented cells in the nucleus dorsalis.

Clarke, Jacob Augustus Lockhart   (1817–1880) English anatomist and neurologist who trained first at Guy's Hospital in London and later at St. Andrews. After his initial anatomical publications, which started in 1851 when he described the nucleus dorsalis, he was elected a Fellow of the Royal Society (1854) and he received thier gold medal 10 years later. Although initially a general practitioner, he was appointed to the staff of the Hospital for Epilepsy and Paralysis in Regent's Park, London (now the **National Hospital,** Queen Square) on the basis of his research output. Most of his other papers were on the subjects of **diabetes,** the muscular atrophies, paraplegias, and tetanus.

clasp-knife rigidity   If the examiner attempts to extend the flexed limb of a patient with a pyramidal lesion, **Gowers** noted that "when near full extension the spasm [of the extensor muscles] suddenly comes on and completes the movement, as the blade of a pocket knife moves under the influence of a spring."[2240] Today it is considered that sudden inhibition of the resistive flexor force is a more likely explanation. This is presumably due to the activation of the Golgi tendon organs by the force of the stretch, leading to the usual generation of their impulses inhibiting activity in the reflex arc.

class hysteria   Contagious behavioral excess. The **dancing mania** is a relatively benign example of such activity; teen behavior at rock concerts is another, and mob violence another still, but more malignant.

classical torsion dystonia   See **dystonia.**

classification of neurologic disease   "It is impossible to base a classification on the pathological evidence alone; this is only part of the clinical picture. Any classification must be based on genealogic, clinical and pathological manifestations."[5800] This excellent advice is not always heeded, and the common phenotypic variability of dominantly inherited diseases provides a rich mine, ripe for eponymous excavations.

Claude, Henri-Charles-Jules   (1869–1945) French neurologist who graduated and then trained further in Paris, at one time being assistant to Raymond and Bouchard. He was later appointed to the staff of the **Salpetrière** in Paris. His earliest contributions were studies in pathology, but he later turned to psychiatry and neurology and was concerned with movement disorders, hysteria, peripheral nerve lesions, epilepsy, and the physical treatment of the psychoses in particular.[1750]

Henri-Charles-Jules Claude

Claude hyperkinesis   Painful stimuli applied to paretic muscles excite reflex flexion or extension movements of those muscles; presented as evidence of organic weakness.

Claude syndrome   The combination of third and fourth cranial nerve palsies with contralateral cerebellar ataxia, rubral tremor, and hemianesthesia, resulting from a paramedian midbrain tegmental lesion involving the red nucleus and the superior cerebellar peduncle. The etiology is usually a stroke, tumor, or aneurysm.[1052] See **cerebellar ataxia with crossed third nerve palsy.**

Claude topoanesthesia   See **Verger-Déjérine syndrome.**

claudication   (from Lat, to halt or be lame) Limping. The word is speculatively considered to have been introduced through the lameness of the Roman Emperor Claudius.

claudication of the cord   Inability to continue the act of walking due to acutely progressive weakness of the legs. See **lumbar spinal stenosis.**

Clauss phenomenon   The toe phenomenon—see **Strümpell sign,** although it was described independently in 1926 by Clauss.

claustrophobia   (from Lat, a bolt + Gr, fear) Mental anguish from being enclosed within a small confining space.

claustrum   (Lat, a barrier or fence) A thin gray-matter strip described by **Meynert,** lying lateral to the lenticular nucleus and beneath the insula.

clavus hystericus   (Lat, a nail + hysterical) Sharp, sudden, stabbing, local head pain, as though a nail were being driven in.[2240] Despite the name, there is no suggestion that this is a psychiatric disorder. See **ice pick pains.**

claw foot   ("le pied en griffe") The position taken up by the foot with paralysis of its intrinsic muscles. The mechanical effect of unopposed action of the long toe extensors is to cause raising of the arch with shortening of the foot, dorsiflexion of the proximal phalanges, and plantar flexion at the distal joints.

claw hand   ("le main en griffe") The position taken up by the hand with paralysis of its small intrinsic muscles such as the interossei and lumbricals; the long finger flexors produce flexion at the proximal and distal interphalangeal joints while extension at the metacarpophalangeal joints is maintained by the long extensors.

CLEAT syndrome   The acronym of **C**erebral infarcts, **L**ivedo reticularis, **E**ndocardial lesions, **A**maurosis fugax, and **T**hrombosis, these comprising selected but characteristic clinical manifestations of the **antiphospholipid antibody (Sneddon) syndrome.**

Cleckley reflex   See **Allen reflex.**

cleft lip–palate and tetraphocomelia   (Apelt-Gerkin-Lenz syndrome) A recessively inherited syndrome characterized by bilateral cleft lip and palate, tetraphocomelia with a reduction in the number of digits, proptosis, hyperteleorism, and dwarfism. Hydrocephalus, encephalocele, spina bifida, and cardiac defects have also been described in association.[195] See **Roberts syndrome.**

clefting   A craniofacial malformation in which there is persistence of epithelium between the borders of the facial bony processes which normally fuse during development. Clefts thus occur at the sites of normal fusion, as between the lateral or medial nasal and the maxillary processes (naso-ocular clefts and cleft lip); between the palatine processes of the maxillae (cleft palate); or between the maxillary and mandibular processes (macrostomia).[4]

clefting with skeletal anomalies   See **Crane syndrome**.

clefting–corneal opacity–retardation syndrome   See **Anyane-Yeboa syndrome**.

Clifton Assessment Procedure for the Elderly (CAPE) A brief mental status examination assessing orientation, mental abilities, and psychomotor abilities in chronic psychiatric and geriatric patients and used to differentiate dementing from functional disorders.

The scale has two parts, the first concerning information/orientation and scored after interview with the subject, while the second is a behavior rating scale in which activities of daily living are also scored.[4366]

Clinical Autonomic Research   A journal communicating data on research and treatment related to autonomic function and dysfunction. It is the official journal of the American Autonomic Society, the Clinical Autonomic Research Society, and the European Federation of Autonomic Societies, and is published by Lippincott Williams & Wilkins.

Clinical Dementia Rating Scale   A composite instrument for the assessment of the severity of dementia on the basis of a semistructured interview procedure with the patient and an informed caregiver. Six areas of functioning (memory, judgement and problem-solving, orientation, community affairs, home/hobbies, and personal care) are each rated on a 5-point scale (0 = none; 0.5 = questionable; 1 = mild impairment; 2 = moderate impairment; and 3 = severe impairment). Language and praxis are not assessed.[487,2691]

Two additional categories have been suggested, to allow a rating of more severely impaired people:

   CDR 4: *Profound* indicates severe impairment of language or comprehension, with inability to walk unaided, and difficulty in feeding, in recognizing family, or in controlling bladder or bowel function.

   CDR 5: *Terminal* is applied to subjects who require total care and are completely uncommunicative, bedridden, vegetative, and incontinent.

Clinical EEG Electroencephalography (*Clin. EEG Electroencephalogr.*) A subspecialty medical journal. Address: American Medical Electroencephalographic Association, 850 Elm Grove Road, Suite #11, Elm Grove, WI 53122.

clinical electromyography (electroneuromyography) A term encompassing all electrodiagnostic studies of peripheral nerves and muscles. See also **electromyography, nerve conduction studies**.

Clinical Journal of Pain   A subspecialty journal published by Lippincott, Williams and Wilkins. Web site: http://www.clinicalpain.com/.

Clinical Neurological Assessment Tool   A 21-item instrument assessing various parameters of activity in patients following head trauma. The scale is strengthened by the incorporation of items relating to brainstem function (see Chart C–22).

The scores attained on this scale correlate well with those of the **Glasgow Coma scale**.

Chart C–22. Clinical Neurological Assessment Tool

   I. *Assessment of patient's response following verbal stimulation*
      1. *Response to verbal stimulation.* Assessor will say, "Hello [patient's nickname or first name]. This is [assessor's name]. How are you?"
         1. No response
         2. Minimally aroused/slight movement
         3. Becomes agitated/startles
         4. Opens eyes, lids fluttering and blinking
         5. Orients toward verbal stimulation/demonstrates signs of recognition
      2. *Eye movement in response to verbal stimulation*
         1. No response
         2. Slight movement of eyelids/eyes
         3. Opens eyes sluggishly
         4. Opens eyes, lids fluttering and blinking
         5. Opens eyes briskly, purposeful blinking
   II. *Assessment of patient's response to tactile stimulation. Firmly grasp left or right arm, and shake it.*
      3. *Body response to touch*
         1. No response
         2. Startles or becomes agitated/demonstrates posturing
         3. Slight movement
         4. Movement away from source
         5. Movement toward source
         6. Movement toward source/attempts to grasp assessor
         7. Able to discriminate areas of light touch
      4. *Eye movement in response to touch*
         1. No response
         2. Slight movement of eyelids
         3. Opens eyes sluggishly
         4. Opens eyes, lids fluttering and blinking
         5. Opens eyes briskly, purposeful blinking
      5. *Response to painful stimulation*
         1. No response
         2. Startles or becomes agitated/demonstrates posturing
         3. Sluggish/delayed motor response
         4. Moves away from source of pain
         5. Localizes to pain source
         6. Purposeful avoidance of pain/grimace
         7. Able to discriminate sharp from dull stimulation
   III. *Assessment of patient's ability to follow commands*
      6. *Request patient to follow movement of finger with eyes:* "[patient's name], follow my finger."

1. No response
2. Opens eyes
3. Follows <30° arc
4. Follows >30° arc but <90° arc
5. Follows 90° arc

7. *Response to command to squeeze and release assessor's hand.* Record best score, right hand versus left hand.
   1. No response
   2. Delayed but slow squeeze
   3. Slow squeeze
   4. Brisk squeeze
   5. Squeeze and release

8. *Demonstrates subjective behavior*
   1. None
   2. Willful uncooperative activity
   3. Willing but unable to cooperate
   4. Willful cooperative activity

IV. *Assessment of patient's muscle tone and resistance*

9. *Muscle tone of biceps.* Record best score, right arm versus left arm.
   1. Flaccid
   2. Rigid
   3. Tense
   4. Normal

10. *Resistance associated with flexion/extension of arms.* Record best score, right versus left.
    1. Flaccid
    2. Rigid
    3. Tense
    4. Normal

11. *Muscle tone of quadriceps.* Record best score, right versus left leg.
    1. Flaccid
    2. Rigid
    3. Tense
    4. Normal

12. *Resistance associated with flexion/extension of legs.* Record best score, right versus left.
    1. Flaccid/no resistance
    2. Inability to flex/fixed
    3. Flexion/rigid (clasp-knife)
    4. Flexion/nonpurposeful resistance
    5. Flexion normal

V. *Assessment of patient's body and extremity position/movement*

13. *Body position in bed*
    1. Motionless/remains stationary
    2. Position secondary to posturing
    3. Skewed/nonaligned
    4. Relaxed/purposeful/sleep-like

14. *Arm activity*
    1. Motionless/flaccid
    2. Both extended and internally rotated (decerebrate)
    3. One arm extended and one arm flexed (decorticate/decerebrate)
    4. Both decorticate
    5. Semiflexed/appears tense
    6. Normal/flexed

15. *Leg activity*
    1. Motionless/flaccid
    2. Both extended (decerebrate)
    3. Semiflexed/appears tense
    4. Normal/flexed

16. *General voluntary body movement*
    1. No voluntary movement or posturing
    2. Slight movement
    3. restlessness, rolling and turning
    4. Aroused/nonpurposeful movement
    5. Purposeful movement

17. *Position of eyelids.* Record best score
    1. Half open
    2. Closed/no movement
    3. Closed with oscillation of eyes
    4. Closed with blinking/fluttering
    5. Tightly closed/purposeful
    6. Open and blinking/fluttering

VI. *Assessment of patient's chewing, yawning, verbalization*

18. *Chewing*
    1. Absent
    2. Nonpurposeful
    3. Grinds teeth
    4. Normal purposeful

19. *Yawning*
    1. Absent
    2. Present
    If chewing and yawning are not observed, consult with person caring for patient. If no one has observed chewing or yawning, mark absent.

20. *Verbalization*
    1. Unconscious/no sound
    2. Moaning and/or babbling
    3. Conscious/no attempts at speech
    4. Single-word answers/nodding or shaking head
    5. Spontaneous communication to self or others
    6. Meaningful communication yet word retrieval problems
    7. Meaningful communication (written, verbal, and/or gestures)

21. *Orientation*
    1. Unable to communicate (this does not mean because of tracheostomy)
    2. Disoriented
    3. Oriented to time, place, person, situation (reason for hospitalization) (if incorrect responses, patient should be classified disoriented)

Adapted from Crosby L, Parsons LC. Clinical neurological assessment tool. Heart Lung 1989;18:121–129.[1194] *Reprinted by kind permission of Elsevier Science.*

Clinical Neurology and Neurosurgery (*Clin. Neurol. Neurosurg.*) A clinical neuroscience Journal. The official publication of the Netherlands Society of Neurology, the Netherlands Society of Neurosurgery, and the Flemish Society of Neurology, published by Elsevier Science. Web site: http://www.elsevier.com/locate/clineuro.

clinically definite multiple sclerosis 1. That form of **multiple sclerosis** fulfilling all of the **Schumacher Criteria.**[5011] 2. A diagnostic category of **multiple sclerosis** characterized by the occurrence of two preceding attacks, with evidence of involvement of two or more sites in the nervous system (clincally probably multiple sclerosis [CPMS]) A1 or with two previous attacks, clinical evidence of one involved site in the nervous system and paraclinical evidence of multiple sclerosis such as positive oligoclonal banding, positive MRI findings, or abnormal evoked responses. See **Poser criteria.** See also **McDonald-Halliday criteria.**[3744]

clinically probable multiple sclerosis A diagnostic category of **multiple sclerosis** characterized by evidence of two preceding attacks with clinical evidence of one abnormal site in the nervous system (CPMS C1); of one prior attack and evidence of two involved sites in the nervous system (CPMS C2); or of evidence of one prior attack, clinical evidence of one site involved in the nervous system and the presence of para-clinical evidence of multiple sclerosis (CPMS C3). See **Poser criteria.** See also **McDonald-Halliday Criteria.**[3744]

Clinician Interview-Based Clinical Impression An FDA-mandated attempt to categorize the physician's gestalt in the context of clinical trials of medications for **Alzheimer disease.** Minimally or very much improved/worsened are the preferred ratings.[3099]

clinocephaly (Gr, bed or inclination + head) A cranial developmental malformation in which there is depression of the cranial vault behind the bregma; the vertex is thus flattened into the shape of a couch.[4]

clinodactyly Incurving and shortening of the little finger; a common feature in developmental diseases such as **Down syndrome.**

clinoid (Gr, in the shape of a bed). Shaped like an antique bed.

clipping Distortion of EEG waves as a result of overload, which makes them appear flat-topped in the paper write-out.

clitoral crises Paroxysms of sexual excitement in females with **tabes dorsalis.**[2240] An unnecessary term for a rare manifestation of an unusual disease in a restricted population.

clivus That part of the sphenoid bone forming the central portion of the base of the skull.

clivus edge syndrome See **Kernohan notch syndrome, transtentorial herniation.** The term is not altogether appropriate since it is the tentorial free edge, not the clivus, which compresses the brainstem.

clonic absence attacks See **myoclonic absence attacks.**

clonic facial spasm See **hemifacial spasm.**

clonic seizures Those forms of seizure in which the muscular contractions are intermittent. In the case of focal seizures, the jerks involve a part of the face or part or all of one limb. Consciousness is preserved.[3720]

clonic status epilepticus See **status epilepticus.**

clonic-tonic-clonic seizures Tonic-clonic seizures preceded by prominent myoclonic jerks.[1361]

clonus (from Gr, a commotion or tumult) Repetitive involuntary alternating contractions of agonist and antagonist muscle groups at about 5 Hz in response to a sudden maintained stretching force. It is due to disinhibition of a spinal generator within the reflex arc at that level, as in pyramidal tract lesions.[5821]

closing-in phenomenon The tendency to draw upon or close to the pattern to be copied in drawing tests, seen in patients with diffuse cortical disease.[3718]

clouding An alteration of consciousness such that perceptions are reduced in number, immediacy, and strength, the speed and clarity of thought are diminished and, in many but not all cases, the patient is abnormally distractible. Clouding is a common sign in the early stages of delirium and in patients with severe dementia.

Clouston disease (hidrotic ectodermal dysplasia) A dominantly inherited syndrome characterized by nail dystrophy, telangiectasias, hair defects, hyperkeratosis of the palms and soles, cataract, and strabismus.[1059]

cloverleaf skull (Holtermuller-Weidermann syndrome) A deformity resulting from premature synostosis of the parietotemporal sutures.[2633]

CLOX An executive clock drawing task that correlates closely with cognitive test scores and discriminates between healthy and demented elderly people. The test is divided into two parts. CLOX1 is an unprompted task that is sensitive to executive control, while CLOX2 is a copied version that is less dependent on executive skills. CLOX1 is more "executive" than several other comparable clock-drawing tasks. CLOX1, but not CLOX2, makes a significant independent contribution to the level of care recieved by elderly retirees.[4835]

club foot Shortening of the foot with elevation of the arch, usually a congenital deformity inherited as a recessive trait, although a majority of patients are male. The problem is usually bilateral.

The term was in use in England in the mid-sixteenth century. The earliest full description was in 1794 by Antonius Scarpa (1747–1832), an Italian anatomist and surgeon who also described (Scarpa's) canal in the inner ear, and the nerve, canal, fascia, and triangle to which his name is also given. He was also the first to identify disease of the medial wall of arteries as the basis of aneurysms.[4723]

cluneal nerve syndrome A myofascial pain syndrome presenting with paravertebral and gluteal pain and stiffness with palpable trigger zones in the affected areas.[5382] See also **piriformis syndrome.**

cluster headache (Bing headache [syndrome]) Attacks of severe, strictly unilateral pain occurring orbitally, supraorbitally, and/or temporally, lasting 15–180 minutes and occurring from once every other day to 8 times a day. The pain is associated with one or more of the following: conjunctival injection, lacrimation, nasal congestion, rhinorrhea, forehead and facial sweating, miosis, ptosis, and eyelid edema. Attacks occur in series lasting for weeks or months (so-called cluster periods) separated by remissions usually lasting months or years. About 10% of patients have chronic symptoms. Even fewer have a preceding aura.

The clinical features suggest excessive cranial parasympathetic discharge and abnormal activation of the suprachiasmatic nucleus has been postulated as a causal factor.

The following diagnostic criteria are suggested by the Headache Classification Committee of the International Headache Society[1051] (see Chart C–23).

Chart C–23. Cluster Headache: Diagnostic Criteria

A. At least five attacks fulfilling B–D below
B. Severe unilateral orbital, supraorbital, and/or temporal pain lasting 15 to 180 minutes untreated
C. Headache is associated with at least one of the following signs which have to be present on the pain side: conjunctival injection, lacrimation, nasal congestion, rhinorrhea, forehead and facial sweating, miosis, ptosis, and eyelid edema
D. Frequency of attacks; from 1 every other day to 8 per day
E. At least one of the following:
History and physical and neurological examinations do not suggest one of the disorders listed in groups 5–11.9 (see **headache** Chart H–5).
History and/or physical and/or neurological examinations do suggest such disorder, but it is ruled out by appropriate investigations.
Such disorder is present, but cluster headache does not occur for the first time in close temporal relation to the disorder.

From the Headache Classification Committee of the International Headache Society. Classification of headache disorders, cranial neuralgias and facial pains; and diagnostic criteria for primary headache disorders. Cephalgia 1988;8(Suppl):1–96. Reproduced (adapted) by kind permission.

In *secondary cluster headache,* the clinical features are the same except for the lack of periodicity seen in the primary form, but follow injury or disease in the trigeminal distribution or vertebral artery dissection.[1159]

See also **episodic cluster headache, chronic cluster headache, chronic paroxysmal hemicrania.**

The tireless reader who has examined the contents of this book from A to C will have found already, and will still find, references to this condition from (in all) about 16 entries, so various are the names which have been given to it. The now-fashionable name **cluster headache** was the happy invention of Kunkle (1954), who remarked on the periodicity of the attacks 80 years after the condition was first described by Eulenberg.[3177] The most arresting descriptions were those of Symonds[5458] and of Horton et al.[2662]

cluster headache variant An alternative name for **chronic cluster headache,** in which atypical cluster headache, multiple jabs of pain, and background vas-

cular headache occur. The headache is atypical in that it occurs several times daily, shifts sides, is less severe and briefer than the typical cluster headache, does not recur in bouts, and is less constantly accompanied by signs of autonomic overactivity.[3801]

cluster headache–like disorder not fulfilling criteria Headache attacks believed to be a form of cluster headache or **chronic paroxysmal hemicrania** but which do not quite meet the operational diagnostic criteria for any of the forms of either condition. This definition and the following diagnostic criteria are suggested by the Headache Classification Committee of the International Headache Society[1051] and are reproduced by kind permission, adapted.

A. Fulfilling all but one of the criteria for **cluster headache** or **chronic paroxysmal hemicrania** (see Charts C–20 and C–23).

cluster minibouts Episodes of **cluster headache** lasting only 1–2 weeks.[5197]

cluster vertigo The association of cluster headaches with episodic vertigo which occurs during the cluster headache periods.[2108]

cluster-migraine A syndrome combining some of the components of cluster headache and of migraine headache, without abnormal findings on neurological examination. An example might be the occurrence of a typical (migrainous) visual aura preceding a cluster headache.[5256]

cluster-tic syndrome A variant of **cluster headache** in which **trigeminal neuralgia** is associated with tic-like pains. The pains respond somewhat to carbamazepine and baclofen but not to methysergide.[5256]

cluttered speech (tachyphemia) A developmental articulatory disorder in which the speed of speech is increased beyond the patient's control, the patient varies the inflexions and division of syllables in a manner which is not euphonious, and speech is arrhythmic and repetitious.

These features may be accompanied by hyperactivity, impaired concentration, poor musical ability, and disturbances of reading and writing. The site and nature of the causal lesion are not known.[208]

Clutton joints Painful (sometimes painless) hydrarthrosis of the knees in children with congenital syphilis. This was first described by Dr. Henry Clutton (1850–1909) in 1886.

CMT International (Charcot-Marie-Tooth Disease International) A charitable organization based at 34-B Bayview Drive, St. Catherines, Ontario, Canada L2N 4Y6.

CNS Drugs A journal reviewing disease management and optimum drug therapy for psychiatric and neurological disease, published by ADIS (New Zealand). Web site: http://biomednet.com/library/jcnd.

CNS hypersomnia syndrome A chronic disorder of excessive daytime somnolence. The cause is not known, but prior infection with Epstein-Barr virus may play a part.

Coats, G. (1876–1915) A Scottish ophthalmologist working in London.

Coats syndrome A syndrome consisting of exudative telangiectasias of the retina, optic atrophy, and sensorineural deafness, sometimes associated with a port wine stain or with **facioscapulohumeral muscular dystrophy.**[5507]

coaxial needle electrode See **concentric needle electrode.**

Cobb, Stanley (1887–1969?) American neurologist and psychiatrist who trained at Harvard and in British and European centers before returning to the United States and serving as Chief of the Neurology Service at Boston City Hospital, from where he published widely on the cerebral circulation and demonstrated the reactivity of its arterial system to carbon dioxide rather than oxygen. He transferred to become Head of Psychiatry at the Massachusetts General Hospital in 1934, from which post he retired in 1954.

Cobb as much as anyone helped to reintegrate neurology and psychiatry, and demonstrated the utility and possibility of running a psychiatric service within a general hospital. His broad training in the basic neurosciences also allowed him an imaginative view of the nervous system which was perhaps unique for a psychiatrist who espoused the psychoanalytical school.[5940]

Cobb syndrome (cutaneomeningospinal angiomatosis) A sporadic **neurocutaneous syndrome** characterized by the association of pial venous hemangiomas of the spinal cord behaving as extradural mass lesions with compression of the spinal cord or nerve roots, and by nevi in the overlying skin of the corresponding dermatomes.[1061] Those nevi in cervical regions may be associated with lesions of the lower cranial nerves. See **cutaneomeningospinal angiomatosis, Klippel-Trenaunay-Weber syndrome.**[3724]

cobblestone complex Forms of lissencephaly (malformations due to abnormal neuronal migration) in which the brain is not abnormally smooth. They have been classified[358] as follows:

Cobblestone Complex Syndromes
1. Congenital muscular dystrophy syndromes
   a. Walker-Warburg syndrome
   b. Muscle–eye–brain (MEB) disease
   c. Fukuyama congenital muscular dystrophy
2. Syndromes with no involvement of muscle
   a. Cobblestone complex MEB pattern with normal eyes and muscle
   b. Cobblestone complex diffuse with normal eyes and muscle

From Barkovich AJ, Kuzniecky R, Jackson GG, et al. Classification system for malformations of cortical development. *Neurology* 2001;**57**:2168–78. Reproduced by permission.

cocaine test One drop of 10% cocaine solution is instilled into each eye, followed by another drop in each eye 1 minute later. A normal pupil will dilate by the time the eyes are reexamined in 45 minutes, but the pupil with loss of sympathetic innervation will not do so.

The mechanism is the prevention by the cocaine of the reuptake of norepinephrine at the sympathetic junctions of the normal iris, leading to an excessive local adrenergic dilator effect; when there is a distal lesion of the sympathetic pathway, less norepinephrine than usual is available. See also **hydroxyamphetamine test.**

coccidioidomycosis An uncommon infection with the soil fungus *Coccidioides immitis,* capable of causing a chronic basal granulomatous leptomeningitis, which usually results from the spread of cranial osteomyelitis, and choroiditis, uveitis, optic nerve granuloma, papilledema, and sixth cranial nerve palsy.[442]

coccydynia (coccygodynia) Persistent pain felt in the coccygeal area, especially on sitting and with local pressure, with no known cause.

coccygodynia See **coccydynia.**

coccyx (Gr, the cuckoo) The four lowest small, fused, triangular vertebrae.

cochlea (Lat, a snail, from Gr, a winding staircase) A tapering, coiled tube in the anterior part of the labyrinth within the petrous temporal bone; the auditory endorgan.

cochlear aplasia Developmental disorders of the inner ear and usually of the seventh cranial nerve. See **Michel, Mondini** and **Scheibe** defects.

cochlear deafness, myopia and oligophrenia syndrome See **Flynn-Aird syndrome.**

cochleo-orbicularis reflex See **cochleopalpebral reflex.**

cochleopalpebral reflex (cochleo-orbicularis reflex) Blinking of the eyes in response to a sudden loud noise.[6064] See also **palpebral reflex.**

cochleopupillary reflex Mydriasis in response to a sudden and unexpected loud noise; a normal phenomenon.

cochleovestibular atrophies A group of inherited disorders, often with congenital onset, manifesting nerve deafness and/or vestibular malfunction.

Cockayne, Edward Alfred (1880–1956) English lepidopterist and physician or pediatrician, to the Middlesex and Great Ormond St. Children's Hospitals, respectively. His major interests were endocrinopathics and genetic diseases.[1750]

Cockayne syndrome (type VI sudanophilic leukodystrophy, dwarfism with retinal atrophy and deafness) A rare, recessively inherited condition, only possibly a leukodystrophy, in which there is failure of DNA repair.[1064] See also **Neill-Dingwall syndrome.**

Clinically, the children appear normal at birth but later develop mental retardation, prognathism, thickened microcephalic skull, an abnormally old facial appearance, anhidrosis, cachexia, skin photosensitivity, kyphosis, dwarfism with large hands and feet, and joint contractures. Neurological features include sensorineural deafness, optic atrophy, cataracts, cerebellar ataxia, demyelinating sensorimotor peripheral neuropathy, and pigmentary retinal degeneration.[3965,5660]

Death occurs by the third decade, by which time marked spasticity and often tremor, nystagmus, ataxia, seizures, choreoathetosis, patchy CNS demyelination, and both basal ganglion and perivascular calcification are usually notable.[5251]

cocktail party deafness   Those forms of minor or moderate nerve deafness in which speech discrimination is markedly diminished as a result of background noise.

cocktail party syndrome   (chatterbox syndrome, chronic brain syndrome of infantile hydrocephalus) A syndrome manifest in children with arrested hydrocephalus who appear bright and very talkative but in whom mental development is profoundly affected.[2740]

codfish vertebrae   Biconcavity of the posterior aspects of the vertebral bodies, seen in homocystinuria.[5555]

coenesthesis   (Gr, common + sensation) Subjective awareness without precision as to the modes stimulated which produce that awareness; the total impression of internal bodily sensations. The reality of such a sensory mode, and the different interpretations placed upon the meaning of the word in the last 200 years, have made the word and possibly the concept obsolescent.[4965]

Coffin syndrome   (lean spastic dwarfism) A familial dysmorphic syndrome characterized also by spastic quadriparesis, seizures, predisposition to infections, congenital cardiac anomalies, and mental and motor delay.[1068]

Coffin-Lowry syndrome   (fifth digit syndrome) A congenital X-linked dysmorphic syndrome mapping to Xp 22.2, characterized by mental and developmental delay, growth retardation, scoliosis, thickened calvarium, hypotonia, lax joints, ptosis, hypertrichosis, and abnormal development of the fifth digits and their nails, and sometimes of other digits as well. The **Dandy-Walker malformation** or other hindbrain abnormalities are associated with unusual frequency.[1323]

Coffin-Siris syndrome   A congenital syndrome comprising mild microcephaly, coarse facial features, absent or hypoplastic fifth digits and their nails, hypotonia, and psychomotor delay, accompanied by the **Dandy-Walker malformation.**[1323]

COFS syndrome   (cerebro-oculofacioskeletal syndrome) See **Pena-Shokeir phenotype.**

Cogan sign (lid twitch sign)   The patient is asked to look down, then up, and down and up twice more. As a result of fatigue of the weaker levator muscle in **myasthenia gravis,** both lids go up, but the weaker one then slowly descends again, as if overshooting and then settling.[1074]

Cogan syndrome   1. (congenital oculomotor apraxia, Wieacker syndrome) An inability to perform voluntary saccadic horizontal eye movements, although spontaneous and reflex movements are possible, described by Cogan in 1953. Thus affected children are unable to deviate their eyes when asked to examine an object set to one side, but rather turn their head, at which the eyes actually deviate the other way because of the integrity of the vestibulo-ocular reflex.[1070]

As a result of the abnormal movements of the head and eyes during attempted changes in the direction of gaze, only delayed and hypometric horizontal jerk saccades can be made when the head is immobilized; when it is not, the subject makes thrusting and overshooting head movements to compensate for the inability to move the eyes voluntarily. A history of prematurity, delayed psychomotor development, strabismus, and slight clumsiness are common accompaniments. The anatomical substrate for the condition is not certainly defined.[6113] See also **ocular apraxia.**

2. *Nonsyphilitic interstitial keratitis* occurring in young adults, who present with photophobia, blurred vision, recurrent attacks of vertigo, vomiting, tinnitus, and deafness, resembling the symptoms of **Ménière disease** but due to diffuse vasculitis.[1069] Other neurological and systemic manifestations are variably present.[559]

3. A congenital syndrome manifesting hemianopia, loss of optokinetic nystagmus, dyslexia, spasm of conjugate gaze, lateral disorientation, finger agnosia, dysgraphia, and dyscalculia.

cognition   (Lat, with + knowledge) A generic term for quality of knowing, which in this context has been said to include abstraction ability, attention, conceiving, imagining, judgement, memory, perception, praxis, problem-solving reasoning, recognizing, sensing, and use of language. This motley collection of mental accomplishments constitutes a summation of adaptive behavior.

Cognitive Capacity Screening Examination   A formalized, short, bedside screening test of cognitive function with adequate reliability but with a substantial false-negative rate. It consists of 30 questions testing orientation to place and time, concentration, short-term memory, abstraction, digit recall, and arithmetic ability.[2781]

cognitive closure   The mental completion of an incomplete stimulus; the ability to perceive a complete pattern where only an incomplete one is presented. Tests of such gestalt operations are considered to give information on right hemisphere functioning. See also **Gollin Incomplete Figures Test.**

cognitive dissonance   The acceptance of both of two opposing viewpoints; a match/mismatch situation in which a subject wishing to believe in a pair of mutually exclusive ideas frequently experiences emotional distress.

cognitive domains   The functions of orientation, attention, language, visuospatial functions, executive functions, motor control, and praxis.

cognitive failures questionnaire   A series of 25 questions to do with minor errors of memory or judgment that subjects may make ("Do you fail to listen to people's names when you are meeting them?") presented as a list for the patient to score between 0 (never) to 4 (very often). In a second part, a relative is asked to rate the patient on a different series with eight questions.[760]

cognitive fatigue   A decline in cognitive performance during a single psychological testing session documented in multiple sclerosis,[3169] but likely to be a nonspecific finding.

cognitive processing epilepsy   A composite of seizure types (generalized tonic-clonic, myoclonic, absence) sharing the common bond of precipitation by higher cortical processes such as performing mathematical problems, making decisions, playing board or card games, drawing, etc.[554] *Epilepsy arithmetices, decision-related epilepsy,* and *drawing-induced seizures* are named examples.

cognitive reserve   A proposed mechanism accounting for the fact that some people show more and some show less cognitive impairment after similar brain injuries; and explaining nicely the protective effect of higher education in the prevention or delay of the symptoms of **Alzheimer disease.**

cogwheel phenomenon   The arrhythmic, repetitive alteration of resistance to passive stretch occurring during passive movement of a joint; a palpable tremor. Such regular involuntary interruptions to the smooth flow of passive movements are a sign of disease of the basal ganglia, as in parkinsonism.

cogwheel (saccadic) pursuit eye movement   The occurrence of **catch-up saccades** during pursuit eye movement in an effort to compensate for a diminished velocity of those eye movements caused by, for example, reduced consciousness from any cause, or diffuse hemispheric or brainstem disease.[3329]

Coh syndrome   A craniofacial malformation characterized by **cloverleaf skull** with fusion of all sutures, polymicrogyria, absent olfactory tracts and bulbs, duplication of the thumbs, micropenis, and bifid scrotum.[4]

Cohen hamartoma syndrome   A congenital dysmorphic syndrome characterized by asymmetrical eyes, heterochromia iridis, epibulbar dermoids, cataract, detached retina, malocclusion of teeth, asymmetrical leg hypertrophy with varicose veins, macrocephaly, hydrocephalus, and mental and developmental delay. Papules, capillary hemangiomas, lipomata, and other tumors of the skin are often present.[337]

Cohen syndrome   A recessively inherited syndrome characterized by facial, oral, and ocular abnormalities, with microcephaly, microphthalmia, myopia, lax joints, brachydactyly, syndactyly, scoliosis, obesity, and hypotonia. The condition may be a manifestation of hyper-β-alaninemia.[1096,2568,3272]

coin-in-the-hand test   A bedside or office test used to determine the organicity of claimed amnesia in which the subject is shown a coin in one of the examiner's hands, and after 10 seconds of eye closure is asked to indicate the hand in which the coin was held, over 10 trials. Malingering patients perform at chance levels, but those with delayed memory failure, as after herpes encephalitis, usually attain a perfect score.[2927]

coital cephalgia   See **headache associated with sexual activity.**

cold   The sensation that an object contacted is at a lower temperature than the self. "In medicine, the sensation was formerly described as having three degrees of intensity: *algor,* when there was merely the feeling of cold; *horror,* when there was the creeping feeling of chilliness; and *rigor* when there was actual shivering."[4512] The phenomenon of cold is of interest in neurology because subjective descriptions of localized sensations of cold are occasionally heard in patients with myelopathy, particularly that due to **multiple sclerosis.** Cold itself may, however, have a beneficial effect in multiple sclerosis, while heat often induces an increase in symptoms, perhaps through alterations in the functioning of the neural potassium pump. With cerebral lesions, such as strokes, the affected limbs, especially the leg, may be several degrees cooler than the unaffected limbs.

cold face test   The measurement of cardiac rate following the application of cold compresses to the face, which induce bradycardia, decreased cardiac output, selective vasoconstriction of the skin and viscera, and maintained blood pressure depending on the function of the trigeminal-brainstem-vagal reflex pathway. The *diving reflex* and the *simulated diving reflex* (for which the stimuli are, respectively, immersion of the body and of the face in cold water) depend upon the same pathways.[3031] See also **cold pressor test.**

cold nerve injury   Nerve damage as a result of nonfreezing cold injury following a period in which temperatures fluctuate, likely because of repeated reperfusion injury.[2859]

cold pain   See **post-traumatic neuralgia.**

cold pressor test   A measure of sympathetic efferent vasoconstrictor activity. When a patient's hand is placed in ice water for 1 minute, or when ice is applied to the neck (**cold face test**), the forearm blood flow diminishes and the blood pressure should rise by 20/15 mmhg,[3777] but it does not do so in the presence of a central or an efferent sympathetic lesion.[3485] Bradycardia also occurs, in the absence of a parasympathetic lesion.

cold reversal   The sensation of heat and pain occurring with cold stimulation of the skin, as in **ciguatera** poisoning.

cold stimulus headache   Headache resulting from the exposure of the head to low temperatures. Generalized headache following exposure of the unprotected head to a low environmental temperature as in sub-zero weather or when diving into cold water. This definition and the following diagnostic criteria are suggested by the headache classification committee of the International Headache Society (from Classification of headache disorders, cranial neuralgias and facial pains; and diagnostic criteria for primary headache disorders. *Cephalalgia* 1988;8[suppl]:1–96):

A. Develops during external exposure to cold
B. Is bilateral
C. Varies in intensity with the severity and duration of the cold stimulus
D. Is prevented by avoiding exposure to cold
E. Is not associated with organic cranial or intracranial disease

The headache was first described by Robert **Whytt.**

A subvariety is *ice-cream headache,* a pain produced in susceptible individuals by the passage of cold material, solid or liquid, over the palate and posterior pharyngeal wall. This definition and the following diagnostic criteria are suggested by the Headache Classification Committee of the International Headache Society (from classification of headache disorders, cranial neuralgias and facial pains; and diagnostic criteria for primary headache disorders. *Cephalalgia* 1988;8[suppl]:1–96[1051]):

A. Develops during ingestion of cold food or drink
B. Lasts for less than 5 minutes
C. Is felt in the middle of the forehead, except in people subject to migraine, in which case the pain may be referred to the area habitually affected by migraine headache (code migraine first)
D. Is prevented by avoiding the rapid swallowing of cold food or drinks
E. Is not associated with organic disease

cold test   Local cooling, which reduces myasthenic fatigability, as is well shown in the ptotic eyelids of the myasthenic patient, which open after ice has been applied to them, until they warm again. The mechanism is not known.[665]

cold vasodilatation   Capillary vasodilation of the skin causing transient rises in the skin temperature follow-ing immersion of the fingers in cold water. This is uninfluenced by sympathetic nerve integrity but is absent after section of the somatic nerves and so is likely to be due to a sensory nerve axon reflex.[2267]

Coleman syndrome   (cervical spine trauma with injury of the head and shoulder girdle) A nonspecific cervical spine injury occurring in association with combined injuries to the head and the shoulder girdle. The lesion may include a fracture of the odontoid process, rotary dislocation of the atlas on the axis, fractured dislocation of the cervical vertebrae, and fracture of the transverse spinal processes. Cervical cord contusion is a possible reason for these features.[3841]

collapse   (from Lat, to fall together) More or less sudden prostration as a result of severe physical or emotional illness such as fever, shock, seizure, or overwhelming affect.

Though formerly a respectable word in medicine, its clear meaning has endeared it to the laity so the profession therefore largely eschews it.

collateral   (Lat, with + the side) 1. That which accompanies or runs beside; an alternate pathway—thus an auxiliary blood supply of a body part. 2. A branch of an axon.

collateral circulation   The auxiliary pathways for blood supply to the brain, comprising extracranial arterial connections, the persistence of vessels running between the extracranial and intracranial circulations (middle–anterior meningeal, facial, anterior choroidal–posterior cerebral) and intracranial cerebral arterial anastomoses, such as the circle of Willis and superficial anastomoses between branches of the three major cerebral arteries.[2922]

collateral reinnervation   The growth of nerve sprouts from a healthy axon's subterminal fiber to innervate a denervated motor end-plate. An indicator of the presence of neurogenic disease.

Collet, Frederic Justin   (b. 1870) French otolaryngologist; he described the following condition in 1915, 2 years before the account by J.A. Sicard, a French radiologist.

Collet-Sicard syndrome   (posterior lacerocondylar syndrome, Bonnet-Collet syndrome, Weisenberg-Sicard-Robineau syndrome) Unilateral paresis of the bulbar nerves IX, X, XI, and XII, from which result loss of taste on the posterior third of the tongue, paralysis of the vocal cords and palate, weakness of the sternomastoid and trapezius muscles, and hemianesthesia of the palate, tongue, and pharyngeal walls. In contradistinction to the findings in **Villaret syndrome,** there is no **Horner syndrome.**[1103]

Although Collet's patient had a bullet lodged in his head, the syndrome is usually due to compression or infiltration by local infection such as tuberculosis or by tumors such as lymphomas, chromaffinomas, or parotid body tumors causing ischemia in the territory of the neuromeningeal trunk of the ascending pharyngeal artery. See also **Vernet syndrome.**

colliculus   (Lat, a little hill) In the CNS, the anterior and posterior quadrigeminal bodies in the midbrain, parts of the optic and auditory reflex pathways, respectively.

Collier, James Stansfield   (1870–1935) English neurologist and neuropathologist who trained at St. Mary's Hospital and who was later on the staffs of the **National Hospital** and St. George's and the Bethlem Hospitals, where he was known as a dramatic and inspiring teacher and a superb diagnostic clinician.

Although he recognized that cerebral palsy was often the result of arrested development in utero, his best known works were his contribution to the study of **subacute combined degeneration of the cord** with **Russell** and **Batten,** and his description of the **superior orbital fissure syndrome,** which he considered to be a periostitis. He was the first to suggest that the dilated lateral ventricles in patients with **hydrocephalus** stretch and displace those descending motor fibers destined to control leg movements, thus explaining the spasticity in the legs in that condition.

Collier sign   (posterior fossa stare, tucked lid sign, lid retraction) Bilateral symmetrical lid retraction in the dorsal midbrain syndrome, resembling that of hyperthyroidism, but here accompanied by light-near dissociation and without lid lag on down-gaze.

Collins, Edward Treacher   (1862–1932) English ophthalmologist who practiced at Moorfields and Charing Cross Hospitals in London. He described what we call **Treacher Collins syndrome** in 1900, but there had been a prior report in 1846.

collision   When used with reference to nerve conduction studies, the interaction of two action potentials propagated toward each other from opposite directions on the same nerve fiber so that the refractory periods of the two potentials prevent propagation past each other.

colloid cyst   (Gr, glue-like + a bag) Benign, thin-walled cysts, usually detected in the anterior end of the third ventricle, with a columnar or cuboidal epithelial wall and soft colloidal contents. They are considered to arise from the embryonic remnant of the stomatodeum.

Their clinical effects result only when the cyst causes obstruction of CSF flow, when they may be manifest by intermittent paroxysms of acute headache with a notable postural factor, and by signs of raised intracranial pressure, coma, and profound mental changes, but usually eventual complete recovery. This classical picture is, however, uncommon; syndromes of raised intracranial pressure without any localizing signs, of sudden

weakness of the legs with falling, or of progressive or fluctuating dementia are at least as common.[6,905,2998]

In a *congenital* form, microphthalmia, seizures, cranial meningocele, hydranencephaly, porencephaly, or aqueduct stenosis may accompany these choroid plexus tumors.[337] See also **neuroepithelial cyst.**

colloidal gold test   An indirect assessment of the amount and nature of gamma-globulin present in a fluid specimen, relying on the tendency of colloidal gold to precipitate in the presence of slowly migrating gamma globulins.

Quantitative tests have largely replaced this measure, which was at one time considered able to differentiate between paretic, luetic, and meningitic reactions in neurosyphilis according to the pattern of precipitation seen in the graded concentrations of colloidal gold test solutions—the early-, middle-, or late-zone rise.[3266]

coloboma   (Gr, the part taken away after mutilation) 1. A sporadic congenital malformation of the optic nerve head or of the iris resulting from developmental arrest (defective closure of the fetal fissure).

Clinically, the disk is usually enlarged, often with a deep cup, abnormally pigmented, and crossed by abnormal glial remnants and embryonic blood vessels. The condition leads to field defects in the region of the disk, and is commonly associated with basal encephalocele, midline facial dysmorphisms, and hypopituitarism.[2133]

2. A developmental defect of the eyelid, affecting primarily the upper or the lower lid margin. At its most severe, the eyelid is absent (*ablepharon*) while minimal degrees lead only to notching of the lid.[4]

coloboma–anal atresia syndrome   See **cat eye syndrome.**

color agnosia   Inability to name colors in the presence of normal color discrimination; impairment in relating a color to its name in the absence of deficits in color discrimination. This is revealed by normal performance on, for example, the Ishihara charts, with difficulty in naming colors at sight and in matching dictated color names to color choices.

color anomia   (color naming disorder) Failure to name a color, or to indicate colors when given their names, in the absence of demonstrable defects in color perception or of aphasia,[1260] as shown by a retained ability to point to and sort colors.

The condition is usually associated with a right homonymous hemianopia and intact color perception in the left half-field; the lesion is subsplenial, lying between the occipital and temporal lobes in the left hemisphere.[3851]

Errors are made when naming colors or when the subject is asked to point to a named color, although color matching and interpretation of the Ishihara pseudoisochromatic plates are normal. The syndrome is usually associated with a right-sided visual defect and with pure alexia caused by infarction in the territory of the left posterior cerebral artery. Two varieties are described—one a primary aphasic disorder, the other a disconnection syndrome separating the visual input and the cerebral structures subserving language function.[4283]

color association   The ability to indicate the color of known common objects, impaired in patients with auditory–verbal deficits but intact in those with color anomia.

color blindness   (deuteranopia) An X-linked recessive trait, in which the subject cannot perceive certain colors. Red-green blindness is the usual form, blue-yellow blindness (**tritanopia**) being less common. It was first described in detail by the color-blind English Chemist John Dalton (1766–1844) in 1794, although there is a report of a letter to Joseph Priestly by Joseph Huddard in 1777 in which the phenomenon was reported. See also **achromatopsia.**

color desaturation   Subjective reduction in the intensity of hue of a perceived object, usually as a result of disease of the optic nerve.

color duplex sonography   A refinement of Doppler sonography in which color-coding systems provide a real-time color image of blood flow in vessels, superimposed on the simultaneously generated B-mode image, so that areas of major blood flow disturbance are readily identified.[4141]

color flickerings   Periodic visual phenomena at the margin of a field defect, as in the auras of migraine.

color naming disorder   See **color anomia.**

color vision   The theory of three types of retinal receptor, each responding maximally to one of three colors. The theory was first suggested by Young, and then developed by Helmholtz in 1852.

Colorado tick fever   A benign acute fever due to infection with a reovirus member of the arbovirus group, seen mainly in the western United States and Canada. It is a rare cause of encephalitis.[5304]

colpocephaly   A dysmorphogenetic condition in which there is enlargement of the occipital horns of the ventricles in underdeveloped brains.

The condition is associated with mental retardation and frequently with varied signs of neurological dysfunction, such as optic atrophy, seizures, and pyramidal signs.[2031]

Columbia Rating Scale   A scale for assessment of change in patients with Parkinson disease.[1726]

The scale rates *tremor* (in the arms, head, and legs); *rigidity* (in the arms, neck, and legs); *bradykinesia* (including gait disturbance, posture, postural stability, and rising from a chair); *functional performance* (finger dexterity, alternating movements, foot tapping, facial ex-

pression, seborrhea, and sialorrhea); and *speech disorder*. See also **Hoehn and Yahr scale, Parkinson Disease Impairment index, Unified Rating scale for parkinsonism.**

coma   (Gr, a deep sleep) the term used by Hippocrates to mean lethargy but now used to describe a state characterized by a reduction of conscious level to a point where the subject is unable to make meaningful responses to environmental stimuli because of either dysfunction of the reticular activating system or widespread depression of cerebral cortical function. The score on the **Glasgow Coma scale** will be 2-4-2 or less.

coma classification   A proposed electroencephalographic classification that has been shown to have high intraobserver reliability.[6090]

Category	Subcategory
I. Delta/theta >50% of record (not theta coma)	A. Reactivity B. No reactivity
II. Triphasic waves	
III. Burst suppression	A. With epileptiform activity B. Without epileptiform activity
IV. Alpha/theta/spindle coma (unreactive)	
V. Epileptiform activity (not in burst-suppression pattern)	A. Generalized B. Focal or multifocal
VI. Suppression	A. <20 uV but >10 uV B. ≤10 uV

From Young GB, McLachan RS, Kreeft JH, et al. An Electroencephalographic Classification for Coma. Can J Neurol Sci 1997;24:320–5. Reproduced by permission.

Coma Outcome scale   A 5-point scale rating the functional outcome from coma, designed to allow comparisons between the results of different treatment plans.[2844]
1. No recovery; comatose until death
2. **Persistent vegetative state**
3. Severe disability; some cognitive function but dependent on others for daily support
4. Moderate disability; independent in activities of daily living but unable to resume normal function
5. Good recovery; able to lead a normal life or to resume normal activity in the presence of a preexisting disability

(Adapted from Jennett B, Bond MR. Assessment of outcome after severe brain damage Lancet 1975;1:480. Reprinted by kind permission of Elsevier Science.)

Coma Recovery scale   A wide-ranging assessment tool designed to predict the outcome in minimally responsive patients.

Six items to do with *arousal and attention,* five with *auditory functions,* seven with *visual functions,* seven with *motor functions,* two with *oromotor functions,* six with *communication abilities,* and two concerned with *initiative* are rated. The possible scores range between 0 and 35.[2093] The scale scores correlate well with those of the **Glasgow Coma Scale.**

coma scales   See **Glasgow Coma scale, Reaction Level scale, Innsbruck Coma scale, Glasgow-Liege**

scale, **Coma Recovery scale, Comprehensive Level of Consciousness scale.**

coma vigil 1. Originally a lethargic delirious state described by French physicians in those moribund as a result of typhoid fever. It was **Osler** who recognized that it also occurred in typhus. 2. For present use, see **persistent vegetative state.**

comatose In a state of coma.

comb rhythm See **mu rhythm.**

combined central and peripheral myelinopathy A syndrome characterized by the occurrence of both a primary demyelinating polyneuropathy and features of a **leukodystrophy** such as **adrenomyeloneuropathy, metachromatic leukodystrophy,** or **Krabbé disease.**[5552]

combined flexion phenomenon See **Babinski trunk-thigh test.**

combined lateral and medial medullary syndrome See **Babinski-Nageotte syndrome.**

combined plantar sign Described as "the simultaneous disappearance of the cortical and spinal plantar reflex met with in hysteria,"[4723] this sign probably requires further verification before it is generally adopted.

combined system diseases Disorders affecting both the lateral and posterior columns of the spinal cord. Although subacute combined degeneration of the cord is now regarded as the classic example, Friedreich ataxia was once so considered, and other hereditary, nutritional, toxic, and other conditions may also be responsible.

comma-shaped degeneration The appearance of the short vertical fibers of the posterior columns in stained preparations of the cord taken from below a transection.[2240]

commissural myelotomy Sagittal incision of the spinal cord made in an attempt to divide the crossing fibers in the anterior commissure destined for the spinothalamic tracts, and thus to relieve pain. This aim has often been achieved, while the absence of permanent alteration in thermal sensitivity remains unexplained.[1122]

The *Bischoff myelotomy* is performed to relieve spasticity; it incises the cord laterally at a number of levels in order to interrupt the fibers of the stretch reflex running from the dorsal root entry zone to the anterior horn cell pool.

commissure (Lat, a joining-together) Those fibers which join the two cerebral hemispheres—the corpus callosum, and the anterior, posterior, habenular, and hippocampal commissures.

commissure aphasia See **conduction aphasia.**

commissurotomy Incision of the anterior or posterior commissures, usually performed in an attempt to reduce the frequency of epileptic seizures.

common EEG input test A procedure in which the same pair of EEG electrodes is connected to the two input terminals of all the channels of an EEG machine as an adjunct to the calibration procedure. See also **calibration.**

common mode rejection A characteristic of differential amplifiers whereby they provide markedly reduced amplification of common mode signals compared to differential signals. It is expressed as the common mode rejection ratio, i.e., the ratio of amplifications of differential and common mode signals. Example:

$$\frac{\text{amplification, differential}}{\text{amplification, common mode}} = 20,000 = 20,000{:}1$$

common mode signal The common component of the two signals applied to the two respective input terminals of a differential EEG amplifier. In EEG recordings, external interference frequently occurs in this way.

common peroneal nerve palsy A mononeuropathy affecting most often the deep branch of the nerve at the fibular head as the result of local compression, prolonged squatting, or direct injury, although more proximal lesions can occur.

Clinically, the usual findings consist of weakness and wasting of the muscles of the anterior compartment (leading to weakness of ankle dorsiflexion and eversion, and of toe dorsiflexion) with altered sensation over the lateral aspect of the shin and the dorsum of the foot. A **Tinel sign** is often elicitable at the site of the nerve lesion. The area of sensory disturbance cannot be differentiated from that associated with a lesion of the L5 root, but lumbar pain or any lower motor neuron signs in the glutei, tensor fascia lata, hamstrings, or tibialis posterior indicates that it is the root rather than the nerve which is involved.

common reference electrode A reference electrode connected to the input terminal 2 of several or all EEG amplifiers.

common reference montage Several referential derivations sharing a single reference electrode. See also **referential derivation, reference electrode**

commotio cerebri Originally, an intracranial hemorrhagic lesion resulting from a blow to the head, or brain injury in the absence of skull fracture as described by Ambrose Paré.

communicating hydrocephalus That form of hydrocephalus in which there is obstruction to the circulation of CSF between the roof of the fourth ventricle and the superior sagittal sinus.

compartment syndromes 1. Disorders resulting from an increase in the interstitial pressure within a closed anatomical space, such as an osseofascial compartment, that leads to microvascular compromise.

2. Compressive ischemia of muscles and nerves lying within a compartment bounded on all sides by muscle, connective tissues, and/or bone and occurring when there is pathological swelling of muscle or with any other cause of increased interstitial pressure within that compartment. Excessive pressure within such enclosed regions leads to pain, edema, muscle necrosis with myoglobinuria, and nerve ischemia, with the expected clinical deficits for each nerve affected.[4031]

In the leg, the *anterior tibial compartment* contains the tibialis anterior muscle, the long ankle and toe dorsiflexors, and the anterior tibial nerve (see **anterior tibial syndrome**); the *peroneal compartment* contains the peroneal muscles and the superficial peroneal nerve; the *deep posterior (tibial) compartment* contains the long plantar flexors of the ankle and toes and the posterior tibial nerve; and the *superficial posterior (triceps surae) compartment* contains the gastrocnemius-soleus muscles and the sural nerve.

In the forearm, the structures anterior to the radius and ulna are within the *volar compartment,* those posterior to the radius are within the *dorsal (extensor) compartment.* In the trunk, the *rectus abdominis* muscle may similarly compress the emerging spinal nerves.[681,5023]

compass gait   Rotation toward the side affected by a cerebellar lesion, best tested by having the patient walk a few steps forward and backward in an open area with the eyes closed.

compelled movements   Involuntary movements arising because of abnormal excitation of some part of the CNS. The term has been supplanted by **dystonia.**

compensation neurosis   Symptoms not of organic origin but produced without conscious intent, determined by an individual's quest for financial reward as a result of injury. Differentiation is made from **malingering,** in which the patient consciously fabricates symptoms and signs for the same purpose. See **disability neurosis.**

compensation syndrome   See **nystagmus-blockage syndrome.**

compensatory nystagmus   See **vestibular nystagmus.**

competency   A legal term, signifying an individual's capacity to make rational medical (and other) decisions that are to be respected unless an opposing view is represented by a better lawyer.

complementary neuromotor examination   A system of examination of neonates and infants in which the active participation of the alerted infant is obtained through close contact and by suppressing the intrusive **Moro reflex,** the latter achieved by fixing the infant's neck so that she reacts as if possessed of the amount of head control that normally appears only by the age of 3 months. Using this method, an 8-week-old infant can be brought actively to raise herself up into the sitting position.[154]

completed stroke   1. A stroke syndrome in which the progression of the deficit has stopped (**stable stroke**). 2. The attainment of maximal impairment such as complete hemiplegia or hemianesthesia, such that the symptoms could not get any worse.[4141]

completion phenomenon   A variety of visual illusion in which there occurs the psychological "filling-in" of images, part of which fall in a hemianopic field; this results in patients reporting that they can perceive, for example, the whole face of the examiner when only half of it can actually be seen, because of the hemianopic defect.[2047]

complex   A sequence of two or more waves having a characteristic form or recurring with a fairly consistent form and distinguishable from background activity.

complex absence   A form of generalized seizure disorder in which prolonged absences occur in conjunction with myoclonic activity or atonic attacks in children with preexisting brain damage.

complex figures test   See **Rey-Osterreith test.**

complex I disease   Rare, recessively inherited, mitochondrial respiratory chain diseases resulting from deficiency of NADH coenzyme Q reductase. Typically they present in infancy or early childhood with features resembling **Leigh disease,** *fatal infantile lactic acidosis, cardiomyopathy and lactic acidosis with or without cataract, macrocephaly and leukodystrophy,* or *hepatopathy with tubulopathy.* See also **mitochondrial diseases.**[3454]

complex II disease   A rare mitochondrial respiratory chain disease due to deficiency of succinate coenzyme Q reductase. See also **mitochondrial diseases.**

complex III disease   A rare mitochondrial respiratory chain disease presenting with ptosis and fatiguable weakness and due to deficiency of coenzyme Q cytochrome-*c* reductase, a respiratory chain enzyme.[2488] See also **mitochondrial diseases.**

complex IV disease   A rare mitochondrial respiratory chain disease due to deficiency of cytochrome-*c* oxidase. See also **mitochondrial diseases.**

complex motor unit action potential   A motor unit action potential that is polyphasic or serrated. See preferred terms, **polyphasic action potential** or **serrated action potential.** (From the 2001 Report of the Nomenclature Committee of the American Association of Electromyography and Electrodiagnosis.[10] Used by permission, copyright © 2001, AAEM.) More than five phases (crossings of the baseline) are required before a motor unit action potential is considered to be polyphasic. The normal proportion of such units recorded is <10%, but it may be higher in some muscles such as the deltoid.

complex partial seizures   Forms of epilepsy originating locally in a limited area of one cerebral hemisphere, presenting most often in adolescence or adult life and manifesting simple or elaborate automatisms (especially of the trunk and limbs), impairment of awareness or responsiveness to externally applied stimuli (including absence attacks), and, in some cases, clonic movements, loss of body tone, and ictal or postictal speech disturbances. They usually last for 1 minute but occasionally for up to 15 minutes and are seldom preceded by an aura. No single typical EEG manifestation is described.[2182,5532]

In brief, these are partial seizures with motor, sensory, and/or psychological manifestations in which there is always some impairment of consciousness.

complex partial status epilepticus   The rare repetition of the manifestations of **complex partial seizures** leading to a confusional state, automatic behavior, and subsequent amnesia, usually seen in children and associated with a variety of cerebral lesions.[2182]

complex regional pain syndrome   (reflex sympathetic dystrophy, RSD; Sudeck atrophy; major causalgia, minor causalgia, mimocausalgia, shoulder-hand syndrome, algoneurodystrophy, reflex neurovascular dystrophy, posttraumatic osteoporosis, pain syndrome, edema or angiospasm; traumatic angiospasm; peripheral acute trophoneurosis; postinfarctional sclerodactlyl; Steinbrocker disease, chronic traumatic edema) A condition of painful swelling, dryness and warmth of the hand not limited to the distribution of a single peripheral nerve, with immobility enforced by the pain and developing osteoporosis.[4997,5404] Two varieties are distinguished, without (type I) and with (type II) a proximate cause in nerve injury.

So-called Type I has been defined by the International Association for the Study of Pain as a pain syndrome:[5316]

1. In the presence of an initiating noxious event or a cause of immobilization (however, this is not always accepted).
2. If the subject manifests continuing pain, allodynia, or hyperalgesia, but the degree of pain experienced appears to be disproportional in severity and duration to the inciting event (if there is one).
3. If there is evidence at some time of edema, changes in skin blood flow, color, and temperature or other abnormal autonomic activity in the region of the body affected by the pain. This is usually the distal aspect of an affected extremity or it may have a distal-to-proximal gradient.
4. If there is a reduction in the range of motion of the affected parts with stiffness, weakness, and tremor.

The diagnosis would be excluded in the presence of other conditions that could otherwise account for the degree of pain and dysfunction experienced.

Other criteria variously suggested have included the presence of pain, allodynia, or hyperalgesia, the pain being disproportional in severity and duration in relation to the inciting event (if there is one); and the presence of edema, changes in skin blood flow, color and temperature, skin mottling, abnormal sudomotor activity in the region of the pain (usually the distal aspect of an affected extremity or with a distal-to-proximal gradient). Reduction in the range of motion of the af-

fected areas with stiffness, weakness and tremor are further common clinical features.

Type II represents what was known formerly as **causalgia,** and in this case prior nerve injury will have occurred.[5316] In association with the intractable pain and trophic changes described above, pareses, incoordination, tremor, myoclonus, and dystonia are also occasionally manifest. The condition is seen after myocardial infarction, injuries to the arm or shoulder, with cervical or shoulder joint disease, and with numerous diseases of both the central and peripheral nervous systems, stroke in particular.[5030] It was once thought to signify damage to the sympathetic innervation of the affected limb but the pathogenesis remains uncertain, although in patients with stroke, avoidance of traction damage to the shoulder may supply some protection.

complex repetitive discharge   A type of spontaneous activity consisting of a regularly repeating series of complex polyphasic or serrated potentials that begin abruptly after needle electrode movement or spontaneously. The potentials have a uniform shape, amplitude, and discharge frequency ranging from 5 to 100 Hz. The discharge typically terminates abruptly. This activity may be seen in both myopathic and neurogenic disorders, and is usually chronic. The discharges are thought to be due to ephaptic excitation of adjacent muscle fibers in a cyclic fashion. This term is preferred to **bizarre high-frequency discharge, bizarre repetitive discharge, bizarre repetitive potential, near-constant frequency trains, pseudomyotonic discharge,** and **synchronized fibrillation.** (From the 2001 Report of the Nomenclature Committee of the American Association of Electromyography and Electrodiagnosis.[10] Used by permission, copyright © 2001, AAEM.)

complex visual hallucinations   Abnormal visual perceptions that affect some normal individuals on going to sleep and are also seen in association with sleep disturbances. The content of the hallucinations is striking and relatively stereotyped, often involving animals and human figures in bright colors and dramatic settings. Causes include the **narcolepsy-cataplexy** syndrome, **peduncular hallucinosis,** treated idiopathic **Parkinson disease, Lewy body** dementia, migraine coma, Charles **Bonnet syndrome,** schizophrenia, hallucinogen-induced states, and **epilepsy.**

Pathogeneses cited include epileptic hallucinations due to a direct irritative process acting on cortical centers integrating complex visual information; visual pathway lesions with defective visual processing or an abnormal cortical release phenomenon, or brainstem lesions affecting ascending cholinergic and serotonergic pathways are considered.[3588]

complicated acrocephalopolysyndactly   See **craniosynostosis.**

complicated amyotrophic lateral sclerosis   The association of dementia, posterior column degeneration, or parkinsonism in patients with familial or classical amyotrophic lateral sclerosis. In sporadic amyotrophic lateral sclerosis, posterior column degeneration is uncommon. Familial amyotrophic lateral sclerosis in children is recessively inherited; that in adults is dominantly inherited. The association of these conditions has been reviewed.[2685] See **amyotrophic lateral sclerosis.**

complicated hemianopias   See **hemianopia.**

complicated hereditary infantile optic atrophy   See **Behr disease.**

compound action potential   A potential or waveform resulting from the summation of multiple individual axon or muscle fiber action potentials. See **compound mixed nerve action potential, compound motor nerve action potential, compound nerve action potential, compound sensory nerve action potential, compound muscle action potential.** (From the 2001 Report of the Nomenclature Committee of the American Association of Electromyography and Electrodiagnosis.[10] Used by permission, copyright © 2001, AAEM.)

compound granular corpuscles   (Gitterzellen) Microglial cells swollen with lipid droplets following local tissue injury and cell breakdown.

compound mixed nerve action potential   A compound nerve action potential recorded from a mixed nerve when an electric stimulus is applied to a segment of the nerve that contains both afferent and efferent fibers. The amplitude, latency, duration, and phases should be noted. (From the 2001 Report of the Nomenclature Committee of the American Association of Electromyography and Electrodiagnosis.[10] Reproduced by kind permission of the Association.)

compound motor nerve action potential   (compound motor NAP) A compound nerve action potential recorded from efferent fibers of a motor nerve or a motor branch of a mixed nerve, elicited by stimulation of a motor nerve, a motor branch of a mixed nerve, or a ventral nerve root. The amplitude, latency, duration, and number of phases should be noted. This should be distinguished from **compound muscle action potential.** (From the 2001 Report of the Nomenclature Committee of the American Association of Electromyography and Electrodiagnosis.[10] Used by permission, copyright © 2001, AAEM.)

compound movements   Those movements which involve change of posture at two or more joints, as bringing a finger to the nose or a heel to the opposite knee.[2625]

compound muscle action potential   (CMAP) The summation of nearly synchronous muscle fiber action potentials recorded from a muscle, commonly produced by stimulation of the nerve supplying the muscle either directly or indirectly. Baseline-to-peak amplitude, duration, and latency of the negative phase should be noted, along with details of the method of stimulation and recording. Use of specific named potentials is recommended, e.g., **M wave, F wave, H wave, T wave, A wave,** and R1 wave or R2 wave (see **Blink responses**). (Adapted from the 2001 Report of the Nomenclature Committee of the American Association of Electromyography and Electrodiagnosis.[10] Used by permission, copyright © 2001, AAEM.)

compound nerve action potential   (compound NAP) The summation of nearly synchronous nerve fiber action potentials recorded from a nerve trunk, commonly produced by stimulation of the nerve directly or indirectly. Details of the method of stimulation and recording should be specified, together with the fiber type (sensory, motor, or mixed nerve). (From the 2001 Report of the Nomenclature Committee of the American Association of Electromyography and Electrodiagnosis.[10] Used by permission, copyright © 2001, AAEM.)

compound sensory nerve action potential   (compound SNAP) A compound nerve action potential recorded from the afferent fibers of a sensory nerve, a sensory branch of a mixed nerve, or in response to stimulation of a sensory nerve or a dorsal nerve root. May also be elicited when an adequate stimulus is applied synchronously to sensory receptors. The amplitude, latency, duration, and configuration should be noted. Generally, the amplitude is measured as the maximum peak-to-peak voltage when there is an initial positive deflection or from baseline to peak when there is an initial negative deflection. The latency is measured as either the time to the initial deflection or the negative peak, and the duration as the interval from the first deflection of the waveform from the baseline to its final return to the baseline. Also referred to by the less preferred terms *sensory response, sensory potential,* or *SNAP.* (From the 2001 Report of the Nomenclature Committee of the American Association of Electromyography and Electrodiagnosis.[10] Used by permission, copyright © 2001, AAEM.)

Comprehensive Level of Consciousness scale (CLOCS) A system for assessing physical signs relating to consciousness[5317] (see Chart C–24). See also **coma scales.**

Chart C–24. Comprehensive Level of Consciousness Scale

1. Posture

4 Posture is under volitional control and is normally flexible.
0 No abnormal posture but muscle tonus is completely flaccid.

2. Eye position at rest

6 Midposition and conjugate
0 Skew deviation

3. Spontaneous eye opening

4 Volitional control of eye opening
0 No spontaneous or elicited eye opening

4. General motor functioning

6 Normal spontaneous movements within the limits of the
   patient's physical abilities
0 No spontaneous motor movements

5. Abnormal ocular movements

6 None
0 Complete absence of ocular motility

6. Pupillary light reflexes

7 Normal direct and consensual light reflexes
0 Wide pupillary dilatation and fixed to all stimuli or bilaterally small (pinpoint) pupils which are fixed to all stimuli

7. General responsiveness

8 The person is fully aroused and alert, or, if asleep, arouses and
   attends to the examiner after only mild or moderate stimulation. The arousal outlasts the duration of the stimulus.
0 Total absence of discernible motor activity even in response
   to noxious stimulation

8. Best communicative effort

7 Normal communication is possible through speech, writing,
   gesturing, etc.
0 No elicited or spontaneous vocalizations, searching behaviors, or eye contact

*From Stanzak et al., 1984,[5317] reproduced from J Neurosurgery by kind
permission.*

Comprehensive Psychopathology Rating Scale   A
scale containing 66 items representing neuropsychological symptoms or signs detected in a clinical interview and rated between 0 and 3; the scale is highly sensitive and specific, particularly for the detection of
depression in elderly patients.[226]

compressed spectral array   A mathematical method
of displaying EEG signals which depicts changes in the
amplitude and frequency of brain activity.[555]

The sequential spectra of the mean frequencies of
EEG activity over a defined period are closely applied
in the printout, creating a graphic pseudo–three-dimensional representation. Analysis of such recordings
taken over a prolonged period may be of value in determining prognosis in comatose patients.

compression neuropathy   Deficits within the territory of a nerve as a result of continued pressure causing ischemic conduction block within the nerve.

compression nystagmus   See **vestibular nystagmus.**

compulsive tics   See **Tourette syndrome.**

computerized axial tomography   (CAT scan) A refinement of plain radiological tomography in which
electronic detectors receive X-rays from a source rotating 180° on the opposite side of the subject, examining
the subject thus from all angles to provide accurate
cross sections in the axial plane. Computer analysis of
the images allows for two-dimensional reconstruction
of the structures irradiated at any number of transverse
levels. Further computer analysis of the data to allow
coronal or sagittal reconstructions is also possible.

Following the initial mathematical work by Allan
Cormack, and by Dr. W.H. **Oldendorf,** Dr. Godfrey
Hounsfield developed the method for CT scanning in
humans, for which he and Prof. Cormack were awarded
the Nobel prize in 1979. The contribution of Dr. Oldendorf was not so recognized.

Computerized Everyday Memory Battery   An automated instrument in which the subject's abilities on
such tasks as telephone dialing with or without interference, name–face association (with both immediate
and delayed recall), recognition of faces with immediate and delayed signal detection, reaction times, selective reminding, tests of associative learning and memory, visual (nonlanguage) memory, and narrative recall.
The battery is used to evaluate potential cognition-en-
hancing pharmaceutical compounds.[3278]

conation   (Lat, to try) The products of thought, as opposed to the **cognitive** powers which allow such exer-
tions to occur.

concentration   The ability to maintain focused attention upon one item or activity over a period of time.
This capacity tends to be lost early in the dementias and
at the outset in delirious states.

Digit-span and serial-seven subtraction tests are
those generally used at the bedside to assess concentration.

concentric lacunar leukoencephalopathy   A subacutely progressive demyelinating disorder of the CNS,
related to **neuromyelitis optica,** in which zones of cavitation alternate with glial septa devoid of axons and
myelin sheaths.

Clinically, the condition presents in adult life with
cortical blindness, seizures, and focal deficits.[1224]

concentric macro-EMG   A technique for studying the
concentric motor unit action potential alongside the
macropotential, using a needle electrode combining
concentric and macro recording surfaces.[2767]

concentric needle electrode   Recording electrode
that measures an electric potential difference between
a centrally insulated wire and the cannula of the needle through which it runs. (From the 2001 Report of
the Nomenclature Committee of the American Association of Electromyography and Electrodiagnosis.[10]
Used by permission, copyright © 2001, AAEM.)

conceptual apraxia A form of apraxia in which the concept of the action is lost. It is characterized by impaired ability to use tools and to understand meaningful gestures.[3138] See **apraxia.**

concussion (from Lat, to shake violently) A clinical syndrome, traumatic in origin, characterized by immediate neurological dysfunction (usually involving at least transient impairment of consciousness and awareness) that is fully reversible and not associated with demonstrable gross changes, though microscopic brainstem and cortical abnormalities may be shown to exist.

Concussion affects the cerebrum and the spinal cord similarly. The mechanism is unknown but is considered to involve shearing stresses on fibers in the brainstem. Cranial impact is not a necessary factor in causation; acute acceleration injury affecting the cervical cord or brainstem have also been held responsible.

The subject has received a superb recent review.[3737]

Stages of recovery from cerebral concussion have been defined:[4338]

4 Respiratory arrest with somatic immobility
3 Shallow, irregular respirations with somatic immobility
2 Normal respiratory movements with inadequate, ineffective, and inappropriate somatic movements
1 Normal posture, gait speed, and attitude but impaired performance of complex tasks
0 Full recovery

Immediate features include headache, dizziness, vertigo, and nausea in the short term and headache, inattention, lightheadedness, impaired memory, fatigability, irritability, light and noise intolerance, anxiety, and sleep disturbances days or weeks later.[2997]

Guidelines for classification of concussion suffered during sports have been defined by a committee of the American Academy of Neurology (AAN):[4554]

Grade 1
  Transient confusion
  No loss of consciousness
  "Bell rung" or "dinged"
  Concussion symptoms or mental status abnormalities on examination resolve in <15 min.
Grade 2
  Transient confusion
  No loss of consciousness
  Concussion symptoms or mental status abnormalities on examination resolve in >15 min.
Grade 3
  Any loss of consciousness, brief (seconds) or prolonged (minutes)

Grade 0 of Nelson (not a part of the AAN classification system above) may be assigned when the athlete's head is struck or moved rapidly, but the athlete is not stunned or dazed initially but subsequently complains of headache and difficulty in concentrating. The range of disabilities caused by minor head injuries has been reviewed.[4699]

See also **second impact syndrome, chronic fatigue syndrome, ding, postconcussional syndrome.**

conditionally responsive extrapyramidal syndrome See **paroxysmal kinesigenic choreoathetosis.**

conditioned insomnia The occurrence of chronic insomnia as a result of a learned negative emotional association between sleeping and a particular environment. (Adapted from Association of Sleep Disorders Centers. Diagnostic classifications of sleep and arousal disorders. *Sleep* 1979;2:1–137.[249])

conditioned reflex Reflex responses to stimuli that do not normally produce such responses, these responses being acquired as a result of training and repetition. The two stimuli must be related in time and the conditional stimulus must precede the unconditional.

Such reflexes are in contradistinction to unconditional reflexes or instincts that are native to the organism. **Pavlov** introduced the concept and the term in 1898, following his research on food rewards and secretion in the canine stomach.

The theory underlying **behaviorism** is that overt human behavior is the result of the building up of series of conditioned reflexes throughout life.

conduction aphasia (central aphasia, Leistungsaphasie, commissure aphasia) That form of dysphasia produced by lesions of the supramarginal gyrus and the subjacent arcuate fasciculus (which extends from the supramarginal gyrus anteriorly to the motor association and Broca areas) in which the auditory language comprehension center is separated from the verbal motor center. Repetition of spoken speech is seriously affected, word-finding and naming are impaired, and there are many circumlocutions and phonemic (literal) paraphasias with self-correction, but there is retention of comprehension, and spontaneous speech and writing are usually fluent and copious. Facial apraxias are commonly found.[3730]

Such fluent paraphasic speech with normal comprehension but severely impaired repetition was described by Wernicke (1874), who recognized that it was due to disconnection of the first temporal and third frontal gyri, and called it *aphasia of the insular region,* later, however, correctly incriminating lesions of the arcuate fasciculus. Goldstein regarded it as a disturbance of **inner speech.**

conduction apraxia A syndrome resulting from damage to the left hemisphere and characterized by good performance to pantomime on verbal command but impaired performance on attempted imitation in the presence of severe ideomotor apraxia to verbal command and naming. Reception of the gestures is apared.[4192]

conduction block Failure of an action potential to propagate past a particular point upon an intact axon in the nervous system as a result of failure of depolarization of the axonal membrane because of the increased capacitance induced by demyelination. Conduction nevertheless is possible below the point of the block. It is documented by demonstration of a reduction in the area of a compound muscle action potential greater than that normally seen with stimulation at two different points on a nerve trunk; anatomic variations of nerve pathways and technical factors related to nerve stimulation must be excluded as the cause of the reduction in area. (Adapted from the 2001 Report of the Nomenclature Committee of the American Association of Electromyography and Electrodiagnosis.[10] Used by permission, copyright © 2001, AAEM.)

The finding of a 50% reduction in such amplitudes with no more than a 15% increase in the duration of the compound muscle action potential is characteristic of demyelinating but not of axonal neuropathies. Conduction block is also documented by demonstration of a reduction in the area of an evoked potential greater than that normally seen with electrical stimulation at two different points on a nerve trunk; anatomical variations of nerve pathways and technical factors related to nerve stimulation must be excluded as the cause of the reduction in area. (From the American Association of Electromyography and Electrodiagnosis (AAEE) glossary of terms in clinical electromyography. *Muscle Nerve* 1987;**10S**:G5–G23.[146] Reprinted by permission of John Wiley and Sons, Inc.)

conduction syndromes   See **disconnection syndromes.**

conduction velocity   (CV) Speed of propagation of an action potential along a nerve or muscle fiber. The nerve fibers studied (motor, sensory, autonomic, or mixed nerve) should be specified. For a nerve trunk, the maximum conduction velocity is calculated from the latency of the evoked potential (muscle or nerve) at maximal or supramaximal intensity of stimulation at two different points. The distance between the two points (conduction distance) is divided by the difference between the corresponding latencies (conduction time). The calculated result is the conduction velocity of the fastest fibers and is usually expressed in meters per second (m/s). As commonly used, conduction velocity refers to the maximum conduction velocity. By specialized techniques, the conduction velocity of other fibers can also be determined and should be specified, e.g., minimum conduction velocity. (From the 2001 Report of the Nomenclature Committee of the American Association of Electromyography and Electrodiagnosis.[10] Used by permission, copyright © 2001, AAEM.)

conduit d'apprendre   (Fr, literally, learning pathway). The struggle of paraphasic subjects to utter the correct word, achieved (or not) after many incorrect attempts.

cone dysfunction syndromes   See **cone dystrophy.**

cone dystrophy   (achromatopsia, cone dysfunction syndromes) Retinal degenerative syndromes character- ized by selective loss of retinal cone function and presenting with bilateral diminution of visual acuity and of color vision, photophobia, day-blindness (**hemeralopia**), central visual field defects, and abnormal single-flash and flicker **electroretinogram** (ERG).

Most cases are dominantly inherited and occur in association with evidence of hereditary **cerebellar ataxias,** but all forms of inheritance have been described.[2196,4710]

Variant forms are *rod monochromatism,* in which there is congenital absence of cones with marked impairment of visual acuity and of color vision, nystagmus, and abnormal photopic (cone-mediated) but normal scotopic (rod-mediated) ERG responses, and the *macular form of pigmentary retinopathy* (inversa form), which is a selective loss of cone function at the macula.

cone-rod dystrophy   See **pigmentary retinal degeneration.**

confabulation   The uttering of statements that are incorrect by a patient who believes them to be true; fabrication of details to compensate for loss of memory.[466]

Two forms have been differentiated: *spontaneous confabulation,* which may result from the superimposition of frontal lobe dysfunction on an organic amnesia, and in which the statements made represent inadvertent displacement to the present of memories taken from the past; and the *provoked form,* which is considered a reasonable response in the presence of a faulty memory.

It is necessary for one to be unaware of the memory deficits suffered in order to confabulate. As Dr. C. Miller Fisher pointed out: "The subject cannot say 'I don't know' if he is unaware of his deficit. His answer is whatever comes to mind. 'I don't know' represents a relatively preserved intellect." Thus he designated confabulation as "false recollections and delusions with anosognosia (various types)."[1860] See also **Wernicke-Korsakoff syndrome.**

confabulation questionnaire   A scale useful in excluding confabulation, as would be common in the **Wernicke-Korsakoff** syndrome and in certain toxic dementias, but rare in **Alzheimer disease.**

confirmed epilepsy   The occurrence of at least two unprovoked seizures separated by more than 24 hours.[3462]

confrontation   An insensitive technique for assessing visual fields in which the examiner stands immediately in front of the patient who is asked to fix her gaze on the examiner and to identify the side on which the latter moves his fingers, placed in various parts of the field, or to count the number of fingers raised.

Suprathreshold techniques involve the stationary presentation of fingers or targets well within the visual field; *threshold* techniques require the patient to identify the point of first awareness as the fingers are brought into the field from outside it. The sensitivity can be improved if colored targets are used.[5639]

confusion   See **confusional state.**

confusional arousals (excessive sleep inertia, Schlaftrunkenheit, livresse du sommeil) Episodes of confusion occurring during and following arousals from sleep, usually from deep sleep in the first part of the night. See **sleep drunkenness.** Diagnostic criteria have been suggested:[234]

A. A complaint by the patient or an observer of recurrent mental confusion upon arousal or awakening.

B. Spontaneous confusional episodes can be induced by forced arousal.

C. Absence of fear, walking behavior, or intense hallucinations in association with the episodes.

D. Polysomnography demonstrates arousals from slow wave sleep.

E. Not associated with the medical disorders such as partial complex seizures.

F. Does not meet the diagnostic criteria for other sleep disorders causing the complaint, e.g., sleep terrors, sleepwalking.

(From ASDA Diagnostic Classification Steering Committee. The International Classification of Sleep Disorders Diagnostic and Coding Manual. Rochester, MN. American Sleep Disorders Association, 1990, by kind permission.)

Confusional Assessment method   An instrument for the detection of delirium, based upon clinical observation, and using a diagnostic algorithm for confusion based on the DSM-IIIR criteria. It depends on the presence of four features:

A. Acute onset

B. Fluctuating course

C. Inattention

D. Disorganized thinking *or* altered level of consciousness

This leads on to the assessment of orientation, memory, perception, psychomotor agitation, and retardation and the sleep-wake cycle. The presence of such features reliably predicts delirium.[2744]

confusional migraine   A migraine syndrome that occurs more commonly in boys, characterized by a typical aura, a headache (which may be insignificant), and confusion (inattention, distractibility, and difficulty maintaining speech and other motor activities) that may precede or follow the headache.

Agitation, memory disturbances, obscene utterances, and violent behavior are not uncommon. Single attacks are typical, multiple attacks are rare. Both may be triggered by mild head trauma. If the level of consciousness is more profoundly disturbed, **migraine stupor** lasting 2–5 days can occur.[2665] See also **dysphrenic migraine.**

confusional state   (confusion, delirium) An alteration in mental state characterized by some degree of reduction in consciousness, in which the most salient deficits are those of attention, leading in turn to impairments in clear thinking, perception, orientation, and memory. The **Glasgow Coma scale** score will be 4-6-4.

Clinically, fluctuating disturbances of vigilance and of attentiveness (i.e., distractibility); impairment of coherence in the stream of thought and of skilled, goal-directed movements; perceptual distortions; disorientation; impaired judgment, blunted insight, and labile affect; apathy or agitation; and anomia, dysgraphia, acalculia, and failure of constructional abilities are the more notable features.[3851]

congenital absence of the pectoral muscles   See **Souques syndrome.**

congenital amaurosis   See **Leber congenital amaurosis.**

congenital analgesia   See **congenital indifference to pain.**

congenital aphasia   See **developmental dysphasia, congenital auditory imperception.**

congenital apnea   A malformation syndrome in which medullary and olivary hypoplasia are associated with periods of apnea in infants.[3051]

congenital ataxia with aniridia   See **cerebellar ataxias** (*variants*).

congenital ataxia with choroidal coloboma   See **Pfeiffer syndrome.**

congenital atlantoaxial dislocation   First observed in 1960 by the Bombay neurologist N.H. Wadia,[5793] this condition is rare in the West but is well recognized in India. Symptoms are precipitated by neck movement and include cervical pain and stiffness, transitory attacks of paralysis, paresthesias, visual loss or loss of consciousness, and progressive pyramidal dysfunction. Young men with short necks are mainly affected. Occipitalization of the atlas, fusion of the second and third cervical vertebrae, and an abnormal odontoid process are the more common structural findings. The treatment is surgical.

congenital auditory imperception (congenital aphasia, developmental aphasia, congenital word deafness) Impaired discrimination of sounds, including speech sounds, leading to reliance on gesture, facial expression and lip reading, and to delayed attainment of speech expression and comprehension with **idioglossia.** The condition is considered to be a developmental speech disorder syndrome.[109] See **Worster-Drought-Allen syndrome.**

congenital bilateral perisylvian syndrome (Foix-Chavanay-Marie syndrome) A familial (probably X-linked dominant) developmental syndrome characterized by the association of facio-pharyngo-glosso-masticatory diplegia and bilateral perisylvian polymicrogyria.

The usual clinical features include pseudobulbar signs, cognitive deficits, epilepsy, and perisylvian abnormalities on imaging studies, but the presentations are variable.[2307] See also **bilateral periventricular nodular heterotopia, anterior operculum syndrome.**

congenital brachial palsy   Intrapartum stretch injury of the (upper) brachial plexus, frequently bilateral though asymmetrical.[4938]

congenital brevicollis   See **Klippel-Feil anomaly.**

congenital bulbar palsy   See **Möbius syndrome.**

congenital cataracts, facial dysmorphism neuropathy syndrome   A recessively inherited disorder of children, detected in Wallachian gypsies, characterized by microcornea and cataracts, a mainly motor neuropathy starting in the legs, mild nonprogressive cognitive impairment, and, in some cases, pyramidal signs and chorea. Short stature, facial dysmorphism, and hypogonadotrophic hypogonadism are other features of the syndrome.[5616]

congenital central apnea   Failure to breathe from birth, associated in one case with medullary hypoplasia and malformations of the inferior olives.[3051]

congenital central hypoventilation syndrome   (central alveolar hypoventilation syndrome, primary alveolar hypoventilation syndrome) A syndrome occurring usually within the first few days of life and characterized by episodes of apnea at sleep onset. It is likely to be due to a defect in the function of central chemoreceptor function.[413] See **Ondine's curse.**

Failure of the autonomic control of ventilation occurs because of a decrease in the density of neurons and myelinated fibers in the medullary respiratory centers, and may lead to a fatal outcome.[3810] The syndrome is characterized by hypoventilation, which is worse during sleep than wakefulness, and is unexplained by primary pulmonary disease or ventilatory muscle weakness. In central alveolar hypoventilation, there is considered to be a failure of the automatic control of breathing.[4361]

Clinical diagnostic criteria have been suggested.[234]

A. Shallow breathing, or cyanosis and apnea, worse during sleep than in wakefulness, which has a perinatal onset

B. Hypoventilation that is worse during sleep than in wakefulness

C. Absent or diminished ventilatory response to hypoxia and hypercapnia

D. Polysomnographic monitoring demonstrates hypercapnia and hypoxia during sleep, predominantly without apnea

E. The absence of primary lung disease or ventilatory muscle dysfunction that can explain the hypoventilation

F. Not due to any other sleep disorder, such as infant sleep apnea

(From ASDA Diagnostic Classification Steering Committee. The International Classification of Sleep Disorders Diagnostic and Coding Manual. Rochester, MN. American Sleep Disorders Association, 1990, by kind permission.)

congenital cerebellar ataxia   See **cerebellar ataxias.**

congenital cerebellar atrophy   See **cerebellar ataxias.**

congenital cerebellar hypoplasia   (ataxic cerebral palsy) A congenital developmental syndrome characterized by colobomas of the retina, strabismus, dysarthria, and cerebellar signs due to cerebellar hypoplasia, sometimes with mental delay. See **cerebral palsy.**

congenital cervical spinal muscular atrophy   A nonfamilial, neurogenic type of **arthrogryposis** limited to the upper limbs, characterized by severe symmetrical muscle wasting with areflexia, and congenital contractures of the shoulders and arms.

Sensory and bulbar symptoms, long tract signs, scoliosis, and leg involvement are absent.[2370]

congenital chiasmal dysplasia   Developmental anomalies usually associated with other midline malformations affecting, for example, the hypothalamus and the lateral or third ventricles. **Optic nerve hypoplasia** is a milder variant. See also **septo-optic dysplasia.**

congenital chorea   See **Vogt syndrome.**

congenital cranial osteoporosis   See **craniotabes.**

congenital cytomegalovirus infection   Infection by this double-stranded DNA herpes virus follows maternal viremia and affects up to some 2% of all live-born children, most, however, remaining asymptomatic.

Clinically, the disease is characterized by multiple organ system involvement, low birth weight, jaundice, a petechial skin rash, and chorioretinitis. Neurologically, microcephaly, ventricular enlargement, periventricular calcification, mental retardation, spasticity, and deafness are the most common features in symptomatic infants.

Some infected children who are asymptomatic at birth develop neurological problems later, particularly behavioral disturbances and arrest of intellectual development, over the course of the next few years. Deafness is also a common complication.[729,4674] The pathology is that of a chronic encephalitis with particular damage to the periventricular subependymal tissues.[6030]

congenital deafness and otitic meningitis   The combination of congenital unilateral deafness and nontraumatic otorrhea due to a malformation of the inner ear, this latter leading on to recurrent episodes of meningitis.[4105]

congenital demyelinating encephalopathy   A syndrome of mental retardation with epileptic seizures and spastic paresis of congenital onset, accompanied by particular damage to CNS myelin with destruction of axis cylinders and with reactive gliosis. The etiology is unknown; perinatal asphyxia may be responsible.[3551]

congenital demyelinating neuropathy with multifocal CNS demyelination   A syndrome combining the features of chronic demyelinating peripheral neuropathy (with slow nerve conduction velocities, peripheral nerve hypertrophy, elevation of CSF protein levels, insidious onset, and continuous progression) and evidence of multifocal lesions in the CNS, including optic neuritis, brainstem involvement, and cerebellar and pyramidal signs, with episodic expression.[5552] The latter fulfil diagnostic criteria for clinically definite **multiple sclerosis.**

The findings suggest the coincidence of a chronic inflammatory demyelinating polyneuropathy and multiple sclerosis, which might represent central and peripheral responses to a common antigen at some time past.

congenital encephalo-ophthalmic dysplasia   See **Krause syndrome.**

congenital end-plate acetylcholine receptor deficiency   A rare variant of congenital myasthenia with electrdcal responses resembling those found in the adult disease.[1658] See also **myasthenia gravis.**

congenital end-plate acetylcholinesterase deficiency   A rare variant of congenital myasthenia manifesting severe weakness and fatigability of all muscles from birth, refractory to anticholinesterase drugs, and with a decrement at all rates of stimulation on electrical testing.[1668]

congenital facial-abducens paralysis   See **Möbius syndrome.**

congenital facial diplegia, congenital nuclear agenesis/aplasia   See **Möbius syndrome.**

congenital facial palsy   A dominantly inherited facial palsy present (usually bilaterally) at birth and due to nuclear agenesis as in **Möbius syndrome** or as a result of more peripheral damage to the nerves, though not occasioned by trauma during birth.[3761] See also **Bell palsy.**

congenital familial fibrosis   A rare form of restrictive ophthalmoplegia characterized by the replacement of the extraocular muscles by fibrous tissue.[2453]

congenital fiber-type disproportion   An idiopathic nonprogressive **congenital myopathy** presenting with hypotonia and weakness in the neonatal period, and in which biopsy changes in muscle include uniform smallness and numerical predominance of type 1 muscle fibers, and hypertrophy of type 2 fibers (particularly of subtype 2b). The finding is also present in some patients with other infantile neuromuscular disease or as a manifestation of a CNS disorder.

The weakness often involves the respiratory muscles; in addition there are delay in achieving motor milestones, short stature, high palate, scoliosis, joint contractures, macrocephaly and the later development of muscle and joint contractures, and skeletal deformities such as congenital dislocation of the hips.[1679,2139] The EMG is usually normal and the serum creatine kinase levels are only slightly, if at all, raised.

In *variant forms,* slowly progressive proximal weakness occurs in children in whom muscle biopsy speci-

mens show the presence of a relative excess of type 1 fibers and minimally enlarged type 2 fibers,[1622] and in **Krabbe disease.**[1336]

congenital hemihypertrophy   (Curtius syndrome) A congenital syndrome manifesting an increase in the size of all or part of one side of the body, including the face and limbs, or of a single system (nervous, vascular, muscular) only, with dilated and tortuous veins, associated variously with hypogenitalism, mental delay, facial dysmorphisms, tumors of the kidney or adrenal glands, cataracts, and psychosis.[1227]

congenital hydrocephalus-hydranencephaly   A syndrome of aqueduct atresia and arthrogryposis, complicated by hydramnios.[1923]

congenital hypomyelination polyneuropathy   (congenital hypomyelination neuropathy) A group of recessively inherited or sporadic neuropathies characterized by the presence in infancy of evidence of a hypertrophic neuropathy in which there is severe hypomyelination or even the complete absence of myelin in all the fibers of peripheral motor and sensory nerves. The condition resembles **hereditary motor and sensory neuropathy (HMSN) type 3** but has the atypical pathological features of absence of myelin breakdown products, of **onion bulbs** and of inflammatory infiltrates.[307] The number of axons is markedly reduced.[2346]

The disease is manifest in infancy with hypotonia, severe distal weakness, and difficulties with feeding and respiration; motor development is retarded in surviving children. Motor nerve conduction speeds are extremely slow. The condition is probably a variant of Déjerine-Sottas disease (HMSN 3, itself probably a form of HMSN 1).[2346]

Variant forms include a form with **arthrogryposis multiplex congenita** in association,[695] as well as *late infantile* and *juvenile* (group 2 and group 3) onset forms. See also **hereditary motor and sensory neuropathy type 3.**

congenital hypotonia-sclerotic muscular dystrophy   A possible variant of **congenital muscular dystrophy** characterized by muscle dystrophy, unimpaired intelligence, and recurrent respiratory infections.[2000] See **congenital muscular dystrophy.**

congenital hypotonia with small type 2 fibers   A **congenital myopathy** distinguished by the presence in muscle biopsy specimens of hypotrophy of the type 2 fibers.

congenital hypotonia with type 1 fiber predominance   A mild and nonprogressive or abating **congenital myopathy** with decreased reflexes and skeletal deformities, distinguished by the presence in muscle biopsy specimens of a relative excess of type 1 fibers.

congenital indifference to pain   (congenital analgesia) A sporadic or dominantly or recessively inherited congenital syndrome in which pain is perceived as a sensation but one to which there is no emotional response, although subjects can differentiate between hot and cold and between sharp and dull. Touch sensation, muscle stretch reflexes, the histamine flare response, and microscopy findings in peripheral nerves are normal (the last not using all modern methods). The corneal responses are absent and itching is not perceived. Some affected subjects also manifest developmental delay and multiple fractures.

One prominent patient reported in the nineteenth century styled himself "The Human Pincushion" and exhibited himself in the United States for a fee; his *pièce de* (non-) *résistance* was his crucifixion on stage, which had to be terminated prematurely, however, on account of the more acute sensibilities of some of the audience.[1321]

See also **hereditary sensory and autonomic neuropathy.**

congenital inflammatory myopathy   A form of myositis with antenatal or neonatal presentation and clinically resembling **congenital muscular dystrophy,** but associated with microcephaly and intellectual impairment. The serum creatine kinase levels are raised. Muscle biopsy findings include inflammatory infiltrates, muscle fiber damage, and class 1 major histocompatibility complex products in the muscle sarcolemma.[5126]

congenital insensitivity to pain   A recessively inherited syndrome present from birth, and manifesting absence of pain sensations throughout the body with minimal or no impairment of other sensory modalities or of the muscle stretch reflexes.

Whether the lesion is in the peripheral nervous system (though undetected in some studies) or is a manifestation of a central disorder remains undetermined; both forms probably occur. Those patients with various forms of **hereditary sensory and autonomic neuropathy** (e.g., types 4 and 5) also present with loss of pain awareness, but in such cases other modalities are clearly affected as well.[5571]

Variants are *congenital insensitivity to pain with anhidrosis* (see **hereditary sensory and autonomic neuropathy type 4**), and *congenital insensitivity to pain, dominant form,* which is a congenital neuropathic syndrome comprising sclerocornea, hyperactivity, self-mutilation, paroxysmal headache, loss of pain and temperature sensation, paresthesia or hyperesthesia, and flushing.[1113]

See **hereditary sensory and autonomic neuropathy** (recessive and *variant* forms). See also **congenital indifference to pain.**

congenital lactic acidosis   The result of an inborn error of pyruvate metabolism with numerous phenotypes.

congenital lower motor neuron disease with arthrogryposis   See **hereditary motor neuropathy.**

congenital muscle fiber-type disproportion   An idiopathic neuromuscular disorder that may be the manifestation of a CNS or a lower motor neuron disorder and which presents with polymorphic features including severe generalized weakness (often involving the respiratory muscles), hypertonia, and a variable outcome.[2139]

congenital muscular dystrophy   1. A heterogeneous group of genetically determined disorders characterized by severe muscle wasting from birth or shortly thereafter. 2. All congenital myopathies, not otherwise specified. 3. (Donner type) Congenital muscle disease manifest by hypotonia, facial and proximal weakness, and often contractures at birth, with biopsy evidence of primary muscle disease. An increased incidence of spinal tumors has been reported, but otherwise CNS or retinal lesions are only occasionally associated.[4150,4821] See also http://www.neuro.wustl.edu/neuromuscular/maltbrain.html.

Diagnostic criteria have been suggested by Fenichel:[1781]

1. Hypotonia, weakness, or arthrogryposis is present at birth. Children who appear normal at birth and develop clinical features of muscle disease during infancy should not be considered to have congenital muscular dystrophy unless there is another family member with a similar disorder whose clinical symptoms were present at birth.

2. The muscle biopsy findings should be consistent with myopathy (that is, spectrum of fiber sizes, degeneration of medium-sized fibers, fat, and collagen replacement of muscle fibers) and should specifically exclude denervation.

3. Other myopathies of the newborn with recognizable clinical or pathological features are excluded.

Brooke[773] distinguishes five subcategories of congenital muscular dystrophy. The first two account for the large majority of cases:

1. *Undifferentiated type* (Batten-Turner syndrome) The classical (occidental form) is a relatively benign, probably autosomal recessive syndrome consisting of hypotonia, girdle weakness, and motor delay in young children whose muscle biopsy findings suggest a primary myopathy.[5670] No evidence of CNS involvement is apparent. Two forms are determined according to the presence or absence of merosin.

   a. *The merosin-negative* type shows marked motor disability with normal mentation but white matter lucencies on MRI scans, and is mapped to chromosome 6q22–23.

   b. *The merosin-positive* type is characterized by reduced fetal movements in the last trimester of pregnancy, poor sucking, hypotonia, and weakness in postnatal life; delayed developmental milestones with psychomotor impairment; and absence of CNS findings.[3107]

2. *Fukuyama type* (congenital muscular dystrophy with CNS involvement, Walker-Warburg syndrome) A recessively inherited congenital or infantile form, in which the features of severe muscle dystrophy with joint contractures in infancy and complex malformations of the brain and the eyes are accompanied by marked mental retardation, seizures, and skeletal deformities.[1988] Bulbar weakness, pyramidal signs, cerebral atrophy, hydrocephalus, lissencephaly, polymicrogyria, and heterotopias are also described. Vision

is normal. The condition maps to 9q31–33. See also **muscle-eye-brain disease.**

3. *Atonic-sclerotic type* (Ullrich syndrome) Congenital muscle dystrophy with proximal joint contractures but with hyperextensibility of the digits, kyphoscoliosis, dysmorphism, hyperhidrosis, and a tendency to recurrent infections.[5684]

4. *Stick man type* A delayed-onset form of congenital muscle dystrophy characterized by atrophy which is disproportionately severe in comparison to the extent of weakness, contractures, and nonrandom distribution of the small muscle fibers.[773,2151]

5. **Rigid spine syndrome** A congenital form of muscular dystrophy with marked limitation of flexion of the spine along its length, in association with kyphosis, myopathic limb weakness and contractures, seizures, and mental and developmental delay.[1531] In a *variant* form, the onset is later in life and spinal extensor contractures are notable.[1882]

Dubowitz has provided a better, genetic, classification:[1532]

Congenital muscular dystrophy (CMD)

CMD (M−) In one form located to 6q2 with a mutation in the merosin (α2-laminin) protein

CMD (M+) (RSS) In one form located to 1q

CMD (M+) Mapped to 12q13 and involving a mutation of the integrin a7 protein

Fukuyama muscular dystrophy Mapped to 9q31–q33 and involving a mutationof the fukutin protein

Muscle-eye-brain disease

Walker-Warburg syndrome

Other *variants* are *cerebro-ocular dysplasia with muscular dystrophy* (muscle-eye-brain disease, Santavuori syndrome), a congenital form of muscular dystrophy complicated by glaucoma, optic atrophy, myopia, choroidal hypoplasia, ophthalmoplegia, seizures, mental and developmental delay, and hypodensities in the white matter on CT scans.[4913] *Congenital muscle disease with abnormal CT findings* is a congenital form of muscular dystrophy with pyramidal signs, hydrocephalus, and hypodensities in the white matter on CT scans, but normal intelligence.[4150]

congenital muscular hypertrophy Abnormal enlargement of skeletal muscles from birth, with development of normal strength. Hypertrophy is also seen in the **de Lange, Debré-Semelaigne,** and other syndromes reviewed by Zellweger.[6118] Such conditions were first described by Bruck in 1889.

congenital myasthenia A generally benign, heterogeneous group of genetically determined forms of myasthenia gravis, present at birth or during the first 2 years of life in children born to women without myasthenia, and manifesting mainly ocular, but also some facial, bulbar, and limb involvement.[1659,4302] Anti-AchR antibodies are typically detected. For a review see Richman et al.[4678]

The oculomotor palsies are sometimes incomplete but tend to be symmetrical and they are permanent. While these clinical features are similar to those in the adult form, no anti-acetylcholine receptor antibodies and no evidence of an immunological defect are detected, and the usual therapies with immunosuppressants and plasma exchange are ineffective.[1780] The problem appears to be one of defective acetylcholine synthesis or mobilization[1669] as a result of presynaptic defects that reduce quantal size or alter quantal release or from postsynaptic defects that impair quantal efficiency.

A *variant* is *congenital myasthenia with facial malformations,* a recessively inherited syndrome described in Iraqi and Iranian Jewish children, characterized by ptosis, face and jaw muscle weakness, and fatigability, responsive to cholinesterase inhibitors, and due to a postsynaptic abnormality.[4870]

Other *variant* forms include **familial infantile myasthenia, congenital end-plate acetylcholinesterase deficiency, congenital end-plate acetylcholine receptor deficiency, refractory congenital myasthenia,** and the **slow channel syndrome.** See **myasthenia gravis.**[1659]

congenital myopathies A group of slowly or nonprogressive diseases of muscle with onset in infancy or at least early childhood, manifesting muscle hypotrophy; weakness of the ocular, bulbar, facial, truncal, or limb muscles; and hypotonia, with a resulting delay in motor milestones. The condition is often accompanied by skeletal deformities and contractures. Members of the group are distinguished by individually characteristic changes on muscle biopsy, although these may overlap. The better-established varieties are listed in Chart C–25 and at http://www.neuro.wustl.edu/neuromuscular/index.html.

Chart C–25. Varieties of Congenital Myopathy

Bender-type myopathy
CAP congenital myopathy
Central core disease
Centronuclear myopathy
Congenital fiber type disproportion
Congenital hypotonia with small type 2 fibers
Congenital hypotonia with type 1 fiber predominance
Congenital myopathies with intracytoplasmic inclusions
Congenital myopathy with cytoplasmic bodies See congenital myopathies with intracytoplasmic inclusions.
Congenital myopathy with multifocal degeneration of muscle fibers See multicore myopathy.
Congenital myopathy with trilaminar muscle fibers
Congenital neuromuscular disease with uniform type 1 fibers
Distal myopathy with onset in infancy
Fatal infantile myopathy
Minimal change myopathy See benign congenital myopathy.[1744]
Multicore myopathy (congenital myopathy with multifocal degeneration of muscle fibers)
Multi-minicore disease
Myopathy with cylindrical spiral inclusions
Myopathy with focal loss of cross striations and multicores
Myopathy with lysis of myofibrils in type 1 fibers
Myopathy with tubulomembranous inclusions
Nemaline (rod) myopathy
Reducing body myopathy
Sarcotubular myopathy
X-linked myotubular myopathies

congenital myopathies with intracytoplasmic inclusions (congenital myopathy with cytoplasmic bodies)

Rare syndromes conforming to the usually benign clinical features of the congenital myopathies, with facial, proximal, and distal myopathic weakness, dysphagia and feeding problems in infants, joint contractures and laxity, chorea, and athetosis; but in which electron microscopy demonstrates characteristic inclusions such as **zebra bodies, fingerprint bodies,** and cytoplasmic bodies, etc. See **zebra body myopathy, fingerprint inclusion myopathy, cytoplasmic body myopathy.**

The diagnosis of such conditions is solely within the purview of the electron microscopist; the functional and pathological significance of the findings are unknown.[1744] See also **neuromyopathy.**

congenital myopathy with multifocal degeneration of muscle fibers   See **multicore myopathy.**

congenital myopathy with trilaminar muscle fibers
A congenital myopathy of unknown cause characterized by muscle rigidity, reduced spontaneous movements, raised serum creating kinase levels, and the presence of muscle fibers with three concentric zones (trilaminar fibers). EMG and nerve conduction studies are normal.[4706]

congenital myophosphorylase deficiency   See **glycogen storage diseases.**

congenital neuroectodermal dysplasia   See **Sturge-Weber syndrome, phakomatoses.**

congenital neuromuscular disease with uniform type 1 fibers   An inherited myopathy characterized by congenital facial, proximal, and distal limb myopathic weakness and changes in muscle biopsy specimens, as suggested by the title.[4212]

congenital neuropathy with absence of myelin in PNS   A rare, fatal disease of infants characterized by hypotonia, areflexia, minimal residual motor activity, and absence of developmental reflexes. Myelin is almost completely absent from the CNS and there is no myelin on the axons in the peripheral motor or sensory nerves.[4305]

congenital nonprogressive external ophthalmoplegia   A rare syndrome of dominantly inherited third, fourth, and sixth cranial nerve pareses.[3546]

congenital nuclear agenesis/aplasia   See **Möbius syndrome.**

congenital nystagmus   (fixation nystagmus, hereditary nystagmus) A form of rhythmic pendular and/or jerk nystagmus that is usually detectable shortly after birth. It is usually horizontal, symmetrical in the two eyes, reduced by convergence but increased by attempts at fixation and abolished in sleep. Horizontal nystagmus on upward gaze is a typical finding. The frequency and amplitude vary in different directions of gaze and there is a **null point.** In most cases, the slow phase has an increasing velocity. The patient's visual acuity is usu-

ally decreased and this may have pathogenetic importance. **Oscillopsia** is absent[2392] but oscillation of the head is usual.

The nystagmus later evolves into a smaller-amplitude, lower-frequency, pendular waveform, the latter itself sometimes changing to a jerky waveform before 18 months of age. The eye movements are commonly in the horizontal plane, but vertical forms are also described.[1368]

The differentiation from nystagmus acquired in infancy is difficult but may be made when pendular nystagmus occurs in the presence of evidence of visual impairment affecting the central part of the field. The several complex waveforms in this condition have been analyzed and reviewed.[1371,6075]

congenital oculobulbar palsy   Selective nonprogressive weakness of the ocular and bulbar muscles with onset before the age of 2 years, accompanied by subclinical myopathic weakness of trunk and limb muscles, not due to myasthenia, giant axonal neuropathy, or **Fazio-Londe disease.**[2840]

congenital oculofacial paresis   See **Möbius syndrome.**

congenital oculomotor apraxia   See **Cogan syndrome** (definition 1).

congenital ophthalmoplegia   A very rare autosomal recessive or X-linked disorder characterized by progressive congenital ophthalmoplegia (without mitochondrial cytopathy seen in a biopsy specimen), myopia, pigmentary retinopathy, pituitary insufficiency, small stature, and muscular hypotonia.[4573]

congenital optic atrophy   (Thompson syndrome) See **Behr disease.**

congenital pain asymbolia   Perception of sensations that would normally be expected to be painful but to which there is indifference on the part of the subject. The condition may be associated with other evidences of higher cortical dysfunction such as auditory imperception, personality disorder, etc., but reports of minor changes on peripheral nerve biopsy and in autonomic tests in some reported cases raise the question of the possible basis of a peripheral neuropathy.

A variant is *pain asymbolia with auditory imperception,* a congenital syndrome characterized by speech delay and pain agnosia.[337] See also **hereditary sensory and autonomic neuropathy, congenital insensitivty to pain.**

congenital paramyotonia   See **Eulenberg disease.**

congenital persistent myasthenia   See **myasthenia gravis.**

congenital Pick cell encephalopathy   A congenital neuronal inclusion disease manifesting amentia, joint contractures, respiratory distress, hypotonia, paroxysmal EEG discharges, and diffuse gliosis.[337]

congenital progressive oculo-acousticocerebral degeneration   See **Norrie disease.**

congenital ptosis   A dominantly inherited syndrome consisting of isolated ptosis, usually unilateral and accompanied in some cases by impairment of upward movement of the eye and due to abnormal differentiation of the levator palpebrae and/or superior rectus muscles.[586]

congenital pure word deafness   See **Worster-Drought-Allen syndrome.**

congenital rod disease   See **nemaline myopathy.** The finding of rods is by itself nonspecific, as they may be secondary to denervation.

congenital rubella embryopathy   (Gregg syndrome) A syndrome consequent upon fetal infection with the rubella virus, and (in infants born alive) characterized by low birth weight, short stature, sensorineural deafness, glaucoma, microphthalmia, iris abnormalities, cataract, coarctation of the aorta, patent ductus arteriosus, hepatosplenomegaly, purpura, neonatal jaundice, microcephaly, pleocytosis in the CSF, wide anterior fontanelle and metopic sutures, mental and developmental delay, and high levels of specific rubella IgM antibodies in the blood at birth and of any rubella antibody after the age of 1 year.[1420]

congenital sensory neuropathies   See **hereditary sensory and autonomic neuropathy, type 2.**

congenital sensory neuropathy with selective loss of small myelinated fibres   See **hereditary sensory and autonomic neuropathy.**

congenital spastic (di-) paraparesis   See **Little disease.**

congenital stiff man syndrome   A dominantly inherited syndrome of continuous motor neuron discharges arising in the CNS.[3079] See **startle epilepsy.**

congenital suprabulbar paresis   A dominantly inherited congenital or childhood dysmorphic syndrome characterized by seizures, microcephaly, pyramidal signs, dysarthria, facial and bulbar weakness, and mental and developmental delay, sometimes complicated by deafness, seizures, and mental retardation.[335] See **Worster-Drought syndrome.**

congenital syphilis   Infection in utero from the mother, leading to skin rash resembling the secondary syphilis in the adult; rhinitis; osteochondritis and periostitis; and chronic meningitis. Manifestations appearing later in life include interstitial keratitis, gummas, Hutchinson teeth, mulberry molars, and numerous other neurological disturbances including vestibular dysfunction, nerve deafness, and further cortical atrophy.

congenital syphilitic paralysis   See **Dennie-Marfan syndrome.**

congenital tilted disk syndrome   See **tilted disks.**

congenital toxoplasmosis   (chronic congenital toxoplasmosis with late degeneration) Infection by *Toxoplasma gondii,* an intracellular protozoan organism existing worldwide.

Transplacental transmission may follow acute infection of the mother during pregnancy, leading to the classic triad of hydrocephalus, intracranial calcification, and chorioretinitis, often accompanied by microcephaly or hydrocephalus in newborn infants.[100,1588] The titer of anti-*Toxoplasma* IgM antibodies is elevated.

In the *acquired form,* infection occurs after ingestion of cysts in undercooked meat or from contamination of food by the feces of cats.

congenital trigeminal anesthesia   Unilateral or bilateral loss of sensation over the face, present from birth. When bilateral, this may be the only problem or focal brainstem signs may be associated; the cause in such cases is assumed to be primary neural hypoplasia. In a second group, congenital mesenchymal anomalies such as oculoauriculovertebral dysplasia are also present.[4785]

congenital tritan defects   Inherited disorders of color vision characterized by normal distant and near vision, normal visual fields, normal-appearing optic nerves, and tritanopia.[3162]

congenital unilateral lower lip palsy   A syndrome of lower quadrant facial weakness occurring in infants who also have congenital heart disease. See **cardiofacial syndrome, asymmetric crying facies.**

congenital universal muscle hypoplasia   A rare, nonprogressive disorder characterized by generalized smallness of muscles from birth without histological evidence of inflammation or myopathy. Clinically, poor power and gait control, hyporeflexia, and easy tiring are the major findings.[3149]

congenital varicella   A **static embryopathy** associated with infections of the mother with the varicella virus and characterized clinically by hypoplasia of the limbs, skin lesions, and cerebral atrophy.[743]

congenital webbed neck   See **Klippel-Feil anomaly.**

congenital word blindness   (developmental dyslexia) A form of pure visual receptive dysphasia occurring as a developmental defect in the region of the left angular gyrus. Visual agnosia for objects is likely to be present as well. The term was coined in 1895 by James Hinshelwood, a Scottish ophthalmologist. See **alexia.**

congenital word deafness   See **congenital auditory imperception, developmental dysphasia.**

congestive brain swelling   An increase in the volume of the brain as a result of an increase in the cerebral blood volume.

congophilic angiopathy   (primary cerebrovascular amyloidosis, familial presenile dementia with spastic paralysis; precocious, juvenile, or atypical Alzheimer disease) A dominantly inherited form of amyloidosis confined to the cerebral blood vessels, characterized pathologically by multiple hemorrhages and softenings in the brain and abundant amyloid-containing plaques, mainly in the hippocampus and cerebellar cortex.

Clinically, the disease appears in adult life as a syndrome consisting of progressive dementia with ataxic dysarthria, spastic paralyses, and frequently multiple lobar intracerebral hemorrhages. The differentiation from **Alzheimer disease** can thus be made clinically, and the histological appearance of the amyloid-containing plaques is also different, although there are definite pathological similarities between the two conditions.[2282] See also **cerebral amyloid angiopathy.**

Congress of Neurological Surgeons   A professional organization based at University of Southern California. Address: 1200 North State St., Los Angeles, CA 90033.

congruence   (congruity) Uniformity of the visual field defect in the two eyes in cases of hemianopia. The more congruent the defects, the more posterior the responsible lesion.

congruity   See **congruence.**

coning   The downward descent of the medulla and cerebellar tonsils into the foramen magnum as a result of increasing intracranial pressure.

The occurrence of coning is a sign of impending catastrophe, the brainstem and its blood supply being compressed and distorted, which may lead eventually to ischemic necrosis.

conjugate eye deviation   (Prévost sign) The lateral deviation of the two eyes in parallel, typically toward the side of a hemispheric stroke but away from the side of a stroke affecting the brainstem. The sign was first noted by Prévost in 1865.

The lesion can occur at various sites in the circuit between the inferior parietal lobule and the frontal eye fields, and their projections to the superior colliculus or the paramedian pontine reticular formation.[5584]

conjugate gaze   (Lat, yoked together) The harnessing of the two eyes so that they normally move with their axes parallel (except during convergence).

conjugate gaze palsy   An inability to turn the eyes past the midline using any mechanism (saccadic, pursuit, optokinetic or vestibular).

conjugate movements   A term generally employed to describe the normal yoking together of the eyes in their movements so that the parallelism of the ocular axes is maintained. The same concept is relevant in regard to the front wheels of steered vehicles.

conjunctival reflex   Blinking in response to conjunctival stimulation; a normal phenomenon.

Conn syndrome   (primary aldosteronism) Excessive secretion of aldosterone by an adenoma or carcinoma or by a hyperplastic adrenal cortex. Hypertension and resultant stroke, hypokalemic myopathy, tetany, and polyuria, and polydipsia are the features most likely to bring the patient to a neurologist.

connectivity   The pattern of interconnection between specific cortical areas. The term can be used anatomically or functionally, or within the context of artificial intelligence.

Conradi-Hünermann syndrome   (multiple epiphyseal dysplasia, chondrodystrophia calcificans punctata congenita, Conradi-Raap disease) A dominant, sexlinked, or recessive condition characterized by facial dysmorphism; short neck, trunk and limbs; mental deficiency; kyphoscoliosis due to asymmetry of the vertebral bodies; and craniosynostosis.

Alopecia, dry skin, muscle fibrosis, hypoplasia of the bones of the hands and feet, cataracts, rhizomelia of limbs with asymmetry, joint stiffness, paraplegia, and other systemic abnormalities may also be found.[1120]

In a *variant* congenital form, microcephaly, nystagmus, and mental and developmental delay are the major neurological manifestations.

Conradi-Raap disease   See **Conradi-Hünermann syndrome.**

conscious level   The vigilance of an individual; the ability to perceive, attend to, memorize, and react to events in the internal and external environments.

consciousness   1. The awareness of being aware. The same neurological mechanisms that support this function also allow awareness of the self and the environment, as well as attention, perception, cognitive functions, motor decisions, and responsiveness. 2. The perception of what passes in a person's own mind (John Locke, 1690). 3. "Consciousness is not something which we can define in terms of anything else; we can only indicate its meaning denotatively, that is by pointing to instances of it. . . . There is no such thing as consciousness apart from conscious states any more than there is a redness apart from red objects" (Lord Brain).

Yet if a thing exists, surely it is definable; since it appears undefinable to some, so they have denied the concept or relegated it to the status of a semantic artifact or an epiphenomenon. The philosophical difficulties of the subject have been reviewed by Gloor.[2140]

consecutive   (Lat, following after). Following in order.

consecutive optic atrophy   1. To ophthalmologists, optic atrophy occurring first in one and later in the other eye. 2. To neurologists, optic atrophy succeeding prior papilledema. 3. To other ophthalmologists and neurologists, optic atrophy following upon retinal or choroidal diseases.

consensual reflex   The occurrence of a bilateral reflex response in response to a unilateral stimulus, as when both pupils constrict in response to the stimulation of one eye only. This response was first remarked upon by **Whytt.**

When one pupil only is illuminated but the other one does not contract equally, a *consensual deficit* is said to exist.

Consortium of Canadian Centres for Clinical Cognitive Research   A professional organization promoting and assisting research into cognitive disorders. Web site: http://www.c5r.ca/.

Consortium of Multiple Sclerosis Centers   A professional organization concerned with the provision of appropriate services in multiple sclerosis clinics. Web site: http://www.mscare.org/.

Consortium to Establish a Registry for Alzheimer Disease   (CERAD) A group of American workers combining in their aim to develop, standardize, and test the reliability of a brief clinical and neuropsychological assessment schedule for patients with **Alzheimer disease.**[3997,3998]

constructional apraxia   A failure of visuoconstructive ability such that the subject is unable to assemble component parts into a coherent whole.[3138] This results in impairment of the ability to construct the copy of a visually presented model by means of assembling objects or drawing; normal visual acuity and perception of the number and relationship of the items to be copied and normal gross motor abilities are assumed. *Apractagnosia* was the term preferred by Lord **Brain** because of the visual perceptive disorder so often associated.

Despite the name (suggested by Kleist in 1923[3857] and more fully described by Mayer-Gross[3718]), the deficit is not truly an apraxia. Lesions of either parietal lobe may be responsible. See also **apraxia.**

contact point headache   A suggested headache/facial pain syndrome resulting from nasal septal spurs or other intranasal pathologies (not including chronic sinusitis) but due to abnormalities of the turbinates that cause "mucosal contacts." Criteria for the diagnosis of this very uncertain syndrome have been suggested by Tosun et al.[5614] (and are adapted) as follows:

Criteria for Contact Point Headaches
1. History of chronic headache
2. Lack of acute or chronic inflammatory findings on the ear-nose-throat examination (clinical, X-ray, and CT)
3. Absence of any other cause of headache after a thorough evaluation by a neurologist, ophthalmologist, dentist, internist or any other related specialist
4. Presence of "contact points" documented by nasal endoscopy, CT, or both
5. Failure of medical therapy for headaches [not further defined]
6. Relief of headache after applying topical anesthesia to the contact points
7. Contact points that still remain after mucosal decongestion.

Contemporary Neurology Series   A neurological review book series, published by Oxford University Press.

continence   1. The physiological capacity to maintain voluntary closure of the urinary or anal sphincter until evacuation of the contents of the bladder or bowel is appropriate. 2. Restriction of sexual activity to one partner.

contingent negative variation   An event-related slow negative potential recorded best in the frontal regions of alert subjects during the 1-second interval between a warning stimulus and a response stimulus, subjects having been primed to make a decision concerning their motor response to the second signal.[5835]

continuous motor neuron discharges   A dominantly inherited syndrome characterized by continuous motor neuron discharges with persistent twitching and episodic stiffness, mainly in the legs. It occurs first in early childhood and remits to some extent in adult life. The discharges disappear during spinal anesthesia, suggesting their generation from the proximal portion of the motor unit.[241] See also the Web site http://www.neuro.wustl.edu/neuromuscular/index.html.

Other conditions in which such continuous motor unit discharges occur may be classified as follows:
1. Central origin
   Congenital stiff man syndrome
2. Peripheral origin
   a. Without overt peripheral neuropathy
      Schwartz-Jampel syndrome[5027]
      Hereditary myokymia[260]
      Hereditary myokymia with episodic ataxia[5725]
      Hereditary persistent distal cramps
      Associated with gold therapy; intrathoracic malignancy or **idiopathic neuromyotonia**
   b. With overt peripheral neuropathy
      Hereditary neuromyotonia[3846]
      Sporadic; **Isaacs syndrome;** associated with exposure to toxins, with inflammatory neuropathy, or with intrathoracic malignancy
   c. Tetany
   d. Following plexus irradiation[241,260]

continuous motor unit activity   See **neuromyotonia.**

continuous muscle fiber activity   See **neuromyotonia.**

Continuous Performance Test   A test of concentration span and vigilance, in which the subject identifies a specific recurring letter randomly presented with others over a 10-minute period.[4808]

continuous-wave Doppler sonography   An early technique used in the diagnosis of carotid artery disease, in which a continuous-wave Doppler probe traverses the line of the carotid arteries; a shift in the Doppler frequency indicates the presence of severe stenosis.[4141]

contraction   (from Lat, shorten or draw together) 1. (muscular) The reversible shortening of the distance between the origin and insertion of a muscle as a result of electrical excitation. A voluntary or involuntary reversible muscle shortening that may or may not be accompanied by action potentials from muscle. (From the 2001 Report of the Nomenclature Committee of the American Association of Electromyography and Electrodiagnosis.[10] Used by permission, copyright © 2001, AAEM.) cf. **contracture.** 2. (visual field) Absolute loss of the visual field, usually peripherally, such that no stimuli are seen in the affected area.

contraction fasciculation   Clinical term for visible twitching of a muscle with weak voluntary or postural contraction that has the appearance of a fasciculation. More likely to occur in neuromuscular disorders in which the motor unit territory is enlarged and the tissue covering the muscle is thin, but may also be observed in normal individuals. (From the 2001 Report of the Nomenclature Committee of the American Association of Electromyography and Electrodiagnosis.[10] Used by permission, copyright © 2001, AAEM.)

The term is employed to refer to the repetitive twitching of the chin with pursing of the lips seen in **bulbospinal muscular atrophy** (neuronopathy), in which they are due to grouped motor discharges, activated by voluntary muscle contraction in some but not all cases.[4233]

contracture   1. Immobility of a joint due to fixed muscle shortening. 2. An electrically silent, involuntary state of semipermanent shortening of the distance between the origin and insertion of a muscle as a result of disease. 3. Fixed resistance to stretch of a shortened muscle due to fibrous connective tissue changes and loss of sarcomeres in the muscle. Limited movement of a joint may be due to muscle contracture or to fibrous connective tissue changes in the joint. Contrast with contraction, which is a rapidly reversible painless shortening of the muscle. 4. The prolonged, painful, electrically silent, involuntary state of temporary muscle shortening seen in some myopathies (e.g., muscle phosphorylase deficiency). (From the 2001 Report of the Nomenclature Committee of the American Association of Electromyography and Electrodiagnosis.[10] Used by permission, copyright © 2001, AAEM.) See also **cramp.**

contractures, muscle atrophy, and ocular lesions syndrome   See **Cogan syndrome.**

contracturing granulomatous myositis   A chronic granulomatous disease of muscles without systemic involvement, presenting in adult life with progressive flexion contractures of the limbs. The condition is thought to differ from **idiopathic granulomatous myositis** and sarcoidosis, mainly on the basis of the clinical features of lack of pain and the absence of systemic involvement.[5167]

contralateral abdominal proprioceptive reflex   See **Tramer reflex.**

contralaterality   The phenomenon of the clinical expression of a motor or sensory function (or functional deficit) on the side of the body opposite to that on which the responsible brain area is situated.

contrapulsion   A disorder of saccadic eye movements due to lesions of the superior cerebellar peduncle and characterized by hypermetric horizontal saccades away from the side of the lesion, hypometric ipsilateral saccades, and diagonal movements of the globes with attempted vertical saccades.[4582] See also **saccadic lateropulsion.**

contrary movement   A distortion of a normal willed movement seen characteristically in **athetosis,** whereby it begins with contraction of the antagonistic muscles.[1900]

contrast   1. A chemical substance given to a subject in order to enhance the visualization of certain structures during radiological imaging procedures such as myelograms or arteriograms, or during MRI. Water-soluble, iodine-containing compounds are usually used in the former case and gadolinium in the latter. 2. A change in brightness across space (visual physiology).

contraversive pushing   (pusher syndrome) A phenomenon seen in some patients after stroke, who actively push away from the unaffected side, leading to lateral postural imbalance and a tendency to fall towards the paralyzed side as a result of an altered perception of the body's orientation in respect to gravity.[2933]

contrecoup injury   (Fr, against + a blow) Contusion or laceration of the brain on the side opposite to that struck, as a result of the delay in deceleration of the brain after it is impelled away from the site of injury. The frontal and temporal poles are most commonly affected. The phenomenon was well known to the ancient Greeks.

Controlled Word Association Test   A measure of semantic information in which the subject is asked to name as many words beginning with *F* as possible in 1 minute. The same is asked for the letters *A* and *S* thereafter.[471]

controller signal   A mechanism whereby signals from the nervous system cause a change of state of part of the effector mechanisms of the body and re-set the system so that the new state is maintained. See **pulse-step control.**

contusion   (Lat, a bruise) Physically inflicted injury to an organ without breach of its surface.

Contusion Index   A semiquantitative account of the number and site of the lesions resulting from cerebral contusions.[6]

conus medullaris   (Lat, a cone + marrow) The inferior tip of the spinal cord, comprising the last few sacral segments located opposite the first lumbar vertebra.

conus medullaris syndrome   The signs resulting from lesions of the lower three sacral and the coccygeal segments of the spinal cord, as by compression from local masses or resulting from infiltration.

These consist of **saddle anesthesia** and **dissociated anesthesia** in the appropriate dermatomal areas, loss of sphincter functions with urinary and fecal incontinence, impotence, wasting and flaccid paresis of the (few) muscles innervated by S3, 4, and 5, and pain in the back and perineum. The syndrome was first described by Roussy and Lhermitte in 1918.[4824]

See also **cauda equina syndrome.** It must be noted that lesions seldom affect the nervous system in this nicely classified manner, so that the features of both of these syndromes often occur together.

convergence   1. The termination of different axons upon the same postsynaptic membrane, allowing integration of activities to occur at synapses. 2. The turning inward of the eyes when focusing on an object brought near to the face; the only physiological situation in which the axes of the eyes are not parallel. This complex function, consisting of pupillary constriction, accommodation, and adduction of both eyes, can be disturbed by various neurological disorders, especially those affecting the dorsal midbrain in the tectal region.[3330]

convergence insufficiency   Impairment of fusional convergence, the near-point of which is abnormally distant, in the presence of exophoria at near distances. The near-point of accommodation, however, is typically normal.[2133]

convergence nystagmus   See **convergence-retraction nystagmus.**

convergence paralysis   An abnormality of the accommodation-vergence system such that there is impairment in adduction of the eyes at near gaze. This may be congenital or the result of **progressive supranuclear palsy** or **Parkinson disease.** See also **convergence insufficiency.**

convergence spasm   Slow, persisting convergence movements of the eyes giving an appearance of sixth nerve palsy or of gaze paresis, but voluntary in nature and accompanied by miosis and often facial grimacing and complaints of blurred vision and ocular pain. Pupillary constriction occurs when the patient attempts to look laterally, but full abduction is seen with the oculocephalic reflex.[1078]

The range of movement of each eye alone is normal when the other is occluded, which with the above features allows the diagnosis of functional eye disease.[2977] See **spasm of the near reflex.**

convergence-evoked nystagmus   Unusual forms of nystagmus in which the variable (up- or downbeating) abnormal movements are provoked by convergent gaze. Some cases are congenital; in others, the causative lesion (such as a multiple sclerosis plaque) is thought to be in the brainstem.[5098]

convergence-retraction   nystagmus   (convergence nystagmus, nystagmus retractorius) Simultaneous contraction of all the extraocular muscles on attempted upward gaze or with a downward-moving optokinetic stimulus, leading to retraction of the eyes into the orbit and to nasal deviation of each eye, and due to the cocontraction of the agonist and antagonist extraocular muscles. The condition is thus not really nystagmus at all but rather an unusual form of saccadic movement.

The presence of the sign indicates a lesion in the pretectal regions of the midbrain; it comprises a part of the **dorsal midbrain–sylvian aqueduct syndrome,** in which it accompanies paresis of upward gaze.[5098]

converse ocular bobbing   See **slow-upward ocular bobbing.**

conversion   The mental mechanism whereby the anxiety or conflict experienced is transformed into a physical manifestation. The nature, rationale, and purpose of such a mechanism are not hereby explained.

conversion disorder   (somatoform disorder) A relatively persistent loss or distortion of function, not fully explained by structural or biochemical disease or pathophysiological mechanisms; and with evidence for linkage of the symptoms to psychological factors; assumption of the sick role in the absence of bodily disease.

The presence of other evidence of somatization disorder, of associated psychopathology, of a model for the symptom and of evidence of recent emotional stress may increase clinical confidence in the diagnosis, but there is almost always a need for neurological investigation in such patients as judged by the follow-up studies of eventual morbidity.[3305] See also **hysteria, somatization disorder.**

convexity block   Obstruction of CSF circulation due to failure of flow over the convexities of the hemisphere, considered to be due to adherence of the pial and arachnoid membranes, especially over the parietal lobes.

convolutions   (from Lat, to roll together) Infolding of the surface of the cerebral cortex, causing a marked increase in its surface area. Their presence was known to the ancient Egyptians, who considered that their greater complexity in humans than in animals reflected our greater intelligence, but this insight was lost thereafter and Galen denied that they had any function. They were drawn by Leonardo da Vinci and others to resemble the coils of the intestines.

convulsion   (from Lat, to tear) 1. Violent agitation of the limbs, face, and trunk with intermittent, involuntary muscle contractions, usually as a result of epilepsy. 2. Episodes of excessive, abnormal, involuntary muscle contractions which may be sustained or interrupted and which may be epileptic or nonepileptic in origin.

convulsive movements of the stump   See **stump spasm.**

convulsive syncope   Convulsive movements (usually tonic extensor spasms) occurring as components of a syncopal reaction in susceptible individuals, due to the cerebral ischemia induced by the hypotension.[3412] See **Adams-Stokes-Morgagni syndrome.**

convulsive tonic-clonic status epilepticus   See **status epilepticus.**

convulsive tremor   See **paramyoclonus multiplex.**

Cooke, John   (1756–1838) English physician who trained in London, Edinburgh, and Leyden and who became physician to the London Hospital. His *Treatise on Nervous Disorders* (1820–1823, and thus preceding **Romberg**) was the first book on neurology. The three parts to the work dealt only with the clinical aspects of apoplexy, palsy, and epilepsy, Cooke having concluded that "the physiology of the nervous system remains involved in impenetrable obscurity."

Cooper, Sir Astley   (1768–1841) English surgeon at Guy's Hospital who first ligated the carotid artery for the treatment of aneurysm (1805).

coonhound paralysis   A demyelinating disease of dogs, resembling **acute inflammatory demyelinating polyradiculoneuropathy.**

coordination   (Lat, with + order) The smooth patterning of voluntary movements. Hughlings-Jackson noted that, "It will not suffice to speak of coordination as a separate faculty, co-ordination is the function of the whole and of every part of the nervous system," and that "Half of the symptomatology of disorders of co-ordination is paralysis (i.e., loss of function) owing to that negative central lesion, But the other half is from forcing of other movements by overactivity of perfectly healthy nervous arrangements. The two elements, negative and positive, constitute the disorder of coordination."

Tests of coordination in the arms include the finger–nose test, rapid alternating movements of the fingers, pronation-supination of the forearms, repetitive hand patting tests, handwriting, and serial approximation of fingers to thumbs. Fisher describes an improvement, in which the patient taps the tip of the flexed index finger against the distal knuckle of the thumb.[1840] In the legs, the heel–knee test with Fisher's modification (tapping the shin with the heel of the other leg as well as running the heel down the length of the shin) is the only test in common usage.[1841]

cop-1   A random polymer simulating myelin basic protein, able to enhance the production of antigen-specific suppressor T cells and thus used in the treatment of **multiple sclerosis.**

coping   The varying cognitive and behavioral attempts to manage those internal or external demands that strain an individual's resources.

coprolalia   (Gr, filth or dung + speech) The compulsive uttering of obscene words, commonly but not exclusively as a complex vocal tic in **Tourette syndrome.**

coprolaliopraxia   See **signing tics.**

coprophemonena   Motor activities that directly or indirectly are reminiscent of fecal functions or of other unclassified filth. They include **coprolalia, copropraxia,** and **mental coprolalia,** all of which are motor or phonic tics or their substitute, and occur in **Tourette syndrome.**

coproporphyria   A dominantly inherited form of porphyria in which the excretion of coproporphyrins is greatly increased. The condition is characterized clinically by the onset in childhood of hirsutism, skin photosensitivity with the formation of bullae or vesicles, depression, sleep disorders, complex partial seizures, cerebellar signs, sensorimotor axonal peripheral neuropathy (which may be acute), and abnormal urinary color on standing.[1164,4756]

copropraxia   Obscene gesturing as a form of motor tic in **Tourette syndrome.**

Copy a Cross test   A test of visuospatial and constructional abilities in which the subject is asked to copy a line drawing of a Greek cross.[2191] Inability to do so appropriately suggests impairment of visuospatial functions.

cor anglais players thumb   An **overuse syndrome** or focal **dystonia** affecting the first digit.

cord bladder   See **automatic bladder.**

cord sign   (dense triangle sign) The CT appearance of a clot in a dural venous sinus or a cortical vein, the thrombosed vein highlighting within an extraaxial fluid collection.[4590]

cordotomy   (myelotomy) Incision of the anterolateral or central parts of the spinal cord in an attempt to reduce the central conduction of impulses allowing pain perception or regulating tone.

The operation was introduced by William G. Spiller and Edward Martin, American physicians, in 1912.[5287] See also **tractotomy.**

corectopia iridis   (ectopia pupillae) Spontaneous, cyclic, independent, and eccentric dilation of the pupils, which are displaced from the center of the iris.

The condition is most often seen in comatose patients with a midbrain lesion. The sign was first reported by Kinnier **Wilson** in 1906. The dilatation may be oval; up-gaze paresis and loss of the pupillary light reflexes are often present as well.[5058]

cores   Areas lying centrally within type 1 myofibrils, which do not take up stains for oxidative enzymes. They are composed of Z-line and granular material. The appearance is seen in certain **congenital myopathies,** but also in denervation, malignant hyperthermia, etc. See also **target fibers.**

Cori, C.F.   (b. 1896) German-American biochemist, professor of biochemistry at Washington University, St. Louis. He and his wife were awarded the Nobel prize for work on glycogen dysmetabolism.

Cori disease   See **Cori-Forbes disease.**

Cori-Forbes disease   (Cori disease) Type III glycogen storage disease, the major features of which are hepatomegaly, hypoglycemia, slight retardation of growth, and a degree of muscle weakness of late onset.[1131] See **glycogen storage diseases, debrancher enzyme deficiency.**

Coriolis effect   Severe spatial disorientation with vertigo induced by the rotation of the head around two axes simultaneously, as in airplane stunt pilots.[727]

corneal reflex   Sudden involuntary blinking as a result of stimulation of the sensitive fibers of the ophthalmic division of the fifth cranial nerve in the cornea, which leads to contraction of the orbicularis oculi muscles bilaterally.

The *eyelash* (**ciliary**) and the *conjunctival* reflexes are similar, travel by almost identical pathways, and are less hazardous to perform, though slightly less sensitive. If either of these are present, however, it may be taken as certain that the corneal reflex will be present as well.

Cornelia de Lange syndrome   See **de Lange syndrome.**

Cornelia de Lange Syndrome Foundation   A charitable support organization. Address: 60 Dyer Ave., Collinsville, CT 06022.

Cornell Scale for Depression and Dementia   A validated scale yielding a quantitative measure of depression in demented patients, but not designed as a diagnostic instrument. A score is assigned on the basis of information obtained after interviewing the patient and a caregiver.

Mood-related signs such as anxiety, sadness, lack of reactivity to pleasant events, and irritability; behavioral disturbances including agitation, retardation, multiple physical complaints, and loss of interest; physical signs including loss of appetite, weight, and energy; cyclic functions such as diurnal variation of mood, difficulty falling asleep, multiple awakenings, and early morning waking; and ideational disturbances such as suicidal thoughts, poor self-esteem, pessimism, and mood-congruent delusions are the items rated on a 3-point scale.[98]

Cornell, Ethel L.   (b. 1892) American psychologist who devised a nonverbal test of intelligence (Cornell-Coxe Performance Ability Scale).

Cornell sign   A variant of the **Babinski reflex** whereby extension of the hallux is sought as a response to scratching the inner side of the dorsum of the foot.

corneomandibular reflex   Closure of the mouth or deviation of the jaw away from the side of corneal stimulation. This is normally not present after infancy and represents one of the primitive or **developmental reflexes** which may appear in association with diffuse cortical dysfunction (especially in ill patients with a reduced level of consciousness, increased intracranial pressure, and transtentorial herniation) but which is also common with advancing age.

It was first described by Von Solder in 1902 but was further discussed by Wartenberg as the winking jaw or reverse **Marcus Gunn phenomenon.**[2301,4370] See also **palpebromandibular synkinesia, Wartenberg winking-jaw phenomenon.**

corneo-oculogyric reflex   Deviation of the eyes upward and away from a corneal sensory stimulus; a normal phenomenon.

Cornil, Lucien   (1888–1959) French neuropathologist who trained in Paris. During and after World War I, he worked with Roussy and Lhermitte, setting up the neuropathology laboratory at the Hôpital Paul-Brusse. He was elected professor of pathological anatomy at Marseille in 1930 and became dean of the faculty in 1937. His neuropathological publications mainly concerned the basal ganglia, cerebral tumors, and hypertrophic neuritis.

Corning, James Leonard   (1855–1923) New York neurologist who trained in Germany and practiced in New York. He introduced the technique of lumbar puncture to America in 1885, 6 years before Wynter and Quincke, but his object was to inject cocaine and he did not draw cerebrospinal fluid; it is thus uncertain whether his needle penetrated the arachnoid membrane at all.[2210]

corona radiata   (Lat, a crown + rays) The term applied by Reil to the fan-like spread of the descending pyramidal fibers when traced upwards from the pyramids through the internal capsules to the cerebral hemispheres.[4512]

coronal bipolar montage   (transverse bipolar montage) A montage consisting of derivations from pairs of electrodes along coronal (transverse) arrays. (Adapted from the report of the Committee on Terminology, IFCN,[989] © 1974, with permission from Elsevier Science.)

corpora amylaceae   (from Lat, bodies + starch) Spherical basophilic, periodic acid-Schiff–positive structures found in astrocytic processes beneath the pia or ependyma in patients with various degenerative diseases and in increasing numbers with advancing age.[3461] See **polyglucosan bodies.** See also **Lafora bodies, Bielschowsky bodies.**

corpora arenacea   See **psammoma bodies.**

corpus callosum   (Lat, a tough body) The term given by Galen to the largest (8-cm-long) interhemispheric commissure. It manifests topographical localization. It is sometimes partially sectioned in cases of intractable epilepsy since its presence is essential for the spread of a bilateral synchronous discharge. **Agenesis of the corpus callosum** may be asymptomatic, or may be associated with a clinical syndrome of mental deficiency, seizures, and hemiparesis, often accompanied by such developmental defects as deficiency of the septum pellucidum and microgyria.[121] See also **Shapiro syndrome.**

corpus callosum agenesis with recurrent hypothermia (Shapiro syndrome) A congenital dysmorphic syndrome characterized also by hypercalcemia, recurrent hypothermia and reduction in consciousness, seizures, and callosal agenesis.[5095]

corpus striatum (Lat, body + furrowed) The basal ganglia include the lentiform nucleus (comprising the putamen and globus pallidus) and the caudate, the claustrum, the subthalamic nucleus, the substantia innominata of Meynert, and the substantia nigra. The striped appearance of the caudate and lentiform nuclei on stained horizontal sections of the brain have led to the term *corpus striatum* (or *striatum* alone) for this region.

corrective catch-up saccades Brief, small-amplitude, conjugate saccades correcting any positional error made in the last major saccade.

Corsi blocks test A test of nonverbal (visual) attention span/memory, in which the subject points to a progressively greater number of blocks in the same order as previously indicated by the examiner, or in reverse. The normal forward span is 6 ± 1 and the reverse span is 2 less.[3897]

cortex (Lat, outer bark, rind) The outer neuronal layer of the cerebrum.

Cortex A neurological subspecialty journal devoted to the study of the interrelations between the nervous system and behavior. Address: Masson SA, Avenue Beauregard 12, CH-1701 Fribourg, Switzerland. Web site: http://www.masson.it/riviste/cortex.html.

Corti, Alfonso Marchese (1822–1888) Sardinian histologist, who worked in Vienna, Berlin, Utrecht, Turin, and Rome. He held no academic appointment but was an amateur in the best sense; he described the spiral organ of the cochlea (the end organ for hearing, which consists of specialized neuroepithelium in the inner ear aligned in rows within the cochlear canal upon the basilar membrane) and the perilymph.

cortical abscess See **subdural empyema.**

cortical anarthria See **aphemia.**

cortical blindness Loss of vision produced by lesions of the geniculocalcarine visual pathways. Denial of such blindness is a rare accompaniment. See **Anton syndrome.** It is seldom complete and macular sparing may occur. The patient recovers poorly when the condition is due to vascular disease, better when it follows cardiac surgery or angiography.[92]

In a *variant* congenital recessively inherited form, the cortical blindness is accompanied by postaxial polydactyly, mental retardation, and growth failure.[2549]

cortical cerebellar degeneration (Déjèrine-Thomas syndrome) A dominantly inherited form of late-onset **cerebellar ataxia** (**olivopontocerebellar atrophy**). See **Déjèrine-Thomas syndrome.** See also **cerebellar cortical degeneration,** which is a **paraneoplastic syndrome.**

cortical deafness The rare occurrence of inability to interpret verbal or nonverbal sounds in the presence of retained hearing, due to a lesion affecting the anterior and posterior transverse temporal gyri of Heschl or their connections bilaterally, while the peripheral pathways are intact. Both verbal and nonverbal sounds are uninterpreted, and the temporal order of sounds and their localization in space are impaired.

Pure word deafness (auditory agnosia) may occur as the result of bilateral infarctions of the superior temporal cortex.[2253]

cortical dementia Dementing diseases presenting with prominent dysphasia, agnosia, and apraxias, reflecting involvement of the association cortex in the pathological process.

See also **subcortical dementia,** in which the major problems are slowness of cognition and impairment of executive function. However, although the distinction is clinically real, the degree of overlap in the presentations of the pathologies leading to dementia limits the diagnostic value of this differentiation.

cortical dumbness See **aphemia.**

Cortical Dysgenetic Index A method of scoring the presence of minor cortical irregularities, dysplasias, and microdysgenesis in brains. **Leptomeningeal glial heterotopias, merged gyri,** and **gray matter heterotopias** score 5; abnormal cortical bundles of myelin, neuronal multinucleation, ballooned cells, and cortical nodules score 3; and neuronal heterotopias; subpial neurons; single-file neuronal radial patterns; abnormal neuronal clusters; large, overabundant, or misaligned neurons; abnormal lamination, or irregular gray/white matter score 2. A total score of 5 or more indicates the presence of cortical microdysgenesis.[417]

cortical dysplasia The presence of large dysplastic neurons and of giant astrocytes in all but the first layer of discrete segments of the cortex, typically the rolandic cortex. **Macrogyria, lissencephaly, unilateral megalencephaly, pachygyria,** and **polymicrogyria** are recognized accompaniments.

The clinical syndrome comprises the onset in childhood of focal cortical myoclonus and focal motor seizures, with mild hemiparesis, widespread cognitive deficits, and a progressive course.[3206]

cortical electrode An electrode applied directly upon or inserted within the cerebral cortex.

cortical function 1. "The whole cortex . . . has no other function but to select, abstract, differentiate, integrate and condense rhythms or patterns of nervous activity (to provide) . . . the basis for the comparison of sensory relationships; for recognition, or memory; for symbols which with notions of space, time direction and many other ideas have enabled man to create calculating machines, symphonies and poems." Dr. William Gooddy (1954).[2188] 2. Those endowments which preferentially serve instrumental functions, such as language, perception, memory, and calculation. Dysfunction thus leads to aphasias, agnosias, acalculia, and amnesia.

cortical mantle The cerebral cortex, so named in appreciation of its position as a covering for the entire brain in the supratentorial compartment.

cortical motor aphasia See **Broca aphasia.**

cortical myoclonus (focal cortical myoclonus, cortical reflex myoclonus) A form of **stimulus-sensitive myoclonus** (the other form being subcortical or reticular) seen in **progressive myoclonic epilepsy, (Unverricht-Lundborg-)Lafora body disease,** lipidoses, and postanoxic states, and also in **Alzheimer** and **Creutzfeldt-Jakob** diseases.

The movement can be considered as a fragment of partial epilepsy in which each myoclonic jerk typically involves only a few adjacent, usually distal, muscles, although many different areas may be involved. Triggers are sensory stimulation or voluntary limb movements. The somatosensory cortex is the likely site of the discharges. The cortical events recorded by EEG are time locked to the jerks, which occur spontaneously or in response to somatosensory stimulation (**reflex myoclonus**) or to voluntary movement (**action myoclonus**).[2384]

In this condition, somatosensory evoked potentials are typically of unusually high amplitude, suggesting pathological hyperexcitabilty of the motor cortex. See also **reticular reflex myoclonus, primary generalized epileptic myoclonus, myoclonus.**

cortical nodules Projections of the pial surface of the brain into the subarachnoid space as a result of cortical dysgenesis.

cortical paralysis of visual fixation See **Balint syndrome.**

cortical receptive aphasia See **Wernicke aphasia.**

cortical reflex myoclonus Generalized myoclonus occuring in response to low-frequency photic stimulation, with an accompanying frontal spike discharge. The condition may complicate numerous diseases affecting the gray matter. See **photomyogenic response.**

cortical sensation Three classes of sensation were defined by **Head;**

1. Recognition of spatial relations, such as the recognition of passive movements, two-point discrimination, or "spot-finding" (topical localization);

2. A graduated response to stimuli of different intensity; and

3. Appreciation of similarity and difference in external objects, brought into contact with the surface of the body—thus appreciation of size, shape, weight, and texture.

He also noted that diminution of sensitivity to pinprick and vibration may result from cortical lesions but to much less extent, and hypotonia is another association. Representation of different areas is separate, so one finger may be affected while another is spared. The palm and sole have the greatest representational areas, "so a cortical lesion may disturb the sensibility of the hand and foot without of necessity affecting the elbow, shoulder or knee."[2494]

cortical sensory aphasia See **Wernicke aphasia, aphasia.**

cortical sensory loss Impairment of the senses of tactile localization; graphesthesia; appreciation of size, shape, weight, or texture; and bilateral simultaneous tactile stimulation.

cortical sensory syndrome An isolated loss of discriminative sensation involving one of two parts of the body, and occurring with infarcts of the superior–posterior parts of a parietal lobe.[383] See also **parietal stroke.**

cortical spreading depression (of Leao) A transient, slowly moving suppression of electrical activity which propagates across (and remains confined to) the cortex at 2–5 mm/min, accompanied by a disruption of ion homeostasis, depolarization of nerve cells, and increased energy metabolism. The depression seldom moves further forward than the central sulcus.

The role of this phenomenon is uncertain, but it has been suggested that the changes in cerebral blood flow in patients with migraine attacks resemble those in animals during the occurrence of spreading depression.[3292]

cortical tremor A variant of cortical reflex myoclonus resembling intractable **essential tremor** and characterized by the electrophysiological findings of cortical reflex myoclonus in which rhythmic but unsynchronized involuntary movements occur distally, particularly in the outstretched hands, and during activity.

The brief movements are accompanied by EMG bursts lasting about 50 msec which result in a fine, shivering-like finger twitching, provoked mainly by action and posture. Giant somatosensory evoked potentials with enhanced long-loop reflexes and pre-movement cortical spikes are the electrical concomitants of the abnormal movement disorder.[2726]

cortical thumb The adducted and flexed position of the thumb, often covered by the flexed fingers, adopted by infants or children with hemiparesis in whom there is always a parietal lobe lesion. See also **fisting, dystonic toe.**

cortical word deafness See **pure word deafness.**

cortical-basal ganglionic degeneration   See **corti-cobasal degeneration.**

corticectomy   The removal of the cortex of a small or large area, usually performed in patients with intractable seizure disorders due to neuronal migration disorders or severe ischemic injury of the cortex.

corticobasal degeneration   (cortical-basal ganglionic degeneration, corticodentatonigral degeneration with neuronal achromasia, Rebeitz-Kolodny-Richardson syndrome) A rare, slowly progressive degenerative tauopathy of unknown cause affecting older adults who present with dementia, slowness, and awkwardness of movements, (limb ideomotor apraxia), superimposed involuntary movements, unilateral parkinsonism (tremor and rigidity) unresponsive to levadopa, and pyramidal signs. The disorder tends to be gradually progressive, the gait disturbances, cortical sensory loss, and stimulus sensitive myoclonus resulting in a "jerky useless hand." Frontal release signs, disturbed balance and gait, progressive external ophthalmoplegia, **alien limb** phenomena, dysphagia, chorea, postural action tremor, fixed limb dystonias, and cortical sensory loss are other features. Cognitive disturbances due to degeneration of the cortical, striatal, and nigral neuronal pathways are also reported later in the course of the disease. The condition leads to death within about 10 years of onset.

The best predictors for the diagnosis have been identified as limb dystonia, ideomotor apraxia, myoclonus, and an asymmetric akinetic-rigid syndrome with the late onset of gait or balance disturbances.[3439] However, there is important clinical (and some genetic) overlap with **primary progressive aphasia** and frontotemporal dementia,[3022] as well as with **progressive supranuclear palsy,** with which this condition shares a common **tau** haplotype.

Neuronal achromasia (swelling of the cell body and resistance to stains), gliosis, and asymmetric degeneration of the frontoparietal cortex and of the striatal and nigral neuronal pathways are notable pathological features.[4617] Pathological criteria for diagnosis have been suggested:[3490]

Cortical degeneration with swollen neurones
Neuronal loss in the substantia nigra (pars compacta) with corticobasal inclusions
Variable involvement of subcortical structures
Extensive neuronal and glial tau immunodeposits.

corticodentatonigral degeneration with neuronal achromasia   See **corticobasal degeneration.**

corticogram   See **electrocorticogram.**

corticography   See **electrocorticography.**

corticoid areas   Parts of the basal forebrain (the septal region, the substantia innominata and part of the amygdaloid complex) which form part of the limbic system. The structures are part of the cortical mantle but their organization is rudimentary.[3851]

corticomeningeal diffuse angiomatosis   See **Van Bogaert syndrome.**

corticopallido(or striato)spinal degeneration   See **Creutzfeldt-Jakob disease.**

corticospinal tract   See **pyramidal tract.**

corticosteroid myopathy   A syndrome of proximal muscle weakness and wasting preferentially affecting the legs. Type II fiber atrophy is the characteristic finding on muscle biopsy. Serum creatine kinase levels are usually at the lower end of the normal range and the EMG is normal or mildly myopathic.[3029]

corticotrophin releasing factor   A peptide secreted by the hypothalamus also inhibitory of the release from that site of gonadotrophic-releasing hormones.

costal arch reflex   See **abdominal reflex.**

costal margin reflex   See **abdominal reflex.**

costal periosteal reflex   See **abdominal reflex.**

costal reflex   (costo-abdominal reflex, costal arch reflex, costal periosteal reflex, costal margin reflex) The **abdominal reflex** obtained by tapping the costal margin medial to the nipple line. The reflex is mediated by cord segments T5–T9.

costalgia   Intercostal neuralgia.

Costen, James Bray   (1895–1962) American otolaryngologist practicing in St. Louis.

Costen syndrome   The association of dull pain in the ear and the region of the temporomandibular joint, with burning in the nose, throat, and tongue, as well as vertical and occipital headache, persistent hearing disorders, tinnitus, vertigo, nystagmus, dryness of the mouth, stuffy ears, reduced mandibular movements, and clicking or snapping of the temporomandibular joint due to overbite (abnormal closure of the mouth with the lower teeth nestling inside those of the upper jaw). Costen considered that the mandibular joint pathology (posterior condylar displacement) was entirely responsible, but it is now thought to be due to occlusal dysfunction of the joint and/or spasm of the masticatory muscles.[1140]

Although such pain felt as a result of misalignment of the temporomandibular joint or overactivity of the temporalis or masseter muscles (or both) is an entity with high face validity, the putative cause has never been proved.

costoabdominal reflex   See **abdominal reflex.**

costoclavicular syndrome   See **thoracic outlet syndrome.**

Cotard syndrome   (*délire de negations*) Paranoia, nihilistic delusions, suicidal ideation, and sensory disturbances, described first by Jules Cotard, a French psychiatrist, in 1880. The syndrome probably represents the occurrence of somatic dysesthesias in psychotically depressed patients. The classic complaint of subjects is that they are dead.[6086] For an account of the accomplished but unhappy life of Jules Cotard, see Pearn J. et al. *Neurology* 2002;**58**:1400–3.

Coté-Katsantoni syndrome   See **Katsantoni syndrome.**

cotton wool spots   1. (cytoid bodies) Aggregates composed of the swollen ends of disrupted retinal nerve fibers, occurring as a result of ischemia and healing with the formation of a glial scar.

2. Infarcts of the retinal nerve fiber layer, typically seen with fully developed **papilledema.**

Cotugno disease   See **sciatica.**

Cotugno, Domenico Felice Antonio   (1736–1822) Neapolitan surgeon, professor at Naples, who described the skin lesions of smallpox, the gut lesions of typhoid, the cerebrospinal and the labyrinthine fluids, and the anatomy of the inner ear (100 years before Helmholtz); he also demonstrated albuminuria, and wrote on sciatica and nephritis in his book *De ischiade Nervosa Commentarius,* published in 1764.

Domenico Felice Antonio Cotugno

cough headache   An uncommon syndrome of brief, severe pain in the head precipitated by coughing or by other maneuvers that raise intracranial pressure, mainly affecting middle-aged men with no organic intracranial lesion.[5458,5459] The headaches disappear after months or years without residua. Most patients are pain-free between attacks of head pain but in some cases the paroxysms are followed by dull, aching pain that may persist for hours. Since brain tumor and the Chiari malformation cause similar symptoms, it has been recommended that magnetic resonance imaging of the head

should be obtained in all cases.[4603] The character of the headache is the same regardless of whether there is an intracranial lesion.

cough syncope   (vertige larynge of Charcot, Charcot vertigo, laryngeal epilepsy, respiratory syncope, post-tussive syndrome, laryngeal vertigo) Dizziness or actual loss of consciousness, sometimes with convulsive movements, occurring in plethoric, bronchitic middle-aged men after coughing, and in others after, for example, trumpet-playing. The cough has been regarded as an aura and the whole condition is thus considered to represent a form of **complex partial seizure,**[5952] although increased intrathoracic pressure and thus decreased venous return and decreased cardiac output are at first sight an obvious cause. Increased CSF pressure and induced cardiac arrhythmias may also be incriminated.[3014]

The term was applied by Liveing to a condition in which patients awaken from sleep, clutch at their neck, and struggle for breath, the attack subsiding in a few minutes.

counter-pressure   See **geste antagonistique.**

counterrotation   A noticeable circular movement of the eyeballs in the opposite direction when the head is tilted from the upright position towards one shoulder. The movement is in the opposite direction and is maximal with the first 20° of tilt.

coup de la chaleur   See **heat stroke.**

coup lesion   The traumatic brain injury (contusion or laceration) directly beneath the point of impact.

coupled discharge   See **satellite potential.**

Courtois, Adolphe   (1903–1935) French psychiatrist who trained in Paris and after graduation worked for Guillain before his appointment as physician to a Parisian mental hospital.

Courtois sign   Flexion of the head on the chest in a comatose patient with a lateralized intracranial lesion producing flexion of only the healthy leg.[1145]

Courville, Cyril   (1900–1968) American neurologist and neuropathologist who trained with **Cushing** and **Bailey** before concentrating on neurology and neuropathology at the Loma Linda University School of Medicine. His most lasting works dealt with cerebral palsy, perinatal brain injuries, and cerebral tumors.[7]

Couvade syndrome   (Fr, to hatch) (married man's toothache) A psychogenic disorder characterized by the occurrence of the symptoms of pregnancy in the husband during the pregnancy of the wife. Nausea, abdominal pain, bulimia or loss of appetite, toothache, and abdominal bloating are typical symptoms.[5632]

The condition was first recorded by Francis Bacon in 1627.

cover test   1. A test of paretic ocular muscles in which the paretic (nonfixating) eye is covered first; the nonparetic eye will not move, nor does it move when the cover is taken away. When the nonparetic eye is covered, the paretic eye deviates in order to attempt fixation, and the nonparetic eye deviates excessively in the same direction (**secondary deviation**). When the cover is taken away, either the normal eye takes up fixation again or the abnormal one retains fixation and the normal eye remains in deviation—if the patient is an **alternate fixator.**[3330]

2. (*alternate cover test*) A test of paretic ocular muscles in which each of the two eyes is covered alternately every second or two, while the subject fixates on an object. The fixating eye will be positioned so that the light from the target falls on the fovea, but the occluded eye may deviate (**primary deviation**), now that it has lost its continuing stimulus to retain parallelism of the ocular axes, if it is subject to strabismus.

When the normal eye is covered and the eye with defective muscle balance fixates on the object, the normal eye will deviate, this time in a direction opposite to that of the paretic eye (**secondary deviation**).

covert dyskinesia Abnormal involuntary movements (**tardive dyskinesia**) which only appear when the dose of the causal drug is reduced or when it is no longer taken.

Cowden disease   See **Lhermitte-Duclos disease.**

COWS The mnemonic for the direction of the normal nystagmoid response to irrigation of the external auditory meatus with water: **C**old **O**pposite, **W**arm **S**ame. Thus, irrigation of the left ear with ice-cold water leads to nystagmus with its fast component to the right. The important ocular movement, the slow deviation is, of course, in the *opposite* direction to that of the nystagmus.

crack dancing Choreoathetosis, akathisia, and parkinsonism with tremor, associated with the repetitive use of the freebase form of cocaine as a recreational drug.[1281]

cracked-pot note (bruit de pot fêlé) The off-key sound heard when the skull of an hydrocephalic child is percussed. It is not a sign of fracture of the cranial vault, but rather of the separation of the sutures in hydrocephalus. Exactly the same sign occurs in cavitating lung disease, such as abscess or tuberculosis, when the cavity contains both air and fluid, and it is also elicited over the chests of crying children. The Scottish surgeon Sir William MacEwen (1848–1924) described it first in 1893.[3548]

Cram test   See **bowstring sign.**

cramp 1. Sudden involuntary, painful shortening of muscle with abrupt onset, attended by visible or palpable knotting of muscle and often leading to abnormal posture of the affected joints.[4826] 2. A painful muscle contraction with an accompanying EMG discharge comprising irregular high-frequency bursts of motor

unit potentials with gradual onset and termination. See also **cramps.**

cramp discharge Involuntary repetitive firing of motor unit action potentials at a high frequency (up to 150 Hz) in a large area of a muscle usually associated with painful muscle contraction. Both discharge frequency and number of motor unit action potentials activated increase gradually during development, and both subside gradually with cessation. See muscle **cramp.** (From the 2001 Report of the Nomenclature Committee of the American Association of Electromyography and Electrodiagnosis.[10] Used by permission, copyright © 2001, AAEM.)

cramp-fasciculation syndrome (**muscle-pain fasciculation syndrome,** benign motor neuron disorder) An acquired syndrome characterized by the sudden onset of muscle aching, cramps, stiffness, limb muscle fasciculations or myokymia, and exercise intolerance without clinical muscle atrophy or weakness, in otherwise healthy adults, due to abnormal excitation of the distal motor axon. Muscle biopsy specimens may show neurogenic changes. Muscle biopsy is normal or shows mild neurogenic changes. The EMG does not show continuous muscle fiber activity as in **Isaacs syndrome,** but showers of afterdischarges are recorded following motor nerve stimulation, as in the latter condition.[260,5467]

cramps (ordinary muscle cramps) Sudden, severe, painful, palpable, involuntary contraction of muscles, most commonly experienced in the calves by elderly people during the night but potentially occurring in any healthy muscle when it is contracted voluntarily for extended periods. They may be relieved by passive stretching.

Cramps typically affect a single muscle, and are thought to follow and spread out from a zone of repetitive fasciculations arising from nerve terminals in that muscle. They are followed by further fasciculations.[3302] Their biochemical basis is uncertain, but dehydration, hemodialysis, hyponatremia, hypomagnesemia, hypocalcemia, dysthyroid states, adrenal insufficiency, and pregnancy are known to be associated, as are all forms of motor neuropathy. Treatment with phenytoin, quinine, or calcium salts is highly effective though seldom prescribed, which is ironic when one considers that therapy for many other neurological conditions is not available.

A *variant condition* is *adolescent familial cramps,* a benign X-linked muscular dystrophy presenting with exercise-induced cramps.[2424] See also **electrically silent cramps.**

cramps, occupational   See **dystonia.**

crampus syndrome The repeated occurrence of cramps without any evidence of neurological or biochemical abnormality.[4826]

Crandall syndrome The association of sensorineural deafness, pili torti, hypogonadism, and alopecia.[1156]

Crane syndrome   (clefting with skeletal anomalies) A congenital dysmorphic syndrome characterized by low birth weight, hypertelorism, micrognathia, cleft upper lip and palate, segmentation defects of the spine, absent or hypoplastic clavicles, syndactyly, club foot, undermineralization of the skull, hydrocephalus, and callosal agenesis.[337]

cranial   (from Gr, the skull). Pertaining to the skull.

cranial aerocele   See **pneumocephalus.**

cranial arteritis   See **giant cell arteritis.**

cranial dystonias   (Brueghel syndrome, Meige syndrome, idiopathic orofacial dystonia, spasme faciale mediane) Dystonias of adult life characterized by prolonged symmetrical contractions of the orofacial musculature with the production of any combination of **blepharospasm, oromandibular dystonias,** and **laryngeal** or **pharyngeal dystonias** often disabling the patient.

The first account of this disorder was that of Henri Meige in 1910, who noted that the blepharospasm was worsened by stress and certain patterns of activity, and disappeared in sleep. Extension to other muscle groups and clinical depressive illness are also common findings in such patients. Familial occurrence of the condition has been recorded.[5601] See **Meige syndrome.** In **Brueghel syndrome** the classic abnormality is wide opening of the mouth rather than blepharospasm.

cranial lacunae (Lückenschadel)   Radiolucent defects seen on plain X-ray studies of the skulls of neonates evidencing a bony dysplasia, but of no significance in diagnosis.[1874]

cranial meningocele   A developmental anomaly characterized by extracranial herniation of the meninges through a cranial defect.

cranial metaphyseal dysplasia   A rare hereditary disorder of bone absorption or remodeling in which hyperostosis and sclerosis of the skull and facial bones cause narrowing of the cranial foramina, which may lead to cranial nerve palsies, especially of the seventh cranial nerve, and which has also been associated with seizures or long tract signs.[4916]

cranial nerves   Those nerves issuing from the skull and emanating from the brain or brainstem.

The number of cranial nerves has never been resolved satisfactorily. **Galen** described 11 pairs, ignoring the first, which was included, however, by **Vesalius.** In 1684 **Willis** described nine pairs, the first six as they are known today, the seventh and eighth together next as the seventh, the next three included by him as the eighth, and the hypoglossal nerve as the ninth. In 1942 Lensell named 16 pairs.

The fact that the first and second are actually clothed not with Schwann cells but with oligodendroglia would merit their classification as central rather than periph-

eral nervous system structures, but today we regard 12 as the correct number, as suggested by **Soemerring.**

cranial neuralgias   Painful states affecting the head as a result of disease usually affecting the fifth, seventh, or ninth/tenth cranial nerve complex. A classification has been proposed by the International Headache Society (see Chart C–26). The individual conditions are entered separately.

Chart C–26. Cranial Neuralgias, Nerve Trunk Pain, and Deafferentation Pain

12.1	Persistent (in contrast to tic-like) pain of cranial nerve origin
	12.1.1 Compression or distortion of cranial nerves and C2.3 roots
	12.1.2 Demyelination of cranial nerves
	12.1.2.1 **Optic neuritis** (retrobulbar neuritis)
	12.1.3 Infarction of cranial nerves
	12.1.3.1 Diabetic neuritis
	12.1.4 Inflammation of cranial nerves
	12.1.4.1 Herpes zoster
	12.1.4.2 Chronic post-herpetic neuralgia
	12.1.5 **Tolosa-Hunt syndrome**
	12.1.6 **Neck-tongue syndrome**
12.1.7	Other causes of persistent pain of cranial nerve origin
12.2	**Trigeminal neuralgia**
	12.2.1 Idiopathic trigeminal neuralgia
	12.2.2 Symptomatic trigeminal neuralgia
	12.2.2.1 Compression of trigeminal root or ganglion
	12.2.2.2 Central lesions
12.3	**Glossopharyngeal neuralgia**
	12.3.1 Idiopathic glossopharyngeal neuralgia
	12.3.2 Symptomatic glossopharyngeal neuralgia
12.4	Nervus intermedius neuralgia
12.5	**Superior laryngeal neuralgia**
12.6	Occipital neuralgia
12.7	Central causes of head and facial pain other than tic douloureux
	12.7.1 **Anesthesia dolorosa**
	12.7.2 Thalamic pain
12.8	Facial pain not fulfilling criteria in groups 11 or 12.

Adapted from Classification of headache disorders, cranial neuralgias and facial pains; and diagnostic criteria for primary headache disorders. Cephalalgia 1988;8(suppl):1–96,[1051] by kind permission.

cranial neuropathies   Disorders that selectively or predominantly involve the cranial nerves, usually the fifth and seventh and less commonly the bulbar (IX–XII) nerves. Autoimmune disease and mitotic lesions are the most common causes.

cranial synostosis and fibular aplasia   See **Lowry syndrome.**

craniocarpotarsal dysplasia   See **whistling face syndrome.**

craniocerebral trauma   Syndromes resulting directly or indirectly from head injury.[415] These include **concussion,** contusion and laceration of the brain, **epidural (extradural) hemorrhage, subdural hemor-**

rhage and **intracerebral hemorrhage,** skull fracture, **CSF rhinorrhea,** and **postconcussional syndromes.**

The severity of the lesions suffered has been graded on CT scans[3651] as follows:

Craniocerebral trauma severity score

Diffuse injury 1. No visible intracranial pathology

Diffuse injury 2. Cisterns present; shift of 0.5 mm and/or lesion densities present; no high- or mixed-density lesion >25 ml; may include bone fragments and foreign bodies

Diffuse injury 3. Cisterns compressed or absent; shift 0–5 mm; no high or mixed-density lesion >25 ml

Diffuse injury 4. Shift >5 mm; no high- or mixed-density lesion >25 ml

Evacuated mass lesion

Non-evacuated mass lesion High- or mixed-density lesion >25 ml; not surgically evacuated

From Marshall LF, Marshall LB, Klauber MR, et al. The diagnosis of head injury requires a classification based on computed axial tomography. J Neurotrauma 1992;9 Suppl.1:S287–S292. Reprinted by permission.

Trauma severity scores[3097] and prognostic scales[2845,4596,5515,6073] have also been created. See **coma, coma scales.**

craniocervical dystonia   That form of **dystonia** in which the muscles of the head and neck are involved, in the former case producing **oromandibular dystonias** and in the latter, **torticollis, retrocollis,** etc.

craniocervical malformation   A congenital syndrome characterized by the presence of a short neck with combinations of cerebellar and pyramidal signs. See **Chiari malformation.**

craniocleidodysostosis   (craniocleidal dysplasia) A dominantly inherited syndrome, characterized by aplasia or hypoplasia of both clavicles with variability in the size of the attached muscles; facial dysmorphisms with frontal bossing, saddle nose, and delayed ossification of the fontanelles; an abnormally wide cranium with brachycephaly; kyphoscoliosis; lax joints; and occasionally paraparesis or hemiparesis.[3036]

Syringomyelia, callosal agenesis, spinal dysraphism, and cervical ribs occasionally complicate the primary features. The condition was first described by Pierre **Marie.**[2219]

craniocleidal dysplasia   See **craniocleidodysostosis.**

craniodiaphyseal dysplasia   A group of diseases within the spectrum of craniotubular dysplasias and including at least the following:

1. A severe recessively inherited bone disorder characterized by massive generalized hyperostosis and sclerosis, especially involving the skull and facial bones, with mental and growth retardation, seizures, visual failure, and deafness.[2219]
2. A dominantly inherited syndrome manifesting hypertrophy of the membrane bones of the face and skull, leading to severe dysmorphism and to second and eighth cranial nerve palsies. Macpherson delineates a spectrum running from metaphyseal dysplasia through craniometaphyseal

dysplasia and leontiasis ossea to craniodiaphyseal dysplasia and progressive diaphyseal dysplasia.[3559]

craniodigital syndrome   The coexistence of mental and growth retardation, unusual facies, syndactyly, mild brachycephaly, and abnormal palmar dermatoglyphics. See also **Saethre-Chotzen syndrome.**[5032]

craniofacial dysostosis   A congenital, dominantly inherited, dysmorphic syndrome characterized by prominent frontal bossing, absent auditory canals, hypertelorism, prominent eyes, strabismus, parrot-beaked profile of the nose, hypoplastic facial bones, high palate, oligodontia and brachycephaly, ossicle malformations and a mixed hearing loss, dwarfism, optic atrophy, micrognathia, nystagmus, hydrocephalus, craniosynostosis involving multiple sutures, callosal agenesis, and mental and developmental delay.[2214] See **Crouzon syndrome.**

craniofacial malformations   Disorders of maturation characterized by abnormalities of body modeling and frequently with associated neurological defects. A classification has been achieved[4] (see Chart C–27).

Chart C–27. Craniofacial Malformations

1. Cerebrocranial dysplasias
   Anencephaly, microcephaly
2. Cerebrofacial dysplasias
   Rhinencephalic dysplasias
   Oculo-orbital dysplasias (anophthalmia)
3. Craniofacial dysplasias
   a. With clefting
   b. With dysostosis
   c. With synostosis
      Craniosynostosis
      Craniofaciosynostosis
      Faciosynostosis
   d. With dysostosis and synostosis
      Crouzon syndrome
      Acrocephalosyndactyly (Apert syndrome)
      Cloverleaf skull
4. Craniofacial dysplasias with other origin
   a. Osseous
   b. Cutaneous
   c. Neurocutaneous (**neurofibromatosis**)
   d. Neuromuscular (Robin syndrome, **Möbius syndrome**)
   e. Muscular (glossoschizis)
   f. Vascular (hemangioma, hemolymphangioma, lymphangioma)

Adapted from Stricker et al. (1990).[4] Reprinted from Stricker et al. Craniofacial Malformations. Edinburgh: Churchill, 1990, by kind permission.

craniofrontonasal dysplasia   A congenital dysmorphic syndrome characterized also by strabismus, syndactyly, broad hallux, sandal gap between the toes, and craniosynostosis with brachycephaly and hypertelorism.[4]

craniohypophysial xanthomatosis   See **generalized xanthomatosis, Hand-Schüller-Christian disease.**

craniology   The study of the comparative sizes and proportions of skulls.

craniometaphyseal dysplasia   A dominantly or recessively inherited congenital dysmorphic syndrome characterized also by prominent eyes, thick calvarium, sclerosis of the skull with underdevelopment of sinuses, osteosclerosis or osteopetrosis and metaphyseal splaying of the long bones, and skull abnormalities leading to headache and cranial nerve palsies (particularly deafness).[2219,4916,5020]

Pyle disease is similar but lacks the orofacial involvement.

craniopathy   Disease of the cranium.

craniopharyngioma   Cystic or solid, benign, multi-loculated tumors arising from the embryonic pouch of Rathke above the sella turcica, composed of sheets of squamous cells with calcification, keratin pearls, and granulomas, and containing glairy "machine-oil" fluid full of cholesterol crystals. They are prone to recurrence after removal.[6] The tumor arises from embryonic squamous cell rests in the site of the obliterated craniopharyngeal duct.

Clinically, craniopharyngiomas present most often in childhood with growth failure or complaints of headache and other evidence of raised intracranial pressure, chiasmal compression, hypopituitarism, or alterations in mental status; in adults, sexual dysfunction, visual deficits, and a syndrome of progressive dementia are the usual symptoms. See also **suprasellar cysts.**

cranioschisis   A severe and potentially lethal developmental defect due to failure of the cranial portion of the neural tube to close. In its most severe form (*cranioschisis aperta with encephaloschisis,* **anencephaly**), there is an absence of the cranial vault and of the cerebral cortex, the basal ganglia forming the most cephalad portion of the nervous system. In *cranioschisis occulta with encephalocele,* the brain herniates through a relatively small defect in the skull.[3624]

cranioscopy   Franz **Gall's** preferred name for **phrenology.**

craniostenosis   See **craniosynostosis.**

craniosynostosis   (craniostenosis) The result of premature fusion of one or more cranial sutures in infancy, leading to a reduction in the volume of the cranium and to diffuse encephalopathies as a consequence of the pressure on the brain.[1088] See Chart C–28.

The sagittal suture is affected most often; the lambdoid, metopic, or coronal sutures less commonly. Characteristic deformities of the skull (**turricephaly, brachycephaly, oxycephaly, pachycephaly**) result and may require early surgical correction, either for cosmetic reasons or because of increased intracranial pressure. The forms of craniosynostosis were first classified by **Virchow** in 1851; he also coined this term and brachycephaly, dolichocephaly, scaphocephaly, and macro- and microcephaly. A newer classification is that of Jacobson.[2787] The condition is not new, having been recorded in the time of the Egyptian pharaohs.[5245]

See also the syndromes of **Apert, Berant, Crouzon, Christian, Carpenter, Pfeiffer,** and **Saethre-Chotzen,** and the **kleeblattschadel anomaly** as well as the following *variants* listed in Chart C–28. See also **Adelaide** and **Boston craniosynostosis, Jackson-Weiss syndrome, Greig syndrome, thanatophoric dysplasia,** and the Web site http://www.ninds.nih.gov/health_and_medical/disorders/craniosytosis_doc.htm.

Chart C–28. Variant Forms of Craniosynostosis

Armendares syndrome[216]

Baller-Gerold syndrome (craniosynostosis and radial aplasia) A recessively inherited congenital syndrome characterized by craniosynostosis and radial aplasia.[309]

Berant syndrome.[480]

Christian syndrome

Complicated acrocephalopolysyndactyly (**Sakati-Nyhan-Tisdale syndrome**) A rare syndrome manifesting polydactyly, premature fusion of all cranial sutures with **acrocephaly,** giantism, and dysmorphism.[4882]

Craniosynostosis, arthrogryposis, and cleft palate syndrome (Christian-Andrews-Conneally-Molar syndrome) A recessively inherited congenital syndrome characterized by craniosynostosis, microcephaly, hypertelorism, antimongoloid slant of the eyes, ophthalmoplegia, and facial dysmorphisms.[1028]

Craniosynostosis, brachydactyly, symphalangism, strabismus, hip osteochondritis, and carpotarsal fusion A rare, probably dominantly inherited syndrome manifesting these features[5747]

Craniosynostosis with 7p-karyotype[2219]

Craniosynostosis with foot anomalies[5903]

Fairbank syndrome

Gorlin-Chaudhry-Moss syndrome A syndrome consisting of dysmorphism with craniosynostosis, facial dysostosis, translucent teeth, congenital cardiac defects, and defective upper eyelids.[2214]

Herrmann-Pallister-Opitz syndrome (craniosynostosis, brachysyndactyly of hands and absence of toes, Herrmann syndrome 1) A sporadic congenital malformation syndrome characterized by facial dysmorphisms including cleft lip or palate, craniosynostosis affecting the coronal suture, hypertelorism, brachysyndactyly of the hands, and absence of some toes. Mental retardation and growth failure are also present.[2553]

Lowry syndrome 1. Premature fusion of the coronal sutures with cryptorchidism.[3495] 2. craniosynostosis and fibular aplasia (Lowry syndrome) A recessively inherited congenital syndrome characterized by these two features.[3495]

Sensenbrenner syndrome A rare syndrome manifesting premature fusion of cranial sutures with **dolichocephaly,** fine hair, impaired tooth formation, and brachydactyly.[3373]

Summitt syndrome A syndrome consisting of craniosynostosis, obesity, strabismus, and syndactyly.[5414]

Woon syndrome The congenital combination of craniosynostosis and absence of the thumbs.

craniosynostosis and fibular aplasia (Lowry syndrome)
A recessively inherited congenital syndrome characterized by synostosis and bilateral fibular aplasia.[3495]

craniosynostosis and radial aplasia (Baller-Gerold syndrome) A recessively inherited congenital syndrome characterized by these two features.[309]

craniosynostosis, severe symmetrically deformed extremities, and cleft lip-palate syndrome See **craniosynostosis.**

craniosynostosis with foot anomalies See **craniosynostosis.**

craniosynostosis with 7p-karyotype See **craniosynostosis.**

craniotabes (congenital cranial osteoporosis) Softening of the infantile skull in parasagittal, parietal, and vertical regions, considered to be caused by prolonged compression of the skull in utero. The condition is common, harmless, and temporary.

craniotelencephalic dysplasia A congenital dysmorphic syndrome characterized also by prominent frontal bossing, microphthalmia, hypoplasia of the optic nerves, trigonocephaly, craniosynostosis, encephalocele, hydrocephalus from aqueduct stenosis, lissencephaly, cerebellar atrophy, agenesis of the corpus callosum, and mental and developmental delay.[337]

craniotubular dysplasias Genetic hyperostotic and osteosclerotic disorders stemming from a defect in bone modeling[2216,3593] with secondary effects upon the nervous system.

craniotubular hyperostoses Genetic hyperostotic and osteosclerotic disorders stemming from an active overgrowth of bone, and including **Camurati-Engelmann disease.**[3593]

craniovertebral anomalies (craniovertebral malformations) Congenitally determined abnormalities of the skull base and upper cervical spine. These include basilar impression, platybasia, occipitalization of the atlas, fusion of cervical vertebrae, and chronic atlantoaxial dislocation. They are common in patients with syringomyelia and cerebellar ectopias but, in other instances, may be asymptomatic or associated with postural loss in the arms, mirror movements, and vertical nystagmus with oscillopsia.[328]

craniovertebral malformations See **craniovertebral anomalies.**

cranium The membrane bones of the skull; all the skull bones above the skull base.

cranium bifidum A failure of fusion of the posterior midline portion of the skull, so that a bony cleft remains through which the brain may extrude (encephalocele).

crash migraine See **thunderclap headache.**

creatine A muscle protein isolated in 1832 by Michel Chevreuil, a French chemist.

creatine kinase (CK) An enzyme catalyzing the reversible reaction: ATP + creatine = ADP + phospho-

creatine, and thus responsible for energy production within muscle. Elevation of its levels in serum is a reliable indicator of damage to muscle membranes resulting from any cause.[4408]

Cree encephalitis A familial disease, possibly a viral infection, manifesting with severe mental retardation from birth, microcephaly, cerebral atrophy with white matter changes of panencephalitis with calcifications, and systemic immunological abnormalities (polyclonal hypergammaglobulinemia) leading to recurrent infections.[594]

Cree leukoencephalopathy A syndrome with neonatal onset described in Cree Indian children in Quebec, and characterized by seizures, pyramidal signs, and mental and developmental delay associated with abnormal CNS myelination.[593]

Cree microcephaly with micromelia A congenital dysmorphic syndrome characterized by low birth weight, mesomelia of upper limbs, synostosis of the elbows, hypoplastic or absent radii and ulnae, absent fingers, and microcephaly.[2761]

creeping palsy See **amyotrophic lateral sclerosis.**

cremasteric reflex Contraction of the cremaster muscle with elevation of the homolateral testicle, in response to a scratch on the inside of the thigh ascending from some 3 inches (7.5 cm) below the inguinal crease and resulting from contraction of the dartos muscles in the overlying skin.

   This superficial reflex is centered on L2 and may be lost in pyramidal tract lesions above that level, as shown by **Romberg** in 1853, as well as with scrotal pathology.

crescendo TIAs Repetitive ischemic attacks, most often due to hemodynamic phenomena in diseased small, penetrating vessels. When cerebral infarction develops, it is usually lacunar and involves a single penetrating vessel, although restricted to the region of the internal capsule. The clinical manifestations usually affect the face, arm, and leg.[1492] See also **capsular warning syndrome.**

cretinism Retardation in physical and mental development due to dysgenesis or inability to synthesize thyroid hormone in utero or in early life.

Creutzfeldt, Hans-Gerhardt (1885–1964) German neuropsychiatrist. He studied medicine at Jena, Rostock, and Kiel and then served as a ship's surgeon. On returning to Germany, he studied psychiatry in Kiel but spent years in practice in Munich and Berlin before returning to Kiel University as professor of psychiatry and neurology in 1938.

   In 1920[1162] he described one case of the disease bearing his name while working with Spielmeyer in Munich. His patient, a 23-year-old woman, manifested tics, myoclonus, focal seizures, and pyramidal tract signs progressively over 1 year; this patient had two siblings who were mentally retarded and the reliability of the diagnosis is open to question, unlike the three patients of Jakob described in the following year, whose features are more in keeping with current concepts of the disease.

Creutzfeldt also published on the psychoses, multiple sclerosis, encephalitis, toxic diseases, and radioactive studies in CNS disease.[3294]

Creutzfeldt-Jakob disease (Jakob-Creutzfeldt disease [CJD], spastic pseudosclerosis, corticopallidospinal degeneration, Heidenhain syndrome, subcaute cerebral degeneration, polio-encephalomyelopathy, subacute spongi-form encephalopathy, subacute presenile polio-encephalopathy, subacute presenile spongy atrophy, subacute degenerative polioencephalopathy of the presenium). A rare, progressive, and fatal spongiform encephalopathy due to infection by a virus particle (**prion**).[4532]

The American Psychiatric Association (DSM-IV TR)[150] suggested that the condition should be suspected in all cases of dementia that progress fairly rapidly over months to 1–2 years and that are accompanied or followed by multiple neurological symptoms and that the triad of rapidly progressing, devastating dementia; pyramidal and extrapyramidal disease with myoclonus; and that a characteristic (triphasic) EEG is highly suggestive.

There is usually progressive spastic paralysis of the limbs, accompanied by extrapyramidal signs with tremor, rigidity and choreoathetoid movements, but numerous phenotypes are recognized, varying with the size of the casual virus particle. In some cases, such as the "amyotrophic" form, the neurological signs may precede the onset of the dementia. Ataxia, visual failure, muscle fibrillations, and atrophy of the upper motor neuron type are also described.

Criteria for the diagnosis have been suggested; (Masters, Harris, et al. 1979) (See Chart C–29). 14-3-3 protein (a cell surface signalling protein) if present is a sensitive but not a specific marker for CJD; any neurological injury such as infarct, tremor, or infection can give a false positive result. The inclusion of this CSF protein in the criteria of Masters and colleagues (1979) improves the accuracy of clinical diagnosis. The presence of 14-3-3 protein in the CSF discriminates better between Creutzfeldt-Jakob disease and other rapidly progressive dementias than does the EEG pattern or the MRI.

Chart C–29. Suggested Criteria for the Diagnosis of Creutzfeldt-Jakob Disease

Diagnostic Criteria for Classical Creutzfeldt-Jakob Disease

A. Sporadic
  1. Definite
     Neuropathologically confirmed and/or
     Immunocytochemically confirmed PrP positive (Western blot) and/or
     SAF (scrapie-associated fibrils)
  2. Probable
     Progressive dementia

  Typical EEG
  At least two of the following clinical features:
     Myoclonus
     Visual or cerebellar signs
     Pyramidal/extrapyramidal signs
     Akinetic mutism
  3. Possible
     Progressive dementia
     Two of the clinical features listed above
     No EEC or atypical EEC
     Duration <2 years
B. Accidental transmission
   Progressive cerebellar syndrome in a pituitary hormone recipient
   Sporadic CJD with a recognized exposure risk
C. Familial
   Definite or probable CJD plus definite or probable CJD in a 1st degree relative.

From Masters CL, Harris JO, Gajusdek DC, et al. Creutzfeldt-Jakob Disease: Patterns of Worldwide Occurrence and the Significance of Familial and Sporadic Clustering. Ann. Neurol. 1979;5:177–88. Reproduced by kind permission.[3689]

Modified criteria are also presented, varying somewhat here from those of Brandel[718] and of Lanska.[718]
  Progressive dementia over <2 years
  At least two of the following:
     Myoclonus
     Visual or cerebellar signs
     Pyramidal or extrapyramidal signs
     Akinetic mutism
  At least one of the two following laboratory features:
     Periodic sharp- and slow-wave complexes on the EEG
     14-3-3 protein present in the CSF
  Pathological hallmarks are neuronal loss, spongy changes in the gray matter, and an astrocytic response.

This is possibly the same condition as the **Stern-Garcin syndrome,** a rapidly progressive dementing illness described first by Dr. K. Stern in a 41-year old patient admitted to the National Hospital under Dr. F.M.R. Walshe (and again by Raymond Garcin in 1962) with severe dementia and bilateral symmetrical degeneration of the thalamus.

Variant forms are described:
1. A form in which the cerebellar signs are preeminent initially[2184]
2. *Familial Creutzfeldt-Jakob disease*, occurring in about 10% of all cases (Baraitser[335] has summarized these reports.)
3. An *Amyotrophic form* presenting with signs of upper and lower motor neuron involvement with early and conspicuous dementia;[110]
4. Forms in which the duration of illness is greater than 2 years (less than 5% of all cases).
5. **New variant Creutzfeldt-Jakob disease**

cri du chat syndrome (Lejeune syndrome, cat cry syndrome) A syndrome of chromosomal dysgenesis (deletion of the short arm of chromosome 5) in which **hypertelorism,** microcephaly, severe mental and physical retardation, and facial dysmorphism are notable, and the child's cry is little more than a distant mew.[3335]

cri hydrencephalique   A brief, shrill wail intermittently uttered by children with hydrocephalus or meningitis, described first by Trousseau.[574]

cribriform   (Lat, like a sieve, perforated) The ethmoid bone with its many holes merits the description, however, no more than the anterior or posterior perforated substance.

cribriform state   A pathological finding, comprising dilatations of the perivascular spaces in the pallidum and putamen with smooth and clearly defined borders, containing one or more vessels which differentiates them from type 1 **lacunes,** which are cavitating infarcts. See also **état marbré.**

Crichton-Brown sign   Tremor of the labial folds and the outer angles of the eyes in **general paresis of the insane.**

Crichton-Brown, Sir James   (1840–1938) Scottish physician who inherited his father's interest in psychiatry and the care of the mentally ill. He was at some time a colleague of Hughlings-**Jackson** at the West Riding Asylum, of which he was superintendent from 1866, and he established the research laboratory at Wakefield, where **Ferrier** performed his early experiments in cerebral localization. He also founded the *West Riding Asylum Reports* (the first English psychiatric journal) in 1871, and with Jackson and others was a founder of **Brain** in 1878. He was elected a Fellow of the Royal Society in recognition of his work on mental disorders.

cricopharyngeal spasm   (pharyngisimus) Spasm of the pharyngeal constrictor muscles, as in **globus hystericus** and **rabies,** and as a result of local irritation. See **pharyngisimus.**

Crighton Royal Assessment Scale   A scale of use for the evaluation of patients whose mental deterioration makes clinical interviewing impossible.

It is also used widely by nonmedical staff for the day-to-day assessment of change in behavior of such patients when undergoing therapy. This scale combines simplicity of completion, high face validity, and interobserver reliability, but is, nevertheless, a relatively coarse measure of abilities.

Crigler-Najar kernicterus   A corencephalopathy associated with an inherited hyperbilirubinemic state. See **kernicterus.**

crises   Commonly applied to acute attacks of pain in certain regions, lasting hours or days in patients with tabes dorsalis. Gastric, rectal, nephralgic, clitoral, vesical, urethral, bronchial, and laryngeal crises were described by Gowers.[2240]

Crisponi syndrome   A lethal congenital syndrome characterized by contraction of the facial and neck muscles with opisthotonus, facial dysmorphism, camptodactyly, fever, and seizures, worsened by touching and with crying. See http://www.wustl.edu/neuromuscular.

cristae ampullaris   Plumes of hair cells on the sensory neuroepithelium located in the dilatations of the three semicircular canals.

Critchley, Macdonald   (1900–1997) Incisive, insightful English neurologist with eclectic interests in neurology and its wider aspects, but specializing in the assessment of cortical functioning. His book on the parietal lobes was a classic from the day of its publication. (Critchley M. The parietal lobes. London: Arnold, 1953.[1171])

critical flicker fusion   See **flicker fusion.**

critical illness myopathy   Type 2 muscle fiber atrophy, loss of myosin-containing fibers, and muscle fiber necrosis presenting as an acute or subacute myopathy with dissuse flacid weakness in severely ill patients in status asthmaticus, following transplants, or with sepsis, all usually requiring intensive care for multiple organ dysfunction. Muscle stretch reflexes are usually depressed. Steroids and perhaps neuromuscular blocking agents appear to be causally related.

Diagnostic criteria emphasizing the electrodiagnostic features for a probable diagnosis and requiring histopathologic identification of myosin loss (as well as supportive nonpathologic features) for a definite diagnosis have been suggested for research protocols.

Three varieties are differentiated: acute necrotizing myopathy; a myopathy with selective loss of myosin filaments presenting as above; and a non-necrotizing cachectic myopathy.[2699]

Suggested diagnostic criteria for critical illness myopathy are as follows. (After Lacomis D, Zochodne DW, Bird SJ. Critical illness myopathy. *Muscle Nerve* 2000;**23**:1785–8. Reproduced by permission.)[3219] The diagnosis of a "motor" variant of critical illness polyneuropathy should not be made without excluding myopathy with myosin loss histopathologically. Some patients may either be unable to recruit motor unit potentials or have a preexisting or coexisting polyneuropathy and still have a myopathy. Therefore, diagnosis of probable or possible critical illness myopathy should be allowed for, on the basis of a combination of major and supportive features even in the presence of low sensory nerve action potential (SNAP) amplitudes or an equivocal needle electrode examination. Direct needle stimulation of muscle may be added in the future as a major diagnostic feature and method of differentiating critical illness polyneuropathy from myopathy, perhaps even in place of histopathologic proof.

Proposed Major Diagnostic Features for Critical Illness Myopathy

1. SNAP amplitudes >80 of the lower limit of normal (LLN) in two or more nerves
2. Needle EMG with short-duration, low-amplitude MUPs with early or normal full recruitment, with or without fibrillation potentials
3. Absence of a decremental response on repetitive nerve stimulation

4. Muscle histopathologic findings of myopathy with myosin loss

Supportive Features

1. CMAP amplitudes <80 LLN in two or more nerves without conduction block
2. Elevated serum CK (best assessed in the first week of illness)
3. Demonstration of muscle inexcitability

By definition, patients are or were critically ill and weakness should have started after the onset of critical illness. For a definite diagnosis of critical illness myopathy, patients should have all four major features. For probable critical illness myopathy, patients should have any three major features and one or more supportive feature. For possible critical illness myopathy, patients should have either major features 1 and 3, or 2 and 3, and one or more supportive feature. One may consider muscle biopsy if another myopathic process such as an inflammatory myopathy is suspected or if the histologic findings may affect management.

See also **acute quadriplegic myopathy, critical illness polyneuropathy, Hopkins syndrome.**

critical illness polyneuropathy   A reversible, acute, or subacute generalized axonal sensorimotor peripheral neuropathy causing marked limb muscle weakness, wasting, and hyporeflexia, affecting also the respiratory muscles and occurring in patients with a systemic inflammatory response (septic syndrome) and multiple organ failure, including septic encephalopathy. The necessary inducing agent is unknown.[6133]

Difficulty in weaning from a ventilator, hyporeflexia, and distal weakness are the usual presenting features. The cranial nerves are relatively spared. Electromyelographic indicators of the condition include the presence of small polyphasic units with early full recruitment; reduced compound motor action potential amplitudes; variable fibrillations; and occasionally reduced sensory nerve action potentials or distal denervation suggesting chronic inflammatory demyelinating polyradioneuropathy or acquired sensorimotor axonal polyneuropathy.[3555]

The spectrum of neuromuscular disorders in such patients has been reviewed.[952,2699] See also **Hopkins syndrome, critical illness myopathy.**

critical perfusion pressure   The difference between the mean systemic arterial pressure and the mean intracranial pressure, giving thus the pressure with which arterial blood is introduced into the cranial cavity.

crocodile tears   (Bogorad syndrome, gustatory lacrimation, gustolacrimal reflex) Lacrimation accompanying eating.

The Arian theologian Asterios, seeking to explain why a crocodile sheds tears while eating, wrote in 340 A.D. that the animal was mourning the fact that the heads of children which he was consuming contained no meat.[5047] In 1600, Hakluyt, in describing Sir John Hawkins' voyage of 1565, embarked upon a flight of fancy, claiming that the crocodile's "nature is ever, when he would have his prey, to cry and sob like a Christian body, to provoke them to come to him, and then he snatcheth at them, and thereupon came this proverb that is applied unto women when they weep, *lachrymae crocodili,* the meaning whereof is that as the crocodile . . . so doth the woman when she weeps." The syndrome was also described by Legendre.

The physiological reason, adduced by the Russian physiologist F.A. Bogorad in 1928,[625] can be found in the identical innervation of the reptile's lacrimal and salivary glands. Following facial palsy in humans, aberrant reinnervation may lead to the shedding of tears while eating, when salivation alone would have been appropriate. Presumably the regenerating parasympathetic fibers have been diverted through the greater superficial petrosal nerve to the otic ganglion, when they should have continued on in the chorda tympani to innervate the submandibular and submaxillary glands. The occurrence of crocodile tears thus indicates that the original lesion of the facial nerve must have been somewhat proximal.

Crome syndrome   (cataracts–renal tubular necrosis–encephalopathy) A fatal congenital dysmorphic syndrome characterized by cataract, seizures, microcephaly, cerebral and cerebellar atrophy, mental and developmental delay, and renal tubular necrosis.[1188]

Cross oculocerebral syndrome   (oculocerebral hypopigmentation syndrome) A recessively inherited congenital dysmorphic syndrome characterized also by generalized depigmentation of the skin and hair, cloudy corneas, microphthalmia, gum hypertrophy, high palate, nystagmus, pyramidal signs, athetosis, and mental and developmental delay.[1197]

cross talk   1. The activation of inactive nerve fibers by an action potential travelling in adjacent active fibers. The electrical transmission between fibers thus occurs at a false synapse (an **ephapse**). This has been proposed as the mechanism responsible for hemifacial spasm, and possibly for some neuralgias, gustatory lacrimation, and sweating.[2022] 2. In **kinesiologic EMG,** signals recorded from adjacent muscles.[10]

crossed adductor reflex   Contraction of the contralateral adductor muscles in response to a tap on the adductor (or quadriceps) tendon. The reflex is evidence of a pyramidal lesion above the L2 segment, but is also normally found in infants between 3 and 8 months of age.

crossed aphasia   The occurrence of aphasia and hemiplegia with a right hemisphere lesion in right-handers (or with a left hemisphere lesion in left-handers), and in subjects without a family history of left-handedness and without any clinical or imaging evidence of a left hemisphere lesion. Other right hemisphere functions may remain as usual.[2531]

This indicates either that handedness and language lateralization are not invariably linked, or that transcallosal **diaschisis** is a mechanism. The condition was known to Hughlings-**Jackson** but the term was introduced by Bramwell in 1899. The characteristics of the dysphasias are not different from those seen with lesions of the more appropriate hemisphere in other patients.

crossed cerebral-cerebellar diaschisis   Reduction of blood flow and energy metabolism in one cerebellar hemisphere following infarction of the contralateral cerebral hemisphere as a result of neuronal depression secondary to damage to the corticopontocerebellar pathways.[369,1760] See **diaschisis.**

This may be the mechanism for homolateral ataxia and crural paresis, formerly regarded as a lacunar syndrome.[2126]

crossed diplopia   That form of diplopia which is the result of **exotropia** and in which the false image is displaced away from the side of the paretic eye. See also **uncrossed diplopia, diplopia.**

crossed extensor reflex   (Philippson reflex) Extension of the hip and knee with plantar flexion of the ankle and toes of the opposite limb when the **flexor reflex** is being elicited. The child is placed in the supine position and the sole of the foot is stroked firmly; the opposite leg flexes and then extends, with adduction of the leg and extension and fanning of all the toes.[6064] The reflex is normally present in infancy but it disappears by 12 months of age.

crossed flexor reflex   Flexion of the hip and knee and dorsiflexion of the foot in the leg opposite to that stimulated in an attempt to elicit the ipsilateral flexor reflex.

crossed hemianopic hemispatial neglect   Failure to copy the left side of drawings and neglect of the items on the left side of the page in the Line Crossing test, occurring when the subject with a severe callosal lesion holds the pencil in the right hand. These errors are not seen when the left hand is used. See also **crossed homonymous hemianopia.**

crossed hemiplegia   See **pyramidal decussation syndrome.**

crossed homonymous hemianopia   A varying hemianopic defect detected using static or kinetic perimetry apparatus, appearing on the side opposite that of the hand being used to push the switch of the perimeter. This (rare) condition has been described with severe callosal lesions.[2912]

crossed leg progression   A peculiarity of gait whereby spasm in the hip adductors due to chronic pyramidal tract lesions (such as **spastic diplegia** and **Little disease**) leads to the subject walking with the legs tightly adducted or actually crossed one before the other.

crossed palsy   See **alternating hemiplegia.**

crossed parabulbar syndrome   Spastic hemiparesis, cerebellar ataxia, and trigeminal thermoanesthesia on one side and thermoanalgesia of the trunk and limbs on the other side, due to a lesion of the high cervical cord.[5599]

crossed reflexes   The appearance of homologous muscle stretch reflex activity on the side opposite to that stimulated. They provide evidence of disinhibition at spinal segmental levels, and thus of bilateral pyramidal tract disease.

crossed spinoadductor reflex   Adduction and inward rotation of the contralateral leg in response to the vibration set up by a tap on the anterior superior iliac spine; present in normal subjects and increased in patients with pyramidal disease.

crossed upgoing toe sign   Dorsiflexion of the hallux on the abnormal side when the opposite, normal leg maintains flexion of the hip against resistance. This sign was described by Hindfelt et al. in 1976, but was only validated recently.[5991] It represents a sign of an early or incomplete upper motor neuron lesion.

Crouzon, Octave   (1874–1938) French physician with interests in pathology, genetics, and neurology, who trained in Paris, where he was influenced by **Babiński, Marie,** and Janet. He was appointed as physician at the Hôtel Dieu and later at the **Salpêtrière,** where he investigated a range of neurological conditions including cerebellar disease, the muscle dystrophies, and topics in psychiatry. His interest in the social and legal aspects of disease led to the creation for him of a special *Chair d'Assistance Medico-sociale* at the University of Paris.[1829] He described la dysostose cranio-faciale hereditaire first in 1906.[1198]

Crouzon syndromes   Congenital, dominantly inherited, dysmorphic syndromes characterized by **craniosynostosis** affecting the coronal suture with resulting acrocephaly, prominent frontal bossing, absent auditory canals, **hypertelorism,** parrot-beaked profile of the nose, hypoplastic facial bones, high palate, oligodontia, malformations of the ossicles with mixed hearing loss, dwarfism, micrognathia, optic atrophy, strabismus, nystagmus, exophthalmos, hydrocephalus, callosal agenesis, and mental and developmental delay.[1199,2214]

Five forms (maxillary, facial, cranial, and two combinations) may be differentiated according to the specific topography of the lesion.[4] The condition was first described by Oribasius (325–403) but may also have been recognized by Homer, whose hero Thersites was described as if so afflicted. See also **acrocephaly, oxycephaly, tower skull, craniofacial dysostosis.**

Crouzon-Crostophy-Gaucher syndrome   See **Sturge-Weber syndrome.**

crowbar case   Mr. Phineas **Gage,** an American railway foreman, was struck in the head by a tamping rod which did not kill him, but entering the anterior cranial fossa from below it extruded superiorly, effectively causing a frontal lobotomy. This led to the first description, by Harlow in 1848, of the **frontal lobe syndrome.** The changes in character and behavior of Mr. Gage as a result of the accident were severe; formerly described as pious, quiet, responsible, and hardworking, he became irreverent, profane, and unable to plan for the future or to hold down a job. He exhibited himself in a circus and was later a stage coach driver in Chile.

crowded orbital apex syndrome   The association of optic nerve lesions, retinopathy, and papilledema secondary to intraorbital hypertension, the visual loss commonly being bilateral and progressive.

Visual evoked responses and color perception tests are those most sensitive in diagnosis.

crowding of the optic disk   Compression of the fibers of the optic nerve as the result of a small scleral canal; such horizontal crowding is considered likely to promote infarction in the case of an already compromised optic disk circulation.[3596]

Crowe, S.J.   (1883–1955) American otolaryngologist who worked with **Cushing** and was later professor at Johns Hopkins.

Crowe (sign) test   1. Swelling of the facial and retinal veins with manual compression of one jugular vein in the neck. A sign of occlusion of the contralateral jugular vein or of the transverse sinus above it. 2. Axillary freckling in **neurofibromatosis** is also known as the Crowe sign, but was described by a different physician of that name.

Crow-Fukase syndrome   A **gammopathic neuropathy** (polyneuropathy with lambda paraproteinemia, edema, clubbing of the digits, organomegaly, endocrinopathy, bone lesions, and hyperhidrosis),[1201] best regarded as part of the **POEMS** syndrome.

Cruchet, Jean-René   (1875–1959) French pathologist and pediatrician, who trained and practiced in Bordeaux. His paper on 40 cases of encephalitis lethargica preceded by 13 days that of **von Economo.** Its clinical detail concerning initial extreme lassitude and expressionless facies, with slow recovery and motor deficits, and the types of the disease (mental, choreiform, convulsive, meningitic, hemiplegic, pontocerebellar, bulbar, and poliomyelitic), is excellent and the series was much larger than that of von Economo, who did, however, also note all the more important features of the disease.

The name of Cruchet has also been applied to **torticollis,** of which he gave a full account in 1907.

cruciate hemiplegia   See **pyramidal decussation syndrome.**

cruciate paralysis   (alternate brachial diplegia) Disproportionate motor deficits involving both arms, with relative sparing of power in the legs, usually resulting from damage to the central part of the cervical spinal cord.[440]

The syndrome is considered to result from involvement of those fibers destined for the cervical segments that decussate in the cord at a higher level than those destined for the lumbar segments.

Cruickshank disease   Olfactory hallucinations, **angor animi,** and facial pallor in partial complex seizures. Presumably the latter features derive from the stimulation of autonomic regulating structures (amygdala) by the seizure discharge.

Cruickshank, William Cumberland   (1745–1800) Scottish-born surgeon, assistant to William Hunter and physician to Dr. Samuel Johnson.

He forecast his own death from apoplexy, being aware of a thrilling sensation in the front of the left side of his head whenever he stooped forward. He had also been prone to attacks of sudden loss of memory and of pallor, sneezing, and olfactory hallucinations, which were precipitated by any form of strong emotional excitement.[5537]

crural monoplegia   Weakness of one leg as a result of stroke, with which a degree of mental confusion and cortical sensory loss are usually associated. The involved vessel is the paracentral branch of the anterior cerebral artery.

crural nerve   The femoral nerve.

crural neuritis   An acute, painful, allergic motor neuropathy affecting nerves branching from the lumbar plexus. See also **acute brachial neuritis, lumbosacral plexopathy.**

crus   (Lat, the leg or shin) A term applied to any leglike structure, often in the form of a *V* or an *X*; thus the **crus cerebri.**

crusta   The lower anterior part of the crus, or cerebral peduncles, separated from the upper part (the tegmentum) by the substantia nigra.

crutch palsy   Paralysis of the deltoid as a result of compression of the axillary nerve, as by a crutch in the armpit.

Cruveilhier atrophy   See **amyotrophic lateral sclerosis.**

Cruveilhier, Jean   (1791–1874) French surgeon and pathological anatomist who was born in Limoges and trained in Paris under Dupuytren. He held chairs in surgery and in descriptive and pathological anatomy, the latter at the **Salpêtrière,** where he established neuropathology as a major resource upon which **Charcot** and others built further.

In so doing, he differentiated intrinsic from extrinsic cord tumors and gave the first descriptions of cerebellopontine angle tumors, the appearances of multiple sclerosis in the spinal cord, red and white infarcts, sinus thrombosis, the Chiari malformation, cerebral tumors, and brainstem hemorrhages, publishing many of these accounts in his monumental book, *The Pathological Anatomy of the Human Body* (Paris, 1829–1842). He also gave a good account of **amyotrophic lateral sclerosis** (once known as Cruveilhier atrophy) in 1853, some 20 years before Charcot's description,[1880] and published an atlas of types of cerebral atrophies, recognizing micro- and hemi-atrophy, porencephaly, hydrocephalus, and cerebral dysgenesis between 1835 and 1842.

Cruveilhier palsy   See **amyotrophic lateral sclerosis.**

crying seizures   See **dacrystic epilepsy.**

cryoglobulinemia   Conditions characterized by the presence of a serum protein, usually IgG or IgM, which precipitates on cooling and dissolves on warming to body temperatures.

In *essential cryoglobulinemia* no associated disease is present; but, in the *secondary* form, the condition is associated with monoclonal or polyclonal gammopathies. Clinically, purpura, Raynaud phenomenon, arthralgia, nephropathy, and neuropathy are the more common manifestations and encephalopathy is rare.

cryoglobulinemic neuropathy   See **gammopathic neuropathy, relapsing ischemic encephalo-enteropathy, and cryoglobulinemia.**

cryptic vascular malformations   Small arteriovenous malformations in the cortex and white matter, considered to be present in the brains of 4% of those suffering intracerebral hemorrhages, but usually destroyed by the bleeding.[3158]

crypto-   (Gr, hidden). Prefix denoting hidden.

cryptococcal meningitis   (Busse-Buschke disease) A chronic leptomeningitis due to blood-borne infection with the yeast *Cryptococcus neoformans,* a common soil organism found in bird excrement. Granulomas may also occur.

Clinically, it is marked by headache, nausea and vomiting, meningism, fever, and disturbance of balance, gait, and vision, with chronically raised intracranial pressure and sometimes seizures and focal signs. The CSF shows pleocytosis and glucose levels are reduced; the yeast is well shown using india ink preparations.[1312]

The condition is unusually common and rapidly progressive among immunocompromised subjects, such as those with HIV infection, in whom the clinical features are relatively silent.[1328] See also **torulosis.**

cryptogenic drop attacks   **Drop attacks** occurring as an isolated symptom while walking in perhaps 3% of adult women. They have no known cause nor associated pathology and bear a good prognosis. Matthews and Stevens noted that "extinction of the ego by intru-

sion of a forbidden erotic thought" had been put forward as being etiologically relevant, but they did not choose to investigate this theory.[5348]

cryptogenic epilepsies   Partial or generalized unprovoked seizures or epilepsies in which no factor associated with increased risk of seizures has been identified. This group includes patients who do not conform to the criteria for the symptomatic or idiopathic categories.[1115]

cryptogenic myoclonic epilepsy   See **myoclonus.**

cryptogenic sensory polyneuropathy   A chronic neuropathy characterized by pain, symmetrical numbness, and paresthesias in the distal extremities, without weakness and with no identified cause. The diagnosis is one of exclusion, and there are likely to be numerous causes for this syndrome.[6021]

cryptophthalmia   A rare, recessively inherited craniofacial malformation characterized by complete fusion of the upper and lower eyelids and absence of the eyelashes, so that there is an unbroken reach of skin between the face and the forehead. The underlying eyes may be well enveloped but are frequently disorganized. Other facial dysmorphisms are commonly present.

The condition was reported first by Zehender in 1872.[4]

cryptophthalmos syndrome   A recessively inherited congenital syndrome characterized by growth of skin down over the eyes, one or both of which are completely covered, with syndactyly of the fingers or toes.[5405,6115]

CT scan   See **computerized axial tomography.**

ctenoids   See **Fourteen and six positive Hz burst pattern.**

C-trigonocephaly syndrome   A congenital dysmorphic syndrome characterized by strabismus, facial hemangiomas, congenital cardiac anomaly, pulmonary segmentation defects, cryptorchid testes, abnormal palmar creases, polydactyly and syndactyly of fingers and toes, joint contractures, multiple joint dislocations, hypotonia, seizures, trigonocephaly, cutis laxa, and mental and developmental delay.[337]

Cuban optic neuropathy   An epidemic neuropathy affecting both the optic and the peripheral, mainly sensory nerves, sometimes associated with deafness, ataxia, and pyramidal signs and likely due to the combination of malnutrition and tobacco smoking in those affected.[1209]

The United States' "Cuban Democracy Act" has been blamed for the occurrence of the condition.[4748]

cubital tunnel syndrome   Compression of the ulnar nerve above, behind or just below the medial epicondyle, with dysfunction of the nerve at that site due to conduction block.

The signs associated are weakness and wasting of the intrinsic hand muscles supplied by the nerve (hypothenar muscles, adductor pollicis and interossei) and numbness of the ulnar 1 1/2 digits and palm on their anterior aspect. The flexor carpi ulnaris and the ulnar half of the flexor digitorum profundus are usually innervated by a branch of the nerve taking off above the cubital tunnel and so are likely to be spared.

Tardy ulnar palsy was the term applied by Mouchet in 1914 to the occurrence of this condition remotely following fracture of the humerus.

Cautions about anterior transposition of the nerve in cases of compression at the elbow sites have been raised and decompression advocated as a safer operation.[883]

cuff compression test   The provocation of symptoms in **carpal tunnel syndrome** by constriction of the upper arm by a blood pressure cuff inflated above systolic pressure.

Cullen, William   (1710–1790) Scottish surgeon who described the bruising behind the ear suggesting the presence of a fracture of the base of the skull.

Cumings, John Nathaniel   (1906–1974) English pathologist at the National Hospital, where he became professor of chemical pathology at the Institute of Neurology. He is best remembered for his studies of the chemical pathology of the lipidoses and leukodystrophies, and for his development of the specialty of clinical chemical pathology as a major area of research and clinical service.

cuneate fasciculus and nucleus   (Burdach's column) The lateral of the two posterior columns of the spinal cord, described in 1806 by Karl Frederich Burdach (1776–1847), a German anatomist and physiologist.[4979]

cupulolithiasis   The aggregation of detached sediment from the macula of the utricle upon the cupula of the posterior semicircular canal, rendering it sensitive to changes in static head position and thus inducing positional vertigo.[727]

Current Neurology   (Curr. Neurol.) A neurological review book series. Address: Mosby-Year Book, Inc. 11830 Westline Industrial Dr., St. Louis, MO 63146.

Current Opinion in Neurology and Neurosurgery (Curr. Opin. Neurol.) A neurological review/update journal. The 2002 website is http://www.co-neurology.com/.

Curry syndrome   See **vertebral dysplasia-spinal dysraphism.**

cursive epilepsy   Seizures with a focus in the temporal lobe, in which the subject runs.[3345,5080]

curtain sign   Displacement of the whole of the posterior pharyngeal wall toward the healthy side when its mucosa is stimulated by the examiner. This is a feature of bulbar weakness, as in **Vernet syndrome.**

Curtius, Friedrich   (1896–1975) German physician.

Curtius syndrome   See **congenital hemihypertrophy.**

curvilinear bodies   Intraneuronal or intramuscular inclusions seen on electron microscopy in **lipofuscinosis.**

Cushing, Harvey Williams   (1869–1939) American neurosurgeon, educated successively at Yale, Harvard, and Johns Hopkins, where his surgical promise led to intensive and personalized training from Halsted and where he learned his neurology from **Osler.** He also trained with Kocher in Berne. Cushing served with the British Royal Army Medical Corps and the American Army Medical Corps during World War I, when ironically he attended Osler's only son at his death in battle. His monumental work was done as Moseley Professor of Surgery at Harvard and as Sterling Professor of Neurology at Yale.

He is regarded as the father of modern neurosurgery, not only for his technical skill and practical innovations but also for his careful research into, among other topics, the pituitary gland and its diseases, cerebellopontine angle tumors, the CSF (*The Third Circulation,* 1926), classification of gliomas and of meningiomas (*Intracranial Tumours,* 1932) and the history of medicine; his life of **Osler** won him a Pulitzer Prize in 1925. Nevertheless, some of his publications incorporated the observations of such associates as **Dandy** and **Bailey** without proper care to acknowledge them. His chapter "Surgery of the Head" was the first major American review of neurosurgery. He was a founder of the Society of Neurological Surgeons and was generally regarded as a leading citizen in medicine, not only in the Americas but throughout the world.[7] The importance of his research is indicated by the next entries.

Cushing response   (reflex) The reflex maintenance of cerebral perfusion pressure by an increase in mean arterial blood pressure in response to a decrease in medullary perfusion.[1228]

Cushing syndrome   1. Hyperadrenocorticism secondary to a chromophobe or basophil adenoma of the pituitary gland, although other causes produce similar features.[1232] *Myopathy* is a complication. See also **Nelson syndrome.** 2. Primary optic atrophy with bitemporal hemianopsia due to a sellar or suprasellar tumor. See **chiasmal syndrome.**[1231] 3. (Cerebellopontine angle syndrome) Nystagmus, tinnitus, deafness, diminished corneal reflex, sixth and seventh nerve palsies, hoarseness, dysphagia, headache, and ipsilateral cerebellar signs due to compression by a mass lesion such as an acoustic schwannoma.[1229]

Cushing triad   The association of systemic hypertension, bradycardia, and slow and irregular respirations seen in patients with increased intracranial pressure, at a late stage.

Cushing tumor   1. **medulloblastoma.** A solid malignant cerebellar neoplasm which consists of spongioblastic and neuroblastic cells.[293] 2. See **meningioma.**[1230]

Cushing-Bailey-Cobb syndrome   See **Sturge-Weber syndrome.**

cutaneocerebral angioma   See **Sturge-Weber syndrome.**

cutaneomeningospinal angiomatosis   A syndrome characterized by vascular malformations in the spinal cord, presenting with spasticity and other evidence of myelopathy, and brain nevi or capillary and cavernous hemangiomas, causing seizures and focal deficits. See **Cobb syndrome.**

cutaneous albinism and deaf-mutism   An X-linked syndrome of sensorineural deafness and hypomelanosis of the skin.[3610]

cutaneous albinism, ataxia, and peripheral neuropathy   A syndrome in which these features occur, sometimes with spastic paraparesis as well.[3428]

cutaneous meningeal melanosis   See **incontinentia pigmenti.**

cutaneous reflexes   Motor activity occurring reflexly in response to stimulation of skin or mucous membranes. They include the palmar, scapular and interscapular, superficial abdominal, gluteal, plantar, and superficial anal reflexes. The first description was that of **Gowers** in 1888.[2240] See **superficial reflexes, cutaneous reflex.**

cutis laxa, retardation, and corneal opacity   See **de Barsy syndrome.**

cutis laxa with mental and physical retardation   A recessively inherited congenital dysmorphic syndrome characterized by low birth weight, dwarfism, hypertelorism, dislocation of the hips, laxity of the skin, delayed closure of the fontanelles with wide cranial sutures, and mental and developmental delay.[4652] See **Ehlers-Danlos syndrome.**

cutis verticis gyrata with acromegaloid appearance and leukoma   A congenital dysmorphic syndrome characterized by tall stature, frontal bossing, cloudy corneas, prominent mandible, large hands with abnormal dermatoglyphic patterns, macrocephaly, and cutis gyrata (abnormal growth of the skin resulting in anteroposterior ridges and furrows) of the scalp.[65] The primary form is associated with a congenital static encephalopathy and manifests chronic seizures. The secondary form occurs as a result of infiltration of the skin in the context of systemic disease without neurological disorder.

In a variant condition, *cutis verticis with Lennox syndrome,* seizures accompany the above findings.

cutis verticis with Lennox syndrome   See **cutis verticis gyrata with acromegaloid appearance and leukoma.**

cycas circinalis   The false sago palm, a tree growing in the Western Pacific, the seeds of which contain a neurotoxin considered a likely cause of **lytico-bodig.**

cycle   The complete sequence of potential changes undergone by individual components of a sequence of regularly repeated EEG waves or complexes, or by physiological functions such as pupillary constriction, sleep, etc.

cyclic eosinophilic myositis   A syndrome characterized by muscular swelling, induration, and discomfort with weight gain and malaise, associated with high levels of IgE, creatinine kinase, and eosinophils and with biopsy evidence of eosinophilic polymyositis. The symptoms recur on a 4- or 5-week cycle.[5454]

cyclic esotropia   A rare circadian form of strabismus characterized by 1- to 3-day-long periods of esotropia, followed by similar periods of normal ocular function. The condition usually occurs spontaneously in small children; its cause is not known.

cyclic insomnia   Periodic and repetitive disturbances in sleeping, usually as a result of psychiatric disturbances, drug abuse, or alcoholism.

cyclic migraine   The occurrence of well-regulated episodes of migraine headaches cycling over time.[3801]

cyclic oculomotor palsy   (Axenfeld-Schurenberg syndrome, cyclic oculomotor paralysis) Periodic contraction and dilation of the pupil on a 1- to 2-minute cycle. It is rare syndrome, occurring particularly in the first year of life in which a complete or partial third nerve palsy alternates with brief spasms of third cranial nerve hyperfunction.[3456]

The periodic paroxysmal unilateral third nerve paresis causes mydriasis, blurred vision, diminution or absence of eye movements, and complete ptosis, occurring for up to 3 minutes at a time in bouts lasting hours or days, while during the periods of overactivity there is lid retraction and miosis.[389]

The condition was first described in 1894 by Rampoldi. See also **misdirection syndrome.**

cyclic oculomotor paralysis   See **cyclic oculomotor palsy.**

cyclic oculomotor spasm   (springing pupil type 3) A rare abnormality characterized by pupillary dilatation, ptosis, and extraocular muscle paresis after congenital or early acquired third nerve palsy, alternating after some years with periods of miosis and retraction of the upper lid during sleep and wakefulness. The cause may be aberrant regeneration.[2388]

cyclic sympathetic spasm   A rare syndrome characterized by periodic dystonia of one limb with homolateral mydriasis, alternating with normal limb tone and a Horner syndrome, described in association with a spinal cord lesion.[3492]

cyclic vomiting   A childhood syndrome of recurrent episodic vomiting often with associated pallor and photophobia,[359] changing into a more typical migraine syndrome with increasing age.

The condition is considered to represent a **migraine equivalent.**

cyclists' palsy   Distal compression of the ulnar nerve, first described in 1896 by Destot. Weakness and wasting of the muscles supplied by the deep branch of the nerve results, presumably from a prolonged period of compression of the nerve (in the region of Guyon's canal) by the handlebars.[4171] Compression more proximally, with damage to the superficial branch, leads to sensory symptoms in the ulnar 1 1/2 fingers.

The syndrome is also known by the name of Ramsay **Hunt,** who described it (not in a cyclist) in 1908.

cyclopia   A developmental malformation in which, as a result of failure of the forebrain to divide into cerebral hemispheres (**holoproscencephaly**), there is a single orbital cavity with a proboscis projecting above it.[335] The lateral ventricles are fused, and midline structures may be either absent or incomplete.

The malformation was described in the character Polyphemus in Homer's *Odyssey.*

cycloplegia   Paralysis of both the pupilloconstrictors and the ciliary body, thus preventing miosis as a result of accommodation or light stimulation.

cyclorotation   See **ocular torsion.**

cylindrocephalic   Having a long (thus cylindrical) head.

cylindroma   (plexiform sarcoma) An adenoid cystic carcinoma arising in the orbit and stomach, which in the former site may present with unilateral cranial neuropathy.[3677]

cylindromatosis   (turban tumors) A syndrome of cystic ear pinnae, with conductive deafness and cysts and tumors of the face and scalp.[337]

cymbal-players shoulder   An **overuse syndrome** presenting with shoulder pain. Deafness is not reported as associated with the syndrome.

cynic spasm   (from Gr, a dog) A snarl, the muscles of one side of the face only being contracted to display the teeth.

cystathionase deficiency   (cystathioninuria) An inherited enzymatic deficiency metabolic disorder leading to a failure to break down cystathionine. The clinical features may include mental and developmental delay, signs of metabolic acidosis, and thrombocytopenia.[2462]

cystathionine beta-synthetase deficiency   See **homocystinuria.**

cystathioninuria   See **cystathionine deficiency.**

cystic dilatation of occipital horn   The occurrence of complex partial seizures associated with cystic dilatation of the posterior part of one lateral ventricle, the initial event occurring in the neonatal period as a result of occlusion of one posterior cerebral artery. The seizure disorder occurs years later.[4659]

cystic myelopathy   (post-traumatic syringomyelia) Cavitations within the spinal cord following serious cord injury. The neurological features of myelopathy are not specific. Cord compression, a tense syrinx at the cervical vertebral fracture site, and kyphosis are associated with enlargement of the intraspinal cyst.[5013]

cysticercosis   A systemic infection frequently causing infestation of the brain with the larvae of *Taenia solium,* the adult pork tapeworm, for which humans are the definitive host. Infection is sometimes asymptomatic but, if the nervous system is invaded, the major clinical results are seizures, intracranial hypertension, dementia, stroke-like syndromes, myelopathy, and evidence of meningeal inflammation, usually occurring only after a long incubation period.[4228]

Multiple intracranial calcifications are often demonstrable on CT scanning. The condition, although uncommon, is nevertheless the most common parasitic disease affecting the CNS and is seen mainly in Hispanic people.[3734,4234]

Criteria for human cysticercosis have been suggested by del Brutto et al.[1357,1358] and are reproduced here (adapted) by kind permission.

Absolute Criteria
Histologic demonstration of the parasite
Direct visualization of the parasite by fundoscopic examination
Evidence of cystic lesions showing the scolex on CT or MRI*
Major Criteria
Evidence of lesions suggestive of neurocysticercosis on neuroimaging studies*
Positive immunologic tests for the detection of anticysticercal antibodies**
Plain X-ray films showing cigar-shaped calcifications in thigh and calf muscles
Minor Criteria
Presence of subcutaneous nodules (without histologic confirmation)
Evidence of punctuate soft-tissue or intracranial calcifications on plain X-ray films
Presence of clinical manifestations suggestive of neurocysticercosis†
Disappearance of intracranial lesions after a trial with anticysticercal drugs
Epidemiological Criteria
Individuals coming from or living in an area where cysticercosis is endemic
History of frequent travel to cysticercosis-endemic areas
Evidence of a household contact with *T. solium* infection

Computed tomography (CT) or magnetic resonance imaging (MRI) showing cystic lesions, ring-enhancing lesions, parenchymal brain calcifications hydrocephalus, and abnormal enhancement of the leptomeninges, and myelograms showing multiple filling defects in the column of contrast medium.

**Serum immunoblot developed by the Centers for Disease Control and Prevention, and CSF immunosorbent assay.*

†Epilepsy, focal neurologic signs, intracranial hypertension, and dementia.

cystinosis   A recessively inherited error of metabolism (a lysosomal storage disorder) characterized by the deposition of cystine crystals in the corneas, white blood cells, and bone marrow, with impairment of water resorption by the kidney leading to renal failure and hypophosphatemic rickets. Retinopathy, growth retardation, and distal vacuolar myopathy are also described in this condition.[984]

cystinuria A recessively inherited inborn error of metabolism in which there is impaired intestinal and renal transport of dibasic amino acids and urinary excretion of excessive amounts of cystine with stone formation.

Neurological complications include myopathy, a syndrome resembling multiple sclerosis, mental retardation, and psychiatric disturbances; pigmentary retinopathy, pyramidal and extrapyramidal degeneration, and deaf-mutism are often associated.[597]

cystometry The graphic representation of pressure as a function of vesical volume; the patient voids and then is catheterized, after which fluid is infused into the bladder. As the fluid goes in, the patient reports in turn the first sensation of bladder fullness, the first urge to urinate, and the time of onset of the first severe urge to void, while the intravesical pressure is monitored throughout.

cytoarchitectonics The design of the cellular characteristics of the cortex, which varies in different brain regions and allows mapping of the cortex and some ascriptions of specialized functions to certain areas. See H. **Vogt.**

cytochrome-*b* (complex III) deficiency A mitochondrial disease marked by deficiency of this enzyme, which normally functions in the respiratory transport chain.

Clinically, exercise-induced muscle pain, cramping, and weakness are present but progressive over years, with a marked increase in serum lactic acid levels following minor exertion.[3980]

cytochrome-*c* oxidase The enzyme responsible for catalyzing the transfer of electrons from cytochrome-*c* to oxygen, resulting in the generation of water. Deficiency of the enzyme causes a backup of electrons to occur, so that substances higher up the metabolic chain remain in a reduced (nonoxidized) form (e.g., NADH rather than NAD^+) and production of ATP is arrested.

cytochrome-*c* oxidase deficiency A mitochondrial disease marked by deficiency of this enzyme normally functioning in the respiratory transport chain. Clinically, severe hypotonia and respiratory muscle weakness affect infants with lactic acidosis, aminoaciduria, glycosuria, and proteinuria.[1448] Other phenotypes include those of **Leigh disease;** transient, chronic, or severe forms of infantile myopathy; **MERRF;** and **Kearns-Sayre syndrome.**

In an autosomal recessive form, stroke-like episodes have been recorded.[3988]

cytoid bodies Retinal swellings due to axonal enlargement within the nerve fiber layer, occurring as a consequence of ischemia. See **cotton wool spots.**

cytomegalovirus infections The organism has been described as an ubiquitous agent with protean clinical manifestations. Infection is a common condition of infants and in some cases leads to microcephaly, psychomotor retardation, seizures, chorioretinitis, or deafness. It is less commonly a cause of neurological problems in adults, but is increasing as a result of infection of the immunocompromised.[729] After childhood, acute infectious polyneuropathy, retinopathy, and meningoencephalitis are the most common neurological presentations.

The role of preceding cytomegalovirus infection in the genesis of many other neurological conditions remains unproved.[306]

cytomegalovirus polyradiculitis See **HIV-associated lumbosacral polyradiculopathy.**

cytoplasmic bodies Small periodic acid-Schiff–positive, eosinophilic masses of actin filaments within myofibrils in normal as well as variously diseased muscles, such as some cases of dermatomyositis and in the following conditions.

cytoplasmic body myopathies (desmin-storage myopathy) An uncommon dominantly inherited **myofibrillar myopathy** characterized by proximal myopathic weakness and the presence of intracytoplasmic inclusion bodies originating from the Z lines in muscle biopsy specimens. The condition presents in later adult life or in childhood with facial, neck, proximal, truncal, spinal, or cardiac muscle weakness, and with a progressive course. The muscle stretch reflexes and serum creatine kinase levels may be normal. Muscle biopsy specimens show fiber variations and displaced nuclei, fibrosis, and cytoplasmic bodies.[4358] The following entries are abstracted from the Neuromuscular Web site at Washington University, St. Louis, http://www.neuro.wustl.edu/neuromuscular/maltbrain.html by courtesy of Dr. Alan Pestronk.

1. *Severe limb-girdle type* A recessively inherited form with onset in infancy or childhood of hypotonia and proximal weakness, skeletal abnormalities, respiratory insufficiency, and death in early adult life.
2. *Mild limb-girdle type* A dominantly inherited form with onset in adolescence of slowly or nonprogressive limb-girdle weakness.
3. *Myopathy with proximal weakness and early respiratory muscle involvement (type 1)* A dominantly inherited form mapped to 2q24–q31 (similar to tibial muscular dystrophy) with onset in adult life of girdle and diaphragmatic weakness and early involvement of the neck flexors. Serum CK levels are normal or slightly elevated. Muscle biopsy shows bodies containing actin in type I muscle fibers.
4. *Myopathy with proximal weakness and early respiratory muscle involvement (type 2)* A dominantly inherited

form mapped to 2q21 with onset in young adult life of girdle and diaphragmatic weakness. Serum CK levels are normal. Muscle biopsy shows the presence of cytoplasmic bodies containing actin and desmin in type I muscle fibers.

5. *Distal type* A dominantly inherited form with onset of proximal and distal weakness in late adult life, progressing to respiratory failure and with cardiomyopathy producing heart block arrhythmias and congestive heart failure. Serum CK levels are nomal or slightly elevated, the EMG is myopathic with complex repetitive discharges, and muscle biopsy is characterized by the presence of myofibrillary inclusions in the cytoplasm of type I muscle fibers. See also **myofibrillar myopathy, distal myopathies**

cytoplasmic body neuromyopathy   A sporadic chronic progressive neuromyopathy characterized by early neck weakness, weight loss, respiratory failure, fatigability, headache with increased intracranial pressure, dyspnea, somnolence, the presence of cytoplasmic bodies in type 1 muscle fibers, and an axonal polyneuropathy.[2852]

The difference between this condition and **cytoplasmic body myopathy** is not clear.

cytosol tyrosine aminotransferase deficiency   A rare diffuse encephalopathy resulting from this enzymatic defect, characterized clinically by midline clefting, microcephaly, and severe mental retardation.[3004]

cytosolic receptors   Receptors found on the surface of some tumor cells, able to bind sex hormones in the cytoplasm.

cytotoxic cerebral edema   Swelling of brain parenchymal cells as a result of damage to the sodium–potassium exchange pump mechanism, leading to the accumulation of intracellular water. This is typically seen following hypoxia-ischemia or metabolic (toxic) damage.

D state   See **REM sleep** (paradoxical sleep).

Da Costa syndrome   See **chronic fatigue syndrome, hyperventilation syndrome.**

Da Vinci, Leonardo   (1452–1519) Italian artist, anatomist, engineer and writer. Analysis of his writing and drawing techniques have suggested that he is the model for disconsolate left-handers, but this may have been an effect of a right hemiparesis acquired later in life. However, most of his script was in mirror writing, regarded by the **Vogts** as the natural form of script for sinistrals.[4994]

His anatomical drawings were lost until discovered by William Hunter, the English surgeon, in 1784.

DACE syndrome   See **dystonia.**

D'Acosta disease   See **altitude sickness.**

dacryo-   (Gr, to weep) A prefix denoting association with the lacrimal gland or tears.

dacrystic epilepsy   (from Gr, shouting out loud) (quiritarian epilepsy) Epileptic attacks in which the patients weeps; described rarely in seizures with temporal lobe foci.[4204,5080]

dactyl-   (Gr, a finger) A prefix denoting an association with the finger.

Daentl syndrome   A congenital syndrome manifesting short stature, blue sclerae, nephropathy, the **Chiari malformation,** and hydrocephalus.

Dagnini, G.   (b. 1905) Italian physician, professor of medical pathology at Bologna.

Dagnini sign   (extension-adduction reflex) Percussion of the radial aspect of the dorsum of the hand leads to extension of the wrist in patients with a pyramidal lesion of that limb.

Dale principle   Any one neuron uses but a single neurotransmitter, the same at every one of its terminals.

The principle was long considered correct but recently has been shown to have exceptions—in the corpus striatum, for example.

Dale, Sir Henry   (1875–1968) English physiologist and pharmacologist who differentiated the nicotinic and muscarinic effects of acetylcholine and clarified the question of the transmission of nerve impulses, demonstrated acetylcholine release at motor nerve endings, and identified oxytocin as an important secretion of the posterior pituitary gland.

Sir Henry Dale

Dalrymple sign   Widening of the palpebral fissure, mainly from retraction of the upper eyelids due to excessive sympathetic stimulation of Müller's muscle initially and later to levator fibrosis. A sign of dysthyroid orbitopathy. See **scleral show.**

John Dalrymple (1804–1852) was an English ophthalmologist.

Dalton, John   (1766–1852) English chemist, who was color-blind himself but who first identified the condition (thereafter called *daltonism*) in 1798.[1254] Joseph Huddart (1741–1816), however, had given an account of "Persons who could not distinguish color" to Joseph Priestly, who in turn communicated it to the Royal Society in 1777.

Charles Loomis Dana

Dana, Charles Loomis   (1852–1935) New York neurologist and classicist who trained at Columbia University after an early career in zoology. He became a professor of physiology and then of diseases of the mind and nervous system in New York before being appointed as professor of neurology at Cornell. He was a cofounder of the New York Neurological Institute and was president of the American Neurological Association in 1892 and again in 1928.

Apart from identifying in 1891 the syndrome to which his name was lent (the same year as J.J. **Putnam** described it), he is remembered for having persuaded a neurosurgical colleague to resect some of the posterior spinal roots for the relief of pain, and also for describing spastic pareses and amplifying Hammond's account of athetosis (1888). He was also a classical scholar with a special interest in Horace. In 1892 he published his acclaimed *Text-book of Nervous Diseases,* which went to 10 editions over the next 33 years.

Dana syndrome   See **subacute combined degeneration of the cord.**

dancing eyes (dancing feet) syndrome   See **opsoclonus.**

dancing larynx   A variant of **palatal tremor** characterized by arrhythmic contractions of the laryngeal and pharyngeal muscles, leading to clicking sounds. The uvula is unaffected.

dancing mania   (St. John dance, St. Vitus dance, danse de St. Guy, tarantism, jumpers, rollers, barkers, leaping ague, astonagaza, chorea germanorum, etc.) Probably a form of mass hysteria and not now reported, this consisted of epidemic propensities to dance experienced by men and women, who circled hand in hand for hours at a time. "They worked themselves up to a pitch of excitement, foamed at the mouth and fell down exhausted and half-fainting."[2764] During the dancing, some saw visions, while others appeared to convulse. As the mania spread, it became more licentious and sexually oriented.

The condition was reported from Aix-la-Chapelle in 1374; in 1418, the Chief Magistrate of Strasbourg ordered dancers in his city to go to the chapel of St. Vitus at Zabern, a remote Alsatian village, for relief from the condition; the name of St. Vitus was thus associated with the dancing mania and by extension with the dance-like movements of chorea, until these were distinguished by Sydenham in 1675.

The tradition continues on Whit Tuesday in Echternach (Luxembourg). See also **epidemic chorea.**

Dandy, Walter Edward   (1886–1946) American neurosurgeon, professor at Johns Hopkins in Baltimore, where he had also been a student and where he trained for a time with his mentor, Halsted, and then with **Cushing,** with whom he did not get on and to whom he would not speak. At Johns Hopkins, he investigated the dynamics of the CSF circulation and as a result devised operations for the relief of hydrocephalus as well

as for trigeminal neuralgia (approaching the nerve roots through the posterior fossa) and for the removal of cerebellopontine angle and pineal tumors, using a transcallosal approach. He introduced the techniques of air encephalography in 1918 and of ventriculography in the following year, and was the first surgeon to clip a cerebral aneurysm.[7]

Dandy-Walker syndrome   A malformation of the fourth ventricle and cerebellum, characterized by atresia of the foramina of Luschka and Magendie[1272] with failure of development of the midline structures of the cerebellum (which form instead a large cyst obstructing the CSF flow and causing hydrocephalus) as well as some bulging of the occiput.[1272]

The cardinal features are malformation of the vermis, a cystic roof to the expanded fourth ventricle, and elevation of the tentorium. Clinically, the syndrome is characterized in its full expression by cleft palate, pyloric stenosis, multiple renal cysts, bilateral pyramidal and cerebellar signs, and mental and developmental delay. Dolichocephaly, scaphocephaly or microcephaly, encephalocele or cranial meningocele, aqueduct stenosis with hydrocephalus, polymicrogyria, heterotopias, and callosal agenesis are the main pathological features. In some cases, congenital cardiac anomalies also occur[2466] and the cyst is also a feature of various other congenital malformation syndromes characterized by facial dysmorphisms, skeletal anomalies, microcephaly, etc.

A.E. Walker (b. 1907) was an American neurosurgeon, a colleague of **Dandy** at Johns Hopkins. The first description of the malformation was actually published by J.B. Sutton in *Brain* (1887).

Danielssen, Daniel   (1815–1894) Norwegian physician who gave the first complete clinical and pathological account of leprosy, which was at that time endemic in the coastal region where he practiced.

Danielssen-Boeck syndrome   See **anesthetic leprosy.**

Danks syndrome   (recessive osteodysplasty) A congenital dysmorphic syndrome manifesting also numerous skeletal malformations and recurrent infections, delayed closure of fontanelles, and hydrocephalus.[337]

Danon disease   An X-linked glycogen (lyosomal) storage disorder resembling Pompe disease but with normal levels of α-glucosidase. Mental retardation, somatic myopathy, and cardiomyopathy are the chief presenting features.[1276]

danse de St. Guy   See **Sydenham chorea.**

danse du ventre   A dystonic syndrome in some elderly people who make repetitive writhing movements resembling an attempt to scratch the abdomen without using the hands.

dark adaptation   (dark response) Progressive improvement of vision in conditions of low illumination, largely due to widening of the pupillary aperture as a result of inhibition of the pupillary sphincter muscles and contraction of the pupillary dilators. The phenomenon was first described by Hermann Aubert (1826–1892), a German physician.[257]

dark response   See **dark adaptation.**

Darkshewitsch fibers   Those fibers running between the optic tract and the habenular ganglion.

Darkshewitsch, Liverij Osipovich (1858–1925) Russian anatomist at the Universities of Moscow and St. Petersburg.

Darkshewitsch nucleus (ganglion)   The nucleus of the posterior commissure, situated within the third ventricle and anterior to the **Edinger-Westphal nucleus.**[1478]

Dartmouth Screening Battery for Diffuse Cerebral Dysfunction   A rating scale shown to be valid and reliable in the diagnosis of diffuse cerebral dysfunction.[2837] It examines 13 functions, including the **nuchocephalic** and **glabellar tap reflexes;** the **sucking** response; **pursuit eye movements;** maintenance of lateral gaze and up- and down-gaze; and **gegenhalten** in both the arms and the legs. The battery also includes some items in the **Mini-Mental State** Exam (three-item recall and some knowledge questions).

Daur-Babinski sign   Dystonic permanent extreme dorsiflexion of the hallux, a sign of chronic pallidal lesions. See **dystonic toe.**

David anomaly   Originally described as the congenital absence of one or both pectoral muscles with syndactyly, but now extended to include congenital absence of muscles (e.g., the abdominals). The condition might be classified as a disorder of muscle, but it is not known whether it represents a developmental failure of the muscle only or whether whole motor units, including the anterior horn cells, are absent as well. See also **thenar hypoplasia, Souques syndrome.**

Davidenkow, S.   (fl. 1926) Russian neurologist, practicing in Moscow.

Davidenkow syndrome   See **scapuloperoneal syndrome.**

Davidsohn, Hermann   (1842–1911) German physician who devised a method for illumination of the sinuses (also showing up the pupils) by shining a bright light into the mouth of the patient in a dark place.[4979]

Dawson encephalitis   See **subacute sclerosing panencephalitis.**

Dawson fingers   Extensions of plaques of demyelination beside blood vessels within the white matter of the brain extending perpendicularly from the walls of the lateral ventricles in **multiple sclerosis,** visible on **MRI** scans.

Dax, Marc   (1771–1837) French general practitioner, who in 1836 noted the relationship between left hemispheric lesions and disturbances of speech, an observation which he did not publicize and which was therefore neglected until republished in 1865 by his son Gustav.[1316]

In his graduation thesis he described postepileptic (**Todd**) paresis.

day blindness   See **nyctalopia.**

dazzling test   Persistent reduction in vision after bright light stimulation, seen in subjects with optic neuritis.

De Barsy syndrome (cutis laxa, retardation and corneal opacity) A congenital dysmorphic syndrome manifesting also short stature, sparse hair, cloudy corneas, premature aging, microcephaly with delayed closure of the fontanelles, involuntary movements, and mental and developmental delay.[1322]

De Clerambault syndrome   A pathological belief that one is loved by another person, whose every action is interpreted in a way that sustains the delusion, despite the attempts of the unfortunate target of that false belief to be rid of his (more rarely her) admirer.[5632]

Dr. G.H.A.E.L.M.G. de Clerambault (1872–1934) was a French physician.

De Grouchy-Royal-Salmon-Lamy syndrome   A heterogeneous entity resulting from deletion of the distal long arm of chromosome 18q and characterized variously by mental retardation, microcephaly, midface hypoplasia, abnormalities of the ears and genitalia, hypotonia, talipes equinovarus, and segmental spinal muscular atrophy.[1331],[5996] See **chromosome 18 partial deletion.**

De Lange, Cornelia   (1871–1950) Dutch pediatrician, practicing in Amsterdam.

De Lange syndrome   1. (Cornelia de Lange syndrome, Brachmann-de Lange syndrome, Amsterdam dwarfism) A sporadic syndrome of growth retardation from conception with severely diminished stature (always below the third percentile) despite congenital muscular hypertrophy. The syndrome also consists of microcephaly, severe mental retardation, nystagmus, initial hypertonicity, extrapyramidal disorders, facial dysmorphism, flexion contractures of the elbows, **clinodactyly,** syndactyly, transverse palmar crease and dermatoglyphic abnormalities, generalized hirsutism, and synophrys. The neck and limbs are broad and thick, the hairline low, and the skull asymmetrical because of porencephaly. Various cerebral dysgenetic malformations are also found.[1355]

Despite the attribution to de Lange, the first report was by Bruck in 1889.

2. (**Bruck–de Lange syndrome**) A syndrome of congenital symmetrical muscular hypertrophy with extra-

pyramidal rigidity and mental retardation, porencephaly, facial dysmorphisms, and decerebrate posturing. Death usually occurs before the end of the second year.[1356]

de Morsier syndrome   1. (posterior diencephalic autonomic epilepsy syndrome) Paroxysmal attacks of muscle rigidity of the trunk and jaws with profuse perspiration.[1381]

2. A syndrome of unilateral disorder of pain and proprioceptive impairment accompanied by photophobia, fatigability, and disturbances of memory and behavior, sometimes with disturbances of the chemical senses, hyperpathia, hallucinations, involuntary movements, and weakness. It is considered to be due to disturbances of the reticular hypothalamic system.[1379]

3. (olfactogenital dysplasia) A rare syndrome characterized by anosmia, seizures, agenesis of the septum pellucidum, optic nerve hypoplasia, pyramidal signs, and neuroendocrine defects such as growth failure, diabetes insipidus, or panhypopituitarism.[1380] See **septo-optic dysplasia.**

De Sanctis, Sante (Carlo)   (1862–1935) Italian neuropsychiatrist born in Umbria and educated in Sienna and Rome. His early career was devoted to studies of neuroanatomy, anthropology, and psychology, after which he trained in psychiatry at the **Salpêtriére** and in Rome, where he eventually became professor of neurology and psychiatry in 1929. He published over 300 papers on the normal and pathological anatomy of the nervous system and on experimental psychology, as well as describing the structure of the mamillary bodies and myelination of the cerebellum. He also studied Down syndrome and childhood epilepsy and schizophrenia in the population of Italy.

De Sanctis–Cacchione syndrome   (xerodermic idiocy) A recessively inherited congenital dysmorphic syndrome manifesting also skin photosensitivity, patchy pigmentation of the skin, telangiectasia, warts and other skin tumors, seizures, microcephaly and cerebral atrophy with ataxia, spasticity, sensory neuropathy, and mental and developmental delay.[1417] See **xeroderma pigmentosum.**

deafferentation   Removal of the afferent processes normally playing upon a nerve cell or neural structure.

deafferentation pain   Dysesthetic pain resulting from incomplete central or peripheral neural injury; pain felt in an area which is partially or completely anesthetic or in the region surrounding it. This implies not only a loss of input but also that actual degeneration has occurred, so that the spinal cord cells are free to act in a pathological way. See **causalgia.**

deafferented bladder   A dilated bladder as a result of, for example, severe autonomic neuropathy, in which the reflex arc maintaining detrusor tone is interrupted on the afferent side, reflex contraction in response to stretch thus being lost.

deafness   Reduction in auditory acuity, due either to abnormality of the afferent nerve pathway (*sensorineural deafness*) or of the mechanically conducting tissue in the middle ear (*middle ear* or *conductive deafness*). See also **cortical deafness, word deafness,** entries listed in Chart D–1, other entries listed under **amyotrophic lateral sclerosis** and **cerebellar ataxia,** and the entries following.

Chart D–1. Hereditary Causes of Deafness

Alport syndrome
Dominant albinism and congenital deafness
Dominant anhidrosis and progressive hearing loss
Dominant congenital severe deafness
Dominant knuckle pads, leukonychia, and hearing loss
Dominant hand weakness with sensorineural deafness
Dominant low-frequency hearing loss
Dominant mid-frequency hearing loss
Dominant photomyoclonus, hearing loss, diabetes, and
  nephropathy
Dominant preauricular pits and neural hearing loss
Dominant progressive nerve deafness
Dominant saddle nose, myopia, cataract, and hearing loss
Dominant unilateral deafness
Familial hemiplegic migraine
Flynn-Aird syndrome
Hereditary motor and sensory neuropathy
Hereditary motor neuropathies
Hereditary photomyoclonus
Hereditary piebaldness and congenital deafness
Hereditary sensory and autonomic neuropathy
Hereditary spastic paraplegia
Herrmann disease
Hittner syndrome
Hutchinson triad
Hyperuricemia, deafness and ataxia
Jervell-Lange-Nielsen syndrome
Mohr-Tranebjaerg syndrome
Mucopolysaccharidoses
Recessive absence of tibia and deafness
Recessive atopic dermatitis and neural hearing loss
Recessive congenital moderate deafness
Recessive congenital severe deafness
Recessive early-onset neural deafness
Recessive goiter and deafness
Recessive malformed low-set ears and conductive deafness
Recessive myopia and deafness
Recessive optic atrophy, hearing loss, and juvenile diabetes
Recessive pili torti and deafness
Recessive retinal changes, deafness, muscular wasting, and
  mental retardation
Red-M syndrome
Richards-Rundle syndrome
Ruzika syndrome
Sylvester syndrome
Usher syndrome
X-linked congenital neural deafness
X-linked early-onset neural deafness
X-linked moderate hearing loss
X-linked pigmentary abnormalities and congenital
  deafness

deafness and atopic dermatitis   A recessively inherited syndrome of moderate congenital neural deafness with the appearance of atopic dermatitis in the second decade.[1117,3124]

deafness and diabetes A progressive but subtotal hearing loss involving first higher then lower frequencies in diabetic subjects. The condition is genetically determined but the association with diabetes may or may not be.[2608]

deafness and ear pits The association of congenital conductive or sensorineural hearing loss inherited as an autosomal dominant characteristic and with the presence of a small pit or sinus present in front of the anterior extremity of the helix on one or both ears.[1918] See **Wildervanck syndrome.**

deafness and goiter See **Pendred syndrome.**

deafness, keratopachydermia, and digital constrictions (Vohwinkel syndrome) A rare syndrome with onset in infancy or early childhood, characterized by palmar and plantar keratoderma with keratosis of the dorsum of the hands and feet, elbows, and knees. Digital bandlike constrictions of the distal interphalangeal creases develop in childhood. High-frequency neural hearing loss is associated.[2104]

deafness, renal and digital anomalies A rare syndrome in which conductive or mixed hearing loss is associated with rudimentary distal phalanges with bifurcations at their distal ends. The condition may be inherited as an autosomal recessive trait. Some members of the single family reported had nephritis.[806]

deafness, stippled epiphyses, and goiter with elevated PBI A congenital metabolic defect characterized by resistance to thyroid hormone action, goiter, profound congenital sensory neural deafness, bird-like facies, pigeon breast, and winged scapulas. Delayed bone age with stippled epiphyses but with normal dental development are reported. The thyroid activity is not associated with high levels of free circulating thyroid hormone.[4630]

deafness-achalasia-vitiligo syndrome A congenital dysmorphic syndrome manifesting also short stature, sensorineural deafness, bulbar palsies, muscle atrophy, and patchy depigmentation of the skin.[337]

deafness-alopecia-hypogonadism syndrome See **Crandall syndrome.**

deafness-ataxia-piebaldness syndrome A congenital dysmorphic syndrome manifesting also patchy depigmentation of the skin and hair, sensorineural deafness, cerebellar ataxia, and mental and developmental delay.[6035]

deafness–diverticulosis–sensory neuropathy syndrome A congenital dysmorphic syndrome manifesting also anencephaly or craniorachischisis, sensorineural deafness, sensorimotor peripheral neuropathy, diverticulosis of the colon, and acanthosis nigricans.[337]

deafness–metaphyseal dysplasia syndrome A congenital dysmorphic syndrome manifesting also short stature, short limbs, coxa valga, genu valgum or varum, brachydactyly, conductive deafness, and mental and developmental delay.[337]

deafness-onychodystrophy-oncholysis-retardation syndrome (DOOR syndrome) A congenital, recessively inherited dysmorphic syndrome manifesting the listed skeletal malformations, profound sensorineural deafness, and mental and developmental delay.[2198]

In a *variant* dominantly inherited form, no seizures occur and the mental status is normal.

deafness-dystonia syndrome (Mohr-Tranebjaerg syndrome) An X-linked disorder characterized by the association of progressive sensoruneural deafness, cortical blindness, dystonia, dysphagia, and paranoia.[5623]

death, cerebral See **brain death.**

debrancher enzyme deficiency See **glycogen storage diseases.**

Debré, Robert (1882–1978) French physician.

Debré-Semelaigne syndrome (Kocher-Debré-Semelaigne syndrome) The association of generalized enlargement of muscles with slow muscle contraction and relaxation and **myoedema** in hypothyroid children.[1324] Intellectual, physical, osseous, and dental development are all retarded and the usual signs of hypothyroidism are usually marked.

The absence of pseudomyotonia and of painful spasms differentiates the condition from **Hoffmann syndrome,** which it otherwise resembles.

decerebrate rigidity An extensor posture of the neck, trunk, and limbs with hyperpronation of the arms and hyperreflexia, adopted by subjects with actual or functional transections of the brainstem below the red nucleus and colliculi but rostral to the vestibular nuclei.

It was first described by **Sherrington** in 1898. See also **decorticate rigidity.**

Dechambre, André (1812–1886) French physician and scientific journalist who graduated from Strasbourg and worked for a period at the Salpêtrière with Cruveilhier. He is remembered for being the first to use the term *lacune* for cystic cavities in the brain (in 1838), and for publication of the *Dictionnaire Encyclopedique des Sciences Medicales,* which ran to 100 volumes. He was elected a member of the French Academie de Médicine in 1875.

declarative learning The learning of facts as opposed to skills, as measured by tests that require explicit recall or recognition of prior events. It is impaired by hippocampal lesions, in **Alzheimer disease,** and as a result of scopolamine administration.

declarative memory The capacity for conscious recollection of previous events and knowledge derived from prior experience.[9] See **explicit memory.**

decomposition See **automatic decomposition EMG.**

decomposition of movement   1. The performance of compound voluntary limb movements slowly, awkwardly, and without the normal flow and smoothness of execution so that the action is separated into its component parts and proceeds joint by joint, leading to the jerky performance of the same. The appearance rather resembles the movements of an unskillfully handled marionette.

It is classically a sign of a lesion of the lateral lobe of the cerebellum, in which case the mechanisms are the same as those for **dysdiadochokinesis.**

2. Delay in the initiation of one component relative to that of another, and excessive range of one element of the movement relative to another, particularly at a proximal joint.[2625]

decompression sickness   (caisson disease, the bends, dysbarism) Diffuse and multifocal disease of the nervous system due to thrombogenic nitrogen emboli forming (particularly in the epidural venous plexuses) as a result of too-rapid decompression after diving or other work done at high levels of atmospheric pressure.[2801]

The condition presents commonly with painful myelopathy but the pathology is widespread within the nervous system. Two types are defined: *type 1* is characterized by fleeting pains in the muscles or joints of the upper more than the lower limbs; pruritus and vascular stasis in the skin; edema; malaise, fatigue and anorexia, and *type 2* represents a far more serious disorder, in which the spinal cord, the brain, or the labyrinths are damaged as the result of gaseous emboli ("air embolism").

Clinical manifestations include altered consciousness, confusion, visual loss, vertigo, weakness, ataxia, sensory loss, and sphincter disturbances. The thoracic cord is the site most frequently affected.[1433]

See also **arterial gas embolism, Divers Alert Network.**

decorticate rigidity   A state of abnormal flexion responses in the arms with or without extensor responses in the legs, resulting from a lesion of the high brainstem.

This modified extensor posture (the neck, trunk, and legs typically being thrust into extension and the arms into flexion) is adopted by subjects with actual or functional transections of the brainstem above the level of the colliculi, or possibly with lesions affecting the cortex diffusely.

decortication   Removal of the cortex from a cerebral hemisphere.

decremental response   See **decrementing response.**

decrementing response   (decremental response) A reproducible decline in the amplitude and/or area of the M wave of successive responses to repetitive nerve stimulation. The rate of stimulation and the total number of stimuli should be specified. Decrementing re-

sponses with disorders of neuromuscular transmission are most reliably seen with slow rates (2 to 5 Hz) of nerve stimulation. A decrementing response with repetitive nerve stimulation commonly occurs in disorders of neuromuscular transmission, but can also be seen in some neuropathies, myopathies, and motor neuron disease. An artifact resembling a decrementing response can result from movement of the stimulating or recording electrodes during repetitive nerve stimulation (see pseudodecrement). cf. **incrementing response.** (From the 2001 Report of the Nomenclature Committee of the American Association of Electromyography and Electrodiagnosis.[10]

decubitus   (from Lat, to lie down) The lying or recumbent posture.

decussate   (from Lat, to divide across) The crossing of fibers such as nerve fibers; the term is usually applied when it is the midline that is crossed.

de-efferented state   See **locked-in syndrome.**

deep cerebral venous thrombosis   Occlusion of the deep internal cerebral vein, the vein of Galen, extending towards the straight sinus. Clinically, headache, altered consciousness, papilledema, hemisensory disturbances, and hemipareses are the usual features and the condition is often lethal. Computed tomography scans show large bilateral thalamocapsular hypodensities.[2374]

deep dyslexia   (phonemic dyslexia, phonological dyslexia) An acquired reading disorder in which patients substitute synonyms for the written words they are reading aloud (**semantic paralexia**). Abundant word substitutions (verbal paraphasias) occur, with a difficulty in linking the visual form of words with their phonological structure as shown by the inability of affected people to read nonsense words, identify homophones, and appreciate rhyme. Dysphasia, dysgraphia, and a variety of parietal lobe signs such as acalculia and constructional apraxia are also commonly associated.[1109]

The syndrome reflects posterior parietal lesions of the dominant hemisphere and may appear during the recovery stage after global alexia.[1109] See also **alexia.**

deep dysphasia   A disorder of language characterized by the making of semantic errors when heard speech is repeated. Errors are most pronounced when single words are repeated, less so during the repetition of phrases.[856]

deep radial nerve paralysis   See **posterior interosseous syndrome.**

deep sleep   1. Sleep in non–rapid eye movement stages 3 or 4. 2. The rapid eye movement sleep state.

deep tendon reflex   One of the most ubiquitous misnomers in clinical neurology, not only because it is the superficial rather than the deep tendons that are tapped in clinical practice, but because stimulation of the afferent neurons from tendons causes inhibition of muscle activity rather than muscle contraction; the tendons have nothing to do with the reflex, except that they provide a site from which to stimulate the muscle stretch receptors. Either *muscle stretch reflex* or (as favored by Sherrington) *myotatic reflex* is a preferable term. See **muscle stretch reflex.**

deep toe reflex   (Rossolimo reflex) Flexion and abduction of the toes in response to percussion of their ends; a minor sign, found in some patients with upper motor neuron lesions.

defecation syncope   A form of situational syncope in which typically the rise in intrathoracic pressure required by those with a tendency to constipation decreases cardiac venous return, cardiac output, and thus cerebral perfusion, leading to syncope.

defense reaction   Threatening, aggressive display as a result of stimulation of the amygdaloid and local limbic circuit nuclei in experimental animals.

deficient sellar diaphragm   See **empty sella syndrome.**

definite multiple sclerosis   See **clinically definite multiple sclerosis.**

definition   A brief description of the consistent attributes of an object which allow it to be differentiated from other objects.

deformation   An abnormal form, shape, or position of a part of the body developing as a result of mechanical force.

degenerate   Departing from the virtues of ones ancestors.

degeneration   (from Lat, changing for the worse) A morbid condition of a body part that becomes less differentiated and eventually undergoes transformation to unspecialized tissue, atrophies, and dies.

degenerative dementias   Disorders of the brain characterized by the decay and death of neurons leading to cognitive impairment. The following listing of these has been suggested:[1772]
1. **Alzheimer disease** (AD)
2. Dementia with Lewy bodies (DLB)
3. **Frontotemporal degenerations**
   i. Pick disease
   ii. Frontotemporal dementia with motor neuron disease (MND)
   iii. Corticobasal degeneration (CBD)
   iv. Primary progressive aphasia (PPA)
4. Vascular dementia (VaD)
   i. Lacunar disease
   ii. Multiinfarct type (large vessel)
   iii. **Binswanger disease**
   iv. Watershed ischemia
   v. Strategic infarcts
   vi. Anoxic encephalopathy
   vii. **Amyloid angiopathy**
   viii. Cerebral angiitis
   ix. **CADASIL**
   x. Other
5. Mixed dementia (more than one of the above)
   i. AD and VaD
   ii. AD and DLB
6. Other degenerative dementias
   i. **Huntington disease**
   ii. **Progressive supranuclear palsy**
   iii. **Parkinson disease**

degenerative spinal stenosis   Narrowing of the diameter of the spinal canal, usually at multiple lumbar levels, due to local degenerative disease. Clinical features include back pain aggravated by standing and relieved by rest and forward flexion, **neurogenic claudication,** and a posture of persistent flexion of the lumbar spine.

degenerative spondylolisthesis   Forward displacement of L4 on L5 without a break in the pars interarticularis, a cause of **lumbar spinal stenosis.**[1974]

deglutition   (Lat, down + swallow) Swallowing.

deglutition syncope   (swallow syncope) Syncope provoked by swallowing, commonly in association with esophageal lesions. Atrioventricular block and sinus bradycardia are the usual mechanisms, triggered by reflexes arising in the esophagus.[5963]

Degos syndrome   See **malignant atrophic papulosis.**

Deiters nucleus   The lateral vestibular nucleus of the pons, which gives rise to the lateral vestibulospinal tract, excitatory to those anterior horn cells innervating extensor muscles.

Deiters nucleus syndrome   See **Bonnier syndrome.**

Deiters, Otto Frederick Karl   (1834–1863) German anatomist. He studied under **Virchow** in Berlin and quickly became professor of anatomy and histology at the University of Bonn, but died young of typhoid. Deiters was the first to identify axons in the anterior roots, which he differentiated from dendrites in 1865. He also identified astrocytes and showed that axis cylinders form the core of the nerve fiber and emanate from the nerve cells.

déjà vécu   (Fr, already lived) A broader experience than **déjà vu** in which the subject falsely recalls having previously experienced a current situation.

Such a symptom (usually due to epileptic discharges in a temporal lobe) is not a misinterpretation of sense impressions but an inappropriate judgment, and thus is better regarded as delusional than as illusory.

déjà vu   (Fr, already seen) A French phrase indicating prior awareness of an event. In neurology it is synonymous with the aura of partial seizures with temporal lobe origin. Phenomenologically, déjà vu can be regarded as a delusion of recognition.

Dejean syndrome (orbital floor syndrome) The occurrence of exophthalmos, diplopia, maxillary pain and trigeminal (maxillary) sensory loss due to a mass lesion or a **blowout fracture** of the orbital floor.[1337]

Déjèrine, Joseph-Jules (1849–1917) Parisian neurologist born in Savoy who lived his early life in Switzerland, later training in Paris under **Vulpian** whose favorite student he became. After internship he was appointed agrégé at the faculty of medicine and eventually professor of diseases of the nervous system at the **Salpêtrière** after **Raymond.** He married Augusta (**Déjèrine-**) **Klumpke,** an American physician whom he met at the Salpêtrière, and she shared fully in all their clinical and research activities, continuing them after his death in 1917 as a result of exhaustion arising from his work in the wards of a military hospital.

His wide experience with neurological conditions is suggested by the following entries; he also classified **alexia** into forms with and without agraphia, and that form accompanying Broca aphasia (**third alexia**).[2532] Less well known but of even greater value was his work on the anatomy of the nervous system, on cerebral localization, and on the clinical features of numerous neurological diseases.

Joseph-Jules Déjèrine

Déjèrine neurotabes A form of combined anterior and posterior radiculopathy in which there is selective initial involvement of large fibers subserving deep sensibility, associated with paraparesis, in patients with syphilis.[1338] See **Déjèrine syndromes,** definition 4.

Déjèrine sign Acute pain in the neck on sneezing, as though something had torn; evidence of the precipitation of radicular pain by sudden changes in intraspinal pressure, usually, in this context, due to cervical radiculopathy.[1340]

Déjèrine syndromes 1. (anterior bulbar syndrome, pyramid-hypoglossal syndrome, alternating hypoglossal-hemiplegia, medial medullary syndrome) A brainstem syndrome due to infarction of the paramedian region of the medulla as a result of occlusion of branches of the vertebral or anterior spinal arteries. The clinical features include homolateral hypoglossal palsy, **alternating hemiplegia,** and sometimes involvement of the medial lemniscus. See also **Jackson syndrome, alternating hypoglossal hemiplegia syndrome.**[2592] It has also been reported in patients with meningovascular syphilis.[5512] A further complete dissection of the syndromes arising with medial medullary strokes has been published.[382]

2. (*parietal lobe syndrome*) Astereognosis and impaired tactile localization and proprioception, with retention of the senses of temperature, crude light touch, and pain.[1339]

3. Diphtheritic neuropathy.

4. (radiculitis, **Déjèrine** *neurotabes*) A form of combined anterior and posterior radiculopathy in which there is selective initial involvement of large fibers subserving deep sensibility, associated with paraparesis in patients with syphilis.[1338]

5. **Facioscapulohumeral muscular dystrophy** (Landouzy-Déjèrine syndrome).

6. See **Verger-Déjèrine syndrome.**

Déjèrine-Klumpke, Augusta (1859–1927) American neurologist from San Francisco, the wife of J-J. **Déjèrine,** who trained and did postgraduate work as the first woman *interne des hôpitaux* in Paris, despite strong resistance from the medical establishment. Her graduation thesis was on lead neuropathy.

Much of the work of her husband reflected her interest and advice; her own report of lower brachial plexus palsy was written in 1885, 3 years before her marriage. With J-J. Déjèrine she published an atlas of cerebral anatomy based on their meticulous dissections. After his death, she worked mainly on spinal cord diseases with her daughter, also a physician.[7]

Déjèrine-Klumpke palsy See **Klumpke palsy.**

Déjèrine-Mouzon syndrome See **Verger-Déjèrine syndrome.**

Déjèrine-Roussy syndrome See **thalamic syndrome.**

Déjèrine-Sottas syndrome See **hereditary motor and sensory neuropathy, type 3.**

Déjèrine-Thomas syndrome (cortical cerebellar degeneration, delayed cerebellar ataxia) A form of **olivopontocerebellar atrophy** occuring in adults, in which imbalance, gait disturbance, hyperreflexia with downgoing plantar responses, truncal ataxia, and eventual immobility develop. Cerebellar intention tremor is not seen, extraocular movements are preserved, and the posterior columns function normally. Histologically, the cerebellum and pons are atrophic.[1346]

The absence of a positive family history in the original report calls into question the familial nature of the condition. See **cerebellar ataxias.**

DeJong, Russel, N. (1906–1990) American neurologist of Dutch ancestry who received his under- and postgraduate training at the University of Michigan, where he later was to become chairman of the department of neurology.

He was a founder of the **American Academy of Neurology** and was a painstaking and successful editor as well as teacher and clinician. He served as the (first) editor of *Neurology,* for 26 years, but is even better remembered as the author of *The Neurological Examination,* a classic text which since its first publication has been the ultimate source of information on the clinical examination of the nervous system.

Delamarre, Georges French physician who described gastric crises in tabes with Pierre **Marie** in his graduation thesis (1866).

de Lange, Cornelia Catherina (1871–1950) Dutch pediatrician who graduated from Amsterdam University and worked in Zurich before returning, eventually becoming professor of pediatrics.

de Lange syndrome 1. (*de Lange–Brachmann syndrome,* Cornelia de Lange syndrome, Amsterdam dwarfism) A sporadic dysmorphic syndrome, characterized by growth retardation from conception and postnatally, with severely diminished stature, always below the third percentile, severe mental retardation, facial dysmorphism, antimongoloid slant to the eyes, syndactyly, flexion contractures of the elbows, **clinodactyly,** microbrachycephaly, transverse palmar crease, synophrys, and generalized hirsutism.[1355]

2. (*Bruck–de Lange syndrome*) Congenital muscular hypertrophy, mental retardation, and extrapyramidal disorders (hypertonia) with broad and thick neck and limbs, low hairline, and asymmetrical skull due to porencephaly. Various cerebral dysgenetic malformations are also found.[1356]

Despite the attribution to de Lange, the first report (acknowledged by her) was that of Dr. Franz Bruck in 1889.

delay The interval between the beginning of the horizontal sweep of the oscilloscope and the onset of an applied stimulus. See also **delay line.**[10]

delay line An information storage device used to display events that occur before a trigger signal. This is a method for displaying repetitive waveforms at the same point on a sweep on a free-running electromyogram.[10]

delayed cerebellar ataxia See **Déjèrine-Thomas syndrome.**

delayed cerebral edema Severe, possibly fatal cerebral edema following relatively minor trauma and after a lucid interval, occurring in young people. The ge-

netic basis for this rare condition is the same as that for **familial hemiplegic migraine** and involves a mutation in the *CACNA1* calcium channel subunit gene on chromosome 19.[3134]

delayed cortical cerebellar atrophy See **Déjèrine-Thomas syndrome.**

delayed cramps and fasciculation A syndrome of benign cramps, exercise-related myalgia, fasciculations, and sometimes denervation hypertrophy but without new weakness, following prior poliomyelitis or myelitis.[1787]

delayed deterioration of consciousness An unusual syndrome seen in infants and small children, characterized by progressive reduction in consciousness hours or days after a trivial head injury.[2351] See **spät-apoplexy.**

delayed measles encephalitis The acute onset of neurological signs with intractable focal seizures and coma and a fatal outcome occurring in children within months of an attack of measles. The anti-measles antibody titers are high and the virus is not recoverable.[3533]

delayed myotonia Myotonia that only appears after a period of muscle contraction, as in **myotonia fluctuans.**

delayed post-traumatic myelitis of Gowers See **railway spine.**

delayed recall A learning test sensitive to left temporal lobe lesions.

delayed recognition span test A memory test in which the subject is required to remember a lengthening series of disks bearing various stimuli (such as words, faces and designs) added to each other upon a board, recognizing each addition as such. The subject then tries to recall the words written on it, both immediately and after a further 2 minutes. The latter part of the test differentiates between patients with **Alzheimer disease** and those with other conditions such as **Huntington disease** and **Korsakoff syndrome.**[4016]

delayed sleep phase syndrome (phase lag, phase delay, sleep-onset insomnia, morning sleepiness) A **circadian rhythm sleep disorder** characterized by a chronic disturbance of circadian sleep scheduling, manifest as a persistent and consistent delay in the times of sleep onset and of waking, but with normal sleep architecture. This leads to complaints of being unable to sleep until, for example, the early morning ("night people"), sleep then continuing unless interrupted for a physiological period,[5907] and of excessive daytime sleepiness when the subject's intrinsic pattern is forced into the conventional scheme. The condition affects mainly adolescents.

Diagnostic criteria have been suggested[234] (see Chart D–2). See also **ASDA** Diagnostic Classification, **sleep disorders.**[234]

Chart D–2. Delayed Sleep Phase Syndrome

A. The patient complains of an inability to fall asleep at the desired clock time, or inability to awaken spontaneously at the desired time of awakening, or excessive sleepiness.

B. There is a phase delay of the major sleep episode in relation to the desired time for sleep.

C. Symptoms are present for at least 1 month.

D. When not required to maintain a strict schedule (e.g., vacation time), patients will
   1. Have a habitual sleep period that is sound and of normal quality and duration;
   2. Awaken spontaneously;
   3. Maintain stable entrainment to a 24-hour sleep–wake pattern at a delayed phase.

E. There is evidence of a delay in the timing of the habitual sleep period illustrated on daily sleep logs for a period of at least 2 weeks.

F. Laboratory evidence of a delay in the timing of the habitual sleep period is given by
   1. Twenty-four hour polysomnographic monitoring (or by means of two consecutive nights of polysomnography and an intervening multiple sleep latency test); or
   2. Continuous temperature monitoring showing that the time of the absolute temperature nadir is delayed into the second half of the habitual (delayed) sleep episode.

G. The syndrome does not meet criteria for any other sleep disorder causing inability to initiate sleep or excessive sleepiness.

Adapted from The International Classification of Sleep Disorders Diagnostic and Coding Manual. *Rochester, MN: American Sleep Disorders Association, © 1990. Reproduced by kind permission of the American Academy of Sleep Medicine.*

delayed-onset cerebellar syndrome   The rare occurrence of ataxia and intention tremor 3 weeks to 2 years after stroke or head injury. Dystonia and myoclonus are other complications known.[3478]

Deléage disease   See **myotonic dystrophy.**

deletion 4p   See **Wolf-Hirschorn syndrome.**

delirium   (Lat, from + a furrow; thus, to deviate from the straight course) A transient disruption of global cognitive functioning characterized by the acute onset of alterations in attention and arousal and disordered thinking, with a fluctuating course. The **Glasgow Coma scale** scores will be 4-5-4.

Characteristic clinical features include inattention, disorganization of thinking shown by rambling and irrelevant speech, clouded consciousness, perceptual disorders (hallucinations), alterations in the sleep–wake cycle and in psychomotor status, disorientation, and impairment of memory, cognition, perception, and behavior (e.g., motor restlessness).

Nocturnal worsening, an inability to grasp and retain information for events, labile emotions, fear and restlessness, auditory and visual hallucinations, insomnia, and paranoid ideation are typical features. Celsus used the term first in this way; today a popular (if inaccurate) name for the syndrome is *confusion.*

It is caused both by primarily neurological disorders such as meningitis, brain tumor, or stroke, and by multitudinous metabolic diseases such as fever, infection, drug administration or withdrawal, vitamin deficiency, liver, lung and renal failure, hypoglycemia, and electrolyte disturbances, and is especially common in the elderly and those recovering from vascular surgery or in pain.[5506] More than one of these causes coexist in most instances. The subtypes of delirium depicted in Mayne's Lexicon[4512] are numerous and include *acute* or *furiosum,* which represent mania; *cum massitania* (muttering, once regarded as specific for typhoid fever); *febrile,* in association with fevers; *ferox,* when accompanied by violent anger; *grandiosum,* in which the delusions are of personal power or riches, as in general paresis; *persecutionis,* in which the patient has delusions that others are conspiring against him; **tremens;** and *sympathetic,* the delirium occurring in the setting of acute general illness. A full description was that of Trenel.[5631] See also **confusional state.**

Two sets of diagnostic criteria have been published, in the International Classification of Diseases (ICD)[6041] (http://www.cdc.gov/nchs/about/otheract/icd9/abticd9.htm) and by the American Psychiatric Association (DSM-IV).[150] See Charts D–3 and D–4.

Chart D–3. ICD-10 Diagnostic Criteria for Delirium

For a definite diagnosis, symptoms, mild or severe, should be present in each one of the following areas:

A. Impairment of consciousness and attention (on a continuum from clouding to coma; reduced ability to direct, focus, sustain, and shift attention)

B. Global disturbance cognition (perceptual distortions, illusions, and hallucinations, most often visual; impairment of abstract thinking and comprehension, with or without transient delusions, but typically with some degree of incoherence; impairment of immediate recall and of recent memory but with relatively intact remote memory; disorientation for time as well as, in more severe cases, for place and person)

C. Psychomotor disturbances (hypo- or hyperactivity and unpredictable shifts from one to the other, increased reaction time; increased or decreased flow of speech; enhanced startle reaction)

D. Disturbance of the sleep–wake cycle (insomnia or, in more severe cases, total sleep loss or reversal of the sleep–wake cycle; daytime drowsiness; nocturnal worsening of symptoms; disturbing dreams or nightmares, which may continue as hallucinations after awakening)

E. Emotional disturbances—for example, depression, anxiety or fear, irritability, euphoria, apathy, or wondering perplexity

The onset is usually rapid, the course diurnally fluctuating and the total duration of the condition less than 6 months. The above clinical picture is so characteristic that a fairly confident diagnosis of delirium can be made even if the underlying cause is not firmly established.

In addition to a history of an underlying physical or brain disease, evidence of cerebral dysfunction (such as an abnormal electroencephalogram, usually but not invariably showing slowing of the background activity) may be required if the diagnosis is in doubt.

Chart D–4. Diagnostic Criteria for Delirium

(Abstracted from the *Diagnostic and Statistical Manual of Mental Disorders, Fourth Edition, Text Revision,* (APA DSM-4 TR[150]) by kind permission of the American Psychiatric Association, Washington, DC. Copyright 2000.

1. Disturbance in consciousness, resulting in
2. Reduced ability to maintain attention to external stimuli and to appropriately shift attention to new external stimuli. Thus there must be present at least 1 of:
   Questions have to be repeated because attention wanders.
   Perseverated answers to previous questions
   Disorganized thinking
   Confusion developed over a short period of time
   Fluctuating severity

And at least 2 of:
Reduced level of consciousness
Perceptual disturbances
Disturbance of sleep–wake cycle
Increased or decreased psychomotor activity
Disorientation to time, place, or person
Memory impairment

And either of the following:
Evidence that an organic factor (a general medical condition) initiated and maintained this confusion, which cannot be accounted for by any non-organic mental disorder

Delirium due to an underlying general medical condition is characterized by;

1. Disturbance of consciousness (i.e., reduced clarity of awareness of the environment) with reduced ability to focus, sustain or shift attention.
2. A change in cognition (such as memory deficit, disorientation, language disturbance) or the development of a perceptual disturbance that is not better accounted for by a preexisting, established, or evolving dementia.
3. The disturbance develops over a short period of time (usually hours to days) and tends to fluctuate during the course of the day.
4. There is evidence from the history, physical examination, or laboratory findings that the disturbance is caused by the direct physiological consequences of a general medical condition.

See also **hepatic encephalopathy.**

delirium alcoholicum   See **delirium tremens.**

delirium cum massitania   See **delirium.**

delirium e potu   See **delirium tremens.**

delirium ferox   See **delirium.**

delirium furiosum   See **mania.**

delirium grandiosum   See **delirium.**

delirium persecutionis   See **delirium.**

delirium potatorum   See **delirium tremens.**

Delirium Rating scale

A symptom rating scale for delirium:[5652]

1. Temporal onset of symptoms
2. Perceptual disturbances
3. Hallucination type
4. Delusions
5. Psychomotor behavior
6. Cognitive state during formal testing
7. Physical disorder
8. Sleep-wake cycle disturbances
9. Lability of mood
10. Variability of symptoms

Items 1–5 and 9 are rated 0–2; items 6, 8, and 10 are rated 0–4; item 7 is rated 0–2.

From Trzepacz PT, Baker RW, Greenhouse JA. A symptom rating scale for delirium. *J. Psychiatr. Res.* 1987;**23**:89–97. © 1987. With permission from Elsevier Science.

See also **Confusional Assessment method.**

delirium tremens   (Lat, trembling) (Saunders-Sutton syndrome, delirium alcoholicum, delirium potatorum, delirium è potu, ebriositatis) An acute organic psychosis characterized by tremors, delirium, visual hallucinations, pallor, sweating, tachycardia, restless excitement and anxiety, anorexia, and mental distress as a result of chronic alcoholism, especially following withdrawal.

Delirium tremens was possibly the basis of the Bacchanalian frenzies described by the ancient Greek writers. The first modern description was that of Samuel Burton Pearson, a physician in Newcastle (fl. 1800), in his privately circulated pamphlet *Observations on Brain Fever* (1801). Pearson advocated treatment with wine, opium, and nourishing soups together with a minimum of restraint.[5429] The English physician Thomas Sutton (1767–1835) gave a fuller description and introduced the term in 1813 for that form of delirium made worse by bleeding and improved by opium. See also **delirium.**

Delleman syndrome   (orbital cysts and cerebral malformation) A congenital dysmorphic syndrome manifesting also microphthalmia, bifid ribs, hydranencephaly, callosal abnormalities, seizures, patchy aplasia of the skin, and mental and developmental delay.[337]

delta band   A frequency band under 4 Hz applied to EEG recordings.

delta rebound   An increase in the amount of delta sleep that occurs after deprivation of this sleep stage.

delta rhythm   (Gr, the letter *D,* a triangle) Slow waveforms on the EEG, at or less than 3.5 Hz. Focal delta activity suggests brain pathology at that site. When diffuse, delta activity usually indicates degenerative or biochemical disease.

delta sleep   The third and deepest stage of non–rapid eye movement sleep, characterized by the appearance of high-amplitude slow waves at 0.5–2 Hz occupying about a fifth of the time of a nocturnal sleep recording.

delta wave   An EEG wave with a duration >250 msec.

deltoid reflex   Abduction of the shoulder in response to a smart tap on the humerus at the level of the insertion of the deltoid. Normally this is not visible, but the amplitude of the reflex is increased in patients with a pyramidal tract lesion above C5.

delusion   (Lat, a deception) An erroneous belief, tenaciously held in the face of logical counterargument. Usually it suggests the presence of a psychiatric disorder such as schizophrenic or depressive illness, but delusions may occur in states of delirium (confusion) and other organic brain diseases causing dementia.

delusional memory   1. A false memory arising in the context of a psychosis. 2. A deluded interpretation of a true memory. In either case, the difference from spontaneous confabulation is hard to determine.

delusional parasitosis   A syndrome in which patients are convinced beyond all logic and persuasion that they are harboring parasites. (HJM)[3526]

demarcation potential   See **injury potential.**

dementia   (Lat, out of + the mind) An acquired, persistent, more or less global impairment of intellectual, emotional, conative and cognitive functioning due to biochemical or diffuse structural disease of the brain, occurring in the alert state and leading to functional incapacity.

Some authorities suggest that any three of language, memory, visuospatial skills, emotion, personality, and cognition should be affected to make the diagnosis. In mental status testing, examination of the level of arousal, orientation, recent and remote memory, language, praxis, visuospatial abilities, calculation and judgment are necessary to make the clinical diagnosis.

The American Psychiatric Association DSM III criteria required the presence of multiple cognitive deficits including memory impairment *and* at least one of:

Aphasia, apraxia or agnosia

A disturbance in executive functioning

The loss of intellectual abilities of sufficient severity to interfere with social or occupational functioning and must represent a decline from a higher level of functioning.

Previous definitions required at least one of the following: Impairment of abstract thinking as manifested by the concrete interpretation of proverbs, inability to find similarities and differences between related words and other similar tasks, impaired judgment, other disturbances of higher cortical function, personality changes, and no clouding of consciousness. See *Diagnostic and Statistical Manual of Mental Disorders, Fourth Edition, Text Revision. American Psychiatric Association Washington, DC.*

The word was first used in the modern sense by the French psychiatrist Pinel, before which time it was taken to mean all kinds of mental disease. Kraepelin (a German psychiatrist) later distinguished the schizophrenias and depressive reactions, while keeping the word *dementia* as their prefix.

The causes of dementia include numerous medical and metabolic diseases, including the effect of toxic agents as well as diseases of the CNS.[1213] **Alzheimer disease** is the most common single cause. The first treatable form recognized was the dementia of **pellagra.**

Dementia Behaviour Disturbance Scale   An instrument designed to measure behavioral disturbances in patients with severe dementia.[396]

dementia guidelines   New dementia guidelines released by the American Academy of Neurology designed to facilitate early detection, diagnosis, and treatment options for dementia patients and their families. The full text with data, tables, and summaries for physicians, patients, family, and friends is available at www.aan.com/public/practiceguidelines.

dementia infantilis   See **Heller disease.**

dementia lacking distinctive histologic features (DLDH) An uncommon primary cerebral degenerative condition involving multiple sites and presenting with memory loss and personality changes, leading to dysphagia and dysarthria after a course of between 2 and 7 years.

Pathologically, the condition is characterized by cell loss and astrocytosis in the frontoparietal cortex, striatum, medial thalamus, substantia nigra, and hypoglossal nucleus; but neuronal inclusions, neurofibrillary tangles, and senile plaques are not seen.

The degree of overlap between this condition and **frontotemporal dementia, Pick disease without Pick bodies, nonspecific degeneration, dementia with ALS,** and **dysphasic dementia** is not defined but is likely to be considerable.[3100]

Dementia Mood Assessment Scale   An objective measure of mood in cognitively impaired subjects, though not a diagnostic instrument for depression. Seven of the 24 items are concerned with providing an indication of the severity of dementia. Scores for the factors of depression, social interaction, anxiety, and vegetative symptoms can be extracted.[5417]

dementia of frontal lobe type   See **frontotemporal dementia.**

dementia paralytica   (general paralysis of the insane, Bayle disease) Tertiary syphilis, first described by Thomas **Willis** and later by Antoine **Bayle,** a French physician in 1822. It was discovered to be a syphilitic affection by Jean Fournier, a French syphilologist in 1894. See **general paralysis of the insane.**

dementia pugilistica   See **punch-drunk syndrome.**

Dementia Rating Scale   (Mattis Dementia Rating Scale) A short, practical, formalized, bedside screening test instrument designed to assess cognitive dysfunction, particularly memory and behavior.[3711]

The scale is a shortened form of Mattis' much longer organic mental syndrome screening test battery, of value in the evaluation of severely demented patients. Five subscales (attention, perseveration and initiation, construction, conceptualization and verbal and nonverbal memory) comprise the test. The perseveration item strengthens it in comparison to almost all others, although there remains a substantial false-negative rate.

See also **Blessed Rating Scale, Mini-Mental State Exam, Wechsler Adult Intelligence Scale, Brief Cognitive Rating Scale, Clinical Dementia Rating Scale, Alzheimer Disease Assessment Scale.**

Dementia Research Group A professional group based at the **National Hospital for Neurology and Neurosurgery** in London. Web site: www.dementia.ion.ucl.ac.uk.

dementia syndrome of depression The occurrence of intermittent confusion and memory impairment in a person (usually elderly) suffering from a primary depressive illness as a complication of the early stages of **Alzheimer disease.** Although these signs are reversible with appropriate antidepressant therapy, other evidence of the underlying dementia surfaces within a year or two.[4624]

dementia, vertical gaze palsy, copper dysmetabolism syndrome See **Willvonseder syndrome.**

dementia with ALS See **frontal lobe dementia.**

dementia with argyrophilic grains A syndrome of progressive dementia resembling **Alzheimer disease** or **Pick disease** but characterized by the presence of argyrophilic grains (granular filaments staining with Alz-50 monoclonal antibody) throughout the cerebral cortex rather than senile plaques, neurofibrillary tangles, or Pick bodies characteristic in such types of dementia.[2759]

dementia with lobar atrophy and neuronal cytoplasmic inclusions See **Pick disease.**

dementia with Parkinson disease See **parkinsonism.**

dementia with widespread neurofibrillary tangles A dominantly inherited, slowly progressive neurodegenerative disease characterized by early-onset dementia resembling that of **Alzheimer disease** but with pathological features resembling **progressive supranuclear palsy.** The condition may be classified as a tauopathy.[4627]

demilunes of Adamkiewicz Crescent-shaped cells lying beneath the neurilemma of medullated nerve fibers, described by **Adamkiewicz** in 1885.

de Morsier syndromes 1. A syndrome comprising mental fatigability, memory disturbances, hallucinations, disorders of perception, hyperosmia, hyperacusis, and gait disturbances, considered by de Morsier to

result from damage to the hypothalamus, but not now known to have any specific pathology.[1394] See **post-traumatic syndrome.** 2. See **sensorimotor psychological syndrome.**[1381] 3. (olfactogenital dysplasia) A congenital dysmorphic syndrome manifesting also agenesis of the olfactory lobe and corpus callosum and eunuchoidism.[1380]

demyelinating motor neuropathy A syndrome of asymmetrical multifocal lower motor neuron lesions closely resembling **multifocal motor neuropathy with conduction block.** In fact, many of the patients have anti-GM_1 antibodies. The following criteria for the diagnosis have been suggested:[3632]

Asymmetric lower motor neuron type limb weakness
Chronic progressive course
Absence of pyramidal and of sensory findings
Electrical evidence of both axonal and demyelinating pathology, and sometimes multifocal conduction block

demyelinating neuropathies One of the two major forms of peripheral neuropathy distinguished by primary and selective attack upon the Schwann cells leading to **segmental demyelination** and sometimes to the formation of **onion bulbs.** See also **axonal neuropathies.**

demyelinating polyneuropathy with IgM binding to GalNAc-GD$_{1a}$ and GM$_2$ gangliosides A rare, distal, symmetrical sensorimotor neuropathy of adult life presenting with gait disorder and distal pan-sensory loss, mild weakness, areflexia, and cerebellar signs. The course is slowly progressive over years. Electrodiagnostic testing shows the demyelinating neuropathy. A serum M protein is detectable. More information is at http://www.wustl.edu/neuromuscular. See **monoclonal gammopathy of uncertain significance.**

demyelination Loss of myelin, which in the CNS is due to disease affecting the oligodendroglia and in the peripheral nervous system, to that affecting the Schwann cells. *Primary demyelination* is due to disorders that selectively damage myelin itself or the cells that form it. *Secondary demyelination* refers to the breakdown of myelin following axonal degeneration (see **Wallerian degeneration**).

The electrodiagnostic criteria[768] for demyelination in peripheral nerves are listed under **acute inflammatory demyelinating polyneuropathy.** They include complete or partial conduction block, slowed conduction, failure to transmit high-frequency impulses, and the occurrence of **ephaptic transmission.**

dendrite (Gr, tree or plant) The small, many-branched afferent processes leading back to the neuronal cell body.

denervation 1. The separation of a structure that is normally innervated from its nerve supply. The term is usually employed for the changes in muscle separated in this way from its motor nerve supply, which include atrophy and loss of contractile ability clinically, an increase in the number of acetylcholine receptor sites on the muscle membrane, and a decrease in the resting membrane potential physiologically.

2. Electromyographically, the presence of increased insertional activity, abnormal spontaneous activity at rest (fibrillations and positive sharp waves), reduced recruitment of **motor unit potentials** with increased amplitude, abnormally long duration, polyphasia, and a high firing rate.

denervation hypertrophy   An increase in the volume of partially denervated muscles, most often seen in cases of long-standing disease of the lower motor neuron, in which muscle biopsy specimens show both myofibrillar atrophy and hypertrophy.

Whether this hypertrophy is due to stretch or to excessive work performed by the residual myofibrils is not known. In cases of **myokymia** or **pseudomyotonia,** continuous muscle work is considered to be the likely explanation.

denervation potential   See **fibrillation potential, positive sharp wave.**

dengue   An infectious disease occurring in the Orient and in Africa, transmitted by mosquitoes and due to members of the dengue group of viruses.

Clinically, it is manifest by a remitting and relapsing course with severe prostrating head and eye pains, chemosis, corneal ulceration, conjunctivitis, lymphadenopathy, desquamating erysipeloid skin rashes, muscle pain, severe malaise, and flitting arthropathy.

denial of illness   Any condition or illness that is not acknowledged by the patient, although a healthy subject could be expected to be aware of it. This suggests an active or almost delusional process, especially since some subjects may be aware, for example, of paresis of an arm but deny any problem in their equally paretic leg. Associated sensory and/or cognitive deficits are also usually present.[1642]

The phenomenon was described first by **Anton** in 1898 with reference to his patients who were unaware of blindness. See **anosognosia,** the term suggested by **Babinski.** See also **neglect.**

Dennie, Charles Clayton   (1883–1917) American dermatologist.

Dennie-Marfan syndrome   (congenital syphilitic paralysis) Incomplete spastic or flaccid pareses of the legs, mental retardation, seizures, nystagmus, and cataracts occurring in children with **congenital syphilis.**[1388]

Dennis syndrome   A congenital dysmorphic syndrome manifesting mental retardation, sparse hair, joint laxity, seizures, early closure of the fontanelles, and developmental delay.

Denny-Brown, Derek Ernest   (1901–1981) New Zealand–born neurophysiologist and neurologist who trained in medicine at Otago and then worked under **Sherrington** at Oxford, where he developed his interest in the control of motor systems, posture, and muscle physiology. After training further in neurology at the **National Hospital** and at Guy's Hospital under **Holmes** and Symonds, he was appointed to the National and to St. Bartholomew's Hospitals as neurologist in 1935, spending the following year at Yale on a Rockefeller fellowship.

He was at first unable to take up the James Jackson Putnam Chair of Neurology at Harvard, which he was offered in 1939, because of his wartime responsibility for setting up the medical side of the Head Injuries Research Unit at Oxford, but did so in 1941, returning to England in 1945 for a year to study nutritional deficits in prisoners of war. Thereafter he continued his clinical and laboratory activities at Boston City Hospital.

Among the areas of his particular research success one may include the treatment of **Wilson disease** with British anti-Lewisite, his description of the **hereditary sensory and autonomic neuropathies,** electromyography, **paraneoplastic syndromes,** parietal lobe functions, and stroke syndromes and his continuing studies on the central and peripheral control of movement. Denny-Brown was also universally respected as a clinician and as an inspiring teacher of undergraduates and of neurologists in training.[1903,2082]

Denny-Brown syndrome   1. **hereditary sensory and autonomic neuropathy, type 1.** 2. **paraneoplastic sensory neuropathy** with polymyositis.[1391]

Denny-Brown-Foley syndrome   A syndrome of benign fasciculations with cramps, unassociated with other evidence of neurological disease, and of unknown cause.[1401] See **benign fasciculations and cramps.**

dens   (Lat, a tooth) The tooth-like process pointing upward from the axis, covered by the transverse ligament of the atlas and helping to maintain stability of the head on the neck.

dense triangle sign   An area of density seen posteriorly within the superior sagittal sinus on an unenhanced CT scan in patients with thrombosis of this sinus. See also **empty delta sign, cord sign.**

dentate gyrus   Three-layered archicortex on the inferomesial aspect of the temporal lobe. With the hippocampus this makes up the hippocampal formation.

dentatorubral atrophy   See **dentatorubropallidoluysian atrophy** and **Ramsay-Hunt syndrome.**

dentatorubro-olivary degeneration   A form of **pallidonigral degeneration** with clinical features resembling those of **Friedreich ataxia.**

dentatorubro-pallidoluysian atrophy   (DRPLA; OMIM 125370) A group of **pallidonigral degenerations** with both dominant inheritance and sporadic occurrence at any age, reported mainly from Japan. Their onset is usually in young- or mid-adult life and they are characterized by dementia, ophthalmoplegias, vertical nystagmus, cerebellar signs, choreoathetosis, ataxia, chorea, dystonia, and sometimes fasciculations and myoclonus in various combinations. Phenotypic variability is extensive and the precise diagnosis is made most often at postmortem,[2725,5664] but there is a trinucleotide repeat expansion at chromosome 12q23-24-1 or 12p13.31. The condition is a cause of **progressive myoclonus epilepsy**[5229,5470] but could equally well be classified as a **cerebellar ataxia.**

The pathological changes involve mainly the dentate nucleus and the external segment of the globus pallidus, and thus the subthalamic and red nuclei.

The following *variants* are described:

Myoclonic form A syndrome with onset in young- or mid-adult life, characterized by choreoathetosis, myoclonus, and dementia.[5470]

Pseudo-Huntington form A dominantly inherited syndrome with onset in young- or mid-adult life, characterized by ataxia, choreoathetosis, dystonias, progressive myoclonic epilepsy, generalized seizures, and dementia.[5470] An identical *sporadic form* is also recorded.

Ataxic-choreoathetotic form A syndrome in which the initial ataxia is overwhelmed by choreoathetosis and dementia.[5229]

dentolabials Those consonants such as *T* and *V,* which depend for their utterance upon pressure of the teeth upon the lips. See also **articulated labials.**

Denver Developmental Screening Test A complex assessment battery assessing personal-social, fine motor–adaptive, gross motor, and language skills in children up to the age of 6 years.[1934]

A refinement has been pubished.[1934]

deorsumduction See **ductions.**

depersonalization (cerebrocardiac neurosis, Krishaber disease) A distressing, insightful illusion of the unreality of the self in an unreal world, but reversible, most easily by external stimulation; the feeling that one is not a real being, or that the mind and body are separated.[3163] "A state in which individuals feel changed throughout in comparison with their former state. This change extends both to the self and to the outer world and leads to individuals not acknowledging themselves as a personality. Their actions seem to them automatic; they observe their own actions like a spectator. The outer world seems strange to them and has lost its character of reality."

It occurs in complex partial seizures and in some depressive and dissociated psychiatric illnesses but also occasionally as a normal phenomenon, mainly in adolescents and young adults.[5140]

depolarization The reduction of the internal negativity of the cell, normally at about −90 mV, by an inward rush of sodium ions because of a sufficiency of excitatory postsynaptic potentials playing upon the cell membrane. If depolarization is adequate, an action potential is generated. See **polarization.**

depolarization block Failure of an excitable cell to respond to a stimulus because of preexisting depolarization of the cell membrane.[10]

depression 1. Sadness. 2. A morbid condition, presumably a biochemical disorder of the CNS, characterized by mental and/or physical symptoms, and signs that frequently suggest the presence of structural neurological disease. See **Hamilton Rating Scale, Zung Self-rating Scale, Depression Adjective Checklist, depression rating scales (CES-D).**

Key *DSM-IV* Diagnostic Criteria for Major Depressive Disorder[150]

Five (or more) of the following symptoms have been present during the same 2-week period and represent a change from previous functioning; at least one of the symptoms is either *(1)* depressed mood or *(2)* loss of interest or pleasure.

1. Depressed mood most of the day
2. Markedly diminished interest or pleasure in all, or almost all, activities most of the day
3. Significant weight loss when not dieting or weight gain or decrease or increase in appetite
4. Insomnia or hypersomnia
5. Psychomotor agitation or retardation
6. Fatigue or loss of energy
7. Feelings of worthlessness or excessive or inappropriate guilt
8. Diminished ability to think or concentrate, or indecisiveness
9. Recurrent thoughts of death (not just fear of dying), recurrent suicidal ideation without a specific plan, or a suicide attempt or a specific plan for committing suicide

Adapted from American Psychiatric Association, Diagnostic and Statistical Manual of Mental Disorders, 4th ed (DSM-IV-TR). *Washington, DC. By kind permission.* © American Psychiatric Association, 2000. See DSM-IV-TR *for full criteria.*

Depression Adjective Checklist A self-report questionnaire appropriate for the repeated assessment of depressive mood.[3498]

depression of visual acuity A loss of visual field that is relative, so that some stimuli are seen but other are not.

depression rating scales Instruments for diagnosing depression or for recording depressive symptomatology to assess the effect of therapy. See **Zung Depression Scale, Hamilton Depression Rating Scale, Depression Center for Epidemiologic Studies Depression Scale (CES-D), Depression Adjective Checklist, Cornell, Beck,** and **Lubin** scales, and the **Geriatric Rating Scale for Depression.**

depressive pseudodementia Reduction of cognitive abilities during a depressive illness. Since dementia is generally considered irreversible but these patients are likely to recover, this cognitive syndrome does not fit the standard definition.

In some cases, the dementia is psychogenic.[521]

depth electrodes Electrodes inserted using stereotactic techniques into the substance of the brain for stimulation or recording. Fine wires are inserted into the substance of the brain to detect and localize abnormal electrical discharges in patients with epilepsy.

depth electroencephalogram (DEEG) The electrical activity of the brain recorded by means of electrodes implanted within the brain substance itself. See also **stereotactic (stereotaxic) depth electroencephalogram.**

depth electroencephalography The technique of recording the electrical activity of the brain by means of electrodes implanted within the brain substance itself.

depth perception The ability to distinguish the relative distances of objects seen. The sense depends upon stereopsis and upon such visual clues as overlap and relative appearance of movement.

depth sense esthesiometry A simple test, invented by Dr. S. Renfrew in 1960, for assessing fingertip sensation using an acrylic plate with a sloping ridge.[4661] The subject passes a finger across the plate and sensation is measured according to the threshold of appreciation of the presence of the ridge.[5212]

deranencephalia (Gr, long + negative + the brain) (derencephalus) A malformation characterized by the total absence of the encephalon, the CNS consisting solely of the spinal cord.

Dercum disease (adiposis dolorosa, Ander disease) The association of headache and depression with voluminous and painful nodular accumulations of fat in the legs of middle-aged women. Peripheral neuropathy is said to be associated.[1406,1407]

Dercum, Francis Xavier (1856–1931) American neurologist and anthropologist, who succeeded C.K. Mills as head of the Neurology Clinic at the University of Philadelphia and was later appointed professor at Jefferson Medical College. His interests were in medical photography and hysteria, and he wrote and edited successful textbooks on neurological therapeutics and on psychiatry.[5047]

derealization The feeling that the world around is unreal and qualitatively different from its normal state. The causes are the same as for **depersonalization.** See also **Alice in Wonderland syndrome.**

derivation 1. The process of recording from a pair of electrodes in an EEG channel. 2. The EEG record obtained by this process.

dermal nerve sheath myxoma See **neurothecoma.**

dermatalgia Skin pain.

dermataneuria Skin anesthesia.

dermatoid (dermoid) Resembling the skin.

dermatoleukodystrophy A congenital dysmorphic syndrome manifesting also cutis laxa and excessive skin wrinkling, neurodegenerative regression, optic atrophy,

grand mal seizures, cerebellar and pyramidal signs, and cerebral atrophy with diffuse gliosis and demyelination.[337]

dermatomal somatosensory evoked potential Scalp-recorded waveforms generated from repeated stimulation of a specific dermatome. These are not the same as the **somatosensory evoked potentials** recorded in response to stimulation of a named peripheral nerve. (From the 2001 Report of the Nomenclature Committee of the American Association of Electromyography and Electrodiagnosis.[10] Used by permission, copyright © 2001, AAEM.

dermatomes The geographical areas of skin whose sensory afferents run to a single cord segment. Developmentally, the pattern can be understood as a result of outpouching of the limb buds, the trunk having a simple banded arrangement of dermatomes (although there is considerable overlap which itself varies according to the sensory modality examined). Their arrangement in the limbs is more complicated, to the extent that no two sources agree precisely. Current views are based largely on the studies of Henry **Head** and Otto **Foerster** on herpes zoster.[1893]

dermatomyositis (Wagner syndrome, Wagner-Unverricht syndrome) An autoimmune acute, subacute, or chronic inflammatory disease of children or adults affecting muscle and skin, both of which show lymphocytic infiltration.

The condition is differentiated from **polymyositis** and from **inclusion body myositis** on the basis of the frequent skin involvement and on variations in the clinical and pathological findings. Various antibodies (Mi-2, Jo-1, EJ, etc.) have been detected in different cases. **Childhood dermatomyositis** has different characteristics and is considered to be a separate condition, as is the form induced by penicillamine.[922]

More females than males are affected. A mauve-colored skin eruption is seen on the eyelids and face, the extensor joint surfaces, and other areas exposed to the sun. Muscle fatigue, dysphagia, and respiratory muscle weakness are common, and involvement of lungs and myocardium is usual. The distribution of weakness is proximal, the course is usually subacute, serum creatine kinase levels are usually greatly raised, and the response to treatment is good unless joint contractures occur. However, in about one-fifth of the cases, a remote carcinoma is present. Retinopathy, conjunctivitis, iritis, uveitis, and small vessel disease (Prinzmetal angina, Raynaud) are other occasional accompaniments.

In adults who are Mi-2 antibody negative, effusions, arrhythmias, interstitial lung disease, sclleroderma, and rheumatoid arthritis and an increased risk of malignancy are added features, while those with this antibody have more pronounced skin involvement. Associated connective tissue disorders are uncommon.

Wagner's original description was in 1863,[5801] Unverricht's was in 1891.[5688] Diagnostic criteria have been suggested[2684] and are listed below:

1. Clinical: proximal muscle weakness, usually symmetrical, progressing over weeks or months, with or without muscle pain. Dermatological manifestations (rash, calcinosis) may be present.
2. Pathological: muscle fiber necrosis and regeneration, mononuclear cell infiltration. Perifascicular atrophy may be present.
3. Biochemical: raised serum CK (MM isoenzyme), aldolase, or myoglobin levels.
4. EMG: multifocal EMG features of myopathy. Spontaneous activity is often present at rest.

The presence of Mi-2 or Jo-1 antibodies, myoglobinuria, and EMG evidence of an irritative myopathy with small-amplitude, brief, polyphasic motor units, fibrillations, and positive sharp waves are other typical laboratory features.

The *adult Mi-2 antibody–negative* form is associated with other connective tissue disorders such as scleroderma and the CREST syndrome, effusions, cardiac arrhythmias, interstitial lung disease, and an increased risk of malignancy.

The *adult Mi-2 antibody–positive* form appears acutely in adults whose skin signs tend to be severe and who all have positive ANA. The HLA type DR7 is overrepresented in this group.

The form associated with *malignancy* is seen in adult females with advanced ovarian carcinoma; or with epithelial nasopharyngeal carcinoma in Oriental subjects. EJ antibodies are detected.

dermatoradiculoneuromyositis See **neuromyositis.**

dermoid See **dermatoid.**

dermoid cyst (embryoma of head or neck, orbital teratoma, teratoid tumor of head or neck) Rare cysts resembling **epidermoid cysts** in their histology and site of growth in the head and neck, but containing also fragments of skin appendages. They occur almost exclusively in infants and young children.

Nasal dermoids are usually found at birth, a small midline pit on the bridge of the nose being marked by local hairiness and representing the opening of a sinus tract extending back to the cribriform plate. *Orbital teratomas* are associated with unilateral exophthalmos and some degree of microphthalmos, commonly visible at birth. The mass lesion may extend into the anterior or middle cranial fossas or into the nasal cavity. *Cervical teratomas* are found in the first year of life, presenting with a mass in the neck frequently compressing the larynx or trachea and the esophagus. *Nasopharyngeal teratomas* are pedunculated or sessile tumors that are present at birth, usually in females, causing airway obstruction, rhinorrhea, and a nasal or retropharyngeal mass; they are sometimes associated with anencephaly or hemicrania.[4112]

dermotrichic syndrome (alopecia-ichthyosis-retardation and seizures) A congenital dysmorphic syndrome manifesting also alopecia, ichthyosis, megacolon or Hirschprung syndrome, aminoaciduria, seizures, and mental and developmental delay.[337] See also **alopecia–mental retardation syndrome.**

desanimania (Lat, down + the mind + madness) Mindless insanity. The term is probably obsolete.

Descartes reflex (retinoorbicular reflex) Involuntary blinking in response to suddenly presented visual stimuli, thus a variant of the **orbicularis oculi reflex.**

Descartes, Renatus (Rene) (1596–1650) French philosopher and scientist. In his magnum opus "De Homine," he considered the pineal to be the seat of the soul, controlling the flow of animal spirits within the ventricles. Because he also enunciated the principle that incoming stimuli to the brain lead to specific outgoing motor effects, he may be said to be the first to delineate reflex activity; his examples were withdrawal from pain and the **menace reflex.** His comparison of the eye to a *camera obscura* and his description of accommodation as an effect of a change in the curvature of the lens in his *Dioptrica* (1637) were also notable contributions.

Descemet, Jean (1732–1810) French professor of anatomy and surgery in Paris. His description of the corneal membrane was actually preceded by that of Benedict Duddell, an English surgeon-oculist (1729).[1478]

Descemet membrane The posterior elastic membrane of the cornea, the site of copper deposition in **Wilson disease.**

descending paralysis Unilateral progressive descending paralysis of the trunk and limbs, first described in 1906 by Charles K. Mills (1845–1931), an American neurologist. This condition might well have been **acute inflammatory demyelinating polyneuropathy, botulism,** or **tic paralysis.**

desensitization 1. The lack of response of the receptor on the muscle membrane to persisting high levels of acetylcholine when that substance has not been hydrolyzed quickly; the muscle cell does not remain depolarized in this state, however. 2. A form of deconditioning therapy introduced by Dr. Joseph Wolpe, in which the subject creates a list of anxiety-provoking items graded in order of severity, and is exposed to these in order, at lessening distances, intensities, or durations, starting with the least anxiety-provoking ones. Such exposure may be either mental as a form of imagery or by actual exposure, as, for example, in the case of the agoraphobic patient who is first taken to the closed door, then the open door, then the doorstep, then the front step, etc., moving only to the next stage when the last is tolerated without excessive anxiety.[6026]

desert blindness   See **photophthalmia.**

desmin   The intermediate filament protein of skeletal and cardiac muscle fibers and of some smooth muscle cells.[2147]

desmin storage myopathy   See **desminopathy, myofibrillar (desmin-storage) myopathy.**

desminopathy   Disorders characterized by abnormal expression of type 3 intermediate filaments (desmin) within the subsarcolemmal regions of muscle cells, expressed clinically as a slowly progressive myopathy with cardiomyopathy. Most of these present in childhood and are familial.[5696]

Three forms are described: a granulofilamentous type with cardiomyopathy; one with cytoplasmic/spheroid inclusion bodies, less often with cardiomyopathy (both autosomal dominant); and a recessive form with Mallory body–like inclusions. A common feature is focal dissolution of myofibrils and accumulation of multiple proteins. Links to chromosomes 2q35, 11q22, and 12 have been mapped.[3816] See **distal muscular dystrophies.**

desmoid tumor   (Lat, like a bundle; tumor) A large, benign growth of fibrous tissue within muscle.

desmoplastic medulloblastoma   See **medulloblastoma.**

desynchronization   An alteration in the pattern of EEG activity as a result of external or internal stimuli. See also **blocking, attenuation.**

desynchronized sleep   Rapid eye movement sleep, in which the regularity of the EEG waveform is disturbed by increased, irregular-frequency waves. See **REM sleep.**

detentio   (Lat, keeping back) Catalepsy.

Determann syndrome   (dyskinesia intermittens angiosclerotica) See **dystonia.**

DeToni-Fanconi-Debré syndrome   Aminoaciduria resulting from dysfunction of the proximal renal tubules. See **mitochondrial cytopathy.**

detrusor   (from Lat, to thrust away) The muscular coat of the bladder.

detrusor–external sphincter dyssynergia   Contraction of the bladder and its sphincters at the same time. See **dyssynergia.**

deuteranopia   See **color blindness.**

deuteropathia   (from Gr, second + disease) A disease induced by another.

deuteropathic lateral sclerosis   An unwarranted distinction made by **Charcot** between tonic and atonic atrophy in lateral sclerosis, "the separation being based on the assumption that in such cases the primary lesion is the degeneration of the pyramidal tracts and that the affection of the grey matter is secondary or deuteropathic."[2240]

developmental aphasia   See **congenital auditory imperception.**

Developmental Assessment   A standardized schedule for assessment of gross motor (60 items) and reflex function (18 items) in infants.[2666] Norms for posture and large movements, vision and fine movement, hearing and speech, and social behaviour and play have been determined by Sheridan.[5116] See also **Denver Developmental Screening Test.**

Developmental Brain Dysfunction   Address: Cambridge University Press, The Edinburgh Building, Shaftesbury Road, Cambridge CB2 2RU, England.

developmental disabilities   Chronic impairments in brain function secondary to maldevelopments or injuries to the developing brain in the perinatal or postnatal periods. The deficits are lifelong and include global cognitive deficits, motor disabilities (cerebral palsy), social and language failures, and specific cognitive deficits.

developmental dyslexia   See **word blindness.**

developmental dysphasia   (congenital aphasia, congenital word-deafness) An isolated developmental deficit or delay in acquiring expressive and/or receptive speech and language for communicative purposes, in the absence of significant hearing loss, emotional disturbance, mental retardation, or aphasia, and resulting from focal pathological lesions usually affecting the left cerebral hemisphere.[1085] See **congenital auditory imperception.**

developmental Foix-Chavany-Marie syndrome   See **bilateral central macrogyria.**

developmental indicators for assessment of learning-revised   (DIAL-R) A developmental screening test designed to assess gross and fine motor activity, academic, expressive, and receptive language skills, and articulation in children aged between 3 and 7 years.

developmental learning disorders   A group of conditions with their onset before puberty, characterized by difficulties in acquisition of speech or certain cognitive functions, or in anomalies of emotional development.

These include stuttering, developmental dyslexia, childhood autism, hyperactivity, and possibly **Tourette syndrome.** They occur more often in males, and left-handedness in unusually common among such people.[467]

Developmental Medicine and Child Neurology. A subspecialty journal published by Cambridge Journals. Web site: http://titles.cambridge.org/journals/journal_catalogue.asp?historylinks=ALPHA&mnemonic=DMC.

Developmental Neuroscience (*Dev. Neurosci.*) A basic neuroscience journal. Web site: http://www.karger.com/journals/dne/dne_jh.htm.

developmental receptive aphasia   See **word deafness.**

developmental reflexes   (fetal or primitive reflexes) Responses to stimulation that are normally present in the early stages of maturation of the nervous system but that disappear at various ages, reappearing when the central nervous system is altered by age or disease. **Sucking, snouting, palmomental, grasp, tonic foot,** and **corneomandibular reflexes, gegenhalten,** and those listed in Chart D–5 are examples.[3,4370] See also **primitive reflexes.**

Chart D–5. Developmental Reflexes

Reflex	Age at Appearance	Age at Disappearance (months)
Adductor spread of knee jerk	Birth	7–8
Landau reflex	10 months	24
Moro	Birth	5–6
Palmar grasp	Birth	6
Parachute	8 to 9 months	Persists
Plantar grasp	Birth	9–10
Rooting	Birth	3
Tonic neck response	Birth	5–6
Truncal incurvation	Birth	1–2

developmental testing   The determination of certain representative motor, sensory, and psychological abilities in children in order to compare them with the average abilities of normal children of the same age.

The procedures were first rationalized by Charles Darwin, who described the **rooting reflex,** the cephalocaudal sequence of development, signs of emotional expression, and other capabilities. Arnold Gesell developed the first "norms" of development in 1925 and numerous others have been published since. The **Denver Developmental Screening Test** appeared in 1967, but was based on a selected and healthy sample of children. It was followed by a briefer, revised version in 1981.[1934]

deviation   See o**ccular motor deviation.**

deviational nystagmus   See **gaze-evoked nystagmus.**

Devic disease   (Devic-Gault syndrome, neuroptic myelitis) See **neuromyelitis optica.** The condition was first described by Albutt in 1870,[106] followed by others, but was redescribed by Devic in 1894 and reviewed in detail by his student Fernand Gault (in his graduation thesis) in the same year.

Devic, Eugene   (1869–1930) French cardiologist practicing in Lyon, remembered for his complete description of **neuromyelitis optica** in 1894, in which he reviewed the reports of the same condition by 16 other authors (not including Albutt, see above).[1424]

Devic-Gault syndrome   See **neuromyelitis optica.**

Devil's grippe   See **pleurodynia.**

Devonshire colic   Abdominal colic due to lead poisoning, described in workers in lead mines.

dexamethasone suppression test   The assessment of baseline plasma cortisol levels before and after the oral administration of 1 mg of dexamethasone. Values >5 μg/DI after administration of the steroid are regarded as abnormal and suggestive of depressive illness so long as primary adrenal disease is not present.[4624]

D-glyceric aciduria   An aminoacidopathy causing very atypical **progressive myoclonus epilepsy.** See **glyceric aciduria.**

Di Ferrante syndrome   See **mucopolysaccharidosis type 8.**

diabetes insipidus   (diabetes neurogenes, spurious diabetes, ureal diabetes) A condition of excessive production of urine and consequent thirst resulting from deficiency of antidiuretic hormone due to lesions of the supraoptic and paraventricular nuclei of the hypothalamus. It was distinguished from diabetes mellitus by **Willis** and shown to be due to a lesion of the posterior lobe of the hypophysis by Alfred Frank (b. 1884), a German physiologist. See also **Wolfram syndrome.**

diabetes insipidus, diabetes mellitus, optic atrophy, and deafness (DIDMOAD) See **Wolfram syndrome.**

diabetes mellitus   (Gr, through + to go on; and Lat, sweet) A common disorder of carbohydrate metabolism leading to high levels of blood glucose, glycosuria, and acidosis.

Apart from the neurological syndromes commonly ascribed to diabetes, it may also be noted that there are some disorders in which diabetes is a recognized associate but in which it is not thought to be causal; **myotonic dystrophy, Louis-Bar syndrome, Huntington disease,** and **progeria** are examples.

diabetes mellitus encephalopathy   Organic mental deterioration, often accompanied by pyramidal signs, as a result of hypoglycemic brain damage.[1218]

diabetes mellitus–optic atrophy syndrome   The occurrence of optic atrophy, sometimes with nerve deafness, vestibulopathy, hypogonadism, congenital cardiac disease, congenital cataracts, and aminoaciduria, in patients with juvenile diabetes mellitus.[281] See also **Wolfram syndrome.**

diabetes neurogenes   See **diabetes insipidus.**

diabetes, obesity, and hearing loss   See **Alström-Hallgren syndrome.**

diabetic amyotrophy   (diabetic myelopathy, Garland amyotrophy, diabetic lumbosacral radiculoplexus neuropathy) A subacute or insidiously progressive, often painful, unilateral or bilateral pure motor neuropathy producing atrophy of the quadriceps and other pelvifemoral muscles without sensory impairment, occurring in older insulin-dependent diabetic patients[2035] and in males with non–insulin-dependent diabetes, most of whom have suffered recent marked weight loss. EMG evidence of bilateral paraspinal and gluteal denervation is commonly reported. The condition shows a tendency to abate over months if diabetic control is attained.

The condition was first described by Dr. Hugh Garland, an English neurologist, who noted the presence of upgoing plantar responses and raised CSF protein levels in many of his patients and concluded that the disease process lay in the spinal cord,[2035] a view no longer held. A similar syndrome was described by Ludwig Bruns in 1890.

The condition is considered to be a variety of diabetic motor neuropathy with a vascular or axonopathic etiology[4879] and the extensor plantar responses are ignored, denied, or ascribed to a vascular lesion at a higher level. See also **diabetic neuropathies.**

diabetic femoral neuropathy   A rare form of nerve involvement affecting mainly male non–insulin-dependent diabetic patients aged over 60 years, characterized by the acute occurrence (often following a period of substantial weight loss) of severe burning dysesthetic anterior thigh pain succeeded by quadriceps weakness and atrophy, loss of the knee jerk, and sensory loss in the painful territory. Incomplete recovery takes place over a year or more.[1125]

However, most diabetic patients with this syndrome actually have more extensive involvement due to **diabetic amyotrophy.**

diabetic lumbosacral radiculoplexus neuropathy See **diabetic amyotrophy**

diabetic myelopathy   See **diabetic amyotrophy.**

diabetic neuropathic cachexia   A condition of male diabetic patients who develop anorexia, extreme weight loss, impotence, malaise, depression, and bilateral symmetrical sensorimotor neuropathy with persistent neuropathic pain, without retinopathy or nephropathy, early in the course of the diabetic disorder.[1635]

diabetic neuropathies (polyneuropathies)   A heterogeneous group of peripheral somatic or autonomic neuropathies united by the common factor of their association with diabetes mellitus and characterized by degeneration of both large and small nerve fibers. They were first described by Pitres in 1917. Chart D–6 is based upon the classifications of Brown and Asbury,[796] of Feldman et al.,[1769] and of the San Antonio Conference.[1121]

Chart D–6. Classification of Diabetic Neuropathies

Class I: Subclinical Neuropathy

A. Abnormal electrodiagnostic tests (EDX) only
  1. Decreased nerve conduction velocity
  2. Decreased amplitude of evoked muscle or nerve action potential
B. Abnormal quantitative sensory testing (QST)
  1. Vibratory/tactile
  2. Thermal warming/cooling

  3. Other
C. Abnormal autonomic function tests (AFT)
  1. Diminished sinus arrythmia (beat-to-beat heart rate variation)
  2. Diminished sudomotor function
  3. Increased pupillary latency

In these forms, neurologic function tests are abnormal but no neurologic symptoms or clinically detectable neurologic deficits indicative of a diffuse or focal neuropathy are present. Class I, subclinical neuropathy, is further subdivided into Class Ia if an AFT or QST abnormality is present, Class Ib if EDX or AFT and QST abnormalities are present, and Class Ic if an EDX and either AFT or QST abnormalities, or both, are present.

Class II: Clinical Neuropathy

A. Diffuse neuropathy
  1. Distal symmetric sensorimotor polyneuropathy
    a. Primarily small fiber neuropathy
    b. Primarily large fiber neuropathy
    c. Mixed
  These are the most common major syndromes of peripheral axonal neuropathy in diabetes. They comprise the following forms.
    A. *Mixed form* An insidiously progressive axonal neuropathy producing any combination of motor, sensory, and autonomic involvement, with variable relative degrees of severity.
      Clinically, this is the most common form of diabetic neuropathy and it presents with complaints of numbness; tingling; burning paresthesia; contact hyperesthesia; aching pain, especially at night; impotence; and depression. Examination reveals loss of the ankle jerks and a symmetrical reduction in distal sensations, especially vibration. In some cases, the manifestations are precipitated by weight loss, unstable diabetes, stress, infections, or insulin therapy.
    B. *Sensory form* An insidiously progressive symmetrical axonal neuropathy affecting large (**diabetic pseudotabes**), small, or mixed sensory fibers. Clinically, the pattern of sensory involvement reflects the fiber types involved. In all, paresthesias, dysesthesias, and pain are common complaints and autonomic symptoms may be present.
    C. *Motor form* An uncommon acute, reversible motor polyneuropathy that may follow ketoacidosis in younger diabetic patients.
  2. Autonomic neuropathy
    a. Abnormal pupillary function
    b. Sudomotor dysfunction
    c. Genitourinary autonomic neuropathy
      1. Bladder dysfunction
      2. Sexual dysfunction
    d. Gastrointestinal autonomic neuropathy
      1. Gastric atony
      2. Gallbladder atony
      3. Diabetic diarrhea
      4. Hypoglycemic unawareness (adrenal medullary neuropathy)
    e. Cardiovascular autonomic neuropathy
    f. Hypoglycemic unawareness
  These forms of selective subacutely evolving autonomic (visceral) neuropathies involve the sympathetic and parasym-

pathetic divisions of the autonomic nervous system in the context of diabetes. Despite the name, features of motor or sensory involvement can often be detected as well. They are most commonly seen in younger insulin-dependent diabetics who presewnt with such problems as pupillary denervation, loss of lacrimal and sweat gland secretions, postural hypotension, cardiac denervation, peripheral edema, intestinal atony, diarrhea, gustatory sweating, loss of respiratory control, bladder atony, retrograde ejaculation, impotence, and unawareness of hypoglycemia. The mortality rate is greatly increased.

B. Focal neuropathy

1. *Mononeuropathy (peripheral entrapment neuropathy)* Mononeuropathies occurring at the more common sites of neural compression as in nondiabetics and carrying a fair prognosis for recovery. Whether this is the same as *diabetic multiple mononeuropathy* is uncertain.

2. *Multiple mononeuropathy*

3. *Plexopathy (proximal symmetrical motor neuropathy)* An acute, asymmetrical, painful motor neuropathy affecting the lumbosacral plexus or the femoral or obturator nerves. The prognosis for eventual recovery is good. See also **diabetic femoral neuropathy, diabetic amyotrophy.**

4. *Radiculopathy* See **diabetic truncal neuropathy.**

5. *Cranial mononeuropathy* This reflects *a*cute ischemic damage to a cranial nerve (usually the third), producing painful ophthalmoplegia with a tendency to spare pupillary reactivity and to abate spontaneously over weeks. The fourth, sixth, and seventh cranial nerves may also be affected.

Diabetic neuropathies have also been classified for research purposes by the American Diabetes Association[147] (see Chart D–7):

Chart D–7. Clinical Assessments of Diabetic Neuropathies for Research Purposes

	Symptom Neurologic Examination		Abnormal Physiological Tests
	Score	Score	
Class 1			
A	0	0	0 or AFT or QST
B	0	0	EDX or AFT and QST
C	0	0	EDX and AFT and/or QST
Class 2			
A	+	0	0 or AFT or QST
B	0/+	+	EDX or AFT and QST
C	0 or +	+	EDX and AFT and/or QST
or	+	0	+

0, Normal; +, abnormal. AFT, autonomic function testing; EDX, electrodiagnosis; QST, quantitative sensory testing.[147,1568]

(Adapted from American Diabetes Association. Report and recommendations of the San Antonio Conference on Diabetic neuropathy. Muscle Nerve 1988;11:661–667,[147] and Dyck PJ. Detection, characteristics and staging of polyneuropathy: assessed in diabetics. Muscle Nerve 1988;11:21–32.[1568] © 1988. All rights reserved. Reprinted by permission of John Wiley and Sons, Ltd.)

For the diagnosis of diabetic polyneuropathy, abnormalities of at least two of the following must be present:

1. Nerve conduction (NCS)
2. Neurological examination (NE)

3. Quantitative motor (QME), autonomic (QAE), or sensory (QST) testing

4. Neuropathic symptoms (NS)

Further staging is based on the results of these assessments, as follows:[1568]

Stage 1 (asymptomatic neuropathy) Two or more abnormalities among NC; NE; or QME, QSE, QAE but no abnormality of NS.

Stage 2 (symptomatic neuropathy) Two or more abnormalities among NC; NE; QME, QSE, QAE; or NS. Neuropathic symptoms are present but are of lesser severity than in stage 3.

Stage 3 (disabling neuropathy) Two or more abnormalities among NC; NE; QME, QSE, QAE; or NS. Disabling neuropathic symptoms are present.

Another alternative classification with diagnostic criteria was suggested by Dyck in 1988 (see Chart D–8).[1568]

Chart D–8. Diabetic Neuropathy—Neurological Symptom Score

Score 1 point for presence of a symptom.

1. Symptoms of muscle weakness
   A. Bulbar
      1. Extraocular
      2. Facial
      3. Tongue
      4. Throat
   B. Limbs
      5. Shoulder girdle and upper arm
      6. Hand
      7. Glutei and thigh
      8. Legs

2. Sensory disturbances
   A. Negative symptoms
      9. Difficulty identifying objects in mouth
      10. Difficulty identifying objects in hands
      11. Unsteadiness in walking
   B. Positive symptoms
      12. Numbness, asleep feeling, "like novocain," prickling at any site
      13. Pain—burning, deep aching, tenderness—at any location

3. Autonomic symptoms
      14. Postural fainting
      15. Impotence in male
      16. Loss of urinary control
      17. Night diarrhea

Abnormality of quantitative nerve tests One or more abnormal results among tests assessing muscle strength (QME), detection threshold of vibratory (VDT), cooling (CDT), or warming (WDT) sensation (QSE), or autonomic function (QAE) serve to fulfil criteria for abnormality of quantitative nerve tests.

Symptomatic neuropathy Occurrence of any symptoms (among the 12 listed below) judged to be due to diabetic polyneuropathy but not disabling (see stage 3 below) is sufficient to fulfil the criteria for stage 2. Patients with questionable degrees of symptoms are staged as 0 or 1.

Motor

1. Symptoms of muscle weakness in acts of daily living

Sensory

1. Absence of feeling: reported deficiency of tactile, thermal, or nociceptive sensation encountered in acts of daily living
2. Sensory ataxia: reported unsteadiness in walking
3. Numbness or paraesthesia ("dead asleep," "prickly asleep," "like novocaine," "like hand gone asleep," "tightly bound feeling," etc.) judged by its distribution, persistence, and duration to be due to neuropathy and not due to physiologic compression as occurs in acts of daily living or entrapment, e.g., carpal tunnel syndrome, or to another condition
4. Neuropathic pain: burning, aching, excessive discomfort of feet or hands with use and lancinating pain

Autonomic

Any of the following symptoms attributed to diabetes mellitus and not due to medications, psychologic disturbance, intercurrent illness, disease of the organ, or previous injury or surgery:

1. Gastric atony
2. Urinary retention
3. Urinary incontinence
4. Rectal incontinence
5. Diarrhea
6. Impotence in males <65 years of age
7. Postural hypotension, light-headedness, or fainting (with postural decrease of systolic BP ≥30 mmHg)

Disabling diabetic neuropathy That degree of diabetic neuropathy in which occurrence of any of the following 10 conditions occurs:

Motor

1. Symptoms of muscle weakness of such severity that the patient cannot walk independently, confirmed by examination

Sensory

2. Symptoms of sensory loss of sufficient severity that the patient cannot walk independently because of sensory ataxia, confirmed by examination
3. Absence of feeling in the hands such that the patient is disabled
4. The presence of disabling neuropathic pain for which the patient has seen physicians for pain relief, work and recreational activities have been curtailed by at least 25%, and medication has been taken for pain on at least half of the preceding 42 days

Autonomic

5. Gastric atony, as demonstrated by gastric retention tests and by exclusion of other gastric or psychiatric causes of emesis, causing emesis of retained (>18 hours) food at least once weekly for at least 6 weeks
6. Urinary retention as demonstrated by manometer evidence of detrusor hypoactivity and not due to psychiatric disturbance or urinary bladder disease, necessitating continuous use of a catheter for 6 weeks or longer
7. Urinary incontinence due to loss of sphincter function, necessitating continuous (>50% of time) use of dia-

pers or a leg urinal for at least 6 weeks, and not due to psychiatric or bladder disease

8. Rectal incontinence due to loss of anal sphincter function of at least 6 weeks duration and not due to psychiatric or rectal disease
9. Diarrhea to the degree that it causes weight loss (>5 kg) and steatorrhea >10 mg/24 hours, and not due to psychiatric disturbance, laxative abuse, or other bowel disease
10. Symptomatic light-headedness or fainting due to orthostatic hypotension (>30 mmHg systolic) with concomitant blood pressure drop, present continuously (light-headedness or fainting weekly) for at least 6 weeks

From Dyck PJ. Detection, characteristics and staging of polyneuropathy: assessed in diabetics. Muscle Nerve 1988;11:21–32. © 1988. All rights reserved. Reprinted by permission of John Wiley and Sons, Inc.

diabetic proximal neuropathy A heterogeneous condition first recognized by Bruns in 1890 but best described by Garland. See **diabetic amyotrophy.**

diabetic pseudotabes The association of **Argyll Robertson pupils** with lightning pains, posterior column dysfunction, neurogenic bladder, neuropathic arthropathy, and areflexia in the legs, the whole resembling the findings in **tabes dorsalis** but in fact due to diabetic peripheral neuropathy (sensory form) and autonomic neuropathies.

diabetic thoracic polyradiculopathy See **diabetic truncal neuropathy.**

diabetic truncal neuropathy (thoracoabdominal neuropathy, diabetic thoracic radiculopathy or polyradiculopathy, truncal mononeuropathy). A common form of diabetic peripheral neuropathy affecting the truncal nerves at various sites and usually causing severe abdominal or chest pain, not always radicular in character, as well as dysesthesia, sometimes with weakness of the abdominal muscles.[3069,5352] The condition is associated frequently with marked weight loss but carries a good prognosis for recovery.

Diagnostic Classification of Sleep and Arousal Disorders A compilation of such disorders first prepared by the American Sleep Disorders Association[3572] but now superseded. See **sleep disorders.**

diagnostic dyspraxia Intermanual conflict occurring as an **alien hand** sign.

diagnostic interview schedule A complex, interview-based, observer-rated measure of depression designed to establish the full range of the American Psychiatric Association DSM-III Depressive disorders.[4725]

diagonal nystagmus See **circular nystagmus.**

diagonal paresis Weakness of one arm and of the opposite leg as a result of a lesion of the highest levels of the spinal cord damaging the corticospinal tract fibers supplying the arm (which at this level have crossed) and those supplying the contralateral leg (which cross one or two segments below).

dialysis cramp   Painful calf cramps occurring in patients during hemodialysis, probably due to temporary hyponatremia.[3301]

dialysis dementia   See **dialysis encephalopathy.**

dialysis dysequilibrium syndrome   An acute delirious state lasting days to weeks, with headache, nausea, muscle cramps, and occasionally seizures, and due to cellular overhydration as a response to the rapid lowering of blood urea by dialysis.[4778] For further data, see http://www.kidneydoctor.com/equilib.htm.

dialysis encephalopathy   (dialysis dementia) A subacutely progressive syndrome lasting 3–15 months in subjects on hemodialysis for over a year, and characterized by increasing dementia, a dysphasic language disorder often accompanied by hesitant, stuttering speech, and distinctive EEG patterns with **FIRDA.** Myoclonic and generalized seizures, behavioral disturbances, and confusional states are less reliable (though common) components of the syndrome.[1016]

The condition is considered to be due to aluminum toxicity.

dianoetic   Capable of thought.

diaphragm reflex of Hess   The **abdominal muscle reflex** obtained by tapping the nipple.

diaphragmatic flutter   (moving umbilicus syndrome) Clonic contractions of the diaphragm occurring at high frequency and without any associated inspiratory sound. The syndrome is uncommon, occurs at any age, and is due to either phrenic denervation or irritation of the diaphragm itself. Patients may complain of respiratory distress, muscular fatigue, or pain in the abdominal wall or precordium, or palpitations of the chest. The condition may also represent a variant of the **palatal myoclonus** syndrome. See also **belly dancers' dyskinesia.**[2730]

diaphyseal dysplasia   See **Camurati-Engelman syndrome.**

diaschisis   (Gr, division or splitting) A sudden abeyance or reduction of motor function following the interruption at a remote site of an afferent pathway that normally supplied background excitation to the neurons in question, keeping them in a state of low activity. "Shock" of the nervous system.[1760]

The concept was introduced first by **von Monakow,** who described *diaschisis corticospinalis* (progression of functional depression of the spinal cord following an injury to the motor cortex); *diaschisis commissuralis* (functional depression of the contralateral cerebral cortex after injury to the cortex of one hemisphere); and *diaschisis associativa* (depression of function in intact cortical areas adjacent to the site of a cortical injury). The term now includes the following *varieties:*[4126]

Corticocerebellar diaschisis (crossed cerebral-cerebellar diaschisis, corticocerebellar diaschisis, transtentorial diaschi-

sis) Reduction of metabolic activity of the cerebellar hemisphere contralateral to the side of a supratentorial ischemic infarct. Clinical signs of this form are few.

Crossed hemispheric diaschisis (cerebellocortical diaschisis, crossed cerebellocortical diaschisis) Hypoperfusion in the contralateral cerebral hemisphere after unilateral cerebellar infarction.

Transhemispheric diaschisis Bilateral reduction of perfusion in subjects after a unilateral hemispheric infarct, and dependent on continuing function of the corpus callosum.

Corticothalamic diaschisis Diminished metabolism and perfusion in the thalamus after an infarct or other lesion has interrupted thalamocortical projection pathways.

Thalamocortical diaschisis A reversal of the latter form, in which there is a reduction in metabolism of the homolateral hemisphere after subcortical/thalamic stroke.

Basal ganglion–cortical diaschisis Hypometabolism in focal or diffuse cortical regions (usually frontal) in the presence of lesions of the lenticular nucleus, globus pallidus, caudate, etc.

diastaltic   (Gr, exciting) The term used by Marshall **Hall** for what is now called *reflex*; today it is seldom employed.

diastasis   Separation of the cranial sutures, as may occur in children with cranial trauma, meningeal tumors, or elevated intracranial pressure.

diastematencephalacia   (from Gr, to separate + the brain) A congenital maldevelopment in which the brain is divided into two by a midline cleft.

diastematomyelia   (Gr, to separate + the spinal cord) (split notochord syndrome) A congenital maldevelopment in which there is splitting of the spinal cord into two dura-enclosed tracts by a midline bony or cartilaginous spicule, usually extending over several segments in the thoracic or lumbar regions, and sometimes associated with spina bifida.

Although the condition is often asymptomatic in youth, symptoms such as gait disturbance, back pain, and motor or sensory disturbances in the legs arise when the greater growth of the vertebrae compared with that of the cord leads to traction on the cord, and subsequently to myelopathy.[470]

diathesis   (Gr, an arrangement) A morbid tendency or susceptibility to a certain type of disease; a vague term, now nearly defunct, although the underlying concept is real enough.

dicephalus   A two-headed monster.

dichotic stimulation   A psychometric localization test using auditory stimulation, whereby different sounds (e.g., numbers) are presented simultaneously to the two ears.

Dide-Botcazo syndrome   A syndrome of the posterior cerebral artery in which bilateral calcarine and posterior temporal infarcts are associated with loss of immediate memory, retrograde amnesia, spatial agnosia, and temporal disorientation.[1437,1438]

DIDMOAD   See **Wolfram syndrome.**

diencephalic amnesia   Deficits in anterograde visual and verbal learning and in retrograde amnesia, with retention of motor learning abilities, due to lesions involving the amygdaloid and hippocampal pathways in the anterior part of the diencephalon surrounding the floor and walls of the third ventricle, and especially of the medial-dorsal thalamic nucleus.[2251,3746]

diencephalic autonomic seizures   (dysautonomia, autonomic dysfunction syndrome, autonomic storm, brainstem attack, hyperpyrexia associated with muscle contraction, hypothalamic-midbrain dysregulation syndrome, acute midbrain syndrome, Penfield syndrome, autonomic diencephalic epilepsy, tetanus-like seizures, cerebellar or tonic seizures, minor epilepsy) An unusual variety of "seizure" in which major autonomic (sympathetic) manifestations occur because of hypothalamic lesions, such as tumors, or associated with severe diffuse axonal injury and cerebral hypoxia following craniocerebral trauma. Manifestations include transient increases in blood pressure and speeding or slowing of respiration such as the Cheyne-Stokes pattern, lacrimation, sweating, shivering, pupillary changes, vasodilatation, lacrimation, salivation, piloerection, tachycardia, hyper- or hypothermia, posturing, exophthalmos, and hiccuping.

Penfield's case[4401] was of a woman who died with an encapsulated tumor that was compressing the thalamus; her attacks were considered to represent epileptic discharges but it seems more likely that they were due to a release phenomenon at the level of the upper brainstem,[833] perhaps witnessing to the effects of plateau waves in patients with acute intermittent hydrocephalus. See also **de Morsier syndrome.**

diencephalic neuronal necrosis   Neuronal injury limited to the thalamus, hypothalamus, and brainstem following hypoxic-ischemic injury in utero.[4333]

diencephalic syndrome   (Batten-Russell-Collier disease) Emaciation and failure to thrive with full alertness but showing minimal neurological signs, occurring in infants or small children in association with a tumor of the diencephalon (usually an anterior hypothalamic glioma).

Alertness and increased vigor and appetite with friendliness (or even elation in the early stages) give way to vomiting, cachexia, and emaciation, pallor, nystagmus, hydrocephalus, optic atrophy, and tremor despite the fact that the child remains bright, cheerful, and active until a late stage. The condition was best described by Russell.[4852]

diencephalon   (Gr, through or between + brain) The caudal end of the forebrain, continuous with the mesencephalon; the thalamus.

differential signal   The difference between two unlike signals applied to the respective two input terminals of a differential EEG amplifier.

differentiation   The process whereby tumor cells acquire unique histological characteristics differentiating them from other types of cells.

diffuse astrocytoma   See **astrocytoma.**

diffuse axonal injury   (diffuse degeneration of white matter, shearing injury, inner cerebral trauma, diffuse white matter shearing injury) The appearance of axonal injury with associated focal lesions in the corpus callosum and rostral brainstem and with intraventricular hemorrhage, occurring in brains subjected to severe angular acceleration but without increased intracranial pressure or hypoxia.[6] This condition and ischemia represent the major mechanisms responsible for neuronal damage following head injury.

This traumatic disorder of CNS axons is shown pathologically by scattered disruptions of the axons with axonal retraction, sometimes in more severe cases associated with focal petechial hemorrhages and larger areas of hemorrhagic necrosis in the dorsal lateral midbrain and corpus callosum. The condition is due to simple forces acting upon the brain and does not require that the head actually make contact with an unyielding surface. Initial coma improving through stages of mutism, hypophonia, cerebellar and pyramidal signs, and vestibular symptoms and signs are the usual clinical concomitants.

diffuse cerebellar cortical hypertrophy   A rare developmental anomaly characterized by the presence of enlarged cerebellar folia with abnormal cells beneath the granule cell layer.[4254] See also **Lhermitte-Duclos disease.**

diffuse cerebral degeneration in infancy   See **Alpers disease.**

diffuse cerebral ischemia   That condition of the cerebral circulation in which the level of blood flow is not sufficient to meet all the metabolic needs of the brain but is sufficient to protect against infarction.

diffuse cerebral sclerosis with pigmentary retinopathy   A sporadic disorder characterized by abnormal phytanic acid storage, bilateral keratopathy, and sudanophilic leukoencephalopathy.[2971]

diffuse cortical dysplasia   (double-cortex syndrome, subcortical band heterotopia, band heterotopia) A genetically determined disorder of neuronal migration characterized by diffuse band heterotopia underlying the cortical mantle and giving the appearance on MRI scans of a double cortex, as a result of the arrest of migration of a population of neurons in subcortical regions on its way to the cortex. It is due to a mutation in the doublecortin gene on chromosome X. A comprehensive review is that of Aicardi.[59]

Clinically, the disorder is usually found in females and presents with various epileptic syndromes, including drop attacks, the **Lennox-Gastaut syndrome,** and

infantile spasms. Some degree of mental retardation is usual.[4311]

See also **lissencephaly,** in which the failure of neuronal migration is more generalized and does not show the same double cortex appearance.

diffuse cortical sclerosis   See **Alpers disease.**

diffuse degeneration of white matter   See **diffuse axonal injury.**

diffuse infiltrative lymphomatosis   An AIDS-related peripheral sensorimotor neuropathy in which the nerves (as well as many other tissues) are infiltrated by CD8 T lymphocytes. The condition is not a lymphoma, despite the name applied.[2089]

diffuse Lewy body disease   (idiopathic Lewy body disease/dementia, dementia with Lewy bodies, [diffuse] Lewy body variant of Alzheimer disease; a dozen other names have been given[2419]) A condition clinically resembling **Parkinson** or **Alzheimer disease** or **progressive supranuclear palsy** in which **Lewy bodies** staining for **ubiquitin** are found in cortical and subcortical regions; there are also spongy changes in the medial temporal lobe and pallor in the substantia nigra, and neuronal loss also occurs in the substantia nigra, locus ceruleus, and substantia innominata.

The features differentiating this condition from other "cortical" dementias are that the dementing features fluctuate, parkinsonism may be present, and there are greater disturbances of attention, fluency, and information processing in this disorder.[862,2094,2098] *Diffuse, transitional,* and *brainstem* types of Lewy body disease have been differentiated on the basis of the distribution of these neuronal inclusions. Signs suggesting **amyotrophic lateral sclerosis** and **multiple-system atrophy** have also been described. A feature differentiating this condition from **Alzheimer disease** is the relatively early occurrence of urinary incontinence.

Consensus guidelines for the diagnosis have been published,[3764] although their sensitivity and specificity have been questioned. Guidelines for brain sampling, for evaluation of the distribution and frequency of the Lewy bodies, and for a diagnostic rating protocol have also been suggested.

Consensus Criteria for Clinical Diagnosis of Probable and Possible Dementia with Lewy Bodies (DLB)

1. The central feature required for a diagnosis of DLB is progressive cognitive decline of sufficient magnitude to interfere with normal social or occupational function. Prominent or persistent memory impairment may not necessarily occur in the early stages but is usually evident with progression. Deficits on tests of attention and of frontal–subcortical skills and visuospatial ability may be especially prominent.
2. Two of the following core features are essential for a diagnosis of probable DLB, and one is essential for possible DLB:

   a. Fluctuating cognition with pronounced variations in attention and alertness
   b. Recurrent visual hallucinations that are typically well formed and detailed
   c. Spontaneous motor features of parkinsonism
3. Features supportive of the diagnosis are
   a. Repeated falls
   b. Syncope
   c. Transient loss of consciousness
   d. Neuroleptic sensitivity
   e. Systematized delusions
   f. Hallucinations in other modalities
4. A diagnosis of DLB is less likely in the presence of
   a. Stroke disease, evident as focal neurologic signs or on brain imaging
   b. Evidence on physical examination and investigation of any physical illness or other brain disorder sufficient to account for the clinical picture

(From McKeith IG, Galasko D, Kosaka K, et al. Consensus guidelines for the clinical and pathological diagnosis of dementia with Lewy bodies. Neurology 1996;47:1113–24. Reproduced by kind permission.)

The clinical phenotypes produced are, however, diverse; they include those of idiopathic and of (dominantly inherited) juvenile Parkinson disease and of Alzheimer disease with added features of Parkinson disease.[2158,2419]

Other published criteria (reviewed by Mega et al.[3805]) require variously a **Clinical Dementia Rating Scale** score of 0.5–2 and extrapyramidal signs, delusions or hallucinations, unexplained falls, transient clouding of consciousness, fluctuating cognition, attention or alertness, failure to respond to levadopa, and/or unusual sensitivity to neuroleptics. Another system[2418] requires a neuropsychological profile.

Diagnostic Criteria for Lewy Body Disease Using Neuropsychological Criteria

A. Severe attention deficit (low total digit-span score),
B. Impaired verbal fluency affecting letter and category fluency tasks equally,
C. Severely impaired visuospatial performance on the Wechsler Intelligence Scale for Children–Revised (WISC-R) block design and on drawing tests, and
D. Difficulty in writing to dictation; with

Signs on neurological examination:

A. Mild extrapyramidal features, particularly masked facies, often combined with bradykinesia, slowing of rapid alternating movements or gait difficulty in the absence of flexed posture, resting tremor, and other classical parkinsonian signs
B. Essential tremor.

Adapted from Hansen L, Salmon D, Galasko D, et al. The Lewy-body variant of Alzheimer's disease. Neurology 1990;40:1–8.[2418]

In another *variant* form, Lewy-body parkinsonism is inherited as an autosomal dominant characteristic in adult life.[5869]

A valuable website is at *www.nottingham.ac.uk/ pathology/lewy/lewyhome.html.*

diffuse neonatal hemangiomatosis   A congenital dysmorphic syndrome manifesting also facial capillary hemangiomas, visceromegaly, hydrocephalus, and skin papules.[337]

diffuse neurofibrillary tangles with calcification   A syndrome of slowly progressive cortical dementia in adult life with temporal and/or frontal lobar atrophy, and widespread neurofibrillary tangles in the cortex.[3137]

diffuse neuronal necrosis   A result of hypoxic-ischemic injury in the neonate.

diffuse poliodystrophy   The condition of diffuse proliferation of microglia and astroglia with some neuronal loss within the brain, as occurs in some patients with **HIV** infection. The condition represents a subacute encephalitis, which was its former name.[3727]

diffuse progressive cerebral cortical atrophy   See **Alpers disease.**

diffuse sclerosis   1. See **Schilder disease.** 2. See **leukodystrophies.** 3. Subacute encephalitis, in the classification of Poser and van Bogaert.[4506]

diffuse white matter shearing injury   See **diffuse axonal injury.**

diffusion weighted imaging   An MRI technique allowing visualization of stroke effects within an hour of their occurrence, and also permitting aging of stoke lesions seen. "Diffusion" here refers to the random translational motion of molecules in a fluid system. In this case it is the diffusion of water itself that is imaged. For further discussion of such MRI techniques, see Filippi M. et al. Neurology 2002;**58:**1147–1153.

digastric line   See **Fischgold line.**

DiGeorge syndrome   (third and fourth pharyngeal pouch syndrome; velocardiofacial syndrome) A chromosomal anomaly (deletion of 22.q11.2) characterized by hypoplasia or absence of the thymus and parathyroid glands. Clinically, the condition presents with neonatal hypocalcemic tetany, delayed mental and neurological development, and frequent infections,[1444] as well as congenital cardiac anomalies, facial dysmorphisms, gastrointestinal malformations, and more.[3000]

digit   (from Lat, a finger) 1. A finger, thumb, or toe. 2. A number from 0 to 9.

digit span test   A subtest of the **Wechsler Adult Intelligence Scale** test of attention span, in which the subject repeats progressively longer lists of numbers read out at 1 per second by the examiner, and then repeats similar lists but in reverse order. The normal forward span is 6 + 1, and the reverse span 2 less.

The test is not significantly affected by normal aging and is not very sensitive to dementia.[3851]

digit symbol test   A part of the **Wechsler Adult Intelligence Scale** in which the subject is required to place the correct number under each of a line of symbols according to a key provided, over a fixed period of time.[5889] The test is sensitive mainly to right hemisphere damage.

digital reflex   See **Hoffman reflex.**

digital subtraction   A technique whereby X-ray information is taken from a fluoroscopic screen by photomultiplier tubes and digitalized. By obtaining information from the screen immediately before passage of the contrast material through the blood vessels, the background information can be mathematically subtracted from that obtained after injection of the dye, so that only the opacified blood vessels are visualized.

digital subtraction angiography   A technique of angiography with intravenous injection of the contrast medium. Enhancement and digitalization of the initial image allows its electronic "subtraction" from the image obtained following injection, done by means of a computer.[4397,5385]

The sensitivity of digital subtraction systems permits a great reduction in the amount of dye injected compared to that required for conventional angiography, such savings being important in patients with congestive heart failure or renal failure. The combination of smaller catheters and digital subtraction equipment may enable the examination to be performed as an outpatient procedure.[4141]

digitalgia paresthetica   The term of **Wartenberg** for tingling suddenly felt in the distribution of the superficial branch of the ulnar nerve and followed by numbness without preceding trauma. Abduction of the little finger precipitates the tingling thereafter. The cause is unknown.[5862]

digiti quinti sign   (fifth finger sign) Slight abduction of the little finger on one side when the arms are outstretched; a sign of mild hemiparesis rather than of cerebellar disease as differentiated by Dr. Milton Alter. When the finger spread occurs bilaterally, however, the sign has no diagnostic significance.[128] See also **Souques sign, Leri sign.**

digitoocular maneuver   See **blindisms.**

digitoocular sign   The tendency of photophobic children to dig their fingers or fists into their orbits, which in time leads to atrophy of the periorbital tissues and sunken eyes.

digitorenocerebral syndrome   A recessively inherited dysmorphic syndrome characterized also by absence of the distal phalanges, renal and cardiac anomalies, seizures, optic atrophy, hypotonia, and mental and motor delay.[1699]

dihydrobiopterin synthetase deficiency   A congenital syndrome manifesting also hypotonia, dystonia, spasticity, neonatal seizures, hyperphenylalaninemia, aminoaciduria, and mental and developmental delay.[2965] See **phenylketonuria.**

dihydropteridine reductase deficiency (phenylketonuria 2) A progressive, congenital, dysmorphic syndrome manifesting also feeding difficulties, hypotonia, dystonia, spasticity, neonatal seizures, hyperphenylalaninemia, aminoaciduria, and mental and developmental delay,[2965] and usually leading to death within 2 years. The condition does not respond to diets with a low phenylalanine content. See also **phenylketonuria.**

dihydropyrimidine dehydrogenase deficiency A syndrome with onset in infancy or childhood, manifesting grand-mal seizures as a result of this metabolic error.

dilatation (from Lat, dilato, or Fr, dilatation, to spread out or widen) Abnormal widening of a structure such as a hollow viscus or artery. The word *dilation* is perfectly adequate but the repetition of the -at- is for some reason now customary, though its Latin derivation is from the transitive verb, or from the noun for an implement which itself does the dilating. Dilatators are not, however, used at all today.

dilatation lag Slowness and delay in dilation of the pupil in dark conditions after a bright light stimulus is withdrawn, as a result of the decreased pull of the radial dilator muscle.

There is less dilation of the affected pupil (>0.5 mm difference at 4 seconds than at 12 seconds) after a light flash. The lag is assessed after 5 seconds of darkness in comparison with the other, healthy pupil, and there should be no further lag between 5 and 10 seconds.[4445]

The presence of such lag is a cardinal feature of the *Horner syndrome*,[5721] although it is almost invisible to the naked eye and can only be demonstrated by in-dark or infrared pupillometry. The appropriate machine (a Polaroid camera), however, can quantitate the rate of dilation accurately, science thus eclipsing art.[4445]

Dimitri-Parkes-Weber disease See **Sturge-Weber syndrome.**

dimorphous leprosy A form of **leprosy** with features of both the lepromatous and the tuberculoid forms, and with both skin and nerve involvement.

dimple sign The presence of a localized, concave, oval area of pressure atrophy of compressed tissues, seen over the fibular head in cases of peroneal nerve pressure palsy, below the medial epicondyle in patients with ulnar neuropathy at the elbow[908] and in the low buttock after local trauma to fibers destined for the pudendal nerve at that site.[5326]

DIMS Acronym for **D**isorders of **I**nitiating and **M**aintaining **S**leep.

DIMS with atypical polysomnographic features A syndrome characterized by complaints of frequent awakenings and of nonrestorative sleep. The EEG shows high-voltage alpha waves superimposed on the non–rapid eye movement sleep delta activity, either persistently or as brief intrusions. See also **ASDA Diagnostic Classification.**[234]

ding (the ding) Mild post-traumatic concussion with brief amnesia but without discernible evidence of alteration in consciousness.

It is an occupational disease of professional football players[6068] but is far more frequently seen in the characters portrayed in children's animated cartoons.

dinitrophenyl hydrazine reaction (DNPH reaction) When equal volumes of a saturated solution of DNPH in 1 N hydrochloric acid and of urine are added together, a yellow or white precipitate is formed if ketoacids or ketones are present.

The test is generally requested as a screen for the presence of ketoacids in **maple syrup urine disease** but is also positive with the ketones produced in **propionic acidemia** and **methylmalonic aciduria.**

Dinno syndrome (pseudo-Marfan syndrome) A congenital dysmorphic syndrome manifesting also dislocation of the lens, arachnodactyly, macrocephaly, hydrocephalus, and osteosclerosis or osteopetrosis.[337]

Diogenes syndrome A literary allusion to the habits of the Greek philosopher who is said to have supplied all of his (minimal) needs for food and clothing by begging. His ideals included living a life according to nature, self-sufficiency, freedom from emotion, lack of shame, outspokenness, and contempt for social organization.[5047] Clark and colleagues reported the cases of 30 people who showed gross self-neglect in old age, living in squalor and filthy domestic and personal disorder, and suggested that this state constitutes a syndrome, to which they gave this name. Most of these people had had successful careers and 15 of the group still had a mean intelligence score of 115, dementing diseases thus being ruled out as causal. Cerebrovascular disease, parkinsonism, and malignancies were detected in some subjects, but vitamin deficiencies were found in almost all.

A conspicuous example of the syndrome was the English aristocrat Lord Rokeby, who allowed his estate to run to seed untended, while he spent much time immersed in water, keeping a piece of meat beside him for occasional sustenance.

diphasic dyskinesia A hyperkinetic form of fluctuation in the severity of dyskinetic movements in parkinsonian patients on long-term levadopa therapy, in parallel with the variations in the levadopa levels in the blood.

diphasic wave (biphasic wave) A wave consisting of two components developed on alternate sides of the baseline.

diphtheria Poisoning with the toxin of *Corynebacterium diphtheriae* (Klebs-Loeffler bacillus), which induces local paralysis of the bulbar, accommodative, external ocular, respiratory, and/or limb muscles in about one in five cases, due to demyelinating motor neuropathy during the third to the twelfth week after healing of the respiratory lesions. Mild sensory and potentially severe autonomic neuropathies may also occur, and optic neuritis and encephalitis have been reported, but rarely. In the majority that survive diphtheritic neuropathy, recovery is eventually complete.

Post-diphtheritic paralysis was the first neuropathy described as such, by Dr. Samuel Bard in 1771, although Hippocrates described nasal regurgitation in what was surely this disease. Lettsom gave an account of alcoholic polyneuritis 8 years after Bard's report.

diphtheritic pseudotabes   The syndrome of severe proprioceptive loss with sensory ataxia occurring in some patients with **diphtheria.**[2378]

diphthongia   The utterance of sounds having two different pitches during phonation, usually as the result of a local lesion of the larynx.

diplacusis   1. A sound being perceived by the two ears as having a different pitch. 2. Perception of a single sound as having two components. In each case, a disorder of the cochlear apparatus is likely to be responsible.

diplegia   (Gr, two + strokes) Weakness of the corresponding part on the two sides of the body, usually of both legs or of both sides of the face. Cerebral diplegia (**Little disease**) is a form of spastic cerebral palsy with involvement of both legs.

Since we also have the term *paraplegia,* the word *diplegia* is only relevant when used to describe strokes occurring in the same site on each side of the body, for example, the arms, which is excessively rare.

In **Foerster atonic diplegia,** the legs are affected more than the arms and a cerebellar syndrome, mental retardation, and hypotonia also occur.

diplegia with dissociation   (pseudoplegia, aphemia) A term denoting dissociation of voluntary and emotional movements, such as those of the face, jaws, throat, and larynx in the **anterior operculum syndrome.**[3601] See also **oral-buccal apraxia.**

diploë   The cancellous bone between the layers of compact bone forming the skull, except in the cribriform plate of the ethmoid and the orbital plates of the frontal bones.

diplomyelia   The longitudinal splitting of the spinal cord, as in **diastematomyelia.**

For this portion of its length, the cord is reduplicated rather than bisected, thus there are frequently two central canals.

diplopia   (Gr, double + vision). The awareness of two objects with but a single stimulus, as a result of lack of parallelism of the ocular axes.

In *crossed diplopia* (double vision caused by exotropia), the false image (from the affected eye) is peripheral to

that from the healthy eye. In *uncrossed* or *homonymous diplopia* (double vision caused by esotropia), the false image (from the affected eye) is on the same side as that eye; the cause is likely to be a sixth nerve palsy.

In *monocular (uniocular) diplopia,* the two images are seen with one eye.[3799] *Binocular diplopia* is that condition in which one of the two images is obliterated when either eye is closed.

See also **cerebral diplopia.**

dipole localization method   A technique under development whereby using computerized processing of scalp-derived recordings of induced spikes on the EEG, the dipole of origin may be localized intracerebrally.[5219]

dipping   (slow-downward **ocular bobbing**) An abnormal ocular condition in which the eye movement is slow downwards with a fast return to the mid-position. It is usually caused by anoxic encephalopathy, the area responsible being in the pons.

dipsomania   (Gr, thirst + madness) (oenomania) A recurrent, overpowering desire to drink alcohol in quantity, followed by periods of abstinence.

direct current amplifier   An amplifier that is capable of magnifying DC (zero frequency) voltages and slowly varying voltages. The direct-coupled amplifier and the chopper amplifier are direct current amplifiers. See also **direct-coupled amplifier, chopper amplifier.** (Adapted from the 1974 report of the Committee on Terminology, IFCN. In: Chatrian GE, Bergamini L, Dondey M, et al. A glossary of terms most commonly used by clinical electroencephalographers. *EEG Clin Neurophysiol* 1974;**37**:538–548.[989] Reprinted by kind permission of Elsevier Science.)

direct-coupled amplifier   An amplifier in which successive stages are connected (coupled) by devices that are not frequency dependent.

directional akinesia   (directional hypokinesia) A reluctance to move the eyes or the hands towards the (left) side, where there is hemispatial neglect as a result of a (right) parietal lobe lesion causing defective organization of movements towards the left half-space.[675]

directional cutaneous kinesthesia   The recognition of the direction in which a cutaneous stimulus is passing; a fundamental requirement for the perception of a complex pattern drawn on the skin such as a letter or number, and a function of the posterior columns in humans.[1295] See **direction-of-scratch test.**

directional continuous-wave Doppler sonography   A test employing ultrasound to assess changes in the periorbital circulation and thus to detect disease in the cervical portion of the internal carotid artery.

In normal supraorbital and frontal arteries, blood flows from within the skull to the surface of the scalp. Direction-sensing continuous-wave Doppler sonography identifies both the amplitude of the pulsations and the direction of the flow. In the presence of severe disease of the ipsilateral internal carotid artery, the direction of blood flow is reversed. The sensitivity of the test can be increased by using a variety of compression maneuvers to determine whether there is a compensatory increase in blood flow from collateral vessels.

The test is relatively simple to perform but is sensitive only to severe stenosis of the internal carotid artery and cannot differentiate this from occlusion.[4141]

directional dermokinesia   The awareness of the direction in which the skin is being pulled by an examiner.

directional hypokinesia   See **directional akinesia.**

directional preponderance   An increase in the duration or amplitude of the nystagmus beating toward one side compared with the other when induced by **caloric testing.** This lateralized difference suggests the presence of imbalance within the vestibular system but has no precise localizing value.

direction-changing nystagmus   That form of jerk nystagmus in which the direction of the fast component is the same as the direction of gaze. Thus the fast component will be to the left with leftward gaze and to the right with rightward gaze. See **central nystagmus.**

direction-fixed nystagmus   That form of jerk nystagmus in which the direction of the fast component is to the same side, whatever the direction of gaze.

Direction-fixed positional nystagmus is a horizontal jerk nystagmus that may occur transiently in normal subjects whose heads are rotated in either direction while they lie supine in darkness, but it always beats to the same side, whereas with *direction-changing positional nystagmus*, the nystagmus changes direction with head rotation, so that it either beats in the direction of the floor (*geotropic nystagmus*) or towards the sky (*apogeotropic nystagmus*). See also **peripheral nystagmus.**

direction-of-scratch test   A test of posterior column (and of cortical sensory) function, in which the examiner demonstrates the direction in which she makes a light scratch on the subject's palm (towards, away, left, right) while the latter watches; and then asks for identification of the direction in which further scratches are made with the subject blindfolded. Rough quantitation can be attained by varying the length of the scratch stimulus.[2415]

disability   The functional consequence of impairment, reducing a patient's capacity to perform the normal activities of daily life within that person's physical and social environment.

Scales for **activities of daily living** and performance scales examine this competency.

disability neurosis   (post-traumatic neurosis, accident neurosis) The persistence of injury-related symptoms beyond the time expected for recovery in the absence of evidence of incapacitating illness sufficient to prevent the patient from returning to work. Such patients are convinced of the reality of their disability and their histories do not suggest previous manipulative or exploitative behavior, but they tend to retain substantial resentment against their employer and, often, their physician. In the words of Ford,[1909] "The physical symptoms are . . . worn as a badge of angry protest for the injustices which they feel they have suffered. To give up these symptoms would mean that their anger had no justification. [When seen in psychiatric consultation they] have long-established patterns of disability and like Humpty Dumpty "all the King's horses and all the King's men' can't put them together again." See **compensation neurosis.**

disability scales   Semiquantitative rating scales of capacity and of performance. See also **stroke scales.**

disability status scale   See **Kurtzke rating scale.**[3198]

disabling (diabetic) neuropathy   See **diabetic neuropathy.**

disabling positional vertigo   A syndrome of persistent positional vertigo with nausea and tinnitus, considered to be caused by ischemia of the eighth cranial nerve.[2813]

discharge   An interpretative term used to designate EEG patterns. See **epileptiform pattern, seizure pattern, action potential.**

discharge frequency   The rate at which a potential discharges repetitively. When potentials occur in groups, the rate of recurrence of the group and rate of repetition of the individual components in the groups should be specified. (From the 2001 Report of the Nomenclature Committee of the American Association of Electromyography and Electrodiagnosis.[10] Used by permission, copyright © 2001, AAEM.

discrete activity   See **interference pattern.**

discogenic pain   Pain felt in radicular distribution as a result of impingement/irritation of a posterior nerve root by a protruded intervertebral disk. Its localization, lancinating quality, and association with activities that stretch the theca (such as coughing and bending over) are suggestive features, but it takes a trained neuroanatomist to distinguish discogenic pain from that due to **myofascial pain syndromes.** As a result, the diagnosis of prolapsed intervertebral disc is made in many patients when the problem is actually resulting from what is presumed to be local muscle spasm.

discography   The injection of contrast medium into an intervertebral disk under fluoroscopic control, in order to visualize extrusion of the disk or another pathology such as **disk disruption** as a cause of pain in the back.

discoid   In the shape of a disk or quoit.

disconnection anomia   See **anomia.**

disconnection syndromes (disconnexion syndromes; transcortical syndromes, conduction syndromes) The effects of lesions of association pathways, connecting separate brain regions, either those which lie exclusively in a single cerebral hemisphere or those which join the two halves of the brain. They include **alexia (word-blindness) without agraphia, pure word-deafness, ideomotor apraxia, tactile aphasia, conduction,** and **transcortical dysphasias.**[2080]

Although **Wernicke** suggested that **conduction aphasia** resulted from damage to the pathways separating the posterior language comprehension center and the speech output center, the concept of disconnection as the basis for certain syndromes of cerebral damage was only fully developed by **Geschwind.**[2080] A recent review is that of Absher and Benson.[29]

disconnexion syndromes   See **disconnection syndromes.**

discrete movements   "A process employing a small field of musculature and producing a single phasic movement of a small movable part against the background of a phasically inert musculature, in an anaesthetized animal" (Sir Francis Walshe).

This represents a laboratory abstraction rather than a clinical reality, since all focal movements occur in association with others in more proximal areas and thus are never truly "discrete," if the word is taken to mean separate or distinct. Nevertheless, with the introduction of **transcranial magnetic stimulation** in the human, the term may have regained both relevance and currency.

disease   The clinical expression of a morbid process.

Disease Steps   An assessment schedule used in patients with multiple sclerosis, relying largely upon motor (ambulatory) functions.[2610]

disinhibition-dementia-parkinsonism-amyotrophy complex (DDPAC) A dominantly inherited disorder with onset in mid-adult life, characterized by dementia, parkinsonism without tremor, and amyotrophy. Personality changes, alcoholism, and hyperphagia are early symptoms, after which the usual features of frontal lobe dementia develop. The gene is mapped to 17q21–22. Pathologically, atrophy and spongy changes are found in the frontotemporal cortex and there is neuronal loss in the substantia nigra and amygdala, without Lewy bodies.[3343] See **frontotemporal dementia.**

disjunctive eye movements   1. Abnormal eye movements resulting from aberrant regeneration of one of the oculomotor nerves, its fibers being directed to the wrong nerve.[449] 2. See **vergence.**

disjunctive nystagmus   Forms of nystagmus in which the eyes do not maintain their normal yoked position. See **dissociated nystagmus.**

disk disruption   A syndrome of persistent low back pain following compressive spinal overload. The diagnosis is made by **discography,** which reproduces the patient's pain and demonstrates disruption of the internal architecture of the disk.[1184]

disk prolapse   Backward herniation of the nucleus pulposus of an intervertebral disk as seen on a **myelogram,** to the extent that nerve roots may be compressed or the spinal canal compromised.

disk protrusion   Bulging of an intervertebral disc, as seen on a **myelogram.** This is a common finding related to age and wear and tear, and has no pathological significance unless it leads to surgery; unlike **disk prolapse,** it is not associated with compression of a spinal nerve root. The problem lies in telling the difference.

disk reabsorption (isolated disk resorption) A variant of **degenerative spinal stenosis** in which chronic low back pain is associated with reduction of the height of the (L5/S1) disc to 3 mm or less, facet joint hypertrophy, and a trefoil appearance of the spinal canal.[1183]

disorders of excessive sleep (DOES) A group of functional and organic conditions in which the chief symptoms are the awareness of inappropriate and undesirable sleepiness during waking hours, often with decreased cognitive and motor performance, excessive tendency to sleep, unavoidable napping, and an increase in total 24-hour sleep with full arousal on awakening. The classification in Chart D–9 is adapted from the 1979 Association of Sleep Disorders Centers Diagnostic Classification,[249] which, although superseded by the American Sleep Disorders Association classification,[234] provides a useful overview of this class of disturbances.

Chart D–9. Disorders of Excessive Sleep

B1. Psychophysiological
    a. **Transient and situational DOES**
    b. **Persistent DOES**
B2. Associated with psychiatric disorders
B3. DOES associated with use or withdrawal from drugs or alcohol
B4. DOES associated with sleep-induced respiratory impairment
    a. **Sleep apnea DOES syndrome**
    b. **Alveolar hypoventilation DOES syndrome**
B5. Sleep-related myoclonus and restless legs
    a. **Sleep-related myoclonus DOES syndrome**
    b. **Restless legs DOES syndrome**
B6. **Narcolepsy**
B7. **Idiopathic CNS hypersomnolence**
B8. DOES associated with other medical, toxic, and environmental conditions
B9. Other DOES conditions
    a. Intermittent DOES (periodic) syndromes
        Kline-Levin syndrome
        Menstrual-associated syndrome
    b. Insufficient sleep

c. **Sleep drunkenness**

B10. No DOES abnormality

   a. **Long sleeper**

   b. Subjective DOES complaint without objective findings

disorders of initiating and maintaining sleep (DIMS) Heterogeneous conditions considered to be responsible for inducing disturbed sleep and for diminishing the amount of sleep experienced. The classification in Chart D–10 is adapted from the 1979 Association of Sleep Disorders Centers Diagnostic Classification,[249] which, although superseded by the American Sleep Disorders Association classification,[234] provides a useful overview of this class of disturbances.

Chart D–10. Classification of Disorders of Initiating and Maintaining Sleep

A1a. **Transient and situational DIMS**

A1b. **Persistent DIMS**

A2. DIMS associated with psychiatric disorders

A3. DIMS associated with use or withdrawal from drugs or alcohol

A4. DIMS associated with sleep-induced respiratory impairment

   a. **Sleep apnea DIMS syndrome**

   b. **Alveolar hypoventilation DIMS syndrome**

A5. Sleep-related myoclonus and restless legs

   a. **Sleep-related myoclonus DIMS syndrome**

   b. **Restless legs DIMS syndrome**

A6. DIMS associated with other medical, toxic, and environmental conditions.

A7. **Childhood-onset DIMS**

A8. Other DIMS syndromes

   a. **Repeated REM sleep interruptions**

   b. Atypical polysomnographic features

A9. No DIMS abnormality

   a. **Short sleeper**

   b. Subjective DIMS complaint without objective findings

disorders of the sleep–wake cycle Conditions sharing the feature that they represent the misalignment of the subject's individual sleeping and waking patterns and the circadian pattern of that individual or society. This group represents the third class of sleep disturbances recognized in the Association of Sleep Disorders Centers Diagnostic Classification[249] (see Chart D–11 but see also the American Sleep Disorders Association Diagnostic Classification[234]).

Chart D–11. Classification of Disorders of the Sleep–Wake Cycle

C1. Transient

   a. **Rapid time zone change syndrome** (jet lag)

   b. **Work shift change** in conventional sleep–wake schedule

C2. Persistent

   a. Frequently changing sleep–wake cycle

   b. **Delayed sleep phase syndrome**

   c. **Advanced sleep phase syndrome**

   d. **Non–24–hour sleep–wake syndrome**

   e. Irregular sleep–wake pattern

disorganization The gross alteration in frequency, form, topography, and/or quantity of physiological EEG rhythms in an individual record relative to previous records in the same subject or to the rhythms of homologous regions on the opposite side of the head. (From Chatrian GE, Gergamini L, Dondey M, et al. A glossary of terms most commonly used by clinical electroencephalographers. *EEG. Clin. Neurophysiol.* 1974; 37:538–48,[989] with permission from Elsevier Science.)

disorientation The lack of ability to define one's position vis-à-vis the environment, or to localize oneself within a place such as a room, house, town, or country, usually due to a lesion in the right parietal lobe.[1852]

dissecting aneurysm See **aneurysm.**

dissection 1. Splitting of the wall of an artery due to disease of the intima, thus opening up a false channel for the passage of blood that compresses the normal channel. 2. The lesion produced by penetration of the circulating blood into the substance of the wall of a vessel with subsequent extension of the effused blood for a varying distance between its layers. Mechanical trauma and an inherent weakness of the arterial wall collagen are thought to be responsible. The presence of the dissection is well shown by magnetic resonance angiography.

Dissections were first recognized by Maunoir, a Swiss surgeon, in 1802. They are important causes of strokes in young adults. In the extracranial carotid artery, the usual clinical picture includes minor strokelike episodes with vascular headaches and an associated **Horner syndrome** due to dissections of the medial coat; the prognosis is commonly good. Intracranially, the dissections are usually subintimal and may lead to subarachnoid hemorrhage. Dissections of the vertebral arteries extracranially are less common; they are more common in women, are often bilateral, and can lead to brainstem strokes and neck pain. Minor trauma is likely to play a part in causation. Intracranial vertebral dissections present with subarachnoid hemorrhage. Basilar dissections are typically lethal but rare. Common carotid artery dissection causes local swelling and pain.

The main neurological syndrome associated with aortic dissections is that of cervical vascular myelopathy, but the cardiac complications often overshadow that.

disseminated encephalomalacia with cavity formation (familial multilocular encephalomalacia) A leukoencephalopathy of unknown cause characterized by the formation of large cavities in the white matter of infants.

Seizures, progressive rigidity, and pareses lead to stupor and early death.[1190]

disseminated intravascular coagulation A syndrome resulting from vascular damage in which there is activation of plasma coagulation factors or entry of tissue thromboplastic material into the blood. The most prominent clinical feature is bleeding, including cerebral hemorrhage, which stems from the consumption of platelets and certain coagulation factors; as a result of this, severe thrombocytopenia and deficiency of fibrinogen arise. The clinical spectrum extends from insignificant laboratory abnormalities to uncontrollable and persistent hemorrhage and thrombosis.

disseminated neurogenic atrophy The occurrence of clusters of three to six small, angulated muscle fibers of the same histochemical type in muscle biopsy specimens. The finding suggests progressive denervation without effective collateral sprouting.

disseminated sarcoid leukoencephalopathy See **neurosarcoidosis.**

disseminated vasculomyelinopathy A term encompassing the para- or postinfectious diseases of the nervous system which takes note of the fact that there is evidence of both demyelination and damage to small blood vessels in these conditions.

Clinically, an abrupt monophasic illness follows common infections with a latent interval of days or weeks and consists of any of the syndromes of clinical encephalitis, aseptic meningitis, ataxia, chorea, myelitis, cranial and peripheral neuropathies (including **acute inflammatory demyelinating polyneuropathy**), and brachial neuritis, in any combination.[4500]

dissociated anesthesia Impairment of some forms of sensation with retention of others in the same area.

A typical form is the loss of the thin-fiber (spinothalamic) functions of pinprick pain, light touch, and temperature sensation, with sparing of the thick-fiber functions such as discriminative light touch, position sense, and vibration, on the body below the level of a cordotomy sectioning the spinothalamic tract. The **lateral medullary syndrome, tabes dorsalis,** vitamin B_{12} deficiency, **diabetes mellitus,** and some forms of **hereditary sensory and autonomic neuropathy** are other examples.

dissociated aphasia See **Wernicke aphasia.**

dissociated nystagmus (disjunctive nystagmus) Those forms of nystagmus in which the movements of the eyes are not symmetrical, the oscillations being greater in amplitude, speed, or direction in one eye, or present only in one eye. Both jerky and pendular forms can occur. **Internuclear ophthalmoplegia, conver-**

gence–retraction nystagmus, spasmus nutans, and see-saw nystagmus are examples. The usual cause is a brainstem lesion. See also **pseudoabducens palsy, divergence nystagmus.**

dissociated vertical divergence A congenital ocular dysmotility syndrome, in which occlusion or dimming of one eye leads to the elevation of that eye. The sign has no localizing value.[1128]

dissociation (conversion) A mental mechanism whereby a subject can suppress awareness of sensation or of mental content, or can inhibit the usual facility for movement of a body part either voluntarily or under the influence of strong emotion. **Head** pointed out that neurologists employ this mechanism every time they look through an ophthalmoscope.

It is defined in the ICD-10 as "a partial or complete loss of the normal integration between memories of the past, awareness of identity and immediate sensations, and control of body movements." Thus included would be dissociative amnesias, fugue states, trance and possession disorders, dissociative anesthesia, sensory losses, motor disorders, convulsions (**nonepileptic seizures**), and other intercurrent and usually unnamed manifestations.[803]

dissociation cytoalbuminologique An euphonious French phrase indicating that the increases in CSF protein levels and in the CSF cell count are not always of the same magnitude; in this case, the protein level is greatly elevated but there is little or no increase in the number of white cells. This may occur in spinal block, in **acute inflammatory demyelinating polyneuropathy,** and with **vestibular schwannoma.**

dissociation of lateral gaze syndrome See **Raymond-Cestan syndrome.**

dissociation of reflexes Absence of the superficial and augmentation of the muscle stretch reflexes, as with pyramidal tract lesions.

dissociative disorder See **somatization disorder.**

dissociative speech syndromes Those varieties of dysphasia in which the relevant cortical areas are partly isolated from the remainder of the brain by virtue of the interruption of afferent, efferent, or associative pathways. **Conduction** and **transcortical dysphasias** are examples.

dissonance (from Lat, to disagree in sound) Discord.

distal (from Lat, to be distant from another thing) The term for those body parts progressively more distant from the trunk or midline—thus the hands and feet and *a fortiori* the fingers and toes—as opposed to **proximal.**

distal acquired demyelinating symmetric neuropathy (DADS) An acquired, symmetrical demyelinating neuropathy with distal sensory or sensorimotor features. The distribution of the weakness and the usual presence of an IgM-κ monoclonal gammopthy help to distinguish this condition from **chronic inflammatory demyelinating polyradiculoneuropathy.**[2953]

distal amyotrophy predominantly of the upper limbs See **monomelic amyotrophy.**

distal and segmental muscular atrophy of upper extremities See **hereditary motor neuropathy.**

distal anterior compartment myopathy A recessively inherited muscular dystrophy (*a dysferlinopathy*) mapped to the 2p13 locus. It resembles *Miyoshi* and *Nonaka myopathies* (see **distal muscular dystrophy**) but is characterized by onset in early adult life, initial weakness, and wasting in the anterior tibial muscles before rapid generalization to all muscle groups, raised serum CK levels, and sparing of the cranial muscles.[2731]

distal axonal degeneration See **distal axonopathy.**

distal axonal spheroids Swellings containing various organelles, occurring at the terminations of axons in a variety of diseases.

distal axonopathy (dying-back neuropathy, distal axonal degeneration, distal lower motor neuron syndrome) Forms of neuropathy in which there is asymmetrical distal but centripetal failure of function due to impairment of the axonal transport mechanisms, in turn usually as a result of damage to the perikaryon of the nerve cell.[940] This leads to secondary myelin breakdown.

High titers of anti-GM$_1$ or other antibodies are found in a majority of cases. See also **multifocal motor neuropathy, proximal lower motor neuron syndromes.**

distal hereditary upper limb muscular atrophy A dominantly inherited neurogenic disorder presenting with weakness and atrophy of the distal arms and hands, brisk reflexes, and minimal sensory findings. Electrophysiological studies do not suggest axonal loss and motor nerve conduction velocities are nearly normal whereas distal motor latencies are prolonged.[2289]

distal latency The interval between the delivery of a stimulus to the most distal point of stimulation on a nerve and the onset of a response. A measure of the conduction properties of the most distal portion of motor or sensory nerves. (From the 2001 Report of the Nomenclature Committee of the American Association of Electromyography and Electrodiagnosis.[10] Used by permission, copyright © 2001, AAEM.)

distal lower motor neuron syndrome See **distal axonopathy.**

distal muscle wasting, nephritis, and deafness See **hereditary motor and sensory neuropathy, type 2.**

distal muscular dystrophy (type 1 distal myopathy, Gowers syndrome, late hereditary myopathy, Welander myopathy) A heterogeneous group of genetic muscle diseases, often dominantly inherited, and characterized by progressive distal weakness and wasting. Creatine kinase levels are slightly raised and in some forms vacuolar changes are seen on muscle biopsy specimens. Cardiomyopathy is also described.[2241] Abnormalities of the genes for dysferlin and desmin are the two best decribed.

In the myopathy described by **Welander,**[5908] progressive distal weakness and wasting with onset in mature adult life affects the hands most of all. The condition is seen almost exclusively in the population of Scandinavian countries. Serum creatine kinase levels are slightly raised and vacuolar changes are seen on muscle biopsy specimens. **Gowers** described a condition such as this in 1902,[2241] but his patients might equally well have had **myotonic dystrophy.** *Variant* forms are listed in Chart D–12.

Numerous distinct predominantly **distal myopathies** have been identified with discrete clinical and genetic patterns. The following descriptive listing owes much to the review by Mastaglia and Laing[3686] and the study by Nonaka.[4152]

Chart D–12. Forms of Distal Muscular Dystrophy

A. *Definite entities*

1. *Welander myopathy* (late adult onset, type 1), with autosomal dominant inheritance, linked to 2p13, as described above.

2. *Nonaka myopathy* (distal myopathy with rimmed vacuole formation; early adult onset, type 1), with autosomal recessive inheritance and molecular localization to 9p1–q1. There is striking distal weakness of the gastrocnemii and peroneal muscles and mild proximal weakness, with onset in early adult life and slightly elevated CK levels. Nonaka myopathy is identical to *quadriceps-sparing familial inclusion body myopathy.* Progression is slow. Pathologically, the condition is characterized by muscle fiber atrophy with rimmed vacuole formation in the cytoplasm.[4153]

3. *Miyoshi myopathy* (early adult onset, type 2), with autosomal recessive inheritance and localization to the 2p13 locus (like limb-girdle muscular dysytrophy type 2b, a *dysferlinopathy*). Onset is in youth or adult life with distal muscle weakness and atrophy. Uniquely in this group, first the gastrocnemii are affected, and there are high serum CK levels. The arms are affected late but the small hand muscles are spared. Muscle biopsy changes are similar to those of Duchenne dystrophy.[367,3921]

4. *Distal myopathy with rimmed vacuole formation,* a recessively inherited myopathy presenting with striking distal weakness of the gastrocnemii and peroneal muscles and mild proximal weakness, with onset in early adult life and with slightly elevated CK levels. It is mapped to 9p1–q1, and is characterized pathologically by muscle fiber atrophy with rimmed vacuole formation in the cytoplasm.[4153]

5. *Tibial myopathy or Markesbery-Griggs/type 2, late-onset hereditary distal myopathy* (Finnish, late adult onset, type 2), with autosomal dominant inheritance and linkage to chromosome 2q31–33. This is a slowly progres-

sive form, with onset in the anterior compartment. Serum CK levels are slightly raised.[3629,3630,5681]

6. *Laing early-onset myopathy* (early adult onset, type 3), with autosomal dominant inheritance and linkage to chromosome 14q11. Initial weakness and wasting are in the anterior compartment. Serum CK levels are slightly elevated.[3227]

B. *Forms reported only in single families*
Adult-onset distal myopathy[1777]
Distal myopathy with pes cavus and areflexia[5077]
Distal myopathy with vocal cord and pharyngeal signs[1768]
Very late-onset distal myopathy[4407]
Variable-onset distal myopathy Sumner (1971) referenced by Udd[5679]

C. *New phenotypes*
Juvenile-onset distal myopathy[6130]
New Finnish distal myopathy[3568]
Distal myopathy with respiratory failure[1012]

D. *Other distal myopathies*
Desmin-related distal myopathy[3873]
Desmin-related myopathy.[5679] See **distal myopathy with desmin storage.**
Desmin-related with sarcoplasmic bodies[1605]
Oculopharyngeal distal myopathy[4925]
Distal myopathy with onset in infancy. An autosomal dominant form has also been described.
A *dominantly inherited nonprogressive form* with onset in early childhood. Clinically, distal involvement of the arms and legs with selective weakness of the deltoid muscles occur in association with scoliosis, genu valgus, and limitation of mobility of some joints. Muscle biopsy specimens show disproportion of fibers with selective atrophy of type 1 fibers.[398]
Distal myopathy with early adult onset A dominantly inherited myopathic syndrome with onset in young or middle adult life. The thenar muscles and hand flexors are affected early and pes cavus is usually present. Muscle biopsy specimens show sarcoplasmal bodies and an abundance of intermediate-sized skeletin filaments.[53]
Double ring myopathy. A myopathy of adult life.
Forms with *autosomal recessive* inheritance[5031] and with more generalized weakness and earlier onset.[3156] In such cases, marked leg plantar flexor weakness is characteristic.
Distal myopathy (New Guinea). A recessively inherited syndrome of distal weakness and wasting with onset in the fourth decade leading to oculopharyngeal symptoms within the next 10 years, reported from New Guinea.

distal myopathy   See **distal muscular dystrophy.**

distal myopathy with desmin storage   A dominantly inherited distal myopathy characterized by onset in early to middle adult life, gait disturbance due to distal leg weakness, and eventual generalization to all body areas, including the heart, leading to premature death. Electrical findings include prominent spontaneous activity, short-duration motor unit potentials, and polyphasia. Muscle biopsy specimens show desmin storage and autophagocytosis.[2657]

distal myopathy with onset in infancy   See **distal muscular dystrophy.**

distal myopathy with proximal weakness and early respiratory failure   A dominantly inherited distal myopathy presenting in mid-adult life with tibialis anterior weakness, proceeding to ventilatory impairment and girdle weakness.[1012] Other, similar phenotypes have also been described.[4129,6057] See **myopathy.**

distal myopathy with rimmed vacuole formation   See **distal muscular dystrophy** (*Nonaka form*).

distal small-fiber neuropathy   A form of generalized peripheral neuropathy affecting the small-diameter, thinly myelinated and unmyelinated fibers.

Clinically, complaints of paresthesias, hyperesthesias, and burning, aching, shooting, or prickling dysesthesias are the usual findings, along with only a minor reduction in temperature and sharp pain sensations, and reduction in distal sweating. Thick-fiber sensory functions, motor power, reflexes, and conventional nerve conduction studies are almost or completely normal.

Amyloidosis, monoclonal gammopathy, and **chronic inflammatory demyelinating neuropathy** are representative causes.[5353]

distal spinal muscular atrophy   A variously inherited syndrome of distal wasting without sensory change, not yet definitively classified between the hereditary motor and the hereditary motor and sensory neuropathies. The clinical manifestations appear in childhood or adolescence and resemble those of **hereditary motor and sensory neuropathy, type 1** or **2** but with less arm weakness, relative preservation of the muscle stretch reflexes, and normal sensory examination.[2445] See **hereditary motor and sensory neuropathy, neuronal form, hereditary motor neuropathies** (*variants*).

distal spinal muscular atrophy with a hoarse voice   See **hereditary motor neuropathy** (*variants*).

distal spinal muscular atrophy with vocal cord paralysis   See **hereditary motor neuropathy** (*variants*).

distal vacuolar myopathy   A severe generalized myopathy affecting distal muscles of the hand at first, and later the bulbar muscles. Sensory functions and muscle stretch reflexes are normal.

The condition is described in patients with nephropathic cystinosis who have received renal transplants.[984]

distance receptors   Those receptors which respond to objects at a distance and upon which the brain is constructed and has evolved. Generally speaking, the channels are physical rather than chemical.

distance shortening   In patients with pyramidal lesions, the distance that the subject extends the paretic arm away from the nose in the finger–nose test progressively shortens with repeated cycles. This may be a useful early sign of an upper motor neurone lesion.[4479]

distant toe flexor reflex   (Schrijver-Bernhard reflex) Plantar flexion of the toes in response to a tap given to a distant part of the body, sometimes seen in patients with extrapyramidal but not with pyramidal lesions.[5858] The mechanism of the sign is not known and its clinical significance is dubious.

distant wounded glioma syndrome   A tumor-induced coagulopathy, leading to hemorrhage within the cavity of partially resected tumors such as multifocal glioblastoma multiforme or within distant tumor nodules following surgical resection, even though the distant sites were not directly manipulated during the surgical procedures. It is postulated that because of their rich vascularity, these distant tumor nodules are more susceptible to hemorrhage, resulting from coagulation changes after tumor resection, than are other sites.[3110]

distortion   An instrumental alteration in waveforms on EEG or EMG recordings.

disturbance   (from Lat, to put in disarray) An interference with the normal physiological functions of the body or of a part of it.

disturbance in visual orientation   See **visuomotor ataxia.**

disuse atrophy   The reduction in size of a body part when its function is impaired as a result of disease. The histological changes accompanying this are minimal, but atrophied groups of fibers may be found in some muscles.[4357]

diurna(l)   (from Lat, a day) 1. Daily. 2. In the daytime.

diurnal dystonia   (dystonia with marked diurnal variation) A dominantly inherited condition in which dystonic movements occur in the evening and night rather than in the morning and in which patients may show evidence of parkinsonism.[4278,5052]

The condition may be a variant of **dopa-responsive dystonia** since it also responds to L-dopa and to bromocriptine in low dosage. See also **dystonia.**

divaricate   (Lat, to stretch apart) Separate.

divebomber sound   The decrescendo whine of myotonic discharges heard on the EMG machine's loudspeaker. Those who have had the dubious privilege of hearing both, however, consider that the sound of a receding motor cycle provides a closer comparison.

divergence   (from Lat, apart + to incline) Separation from a common point.

divergence nystagmus   A form of nystagmus complicating congenital adduction palsy or hindbrain lesions such as the **Chiari malformation,** in which the affected eye moves into abduction on attempted adduction. The associated nystagmus is of jerk type, the fast component of the two eyes being to their respective sides.

divergence paralysis   See **dorsal midbrain syndrome.**

Divers Alert Network   (Duke University, Durham, NC) A central facility offering advice on the management of diving accidents. Tel: 919–684–8111. Web site: http://diversalertnetwork.org/.

divination   (from Lat, to foresee) Prognostication without medical evidence.

divisional paresis   Weakness of the muscles supplied by the superior or by the inferior branches of the third cranial nerve.

The causal lesion will usually be found in the anterior cavernous sinus (where the two divisions separate) or in the posterior orbit, but may be in the brainstem. The superior division innervates the levator palpebrae superioris and the superior rectus (in the latter case by fibers from the contralateral side), while the inferior branch supplies the inferior and medial rectus, the inferior oblique, and the iris sphincter.[3172]

Divry–van Bogaert syndrome   (familial capillary-venous leptomeningeal angiomatosis) See **van Bogaert syndrome.**

dizziness   A disturbance in the sense of a person's subjective relationship to the exterior environment (subjective awareness of instability) resulting from impairment of proprioception, vision, vestibular function, or global cerebral blood flow and used in the vernacular for vertigo, light-headedness, faintness, and the awareness of being liable to fall.

DNPH reaction   See **dinitrophenylhydrazine reaction.**

Doctrine of the Nerves   The phrase of Thomas **Willis** denoting "neurology," adopted by Spillane for his masterly review of the history of this subject.[5280]

DOES   Acronym for **D**isorders **O**f **E**xcessive **S**leep.

dogmatics   An ancient Greek sect of physicians who attempted to discover the causes of disease by using reasoning, and recommended the study of anatomy and the basic sciences. Their opponents, the **Empirics,** denied the value of such study.[4512]

Only when curriculum committees are composed of members of these two sects in equal numbers is the dean able to exert some influence on the teaching methods employed within a medical school.

dolichocephaly   (Gr, long + head) A developmental defect in skull shape in which there is abnormal length of the head in its anteroposterior diameter, due to premature fusion of the sagittal suture.

In lesser degrees, this also represents one physiological skull shape as defined in 1842 by Anders Adolf Retzius (1769–1860), a Swedish anatomist, on the basis of the cranial index; the length/breadth ratios were said to be in the proportion 9:7 or more. The converse form, in which the skull is abnormally wide, is **brachycephaly.**

dolichoectasia   Fusiform dilatation of an artery. *Intracranial arterial dolichoectasia* is a condition in which such enlargement and tortuosity exist in vessels coming off the circle of Willis. Atherosclerosis is the most common cause, but it is also seen in **Fabry disease.** Clinical features reflect the occurrence of stroke, local compression of neurological structures by the enlarged vessels, or increased intracranial pressure.[2734]

Dollinger-Bielschowsky syndrome   See **neuronal ceroid lipofuscinosis.**

doll's eye movements   See **oculocephalic reflex.**

doll's eye response   See **oculocephalic reflex.**

doll's eye sign   See **Cantelli sign.**

doll's eyelids   Reflex opening of the eyelids when the neck is briskly flexed in comatose patients; a phenomenon largely confined to cases of subarachnoid hemorrhage with stupor.[1847]

This is the only one of the commonly described "doll signs" in which the clinical phenomenon is actually the same as that seen in the toy.

doll's head response   See **oculocephalic reflex.**

dolor capitis/cephalicus   (Lat, pain + of the head) Headache.

Dolman-Delcato treatment   An exclusive system of treatments involving passive exercises, promoted for the management of children suffering from brain damage and other conditions but condemned because of the lack of scientific substantiation provided by its proponents.[140]

dominance   The particular responsibility for a function invested in one or other of the cerebral hemispheres; a concept remarked upon by Marc Dax in 1836 where even Gall was silent. (Gall had localized speech functions in the anterior part of the frontal lobes by 1819 but made no comment about lateralization.) It was introduced as a truth by Broca in 1865, who correlated aphasia, right-handedness, and lesions of the left hemisphere.[473]

Deficits that indicate dominant responsibilities of the left hemisphere are disorders of gesture; ideational and ideomotor apraxias; agnosias for reading and writing, objects, and colors; and somatognosis; bilateral asomatognosia also follows a left hemisphere lesion.

Hughlings-**Jackson** made the perceptive comment in 1864 that if "the faculty of expression resides in one hemisphere, then there is no absurdity in raising the question as to whether perception—its corresponding opposite—may not be seated in the other." Indeed, nondominant hemisphere lesions do lead to visuospatial disturbances, including unilateral **asomatognosia,**

dressing apraxia, some forms of **dyslexia, dysgraphia** and **dyscalculia,** and the inability to recognize faces (**prosopagnosia**) as suggested first by Hughlings-**Jackson,** who also correctly assigned to the right hemisphere a role in automatic and emotional speech. **Babinski** noted first the occurrence of anosognosia following right hemisphere lesions in 1914, while Dide[1438] considered that visuoconstructive disorders (**constructional apraxia**) reflected a posterior right hemisphere lesion.

dominant albinism and congenital deafness   (Tietz syndrome) A dominantly inherited syndrome of complete albinism except for the optic fundi and irides, scanty eyebrows, and congenital severe neural hearing loss.[5583]

dominant anhidrosis and progressive hearing loss A dominantly inherited syndrome of congenital anhidrosis with progressive neural hearing loss in middle age.[2530]

dominant ataxia   See **cerebellar ataxias.**

dominant basal ganglion calcification   See **striatopallidal calcification.**

dominant cerebellar ataxia plus   See **cerebellar ataxias** (*variants*).

dominant congenital severe deafness   A dominantly inherited syndrome characterized by congenital severe deafness but normal vestibular responses.[3124]

dominant hand weakness with sensorineural deafness   A rare congenital familial syndrome of unilateral or bilateral neural deafness with contractures of the digits and wasting of all the small hand muscles. Flexion creases are absent over the interphalangeal joints, and there is a single vertical palmar crease. There is no abnormality on X-ray studies of the affected hand joints.[5354]

dominant knuckle pads, leukonychia, and hearing loss   (Bart-Pumphrey syndrome) A rare, nonprogressive, dominantly inherited syndrome characterized by congenital leukonychia, childhood onset of knuckle pads, progressive neural deafness, and diminished vestibular responses.[377,3124]

dominant leukodystrophy showing cerebellar deficits and spastic paraparesis   A dominant hereditary disorder with onset in early childhood, showing progressive spastic paraparesis with cerebellar deficits and mild mental deterioration, and the subsequent appearance of limb spasticity. It results in severe disability by the fourth decade of life. Brain MRI shows diffuse white matter involvement. No biochemical or gene deficits characteristic of other leukodystrophies are present.[1981]

dominant low-frequency hearing loss   A dominantly inherited syndrome with variable penetrance, characterized by moderate low-frequency hearing loss appearing at any time in life, with slow progression to moderately severe deafness involving all frequencies but with normal vestibular function.[3124]

dominant mid-frequency hearing loss A dominantly inherited syndrome characterized by progressive mid-frequency hearing loss in childhood and eventually loss at all frequencies, especially high tones, but with normal vestibular function.[3652]

dominant muscular dystrophy with humeropelvic distribution A slowly progressive myopathy presenting with humeropelvic weakness and contractures in childhood and cardiomyopathy after the age of 20. The syndrome is dominantly inherited but otherwise resembles the **Emery-Dreifuss** form of X-linked dystrophy.[1784]

dominant myopia, hearing loss, peripheral neuropathy, and skeletal abnormalities syndrome See **Flynn-Aird syndrome.**

dominant nephritis and hearing loss See **Alport syndrome.**

dominant optic atrophy A syndrome with adult onset, characterized by ptosis, ophthalmoplegia, optic atrophy, ataxia, nerve deafness, and myopathic weakness.[5628]

dominant osteosclerosis See **hyperostosis corticalis generalisata congenita.**

dominant otofaciocervical abnormalities A dominantly inherited syndrome characterized by hypoplasia of the maxillofacial complex, preauricular pits and fistulas, hypoplasia of the cervical muscles, resulting in lowering of the shoulder girdle, and conductive hearing loss.[1742]

dominant photomyoclonus, hearing loss, diabetes, and nephropathy A dominantly inherited condition characterized by neural deafness in association with bilateral neurofibromas of the eighth cranial nerve (usually unassociated with other evidence of **neurofibromatosis**) and seizures.[2551]

dominant preauricular pits and neural hearing loss A dominantly inherited syndrome with variable penetrance, manifesting mild to severe progressive neural hearing loss with onset in childhood or youth, unilateral or bilateral preauricular pits, and unilateral or bilateral branchial fistulas in a few cases.[1918]

dominant progressive nerve deafness A dominantly inherited syndrome characterized by childhood onset of a progressive symmetrical neural hearing loss beginning with high frequencies and leading to moderately severe hearing loss in later life.[5333]

dominant saddle nose, myopia, cataract, and hearing loss (Marshall syndrome) A dominantly inherited syndrome consisting of myopia, cataracts, saddlenose, and early-onset progressive neural deafness.[3649]

dominant stroke-like episodes and leukoencephalopathy A dominantly inherited syndrome characterized by recurrent subcortical stroke-like episodes in adult life, and with leukoencephalopathy, muscular lipidosis, and immunological abnormalities.[5617]

dominant unilateral deafness A dominantly inherited syndrome with variable penetrance, characterized by congenital moderate to severe unilateral or bilateral hearing loss and normal vestibular function.[5215]

domoic acid encephalopathy A syndrome comprising acute gastrointestinal upset followed by neural hyperexcitability and chronic loss of function following the ingestion of domoic acid, a naturally occurring toxin that is related to glutamate and that caused an outbreak of poisoning in Canada in 1987.

Initial symptoms include abdominal discomfort, vomiting, diminished consciousness, short-term memory loss, confusion, headache, seizures and myoclonus, autonomic disturbances, and variable pareses, including ophthalmopareses. In the long term, anterograde-term memory loss and chronic anterior horn cell lesions may persist.[5517]

Donaldson syndrome (nephrolithiasis-mitochondrial cytopathy) A congenital dysmorphic syndrome manifesting also short stature, cataract, retinitis pigmentosa, strabismus, cardiomyopathy, nephropathy, diabetes, red cell abnormalities, cerebral atrophy, seizures, ataxia, and distal myopathic weakness.[337]

Donner muscular dystrophy See **congenital muscular dystrophy.**

Donohue syndrome A rare, autosomal recessive, congenital encephalopathic and dysmorphic syndrome characterized by facial and generalized hirsutism, marasmus, hypoglycemia, hypotonia, microcephaly, prenatal growth defect, failure of bony maturation, lipodystrophy, enlarged genitalia, and mental and motor delay. It usually leads to death in infancy.[1494] See **leprechaunism.**

DOOR syndrome See **deafness-onychodystrophy-onycholysis-retardation syndrome.**[891]

Doose syndrome See **centrencephalic myoclonic-astatic epilepsy.**

dopamine A neurotransmitter with particularly high levels in certain neurons of the neostriatum, derived from L-dopa by dopa-decarboxylase and greatly reduced in parkinsonian syndromes.

dopamine receptors D_1 and D_2 receptors are recognized, the former stimulating and the latter inhibiting adenylate cyclase and both together thus regulating dopamine metabolism.

dopa-responsive dystonia (autosomal dominant torsion dystonia, dopa-sensitive progressive dystonia of childhood, dystonia musculorum deformans, dystonia with marked diurnal variation associated with biopterin deficiency, fluctuating dystonia, hereditary parkinsonism-dystonia, hereditary dystonia-parkinsonism syndrome of juvenile onset) A dominantly inherited (or recessively inherited or sporadic) variant of idiopathic (torsion) dystonia, due to a mutation of the GCH1 locus on chromosome 14q, manifesting foot and dystonia and gait disorder in children before the age of 12 years, and marked by worsening as the day progresses, unusual responsiveness of the symptoms to oral L-dopa in low dosage, and by the frequent presence of parkinsonian features, at least later in life.[4181] See also **dystonia, Segawa dystonia.**

dopa-sensitive progressive dystonia of childhood See **dopa-responsive dystonia.**

doppelgänger An hallucinated representation of oneself. See **heautoscopy.**

Doppler, C.J. (1803–1853) Austrian mathematician, professor of experimental physics at Vienna University.

Doppler effect When a source of sound is approaching an observer, the wave length of the sound decreases and so the pitch increases. This effect is used in angiology, when ultrasound waves are reflected toward a transducer by the moving column of blood, which allows both an estimate of the speed of the blood flow and (with the aid of certain scanning devices) generation of a two-dimensional map of the anatomy of the reflecting surfaces.

Doppler's original experiments which led to the discovery of the effect were conducted with the assistance of the brass section of the Vienna Symphony Orchestra, which played while on a rolling railroad flat-car.

dorsal columns (Lat, of the back) (posterior columns, Goll columns, Burdach columns) Symmetrical pathways ascending on the posterior aspect of the spinal cord and terminating in the gracile and cuneate nuclei.

Their functional responsibilities are still disputed, but selective section in humans leads to loss of the ability to carry out tasks in which simultaneous spatial and temporal analysis of the stimulus is required, such as figure identification; however, sensations of pressure, localization, passive movement, and speed of movement remain intact.[5814]

dorsal enteric cyst See **neurenteric cyst.**

dorsal foot response (tarsophalangeal response, Mendel-Bekhterev response #1) Plantar flexion of the toes, seen in patients with pyramidal tract lesions when the lateral aspect of the dorsum of the foot is struck.

dorsal interosseous syndrome See **posterior interosseous syndrome.**

dorsal midbrain syndrome 1. (Parinaud syndrome, pretectal syndrome, sylvian aqueduct syndrome, Koerber-

Salus-Elschnig syndrome, syndrome of the posterior commissure) The association of impairment of voluntary vertical gaze, especially upward; skew deviation; paralysis of upward and sometimes of downward saccades and of pursuit; convergence–retraction nystagmus on attempted up-gaze; ptosis; eyelid retraction (Collier sign); corectopia; spasm and paralysis of accommodation and convergence; and light–near dissociation of the pupillary response.[246]

The syndrome is commonly caused by tumors of the pineal region or by intrinsic lesions of the dorsal midbrain. Reflex eye movements are relatively preserved.[317] However, paralysis of up-gaze is probably a result either of bilateral lesions within the pretectum or of sectioning the posterior commissure.[4331,4332] The best of the original descriptions was that of Salus,[4891] a pupil of Elschnig.

2. **Benedikt syndrome** has also been known by this name.

dorsal rhizotomy Surgical section of posterior roots, used formerly for pain control and currently under investigation as a treatment in cerebral palsy.

dorsal root entry zone lesions (DREZ lesions) Surgical lesions placed in the dorsal root entry zones in order to alleviate **deafferentation pain.**[4075]

dorsal tegmental syndrome See **dorsal midbrain syndrome.**

dorsocuboidal sign See **Mendel-Bekhterev sign** #2.

dorsolateral frontal epilepsy (Lat, of the back and of the sides) (dorsolateral region seizures) Seizure patterns which may be tonic or, less commonly, clonic with versive eye and head movements and speech arrest. (Adapted from Commission for classification and terminology, ILAE. Proposal for Revised Classifications of Epilepsies and Epileptic syndromes. *Epilepsia* 1989;30:389–399.[1114]) With kind permission from Blackwell Cell Science.

dorsolateral midbrain syndrome A vascular brainstem syndrome characterized by rubral tremor, ipsilateral **Horner syndrome,** and contralateral anesthesia for all modalities. It is due to infarction of the mesencephalon supplied by a short circumferential artery.

dorsolateral region seizures See **dorsolateral frontal epilepsy.**

dorsum The vertebral column or the back of any body part.

Dostoevsky, Fyodor Mikhailovitch (Dostoiewsky) (b. 1821) Russian novelist who suffered from epileptic seizures of various kinds, including some heralded by ecstatic auras. A number of the characters in his books (for example, *The Idiot*) are similarly afflicted.[2050]

Dostoevsky, commenting on the pleasurable sensations as the first expression of some of his seizures, wrote that he would have given all that he had for the enjoyment of another.[70]

double athetosis   Abnormal myelination of the basal ganglia due to anoxic birth injury, giving them a marbled appearance. The clnical syndrome comprises dystonia, choreoathetosis, speech disturbances, pyramidal dysfunction (cerebral palsy), seizures, and mental retardation.[4253] See also **Vogt syndrome, état marbré, status marmoratus, status dysmyelinatus.**

double discharge   (doublet) The appearance of two motor unit action potentials or fibrillation potentials of similar form and amplitude, occurring consistently in the same relationship to one another at intervals of 2 to 20 msec.[10] See also **paired discharge, multiple discharge, triple discharge.**

double saccadic pulse   A saccadic intrusion into fixation characterized by the presence of two back-to-back saccades without any intervening delay, occurring in single pairs or in runs. The condition represents a diluted form of **ocular flutter.**[23]

double whammy   The ability to cause protrusion of one or both of the eyes at will, the upper and lower lids being withdrawn behind the coronal equator of the eye.[513]

double-cortex syndrome   See **diffuse cortical dysplasia, heterotopias.**

double-crush syndrome   The existence of two separate lesions of nerve fibers, one proximal and the other distal, which together lead to symptoms of nerve compression where either alone is considered unlikely to do so.

An example would be compression of the C8 OVT1 nerve roots in association with a mild carpal tunnel syndrome, producing a sensory or motor variety of the syndrome, respectively, in each case as a result of serial constraints of axoplasmic flow in nerve fibers.[5691]

Unfortunately, although it is logical and inherently likely, there is no evidence that the phenomenon exists[4676] (although absence of proof is not proof of absence).

double-elevator palsy   A congenital anomaly consisting of paresis of the two muscles (inferior oblique, superior rectus) controlling elevation of one eye as the result of a pretectal lesion in the brainstem on either side,[3361] causing a supranuclear paresis of monocular elevation.[441]

The same may occur in adult life as a result of a small pretectal vascular lesion.

doublet   See **double discharge.**

double-stimulation evoked responses   A technique for assessing cerebral cortical excitability by means of giving double stimuli at varying short interstimulus intervals; in some forms of cortical reflex myoclonus, there is marked enhancement with the second stimulus of the pair when the interval between them is 60–100 msec.

doughnut sign   The ring of isotope uptake seen on radionucleide brain scans in cases of necrotic tumor, abscess, or (occasionally) cerebral infarction.

Down, James Langdon Haydon   (1828–1896) English physician who trained initially as a pharmacist and so entered medical school late, but graduated with honors. He was eventually appointed to the staff of the London Hospital, where he lectured mainly on therapeutics, and to the staff of the Earlswood Asylum, where he organized a model unit for the care of the mentally retarded. He championed the cause of establishing humane and productive care for mentally retarded people for the whole of his life. The syndrome named for him was described briefly in 1866 (in the same year as a similar report on this syndrome was published by Séguin in Paris) but in full detail in his Lettsomian lectures to the Royal College of Physicians in 1887.

Down tried to classify mental defectives on the basis of their regression from one of the five ethnic groups to another and he considered that "a considerable proportion can be fairly referred to one of the great divisions of the human race other than the class from which they have sprung." Thus he tried to classify subjects as regressing to the Caucasian, Ethiopian, Malay, American, or Mongolian races, substantially on the basis of their facial appearance.

John Langdon Haydon Down

Down syndrome   (trisomy 21, mongolism; OMIM 190685) A genetically determined syndrome comprising amentia, growth deficiency, and abnormal morphogenesis existing as a result of either of two abnormalities—

trisomy of chromosome 21 or translocation of chromosomal material (D/G or G/G) onto that chromosome.

The hallmarks of the disorder are mental retardation; a characteristic facial appearance with small skull, flat occiput, fissured tongue, epicanthic folds, short flat nose, small ears, and eyes slanting upward laterally; an increased incidence of congenital cardiac lesions; and skeletal abnormalities such as a short, broad neck and limbs, broad, flat hands, an incurving little finger, and a single transverse palmar crease. Hypogonadism is common. Ocular features include hypertelorism, strabismus, high myopia, **Brushfield spots** (yellow spots on the irides), and cataracts. Infantile spasms and mixed seizures are also reported.

The incidence of the trisomic form increases with maternal age. Those afflicted who live on to the fifth decade develop a syndrome that is clinically and pathologically indistinguishable from **Alzheimer disease;** the import of this for the understanding of the latter condition is appreciated.

The condition was described in 1866 by James Langdon **Down,** who named it "Mongolism."[1505] A starter Web site is at http://www.downsyndrome.com/.

downbeat nystagmus (downbeating fixation nystagmus) A form of vertical jerk nystagmus due to dysfunction of central vestibular systems, in which the fast component beats downward. It is present in the primary position, but is typically increased by lateral gaze or convergence.

Its presence strongly suggests the existence of disease of the central vestibular connections; it may occur with the **Chiari malformation,** but other lesions at the cervicomedullary junction such as dolichoectasia of the vertebral artery, **cerebellar ataxic syndromes,** paraneoplastic conditions, and intoxications (e.g., lithium) can also be responsible.[2393] See also **ocular dipping.**

In clinical practice, most cases are accompanied by cerebellar signs and the complaint is of **oscillopsia.**

In *variant inherited forms,* vertical nystagmus and ataxia are the main features[337] or the condition occurs only periodically, perhaps in association with thiamine deficiency.[1553]

downbeating fixation nystagmus See **downbeat nystagmus.**

downgaze palsy Selective impairment of downward gaze, following damage to the fasciculus retroflexus in the subthalamic region, usually due to embolic infarction in the territory of the posterior thalamosubthalamic artery.[2394] Paralysis of horizontal gaze may accompany this.

downgaze paralysis, ataxia, foam cell syndrome (DAF syndrome) See **sphingomyelin storage disorders.**

Dracula's teeth syndrome A syndrome of facial pain, ipsilateral facial dystonia, and phantom supernumerary (canine) teeth, beginning after a dental procedure.[2790]

dracunculiasis A nematodal infection occurring in the populations of Asia and Africa in which the infestation rarely leads to mononeuropathy resulting from compression, abscesses (including extradural abscesses), and scarring.[304]

drainage headache See **post–lumbar puncture headache.**

Drake, Charles G. (1920–1998) Canadian neurosurgeon who studied at the Universities of Western Ontario and Toronto and with Fulton at Yale. Though self-described as "just a simple surgeon poking at the edges of knowledge," he was a brilliant technician, an incisive thinker, and an accomplished administrator as the first chairman of the Department of Clinical Neurological Sciences at the University of Western Ontario. He is best remembered internationally for his approaches to the management of aneurysms, particularly those in the posterior fossa, taking these procedures "from the realm of the daring to the domain of the routine." (Dr. Vladimir Hachinski)

Drayer syndrome A congenital dysmorphic syndrome manifesting short stature; hirsutism; strabismus; blepharophimosis; genital, skeletal, and dermal lesions including absence of phalanges; and atrial septal defect with microcephaly and mental and developmental delay.[337]

dream A train of thoughts, images, or fancies passing through the mind during rapid eye movement (less often non–rapid eye movement) sleep. The history of humankind's attitude to and interpretation of the significance of dreams has been reviewed.[4966]

dream anxiety attacks The occurrence of an awakening from rapid eye movement sleep with full factual recall of a disturbing dream and with subjective and autonomic evidence of marked anxiety or disquiet such as tachycardia, sweating, and tachypnea. See also **sleep disorders, nightmares.**

dreamy state The epileptic manifestation described by Hughlings-**Jackson** in his paper "On A Particular Variety of Epilepsy,"[2777] in which he expanded on the "intellectual aura" (a term that he disliked) in which smell, taste, reminiscence (déja vu), and epigastric sensations may occur in company with chewing movements and a defect (though not a loss) of consciousness.

He first described this condition in 1876 in a physician, Dr. Z, who was Jackson's neighbor and patient. In 1898 Dr. Z. died from an overdose of chloral, and there was found at autopsy a small patch of softening in the left uncinate region. Jackson applied the term *uncinate fits* to this form of epilepsy in 1899. See also **affective-psychic seizures.**

dressing apraxia Impairment in fitting the form of a garment to the form of the body, in the absence of significant motor or sensory impairment; and usually as-

sociated with a right-sided or bilateral parieto-occipital lesion producing neglect of left-sided space and
to impairment in visuospatial judgment (**visuospatial
agnosia**).[707]

Despite the name, the condition is not truly an
apraxia. It was known to Hughlings-**Jackson** but was
first described fully by **Brain** in 1941. See **apraxia for
dressing.**

Drew family disease   A dominantly inherited syndrome with early adult onset, characterized by progressive euphoria, optic atrophy, lost up-gaze, nystagmus,
pyramidal and cerebellar signs, parkinsonism, loss of
light touch, and impaired sphincter control.[1788] The condition may be a form of **olivopontocerebellar atrophy.**

drift   The tendency for a limb to sink slowly when
held horizontally against gravity.

The sign is examined with the patient's eyes closed
and the arms held straight out in front. Drifting downward occurs within 15 seconds or so in patients with
cerebellar disease, but also in those with weakness of
shoulder flexion, contralateral parietal lobe disease, and
disease of the shoulder joint.

Drilled Word Span test   A test of memory in which
subjects learn to criterion a list of words one shorter in
length than their forward digit span; their delayed recall is tested after further unfilled or filled intervals.[3851]

dromedary gait   A rolling, high-stepping gait with
protrusion of the buttocks due to excessive lordosis,
seen in dystonic patients.

droopy shoulder syndrome   A syndrome of women
that is characterized by the association of low-set shoulders; long neck (as shown by the appearance of T2 on
lateral cervical radiographs); pain in the neck, shoulder, chest, arms, or hands made worse by downward
traction of the arms and alleviated by elevation of the
shoulders; and a positive **Tinel sign** over the brachial
plexus.

There are no hard neurological or vascular signs and
EMG and nerve conduction study findings are normal.[5450]

drop attacks   Sudden weakness of the legs without
loss of consciousness and causing an immediate fall to
the ground; vision, hearing, and speech remain intact.

The attacks may occur as a result of myoclonus,
abrupt cortical inhibition, cataplexy, or impairment of
the integrity of brainstem structures (vertebrobasilar
insufficiency, colloid cyst, etc.) causing brief interruption of the functions of the reticular activating system.
In the latter cases, brief alteration of consciousness may
occur, however.

The term was introduced by Sheldon[5111] to describe
a sudden, unheralded fall to the ground, usually in the
elderly, without alteration in consciousness or any postictal residuum and with immediate righting. See also
otolithic crisis.

drop finger   Weakness of extension of a digit at the
metacarpophalangeal joint due to a lesion of the posterior interosseous nerve with pareses of extensors in-
dicis, digitorum, and pollicis. Drop thumb and **drop
wrist** have similar connotations.

drop seizure   Abrupt loss of postural tone without
any change in the sensorium occurring as a manifestation of a seizure discharge ("astatic seizure" in the
words of **Ramsay Hunt**).

drop wrist   Inability to maintain extension of the
wrist, such that it falls into a position of flexion, as with
paresis of the radial extensor muscles of the wrist and
fingers.

dropped head syndrome   (Suarez-Kelly syndrome)
Involuntary forward flexion of the neck as a result of
particular weakness of the neck extensor muscles, as in
**myasthenia gravis, facioscapulohumeral dystrophy,
polymyositis, amyotrophic lateral sclerosis, carnitine deficiency, nemaline myopathy, chronic inflammatory demyelinating polyneuropathy, focal
steroid-responsive myositis,** in severe hypokalemia,
and in a restricted, nonspecific cervical myopathy.[5400]
Some shoulder-girdle weakness may also be noted. Similar weakness of the thoracic paraspinal muscles may
cause "bent spine syndrome." An EMG of the paravertebral muscles may suggest either neurogenic or myogenic disease.[4203] See also **camptocormism.**

dropsy   (short for hydropsy: from Lat, watery) An abnormal accumulation of fluid. Thus cerebral dropsy is
hydrocephalus.

drowsiness   (Saxon, sluggishness) The earliest stage
of that physiological depression of consciousness which
is likely to lead to sleep.

drug holiday   A period of transient (up to 7 days)
drug withdrawal during hospitalization, as used in
some patients with complications of long-term levadopa therapy, in an attempt to enhance motor performance and to diminish these side effects.[5895]

Although successful to a degree in achieving these
goals for a limited period after the restoration of therapy, the régime is associated with the dangers of greatly
decreased mobility during the holiday and is viewed
with circumspection by many physicians.

drug-induced headache   1. See **analgesic rebound
headache, ergotamine withdrawal headache, medication-induced headache.** 2. Headaches typically and
only occurring following the ingestion of certain agents
such as indomethacin, nifedipine, and cimetidine, etc.

drug-induced nystagmus   See **induced nystagmus.**

drug-induced refractory headache   See **rebound
headache.**

drug-resistant intractable seizures   (OMIM 171050)
A rare disorder of the p-glycoprotein mechanism char-

acterized by multiple seizures, unresponsive to anti-convulsants.

Drummond syndrome   See **blue diaper syndrome.**

drusen   (from Ger, a rock cavity lined with crystal) 1. Hyaline-like pallid nodular debris derived from the pigmented retinal layers (**Brusch's membrane**), perhaps as a result of axonal degeneration.

In this dominantly inherited abnormality, the deep yellowish lesions, usually round or oval in shape, are mainly in the posterior polar region of the eye and sometimes widely spread over the retina. They possibly represent a secretion of the abnormal pigmentary epithelium. Drusen are also seen in numerous diseases of the choroid. They usually appear in early adult life and are symptomless unless there is secondary macular degeneration.[3161]

2. The same, seen on and in the region of the optic disk, where their presence causes elevation of the disk head (and thus the obliteration of the cup and the appearance of papilledema, especially if prepapillary hemorrhages are also present[2590]). Arcuate scotomas may also be found. See **pseudopapilledema.**

3. Senile plaques (in the German literature).

dualism   (Lat, containing two) The system of Descartes in which he tried to explain all the phenomena of human nature on the basis of principles of the essential separateness of body and mind. Thus *mind* here represents more than mere expression of the function of the brain.

Duane, Alexander   (1858–1926) American ophthalmologist, practicing in New York.

Duane syndrome   (ocular retraction syndrome, Stilling-Turk-Duane syndrome) A congenital, dominantly inherited brainstem disorder with aberrant innervation of the lateral rectus by the inferior division of the third cranial nerve, with maximal clinical effects upon eye movements.[1522]

Three types are described: *type 1* in which there is narrowing of the palpebral fissure and retraction of the globe on adduction of the eye, with limitation of abduction; *type 2,* in which there is narrowing of the fissure, retraction, and limited adduction but full abduction; and *type 3,* consisting of deficiency of both ocular abduction and adduction due to fibrosis of the lateral rectus muscle, leading to retraction of the globe by 2–10 mm with narrowing of the palpebral fissure during attempted adduction.

Convergence failure and both brainstem and musculoskeletal abnormalities may coexist. The syndrome is more common in females. It was first described by Stilling in the German literature in 1887.

Variants include an *acquired form,* described in patients with brainstem and third cranial nerve pathology, and *Okihiro syndrome,* a dominantly inherited form in which the typical features of Duane syndrome are accompanied by congenital bony anomalies of the arm and cervical spine.[4230]

See also **Wildervanck syndrome.**

Dubini, Angelo   (1813–1902) Italian physician, practicing in Lombardy.

Dubini disease   (electric chorea) A rare and fatal form of chorea described by Dubini in 1846, but not now reported; as a result, it cannot in retrospect be classified with confidence. The disease was said to have been marked by spasmodic movements in one limb, progressing to involve others, and sometimes characterized by seizures, progressive paralysis, and muscle wasting.[1523]

The nature of the disorder remains uncertain; both a myoclonic form of epidemic encephalitis and hysteria have been suggested as its cause. Though its organicity seems dubious by description, some patients appear to have died from it (or at least with it), and it has been considered by some to be a myoclonic form of epidemic encephalitis. See also **Bergeron disease.**

DuBois-Reymond, Emil   (1818–1896) The father of modern electrophysiology who devoted his whole clinical life to this subject. He was a pupil of Johannes Müller, whom he succeeded as professor of physiology at Berlin University. He demonstrated the polarized state of nerves and muscle fibers and showed that the peripheral passage of a nerve impulse was accompanied by an electrical discharge—the action potential. He was also the first to describe the electrical and mechanical properties of muscle **tetanus.**

His collection of works was translated into English and published by Charles Morgan under the title *Electrophysiology and Therapeutics* (New York: William Wood, 1868), a book regarded by most reviewers at the time as being unreadable. His clinical contributions are less well known, but he gave good accounts of the symptoms of migraine from personal experience.

Dubowitz syndrome   A congenital dysmorphic syndrome manifesting also short stature, eczema, skeletal abnormalities, ptosis, blepharophimosis, microcephaly, and mental and developmental delay.[1529]

Duchenne de Boulogne, Guillaume-Benjamin Armand (1806–1875) French neurologist, who had no permanent hospital appointment in Paris, although he found cases of neurological disease in the wards of hospitals all over the city. In his early years he used faradic currents to assist in diagnosis and recorded his experiences in his book *De l'-electricisation localisée,* of which three editions were published (in 1855, 1861, and 1872.)[1538]

Duchenne described spinal muscular atrophy as a form of **amyotrophic lateral sclerosis** (but passed on publication to Aran) in 1849. He described **progressive bulbar palsy** 9 years later, and **pseudohypertrophic muscular dystrophy** first in 1861 and more fully in 1868, the same year as he introduced the technique of needle muscle biopsy, which he had employed in the diagnosis of the boys in his paper and described in this report. The name of Aran is also linked to this condition, but he reported on patients with a variety of muscle disorders, some of them patients referred to him by Duchenne himself. Dr. Edward Meryon did, however, describe the condition in England in 1852.[7]

In other contributions, Duchenne described upper brachial plexus palsy in 1872, some years before **Erb's** report; distinguished between upper and lower motor neuron facial palsies; described locomotor ataxia (**tabes dorsalis**), lead paralysis, and poliomyelitis; and in 1872 recorded cases of what is now called **facioscapulohumeral dystrophy,** 12 years before **Landouzy** and **Déjèrine** published their description.

McHenry[3760] describes him as unworldly, naïve, absent-minded, and inarticulate, which may explain why his contributions to many areas of neurology were overshadowed so completely by those of colleagues such as **Charcot,** who nevertheless regarded Duchenne as his master in neurology.

Duchenne disease   See **tabes dorsalis.**

Duchenne muscular dystrophy (pseudohypertrophic muscular dystrophy) A progressive and still fatal X-linked recessive disorder affecting young boys in which the affected gene at Xp21.2 on the short arm of the X chromosome fails to produce dystrophin, an essential protein. The same protein is deficient in quantity or altered in composition but not absent in **Becker muscular dystrophy,** which is allelic.

Boys with Duchenne muscular dystrophy have high levels of **creatine kinase** from birth and manifest the signs of the disease as soon as they would normally start to walk. Proximal weakness, affecting first the pelvic girdle muscles (see **Gowers sign**), and fatty replacement of the calf and tongue muscles, making them firm and rubbery ("pseudohypertrophy"), are the leading characteristics. Eventually, kyphoscoliosis, areflexia, and cardiac failure occur.[1537] A wheelchair is needed by the time patients reach early adolescence and the patients die in their early twenties, usually of pneumonia.

The recent triumphant determination of the site[694] and nature of the defect gives some hope that the foregoing description may be out of date when this book is but a year or two old; if the protein can be synthesized and replaced, the fatal prognosis may be tempered.[2600] Duchenne dystrophy was also described by Aran and by Wilhelm Griesinger (1817–1868) in 1865.[2280]

A *variant* is *autosomal recessive Duchenne-like muscular dystrophy*, in which females are affected by a disease exactly mimicking Duchenne dystrophy, as a result of inheritance of a different allele for a polymorphism within the dystrophin gene.[3757] A useful starter web site is at http://www.mdausa.org/. See also http://www.neuro.wustl.edu/neuromuscular/index.html.

Duchenne paralysis   See **progressive bulbar palsy, amyotrophic lateral sclerosis.**

Duchenne sign   Indrawing of the epigastrium with inspiration, a sign of diaphragmatic palsy.

Duchenne-Aran disease   See **progressive bulbar palsy, amyotrophic lateral sclerosis.**

Duchenne-Erb palsy   See **upper brachial plexus palsy.**

ductions   The movements of one eye, the other being covered. The possible movements are *adduction* and *abduction* (toward or away from the nose, respectively); *sursumduction* (elevation) and *deorsumduction* (depression); *incycloduction* (intorsion with the upper pole turned toward the nose); and *encycloduction* (extorsion with the upper pole turned toward the temple).[3330] See also **forced duction** test.

dumb   (Saxon, silent) Unable to make articulate sounds.

dumb rabies   (paralytic rabies) A form of **rabies** producing polyneuropathy rather than encephalitis, the latter producing the "furious" form.[3301]

dumbbell tumors   (hour-glass tumors) Extra- and intradural masses joined by a narrow pedicle passing through an enlarged intervertebral foramen at any level. Less commonly, tumors which are wholly intraspinal with intra- and extradural masses similarly joined. Many are meningiomas or neurofibromas.

dumbness   The inability to make vocal sounds. The condition includes **aphthongia, alalia,** and **anarthria.**

Duplay syndrome   (frozen shoulder, adhesive capsulitis of the shoulder) Pain-limiting rotation and abduction of the shoulder with disuse atrophy of periscapular muscles due to soft tissue inflammation and fibrosis, often following cervical injury, stroke, or myocardial infarction.[1555]

duplex ultrasonography   A noninvasive scanning technique combining B-mode imaging with pulsed Doppler technology to produce an image of blood flow through a vessel.

It allows differentiation of occluded from patent arteries and provides a method of grading the severity of arterial disease based on changes in the blood flow pattern distal to stenosis.

Continuous-wave systems give an average of the cross-sectional velocity in the area examined, while pulsed systems enable more discrete examination of the blood flow pattern in the area of disease.[4141]

duplicity theory of vision   The contention that color vision is a function of the retinal cone receptors and that grayscale tones are recognized by the rods.

Dupré, Ernest   (1862–1921) French physician.

Dupré syndrome   (serous meningitis, toxic encephalopathy) A syndrome of meningeal irritation, sometimes progressing to headache, convulsions, diffuse encephalopathic signs, and coma, following distant infection or as an autoimmune phenomenon after infection, more commonly seen in children.[1556,4763] See **parameningeal infections, idiopathic intracranial hypertension.**

Dupuy syndrome   See **gustatory sweating.**

Dupuy-Dutemps and Cestan sign   Incomplete peripheral paralysis of the face; when the patient is asked to look forward and to close both eyes slowly, the upper lid on the paretic side moves upward a small amount, because of the action of the levator palpebrae superioris.[4723]

Dupuytren, Baron Guillaume   (1777–1835) French surgeon. Dobson[1478] remarks that he "had a remarkable childhood, being kidnapped when three years old by a rich woman of Toulouse. Was returned by her but subsequently taken to Paris (1789) by a Cavalry officer who took a fancy to him." He was educated in Paris and became surgeon to the Hôtel-Dieu and professor at the University of Paris, publishing almost nothing and becoming a huge success.

Dupuytren canals   The diploic spaces in the cranial bones.

Dupuytren contracture   Contracture of the palmar (Dupuytren's) fascia with tight bands of fibrous tissue radiating distally under the palm, causing flexion deformities of the fingers.

dura mater   (Lat, hard + mother; the latter as the Arabians considered that all tissues of the body were derived from the meninges) The tough, fibrous outer layer of the meninges enveloping the brain and spinal cord.

dural arteriovenous fistula   An abnormal connection between the branches of the external carotid artery and the venous sinuses, sometimes caused by sinus thrombosis. Its clinical presentations include complaints of headache, bruit, and imbalance; cranial neuropathies and ischemic and hemorrhagic strokes may also occur. Cervical myelopathy is a rare presentation. The fistulae may disappear spontaneously or may be occluded by arterial compression or embolization.[156]

Durand-Zunin syndrome   The association of agenesis of the septum pellucidum, lacunar skull deficits, dysraphism, hydrocephalus, and pes cavus.[1560]

duration   1. The time during which something exists or acts. In electromyography, the interval from the beginning of the first deflection from the baseline to its final return to the baseline of an action potential or waveform, unless otherwise specified. If only part of the waveform is measured, the points of the measurement should be specified. For example, the duration of the M wave may be measured as the negative phase duration and refers to the interval from the deflection of the first negative phase from the baseline to its return to

the baseline. 2. The interval of the applied current or voltage of a single electric stimulus. 3. The interval from the beginning to the end of a series of recurring stimuli or action potentials. (From the 2001 Report of the Nomenclature Committee of the American Association of Electromyography and Electrodiagnosis.[10] Used by permission, copyright © 2001, AAEM.

Duret hemorrhages   Intrinsic bleeding into the upper (rostral) brainstem resulting from its compression, as by the medial part of the temporal lobe in the **uncal syndrome.**[1562]

Duret, Henri   (1849–1921) French neurologist who trained under **Charcot,** with whom he described the lenticulostriate arteries as the "arteries of cerebral hemorrhage." He is also remembered for his precise mapping of the territories supplied by the anterior, middle, and posterior cerebral arteries[1561] and for noting the brainstem hemorrhages complicating its compression.

Dutch cerebral hemorrhage   (hereditary cerebral hemorrhage with amyloidosis–Dutch type) A dominantly inherited predisposition to multiple large or small cerebral or cerebellar cortical hemorrhages occurring in mid-adult life, arising from a mutation at chromosome 21q21 and leaving as residua focal and global impairments and, frequently, dementia.[2348] Subcortical hemorrhages occur later in many cases. In a variant, the similar *Icelandic form*, it is not the amyloid precursor protein but cystatin C that is mutated.

Duval's nucleus   A small mass of multipolar ganglion cells situated just ventral to the hypogloossal nucleus in the medulla, described in 1883 by Mathias Marie Duval (1844–1907), a French anatomist.[4979]

dwarfism with microcephaly and hydrocephaly   A congenital dysmorphic syndrome manifesting also platyspondyly, microcephaly, hydrocephalus, and callosal abnormalities.[337]

dwarfism with retinal atrophy and deafness   See **Cockayne syndrome.**

Dyel phenomenon   If, in a patient with papilledema, light compression of the eyeball elicits visible pulsations of the retinal arterioles at the optic nerve head, this suggests that the cause is a mass lesion rather than chronic renal disease and hypertension.[1582]

Dyggve-Melchior-Clausen syndrome   A heterogeneous, congenital, recessively inherited dysmorphic syndrome manifesting also skeletal abnormalities, short stature, atlanto-occipital subluxation, platyspondyly, J-shaped sella turcica, and mental and developmental delay.[1583]

dying-back   The process whereby metabolic disturbances of the perikaryon of the largest and longest axons in peripheral nerves lead to a failure of the soma to maintain lines of nutrient supply to distal but progressively more proximal regions of its axon.[939] The degeneration of the axons starts with the longest fibers and the lesion progresses from distal to proximal. Empires in decay similarly lose first those of their possessions which are linked to them by the longest lines of communication.

dying-back neuropathy   See **distal axonopathy.**

Dyke-Davidoff-Masson syndrome   A congenital dysmorphic syndrome manifesting an asymmetrical face, thickening of the cranial vault, overdevelopment of the frontal and ethmoidal sinuses, and elevation of the petrous pyramid of the temporal bone on the side of hemispheric atrophy in children with seizures and hemiplegia.[1584]

dynamesthesia   The appreciation of force or tension during the performance of a voluntary muscle contraction.

dynamic   (from Gr, power) Relating to strength or force. *Sthenic* is a synonym.

dynamic aphasia   (verbal adynamia) A condition in which spontaneous speech is markedly reduced in the absence of any syntactical impairment while naming, repetition and reading skills are normal. Verbal generative and verbal planning skills are normal when the subject is asked to describe pictorial scenes and complex actions. The condition may progress to mutism when it occurs, e.g., in the context of progressive supranuclear palsy.[4729]

dynamic EMG   See **kinesiologic EMG.**

dynamic overshoot   (ocular quiver) 1. A form of saccadic intrusion or oscillation characterized by involuntary deviation of the eye in the direction of gaze, requiring a saccade to restore it to the appropriate position. 2. A corrective movement occurring at the end of a normal saccade and in the opposite direction, greater in degree than the normal reversal of direction that would be required to bring the eye to a halt.[3330]

dynamic saccade   The fast, first part of the saccadic eye movement.

dynamic spelling alexia   The occurrence of **spelling alexia** with relative sparing of writing and of the identification of letters printed in view of the patient by the clinician.

This rare condition was detected in a patient with a large left hemisphere lesion also compressing the corpus callosum.[2655]

dynamic vestibular imbalance   Asymmetrical activity of the vestibular apparatus apparent only with movement. Head shaking and single, rapid head turns are used to demonstrate this. In the former case, jerk nystagmus is produced, usually with its slow phase directed toward the side of the vestibular lesion. Sudden, passive turning of the head with maintained fixation will normally allow fixation to persist; with vestibular imbalance, deviation will occur and a corrective saccade will be seen.[3330]

dynamite encephalosis   Headache, sweating, coughing, vomiting, fatigue, irritability, depression, and impaired concentration up to confusion as a result of chronic toxic exposure to glyceryl trinitrate.[2073]

dynamometer   (Gr, power + measure) An instrument for measuring the strength of contraction of muscles. The *Mathieu dynamometer* consists of a metal ellipse, the two sides connected by a spring with a scale upon which a pointer rotates to indicate the force of manual compression applied to the ellipse. Some methods prescribe precise placement of the limbs of the examiner or the subject in the performance of the tests.[5970]

dynorphin   A peptide neurotransmitter complex, containing leukoencephalins.

dys-   A Greek prefix signifying bad, difficult, or painful.

dysapocatastasis   (Gr, disturbance of + complete restoration) A feeling of morbid discontent with restlessness of mind.

The word is not in general usage, but, even though it has seven syllables, it is still shorter than the definition (which requires nine words). The disorder must represent one of the more common reasons underlying visits to physicians and is otherwise unnamed.

dysarthria   (Gr, difficulty + a joint) (dyslalia) 1. The indistinct pronunciation of words. 2. A group of speech disorders resulting from disturbance in the muscular control of the speech mechanisms due to damage to the central or peripheral nervous systems.

While typically evidence of either upper or lower motor neuron lesions (the latter affecting the fifth, seventh, or the bulbar nerves, the end-plates or the muscles), it may also be caused by local mechanical problems and is heard accompanying dysphasias.[1284]

Spastic, ataxic, and hypokinetic forms are differentiated, due respectively to corticobulbar, cerebellar, and basal ganglion lesions. Their characteristics have been reviewed.[3092] Mechanical and flaccid forms result from local structural and lower cranial motor nerve disorders. In addition, aphasic patients also frequently manifest dysarthria.

dysarthria–clumsy hand syndrome   A **lacunar syndrome** in which mild dysphagia, some dysarthria, tongue deviation on protrusion, and clumsiness of the hand are associated with slight "central" weakness of the face and arm and a positive Babinski sign. Truncal ataxia may also be present. The lesion is most often in the upper part of the internal capsule or in the basis pontis.[1846]

It may be impossible to differentiate this syndrome from **homolateral ataxia and crural paresis** or **ataxic**

hemiparesis clinically except that in the latter, dysarthria is not a feature and hemiparesis and sensory changes are.[2137] See **ataxic hemiparesis.**

dysautonomia 1. Any disorder of the autonomic nervous system, sympathetic or parasympathetic, including hyper- as well as hypofunction. 2. See **diencephalic autonomic seizures.** 3. *Primary dysautonomia* (comprising **pure autonomic failure, Parkinson disease** with autonomic failure, and **multiple-system atrophy**).

Dysautonomia Foundation Inc. A charitable foundation. Address: 633 Third Ave., 12th Floor, New York, NY 10017–6706. Tel: 212–949–6644. Website: http://www.familialdysautonomia.org/aboutfd.htm.

dysautonomic cephalalgia A syndrome of posttraumatic headaches associated with excessive sweating and pupillary dilatation due to partial sympathetic denervation, the injury having been to the anterior triangle of the neck.[5763]

dysbarism See **decompression sickness.**

dysbasia lordotica progressiva See **dystonia.**

dysbulia Difficulty in the exercise of the will; mental torpor. When pathological, there is also evidence of metabolic disease or of lesions affecting the deep frontal regions. See **abulia.**

dyscalculia Disturbance in mental reckoning and in enumeration and calculation on paper, as in **Gerstmann syndrome.**

In *primary dyscalculia*, this deficit stands out in comparison to the disturbance in other skills such as language, memory, attention, or perception, which are equally or more obviously affected in *secondary dyscalculia*. A medial left frontal lesion is suggested as the necessary cause.[3502]

dyschondroplasia See **Ollier disease.**

dyschromatopsia (Gr, difficulty + color + sight) Disturbance of color vision; a distortion of the hue or color of objects seen, as though the observer were looking through a colored filter (e.g., erythropsia, xanthopsia), possibly as a result of lesions of the visual cortex or due to toxic disease.

dysconjugate Not yoked together; or, in the case of the eye movements, not moving in parallel.

dyscoria Abnormal pupillary shape, the pupil being slit-like, oval, hourglass, or irregular. The syndrome is generally benign and may be dominantly inherited.[2535]

dysdiadochokinesis (Gr, difficulty + a follower + movement) Impairment in the speed, precision, and rhythmicity of rapidly performed movements in alternating directions by virtue of irregularities in their force and an inability to change rapidly the patterns of contraction and relaxation of the muscles involved. Rapid repetitive tapping of the back of one hand alternately with the palm and the back of the other one is the test most commonly employed.

The term was originally applied by **Babinski** to such a disturbance of coordinated movement in patients with a cerebellar disorder. This is still considered to be an important sign of a cerebellar lesion on the same side, but pyramidal and basal ganglion disease and local factors may produce a similar difficulty.

dysembryoma (neuroepithelioma) A heterogeneous group of primary malignant tumors arising from peripheral nerves and characterized by the presence of spaces lined by cuboidal or columnar epithelium.[2932]

dysencephalia splanchnocystica (Gruber syndrome, Meckel-Gruber syndrome) A recessively inherited, congenital **neurocutaneous syndrome** characterized by microcephaly, occipital encephalocele, meningocele, ocular abnormalities and facial clefting, polydactyly, and polycystic kidneys, liver, and pancreas.[3,1937] Micropthalmia, congenital heart defects, cleft lip and palate, internal hydrocephalus, anencephaly, and cerebellar aplasia have also been described.[2674] See **Gruber syndrome.**

dysequilibrium syndrome 1. An unusual autosomal recessive syndrome, manifesting the combination of marked motor delay with hypotonia, nystagmus, ataxia, mental retardation, and frequent falls when at last the child attains the standing position.[2368] See **cerebellar ataxias.** 2. See **dialysis dysequilibrium syndrome.**

dysesthesia 1. Painful sensations resulting from stimuli that are not normally painful, in the presence of alterations in the quality of other sensations. They occur commonly in the territory of a partially damaged peripheral nerve. **Charcot** described under this term a distressing pain resembling vibration, which travels up and down a limb when it is touched or stimulated by cold.[4512] 2. Dullness or perversion of sensation; this, however, is an older meaning for the word and does not represent current usage. 3. Disorders of the senses (**Cullen**).

dysesthesia-dysautonomia-hypertension syndrome A syndrome with childhood onset characterized by paresthesias, spontaneous pains, and autonomic dysfunction. The cause is not known.

dysesthetic pain A form of centrally derived pain resulting from spinal pathology (such as an intrinsic or extrinsic spinal tumor, or transverse myelitis stemming from any cause) in which the dysesthesias are in the territory of one or a few dermatomes at the level of the lesion, within a region of altered skin sensation.

dysexecutive syndrome Impairment of goal formulation, planning, execution of plans, and shifting of mental set, frequently in association with dysphasic speech disturbances and impairment of new learning and changes in personality, social skills, and initiative. The syndrome is notable for the retention of general intelligence and of remote memory. It is seen in patients with orbitofrontal lobe lesions or subcortical dementias and in some patients with alcoholism in whom a loss of social control, inaability to abstain, and repetitive habitual behavior are also characteristic.[3392] See also **Behavioral Assesment of Dysexecutive syndrome,** a test devised to assess the magnitude of these problems.

dysferlinopathies   Proximal or distal muscular dystrophies resulting from mutations of the dysferlin gene at 2p12–14. See **distal muscular dystrophy.**[5057]

dysgerminoma   (atypical teratoma, ectopic pinealoma) A tumor of childhood or youth, arising from cell rests in the anterior part of the third ventricle or in the suprasellar region, and histologically resembling a seminoma or an atypical pinealoma. Typical clinical features are hypopituitarism with growth retardation, diabetes insipidus, and visual field loss.[879]

dysgeusia   A distortion of the sense of taste, usually resulting either from the ingestion of toxins, partial damage to the chorda tympani, or lesions in the brainstem. As with similar distortions of smell, the distorted taste is always interpreted as unpleasant.

dysglobulinemic neuropathy   Motor neuropathies with onset in young adult life, leading to complaints of paresthesia and accompanied by paraproteinemias. See **gammopathic neuropathy.**

dysgraphia   Impairment of utilization of writing tools, usually coupled with a tendency to malform individual letters and words—a state which may include features of both dyspraxia and dysphasia, especially if there are also semantic and syntactical errors, misspellings, and neographisms.

dyshoric angiopathy   See **cerebral amyloid angiopathy.**

dyskinesia   (Gr, difficulty + movement) Abnormal involuntary movements, classified as **tremors, chorea** and **ballism, myoclonus, tics,** and **dystonias.**
   Paroxysmal dyskinesias have been classified as follows:[1378]
   Paroxysmal kinesigenic dyskinesia
   Paroxysmal nonkinesigenic dyskinesia, precipitated by stress, menses, heat, and fatigue, occurring at any age and often intermixed with choreoathetosis
   Paroxysmal exertion-induced dyskinesia, characterized by brief episodes of dystonia induced by physical exertion
   Paroxysmal hypnogenic dyskinesia, characterized by intermittent attacks lasting minutes or less, with onset in early childhood and occurring both by day and at night

dyskinetic cerebral palsy   A form of cerebral palsy in which X-linked inheritance has been found occasionally.[335] See **cerebral palsy.**

dyskinetic gait   (dystonic gait) No single pattern of movements can be described in patients with dystonias, the picture varying widely, although plantar flexion at the ankle and extension of the hallux are commonly found.

dyslalia   See **dysarthria.**

dyslexia   (from Gr, difficulty + reading) An innate constitutional difficulty in learning to read; a disorder of phonemic awareness leading to impairment of reading skills in the absence of other disorders of language.
   This term for what had formerly been called *word blindness* (on the supposition that it was intrinsically a visual disorder) was introduced by Rudolf Berlin (1833–1897) in 1887.[511] The condition is frequently familial but the transmission method not always certain. In *dyslexia-1,* however, the gene is mapped to 15q11. See **word blindness.**
   A variant is *spelling dyslexia,* in which the subject with dyslexia without dysgraphia can read single letters aloud, and adopt a letter-by-letter reading strategy, spelling the word aloud.[5851]

dyslogia   (from Gr, difficulty + a word) Speech which is normally formed, but the content of which indicates the presence of a disorder of thought.

dyslysis   See **restless legs syndrome.**

dysmetria   (from Gr, difficulty + distance) 1. The occurrence of errors in judgment of distance when a limb is made to perform a precise movement. The movements usually tested are those of extension and withdrawal of the arm with a finger outstretched, with the intention of touching successively first the examiner's finger held away from the patient at arm's length and then the patient's own nose, repetitively. Classically, the finger overshoots (*hypermetria*) or undershoots the target (*hypometria*) with disease of the cerebellum, and often shows an **action tremor.**
   2. See **ocular dysmetria.**

dysmetric saccades   The ocular equivalent of limb dysmetria, in which the gaze is not accurately brought to bear upon the target but over- (or under-) shooting occurs, with the need for corrective **catch-up saccades** to be made. Either cerebellar or hemispheric lesions may be responsible.[1077] When the deviation is in the line of the eye movement, the term *amplitude dysmetria* may be used; movement at right angles to that line merits the term *direction dysmetria.*[3330] See **ocular dysmetria.**

dysmnesia   (from Gr, difficulty + memory) Any disturbance of memory including flashbacks, déja vu, jamais vu, experiential hallucinations, or panoramic experiences but not including amnesia.

dysmorphism   (craniofacial malformations) Abnormal facial appearances, including low-set ears, flared nostrils, an antimongolian slant to the eyes, extruded lips, etc., occurring as part of a congenital, usually genetic, disorder.[1587]

The following classification has been suggested[4] (see Chart D–13).

Chart D–13. Classification of Dysmorphisms

I. *Cerebrocranial dysplasias*
   Anencephaly
   Microcephaly
   Others
II. *Cerebrofacial dysplasias*
   Rhinencephalic dysplasias
   Oculo-orbital dysplasias (anophthalmia)
III. *Craniofacial dysplasias*
   a. With clefting
   b. With dysostosis
   c. With synostosis
      Craniosynostosis
      Craniofaciosynostosis
      Faciosynostosis
   d. With dysostosis and synostosis
      Crouzon
      Cloverleaf skull
IV. *Craniofacial dysplasias with other origin*
   a. Osseous
   b. Cutaneous
   c. Neurocutaneous
      Neurofibromatosis
   d. Neuromuscular
      Pierre Robin syndrome
      Möbius syndrome
   e. Muscular
      Glossoschizisis
   f. Vascular
      Hemangioma
      Hemolymphangioma
      Lymphangioma

Adapted from Stricker (1990). Reprinted by kind permission of Elsevier Science.

Dysmorphology Database   See **London Neurogenetic Database.**

dysmorphopsia   A distortion of shape perceived.

dysmyelination   An inborn error of metabolism affecting myelinogenesis that causes the process to be delayed or arrested, or the myelin to be abnormal in its constituents. The leukodystrophies, many aminoacidopathies, and the gangliosidoses are examples.[4500,4501]

dysmyelinogenic leukodystrophy   See **Alexander disease.**

dysnomia   Difficulty in naming objects; a dilute form of **anomia.**

dysodia   (dysodes) Hippocrates' term for smelling bad; also used as a collective term for those diseases characterized by such odours.

dysopsia algera   Pain from eye movement in the absence of detectable ocular disease. As with **akinesia algera,** the condition is considered to be functional or psychogenic in such cases.[5286]

dysorthographia   Impairment in the ability to spell, as may occur in the **developmental dyslexias.**

dysosmia   Distorted perception of odors, the sensation being almost invariably unpleasant. Head trauma, viral infections, and other causes of damage to the first cranial nerve, and depressive illnesses are the more common causes.

dysosteosclerosis   A congenital dysmorphic syndrome, a form of craniotubular dysplasia, manifesting also short stature, skeletal, and dental abnormalities, blindness due to optic nerve atrophy, mental delay, and fragile bones.[1810]

dysphagia   (from Gr, difficulty + to swallow) A subjective sensation that swallowing is difficult or painful. When caused by a unilateral cerebral lesion, this is usually in the lowest part of the precentral gyrus or the posterior part of the inferior frontal gyrus. In most cases with a neurological cause, however, bilateral cerebral, bulbar or neuromuscular lesions are required to produce the symptom.[3798]

dysphasia   Disturbance of communication involving language due to disturbance of specific brain regions but in the absence of primary disturbance of the subcortical motor or sensory pathways. It is manifested by difficulties, variously, in fluency, repetition, comprehension, and naming according to the type of dysphasia present. **Global aphasia, Broca aphasia, transcortical aphasias, Wernicke aphasia, conduction aphasia,** and **anomic aphasias** are those most precisely described. See **aphasia.**

dysphatic stuttering   A form of dysfluency of speech related to impairment of sensory input, as with receptive dysphasia or deafness.

dysphonia   (from Gr, difficulty + utterance) Abnormal production of vocal sounds, typically caused by local lesions of the larynx or of its motor nerve supply.

   Dysphonia clericorum was the term given to that form of chronic laryngitis which affected those who said too much, too loudly. In these days of shorter sermons, the condition would be more appropriately named with reference to the legislature, the racecourse, or the auction house.

dysphoria   Hippocrates' term for the restlessness and anxiety that accompany disease states.

dysphrasia   (from Gr, difficulty + speech) Disturbance of speech due to inadequacy of underlying ideation, as in dementia.

dysphrenia   (from Gr, difficulty + the mind) The term of Kahlbaum for disturbance of the intellect resulting from organic disease of the brain.

dysphrenic migraine   A migrainous accompaniment characterized by confusion and amnesia for current events, but not necessarily by headache.[4377] See **confusional migraine.**

dysplasia   The abnormal organization of cells into tissue as a result of abnormal histogenesis. Thus, focal cortical dysplasia is a cause of otherwise unexplained focal cortical myoclonus.

dysplasia of ears, sensorineural and conductive deafness, and retardation syndrome   A congenital dysmorphic syndrome manifesting also psychomotor retardation.[337]

dysprosody   (speech dyspraxia) Loss of the melodic intonations of cultured speech. A feature of all forms of **dysphasia** but especially of **Broca aphasia,** in which incorrect emphases, hesitations, awkward phrasing, and dysmelodic intonation are detectable.[3952]

dysproteinemic neuropathy   A syndrome of acquired demyelinating motor neuropathy resembling **chronic inflammatory demyelinating polyneuropathy** but occurring in the presence of an underlying systemic illness such as plasma cell dyscrasia (including primary systemic amyloidosis), POEMS, **Waldenstrom macrogobulinemia,** gamma heavy-chain disease, **cryoglobulinemia, lymphoma, systemic lupus erythematosus,** Castleman disease, **HIV** infections, or an occult malignancy.[77] See also **paraneoplastic neuropathy, gammopathic neuropathy.**

dysraphism   (Bremer syndrome) Axial skeletal anomalies due to improper closure of the neural tube. The severity of the resulting defect varies widely from the most minor **spina bifida occulta** to **meningomyelocele** or **cranioschisis.**

dysrhythmokinesis   A disorder in the execution of regular or syncopated movements, as is seen with cerebellar lesions.

dyssomnias   Disorders characterized by disturbance of the initiation or maintenance of sleep, or by excessive sleepiness. They include **intrinsic sleep disorders, extrinsic sleep disorders,** and **circadian rhythm sleep disorders.** See also **parasomnias, sleep disorders.**

dyssynergia   1. (detrusor-sphincter dyssynergia) Disturbance in the reciprocal innervation of the detrusor muscle and the internal sphincter, which should allow the former to contract while the latter relaxes, or vice versa. Sphincter-detrusor dyssynergia occurs with pyramidal lesions and leads to complaints of urgency, frequency, and dribbling of urine. 2. (asynergia) A failure of the coordination of contraction or relaxation of muscles which normally act together in a group to produce a smoothly programmed movement. This is classically regarded as a sign of cerebellar disease, but other disorders of motor or sensory pathways and local disease may produce similar findings. 3. A term encompassing all the disturbances of movement occurring as a result of cerebellar disease.

dyssynergia cerebellaris myoclonica   (Ramsay Hunt syndrome) A rare, dominantly or recessively inherited syndrome of olivodentatorubral degeneration with progressive myoclonus epilepsy and intense action and intention myoclonus, tonic-clonic seizures, cerebellar signs, and sometimes mental deterioration. It was described by Ramsay Hunt in 1921.[2704]

The main clinical features are onset in infancy or childhood, generalized seizures, action myoclonus, truncal ataxia, and limb tremor, but no other neurological signs. A variety of EEG patterns (photosensitive responses, paroxysmal discharges, and fast polyspike discharges over central regions during rapid eye movement sleep) is found. Somatosensory evoked responses are unusually large.[4741]

The combination of myoclonic epilepsy and cerebellar signs also occurs in storage diseases such as the **lipidoses, sialidosis** and **lipofuscinosis, Lafora body disease, Baltic myoclonus,** and **mitochondrial encephalomyelopathy.** Another form shows dominant inheritance. Some of Ramsay Hunt's patients developed a cerebellar syndrome before, some after the onset of myoclonic epilepsy and he did not claim that this condition was a single disease *sui generis* (although it has been convincingly distinguished from **MERFF**).[5496] See also **hereditary dentatorubropallidoluysian atrophy.**

In a *variant* form, peripheral neuropathy is detected.[5238]

dyssynergia cerebellaris progressiva   A clinical syndrome of chronic, progressive severe, local, and later generalized intention tremors with dyssynergia, dysmetria, hypotonia, adiadochokinesis, and asthenia but without vertigo, nystagmus, optic atrophy, or dysequilibrium. The muscle stretch reflexes are normal.[2702]

It was described by **Hunt** as a pure cerebellar degeneration but it has been thought likely by others to have been **Wilson disease** (though Hunt considered this and found no corneal pigmentation), **mitochondrial encephalopathy,** or dystonic tremor.

dystasia, hereditary areflexic   See **Roussy-Levy syndrome.**

dysthymia   (Gr, bad + mind) Melancholy.

dysthymia, somatic   Yet another neologistic attempt, this time to name the syndrome in which the somatic manifestations of depression are presented in the absence (or at least in the presence of denial) of affective disturbance. Thus this is possibly one of the most common diseases presenting to neurologists.

dysthyroid orbitopathy   (Graves ophthalmopathy, thyroid ophthalmopathy, endocrine exophthalmos) A varied group of symptoms that are causally related to thyroid disease but that are not always associated with systemic clinical evidence of this. They include orbital and conjunctival congestion and edema, lid retraction, lid lag, proptosis, restrictive extraocular myopathy, and optic neuropathy.[6001] Central scotomas, arcuate or inferior altitudinal defects, and generalized field constriction may be due to optic nerve compression by swollen muscles at the orbital apex.

dystonia (idiopathic torsion dystonia, Oppenheim disease, Ziehen syndrome, tonic torsion neurosis, Gowers tetanoid chorea, paraspasm, dystonia musculorum deformans) Sustained and patterned muscle contractions of agonist and antagonist muscles, usually leading to twisting involuntary movements that are frequently repetitive and that may progress to fixed abnormal postures or to repetitive twisting or squeezing movements. Their speed varies from creeping to myoclonic, but their range is usually limited. Thus, the movements represent an unusually slow and persistent form of **athetosis.** Fixed dystonia also occurs, in which the muscular contraction leads the trunk, limbs, or face to assume a fixed posture. The underlying lesion is usually of the putamen, less often of the brainstem or thalamus, and the mechanism for their production is likely to be a deficiency of the cortical inhibition of subcortical motor pathways.

The clinical condition was first described in an MD thesis by Marcus Walter Schwalbe (b. 1883), a German physician, in 1908,[5016] and then by Georg Theodor Ziehen, a German psychiatrist, in 1911. It was more fully delineated and named by Hermann Oppenheimer in that same year.[4252] However, subjects with what appear to be dystonic postures had been painted by Peter **Brueghel** the younger and by William Blake.

An etiological classification, recognizing *idiopathic (primary)* and *symptomatic (secondary)* forms, has been suggested,[6038] the primary dystonias being further classified as hereditary forms, those associated with other hereditary neurological diseases, and those which are sporadic. A simple clinical classification is that of Warner and Jarman,[5847] adapted here:

Form	Description
1. Primary dystonia	Phenotype of dystonia alone (with or without tremor; see below)
A. Dystonia-plus syndromes	Phenotype of dystonia + additional neurological features (e.g., parkinsonism, myoclonus, (**dopa-responsive dystonia,** rapid-onset dystonia-parkinsonism; see below). See also **deafness-dystonia syndrome.** Plus myoclonus (**myoclonic dystonia;** see below)
B. Paroxysmal dystonia	**Paroxysmal kinesigenic dystonia** **Paroxysmal dystonic choreoathetosis**
2. Secondary dystonias	A. Resulting from structural CNS disease (e.g., craniocerebral trauma, drugs, encephalitis, multiple sclerosis, toxins, perinatal asphyxia, stroke) B. Heredodegenerative diseases Dystonia-plus syndromes occurring in the context of an underlying neurodegenerative disease. These include **X-linked parkinson**ism-dystonia (Lubag); **ataxia-telangiectasia;** biopterin deficient states; dopamine agonist–responsive dystonia caused by decarboxylase deficiency; **dopa-responsive dystonia;** dystonic lipidosis; **striopallidal calcification; gangliosidoses; glutaric acidemia; Hallervorden-Spatz disease; Hartnup disease; homocystinuria; Huntington disease;** *intraneuronal inclusion disease;* **Leigh disease; Lesch-Nyhan syndrome; Machado-Joseph cerebellar ataxia; metachromatic leukodystrophy; mitochondrial encephalomyopathies** such as **Leber disease; myoclonic-dystonia; neuro-acanthocytosis; neuronal ceroid-lipofuscinosis; rapid-onset dystonia-parkinsonism;** mutations of tyrosine hydroxylase and **Wilson disease.**
3. Psychogenic dystonia	

Another classification is based on age at onset; early-onset dystonias usually start in a leg or arm and frequently progress to involve other limbs and the trunk, while late-onset dystonias usually start in the neck, cranial muscles, or arm and tend to remain localized.

A third classification is based on the distribution of the parts affected:

- *Focal dystonias* affect a single body part. They comprise **blepharospasm, oromandibular dystonia, laryngeal** and **pharyngeal dystonias; spasmodic torticollis** (*cervical dystonia*), **truncal dystonia,** writers' cramp and other **occupational cramps, foot dystonia,** adult-onset and childhood-onset **segmental dystonias, generalized dystonias,** and some *symptomatic dystonias.*
- *Multifocal dystonias* affect more than one noncontiguous body part (arm + leg, blepharospasm with writer's cramp).
- *Segmental dystonias* affect two or more adjacent body parts (e.g., neck and trunk, face and jaw, or neck and arm as with torticollis and writer's cramp). **Hemidystonia** affects the face and limbs of one side.
- *Generalized dystonias* affect two or more noncontiguous body parts.[1730]

A fourth classification is based on age of onset: it is not reproduced here in order to preserve the composure of the reader.

However, compounding the confusion is the fact that certain forms of dystonia with unique characteristics pertaining to their site, precipitation or occurrence, age of onset, speed, or response to therapy are described. Thus the idiopathic dystonias include classical torsion dystonia (see Chart D–14), **paradoxical dystonia,**

myoclonic dystonia, diurnal dystonia, and **dopa-responsive dystonia.**

Other dyskinesias include **dystonic dysphagia, dystonic tics, paroxysmal dystonia, hypogenic dystonia, spasmodic and axial dystonia,** and **tardive dystonia.** These are entered elsewhere.[1732,1733,3754] Dystonia can also be psychogenic.[3262]

A classification of the dystonias is provided in Chart D–14.

Chart D–14. Classification of the Dystonias

1. *Primary idiopathic dystonia* (no identifiable exogenous cause or other inherited or degenerative disease)

   A. Inherited (*hereditary torsion dystonia*) (autosomal dominant, recessive, pseudodominant or X-linked recessive)

   The *dominant syndrome* (*idiopathic primary torsion dystonia*) is the most common form and is characterized by the onset in youth or young adult life of torticollis, blepharospasm, or truncal dystonia, although cranial involvement is infrequent, progressing to athetosis, dystonia, and muscle hypertrophy, starting later and of less severity than the recessive form. In this form, the younger the age of onset the greater the chance of generalization. It is common in Ashkenazi Jews, among whom the symptoms rather resemble those of the recessive form. The gene *DYT1* maps to 9q34,[836,4563] and *DYT13* to 1p36.13–36.32.

   A mixed phenotype has onset in childhood or adult life, may begin anywhere, and is dominantly inherited with incomplete penetrance. Cranial involvement with dysarthria and dysphonia is common. This form is mapped to chromosome 8 in Mennonite/Amish families.

   A third phenotype has onset in adult life, with cervical, cranial, or brachial involvement and again is inherited as an autosomal dominant trait but with very reduced penetrance. The dystonia tends to remain localized. This form has been mapped to chromosome 18p but is likely to be genetically heterogeneous.

   Criteria for the diagnosis of have been suggested[3642] and include the following:

   The presence of dystonic movements and postures

   A normal perinatal history

   The absence of any history of precipitating illness or of exposure to drugs known to provoke torsion dystonia before the onset of the illness

   The absence of intellectual, pyramidal, cerebellar, or sensory abnormalities on examination

   A normal laboratory evaluation, including serum copper studies

   For other forms of dystonia, the molecular genetics are less clear. See also **dopa-responsive dystonia.**

   A *recessive form* is characterized by the onset in youth or young adult life of athetosis, dystonia, and muscle hypertrophy. Starting in one limb, symptoms extend to other limbs and the trunk at variable rates.

   The following *variants* have been described:

   Adult-onset axial dystonia A focal dystonic syndrome mapped in some cases to 18p and which starts in adult life, does not affect the legs, and progresses little. Prior trauma may be a factor in a third of cases.[542]

   Deafness-dystonia syndrome

   Dopa-responsive dystonia This form has been mapped to chromosome 14q22.

   Dystonia with marked diurnal variation (diurnal dystonia,

Segawa disease) A dominant or recessive dystonic syndrome with onset in childhood, characterized by initial involvement of one limb, deterioration during the day, abatement with sleep, and complete responsiveness to L-dopa.[5052] Like **dopa-responsive dystonia,** this condition has been mapped to chromosome 14q.

Hereditary myoclonic dystonia (hereditary dystonia with lightning jerks, responsive to alcohol) A dominantly inherited dystonic and myoclonic syndrome with onset in childhood and affecting mainly the neck and arms and sparing the legs. The lightning jerks occur spontaneously, with movement and as a response to startle, with variable symmetry and synchrony, and abate with alcohol ingestion. In some cases, abnormal EEG activity precedes the jerks.[4563]

Myoclonic dystonia (hereditary essential myoclonus, hereditary myoclonic dystonia) A dominantly inherited, rather benign form of idiopathic dystonia with onset in childhood or young adult life, characterized by dystonia of the face, arms, and trunk, upon which is superimposed proximal, action-induced myoclonus affecting mainly the arms and trunk and which is present at rest, worsened by exercise, and substantially relieved by alcohol.[4187] The genetic abnormality is not yet mapped.

Paradoxical dystonia

Paroxysmal kinesigenic and nonkinesigenic dystonias in which dystonic attacks are precipitated by prolonged muscular exertion and last from 5 to 30 minutes. In some families there is an association with migraine.[4041] These conditions are sometimes dominantly inherited (mapped to chromosome 16) but may also occur sporadically.[3859] See also **dyskinesias.**

Paroxysmal nocturnal hemidystonia A syndrome characterized by the occurrence of paroxysmal dystonic-dyskinetic movements during stages 2–3 of non–rapid eye movement sleep. These are actually more likely to represent seizure manifestations.

Rapid-onset dystonia-parkinsonism A dominantly inherited form mapping to chromosome 19q13, with onset in youth or early adult life, in which these motor features affect bulbar and upper limbs especially, with an onset first over hours or days, progressing slowly thereafter.[1483,4457]

X-linked dystonia-parkinsonism (Lubag) An X-linked recessive (Xq21) or codominant syndrome recorded originally in adult male Filipinos; elsewhere, linkage to Xq12–13.1 has been described. Clinically, this form has a gradual onset, but continues rapidly to a state of severe involvement,[335] initially with dystonia; the signs of parkinsonism appear later in life and respond poorly to levadopa therapy.[335, 5870] The word *lubag* is that used in the Philippines for this condition.

   B. Sporadic dystonia (*idiopathic or symptomatic dystonia*)

      1. Generalized

      2. Segmental or limb dystonia (usually secondary dystonias). A dominantly inherited syndrome linked in some cases to a site on chromosome 8.

      3. **Hemidystonia**

      4. Multifocal

      5. Focal *torticollis*, **occupational cramps, oromandibular dystonia, blepharospasm, spasmodic dysphonia**

   Other *variants* include the following:

   Benign idiopathic dystonia A dystonic state occurring in infancy and clearing by the age of 18 months.[5979]

   Dystonia with multiple contractures: A rare syndrome of

chorea and dystonia in the setting of multiple nonprogressive contractures of muscle with childhood onset.[1783]

Determan syndrome Intermittent dystonic movements resulting from cerebrovascular disease affecting the basal ganglia.

2. *Secondary dystonia*

A. Associated with other hereditary neurodegenerative or metabolic disorders such as **ataxia-telangiectasia**; *dystonic juvenile lipidosis*; **Huntington disease; neuronal ceroid lipofuscinosis; GM$_2$ and GM$_1$ gangliosidoses; glutaric aciduria type 1; Leigh disease; metachromatic leukodystrophy; Leber optic atrophy** and other **mitochondrial diseases; Hartnup disease; homocystinuria**; *intraneuronal inclusion disease*; **juvenile dystonic lipidosis; Lesch-Nyhan syndrome;** Lubag (X-linked parkinsonism-dystonia); **Machado-Joseph disease (SCA3); Martha-Alma** (Hallervorden-Spatz) **disease; methylmalonic academia; myoclonic dystonia; neuronal ceroid lipofuscinosis; neurovisceral storage disease; phenylketonuria** and other biopterin deficient states; **supranuclear ophthalmoplegia; tardive dystonia**;[5478] **triosephosphate isomerase deficiency; tyrosinosis**; *tyrosine hydroxylase mutations*; and **Wilson disease.**

Dystonia and basal ganglion calcification A dominantly inherited dystonic syndrome of childhood or early adult life characterized by dysarthria, dementia, resting tremors, dystonia, chorea, and athetosis and with intracranial calcification in the basal ganglia.[337] See also *DACE syndrome* (below).

Torsion dystonia with basal ganglion lucencies A slowly progressive dystonic syndrome without intellectual failure, beginning in infancy or early childhood.[4386]

Idiopathic dystonia–parkinsonism A form of juvenile parkinsonism with a benign and chronic course, characterized by dystonic movements and parkinsonism with marked diurnal fluctuation of symptoms, a marked response to low doses of antiparkinsonian drugs, and EMG findings of continuous discharges of antagonistic muscles.[5419]

Rapid-onset dystonia-parkinsonism A dominantly inherited disorder characterized by the rapid onset of symptoms (of dystonia more than of parkinsonism) in youth or adult life, with little succeeding progression but with minimal response to treatment with L-dopa or dopamine agonists.[1483]

Flexion dystonia in paralysis agitans A syndrome manifesting slowly progressive, persistent, flexed postures of the limbs, especially of the hands and wrists,[1397] accompanied by synchronous grouped discharges of antagonistic muscles.

Dystonia, blepharospasm, and pigmentary retinopathy An inherited syndrome of prominent extrapyramidal dysfunction, retinal pigmentary changes, pyramidal and cerebellar signs, and high-arched palate, with unimpaired intellect.[1126]

DACE syndrome (**D**ystonia, **A**canthocytosis, basal ganglion **C**alcification, and **E**ye abnormalities) A rare syndrome with onset in childhood, characterized by the presence of these features, the dystonia being severe and progressive and the eye disorders comprising nystagmus in the primary position and limitation of vertical movements. Because the high-density signals from the globus pallidus suggest the presence of iron deposits, the condition may be a variant of **Hallervorden-Spatz disease.**[1222]

Post-traumatic cervical dystonia The occurrence of cervical dystonia following neck injury. The syndrome is said to manifest marked limitation in the range of movement of the neck; failure of relief from *gestes antagonistiques* and from sleep; tonic rather than phasic neck muscle contraction; and poor response to treatment.[4892]

B. Associated with other disorders

C. Due to other known acquired (?) metabolic or structural neurological disease, including parkinsonism
Hypoparathyroidism
Encephalitis
Postinfectious states
Toxins—manganese, carbon monoxide, carbon disulfide, L-dopa, D$_2$ receptor agonists
Perinatal cerebral injury, head trauma, brain tumor, stroke

D. Psychogenic

Adapted from Fahn S. Generalized dystonia: concept and treatment. Clin Neuropharmacol *1986;9(**suppl** 2):S37–S48,[1730] Bressman (1998) and other sources referenced.[738]

dystonia and basal ganglion calcification   See **dystonia.**

dystonia, blepharospasm, and pigmentary retinopathy   See **dystonia.**

dystonia, deafness, and mental retardation   An X-linked syndrome with onset in early childhood, characterized by these features and a tendency to self-mutilation.[5040]

Dystonia Disability Scale   An assessment instrument quantifying the disturbance in functioning produced by dystonic disorders. The scale is reproduced as Chart D–15 by kind permission from Burke RE, Fahn S, Marsden CD, et al. Validity and reliability of a rating scale for the primary torsion dystonias. *Neurology* 1985;35:73–7.

Chart D–15. Dystonia Disability Scale

A. Speech

0. Normal
1. Slightly involved; easily understood
2. Some difficulty in understanding
3. Marked difficulty in understanding
4. Complete or almost complete anarthria

B. Handwriting (tremor or dystonia)

0. Normal
1. Slight difficulty; legible
2. Almost illegible
3. Illegible
4. Unable to grasp or maintain hold on pen

C. Feeding

0. Normal
1. Uses tricks; independent
2. Can feed but cannot cut
3. Finger food only
4. Completely dependent

D. Eating/swallowing

0. Normal
1. Occasional choking
2. Chokes frequently; difficulty swallowing
3. Unable to swallow firm foods
4. Marked difficulty swallowing soft foods and liquids

E. Hygiene

0. Normal
1. Clumsy; independent
2. Needs help with some activities
3. Needs help with most activities
4. Needs help with all activities

F. Dressing

0. Normal
1. Clumsy; independent
2. Needs help with some activities
3. Needs help with most activities
4. Helpless

G. Walking

0. Normal
1. Slightly abnormal; hardly noticeable
2. Moderately abnormal; obvious to naive observer
3. Considerably abnormal
4. Needs assistance to walk
5. Wheelchair bound

Adapted from Burke et al. (1985).[842]

Dystonia Medical Research Foundation   (USA) Address: One East Wacker Dr., Ste. 2430, Chicago, IL 60601–2001. Tel: 312–755–0198. (Canada) Address: 777 Hornby St., #1800, Vancouver, BC V6Z 1S4, Canada. A charitable organization, in each case seeking to determine the cause and cure of involuntary movement disorders through the provision of research funding, and undertaking patient support work and both professional and patient information services. Web site: www.dystonia-foundation.org.

Dystonia Movement Scale   A rating scale used for the assessment of the scope and severity of the signs of *primary torsion dystonias*.[842] The scale is reproduced here by kind permission of the authors and of the editor of *Neurology* (see Chart D–16).

Chart D–16. Dystonia Movement Scale

Region	Severity Factor		Factor Weight		Product
Eyes	0–4	×	0–4	0.5	0–8
Mouth	0–4	×	0–4	0.5	0–8
Speech	0–4	×	0–4	1.0	0–16
Neck	0–4	×	0–4	0.5	0–8
Right arm	0–4	×	0–4	1.0	0–16
Left arm	0–4	×	0–4	1.0	0–16
Trunk	0–4	×	0–4	1.0	0–16
Right leg	0–4	×	0–4	1.0	0–16
Left leg	0–4	×	0–4	1.0	0–16

SUM (Maximum = 120)

I. *Provoking factor*
  A. General
    0. No dystonia at rest or with action
    1. Dystonia on particular action
    2. Dystonia on many actions
    3. Dystonia on action of distant part of body or intermittently at rest
    4. Dystonia present at rest
  B. Speech and swallowing
    1. Occasional, either or both
    2. Frequent either
    3. Frequent one and occasional other
    4. Frequent both
II. *Severity factors*
  A. Eyes
    0. No dystonia
    1. Slight, occasional blinking
    2. Mild; frequent blinking without prolonged spasms of eye closure
    3. Moderate; prolonged spasms of eyelid closure, but eyes open most of the time
    4. Severe; prolonged spasms of eyelid closure, with eyes closed at least 30% of the time
  B. Mouth
    0. No dystonia present
    1. Slight; occasional grimacing or other mouth movement (e.g., jaw open or clenched; tongue movement)
    2. Mild; movement present less than 50% of the time
    3. Moderate dystonia movements or contractions present most of the time
    4. Severe dystonic movements or contractions present most of the time
  C. Speech and swallowing
    0. Normal
    1. Slightly involved; speech easily understood or occasional choking
    2. Some difficulty in understanding speech or frequent choking
    3. Marked difficulty in understanding speech or inability to swallow firm foods
    4. Complete or almost complete anarthria, or marked difficulty swallowing soft foods and liquids
  D. Neck
    0. No dystonia present
    1. Slight; occasional pulling
    2. Obvious torticollis, but mild
    3. Moderate pulling
    4. Extreme pulling
  E. Arm
    0. No dystonia present
    1. Slight dystonia; clinically insignificant
    2. Mild; obvious dystonia, but not disabling
    3. Moderate; able to grasp, with some manual function
    4. Severe; no useful grasp
  F. Trunk
    0. No dystonia present
    1. Slight bending, clinically insignificant
    2. Definite bending, but not interfering with standing or walking
    3. Moderate bending; interfering with standing or walking
    4. Extreme bending of trunk preventing standing or walking
  G. Leg
    0. No dystonia present
    1. Slight dystonia, but not causing impairment; clinically insignificant
    2. Mild dystonia; walks briskly and unaided
    3. Moderate dystonia; severely impairs walking or requires assistance
    4. Severe; unable to stand or walk on involved leg

Adapted from Burke et al. (1985)[842] *and reproduced by kind permission.*

dystonia musculorum deformans   See **dystonia, dopa-responsive dystonia.**

dystonia musculorum deformans with hyperuricemia   A congenital syndrome with childhood onset, manifesting dystonia, athetosis and hyperuricemia. See also **Lesch-Nyhan syndrome.**

dystonia rating scales.   See **United Dystonia Rating Scale, Dystonia Movement Scale, Burke-Fahn-Marsden Scale.**

Dystonia Society   (UK) A charitable organization. Address: 46-47 Britton Street, London EC1M 5UJ, UK. Tel: 0171 490 5671. Website: http://www.dystonia.org. uk/dystoniasocietyh.html.

dystonia with contractures and abnormal muscle   An inherited congenital syndrome characterized by joint contractures, chorea, dystonia, and muscle fiber hypotrophy with ring fibers.[337]

dystonia with marked diurnal variation   See **diurnal dystonia.**

dystonia with marked diurnal variation associated with biopterin deficiency   See **dopa-responsive dystonia.**

dystonia with multiple contractures   See **dystonia.**

dystonic choreoathetosis induced by exercise   An inherited syndrome characterized by onset in childhood or youth of athetosis and dystonia which are precipitated by muscular activity.[2189]

This condition and **dopa-responsive dystonia** may be the same. See also **paroxysmal kinesigenic choreoathetosis.**

dystonic cramps   Muscle spasms complicating manual tasks—a form of focal hand cramps.[5110]

dystonic dysphagia   Focal dystonia affecting the pharyngeal muscles.

dystonic foot response   (striatal foot, grasp reflex of the foot, myokymia of Kny and Schultze) Stereotyped, tonic, painful extension of the hallux with flexion of the other toes, arching of the sole, and inversion at the ankle associated with extrapyramidal disease but not with frontal lobe lesions, and worsened by levadopa therapy.[4081] See also **dystonic toe.**

dystonic gait   See **dyskinetic gait.**

dystonic juvenile lipidosis   A rare syndrome comprising mental deterioration, vertical gaze palsy, seizures, dyskinesias, and pyramidal signs, with hepatosplenomegaly. Sea-blue histiocytosis is found in the bone marrow. The condition may be a form of **sphingomyelin storage disorder.**[3034]

dystonic spasms   Forceful and accelerated dystonic movements, with the same implications as other dystonic manifestations.

dystonic stridor   A form of **segmental dystonia** affecting the vocal cords.[1130]

dystonic syndrome of senility   See **danse du ventre.**

dystonic tics   See **tics.**

dystonic toe   The semipermanent dorsiflexed posture of the hallux seen in some patients in whom dystonia affects the leg. See also **dystonic foot response.**

dystonic tremor   Forms of **action tremor** in patients with dystonias.[1422] One form is a postural/kinetic tremor indistinguishable from **essential tremor;** a second is an irregular, jerky action tremor interposed between the involuntary dystonic movements; and a third is an irregular **task-specific tremor.**

dystrophia muscularis progressiva   See **limb-girdle muscular dystrophy.**

dystrophia myotonica   See **myotonic dystrophy.**

dystrophin   A large intracellular protein, coded at Xp21.2, which has recently been shown to be a component of the sarcolemmal plasma membrane (transverse tubule) system. The absence of dystrophin leads to the muscular symptoms of **Duchenne muscular dystrophy.** In **Becker dystrophy,** the protein is present but abnormal in either quantity or composition.[2600]

dystrophin test   A Western blot analysis of dystrophin protein from a muscle biopsy specimen, allowing characterization of the abnormal protein alleles in Duchenne and Becker muscle dystrophies.[2600]

dystrophinopathies   A group of clinicopathological disorders resulting from mutations of the dystrophin gene. They include **Duchenne muscle dystrophy** (and its dilute manifestation in female carriers); **Becker muscle dystrophy;** cardiomyopathy with or without proximal weakness; a syndrome of myalgia and cramps; and hyperCKemic states. See also **sarcoglycanopathy, desminopathy, dysferlin.**

dystrophy   (Gr, difficulty + nourishment; and thus bad growth) The term arbitrarily used for those (usually progressive) diseases of muscle which have a genetic basis, the remainder being called *myopathies*, which just means diseases of muscle. It would have been simpler to call them all either *genetic* or *acquired* myopathies, but it is too late now.

dysversion   Congenital structural abnormalities of the eye, including tilted disks, occurring alone or in association with craniofacial syndromes.

Dzerzhinskii syndrome   A familial syndrome, a form of craniomandibularfacial dysostosis, marked by acrocephaly, scaphocephaly, lordotic curvature at the base of the skull, premature closure of the cranial sutures, dysmorphism, protruding nose, and thickening of the phalanges, sternum, and clavicles.[1589]

E

E-1 See **recording electrode.**

E-2 See **recording electrode.**

Eagle syndrome (stylohyoid process syndrome) Pain in the face or in the floor of the mouth, presumably brought about by trauma to a congenitally elongated or calcified styloid process[1591] or resulting from pressure on local structures (including the carotid artery) exerted by the long styloid process.

The syndrome appears to be confined to adults, in whom the pain is brought on by jaw or neck movements, swallowing, or local pressure.[3679]

Eales disease (retinitis proliferans, periphlebitis retinae, angiopathia retinae juvenalis) The occurrence of retinal periphlebitis, neovascular formation, and recurrent vitreous and retinal hemorrhages in young people.[1593]

The acute ocular events may be followed by severe acute or subacute myelopathy, seizures, and focal neurological deficits. Eales considered that constipation was a likely cause; no better guess has been suggested since.

Eales, Henry (1852–1913) Ophthalmologist, practicing in Birmingham, England.

ear wagging See **Hassin sign.**

ear wiggling Bilateral intermittent movements of the ears due to contractions of the auricular muscles, accompanied usually by scalp movements and considered to have a psychological basis,[3026] although the phenomenon was also displayed by Dopey, one of the seven dwarfs in the Walt Disney movie "Snow White," whose perceived stress level was likely to have been low.

earlobe reflex A normal sign in infants; rubbing the earlobe lightly causes rotation of the head toward the opposite side.[6064]

early infantile epileptic encephalopathy with suppression burst (Ohtahara syndrome) A seizure syndrome with onset within the first few months of life, characterized by frequent tonic spasms and a suppression–burst EEG pattern in both the waking and sleeping states. Partial seizures may occur but myoclonic seizures are rare.[612,4226]

The etiology and underlying pathology are obscure. The prognosis is serious, with severe psychomotor retardation and seizure intractability; often there is evolution to the **West syndrome** at age 4–6 months. (From the revised ILAE Classification,[1114] reproduced by kind permission from Blackwell Science.)

Electrographically, bursts of irregular spikes, sharp waves and slow waves, lasting up to several seconds and occurring over both hemispheres, are separated by periods of marked diminution of activity on the EEG. The syndrome is caused by a variety of early and extensive brain insults, especially brain malformations, and is considered to represent a specific type of epileptic encephalopathy in the neonatal period and early infancy, resembling infantile spasms in older children.[4227] See also **Aicardi syndrome.**

early language milestone scale An instrument assessing all the components of visual and auditory language in infants from birth to 3 years of age, including auditory expressive, auditory receptive, and visual functions.[1124]

early morning akinesia A hypokinetic form of fluctuation in parkinsonian patients on long-term l-dopa therapy in which disability is increased on waking, by which time the previous night's dose has lost its effect.

early morning dystonia A dystonic form of fluctuation in parkinsonian patients on long-term l-dopa therapy in which dystonic movements accompany the morning fall in l dopa to low levels.

early morning waking The inability to fall asleep after unusual and inappropriately early waking from nocturnal sleep. It is usually a symptom of depressive or hypomanic illness.

early multiple sclerosis A diagnostic category in the 1954 definitions of **Allison and Millar,** now largely replaced by the **McDonald** or the **Poser** criteria.

early myoclonic encephalopathy An epileptic syndrome of childhood in with onset before age 3 months, characterized initially by fragmentary myoclonus and then by erratic partial seizures, massive myoclonia, or tonic spasms. The EEG shows suppression–burst activity, which may evolve into **hypsarrhythmia.** The course is severe, psychomotor development is arrested, and death may occur in the first year. Familial cases are frequent, which may suggest the influence of one or several congenital metabolic errors, but there is no constant genetic pattern. (From the revised ILAE Classification,[1114] reproduced by kind permission from Blackwell Science.)

early post-traumatic epilepsy Seizures occurring in the week following craniocerebral trauma. In adults, this is usually associated with severe or complicated cerebral injury. See also **late post-traumatic epilepsy.**

early probable (latent) multiple sclerosis See **McDonald-Halliday criteria.**[3744]

early recruitment A recruitment pattern that occurs in association with a reduction in the number of muscle fibers per motor unit or when the force generated by the fibers is reduced. At low levels of muscle contraction more motor unit action potentials are recorded than expected, and a full interference pattern may be recorded at relatively low levels of muscle contraction.

This is most often encountered in myopathy. (From the 2001 Report of the Nomenclature Committee of the American Association of Electromyography and Electrodiagnosis.[10] Used by permission, copyright© 2001, AAEM.)

early-onset autosomal dominant dementia with ataxia, extrapyramidal features, and epilepsy A rare syndrome with these manifestations, not linked to currently known dementias.[1816]

early-onset spinal muscular atrophy See **hereditary motor neuropathy, type 2.**

early-onset cerebellar ataxia with retained reflexes Recessively inherited cerebellar ataxic syndromes with onset in youth which resemble **Friedreich ataxia** but in which areflexia, optic atrophy, heart disease, diabetes, and skeletal deformity do not occur.[2439]

A *variant* is an *X-linked recessive form.*
Other recessively inherited forms are mainly reported from Quebec;[340] in these the following features are seen, variously: hypogonadism and normal muscle stretch reflexes; myoclonus (Ramsay Hunt syndrome); pigmentary retinal degeneration and mental retardation; optic atrophy and mental retardation; cataracts and mental retardation; deafness alone or with mental retardation; and extrapyramidal features.

See also **cerebellar ataxias.**

earth See **ground electrode.**

earthbound astronaut syndrome A fanciful name applied to an acquired state of dysequilibrium.[1511]

ease-of-falling syndrome Probably the same as **thalamic astasia,**[3668] in which a patient is unable to stand after a unilateral thalamic lesion or a lesion in the superior part of the internal capsule, as described by Miller **Fisher.**[1853,1866] The astasia, in which the patient falls repeatedly to the side of the weakness, appears out of proportion to the mildness of the pyramidal motor deficit.

eastern equine encephalitis An uncommon mosquito-borne arbovirus infection with its reservoir among wild birds living along the American, Atlantic, and Caribbean coasts, usually occurring as sporadic infections, most commonly in children.

Clinically, the encephalitis is severe, with a mortality of up to 70%, leaving neurological sequelae in most survivors. High fevers, seizures, facial edema, signs of raised intracranial pressure, and evidence of severe progressive neurological impairment are the usual clinical features.[2166] Since the routine immunization of horses, equine infection and thus the disease in humans have become uncommon.[4540]

eating epilepsy (prandic epilepsy) Seizures (usually of complex partial type) provoked by the act of eating and associated with a lesion of the deep frontal lobes or rhinencephalon which appears to activate diencephalic structures involved in the cephalic phase of digestion.[4722]

The seizures represent a form of **reflex epilepsy.** There is frequently a positive family history of seizures in affected subjects. This is a disorder of young adults, especially in India, in whom some aspect of eating (hunger, site, smell, taste, chewing, or swallowing) acts as a precipitant of seizures.[3463]

Eaton, L.M. (1905–1958) American neurologist at the Mayo Clinic, where he developed an extensive interest in neuromuscular disease.

Eaton Lambert syndrome See **Lambert-Eaton myasthenic syndrome.**

ebriositatis See **delirium tremens.**

ecchordosis physaliphora A jelly-like excrescence occurring anywhere along the axial skeleton and considered to be a non-neoplastic hamartoma. The lesion is usually clinically silent and rarely leads to the growth of a **chordoma.** Like chordomas, however, these lesions stain positively for cytokeratin and epithelial membrane antigen.[3544]

echenne muscular dystrophy–white matter spongiosis A congenital dysmorphic syndrome characterized by feeding problems in infancy, joint contractures and arthrogryposis, grand mal and absence seizures (including reading epilepsy), dolichocephaly, scaphocephaly or macrocephaly, and myopathic weakness.[337]

Echner, Alexander (1816–1887) German anatomist in Freyburg whose precise and detailed drawings of the cortex in 1869 established the form of the sulci, gyri, and fissures (and thus the lobes) of the cerebrum.

Echner inferior parietal lobule The supramarginal and angular gyri, identified by Alexander Echner (1816–1887) in 1869.[4979]

echo actions The precise repetition by the patient of what the examiner has just said or done. Occasionally a feature of late-stage dementias, it is more often evidence of schizophrenia.

echographia The repetition in writing of what is presented in speech or writing to a subject who is usually aphasic or (as in the first reported cases of **Pick**) is suffering from mental retardation. See **hypergraphia.**

echolalia The involuntary, automatic, precise repetition of the words or phrases said to the patient without change in pronoun, in the presence of gross difficulty in comprehension. The condition is typically due to isolation of the speech areas by a large parietal lesion.[2080]

echolaliopraxia See **signing tics.**

echopraxia The involuntary repetition of the actions or speech of another person.

EC/IC bypass surgery (extracranial–Intracranial bypass) Surgical anastomosis of the superficial temporal artery with a branch of the middle cerebral artery in order to improve blood flow through the latter vessel. Theoretically and technically this is a superb operation, for which an appropriate disease is keenly being sought.

eclampsia   A severe hypertensive state with widespread vasospasm peculiar to women in the peripartum state, up to 2 weeks after delivery. Evidence of hemolysis, elevated liver enzymes, and low platelets (the HELLP syndrome) may be found, associated with cerebral edema and hemorrhage in severe cases. Neurological features include grand mal seizures, headache, and other evidence of raised intracranial pressure, **posterior leukoencephalopathy,** and acutely appearing focal deficits such as stroke-like syndromes and ischemic optic neuropathy. Association with the Leiden Factor V has been shown.[5556]

Economo, Konstantin von   See **Von Economo, Konstantin.**

Economo disease   See **encephalitis lethargica.**

economy class syndrome   The occurrence of venous thromboembolism (usually leading to pulmonary venous infarction) as a result of prolonged relative immobility in an aeroplane seat allowing little opportunity for leg movement and requiring almost a Valsalva maneuver in order to escape from the seat. The migrant emboli may also pass through a patent foramen ovale to cause stroke. The existence of the condition may suggest yet another indication for prophylactic ASA.

ecstasy   3,4-methylenedioxymethamphetamine,   an agent capable of causing the undesired effects of metabolic stimulation and muscle necrosis with hyperthermia, as well as the desired mood alterations.

ectasia, ectasis   (from Gr; to stretch out) Dilation, usually applied to a hollow channel such as a blood vessel.

ectodermal calcification–basal ganglion calcification syndrome   A congenital dysmorphic syndrome manifesting also short stature, alopecia, microcephaly, calcification of the basal ganglia, and mental and developmental delay. See **striatopallidal calcification.**

ectodermal dysplasia   Inherited syndromes comprising abnormalities both of the skin and of the nervous system.[601,1059,2883,4850,5690] Both **neurocutaneous syndromes** and mesodermal disorders such as **Sturge-Weber syndrome** and **Lindau disease** are subsumed under this heading.

See also: **anhidrotic ectodermal dysplasia; hidrotic ectodermal dysplasia; von Recklinghausen disease; tuberous sclerosis; xeroderma pigmentosum; Rud syndrome; Berier disease; Kaposi disease; poikiloderma congenitale; progeria; Bardet-Bledel syndrome; Klippel-Trenaunay-Weber syndrome,** and **Sjögren-Larsson syndrome.**

ectodermal dysplasia–olivopontocerebellar degeneration   A congenital dysmorphic syndrome with mid-face hypoplasia manifesting also short stature, deafness, hypogonadotrophic hypogonadism, cerebellar and pyramidal signs, and mental and developmental delay.[4850]

ectomesodermal blastomatoses   See **phakomatoses.**

ectopia   See **heterotopia.**

ectopia pupillae   See **corectopia iridis.**

ectopic   In an abnormal place.

ectopic intracranial retinoblastoma   The combination of **pinealoblastoma** and **retinoblastoma.**

ectopic pinealoma   See **dysgerminoma.**

ectropion   (Gr, a bending outward) Outward-turning of the eyelids.

Eddowes syndrome   See **Apert syndrome.**

Edelmann great toe phenomenon   Dorsiflexion of the hallux occurring when the leg is maintained straight and the hip is flexed. This is usually a sign of meningeal irritation, but it is also present in some patients with raised intracranial pressure.

edema   See **cerebral edema.**

Edinburgh syndrome   A dominantly inherited, lethal congenital dysmorphic syndrome characterized by hydrocephalus, hyperbilirubinemia, and mental and motor delay.[2353]

Edinburgh-2 Coma scale   A scale measuring consciousness as manifest through patients' best response to maximal stimuli. Subjects are asked the month and their age and to close and open their hand and eyes; and their response to strong pain is assessed.[5407]

Despite the name, the test is actually Japanese; its place in practice in relation to the **Glasgow Coma scale** is uncertain.

Edinger, Ludwig   (1855–1918) German professor of anatomy and neurology at Frankfurt University, who differentiated the palaeo- and neo-cerebellum in 1885 on the basis of the number of cortical layers possessed by each; and the **Edinger-Westphal nucleus,** 2 years before Westphal. He also gave the first complete account of thalamic pain.

Edinger-Westphal nucleus   The   parasympathetic nucleus of the third cranial nerve.

EDMUS   A computerized minimal descriptive record documenting clinical and laboratory data in patients with multiple sclerosis, developed and mainly used in Europe.[1116] A scale of impairment is incorporated. See also **COSTAR, Minimal Record of Disability.**

edrophonium   (tensilon) A synthetic substance with a transient cholinergic effect at the motor end-plate. See **Tensilon test.**

EDS   See **excessive daytime sleepiness.**

Edwards syndrome   A congenital dysmorphic syndrome manifesting also generalized obesity, deafness, retinitis pigmentosa, pendular nystagmus acanthosis nigricans, hypogonadism, glucose intolerance, and mental and developmental delay.[1606] See **trisomy 18 syndrome.**

EEG   Abbreviation for **electroencephalogram.**

EEG coma patterns   A system of grading the EEG records in comatose patients. The original form of Synek[5462] listed 165 categories; a simpler one published more recently has only nine.

Category	Subcategory
I. Delta/theta >50% of record (not theta coma)	
II. Triphasic waves	
III. Burst–suppression	A. With epileptifom activity
	B. Without epileptiform activity
IV. Alpha/theta/spindle coma (unreactive)	
V. Epileptiform activity (not in burst–suppression pattern)	A. Generalized
	B. Focal or rnultifocal
Suppression	A. <20 uV but >I0 uV
	B. ≤ 10 uV

Burst–suppression pattern should have generalized flattening at standard sensitivity for ≥1 second at least every 20 seconds. 2. Suppression for this category; voltage criteria should be met for entire record. 3. When more than one category applies, select the most serious: suppression is the most serious and epileptiform activity is more serious than categories I or II. (From Young GB, McLachan RS, Kreeft JH, et al. An Electroencephalographic Classification for Coma. *Can. J. Neurol. Sci.* 1997;**24**:320–5. Reproduced by permission.)

See also **coma.**

EEG telemetry   Techniques that enable the recording of the EEG for long periods on equipment remote from the patient, transmitted usually by cable, radio, or telephone systems.

effective osmolarity   (in mOsm/L) $2[Na^+ + K^+ (mEqL)] + $ plasma glucose (mg/dl) $\div 18$ A value >320 mOsm/liter reflects hyperosmolarity and >350 mOsm/liter indicates a severe hyperosmolar state with lethal potential. Poor outcome is related to age as well as elevated BUN and sodium concentrations. The syndrome may be complicated by thromboembolic events, aspiration, and rhabdomyolysis.

efferent   (from Lat; to bring out) Bearing something away from a site, as with motor nerves in which electrical impulses pass from the center to the periphery.

efferent nerve   A nerve in which the direction of physiological conduction is away from the central nervous system and towards a muscle or sweat gland.

effort headache   See **benign exertional headache.**

effort syndrome   See **chronic fatigue syndrome.**

Egger syndrome   (Joubert syndrome with orofaciodigital anomalies) A congenital dysmorphic syndrome manifesting also apnea or tachypnea, polydactyly, brain tumors, cerebellar ataxia, and mental and developmental delay. See also **Joubert syndrome.**

Ehlers Danlos syndrome   (cutis laxa, Chernogubov syndrome) A dominantly inherited syndrome of mesodermal lesions of the collagen and elastic tissues, comprising narrow face, hyperelasticity and fragility of the skin, hypermobility of joints, easy bruising, spontaneous rupture of the heart or lung and arterial aneurysms, such as carotid-cavernous fistulase.[1614,2249] Among the seven subvarieties distinguished, X-linked and recessive forms are also recorded. In the genetically heterogeneous type 4, aneurysms, dissections, and spontaneous arteriovenous fistulae are potential complications.

The first reports were by Van Meekeren in 1682 and by A.N. Chernogubov, a Russian physician, in 1892. E. Ehlers (1863–1937) was professor of clinical dermatology in Copenhagen, Denmark; H-A. Danlos (1844–1912) a French dermatologist.

Ehret syndrome   Paralysis following a painful injury leading to the persistent assumption of the least painful posture, resulting in muscle atrophy and contractures. The condition was described by Ehret in 1898[1617] among patients with peroneal weakness after trauma. Its etiology is considered to be conditioning rather than hysteria.[2764]

Ehrlich, Paul   (1854–1915) German physician who demonstrated the existence of a blood–brain barrier in 1885, when he found that every organ in the body except the brain took up vital stains injected into the blood. As a neurohistologist, he introduced methylene blue as an intra vital stain for nervous tissue.

ehrliciosis   (human monocytic ehrlicoisis) A tickborne infection due to the rickettsial bacterium *E. chaffeensis* producing clinical signs of infection, multisystem involvement, pancytopenia, raised BUN, hepatitis, and, in the nervous system, evidence of meningoencephalitis with meningism, seizures, and coma. The CSF contains increased protein and neutrophilic or lymphocytic pleocytosis. Perivascular and intramural mononuclear cell infiltrates are found in the leptomeninges and Virchow-Robin spaces.[2257]

E:I ratio   In autonomic testing, the ratio of the longest electrocardiographic R–R interval during expiration to the shortest during inspiration. Primarily a measure of parasympathetic control of heart rate. See **expiration/inspiration ratio.**

Eichorst, Herman Ludwig   (1849–1921) German physician who graduated from Königsberg University. After posts held in Germany he was appointed professor of medicine at Zurich.

In 1873 he described a form of peripheral motor

neuropathy (Eichorst neuritis) affecting the legs only, which was probably a **hereditary motor and sensory neuropathy.**

18q syndrome   A leukodystrophy due to a deletion of part of the long arm of chromosome 18, which includes the region coding for myelin basic protein (18q22–3–qter). Dysmorphisms, mental retardation, hyperactivity, and aggressivity are associated. The condition has been reported to have its onset in adult life.[395]

Eisenson examination for aphasia   A clinical instrument comprising 37 subtests, designed to provide a protocol for examining the type and severity of language and related deficits.[1621]

Ekbom, Karl Axel Sr.   (1907–1977) Swedish neurologist at Uppsala.

Ekbom syndrome   1. See **restless legs syndrome.** 2. Delusional parasitosis.

Ekman-Lobstein syndrome   A dominantly inherited cochleo–vestibular atrophy with onset in young adult life. See **Van der Hoeve phakomatosis.**

elderly gait   See **cautious gait.**

electric chorea   See **Dubini disease.**

electric feet syndrome   See **burning feet syndrome.**

electrical inactivity   See **electrical silence.**

electrical nystagmus   See **vestibular nystagmus.**

electric shock   Exposure of the body to high-voltage electrical currents, which may lead in the acute phase to local burns, ventricular fibrillation, and such neurological complications as respiratory center paralysis, spinal atrophic paresis, cerebral edema, intracranial hematoma, brainstem syndromes, myelopathic spastic paraplegia,[5636] hemiplegia, radiculopathy, severe axonal neuropathy, or heat-induced myopathy,[1748] and in the longer term to syndromes resembling **amyotrophic lateral sclerosis**[2795] as well to as optic atrophy, retinopathy, cataract, involuntary movement disorders, and various patterns of upper or lower motor neuron lesions, from which latter recovery may not occur. See also **lightning encephalopathy, lightning polyneuropathy.**

electrical silence   The absence of measurable electric activity in a tissue.

electrical status epilepticus in sleep   (ESES, epilepsy with continuous spike–waves during sleep) The occurrence of continuous and diffuse spike and slow wave complexes persisting through non–rapid eye movement sleep. The disorder is most commonly seen in children before the age of 4 years and is not directly associated with clinical features. It continues for months or occasionally for over a year, and is usually seen in subjects with some seizure type, including almost all forms of generalized or partial motor seizures and brief absence attacks. These frequently disappear around the time of puberty. The EEG during wakefulness may show a combination of focal and generalized spikes

Withdrawal, impaired language development, memory and orientation, and a global reduction in intelligence are notable for a few years, after which the electrical and clinical features remit and the child's behavior returns toward normal.[4362] However, despite the usually benign evolution of seizures, the prognosis is guarded because of the occasional later appearance of neuropsychological disorders.[1114]

This seizure syndrome results from the association of various seizure types, partial or generalized, occurring during sleep, and atypical absences when awake. Tonic seizures do not occur.

Diagnostic criteria have been suggested by the American Sleep Disorders Association[234] (see Chart E–1).

Chart E–1. Diagnostic Criteria for Electrical Status Epilepticus in Sleep

A. The disorder is usually asymptomatic, but there may be a complaint of difficulty in awakening in the morning.

B. There is frequent, but not constant, association with epilepsy, particularly typical absences or infrequent partial or generalized motor seizures.

C. The age of onset is typically in childhood.

D. Polysomnographic monitoring demonstrates:
1. Continuous, generalized spike- and slow-wave discharges persisting through non–rapid eye movement sleep stages;
2. A spike/wave (SW) index ranging from 85% to 100%;
3. Disappearance of the electrical status during REM sleep.

E. Other medical or psychiatric disorders can be present, particularly other seizure disorders.

F. The disorder does not meet the diagnostic criteria for other sleep disorders that occur during sleep.

Adapted from The Interntional Classification of Sleep Disorders Diagnostic and Coding Manual. Rochester, MN: American Sleep Disorders Association, © 1990. Reproduced by kind permission of the American Academy of Sleep Medicine.

See also **sleep disorders.**

electrically silent cramps   Painful prolonged muscle contractures provoked by depletion of muscle energy stores unaccompanied by EMG activity. See **glycogenoses; rippling muscle syndrome, Brody syndrome, myoedema, electrically silent cramps.**

electroanalgesia   The reduction of pain by stimulation of sites in the central or peripheral nervous systems.

electrocochleography   A technique for assessing the electrical output of the cochlea and eighth cranial nerve in response to auditory stimulation, by means of a recording needle electrode inserted through the tympanic membrane.[4497] The test has been considered to be of value in the diagnosis of **vestibular schwannomas** (acoustic neuromas), but **MRI scanning** and **brainstem auditory evoked responses** are much better.

electrocorticogram (corticogram) The record of EEG activity obtained by means of electrodes applied directly over or inserted into the cerebral cortex.

electrocorticography (corticography) The technique of recording the electrical activity of the brain by means of electrodes applied over or implanted into the cerebral cortex.

electrode A conducting device used to record an electric potential (recording electrode) or to deliver an electric current (stimulating electrode). In addition to the ground electrode used in clinical recordings, two electrodes are always required to either record an electric potential or deliver a stimulus. See **ground electrode, recording electrode,** and **stimulating electrode.** Also see specific needle electrode configurations: **monopolar, unipolar, concentric, bifilar recording, bipolar stimulating, multilead, single fiber,** and **macro-EMG needle electrodes.** (From the 2001 Report of the Nomenclature Committee of the American Association of Electromyography and Electrodiagnosis.[10] Used by permission, copyright © 2001, AAEM.)

electrode impedance The opposition to the flow of an AC current through the interface between an electrode and the scalp or brain, expressed in ohms (generally kilohms). This is measured between pairs of electrodes or, in some EEG machines, between each individual electrode and all the other electrodes connected in parallel. Over the EEG frequency range, because the capacitance factor is small, electrode impedance is usually numerically equal to electrode resistance. The term is not a synonym for **input impedance.**

electrode resistance The opposition to the flow of a DC current through the interface between an EEG electrode and the scalp or brain, expressed in ohms (generally kilohms). This is measured between pairs of electrodes or, in some EEG machines, between each individual electrode and all the other electrodes connected in parallel.

Measurement of electrode resistance with DC currents results in varying degrees of electrode polarization. See also **electrode impedance.**

electrodermal response See **Galvanic skin response.**

electrodiagnosis (EDX) The recording and analysis of biologic electrical potentials from the central, peripheral, and autonomic nervous systems and from muscles, for medical purposes. See also **electromyography, electroneurography, electroneuromyography, evoked potential studies.**

electrodiagnostic medicine An extension of the clinical examination of the patient, in which the physician integrates information obtained from the clinical history and physical examination of the nervous, muscular, and other systems to diagnose and treat diseases of the central, peripheral, and autonomic nervous systems, neuromuscular junctions, and muscles.[10]

electroencephalogram The record of electrical activity of the brain made by means of electrodes placed on the scalp or from implanted electrodes.

Although this represents the hallowed use of the word that will not now be changed, *electroencephalogram* is by derivation the correct term for the machine and *electroencephalograph* properly used for the printout.

electroencephalography (EEG) The procedure of recording cerebrally derived potential changes, using electrodes placed either on the surface of the scalp, upon the dura, or within the brain, with huge amplification.

Richard Caton (1842–1926), professor of physiology in Liverpool, England, first made recordings of the action currents from the brains of rabbits in 1875, but Johannes (Hans) Berger (1873–1941) recorded the alpha and beta rhythms from humans in 1929.[4979] He received, however, less credit than did Lord **Adrian,** who was awarded the Nobel prize for his confirmation of 'Berger rhythms' in 1934.

The basic science and clinical utilization of the EEG were succinctly reviewed in 1994.[576]

Electroencephalography and Clinical Neurophysiology (EEG Clin. Neurophysiol.) A neurological subspecial journal. Address: Elsevier Scientific Publishers Ireland Ltd., Bay 15, Shannon Industrial Estate, Co. Clare, Ireland.

electromagnetic flowmeter A device able to measure the direction and volume of flow through blood vessels, but not now in use.[2433]

electromyelography The recording and study of electrical activity from the spinal cord and/or from the cauda equina.[146]

electromyogram Equipment used to activate, record, process, and display nerve and muscle action potentials for the purpose of evaluating nerve and muscle function. The machine used to perform **electromyography.**

As with **electroencephalogram,** the terms generally employed represent a reversal of the correct usage; -*gram* properly denotes recording equipment and -*graph*, writing. The small lapse is regrettable but there is nothing that mere writers of books can do about it.

electromyograph The record obtained in electromyography. See comment on **electromyogram.**

electromyography (EMG) Strictly defined, the recording and study of insertional, spontaneous, and voluntary electrical activity of muscle by means of mono- or bipolar needle electrodes, but commonly used to refer to nerve conduction studies as well.

The myofibrillar or motor unit action potentials are amplified and recorded on a cathode ray oscilloscope, a parallel lead to a loudspeaker allowing auditory as well as visual sampling by the electromyographer. The test is slightly painful, but, unless a vital organ or nerve is punctured by the needle, and provided absolute sterility is maintained, it represents a safe and valuable extension of the clinical examination.

The procedure can demonstrate which muscles have lost all or part of their nerve supply (thus permitting an accurate determination of the extent of the root or nerve lesion); can determine the amount of denervation or of the degree of recovery from that; and can inform about the presence of signs of end-plate or primary muscle diseases. A handful of the latter present characteristic electrical features, most show nonspecific evidence of myopathy only, and some are not accompanied by electrical abnormalities. Pathological diagnosis is almost never possible with EMG alone. **Single-fiber EMG** is a refinement of the technique.[3045]

The first EMG was recorded in humans by Probster in 1928; **Adrian** introduced coaxial needles in the following year.

electroneurography   The recording and study of the action potentials of peripheral nerves. See **nerve conduction studies.**

electroneurography index   An index based on 12 electrophysiological parameters such as conduction velocities, F-wave latencies, and amplitudes providing an overall assessment of peripheral nerve function longitudinally.[5253]

electroneuromyography   (ENMG)   The combined studies of electromyography and electroneurography. Synonymous with clinical electromyography. "Electrodiagnostic medicine consultation" is the currently favored term.[10]

electronystagmography   The detection and recording of the movement of the dipole nomally arising from the slight electric field (1 mV) between the cornea and the retina, as a subject follows a target. This is the electrophysiologic equivalent of visual inspection of eye movements while obscuring fixation with high diopter or Fresnel lens and is useful to confirm the presence of nystagmus in the "dizzy" patient.

electro-oculogram   (corneoretinal potential) A record of the standing potential between the cornea and the posterior pole of the eye, measuring a function of the photoreceptors and the pigment epithelium. The test is of some value in the determination of the state of the retina but the **electroretinogram** gives more information.[206]

electro-olfactogram   A record of the potential changes in the olfactory mucosa in response to a stream of air charged with odoriferous particles.

electroretinogram   (ERG)   A recording of the voltage change in the retinal cells in response to a flash (FERG) or changing pattern (PERG) stimulus.

Because the FERG is not affected by ganglion cell disease and is thus normal in disorders affecting the afferent visual pathway, it is an indicator of the presence of lesions of the retinal cells. Although the PERG does appear to depend on the integrity of these cells, its clinical utility is marginal because of reduced reliability of the results. By varying the frequency or wavelength of the stimulus, the test can distinguish between disease of the rods and of the cones, or it can assess the retinal adaptation of the subject.[4295]

electrotonus   The condition of a muscle caused to contract by a Galvanic current, described in 1843 by Émile du Bois-Réymond (1818–1896), a German physiologist.

elementary tics   (Simple tics) See **tics.**

elephantiasis anesthetica   See **leprosy.**

Elevated Arm Stress test   (EAST) Elevation of the arms for 3 minutes (in the surrender position) induces the symptoms of **thoracic outlet syndrome.**[4761] What this means is terms of the underlying pathology is quite uncertain. See also **Wright maneuver.**

elevator nystagmus   See **optokinetic nystagmus.**

elfin face syndrome   See **Williams syndrome.**

Elithorn perceptual maze test   A nonverbal intelligence test in which the subject is required to trace a pathway with a pencil through a lattice, covering as many of the dots randomly placed on the intersections as possible.

Untimed, the test distinguishes subjects with right hemisphere damage; with time constraints, those with aphasia do especially poorly.[3392]

elk   (*Alces malchis*) A species of antelope, once thought to be especially susceptible to epileptic seizures which it was, however, able to cure by putting the hoof of its left foot into its ear.

Ellenberg syndrome   See **diabetic neuropathies.**

Elliott syndrome   A congenital dysmorphic syndrome manifesting also short stature, deafness, blepharophimosis, disordered sexual differentiation, delayed closure of fontanelles, and mental and developmental delay.

Elliptic nystagmus   See **circular nystagmus.**

Ellis gargoylism   See **mucopolysaccharidoses.**

Ellis–van Creveld syndrome   (chondroectodermal dysplasia) A congenital recessively inherited dysostosis (a disturbance in bone form or modeling due to a disturbance in developmental ectodermal or mesenchymal tissues).[1641]

The clinical features include shortening of the tubular bones, especially distally, with resultant dwarfism; polydactyly; small, delayed, and defective teeth and nails; congenital heart disease; and cataract and strabismus. Mental delay has also been described.

The condition has been found mainly in an Old Order Amish kinship in Pennsylvania,[3769] but it has been suggested that the English king Richard III suffered from it too.[63]

eloquent cortex   Those parts of the cerebral cortex concerned in the faculty of speech.

Elpenor syndrome   An allegorical name for the behavior of people who become somnolent after ingesting alcohol or drugs and awaken in unfamiliar surroundings where they commit acts that are destructive, antisocial, or frankly illegal. After regaining awareness, the patients have only vague recollections of the events that transpired.

The syndrome was first described by Benjamin-Joseph Logre, a French psychiatrist who reported the case of Paul-Eugene-Louis Deschanel, the then President of the Republic of France, in the French newspaper *La Monde* (May 1–3, 1948). Decharnel had taken barbiturates on a train journey, lost consciousness, and fell out of the carriage window without noticing it; he regained consciousness in a ditch and was eventually restored to the Elysée Palace where he presided with his customary lucidity. Logre detected a similarity between this incident and one related in the *Odyssey*—the story of Elpenor, the youngest companion of Ulysses, who, according to legend, fell off a terrace and broke his neck on awakening from a drunken sleep. Logre advised that hosts who offer their guests a bed for the night after a convivial evening should provide them with a ground floor room, but today the offer of a taxi is deemed adequate.

Elsahy-Waters branchioskeletogenital syndrome A congenital, autosomal, or X-linked recessively inherited dysmorphic syndrome manifesting also strabismus, ptosis, nystagmus, fusion of vertebrae, genital and skeletal maldevelopment, seizures, and mental and developmental delay.[1645]

Elsberg syndrome   Polyradiculitis of the cauda equina, with urinary retention and CSF pleocytosis.[1646]

The condition may complicate genital herpes, **borreliosis,** or **isolated angiitis of the nervous system,** but is probably most often a variant of **acute inflammatory demyelinating neuropathy** with particular autonomic involvement.

Ely sign   A test in which the knee is flexed and the hip hyperextended with the patient lying prone. L.W. Ely (1868–1944), an American orthopedic surgeon, showed that the elicitation of pain by this maneuver indicates the presence of psoas irritation or hip joint disease. See also **femoral stretch test.**

embolalia   The interposition of meaningless words into spoken speech; two subtypes are distinguished: **angiophrasia** and **logospasmus choreiformis.**

embolism   (from Gr, to throw in) Vascular obstruction by a blood clot or other material (such as air, amniotic fluid, cholesterol, cardiac valvular material, fat, or tumor cells) carried to the site of obstruction in the circulation. The concept was first enunciated by **Virchow.**

embolization   A technique in surgery or interventional radiology whereby inert spheres are introduced into the artery supplying an **arteriovenous malformation** in order to reduce the blood flow within it and to effect shrinkage of the lesion.[1925]

embrace reflex   See **Moro reflex.**

embryoma of head and neck   See **dermoid cyst.**

emergency light reflex   Constriction of the pupils, tight closure of the eyes, flexion of the neck, and sometimes elevation of the arms in response to a sudden threatening stimulus.

Emery-Dreifuss humeroperoneal muscular dystrophy   See **Emery-Dreifuss syndrome.**

Emery-Dreifuss syndrome   (Emery-Dreifuss humeroperoneal muscular dystrophy, Cestan-Lejonne syndrome) Heterogeneous, uncommon, slowly progressive X-linked muscular dystrophies with childhood onset, exhibiting initially biceps and triceps, then pelvic and later pectoral girdle weakness; facial weakness; rigidity of paraspinal muscles; cardiac muscle involvement with conduction defects including complete heart-block; features of the **scapulohumeroperoneal syndrome;** and early muscle contractures at the elbow, ankle, and neck without muscle pseudohypertrophy.[1650,4827] The responsible (emerin) gene is localized at Xq28.

A neurogenic basis has been considered likely in some of the reported cases, a myopathic cause in others; the clinical pattern is constant, however.

Variant forms include the following:

Benign muscular dystrophy with contractures[295]

Benign X-linked muscular dystrophy with cardiomyopathy.[5798]

Emery-Driefuss syndrome with dominant inheritance (see **autosomal dominant humeroperoneal myopathy**) A dominantly inherited proximal myopathy which in every other way resembles this condition but is due to a mutation on the laminin A/C gene at 1q21.2–q21.3.[1779,2113,3886]

Rigid spine syndrome A forme-fruste of the same condition, manifested sporadically.

X-linked muscular dystrophy with humeropelvic distribution, contractures and cardiomyopathy. A similar condition with infantile onset[2874]

X-linked scapuloperoneal syndrome.

EMG   See **electromyography.**

emmetropia   Normal ocular refraction, such that the image of an object at infinity is focused naturally and precisely on the retina.

emotion   (from Lat, to move away) A moving of the mind; conscious or unconscious stimulation to perform some action. "Emotion moves us; hence its name" (Sir Charles **Sherrington**).

emotional facial palsy (mimetic facial palsy) Loss of movement of the lower quadrant of the face during emotional movements (such as laughter), although such movements can be made voluntarily.

The condition is rare; it may be explainable if the descending fibers to the facial nerve nucleus and regulating emotional movements arise in the basal ganglia and descend in pathways other than the corticobulbar tracts.

emotional incontinence See **emotionalism.**

emotionalism (involuntary crying, pathologic emotionality, forced crying, pseudobulbar affect, organic emotionalism, emotional incontinence, spasmodic crying, inappropriate crying, pathological affect) The involuntary expression of emotion without the experience of it. The use of this word is advocated in preference to the alternatives proposed.[116]

Crying, laughter, and rage are the emotions most often expressed, usually in the context of brain disease from any cause affecting the descending motor pathways bilaterally and accompanying depression.

empiric (from Gr; deduced from experience alone) A practitioner whose skills are derived from experience. The Empirics were an ancient sect of physicians opposed to the Dogmatists; they admitted experience as the sole basis of medicine, as determined by chance observation or reporting, trials, and imitation. They dismissed speculation and also rejected the value of anatomy and physiology.[4512]

emprosthotonos The converse of **opisthotonos,** in which tonic flexor rather than extensor spasms occur in patients with tetanus, leading to truncal hyperflexion.[2240]

empty delta sign (negative delta sign) The appearance on enhanced CT scans in a patient with occlusion of the superior sagittal sinus; normally the sinus represents a triangle with its base upward, but in this case the surrounding area is enhanced but the sinus fails to fill, leaving this pale triangular area in contrast. See also **dense triangle sign.**

empty sella headache Typically, a chronic, unilateral frontotemporal headache with facial and laterocervical dysesthesias,[3974] but variable in nature and differentiated from migraine and tension-type headaches by exclusion or in retrospect.

empty sella syndrome (intrasellar arachnoid diverticulum, deficient sellar diaphragm, intrasellar cyst, intrasellar cistern) Herniation of the arachnoid containing CSF through a defect in the diaphragm sella, leading to compression of the pituitary gland.[2960]

The optic nerve may also herniate, with the production of a visual field defect, and there is a possible association with complaints of headache, papilledema, and endocrine disorders,[3974] but otherwise the condition is asymptomatic and detected by chance.

The primary empty sella was defined as that which admitted significant amounts of air at pneumoencephalography in the absence of prior surgery or radiation therapy.[4085] The *secondary type* was that in which such procedures had been undertaken or in which there had been prior raised intracranial pressure or shrinkage of a pituitary adenoma. Today the demonstration of low attenuation in the sella on CT scans would suffice for the diagnosis,[1095] but while radiologically dramatic and sometimes associated with increased intracranial pressure, this appearance is also found in some normal subjects whose headaches it does not explain unless there are other signs of increased intracranial pressure.

The condition may present in infancy or childhood, when pituitary–hypothalamic dysfunction, short stature, facial dysmorphism, spina bifida occulta, hydrocephalus, mental or developmental delay, and delayed skeletal maturation may also be found.[5143]

empty speech That type of conversation which communicates nothing in faultless grammar. When spoken in private circumstances it is suggestive evidence of dementia, but it is commonplace in official utterances, in which context it has no diagnostic value. See also **cocktail party syndrome.**

enabling synkinesis The situation in which one arm can carry out an act only if the other one does the same thing. See also **alien hand syndrome.**

enantesis (from Gr, to meet) The confluence of ascending and descending blood vessels, as with the internal mammary and the anterior spinal arteries.

encapsulation 1. The process whereby bits of words are fused to form a neologism.[1179] 2. The distinction and investment of a pathological lesion by a layer of tissue, either inflammatory or derived from the surrounding tissues.

encephalalgia An old term for head pain, wrongly used since the word derives from that for *brain,* which, unlike other cranial structures, is generally insensitive to pain.

Encéphale A neurological journal. Address: Doin Editeurs, 8 Place de l'Odeon, F 75006 Paris, France.

encephale isolé An experimental physiological preparation, the transverse cut being at the level of the low medulla. The EEG of the animal shows a wakeful pattern.

encephalic Within the head.

encephalion Diminutive of **encephalon,** and applied to the cerebellum.

encephalitis (Gr, brain + inflammation) 1. Inflammation of the substance of the brain, as opposed to its meninges only: a heterogeneous collection of diseases, classified by Greenfield[2269] in 1950.

2. Nonsuppurative inflammation, usually diffusely affecting the substance of the brain with emphasis on the gray matter, producing perivascular and parenchymal infiltration with inflammatory cells and neuronophagia; and due to any infectious or chemical agent or to autoallergic attack.

Clinically, fever, headache, reduced levels of consciousness, seizures, and mononuclear pleocytosis in the CSF are the classic features.

Focal suppurative encephalitis is also described, rarely; it is properly known as **cerebral abscess.** Diffuse infiltrations (e.g., encephalitis periaxialis diffusa) are not truly classified here, despite the name.[2869]

See also **herpes simplex encephalitis, Japanese encephalitis, shiga toxin encephalitis, Nipah virus encephalitis, West Nile encephalitis, Lassa fever.**

encephalitis lethargica   (von Economo disease, epidemic encephalitis, sleeping sickness) A polymorphic epidemic encephalitis that was recorded in Germany in 1712 and was widespread for a decade following the influenza pandemic of 1915–1924, affecting the population of the United States after 1918. Both before and since that time, sporadic cases of this disease have been recorded.

The nature of the causative agent remains uncertain. Von Economo's account,[5780] though based on fewer cases, is fuller than that of Jean Cruchet,[1204] which was actually published 2 weeks before; priority of publication led to a regrettable dispute. The tendency for parkinsonian signs to follow encephalitis lethargica was reported first by Achille Alexandre **Souques** (1860–1944), a French neurologist, in 1921.[5266]

Clinically, the disease was marked by fever, generalized pains, skin rashes, malaise and gastrointestinal complaints, and by such signs as extreme drowsiness, oculomotor pareses, delirium, and catatonia. Other presentations included an acute parkinsonian state; and a hyperkinetic syndrome with chorea and myoclonus.[2375,4571] The pathology was described by Lhermitte.[3396]

The sequelae affected about 40% of those afflicted and included tics, dystonias, akathisia, seizures, ataxia, and pareses; a parkinsonian syndrome with oculogyric crises and narcolepsy, amyotrophy, emotional disturbances, and persistent sleep disorders were also recorded. About 40% of these patients succumbed.[6000]

encephalitis periaxialis concentrica   See **Balo concentric sclerosis.**

encephalitis periaxialis diffusa   See **Schilder disease.**

encephalitis subcorticalis chronica progressiva   See **Binswanger disease.**

encephalitis tremens   A rare condition described once in epidemic form in Nigeria[6047] but not encountered since.

encephalocele   (Gr, the brain + a tumor) A rare congenital maldevelopment characterized by extracranial herniation of part of the cerebral hemispheres such as the occipital lobe, or of the cerebellum, through a midline cranial defect. *Anterior encephaloceles* represent the same maldevelopment in the frontal region.[5237] See also **cephalocele.**

encephalocraniocutaneous lipomatosis   A congenital syndrome consisting of localized scalp alopecia, craniofacial lipomas, eyelid papules, conjunctival nevi, porencephalic cysts, seizures and mental retardation.[99]

encephalocutaneous lipomatosis   A congenital neurocutaneous dysmorphic syndrome characterized by cerebral atrophy with intracranial calcification, hydranencephaly or porencephaly, hydrocephalus, seizures, soft tissue tumors of the cranium and eyes, and mental and developmental delay.[2354]

encephalofacial angiomatosis   See **Sturge-Weber syndrome.**

encephalography   A radiological method for estimating the size of the ventricles at **pneumoencephalography;** now obsolete.

encephaloid   Resembling a brain.

encephalolith   A calcareous structure within the brain. *Encephalolithiasis* is that condition in which such accretions occur.

encephalomalacia   An area of softening of brain tissue occurring in the period immediately following its infarction.[JF] See **multicystic encephalopathy.**

encephalomyelitis   Inflammation of the substance of the brain and of the spinal cord.

encephalomyelitis with carcinoma   Forms of **paraneoplastic syndrome** including limbic (**limbic dementia**) and bulbar encephalitis, myelitis with predilection for the anterior horn cells, and ganglioradiculitis; usually with subacute progression and occurring in older adults with bronchogenic (and less often with stomach, breast, or ovarian) carcinomas.[2543]

Clinically, an initial painful neuropathy is usually followed by the development of any combination of dementia, cerebellar and pyramidal signs, extrapyramidal findings, and brainstem dysfunction with multifocal myoclonus, leading to death within 2 years.

encephalomyeloneuritis   Usually a **paraneoplastic** syndrome (see **encephalomyelitis with carcinoma**) but an identical syndrome is reported in subjects without detectable malignancy.[3269]

encephalomyelopolyradiculopathy   A febrile illness of unknown cause characterized by evidence of involvement of all the structures suggested in the title and leading to confusion, pain, paraparesis, and loss of sphincter control.

encephalomyeloradiculitis See **acute inflammatory demyelinating polyneuropathy.**

encephalomyopathy with epilepsy, chorioretinitis, basal ganglion involvement, and muscle minicores A congenital muscular dystrophy complicated by psychomotor retardation, seizures, rigidity, chorioretinitis, and bilateral basal ganglion, thalamic, cerebellar, and cerebral cortical MRI abnormalities.[273]

See also **muscle-eye-bain disease, Fukuyama muscle dystrophy.**

encephalon (Gr, in + the head) (encephalos, encephalus, encephalum) Used synonymously with "the brain."

encephalo-ophthalmic syndrome See **Krause disease.**

encephalo-optic dysplasia See **Walker-Warburg syndrome.**

encephalopathie saturnine Lead encephalopathy.

encephalopathy/encephalopathia Disease of the brain. In general usage, diffuse disorders affecting the greater part of the cortex and/or subcortical regions.

See also **dialysis encephalopathy, Dupré syndrome, hypertensive encephalopathy, metabolic encephalopathy, portosystemic encephalopathy, rejection encephalopathy, parainfectious noninflammataory encephalomyelitis, Shiga toxin encephalopathy, uremic encephalopathy, Wernicke-Korsakoff encephalopathy.**

encephalopathy of sepsis Diffuse cerebral disease producing depression in conscious level, multifocal EEG abnormalities, seizures, and focal neurological signs in the presence of chronic, severe, disseminated infection.

The underlying pathologies include bacterial invasion of the brain with the formation of disseminated microabscesses, cerebral infarction, multiple small white matter hemorrhages, **central pontine myelinolysis,** and possibly disturbances in cerebral synaptic transmission as a direct result of toxicity from the infecting agent.[2770]

encephalopathy with fatty degeneration of the viscera See **Reye syndrome.**

encephalorrhagia Purpura of the brain, the blood damaging both myelin and axons.

encephalos See **encephalon.**

encephalosyncope (vasovagal attacks) Syncope, blurred vision, dizziness, abdominal sensations, or weakness with or without loss of consciousness occurring in subjects with abnormal EEG records and considered to represent a minor seizure disorder triggered by cerebral ischemia.

The term was suggested by Kershman in 1949 but did not find favor.

encephalotrigeminal angiomatosis See **Sturge-Weber syndrome.**

encephalum See **encephalon.**

encephalus See **encephalon.**

enchondromatosis A dysmorphic syndrome characterized by short stature, scoliosis, platyspondyly, mental and developmental delay, sclerosis of the skull with enchondromata, and skeletal cysts or tumors. See **Maffucci syndrome.**

encycloduction See **duction.**

end artery An artery which, uniquely, supplies a volume of tissue.

end bulb (Bouton terminale) The term employed by Krause for the expansions of the distal ends of sensory nerves.

endarterectomy An open surgical procedure whereby the stenotic or atheroma-encrusted lining of the cervical carotid artery is reamed out or dissected to reduce turbulence and future platelet deposition and to increase flow. The procedure has been shown to reduce a symptomatic patient's risk of stroke when the stenosis is between 70% and 99% of the lumen, but, with lesser degrees of narrowing and in asymptomatic people, the benefit derived is not yet determined.

endarteritis obliterans (Heubner endarteritis) An inflammatory condition of the media and adventitia of the walls of large and medium-sized arteries, associated with fibroblastic proliferation of the intima, and thus liable to cause occlusion of the vessel and distal infarction.

This is a typical finding in secondary or meningovascular syphilis.

endocranium The inner surface of the skull bones.

endocrine candida syndrome The association of candida with idiopathic hypoparathyroidism and Addison disease, together with defective delayed hypersensitivity.[2043]

Neurological features include increased intracranial pressure with papilledema and intracranial calcification, seizures, mental retardation, muscle twitching, cramps and rigidity.[2881]

endocrine exophthalmos See **dysthyroid ophthalmopathy.**

end-of-dose deterioration (wearing-off effect) A hypokinetic form of fluctuation in parkinsonian patients on long-term l-dopa therapy in which disability increases as the l-dopa levels fall.

end-of-dose dystonia A form of fluctuation in parkinsonian patients taking long-term l-dopa therapy, in which dystonic movements appear as the l-dopa levels fall.

endolymphatic hydrops See **Ménière disease.**

endomysium   (Gr, within + muscle) The connective tissue investing each myofibril.

endoneurial area   The total area of the nerve fascicles encompassed by the perineurium.

endoneurium   (Gr, within + nerve) The connective tissue investing each nerve fiber within a funiculus.

endophasy   The unspoken language of thought.

endorphins   Opioid peptides. Among these, beta endorphin is a mediator of pain perception.

endosteal hyperostosis   (van Buchem disease) A genetic craniotubular hyperostotic syndrome existing in two forms. *Autosomal dominant osteosclerosis* presents with hyperostosis and osteosclerosis of the skull, mandible, clavicles, and ribs and long bone diaphyseal hyperplasia; seventh and eighth cranial nerve deficits may occur.[6044]

In the *autosomal recessive* form the symptoms are similar but more severe.[5710]

end-plate   The specialized receptor area on the muscle membrane at the neuromuscular junction.

end-plate acetylcholine receptor deficiency   A congenital myasthenic syndrome.[1658] See **myasthenia gravis.**

end-plate acetylcholinesterase deficiency   A congenital myasthenic syndrome.[1658] See **myasthenia gravis.**

end-plate activity   Spontaneous electric activity recorded with a needle electrode close to muscle endplates. These potentials may have several different morphologies.

1. Monophasic: Low-amplitude (10 to 20 uV), short-duration (0.5 to 1.0 msec) negative potentials occurring in a dense, steady pattern, the exact frequency of which cannot be defined. These nonpropagated potentials are probably miniature end-plate potentials recorded extracellularly. Referred to as end-plate noise or seashell sound (sea shell roar or noise).
2. Biphasic: Moderate-amplitude (100 to 300 uV), short-duration (2 to 4 msec), initially negative spike potentials occurring irregularly in short bursts with a high frequency (50 to 100 Hz). These propagated potentials are generated by muscle fibers excited by activity in nerve terminals. These potentials have been referred to as biphasic spike potentials, end-plate spikes, and, incorrectly, nerve potentials. They may also have a biphasic (initially positive) morphology.
3. Triphasic: Similar to biphasic potentials, but the waveforms have three phases with an initial positive deflection. These fire in an irregular fashion; contrast with fibrillation potential.

From the 2001 Report of the Nomenclature Committee of the American Association of Electromyography and Electrodiagnosis.[10] Reproduced by permission of the Association and of John Wiley and Sons, Inc.

end-plate noise   See **end-plate activity** (monophasic).

end-plate potential (EPP)   The graded nonpropagated membrane potential induced in the postsynaptic membrane of a muscle fiber by release of acetyl choline from the presynaptic axon terminal in response to an action potential. (From the 2001 Report of the Nomenclature Committee of the American Association of Electromyography and Electrodiagnosis.[10] Used by permission, copyright © 2001, AAEM.)

end-plate spike   See **endplate activity** (biphasic).

end-plate zone   The region in a muscle where neuromuscular junctions are concentrated.

end-point nystagmus   (end-position nystagmus) A form of ill-sustained, irregular, low-amplitude, physiological, gaze-evoked, jerk nystagmus of small (0.5–3 uV) amplitude, at a frequency of 1–3 Hz, seen best in the abducting rather than the adducting eye during maintained far lateral gaze. It probably represents physiological fatigue in the oculomotor muscles.[22] If far lateral gaze is prolonged, **fatigue nystagmus,** a different phenomenon, may also ensue. See also **physiological nystagmus.**

end-position nystagmus   See **end-point nystagmus.**

enervate   (from Lat, to weaken) To be without energy; the state of weakness.

ENG   See **electroneurography.**

Engelhard syndrome   A dysmorphic syndrome characterized by ptosis polydactyly, syndactyly, microcephaly, intracranial epidermoid and other tumors, and a liability to meningitis.[337]

Engelmann disease   See **progressive diaphyseal dysplasia.**

English Malady   See **Cheyne disease.**

engram   1. The permanent impression left behind by psychical experience in the brain's cellular network. A latent memory-picture, a trace of things experienced, in the words of **Penfield,** "The writing left behind in the brain by conscious experience,"[4402] or, as put by **Critchley**, "a memory tracer in a conception of a word or phrase."[1172]

2. A functional template, directing the performance of skilled movements.

enhanced physiological tremor   A physiological tremor of greater than normal amplitude but of normal frequency (8–12 Hz), resulting from unusual synchronization of motor unit discharges and frequently associated with hyperadrenergic states.[1819]

enhanced ptosis   Relatively increased drooping of one eyelid when the subject with myasthenia gravis looks upward while the other eyelid is also elevated but is maintained in that position by the examiner's finger.

In a variation of the response, the descending eyelid oscillates to a point of complete closure.[2208] See **eyebrow lifting test.**

enkephalins   A class of opioid pentapeptides (meta- and leuenkephalins) widely distributed in the brain and spinal cord (nucleus of the fifth nerve, substantia gelatinosa) in areas relevant to the transmission of pain impulses.

ENMG   See **electroneuromyography.**

enolases   A family of glycolytic dimeric enzymes. Neuron-specific enolase is usually found in ganglion cells, but is not restricted to them.

enteric brain   (enteric nervous system) Networks of ganglion cell bodies and preganglionic parasympathetic and postganglionic sympathetic fibers with their interneurons, arising from the neural crest and forming the myenteric and submucosal plexuses of the gastrointestinal tract. It can function independently of the central nervous system. Disorders arising from he enteric nervous system include achalasia, **Hirschprung disease,** acute intestinal ileus, and intestinal pseudo-obstruction.[2244]

enteric cysts   See **enterogenous cysts.**

enteric nervous system   See **enteric brain.**

enterogenous cysts   (enteric cysts) Extrinsic intra-spinal cysts containing elements of gut (such as a mucin-secreting mucous membrane), situated usually in the subarachnoid space and associated often with local defects in the vertebral bodies. See **neurenteric cyst.**

entomopia   (from Gr, insect + eye) A rare form of polyopia in which the subject sees multiple reduplicated images in rows and columns, as one supposes to be the experience of those insects possessing compound eyes. The phenomenon has been reported as a result of lesions of the cornea or lens, and with lesions of the occipital lobe.[3469]

entonia   (Gr, tension) Tonic spasm.

entopic images   See **entoptic images.**

entoptic images   (entopic images) Those images that arise from within the optic globe itself.

entorhinal cortex   The parahippocampal area.

entrainment   Synchronization to external time cues.

entrapment neuropathy   Neural deficits consequent upon nerve compression.[3128]

entrapped temporal horn   "Obstruction of the trigone of the lateral ventricle which seals off the temporal horn from the rest of the ventricular system" causing hemiparesis, homonymous hemianopia, and memory disturbances due to compression of the internal capsule.[5867]

entropion   Inward-turning of the eyelids. cf. **ectropion.**

enuresis   Recurrent involuntary micturition occurring during sleep in the absence of any urologic, medical, or psychiatric pathology. Diurnal and nocturnal forms relate to the time of occurrence of enuresis, par-

alytic and spastic forms to the lower or upper motor neuron lesions causing it, respectively. In a more restricted sense, the word is applied only to involuntary micturition during any phase of sleep in subjects with normal daytime bladder control. It is considered abnormal in most cases after the age of 10 years.

In *primary enuresis,* the child never achieves continuous dry nights, while in *secondary enuresis* the child has had at least 3 months of dryness then reversed to the pattern of enuresis, usually in the first third of the night. The episodes can also occur during nocturnal wakefulness.

environmental dependency syndrome   Complex behavioral sequences in which patients recognize the environmental situation in which they find themselves (or accept a suggestion as to its nature) and act out behavior which would be appropriate in that situation, but which in fact is inappropriate for the patient to perform—thus, for example, watering someone else's garden, examining the physician's throat, etc. In a *variant* form, patients are 'forced' to comment verbally on situations and activities occurring around them (*forced hyperphasia*).[5482] The syndrome is considered to represent a failure of personal autonomy, secondary to unilateral lesions of the frontal lobe.[3393a,3394]

environmental sleep disorder   A sleep disturbance due to a disturbing environmental factor that causes a complaint of either insomnia or excessive sleepiness. Sleep efficiency and duration are normal, there are no psychological factors that induce the disturbance of sleep, and removal of the disturbing stimulus leads to eventual restoration of normal sleep patterns.

The American Sleep Disorders Association has suggested following diagnostic criteria:[234]

A. The patient complains of insomnia or excessive sleepiness.

B. The complaint is temporally associated with the introduction of a physically measurable stimulus or environmental circumstance that disturbs sleep.

C. The physical properties of the environmental factor account for the sleep complaint; the psychological meaning of the environmental factor does not account for the complaint.

D. Removal of the causative environmental factor results in immediate or gradual restoration of normal sleep.

E. The disorder has been present for more than 3 weeks.

F. Polysomnographic monitoring demonstrates normal sleep efficiency and duration.

G. There is no evidence of significant underlying medical or psychiatric disorder accounting for the complaint.

H. The disorder does not meet the diagnostic criteria for any other sleep disorder causing a complaint of insomnia or excessive sleepiness, for example, toxin-induced sleep disorder.

From ASDA Diagnostic Classification Steering Committee. *The International Classification of Sleep Disorders Diagnostic and Coding Manual.* Rochester, MN: American Sleep Disorders Association, 1990. Reproduced by kind permission of the American Academy of Sleep Medicine.

environmental status scale   A rating scale designed to quantify the handicap experienced by patients with **multiple sclerosis.**[3820] See **socioeconomic scale.** See also **Kurtzke disability status scale.**

eosinophilia-myalgia syndrome   The occurrence of joint pain, generalized myalgias that limit the subject in the activities of daily living, and eosinophilia ($>1 \times 10^9$ cells/liter) in the peripheral blood and muscle infiltrates, in the absence of other (infectious or allergic) disease.[184]

Weakness, a scleroderma-like skin rash, pruritus, angioedema, fever, abdominal pains, and subcutaneous nodules also occur. Evidence of myopathy or peripheral axomnal polyneuropathy is found in a quarter of the subjects and cognitive complaints (of fatigue, impaired memory and attention, representing a selective **dysexecutive syndrome**) may persist long into the recovery period. The erythrocyte sedimentation rate is normal.

The syndrome has most commonly been found in women who had taken (allegedly contaminated) oral L-tryptophan for premenstrual complaints, insomnia, or depression.[2559] See also **eosinophilic fasciitis, eosinophilic perimyositis, eosinophilic polymyositis.**

eosinophilic adenoma   A benign tumor of the pituitary gland with a propensity to secrete growth hormone, and thus the usual lesion in patients with **gigantism** or **acromegaly.**

eosinophilic fasciitis   (Schulman syndrome) A syndrome of tenderness and edema of the skin of the neck, trunk, and proximal limbs, which later becomes indurated or even leathery with patchy hyperpigmentation; interstitial myositis of subjacent muscles; eosinophilia; and joint contractures, synovitis, and nerve compression syndromes in many cases. The clinical features may be precipitated by vigorous exercise.[5144]

Accompanying blood dyscrasias are not unusual. The presence of the **groove sign** strongly suggests the diagnosis.[5168] See also **eosinophilia-myalgia syndrome.**

eosinophilic granulomatous vasculitis   See **Churg-Strauss syndrome.**

eosinophilic perimyositis   A syndrome of relapsing myalgia accompanied by nonspecific inflammatory features with a perimysial infiltrate consisting of eosinophils in muscles, but with minimal peripheral eosinophilia. Biopsy evidence of fascitis is not found, there are no skin changes, and the response to anti-inflammatory agents is prompt, although relapses can occur.[5073] See also **eosinophilia-myalgia syndrome, eosinophilic polymyositis, eosinophilic fasciitis.**

eosinophilic polymyositis   A rare inflammatory disease of muscle in which systemic visceral manifestations, including encephalopathy and neuropathy, occur in conjunction with severe proximal or generalized muscle weakness or tenderness, localized painful swelling of muscles, and features of the hypereosinophilic syndrome.

Myocarditis, pericarditis, and multiple mononeuropathy have been reported to occur in association with the disorder.[3304] The condition may be a variant of the **Churg-Strauss syndrome.**[3304] It differs from **polymyositis** in the number of eosinophils in the inflamed muscles. See also **eosinophilia-myalgia syndrome** and the preceding entries.

epaxial muscles   (Gr, upon + Lat; an axis) Those muscles which lie above the central axis of the embryo, divided between dorsolateral and ventrolateral groups.

ependyma   (Gr, a cloak or upper garment) The epithelial membrane lining the ventricles and the central canal of the spinal cord, named by **Virchow.**

ependymitis   Inflammation of the ependyma, either as part of a generalized **meningitis** or due to specific infections with, for example, *Toxoplasma.*

ependymoblastoma   A poorly differentiated primary neuroectodermal tumor arising in the fourth ventricle in children, characterized by the prominent formation of perivascular **pseudorosettes.**[6]

ependymoma   A primary neuroectodermal malignant but slowly growing glial tumor arising from the ependymal lining of the ventricles, spinal cord or cauda equina occurring in childhood, and occasionally in adult life.

Their histological characteristics vary, but include the presence of ciliated cuboidal epithelial cells, rosettes of ependymal cells, **pseudorosettes, Rosenthal fibers,** positive staining for S-100 protein and **glial fibrillary acidic protein** but not carbonic anhydrase C, absence of a collagenous stroma, and, in well-differentiated forms, uniformity of nuclear morphology. **Ependymoblastoma, subependymoma,** and *well-differentiated, poorly differentiated, anaplastic,* and *myxopapillary* types are distinguished, the latter arising from the filum terminale and characterized by the presence of columnar cells surrounding mucoid zones.[6]

ephapse   A point of abnormal communication at which an action potential in one muscle fiber or axon can cause depolarization of an adjacent muscle or axon, generating an action potential in it. Such abnormal electrical cross-communications are supposed to represent the result of prior local trauma.

ephaptic transmission   (axonal cross-talk) The transmission of nerve impulses across artificial synapses (**ephapses**) spontaneously created between axons following local injury. This may lead to pain (e.g., **trigeminal neuralgia, complex regional pain syndrome**) or motor manifestations (e.g., **hemifacial spasm**). It has also been invoked to explain the repetitive firing of neurons in other chronic denervating states such as radiculopathy.[5603] See also **myokymic discharge, complex repetitive discharge.**

epi-   Greek prefix, signifying "upon."

epiblepharon   A craniofacial malformation, sometimes dominantly inherited, in which there is absence of the palpebral groove because of maldevelopment of the insertion of the levator palpebrae superioris muscle, with a horizontal fold of skin over the tarsal region. It is best seen on downward gaze.[4]

epicanthis   See **epicanthus.**

epicanthus   (epicanthis) 1. The inner angle of the eye. 2. A dominantly inherited craniofacial malformation in which a bilateral symmetrical skin fold (the *epicanthal fold*) runs vertically at the naso-orbital angle.[4]

epicranium   The soft tissues attached to the outer surfaces of the skull bones below the **pericranium.**

epicritic   (from Gr, discernment or judgment) Superficial sensations, capable of precise appreciation and localization. This implies cortical assessment and perception of the stimulus—for example, discriminative light touch, direction of scratch, and the recognition of the finer gradations of temperature into warm and cool. It is characterized by low threshold, short latency, high adaptability, and accurate localization and discrimination.[2540] It returns later than protopathic sensation during the process of recovery from a nerve injury.

The word was employed by Sir Henry **Head;** the other class of sensation that he defined he called **protopathic.**

epidemic chorea   See **hysteria.**

epidemic convulsions   Hysterical, seizure-like movements (the *jerks* and the *barks*) witnessed during a period of fundamental religious fervor in Tennessee and Kentucky during the mid-eighteenth century and regarded then either as tokens of divine favor or as a form of chorea.[6063] See **pseudoseizures.**

epidemic encephalitis   See **encephalitis lethargica.**

epidemic myalgia   See **pleurodynia.**

epidemic myalgic encephalomyelitis   (epidemic myalgia) See **chronic fatigue syndrome.**

epidemic neurolabyrinthitis   See **epidemic vertigo.**

epidemic neuromyasthenia   See **postinfection fatigue syndrome.**

epidemic neuromyelitis   An acute illness resembling ascending infectious polyneuritis, seen in Rio de Janeiro in 1931 but not reported since.

epidemic paralytic vertigo   See **Gerlier disease.**

epidemic pleurodynia   (Bornholm disease) A benign sporadic or epidemic localized inflammatory myopathy resulting from infection by coxsackie B viruses.

Clinically, children are affected more often than adults, and complain of headache, fever, and severe localized pain and tenderness in the muscles of the chest wall, shoulders, or back.

epidemic spastic paraparesis   The sudden onset of spastic paraparesis associated with speech disturbances and visual complaints, occurring epidemically (and also sporadically) in central Africa. Recovery may be complete or dysarthria and paraparesis may remain. Both infectious and toxic causes have been suspected.[930]

epidemic vertigo   (epidemic neurolabyrinthitis) Small epidemics characterized by the sudden onset of vertigo with accompanying nausea and vomiting which become paroxysmal but with decreasing frequency and intensity; many attacks follow upper respiratory or gastrointestinal symptoms, and a chronic asthenic phase is reported in a minority of cases. The etiology is not known.[4387] See **vestibular neuronitis.**

epidermal nevus syndrome   (nevus unis lateralis, epidermal nevus, ichthyosis linearis neuropathica, Feuerstein-Mills syndrome, linear nevus sebaceus syndrome) A rare, sporadic, congenital **neurocutaneous syndrome.**

The skin lesions include raised, yellow-brown, verrucous skin lesions and orange-brown waxy plaques; nevus unis lateralis; ichthyosis hystrix; acanthosis nigricans; and midline linear sebaceous nevi on the scalp, neck, or face, with later hyperkeratosis, and verrucous transformation. The associated neurological disorders are due to cortical dysgenesis and include mental retardation, cortical atrophy, seizures, hydrocephalus, hyperkinesis, and a variety of focal signs signifying cortical dysfunction, usually on the same side as any skin lesions present on the face or head.[303,1806]

Colobomas of the iris, congenital cardiac anomalies, renal tumors, porencephaly, megalencephaly, sebaceous adenomas, skin pigmentation, asymmetrical limbs, and cerebral neoplasms are also described in this condition.

A *variant* form comprises facial epidermal nevus, ipsilateral hemimegalencephaly and gyral malformations, mental retardation, seizures including early infantile spasms, and sometimes facial hemihypertrophy.[4373]

epidermoid cyst   (epidermoid tumor) A cyst composed of squamous epidermal cells in a fibrous and keratinized wall containing cholesterol, situated usually in the cisterns at the skull base, in the cerebellopontine angle, at the cauda equina level, or within the substance of the cord.[495] See also **dermoid cyst.**

epidermoid tumor   See **epidermoid cyst.**

epidural abscess   Pyogenic infection of the cranial or spinal meninges in which the pus lies external to the dura and adjacent to the bone, mainly posteriorly and usually at thoracic levels.

The infection reflects dissemination of local (vertebral) disease or results from hematogenous spread and occurs most commonly in the immunocompromised or chronically sick. The major clinical features are rapidly progressive myelopathy with progressive paraparesis and sphincter involvement, and severe local and radicular pain with local tenderness.

epidural ascending spinal paralysis See **hypertrophic spinal meningitis, Spiller syndrome.**

epidural block The injection of anesthetic solutions into the epidural space in order to produce regional anesthesia. The neurological complications of this technique have been reviewed.[2913]

epidural blood patch A technique of injecting autologous whole blood into the epidural space under sterile conditions in order to relieve post–lumbar puncture headache, which it does safely and effectively in a high proportion of cases.[2224]

epidural electrode A recording electrode placed upon the dural covering of the cerebrum.

epidural hematoma See **epidural hemorrhage.**

epidural hemorrhage (epidural hematoma, extradural hemorhage or hematoma) Bleeding outside the outermost layer of the dura mater, which is thus stripped away from the inner table of the skull or spinal canal.

In almost all cases of *intracranial epidural hemorrhage,* the cause is traumatic, most often with rupture of the middle meningeal artery as a result of a fracture of the temporal bone.

Traumatic spinal epidural hematomas are associated with fracture-dislocations of the spine and cause acute or subacute myelopathy. *Nontraumatic (spontaneous) spinal epidural hematomas* are usually venous in origin and occur in the setting of minor trauma, pregnancy, physical exertion, abnormal bleeding tendencies, etc.[3293]

epigastric aura An indescribable sensation in the pit of the stomach, sometimes rising to the head, occurring as the initial manifestation of some forms of complex partial seizure with origin in the temporal lobe.

The lack of appropriate words that can be summoned up by the patient to describe the experience is a characteristic finding.

epigastric reflex Light stroking of the skin downward from the nipple normally leads to contraction of the epigastric muscles. The reflex informs on the reflex arcs T5–T7 but as a superficial reflex it is lost with upper motor neuron lesions above these levels.

Epilepsia A neurological subspecialty journal, the official organ of the International League Against Epilepsy. Web site: http://www.epilepsia.com/.

epilepsia arithmetices The precipitation of epileptic seizures as a result of performing mental arithmetic.[2741]

A similar condition occasionally affects computers.

epilepsia cursiva (running fit) See **cursive epilepsy.**

epilepsia larvata A postepileptic phenomenon that Esquirol called "masked" epilepsy, referring to the confused speech and automatic movements made following a tonic-clonic seizure, which was in those days thought to be itself a seizure manifestation.

epilepsia minoris continua See **status epilepticus.**

epilepsia nutans A discarded term for **myoclonic epilepsy.**

epilepsia partialis continua See **partial continuous epilepsy.**

epilepsie rotatoria See **tornado epilepsy.**

epilepsy (Gr, a seizure) 1. A tendency to recurrent epileptic seizures. This definition is not as silly as it sounds, one seizure not constituting epilepsy. 2. A condition characterized by recurrent (two or more) epileptic seizures, unprovoked by any immediate identified cause. Multiple seizures occurring in a 24-hour period and an episode of status epilepticus are considered to represent a single event. Those who have had only febrile seizures or only neonatal seizures as defined here are excluded from this category.[1115]

The condition was known to Hippocrates who recorded it in children as "The Sacred Disease"[2579] epilepsy then being considered a temporary departure of the soul from the body. Even in the past 100 years, the attempt to call the soul back by waving a garment of the patient from the rooftops and banging gongs has been recorded in China. Hippocrates argued that it was a malady affecting the whole constitution and rejected the concept that it was a divine malediction. He also recognized that injury to one side of the brain may cause a seizure to occur on the other side of the body.[1104]

The word *epilepsy* was the invention of the Arab physician **Avicenna.** Previous names had included *hieron nosema, nosema paideon, morbus lunaticus, morbus major sonticus, morbus caducus, Herculean disease* (perhaps because of the strength of the convulsive movements) and the *great evil.* In England, Germany, and France it came to be known as the *falling evil.*

Focal, partial, or localization-related epilepsies were described by **Bravais** and later by **Jackson,** but had actually been recorded by **Arataeus** nearly 1800 years before.[209] The condition was well known in biblical times, accounts of the epileptic boy's presentation to Christ appearing in the gospels of St. Luke and of St. Mark (chapter 9). At this time, the condition was popularly regarded as evidence of demoniacal possession, and in Rome gatherings were discontinued when an attender had a seizure, and Romans spat in the street when they passed an epileptic person, a custom which survived until the end of the eighteenth century in France. With medicine impotent to help, such reactions may have prompted the frequent appeals made to many saints, of whom 37 (ranging from Saints Sebastian and Valentine to St. Edward the Confessor) have been considered to have a particular interest in the subject. In 1750 Sauvage collected all extant work on the subject, including

Boerhaave's classification of the causes and description of the signs, in his book *Nosologie d'Epilepsie*. Pinel (who regarded epilepsy as a neurosis, i.e., something caused by a neurological disorder) established a hospital for epileptics at the **Salpêtrière** in 1795, generating a large body of research on the subject. Effective treatment began with Sir Charles Locock's introduction of bromides; Hauptmann's publication on phenobarbitone occurred in 1910,[2476] and Merritt and Putnam synthesized phenytoin in 1934.

Among those claimed to have been subject to seizures (not always on good evidence) are St. Paul, Julius Caesar, Caligula, Germanicus Brittanicus, Mahomet, Charles V, at least one Holy Roman emperor, Peter the Great, the Duke of Marlborough, Balzac, the Emperor Napoleon, the Duke of Wellington, Lord Byron, Schiller, Handel, Mendelssohn, **Dostoevsky,** and Mozart.[1104] Among Shakespearean characters, Henry IV and Julius Caesar were depicted as suffering generalized, and Othello and Macbeth, complex partial seizures.

Classification of Epilepsies and Epileptic Syndromes

A distinction is drawn between the various types of seizure and the syndromes of which such seizures are a manifestation. The former may be seen as colors on the palette of an artist, the latter as a painting; the different epileptic syndromes are composed of various kinds of seizure.[1516] Those printed in bold face in Chart E–2 are defined or described in the place appropriate to their alphabetization. See also the dictionary of Gastaut[2049] and the discussion of epileptic syndromes by Delgado-Escueta.[1361]

Generalized epileptic disorders are characterized by seizures in which there are symptoms suggesting bilateral cerebral involvement, reflected clinically and in the bilateral abnormalities of the EEG at the onset of the seizure. They reflect dysfunction of the whole brain or of major brain systems. In the so-called *partial epilepsies,* the clinical and electrographic features indicate that the seizure originates in one or more discrete brain regions.

The 1989 revision of the International League Against Epilepsy's classification of the *epileptic syndromes* is given in Chart E–2. It differs from the classification designed for genetic studies[1362] (see Chart E–3) and from the classification of **epileptic seizures.**

Chart E–2. ILAE Classification of Epilepsies, Epileptic Syndromes, and Related Seizure Disorders (adapted)

1. *Localization-related (focal, local, partial) epilepsies and syndromes*
   1.1. Idiopathic (primary)
      Benign childhood epilepsy with centrotemporal spikes
      Childhood epilepsy with occipital paroxysms
      Primary reading epilepsy
   1.2. Symptomatic
      Chronic progressive epilepsia partialis continua of childhood (**Kojewnikow syndrome**)
      Temporal, frontal, parietal, and occipital lobe epilepsies
      Syndromes characterized by seizures with specific modes of precipitation
   1.3. Cryptogenic
      Cryptogenic epilepsies are presumed to be symptomatic and the etiology is unknown. This category thus differs from the previous ones by the lack of etiological evidence. These epilepsies are defined by seizure type, clinical features, anatomical localization, and etiology (where known).
2. *Generalized epilepsies and syndromes*
   2.1. Idiopathic (with age-related onset, listed in order of age)
      Benign neonatal convulsions
      Benign neonatal familial convulsions
      Benign myoclonic epilepsy in infancy
      Childhood absence epilepsy (pyknolepsy)
      Juvenile absence epilepsy
      Juvenile myoclonic epilepsy (impulsive petit mal)
      Epilepsy with grand mal (generalized tonic-clonic) seizures on awakening
      Epilepsies with seizures precipitated by specific modes of activation
      Other generalized idiopathic epilepsies
   2.2. Cryptogenic or symptomatic (in order of age)
      West syndrome (infantile spasms, Blitz-Nick-Salaam Krämpfe)
      Lennox-Gastaut syndrome
      Epilepsy with myoclonic-astatic seizures
      Epilepsy with myoclonic absences
   2.3. Symptomatic
      2.3.1 Nonspecific etiology
         Early myoclonic encephalopathy
         Early infantile epileptic encephalopathy with suppression burst
         Other symptomatic generalized epilepsies not defined above
      2.3.2 Specific syndromes
         Epileptic seizures may complicate many disease states. Under this heading are included diseases in which seizures are a presenting or predominant feature.
3. *Epilepsies and syndromes undetermined, whether focal or generalized*
   3.1. With both generalized and focal seizures
      Neonatal seizures
      Severe myoclonic epilepsy in infancy
      Epilepsy with continuous spike-waves during slow wave sleep
      Acquired epileptic aphasia (**Landau-Kleffner-syndrome**)
      Other undetermined epilepsies not defined above
   3.2. Without unequivocal generalized or focal features. All patients with generalized tonic-clonic seizures (GTCS) in which clinical and EEG findings do not permit classification as clearly generalized or localization related, such as in many cases of sleep grand mal (GTCS), are considered not to have unequivocal generalized or focal features.

4. *Special syndromes*
   4.1. Situation-related seizures (Gelegenheitsanfälle)
      Febrile convulsions linked to 8q or 19p
      Isolated seizures or isolated status epilepticus
      Autosomal dominant nocturnal frontal lobe epilepsy
      Seizures occurring only when there is an acute metabolic or toxic event due to factors such as alcohol, drugs, eclampsia, or nonketotic hyperglycemia

*From Commission for Classification and Terminology, ILAE. Proposal for Revised Classifications of Epilepsies and Epileptic syndromes. Epilepsia 1989;**30**:389–399. Reproduced by kind permission of Dr. F. Dreifuss, the ILAE, and Blackwell Science.*

Chart E–3. ILAE Research Classification of the Epilepsies[1362] (adapted)

I. *Primary generalized epilepsies* (genetically determined with specific age penetrance)
   A. *Absence epilepsies*
      1. Classic absence of childhood with diffuse 3–Hz spike–wave complexes
      2. Absence in **juvenile myoclonic epilepsy:** staring, with diffuse 3- to 6-Hz multi-spike–wave complexes during adolescence
      3. Juvenile absence with diffuse 8- to 12-Hz rhythms
      4. Myoclonic absence with diffuse 3- to 6-Hz multi-spike-wave complexes
      5. Myoclonic absence, staring, fragmentary myoclonus, automatisms, and diffuse 8- to 12-Hz rhythms
   B. *Myoclonic epilepsies*
      1. Benign myoclonic epilepsy of infancy
      2. **Benign familial infantile (or neonatal) convulsions**
      3. **West syndrome**
      4. Myoclonic seizures of early childhood with 3- to 6-Hz multi-spike–wave complexes and without mental retardation (**Doose syndrome**)
      5. Juvenile myoclonic seizures of Janz or benign myoclonic seizures of adolescence and late childhood with diffuse 4- to 6-Hz multi-spike–wave complexes; impulsive petit mal; Herpine-Janz syndrome limked to chromosome 6p
II. *Primary partial epilepsies* (genetically determined with specific age penetrance)
   A. **Benign childhood (Rolandic) epilepsy with centro-temporal spikes** linked to 15q
   B. **Autosomal dominant rolandic epilepsy with speech dyspraxia**
   C. **Benign occipital epilepsy** with occipital spike–wave complexes
   D. **Autosomal dominant nocturnal frontal lobe epilepsy**
   E. **Familial temporal lobe epilepsy** [506]
   F. **Autosomal dominant partial epilepsy with variable foci**
III. *Secondary or symptomatic partial epilepsies* (caused by structural lesions)
   A. Secondary or symptomatic partial epilepsies without loss or impairment of consciousness
      1. Sensorimotor epilepsies
      2. Partial or focal motor epilepsies (**epilepsy with evoked parietal spikes**)
      3. **Kojewnikow syndrome**
      4. Occipital epilepsies
      5. **Partial epilepsy with auditory features**
      6. **Partial epilepsy with variable foci**
   B. Secondary or symptomatic partial epilepsies with loss or impairment of consciousness
      1. Temporal lobe epilepsies
         a. Medial basal limbic or hippocampal epilepsy
         b. Amygdaloid and anterior temporal polar epilepsy
         c. **Lateral posterior temporal epilepsy**
         d. Opercular or island of Reil epilepsy
      2. Frontal lobe epilepsies
         a. Cingulate epilepsies
         b. Supplementary motor epilepsies
         c. Orbitofrontal and prefrontal epilepsies
         d. Dorsolateral frontal epilepsies
            See also **nocturnal frontal lobe epilepsy, epileptic negative myoclonus**
      3. Medial occipital-hippocampal epilepsies
IV. *Secondary generalized epilepsies* (caused by structural lesions)
   A. Simple partial epilepsy, evolving to tonic-clonic epilepsy (secondary tonic-clonic epilepsy)
   B. Infantile spasms (propulsive petit mal, infantile myoclonic encephalopathy with **hypsarrhythmia, West syndrome**)
   C. Myoclonic astatic or atonic epilepsies (epileptic drop attacks, atypical absence, tonic seizures of **Lennox-Gastaut syndrome** in children with mental retardation)
   D. Progressive myoclonic epilepsies in adolescents and adults with dementia (myoclonic epilepsies of **Lafora, Unverricht-Lundborg-Hartung, Ramsay Hunt,** or **Kufs**)
V. *Unclassified epilepsies or syndromes not included in the above list*
      Rolandic epilepsy and speech dyspraxia
      Generalized epilepsy with febrile seizures plus
      Partial epilepsy with auditory features
      Autosomal dominant) nocturnal frontal lobe epilepsy
      Nocturnal paroxysmal dystonia *and nocturnal wandering*

*Adapted from Delgado-Escueta AV, Greenberg D. Classification of the epilepsies for genetic studies. Ann Neurol 1984;**16**(Suppl): 1–11. Reproduced by permission.*

epilepsy and febrile seizures-plus   A benign, dominantly inherited syndrome of febrile convulsions and various other (usually generalized tonic-clonic) seizure types, occurring in children and in the absence of fever. Absences or myoclonic or atonic seizures can also occur. Various chromosomal linkages have been determined; the condition is genetically heterogeneous.[3352]

epilepsy and mental retardation limited to females   A dominantly inherited seizure disorder with onset in early childhood, in which half of the affected females are also mentally retarded.[2889]

Epilepsy Canada   A national, non-profit organization dedicated to improving the quality of life for people with epilepsy and their families. Address: 745 1470 rue Peel, Montreal, QC, Canada H3A 1T1. Email:

epilepsy@epilepsy.ca. Web site: http://www.epilepsy.ca/eng/mainSet.html.

Epilepsy Foundation of America   A charitable organization. Address: 4351 Garden City Dr., Landover, MD 20785. Tel: 301-459-3700, 301-577-9056. Web site: http://www.efa.org/.

epilepsy, heterochromia iridis, and deafness   A rare variant of **Usher syndrome** in which the iris changes are added features.

epilepsy in remission with treatment   A prevalent case of epilepsy with no seizures for 5 or more years and receiving antiepileptic drugs at the time of ascertainment.[1115]

epilepsy in remission without treatment   A prevalent case of epilepsy with no seizures for 5 or more years and not receiving antiepileptic drugs at the time of ascertainment.[1115]

Epilepsy Research (incorporating the *Journal of Epilepsy*) A subspecialty journal published by Elsevier. Web site: http://www.elsevier.com/locate/epilepsyres.

epilepsy seizure scales   See **Chalfont scale; Hague scale; VA scale.**

epilepsy with continuous spike-waves during slow-wave sleep   See **electrical status epilepticus during sleep.**

epilepsy with evoked parietal spikes   An uncommon seizure disorder characterized by the presence of focal attacks without loss of consciousness, or with generalized seizures. Parietal spikes or spike-wave discharges are recorded on the EEG. In some cases, a similar EEG occurs but only when the contralateral foot is tapped. Thus it appears that the condition may or may not find any clinical expression.[1374]

epilepsy with generalized tonic-clonic seizures on awakening   A syndrome with its onset occurring mostly in the second decade of life. The seizures occur exclusively or predominantly (>90% of the time) shortly after awakening, regardless of the time of day, or in a second seizure peak in the evening period of relaxation. If other seizures occur, they are mostly absence or myoclonic, as in **juvenile myoclonic epilepsy.** Seizures may be precipitated by sleep deprivation and other external factors. Genetic predisposition is relatively frequent. The EEG shows one of the patterns of idiopathic generalized epilepsy. There is a significant correlation with photosensitivity. (From the revised ILAE Classification,[1114] reproduced by kind permission from Blackwell Science.)

epilepsy with infantile baldness and mental retardation   A syndrome characterized by such features from birth. Both major motor and complex partial seizures are described in the few kinships reported.[4024]

epilepsy with myoclonic absences   A syndrome clinically characterized by absences accompanied by severe bilateral rhythmical clonic jerks, often associated with a tonic contraction, in children aged between 2 and 12 years, with male preponderance. On the EEG, these clinical features are always accompanied by bilateral, synchronous, and symmetrical discharge of rhythmical spike–waves at 3 Hz, similar to childhood absence. Seizures occur many times a day.[4207]

Awareness of the jerks may be maintained. Associated seizures are rare. The prognosis is less favorable than in pyknolepsy, owing to resistance to therapy of the seizures, mental deterioration, and possible evolution to other types of epilepsy such as **Lennox-Gastaut syndrome.** (From the revised ILAE Classification,[1114] reproduced by kind permission from Blackwell Science.)

epilepsy with myoclonic-astatic seizures   Manifestations of myoclonic-astatic seizures begin between the ages of 7 months and 6 years (mostly between the ages of 2 and 5 years), with (except if seizures begin in the first year) twice as many boys affected. There is frequently a hereditary predisposition and usually a normal developmental background. The seizures are myoclonic, astatic, myoclonic-astatic, absence with clonic and tonic components, and tonic-clonic. Status frequently occurs. Tonic seizures develop late in the course of unfavorable cases.

The EEG, initially often normal except for 4- to 7–Hz rhythms, may have irregular fast spike–wave or polyspike waves. The course and outcome are variable. (From the revised ILAE Classification,[1114] reproduced by kind permission from Blackwell Science.)

epilepsy-telangiectasia syndrome   A recessively inherited dysmorphic syndrome characterized by conjunctival telangiectasias, brachydactyly, seizures, and mental retardation. See **ataxia–telangiectasia-like syndrome.**

epileptic amnesia   See **transient epileptic amnesia.**

epileptic aphasic syndrome   (see **Landau-Kleffner syndrome**) A syndrome of acquired temporary aphasia lasting days to months, in the absence of any detectable focal cerebral disease but associated with heterogeneous clinical seizures and with generalized spike and wave discharges on the EEG, the clinical and electrographic abnormalities abating together.[2182]

The following criteria for the diagnosis of *ictal aphasia* have been defined;[4782] the patient must be alert and speaking during the ictus; the speech produced must be dysphasic (dysnomic, non-fluent, paraphasic); and simultaneous EEG demonstrates seizure activity that comes and goes with the seizure events.

epileptic cephalea   Headache occurring as the only manifestation of a seizure disorder.[2397]

epileptic discharge   A diffuse or localized but temporary paroxysmal change in EEG activity, characterized by high-amplitude rhythmic discharges due to excessive synchronization of potentials in an aggregation of neurons and less frequently by high-frequency, low-amplitude discharges.

epileptic drop attacks   See **atonic seizures.**

epileptic encephalopathy   A syndrome comprising daytime absence-type seizures and nocturnal orofacial seizures during slow-wave sleep, mental impairment, aphasia, or speech arrest, with EEG activation during non–rapid eye movement sleep and the disappearance of the worst of the abnormalities during periods of rapid eye movement sleep.[4362]

epileptic endocrine syndrome   (Bondin-Barbizet syndrome) Mental retardation and precocious puberty with accelerated growth in epileptic children, due in most cases to a hypothalamic or diencephalic lesion.[651]

epileptic forced thinking   See **forced thinking**

epileptic mydriasis   Temporary unilateral fixed dilatation of a pupil after an epileptic seizure.[4322]

epileptic myoclonus   1. Those forms of **myoclonus** which are related to some **epileptic syndrome.** These include **cortical reflex myoclonus; reticular reflex myoclonus;** and **primary generalized epileptic myoclonus.** In all forms, the EMG burst length is less than 50 msec., the muscles are synchronously activated by the same discharge, and a correlated discharge, is recordable on the EEG.[2384] See also **nonepileptic myoclonus.**

2. (*petit mal triad*) The concurrence of absence or generalized tonic-clonic seizures, akinetic attacks, and myoclonus. See **myoclonus.**

epileptic negative myoclonus   A phenomenon related to epileptiform discharges located in contralateral central regions, occurring in a variety of epileptic syndromes and presenting as brief postural lapses of muscle tone in a body segment time-locked to a train of spike discharges in the contralateral hemisphere and accompanied by periods of EMG silence lasting up to 400 msec. Giant somatosensory evoked potentials may be recorded in such patients.[4146] See also **asterixis.**

epileptic nystagmus   (ictal nystagmus) Pendular, torsional, retraction or **central (jerk) nystagmus** occurring in association with paroxysmal discharges from a contralateral parietal focus, as shown on the EEG.[1993]

The phenomenology of the eye movements and the nature of the discharging lesion vary, so much so that no further definition is offered. The subject is reviewed by Leigh and Zee.[3330]

epileptic psychosis   Functional alteration in mental status in patients with seizure disorders, usually of the partial variety. These are classified in Chart E–4 as follows:

Chart E–4. Classification of Epileptic Psychoses

1. Brief psychoses in the context of altered consciousness related to an ictus
   A. Nonconvulsive status
      Absence status.
      Psychomotor status.
   B. Postictal 'twilight states' (brief, mild confusion)
   C. Postictal hypomania.
   D. Fugue states
   E. Alternating psychoses with 'forced normalization' of the EEG
   F. Transient ictal depression, dysphoria or hypomania
2. Chronic psychoses without known relationship to seizure activity and with normal conscious level
   A. **Schizophrenia-like psychoses of epilepsy**[5208]
   B. Paranoid states
   C. Bipolar affective disorder

---

epileptic recruiting rhythm   (fast rhythmic waves) Bursts of sinusoidal waves at 8–30 Hz, widespread over the scalp, resembling beta activity and presaging the occurrence of tonic seizures or absences.[612]

epileptic seizure   1. A paroxysmal clinical event reflecting the occurrence of an epileptic discharge. Such events are the building blocks of the **epileptic syndromes.** The International League Against Epilepsy classification is given in Chart E–5.

2. A clinical manifestation presumed to result from an abnormal and excessive discharge of a set of neurons in the cortex of the brain. The clinical manifestation consists of sudden and transitory abnormal phenomena that may include alterations of consciousness, motor sensory, autonomic, or psychic events, perceived by the patient or an observer.[1115]

Chart E–5. Classification of Epileptic Seizures

I. *Partial seizures* (seizures beginning locally)
   A. Simple partial seizures (consciousness not impaired)
      1. With motor symptoms
      2. With somatosensory or special sensory symptoms
      3. With autonomic symptoms
      4. With psychic symptoms
   B. Complex partial seizures (with impairment of consciousness)
      1. Beginning as simple partial seizures and progressing to impairment of consciousness
         a. With no other features
         b. With features as in A.1–4
         c. With automatisms
      2. With impairment of consciousness at onset
         a. With no other features
         b. With features as in A.1–4
         c. With automatisms
   C. Partial seizures, secondarily generalized
II. *Generalized seizures* (bilaterally symmetrical and without local onset)
   A. Absence seizures
      1. Typical absence seizures
      2. Atypical absence seizures

B. Myoclonic seizures

C. Clonic seizures

D. Tonic seizures

E. Tonic-clonic seizures

F. Atonic seizures

III. *Unclassified epileptic seizures (inadequate or incomplete data).*[1516]

From Driefuss FE. *The epilepsies: clinical implications of the international classification.* Epilepsia *1990;31:S3–S10. Reproduced by kind permission of Dr. F. Driefuss and Blackwell Science.*

epileptic syndrome   An epileptic disorder characterized by a characteristic individual cluster of signs and symptoms customarily occurring together; these include such items as type of seizure, etiology, anatomy, precipitating factor, age of onset, severity, chronicity, diurnal and circadian cycling, and sometimes prognosis. A single syndrome may have different etiologies and prognoses.[56] A classification is given under **epilepsy.**

epileptic twilight state   See **status epilepticus.**

epileptiform   Resembling epilepsy, or, by extension, things that are often associated with epilepsy, such as certain EEG rhythms. The word means neither **epileptogenic** nor epileptic, in any context. In using the term epileptiform discharges, electroencephalographers wish to convey the presence of spikes, sharp waves, or spike–wave complexes which, by their morphology, frequency, or distribution, suggest to them that such waveforms are associated with a clinical seizure disorder.

epileptiform pattern   An EEG pattern that applies to distinctive waves or complexes, distinguished from background activity and resembling those waves or complexes recorded in a proportion of human subjects suffering from epileptic disorders and in animals rendered epileptic experimentally. Epileptiform patterns include spikes and sharp waves, alone or accompanied by slow waves that follow, occurring singly or in bursts lasting at most a few seconds.

The term refers to interictal paroxysmal activity and not to seizure patterns. The probability of association with clinical epileptic disorders is variable. See also **seizure pattern.** (Adapted from the report of the Committee on Terminology, IFCN,[989] © 1974, with permission from Elsevier Science).

epileptogenic   (epileptogenous) Capable of provoking epileptic seizures.

epileptogenous   See **epileptogenic.**

epileptogenous encephalopathy   Intellectual deterioration and transient neurological signs occurring in children with no past history or family history of epilepsy, after a sudden and dramatic illness marked by repeated convulsions and without current evidence of encephalitis.[740]

epileptoid   Resembling epilepsy.

epiloia   The term suggested by E.B. Sherlock in 1901 for **tuberous sclerosis.**

epimysium   The connective tissue investing muscle fascicles.

epineurium   Areolar connective tissue that loosely holds together bundles of funiculi to form a nerve trunk.

epipaxic postural tremor   See **cerebellar tremors.**

epiphysis cerebri   The pineal gland.

episodic ataxia   Inherited syndromes of early onset in which the ataxia is the most obvious clinical feature. Most patients recover fully between attacks, but some may develop progressive ataxia with cerebellar atrophy.

Type 1 (EA1) is a dominantly inherited potassium channelopathy, characterized by attacks of cerebellar ataxia triggered by startle or exercise lasting minutes, and continuous interictal myokymia, as a result of mutations of the voltage-gated potassium channel gene on chromosome 12p.13.[1711]

Type 2 (EA2) is also dominantly inherited but is a calcium channelopathy mapped to chromosome 19p13, at the same locus as familial hemiplegic migraine and cerebellar ataxia (SCA6). It is characterized by attacks of cerebellar ataxia lasting hours to days, provoked by stress rather than by startle and responsive to acetazolamide. Dysarthria, nystagmus, vertigo, diplopia, and headache also occur in the attacks. Interictal nystagmus is another feature.[1386]

See also **cerebellar ataxias.**

episodic autonomic dysreflexia   (autonomic storm) The occurrence in patients with severe thoracic cord lesions of excessive sympathetic discharge (manifested by flushing and sweating rostral to the level of the cord lesion, headache, hypertension, and reflex bradycardia) in response to visceral stimuli such as bladder distension.

episodic cluster headache   A headache that occurs in periods lasting 7 days to 1 year, separated by pain-free periods lasting 14 days or more. This definition and the following diagnostic criteria are suggested by the Headache Classification Committee of the International Headache Society.[1051]

A. All the letter headings of **cluster headache.**

B. At least two periods of headaches (cluster periods) lasting (untreated patients) from 7 days to 1 year, separated by remissions of at least 14 days.

From Classification of headache disorders, cranial neuralgias and facial pains; and diagnostic criteria for primary headache disorders. *Cephalalgia* 1988;**8** (suppl): 1–96.[1051] Reprinted by kind permission of Blackwell Science.

episodic hyperhidrosis   An uncommon manifestation of diencephalic dysfunction, usually associated with both hypothermia and reduction in conscious level. Causative pathologies have included primary and infiltrating tumors of the hypothalamus, epilepsy, and agenesis of the corpus callosum.[1286]

episodic memory The mechanism whereby events, places, dates, faces, and facts that were personally experienced are remembered. cf. **semantic memory,** the remembering of words. A type of long-term memory containing information about the ordering of events in time; it is thus memory for personal history. This memory store is somewhat more fragile that semantic memory, perhaps because the data within it constantly change.[3076]

episodic nocturnal wanderings Nocturnal behavioral disturbances characterized by abrupt arousal, followed by violent stereotyped complex automatisms, including walking, screaming, yelling and unintelligible speech, kicking, leaping, and head banging within the context of expressed fear and unresponsiveness to the environment and with a tendency to semidirected violence. They occur mainly in adolescents and young adults, many of whom have interictal seizure discharges.

The attacks usually last for minutes and occur in clusters during non–rapid eye movement sleep stage 2. They are unaccompanied by pathological behavior by day.[4388] They resemble night terrors or sleepwalking, except that they are suppressed by anticonvulsants.[3672,3954,5291]

episodic paroxysmal hemicrania A syndrome in which the bouts of otherwise typical **chronic paroxysmal hemicrania** last for weeks without progressing to a chronic phase. Responsiveness to indomethacin is near-complete.[3178]

episodic spontaneous hypothermia with hyperhidrosis A rare condition seen at any age and characterized by unprovoked hypothermia with diaphoresis lasting minutes to months with eventual remission. It is associated with the presence of congenital CNS anomalies or hypothalamic disorders. See **corpus callosum agenesis with recurrent hypothermia.**

episodic tension-type headache (tension, muscle contraction, psychomyogenic, stress, ordinary, headache, idiopathic or psychogenic headache) Recurrent episodes of headache lasting minutes to days. The pain is typically pressing/tightening in quality, of mild or moderate intensity, and bilateral in location and does not worsen with routine physical activity. Nausea is absent, but photophobia or phonophobia may be present. This description and the diagnostic criteria in Chart E–6 are suggested by the Headache Classification Committee of the International Headache Society.[1051]

Chart E–6. Features of Chronic Tension-type Headaches

A. At least 10 previous headache episodes fulfilling criteria B-D listed below. Number of days with such headache is <180/year (<15/month)

B. Headache lasting from 30 minutes to 7 days

C. At least 2 of the following pain characteristics:
Pressing/tightening (nonpulsating quality)
Mild or moderate intensity (may inhibit but does not prohibit activities)
Bilateral location
No aggravation by walking stairs or similar routine physical activity

D. Both of the following:
No nausea or vomiting (anorexia may occur)
Photophobia and phonophobia are absent, or one but not the other is present

E. At least one of the following:
History, physical, and neurological examinations do not suggest one of the disorders listed in groups 5–11 (see **headache**)
History and/or physical and/or neurological examinations do suggest such disorder, but it is ruled out by appropriate investigations
Such disorder is present, but tension-type headache does not occur for the first time in close temporal relation to the disorder

Two varieties are described:

1. *Episodic tension-type headache associated with disorder of pericranial muscles* (muscle contraction headache) Episodic tension-type headache with increased levels of tenderness and/or EMG of pericranial muscles, with features that meet the following diagnostic criteria:
A. Fulfils criteria for **episodic tension-type headaches**
B. Presence of at least one of the following:
Increased tenderness of pericranial muscles demonstrated by manual palpation or pressure algometer
Increased EMG level of pericranial muscles at rest or during physiological tests

2. *Episodic tension-type headache unassociated with disorder of pericranial muscles* (idiopathic headache, essential headache, psychogenic headache) Episodic tension-type headache with normal levels of tenderness and/or EMG of pericranial muscles, with features that meet the following diagnostic criteria:
A. Fulfilling criteria for **episodic tension-type headaches**
B. No increased tenderness of pericranial muscles. If studied, EMG of pericranial muscles shows normal levels of activity.

From Classification Committee of the International Headache Society. Classification of headache disorders, cranial neuralgias and facial pains; and diagnostic criteria for primary headache disorders. Cephalalgia 1988;8 (suppl):1–96,[1051] *Reprinted by kind permission of Blackwell Science.*

See also **chronic daily headache, new daily persistent headache, medication-induced headache.**[5156]

episodic unilateral mydriasis A syndrome characterized by the spontaneous occurrence of unilateral fixed pupillary dilatation associated with homolateral headache, lasting from minutes to weeks in young people, without ptosis or diplopia, with eventual remission, and without residua.

A similar syndrome occurs in **Horner syndrome,** with **springing pupils,** and in **cyclic oculomotor paralysis.**[2388]

episodic vertigo A feature of various conditions including **benign paroxysmal positional** and **benign**

recurrent vertigo, vertebrobasilar insufficiency, **migraine,** and **episodic ataxia type 2,** as well as the following.

episodic vertigo and hearing loss   A dominantly inherited syndrome of fluctuating nerve deafness with episodic tinnitus and vertigo. See **Ménière disease.**

Epley maneuver   An effective bedside method for repositioning the otolith particles in the semicircular canals as treatment for patients with **benign positional vertigo.**[1684] The actual method is superbly demonstrated at http://www.emedicine.com/emerg/topic57.htm. See **also Semont liberatory maneuver.**

epoch   A period of time in an EEG record or other physiological recording session, its duration determined arbitrarily.

EPP   See **end-plate potential.**

EPSP   See **excitatory postsynaptic potential.**

Epworth Sleepiness Scale   A subjective tool for the evaluation of sleepiness, though it was the Maintenance of Wakefulness test that was adopted by the U.S. Federal Aviation Administration as the standard for measuring treatment efficacy when testing pilots with sleep apnea.

EQ-5D   A generic quality-of-life measure assessing self-care, mobility, usual activites, pain/discomfort, and anxiety/depression and found valuable in the assessment of people with Parkinson disease.[5000]

equal loudness balance test   A localizing test in auditory dysfunction, in which pure tones at various frequencies are delivered to the two ears alternately, the subject signifying when the sound in the two ears is of equal intensity. With cochlear dysfunction, the loudness in the affected ear approaches, equals, or exceeds that in the normal ear at high-intensity levels; with conductive deafness or retrocochlear lesions, no such recruitment occurs; and with neural lesions, the sensation of loudness in the deaf ear grows more slowly than that in the normal ear with increasing intensity of stimulation.[1921]

equine gait   The "steppage" gait of drop foot due to weakness of the ankle dorsiflexor and evertor muscles.

equipotential   A term that applies to regions of the head or to electrodes that are at the same potential at a given instant in time.

equipotential line   An imaginary line joining a series of points that are at the same potential at a given instant in time.

equivocal signs   Signs that suggest the presence of neuropathology but that are either so slight as to generate uncertainty or are inconsistently present. In other situations, the sign is not confirmed by the presence of other signs ordinarily present, given the lesion suggested by the original finding.

Eramo syndrome   A dysmorphic syndrome characterized by short stature, dry skin, hyperkeratosis or ichthyosis, alopecia, absent eyebrows and sparse eyelashes, corneal ulceration and photophobia, mental and developmental delay, seizures, and nystagmus.[337]

Erb, Wilhelm Heinrich   (1840–1921) The leading German neurologist of his time, Erb graduated from Munich University and trained with **Friedreich** at Heidelberg University, succeeding him there as professor after some years spent in Heidelberg and Leipzig. He is best remembered for his initial classification of the muscular dystrophies which he also distinguished from spinal muscular atrophies; and for his work on the tendon reflexes. He was the first to employ a hammer to elicit these, the hammer formerly having been used to percuss the chests of humans and the heads of cows (in the latter case, to detect the presence of echinococcal cysts).[4964]

Erb was one of the first neurologists to stress the value of the neurological examination; he and **Westphal** showed at the same time that the knee jerk was absent in **tabes dorsalis.** He succeeded in getting adequate training in neurology into the undergraduate medical curriculum in Germany, an advance that has sadly proved temporary, at least in North America. The syndromes, etc. for which he is remembered (from over 270 of his publications) are listed in the following entries.

Erb dystrophy   See **limb-girdle muscular dystrophy.**

Erb myotonic reaction   The prolonged contraction of muscle resulting from faradic stimulation applied at the motor point.

Erb palsy   See **upper brachial plexus palsy.**

Erb phenomenon   The increased excitability of the peripheral motor nerves in tetany.

Erb's point   That point behind the insertion of the sternomastoid muscle into the clavicle where percutaneous nerve stimulation activates the axons of the upper trunk of the brachial plexus.

Erb reaction of degeneration   The persisting sensitivity of muscle to galvanic but not to faradic stimulation following denervation.

Erb sign   Hyperexcitability of the nerves in tetany.

Erb spastic paraparesis   See **Erb-Charcot syndrome.**

Erb-Charcot syndrome   (spastic spinal paralysis, Erb spastic paraparesis, syphilitic myelitis) Syphilitic myelopathy with the usual pyramidal signs, sphincter disturbances, muscle atrophy at the level of the cord lesions, and long-tract sensory changes, due to syphilitic endarteritis of the thoracic cord.[1688] Syphilitic myelopathy can similarly be caused by pachymeningitis. The name given here is that by which the disease is better known, but Erb gave primacy to **Charcot** in its description.[1689]

Erb-Duchenne syndrome See **upper brachial plexus palsy.**

Erb-Goldflam syndrome See **myasthenia gravis.**[1690]

Erb-Landouzy syndrome See **limb-girdle muscular dystrophy.**

Erb-Westphal sign Absence of the knee jerk in **tabes dorsalis.**

Erdheim, Jakob (1874–1937) Viennese physician who described parathyroid adenoma and medial necrosis of the aorta as well as the tumor once named for him.

Erdheim syndrome Cervical spondylosis with hyperplasia of the intervertebral disks associated with acromegaly and leading to pain and restriction of cervical mobility.[1695]

Erdheim tumor Craniopharyngioma, described by Erdheim in 1904.

Erdheim-Chester disese A rare form of systemic histiocytosis with widespread tissue infiltration, especially shown as metaphysial sclerosis, and with retroperitoneal, cardiac, and pulmonary involvement but also capable of causing neurogenic diabetes insipidus, orbital lesions, and pyramidal and cerebellar signs, the latter being due mainly to extraaxial infiltration.[6048]

ergotamine tartrate A serotonin receptor agonist and vasoconstrictor isolated by Stoll in 1918 and first used for the treatment of migraine by Maier in 1926.

ergotamine withdrawal headache A form of **rebound** or **medication-induced headache** in subjects with a prior headache syndrome, its characteristics resembling both those of migraine and of tension-type headaches, preceded by chronic daily ergotamine intake (oral ≥2 mg, rectal ≥1 mg) and occurring within 48 hours after ergotamine withdrawal.[1051]

ergotism (from Fr; a cock spur, which resembles the spike on the fungus *Claviceps purpurea* which may infest spoiled rye grain) Poisoning by the toxin of the ergot fungus, the disease known in the Middle Ages as *Holy, St. Anthony's,* or *St. Martial's fire,* and often appearing then in epidemics.

Neurovascular (gangrenous) and *spasmodic* or *convulsive* forms are recognized, the latter presenting with limb pains, paresthesias, intermittent strong muscular contractions, seizures, psychoses, and signs resembling those of peripheral neuropathy or tabes.[6000]

Erichsen, Sir John Eric (1818–1896) English surgeon (born in Copenhagen) who described **railway spine** (a condition which does not exist) in 1866.

Erisistratos (d. circa 250 B.C.) Alexandrian anatomist, physician, and surgeon who was possibly the grandson of Aristotle. He named the cerebrum and the cerebellum and described the convolutions of the brain.

Erlanger, Joseph (1874–1965) American neurophysiologist who established the nature of the nerve action potential using a cathode ray oscilloscope, and took the 1944 Nobel prize (with H. Gasser, a former student of his) for work on the differentiation of nerve fiber functions.

Ernest syndrome A syndrome of facial pain considered to be due to inflammation of the tendon of the temporalis muscle, and characterized clinically by pain felt in and about the ear, temporomandibular joint, anterior temple, mandible and adjacent teeth, throat, and/or eye. The pain is exacerbated by digital compression of the insertion of the stylomandibular ligament and relieved by local anesthetic injection at that site.

erratic seizures See **fragmentary seizures.**

erythema chronicum migrans Classically, an expanding red or bull's eye annular "target" lesion typically associated with B. burgdorferi tick bites and the most common manifestation of early Lyme disease. Variations such as uniform coloration, lesions with necrotic or vesicular centers, and lesions with shapes that are not circular or oval also occur. The classic lesion was first described by Arnold **Pick.**

erythism Redness of the skin, as part of the syndrome of poisoning with inorganic mercury. The term became generalized to describe the associated emotional irritability.

In retrospect, it is surprising that the similarity of the signs of **pink disease** to those of erethism was not recognized earlier.

erythrokeratodermia with ataxia A rare, recessively inherited syndrome of congenital ichthyosiform erythroderma, clearing by the age of 25 years, with adult-onset gait ataxia, pyramidal signs, and myalgia.[2127]

erythromelalgia A chronic condition characterized by burning and erythema of the involved extremity. When the extremity is lowered, or heat is applied, the pain is intensified. The application of cold or elevation of the extremity will have the opposite effect of decreasing the pain. Sympathetic vasoconstrictor responses are diminished, perhaps as a result of denervation supersensitivity causing increased vasoconstrictor responses to circulating catecholamines, leading to a reduction in skin blood flow.[2558]

In primary erythromelalgia there is no accompanying disease process. Secondary erythromelalgia is associated with myeloproliferative syndrome-related thrombocythemia. Silas Weir Mitchell first suggested the term in 1878. When affecting the face or head, the term refers to **cluster headache.** See **Weir Mitchell syndrome, thrombocytosis.**[4167]

erythropia The abnormal perception of redness in objects seen; an occasional complication of lens extraction.

erythroprosopalgia A redundant term for **cluster headache.**

Escherich sign Periorbital and perioral muscle contraction induced by percussion of the lips or tongue; seen in tetany.[4723]

esodic Afferent.

esophoria (latent convergent strabismus) A tendency for the visual axes to deviate medially; a predisposition to ocular convergence. See also **esotropia.** cf. **exophoria.**

esotropia (convergent strabismus) A visible turning-inward of the visual axis of an eye. See also **cyclic esotropia, thalamic esotropia.**

esphlasis (from Gr, a pressure inwards) A comminuted fracture of the skull.

Espildora-Luque syndrome Unilateral blindness with contralateral hemiplegia due to an embolism in the ophthalmic artery which, it is supposed, induces reflex spasm in the middle cerebral artery on the same side.[1704] See **amaurosis-hemiplegia syndrome.**

Esquirol,   Jean-Etienne-Dominique (1772–1840) French physician, psychiatrist at the **Salpêtrière,** who first brought rational and humanistic ideas to the management of patients with mental disorders[1705] and who introduced the terms *grand mal* and *petit mal* to neurology in 1838.

essential anisocoria Benign pupillary inequality of unknown cause, in which the difference in sizes of the pupils is maintained under different conditions of illumination, responses to light and accommodation are present, and eye movements are full. See **anisocoria.**

essential benign myoclonus See **myoclonus.**[1299]

essential blepharospasm A common **dystonia** in adults, presenting as blepharospasm with no known cause, often without any other dystonic manifestations.

essential chorea A rare disorder of unknown cause manifesting nonprogressive chorea with onset in adult life, with no associated neurological deficit, positive family history, or abnormality on cerebral imaging.[1731]

See also **hereditary nonprogressive chorea, senile chorea.**

essential headache See **episodic tension-type headache.**

essential myoclonus A disorder characterized solely by the occurrence of myoclonus. Both *hereditary* (paramyoclonus multiplex) and *acquired* forms have been described, but, even in the latter, no preceding causal event can be determined.[739]

The acquired, sporadic condition is heterogeneous and may represent a variant of idiopathic epilepsy in which myoclonus occurs in subjects with no other form of epilepsy and who show no neurological deficit. In some cases, malignancies are associated. See **my-**oclonus, hereditary essential myoclonus, ballistic movement overflow myoclonus.**

essential tremor (benign essential familial tremor, minor tremor, familial tremor) A dominantly inherited or sporadic syndrome of postural and kinetic tremor, worst in the arms with actions such as writing or lifting a cup but frequently also affecting the head, jaw and vocal apparatus; in the absence of signs of Parkinson disease or of other causes of tremor. Mapping to chromosomes 2p22–25 and 3q13 has been achieved.

The tremor is absent at rest. It may affect other areas of the body as well as the arms and is usually most pronounced distally, and present during both maintenance of posture and performance of an action. In elderly people, a rest component may be seen. Eye movement abnormalities are not present in association with this kind of tremor. As first recorded by Robert **Whytt,** alcohol consumption may relieve the tremor of the hands. The condition was first described in full by Lazar **Minor.** Hubble et al.[2678] have published a complete review.

Criteria for the diagnosis of essential tremor have been suggested[1423] (see Chart E–7).

Core criteria[300,1630] are the presence of bilateral tremor of the hands and forearms (but not rest tremor); the absence of other signs apart from the cogwheel phenomenon; and head tremor in the absence of signs of dystonia (the tremor should be postural/kinetic in type). Secondary criteria supporting but not required for the diagnosis are long duration (>3 years); a positive family history; and a beneficial response to alcohol.

Exclusion criteria for this tremor, suggested by Dr. Joseph Jankowicz (personal communication; 1994, and reproduced by kind permission), are the presence of neurological signs; the causes of accentuated physiological tremor; current or recent exposure to tremor-genic drugs; direct or indirect trauma to the CNS or PNS; historical or clinical evidence of a psychogenic origin for the tremor; or convincing evidence of sudden onset or of stepwise deterioration.

Chart E–7. TRIG Classification of Essential Tremor

A. *Definite essential tremor*
  1. Inclusion criteria
     i. Tremor: Bilateral postural tremor with or without kinetic tremor, involving hands and forearms, that is visible and persistent (Tremor of other body parts may be present in addition to upper limb tremor. Bilateral tremor may be asymmetric. It is reported by the patient to be persistent, although the amplitude may fluctuate, but it may or may not produce disability.)
     ii. Duration: longer than 5 years
  2. Exclusion criteria
     i. Other abnormal neurologic signs (with the exception of the presence of tremor and **Froment sign,** the full neurologic examination should be normal for age)
     ii. Presence of known causes of enhanced physiologic tremor

iii. Concurrent or recent exposure to tremorogenic drugs or the presence of a drug withdrawal state (Many drugs acting on the central nervous system can produce tremor as a side effect. In people, drug-induced tremor is most often in the form of action tremor. Subjects should be drug-free for a period exceeding the known biologic effect of the drug.)

iv. Direct or indirect trauma to the nervous system within 3 months preceding the onset of tremor (This includes head injury [direct or indirect] and peripheral injury, if the anatomic distribution is the same as that of the tremor.)

v. Historic or clinical evidence of psychogenic origins of tremor (The definition of psychogenic tremor is itself open to debate. Clinical features that may suggest psychogenic tremor are unphysiological variations [>1 Hz] in tremor frequency, unusual and inconsistent behavioral characteristics, and spontaneous remission. Psychiatric or social factors [multiple somatization, secondary gain, litigation or compensation pending] may support the diagnosis of psychogenic tremor.)

vi. Convincing evidence of sudden onset or evidence of stepwise deterioration

B. *Probable essential tremor*

1. Inclusion criteria

i. The same as those for definite essential tremor (Tremor may be confined to body parts other than hands. These may include head and postural tremor of the legs. However, abnormal posture of the head would suggest the presence of dystonic head tremor.)

ii. Duration longer than 3 years

2. Exclusion criteria

i. The same as for definite essential tremor

ii. Primary orthostatic tremor (isolated, high-frequency [14–18 Hz] bilaterally synchronous tremor of the lower limbs on standing)

iii. Isolated voice tremor (because of the clinical difficulty of separating essential tremor of the voice from the speech disturbances of laryngeal dystonia and other dystonias of the vocal apparatus)

iv. Isolated position-specific or task-specific tremors, including occupational tremors and primary writing tremor

v. Isolated tongue or chin tremor

C. *Possible essential tremor*

1. Inclusions

i. Type I

a. Subjects who satisfy the criteria of definite or probable essential tremor but exhibit other recognizable neurologic disorders, such as parkinsonism, dystonia, myoclonus, peripheral neuropathy, or restless leg syndrome

b. Subjects who satisfy the criteria of definite or probable essential tremor but exhibit other neurologic signs of uncertain significance not sufficient to make the diagnosis of a recognizable neurologic disorder. Such signs may include mild extrapyramidal features, such as hypomimia, decreased arm swing, or mild bradykinesia.

ii. Type II

Monosymptomatic and isolated tremors of uncertain relation to essential tremor. This includes posi-tion-specific and task-specific tremors, such as occupational tremors, primary writing tremor, primary orthostatic tremor, isolated voice tremor, isolated postural leg tremor, and unilateral postural hand tremor.

2. Exclusions

The exclusions are the same as item 2 under *definite essential tremor.*

The following subgroups of essential tremor were differentiated by Marsden et al.:[3643]

Type 1, *benign exaggerated physiological essential tremor* A nonfamilial postural tremor at 8–12 Hz, seen in the arms and due to enhancement of the normal stretch reflex. See also **physiological tremor.**

Type 2, *benign pathological essential tremor* A frequently familial postural tremor at 5–7 Hz, seen in the arms and perhaps in the head and legs as well, and considered to be due to dysregulation of a central oscillator.

Type 3, *severe pathological essential tremor* A frequently familial postural tremor at 5–9 Hz, that is more marked than type 2, seen in the arms and perhaps also in the head and legs, and considered to be due to dysregulation of a central oscillator.

Type 4, *symptomatic essential tremor* A frequently familial postural tremor at 5–7 Hz, seen in the arms only, in association with peripheral neuropathy or with basal ganglion disorders.

Orthostatic and *primary writing tremor* and *tremor of the smile* are *variants* of the same condition,[1820] which is itself heterogeneous as judged by electrophysiological study.

esthesioneuroblastoma An invasive malignant tumor of the nasal cavity derived from the olfactory mucosal receptor cells. Microscopically, the tumor resembles a neuroblastoma. It occurs mostly in young adults and invades locally, giving rise to cranial nerve pareses, but may occasionally metastasize locally or may spread intracranially.[494,1634]

état criblé 1. The normal open-weave appearance of the anterior and posterior perforated substances through which small arteries pass into the brain.

2. The abnormal sieve-like appearance of the brain in areas of vascular ectasia, usually the centrum semiovale and the basal ganglia, due to dilatation of the perivascular spaces, thickening of the walls of the smaller arteries, and perivascular demyelination. This condition was reported by Dechambre in the same paper in which he published his observations of lacunes.[1325]

3. The occurrence of multiple type 3 **lacunes** in the brain.

état lacunaire The occurrence of multiple type 1 **lacunes** in the brain, often associated clinically with progressive neurological deterioration, *marche à petits pas,* pseudobulbar palsy, and incontinence.

état marbré (Fr, marbled state) (status marmoratus) Scarring of the putamen and other basal ganglia with prominence of myelinated fibers in the gray matter, giving rise to a marbled appearance. It is seen in neonates following **hypoxic-ischemic encephalopathy** and clinically is usually associated with athetosis. See **double athetosis, Vogt syndrome.**

Ethan syndrome See **nystagmus-blockage syndrome.**

ethmocephaly (from Gr, a sieve + brain) A developmental malformation in which the two orbits are placed unusually close together. The nose, when present, is normally sited between them.[335] The nasal cavities, nasal bones, ethmoid, and premaxilla are usually missing.[4]

ethmoid (Gr, resembling a sieve) A thin, cavitated, unpaired bone in the midline beneath the frontal and anterior to the sphenoid bones and forming parts of the cranium, the orbits, and the nasal fossae. Its upper border forms the cribriform plate. The bone was known to Celsus and was named by Galen.

ethnology The science of the physical and mental differences between the races of humanity.

ethology The scientific study of the structure of animal behavior by observation; an activity, in Medawar's phrase, "which only simpletons think simple." This is a modern science, dating from the paper by Julian S. Huxley, "The Courtship Habits of the Great Crested Grebe" in the *Proceedings of the Zoological Society of London* in 1914.

That the behaviors of humans resemble those of animals should come as no great surprise; that there are differences allows a measure of reassurance.

Étienne, Charles (1503–1564) French physician who gave the first account of the anatomy of the spinal canal.

Albert Eulenberg

Eulenberg, Albert (1840–1917) German professor of neurology in Greifswald and Berlin. He described pe-

riodic attacks of myotonia and paralysis in six generations of one family in 1886,[1710] wrote extensively on the autonomic nervous system, and introduced ergot therapy for the treatment of migraine.

Eulenberg disease See **paramyotonia congenita.**

euphoria (Gr; easily carried) Originally, well-being, the perfect ease and comfort of healthy people.[4512] Now used (improperly) to refer to a state of unwarranted, insightless cheerfulness, optimism, and jollity of mood with the 'appropriate' (actually inappropriate) verbal and behavioral accompaniments.

eupraxic centers Centers in the brain for the ideational combination of movements.

European Federation of Neurological Societies A professional organization with the aim of advancing the neurological sciences and clinical and experimental research within Europe and of fostering international exchange. Address: University Campus, Alser Strasse 4, A-1090 Vienna, Austria. Tel.: +43 1 889 05 03. E-mail: headoffice@efns.org. Web site: http://www.efns.org/

European Journal of Neurology The official journal of the European Federation of Neurological Societies (EFNS). Web site: http://www.blackwell-science.com/~cgilib/jnlpage.asp?Journal=ene&File=ene&Page=aims.

European Journal of Neuroscience (*Eur. J. Neurosci.*) A subspecialist journal published by Blackwell Science. Web site: http://www.neurosciences.asso.fr/Annonces/A07032000_1.html.

European Neurological Society (ENS) A professional neurological organization. Web site: www.ensinfo.com.

European Neurology (*Eur. Neurol.*) A neurological journal. Address: S. Karger AG, P.O. Box 10, Allschwilerstrasse, CH-4009 Basel, Switzerland. Web site: http://www.karger.com/journals/ene/ene_jh.htm.

European Neuromuscular Centre A center for coordinating the various medical and scientific affairs of the European Alliance of Muscular Dystrophy Associations. The center provides some research funding. Address: European Neuromuscular Centre, Lt. General van Heutszlaan 6, NL-3743 JN Baarn, The Netherlands. Web site: http://www.enmc.org/ The ENMC published the first edition of *Diagnostic Criteria for Neuromuscular Disorders,* edited by Prof. A.E.H. Emery in 1994. A digital version of the second edition (1988) is now available on the ENMC site http://www.enm.org/nmd/diagnostic.cfm by kind permission of the *Royal Society of Medicine Press.*

euroquol See **quality of life.**

euryblepharon (Gr, wide + the eyelid) A craniofacial malformation in which there is abnormal widening of the palpebral aperture due to deficiency of the palpebral skin.[4]

eurycephalous (Gr, wide + the head) Having a large, broad head.

euryopia See **Greig syndrome.**

Eustachius (Bartolommeo Eustachio, 1524–1574) Italian physician, professor of anatomy at Rome University. He was a contemporary of Vesalius, whose discoveries overshadowed his, not least because Eustachius' illustrations were only discovered and published 140 years after his death. They showed that he had defined numerous anatomical structures not formerly recognized, including the optic and abducens nerves and much of the anatomy of the sympathetic chain.

Evans index The ratio of the transverse diameter of the anterior horns of the lateral ventricles measured at pneumoencephalography to the greatest internal transverse diameter of the skull.

Since pneumoencephalography is now obsolete, so is the index; the CT scan allows far better estimation of the size of the ventricles.

event-related potentials Cortically derived voltage shifts seen when a subject is selectively attentive to a provided stimulus and is required to distinguish a specific stimulus from others. They are relatively independent of the physical characteristics of the stimulus and appear to monitor a substage of information processing. See **contingent negative variation, alpha rhythm.**

evoked potential (evoked response) 1. The potential shift in the cortical dendritic population underlying surface electrodes placed on the scalp, occurring in association with the arrival of impulses signifying peripheral or central stimulation. A wave or complex elicited by and time-locked to a physiological or other stimulus; for instance, an electrical stimulus delivered to a sensory receptor or nerve, or applied directly to a discrete area of the brain and usually requiring computer summation techniques for their detection. (Adapted from the 1974 report of the Committee on Terminology, IFCN. In: Chatrian GE, Bergamini L, Dondey M, et al. A glossary of terms most commonly used by clinical electro-encephalographers. *EEG Clin Neurophysiol,* 1974;**37**:538–548.) Reprinted by kind permission of Blackwell Science.

2. An electrical waveform elicited by and temporally related to a stimulus, most commonly an electrical stimulus delivered to a sensory receptor or nerve, or applied directly to a discrete area of the brain, spinal cord, or muscle. See also **auditory EP, brainstem auditory evoked potential, spinal evoked potential, somatosensory evoked potential, visual evoked potential, compound muscle action potential, compound sensory nerve action potential.**[146] (Adapted from the 1987 Report of the Nomenclature Committee of the American Association of Electromyography and Electrodiagnosis. Used by permission, coyright © 2001, AAEM).

In clinical practice, visual, auditory, somatosensory, and cognitive potentials are those usually recorded, and are regarded as providing reproducible information about the functional status of the relevant afferent sensory channel and as being capable of showing abnormalities where none can be ascertained clinically. Their clinical value has been reviewed.[1008]

Castigated as lucrative, nonspecific, and uninformative by the unconvinced but defended as accurate, relevant, and underused by their champions, the tests in general inform about electrical disturbances within a sensory pathway, assist not at all in pathological diagnosis, and, if regarded as extensions of the clinical examination, provide data that the experienced clinician may find valuable when they confirm his or her clinical impressions, the errant excreta of machines being generally more acceptable to the naïve than are the judgments of experienced physicians.

evoked potential studies The recording and analysis of electrical waveforms of biological origin elicited in response to electrical or physiological stimuli in the peripheral and central nervous system, whereas *nerve conduction studies* refers to studies of waveforms generated in the peripheral nervous system.

There are two systems for naming complex waveforms in which multiple components can be distinguished.

A. The different components are labeled P1 or N1 for the initial positive and negative potentials, respectively, and P2, N2, P3, N3, etc., for subsequent positive and negative potentials.

B. The components are specified by polarity and the average peak latency in normal subjects to the nearest millisecond.

The first nomenclature principle has been used in an abbreviated form to identify the seven positive components of the normal brainstem auditory evoked potential, customarily given in Roman numerals for no obvious reason; thus, I–VII. The second nomenclature principle has been used to identify the positive and negative components of visual (N75, P100) and somatosensory evoked potentials (P9, P11, P13, P14, P20, P23). Regardless of the system of nomenclature employed, it is possible under standardized conditions to establish normal ranges of amplitude, duration, and latency of the individual components of these evoked potentials. The difficulty with the second system is that the latencies of components of evoked potentials depend upon the length of the pathways in the neural tissues.

Thus the components of a somatosensory evoked potential recorded in a child have different average latencies from the same components of one recorded in an adult. Despite this problem, there is no better system available for naming these components at this time. (Adapted from the 1987 Report of the Nomenclature Committee of the American Association of Electromyography and Electrodiagnosis. AAEE glossary of terms in clinical electromyography. *Muscle Nerve* 1987;**10S**:G5-G23. © 1987. Reprinted by permission of John Wiley and Sons, Inc.)

evoked response   See **evoked potential.**

evoked seizures   (reflex epilepsies) Those seizures regularly provoked by physiological or psychic stimuli. The specific external stimuli include sounds or lights, the internal ones, thoughts or memories.

The term was first introduced by Prochaska in the latter part of the eighteenth century but these events were also recognized by Hughlings-**Jackson** and were fully described by **Gowers** (1901). Abrupt changes in illumination, reading, music or other sounds, odors, particular movements, eating, startle, noise, pain, touch, emotional upsurges, and complex activities such as playing cards or chess have been described as precipitants.[5460] Reflex epilepsy is perhaps not the best or most precise term but is in current usage.[3442] See also **eating epilepsy.**

Evoked seizures are classified in Chart E–8.

Chart E–8. Types of Evoked Seizures

1. *Reflex epilepsy syndromes*
   A. Simple stimuli
      i. **Photogenic epilepsy**
         a. Television epilepsy
         b. Self-induced photogenic seizures
      ii. **Startle epilepsy**
      iii. **Hot water epilepsy**
      iv. **Eating epilepsy**
      v. Rubbing the skin
      vi. Tooth-brushing
   B. Complex stimuli
      i. **Primary reading epilepsy**
      ii. **Musicogenic epilepsy**
      iii. Cognitive processing epilepsy
      iv. Playing Mah-Jong
      v. Speech/language
2. *Secondary epilepsy with stimulus evoked seizures*
   A. Simple stimuli such as visual sound stimuli, or bodily movement
      i. Visual input
      ii. Sound
      iii. Movement
      iv. Eating epilepsy
   B. Complex stimuli such as reading or listening to music.
      i. Reading
      ii. Music

evolution   Change in form over generations; descent with modification.

evolution of the nervous system   A concept of Hughlings-**Jackson** regarding the increasing specialization of the nervous system, both up the evolutionary scale and within a hierarchy of organized activity in the human CNS. Evolution consists of a passage from the lowest, most organized centers up to the highest centers, which are constrained by the least organization; from the most simple to the most complex; and from the most automatic to the most voluntary.[47] See also **levels of organization.**

evolving stroke   (stroke-in-evolution) Stroke that is seen to be producing progressive impairment of function with time.

Ewald's Laws   1. A horizontal semicircular canal is maximally stimulated by movement of the endolymph that it contains away from its ampulla. 2. Maximal stimulation of a semicircular canal results in nystagmus with its fast component toward the side which is stimulated, but minimal stimulation produces nystagmus in the other direction.

Ewart phenomenon   The elevation of a ptotic eyelid on swallowing—a synkinesis due to aberrant regeneration of fibers from the seventh to the third cranial nerve, joining fibers innervating the levator palpebrae superioris.[411]

exercise-induced muscle pain and stiffness   A sporadic condition presenting with muscle pain and cramps but with minimal weakness, affecting males more often than females. Serum CK levels are slightly raised, especially after exercise. See http://www.neuro.wustl.edu/neuromuscular/maltbrain.html.

Excerpta Medica; Neurology and Neurosurgery   A neurological review book series. Address: Excerpta Medica, Marketing and Sales Department, P.O. Box 548, 1000 AM Amsterdam, The Netherlands. Web site: http://www.empublications.com/catalogue/titlesearch.cmf.

excessive daytime drowsiness   See **hypersomnolence.**

excessive daytime sleepiness   (EDS, somnolence) Subjective difficulty in maintaining the awake state, coupled with a ready entry into sleep when possible.[249]

The most common cause is **sleep apnea,** but in some cases, the phenomenon represents only an augmentation of the normal tendency to be sleepy in the afternoons, though it can progress to a stage in which the need to sleep during this period is paramount. The result in all cases is lethargy, automatic behavior, fatigue, visual problems, and daytime sleep attacks. The symptoms also appears in Parkinson disease, encephalopathies, the Kline-Levin syndrome, and with other diencephalic lesions. See **hypersomnolence.**

excessive eye blinks   Repetitive blinking either as a result of local ocular irritation or as a prodromal sign of essential blepharospasm, when it is usually bilateral, variable, and associated with ocular irritation and photophobia.[1649]

excessive sleep inertia   See **confusional arousals.**

excitability   The capacity to be activated by or to react to a stimulus.

excitability of nerve   The property of accepting and transmitting an electrical stimulus.

excitable cortex   The motor and premotor regions.

excitation contraction coupling   The series of events whereby the propagated action potential on the muscle fiber surface membrane leads to the twitch contraction of the fiber.

excitatory postsynaptic potential   (EPSP) A local, graded depolarization of a neuron in response to activation by a nerve terminal. cf. **inhibitory postsynaptic potential.**

excitomotor system   That part of the nervous system concerned in the production of reflex action. The term was applied by Marshall **Hall.**

excitotoxins   Substances that cause neuronal death as a result of excessive prolonged membrane depolarization. Examples include glutamate, domoic acid, kainic acid, quisqualate, N-methyl-D-aspartame and biculline, a gamma-aminobutyric acid antagonist.

excyclotropia   Rotation of the eye during attempted downward gaze (as with a fourth cranial nerve palsy).

executive cognitive functions   Royall et al., define these as follows: "The processes that orchestrate relatively simple ideas, movements or actions into complex goal-directed behaviours. Without them, behaviours important for independent living such as cooking, dressing or self-care . . . break down into their component parts."[4836] Conceptual reasoning, inhibition of overlearned patterns of behavior, inhibition of responses to salient stimuli, mental flexibility, set-shifting, organizational ability, planning, regulation of working memory, and fluency of thought are examples.[3151] Loss of executive control produces apathy, irritability, and impaired spontaneity, and self-neglect is considered to reflect frontal lobe dysfunction at either cortical or subcortical levels. See also **Stroop test.**

Executive Interview (EXIT25)   A 25-item instrument providing a standardized assessment of executive control functions and designed to elicit signs of frontal system pathology such as imitation, intrusions, disinhibition, environmental dependency, perseveration, and frontal release, etc. Scores correlate strongly and specifically with left mesiofrontal cerebral blood flow by single photon emission computerized tomography (SPECT) and left frontal system pathology on MRI and are significant independent predictors of level of care among elderly retirees. High scores indicate impairment. A cut-point of 15/50 is recommended.[4833,4836] See also **CLOX, Behavioral Dyscontrol Scale.**

exercise   (from Lat; to drive on or keep occupied) Voluntary muscular activity.

exercise test   Serial electrodiagnostic measurements of the compound muscle action potential (CMAP) every 60 seconds after a 2- to 5-minute period of exercise of the muscle examined.

The test is performed between episodes of weakness in patients with thyrotoxic or **familial periodic paralysis,** in whom there is usually an initial increase in the amplitude of the CMAP immediately after exercise, followed by a progressive decrease.[2772]

exertional headache   See **benign exertional headache.**

Exner, Sigmund   (1846–1926) Austrian physiologist who described a fiber layer near the surface of the cerebral cortex.

exodic   1. Efferent. 2. (Gr, out of + a way—in this case the spinal cord) Marshall **Hall**'s preferred term for reflex motor activity. It has not found favor generally.

exogenous psychosis   See **Bonhoeffer syndrome.**

exophasy   Thoughts uttered; vocal, audible language.

exophoria   A predisposition to ocular divergence as a result of impaired fusion, and shown by the **alternate cover test.**

exophthalmic ophthalmoplegia   The occurrence of proptosis and extraocular muscle pareses in hyperthyroidism. See **dysthyroid ophthalmopathy.**

exophthalmos   (Gr, out + eye) Protrusion of the eye.

exotropia   (divergent strabismus) A condition in which the visual axes of the eyes diverge. See also **WEBINO syndrome.**

expanded disability status scale   See **Kurtzke scale.**

experiential hallucination   The term of **Penfield** for hallucinations of things formerly seen or heard or experienced, occurring as manifestations of spontaneous epileptic seizures.[4403]

experiential illusions   The vivid re-experience of past events in which, as **Penfield** put it, "the subject discovers himself on the stage of the past as well as in the audience of the present."

These illusions were noted by Penfield during electrical stimulation of the upper and lateral parts of the temporal lobe at open operation in conscious epileptic patients, but it was also realized that they occur as components of the syndrome of **partial complex seizures.**

experiential responses   The term of Penfield for hallucinations of things formerly seen, heard, or experienced, and reproduced by stimulation of the cortex at operation.[4403]

experimental allergic encephalomyelitis   A monophasic but sometimes relapsing form of encephalitis induced by a combination of cell-mediated immunity to myelin basic protein and an antibody-mediated reaction to galactocerebroside, etc., in which the pathology closely resembles that of **multiple sclerosis.**

expiration/inspiration ratio   (E:I ratio) The ratio of the heart rate measured on the electrocardiogram during expiration to the rate during inspiration. This is a reliable measure of parasympathetic activity.[2736]

explicit memory   (declarative memory) That form of memory which requires the conscious recall/recognition of specific information which has recently been presented. This is what is asessed by most of the traditional bedside or office memory tests. See also **implicit memory, working memory.**

explicit memory tests   Memory tests which require conscious recall/recognition of specific information which has recently been presented. Memory instructions are usually given at the time of presentation and the time of retention testing to indicate clearly the nature of the task. These tests correspond to most traditional forms of memory tests. See also **implicit memory, working memory.**

exploding head syndrome   The occurrence of the sensation as of a loud noise in the head during sleep onset (non–rapid eye movement sleep stages 1 and 2) in normal people.

The sensation has been likened to a crack, a loud snap, or a bang, often waking the subject who is usually elderly and female. The phenomenon is sometimes familial, occurs over years, and is benign.[4379]

exploring electrode   Any electrode over the scalp or within the brain substance intended to detect EEG activity. Such an electrode is customarily connected to either input terminal 1 or input terminal 2 of an EEG amplifier in bipolar derivations and to input terminal 1 of an EEG amplifier in referential derivations. See also **active electrode, recording electrode, bipolar derivation, referential derivation.** (Adapted from the report of the Committee on Terminology, IFCN,[989] © 1974, with permission from Elsevier Science.)

express saccades   Saccades with unusually short latencies (even of 100 msec) as may occur when the fixation target is extinguished before the new peripheral target appears.[3330]

expressive amusia   Loss of a previously possessed ability to play a musical instrument, to sing, or to reproduce musical themes.

expressive aphasia   See **Broca aphasia, aphasia.**

extended arms test   A test of vestibular system function, in which the subject stands with the arms outstretched and index fingers pointing at those of the examiner similarly held up. Deviation of the subject's fingers on eye closure (in the direction of the slow component of any nystagmus present) suggests vestibular system abnormality.

Extended Scale for Dementia   An expanded version of the **Mattis Dementia Rating Scale.**[2555]

extensive (extended) large subcortical infarcts   Large infarcts of the hemispheric white matter, internal capsule, and basal ganglia due to disease of the internal carotid and/or middle cerebral arteries. The clinical features resemble those of large middle cerebral artery territory infarcts with dense hemiplegia and neuropsychological dysfunctions appropriate to the affected hemisphere. CT and MRI show extensive involvement of the hemispheric white matter and basal ganglia with cortical sparing.

extension-adduction reflex   See **Dagnini sign.**

extensor   (from Lat, to stretch out) That which stretches out; the word applies to those muscles which antagonize the flexors and in general act to lengthen the body (or a part of it) by straightening it.

extensor digitorum brevis reflex   Contraction of this muscle with dorsflexion of the second to fifth toes following a tap on its tendons distally on the dorsum of the inverted and plantar flexed foot. The reflex does not discriminate between L5 and S1 radiculopathies.[3620]

extensor reflex   See **extensor response.**

extensor response   (extensor reflex) Extension of the hip and knee and plantar flexion of the foot with stimulation of the buttock, perineum, and upper thigh on that side.[3648] The **Babinski reflex** is actually an integral part of the flexion reflex, never occurring without reflex contraction of the proximal limb flexors. Accessory to this is reflex extension of the crossed limb, which includes plantar flexion of foot and toes.[5829]

extensor spasms   An epileptic syndrome characterized by abrupt extension of the neck and trunk with extension and abduction of the arms. They are seen typically in the syndrome of **infantile spasms** but are less common than flexor spasms in that condition.[56]

extensor thrust   Reflex extension of the hip and knee with plantar flexion of the foot and toes in response to pressure upwards on the plantar surfaces of the toes; seen in patients with severe but incomplete spinal cord injuries. Flexion may follow each extensor movement, giving the appearance of marching.[3648]

external carotid steal   Diversion of blood from the vertebral and internal carotid systems to supply the territory of an occluded external carotid artery.[365]

external compression headache   (swim-goggle headache) Headache resulting from continued stimulation of cutaneous nerves by the application of pressure, for example, by a band around the head, a tight hat, or goggles worn for the protection of eyes during swimming training. This definition and the following diagnostic criteria are suggested by the Headache Classification Committee of the International Headache Society (Classification of headache disorders, cranial neuralgias and facial pains; and diagnostic criteria for primary headache disorders. *Cephalalgia* 1988;**8**[suppl]: 1–96).

   A. Results from the application of external pressure in the forehead or the scalp
   B. Is felt in the area subjected to pressure
   C. Is a constant pain
   D. Is prevented by avoiding the precipitating cause
   E. Is not associated with organic cranial or intracranial disease

external hamstring reflex   (biceps femoris reflex, lateral hamstring reflex, posterior peroneofemoral reflex) Contraction of this muscle in response to a tap on its tendon in the lateral part of the popliteal fossa. It is normally just palpable, but is increased with pyramidal lesions above the L5 level.

The reflex informs on the state of the L5 and S1 reflex arcs. The **fibular reflex** is similar.

external hydrocephalus   Expansion of the subarachnoid space over the surface of the cortex. See also **internal hydrocephalus, communicating hydrocephalus.**

external malleolar sign   See **Chaddock reflex.**

exteroceptive reflex myoclonus   Reflex myoclonus triggered by exteroceptive rather than proprioceptive afferent discharges, the latter being more commonly identified.[2185]

exteroceptive sensations   Those sensations dependent upon receptors in the skin and comprising touch, temperature, and surface pain. The other group of sensations defined by **Sherrington** was **interoceptive,** now better known as **proprioceptive.**

extinction   (from Lat, to quench or destroy) 1. The failure of sensory events from one side to reach awareness, while the subject is perfectly aware of similar events occurring simultaneously on the other side.

2. The inability to perceive both of two stimuli in the same sensory channel (visual, auditory, tactile) when they are presented simultaneously.

Although testing is usually performed by, e.g., touching the patient on the same spot on each side of the body, touching two places on the *same* side (for example, the face and the hand) may also demonstrate that only one of these can be perceived.[450] See also **sensory competition, simultagnosia.**

Any modality (or modalities) may be affected, both from personal and extrapersonal space. The lesion is usually of the right hemisphere, less commonly affecting the corpus callosum. Reduced motor activity on or toward the neglected side, dressing and constructional apraxias, and denial of illness are often notable when the lesion is of the right hemisphere. See **neglect.**

extraabdominal paraganglionic system   A group of cell masses associated with the autonomic nervous system, characterized by the storage of catecholamine granules and exhibiting chemoreceptor function. They may be situated in the adrenal medulla, glomus jugulare, or carotid body, around the aortic arch, or on the abdominal aorta. They are generally of low malignancy but may metastasize.[6]

extracerebral potential   Any potential that does not originate in the brain and is regarded as an artifact in the EEG record. It may arise from electrical interference external to the subject and recording system, from the subject, from the electrodes and their connections to the subject and the electroencephalograph, and from the EEG machine itself. See **artifact.** (Adapted from the report of the Committee on Terminology, IFCN[989] © 1974, with permission from Elsevier Science.)

extracranial–intracranial bypass surgery   See **EC/IC bypass surgery.**

extradural hemorrhage   See **epidural hemorrhage.**

extramedullary   (Lat, outside + marrow) Outside the spinal cord.

extraocular palsy   Paresis of the extraocular muscles as a result of damage to cranial nerves III, IV, or VI, the motor end-plates, or the muscles themselves, and commonly associated with the complaint of diplopia if vision is retained in both eyes.

extrapyramidal pathways   Efferent cortical neuron systems other than the pyramidal pathways, and all subcortical efferent neuron systems that subserve movement.

extrapyramidal seizures   See **paroxysmal choreoathetosis.**

extrapyramidal signs and cataract   See **Waardenburg syndrome.**

Extrapyramidal Symptom Rating Scale   A 55-item instrument assessing such symptoms.[1023]

extrapyramidal syndromes   Syndromes manifesting excessive involuntary movements (such as **chorea, athetosis, dystonia,** or **tremor**) or deficiency of movement, as in **parkinsonism,** in which the pathology is considered to involve the basal ganglia or their connections.

Diseases of the cerebellum are arbitrarily excluded from this category.

extrapyramidal system   The term of Kinnier **Wilson** for all those efferent mechanisms, apart from the pyramidal tract, which have to do with the control of motor activity. A complex of deep motor nuclei (the basal ganglia) including the striatum, globus pallidus, and substantia nigra, which project through the thalamus to the cortex. Less formally, he referred to these as "the dark basement of the brain."

Although the term is in very general use, the system has no rigid anatomical boundaries, but extends from at least the olives to the cortex; it functions in ways other than those affecting motor control, and how these are achieved remains unknown. The very obvious contribution to motor control of the cerebellum and its pathways nevertheless does not gain it admittance.[3862]

extreme somatosensory evoked potential   High-voltage somatosensory action potentials in response to tactile stimulation of the feet, recorded over the scalp in a small minority of apparently normal children who within 2 years may go on to suffer partial motor seizures for a limited period.[1374]

extrinsic sleep disorders Dyssomnias that are causally related to factors outside the body. They are classified by the **ASDA** as follows:[234]

1. Inadequate sleep hygiene
2. Environmental sleep disorder
3. Altitude insomnia
4. Adjustment sleep disorder
5. Insufficient sleep syndrome
6. Limit-setting sleep disorder
7. Sleep-onset association disorder
8. Food allergy insomnia
9. Nocturnal eating (drinking) syndrome
10. Hypnotic-dependent sleep disorder
11. Stimulant-dependent sleep disorder
12. Alcohol-dependent sleep disorder
13. Toxin-induced sleep disorder
14. Extrinsic sleep disorder not otherwise specified

From *The International Classification of Sleep Disorders Diagnostic and Coding Manual*. Rochester, MN: American Sleep Disorders Association. © 1990. Reproduced by kind permission of the American Academy of Sleep Medicine.

See also **sleep disorders.**

eye blinks Spontaneous blinks are bilateral, paroxysmal, brief, repetitive eye closures occurring continuously and in the absence of obvious external stimuli, their rate correlating with level of central dopaminergic activity.[2944]

eyebrow lifting test A bedside maneuver differentiating ptosis due to facial muscle weakness from that due to paresis of the levator palpebrae superioris. When the eyebrow is pushed up by the examiner's thumb, the narrowing of the palpebral fissure is abolished only in cases of VII palsy.[4222]

eye–jaw synkinesis Movement of the jaw in the direction of gaze; often a normal phenomenon.

eyelid apraxia Difficulty in the voluntary opening or closing of the eyelids, while such movements are possible involuntarily. It is reported in extrapyramidal and motor neuron diseases.[21]

eyelid freezing See **apraxia of eyelid opening.**

eyelid myoclonia with (typical) absences An unusual photosensitive myoclonic epilepsy of childhood and adolescence characterized by marked jerking of the eyelids with upward deviation of the eyes following eye closure, in association with what is otherwise a typical absence attack. The EEG shows 3–5 Hz paroxysmal generalized discharges and irregular 3-Hz spike-and-wave complexes seen especially after eye closure but absent in darkness.[202,2820] See also **photosensitive epilepsies.**

eyelid twitch sign See **Cogan signs.**

eye-of-the-tiger sign Marked decrease of the T2-weighted MRI signal in the pallidal nuclei, with a centrally located area of increased signal, described in **Hallervorden-Spatz disease with acanthocytosis.**[2570]

eye-winking tics Rapid, exaggerated coordinated contractions of the orbicularis oculi muscles, under a degree of voluntary control, increased by boredom or anxiety, and usually occurring in boys. They disappear after a few years.[3320]

Eysenck Personality Inventory A self-administered scale yielding scores on two dimensions of personality: neuroticism–stability and extraversion–intraversion.[1725a]

F wave A compound action potential evoked intermittently from a muscle by a supramaximal electrical stimulus to the nerve. Compared with the maximal amplitude M wave of the same muscle, the F wave has a smaller amplitude (1%–5% of the M wave) and more variable configuration and latencies.

The F wave (so named by Magladery and McDougal in 1950 because they first identified it in muscles of the foot) can be found in many muscles of the upper and lower extremities, and its latency is longer with more distal sites of stimulation. It is due to antidromic activation of motor neurons. (Adapted from the 1987 Report of the Nomenclature Committee of the American Association of Electromyography and Electrodiagnosis. AAEE glossary of terms in clinical electromyography. *Muscle Nerve* 1987;**10S:**G5–G23. Copyright 1987. All rights reserved. Reprinted by permission of John Wiley and Sons, Inc.)

These small, variable, and delayed electrical accompaniments of the muscle potentials are evoked by stimulation of a motor nerve. They do not represent reflexes but are due to the antidromic activation of motoneuron cell bodies in the anterior horn cell pool as a result of a supramaximal electrical stimulus that passes both distally to activate the muscle and proximally back to the spinal cord, evoking the F waves irregularly. The F wave almost always evaluates more than one segmental level. It traverses only the ventral root

Prolonged minimal latency, chronodispersion, persistence, and impersistence or absence of the wave have all been studied, but the parameter most useful in diagnosis remains undetermined[1938] and its methodology unstandardized.[4319] Although routinely performed, this appears to be a test still in search of an application.

F wave tacheodispersion The distribution of the conduction velocities of individual nerve fibers, or of small groups of nerve fibers, as estimated from repetitive recording of 30 or more consecutive F waves in a given nerve. The technique may be more sensitive than routine motor nerve conduction velocity recordings in detecting motor neuropathies.[1030]

FABERE test (**F**lexion, **AB**duction, **E**xternal **R**otation, **E**xtension), See **Patrick test.** Pain during this test suggests sacroiliac or hip joint disease.

Fabry disease (Fabry-Anderson syndrome, angiokeratoma corporis diffusa, trihexose ceramide lipidosis, hereditary dystopic lipidosis) An X-linked recessive lysosomal storage disease (a sphingolipidosis) affecting glycolipid metabolism in which there is abnormal accumulation of ceramide trihexoside in the ganglion cells, the blood vessels, kidneys, corneas, and heart due to deficiency of α-galactosidase A. The genetic defect maps to chromosome Xq21.3q22.

Its major features appear in young adult life and include a deep red papulomacular skin rash mainly involving the swim shorts area and thighs, crises of burning pain in the limbs, edema, hyperhidrosis, fever, corneal opacities, renal impairment, strokes, and peripheral neuropathy, all due to deposition of the abnormal glycolipids.[588,1728]

Fabry in Germany[172] and Dr. W. Anderson in England described the disease in the same year (1898).

Fabry, Johannes (1860–1930) German dermatologist.

Fabry-Anderson syndrome See **Fabry disease.**

face-hand extinction When the subject's face and hand on one side are touched simultaneously by the examiner, the face is dominant—i.e., it is likely to be the touch on the face that is felt rather than that on the hand.

face-hand test A test of tactile inattention in which the subject is touched on one or two points of the body simultaneously and asked to report the location of the stimuli.[1827]

Simultaneous touch stimulations of the cheek and hand on one side are normally both appreciated; children and patients with organic mental syndromes tend not to be aware of the touch on the hand (**extinction**) while they do appreciate that on the face.

In a *variant* of the test, the hand and foot are touched simultaneously. In organic mental disease, the foot "dominates" and the touch on the hand is again "extinguished."[1827]

facet (Lat, a small plane surface) A circumscribed articular surface, as in the vertebral column.

facet syndrome (facet tropism) A developmental or acquired degeneration of the cartilage with subluxation of the facet joints (posterior zygoapophyseal joints) of the vertebrae so that they are aligned in different planes (coronal and sagittal).

This usually occurs at lumbosacral levels, leading to muscle spasm and local pain, aggravated by twisting and extension, referred to the buttocks and the posterior thigh, with stiffness and scoliosis.[2225]

facet tropism See **facet syndrome.**

facial arthromyalgia See **Costen syndrome.**

facial asymmetry A minor dysmorphism recognized in some healthy people and in a proportion of patients with complex partial seizures of temporal lobe origin. Unilateral facial weakness during emotional expression on the side contralateral to the cerebral lesion is the usual sign.[4658]

facial chorea (chronic chorea) See **trigeminal neuralgia.**

facial diplegia   A benign variant form of the syndrome of **multiple cranial nerve palsies** in which bilateral facial weakness is associated with little if any detectable weakness of the limbs, nor sensory loss.[986,5141]

facial hemiatrophy   See **Parry-Romberg syndrome.**

facial hemihypertrophy   See **Friedreich disease.**

facial migraine   See **carotidynia.**

facial myokymia   Worm-like writhings of the facial muscles, usually in the orbicularis oculi, most commonly due to anxiety or overtiredness but sometimes associated with brainstem lesions, as in multiple sclerosis. The definitive diagnosis is made using the EMG, which shows double discharges variably appearing in a regular pattern at 6–100 Hz.[2591]

facial nevi, anomalous cerebral venous return, and hydrocephalus   A rare syndrome manifesting macrocrania, bilateral facial nevi, and anomalous intracerebral venous drainage, described in infancy and once in an adult, suggesting that the prognosis is benign.[5093]

facial palsy   Weakness of the muscles of the face, including the periorbital muscles, as a result of a lesion of the seventh cranial nerve, first described by Nicolaus Friedreich (1761–1836), a German physician, in 1797[583] and thereafter by Sir Charles **Bell** in 1821. In 1903 Cushing reported successful reinnervation after anastomosis with the accessory nerve. See **Bell palsy.**

The nerve was first noted by Thomas **Willis** to be a separate structure from other cranial nerves (the "portio dura"), but was named and numbered by **Soemerring.**

facial paraspasm   See **blepharospasm.**

facial recognition test   A non-memory matching task, used as a test of visual perceptual function.[474]

facial reflex   Visible contraction of the orbicularis oris muscle in response to stretch applied when the examiner's finger is tapped by a reflex hammer while pulling gently on the side of the mouth. The contraction is seen in patients with bilateral, diffuse lesions of the cortex and in those with damage to the corticobulbar fibers from the contralateral hemisphere.

The subject of facial reflexes was reviewed by Kugelberg.[3181]

facial vision of the blind   (fersinn, sixth sense, sense of obstacles) The unexplained ability of the blind to be at least partially aware of the presence of certain objects before them. This might however, be due to aural or thermal cues.

facies paralytica   The facial expression encountered rather constantly in patients with **general paresis;** lack of activity in the muscles of facial expression, asymmetrical and variable facial weakness, and lack of wrinkling of the forehead are described as characteristic.

facilitation   An increase in an electrically measured response following identical stimuli. This occurs in a variety of circumstances:

1. Improvement of neuromuscular transmission resulting in activation of previously inactive muscle fibers. This may be identified in several ways:

   Incrementing response–reproducible increase in the amplitude and area of successive M waves during repetitive nerve stimulation.

   Postactivation or post-tetanic facilitation. Nerve stimulation studies performed within a few seconds after a brief period (2 to 60 seconds) of nerve stimulation producing tetanus or after a strong voluntary contraction may show changes in the configuration of the M wave(s) compared to the results of identical studies of the rested muscle as follows:

   a. Repair of the decrement. A diminution of the decrementing response with slow rates (2 to 5 Hz) of repetitive nerve stimulation.

   b. Increment after exercise. An increase in the amplitude and area of the M wave elicited by a single supramaximal stimulus. Distinguish from pseudofacilitation, which occurs in normal individuals in response to repetitive nerve stimulation at high rates (20 to 50 Hz) or after strong volitional contraction. It probably reflects a reduction in the temporal dispersion of the summation of a constant number of muscle fiber action potentials and is characterized by an increase in the amplitude of the successive M waves with a corresponding decrease in their duration. There is no net change in the area of the negative phase of successive M waves.

2. An increase in the amplitude of the motor evoked potential as a result of background muscle activation.

(From the 2001 Report of the Nomenclature Committee of the American Association of Electromyography and Electrodiagnosis.[10] Used by permission, copyright © 2001, AAEM.)

facilitatory paratonia   A variant of **paratonia** in which the patient acts in the same direction as the passive movement, rather than in the opposite direction. Its presence predicts lower scores on tests of cognitive function.[537]

faciocardiorenal syndrome   A recessively inherited dysmorphic syndrome in which numerous skeletal and visceral abnormalities are associated with mental and developmental delay.[1596]

faciolingual syndrome   A clinical combination of hemiparesis affecting the lower face and the tongue with some degree of dysarthria but without any aphasia. This was first described by Déjèrine and Klumpke[1342] in 1901, who identified the presence of a small infarct in the genu of the contralateral internal capsule. See also **capsular genu syndrome.**

faciolinguopharyngomasticatory diplegia   See **anterior operculum syndrome.**

facioscapulohumeral atrophy   See **hereditary motor neuropathy** (*variants*).

facioscapulohumeral dystrophy   (Landouzy-Déjèrine syndrome) A group of relatively common, slowly progressive, dominantly inherited muscular dystrophies with onset in childhood or youth, in which the common factor is weakness and wasting of the muscles of the shoulder girdle (especially the periscapular and humeral muscles), the face, and the proximal leg muscles, eventually accompanied in most cases by peroneal weakness.[3255] The responsible gene is commonly located at chromosome 4q35, where there is a deletion of a fragment of DNA. Despite the accepted eponym, **Duchenne** described the condition in 1868 (as occurring congenitally).

Both neurogenic[1782] and myopathic diseases with facioscapulohumeral distribution have been identified and in some cases mitochondrial changes have been detected.[5499]

The numerous *variants* include the following:

A lethal, dominantly inherited *infantile* form in which there is a severe muscular dystrophy with onset in infancy and death in adolescence. Although the disease is dominantly inherited, the parent may be only minimally affected. Facial weakness is the first sign, while bulbar dysfunction, hypotonia, progressive proximal weakness, and subsequent respiratory insufficiency follow.[296]

A form with *late exacerbation*

A form with facial sparing[1778]

A disputed *form with recessive inheritance*[335]

A *childhood form* in which features of **Möbius syndrome** are also present[2425]

Facioscapulohumeral dystrophy and deafness A congenital myopathic syndrome characterized by proximal and facial myopathic weakness and deafness. This may be an integral part of the basic syndrome.[788]

Facioscapulohumeral dystrophy and Coats syndrome A dysmorphic syndrome with onset in infancy manifesting also sensorineural deafness, exudative retinal telangiectasias, detached retina and tortuosity of the retinal vessels, ptosis, facial, proximal and distal myopathic weakness, and mental and developmental delay.[2106,5507]

An early-onset form with added *epilepsy and mental retardation*[1992]

A form with hearing loss and tortuosity of the retinal vessels.[2106]

facioscapulohumeral spinal muscular atrophy A variant of the usual proximal pattern of **hereditary motor neuropathy** in which dominantly inherited weakness and wasting occur in the above distribution.[1782] Nevertheless, whether this syndrome represents a neuropathic rather than a dystrophic disorder is not firmly established.

factitious disorder The conscious fabrication of symptoms and signs, regardless of whether the motivation to do so is perceived by the patient. Clues to the presence of this disorder have been suggested by Eisendrath et al.[1620] See also **hysteria.**

faculty (from Lat, capability) 1. A special power or ability of the mind. 2. The academic staff of an institution of learning.

fading athlete syndrome The ascription of declining performance by skilled athletes to neuromuscular disease, a reaction considered to be psychogenic.[4829]

Fahr syndrome See **striatopallidal calcification.**

Fahr, Theodor (1877–1945) German pathologist who graduated at Giessen University and eventually became professor of pathology in Hamburg. His publications concerned mainly renal and vascular diseases. He was not the first to describe familial calcifications of the basal ganglia, nor, in retrospect, have his observations been regarded as completely accurate.

Theodor Fahr

failure of visuoconstructive ability See **constructional apraxia**

faint 1. Weak or languid. 2. (syncope, swooning) Reduction in consciousness with loss of power of the body and the mind as a consequence of reduced cerebral blood flow. See *syncope.*

fainting (from Gr, cut short) A sense of impending dissolution, usually with dimming or loss of vision and eventually loss of consciousness and motor tone, leading to loss of the upright posture and due to reduction in cerebral blood flow.

Fairbank syndrome A developmental anomaly, characterized by facial dysmorphism, short hands and digits, turribrachicephaly, exophthalmos, enlarged sella turcica, and metaphyseal and epiphyseal changes.[2219] See **craniosynostosis.** See **syncope.**

Fajersztajn crossed sciatic sign In sciatic root irritation, the hip can only be flexed when the knee is flexed, not when it is held straight, and pain is felt on the side of the root irritation during performance of the **Lasègue maneuver** on the healthy side.

This amounts to the straight-leg raising test from a different aspect.

fakirism Control of the body's motor and sensory processes as a result of mental concentration. Thus, for example, pain may not be felt in circumstances that would otherwise be extremely unpleasant. During such times the EEG records generalized theta activity.

falciform lobe (from Lat, resembling a sickle) **Schwalbe's** term for the limbic lobe.

Falconer, Murray (1910–1988) Neurosurgeon, born in New Zealand. He practiced at the Guy's-Maudsley Unit in London, where he specialized in the surgical treatment of epilepsy.

Falconer-Weddell syndrome See **thoracic outlet syndrome.**

fall risk index A standardized tool to assess the risk of falling in patients with dysequilibrium.[5591]

fallen fontanelle (caida de mollera) Depression of the anterior fontanelle, a sign of childhood trauma, as in the **battered baby syndrome.**[2299]

Fallopius (Gabriel Fallopio, 1523–1563) Italian professor of anatomy and botany at Padua University. His observations of greatest relevance to neurology were his descriptions of the facial canal in 1561 and of cranial nerves IV, V, IX, and X. His drawings demonstrate that he had noted the anatomy of the arterial circle at the base of the brain well before **Willis.**

false image The less distinct and more peripheral image, coming from the affected eye of a patient with diplopia. The mechanism responsible for the loss of clarity is the reception of light from the object by a part of the retina other than the macula.

false localizing signs Clinical neurological signs which do not arise from damage to the area of the primary lesion in question, and which suggest incorrectly that the mass is situated at a certain site.

The lesion itself is usually a tumor causing increased intracranial pressure, either the mass or more often its pressure effect leading to traction upon, or displacement or compression of, other intracranial structures, or leading to interruption of their blood supply.

The classic example is the unilateral sixth cranial nerve palsy due to stretching of the nerve as a result of increased intracranial pressure rather than as a result of the direct compressive effect of the mass. Other examples include dementia with temporal lobe tumors; anosmia; visual field defects; anisocoria, pupillary paresis, nystagmus, ptosis, sixth nerve palsy, and gaze palsies; initial contralateral mydriasis with frontal lobe hemorrhage;[997] fifth nerve paresthesia or pain; cerebellar signs; pyramidal deficits; neck stiffness; proptosis; hypothalamic disturbances; and decerebrate rigidity, all associated with increased intracranial pressure.

Signs referable to dysfunction of regions in immediate proximity to a lesion are considered to be "neighborhood" signs and not falsely localizing.[2046]

false Rombergism Wildly excessive swaying without falling, seen when the **Romberg test** is performed by subjects with psychogenic complaints of imbalance.

The remarkable gyrations occasionally witnessed actually indicate superior balance.

false sago palm A tree growing in the Western Pacific region, the seeds of which contain the neurotoxic agent *Cycas circinalis* considered responsible for **Lytico-Bodig.**

falx cerebri, falx cerebelli (Lat, sickle + brain or little brain) Condensations of the dura mater which divide and support the two lobes of each structure.

falx syndrome Acute and severe paresis and/or simple motor seizures of one or both legs as a result of an interhemispheric subdural hematoma or empyema.[3431]

familial acephalgic migraine The occurrence of migraine auras (usually visual and paresthetic and precipitated by bright lights) in the absence of headache. The condition has been reported as dominantly inherited.[6125]

familial acoustic neuroma See **neurofibromatosis 2.**

familial adult myoclonic epilepsy (FAME) A dominantly inherited variant of progressive myoclonic epilepsy or juvenile myoclonic epilepsy reported first from Japan.[4459] It differs from these conditions in its onset in adult life and usual genetic locus at chromosome 8q24, but like them presents with variable limb myoclonus, some tonic-clonic seizures, and a benign course.

familial Alzheimer disease See **Alzheimer disease.**

familial amaurotic idiocy (Tay Sachs disease) See **GM$_2$ gangliosidoses.**

familial amyloid neuropathy A group of variously inherited inherited diseases characterized by the deposition of fibrillar material in body tissues, predominantly in the nutrient blood vessels of the peripheral nervous system. Mutations in the transthyretin protein are responsible for the sensory or autonomic neuropathies that constitute the major clinical syndromes, though ocular and cardiac manifestations are also common.

Forms that have been identified are listed in Chart F–1. See also **amyloid neuropathy.** For a recent review, see Adams (2001).[35]

Chart F–1. Forms of Familial Amyloid Neuropathy

Amyloidosis type 1, dominant (Andrade, Portuguese type) A dominantly inherited syndrome due to an abnormality of the plasma protein transthyretin (prealbumin), for which the abnormal gene maps to 18q11.2q12.1. Clinically, the condition manifests an axonal thin-fiber neuropathy that presents with spontaneous pains in youth, and with more generalized motor, sensory, and autonomic dysfunction plus cardiac, renal, and ocular involvement later. Selective early losses of A-delta and C fibers in the peripheral nerves are characteristic.[174,175] At least 40 other transthyretin mutations producing amyloidoses are also described.

Amyloidosis type 1, recessive type (Portuguese type) A recessively inherited syndrome also due to transthyretin abnormalities, characterized by the onset in mature adult life of axonal thick- and thin-fiber sensorimotor and autonomic neuropathy (often presenting as carpal tunnel syndrome) with vitreous opacities and cardiac involvement.[6103]

Amyloidosis type 2 (Rukavina or Indiana types) A dominantly inherited acropathic sensorimotor axonal neuropathy with adult onset, mainly affecting the arms. The early symptoms are those of **carpal tunnel syndrome,** evidence of generalized polyneuropathy appearing years later. Sclerodermatous skin thickening and both corneal and vitreous opacities are common early and cardiac involvement is a late complication.[3572,4848] Apolipoprotein-A1 is the mutated protein in this case.

Amyloidosis type 3 (Van Allen or Iowa type) A dominantly inherited syndrome with young adult onset of severe and widespread sensorimotor neuropathy with associated cataracts, deafness, peptic ulcer disease, and later autonomic effects, due to widespread deposition of amyloid which eventually leads to renal failure. Type 3 familial amyloid polyneuropathy is thus similar to type 1, but has a later age of onset.[5700,5701] The genetic defect maps to 11q23–q24.

Amyloidosis type 4 (Finnish type, Gelsolin variant, cranial neuropathy) A dominantly inherited form characterized by the onset in mature adult life of facial and bulbar cranial neuropathies, followed years later by mild thick- and thin-fiber sensorimotor and autonomic neuropathy, atrophy of the skin, corneal lattice dystrophy, and renal and cardiac involvement.[3843] The genetic base substitution responsible is located at 9q33, codon 187 of plasma gelsolin complementary DNA.[3070]

Amyloidosis type 5 with cranial neuropathy and corneal lattice dystrophy (Jewish type) A variant due to abnormality of gelosis, for which the responsible gene maps to 9q32–q34.[2003]

Amyloidosis type 6 with variant prealbumin (Appalachian type) A dominantly inherited form with late onset.[5815]

Amyloidosis type 7 (oculomeningeal or Ohio type) A form characterized by the onset of cerebrovascular changes in young adult life, leading to emotional lability, abnormality in consciousness, seizures, dementia, and pyramidal and cerebellar signs.[2211]

Other *variants* are *trigeminal neuropathy with nasal ulceration,*[5283] and *dominant familial amyloid neuropathy with severe cardiac involvement,* an unusually early and severe cardiomyopathy occurring in the setting of familial amyloidosis,[4933] and a *dominantly inherited form* mapping to chromosome 20.[3050]
See also **Dutch cerebral hemorrhage.**

familial amyotrophic chorea with acanthocytosis See **neuroacanthocytosis.**

familial amyotrophic lateral sclerosis See **amyotrophic lateral sclerosis.**

familial antiphospholipid antibody syndrome A genetically determined disorder of blood predisposing to stroke, and as yet unmapped.

familial apoceruloplasmin deficiency A rare, inherited dysmetabolic state that presents with dystonias and retinal degeneration.[3920]

familial ataxic diplegia See **Fanconi-Turler syndrome.**

familial benign essential chorea See **hereditary nonprogressive chorea.** See also **Huntington disease.**

familial benign neonatal convulsions An inherited tendency to generalized tonic-clonic seizures in the neonatal period. The responsible gene maps to chromosome 20.

familial bilateral striatal necrosis (infantile bilateral striatal necrosis, familial holotopistic striatal necrosis, juvenile Leigh disease, familial cerebral degeneration affecting chiefly the lenticular nucleus, symmetrical degeneration of the neostriatum, familial striatal degeneration) A rare, maternally inherited, missense mitochondrial ATPase mutation causing a pallidonigrostriatal degeneration resembling **Leigh disease** without the progression. The condition is characterized by childhood onset of an acute disturbance of consciousness followed by progressive rigidity with pyramidal signs, hyperactivity, involuntary movements such as athetosis, tremor and myoclonus, and dysphasia. Loss of spontaneous movements, seizures, mental retardation, and stereotyped responses to all stimuli are also described. Subacutely progressive athetosis and rigidity lead to hypotonia, dysarthria and dysphagia, and mental retardation.

Pathologically there is marked symmetrical neuronal loss in the caudate nucleus and putamen. The brainstem is spared.[4359,4739,5578] The condition might represent a form of parainfectious encephalitis,[1955] but an X-linked form is considered to be a variant of Leigh disease.[3754]

familial brachial plexus palsy See **neuralgic amyotrophy.**

familial British dementia with amyloid angiopathy An autosomal dominant condition characterized by a dementia, progressive spastic tetraparesis, and cerebellar ataxia with onset in the sixth decade and due to a point mutation in the BRI gene. A common ancestor has been identified between the large pedigree and a case report of "familial cerebellar ataxia with amyloid angiopathy." Neurological examination was abnormal in three patients, with limb and gait ataxia and mild spastic paraparesis. Three patients had impaired recognition and recall memory and another had mild impairment of delayed visual recall. All affected individuals had an abnormal MRI of the brain, consisting of deep white-matter hyperintensity (T2-weighted scans) and lacunar infarcts, but no intracerebral hemorrhage. The corpus callosum was affected particularly, and in one patient it was severely atrophic.[3792]

familial calcification of the basal ganglia   See **striatopallidal calcification.**

familial calcification of the brain, iron storage, and porphyria   See **striatopallidal calcification.**

familial calcifying polioencephalopathy   See **striatopallidal calcification.**

familial capillary-venous leptomeningeal angiomatosis   See **Divry–van Bogaert syndrome.**

familial carpal tunnel syndrome   See **carpal tunnel syndrome.**[1278]

familial cavernous angioma/hemangioma of the retina   (Gass syndrome) A dominantly inherited syndrome of retinal cavernous angioma and/or skin hemangiomas.[1482]

familial cerebellar ataxia and hypogonadism   The association of cerebellar ataxia with primary hypogonadism. Whether this is fortuitous or etiologically meaningful is not clear.[3710]

familial cerebellar ataxia with cerebrovascular amyloid   See **cerebellar ataxias** (*variants*).

familial cerebral amyloid angiopathy   (Dutch type) A dominantly inherited condition mapped to 21q–21.3q22.05 and leading to cerebral hemorrhages.

familial cerebral amyloidosis with spongiform encephalopathy   A dominantly inherited infiltrative spongiform encephalopathy, also involving the peripheral nervous system and affecting mature adults who develop dementia; apraxias; ophthalmoplegia; nystagmus; pyramidal; extrapyramidal, and cerebellar signs; and both sensory and autonomic neuropathies. See **Gerstmann-Straussler-Scheinker syndrome.**

familial cerebral cavernous hemangiomas   See **cavernous angioma.**

familial cerebral degeneration chiefly affecting the lenticular nucleus   See **infantile bilateral striatal necrosis.**

familial cerebral sarcoma   The rare occurrence of cerebral fibrosarcomas in more than one family member.[2006]

familial cerebromeningeal angiomatosis   See **Divry–van Bogaert syndrome.**

familial chorea with acanthocytosis   See **neuroacanthocytosis.**

familial chorea with myoclonic epilepsy   A dominantly inherited syndrome consisting of chorea, ataxia, myoclonus, seizures, and dementia.[5471] See **myoclonus.**

familial congenital corneal anesthesia   A rare, dominantly inherited syndrome of isolated corneal anesthesia with secondary trophic lesions.[3106]

familial cortical tremor, epilepsy, and mental retardation   A rare, dominantly inherited syndrome manifesting action tremor, seizures and mental retardation with diffuse spike-and-wave EEG activity and photoparoxysmal responses as well as the usual features of **cortical reflex myoclonus.**[1633]

familial cramps and muscle pain   A syndrome with its onset in youth, characterized by muscle pain or cramps, incontinence, and the clinical and pathological features of mild myopathy. See **adolescent familial cramps.**

familial Creutzfeldt-Jakob disease   See **Creutzfeldt-Jakob disease.**

familial Cushing syndrome   (Swiss syndrome, Carney complex) A rare autosomal dominant disorder characterized by mesenchymal tumors including cardiac and cutaneous myxomas, and by spotty skin pigmentation, functional endocrine overactivity, and schwannomas of the peripheral nerves.[907]

familial cutaneous amyloidosis with systemic manifestations   A congenital syndrome manifesting cloudy corneas, malabsorption, recurrent infections, hyperkeratosis, patchy skin pigmentation, seizures, and mental and developmental delay. See also **familial amyloid neuropathy.**

familial degeneration of the pallidonigral system   A fatal degenerative disorder of early childhood, manifesting febrile episodes, hepatosplenomegaly, anemia, pyramidal signs, and seizures. Pathological findings include degeneration of the globus pallidus, subthalamic nucleus, and substantia nigra.[3736]

familial distal dysautonomia   A familial syndrome of autonomic dysfunction affecting the hands and feet as well as vasomotor, pilomotor, and sudomotor function, without other evidence of peripheral somatic neuropathy. The condition may be dominantly inherited.[4726]

familial dysautonomia   See **hereditary sensory and autonomic neuropathy type 3** and **Riley-Day syndrome.**

familial dyskinesia and facial myokymia   A dominantly inherited disorder characterized by involuntary chorea-like movements and perioral and periorbital myokymia with onset in early childhood or adolescence. The movements are paroxysmal initially but increase in frequency and severity, and may become constant in the third decade, stabilizing or even improving thereafter. The adventitious movements are worsened by anxiety but not by voluntary movement, startle, caffeine, or alcohol. The disease is socially disabling, but there is no intellectual impairment or decrease in lifespan. Its genetic basis is not yet determined.[1794]

familial dyslexia   See **dyslexia.** The genetic abnormality in this familial form has been localized to the short arm of chromosome 15.

familial dystonic choreoathetosis (syndrome of Mount and Reback) see **familial paroxysmal dystonic choreoathetosis.**

familial encephalopathy and basal ganglion calcification   See **striatopallidal calcification.**

familial epilepsy and yellow teeth   A syndrome of severe seizures in infancy, with mental and motor delay, pyramidal signs, and unusually colored teeth.[3114]

familial episodic ataxia   See **cerebellar ataxia.**

familial erythrophagocytic lymphohistiocytosis (Omenn syndrome) A lethal, recessively inherited, congenital dysmorphic syndrome manifesting also visceromegaly, anemia, low white blood cell and platelet counts, recurrent infections (including meningitis and encephalitis), seizures, ataxia, pyramidal signs, and neurodegenerative regression. Widespread infiltration with reticulum cells is usually found. Low-density areas due to gliosis and demyelination are seen in the white matter on CT scanning.[4237]

familial essential benign chorea   See **hereditary essential chorea, Huntington disease.**

familial essential myoclonus   A dominantly inherited syndrome of stimulus- and movement-sensitive myoclonic jerks associated with rhythmic discharges alternating with asynchronous, dysrhythmic complexes on the EEG, alleviated by alcohol consumption and sometimes associated also with **essential tremor.**[3136]

familial extrapyramidal disease with polyneuropathy   A dominantly inherited syndrome characterized by symptoms of **Parkinson disease** with onset in mature adult life. The disorder is also characterized by the delayed development of an axonal or demyelinating sensorimotor peripheral neuropathy with distal weakness, ataxia, muscle wasting, and loss of reflexes.[860]

In *variant* forms, postencephalitic parkinsonism is accompanied by amyotrophy.

familial frontotemporal dementia   A dementing illness with parkinsonism, due to mutations in the tau gene on chromosome 17.[6072] See **frontotemporal dementia.**

familial hearing loss, polyneuropathy, and optic atrophy   An autosomal or X-linked recessively transmitted syndrome manifesting progressive neural deafness from childhood with polyneuropathy and optic atrophy.[2541]

familial hemiplegic migraine   (cerebellar migraine) A dominantly inherited or sporadic form of **migraine with aura** occurring first in youth and characterized by paroxysmal headaches, many with hemiplegia occurring before, during, or after the headache phase and lasting for hours or days. Attacks may be precipitated by head trauma. The attack is usually part of the aura of migraine and lasts less than an hour (migraine with typical aura). Typically, there is a visual aura that is fol-lowed by the onset of slowly progressive unilateral sensory or motor symptoms. Fever, dysarthria, aphasia, and reduction in consciousness are common associated symptoms. Rarely, symptoms can last up to a week (migraine with pronounced aura).[2665]

The condition is due to missense mutations in the *CACNA1A* gene on chromosome 19p13 in half the cases, and in a fifth there are permanent cerebellar signs, indicating genetic heterogeneity.[2886] Various mutations at the same site are associated with **episodic ataxia** type 2 and delayed cerebral edema and with fatal coma after minor head trauma.

The following diagnostic criteria are suggested by the Headache Classification Committee of the International Headache Society[1051] (Classification of headache disorders, cranial neuralgias and facial pains; and diagnostic criteria for primary headache disorders. *Cephalalgia* 1988;**8**[suppl]:1–96.[1051] Reprinted by kind permission of Blackwell Science.)

A. Fulfils criteria for **migraine with aura.**
B. The aura includes some degree of hemiparesis and may be prolonged.
C. At least one first-degree relative has identical attacks.

Variants include the following:

Hemiplegic migraine and ataxia A dominantly inherited syndrome with onset in youth, characterized by paroxysmal headaches, ophthalmoplegia, nystagmus, ataxia, hemiplegia, and tremor.

Hemiplegic migraine, nystagmus, and deafness A rare, presumably dominantly inherited syndrome comprising these features.[6091] Associations with ataxia (cerebellar migraine), tremor, and retinal degeneration have also been reported.[335,6127]

A form in which *hemihypesthesia* occurs instead of hemiplegia

familial holotopistic striatal necrosis   See **infantile bilateral striatal necrosis.**

familial hyperkalemic periodic paralysis   See **familial periodic paralysis.**

familial hyperthyroidism   See **Frank syndrome.**

familial hypertrophic interstitial neuropathy   See **hereditary motor and sensory neuropathy type 3.**

familial hypertrophic neuropathy with gammopathy (familial hypertrophic paraprotein polyneuritis) A dominantly inherited hypertrophic polyneuropathy with slow progression and both motor and sensory features, accompanied by a gammopathy.

familial hypertrophic paraprotein polyneuritis   See **familial hypertrophic neuropathy with gammopathy.**

familial hypoparathyroidism, sensorineural deafness, and renal dysplasia   A rare, dominantly inherited syndrome characterized by these features.[570]

familial hypoplasia of the carotid arteries   (carotid hypoplasia) A developmental dysgenetic syndrome with onset in youth; a rare cause of atherothrombotic brain infarction.[337]

familial idiopathic brain calcification A dominantly inherited syndrome characterized by calcification within the basal ganglia associated with slowly progressive intellectual decline, parkinsonism, seizures and mild cerebellar ataxia.[3105]An X-linked dominant form is also described.

familial inclusion body myositis See **inclusion body myositis.**

familial infantile myasthenia A recessive variant of childhood **myasthenia gravis,** in which the mother is unaffected; weakness after activity is more severe than in the classic form and leads to severe respiratory and feeding difficulties from birth but does not involve the extraocular muscles. Fatigability occurs with the usual decrementing response to repetitive stimulation on EMG, and there is a tendency to later recurrence of apnea caused by crying, vomiting, or fever. There is nevertheless a trend toward spontaneous remission.

The pathogenesis is a defect in acetylcholine resynthesis. The motor end-plate potential amplitude is normal in rested muscle with stimulation but a decrement is seen after exercise or electrical stimulation of muscle. The synaptic vesicles are abnormally small.[773,1658,3964]

familial infantile myopathy A **mitochondrial** disorder due to cytochrome-*c* oxidase deficiency, presenting in early childhood with proximal muscle weakness and wasting.

familial intermittent ataxia An X-linked syndrome in which the intermittent ataxia is accompanied by abnormalities of pyruvate metabolism, and with cerebral pathology resembling that of **Leigh disease.** There is response to acetazolamide.

It is likely that this represents more than one condition.[3444] See **cerebellar ataxias.**

familial inverted chorea A rare, dominantly inherited condition with the onset in infancy of chorea and athetosis of the legs only, with added pyramidal signs.[1870]

familial juvenile macular degeneration See **Stargardt syndrome.**

familial juvenile motor neuron disease See **amyotrophic lateral sclerosis.**

familial limb-girdle myasthenia A form of **myasthenia gravis** in which there is selective muscle involvement, giving the appearance of muscular dystrophy. Proximal weakness without atrophy or bulbar or ocular involvement is notable, but there is a good response to anticholinesterase drugs.[3790]

familial lumbosacral syringomyelia See **hereditary sensory and autonomic neuropathy.**

familial lysis of type 1 fibers A rare form of congenital myopathy in which **cores** extend across the whole width of a muscle fiber.[6] See also **multicore myopathy, congenital myopathy.**

familial macrocephaly See **familial megalencephaly.**

familial megalencephaly (familial macrocephaly) A congenital syndrome of uncomplicated macrocephaly.[337]

familial meralgia paresthetica See **meralgia paresthetica.**[3675]

familial methemaglobinemia A recessively inherited diffuse encephalopathy presenting with mental retardation as a result of deficiency of methemaglobin reductase.

familial migraine with vertigo and essential tremor A dominantly inerited syndrome of episodic vertigo, migraine headaches, and essential tremor, with onset in youth and with no defined genetic linkage.[313]

familial mitochondrial myopathy A dominantly inherited myopathy associated with single large or multiple deletions of mitochondrial DNA manifesting bulbar and girdle weakness, progressive external ophthalmoplegia, and sensorineural deafness.[6124]

familial motor neuron disease A dominantly inherited syndrome of adult onset with features resembling those of acquired **amyotrophic lateral sclerosis** but with a somewhat younger onset.

Variant forms with associated sensory loss or deafness, or with onset in youth, have also been described.

familial moyamoya disease A dominantly inherited polygenic disorder mapped to 3p24.2–p26, predisposing to stroke. See **moyamoya disease.**

familial multicore disease with focal loss of cross-striations and ophthalmoplegia (familial myopathy with focal loss of cross-striations) A congenital myopathy, considered to be a subvariety of **multicore disease,** presenting with ptosis and ophthalmoplegia from birth, proximal muscle weakness with delayed motor development, hypotonia and hyperreflexia, and with muscle biopsy findings of multicores and a focal loss of cross striations.[1663,5442]

familial multi-infarct dementia (familial vascular encephalopathy, familial spastic paraparesis and dementia) An inherited syndrome of young adult life characterized by vascular dementia with facial weakness, pseudobulbar and limb pyramidal signs, and cerebral atrophy. See also **familial subcortical dementia with arteriosclerotic leukoencephalopathy, Worster-Drought syndrome.**

familial multilocular encephalomalacia See **disseminated encephalomalacia with cavity formation.**

familial multiple symmetric lipomatosis with peripheral neuropathy (Madelung disease, Launois-Bensaude syndrome, benign symmetric lipomatosis) A rare, dominant or recessively inherited condition affecting mainly middle-aged males and characterized by the development of large, non-encapsulated lipomata on the neck, shoulders, and proximal arms, with an axonal polyneuropathy affecting mainly the larger myelinated fibers. It was first described by Sir Benjamin Brodie in 1846.[956]

familial multisystem atrophy A dominantly inherited syndrome, different phenotypes exhibiting combinations of clumsiness, spasticity, optic atrophy, and mental deterioration resembling that of **thalamic dementia.**[2950]

familial myasthenia gravis See **myasthenia gravis.**

familial myoclonic dementia (Stern-Garcin syndrome, subacute degeneration of the thalamus) A dominantly inherited form of **thalamic dementia** characterized by having a subacute course of progressive dementia (memory loss, psychotic behavior, frontal release signs, and hallucinations) occurring over a period of up to 2 years, associated with myoclonus.[3433,5341] See **fatal familial insomnia.**

familial myoclonic epilepsy See **Unverricht-Lundborg-Lafora syndrome.**

familial myoclonus epilepsy and choreoathetosis See **hereditary dentatorubropallidoluysian atrophy.**

familial myofibrillar inclusion body myopathy A dominantly inherited myopathy with these microscopic features. The disorder is not always symptomatic.[1044]

familial myoglobinuria See **myoglobinuria.**

familial myopathy with focal loss of cross-striations See **familial multicore disease with focal loss of cross-striations and ophthalmoplegia.**

familial myopathy with muscle cramps A hereditary nonprogressive muscle disorder with adult onset presenting with mild proximal muscle weakness and painless muscle cramps following exercise, associated with the finding of multiple cores in muscle biopsy specimens low in oxidative enzymes.[533]

familial myopathy with myofibrillar lysis A hereditary myopathy presenting with hypotonia in the infant and later with proximal weakness. Muscle biopsy findings are of accumulations of subsarcolemmal granules.[888]

familial myopathy with thrombocytopenia A hereditary nonprogressive muscle disorder with onset in childhood, comprising proximal and distal myopathic weakness and thrombocytopenia.[337]

familial myosclerosis (myodysplasia fibrosa multiplex) A condition marked by the replacement of muscle by fibrous issue, giving it a hard consistency on palpation. It is probably not a single entity, but represents the end stage of various primary neurogenic and primary myopathic disorders.[701]

familial myotubular myopathy A nonprogressive, X-linked recessive myopathic syndrome presenting with hypotonia and respiratory difficulty in the postnatal period, with subsequent involvement of the extraocular, facial, and neck muscles and with areflexia. Muscle biopsy findings include small muscle fibers with a peripheral rim of myofibrils in the central zone containing either a single nucleus or a collection of sarcoplasmic components.[5741] See also **centronuclear myopathies.**

familial neuroacanthocytosis See **neuroacanthocytosis.**

familial neuromuscular disease with type 1 fiber hypoplasia, tubular aggregates, cardiomyopathy, and myasthenic features A recessively inherited syndrome comprising these manifestations, with lordosis, joint contractures, and normal anti-acetylchline receptor antibody levels, and with onset in childhood.[1477]

familial neuropathy with dementia A slowly progressive syndrome of cerebral atrophy associated with visual loss resulting from both pigmentary retinal degeneration and optic atrophy, accompanied by the clinical features of hereditary motor and sensory neuropathy and by attacks of vomiting and a labile blood pressure, indicating autonomic involvement.[4286] See also **NARP syndrome.**

familial normokalemic periodic paralysis See **familial periodic paralysis.**

familial occipital calcifications, hemorrhagic strokes, leukoencephalopathy, dementia, and external carotid dysplasia (FOCHS-LADD) An inherited cerebrovascular disease with these features.[2724]

familial occipital dysplasia See **Chiari malformation.**

familial olivopontocerebellar degenerations See **cerebellar ataxias.**[3125]

familial opticoacoustic nerve degeneration and polyneuropathy A syndrome of progressive optic atrophy and sensorineural deafness complicating **hereditary motor and sensory neuropathy type 2** and with probably X-linked inheritance.[4791]

familial orthochromic leukodystrophy A rare, inherited degeneration of white matter resembling **Pelizaeus-Merzbacher disease.** Clinical features include early onset, psychomotor decline, pyramidal signs, progressive loss of vision, speech, and hearing, and eventual decerebration and death.

familial orthostatic hypotension See **progressive autonomic failure.**

familial paralysis of horizontal gaze A recessively inherited syndrome consisting of paretic horizontal gaze and progressive scoliosis, sometimes associated with bilateral facial myokymia. Convergence, vertical gaze, and pupillary constriction are normal.[5101]

familial parkinsonism-dementia syndrome A recessively inherited syndrome characterized by mental retardation, parkinsonism, pyramidal signs, and external ophthalmoplegia beginning in the third decade and progressing for many years.[3692]

familial paroxysmal ataxia (familial periodic ataxia, familial vestibulocerebellar ataxia) A rare, dominantly inherited syndrome in which patients experience recurrent attacks of vertigo, nystagmus, or cerebellar incoordination in the absence of multiple sclerosis and without detectable inborn errors of metabolism.

Clinically, the attacks are accompanied by rotary, dissociated, vertical, or downbeating nystagmus, the latter suggesting the presence of a medullary lesion.[1490] See also **cerebellar ataxias** (*variants*).

In another dominantly inherited *variant* form, myokymia is associated.[5725] It responds to acetazolamide.[2284] Yet another form, in which the movements are induced by exercise, is also differentiated.

familial paroxysmal choreoathetosis See **paroxysmal kinesigenic choreoathetosis.**

familial paroxysmal dystonia See **paroxysmal kinesigenic choreoathetosis.**

familial paroxysmal dystonic choreoathetosis (syndrome of Mount and Reback, familial paroxysmal dystonia) A rare sporadic or dominantly inherited involuntary movement disorder, usually with childhood onset, in which frequent and prolonged attacks of dystonic posturing, choreoathetosis, or ballism are induced by exercise, emotion, coffee or tea, or alcohol consumption without alteration in consciousness or on the EEG, but not induced by startle.[3234,4019]

Attacks similarly produced but lasting less than 5 minutes are known as **paroxysmal kinesigenic choreoathetosis.**[3017]

Variants are similar disorders in which the attacks are induced by startle, exercise, or other stresses (*kinesigenic*[2189] and *nonkinesigenic*[4019] varieties are reviewed by Baraitser[335]); *familial paroxysmal hypogenic dystonia,* a dominantly inherited syndrome of painful dystonic flexion spasms occurring during non–rapid eye movement sleep;[3314] and a form in which myokymia also occurs and the other symptoms are relieved by brief periods of sleep.[861]

familial paroxysmal kinesigenic ataxia A familial syndrome consisting of paroxysmal ataxia, shaking, or titubation, lasting minutes and repeated many times each day, with evidence of continuous abnormal motor unit activity (**myokymia**), the impulses being generated in peripheral nerves.

familial partial epilepsy with variable foci A dominantly inherited seizure disorder with onset in youth presenting varied clinical and EEG manifestations within the same kinship, and possibly linked to a mutation on chromosome 2.[4948]

familial periodic ataxia See **familial paroxysmal ataxia**

familial periodic paralysis Dominantly inherited sodium- or calcium channelopathies in which episodic bouts of weakness occur because of genetically determined abnormalities in potassium metabolism; these are followed by recovery of strength. During the paralytic episodes, muscle fibers are refractory to any form of electrical stimulation. Two (perhaps three) major forms are described in Chart F–2.

Chart F–2. Forms of Familial Periodic Paralysis

Type 1: hypokalemic A rare, dominantly inherited disease seldom expressed in females, manifest by episodes of flaccid paralysis of limb and trunk muscles and areflexia lasting from 12 to 24 hours, in association with reduced serum potassium levels at 1.5–2.5 mEq/L and the usual ECG changes of hypokalemia.[4385] The responsible gene is mapped to 1q32, the site of the *CACN1S* dihydropyridine receptor calcium channel á-subunit.

Provocative factors include rest after exercise, carbohydrate ingestion, alcohol ingestion, physical or emotional trauma, cold, epinephrine, and steroids. Eyelid myotonia and permanent mild proximal weakness are often noted.

A similar syndrome (*thyrotoxic periodic paralysis*) is yet another type; described mainly in the Orient, it may complicate hyperthyroidism, particularly in Japanese people.[4166] See also **potassium exercise test.**

Type 2: hyperkalemic (adynamia episodica hereditaria, paramyotonia congenita, Gamstorp syndrome) A dominantly inherited sodium channel disorder with onset in early childhood, (abating in adult life), manifesting recurrent brief attacks of proximal muscle weakness and flaccidity and myotonia markedly increased by cold, and with elevated serum potassium levels during the attacks in about half of the subjects. Cardiac rhythm disturbances may occur.[3424] The attacks are provoked by rest after exercise, hunger, exertion, or potassium administration, and are aborted by intravenous calcium, but in some cases are allayed by further activity or by eating.

As in the hypokalemic form, permanent mild proximal weakness is often noted. Myotonia of the tongue, face, and thenar muscles and lid lag may also be found. Raised serum potassium levels are characteristic during the attacks.[2014] The responsible gene maps to 17q13.1–ql3.3, where there are various *SCN4A* point mutations affecting the sodium channel á-subunit.

In an *acquired form,* chronic hyperkalemia produces the same clinical picture. *Myotonic periodic paralysis* may be another variant.

See also **myotonia fluctuans, myotonia permanens, paramtotonia congenita.**

Type 3: normokalemic A dominantly inherited syndrome characterized by onset during the first decade of life, episodes of often severe paralysis occurring at intervals of 1 to 3 months lasting from 2 days to 3 weeks, leading to quadriplegia and weakness of the masseter muscles, but not affecting facial expression, bladder and bowel function, or respiratory muscles. The episodes are provoked by rest after exertion, prolonged inactivity, alcohol consumption, cold, and dampness. Administration of potassium chloride brings on an attack or worsens the symptoms, but the plasma potassium level is normal during the attacks.[4507]

The position of this rare syndrome is uncertain, because its manifestations closely resemble those of the *hyperkalemic* form, and it is recognized that serum potassium levels vary according to the part of the body from which the blood is drawn.

familial peroneal atrophy and ataxia   A form of **hereditary motor and sensory neuropathy** manifesting also cataract and both cerebellar and pyramidal signs.

familial poliodystrophy, mitochondrial myopathy, and lactic acidemia   A rare form of **mitochondrial encephalomyelopathy.**

familial polyradiculopathy syndrome   A dominantly inherited syndrome with adult onset characterized by painful paresthesias, progressive centripetal sensory loss, fasciculations, and severe muscle wasting. The cause is unknown.[1138]

familial posterior column ataxia   See **Biemond ataxia.**

familial presenile dementia with psychosis   A dominantly inherited, slowly progressive, dementing disease characterized by initial belligerent antisocial behavior and later dementia, distinct from **Alzheimer disease,** with which, however, it shares some pathological features.[5411]

familial presenile dementia with spastic paralysis   See **congophilic angiopathy.**

familial prion disease   See **Creutzfeldt-Jakob disease, Gerstmann-Scheinker-Strauss syndrome.** The responsible gene maps to 20pter-p12.

familial progressive bulbospinal muscular atrophy   See **X-linked bulbospinal neuronopathy.**

familial progressive myoclonus and ataxia   A dominantly inherited syndrome of childhood, characterized by slowly progressive motor impairment (limb ataxia and tremor) with intermittent myoclonic and generalized tonic-clonic seizures but without intellectual impairment.[2110]

familial progressive subcortical gliosis   See **progressive subcortical gliosis.**

familial protein intolerance   (lysininuric protein intolerance, dibasic aminoaciduria II) A rare, diffuse encephalopathy characterized by recurrent vomiting, diarrhea, hepatic cirrhosis, severe physical and mental retardation, mild intestinal malabsorption, and increased urinary excretion of lysine, ornithine, and arginine. Protein feeding causes hyperammonemia, asterixis, and attacks of stupor.[5166]

familial Q-T prolongation syndrome   A rare syndrome with two *variants*: a *dominant form* (Romano-Ward syndrome), consisting of prolongation of the Q-T interval on the ECG, giving rise to syncopal attacks,[4832] and a *recessive form* (Jervell and Lange-Nielsen syndrome), which is identical to the dominant form but with the addition of congenital deafmutism.[2854]

familial rectal pain   A dominantly inherited syndrome characterized by episodes of burning rectal pain followed by flushing of the legs and provoked by defecation. Associated features include ocular pain (caused by cold wind or other irritants) and jaw pain, triggered by the sight of food. The findings from the neurological examination and all laboratory studies including EEG are normal. The attacks might represent forms of dysautonomia, migraine, or epilepsy; the cause is not known.[5005]

familial recurrent brachial plexus neuropathy   See **hereditary brachial plexopathy.**

familial recurrent polyneuropathy   See **hereditary pressure-sensitive neuropathy.**

familial recurrent pressure palsies   See **hereditary pressure-sensitive neuropathy.**

familial renal-retinal dystrophy   See **Senior-Loken syndrome.**

familial restless legs syndrome   See **restless legs syndrome.**

familial sleep apnea–plus syndrome   A dominantly inherited syndrome consisting of sleep apnea with anosmia, color blindness, partial complex seizures, and cognitive dysfunction.

Variants of the syndrome include forms manifesting **multiple system atrophy, myotonic dystrophy, olivopontocerebellar atrophy, cervicomedullary lesions, glaucoma,** or **ophthalmoplegia.**[3594]

familial sleep paralysis   An X-linked recessive syndrome seen at any age and characterized by the occurrence of **sleep paralysis** without other features of the **narcolepsy** complex.[4811] See **ASDA** diagnostic classification, **sleep disorders.**[234,4337]

familial spasmodic torticollis   A dystonic syndrome inherited either dominantly or recessively and characterized by the onset in youth or early adult life of torticollis without progression of the dystonia to other regions.[5579]

familial spastic ataxia   A dominantly or recessively inherited syndrome characterized by the variable appearance of slowly progressive cerebellar and pyramidal signs and optic atrophy in childhood or adult life. See **cerebellar ataxias** (*variants*).

familial spastic paralysis/paraparesis   See **hereditary spastic paraplegia.**

familial spastic paraparesis and deafness   See **hereditary spastic paraplegia.**

familial spastic paraparesis and dementia See **familial multi-infarct dementia, Worster-Drought syndrome.**

familial spastic paraparesis, peroneal neuropathy, and crural hypopigmentation See **hereditary spastic paraplegia.**

familial spastic paraplegia with amyotrophy of the hands See **hereditary spastic paraplegia.**

familial spinocerebellar ataxia See **cerebellar ataxias** (*variants*).

familial spinocerebellar degeneration with corneal dystrophy See **cerebellar ataxias** (*variants*).

familial static ophthalmoplegia A rare, dominantly inherited (occasionally recessive or X-linked) syndrome of pure external ocular muscle weakness, presenting as ptosis with or without ophthalmoparesis.[3319] The cause may be either a myopathy or nuclear agenesis. See **Möbius syndrome.**

familial stiff man syndrome See **neuromyotonia.**

familial striatal degeneration See **familial bilateral striatal necrosis.**

familial subcortical dementia with arteriosclerotic leukoencephalopathy (chronic familial vascular encephalopathy, hereditary multi-infarct dementia) A dominantly inherited syndrome of mid-adult life characterized by recurrent attacks of focal neurological deficits including **subcortical dementia** and pseudobulbar palsy, due to multiple small infarcts in the white matter, basal ganglia, thalamus, and brainstem. Their appearance resembles that of leukoencephalopathies on CT or MRI scans.[3666] See also **familial multi-infarct dementia, Worster-Drought syndrome.**

familial tapetoretinal degeneration and epilepsy A rare inherited childhood syndrome of retinitis pigmentosa, generalized tonic-clonic seizures, and mental and developmental delay.[1089]

familial temporal lobe epilepsy A dominantly inherited syndrome of simple (seldom complex) partial seizures with psychic and autonomic manifestations, and occasional secondary generalization, with onset in youth or early adult life. The condition appears to be genetically heterogeneous.[506]

familial tremor See **essential tremor.**

familial vascular encephalopathy See **familial multi-infarct dementia.**

familial vestibulocerebellar ataxia See **familial paroxysmal ataxia.**

familial vestibulocerebellar dysfunction A syndrome characterized by motion sickness and rebound nystagmus in which the nystagmus is of the type 1 vestibular form, the slow phase of the optokinetic response is defective, and the vestibulo-optic reflex fails to be suppressed.[5533]

familial visceral myopathy (oculogastrointestinal muscular dystrophy) A group of rare genetic diseases of childhood or youth characterized by degeneration, atrophy, and fibrosis of the intestinal muscles, with or without diffuse neurological abnormalities, autonomic insufficiency, and denervation hypersensitivity of the pupil and esophageal smooth muscle. Chronic intestinal pseudo-obstruction is a common presentation. Neuronal intranuclear inclusion bodies are found in the submucosal and myenteric neurons as well as in the brain, spinal cord, autonomic nervous system, and peripheral nerves. The detrusor muscle may also be affected.[5007]

Type 1 is dominantly inherited, and the upper intestine is affected; *type 2* is recessive, and the stomach and small bowel are involved; *type 3*, also recessive, affects the whole length of the alimentary tract.[3913]

The recessive forms have also been associated with progressive external ophthalmoplegia, and a severe sensorimotor peripheral neuropathy.[6044]

familial visceral neuropathy A recessively inherited syndrome characterized by chronic intestinal pseudo-obstruction, with or without diffuse neurological abnormalities, autonomic insufficiency, and denervation hypersensitivity of the pupillary and esophageal muscles but with neuronal intranuclear inclusions in the submucosal and myenteric neurons and in the brain.[3717]

In a *variant* dominantly inherited form, the small bowel is affected in isolation and intranuclear inclusions are not found.

familial X-linked myalgia and cramps A nonprogressive myopathy associated with a deletion in the dystrophic gene.

Clinically, the condition presents with muscle cramps and myalgia, especially following activity, and with raised serum levels of creatine kinase.[2227]

Families Of Spinal Muscular Atrophy A charitable organization in this field with chapters in many of the United States, Canada, Australia, and Italy. Web site: http:/www.fsma.org/interact.shtml.

famous faces test A test of remote memory in which the subject is asked to name celebrities from previous years, shown in photographs.[85] See also **Wechsler Adult Intelligence Scale.**

Fanconi pancytopenia A recessively inherited, congenital dysmorphic syndrome manifesting also short stature; congenital cardiac anomalies; hematological, dermal, skeletal, and genital maldevelopments; asplenia; recurrent infections; nystagmus; strabismus; microcephaly; and mental and developmental delay.[1740]

Fanconi-Turler syndrome (familial ataxic diplegia) A congenital syndrome consisting of nonprogressive cerebellar ataxia, uncoordinated eye movements, and mental retardation; it is probably a form of olivopontocerebellar atrophy.[1741] See also **cerebellar ataxias.**

fantaisiste ataxia   Variability of voluntary limb movement from one moment to the next, as may be seen in patients with **sensory ataxia.**

far point   That most distant place from which rays of light entering the eye are focused upon the retina rather than anterior or posterior to it. In the emmetropic (normally refracting) eye, this point is at infinity; but in myopia, it may be only inches away from the cornea. The nearer the far point, the greater the degree of myopia.

Faraday, Michael   (1791–1867) English physicist who discovered inductive electricity.

faradic nystagmus   See **vestibular nystagmus.**

faradism   The term suggested by **Duchenne** de Boulogne for the application of induced currents to cause muscle excitation, in honor of Michael **Faraday.**

Farber disease   (lipogranulomatosis, ceramidase deficiency, ceramide lactoside lipidosis) A rare, recessively inherited lysosomal storage disease in which a deficiency of ceramidase is the key biochemical abnormality, leading to the deposition of chondroitin sulfate B.

It is manifest in infants by joint swelling and stiffness, mainly at the wrists and ankles, with the development of contractures, mental retardation, short stature, skin pigmentation, hepatomegaly, respiratory distress, hoarseness, diarrhea and vomiting, inanition, and early death.[1743] Cloudy corneas or sclerocornea and a macular red spot may be seen.

far-field   A region of electrical potential where the isopotential voltage lines associated with a current source change slowly over a short distance. Some use the term *far-field potential* to designate a potential that does not change in latency, amplitude, or polarity over infinite distances; alternative designations include *boundary potential* and *junctional potential.* The terms *near-field* and *far-field* are arbitrary designations as there are no agreed-upon criteria defining where the near-field ends and the far-field begins. Compare with **near-field.** (From the 2001 Report of the Nomenclature Committee of the American Association of Electromyography and Electrodiagnosis.[10] Used by permission, copyright © 2001, AAEM.)

Farnsworth-Munsell 100 hue test   A test in which movable disks of different hues but with the same saturation and brightness, arranged in trays, are to be sorted along the continuum red–yellow–blue/green–blue–purple/red, as a test of color discrimination.

FAS test   A test of the ability to generate words, and of controlled word association, in which the subject is asked to think of as many words as possible, beginning with the letter *F,* then with *A,* and finally with *S.* This is said to be a sensitive indicator of lesions of the frontal lobes.

fascicle   See **fasciculus.**

fasciculation potential   The electric activity associated with a fasciculation which has the configuration of a motor unit activation potential but which occurs spontaneously. Most commonly occur sporadically and are termed "single fasciculation potentials." Occasionally the potentials occur as a grouped discharge and are termed a "brief repetitive discharge." The repetitive firing of adjacent fasciculation potentials, when numerous, may produce an undulating movement of muscle (see myokymia). Use of the terms *benign fasciculation* and *malignant fasciculation* is discouraged. Instead, the configuration of the potentials, peak to-peak amplitude, duration, number of phases, stability of configuration, and frequency of occurrence should be specified. (From the 2001 Report of the Nomenclature Committee of the American Association of Electromyography and Electrodiagnosis.[10] Used by permission, copyright © 2001, AAEM.)

fasciculations   1. Clinically, spontaneous contractions of all of the myofibrils comprising a motor unit and most likely arising from the intramuscular motor nerve terminal.[3302] The twitches do not move joints but can be seen and felt by the subject or by an observer. Most arise from the distal part of the axon. Unless accompanied by wasting and weakness, they may be considered benign, and are extremely common in normal subjects. The word is presumably derived from the following entry, a bundle of muscle fibers contracting in this instance. The term was coined by **Denny-Brown.**

2. The random, spontaneous twitching of a group of muscle fibers belonging to a single motor unit. The twitch may produce movement of the overlying skin (if in limb or trunk muscles) or mucous membrane (if in the tongue). If the motor unit is sufficiently large, an associated joint movement may be observed. The electric activity associated with the twitch is termed a "fasciculation potential." See also **myokymia.**[10]

fasciculus   (Lat, a little bundle) (fascicle) The term is synonymous with *tract, crus, column, funiculus and fillet,* or *lemniscus,* all being variously employed in anatomy to add a little interest to an otherwise dry subject. The word *fasciculus* is usually used with reference to a bundle of nerve fibers (e.g., the spinothalamic tract) and tends to be succeeded by geographical directions in Latin and an eponym; thus fasciculus anterolateralis superficialis of Gowers.

fasciculus cuneatus   See **Burdach column.**

FAST   See **Frenchay aphasia screening test.**

fast activity (beta activity)   EEG activity of a frequency higher than that of the **alpha rhythm.**

fast alpha variant rhythm   A characteristic rhythm at 14–20 Hz, detected most prominently over the posterior regions of the head which may alternate or be intermixed with **alpha rhythms.** It is blocked or attenuated by attention (especially visual) and by mental effort. (Adapted from the report of the Committee on Terminology, IFCN,[989] © 1974, with permission from Elsevier Science).

fast pain (first pain) A bright, sharp, pricking, painful sensation following almost immediately upon discrete local nociceptive stimulation. This is presumably related to that sensation called **epicritic** by **Head;** the second pain felt was **protopathic pain** in Head's terminology.

fast paroxysmal rhythms   See **generalized paroxysmal fast activity.**

fast spike–wave   See **Six-Hz slow spike-and-waves.**

fat embolism   A clinical syndrome occurring 1–3 days after severe trauma in a small minority of subjects. The clinical features include petechiae, pulmonary insufficiency, retinal hemorrhages, and an encephalopathy with confusion, reduced conscious level, seizures, and focal signs.[1727]

fat stains   Dyes such as Sudan IV and Oil Red O, which preferentially stain neutral fat bright red in histological specimens.

fatal cutaneo-intestinal syndrome   See **Degos syndrome.**

fatal familial infantile glycogen storage disease   See **glycogen storage diseases.**

fatal familial insomnia (subacute degeneration of the thalamus, familial myoclonic dementia) A rapidly progressive, dominantly inherited prion disease of middle and late adult life beginning with difficulty in initiating sleep and leading within a few months to a total lack of non–rapid eye movement sleep, and later to spontaneous lapses from quiet wakefulness into a sleep state with enacted dreams; memory deficits with **chronotaraxis,** dysautonomia, and motor signs. Mutation of a prion protein gene at codon 178 has been detected. A sporadic form is also reported

The above findings are accompanied by autonomic hyperactivity, with salivation, fever, hyperhidrosis, hypertension, tachycardia, and tachypnea. In late stages of the disorder, dysarthria, tremor, spontaneous and reflex myoclonus, ataxia, dystonic posturing, and pyramidal signs supervene and lead to coma and finally death. There is no alteration in cognitive function until the patient's alertness is impaired. Thalamic atrophy may be detected, and spongiform encephalopathy and, clinically, cerebellar ataxia and features suggesting Creutzfeldt-Jakob disease have been found in association. Diagnostic criteria are given in Chart F–3.[234,4805]

Chart F–3. Diagnostic Criteria for Fatal
Familial Insomnia

A. A complaint of insomnia is initially present.
B. Autonomic hyperactivity is present, with pyrexia, excessive salivation, hyperhidrosis or anidrosis, and cardiac and respiratory dysfunction.
C. A familial pattern is present.
D. There is progression to stupor, coma, and death within 24 months.
E. Pathological examination demonstrates degeneration of anterior and dorsomedial thalamic nuclei.

F. Polysomnograhic monitoring demonstrates one or more of the following:
 1. Absence of slow-wave sleep
 2. Dissociated rapid eye movement sleep
 3. Myoclonus and tremor-like muscle activity
G. The insomnia is not the result of another medical or psychiatric disorder, for example, Alzheimer dementia, Creutzfeldt-Jakob disease, or schizophrenia.
H. It does not meet the diagnostic criteria for other sleep disorders, e.g., REM sleep behavior disorder.[3803]

Adapted from The International Classification of Sleep Disorder Diagnostic and Coding Manual. *Rochester, MN: American Sleep Disorders Association,* © *1990. Reproduced by kind permission of the American Academy of Sleep Medicine.*

fatal infantile encephalomyopathy   See **acute encephalopathy of infancy.**

fatal infantile leukodystrophy (childhood ataxia with diffuse CNS hypomyelination, CACH, myelinopathia centralis diffusa, vanishing white matter (VWM) disease; OMIM 603896) A genetically determined progressive leukodystrophy with a relapsing–remitting course and an unknown molecular basis, although the VWM locus has been mapped to chromosome 3q27.4.

Clinical characteristics are progressive ataxic diplegia starting between the ages of 1.5 and 5 years after normal early neurologic development and with rapid progression. Seizures, dysarthria, and optic atrophy are frequently found. In some patients, the disease starts acutely, progressing with recurrent episodes of neurologic deterioration and lethargy, exacerbated by febrile illness and minor head trauma.[1927]

fatal infantile mitochondrial disease   See **acute encephalopathy of infancy.**

fatal infantile mitochondrial myopathy and hepatopathy (fatal infantile myopathy) A fatal expression of inherited deficiency in cytochrome-*c* oxidase (complex IV) with by the complete absence of activity of this enzyme in all muscle fibers, occurring with or without cardiomyopathy and renal and hepatic dysfunction. Type 1 fibers have central nuclei while a focal decrease in oxidative enzymes affects mainly the larger type 2 fibers.[3317]

Clinically, hypotonia, myotonia, weakness, ophthalmoplegia, and both feeding and respiratory difficulties are noted shortly after birth; aminoaciduria and lactic acidosis are later detected. Death occurs before the end of the first year.[1448] See also **acute encephalopathy of infancy.**

fatal infantile muscle phosphofructokinase deficiency   See **glycogen storage diseases.**

fatal infantile myopathy   See **fatal infantile mitochondrial myopathy and hepatopathy.**

fatigability   1. Failure to maintain the required maximum force or output of power during sustained or repeated muscle contractions. Central and peripheral forms are recognized. 2. Slow recovery after a period of activation of muscles.

When referring to unusually early tiring after muscular activity, this is the cardinal sign of **myasthenia gravis,** but when (and more commonly) accompanied by a feeling of lack of energy to accomplish such tasks so that they are not attempted in the first place, this is the **chronic fatigue syndrome,** of which **somatic dysthymia** (masked depression) is a far more common cause. Both **central fatigue** and **psychological fatigue** are recognized.[777]

fatigue   1. A sense of weariness and inertia complicated by sleepiness, perceived weakness, and often subjective dyspnea, usually accompanying disorders of the upper motor neuron such as **Parkinson disease** and **multiple sclerosis,** in **chronic fatigue syndrome,** and in the presence of severe systemic disease. 2. In EMG practice, a state of depressed responsiveness resulting from protracted activity and requiring an appreciable recovery time. 3. (muscle fatigue) A state of depressed responsiveness resulting from activity. Muscle fatigue is a reduction in contraction force following repeated voluntary contraction or electric stimulation.[10] See also **central fatigue, Piper instrument,** and the following entries of fatigue scales, none of which has obvious advantages over the others.

Fatigue Assessment Instrument   A self-report tool used to evaluate the severity and quality of fatigue in patients with multiple sclerosis.[3171]

Fatigue Descriptive Scale   A self-report tool used to evaluate the severity and quality of fatigue.

fatigue failure   Fracture of a vertebral neural arch as a result of repetitive stress, as in athletes. The usual result is **spondylolysis,** presenting clinically as subacute low back pain.[1974]

Fatigue Impact Scale   A 40-item inventory assessing the effects of pathological fatigue upon the physical, cognitive, and psychosocial aspects of daily living. The scale has been used mainly in studies of patients with the **chronic fatigue syndrome** and **multiple sclerosis.**[1876]

fatigue nystagmus   A form of **end-point nystagmus** appearing after prolonged maintenance of lateral gaze. See also **physiological nystagmus.**

fatigue paresis   Weakness noted at night in comparison with recovery from paresis in the morning immediately after sleep. The difference in size is obtained by measurement of photographs.

Fatigue Severity Scale   A tool used to evaluate the severity and quality of fatigue in patients with multiple sclerosis.[3170]

fatigue testing   Methods of testing for fatigue: (*1*) the output of a subject is measured while exercising at 10% of maximum capacity, the load increasing by a further 10% every minute; and (*2*) direct electrical stimulation of a contracting muscle is performed, and any increase in the mechanical twitch response so produced is recorded.[777]

Functional grades can be assigned to patients on the basis of their scores on these tests.

Fatty Oxidation Disorders Network   A charitable organization. Tel: 910-547-8682, 513-574–7150. Web site: http:/www.fodsupport.org/.

faucial reflex   The gag reflex.

Fazio, E.   (1849–1902) Italian physician.

Fazio-Londe syndrome   (progressive bulbar paralysis of childhood, bulbar spinal muscular atrophy of childhood) A dominantly inherited progressive bulbar palsy in children or young adults, presenting with facial weakness, dysphagia, drooling, dysarthria, and dysphonia, with later progression to the involvement of other cranial and spinal nerves.[3628,4796] See **amyotrophic lateral sclerosis, hereditary motor neuropathy.**

The condition was described independently by the Italian and French authors in 1892–3; it may represent a variant of amyotrophic lateral sclerosis. P.F.L. Londe (1865–1944) was a French neurologist.[1750]

Variants include a *recessive form* with onset in infancy, in which involvement of the oculomotor nerves and pyramidal system occur as well as the bulbar palsy; a form with *juvenile onset and slow progression,* which may be a genetically determined form of amyotrophic lateral sclerosis;[2874] *progressive adult-onset bulbar paresis,* a dominantly inherited syndrome of pure lower motor neuron bulbar palsy;[3483] **Vialetto–van Laere syndrome;** and *spinal muscular atrophy with optic atrophy and deafness* (see **hereditary motor and sensory neuropathy, type 6**).[335]

febrile convulsions   (seizures) A common "location-related" epileptic disorder occurring in children between the ages of 6 months and 5 years, characterized by the occurrence of occasional epileptic seizures only during the course of rising fever, in children without intracranial infection or other definable cause. Most febrile convulsions are brief and uncomplicated, but some may be more prolonged (over 15–30 minutes) and these may be followed by transient or permanent neurological sequelae, such as the **HHE syndrome.** Risk factors for subsequent epilepsy include seizures lasting longer than 15 minutes; recurrence of a seizure within 24 hours, and focal neurologic features following a seizure. The condition is thought to be dominantly inherited with reduced penetrance. A locus (FEB3) maps to 2q23–24.

Children may also convulse as a result of brain injury caused by an infection also causing fever, or when fever unmasks a preexisting tendency to suffer recurrent seizures.[56]

febrile delirium   See **delirium.**

febrile reflex anoxic seizures   (febrile syncope) Brief tonic seizures resembling **anoxic seizures** but occurring during the course of a febrile illness at the stage of rising temperature. They can be induced by eyeball compression and are thus likely to represent the effect of an excessive vagal response. The diagnosis of **febrile convulsions** has often been made in such cases.[2056]

febrile seizure   An **epileptic seizure** occurring in childhood after age 1 month, associated with a febrile illness not caused by an infection of the CNS, without previous neonatal seizures or a previous unprovoked seizure, and not meeting criteria for other acute symptomatic seizures.[1115]

febrile seizure with neonatal seizure   One or more neonatal seizures in a child who has also experienced one or more febrile seizures as defined here.[1115]

febrile syncope   See **febrile reflex anoxic seizures.**

feeling-tone   See **affect.**

Feer disease   See **pink disease.**

Fegeler syndrome   The association of a port-wine nevus in the distribution of the fifth cranial nerve, with weakness and hyperesthesia in the ipsilateral arm and leg. This would be diagnosed as **Sturge-Weber syndrome** were it not that the features appear for the first time following a head injury.[1750]

Feil, Andre   (b. 1884) French neurologist. See **Klippel-Feil anomaly.**

Feingold syndrome   1. (*deafness-oligo/syndactyly*) A congenital dysmorphic syndrome manifesting also numerous skeletal malformations, sensorineural deafness, and plagiocephaly.[337] 2. (*microcephaly–hand abnormality–fistula*) A congenital dysmorphic syndrome manifesting also duodenal atresia, skeletal abnormalities, tracheooesophageal fistula, rockerbottom feet, and microcephaly.[337] 3. (*retardation–short stature–cleft palate–abnormal ears*) A congenital dysmorphic syndrome manifesting also short stature, hoarse voice, spina bifida occulta, brachycephaly, macrocephaly, distal and proximal myopathic weakness, and mental and developmental delay.[337]

femoral neuralgia   Constant, aching pain within the distribution of the femoral nerve. The character of the pain differs from that of the more classic cranial neuralgias, and unlike in them, motor or sensory deficits may be present. Although listed in the IASP taxonomy, the description is also accurate for any femoral neuropathy.

Depending on the severity of the damage to the nerve, weakness of the quadriceps and reduction in the knee jerk and sensory disturbances on the anterior and medial aspects of the thigh may or may not be present.

femoral neuropathy   Damage to this nerve as a result of compression, stretch, direct injury, radiation, or ischemia, with resultant weakness of the quadriceps, iliacus, and sartorius muscles and usually sensory loss in the territories of the medial and intermediate cutaneous nerves of the thigh and saphenous nerve.[3191]

femoral reflex   Extension of the hip and knee in response to irritation of the skin of the upper thigh; a sign of a pyramidal tract lesion.

femoral stretch test   (Ely test) Passive extension of the hip of a patient lying prone with the knee straight, or flexion of the knee of the prone patient; in each case, maneuvers that put traction on the femoral nerve, causing pain in the anterior thigh in patients with L3 root irritation, but also with tight hamstring muscles. The test was described by Wassermann in 1918. See **reverse straight leg raising.** See also **bent-knee pulling.**

fenestra parietalia symmetricae   See **Catlin mark.**

fenestrations   Spaces between capillary cells, not present within the blood–brain barrier, where these cells are joined by tight junctions.

Fenton syndrome   A congenital or childhood dysmorphic syndrome manifesting ataxia, skin photosensitivity, short stature, skeletal abnormalities, ichthyosis, and mental and developmental delay.[337]

Ferguson-Critchley syndrome   (autosomal dominant cerebellar ataxia, type I, hereditary spastic paraplegia with ocular and extrapyramidal symptoms) See **cerebellar ataxias.** This is the condition suffered by the Drew family of Walworth.

Fernel, Jean-Francois   (1506–1588) French physician to King Henri II, memorable because he gave the first intimation of the existence of reflex activity in the nervous system.

Fernhoff syndrome   A congenital dysmorphic syndrome characterized also by microcephaly.[337]

ferric chloride reaction   A urine test based upon the fact that at a pH below 7, the ferric iron reacts with a variety of drugs having a cyclic structure, and with ketones, to produce a color change (usually green).

Sir David Ferrier

Ferrier, Sir David   (1843–1928) Scottish neurophysiologist and neurologist who graduated from Edinburgh in 1868. His studies of animals and patients at the West Riding Lunatic Asylum led to his demonstration that functions such as speech and motor activity are precisely localized in the human cerebral cortex (though not in the areas corresponding to those suggested by the phrenologists). He later moved to London, where he was a colleague of Hughlings-**Jackson** on his appointment to the **National Hospital** in 1880; he was also on the staff at Kings College Hospital, where he performed new, precise experiments in animals.[1800]

His localization of auditory function to the superior temporal gyrus, using faradic (alternating) currents or ablation experiments,[2511] led to his remarkable definition of the cerebral motor and sensory areas in his book *The Functions of the Brain* (London, 1876, dedicated to Hughlings-Jackson), although his conclusions were at first widely criticized. In a second book, *The Localisation of Cerebral Disease* (dedicated to Charcot), he analyzed in some depth the case of Phineas **Gage** and refined his original observations on the regionalization of cerebral function at a time when, despite **Hitzig** and **Gall** or because of **Spurzheim,** such considerations were not widely accepted. His cavalier attitude toward the preceding work of others was, however, a cause of controversy. Combining the results of his and Hughlings-**Jackson**'s clinical cases, he delivered the Croonian lectures for 1890 on the topic of cerebral localization. He was elected a Fellow of the Royal Society and, continuing the tradition of the regular publication of neurological reports from the West Riding Asylum, to which he had contributed, was a founder of *Brain*.

fersinn   See **facial vision of the blind.**

festination   (from Lat, to hurry) Acceleration of the rate of activity. In neurology, the word is usually used to describe the rapid but small paces of patients with **Parkinson disease.**

fetal akinesia deformation sequence   A collection of developmental anomalies that can be associated with decreased fetal motility in utero as a result of any neuromuscular, connective tissue, or other disease.[3931] See also **Pena-Shokeir phenotype.**

fetal alcohol syndrome   A dysmorphic syndrome also manifesting growth retardation, hypotonia, and cardiac and skeletal abnormalities in infants born to between 2% and 30% of mothers who have ingested excessive alcohol during pregnancy.[1050] Other neurological features include microcephaly, tremor, cavernous hemangiomas, and mental and developmental delay.[1824]

The following diagnostic criteria have been suggested:[1799]

A. Growth retardation
   Prenatal or postnatal weight or length (below the tenth centile) corrected for gestational age
B. Central nervous system
   Microcephaly (below the third centile); brain malformations; developmental delay; behavioral disorders; cognitive impairment
C. Dysmophism
   Short palpebral fissures, elongated mid-face, long and flat philtrum, thin upper lip, flattened maxilla

fetal aminopterin/methotrexate syndrome   The occurrence of short stature, dysplastic low-set ears, hypertelorism, prominent eyes, small mandible, cleft palate, absent fingers, syndactyly, ossification defects of the skull, and hydrocephalus in babies born to women exposed to methotrexate in pregnancy.[5103]

fetal anticonvulsant syndrome   Dysmorphic syndromes with certain other features occurring secondary to intrauterine exposure to certain anticonvulsant agents, although the linkage is not precise. See **fetal trimethadione syndrome, fetal hydantoin syndrome, fetal valproate syndrome.**

fetal hydantoin syndrome   (acrofacial syndrome) The occurrence of any of the following abnormalities in babies born to women exposed to hydantoins during pregnancy: short stature, generalized hirsutism, low frontal hairline, metopic ridges, small nose with a depressed nasal bridge, ptosis, mild hypertelorism, cleft lip and palate, congenital cardiac anomalies, hypoplastic phalanges and nails, dislocation of the hip, delayed closure of the fontanelles, and mental and developmental delay.[3001]

Craniosynostosis affecting the sagittal and coronal sutures is also reported.

fetal nigral transplantation   The instillation of nigral cells from aborted fetuses into the caudate/lenticular nuclei of patients with severe **Parkinson disease** in an attempt to relieve symptoms, especially rigidity and akinesia, tremor being unaffected by the procedure.

fetal reflexes   See **developmental reflexes.**

fetal toluene syndrome   The occurrence of unusual hair whorls, narrow forehead, low-set and prominent ears, deep-set eyes, short palpebral fissures, epicanthic folds, depressed nasal bridge, small mandible, simple philtrum, thin upper lip, abnormal palmar creases, hypoplastic nails, microcephaly, spasticity, and mental and developmental delay in babies born to women exposed to toluene during pregnancy.[337]

fetal trimethiadone syndrome   A prenatal syndrome comprising any of the following abnormalities in babies born to women exposed to trimethadione during pregnancy: short stature, overfolded ear helix, ptosis, epicanthic folds, small upturned nose, wide nasal bridge, micrognathia, cleft palate, congenital cardiac, skeletal or genital anomalies, brachycephaly, and mental and developmental delay.[1771]

fetal valproate syndrome   A prenatal syndrome seen in an infant whose mother ingested sodium valproate during the pregnancy. It comprises any of the following abnormalities: infraorbital creases, epicanthic folds, upturned nose, depressed nasal bridge, psychomotor delay, and spinal dysraphism.[1446]

fetal vitamin A syndrome   A congenital dysmorphic syndrome characterized by absence of the auditory canal, microphthalmia with blindness, micrognathia, cleft palate, congenital cardiac anomalies, mental and developmental delay, microcephaly, cerebral atrophy, porencephaly, hydrocephalus, and the **Dandy-Walker malformation.**

fetal warfarin syndrome   A dysmorphic syndrome of mental and physical delay with optic atrophy, seizures, hypotonia, and skeletal anomalies occurring in infants born to mothers who took anticoagulants during pregnancy.[1467]

Feuerstein-Mills syndrome   See **epidermal nevus syndrome.**

feverfew   An herb, the leaves of which contain parthenolide, a butyrolactone that prevents the secretion of serotonin from platelets and leukocytes and suppresses prostaglandin release. This may explain why it is at present a popular herbal remedy for migraine.[274]

FG syndrome   (of Opitz) A congenital, X-linked, recessive dysmorphic syndrome characterized by dolichocephaly or scaphocephaly resulting from synostosis affecting the sagittal suture, joint contractures, macrocephaly, hypertelorism, hydrocephalus, callosal agenesis, seizures, antimongolian slant to the eyes, strabismus, severe hypotonia, sensorineural deafness, congenital cardiac anomalies, anal atresia, and mental and developmental delay.[4248]

fiber   (from Lat, a thread) An elongated cell, usually an axon or a myofibril.

fiber density   1. Anatomically, a measure of the number of muscle or nerve fibers per unit area. 2. In single fiber electromyography, the mean number of muscle fiber action potentials fulfilling amplitude and rise time criteria belonging to one motor unit within the recording area of a single fiber needle electrode encountered during a systematic search in a weakly, voluntarily contracting muscle. See also **single fiber electromyography, single fiber needle electrode.** (From the 2001 Report of the Nomenclature Committee of the American Association of Electromyography and Electrodiagnosis.[10] Used by permission, copyright © 2001, AAEM.)

fiber splitting   A histological feature in muscle biopsy specimens in which the myofibril is split from its circumference peripherally toward an abnormally sited central nucleus. The finding is nonspecific, occurring because of age or an excessive workload, and is seen in both primary myopathies and neurogenic atrophies.

fiber-type atrophy   Selective atrophy of either type 1 or type 2 myofibrils. The former occurs in **myotonic dystrophy** and in some **congenital myopathies,** the latter with disuse and myasthenia, and with pyramidal lesions.

fiber-type grouping   A finding in muscle biopsy specimens in which two or more muscle fibers of one histological type are enclosed at all points on their circumference by other fibers of the same histochemical type. In some unusually large areas, a hundred or more myofibrils are of the same fiber type, as a result of the reinnervation of myofibrils of one type by a motor axon of another. This leads to their conversion to the type determined by that motor unit. The checkerboard appearance of the normal muscle with adenosine triphosphatase or lactic dehydrogenase stains is thus lost.

The finding is evidence of denervation with reinnervation, probably by collateral axon sprouts, and is a feature of chronic motor neuropathies. See **group atrophy.**

fiber-type predominance   Changes in the relative proportions of myofibrils of type 1 and type 2 in a muscle biopsy specimen.

The proportions vary normally in different muscles. Type 2 fibers predominate normally in the biceps brachii and quadriceps, and a finding >55% of type 1 fibers in those muscles is considered abnormal, while type 2 predominance is said to occur when the proportion of such fibers is >80%.[1533]

fibrillary astrocytoma   See **astrocytoma.**

fibrillary chorea   See **Morvan chorea.**

fibrillary contractions   See **myokymia.**

fibrillary gliosis   Infiltration of neural tissue with hyperplastic and hypertrophied astrocytes (including **gemistocytic astrocytes**) as seen in the plaques of **multiple sclerosis.**

fibrillation   The spontaneous contractions of individual muscle fibers, not visible through the skin nor even in the tongue.

fibrillation potential   The action potential of a single muscle fiber occurring spontaneously or after movement of a needle electrode. It usually fires at a constant rate. It consists of biphasic or triphasic spikes of short duration (usually <5 msec) with an initial positive phase and a peak-to-peak amplitude of <1 mV. It may also have a biphasic, initially negative phase when recorded at the site of initiation. It has an associated high-pitched regular sound described as "rain on a tin roof." In addition to this classic form, positive sharp waves may also be recorded from fibrillating muscle fibers when the potential arises from an area immediately adjacent to the needle electrode. (From the 2001 Report of the Nomenclature Committee of the American Association of Electromyography and Electrodiagnosis.[10] Used by permission, copyright © 2001, AAEM.)

fibrinoid degeneration of astrocytes   See **Alexander disease.**

fibroblastic meningioma   See **meningioma.**

fibrocartilaginous embolism of the spinal cord   A rare cause of anterior spinal artery occlusion, presenting with sudden, severe pain at onset, the interval from pain to maximal neurologic deficit ranging from 15 min to 23 days. The precipitating factors sometimes recorded include minor trauma such as falls and jumps, physical effort, and performance of the Valsalva maneuver. Recovery is poor. Pathologically, fibrocartilaginous emboli are found in the arterial bed and/or venous beds.[5613]

fibrodysplasia ossificans progressiva   See **myositis ossificans.**

fibroma   An unencapsulated benign tumor arising within peripheral nerves, fibers of which traverse the substance of the lesion.

Clinically, a painful swelling in the vicinity of a nerve is the usual presenting complaint; motor and sensory deficits appropriate to the nerve ensue. Such tumors occur particularly but not uniquely in **neurofibromatosis,** in which condition they are usually multiple.

fibromatosis of the optic nerve sheath   See **orbital pseudotumor syndrome.**

fibromuscular dysplasia   (FMD)   A segmental, nonatheromatous and noninflammatory disorder of the muscular arteries (including the carotid and renal arteries) characterized by irregular fibrous or fibromuscular thickening of all coats of the arterial wall causing alternating rings of constriction and dilatation as seen on arteriograms. *Intimal, medial,* and *adventitial* forms are described.[1118,3524]

Females are much more commonly affected; the condition may be dominantly inherited with reduced penetrance in males; it remains unmapped. Clinically, neck pain, transient ischemic attacks, and a carotid bruit are the most constant findings, sometimes due to dissection of the affected vessel. The condition is diagnosed at arteriography, which has usually been performed in the course of the investigation for transient ischemic attacks or subarachnoid hemorrhage. The arteries involved include the cervical, mesenteric, and renal vessels; irregular corrugations of the wall are noted on angiography ("*string of beads sign*"). Intracranial aneurysms are associated in a proportion of cases of cervical fibromuscular dysplasia.[3855,4907]

fibromyalgia   See **myofascial pain syndromes.**

fibromyositis   See **myofascial pain syndromes.**

fibrosarcoma   Large, circumscribed tumors arising from the meninges, often characterized by necrosis, hemorrhage, and cyst formation. Histologically, long spindle cells are found in parallel rows with substantial amounts of supporting reticulin connective tissue. Various grades of malignancy occur.

In a rare *variant* form, *primary diffuse meningeal sarcomatosis,* the highly malignant tumor infiltrates the meninges widely and no single originating tumor mass can be identified.

fibrosing myositis   See **myosclerosis.**

fibrositis   See **myofascial main syndromes.**

fibrous dysplasia   A nonhereditary, localized developmental disorder presenting in youth, in which dense fibrous tissue replaces bone. The craniofacial bones are involved in half of all cases.

Bone pain is a constant symptom and pathological fractures are common. When dysplasia affects the base of the skull and the temporal bones, dysmorphism, skull deformity, proptosis, optic atrophy, visual disturbance, deafness, headache, and cranial nerve compression syndromes result.[2796]

In the *polyostotic* form (McCune-Albright syndrome), skeletal anomalies leading to short stature and bone deformities, sexual precocity, and café-au-lait spots are additional features.

In another *variant* form, fibrous dysplasia of the skull is complicated by encephalopathy with seizures. See **Albright syndrome.**

fibrous dysplasia of the skull with encephalopathy. See **Albright syndrome.**

fibular reflex   Tapping the head of the fibula leads to contraction of the hamstrings, inducing slight flexion of the knee. Presumably, this is due to percussion of the tendon of the lateral hamstrings, which inserts here. See **lateral hamstring reflex.**

fibular tunnel   An arch formed by the insertion of the peroneus longus to the head of the fibula, through which passes the common peroneal nerve.

Fick, Adolf   (1829–1901) German medical physicist. He developed the principle that the blood flow of an organ can be determined if the oxygen consumption and the arteriovenous oxygen difference are known. This led to successful measurement of the rate of cerebral blood flow, initially by Kety and Schmidt.

fictitious epilepsy   The reporting of nonexistent seizures, usually by a parent in a child, or the induction of seizures by wilful abuse.[3796]

fidgety feet   See **restless legs syndrome.**

field of vision   (visual field) That area in space from all points of which light rays can travel to the retina of the immobile eye.

field-holding reflex   A visual fixation mechanism preventing the slow drift of the eyes from a target, which would thus require corrective saccades.[3330]

fifth day seizures   A benign syndrome characterized by the occurrence of repetitive seizures in full-term neonates who on examination are found to have have neither detectable risk factors nor neurological abnormalities. Clonic focal or multifocal convulsions and apneic spells are the usual expressions. Bursts of alternating rhythms on the EEG are common and characteristic but not invariable. The syndrome may be caused by zinc deficiency.[1335]

fifth finger sign   See **digiti quinti sign.**

fifth ventricle   See **cava septi pellucidi et vergae.**

fight-or-flight reaction   The name given by Dr. W.B. Cannon to the combined sympathetic reaction that takes place in response to threatening situations.

Figueira syndrome   A syndrome of subacutely developing but reversible weakness of the neck muscles with increased tone and often hyperreflexia in the legs in small children, usually following an intestinal upset. The nature of the condition is uncertain; it may be an attenuated form of acute poliomyelitis.[1808]

filamentopathies   Disorders primarily resulting from malfunction of muscle or nerve intermediate filaments, usually genetically-determined. See **giant axonal neuropathy; hereditary motor and sensory neuropathy (type 2E); familial ALS; myofibrillar myopathy; Emery-Dreifuss muscular dystrophy, congenital muscular dystrophy with epidermolysis bullosa. Amyotrophic lateral sclerosis, glue-sniffers neuropathy** and iminodiproprionitrile neuropathy are other conditions affecting intermediate filaments.[2551a]

Filippi syndrome   (microcephaly-syndactyly syndrome) A congenital dysmorphic syndrome characterized by short stature, dysarthria syndactyly of the fingers and toes, microcephaly, and mental and developmental delay.[337]

fillet   (from Lat, a thread) A thin **lemniscus,** though usually wider than a **fasciculus** or a tract.

fine motor functions   Movements performed with distal muscles, such as forming a pincer grip, finger manipulations, and the handling of small objects; a measure of both motor pathway integrity and intelligence.

fine syndrome   A congenital dysmorphic syndrome characterized by deafness, glaucoma, cataract, blindness, scoliosis, cryptorchidism, inguinal hernia, cleft palate, brachycephaly, macrocephaly, plagiocephaly, delayed closure of the fontanelles, callosal abnormalities, cavernous hemangiomas, and mental and developmental delay.[337]

finger agnosia   The term employed by Gerstmann to refer to a fragment of **autotopagnosia** (the inability to indicate body parts), with the loss of ability to recognize, identify, differentiate, name, select, indicate, or orient the individual fingers of either hand, the patient's or the examiner's.

Those affected are unable to appreciate the position of individual fingers among their fellows, to point to a named finger, or to move it when it is named by the examiner. The phenomenon was first described by Gerstmann in 1924 as one of the components of the syndrome of the angular gyrus, but the ability was later considered nonspecific (and indeed as evidence of dysphasia by Schilder). More recent studies suggest that "finger sense" is a real faculty and that the association of finger agnosia with the other elements of **Gerstmann syndrome** is more than coincidental,[3055] although Critchley has attacked the concept, contending that the faculty of finger gnosis does not exist.[1177]

finger flexor reflex   (Wartenberg sign) Further flexion of the semiflexed fingers and of the thumb of the supinated hand in response to a tap on the examiner's fingers lying across them. The contraction is enhanced in cases of pyramidal lesions above C6 and also in states of emotional tension.

See also **Rossimolo reflex, Tromner reflex, Hoffmann reflex.**

finger oscillation test   Part of the **Halstead-Reitan Battery** of psychological tests, in which the subject must press a key with the index finger as many times as possible within a specified period of time. The speed of performance of this task is slowed with aging and in the setting of dementia.[2398]

finger sign   See **Gordon sign.**

finger tapping test   A test of motor control (manual dexterity) in which the subject is required to tap a surface with the index finger of each hand as fast as possible.[4654,4655]

Reduction in rate compared to that of the normal age-matched control series suggests the presence of lesions of the contralateral motor areas.

fingerprint bodies   An ultrastructural abnormality of muscle consisting of concentric lamellae arranged in whorls and loops, resembling fingerprints. The finding is not specific for any one disease, having been described in the setting of congenital myopathies, oculopharyngeal muscle dystrophy, myotonic dystrophy, and dermatomyositis.

fingerprint body myopathy   A rare, nonprogressive, congenital myopathy characterized by the presence of subsarcolemmal whorled bodies on muscle biopsy specimens. Clinically, the condition presents in childhood with proximal weakness and hypotonia of limb and truncal muscles with areflexia and tremor but without wasting.[1661] Mental subnormality has also been associated with the disorder.

Similar inclusions are also found in other muscle diseases.[773]

fingerprint inclusion myopathy   A congenital myopathy with intracytoplasmic inclusions. See **fingerprint body myopathy.**

finger-thumb reflex   Opposition and adduction of the thumb with flexion at the metacarpophalangeal joint in response to firm passive flexion of a finger. A postural rather than a muscle stretch reflex, it is normally present, disappearing in patients with pyramidal lesions.

Finkel late-onset type spinal muscular atrophy   See **hereditary motor neuropathy** (*variants*).

Finnish amyloidosis   See **amyloidosis.**

Finnish lipofuscinosis   See **neuronal ceroid lipofuscinosis.**

FIRDA   See **frontal intermittent rhythmic delta activity.**

firearm recoil palsy   Symptoms resulting from entrapment of the upper fibers of the brachial plexus between the clavicle and the underlying scalene muscles as a result of backward compression exerted by the stock of a gun.[5841]

firing pattern   Qualitative and quantitative descriptions of the sequence of discharge of electric waveforms recorded from muscle or nerve. (From the 2001 Report of the Nomenclature Committee of the American Association of Electromyography and Electrodiagnosis.[10] Used by permission, copyright © 2001, AAEM.)

firing rate   The frequency of repetition of a potential. The relationship of the frequency to the occurrence of other potentials and the force of muscle contraction may be described. See also **discharge frequency.** (From the 2001 Report of the Nomenclature Committee of the American Association of Electromyography and Electrodiagnosis.[10] Used by permission, copyright © 2001, AAEM.)

first and second branchial arch syndrome   See **oculoauriculovertebral dysplasia.**

first arch syndrome   See **hemifacial microsomia.**

first pain   See **fast pain.**

Fischer syndrome   (hyperkeratosis-syringomyelia) A dominantly inherited congenital dysmorphic syndrome characterized by keratosis of the palms and soles, sparse hair, thickened eyelids, clubbing of the fingers, spasticity, changes resembling those of progeria, and physical and mental delay.[1832]

Fischgold line   A line joining the lower margins of the mastoid processes on anteroposterior or transoral skull X-ray films. The line normally passes through the atlanto-occipital articulations and the tip of the odontoid is often situated on the same line; both structures are situated above it in **basilar impression.** The *digastric line* (drawn between the medial aspect of the mastoid processes at their junctions with the remainder of the skull) may be as useful,[5282] but CT scanning is much better.

fish odor syndrome   A dysmetabolic, dysmorphic syndrome characterized also by a most unpleasant body smell, hydrocephalus, short stature, hypertelorism, and cortical blindness.[5112]

Fisher sign   When the tip of the index finger is tapped repeatedly upon the middle joint of the thumb, the remaining fingers cannot be held still but move in synchrony; this is seen in patients with a mild corticospinal tract lesion on that side.

A degree of difference is also present according to the handedness of the subject.

Fisher syndrome   See **Miller Fisher syndrome.**

fissure   (Lat, a cleft) A long, narrow crack or cleft such as the deeper sulci, thus delineating the cerebral or cerebellar lobes. The interhemispheric, callosal, calcarine, entorhinal, longitudinal, and transverse fissures are some named examples.

fissure of Rolando   The central fissure of the hemispheres, separating the anterior motor from the posterior sensory cortex, described by Luigi **Rolando** in 1825.

fissure of Sylvius   The lateral fissure, demarcating the superior extent of the temporal lobes, and described by **Sylvius** in 1641.

fisting   Persistent clenching of the fist by an infant with a hemiparesis on that side.

fist-palm-side test   A test of motor control, in which the subject is asked to tap the table repeatedly with the fist, then with the palm, and then with the side of his hand. Errors in the fluent repetition of this sequence suggest the presence of bilateral frontal lobe disease.

fist-ring test   The subject is asked to make a fist, then to oppose the tips of the thumb and index finger, alternating between the actions; with a contralateral premotor lesion, the smoothness of execution is lost and perseveration of one posture may occur. See also **fist-palm-side test,** which is more sensitive.

fistula sign   Increase in the pressure in the external auditory meatus leads to vertigo and brief horizontal nystagmus, as a result of the presence of a fistula in the bony labyrinth of the lateral semicircular canal, usually as a result of chronic otitis media.

fit   The vernacular term for a seizure.

Fitzsimmons syndrome   A congenital X-linked dysmorphic syndrome characterized by hyperkeratosis of the palms and soles, spastic paraparesis, and mental and developmental delay.[1878]

fixation   Direction of the gaze upon an object so that the image of the object falls steadily upon the two foveas. See also **field-holding reflex, smooth pursuit system.**

fixation disparity   The minimal, varying imprecision of the **fusional vergence** system in holding images precisely on the foveas of the two eyes, triggering further corrective movements initiated by that system to align the images so closely that central fusional mechanisms prevent the awareness of any blurring.

fixation index The ratio of the frequency and amplitude of the beats of nystagmus occurring when the eyes are open and when they are closed; with greater suppression, the value of the index rises. In darkness and other situations when no fixation is possible, cerebellar influences on eye movements are minimal, as the cerebellum is concerned with the control of eye movements during fixation. Fixation is the usual method by which ice skaters and ballet dancers reduce vertigo during rapid spins.[2637]

fixation instability Inability of the eyes to maintain stillness during fixation on a target, usually as a result of small horizontal saccades that result in ocular flutter when there is no delay between one saccade and the next one in the other direction, or result in square wave jerks when such a delay does exist.

fixation nystagmus The term of Gordon **Holmes** for that form of nystagmus which is enhanced by visual fixation on an object and inhibited to some degree in its absence; a characteristic of nystagmus of central origin. See **acquired nystagmus.**

fixation point The point at which the visual axes of the two eyes meet; the object of gaze.

fixation spasm A reflex fixation of gaze upon an object in space, from which the gaze cannot be transferred voluntarily. The phenomenon is described in subjects with visual impairment or with bilateral frontal or parietal lesions.[2622]

fixation suppression Suppression of the vestibulo-ocular reflex or of caloric nystagmus by visual fixation.

Failure of this mechanism suggests the presence of a metabolic encephalopathy or posterior fossa disease, including tumor.[123]

flaccid (Lat, flabby) Drooping or lacking in stiffness, but, in neurology, synonymous with hypotonic.

flail arm syndrome Symmetrical wasting and weakness of the arms without similar involvement of other body parts, although pyramidal signs may be found in the legs. The most common cause is a variant of **amyotrophic lateral sclerosis** (ALS), but cervical cord disease and brachial plexopathies can also present with this picture. In the context of ALS, men are more commonly affected with this form than are women.

flail foot Loss of both dorsiflexion and plantar flexion at the ankle as a result of a sciatic nerve injury. The intrinsic foot muscles will also be paretic.

flapping tremor A bilateral but asymmetrical abnormality seen in the outstretched hands, in which involuntary repetitive brisk extension of the wrist (akin to

asterixis) is followed by relaxation and dropping of the hand in patients with a metabolic encephalopathy, such as that due to hepatic failure.

flashbacks The recurrence of sensations formerly experienced while under the influence of lysergic acid diethylamide, now re-evoked by use of other drugs such as cannabis. A panic state often accompanies the experience.

flash-induced nystagmus See **induced nystagmus, flicker-induced nystagmus.**

Flatau, Eduard (1869–1932) Polish neurologist, who trained in Moscow and Berlin. After a career in neurology and comparative anatomy, he returned to private practice in Poland. Among his many publications were important contributions on disseminated encephalitis (Flatau-Redlich disease), tumors of the neuraxis, tuberculous meningitis, and migraine, but he is best remembered for his description of torsion spasm, now known as **dystonia.**

Flatau law The greater the length of the fibers in the spinal cord, the more peripherally they are sited.[1883] This is correct for the pyramidal and spinothalamic tracts but not in the case of the posterior columns.

Flatau sign Pupillary dilation in response to stretching of the neck muscles, described in meningococcal meningitis. The genesis of the sign is unknown and its value is minimal.

flavi- (Gr, yellow) Prefix denoting yellow.

Flechsig loop See **Meyer loop.**

Flechsig, Paul Emile (1847–1929) Bohemian neurologist and professor of psychiatry in Leipzig, who defined the dorsal spinocerebellar tract (Flechsig's tract) in 1876, identified motor and sensory projection areas in the cortex, and named the parts of the internal capsule and the anterior and lateral "ground-bundles" (the former being the pyramidal tract).

Flechsig principle The primary receptive areas of the cerebral cortex have no direct neocortical connections, except with immediately adjacent parasensory (association) areas.

fleece of Stilling The interlaced fibers running to the dentate nucleus from the cerebellar cortex.

Fleischer, Bruno (1874–1965) German ophthalmologist in Erlangen, best remembered for his original account of the corneal pigmentation in **Wilson disease,** published in 1903.

flexibilitas cerea (Lat, waxy flexibility) Unvarying increased resistance to passive movement of a limb which, when overcome, is followed by the patient's maintenance of any posture in which his limb was placed by the examiner. The phenomenon is usually encountered in schizophrenics but is also a manifestation of depression or of drug-induced dyskinesia.

flexion   (Lat, a bending) The state of being bent or the act of bending.

flexion dystonia in paralysis agitans   See **dystonias.**

flexion reflex   1. Dorsiflexion of the hallux with flexion at the ankle, knee, and hip occurring with noxious stimulation of the skin of the foot or leg, seen in some neonates after severe perinatal asphyxia. The Babinski reflex is but a fragment of this full reflex response. 2. Tapping the long flexor tendons at the wrist leads to contraction of the long flexor muscles in patients with a corticospinal tract lesion on that side.

flexion spinal defence reflex   See **flexor reflex.**

flexion-adduction sign   The characteristic posture of patients with **neuralgic amyotrophy,** in which the arm is maintained in flexion at the elbow and adduction at the shoulder. Abduction and lateral rotation of the arm with the elbow extended may result in radicular pain in such patients.[5877]

flexor   A bender; in neurology applied to muscles that are antagonists to extensors and that tend by their action to shorten a limb or to reduce the length of the trunk.

flexor reflex   (flexor withdrawal reflex, flexion spinal defence reflex, réflexe des raccourcisseurs, reflex of spinal automatism) Flexion of the hip and knee with dorsiflexion of the ankle and toes elicited and steadily maintained by a noxious stimulus applied to the sole of the foot, particularly on its lateral side, but also from a wider area. A reflex produced by a noxious cutaneous stimulus, or a train of electrical stimuli, that activates the flexor muscles of a limb and thus acts to withdraw it from the stimulus. In humans, it is well characterized only in the lower extremity.[10]

The **Babinski response** represents part of this reflex, which is a typical finding in the lower limbs in cases of spastic paresis, especially "paraplegia-in-flexion."[3648,5828] When the response is bilateral, this is known as the **crossed flexor reflex.**

flexor spasms   (syndrome de spasmes en flexion, jackknife convulsions, jack-knife spasms, grusskrampfe) A characteristic bilateral symmetrical contraction of the muscles of the neck, trunk, and extremities, leading to sudden flexion of the head and trunk and abduction of the legs (**salaam attacks**). These are characteristically seen in the syndrome of **infantile spasms.** 2. Flexion of the hip and knee and dorsiflexion of the ankle in patients with spastic paraparesis when proprioceptive innervation is lacking, sometimes leading to "paraplegia-in-flexion."

flexor withdrawal reflex   See **flexor reflex.**

flick sign   A shaking of the hands performed spontaneously by patients with **carpal tunnel syndrome** as they demonstrate their reactions to the hand paresthesias that they typically note on waking.[4538]

flicker fusion   (critical flicker fusion) A test of visual function and arousal in which subjects observe a flickering light, speeding up the flicker rate until they perceive it to shine constantly. The test and its modifications have been reported to show abnormalities in patients with multiple sclerosis in the absence of other evidence of visual disturbance.[1250]

flicker-induced nystagmus   (flash-induced nystagmus) A form of conjugate horizontal jerk nystagmus induced by intermittent photic stimulation of one eye. The slow phase beats away from the stimulated eye.[5169] See also **induced nystagmus.**

Flier syndrome   A syndrome of disabling muscle pain with elevation of serum creatine kinase levels, enlargement of the hands and feet, acanthocytosis nigricans, hirsutism, and resistance of target cells to insulin.[3049]

flight of colors   The perception of afterimages such as halos or discs which repeatedly change in color following 10 seconds of bright-light stimulation of the eye and persist for at least 1 minute with at least two color changes in normal subjects.

They are abolished or altered with disease affecting any part of the visual system concerned with central vision, and the test has been claimed to detect optic neuropathy with greater accuracy than visual evoked responses.[1774,4744]

flip sign   Weakness in performance of quick movements of the fingers, such as flicking the finger against an object; a feature of both radial and ulnar nerve (as well as of basal ganglion and pyramidal) lesions.

flip test   Straight-leg raising is performed with patients supine, and they are then asked to sit up and to extend a leg, as if for testing of the plantar response. The ability to flex the hip in the sitting position but not when supine suggests the presence of nonorganic causes of back pain.[5791] See **Waddell signs.**

floaters   Mobile vitreous opacities appearing as gray or black specks obscuring tiny arcs of vision and drifting about in the visual field; they lag behind as the individual moves the head or eyes. Though quite benign, they irritate or worry some patients.

They represent condensations of collagen fibrils within the vitreous humor of the eye. Rarely, they appear with retinal detachment or intraocular hemorrhage.

floating harbor syndrome   A congenital dysmorphic syndrome characterized by aphasia, skeletal anomalies such as micrognathia and clinodactyly, and delay in physical maturation.[3334]

flocculus   (Lat, a small tangle of wool) Part of the paleocerebellum concerned with the maintenance of posture.

floppy infant syndrome   Generalized hypotonia, weakness, and lack of muscle development in neonates and small infants, usually due to central (e.g., cerebral palsy) or metabolic causes and less often to peripheral lesions such as anterior horn cell disease, myopathy, or muscular dystrophy. The causes have been reviewed.[2879] See **benign congenital hypotonia.**

floppy person syndrome   See **quadriplegic myopathy.**

Flourens law   Stimulation of a semicircular canal excites nystagmus in the plane of that canal.

Flourens, Marie-Jean-Pierre   (1794–1867) Parisian, professor of comparative anatomy who suggested, on the basis of stimulation and extirpation experiments in pigeons, that functions were precisely located in many parts of the cortex, though he supposed the cerebrum to be inexcitable.[1889] He correctly identified the cerebellum as being concerned with the coordination of muscular activity (although he supposed this to be exerted contralaterally), and he ascribed to the vestibular system responsibility for vertigo and nystagmus. He also confirmed in 1837 the presence of a center in the floor of the medulla (the *noeud vital*) that controls respiratory activity (although this had previously been suggested by Legallois), and showed that vision depends upon an intact cortex.

flow void   Absence of the normal flow pattern on MRI scanning in **arteriovenous malformations** or within the intracranial venous sinuses in cases of **sinus thrombosis.**

fluctuating dystonia   See **dopa-responsive dystonia.**

fluctuations   Variability in the severity of movement disorder in parkinsonian patients on chronic levadopa therapy, in many instances associated with variability of the levadopa levels. Hyperkinetic forms include *peak-dose chorea* and *diphasic dyskinesia*. Dystonic forms are *early morning, end-of-dose,* and *peak-dose dystonias*; and hypokinetic forms include *akinetic freezing of gait, early morning akinesia, end-of-dose deterioration* (wearing-off effect), and sudden *switching-off or on–off* effects.[2434]

Using a different system of classification, Quinn[4562] suggests the following categorization:

Short-duration motor fluctuations (lasting minutes or less)
　Sudden transient freezing (motor blocks) occurring late in the course of the disease, often provoked by external stimuli, relieved by certain rituals and related to the occurrence of on–off events. This is a common cause of falls in this population.
　Paradoxic kinesis. Sudden and brief relief of the symptoms of parkinsonism provoked by an urgent external stimulus or by rituals.
Medium-duration motor fluctuations (lasting hours or less)
　Beginning of dose worsening
　End of dose rebound
　Wearing off/on–off/yo-yoing
　Diurnal
Long duration (days)
　Slow variations in response to L-dopa therapy

Fluctuations in mood, pain perception, cognitive abilities, and autonomic functions also occur.[4562]

fluent dysphasias   Those forms of dysphasia characterized by empty speech that is still grammatical but in which there is a deficiency of substantive words. Many literal and paraphasic errors occur in speech, of which the patient is unaware. See **dysphasias.**

fluorescein angiography   The observation of the retinal arterioles and venules following the intravenous injection of fluorescein. The morphology of the vessels, the time taken for the agent to arrive at the eye, and the subsequent appearance of the optic nerve head can be assessed safely by repetitive retinal photography, thus providing useful information in cases of retinal vessel disease, arterial occlusion, and, for example, papilledema.[4176]

fluorescent treponemal antibody test   See **FTA-abs test.**

fluorosis   A syndrome of bony distortion as a result of long-term excessive ingestion of fluoride. The vertebral column becomes stiff and distorted by osteophytes, which leads to compression of spinal nerves and, in time, to spinal cord compression as well.[5182]

flutter   See **ocular flutter.**

flutter dysmetria   A form of saccadic intrusion characterized by **ocular flutter** (back-to-back saccades) occurring at the completion of a refixational saccade in some patients with cerebellar disease.[6111]

flutter-like oscillations   To-and-fro pendular oscillations of the eyes at about 10 Hz, associated with a change in fixation in patients with cerebellar disease.[1071]

flycatcher tongue   Sudden irregular protrusion of the tongue, seen in subjects with dystonias or choreic states; an orobuccolingual dyskinesia.

flying saucer syndrome   The tendency for those with chorea or myoclonus to lose control of, drop, or fling away the objects in their hands involuntarily.

The term was first used for the morning catastrophes of patients with **juvenile myoclonic epilepsy,** whose jerks are maximal within the first hour or so after rising.

Flynn phenomenon   Constriction of the pupils in darkness. This inversion of the normal response occurs in some cases of chronic disease of the optic nerve and in congenital achromatopsia.[1932]

Flynn-Aird syndrome   (cochlear deafness, myopia and oligophrenia syndrome, dominant myopia and hearing loss, peripheral neuropathy and skeletal abnormalities syndrome, neuroectodermal syndrome) A dominantly inherited syndrome consisting of progressive sensorineural deafness with myopia, painful sensorimotor peripheral neuropathy, bony cysts and osteoporosis, cataract, pigmentary retinopathy, kyphoscoliosis, mental and developmental delay, seizures, osteoporosis, and distal weakness.

Ataxia, baldness, dental caries, dermal atrophy, joint stiffness, abnormal EEG findings, and elevated CSF protein levels are also described.[1891]

FMD   See **fibromuscular dysplasia.**

focal   Originating from, or to do with, a particular point in space.

focal asymmetric cortical degeneration syndromes Dementing diseases primarily affecting the cortex, still in the process of classification in the presence of different histological and clinical findings. The conditions currently subsumed are the following:

Primary progressive aphasias (fluent, nonfluent, anomic, and mixed) (see also **Pick disease**)

Perceptual-motor disorders (visual, motor, or both) (see also **cortical basalganglionic degeneration, progressive asymmetric rigidity and apraxia syndrome**)

Frontal or frontotemporal atrophies (see also **Pick disease**)

Bitemporal atrophies[934,935]

focal cervical poliopathy of distal arm   See **hereditary motor neuropathy** (*variants*).

focal cervical poliopathy of distal upper extremity causing juvenile muscular atrophy   See **monomelic amyotrophy.**

focal cortical dysplasia   A malformation characterized by congregations of large, bizarre neurons and glial cells through all but the first cortical layer within the temporal lobe. The clinical presentation is usually in youth, with refractory epilepsy. A transmantle form is also described and thought to be due to abnormal stem cell development.[357]

The condition is detected in some specimens resected surgically in the management of intractable seizure disorders.[168,5505] See also **heterotopia.**

focal cortical myoclonus   See **cortical myoclonus.**

focal dermal hypoplasia   (Goltz syndrome) A diffuse congenital encephalopathy inherited as an X-linked dominant (lethal in males) trait characterized by linear pigmentation of the skin, focal areas of skin aplasia, mucosal papillomatosis, hypoplasia of the dental enamel and nails, alopecia, iris colobomas, microcephaly, microphthalmia, scoliosis, spina bifida, and mental retardation.[2177]

focal dystonia   See **dystonia.**

focal eyelid dystonia   See **apraxia of eyelid opening.**

focal inhibitory seizures   See **hemiparetic seizures.**

focal levator atrophy   A rare condition of ptosis as a result of disease of the levator palpebrae muscle, uniquely or as part of a generalized myopathy.[5138]

focal motor neuron disease   Weakness, wasting, and fasciculations in a discrete body region, which is progressive for some months before arresting. This is a residual diagnosis, other focal pathologies requiring exclusion before it can be considered.[5250]

focal myoclonus   See **spinal myoclonus.**

focal necrotizing myopathy   Muscle necrosis, fibrosis, and calcification in the region of repeated intramuscular injections of drugs such as pentazocine or local anesthetics.[3188]

focal neuronal migration disorders   A group of developmental structural lesions characterized by disorganization of the cortical architecture with an aberrant columnar and laminar neuronal arrangement, leading to macrogyria or polymicrogyria. The degree of cytoarchitectonic disorganization and the extent of the brain involved vary widely.

The clinical features usually include mental retardation, intractable seizure disorders, and severe motor dysfunction in infancy; survival seldom exceeds two decades.[4311] See **heterotopias.**

focal nodular myositis   A *variant* form of polymyositis.[1212] See **idiopathic inflammatory myopathy.**

focal reflex myoclonus   (pyramidal myoclonus) A form of myoclonus affecting a single body part and activated by a specific stimulus such as movement. The responsible lesion is thought to involve the cortical and subcortical area of the contralateral cerebral hemisphere.[5427]

focal steroid-responsive myopathy   A rare inflammatory muscle disorder that affects usually the legs, trunk, arms, or neck; in the case of the latter it may cause the **dropped head syndrome.**[580] The presentation is typically with weakness and local muscle swelling.

focal upper limb demyelinating neuropathy   A form of **chronic inflammatory demyelinating polyneuropathy** restricted to the arms, usually motor or mixed motor and sensory, seldom only sensory, and with reduced motor nerve conduction velocities and conduction block and a tendency to nerve hypertrophy.[5545]

focus   A limited region of the scalp, cerebral cortex, or depth of the brain displaying a given EEG activity, whether normal or abnormal.

Foerster, Otfried   (1873–1941) German neurosurgeon who graduated from Breslau University, studied in Paris at the Salpêtrière, and returned to Breslau in **Wernicke**'s clinic, becoming professor in 1922. His clinic received funds from the Rockefeller Foundation and became an independent institute in 1934.

He pioneered the methods of stimulation of the cerebral cortex at open operation in attempts to localize foci of epileptic discharge and trained **Penfield** and others in these techniques. As a result of his studies, mapping of the functions of human cortical areas was begun, previous workers such as the **Vogts** having worked on primates. He advocated section of some thoracic nerve roots to treat the lightning pains in **tabes dorsalis** and also described atonic diplegia (cerebral palsy) in 1909 and the use of tractotomy for the relief of chronic pain.

Foerster demonstrated the effect of hyperventilation in precipitating seizures in 1925, "in showing that a row of institutional epileptics, when ordered to stand still and breathe as fast as possible, would go down one after another in a fit, like soldiers shot down by machine gun fire."[1104] He contributed over 300 papers to the literature on many neurological as well as neurosurgical topics; in the latter area his work concentrated on localization in the brain, epilepsy, and cerebral tumors.[185]

Otfried Foerster

Foerster syndrome   1. (arteriosclerotic rigidity) Generalized but variable increase in tone in subjects with severe and chronic cerebral ischemia, described by Foerster in a 169-page paper in 1921.

2. (Foerster atonic diplegia, atonia-astasia, generalized amyotonia, cerebral atonic-astasic syndrome) A congenital hypotonic diplegic form of **cerebral palsy** with mental and motor delay, muscle weakness, and hypotonia with laxity of ligaments, often with accompanying seizures and later mental retardation and cerebellar ataxia, described by Foerster in 1909.[1892] It is now thought that this was a form of congenital syphilis.

Foerster test   The identification by a patient of numerals traced on his skin; topognosis.

fogging effect   A transitional phase in the second and third weeks after an ischemic infarct, following the early unenhanced CT scan appearance of hypodensity and prior to the late findings of encephalomalacia.[955]

Foix, Charles   (1882–1927) French neurologist who trained on the service of **Marie** at the **Salpêtrière,** where,

after winning the gold medal in his class, he himself was later appointed. He died young, but his publications on the anatomy of Parkinson disease, on the syndromes of the cerebral arteries, and on the following conditions witness his remarkable productivity.[900,2575]

Foix syndrome   1. (red nucleus syndrome) A vascular syndrome of rubral tremor and hyperkinesia in which the fibers of the third cranial nerve are spared following infarction limited to the anterior part of the red nucleus.[1895] 2. See **Foix-Jefferson syndrome.**

Foix-Alajouanine syndrome   (angiodysgenetic myelomalacia, hypertrophic myelomalacia) An ischemic myelopathy leading to insidiously progressive amyotrophic paraplegia with dissociated sensory loss, areflexia, and loss of sphincter control. In the original cases, the paraparesis ascended from the lumbar regions and was at first spastic, but later flaccid.

The myelopathy is due to the primary obliterative sclerosis of abnormal, dilated intramedullary or meningeal vessels in the lower segments of the spinal cord, with thickening of the walls of the meningeal veins and often of the arteries, or it is due to thrombosis of a spinal dural arteriovenous malformation, leading in either case to an ischemic myelopathy.[2272] See also **subacute necrotizing myelopathy, subacute necrotizing myelitis.**

Foix-Chavany-Marie syndrome   (faciolinguopharyngomasticatory diplegia or syndrome, operculum syndrome) See **anterior operculum syndrome.**

Foix-Jefferson syndrome   (Foix syndrome, sphenopetrosal fissure syndrome, cavernous sinus syndrome [of Raeder], syndrome of Bonnet and Bonnet, cavernous sinus-lateral wall syndrome) The **superior orbital fissure syndrome** produced by a tumor or aneurysm in, or thrombosis of, the cavernous sinus and leading to the combination of lesions of the third, fourth, fifth, and sixth cranial nerves, exophthalmos, and eyelid edema.[1894]

Foley syndrome   See **benign fasciculations and cramps.**

folie à deux   Delusions shared by two people, who are usually related.

folie musculaire   See **chorea.**

Fölling, Asbjorn   (1888–1972) Norwegian physician who trained in Olso but, after receiving a Rockefeller Foundation award, studied metabolic disease in the United States. On his return to Norway he became professor of nutritional medicine at Oslo University and later professor of biochemistry at the Oslo Veterinary College, where he determined that the abnormal urinary constituent of the two retarded children of an Oslo dental colleague was phenylpyruvic acid, that this substance could be found in the urine of other mentally retarded children, and that the disorder was a recessively transmitted error of phenylalanine metabolism.

Fölling disease (phenylpyruvic oligophrenia) A recessively transmitted disorder in which phenylalanine cannot be converted to tyrosine. The clinical syndrome includes fair hair, blue eyes, mental retardation, incoordination, athetosis, dystonias, and seizures. The presence of the disease can be determined by screening a urine sample at 3 weeks of life. See **phenylketonuria.**

fontanelle (Lat, a small fountain) The anterior and posterior meeting points of the cranial bones (frontal-parietal, parietal-occipital) and the same in sphenoid and mastoid regions.

They are probably so named because of the welling-up that may be seen or felt there, or because, when trephined, the CSF gushes forth from such areas, which in infants are soft and pulsatile owing to the incomplete ossification of the bones at these sites at this age.

fontanelle reflex See **Grünfelder reflex.**

food allergy insomnia A disorder of initiating and maintaining sleep due to an allergic response to food allergens (usually milk products, eggs, or fish) in which the sleep disorder remits within 4 weeks of the elimination of the allergen from the diet. Psychomotor agitation, daytime lethargy, respiratory difficulties, and skin or gastrointestinal disorders are frequently present in addition.[2901]

food-elicited cataplexy A condition of dogs, best tested for by timing a dog's ability to eat all of 10 pieces of food placed in a row; cataleptic attacks will prolong the time that the affected dog takes to eat them all to a period greater than 45 seconds.

foolishness A defect of judgment in the presence of normal apprehension and memory, leading to improper inferences, often risible. (Thomas **Willis**, ascribed.)

foot drop Weakness of dorsiflexion of the ankle as a result of a lesion of the common peroneal nerve, or of the sciatic nerve at a higher level. In the former case, unopposed plantar flexion and function in the intrinsic muscles of the foot allow some voluntary movement at and distal to the ankle. Compare **flail foot.**

foot dystonia A rare focal dystonia, sometimes provoked by movement, in which abnormal postures of the foot are the only manifestation, unless **parkinsonism** develops later.[3320]

footballer's migraine Vascular headaches induced by repeated mild to moderate head trauma, in this case from heading soccer balls for a living.[3707]

foramen (Lat) A hole.

foramen lacerum syndrome The combination of headache, periorbital pain, palsies of cranial nerves III, IV, and VI, optic atrophy, and trigeminal anesthesia (ophthalmic division), indicating the presence of a posterior cavernous sinus lesion—in this case an aneurysm of the intradural portion of the internal carotid artery.

foramen magnum The large aperture in the base of the skull through which the uppermost part of the cervical spinal cord passes.

foramen of Luschka Paired openings in the lateral recesses of the arachnoid roof of the fourth ventricle allowing egress of CSF.

foramen of Magendie A single medial opening in the arachnoid roof of the fourth ventricle allowing egress of CSF.

foramen of Monro The communication between the lateral and the third ventricles.

foramen ovale A small opening in the skull base through which the mandibular (third) division of the fifth cranial nerve passes.

foramen rotundum A small opening in the skull base through which the maxillary (second) division of the fifth cranial nerve passes.

foramina parietalia permagna See **Catlin mark.**

foraminobasilar angle See **Boorgard angle.**

Forbes disease See **glycogen storage diseases** (type 3).

forced crying See **emotionalism.**

forced duction Mechanical traction of the globe of the eye, using forceps to grasp a fold of the anesthetized conjunctiva.

The test is performed to determine the presence of any restriction to free rotation of the globe of the eye in the orbit, and is thus useful in the diagnosis of, for example, **dysthyroid ophthalmopathy** and **Brown syndrome,** where traction in the direction of action of an apparently weak muscle may not be possible.

forced elbow extension test Passive elbow flexion with the forearm fully pronated and the wrist maximally flexed induces pain felt in the lateral part of the elbow in the presence of **lateral epicondylitis.**

forced grasping See **grasp reflex.**

forced groping See **groping.**

forced hyperphasia Compulsive, involuntary, environmentally dependent speaking; a form of **imitation behavior.**

forced normalization The tendency for patients with partial (focal) epilepsies who develop schizophrenic psychoses to achieve better seizure control; the EEG tends toward a more normal pattern at these times, reverting to its former abnormal state as the psychosis clears.[4299]

forced thinking (intellectual aura) A variety of epileptic aura comprising the experience of repetitive intrusive thoughts, ideas, or the crowding of thoughts at the beginning of a seizure and arising in most cases from a focus in the left frontal lobe.[3831]

Ford, Frank Rodolph (1892–1970) American neurologist who trained at Johns Hopkins and then at

Bellvue, before returning to Baltimore where he quickly became chief of the neurology service. His special interest in pediatric neurology was evinced by his *Diseases of the Nervous System in Infancy and Childhood,* a classic text for many years after its first publication in 1937.

forearm reflex   See **brachioradialis reflex.**

forearm rolling test   Asymmetry of forearm rolling (rotation of one forearm around the other in front of the body). This is a sensitive indicator or sign of unilateral cerebral dysfunction, although there may be false-positive results in Parkinson disease, other extrapyramidal disorders, and local musculoskeletal disorders.[4934] It was probably first described by Prof. G.H. Monrad-Krohn of the University of Oslo in the mid-twentieth century.[2958]

The sensitivity of the sign is further increased if the subject is asked to roll the index fingers around each other.

forearm sign   Stroking of the radial aspect of the semiflexed and semipronated arm normally leads to further flexion of the elbow and to radial deviation of the hand. With pyramidal lesions, only the elbow flexion is seen; when there is psychogenic hyperactivity of the response, elevation of the hand is the most prominent motor reaction.[1349]

foreign accent syndrome   A rare speech output disorder characterized by aprosodic spoken speech with normal syntax and word choice, evolving usually after initial **aphemia,** in which the deficit in prosody leads to the speech sounding as though the patient had a foreign accent.[615] Limited motor cortex damage (to the posterolateral part of the left precentral gyrus) has been considered responsible.

Forel, August   (1848–1931) Swiss psychiatrist, neurologist, and anatomist, working in Zurich. He is best remembered for his anatomical studies of sections of the basal ganglia and subthalamic region. These he performed using the technique of secondary degeneration and with the microtome newly invented by **von Gudden.**

Forel's decussation   The ventral tegmental decussation between the red nuclei.[1478]

formed hallucinations   Hallucinated auditory or visual images which are so structured as to have meaning.

formication   A sensation as of ants crawling on the skin, experienced in the territory of regenerating nerves (when it is a microversion of **Tinel sign**), or occurring with disorders affecting the posterior columns. See also **Lhermitte sign.**

formula speech   See **stereotypies.**

fornix   (Lat, an arch) A long, curved, fiber pathway below the corpus callosum, carrying impulses from the hippocampal formation to the mammillary bodies. Its existence was first described by Vesalius.

Forst, J-J.   French neurologist who gave a modern account of sciatica in his Paris graduation thesis in 1881, including a description of the **Lasègue sign.**

Forster, O.   See **Foerster, O.**

fortification spectra   Common visual auras in migraine, so named (by John **Fothergill** in 1778) because the patterns seen resemble a plan of the fortifications of medieval walled cities (such as Naarden in Holland).[4458] By extension, the patterns of shimmering or flashing lights seen in the same condition have also been given this name. See **teichopsia.**

forty-five-degree test   A method of standardizing muscle contraction force to estimate the number of motor unit action potentials firing during electromyography with reference to the values found in a normal population.

The subject lies with the elbow supported and the forearm raised 45°. Recordings are made from the triceps muscle.[4419]

Robert Foster Kennedy

Foster Kennedy, Robert   (1884–1952) Irish-American neurologist, whose early medical training was at Queen's University, Belfast, and then at the **National Hospital,** Queen Square. After some wartime experience, in 1915 he joined the staff of the Bellvue Hospital in New York and was appointed professor of neurology at Cornell.

In his early papers he addressed topics of current importance, such as the nature of shell shock in World War I as well as of epidemic encephalitis and other encephalopathies, following an outbreak in New York. He is best remembered for his sign, described in 1911 and observed during the analysis of patients with cerebral tumors (but already described by **Gowers** 2 years before, as he acknowledged). He drew attention to the occurrence of "true" retrobulbar neuritis with a central scotoma and optic atrophy on the side of the tumor, with papilledema on the opposite side. All of his patients also had anosmia.

He died shortly after correctly diagnosing **Brown-Séquard syndrome** (secondary to polyarteritis nodosa) in himself.[3682]

Foster Kennedy syndrome (Gowers-Paton-Kelly syndrome, basal-frontal syndrome) Unilateral optic atrophy and contralateral papilledema, commonly with anosmia, mentioned by **Gowers** in 1893 with a description published in 1909 by him and by Paton, but described more fully by Kennedy in 1911.

The typical cause is a tumor on the lesser wing of the sphenoid bone that compresses the first and second nerves and induces papilledema by raising intracranial pressure,[3005] but many other anteriorly sited tumors and other nontumor pathologies can also produce the sign.[3682]

Fothergill, John (1712–1780) English physician and accoucheur who trained in Edinburgh (as a Quaker he was disbarred from entering any English University) and at St. Thomas' Hospital in London. He practiced with great success in London.

Fothergill was the first to give an account of trigeminal neuralgia, in 1773.[1914] "In a moment she would be seized with the most acute excruciating pain affecting the inner canthus of the eye; it lasted but a few seconds, forced out the tears, and gradually went off. In a few minutes the same thing happened and in like manner at unequal distances during the day, so as to occasion a great misery."

He described the migraine aura from personal experience in his *Remarks on that complaint commonly known under the name of sick headache* (1777 *et seq.*). He also described coronary artery sclerosis as the cause of angina, and diphtheritic sore throat.

He put into practice the teachings of his faith; he was active in prison reform and in the abolition of slavery and treated patients at no charge in the free hospital (but charged for home visits, remarking that he climbed on the backs of the poor to the pockets of the rich.) He was a friend of both Lord North, the British prime minister, and Benjamin Franklin; with them, he attempted to reconcile the political differences between England and the North American Colonies, but failed. He entertained visiting Americans after the secession of the United States and gave money and teaching materials to the Pennsylvania Hospital.[1829]

Fothergill syndrome See **trigeminal neuralgia.**

Fotopoulos syndrome The association of chorea and lower motor neuron disease (periscapular weakness

and wasting) appearing in adult life.[4294] See also **neuroacanthocytosis.**

fou rire prodromique A rare form of **pathological laughter**[1786] preceding an intracranial hemorrhage[1786] or brainstem infarct. The neuroanatomical basis for this phenomenon is not known.

Fountain syndrome A recessively inherited congenital dysmorphic syndrome characterized by short stature, thick calvarium, seizures, sensorineural deafness, and mental and developmental delay.[1917]

Fournier test A comprehensive test of gait in which the subject is asked to stand up from a sitting position, walk, stop, and turn quickly on command.

Fourier transformation A mathematical process or technique whereby any wave form is assembled by the addition or superimposition of a number of sine waves.

fourteen- and six-Hz positive burst (14- and 6-Hz positive spikes, ctenoids) A burst of arch-shaped waves at 13–17 Hz and/or 5–7 Hz, but most commonly at 14 and/or 6 Hz, seen generally over the posterior temporal and adjacent areas of one or both sides of the head during sleep. The sharp peaks of its component waves are positive with respect to other regions and their amplitude varies but is generally below 75 uV.

Such bursts are best demonstrated by referential recording using contralateral earlobe or other remote reference electrodes. The clinical significance of this pattern is controversial. (Adapted from the report of the Committee on Terminology, IFCN,[989] © 1974, with permission from Elsevier Science.)

This EEG pattern is commonly found in normal children after the age of 3 years, in whom variable unilateral bursts of positive spikes, lasting a second or so, appear mainly over posterior temporal regions.[5412]

fourteen- and six-Hz positive spikes See **fourteen-and 6-Hz positive burst.**

14-3-3 test Estimation of the quantity of this protein in the CSF undergoing evaluation in the diagnosis of **Creutzfeldt-Jakob disease (CJD).** It appears to be positive in all cases of the sporadic form, but also in some other dementing conditions, including variant CJD.[2263]

fourth of July tetanus Tetanus contracted from the horsehair wadding of blank cartridges fired off in Independence Day celebrations in the United States.[6000]

fovea (Lat, a small hollow) That part of the macula which receives light rays from the central part of the visual field and which is endowed with a high concentration of cone receptors.

foveate To bring a peripheral retinal image onto the fovea by means of a saccade, or to maintain such an image upon the fovea through pursuit movements.

foveation period   A brief instant between the jerk and drift phases of nystagmus, during which time the image of the object of gaze actually lights upon the retina.

foveola   (Lat, diminutive of fovea) The dark central part of the fovea at which point the retinal pigment shows through the retina.

Foville, Achille-Louis-Francois   (1831–1887) French neurologist, anatomist, and physiologist, who trained at the **Salpêtrière** and practiced in the asylum in Rouen where he was appointed superintendent before becoming professor of physiology at Rouen. He later resigned from there and after a period of ill health, went again to Paris as head of the Sharenton, succeeding Esquirol. He was dismissed during the revolution but practiced privately in Paris and finally in Toulouse.

He is credited with a description of **internuclear ophthalmoplegia** (once known as *Foville-Wilson syndrome*) and with important studies of neuroanatomy including the identification of the direct spinocerebellar tract and cranial deformities; he also contributed substantially to the psychiatric literature.[5047] His father, Achille-Louis (1799–1878), described the stria terminalis.

Foville syndrome   A syndrome of infarction within the caudal tegmental pons, the major clinical features being variously described but usually including homolateral nuclear seventh nerve palsy and conjugate gaze palsy toward the side of the lesion, with a contralateral hemiparesis. It is thus a form of **alternating hemiplegia.**

Foville[1920] described a sixth cranial nerve palsy in his patient, whose tongue was also weak on the same side as the facial paresis, in 1858. Except for the latter two findings, the **Millard-Gubler** syndrome is thus almost identical.[4818]

Foville also described variations, according to the involvement of the sixth and the seventh cranial nerves, and the presence of a conjugate gaze palsy resulting from involvement of the peripontine reticular formation.[4723]

Fowler equal-loudness balance test   A test of auditory recruitment using pure tones of varying intensities delivered alternately to either ear, the patient signaling the point at which they are perceived to be equally loud, thus allowing a quantitative measure of unilateral deafness.

Fowler syndrome   A recessively inherited dysmorphic syndrome characterized by intracranial calcification and hydrocephalus.[337]

Fracastoro, Girolamo   (1453–1553) Veronese physician who first applied the word *syphilis* in his poem *Syphilus, sive morbus Gallicus*, published in 1530. In this the poet recounted how Syphilus, a shepherd, abused the sun god when prostrated by heat and was punished by being given a foul and contagious disease.

Fracastoro was particularly interested in infectious diseases, and gave the first accurate account of typhus.

fragile X syndrome   (Martin-Bell syndrome, FRAXA: OMIM 309550) A relatively common X-linked neurodevelopmental disorder, the responsible gene mapping to Xq27.3 or to Xq29. Clinically, nonprogressive mental retardation, large testes, optic atrophy, cerebellar hypoplasia, mitral incompetence, flat feet, and hyperextensible fingers are the usual features.

Delayed motor development, **autism,,** generalized tocin clonic seizures, myhoclonus, and minor neurological signs are also sometimes present.[6011] Some 10% of female carriers manifest evidence of the disease. The name derives from the instability shown by the X chromosome when incubated in a medium deficient in folate. See also **FRAXE.**

fragmentary myoclonus   Brief, fine, twitch-like movements involving various body areas in an asynchronous and asymmetrical fashion and occurring at the onset of sleep and during all sleep stages. The phenomenon is seen in males with fragmented sleep and a variety of sleep disturbances.[783]

See also **periodic limb movement disorder in sleep, hypnic jerks, sleep myoclonus.**

fragmentary seizures   (migratory seizures, erratic seizures) Multifocal clonic seizures occasionally seen in newborns with shifting between locations in the body. Consciousness is usually preserved.[2055]

fragmentation   (of sleep architecture) The interruption of any stage of sleep due to the appearance of another sleep stage or waking, and leading to disrupted non–rapid eye movement–rapid eye movement cycles. Thus, rapid eye movement sleep is interrupted by movement arousals or by non–rapid eye movement stage 2 activity.[249]

Fragoso syndrome   A congenital dysmorphic syndrome of dolichocephaly or scaphocephaly, other skeletal abnormalities resembling those of Marfan syndrome, strabismus, and mental and developmental delay.[337]

Framingham disability scale   An interviewing instrument for the assessment of self-care and physical functioning in the elderly.[4799]

Franceschetti syndrome   See **mandibulofacial dysostosis.**

Franceschetti-Klein-Wildervanck syndrome   See **Wildervanck syndrome.**

Franceschetti-Zwahlen-Klein syndrome   See **mandibulofacial dysostosis.**

Frank syndrome   (familial hyperthyroidism) A congenital dysmorphic syndrome characterized by brachydactyly, clinodactyly, seizures, hyperthyroidism, and mental and developmental delay.[337]

Frankel scale   A global assessment scale for patients with spinal injury.[1933]

Chart F–4. Frankel Scale

Score	Description
A	*Complete injury*; no motor or sensory function below the level of injury.
B	*Sensation only*; some preserved sensation below the level of injury; this does not apply to a slight discrepancy between the motor and sensory level, but does apply to sacral sparing.
C	*Motor function useless*; some preserved motor function below the level of injury, but it is of no practical use to the patient.
D	*Motor function useful*; preserved useful motor function below the level of the injury; patients in this group can walk with or without aids.
E	*Recovery*; normal motor and sensory function; abnormal reflexes may be present.

From Frankel HL, Hancock DO, Hyslop G, et al. The value of postural reduction in the initial management of closed injuries of the spine with paraplegia and tetraplegia. Paraplegia 1969;7:179–192.

Frankl-Hochwart, Lothar von (1862–1915) Austrian neuropathologist who worked with Nothnagel after completing his studies in Vienna. He became professor of neuropathology at the Vienna Polytechnic but died shortly thereafter.

He wrote extensively on the neuropathology of bladder disorders, endocrinology, and **Ménière disease.**[5047]

Frankl-Hochwart syndrome 1. **Ménière disease** with unilateral polyneuritis; a rarity, seldom since detected. 2. Sexual precocity, impairment of upward gaze, evidence of raised intracranial pressure, and hypopituitarism, occurring as a result of a pineal tumor.[1935] 3.The occurrence of lesions of divisions of both the eighth, and the seventh and fifth cranial nerves as manifestations of early neurosyphilis.[4723]

FRAXE A variant of **fragile X syndrome** in which there is mild mental retardation.[3212]

free fraction That portion of a drug which is not bound to plasma proteins and thus is able to cross plasma membranes.

free radicals Momentary chemical substances such as superoxide and hydrogen peroxide and hydroxyl radicals, which have an unpaired electron in their outer shell and which are highly active biologically, especially through their ability to induce the formation of lipid peroxides that damage cell membranes.

They are normally produced by mitochondrial metabolism within all aerobic cells, but are quickly reduced to water by enzymes such as peroxidase, catalase, and superoxide dismutase and are scavenged by vitamins E and C. They are considered to have a role in reperfusion injury, cancer, atheroma, ageing, inflammatory disease, and toxic states.

Freeman-Sheldon syndrome See **whistling face syndrome.**

freezing Brief, sudden, and complete suppression of motor functions, arising typically in patients with **Parkinson disease** and occurring at random or provoked by emotion or by the perception of obstacles to progress in walking.

Fregoli syndrome A delusional misidentification syndrome in which the subject misidentifies a person seen as somebody else, even though that person has a completely different appearance. Lesions in the fusiform gyrus, temporal cortex, and hippocampus are likely to be responsible.[2687] See also **reduplicative paramnesia.**

Freiberg sign (test) Passive, forceful, internal rotation of the extended thigh at the hip causes pain in that area with L5, S1 radiculopathy, but also with in local structural disorders of the hip and buttock. This may be observed in the piriformis syndrome.

French Foundation for Alzheimer Research A charitable organization funding basic research. Address: 11620 Wilshire Blvd Ste., 270, Los Angeles, CA 90025. Web site: http:/www.jdfaf.org/.

Frenchay activities index A **quality-of-life** assessment tool, assessing activities performed over the previous 3–6 months.[2612]

Frenchay Aphasia Screening Test (FAST) A validated and reliable screening test for the presence and nature of aphasia.[1652]

Frenkel sign Hypotonia of the legs in tabes dorsalis.[5047]

Frenkel-Heiden, Heinrich (1860–1931) Swiss psychiatrist who became professor of syphilology at Berlin.

frequency Number of complete cycles of a repetitive waveform in 1 second, measured in hertz (H) or in cycles per second (cps or c/s).[10]

frequency analysis Determination of the range of frequencies composing a waveform, with a measurement of the absolute or relative amplitude of each component frequency. (From the 2001 Report of the Nomenclature Committee of the American Association of Electromyography and Electrodiagnosis.[10] Used by permission, copyright © 2001, AAEM.)

frequency response curve A graph depicting the relationships between the output pen deflection or amplifier output and the input frequency in an EEG channel, for a particular setting of low- and high-frequency filters (Adapted from the report of the Committee on Terminology, IFCN,[989] © 1974, with permission from Elsevier Science.)

Frerichs, Friedreich (1819–1885) German physician who gave the first accounts of both **Wilson disease** (1861) and **multiple sclerosis** (1849).[4979]

Fresnel, Augustin-Jean (1788–1827) French physicist who described the use of glasses with spheres of 20 diopters in order to magnify the eye to the observer when worn as spectacles, but preventing the wearer from focusing on anything and thus from fixating, which encourages the appearance of nystagmus of peripheral (vestibular) origin.

The use of 15 diopter Fresnel prisms in patients with unilateral visual neglect or homonymous hemianopia helps visual perception but does not improve the patient's quality of life,[4806] whatever that may be.

Freud, Sigmund (1856–1939) Austrian physician, born in Moravia, who trained in medicine in Vienna and undertook studies in comparative neuroanatomy and histology until 1882, when financial circumstances drew him to clinical medicine. He combined this with human neuranatomical studies performed in **Meynert**'s laboratory. By then his neurological diagnostic skills were of a high order, but they were further refined as the result of a period spent working with **Charcot** in 1885–86, after which he returned to Vienna to continue his work as a lecturer in pathology and a physician, by now with an interest in hysteria. His views were unacceptable to his former teachers in Vienna, however, and he entered private practice, from which he gained experience to write, with Joseph Breuer, *Studies in Hysteria* and, 5 years later, *The Interpretation of Dreams.*

By the time of his elevation to full professor of neuropathology in 1905, he had over 40 publications, mainly in the basic neurosciences, but his studies on cerebral palsy and his analysis *On Aphasia* (1891) were also notable.[5634] He was the first to distinguish ataxic cerebral palsy, and in 1897 he gave the name *cerebral diplegia* to cerebral palsies with bilateral motor involvement. Freud also translated Charcot's lectures into German, to Charcot's gratification. During the remainder of his life he laid the foundations of psychoanalytic theory, aided by such students as Adler and Carl Jung.[2826]

Frey, Lucja (1889–1944) Polish physician who was born in Lwow, and trained in mathematics and philosophy before entering medical studies in Lwow. She practiced in Warsaw until her death during World War II as a victim of the Nazi régime.

She described the phenomenon of gustatory sweating or sweating of the skin over the parotid gland during salivation (Frey syndrome), which she called the *auriculotemporal nerve syndrome,*[1953] although an account of the same condition had been published in 1757 in France by Dr. M. Duphenix.[850]

Frey, Max von (1852–1932) German physician.

Frey syndrome See **gustatory sweating.**

Frey's hairs Hairs of different diameters mounted on wood and pressed on the skin so that they bend slightly; thus used to determine sensory thresholds for cutaneous touch.

friable (Lat) Easily crumbled.

Fried syndrome A congenital dysmorphic syndrome characterized by syndactyly microcephaly, encephalocele or cranial meningocele, holoprosencephaly, and arhinencephaly.[337]

Friedenwald syndrome Elevation of a ptotic eyelid on turning the eyes to the right, opening the mouth wide,

and protruding the tongue.[2764] This must be rather uncommon. The significance of the sign is not clear.

Friedmann, Max (1858–1925) German neuropsychiatrist, working in Vienna. He described **pyknolepsy** and the following syndromes.

Friedmann syndromes 1. Fullness in the head, irritability, vertigo, insomnia, rapid fatigue, and defective memory following trauma or chronic encephalitis; a set of features which probably represent postconcussional syndrome. 2. (Friedmann-Schultze syndrome) Relapsing infantile spinal paralysis, a variant form of Erb spinal syphilis.[1956] 3. See **pyknolepsy**.[1957] 4. See **pure typical absence epilepsy of childhood.**

Friedman-Roy syndrome An unusual familial syndrome consisting of retardation of both motor and psychomotor development, lalling speech, convergent strabismus, hyperreflexia, upgoing plantar responses, pes cavus, calcification of the choroid plexus, and raised CSF protein levels.

The authors published their findings in a family of six feebleminded children born to normally intelligent parents (cousins) in 1944. The precise nature of the condition is unexplained.[1563]

Friedmann-Schultze syndrome See **Friedmann syndromes.**

Friedreich ataxia The archetypical, recessively inherited spinocerebellar degeneration, described in a series of papers published between 1863 and 1867.[1958] Manifestations occur by puberty and are progressive, so that patients are usually chairbound within 20 years of the onset of the disease.[3222] The defect (an unstable expansion of GAA repeats) is mapped to the frataxin site at 9q13–9q21 and leads to accumulation of iron. Diagnostic criteria have been formulated by Harding[2439] and are given in Chart F–5.

Chart F–5. Diagnostic Criteria for Friedreich Ataxia

1. *Essential criteria for diagnosis*
   i. Within 5 years of onset of symptoms
      Onset before age 25 years
      Progressive ataxia of limbs and gait
      Absent knee and ankle jerks
      Extensor plantar responses
      Motor nerve conduction velocity >40 M/s, with small or absent sensory action potentials
   ii. After 5 years since onset of symptoms
      The above plus dysarthria
2. *Additional features present in over 60% of cases*
   Scoliosis, upper motor neuron weakness of legs, leg areflexia, distal loss of proprioception and vibration, abnormal electrocardiogram (mainly inverted T waves)
3. *Additional features present in less than 50% of cases*
   Nystagmus, optic atrophy, deafness, distal weakness and wasting, pes cavus, diabetes

From Harding AE. The Spinocerebellar Degenerations and Related Disorders Edinburgh, Churchill-Livingstone, 1983. Reprinted by kind permission of Elsevier Science.

Pes planus, equinovarus deformities, and numerous disorders of eye movement control other than nystagmus (slow saccades, jerky pursuit) are also recorded. There is an increased incidence of diabetes and of cardiomyopathy, which is manifest by palpitations and dyspnea, in these patients.

Pathologically, nerve fiber atrophy and demyelination occur mainly in the posterior columns and direct spinocerebellar and lateral corticospinal tracts. The anterior horn cells and the posterior root ganglion cells are also atrophic, the latter resulting in both the posterior column shrinkage and the loss of thick fibers in the peripheral sensory nerves—the prototypic **dying-back** process.[2437] See also **cerebellar ataxias.**

In *variant* forms, also recessively inherited, the same phenotype is associated with selective vitamin E deficiency but without fat malabsorption,[456] the condition occurs at a later age than usual, or linkage to chromosome 9 is absent.[456] A further variant form is *early-onset ataxia with cardiomyopathy and retained reflexes,* which phenotypically differs from Friedreich ataxia but maps to the same locus on chromosome 9q.[4304]

Friedreich Ataxia Group   A charitable organization, affiliated with *Ataxia UK.* Address: 10 Winchester House, Kennington Park, Cranmer Rd., London SW9 6EJ, England. Tel: 020 7582 144. E-mail: office@ataxia.org.uk.

Friedreich disease   1. (polyclonia) A syndrome of bilateral rapid asymmetric muscle contractions which may be inhibited by voluntary muscle contraction.[1960] See **paramyoclonus multiplex.**

2. (facial hemihypertrophy) Asymmetrical enlargement of the facial structures, either alone or with hypertrophy of the remainder of the body on that side.[2764]

Friedreich foot   Pes cavus, described by Friedreich in 1863.[1958]

Friedreich, Nicolaus Anton   (1761–1836) German physician who gave a complete account of facial paralysis in 1797, 24 years before that of Sir Charles **Bell.**

Friedreich, Nikolaus   (1825–1882) German pathologist and physician, born in Wurzburg, where he studied medicine and came under the influence of **Virchow.** He became professor of pathological anatomy in Berlin in 1857 and of medicine at Heidelberg in the following year at the age of 32 and remained there for the rest of his life.

He made contributions in many fields of medicine, but is best remembered for his description of the hereditary ataxia which he first described in 1863[1958] and for his description of **paramyoclonus** (1881).

The independence of the ataxic condition was at first widely disputed, but **Charcot** ultimately gave the disorder the seal of his approval, referring to it as "hereditary ataxy or Friedreich disease" in 1884. Charcot-Marie-Tooth disease (**hereditary motor and sensory neuropathy**) was described by the first two and by the last of these authors 2 years later; the points on which this condition overlaps with Friedreich ataxia may have influenced Charcot to change his opinion to favoring that of Friedreich.[164]

Fritsch, Gustav Theodor   (1838–1927) German neurosurgeon, who demonstrated in 1870 that, in contradiction to currently held opinion, the cerebral cortex is indeed excitable and its stimulation may provoke movement on the other side of the body.[1966]

Fröhlich, Alfred   (1871–1953) Viennese neurologist and pharmacologist who worked with **Sherrington** in Liverpool and with Langley in Cambridge, where he became interested in the autonomic nervous system, which remained a major topic of his research on his return to Vienna as professor. He emigrated to the United States when Austria was invaded in 1939 and worked in Cincinnati. During his life in Europe, he was a friend of Rudyard Kipling and Anton Bruckner, his talents as a writer and pianist being recognized by each.[1829]

Fröhlich syndrome   (adiposogenital dystrophy) A syndrome consisting of obesity, hypogonadism, and bitemporal hemianopia resulting from hypothalamic lesions such as trauma, craniopharyngiomas, and pituitary adenomas.[1967]

Despite the eponym, Berhard Mohr (a German physician) had already described the main features in 1840.[4979]

Froin, Georges   (b. 1874) French physician.

Froin syndrome   (Nonne syndrome) Exceptionally high protein levels in the CSF, causing **xanthochromia** and a tendency for the CSF to clot.[1968] Spinal block, **acute inflammatory polyneuropathy** and vestibular schwannomas are the more common causes. In the complete syndrome, the CSF is under low pressure.

Froment, Jules   (1878–1946) French neurologist practicing in Lyon.

Jules Froment

Froment nerve   (Froment-Rauber nerve) A branch of the radial nerve which innervates (anomalously) the first dorsal interosseous muscle.

Froment sign   1. (signe de journal) Involuntary flexion of the thumb when a piece of paper is held between the finger and thumb of each hand and pulled. The sign indicates ulnar nerve paresis with weakness of the adductor pollicis, for which the long flexor tries to compensate.[1969]

2. (*circle sign*) Lack of flexion at the distal interphalangeal joints of the first and second digits, as would normally be seen when a subject grips a piece of paper between the finger and thumb; a sign of weakness of the flexor digitorum profundus and the flexor pollicis longus, both of which are supplied by the anterior interosseous nerve. This sign, more or less the opposite of the first, is also attributed to Froment.

3. (*Froment maneuver*) Resistance to passive movement of muscles about a joint specifically detected only during voluntary activity of a distant body part. This is not a specific sign and occurs in a number of different disorders manifesting tremor.[1970]

Froment-Rauber nerve   See **Froment nerve.**

Frommann lines   Transverse striae on the axons of myelinated nerve fibers, described by Carl Frommann (1831–1892), a German obstetrician.[4979]

frons   (Lat, the forehead).

frontal alexia   See **alexia.**

frontal apraxia   See **apraxia.**

Frontal Assessment Battery   A tool for the assessment of frontal lobe dysfunction, comprising questions on abstract thought, mental flexibility, motor programming, sensitivity to interference, inibitory control, and environmental autonomy.[1524]

frontal association areas   Areas 9 to 12 of Brodmann.

frontal ataxia   See **frontal disequilibrium.**

Frontal Behavioural Inventory   A validated assessment instrument assisting in the diagnosis of frontotemporal dementia by examining apathy, aspontaneity, indifference, inflexibility, concreteness, personal neglect, distractibility, inattention, loss of insight, logopenia, verbal apraxia, and the alien hand syndrome.[3020]

frontal cortex   The anterior major lobe of the cerebrum, comprising one-third of the hemispheres, and divisible into three zones:

1. The motor–premotor component (Brodmann areas 4 and 6, the supplementary motor area, and parts of the frontal eye fields and Broca's area 44). Lesions here result in contralateral weakness, release of grasp reflexes, altered muscle tone, incontinence, akinesia and mutism, aprosody, apraxia, some of the motor components in unilateral neglect, and **Broca aphasia.**

2. The caudal–mesial–basal part, containing the paralimbic cortex of the anterior cingulate gyrus, and the paraolfactory and caudal orbitofrontal region.

3. The rostral "heteromodal" cortex, comprising Brodmann's areas 9 to 12 and 45 to 47.

The **prefrontal cortex** comprises the latter two of these three divisions, lesions of which lead to manifestations that, taken together, constitute the **frontal lobe syndrome.**

Ablation of the anterior portion leads to loss of recent memory, initiative, and foresight, and indifference or euphoria. Ablation of the posterior part leads to deficits in voluntary movements, expressive aphasia (left second and third convolutions), and motor amusia (right second and third convolutions).

frontal dementias of the non-Alzheimer type   See **frontotemporal dementia.**

frontal disequilibrium   (Bruns gait apraxia, frontal ataxia, astasia-abasia, frontal gait apraxia) A gait pattern dominated by disequilibrium, frequently with inappropriate or counterproductive postural and locomotor synergies. Patients cannot stand (or sometimes sit) unsupported and are unable to organize trunk and leg movements to rise; thus when trying to rise from a chair they may lean back and do not bring their legs in underneath their center of gravity. Nor can they walk because if they step, their feet frequently cross or move in an inappropriate direction.

The pattern is associated with lesions of the frontal lobes or their connections. Associated clinical signs may include dementia, frontal lobe release signs, motor perseveration, urinary incontinence, and extensor plantar responses. (Adapted from Nutt JG, Marsden CD, Thompson PD. Human walking and high-level gait disorders, particularly in the elderly. *Neurology* 1993;**43:**268–279.)

frontal gait apraxia   See **frontal disequilibrium, gait apraxias.**

frontal gait disorder   (magnetic gait apraxia, arteriosclerotic parkinsonism, parkinsonian ataxia, lower half parkinsonism, lower body parkinsonism) A gait pattern characterized by a variable base (narrow or wide), short steps, shuffling, start and turn hesitation, and moderate dysequilibrium.

Patients with this gait syndrome frequently have lesions of the frontal lobes or of their connections, or have multiple hemisphere lesions due to cerebrovascular disease. Associated signs may include cognitive impairment, pseudobulbar palsy with dysarthria, frontal release signs, paratonia, pyramidal signs, and urinary disturbances. (Adapted from Nutt JG, Marsden CD, Thompson PD. Human walking and high-level gait disorders, particularly in the elderly. *Neurology* 1993;**43:** 268–279.) See also **marche à petits pas.**

frontal intermittent rhythmic delta activity (FIRDA) A pattern of fairly regular or approximately sinusoidal waves mostly occurring in bursts at 1.5–3 Hz over the frontal areas of one or both sides of the head but not due to potential changes generated by vertical eye movements. (Adapted from the report of the Committee on Terminology, IFCN,[989] © 1974, with permission from Elsevier Science.)

frontal lobe dementia   See **frontotemporal dementia.**

frontal lobe epilepsies   Location-related seizure disorders characterized by simple partial, complex partial, or secondarily generalized seizures or by combinations of these, emanating from a frontal lobe.

Seizures often occur several times a day and frequently occur during rapid eye movement sleep. Frontal lobe partial seizures are sometimes mistaken for psychogenic seizures. Status epilepticus is a frequent complication. Features strongly suggestive of the diagnosis include:

1. Generally short seizures (<30 seconds)
2. Complex partial seizures arising from the frontal lobe, often with minimal or no postictal confusion
3. Rapid secondary generalization (more common in seizures of frontal than of temporal lobe epilepsy)
4. Prominent motor manifestations which are tonic or postural
5. Complex gestural automatisms frequent at onset
6. Frequent falling when the discharge is bilateral

The attacks tend to be stereotyped and have sudden onset and termination with rapid recovery of consciousness and sometimes violent motor automatisms. Patients are at increased risk for complex partial status epilepticus. The condition is the second most common type of localization-related epilepsy.

Many different frontal lobe seizure subtypes (**cingulate, orbitofrontal, dorsolateral, opercular,** and **motor cortex seizures** and **Kozhevnikoff syndrome**) are described elsewhere; however, multiple frontal areas may be involved rapidly and specific seizure types may not be discernible.[1114,5986] (From Commission for Classification and Terminology, ILAE. Proposal for Revised Classifications of Epilepsies and Epileptic syndromes. *Epilepsia* 1989;**30**:389–399.[1114] By kind permission of Blackwell Science.) See also **autosomal dominant nocturnal frontal lobe epilepsy.**

frontal lobe syndrome   A combination of defects following upon damage to the frontal lobes. Some defects are easily classified and specific, such as aphasia and disturbance of gaze or of motor power; such functions are associated with normal activity in defined, rather more posterior frontal areas. Others, associated with normal function in the frontal association areas, are less specific and include loss of consciousness of the self and its attitude toward the future; loss of coordination and fusion of the incoming and outgoing products of the several sensory and motor areas of the cortex; loss of synthesis; loss of abstract attitude; and loss of execution of visually directed behavior, in the words of several analysts.[3857]

frontal reflex   See **orbicularis oculi reflex.**

frontal release signs   See **primitive reflexes.**

frontofacionasal dysostosis   A recessively inherited congenital dysmorphic syndrome with hypertelorism and characterized also by ptosis, blepharophimosis, brachycephaly and encephalocele, or cranial meningocele.[2011]

frontometaphyseal dysplasia syndrome   (Gorlin syndrome) A congenital, dominantly inherited dysmorphic syndrome characterized by enlarged supraorbital ridges, wide foramen magnum and other cerebral anomalies, generalized hirsutism, distal muscle wasting, and progressive mixed deafness.[2215]

frontonasal dermoid cyst   A dermoid cyst in or abutting the anterior cranial fossa and presenting in childhood with seizures, anosmia, or meningitis.[337]

frontonasal dysplasia   (median cleft face syndrome, median facial cleft syndrome) A congenital, sporadic, or dominantly inherited dysmorphic syndrome characterized by ocular hypertelorism, anterior cranium bifidum occultum, and other inconstant defects, including craniosynostosis, polydactyly, hydrocephalus, stroke syndromes, and agenesis of the corpus callosum.[2219]

frontotemporal dementia   (Pick disease, frontal lobe dementia, Pick-complex disorder, frontotemporal lobar degeneration, progressive subcortical gliosis, frontal dementias of the non-Alzheimer type, dementia lacking distinctive histology, frontal lobe degeneration, disinhibition-dementia-parkinsonism-amyotrophy syndrome, primary progressive aphasia, corticodentatonigral or corticobasal degeneration) Dementing illnesses somewhat resembling **Alzheimer disease,** linked to chromosome 17. Numerous clinical varieties are distinguished: a syndrome of nonspecific frontal lobe degeneration, known also as the frontal variant of frontotemporal degeneration and presenting with marked changes in personality and behavior; the form once known as Pick disease; another in which there is major temporal lobe pathology and clinical evidence of progressive fluent aphasia ("semantic dementia"), and a form with added anterior horn cell loss. Clinically, cognitive, behavioral, aphasic, and extrapyramidal manifestations merge in the various subtypes of the disorder. The pathological characteristics of most of them are listed below.

In many of the subtypes there are prominent accumulations of **tau** protein.

The clinical features that best differentiate the typical condition from Alzheimer disease are social conduct disorders, hyperorality, akinesia, and lack or amnesia or perceptual difficulties. A more formal listing can be synthesized from recent reports[2972,3878] as follows:

Onset is insidious, with slow progression.

Dominant deficits in behavior and conduct appear early in the course of the disease:

Loss of personal awareness (neglect of hygiene and grooming)

Loss of social graces and awareness

Disinhibition (sexually provocative or demanding, inappropriate jocularity)

Impulsivity, distractibility

Hyperorality (dietary changes, excessive eating, smoking, or alcohol consumption)

Withdrawal from social contact

Stereotyped or perseverative behaviors (wandering, repetitive clapping, humming, or singing, ritualistic toileting, dressing)

Speech output changes

Progressive reduction of speech (late mutism)

Stereotypy of speech (few repeated phrases or themes)

Echolalia

Physical signs

Early or prominent primitive or "frontal" reflexes

Early incontinence

Late akinesia, rigidity, tremor

Deficits in social comportment, behavior, judgment, or language are out of proportion to memory deficit.

A major advance was the publication of a consensus statement on the clinical diagnostic criteria for the condition(s) reproduced in an amended form below.

Clinical Diagnostic Features of Frontotemporal Dementia

Behavioral disorder

Core features

Insidious onset and slow progression

Early decline in regulation of personal conduct

Early decline in social interpersonal contact (lack of social tact, misdemeanors such as shoplifting)

Early emotional blunting despite such signs of disinhibition as unrestrained sexuality, violent behavior, inappropriate jocularity, restless pacing, etc.

Early loss of insight into the fact that the altered condition is due to a pathological change of the subject's own mental state

Supportive features

Neglect of personal hygiene and grooming

Mental rigidity and inflexibility

Distractibility, impulsivity, and impersistence

Hyperorality (oral/dietary changes, overeating, food fads, excessive smoking and alcohol consumption, oral exploration of objects)

Stereotyped and perseverative behavior (wandering, mannerisms such as clapping, singing, dancing, ritualistic preoccupation such as hoarding, toileting, and dressing)

Utilization behavior (unrestrained exploration of objects in the environment)

Speech disorder

Progressive reduction of speech (lack of spontaneity and economy of utterance)

Press of speech

Sterotypy of speech (repetition of limited repertoire of words, phrases, or themes)

Echolalia, perseveration or mutism

Affective symptoms

Depression, anxiety, excessive sentimentality, suicidal and fixed ideation, delusion (early and evanescent)

Hypochondriasis, bizarre somatic preoccupation (early and evanescent)

Emotional unconcern (emotional indifference and remoteness, lack of empathy and sympathy, apathy)

Amimia (inertia, aspontaneity)

Spatial orientation and praxis are preserved

Physical signs

Early appearance of primitive reflexes, incontinence

Akinesia, rigidity, tremor (late)

Low and labile blood pressure

Investigations

Normal EEG despite clinically evident dementia

Brain imaging (structural, functional, or both): predominant frontal and/or anterior temporal abnormality

Neuropsychology; profound failure on "frontal lobe" tests in the absence of severe amnesia, aphasia, or perceptual spatial disorder

Supportive diagnostic features

Onset before 65

Positive family history of similar disorder in a first-degree relative

Bulbar palsy, muscular weakness and wasting, fasiciculations (motor neuron disease)

Excluding features

Abrupt onset with ictal events

Head trauma related to onset

Early severe amnesia

Early spatial disorientation, lost in surroundings, defective localization of objects

Early severe apraxia

Logoclonic speech with rapid loss of train of thought

Myoclonus

Cortical bulbar and spinal deficits

Cerebellar ataxia

Choreoathetosis

Early, severe, pathological EEG

Brain imaging (predominant post-central structural or functional deficit; multifocal cerebral lesions on CT or MRI)

Laboratory tests indicating brain involvement or inflammatory disorder (such as multiple sclerosis, syphilis, AIDS, and herpes simplex encephalitis)

Relative diagnostic exclusion features

Typical history of chronic alcoholism

Sustained hypertension

History of vascular disease (such as angina, claudication)

Adapted from Brun A, Englund B, Mann DMA, Neary D, et al. Consensus on Clinical and Neuropathological Criteria for Fronto-Temporal Dementia. J. Neurol. Neurosurg. Psychiatry 1994;**57**;416-418[814] *and Neary D, Snowden JS, Gustafson L, et al. Frontotemporal lobar degeneration.* Neurology 1998;**5157**:1546-54,[4083] *by kind permission.*

Other clinical subtypes have been differentiated as follows: an *orbitobasal* variety characterized by disinhibition, impulsiveness, confabulation, and antisocial behavior; and a *dorsolateral* form with poor attention and focus, working memory deficits, poor organization, planning and word/design generation, poor insight, and abnormal expression of affect. A *medial frontal* form is also described. Variant familial forms, one with added parkinsonian features and another named *hereditary dysphasic disinhibition dementia*[3343] have been mapped to 17q21–22. At least the first of these is associated with multiple tau gene mutations.[3423] The condition also overlaps **corticobasal degeneration syndrome.**[3022] See also **progressive subcortical gliosis.**

Neuropathological Diagnostic Features of Frontotemporal Dementia

1. Frontal lobe degeneration type

Gross changes
These include slight symmetrical convolutional atrophy in frontal and anterior temporal lobes, neither circumscribed nor of a knife blade type; atrophy can be severe in a few cases. The ventricular system is widened frontally. Usually there is no gross atrophy of the stratum, amygdala, or hippocampus, although, in some instances, severe involvement of these regions can occur.

Distribution of microscopic changes
Changes are seen in the frontal convexity cortex, sometimes in the orbitofrontal cortex, often in the anterior third of the temporal cortex and the anterior, but rarely the posterior, cingulate gyrus. The superior temporal gyrus is conspicuously spared. The parietal cortex is mildly involved in a few patients, more so in rare, advanced cases. In some patients with pronounced stereotypic behaviors, there is less neocortical involvement, with mostly striatal, amygdala, and hippocampal changes. These may represent a possible subtype.

Microscopic characteristics, gray matter
Microvacuolation and mild to moderate astrocytic gliosis affecting chiefly laminae I–III are seen, sometimes one or the other change prevailing. There is atrophy/loss of neurons in laminae II and III, whereas those of lamina 5 are mildly affected, being atrophic rather than lost. Occasionally there are a few dystrophic neurites. There are no Pick bodies, inflated neurons, or Lewy bodies. Immunohistochemistry for tau or ubiquitin reveals no distinctive features. In the substantial nigra of some patients, there is mild to moderate loss of pigmented neurons.

Microscopic characteristics, white matter
White matter astrocytic gliosis, moderate to mild, is seen in subcortical U fibers. There is very mild astrocytic gliosis in deeper white matter, sometimes with slight attenuation and loss of myelin. The distribution is related to gray matter changes. Sometimes there is also ischemic white matter attenuation.

2. Pick type

Gross changes
These have the same topographic localization as for frontal lobe degeneration, but are generally more intense and usually more circumscribed. Asymmetry and striatal atrophy are common.

Distribution of microscopic changes
These are the same as in frontal lobe degeneration, in agreement with the gross distribution.

Microscopic characteristics, gray and white matter
The main characteristics are the same as those of frontal lobe degeneration, but with intense involvement of all cortical layers. Inflated neurons and Pick bodies, which are silver positive, tau and ubiquitin immunoreactive, are present. There is more intense white matter involvement. Patients with intense astrocytosis but without inflated neurons or inclusions or both may for the present be included.

3. Motor neuron disease type

Gross changes
These are the same as in frontal lobe degeneration, although usually less severe.

Distribution of microscopic changes and microscopic characteristics in gray and white matter
These are the same as for frontal lobe degeneration. There is spinal motor neuron degeneration, affecting cervical and thoracic levels more than lumbar or sacral. There is greater cell loss in medial than lateral cell columns. Motor neurons, layer II neurons in frontal and temporal cortex, and hippocampal dentate gyrus neurons show inclusions that are ubiquitin positive but not silver or tau reactive. Nigral cell loss is severe in many patients. There is also hypoglossal degeneration in some patients.

Diagnostic exclusion features
These include senile plaques, diffuse amyloid deposits, and amyloid angiopathy with anti–B-protein antibodies, tangles, and neuropil threads, with more anti-tau and ubiquitin antibodies than normal for age. Prion protein is present with anti-prion antibodies. (Adapted from Brun et al.[814])

frontotemporal lobar degeneration   See **frontotemporal dementia.**

frontotemporoparietal encephalitic syphilis   See **general paresis of the insane.**

Froriep, August von   (1849–1917) German anatomist who first described a form of myositis in which connective tissue takes the place of muscle—a chronic polymyositis.[4979]

Froriep induration   Chronic atrophic myositis with marked intramuscular fibrosis.[4979]

frozen shoulder   See **Duplay syndrome.**

fructose 1,6-diphosphatase deficiency   A rare inborn error of metabolism which may be associated with atypical **central core disease** of muscle.[2929]

fructose intolerance   A diffuse encephalopathy inherited as a recessive trait and characterized by hypoglycemia (which may induce seizures) and recurrent abdominal pain, nausea, vomiting, and diarrhea resulting from the ingestion of fructose and related sugars in the presence of a deficiency of the enzyme aldolase B.[1152]

fructosemia   A recessively inherited disease due to deficiency of fructose-1-phosphate aldolase and characterized clinically by the congenital onset of failure to thrive, hypoglycemic episodes, hepatic and renal impairment, and axonal motor neuropathy.[4662]

Fryns syndrome   A lethal, recessively inherited, congenital dysmorphic syndrome manifesting also short stature, anterior chamber abnormalities, cloudy corneas, microphthalmia, ptosis, aortic stenosis, brachydactyly, and mental and developmental delay.[1976]

FTA-Abs   (fluorescent treponemal antibody absorption test) A treponemal test for syphilis, which remains permanently reactive after infection.

Fuchs sign   1. See **Gowers signs.** 2. Uncoordinated movements of the upper eyelid following damage to the third cranial nerve, considered to be the result of anomalous reinnervation. See **pseudo-Graefe phenomenon.**

fucosidosis   A rare inherited, neuronal storage disease (an oligosaccharidosis) resulting from a deficiency of α-fucosidase, which leads to the accumulation of H-isoantigen. Intralysosomal laminated structures and axonal spheroids are detectable by electron microscopy in skin biopsy specimens.[1559] Two forms of the disease are recognised: *type 1* (*infantile*) is characterized by psychomotor deterioration, cloudy corneae, dry skin, telangiectasia, mucopolysaccariduria, hypotonia, and later spasticity, myoclonic seizures, coarse facies, hepatosplenomegaly, cardiomegaly, and dysostoses. The sweat chloride test result is abnormal. In *type 2* (*juvenile*) the onset of similar but milder signs occurs in the first 2 years of life; the sweat chloride test result is normal.

Unnumbered is a *variant* adult form, characterized clinically by gargoyle-like facies, psychomotor retardation, and angiokeratoma corporis diffusum.[2729]

fugax   (Lat) Fleeing or fleeting.

Fugl-Meyer scale   A system of evaluation of motor function, balance, and some qualities of sensation and joint function in hemiplegic patients, in which a cumulative numerical score is assigned. The scale was designed to assess the progressive return of physical performance following the occurrence of stroke.[1977]

fugue state   See **twilight state.**

Fukada stepping test   A test for vestibular dysfunction, in which blindfolded subjects mark time for 1 minute and the degree of rotation on their own axis is assessed. Normally there should be none.

Fukayama congenital muscular dystrophy   A recessively inherited muscular dystrophy presenting in infancy, found almost exclusively in the Orient. This merosin-positive form is characterized by muscle weakness and hypotonia with delayed motor developmental milestones, severe contractures, and only mild mental retardation. The CT and MRI may show some white matter lucencies and micropolygyria.[3107] The homogeneous merosin-negative form is characterized by marked motor disability, seizures, hydrocephalus, Dandy-Walker malformation, cerebral cortical malformations (including heterotopias and pachygyria or microgyria), and skull deformities,[1988] but mentation is relatively unaffected. Serum CK levels are raised and there are numerous areas of low signal intensity on MRI scans. It is mapped to chromosome 6q22–23 and is genetically identical to the **Walker-Warburg syndrome.** See also **congenital muscular dystrophy.**

Fukuhara syndrome   See **MERRF.**

full interference pattern   See **interference pattern.**

full wave rectified EMG   The absolute value of a raw EMG signal, which involves inverting all the waveforms below the isopotential line and displaying them with opposite polarity above the line. This technique is used to analyze kinesiologic EMG signals. (From the 2001 Report of the Nomenclature Committee of the American Association of Electromyography and Electrodiagnosis.[10] Used by permission, copyright © 2001, AAEM.)

full-field stimulation   Excitation of the retina by visual stimuli which occupy all or most of the visual field.

Such a condition is required for the appearance of the **optokinetic reflex.**

fullness of the ears   One of the symptoms that leads to sinking of the heart because of its nonspecificity. The complaint, however, is common in patients with **Ménière syndrome** and in those with cluster headache, so it may truly have some diagnostic value.

Fulton, John Farquar   (1899–1960) American neurophysiologist born in Minnesota. After service in World War I, he entered Harvard as a veteran and, in 1921, graduated with the highest honors in science, proceeding then to Oxford as a Rhodes scholar and later as demonstrator in physiology. At Oxford he came under the influence of **Sherrington,** which turned him in the direction of neurophysiology and medical history;

while at Oxford he compiled the catalogue of **Osler**'s historical library.

After further periods at Yale and Oxford, he returned to assume the Sterling Chair of Physiology at Yale, where he undertook and encouraged studies in aviation physiology, neurophysiology, endocrinology, electro-cardiology, and endocrinology, and where he worked with **Cushing** on the study of cerebral physiology and the compilation of medical history. In 1935 he refused the appointment as successor to Sherrington at Oxford, preferring to remain at Yale. His best-known works were his *Physiology of the Nervous System* (London, 1938), *Readings in the History of Physiology*, and his biography of **Cushing.**

The personal charm and commitment that inspired so many of his students at all levels cannot be depicted adequately in a mere dictionary.

fumarase deficiency   An inherited cause of mito-chondrial encephalopathy in which this enzyme defi-ciency leads to dysfunction within the tricarboxylic acid cycle as a result of an inability to convert fumaric acid to malic acid.

Clinically, this early infantile encephalopathy pres-ents with microcephaly, failure to thrive, profound de-velopmental delay, seizures, hypotonia, facial dysmor-phisms, and cerebral atrophy and leads to death in the first year; polycythemia, lactic and pyruvic aciduria, and fumaric acidemia are other characteristic fea-tures.[3016,6131]

fumaric aciduria   A mitochondrial encephalopathy caused by a deficiency of mitochondrial cytosolic fu-marase.[6131]

functional assessment staging   (FAST) A 16-item scale derived from the self-care axis of the **Brief Cog-nitive Rating Scale.** It is of use in the diagnosis and staging of patients with any type of cognitive disorder and for assessing functional capacity at the severe ex-treme of **Alzheimer disease.** Activities rated include memory, functioning at work and socially, self-care, and speech/language. Seven stages are defined and their dates recorded. Assessment runs from normality through complaints of forgetting the location of ob-jects; decreased job functioning evident to co-workers; decreased ability to perform complex tasks; difficulty in choosing proper clothing; difficulty dressing; and fail-ure in self-care and communication.[4644,4649]

functional bent back   See **camptocormia.**

Functional Composite   An outcome measure for clinical trials of therapies in multiple sclerosis, examin-ing arm/hand function, leg function/ambulation, and cognition.[2909]

functional disease   Disturbance of body functions for which no responsible disturbance of structure can be detected. In this context, the word *structure* includes

pathophysiology and abnormal chemistry within the nervous system.

The similarity of this definition to that of **hysteria** will be noted, but, although the physician using the latter term usually considers that the patient is manifesting a disorder that is rooted in psychopathology, use of the former commonly indicates that a nonpsychiatric cause of the disease state may be incriminated, as, for exam-ple, in the case of *functional hypoglycemia.* See **hysteria.**

functional grading   The scores assigned to patients as a result of **functional muscle testing.**[4796,5589] The scheme of Brooke et al.[775] is given in Chart F–6. Appel et al.[194] have defined similar grades for the bulbar mus-cles (Chart F–7).

Chart F–6. Functional Grades

Arms

1. Starting with arms at the sides, patient can abduct the arms in a full circle until they touch above the head.
2. Can raise arms above the head only by flexing the elbow (i.e., shortening the circumference of the movement) or by using accessory muscles.
3. Cannot raise the hands above the head but can raise an 8 ounce (240 ml) glass of water to mouth (using both hands if necessary).
4. Can raise hand to mouth but cannot use hands to hold pen or pick up pennies from table.
5. Cannot raise hands to mouth and has no useful function of hands.

Hips and legs

1. Walks and climbs stairs without assistance.
2. Walks and climbs stairs with aid of railing.
3. Walks and climbs stairs slowly with aid of railing (over 12 seconds for four standard stairs).
4. Walks unassisted and rises from chair but cannot climb stairs.
5. Walks unassisted but cannot rise from chair or climb stairs.
6. Walks only with assistance or walks independently with long leg braces.
7. Walks in long leg braces but requires assistance for bal-ance.
8. Stands in long leg braces but unable to walk even with assistance.
9. Is in wheelchair.
10. Is confined to bed.

Chart F–7. Functional Grading for Bulbar Muscles

Action	Points
Swallowing	
General diet	3
Soft diet	6
Mechanical soft diet	9
Strained or pureed diet	12
Tube feeding	15

Speech

Clear	3
Pa-Ta-Ka slightly slurred	6
Slurred	9
Unintelligible	12
None	15

From Appel V, et al. A rating scale for amyotrophic lateral sclerosis. Arch Neurol 1987;**22**:328–333. © American Medical Association.

functional hemianopia See **hemianopia.**

functional imaging Noninvasive methods (such as SPECT, MRI, or PET scanning) that allow visualization of neural activity in brain regions during the performance of specific tasks or when treated with extraneous molecules.

Functional Independence Measure An 18-item functional disability scale, of value in the determination of disability in patients with stroke, multoiple sclerosis, or other chronic neurological conditions. The degree of dependence and independence in *personal care, sphincter control, mobility, locomotion, communication, and social cognition* are assessed, with scores of between 1 (requiring full assistance) and 7 (independent) being applied.[2991]

Functional Limitations Profile A British scale containing 136 questions designed to assess the limitations imposed by disease on various categories of activity, such as *ambulation, body care and movement, mobility, household management, recreation and pastimes, social interaction, affect, alertness, sleep, eating, communication, and work.* Individual scores are given on each of these items.

functional localization The localization of particular motor or sensory properties within specific cell groups within the CNS.

functional muscle testing Techniques for evaluating the strength of muscle contractions using the subjective judgments both of the examiner and the patient as regards the capacity of the latter to perform specified motor tasks. As a result of such an evaluation, the patient is assigned a **functional grade,** which with **timed functional testing** allows accurate documentation of the course of a progressive neuromuscular disease.[178,4022]

functional neurosurgery Nondestructive surgery, such as the implantation of neurostimulating electrodes.

Functional Rating Scale A multidimensional rating instrument derived from the **Clinical Dementia Rating Scale** with the addition of the two domains of language and behavior.[1773]

functional refractory period See **refractory period.**

functional seizures See **pseudoseizures.**

functional somatic syndromes A term applied to several related syndromes characterized more by symptoms, suffering, and disability than by consistently demonstrable tissue abnormality. These syndromes include multiple chemical sensitivity, the sick building syndrome, repetition stress injury, the side effects of silicone breast implants, Gulf War syndrome, whiplash, the fatigue syndrome, the irritable bowel syndrome, and fibromyalgia. Common symptoms include fatigue; weakness; sleep difficulties; headache; muscle aches and joint pain; problems with memory, attention, and concentration; nausea and other gastrointestinal symptoms; anxiety; depression; irritability; palpitations and "racing heart"; shortness of breath; dizziness or lightheadedness; sore throat; and dry mouth. Patients often proffer explicit, highly elaborated diagnoses, and they are often refractory to reassurance, explanation, and standard treatment of symptoms. They share similar phenomenologies, high rates of co-occurrence, similar epidemiologic characteristics, and higher-than-expected prevalences of psychiatric comorbidity. Although discrete pathophysiological causes may ultimately be found in some patients with functional somatic syndromes, the suffering of these patients is exacerbated by a self-perpetuating, self-validating cycle in which common, endemic, somatic symptoms are incorrectly attributed to a serious abnormality, reinforcing the patient's belief that he or she has a serious disease. Four psychosocial factors propel this cycle of symptom amplification: the belief that one has a serious disease; the expectation that one's condition is likely to worsen; the "sick role," including the effects of litigation and compensation; and the alarming portrayal of the condition as catastrophic and disabling. Patients with functional somatic syndromes have elevated rates of psychiatric disorders, particularly anxiety, depressive, and somatoform disorders.[376] See also **factitious disease, hysteria.**

Funderbunk syndrome (mesomelia and nephritis) A dysmorphic syndrome characterized by short stature and limbs, strabismus, small widely spaced teeth, nephropathy with hematuria and proteinuria, mesomelia of the upper and lower limbs, Madelung deformity, cortical hyperostosis, and mental and developmental delay.[4360]

fundus oculi (Lat, the bottom or base + eye) That portion of the retina (in the depths of the eye) visible with the ophthalmoscope.

fungal myositis The rare direct infection of muscles with fungi, particularly *Candida albicans.* Immunocompromised subjects are those most likely to be affected.

funicular pain See **central pain.**

funiculus (Lat, a small rope) A group of nerve fibers invested in a sheath of connective tissue, the perineurium, the whole varying in size from 0.04 to 3 mm. Bundles of funiculi form the nerve trunk.

funnel vision The physiological increase in the diameter of the visual field as the test object is taken farther away from the subject; a cone of vision is thus produced. See also **tunnel vision.**

Furukawa syndrome A syndrome characterized by the onset in childhood of optic atrophy, chorioretinitis, retinitis pigmentosa, kyphoscoliosis, diabetes, cerebellar ataxia, myopathic weakness, and sensorimotor neuropathy.[1999]

fusiform (from Lat) Elliptical or spindle shaped.

fusiform aneurysm See **aneurysm.**

fusimotor neurons Gamma efferent fibers that innervate **fusimotor spindles.**

fusimotor spindles Specialized muscle fibers within voluntary muscles which are sensitive to stretch and which send impulses centrally along fast-conducting 1a afferent fibers to assist in the regulation of muscle tone.

fusion (fusion reflex) A cortically mediated mechanism whereby the eyes are directed toward an object in such a manner that this image of the object falls upon the two maculas and any imbalance is corrected for through the working of the occipital cortex to suppress the awareness of blurring of the images perceived, which are now seen as one.

fusion reflex See **fusion.**

fusional adaptation A brainstem mechanism whereby the positions of the eyes are reset to minimize the effect of a disparity in retinal imaging, as might occur if a prism were placed before one eye.

Both *fast* and *slow* adaptive mechanisms are described.[3330]

fusional vergence (disparity-induced vergence) Movements of the eyes which rotate them in opposite directions to minimize any disparity in the direction of visual images on corresponding points of the foveas of the eyes.

G

G syndrome (hypospadias-dysphagia syndrome) A rare, dominantly inherited congenital syndrome characterized by hypertelorism, slit-like palpebral fissures and other facial dysmorphisms, pigmentary retinal degeneration, hypospadias, dysphagia with aspiration and respiratory distress, anosmia, achalasia, pulmonary malformations, and malformations of the alimentary tract.[3435,4246] See also **hypertelorism-hypospadias syndrome.**

G1 See **active electrode.**

GABA Gamma-amino butyric acid, an inhibitory neurotransmitter found mainly in the central nervous system but also in the pancreas.

GABA transaminase deficiency A congenital dysmorphic syndrome manifesting also aminoaciduria, hyperpituitarism, focal CNS demyelination with diffuse gliosis, seizures, dysphagia, and mental and developmental delay.[337]

gabapentin An experimental GABA-related amino acid that may antagonize the action of aspartate, thus acting as an inhibitor of neurotransmission and in turn as an anticonvulsant.

gadolinium A paramagnetic agent used with MRI scanning. It shortens the half-life of relaxation and leads to enhancement of demyelinating lesions.

gag reflex Elevation of the soft palate and contraction of the pharyngeal constrictors in response to tactile stimulation of the pharyngeal mucosa. The afferent arc of the reflex travels via the ninth and the efferent via the ninth and tenth cranial nerves.

Gage, Phineas P. An American railway foreman described as honest and industrious until in 1848 a 3-foot (0.9 meter) tamping iron was accidentally blown through his frontal lobes while he was at work, effecting a frontal lobotomy from which he did not die at once; but the subsequent alteration in his personality (he exhibited himself in a circus for some years and later became a stagecoach driver in Chile) provided the first clue to the highest functions of the prefrontal lobe. He died in status epilepticus 12 years after the accident.

His case was recorded in the *Boston Medical and Surgical Reporter* by Dr. J.M. Harlow, a general practitioner in the same year, and further described by H.G. Bigelow, a Boston surgeon in 1850.[420]

gain The ratio of the output signal voltage to the input signal voltage of an EEG channel. For example:

$$\text{Gain} = \frac{\text{Output Voltage}}{\text{Input Voltage}} = \frac{10 \text{ V}}{10 \text{ uV}} = 1,000,000$$

This is often expressed in decibels (dB), a logarithmic unit; thus a voltage gain of 10 = 20 Db, of 1000 = 60 Db, or of 1,000,000 = 120 Db. See also **sensitivity.**

(Adapted from the 1974 report of the Committee on Terminology, IFCN. In: Chatrian GE, Bergamini L, Dondey M, et al. A glossary of terms most commonly used by clinical electroencephalographers. *EEG Clin Neurophysiol* 1974;37:538–548.[989])

gain of pursuit eye movements (pursuit gain) The relationship between the velocity of a visual target and that of the tracking eyes. It is typically reduced in Parkinson disease, older age, and progressive supranuclear palsy, and may be increased in an eye when the other eye has a paretic muscle.

gait The manner or pattern of walking. **Apraxic, ataxic, dyskinetic, hysterical, magnetic, parkinsonian, spastic,** and **steppage** gaits are described.

gait apraxia (frontal gait apraxia) An entity of doubtful validity in which patients fail to perform whole-body movements in response to command or on imitation, but can do so spontaneously.

This syndrome was dismissed by Geschwind,[2080] who emphasized that most patients diagnosed with gait apraxia have fixed disturbances in the performance of whole-body movements because of lesions at a lower level. See **isolated gait ignition failure.**

However, this has been presented as an inability to stand up or move the feet along the floor while seated, in the absence of ataxia, limb apraxia, or buccofacial apraxia, and despite the retained ability to pantomime walking and peddling movements when supine. The responsible lesion is thought to be bilateral in posterior subcortical regions or in the thalamus.[5114]

gait ignition A starting signal sent to those muscles responsible for ambulation when the appropriate preliminary shifts in the center of gravity have occurred.[4180]

gait ignition failure A term used for by difficulty in initiating walking. The gait has elements of parkinsonism with start and turn hesitation, shuffling, and freezing but is relatively normal once entrained; the posture is upright, with good arm swing, a normal stride length, and no festination. Equilibrium is near normal, and when seated or lying, rhythmic leg movements are generated normally. Facial expression, upper limb mobility, and whole-body movements are well preserved. The lesions causing this syndrome include frontal lobe vascular disease and focal degeneration of the frontal lobes.[252]

galactocerebroside (from Gr, milk + brain) The abnormal substance stored in **Krabbe disease.**

galactokinase deficiency A recessively inherited syndrome resembling **galactosemia** but found only in the Eastern European gypsy population and characterized by hepatosplenomegaly, cataract, and sometimes seizures and mental retardation.[2130]

galactosemic encephalopathy A syndrome of cortical neuronal degeneration with spongy changes occurring in infants with untreated galactosemia (galactosephosphate uridyltransferase deficiency); the gene responsible for this recessive condition maps to 9p13.

Clinically, it presents after the introduction of milk into the diet, with jaundice and other manifestations of hepatic insufficiency, cataract, hypoglycemia, cerebral edema, and early death. Sensorineural hearing loss, mental and motor retardation, and tremors may occur in children when the delayed-onset form is treated.[111] The condition is also rarely reported in adults.

galactosialidosis (β-galactosidase-neuraminidase deficiency) An inherited condition clinically resembling **mucolipidosis type 1.** The responsible gene maps to chromosome 20.

Clinically, the condition has its onset in early adult life, and manifests optic atrophy, ataxia, seizures, stimulus-sensitive myoclonus, and muscle atrophy, hypotonia, and weakness. Angiokeratomas, gargoyle facies, and vertebral changes have also been noted.[4883]

galactosidases Intracellular enzymes required for the metabolism of ceramide (α-galactosidase) or keratan (β-galactosidase), and diminished or absent in **Fabry disease** and **mucopolysaccharidosis type IVb,** respectively.

galactosylceramide lipidosis See **Krabbe leukodystroophy.**

galanin A neuropeptide, found in high concentration in the basal nucleus of Meynert, where, with choline acetyltransferase, its concentration is diminished in **Alzheimer disease.**

Galant reflex (trunk incurvation) When the examiner's finger presses on one side of the back of the prone baby, the infant flexes the trunk so that the spine is concave to that side. The sign is normally present between birth and 4 months of age.

galea (Lat, a helmet) The sheet of connective tissue stretching across the scalp like a cap, into which are inserted the frontalis, temporalis, and occipitalis muscles.

Galen, Claudius (or Clarissimus) (130–200 A.D.) A Roman, born in Pergamum, Asia Minor, studying there and at Smyrna, Corinth, and Alexandria. He became physician to Marcus Aurelius in Venice.

Galen was the founder of the galenic system of medicine, utilizing plants and minerals, and reputedly published over 500 works, although many were lost when his house burned down. His studies of the nervous system were probably facilitated by his responsibility for attending to the wounds of gladiators; he described head and spinal injuries in some detail and, in the latter case, partially anticipated the description of **Brown-Séquard.** His name is given to the great vein of Galen and to the choroidal veins, but he also described and named many parts of the brain and about 300 muscles, demonstrated the origin of nerves from the brain and spinal cord, described seven pairs of cranial nerves, and elucidated the function of the recurrent laryngeal nerve (by cutting it in a pig).

Galen considered that the choroid produced CSF, with contributions of pneuma from air passing through the cribriform plate and from the rete mirabile. He described flow from the lateral ventricles through the third and fourth ventricles to the outlet in the roof, draining from there through the cribriform plate and to the palate.[5608]

Galen has been regarded as the Prince of Physicians on account of his observations in almost all fields of medicine; his works constituted the leading medical authority for 1400 years. He localized mental functions in the cerebrum rather than in the ventricles[5204] and stated that seizures affecting the face were due to disease in the brain, and, when the face was spared, the lesion was in the upper part of the spinal cord. He also described the aura, the facial appearance of chronic epileptic people, the periodicity of the attacks, and focal sensory seizures.

Gall, F.J. (1758–1828) Viennese physician and neuroanatomist, the founder of the discipline of phrenology and the father of cerebral localization. As a boy he noted the different aptitudes of schoolfellows and compared these with their facial and cranial peculiarities. After completing medical studies in Strasbourg and Vienna, he continued to study the relationship between aptitudes and morphology with a series of dissections of the brain; he described first the cervical and lumbar enlargements of the cord, differentiated gray from white matter, and described the origins of cranial nerves II, III, IV, and VI.

This work culminated in his monograph *Anatomie et Physiologie du Systeme nerveux en general, et du Cerveau en particulier,* published after he was prevented from further experimentation in Vienna by the offices of the Church. In this work, he localized certain functions to specific brain areas—a major advance, since Cullen, in his *Practice of Physic* (1776–1784), had written, "nor have we been able to perceive that any particular part of the brain has more concern in the operations of our intellect than any other. Nor have we attained any knowledge of what share the several parts of the brain have in that operation."

Gall isolated 27 cranial areas which he believed corresponded with as many mental attributes—the Propensities, the Sentiments, and the Intellectual Faculties. He was unaware of the asymmetries of brain function and many of the localizations ascribed (for example, he considered that the cerebellum was the seat of the sexual impulse) were ill founded, although in many ways, conventional at the time. The theories which he propounded, the style with which he propounded them, and the influence of his enthusiastic disciples such as J.G. **Spurzheim** led to huge popular support for the cult over some decades. It was when excessive claims were made—such as the ability of phrenology to divine character, and thus its adequacy as a method for selecting members of Parliament—that the movement fell into disrepute and attracted ridicule. Yet, as Edwin G. Boring wrote, his was "an instance of a theory which, while essentially wrong, was just right enough to further scientific thought."

Phrenology helped to move ideas concerning the mind "away from the concept of the unsubstantial Cartesian soul to the concept of the more material nerve function . . . (and thus) . . . was wrong only in detail and in the enthusiasm of its supporters." The best recent critiques of Gall's life and teaching are those of Critchley[1176] and of Temkin.[5520]

GALOP syndrome (**G**ait disorder, **A**utoantibody, **L**ate-age **O**nset **P**olyneuropathy) A symmetric sensorimotor demyelinating polyneuropathy of older adults producing marked gait disorder with ataxia and positive Romberg sign associated with the presence of serum IgM autoantibodies.

galloping tongue Episodic, involuntary, rhythmic, and wave-like tongue movements at 3 Hz and lasting 10 seconds with 20-second periods of rest between, starting posteriorly in the midline and extending laterally, seen rarely following pontine lesions, as after head injury.[2978]

Galton, Francis (1822–1911) English scientist and geneticist, a cousin of Charles Darwin, who founded the statistical school of genetics. Some of his work was concerned with dermatoglyphics (fingerprints and palm prints), a subject which is again becoming of interest to geneticists.

Galton whistle A whistle with a high pitch, once used to detect high-tone hearing loss.

Galvani, Luigi or Aloysio (1737–1798) Italian physician, physiologist, and physicist, and professor of anatomy and operative surgery at Bologna. He was first impelled to study the electrical reactions of the body when his wife Lucia told him that the frog legs that she had prepared for a meal "came alive" when set upon the copper wires of the grill. By connecting the exposed spinal cord of a decapitated frog with a metallic arc to the gastrocnemius muscle, he demonstrated that animal muscles contract as a result of electrical stimulation, but erred in considering that this was derived only (as in his later experiments) from the animals' brains, conducted by the nerves to the muscles rather than from the dissimilar metals with which the apparatus was constructed from which he suspended them.[646]

Through the studies of Galvani which suggested synaptic transmission, the concept of transient electrical potentials traveling in the fibers of the nervous system replaced that of the spirits of the anima in the understanding of scientists.

It was Galvani's nephew, Aldini, who first used electricity medically on humans in attempts to revive the dead, to alleviate melancholia, or to cure paralysis. **Duchenne** was the first to use electrical stimulation for diagnostic purposes.

galvanic current That constant electrical current produced by chemical action.

galvanic nystagmus See **vestibular nystagmus.**

galvanic skin response See **psychogalvanic reflex.**

galvanic tests (galvanic vestibular stimulation) Tests of the adequacy of labyrinthine function, involving stimulation of the standing subject using a small (5–7 mA) direct current, with the anode on the mastoid and the cathode over the sternum. Normally, mixed horizontal and rotatory nystagmus is produced, with its fast phase away from the side of the mastoid examined. The requirement for larger or smaller currents gives some indication of the state of labyrinthine excitability.[1349a]

Galveston orientation and amnesia test A test used in the assessment of patients after head injury (see Chart G–1). It can be administered daily. A score of 78 or more on three consecutive occasions is considered to indicate that the patient has recovered from **posttraumatic amnesia.**[3371]

Chart G–1. Galveston Orientation and Amnesia Test

Question	Error Score	Notes
What is your name?	2	Must give both first and surname
When were you born?	4	Must give day, month, and year
Where do you live?	4	Town sufficient
Where are you now?	5	Must give actual town
What is this building?	5	Usually hospital or rehab center; actual name unnecessary
When were you admitted to this hospital?	5	Date
How did you get here?	5	Mode of transport
What was the first event you remember after injury?	5	Any plausible event is enough; record answer
Can you give some detail?	5	Must give relevant detail
Can you describe the last thing you can recall before the accident?	5	Any plausible event is enough; record answer
Can you give some detail?	5	Any relevant detail
What time is it now?	5	−1 for each half-hour error
What day of the week is it?	3	−1 for each day error
What day of the month is it? (i.e., the date)	5	−1 for each day error
What is the month?	15	−5 for each month error
What is the year?	3	−10 for each year error

Score = (100 − total error). (From Levin HS, O'Donnell VM, Grossman RG. The Galveston orientation and amnesia test. J Nerv Ment Dis 1979;**167**:675–684, reprinted by permission.)

gamma-aminoisobutyric acid A small, neutral amino acid taken up by cerebral tumors, allowing it to be employed in the measurement of tissue permeability.

gamma-glutamylcysteine synthetase deficiency A rare aminoacidopathy of infancy characterized by low levels of glutamate in red blood cells, generalized aminoaciduria, and hemolytic anemia.

The clinical manifestations include ataxia and peripheral neuropathy.[3127]

gammopathic neuropathy Motor, sensory, or mixed neuropathies, often complicated by Raynaud phenomenon, tremor, or ataxia, occurring in association with monoclonal proteins and plasma cell dyscrasias (dysglobulinemias, gammopathies) such as multiple myeloma, amyloidosis (light-chain type), Waldenstrom macroglobulinemia, gamma heavy-chain disease, cryoglobulinemia, and benign immunoglobulin M (IgM), IgA, or IgG gammopathies "of uncertain significance."[2996]

The syndrome is considered to be due to the remote effects of a humoral factor secreted by neoplastic immunocytes.[5226]

Immunoglobulin M paraproteinemia produces a fairly characteristic syndrome of insidiously progressive chronic sensorimotor polyneuropathy in elderly people, who complain of numbness and paresthesias and who are found to have sensory ataxia, static tremor, and minor distal weakness. Both axonal degeneration and demyelination are notable in nerve biopsy specimens. The serum IgM fraction may demonstrate activity against myelin associated glycoprotein (MAG).

Variants include the following:

Anti-MAG antibody-associated polyneuropathies Slowly progressive but eventually disabling disorders with weakness, sensory loss, and gait disorder.[608]

Hereditary hypertrophic neuropathy with paraproteinemia A dominantly inherited, slowly progressive polyneuropathy resembling **hereditary motor and sensory neuropathy type 3,** associated with some degree of nerve hypertrophy and accompanied by the presence of abnormal protein (IgD) in the serum and the CSF.[2100,2996]

Neuropathy associated with monoclonal gammopathy of uncertain significance (MGUS) Acquired sensorimotor polyneuropathies appearing in adult life, associated mainly with serum and urine monoclonal IgM (less often IgG or IgA) protein expression and characterized by sensory loss, ataxia, and marked nerve conduction abnormalities.[2128]

Gamper bowing reflex Flexion of the neck and trunk in response to extension of the hips, a response seen in infants with severe brain damage and corticospinal tract disease.[1829]

Gamper, E. (1887–1938) Austrian professor of psychiatry and neuropathology at Innsbruck, later working in Prague and Munich.[1829]

Gamstorp, Ingrid Swedish pediatric neurologist.

Gamstorp syndrome See **familial periodic paralysis** (*hyperkalemic* form).[2014]

ganglioblastoma A rare, primary, malignant tumor of the CNS composed of mature ganglion cells and glial cells and occurring in childhood or youth, mainly in the region of the third ventricle.[6017]

gangliocytoma A rare, primary, malignant **neuronal tumor** of the CNS occurring in childhood or youth and characterized by the presence of mature neurons with Nissl substance in the cytoplasm and the nuclear characteristics of normal neurons, and supporting glial cells, mainly in the region of the third ventricle. They may stain positively for **glial fibrillary acidic protein** or neurofilament protein. Most are well differentiated.[6017]

ganglioglioma A rare, malignant, slowly growing, circumscribed tumor of the CNS containing both neoplastic astrocytes and neoplastic neuronal cells, found usually in the frontal or temporal lobes.[938] They present most often with seizures, and some patients have focal neurological deficits.[6123]

ganglion (Gr, a mass beneath the skin or close to tendons) A swelling along the course of a nerve, normally produced by the presence of synapses in cell relay stations as in the autonomic nervous system, and abnormally by a nerve tumor or tissue laid down locally in the process of nerve regeneration. The basal ganglia are those cell masses such as the caudate and lenticular nuclei, responsible for initiating voluntary motor activity. See also **pseudocyt.**

ganglion nodosum tumor See **carotid body tumor.**

ganglioneuroblastoma An uncommon primary, malignant, neuronal tumor occurring in the retroperitoneal or thoracic regions of children or young adults and characterized histologically by the presence of cells showing profuse fibril formation and with fibrovascular strands of tissue running through sheets of cells with small round nuclei, and frequently both astrocytes and ganglion cells.

In the *imperfect type*, all stages of differentiation are seen; while in the *immature ganglioneuroblastoma*, different areas suggest **ganglioneuroma** or **neuroblastoma** histologically.[6]

ganglioneurocytoma A rare mixed neuronal and glial tumor that arises in the periventricular regions in and above the posterior fossa.

ganglioneuroma Circumscribed benign tumors consisting of a mixture of neurons, capsule cells, connective tissue, ganglion cells, Schwann cells, and reticulin. Most arise in the posterior mediastinum, on the posterior abdominal wall, or from paraspinal autonomic ganglia.[5374] See **gangliocytoma.**

ganglionitis Inflammatory disease of the dorsal root ganglia, occurring as a result of infection or autoimmune attack or as a **paraneoplastic syndrome.**

ganglionopathy See **paraneoplastic sensory neuronopathy.**

ganglioradiculitis See **subacute sensory neuropathy.**

gangliorhizolysis A technique using radiofrequency waves to induce thermocoagulative lesions in neural structures, such as the fifth cranial nerve in the management of trigeminal neuralgia or chronic cluster headache. The smaller pain fibers are selectively destroyed by this method, the larger fibers subserving touch sensation being less or not at all affected.[3714]

gangliosialidosis, dysmorphic type See **sialidosis.**

gangliosides Water-soluble glycosphingolipid components of cell membranes. They have been classified as GM_1, GM_2, GM_3, etc. on the basis of their mobility on thin-layer chromatography and are normally degraded by the hexosaminidase enzymes.

gangliosidoses A group of recessively inherited **lysosomal storage disorders** in which the substances accumulating are **gangliosides** when due to deficiencies of β-galactosidase (**GM_1-gangliosidoses**) or of N-acetyl galactosaminidase (**GM_2-gangliosidoses**). These lead to the accumulation of excessive amounts of ganglioside in neurons ("ballooned cells") and to the neurological manifestations.

Disorders included are **GM_1 and GM_2 gangliosidoses, sulfatide lipidosis, trihexosamide ceramide lipidosis, galactosylceramide lipidosis, glucosyl-ceramide lipidosis, sphingomyelin lipidosis,** and **Kufs disease.**[3180] See also **neuronal ceroid lipofuscinosis.**

GANS syndrome 1. A syndrome presenting in the elderly in which the clinical features of dementia are accompanied by the pathological appearances of **Pick disease,** the atrophic process, however, being confined here to the frontal lobes.[5047]

2. (granulomatous angiitis of the nervous system) See **isolated angiitis of the nervous system.**

Gans-Rodiet sign Hemianesthesia of the lateral part of the sclera in cases of chronic alcoholism.[5047]

Ganser, Sigbert Josef Maria (1853–1931) German psychiatrist and neurologist, born in the Rhineland. He trained in Medicine in Wurzburg and Strasburg and, after further training in Munich and practice there and at Sorau, he succeeded Kraepelin as head of the department in Dresden, where he remained for the rest of his life. Apart from the syndrome by which his name is remembered (1897), he also described the basal nucleus (named for Meynert) and twilight states, and contributed studies on alcoholism.

Ganser syndrome (hysterical pseudodementia, hysterical twilight state, syndrome of approximate answers, Balderdash syndrome) A manifestation of a dissociative reaction in some patients, of willful malingering in other patients, but not evidence of dementia.[2018] The answers given are often nonsensical but do at least have some relationship to the question ("How many legs has a horse?"—"Four." "And a cow?"—"Four." "And an ox?"—"I don't know." "Do you know any other animals?"—"Elephant." "How many legs has it got?"—"Three.") The abnormal verbal responses are always in reply to questions, are not spontaneous, and indicate that the patient has actually grasped the nature and content of the question.

Ganser's patients were all criminals (or at least accused people in custody) and many also complained of headaches and manifested auditory and visual hallucinations, delusions, and patchy sensory loss. Consciousness was described as normal or clouded. Ganser noted that the syndrome was self-limited, the patients returning to normal in a few days with amnesia for the period, and he thought that this was a form of encephalitis. See also **vorbeireden.**

Ganzfeld electroretinography The recording of the electrical potential changes emanating from the retina by means of corneal surface electrodes, the patient receiving flashes of light filtered or not according to whether rod or cone activity is sought.

GAPO syndrome See **growth retardation, alopecia, pseudoanodontia, optic atrophy.**[2004]

Garcia-Lurie syndrome See **aproscencephaly.**

Garcin syndrome (syndrome paralytique unilateral global des nerfs craniens, hemibasal syndrome, Guillain-Garcin syndrome, Bertoletti-Garcin syndrome, Guillain-Alajouanine-Garcin syndrome) Dysfunction of all or nearly all of the cranial nerves on one side, without long tract signs or evidence of increased intracranial pressure, and due to infiltration by a local malignancy such as a lymphoepithelioma or sarcoma of the nasopharynx.

The syndrome was described briefly by Guillain in 1926[2315] but more completely by Garcin in his graduating thesis in the following year.

gardeners' migraine Vascular-type headaches, repetitively experienced on bending down.

Gardner neuralgia See **petrous neuralgia.**

Gardner syndrome (central or type 2 neurofibromatosis) A syndrome of dominantly inherited bilateral vestibular neurofibromas without notable peripheral manifestations of von Recklinghausen disease.

Clinically, progressive deafness, tinnitus, and imbalance are the major features. Although the syndrome had been described before, Gardner presented a large series of cases and delineated the condition as closely resembling, but consistently different from, the more common peripheral or type 1 **neurofibromatosis.**[2023]

Dr. W.J. Gardner is an American neurosurgeon.

Gareis syndrome The association of mental retardation with absence of the extensors pollices longus, the latter resulting in permanent flexion of the thumbs, with X-linked inheritance.[2028]

Garel syndrome A brainstem vascular syndrome.[374]

gargoyle   A carved face on a waterspout, commonly a hideous caricature of a real or mythical being; hence the origin of the pejorative name for patients with dysmorphism due to **mucopolysaccharidoses.**

gargoylism   See **Hunter syndrome, mucopolysaccharidosis.**

Garland amyotrophy   See **diabetic neuropathies.**

Garland, Hugh Gregory   (1903–1967) English neurologist in Leeds who trained at the **National Hospital.** He set up an active neurological department in his home city, where he was recognized as a unique clinical teacher and diagnostician. He is remembered best for his description of proximal **diabetic neuropathy** (diabetic amyotrophy).

Garrod, Sir Archibald   English physician and chemist who introduced the concept of inborn errors of metabolism in 1908, regarding alkaptonuria, albinism, cystinuria, and pentosuria as fulfilling the criteria.

gas gangrene   See **myonecrosis.**

Gaskell, W.H.   English physiologist whose research helped to lay the foundations of knowledge on the functions of the autonomic nervous system, compiled in his book, *The Involuntary Nervous System* (London, 1916).

gasoline-sniffing myopathy   A subacutely progressive syndrome of proximal weakness and wasting as a result of intoxication with gasoline.[3145]

Gasparini syndrome   Paralysis of cranial nerves V, VI, and VII on one side, with contralateral thermoanalgesia; a condition due to a lesion of the pontine tegmentum.[374]

Gass syndrome   A neurocutaneous syndrome characterized by retinal and intracranial cavernous hemangiomas and angiomatous hamartomas of the skin.[2044]

Gasser, Johann Lorenz   (1702–1777) Viennese anatomist who, in his graduation thesis, described the sensory ganglion of the trigeminal nerve. The appellation was bestowed in 1765 by Antonius Hirsch, an Austrian anatomist and student of Gasser, in honor of Gasser.

gasserian ganglion   (semilunar ganglion) The sensory ganglion of the fifth cranial nerve.

Gastaut, Henri   (1915–1995) French neurologist and neurophysiologist in Marseille and University President in Aix, whose major and seminal contributions were in the realm of epilepsy and the EEG. He was the first to describe photosensitive epilepsy and the following syndrome.

Gastaut syndrome   Unilateral convulsions associated with hemiparesis and generalized seizures with epigastric, pharyngeal, or abdominal auras, occurring in children.[2048]
    See also **Lennox-Gastaut syndrome.**

gastric crises   (gastrodynia) Acute, severe attacks of abdominal pain occurring in tabes dorsalis. Neuralgia resulting from irritation of the dorsal roots by spirochetes seems the most likely cause. At thoracic levels, a similar pain occurs in some patients with postherpetic neuralgia.

gastrodynia   See **gastric crises.**

gate-control theory   (of pain) This theory, propounded by Melzack and Wall in 1966, accounts for the fact that, if one rubs a painful place, the pain is lessened. They postulated the existence of a functional "gate" in the region of the substantia gelatinosa of the cord, which closes during thick-fiber activity and opens with thin-fiber activity, allowing onward passage of impulses destined to induce the perception of pain. A central modulating influence was acknowledged as part of the regulatory system, to accommodate the everyday observation that distraction diminishes the perception of pain. Proof of the existence of such a mechanism is still wanting, and the theory has been severely criticized but remains acceptable to a large majority of neuroscientists.[3826]

Gates-MacGintie reading test   A standardized test allowing the quantitative assessment of reading ability, used in the examination of patients with dysphasias and to form an estimate of prior intellectual functioning.[2059]

Gaucher cells   Cells swollen by the intracytoplasmic accumulation of cerebrosides, giving a foamy appearance in glucosylceramide lipidosis.

Gaucher disease   See **glucosylceramide lipidosis.**

Gaucher, Philippe Charles Ernest   (1854–1918) French physician who trained in Paris, where, as an intern, he described the disease named for him. He was later professor of dermatology at the Hôpital St. Louis in Paris, his research being mainly concerned with the manifestations of tuberculosis, syphilis, and pellagra. See **glucosylceramide lipidosis.**

Charles-Jules-Alphonse Gayet

Gayet, Charles-Jules-Alphonse   (1833–1904) French neurologist whose description of "acute superior hemorrhagic polioencephalitis" preceded that of **Wernicke** by 6 years.

Gayet disease See **Wernicke-Korsakoff encephalopathy.**

Gayet-Wernicke syndrome See **Wernicke-Korsakoff encephalopathy.**

gaze The persistent fixation of vision on an object.

gaze apraxia Inability to direct the eyes in response to a command or to a stimulus presented in visual space. The oculocephalic responses are preserved. The phenomenon is usually seen in the context of **Balint syndrome,** when the lesion is in posterior parietal regions bilaterally; when occurring in isolation, the lesion responsible is thought to be in the frontal eye fields.[2624]

In cases of gaze apraxia, the eyes tend to wander randomly, then either fixate poorly on the target when it is achieved or lock onto the target (*fixation spasm*); pursuit movements and convergence may also be impaired.

gaze palsy A deficit in the yoked deviation of the eyes in any direction as a result of a lesion above the cranial motor nerve nuclei.

gaze-evoked blepharoclonus Repetitive contractions of the facial muscles, with or without associated ocular nystagmus but including bilateral orbicularis spasms, occurring on lateral gaze, reported in some subjects with brainstem multiple sclerosis.[2976]

gaze-evoked nystagmus (gaze-paretic nystagmus, gaze-modulated nystagmus, deviational nystagmus, neurasthenic nystagmus, seducible nystagmus, setting-in nystagmus) Those forms of acquired, conjugate, symmetrical, and horizontal jerk nystagmus that only appear when the eyes are deviated from the primary position (and which are thus absent *in* the primary position of gaze). The slow phases show a declining time course. The patients are unable to maintain eccentric fixation, the eyes drifting centrally and jerking laterally. A defect in the step function of the neural firing frequency is considered to be the pathophysiological mechanism.[5]

This represents the most common variety of nystagmus, in which the direction (fast phase) of the nystagmus is in the direction of gaze and which is most often due to sedative or anticonvulsant usage, or to various brainstem or cerebellar lesions. Such a nystagmus may be attributed to nerve lesions (gaze-paretic nystagmus) or to muscle disease (muscle-paretic nystagmus).

Gaze-modulated nystagmus is a form of jerk nystagmus that is present in the primary position of gaze but is increased when the subject attempts to maintain an eccentric eye position. **Vestibular nystagmus, latent/manifest latent nystagmus,** and **congenital nystagmus** are of this nature.

gaze-evoked tinnitus The occurrence of tinnitus with most or all forms of eye movement but especially far-lateral gaze and presumably stemming from abnormal new connections between the cochlear and vestibular nuclei due to aberrant sprouting of nerve fibers, since it has been reported after, for example, removal of a cerebellopontine mass with sacrifice of the eighth cranial nerve.[5812]

gaze-modulated nystagmus See **gaze-evoked nystagmus.**

gaze-paretic nystagmus (integrator nystagmus) A form of **gaze-evoked nystagmus** seen in subjects recovering from a transient central paralysis of gaze, in which the deviated eyes show fatigue, drifting toward the midline, and then abruptly repositioning with a laterally directed corrective saccade. See also **gaze-evoked nystagmus.**

gegenhalten (Ger, counter-holding) See **paratonia.**

gegenrucke See **square-wave jerks.**

Gehrig, Henry Louis (Lou) (1903–1941) American baseball player who succumbed to **amyotrophic lateral sclerosis** after a spectacular playing career. His name is often applied to the disease.[2945,4078]

gelasmus (from Gr, laughter) Spasmodic or convulsive laughter.

gelastic epilepsy (from Gr, laughter) A form of seizure disorder characterized by bursts of compulsive laughter or giggling, with or without the appropriate affective tone. It was recognized first by **Trousseau** in 1873.

The same phenomenon also occurs in **multiple sclerosis, amyotrophic lateral sclerosis,** lacunar states, and other causes of spastic bulbar palsy (when it appears to suggest the presence of a lesion in or near the hypothalamus[2333]), as well as in bilateral frontal lobe disease and schizophrenia. Hypothalamic **hamartomas** are characteristically associated with seizures of this type; in these situations precocious puberty and behavioral problems are often also present.

Criteria for the diagnosis have been suggested by Gascon and Lombroso[2041] and consist of the following: stereotyped recurrences; no external precipitants; concomitance of other manifestations generally regarded as epileptic, such as tonic or clonic movements, automatisms, or loss of consciousness; presence of interictal/ictal epileptiform discharges; and absence of neurological signs of other conditions (as above) in which pathological laughter is recorded.

gelatio (Lat, freezing) The rigid state of the body in **catalepsy.**

Gélineau, Jean-Baptiste-Edouard (1828–1906) French surgeon and neuropsychiatrist, born near Bordeaux. He trained at the naval medical school in La Rochelle and from 1850 sailed with the French Navy in the Indian Ocean as surgeon, third class. When his thesis on diseases of black and white people on the Comorro Islands was accepted by the University of Montpelier he achieved naval promotion, but he relinquished his commission in 1860. Thereafter, he practiced first in southern France and later, after the Franco-Prussian War and with far more success, as a specialist in nervous diseases in Paris, where he made his numerous contributions to the literature of both medicine and the stage. His full description of narcolepsy was published in 1880.[2067] He also wrote an autobiography and invented and marketed his own pills for epilepsy, with reported success. In 1900, wearying of the profession, he retired to his birthplace, publishing a final book on epilepsy and thereafter devoting himself to viticulture, thus completing an enviably balanced and successful career.[4354]

Gélineau syndrome   See **narcolepsy.**

Gelle syndrome   The effect of infarction of the caudal ventral lateral pons, comprising homolateral VII and VIII palsies and crossed hemiparesis.[5162]

gemistocytic   (Lat, goose-grease + cell) Cells having the appearance of goose grease, such as the plump reactive or hypertrophic astrocytes, the cytoplasm of which is filled with filaments and glial fibrillary acidic protein; the nucleus is displaced eccentrically. Such cells are seen most commonly in the white matter in early cases of demyelinating disease.

The degree to which animal husbandry has influenced neuropathology has never been recognized appropriately.

gemistocytic astrocytoma   See **astrocytoma.**

general acoustic muscle reflex   A startle response, manifest by widespread jerking of the body in response to a sudden and unexpected loud sound.

general adaptation syndrome   The sum of all the nonspecific systemic reactions of the body which ensue upon long-continued exposure to stress; the staged responses to stress shown by an organism.

The first response, the *alarm reaction*, begins with increased sympathetic and adrenal cortical activity. Selye[5060,5061] described it as the sum of all nonspecific systemic phenomena elicited by sudden exposure to stimuli to which the organism is qualitatively or quantitatively nonadapted. The second stage is the *stage of resistance*, and the third, the *stage of exhaustion*, in which the mechanisms called into play to resist the stress in the first place break down.

general paresis of the insane   (Bayle disease, frontotemporo-parietal encephalitic syphilis) A form of subacute encephalitis occurring in patients with tertiary syphilis up to 30 years after the primary infection and characterized by dementia, irritability, a decline in self-care, and later psychotic signs. Intention tremors of the limbs, face, and tongue are common but focal signs rare. The classic grandiose delusional state occurs

in no more than 20% of cases. Blood and CSF serology findings invariably confirm the diagnosis. Pathologically, cortical atrophy with gliosis and perivascular mononuclear cell infiltration are typical changes. The organism is sometimes recoverable from the brain.

The condition was first described in detail by **Bayle** in his graduation thesis of 1822,[402] although Esquirol had referred to it in his book on dementia in 1826 and Thomas **Willis** had described many of its features in *De anima brutorum* in 1672. The disease appears to have reached epidemic proportions in northern France after the Napoleonic wars, but was probably rare before then. The name is a translation of the French *paralysie générale des aliénés,* the term used by Calmeil (1826).[5047] The Germans used the term *dementia paralytica,* the English and Americans, *general paresis.* Treatment with mercury was all that was available until **Wagner von Jauregg** [5802] introduced malarial (hyperpyrexia) treatment in 1917, for which he was awarded the Nobel prize in 1927.

generalization   The propagation of EEG activity from limited areas of the head to all regions of the head.

generalized amyotonia   See **Foerster syndrome.**

generalized epilepsies and syndromes   Epileptic disorders with generalized seizures, that is, "seizures in which the first clinical changes indicate initial involvement of both hemispheres . . . the ictal encephalographic patterns initially are bilateral." (From Commission for Classification and Terminology, ILAE. Proposal for Revised Classifications of Epilepsies and Epileptic syndromes. *Epilepsia* 1989;**30**:389–399.[1114]) See **absence seizures, generalized tonic-clonic seizures.**

generalized epilepsy with febrile seizures plus Dominantly inherited forms of epilepsy characterized by the first occurrence of febrile seizures around the end of the first year of life. These persist after the age of 6 years and may be associated in *variant* forms with tonic-clonic seizures, myoclonus, or absences in the absence of fever. The seizures usually desist in adolescence. Various other seizure types were recorded in the original kinship.[5187]

FEB 1 (OMIM 602476) manifests myoclonus and is linked to 8q. FEB 2 (OMIM 602477) manifests atonic seizures and myoclonic astatic seizures; it maps to 19q 13.1. Another *variant* (OMIM 121210) manifests absences in addition to the febrile seizures.[4516]

generalized gangliosidosis   See **GM₁ gangliosidosis.**

generalized hyperhidrosis   An abnormal tendency to sweat over the whole of the body surface, as in cases of chronic infection, hyperthyroidism, autonomic neuropathy, pheochromocytoma, carcinoid, diabetes, acromegaly, gout, or hyperpituitarism.

generalized multiple spikes   (polyspikes) Multiple spikes or multiple spikes and waves occurring during wakefulness, classically seen in patients with myoclonic epilepsy.

generalized myokymia   See **neuromyotonia.**

generalized paroxysmal fast activity   (fast paroxysmal rhythms, generalized repetitive fast discharge, runs of rapid spikes, generalized rhythmic 15–20 Hz activity, beta band seizure pattern) A rare form of paroxysmal bilateral discharge at high frequency found during sleep in patients who have seizures of various types and who are usually mentally retarded.

Clinically, tonic seizures commonly accompany this activity pattern.[736]

generalized repetitive fast discharge   See **generalized paroxysmal fast activity.**

generalized rhythmic 15–20 Hz activity   See **generalized paroxysmal fast activity.**

generalized seizures   A seizure is considered generalized when clinical symptomatology provides no indication of an anatomical localization and no clinical evidence of focal onset. When possible, three main seizures subtypes may be categorized:[1115]

- Generalized convulsive seizures with predominantly tonic, clonic, or tonic-clonic features
- Generalized nonconvulsive seizures represented by absence seizure
- Myoclonic seizures

generalized sharp and slow-wave discharges   (slow spike-and-wave activity) The presence on the EEG of generalized sharp- and slow-wave complexes occurring at 2–2.5 Hz, frequently with some accompanying behavioral change and seen in patients with the **Lennox-Gastaut syndrome.**

generalized spinal muscular atrophy   A variant of the usual proximal pattern of spinal muscular atrophy.[3800] See **hereditary motor neuropathy.**

generalized tics   Those tics in which the movements affect more than one noncontiguous body part. The disorder may or may not involve vocal tics in a particular case. *Elementary (simple)* and *complex* tics are the other two categories in this classification.

generalized tonic-clonic seizure   (grand mal seizure, major motor seizure, convulsive fit) A common form of seizure characterized typically by initial loss of consciousness with falling, followed by maximal symmetrical tonic contraction of all the somatic and autonomic muscles. This gives way to clonic contractions after 30–60 seconds; thereafter, a flaccid phase ensues before automatic (e.g., ventilatory) and voluntary muscle activity and consciousness are reestablished over the next few minutes.

generalized xanthomatosis   (Hand-Schüller-Christian disease, histiocytosis X, lipoid granulomatosis, craniohypophysial xanthomatosis) See **Hand-Schüller-Christian disease.**

generator   The source of an electrical signal.

GeneTests·GeneClinics   A free, publicly funded (University of Washington, Seattle; NIH) medical genetics information resource developed for physicians, other health-care providers, and researchers, accessible at www.geneclinics.org/profiles.

genetic ataxias   A large complex of disorders which have in common the signs of ataxia and the pathology of degeneration of the cerebellum and/or its connections, as well as of other CNS areas in some cases. There is often pathological and phenotypic variability and overlapping, and biochemical markers are only available in a few cases. See **cerebellar ataxias** and their *variants.*

geniculate herpes   See **Ramsay Hunt syndrome.** Hunt's supposition of the site of the lesion has not been verified pathologically.

geniculate neuralgia   See **Ramsay Hunt syndrome.**

geniculocalcarine blindness   Loss of vision due to bilateral lesions of the occipital lobes, as may result from bilateral posterior cerebral artery infarction, anoxia, trauma, migraine, demyelination, etc. See **Anton syndrome.**

geniculocalcarine pathways   The fiber tracts passing from the lateral geniculate bodies to the occipital lobes, some through the temporal lobe and some through the parietal.

geniospasm   A dominantly inherited syndrome with onset in infancy or early childhood, mapped to chromosome 9q13–q21. Clinically, it is characterized by vertical movements of the tip of the chin and quivering of the lower lip occurring spontaneously or with stress, concentration, or emotion and lasting minutes at a time. Nocturnal tongue biting may also occur. See also **oral-facial-digital syndrome.**

genital reflexes   Penile erection and ejaculation produced by cerebral inducement or as a result of stimulation of the penis. Exaggeration of the reflex in response to peripheral stimulation occurs as part of the **mass reflex.**

The **superficial anal, internal anal, cremasteric, scrotal,** and **bulbocavernosus reflexes** are also so classified.

genitofemoral neuralgia   See **ilioinguinal neuralgia.**

genitofemoral neuropathy   A rare entrapment syndrome causing pain and paresthesia in the territory of the genitofemoral nerve, and possibly loss of the cremasteric reflex, usually as a result of tight compression from clothing, following appendicitis or with other local pathology.[3564] See also **blue jeans syndrome.**

genius   (Lat, the tutelary spirit of a person—or guardian angel) 1. An inborn faculty for an aspect of mental activity; a special or peculiar characteristic. 2. A person possessed of such attributes to an exceptional degree.

Gennari, Francesco (1750–1795) A physician in Padua whose name is given to the striated occipital cortex (the striae genarii), which represents the outer portion of the **Baillarger** line and which he described in 1782 (while still a medical student) as the *lineola albidor*.[1478]

genomic imprinting Variability of the clinical features of a heritable disease according to which parent supplied the defective gene.

genoneurodermatoses See **phakomatoses.**

genu (Lat, knee) A bend in part of an anatomical structure. Derivations from the word are applied to the geniculate bodies, to part of the internal capsule, and to the geniculate ganglion on account of their curvatures or their situation within another curved structure.

genu inversum See **genu valgum.**

genu recurvatum Hyperextension of the knee.

genu valgum (genu inversum, knock-knees) Lateral flexion of the knee such that the two knees approximate and the ankles are separated.

genu varum (bow-leggedness) The opposite of **genu valgum,** in which the knees are separated and the ankles approximate.

genus A class of organisms with similar characteristics within which subclasses called *species* exist.

geophagy (Gr, earth + pagein, to eat) (pica) A tendency to eat earth.

geotropic (earthward) eye and head movements Head and eye deviation remains downward with axial turning 180°. When one has the presence of mind to undertake this it is dramatic. Hemibody tone or posture disparity could be similarly utilized.

geotropic nystagmus A form of nystagmus in which the direction of the fast phase is toward the center of the earth. See **vestibular nystagmus.**

Gerhardt, Karl Adolf Christian Jacob (1833–1902) German physician, professor of medicine successively at Jena, Wurzberg, and Berlin. Although he was particularly interested in croup and laryngeal lesions, he also described **erythromelalgia** and wrote on aspects of the physical examination.

Gerhardt law In paralysis of vocal cords due to lesions of the recurrent laryngeal nerve, the cords assume a position midway between adduction and abduction.[2995]

Gerhardt syndrome Bilateral adductor paralysis of the larynx due to bilateral lesions of the tenth cranial nerve at the brainstem or skull base and leading to severe dysphonia and dyspnoea.[2072] Familial forms have also been described.

In a *variant* form, cerebellar atrophy and pure motor neuropathy are associated.[342]

Geriatric Depression Scale A 30-item self-report questionnaire developed from 100 questions commonly used to diagnose depression and used for that purpose in elderly people. The ratings are performed by the patient or by an observer. A short form is also available for subjects to score themselves.[6078]

A screening test for depression in the elderly is also available.[589]

Geriatric Evaluation by Relatives Rating Instrument (GERRI) A rating scale in which "significant others" can rate attributes of elderly outpatients who show symptoms of mental decline. The instrument includes 49 sentences describing potential cognitive, emotional, or behavioral abnormalities; items are rated on a 5-point frequency scale.[5021]

Geriatric Rating Scale Designed for use by nonprofessional ward staff, this reliable 31-item scale rates patients' behavior in the activities of daily living. The scale yields seven factors, including confusion, memory and orientation, activity and communications, sleep, mood, eating, and psychotic symptoms and also notes disturbing behavior. It is of greatest value in the assessment of a change in behavior in severely demented inpatients.[4468]

Geriatric Self-care Scale An instrument for assessing the residual capacities of elderly infirm people.[3192]

Gerlach, Joseph von (1820–1896) German histologist in Mainz who in 1858 introduced the carmine stain for neuronal cell bodies, the first specific stain discovered.

Gerlier disease (kubisagari, paralytic vertigo) An epidemic summer disorder in Alpine areas described first by Felix Gerlier. It is manifest by transient headache, vertigo, photophobia, nerve trunk pain, and weakness of the oculomotor muscles, the neck extensors, and muscles of the face, larynx, pharynx, and back.

Its occurrence in people exposed to cattle or horses suggests that this may have been a form of brucellosis.[2074] The disease now seems to have disappeared from Europe but has been noted in Japan. See also **vertige paralysant.**

Gerlier, Felix (1840–1914) Swiss physician.

germ cell tumor Potentially malignant tumors of the pineal region, including **teratomas, germinomas, embryonal carcinomas, choriocarcinomas** and **endodermal sinus tumors.** In each case, the tumor is characterized by an elevation of CSF α-fetoprotein and plasma β-human chorionic gonadotrophin or melanotonin levels.[596]

germinal zone (ventricular germinal zone, subependymal zone, subependymal cell plate) That part of the neural tube which generates neuronal and glial precursors destined to migrate and become the cortex and white matter, respectively.

germinoma (seminoma-like tumor, atypical teratoma) A tumor of the pineal gland or of the suprasellar space, composed of large, polygonal cells with large nuclei, coarse chromatin, prominent nucleoli, and eosinophilic cytoplasm, and small T-cell lymphocytes.

The tumor occurs mainly in young adult males and is capable of metastasis within the nervous system.[6]

geromarasmus (Gr, old age + decay) The muscle thinning and weakness found in many aged people.

GERRI See **Geriatric Evaluation by Relatives Rating Instrument.**

Josef Gerstmann

Gerstmann, Josef (1887–1969) Austrian neuropsychiatrist who studied at Vienna and then became first assistant to von Jauregg in the Viennese Psychiatric Clinic. During the World War I, he served in the medical corps in the Italian Alps, attending to a number of soldiers and others who had suffered brain damage incurred in avalanches. He later became professor and head of the neuropsychiatric unit in Vienna in 1928 but emigrated to America 10 years later to escape Nazi persecution. There he held senior posts in clinical and research psychiatry in Maryland, Washington, and New York.

His earlier work was on the cerebral pathology accompanying paralyses, and he published a book on the malarial treatment of **general paresis of the insane.** He described finger agnosia in 1924, and the full syndrome, now named for him, 6 years later. The French ophthalmologist Antoine-Jules Badal (1840–1929) had reported (in 1888) on finger agnosia with inferior quadrantanopia, right–left disorientation, alexia, agraphia, and visual disorientation, but he regarded all of these as manifestations of psychic blindness.

Gerstmann also published an account of frontal gait ataxia, which he considered was due to damage of the frontopontocerebellar tract. He also published descriptions of the following conditions.

Gerstmann syndromes 1. (Badal-Gerstmann syndrome, angular gyrus syndrome) The combination of right–left disorientation, acalculia, agraphia, and finger agnosia, due to a lesion of the left angular gyrus. **Asymbolia** for pain and constructional apraxia are possible additional features.

The association of these four main features has consistent localizing value to the angular gyrus, but whether the appearance of fragments of the syndrome has the same meaning is disputed.[468] Gerstmann developed the concept of a body image with visual, tactile, and somatesthetic components at the start of his 1927 paper, and considered that the cortical representation of at least part of this was in the left angular gyrus.[2076] Badal's description in 1888 was less complete but his name is sometimes added.

2. A paranoid psychosis with auditory hallucinations in patients with **general paresis of the insane,** as a result of malarial therapy, described by Gerstmann in 1924.

Gerstmann-Schilder syndrome Gait apraxia and dysequilibrium as a result of frontal lobe lesions but resembling cerebellar ataxia. The difference between their findings and those of Bruns (which they acknowledge) is unclear. They ascribed the clinical disturbances to damage to the endings of the frontopontocerebellar tracts.

Gerstmann-Straussler-Scheinker syndrome (spinocerebellar ataxia with dementia and plaque-like deposits) A rare, transmissible, and usually familial spongiform encephalopathy marked by amyloid deposits associated with any one of many potential prion protein mutations and presenting in early adult life with progressive spinocerebellar ataxia, parkinsonism, pyramidal signs, impaired smooth pursuit eye movements, and dementia. Numerous mutations are described on the prion protein gene at chromosome 20pter–p12 in this, as in **Creutzfeldt-Jakob disease** and **fatal familial insomnia,** but in most cases there is a mutation at codon 102 of the PNRP amyloid gene on chromosome 20.

Pathologically, there are plaque-like deposits in the cerebral and cerebellar cortex and in the central gray nuclei. These contain the **kuru**-type amyloid protein and thus resemble the plaques of **Alzheimer disease.** This condition, described first by **Gerstmann** et al. in 1936,[2077] has also been considered to be a familial (dominantly inherited) *variant* of **Creutzfeldt-Jakob disease.**[3207] See also **cerebral amyloid angiopathy.**

In a *variant* of the condition itself, an inherited prion disease with codon 105 (Pro to Leu) mutation, progressive dementia, spasticity, and gait disturbance occur without myoclonus, cerebellar signs, or periodic synchronous discharges; amyloid plaques are found throughout the cerebral cortex but there are no spongiform changes.[3067]

Geschwind, Norman   (1926–1984) American neurologist who, before and after war service, trained in neurology at Harvard and thereafter at the **National Hospital** and in Boston, eventually being appointed James Jackson Putnam Professor of Neurology at Harvard, professor of psychology at the Massachussetts Institute of Technology, and chief of neurology at the Boston City Hospital, and then at the Beth Israel Hospital in Boston.

In Boston, he established the Aphasia Research Center (this reflecting both his administrative powers and his particular interest in behavioral neurology). The breadth of scope of his publications revealed his eclecticism and wide-ranging expertise in many areas of neurology. His particular contributions concerned the **disconnection syndromes** (which he identified and named), epilepsy, the organic basis of some psychiatric phenomena, lateralization, cerebral dominance and brain asymmetries, and the apraxias and aphasias. He revitalized the field of aphasiology in the 1960s and created the current school of behavioral neurologists in the United States. A renowned teacher with a skill for synthesis, he simplified the literature on aphasia and returned the field to its original clinicopathological methods.

In addition, he was revered in his lifetime for his personal qualities and as a teacher and clinician. He was blessed both with insatiable curiosity and with the ability to nourish its fruits.[1264,3850]

Gesner, Johann August Philipp   (1738–1801) Physician in Rothenburg who in 1769 produced the first modern account of dysphasia, which he called "speech amnesia."

gestalt   An unverbalized mental impression of the totality rather than the ingredients of a situation or event, whereby the whole is seen as greater than the sum (or indeed the nature) of its parts.

gestational age   Age since conception. The neurological signs allowing estimation of gestational age have been standardized by Dubowitz, Dubowitz, and Goldberg.[1528]

gestational assessment   A systematized evaluation of body and neurologic characteristics, the latter including posture, **square window,** ankle dorsiflexion, arm recoil, leg recoil, popliteal angle, **heel-to-ear flexion, scarf sign, head lag,** and **ventral suspension** on all grades between 0 and 5.[1528]

gestational epilepsy   The occurrence of seizures exclusively during (usually the first) pregnancy or in the postpartum period.

geste antagonistique   (counterpressure) Stimulation of a body part in order to reverse persistent wayward muscle contractions producing an abnormal posture, as in the expression of a focal **dystonia.**

An example of such a trick movement is putting a finger lightly on the chin, a maneuver that may be used to straighten the head on the neck in some patients with **spasmodic torticollis.**

gestures   Within the context of communicating information, movements used to lend further emotional tone to speech.

The comprehension of the message in such movements is largely a function of the right hemisphere. In short, this is a movement made to emphasize verbal utterances, regardless of whether the latter are actually expressed.[1179]

geusis   (Gr, tasting) The sense of taste.

Geyelin-Penfield disease   Dominantly inherited calcific endarteritis affecting the brain arterioles in the region of the junction between the gray and white matter.

Mental retardation after the age of 2 years, polymorphic seizures patterns, and pupillary constriction or dilatation are the main clinical features. The condition sometimes leads to early death.[2085]

GFAP   See **glial fibrillary acidic protein.**

ghost fibers   Myofibrils that do not react in any histochemically stained enzyme preparations. These are occasionally seen in cases of polymyositis.

ghost image   The blurred appearance of an object viewed by a person with monocular diplopia resulting from refractive errors of the ocular media.

Giacci syndrome   The **mutilating acropathy** resulting from a sensory neuropathy or myelodysplasia.

Gianelli sign   See **Tournay sign.**

giant axonal neuropathy   A rare, recessively inherited disorder characterized by accumulations of 10 nm peripheral cytoplasmic neurofilaments within Schwann cells and peripheral nerves, giving rise to focal axonal swellings (spheroids), which may also be found in the CNS and in skin fibroblasts. The responsible gene maps to 16q 24.

The typical clinical presentation is in a child with gait disorder and ichthyosis, unusually kinky hair and the progressive development of seizures, sensory neuropathy, ophthalmoplegia, bulbar weakness, ataxia, intellectual failure, optic atrophy, nystagmus, and pyramidal signs. A slowly progressive mixed axonal and demyelinating sensorimotor peripheral neuropathy,[486] EEG abnormalities, nephropathy, and precocious puberty are less often recorded.

giant cell arteritis   (cranial arteritis, temporal arteritis, Horton arteritis) A systemic vasculitis with a particular predilection for the branches of the external carotid artery and the ophthalmic and posterior ciliary arteries, which show a segmental panarteritis. Clinically, it may cause malaise, fever, weight loss, generalized or localized headaches, and permanent or temporary visual loss, diplopia, jaw muscle ischemia, neuropathies, and stroke syndromes in patients over the age of 55 years, many of whom have symptoms of **polymyalgia rheumatica.**[2195] **Ischemic optic neuritis** and central artery occlusion are potential causes of permanent blindness.[933,2662] In some cases, recessive inheritance is noted.

In a *variant* form, peripheral neuropathy also occurs and responds equally well to steroids.[5848]

giant cell astrocytoma   See **astrocytoma.**

giant cell fibrosarcoma   (monstrocellular sarcoma) See **astrocytoma.**

giant cell myositis, myasthenia, and myocarditis   A rare syndrome in which these features occur in the presence of thymoma.[4071]

giant Lambl excrescences   Unusually large filiform outgrowths from the free borders of cardiac valves, able to act as a source of cerbral or peripheral emboli. Normally such outgrowths are small and innocuous.[4135]

giant motor unit action potential   Use of this term is discouraged. It refers to a motor unit action potential with a peak-to-peak amplitude and duration much greater than the range found in corresponding muscles in normal subjects of similar age. Quantitative measurements of amplitude and duration are preferable. (From the 2001 Report of the Nomenclature Committee of the American Association of Electromyography and Electrodiagnosis.[10] Used by permission, copyright © 2001, AAEM.)

giant pyramidal cells   (Betz cells) Large, triangular cells in the fifth layer of the motor cortex described in 1874 by Vladimir Betz (1834–1894), a Russian anatomist.[4979]

giant somatosensory evoked potential   Enlarged somatosensory evoked potentials seen as a characteristic of cortical reflex myoclonus and reflecting cortical hyperexcitability.[10] Such large cortically recorded potentials occur 40–60 msec before the EMG activity in patients with **minipolymyoclonus** or **cortical tremor** and are best revealed in frontal or parietal regions by **jerk-locked averaging.**[2905]

Gibbon classification   A widely accepted proposal for the classification of micturition disorders on a neurological basis, adapted by Gibbon from the classification of Bors[2101] (see Chart G–2).

Chart G–2. Gibbon Classification of Micturition Disorders

1. Suprasacral (upper motor neuron) lesion
   a. *Uninhibited neurogenic bladder* The result of an incomplete lesion, leading to early detrusor contractions and desire to void with low residual urine. The sacral reflex arc is preserved.
   b. *Reflex neurogenic bladder* The result of a complete lesion, with early detrusor contractions but without a desire to void. Residual urine volumes may be high. The sensation of a full bladder may be retained through sympathetic afferent pathways. Again, the sacral reflex arc is preserved.
2. Sacral lesion
   a. Motor (lower motor neuron) (*motor neurogenic bladder*) There are no detrusor contractions but the desire to void and the sensation of a full bladder are retained. The residual urinary volume is large.
   b. Sensory (*sensory neurogenic bladder*) There are neither detrusor contractions nor any desire to void. Residual urine volumes may be high. The sensation of a full bladder is lost.
   c. Motor and sensory (*autonomous neurogenic bladder*) There are neither detrusor contractions nor any desire to void. Residual urine volumes may be high. The sensation of a full bladder is retained through sympathetic afferent pathways.
3. Mixed.

From Gibbon, NO. Nomenclature of neurogenic bladder. J. Urology *1976;8:423–431. Reprinted by kind permission.*

See also **Bors-Comarr** system. Reproduced by permission.

Gibbs, Frederick   American electrophysiologist. He was the first to describe (in 1935) the 3-Hz spike-and-wave EEG pattern of petit mal epilepsy.[2103]

gibbus   (Lat, a hump) The acute flexor angulation of the vertebral column in destructive diseases of the spine.

giddy   (from Saxon, to be merry) Having the sensation of turning or of unsteadiness. A popular term for many sensations including vertigo, light-headedness, imbalance, etc.

Gifford, H.   (1858–1929) American ophthalmologist who trained with **Horner** in Zurich and practiced in Omaha. He described lid-lag in hyperthyroidism independently of **von Graefe,** as well as the following phenomenon.

Gifford reflex   Pupillary constriction with attempted tight eye closure (a normal phenomenon). See **Westphal-Piltz phenomenon.**

Gigli, Leonardo   (1863–1908) Italian surgeon-gynecologist who, in 1894, invented the flexible wire saw named for him for the performance of pubiotomy, although the saw is now used instead for craniotomy.

Gignoux syndrome   A syndrome of the low brainstem.[374]

Gilford, Hastings   (1861–1941) English obstetrician and pediatrician whose paper on **progeria** appeared in 1914.

Gilles de la Tourette, Georges   See **Tourette.**

Gilles de la Tourette syndrome   See **Tourette syndrome.**

Gillespie syndrome   A congenital cerebellar ataxic syndrome due to cerebellar and brainstem hypoplasia. Associated features include dilated pupils due to partial aniridia, delayed milestones, and mental retardation.[2118]

Both sporadic and dominantly inherited cases have been reported; recessive transmission is rare.

Gilliatt, Roger William   (1922–1991) English neurologist, first professor of clinical neurology in the Institute of Clinical Neurology at the **National Hospital** in London. His work centered upon the morphology and electrophysiology of the peripheral nervous system.

ginklose   An Icelandic term for neonatal tetanus.[4512]

girdle   (from Saxon, a waistband) 1. The parts of the body centered upon the pelvis or the shoulder, with particular reference to the muscles that move, respectively, the femur and the humerus. 2. A band around any part of the trunk, in which case the term is usually employed to describe the distribution of a radicular pain, as in diabetic truncal neuropathy, tabes dorsalis, or herpes zoster.

Giroux syndrome   A dominantly inherited congenital dysmorphic syndrome manifesting also skin erythema, papules, and hyperkeratosis. Dysarthria, gait and limb ataxia, and hyporeflexia appear later, in adult life.[2127]

gitterzellen   See **compound granular corpuscles.**

glabella   (from Lat, smooth, bald) The hairless space between the eyebrows. In **synophrys,** hair grows right across this space.

glabellar tap   See **orbicularis oculi reflex.**

glairy   (from Lat, egg-white) Slimy. The fluid contents of some cysts (such as **craniopharyngiomas**) are described by this.

Glasgow Assessment schedule   A simple, brief, problem-oriented scale assessing impairments and disabilities in the fields of *personality change, subjective complaints, occupational functioning, cognition, neurological deficits,* and *activities of daily living.* The cognitive and neurological assessments are abbreviated, most items being rated only as normal, moderately severe, or severe, but are probably very reliable.[3445]

Glasgow Coma scale   A novel and widely adopted scale for assessment of the depth and duration of impaired consciousness and coma. The features in Chart G–3 are scored.[5515]

Chart G–3. Glasgow Coma Scale

Ability to open the eyes

4 Spontaneously
3 To speech
2 To pain
1 None

Best motor response

6 Obeying commands
5 Localizing stimuli
4 Withdrawal
3 Flexor posturing
2 Extensor posturing
1 No movement

Best verbal response to stimulation

5 Oriented
4 Confused, inappropriate
3 Incomprehensible words
2 Sounds only
1 None

Variants of the scale include the **Glasgow-Liège scale** and the **Reaction Level scale.**

(From Teasedale G, Jennett B. Assessment of coma and impaired consciousness. A practical scale. *Lancet* 1974;**2**:81–84. Reprinted with permission from Elsevier Science.)

The scale has been modified for children, as shown in Chart G–4.

Chart G–4. Modification of the Glasgow Coma Scale for Children

Best verbal response

Appropriate words or social smiles, fixes on and follows objects	5
Cries but is consolable	4
Persistently irritable	3
Restless, agitated	2
Silent	1

The remainder of the scale is scored as for adults. See also **Childrens Coma scale.**

Glasgow Head Injury Outcome Prediction Program   A prognostic tool based upon an algorithmic evaluation of the outcomes in head-injured subjects.[4144]

Glasgow Outcome scale   A tool for categorizing the outcome in patients after severe head injuries with the following categories:

1. *Death*
2. *Persistent vegetative state*: no evidence of meaningful responsiveness.
3. *Severe disability* (conscious but disabled): patients who are dependent for daily support by reason of mental or physical disability or both.
4. *Moderate disability* (disabled but independent): patients with intellectual, personality and neurological deficits who nevertheless are capable of traveling by public transport and who can work in a sheltered environment.
5. *Good recovery*: resumption of normal life despite minor neurological and psychological deficits.[2844]

From Jennett B, Bond M. Assessment of outcome after severe brain damage. *Lancet* 1975;**1**:480–482. Reprinted with permission from Elsevier Science.

Glasgow-Liège scale   A variant of the **Glasgow Coma scale** in which a six-point scale recording the status of certain brainstem reflexes (such as the presence of vertical **doll's eye movements**) is added to the original.[667]

glaucoma   (from Gr, silvery-green) A disease characterized by increased intraocular pressures, often with vitreous opacities. Open-angle and closed-angle glaucoma are described.

The word was used by Hippocrates probably to describe cataract, and it continued in that role until Brisseau defined the difference between cataract and glaucoma in 1709. Von Graefe devised iridectomy for its relief in 1855.

Glees stain   A silver salt method of staining axons and their terminations.

glia   A term for those cells interspersed between the neurons within the CNS, comprising protoplasmic and fibrous astrocytes, oligodendroglia (collectively known as *neuroglia*), and microglial cells. The term was introduced by **Virchow** in 1854.

glial degenerations   See **glioneuronal dystrophies.** Conditions with their onset in infancy or childhood, and characterized by seizures, myoclonus, mental deterioration, nystagmus, blindness, and deafness.

glial fibrillary acidic protein   (GFAP) Normally a protein present only within astrocytes in the CNS, but also immunohistochemically demonstrable in the cells of astrocytomas, ependymomas, papillomas, and oligodendrogliomas but not in those of brain metastases.[1655]

In neuropathology, the protein is used as a marker for astroglia.

glial star   Microglial ingestion of, e.g., dead anterior horn cells.

glioblastoma multiforme   A rapidly expanding, malignant, invasive neuroectodermal tumor of the cerebral hemispheres arising in adult life and characterized histologically by the presence of small bipolar anaplastic cells, pleomorphism, necrosis, lack of areas of differentiation of the tumor cells, **pseudopalisading,** and capillary endothelial proliferation.

Monstrocellular glioblastomas are characterized by the presence of bizarre eosinophilic giant cells in addition to the ones just described. *Gliosarcomas* are further variants in which reticulin-containing spindle cells and poorly differentiated astrocytic cells are intermixed. *Gliomatosis cerebri* is characterized by the diffuse invasion of wide areas of the brain by small, spindle-shaped, anaplastic glial cells.[6] In all cases, death occurs within 2 years.

In a *variant familial form*, the responsible gene maps to 10p12–q23.2.

glioma   (from Gr, glue + tumor) Histologically malignant tumors of the neuroglial elements of the central nervous system, the "glue" here referring to the glial matrix of the CNS. The name was applied by Virchow in 1869.[5204]

According to Bailey,[294] the term includes astroglial gliomas (astrocytomas, anaplastic **astrocytomas,** and **glioblastoma multiforme,** spongioblastoma multiforme, gliosarcoma), oligodendrogliomas, **gangliogliomas,** ependymomas, and medulloblastomas.

See also **grading, brainstem glioma.**

gliomatosis cerebri   A rare form of astrocytoma characterized by the diffuse cellular overgrowth of neoplastic neuroglial elements throughout the cerebral hemispheres, brainstem, and spinal cord.

Clinical features of note are a long history of seizures, later memory loss, and eventually increased intracranial pressure but with few focal signs. This name has replaced the former term for the condition *reticulum cell sarcoma.*[4109] See also **primary diffuse leptomeningel gliomatosis.**

gliomesodermal reaction   Formation of a fibrous capsule in which there is a predominance of astrocytes, as occurs around a cerebral abscess.

gliomyosarcoma   An intracranial tumor composed of mixed glial and sarcomatous elements and containing rhabdomyoblasts. The tumor constitutes some 8% of all glioblastomas.[2171,5318]

glioneuronal dystrophies   (Seitelberger disease) Conditions with onset in infancy or childhood that are characterized clinically by seizures, myoclonus, progressive psychomotor deterioration, nystagmus, hypokinetic movements, hypotonia, limb and cranial nerve palsies, deafness, and optic atrophy with blindness. The condition may be a variant of **Hallervorden-Spatz disease.**

The prototype is a progressive neurodegenerative condition of unknown cause characterized by early delay in mental and motor milestones, and the presence of myoclonic, focal, and generalized seizures. Spastic or flaccid motor weakness, abnormal movements, cerebellar ataxia, blindness, deafness, decerebration, and death before the age of 7 years are the usual features.[2832]

Pathologically, the condition is notable for spongy degeneration of the gray matter, especially of the isocortex, with neuronal loss, diffuse astrogliosis, spongy changes in the deep gray nuclei, and atrophy of the cerebellum.

Other disorders subsumed under this heading include *spongy degenerations* such as **Canavan disease;** recessively inherited *progressive neuronal degenerations* such as **Alpers disease;** and *gliovasal diseases,* in which the process initially affects the astroglia but also engenders an inflammatory reaction leading outside the CNS to hepatopathy. **Zellweger disease** is an example of the last disorder.

gliosis   (astrocytosis, astrogliosis) The process of structural repair within the CNS whereby astrocytes produce intracytoplasmic filaments, leading to a local increase of neuroglial fibers in response to local tissue destruction.

The severity of the process is in proportion to the proximity of the reacting cells to any form of brain injury. Edema and minor degrees of ischemia are also associated with swelling of the astrocytes and the formation of new neuroglial fibers.

glissade (postsaccadic drift) A slow, smooth sliding or drift of the eyes following a voluntary saccade, in which failure of the pulse part of the **pulse-step** signal leads to a hypometric **saccade,** the remainder of the required movement being engineered by the step portion of the signal.[290]

Disease of the vestibulocerebellar connections, as in internuclear ophthalmoplegia, is usually responsible, but glissades also occur in fatigued normal subjects.[290]

glissadic overshoot   See **saccade.**

global aphasia   The most severe form of aphasia, characterized by severe impairment of *fluency* with sparse, short, perseverated, and stereotyped phrases and also of *naming, comprehension,* and *repetition,* such that the patients can neither formulate speech nor comprehend language. The features are thus those of a combination of **Broca** and of **Wernicke** aphasia. Automatic speech may be preserved.

The condition is due to a large lesion of the entire perisylvian region damaging both frontal and parietal language areas, as with mainstem middle cerebral artery infarction. In the classic form, there is an associated right hemiplegia.

In a *variant* subgroup, the temporal and parietal regions are unaffected, and the language disorder evolves into a **Broca aphasia.**[1261]

global aprosodia   See **aprosodia.**

global assessment of psychiatric symptoms   A scale developed to measure changes in the symptoms and behavioral characteristics of problems in elderly people.

Global Deterioration Scale   A descriptive scale rating the severity of cognitive decline and functional impairment in normal aging and in subjects with **Alzheimer disease,** using information obtained both from the patient and from a caregiver. Strong, significant relationships between decline on this scale and numerous behavioral or investigational abnormalities have been demonstrated.

Seven levels of cognitive functioning are rated, extending from 1. no cognitive decline; 2. mild decline (with subjective forgetfulness); 3. moderate decline (early confusion—difficulty at work, in speech, or when traveling in unfamiliar areas, detectable by family, and with a subtle deficit in memory on examination); 4. moderately severe decline (late confusion—decreased ability to travel, count, and remember current events); 5. severe decline (early dementia—needing assistance to choose clothes, disorientation to time or place, and decreased recall of the names of grandchildren); 6. very severe decline (needing supervision in eating and toileting, in-

continence, and disorientation to time, place, and perhaps person); and 7. late dementia (with incontinence, severe loss of speech and motor rigidity). For each of these stages full definitions are given. The scale is not specific for any form of dementia and is best used for staging and the follow-up evaluation of therapy.[4647,4648]

global inattention   See **motor impersistence.**

globoid-cell leukodystrophy   See **Krabbe leukodystrophy.**

globus hystericus   (Lat, globus, a ball) A sensation of choking as if upon a ball lodged in the throat, with tightness at the level of the larynx and sometimes accompanied by actual spasm of the pharyngeal muscles.[2240] The complaint is a classic symptom of **conversion reactions.**

glomus jugulare   (Lat, a ball of thread + neck) The region below the base of the skull where chemoreceptor chromaffin cells are sited within a dilatation of the internal jugular vein.

glomus jugulare tumor   A highly vascular tumor derived from the nonchromaffin chemoreceptor cells of the jugular bulb or along the ninth or tenth cranial nerves, described by Masson in 1924.

Adult females are most often affected. Clinical features include complaints of pulsating tinnitus and pain below the ear, evidence of damage to cranial nerves VII, VIII, IX, and XII, and a mass over which a bruit may be heard. Extension of the tumor into the posterior fossa leads to evidence of cerebellar disease, a Horner syndrome, and/or pareses of the fifth and the phrenic nerves, depending upon the direction of tumor growth. A vascular polyp may be seen in the external auditory meatus.[4185, 5270] See **chemodactoma.**

glossa   (Gr, the tongue) 1. The tongue. 2. The faculty of speech.

Glosso- is the usual prefix to words signifying conditions that relate to the tongue.

glossagra   See **glossalgia.**

glossalgia   (glossagra) Pain in the tongue.

glossodynia   Pain felt in the tongue, an occasional symptom of vitamin B deficiency but sometimes a manifestation of psychopathology. See **burning mouth syndrome.**

glossolabiolaryngeal palsy   See **bulbar palsy.**

glossolalia   "Speaking in tongues"; the enunciation of sentences using strings of words that are not part of the subjects' normal language. This occurs in both schizophrenia and nonschizophrenic states, such as those of religious or other ecstatic experience.

glossolaryngoscapulopharyngeal hemiplegia   See **Collet-Sicard syndrome.** It is this kind of compound word which provides the justification for eponyms.

glossopharyngeal nerve   (Gr, the tongue + the throat) Galen's sixth pair of cranial nerves, but thought to be part of the vagus by Willis and defined as the ninth pair by **Soemerring.**

glossopharyngeal neuralgia (Reichert syndrome, tympanic plexus neuralgia) Brief paroxysms of lancinating or burning pain in the throat, posterior tongue, and ear, often intense and with trigger zones in the throat but also precipitated by talking, chewing, or swallowing. In severe cases, the subject may become emaciated on account of the pain; in even more severe cases, cardiac irregularities such as profound bradycardia may lead to loss of consciousness or even death. It is seldom seen in people aged less that 40. The pathophysiology and treatment are the same as those for **trigeminal neuralgia.**[4634]

In a partial form, the nerve of Jacobsen is involved, leading to pain felt in the external auditory meatus only. The symptomatic form was first described by Weisenberg in 1910, the idiopathic form by Wilfred Harris 11 years later.[640]

Two major forms of the complete syndrome are defined by the International Headache Society[1051] and are given in Chart G–5.

Chart G–5. Forms of Glossopharyngeal Neuralgia

Idiopathic glossopharyngeal neuralgia A severe, transient, stabbing pain experienced in the ear, base of the tongue, or tonsillar fossa or beneath the angle of the jaw. The pain is therefore felt in the distribution of the auricular and pharyngeal branches of the vagus nerve as well as that of the glossopharyngeal nerve. It is commonly provoked by swallowing, talking, and coughing, and may remit and relapse in the fashion of trigeminal neuralgia.

A. Paroxysmal attacks of pain which last a few seconds to less than 2 minutes

B. Pain has at least four of the following characteristics:
1. Unilateral location
2. Distribution within the posterior part of the tongue, tonsillar fossa, or pharynx, or beneath the angle of the lower jaw or in the ear
3. Sudden, sharp, stabbing or burning in quality
4. Pain intensity severe
5. Precipitation from trigger areas or by swallowing, chewing, talking, coughing or yawning

C. No neurological deficit

D. Attacks are stereotyped in the individual patient

E. Other causes of pain ruled out by history and physical and special investigations

Symptomatic glossopharyngeal neuralgia The features are the same as those for glossopharyngeal neuralgia with the provision that aching pain may persist between paroxysms and sensory impairment may be found in the distribution of the glossopharyngeal or vagus nerves.

A. Pain as described above, with or without persistence of aching between paroxysms and signs of sensory impairment in the distribution of glossopharyngeal or vagus nerves.

B. Demonstration of a causative lesion by special investigations or operation.

*From Classification of headache disorders, cranial neuralgias and facial pains; and diagnostic criteria for primary headache disorders. Cephalalgia 1988;**8**(suppl):1–96). Reprinted by kind permission of Blackwell Science.*

glossoplegia Paralysis of the tongue.

glossoptosis The tendency for the tongue to fall back into the hypopharynx, as with hypognathism.

glossopyrosis See **burning mouth syndrome.**

glottal stop A brief, audible click normally preceding a cough and following pronunciation of words ending in *a* or *e*. Its loss in bulbar weakness is an early sign.

glottis (Gr, the mouth of the windpipe)

glucocerebrosidase The deficient enzyme in **Gaucher syndrome.**

glucocorticoid deficiency, achalasia, and deficient tear production A syndrome with childhood onset characterized by corneal and pupillary abnormalities, sparse tears, abnormal motility of the esophagus, achalasia, adrenal hypoplasia, hypoglycaemia, abnormality in consciousness, seizures, and diffuse depigmentation of the skin.[337]

glucosidase (β-glucosidase) An enzyme normally active in the chain of glycogen degradation to lactate, the absence of which produces the features of **Pompe disease.**

glucosylceramide lipidosis (Gaucher disease, cerebroside lipidosis; OMIM 231000) A sphingolipidosis, in which there is generalized deposition of galactosylceramide in the nervous system, due to a deficiency in galactosylceramide β-galactosidase activity. The disease is recessively inherited and has three forms defined according to age of onset.[2061] All occur more commonly in Jewish people; **Gaucher cells** are detectable in all patients and all show hepatosplenomegaly.

Type 1 (adult form) is characterized by hypersplenism, jaundice, thrombocytopenia, anemia, arthropathy, and retinal and skin pigmentation. Dementia, generalized seizures, myoclonus, rigidity, ataxia, and sensory neuropathy have been reported occasionally, but this type is not ordinarily associated with neurological dysfunction.

Type 2 (acute infantile neuronopathic form) is a rare form characterized by mental and motor failure, macular pigmentation, seizures or myoclonus, ataxia, extensor hypertonia, and laryngospasm, with onset at about 6 months of age; it leads to early death.

In *type 3 (juvenile or subacute neuronopathic form)*, the findings include ophthalmoplegias (notably a failure of ocular adduction), pyramidal signs, generalized seizures, myoclonus, and progressive dementia, but onset is usually during the second or third decades.[4142] It is mapped to 1q23.

glucuronidase (β-glucuronidase) An enzyme coded for on chromosome 7. Deficiency leads to the accumulation of dermatan sulfate and heparan sulfate in the Sly syndrome (**mucopolysaccharidosis VII**).

glue-sniffer's neuropathy A progressive, mainly motor neuropathy caused by inhalation of N-hexane or toluene, the organic solvents in some commercial glues.[5618]

Gluszcz syndrome   A congenital syndrome characterized by nystagmus, dermal abnormalities, cerebral and spinal tumors, and vascular malformations.[337]

glutamate   (dicarboxylic amino acid) An excitatory neurotransmitter.

glutamate dehydrogenase deficiency   A recessively inherited or sporadic progressive ataxic syndrome characterized by deficiency of this enzyme in association with the onset in young adult life of features suggesting **olivopontocerebellar atrophy.**

Clinically, progressive external ophthalmoplegia, ataxia, pyramidal signs, parkinsonism, and a motor neuropathy are the main features.[1017]

glutamic acid   (glutamate) An excitatory amino acid, toxic to neurons in high concentrations. Glutamic acid decarboxylase catalyses the conversion of glutamate to GABA and is the autoantigen responsible for the manifestations of **stiff person syndrome** and of insulin-dependent diabetes mellitus (IDDM).

A related syndrome of progressive cerebellar ataxia, late-onset IDDM, and various endocrine defects is described.[4880]

glutamylribose-5-phosphate storage disease   An aminoacidopathy characterized by mental deterioration, seizures, microcephaly, and proteinuria with dysmorphism. Excessive glutamylribose-5-phosphate is found in the brain and kidneys.[5982]

glutaric acidemia   See **glutaric aciduria.**

glutaric aciduria   (glutaric academia, multiple acyl-CoA dehydrogenase deficiency) A rare recessive disorder with onset in early childhood. It is due to a severe defect of mitochondrial oxidation of fatty acids as a result of deficiency of glutaryl coenzyme A dehydrogenase (type 1) or acyl-coenzyme A dehydrogenase (type 2) and is diagnosed by the detection of glutaric acid in plasma or urine.

Type 1 is a dysmorphic syndrome with congenital or early childhood onset due to disordered lysine and tryptophan metabolism. It is characterized by emotional lability; seizures; cerebellar, pyramidal and extrapyramidal signs (dystonias); myoclonus; dementia; and aminoaciduria.[722] The patients may also have acidotic crises resembling those of **Reye syndrome.**

Type 2 presents a heterogeneous collection of phenotypes, including neonatal hypoglycemia and infantile episodic vomiting with hypoglycemia; multiple dysmorphisms; renal cysts; severe hypotonia; and lethal cardiomyopathy. Numerous developmental brain disorders are also associated. Affected children may emanate the odor of sweaty feet.[1024] This form has also been described with onset in adult life and with features of a lipid myopathy.[1425]

See also **Jamaican vomiting sickness.**

glutathionine synthetase deficiency   See **5-oxoprolinemia.**

glutathionuria   A rare, diffuse encephalopathy due to gammaglutamyl peptidase deficiency, characterized clinically by mental retardation in isolation.[2199]

gluteal compartment syndrome   A rare disorder that most often occurs in conjunction with prolonged immobility in the lateral decubitus position after a sedative overdose, but also may result from direct trauma. Patients present with localized tenderness, induration, and pain with passive flexion of the gluteal muscles. Signs of sciatic nerve compression occur frequently, and rhabdomyolysis may be associated with the syndrome. If the diagnosis of gluteal compartment syndrome is suspected, intracompartmental pressures should be measured. If pressures are high or if sufficient clinical suspicion remains, the patient should undergo prompt fasciotomy. See also **blue jeans syndrome, ilioinguinal neuropathy.**[602,4282,4535]

gluteal neuropathy   Damage to the superior or inferior gluteal nerves, usually occurring as a result of local distortion following a femoral fracture or a misplaced injection or due to compression by the piriformis muscle (**piriformis syndrome**) and leading to weakness of the gluteal muscles.[4599]

gluteal reflexes   1. Stroking of the buttock of the prone subject leads to contraction of the gluteal muscles. 2. Tapping the gluteal muscles at their origin from the lateral part of the sacrum leads to their contraction. These reflexes are hard to elicit and almost impossible to interpret; their absence is not alone a sign of lesions of the L5–S1,2 reflex arcs, and their hyperactivity is never found in isolation.

gluteal syndromes   Myofascial pain syndromes consisting of back pain and trigger points in the buttocks, the pain radiating in a sclerotomal distribution and unaccompanied by neurological deficits. See **piriformis syndrome; gluteus medius syndrome.**

Such disorders are often apparent to physicians but less so to their surgical colleagues.

gluten ataxia   A subacute, progressive cerebellar syndrome, especially manifesting gait ataxia, occurring in subjects with gluten sensitivity and clinical evidence of celiac disease in whom there may be found antibodies to Purkinje cells.[2363a] Motor and sensorimotor axonal or demyelinating neuropathies, multiple mononeuropathy, myopathy, leukoaraiosis, neuromyotonia, and stiff-person syndrome are other neurological complications described.

gluteus medius syndrome   A myofascial pain syndrome characterized by pain felt persistently in the medial aspect of the buttock (especially just below the S1 joint), radiating to the upper thigh posterolaterally to the level of the knee, accompanied by trigger zones causing local muscle tenderness, restricted straight leg raising, and discomfort with hip and knee flexion and with medial rotation of the leg. No objective reflex or sensory changes are present.

gluts   A class of stereospecific proteins responsible for transporting glucose across tissue barriers. One form of disturbance of the system (glut-1 deficiency) is dominantly inherited and presents with seizures, developmental delay, ataxia, and low CSF glucose levels.[765]

glycerol kinase deficiency   An X-linked recessive systemic disease manifesting as a myopathy with histological changes similar to those of **Duchenne dystrophy,** accompanied clinically by psychomotor retardation, growth failure, osteoporosis, and hypoadrenalism. The serum levels of glycerol are high and those of glycerol kinase in leukocytes and cultured fibroblasts are low.[2312] The responsible gene maps to Xp21.1.

glycine encephalopathy   (nonketotic hyperglycemia) A fatal autosomal recessive disorder manifested in infancy in which glycine levels are high in the brain, serum, and CSF, because of a defect in the glycine cleavage enzyme.

The condition is characterized clinically by intractable seizures, lethargy, spasticity, failure of mental development, and early death.[3063] The EEG shows a burst–suppression pattern. Eventually the syndrome is one of psychomotor delay with axial hypotonia but peripheral spasticity, poor head control, and severe seizures; hydrocephalus is also described.[5732]

glycogen storage diseases   (glycogenoses) Autosomal recessive diseases characterized by deficiency of muscle phosphorylase, an enzyme required for the breakdown of glycogen into simpler substances to be metabolized by the tricarboxylic acid cycle, with the production of that energy required for muscle contraction. As a result of the deficiency, glycogen is permanently laid down in tissues such as liver and muscle. See also **forearm exercise test.**

Ten enzyme deficiencies, and thus 10 types of glycogen storage disease, are recognized, among which many lead to neurological disease as described in Chart G–6. In most the onset is in adolescence with exercise intolerance, painful muscle cramps, weakness, and occasionally myoglobinuria following exercise. Rarely, the condition manifests first in later adult life with progressive generalized muscle weakness. The muscle contractures that occur are electrically silent. Myoglobinuria is common and may lead to initial presentation with acute renal failure. The "**second wind**" phenomenon described in muscle phosphorylase deficiency has been attributed to increased utilization of free fatty acids as an energy source or increased muscle blood flow. Muscle biopsy shows the presence of excessive glycogen in subsarcolemmal vacuoles. Failure of serum lactate elevation following ischemic exercise is the usual diagnostic test but is not specific.

Chart G–6. Types of Glycogen Storage Disease

Type 1 glycogenosis (von Gierke disease, hepatorenal glycogenosis) A syndrome due to glucose-6-phosphatase deficiency with the resultant deposition of normal glycogen in the liver and inability to process glycogen to glucose.

Clinically, the condition is characterized by hepatosplenomegaly, renal enlargement, hypoglycemic attacks leading to seizures, hyperlipidemia, xanthomas, and ketoacidosis. Hypotonia is detectable but there is no evidence of myopathy.

Type 2 glycogenosis (Pompe disease, acid maltase (α-1,4-glucosidase) deficiency, idiopathic generalized glycogenosis) A recessively inherited syndrome occurring in childhood or adult life in which, due to absence of lysosomal acid α-glucosidase, failure to utilize glycogen leads to accumulation of that substance in cardiac and/or skeletal muscle, liver, kidneys, and nervous system. The condition presents with different features at different ages.[4488,5228] The responsible gene maps to 17q23.

Infantile form (Pompe disease of infants) A fatal glycogen storage myopathy of infants with bulbar, proximal, and distal myopathic weakness; atrophy and pseudohypertrophy; myotonia; macroglossia; cardiomyopathy; hepatomegaly; and scoliosis.[4488,5481] Death is usually due to cardiorespiratory failure and occurs within the first 2 years of life.

The same phenotype has also been reported in children with normal levels of acid maltase.[773]

Juvenile or childhood form (Pompe disease of children) A proximal glycogen storage myopathy (a lysosomal storage disease) presenting in early childhood or youth with proximal and distal myopathic weakness, atrophy and pseudohypertrophy, macroglossia, myotonia, cardiomyopathy, enlarged liver, and scoliosis.[1657] This type is more benign, but still fatal within 20–30 years.

Adult form (*acid maltse deficiency myopathy*) A proximal glycogen storage myopathy of adults, presenting in the third or subsequent decades with slowly progressive proximal weakness, atrophy and pseudohypertrophy, and myotonia.[1657,4813] The syndrome may thus resemble **polymyositis** or **myotonic dystrophy** and may also present as a **scapuloperoneal syndrome** or **rigid spine syndrome.** Typically, patients complain of excessive daytime sleepiness with nocturnal sleep disruption resulting from intermittent apneic spells accompanied by repetitive brady-tachycardia and considered to be due to failure of the other respiratory muscles to suffice during periods of physiological sleep-related atonia in the presence of the severe myopathic weakness of the diaphragm.[1667,2325]

The abnormal gene is located on chromosome 17. The glycogen content in muscle is only slightly increased or normal, there is no cardiomegaly, and death in respiratory failure only occurs very late. Both phenotypes may occur in the same family.[3468] A *variant form* is *acid maltase deficiency type 2,* which is a lysosomal glycogenosis causing proximal muscle weakness, hypertrophic cardiomyopathy, probable intellectual impairment and possible liver involvement occurring in the absence of any deficiency of acid maltase.[1275,4694]

Type 3 glycogenosis (Cori-Forbes disease, amylo-1,6-glucosidase (debrancher) deficiency, limit dextrinosis) A proximal glycogen storage myopathy of infancy, childhood, or adult life, transmitted as a recessive trait (at least in infants) with a tendency to improve at puberty. This is the most common glycogen storage disease, and is a relatively benign metabolic disorder due to deficiency of the enzyme amylo-1,6-glucosidase.

Infants present with hepatomegaly, hypoglycemia, seizures, growth delay, fasting hypoglycemia, and hypotonia, and cardiomyopathy may develop. In older children, cardiomyopathy and somatic muscular exercise intolerance are the main features. Adults may complain of fatigability with proximal myopathic weakness, generalized atrophy, calf pseudohypertrophy, and myotonia.[1454]

In *variant* forms, a gradually progressive polyneuropathy is caused by accumulation of glycogen within all the elements of the peripheral sensory nerves[5682] or gradually progressing polyneuropathy is caused by accumulation of glycogen within all the elements of the peripheral sensory nerves.[5682]

Type 4, brancher enzyme deficiency (Andersen disease, adult amylopectinosis, amylo-transglucosidase [brancher enzyme] deficiency) A recessively inherited glycogen storage disease presenting in infancy with motor delay, hypotonia, calf pseudohypertrophy, proximal myopathic weakness, and atrophy. In some cases, hepatomegaly is present.[1789]

A *variant* form (adult polyglucosan body myopathy) presents in adult life with progressive asymmetrical weakness; the muscle biopsy specimen appearances are those of a vacuolar myopathy, the periodic-acid Schiff–positive vacuoles lying in a subsarcolemmal position.

Type 5, myophosphorylase deficiency (McArdle disease) A recessively inherited glycogen storage disease with childhood or juvenile onset, due to muscle phosphorylase deficiency that results in the accumulation of unusable glycogen in muscles and leads to a failure of the muscles exercised to produce lactic acid. The clinical syndrome has its onset in childhood and comprises muscle stiffness, proximal myopathic weakness and fatigability with painful cramp contractures on exercise, the cramp being chemically and not electrically induced. Myoglobinuria follows in severe attacks. The symptoms may be relieved during exertion by a gentle decrease in the energy expended, which leads to the "second wind" effect.[697]

This was the first of the glycogen storage diseases to be predicted (in 1957 by Dr. Brian McArdle of Guy's Hospital, London) and detected.[3726] The responsible gene maps to 11q13.

The *infantile form* (fatal infantile glycogen storage disease) is an inherited multisystem storage disease presenting with mental retardation, corneal ulceration, and congenital hypotonia and severe myopathic limb weakness with respiratory distress and cardiomyopathy leading to death in childhood. Histochemistry of muscle shows a nonspecific myopathy with the subsarcolemmal accumulation of glycogen. Phosphorylase *b* kinase and phosphofructokinase-1 activities are low or absent.[159,1275,1453] An *intermediate* form is characterized by early childhood onset with proximal myopathic weakness and mental and developmental delay.

A *late adult* form is characterized by onset during adult life with bulbar weakness and facial and proximal myopathy.[1452]

Variants are *muscle phosphorylase b kinase deficiency*, a glycogen storage disease with onset in childhood or adult life with muscle pain, exercise intolerance, cramp, and fatigability. Autosomal and X-linked recessive forms are also described;[18] one form presents with late-onset cramps, stiffness, and muscle swelling and an abnormal ischemic forearm test.[3140] In other forms, dominant inheritance and a diffuse pattern dystrophy of the retinal pigment epithelium are described.

Type 6, Hers disease A glycogen storage disease without neurological features.

Type 7, muscle phosphofructokinase deficiency (Tarui disease) A recessively inherited proximal myopathy with young adult or late adult onset, presenting with muscle pain and decreased exercise tolerance, proximal muscle atrophy and weakness, increased creatine kinase levels, and myoglobinuria.[3303,5492] The responsible gene maps to 1cnq32.

Variants are *fatal infantile muscle phosphofructokinase deficiency*, a congenital form characterized by corneal cloudiness and ulceration leading to blindness, high palate, club foot, joint contractures, respiratory distress in neonates, mental and developmental delay, dolichocephaly, scaphocephaly or microcephaly, pendular nystagmus, proximal and distal myopathic weakness, multifocal paroxysmal EEG discharges, and cerebral atrophy;[159,5493] and an *inherited erythrocyte PFK deficiency* without myopathy.[1709]

Type 9, phosphoglycerate kinase deficiency An X-linked form in which both phosphoglycerate kinase and phosphorylase *b* kinase are deficient; this syndrome presents in childhood with congenital limb weakness, mental retardation, and corneal ulceration, the weakness progressing to truncal weakness and respiratory insufficiency. Short stature, enlarged liver, and arthropathy are also described. The responsible gene maps to Xq13.[737]

Type 10, phosphoglycerate mutase deficiency (Thompson disease, phosphoglucomutase deficiency) A rare glycogenosis presenting in childhood or youth with tight heel cords, calf hypertrophy and muscle cramps, and pigmenturia after exercise. The forearm ischemic lactate test shows little increase in lactate production with ischemic exercise.[1457] The responsible gene maps to 7p13–p12.

Other forms of glycogen storage diseases are *phosphohexoisomerase deficiency* (Satoyoshi disease), a rare variant, characterized by the late onset of myopathy with exertional muscle cramps and impaired stamina;[4926] *glycogen synthetase deficiency*, a rare congenital variant, characterized by lethargy, coma and seizures in recurrent hypoglycemic attacks with the later development of failure to thrive, microcephaly, and mental and motor delay;[4342] **lactic dehydrogenase deficiency;** and mixed enzyme deficiencies.

glycogen storage myopathy with cardiac involvement   See **glycogen storage disease, type 2.**

glycogen synthetase deficiency   See **glycogen storage diseases.**

glycogenosis   The accumulation of intracellular glycogen as a result of a **glycogen storage disease.**

glycogenosome Membrane-bound sacs of glycogen (distended lysosomes), seen in patients with **glycogen storage diseases.**

glycolic aciduria See **hyperoxaluria type 1.**

glycolytic myopathy A familial myopathy of late onset, characterized by normal work capacity for a brief period, delayed muscle pain and stiffness with exertion, absence of contractures or muscle weakness, and failure of lactate production in the blood. The condition is considered to be due to a metabolic defect occurring in glycolysis at the level of phosphohexoisomerase.[4926] See **glycogen storage diseases** (*phosphohexoisomerase deficiency*). See also DiMauro et al.[1449] on distal glycolysis.

glycopeptidosis A diffuse encephalopathy characterized by progressive myoclonic epilepsy and disorders of glycoprotein metabolism with abnormal urinary glycopeptide excretion.[1759]

glycoprotein disorders A group of inherited dysmetabolic states characterized by deficiency of glycoproteins. These include **fucosidosis types 1 and 2, mannosidosis, sialidosis** (congenital, and infantile types), and **aspartyl-glycosaminiduria.**

glycosylation disorders Genetic defects in the synthesis of the glycan moiety of glycoconjugates or in the attachment of glycans to macromolecules.[2794] Standard screening has relied upon the isoelectrofocusing of serum transferrin, but more sensitive genetic methods are now available.

Most of the phenotypes (of which there are many known and many more to be discovered) affect the nervous system; they include microcephaly, brain malformations, psychomotor retardation, behavioral abnormalities, seizures, strokes, ataxia, ocular lesions and abnormalities of eye movement, brain demyelination, peripheral neuropathy, hypotonia, and hyporeflexia.

GM₁ gangliosidosis (generalized gangliosidosis, neurovisceral lipidosis, Hurler syndrome variant, pseudo-Hurler disease, systemic late infantile lipidosis) A recessively inherited progressive and fatal neurovisceral storage disease due to deficiency of lysosomal acid β-galactosidases A and B, in which gangliosides accumulate in the CNS and keratan sulfate–like material, in the viscera. The responsible gene maps to p3p21-p14.2. There are three main phenotypes.

The *type 1 infantile form* (pseudo-Hurler disease or Landing syndrome) shows mental retardation, coarse facial features, macrocephaly, multiple dysostoses, hepatosplenomegaly, seizures, severe and progressive neurological disturbance with dementia and chorea, dysostosis, and blindness. A cherry-red spot may be present. Death usually occurs within 2 years.[4068,4188]

The *type 2 late infantile/juvenile* form manifests after 6 months of life. Somatic and skeletal deformities are absent and the hepatosplenomegaly is less severe, but mental deterioration, ataxia, pyramidal signs, dysarthria, weakness, **hyperekplexia,** and seizures occur. Death occurs before the age of 10 years.[4188,4189]

The *type 3 (adult or chronic)* form presents in infancy, childhood, or adult life with coarsening of the facial features, without visceromegaly or skeletal signs. Chorea, tics, dystonia, parkinsonism, dementia, and spasticity are occasionally concomitant signs.[2300,4068]

GM₂ activator deficiency See **GM₂ gangliosidosis.**

GM₂ gangliosidosis A group of **sphingolipidoses** in which there is generalized deposition of gangliosides in both neuronal and other tissues. The diseases are recessively inherited and have three forms defined according to onset: late infantile (Tay-Sachs disease), juvenile, and adult, as well as a number of *variants*. Deficiency of hexosaminidase A, hexosaminidase A and B deficiency or of the GM₂ activator protein are the underlying metabolic problems. See also **hexosaminidase deficiency.**

The variable phenotypes of GM₂ gangliosidosis have been reviewed[2871] and are described in Chart G–7.

Chart G–7. The Phenotypes of GM₂ Gangliosidosis

1. Alpha locus mutations (deficiency of hexosaminidase A)
Type 1, infantile (classical Tay-Sachs disease, B variant, amaurotic familial idiocy) This form is due to lesions at the alpha locus on chromosome 15 (15q22–q25.1) or at the beta locus on chromosome 5, causing total deficiency of *N*-acetyl β-hexosaminidase A. It affects mainly Ashkenazi Jewish infants, who show macrocephaly and megalencephaly, mental and motor failure, optic atrophy, spasticity, excessive startle responses, seizures, mental and developmental delay, and a cherry-red macular spot. Death occurs within a few years.

The macular findings were first described by Warren Tay, an English ophthalmologist in 1880,[5503] 6 years before a fuller clinical and pathological account was reported by the American Bernard Sachs,[4867] who also coined the term "amaurotic familial idiocy."

Partial deficiency of the enzyme leads to the later appearance of similar signs, but even more rarely, the adult form is described by O'Neill et al.[4240.] The responsible gene maps to 15q22–q25.1. The condition was redescribed by Vogt in 1905.[5777]

Juvenile (partial) type A recessively inherited syndrome manifesting signs of damage to motor and cerebellar systems, dementia, convulsions, and arrest of psychomotor development from the age of 4 years, in which the enzyme deficiency is but partial.[2170] This form is characterized by more slowly progressive mental decline. The main phenotypes are syndromes of slurred speech, spasticity, and ataxia[2872] and of pure ataxia, and those phenotypes resembling **hereditary motor neuropathy type 3, X-linked bulbospinal neuronopathy, neuronal ceroid lipofuscinosis,** and **amyotrophic lateral sclerosis.** In a *late-onset form,* similar symptoms occur in youth or early adult life.[1327]

Chronic type A heterogeneous collection of phenotypes reflecting partial deficiency of Hexosaminidase A and inherited recessively. They include a syndrome resembling

amyotrophic lateral sclerosis,[6058] a syndrome resembling **hereditary motor neuropathy type 3**,[2871] and a variant with manifestations of each of these conditions as well as dystonia, dementia, seizures, sensory neuropathy, internuclear ophthalmoplegia, or psychiatric disorders.[362]
Atypical spinocerebellar degeneration [4594]
Normal adults may have biochemical evidence of the disorder.[2871]

2. Beta locus mutations (deficiency of hexosaminidase A and B)

The *type 2 form* (*O variant, Sandhoff-Jatkiewicz disease, Sandhoff variant*) This form resembles the late infantile form clinically (with the addition of cardiac dysfunction), but the enzyme defect is partial and of both hexosaminidases A and B; the aminoglycolipid globoside accumulates in the viscera and GM₂ ganglioside and asialo-GM₂ ganglioside accumulate in the nervous system.

This recessively inherited sphingolipidosis occurs in non-Jewish infants and is associated with total deficiency of hexosaminidases A and B with some residual hexosaminidase S activity.[4905] Otherwise it is similar to *Tay-Sachs disease* in producing hepatosplenomegaly, cardiomyopathy, bony deformities, myoclonic seizures, macrocephaly, optic atrophy with a macular red spot, pyramidal signs, and mental and motor regression, with a progressive course to death in 2–5 years. The responsible gene maps to 5q13.

Variants include the following:
Juvenile Sandhoff disease[2170]
Chronic GM₂ gangliosidosis with hexosaminidase A and B deficiency
A multisystem disorder with ataxia, dementia, pyramidal signs, and amyotrophy in varying combinations
Juvenile cerebellar ataxia[2872]
Adult-onset spinocerebellar ataxia[4244]
Hereditary motor neuropathy (juvenile-onset spinal muscular atrophy)[2873]
Neuromuscular disease resembling **Kennedy syndrome**[5554]
The biochemical disorder may also be detected in some normal adults.

3. Activator factor mutations (normal hexosaminidase A and B activity). This form of hexosaminidase deficiency may be associated with any of the following syndromes:
The *AB variant* (GM₂ activator deficiency) This form is due to deficiency of the activator protein required for the interaction of hexosaminidase A and GM₂ ganglioside. The responsible gene maps to 5q. The disorder presents in infancy with microcephaly, blindness, and a macular red spot. Grand mal and myoclonic seizures, dementia, nystagmus, and pyramidal signs appear next.[4906]
A form resembling *Tay-Sachs disease,* but milder
An adult GM₂ gangliosidosis with seizures, dementia, and **normal-pressure hydrocephalus**
The biochemical disorder may also be detected in some normal adults[5554]

GM₃ gangliosidosis   A congenital dysmorphic syndrome manifesting also coarse facial features, visceromegaly, seizures, a muscular build, respiratory distress in the neonate, and spongy, cavitating, and cystic changes in the brain.[3556]

gnathalgia   (from Gr, the cheek + pain) Facial neuralgia—pain in the cheek.

gnathic   To do with the upper jaw or cheek.

gnathostomiasis   A rare parasitic nematode infection found usually in the people of Asia. The leading clinical features are fever, subcutaneous swellings, and abdominal pain with eosinophilia; subarachnoid hemorrhage, myelitis, and eosinophilic encephalomyelitis with coma are the neurological syndromes most often described.[1014]

gnomes' calves   Calf pseudohypertrophy as seen in **Duchenne muscular dystrophy.**

gnosanopsia   The faculty of awareness without discrimination.

gnosis   The faculty of knowing and comprehending the significance of what is perceived.

gnostic sensations   Those sensations that require and implicate cortical discriminative processes. These include stereognosis, discrimination of weight, surface, form, and texture; and the senses of passive movement and of the position of joints in space and possibly of vibration.

Godfried-Prick-Carol-Prakken syndrome   The combination of the signs of neurofibromatosis with mongoloid facies, areas of dermal atrophy, mental retardation, and cardiac conduction defects.[910] See **neurofibromatosis.**

Godin syndrome   Intermittent localized headache evoked by compression of the carotid arteries.

Godlee, Sir Rickman John   English neurosurgeon who successfully removed a cerebral tumor in 1884, although the patient died later of sepsis.

Godtfredsen syndrome   (cavernous sinus-nasopharyngeal tumor syndrome) The concurrence of oculomotor palsies and trigeminal numbness and pain due to infiltration of the cavernous sinus region by a nasopharyngeal tumor, with the addition of hypoglossal paresis due to compression of that nerve by enlarged retropharyngeal lymph nodes.[2144,2145]

Goeminne syndrome   A congenital X-linked syndrome consisting of torticollis, facial asymmetry, keloids of the trunk and limbs, crytorchidism, renal failure, testicular failure, respiratory complaints, and renal dysplasia.[2153]

goggia   Local contraction of muscle fibers when they are tapped, seen in prolonged debilitating illnesses.[4723]

The origin of the term is uncertain but the condition is almost certainly **myokymia.**

gogi aphasia   Selective impairment of the processing of semantic Chinese-type characters and difficulty in finding access to the lexicon in terms of both production and reception, with retention of the ability to process phonetic signs and with fluent oral repetition.[4921]

goiter headache   Headache resulting from venous distention in subjects with goiters, the tumor compressing the internal jugular veins at the level of the thoracic inlet.[3237]

Golabi syndrome   A congenital X-linked dysmorphic syndrome manifesting also dwarfism, brittle hair, atrial septal defect, gastrointestinal anomalies, deafness, strabismus, microcephaly or macrocephaly, and mental and developmental delay.[2156]

Goldberg syndrome   (juvenile type 2 sialidosis, mucolipidosis 1) A recessively inherited dysmetabolic state resulting from deficiency of d-N-acetylneuraminidase and β-galactosidase leading to the accumulation of sialyl-oligosaccharides.

Clinically, the onset is after the age of 2 years, with mental retardation, seizures and myoclonus, a cherry-red macular spot, deafness, ataxia and short stature, angiokeratoma, and vacuolated lymphocytes in the peripheral blood.[2161] See also **sialidosis.**

Goldenhar syndrome   See **oculoauriculovertebral dysplasia.**

Goldenhar-Gorlin syndrome   See **oculoauriculovertebral dysplasia.**

Goldflam, Samuel Vulfovich   (1852–1932) Polish neurologist who trained with **Charcot** and **Westphal** and thereafter practiced in Warsaw. He gave an early account of **myasthenia gravis** ("myasthenia pseudoparalytica," once known as Erb-Goldflam disease) in 1893, **Erb** having written on a similar topic in 1879.

Kurt Goldstein

Goldman-Offner reference   See **average potential reference.**

Goldstein, Kurt   (1878–1965) German-American physician who trained with **Wernicke** and **Edinger** and later worked in Frankfurt, Berlin, and, after 1935, in New York. He gave the first description of the catastrophic (anxiety/outrage) reaction seen in demented patients faced with the impossibility of completing an assigned task, as well as a description of the following syndrome. He wrote widely on the topic of dysphasia, introduced a sorting test for the localization of cerebral injuries, and advanced the concept of the difficulty in changing mental "sets" as a basis for understanding the cognitive problems of the brain injured.

Goldstein syndrome   Acute cerebellitis—a postinfectious and probably autoallergic self-limited condition.[2173]

Goldstein-Schirer test   An instrument for the detection of right posterior parietal lesions, in which the subject is asked to sort solid objects by their shape and color.

golf ball epilepsy   Acute post-traumatic and later seizures following cranial trauma from these objects. [954]

Golgi apparatus   A perinuclear assembly of membranes, important in the processes of excretion by the cell.

Golgi, Camillo   (1844–1926) Italian anatomist, born in Lombardy and trained in Pavia, where he eventually became professor of histology and anatomy, dean of medicine, and rector of the university. His staining methods allowed for the first time a full description of the morphology of the neuron.

He introduced silver chromate or nitrate and osmic acid staining (to show neurons and myelin, respectively) in 1873 while in practice as a hospital physician, the work being done in his kitchen; and he was the first to describe dendrites within what he wrongly considered to be a nutritive reticulum. He nevertheless shared the Nobel prize for 1906 with **Ramon y Cajal,** who supported the rival **neuronal theory,** and with whom his relationship was poor.

Golgi also differentiated type 1 neuroglial cells with long axons from the type 2 cells with shorter axonal processes, the Golgi tendon organs; and the intracytoplasmic Golgi apparatus. His later work was largely on malaria.[1829]

Golgi cells   Golgi defined two forms of cortical cells in 1880: type 1 neurons with long axons which terminate at a distance, and type 2 neurons with short axonal processes which terminate in the gray matter close to the nerve cell body; internunciate cells and the stellate cells of the cerebellar cortex are of this type.

Golgi corpuscles   The cutaneous end-organs for touch.

Golgi stain   A silver stain for astroglia, the basis of the success of **Cajal** in neurohistology.

Golgi tendon organs   Specialized stretch receptors in the tendons which discharge when stimulated by excessive tension. This causes inhibition of the α-motor neurons and thus the "give" after increasing resistance felt during assessment of tone in patients with pyramidal lesions.

Goll, Friedrich (1829–1903) Swiss anatomist, physiologist, and neurologist, who eventually became professor of anatomy at Zurich.

Gollin incomplete figures test A test of right hemisphere visual perceptual processing using incomplete images to examine the subject's perceptual organizational skills. [2176]

Goll's columns The fasciculus gracilis, the medial fasciculus of the posterior columns, described in 1860.

Goltz, Friedrich Leopold (1834–1902) Professor of physiology at Halle and Strasburg, whose experimental results led him (incorrectly) to deny the theories of **Ferrier** that suggested that localization of function existed within the nervous system.

Goltz syndrome See **focal dermal hypoplasia.**

Gombault, F.A.A. (1844–1904) French neurologist.

Gombault neuritis Periaxial segmental degeneration of peripheral nerves, described in 1880; it is unlikely that this condition represents a single syndrome, but the eponym has been applied to all forms of segmental demyelination. See **hereditary motor and sensory neuropathy, type 3.**

Gomori, Georg (1904–) Hungarian-American neuropathologist, who introduced a number of stains into pathology, the best-known of which is the Gomori trichrome technique for differential staining; in muscle, connective tissue stains green; muscle and cytoplasm (and myelin) stain red; and nuclei, gray-blue. [2296]

gonadotrophin-releasing hormone A hypothalamic hypophysiotrophic hormone.

Gonda sign See **Allen sign.**

goniometer (Gr, an angle + a measure) An instrument for measuring the cranial or facial angles, now little used, although **Broca** designed one for this purpose. Such instruments are, however, still commonly employed by orthopedic surgeons and psychiatrists.

go–no-go paradigm A simple clinical test of resistance to interference and thus of concentration, in which the subject makes a simple motor response to only one of the two stimuli randomly generated by the examiner.

gonyalgia paresthetica (Gr, knee + abnormal sensation) **Wartenberg**'s term for tingling suddenly felt in the region of the patella when local trigger zones are lightly touched, accompanied by persistent numbness of the region supplied by the infrapatellar branch of the saphenous nerve. The cause is unknown. [5862]

Goodenough "draw a man" test A test in which a child is asked to draw a man as well and as completely as possible, with no time limit. The items included in the child's drawing are scored, the score for the test correlating with those of intelligence tests. [4433]

goosey A chronic, familial, involuntary movement disorder of children seen in the southern United States in which the sudden brief movements occur in response to startle and are accompanied by echolalia. [2450]

Gopalan syndrome See **burning feet syndrome.**

Goppert sign Pupillary dilation in response to minor peripheral sensory stimulation, described in meningococcal meningitis.

Gordon, A.M. (1874–1953) French-American neurologist and psychiatrist who was born in Paris, where he graduated in medicine before emigrating eventually to Philadelphia, where he was on the staff of Jefferson Medical College. His main interest was the study of the reflexes.

Gordon extension sign See **Gordon reflex.**

Gordon reflex 1. A variant method of eliciting the **Babinski** response, in which the deep flexor muscles of the calf are squeezed; as usual, the upgoing toe indicates the presence of a pyramidal tract lesion. [2203] 2. The *tonic reflex;* the leg does not immediately fall back after the patellar tendon has been tapped. [2202] 3. (*Gordon extension sign*) Extension and perhaps fanning of the flexed fingers follows deep pressure exerted upon the radial side of the pisiform bone. [1349a]

Gordon sign 1. (Souques sign, finger sign) Compression over the pisiform bone at the wrist leads to flexion of the thumb and index finger in the presence of pyramidal tract disease. 2. Spreading of the fingers and extension at the elbow when the arm is passively raised, occurring normally but to a much greater extent in patients with hemiparesis.

Gordon syndrome 1. A congenital dysmorphic syndrome manifesting also retinitis pigmentosa, sensorineural deafness, pyramidal signs, joint contractures, and mental and developmental delay. [2204] See also **Alstrom-Hallgren syndrome.** 2. Hypertension, renal tubular acidosis, and hyperkalemia with normal glomerular filtration. A syndrome of secondary **hyperkalemic periodic paralysis** may be associated. [1013]

Gordon-Hay sign The "hung-up" knee jerk, in chorea.

Gorham proverbs test A test of reasoning in which the subject is required to interpret a proverb, spontaneously or by multiple choice. [2212] The instrument is used mainly to assess frontal lobe functions.

Gorlin syndrome See **frontometaphyseal dysplasia syndrome.**

Gorlin-Chaudhry-Moss syndrome A recessively inherited congenital dysmorphic syndrome manifesting craniofacial dysostosis, craniostenosis affecting the coronal sutures, brachycephaly, microphthalmia, astigmatism, corneal scarring, anti-mongolian slant to the eyes, short stature, weakness of eye closure, nystagmus on lateral gaze, dental anomalies, patent ductus arteriosus, hypertrichosis, and mental and developmental delay.[2214] See also **craniosynostosis.**

Gorlin-Goltz syndrome   (Jarisch syndrome, multiple basal cell nevi syndrome) A dominantly inherited syndrome characterized by multiple basal cell nevi, hypertelorism, strabismus, vertebral anomalies with scoliosis, frontotemporal skull bossing, mandibular cysts, and a tendency toward the development of medulloblastoma. The syndrome is also distinguished by a lack of responsiveness to injections of parathyroid hormone, as shown by reduced phosphate excretion.[2223] See **nevoid basal cell carcinoma syndrome.**

Gould sign   See **bowed head sign.**

gourmand syndrome   A benign eating disorder associated with lesions of the right anterior cerebral hemisphere and characterized by a preoccupation with food, a passionate preference for finer quality food, and a craving for food despite normal hunger and satiation signals.[4632]

Gowers ataxic paraplegia   A myelopathy with the combination of a posterior and lateral column disorder which is nonsyphilitic[2240] and probably represents subacute combined degeneration of the cord as a result of vitamin B_{12} deficiency.

Gowers frontal tap   An alternative method of eliciting the **ankle jerk,** in this instance by tapping the belly of the tibialis anterior muscle. It probably works by setting up vibrations transmitted to the posterior compartment of the leg.

Gowers local panatrophy   Areas of wasting of the skin, subcutaneous tissues, and underlying muscles down to bone, varying in diameter from the size of a nut to that of an orange, described by Gowers in his textbook.[2240]

The cause is uncertain; scleroderma may be responsible.

Gowers maneuver   A method of determining that apparent paraplegia is hysterical, whereby the examiner grasps and smartly pulls the pubic hair of the seemingly paraparetic subject. When the condition is indeed not the result of a structural lesion this leads the subject to adduct the legs at once.

Gowers paraplegia   Myelopathy secondary to vertebral osteitis.[2240]

Gowers signs   1. The classic, heart-rending sign of pelvic girdle weakness in young boys who, on getting up from a recumbent position, stand with the trunk in full flexion and their hands on the floor, from which position they proceed to "walk" their hands up their legs in order to attain the erect posture. Though characteristic of every cause of pelvic muscle weakness, the sign was first described in, and still most often leads to the diagnosis of, **Duchenne dystrophy.**[2240]

2. Intermittent oscillation in pupillary size with light stimulation, occurring in early neurosyphilis.[2240]

3. Pain produced along the whole course of the sciatic nerve when the ankle is passively dorsiflexed, in cases of sciatic nerve irritation.

4. Incomplete recovery from a third cranial nerve palsy (pseudo-Graefe sign, Brixa-Koppens sign, Fuchs sign).

5. Inability of a patient with pelvic girdle weakness to rise from a sitting position with the arms outstretched.

Gowers, Sir William Richard   (1845–1915) A leading neurologist in 19th century England, who was house physician to Jenner (and later his secretary) before appointment to the staff of University College Hospital and the National Hospital, Queen Square, in 1872. He later became professor of clinical medicine at the University of London. He was elected a Fellow of the Royal College of Physicians in 1879 and of the Royal Society. He was knighted in 1897.

Despite the success of his *Diagnosis of Diseases of the Spinal Cord* (London, 1880) and of *Epilepsy and Other Chronic Convulsive Diseases* (London, 1881), his greatest work was his magnificent two-volume *A Manual of Diseases of the Nervous System* (1886),[2240] in which he distilled his own and others' clinical wisdom into a work that became in successive editions the bible of neurologists worldwide and is still read with pleasure and profit for the physiological and clinical insights that it contains; it remains in print in a limited edition. He himself etched many of the illustrations, and it is likely that the original drafts were written in shorthand, of which he was a strong proponent.

His studies of epilepsy[2239] are perhaps his best known single area of clinical observation and analysis, but he also devised a hemocytometer; published an atlas of ophthalmoscopy; described distal myopathy (1902), pseudohypertrophic muscular dystrophy, local panatrophy, myotonic dystrophy, sleep paralysis, and vasovagal attacks; differentiated choreic from dystonic forms of cerebral palsy; and defined the dorsal spinocerebellar tract.

Gowers did not publish in *Brain,* as he disliked the editor, who responded with a review of his textbook which offended Gowers even more.[2542]

Gowers syndromes   1. (hereditary distal muscle dystrophy) A dominantly inherited dystrophy with onset in the small muscles of the hands and feet, thereafter spreading proximally. It is more common in adults but can occur also in childhood.[2241] See **distal muscular dystrophy.** 2. (vasoconstriction syncope) Attacks of paresthesia, dyspnea, precordial discomfort, reduced pulse volume, and cramps occurring mainly in women. The resemblances to the **hyperventilation syndrome** are close.[2242] 3. **Saltatory spasm.**

Gowers tetanoid chorea   See **Wilson disease, dystonia.**

Gowers tract (column)   The superficial (anterior) spinothalamic tract, defined in Gowers' textbook *The Diagnosis of Diseases of the Spinal Cord* (London, 1880).

Gowers-Paton-Kelly syndrome   See **Foster Kennedy syndrome.**

Goyer disease   A dominantly inherited syndrome of children, characterized by ichthyosis, progressive deafness, and renal failure in association with hyperprolinemia.[2245]

Gradenigo, Giuseppe   (1859–1926) Italian otolaryngologist who studied in Padua, Venice, Paris, London, and Berlin. He became professor at the University of Naples and wrote widely on otolaryngology. He published an account of the following syndrome in 1904.

Gradenigo syndrome   (Gradenigo-Lannois syndrome, petrous apical syndrome) Painful anesthesia in the territory of the first division of the fifth cranial nerve with sixth nerve palsy and possibly involvement of other oculomotor nerves and of the seventh nerve, stemming from irritation of these structures as a result of osteitis of the petrous portion of the temporal bone, or of their infiltration by a tumor at the skull base, such as a nasopharyngeal carcinoma.[2247]

The classic clinical triad consists of deep retro-orbital pain, paralysis of the ipsilateral lateral rectus muscle from involvement of the abducens nerve as it crosses the petrous bone, and otitic infection with purulent discharge from the ear. The syndrome may be associated with vertigo and hearing loss, either from a concomitant bacterial labyrinthitis or from involvement of the eighth cranial nerve in its bony canal. Unfortunately, radiologic evidence for infection of the petrous apex can be difficult to establish even with high-resolution CT scanning.

Gradenigo-Lannois syndrome   See **Gradenigo syndrome.**

grading   1. (of reflexes) A semiquantitative score assigned to the speed and excursion of the reflex movement made in response to the percussion of tendons. The system in common usage is as follows: 0 = absent; + = reduced; ++ = normal; +++ = hyperactive; ++++ = hyperactive with sustained **clonus.** (+) is written when the reflex is obtained only with **reinforcement.** 2. (of gliomas) Methods of characterizing the attributes of tumors to achieve some idea of their prognosis.[294]

Histological methods based on the features of anaplasia such as necrosis and mitosis, and on cellular differentiation[3011] have been employed for 40 years; gliomas were divided among astrocytomas, oligodendrogliomas, and ependymomas and subdivided among four grades of malignancy. Such gradings are considered to be of utility only in the case of astrocytomas[1303] but are still employed, as modern kinetic techniques are yet under development.

Graefe, Friedrich Wilhelm Ernst Albrecht von (1828–1870) German ophthalmologist who trained in Berlin and later in Prague. He studied extensively in Europe before returning to Berlin, where he became professor of ophthalmic surgery in 1857.

He introduced the operation of iridectomy for glaucoma and refined the procedure of lens extraction. He is also remembered for having described sympathetic ophthalmia, retinal embolism, progressive external ophthalmoplegia, and some of the ocular signs in **dysthyroid ophthalmopathy.**[5047]

Graefe sign   (lid lag) The delay in descent of the upper eyelid on looking down, as in dysthyroid ophthalmopathy and myotonic disorders.

The *pseudo-Graefe sign* consists of elevation of the upper eyelid on looking down, the result of aberrant regeneration of the third cranial nerve after injury.

Gram, Hans C.J.   (1853–1938) Danish bacteriologist who invented the stain named for him in 1884.

grand mal seizures   See **generalized tonic-clonic seizures.**

granular cell hyperplasia   See **cerebellar ataxias, Lhermitte-Duclos disease.**

granular cell myoblastomas   Small dermal nodules derived from Schwann cells, characterized histologically by the presence of sheets of cells with small round nuclei and copious cytoplasm containing basophilic granules.[6,1807] They are usually benign.

granular cell schwannomas   See **granular cell myoblastoma.**

granular cell tumor of the hypophysis   See **choristoma.**

granular cortical atrophy   Multiple, small, cortical infarcts associated with narrowing of the cortical vessels and clinically accompanied by evidence of dementia.[66]

granular ependymitis   A proliferative inflammatory reaction of the ependyma as a response to local viral, bacterial, or spirochetal inflammation.

granular nuclear inclusion body disease   A slowly progressive multisystem disorder of the CNS and of muscles, presenting clinically with dysarthria, gait disturbance, increased reflexes, akinesia, spasticity, and other pyramidal signs. Muscle and nerve biopsy specimens show hyaline nuclear inclusion bodies staining for iron. The condition may be secondary to a virus infection.[5002]

granule cell layer hypoplasia   An uncommon syndrome in which this abnormality affects the cerebellum. Mental retardation, short stature, and delayed milestones accompany the limb and gait ataxia.[2439]

granulomatous angiitis   See **isolated angiitis of the nervous system.**

granulomatous hypophysitis   A rare chronic inflammatory disorder of the pituitary gland that presents clinically as a sellar mass lesion with pituitary insufficiency and/or hyperprolactinemia, headache, ophthalmoplegia, and possibly optic neuritis. Typical MRI findings are of an intensely enhancing pituitary mass with local dural enhancement, radiologically indistinguishable from a pituitary tumor. The etiology is usually undetermined.

Variants are lymphocytic and xanthomatous hypophysitis and the condition has been recorded as a complication of **aortic arch disease.**

granulomatous myositis   Symptomatic muscle infiltration with noncaseating granulomatous tissue in sarcoidosis, Crohn disease, or other autoallergic diseases.

Such infiltration is usually asymptomatic; but syndromes consisting of chronic myopathic weakness, painful cramps, and stiffness,[1502] and acute weakness resembling polymyositis have been described.[5163]

granulomatous neuropathy   A form of multiple mononeuropathy due to sarcoidosis. The seventh and eighth cranial nerves and thoracic spinal roots are most commonly involved; peripheral neuropathy is rare.[1354]

granulomatous polymyositis   A slowly progressive inflammatory disorder of muscle occurring in elderly people who complain of aching and girdle weakness over the course of years. The diagnosis is made on the basis of the finding of noncaseating granulomas on muscle biopsy specimens.

The condition may be a form of sarcoidosis but also appears with Crohn disease and follows intramuscular injections.[3530,3687] See **sarcoid myopathy.**

granulome bizarre de l'orbite   See **orbital pseudotumor syndrome.**

granulovacuolar degeneration   The presence of 3- to 5-μm argyrophilic electron-dense intracytoplasmic granules in vacuoles within the pyramidal neurons of the hippocampus, occurring in relation to advancing age and in greater concentration in **Alzheimer disease, progressive supranuclear palsy, Down syndrome, tuberous sclerosis,** and in the **ALS-parkinsonism-dementia complex of Guam.**[6]

granulovacuolar myopathy   A myopathic disease characterized by profound selective muscle wasting and weakness, electrical myotonia without clinical evidence, and muscle biopsy appearances in which a number of type 1 fibers show sarcoplasmic lobulation.[2890]

graphesthesia   The facility of interpreting letters or figures traced upon the skin. This **gnostic** sensation is mediated by the parietal cortex.

graphogenic epilepsy   A form of **reflex epilepsy** in which the seizures are triggered by writing.[231]

graphology   The study of handwriting; popularly used in the divination of attributes of character.

graphomania,   See **hypergraphia.**

graphoreé   See **hypergraphia.**

graphospasm   See **writer's cramp.**

grasp reflex   Flexion of the fingers over an object placed gently in the palm; a reflex normally present in babies up to 5 months of age.[6064] It is asymmetrical in hemiplegia and increased in spastic and rigid states. It is also found in adults with bifrontal lesions.

The reflex was first described for the adult hand by Janischewsky in 1909 and 1914 and for the foot by Schuster in 1926. The **Hoffman** and **Tromner** signs are pathologic variations of this response.

grasp reflex of the foot   (plantar grasp reflex) A reflex seen in normal infants up to the age of 1 year, consisting of tonic flexion and adduction of the toes in response to light pressure upon the ball of the big toe, whereas a scratch on the sole evokes the usual brief extensor plantar response. The foot grasp persists in patients with **Down syndrome** and in some patients with contralateral frontal lobe lesions.[709]

grasp response   (forced grasping) A stereotyped prehensile reaction of the flexors and the adductors of the fingers and the flexor muscles of the wrists which can be elicited in fractional parts by appropriate localization of the stimulus. The *catching phase* is elicited by distally moving deep pressure over the palmar surface of the hand, the *holding phase* by traction on the flexor tendons. **Denny Brown** distinguished from this an *instinctive grasp reaction*, a deliberate progressive closure of the whole hand made in a series of small movements upon a stationary contact within the palm, terminating in a final complete grip and leading to pursuit (the *magnet reaction*) when attempts are made to remove the stimulus. Groping in response to a visual stimulus is an extension of this tactile response.[5084]

Walshe regarded the reflex as comprising the patient's closure of the hand over an object placed in it when the patient's attention is distracted but not when it is directed to the stimulus, and considered it to represent evidence of a mild pyramidal lesion, resulting from contralateral frontal lobe pathology. The stretch of the flexor tendons leads, in his term, to **tonic innervation,** over which the patient has no control; this represents the holding part of the reflex described by Denny Brown.[5833]

Grasset, Jean   (1849–1918) French neurologist.

Grasset sign   1. The inability of hemiparetic patients to raise both legs together by flexion at the hip, while remaining able to raise either one separately.[5047] 2. (Grasset-Gaussel sign, Hoover sign) When the patient with hemiparesis attempts to raise the weak leg, excessive downward pressure can be felt on the examiner's hand placed under the heel of the healthy leg. Either leg may be lifted independently but they cannot be elevated together. If the paretic leg is elevated, and the normal leg is elevated next, then the paretic leg will fall back to the bed; but if the healthy leg is elevated first, and the paretic leg is then passively raised, then the normal leg will remain in position.[1349a]

Grasset-Gaussel sign   See **Grasset sign.**

Graves, Robert James   (1797–1853) Irish physician practicing in Dublin who first recognized that diseases could affect the peripheral nerves, having attended Parisian patients during an epidemic of "neuritis" in 1828.

Graves ophthalmopathy   See **dysthyroid orbitopathy.**

gray matter heterotopias   Nodules of neuropil, composed of astrocytes and neurons, located in the white matter of the brain.

gray rami   The C fibers.

gray spinal syndrome   An anique term for lesions of the central cord.

great toe phenomenon of Edelmann   See **toe reflex.**

great vein of Galen   A major intracerebral vein, draining into the straight sinus. It was once thought to cause hydrocephalus when occluded, but this is disproved.

greater auricular neuralgia   A syndrome of intermittent painful paresthesias in the distribution of this nerve, not precipitated by touch, and likely to be caused by partial damage to the C3 nerve root.[614]

Greenfield disease   See **metachromatic leukodystrophy.**

Joseph Godwin Greenfield

Greenfield, Joseph Godwin   (1884–1958) British neuropathologist who trained in Edinburgh and at the

National Hospital, Queen Square, where he was appointed neuropathologist in 1914. From his laboratory there emanated a steady output of important papers, their clarity enhanced by brevity, and his book on neuropathology, which was the gold standard during his lifetime. As dean of the Institute of Neurology he fostered the careers of many young physicians. His books *The Pathology of the Nervous System* (1921), *The Cerebrospinal Fluid* (1925, in collaboration) and *Neuropathology* (1958) were acclaimed for presenting the most modern information in a readable style. His contributions to the clinical practice of neurology were recognized by his presidency of the Association of British Neurologists (1954–56).

Gregg syndrome   (maternal rubella syndrome) A syndrome of multiple congenital anomalies as a result of infection of the mother with rubella during the first trimester. Characteristic findings include congenital cataract, microphthalmos, deafness, microcephaly, hydrocephalus, and congenital cardiac anomalies.[2276] See **congenital rubella embryopathy.**

Greig, David Middleton   (1864–1936) Scottish surgeon working in Dundee, where he was concerned with the management of mentally retarded children as well as with a wide range of topics in clinical surgery. He was the first to describe **hypertelorism,** both isolated and as part of the following syndrome.

Greig syndrome   1. (ocular hypertelorism, euryopia) An autosomal dominant, X-linked, or sporadic syndrome of unusually wide spacing between the eyes, frequently in association with other developmental defects.[2277] 2. (cephalopolysyndactyly) A dominantly inherited congenital maldevelopment mapped to chromosome 7p and characterized by the association of hypertelorism, a vertical ridge in the forehead often with brachycephaly or scaphocephaly, flattening of the occiput and bulging of the temporal bones, optic atrophy, bilateral sixth cranial nerve palsies in the event of raised intracranial pressure, polysyndactyly, and frequently mental retardation. See **hypertelorism.**

Grenet syndrome   (crossed-sensory paralysis) Bilateral facial thermoanalgesia, unilateral truncal thermoanalgesia, and homolateral fifth cranial nerve motor involvement due to a lesion of the tegmentum of the pons such a tumor or stroke. Homolateral ataxia, a coarse tremor, and a contralateral hemiparesis may also be present. [5162]

Grey-Walter, W.   English neurophysiologist at the Burden Neurological Institute in Bristol, U.K., who first described **contingent negative variation.**

grid 1   (G1, input terminal 1 [E-l] active or exploring electrode) See **recording electrode.**

grid 2   (G2, input terminal 2 [E-2], or reference electrode) See **recording electrode.**

Griesinger sign   Edema and tenderness over the mastoid process (the point of exit of an emissary vein) as evidence of thrombosis of the lateral sinus.

Griesinger, Wilhelm   (1817–1868) German neurologist and psychiatrist who gave a good account of pseudohypertrophic muscular dystrophy well before **Duchenne**,[2280] and introduced the concept of outpatient psychiatric care to clinical practice.

grip sign   If the examiner's fingers are inserted between the flexed fingers of the subject, the subject's grip is normally increased by wrist extension and decreased by wrist flexion.[1349a]

Grisel syndrome   (nasopharyngeal torticollis) Nontraumatic atlantoaxial dislocation with resultant torticollis, occurring after oronasopharyngeal inflammation.[4326]

Groll-Hirschowitz syndrome   A congenital, recessively inherited, maldevelopmental syndrome manifesting also acanthosis nigricans, a malabsorption syndrome, sensorineural deafness, strabismus, ptosis, pes cavus, sensorimotor neuropathy (perhaps due to vitamin E deficiency), and anencephaly or craniorachischisis.[2588]

Gronblad, Ester Elizabeth   (b. 1898) Swedish ophthalmologist.

Gronblad-Strandberg syndrome   A rare, recessively inherited syndrome due to a widespread disorder of collagen formation and characterized by pseudoxanthoma elasticum in the skin, angioid streaks of the retina, macular and frequently gastrointestinal bleeding, accelerated atherosclerosis, and a tendency to intracranial aneurysm formation.[2286]

Groote syndrome   A congenital dysmorphic syndrome manifesting also visceral maldevelopments, holoprosencephaly or arhinencephaly, polydactyly, hydrocephalus, and callosal abnormalities.[337]

groove sign   Absence of dermal fibrosis overlying veins, leading to grooving over their surface when they collapse as the limb is elevated; a sign of **eosinophilic fasciitis.**

groping   (instinctive grasp reaction, forced groping) The movement of pursuit of a patient's hand towards an object that has touched the hand or crossed the patient's field of vision, as if to retain it. Further searching movements are made when the object has been removed from the palms.

Like grasping, this is evidence of a mild pyramidal lesion, resulting from contralateral frontal lobe pathology.[5833]

Gross Motor and Reflex Development test   A 60-item scale for the assessment of reflex and voluntary motor functions up to the age of 5 years. See also **Denver Developmental Screening test.**

gross motor functions   Those functions that are mainly performed with the aid of proximal muscles, which allow, for example, head control, the sitting posture, and walking. See also **fine motor functions.**

ground connection   The conducting path between the subject and the EEG machine, and between the EEG machine and the earth.

ground electrode   A connection from the patient to earth. Used as a common return for an electric circuit and as an arbitrary zero potential reference point. (From the 2001 Report of the Nomenclature Committee of the American Association of Electromyography and Electrodiagnosis.[10] Used by permission, copyright © 2001, AAEM.)

group atrophy   Atrophy of large groups of contiguous muscle fibers, characteristically seen in neurogenic muscle diseases. Both large groups of some hundreds of myofibrils and small groups of only a dozen or so are seen at different stages.

grouped denervation atrophy   The occurrence of large groups of small, angulated muscle fibers of the same histochemical type in muscle biopsy specimens. The finding suggests severe denervation. See also **disseminated neurogenic atrophy.**

grouped discharge   1. Irregular, voluntary grouping of motor unit action potentials as seen in a tremulous muscular contraction. 2. Involuntary grouping of motor unit action potentials as seen in myokymia. 3. A general term to describe repeated firing of motor unit action potentials. See **repetitive discharge.** (After the 2001 Report of the Nomenclature Committee of the American Association of Electromyography and Electrodiagnosis.[10] Used by permission, copyright © 2001, AAEM.)

Grove sign   Abnormal resistance felt when a retracted eyelid is grasped and gently pulled downward, much as occurs with a forced duction test of the extraocular muscles. This is evidence of dysthyroid lid retraction.[2292]

growing pains   Isolated nocturnal leg pains experienced by healthy children, particularly following a day of strenuous exercise. The nature of the cause is undetermined, but a family history of migraine is commonly noted.[4270]

growth cone   Expansions at the head of newly sprouting axons at the site of nerve injury.

growth deficiency–clefting–retardation   See **Myhre syndrome.**

growth retardation, alopecia, pseudoanodontia, and optic atrophy   (GAPO syndrome) A congenital recessively inherited dysmorphic syndrome characterized by the coexistence of growth Retardation, alopecia, pseudoaniodontia and pseudo-optic atrophy.

Skeletal and dermal anomalies, frontal bossing, midface hypoplasia, hepatomegaly, macrocephaly, pendular nystagmus, papilledèma, cerebral atrophy, and mental and developmental delay are other features described.[5594]

Grox syndrome   A congenital dysmorphic syndrome manifesting also cardiac and skeletal abnormalities, seizures, microcephaly, pyramidal signs, and mental and developmental delay.[337]

Gruber syndrome   (dysencephalia splanchnocystica, Meckel-Gruber syndrome) A recessively inherited congenital dysmorphic syndrome characterized by microcephaly, occipital exencephalocele, micropthalmia, hypertelorism, exophthalmos, polydactyly, polycystic kidneys, liver, and pancreas, congenital heart defects, and cleft lip and palate.[2294] Internal hydrocephalus, anencephaly, and cerebellar aplasia are also described.[2674]

Grüelder reflex   (Fontanelle reflex) Extension of the hallux with pressure on the fontanelle, seen in young children with increased intracranial pressure.

Gruner-Bertolotti syndrome   The association of impairment of conjugate upward gaze, loss of pain and temperature sensations, tremor, and hemiparesis, the effects of a mesencephalic lesion. Readers who enjoy eponyms will be pleased to learn that this condition has been regarded as the combination of Parinaud and von Monakow syndromes.[1563]

grusskrampfe   See **flexor spasms.**

gryposis   (Gr; crooked) Crookedness of a part, a term usually applied to the nails when they curve excessively or to joints (**arthrogryposis**).

Guam parkinsonism-dementia complex   (Guamanian neurodegeneratrive disease) A neurodegenerative disease resulting from ingestion of the seed of the neurotoxic plant *Cycas circinalis,* a traditional source of food and medicine of the Chamorro people. This causes cortical motor neural dysfunction, parkinsonian features, and behavioral abnormalities with chromatic and degenerative changes of motor neurons in the cerebral cortex and spinal cord and an excess of cerebral neurofibrillary tangles.[5271] See **Lytico-Bodig.**

Guamanian neurodegenerative disease   See **Guam parkinsonism-dementia complex.**

Gubler, Adolphe-Marie   (1821–1879) French physician and professor of therapeutics, whose first publications were on liver disease and syphilis. He recognized paralysis occurring after infections, which may have suggested the topic to **Landry,** his student. Gubler produced a series of publications on alternating hemiplegia between 1856 and 1858.[2995] See **Millard-Gubler syndrome.**

Gubler paralysis   see **Millard-Gubler syndrome.**

Gudden atrophy   Secondary degeneration of the thalamic nuclei following destruction of certain cortical areas.[2305]

Gudden, Bernhard Aloys von   (1824–1886) Swiss psychiatrist, professor at Zurich, and then at Munich. He was drowned in a lake by the actions of his patient, the insane King Ludwig II of Bavaria.[4979]

Bernhard Aloys von Gudden

Gudden commissure   A fiber tract between the inferior corpora quadrigemina and the medial geniculate bodies of the two sides, running closely with the optic tracts.

Gudden law   The degeneration of the proximal end of a divided peripheral nerve proceeds centripetally.

Guerin-Stern disease   See **arthrogryposis multiplex congenita.**

Guignon, Georges   (1859–1932) French neuropsychiatrist, a pupil of **Charcot,** who, however, drifted away from neurology and into the specialty of tuberculosis therapy. He published a full account of convulsive tic (see **Tourette syndrome**) in 1886, a year after Tourette, whose work he acknowledged, but the condition has occasionally been called Guignon disease.

Guild Memory test   A compound test including measures of immediate and delayed recall of paragraphs and paired associates, and of immediate recall of designs, used to study changes in normal aging and Alzheimer disease.[2111]

Guillain, Georges   (1876–1961) French physician who trained in Rouen and Paris and was intern under Raymond at the **Salpêtriére,** taking further training in America and Germany. In 1923 he became professor and chairman of neurology at the **Salpêtrière** after

Charcot, Raymond, Déjèrine, and **Marie,** and held the post until 1947 when Alajouanine took it over.

With Barré and Strohl, he published the classic account of **acute inflammatory demyelinating polyneuropathy,** their patients being soldiers who developed the disease during World War I.[2316] A few years later he described the first test for CSF protein. His other areas of research were neuroanatomy, multiple sclerosis, the reflexes, brainstem vascular and other syndromes, hereditary ataxias, and the conditions described in the following entries.

Guillain sign   In cases of meningitis, pinching one quadriceps muscle produces abrupt flexion of the hip and knee on the other side.[374,1341]

Guillain-Alajouanine-Garcin syndrome   See **Garcin syndrome.**

Guillain-Barré syndrome   See **acute inflammatory demyelinating polyneuropathy.**

Guillain-Barré Syndrome Foundation International   A foundation founded in 1980 to assist patients with this condition. The goals of the foundation are support (contacts and personal visits to patients and their families), education (printed materials, meetings, newsletters, international symposia), and research. Address: PO Box 262, Wynnewood, PA 19096. Tel: 610–667-0131. Web site: http://www.guillain-barre.com.

Guillain-Barré Support Group   A British charitable organization providing information and support. Address: LCC Offices, Eastgate, Sleaford, NG34 7EB. Tel/Fax: +44 1529 304615. Support helpline: 0800 374 803 (UK); 0044 1529 415278 (Rol). E-mail: admin@gbs.org.uk. Web site: http://www.gbs.org.uk/.

Guillain-Barré Syndrome Support Group of the United Kingdom   A charitable organization. Address: Foxley, Holdingham, Sleaford, Lincolnshire, UK NG3R 8NR. Web site: http://www.gbs.org.uk/.

Guillain-Bertrand syndrome   Unilateral arrhythmic myoclonus in the limbs as a result of a lesion of the dentate nucleus.[2317]

Guillain-Garcin syndrome   See **Garcin syndrome.**

Guillain-Mollaret triangle   A supposed brainstem pathway connecting the olive, the contralateral dentate nucleus, and the homolateral red nucleus, the circuit being completed by the posterior longitudinal bundle running between the red nucleus and the olive. Lesions of this circuit were determined by Guillain and Mollaret[2318] to result in **palatal myoclonus.** See **myoclonic triangle.**

Guillain-Thaon syndrome   Spastic paraplegia as a result of meningomyelitis in tertiary syphilis.[2314]

Guinea worm   (*Dracunculus medinensis*) A filarial parasite of humans that typically resides in the subcutaneous tissues and protrudes through an ulcer in the skin. At this interface, the female nematode releases her larvae on contact with water, and these are ingested by crustacean animalcules of the genus *Cyclops,* which live in stagnant pools. When the *Cyclops* are inadvertently ingested in drinking water, the life cycle of the parasite is completed. Aberrant migration of the parasite (dracontiasis, dracunculiasis) may rarely result in an epidural abcess with compressive myelopathy. Ocular involvement is also described.[304] It is conceivable that the infestation could be eradicated globally by improvements in drinking water sanitation. (HJM)

Gulf War syndrome   A selection of symptoms, sometimes bizarre and not allowing diagnosis of any known neurological disorder, occurring in some veterans of the 1991 Gulf War. Fatigue, paresthesias, numbness, headache, skin rashes, myalgia, arthralgia, chest pains or discomfort, dyspnea, impaired sleep and memory, and diarrhea are the more common symptoms. Objective signs are few, but evidence of peripheral aneuropathy has been put forward.[2799]

Gull disease   (adult cretinism) Acquired hypothyroidism with enlargement of the tongue, mental slowing, and the usual ectodermal and other systemic changes of **myxedema.**

The condition was described by Gull in 1874;[2330] in the same issue of the Medical Society's transactions he described **anorexia nervosa.**

Gull, Sir William Withey   (1819–1890) Physician to Guy's Hospital, London, and a leading physician in England. He gave the first precise descriptions of anorexia nervosa, myxedema, intracranial aneurysm, and syringomyelia (1856–1862) and, in his Goulstonian Lectures of 1848, he dealt at length on the clinical features of cord compression and the paraplegias. Gull was also the first to recognize the lesions of **tabes dorsalis** in the posterior columns (1856).

Gullstrand, Alivar   (1862–1934) Swedish ophthalmologist who received the Nobel prize in 1911 for his work on "the dioptrics of the eye."

Gullstrand law   When a patient is made to turn the head when fixing on a distant object, if the corneal reflex (corneal light reflection) from either eye moves in the direction in which the head is turning, it moves toward the weaker muscle.[2331]

gum hypertrophy   A classic sign of chronic phenytoin toxicity in those with teeth, which the overgrowth of gingival tissue may hide so that gum excision is necessary.

gumma   (from Lat, gum) Inflammatory granulation tissue composed of fibrosis, mononuclear cell infiltration, and necrosis resulting from obliterative endarteritis, forming an irregular nodular tumor in the cerebral hemispheres, pons, or elsewhere in the brain or the rest of the body in patients with tertiary syphilis.

The term was introduced early in the sixteenth century.

gun-barrel constriction of the visual fields   (tubular constriction) Marked and usually symmetric constriction of the fields, typically found in patients with glaucoma or **pigmentary retinal degenerations.**

The term is unfortunate, because the diameter of the field perceived does in fact increase with distance from the subject in the above conditions, though not in the setting of malingering nor in hysterical visual field constriction.

Gunn pupil   (Marcus Gunn pupil, relative afferent pupillary deficit) Constriction followed by redilation of the pupil with continued exposure to direct light stimulation, in an eye affected by an optic nerve lesion (but also in the other eye consensually).[5861]

When there is pathological attrition of functioning optic nerve fibers, the residual input to the pupilloconstrictor center after several seconds of constant stimulation is much the same as that resulting from the background illumination, so the pupil dilates again.

Levatin rather than Marcus Gunn described the **swinging flashlight test;** Gunn observed the reactions of both eyes to stimulation of one of them, while Levatin observed the paradoxical dilation of the pupil of the affected eye when the flashlight is swung across to it from the normal eye.

Gunn phenomenon   (Marcus Gunn phenomenon, jaw winking, trigemino-ocular synkinesis) A congenital syndrome of marked unilateral ptosis with elevation of the eyelid when the mouth is opened, further increased by deviation of the jaw to the other side. Less typical clinical features include elevation of the lid on protrusion of the jaw or tongue, clenching the teeth or swallowing, inspiration, or smiling. Despite the name, the syndrome does not include a wink at all but rather ocular "mooning," to coin a phrase. It was described by Marcus Gunn in 1883.

This is thus the opposite of the **Marin-Amat syndrome** (inhibition of the levator palpebrae with jaw-opening, usually a developmental anomaly).[2335] Both conditions are usually seen as developmental anomalies, although the syndrome may be recessively inherited or occur as an irregular dominant characteristic, when a supranuclear cause is postulated. When acquired, it may indicate anomalous reinnervation of the levator palpebrae muscle after third nerve injury but it may also occur after seventh nerve lesions[2335] or as the result of abnormal innervation by the motor division of the fifth cranial nerve to the ipsilateral levator palpebrae superioris.[1719]

Gunn, Robert Marcus   (1850–1909) Scottish ophthalmologist who trained in Edinburgh and Vienna and at Moorfields Eye Hospital in London, where (as at the National Hospital and the Hospital for Sick Children)

he was later appointed surgeon. He introduced substantial improvements in the methods of examination of the eyes and ocular surgery. He also wrote on the topics of the retina, optic atrophy, nystagmus, retinal vascular disease, and comparative anatomy.

gustatory   (from Lat, taste) Relating to the sense of taste.

gustatory lacrimation   See **crocodile tears.**

gustatory piloerection   Gooseflesh provoked by eating. This occasionally occurs in an upper limb following surgical injury to a cervical sympathetic ganglion. Evidently the phenomenon is the result of aberrant reinnervation. (HJM)[607,2561]

gustatory reaction   Normal infants will force the salt-coated finger away with their tongue.[6064]

gustatory sweating   (Frey syndrome, Baillarger syndrome, Dupuy syndrome, auriculotemporal syndrome, Salivo-Sudipar syndrome) Localized sweating and flushing of the face in response to acid or spicy tastes, occurring after damage to the parasympathetic fibers in the auriculotemporal nerve as a result of parotid gland disease or from iatrogenic causes. The signs result from cross-stimulation of sympathetic by parasympathetic fibers which have regenerated in an improper direction after injury.[1953]

The syndrome was first described by Duphenix in 1757; Dupuy in 1816 and Parkes-Weber in 1897 gave further accounts before the modern one.

While occasionally seen in normal people (Claude Bernard experienced it when he ate chocolate), it is usually due to damage to the auriculotemporal nerve (**auriculotemporal syndrome**) when the area of sweating is localized to a small region anterior to the ear, or it is due to incomplete damage to the sympathetic pathways, which still allows innervation of a region in which there is a degree of denervation hypersensitivity.[2485]

Foix found the first reported description to have been that of Duphenix in 1757. A dominantly inherited *variant* is also described.[3579]

gustolacrimal reflex   See **crocodile tears.**

Guttmann sign   Autonomic overactivity occurring following a high thoracic cord lesion, with piloerection, sweating, vasoconstriction, hypertension, bradycardia, mydriasis, and blockage of nasal air passages, occurring paroxysmally on the occasions of excessive stimulation of the automatic bladder by urine. See also **Harlequin syndrome.**

Guttmann sweat test   The color change produced when quinizarin powder is placed on sweating skin.[2342]

Guyon canal   A short, oblique, fibro-osseous space medial to the pisiform bone in the hand and bounded by this bone, the hook of the hamate, the transverse carpal ligament, and a ligament between the hamate and the pisiform. The ulnar nerve divides into its deep palmar branch and the hypothenar motor and cutaneous sensory branches to the medial 1 1/2 digits within the canal.

Compression of the nerve at this site is a well-recognized occupational hazard in carpenters, cobblers, cyclists, and others.

Guyon, Jean-Casimir-Felix (1831–1920) French surgeon who studied in Paris, where he later became professor of surgical pathology. He described the canal named for him in 1861.

gyrate atrophy of choroid and retina A recessively inherited congenital tapetoretinal degeneration manifesting also retinal lesions, night blindness, myopia, seizures, myopathic weakness with type 2 fiber atrophy, and hyperornithinemia.[5192]

gyratory nystagmus See **circular nystagmus.**

gyrus (from Lat, a circuit or ring) The convolutions of the surface of the brain, ignored in Greek and Roman writings and only appearing in works during the Renaissance. Most are small and somewhat variable in position, but a few are constant in position, such as the hippocampal, cingulate, angular, transverse (Heschl), precentral and postcentral, subcallosal, superior, middle and inferior temporal, cuneate, and dentate gyri.

The spirals of the cochlea are also named thus.

gyrus rectus syndrome Compression of the optic nerve at the anterior cranial fossa by a frontal mass, with the clinical features of visual loss and papilledema.[5823]

H reflex (H wave, Hoffmann reflex) A compound muscle action potential having a consistent latency evoked regularly, when present, from a muscle by an electrical stimulus to its nerve. It is regularly found only in a limited group of physiologic extensors, particularly the calf muscles with tibial nerve stimulation.

The H wave is most easily obtained in calf and forearm muscles with the cathode positioned proximal to the anode. Compared with the maximum amplitude M wave of the same muscle, the H wave is smaller, and has a longer latency and a lower optimal stimulus intensity. The latency is longer with more distal sites of stimulation. A stimulus intensity sufficient to elicit a maximum-amplitude M wave reduces or abolishes the H wave. An abnormal H reflex results from a lesion anywhere along the reflex pathway with either dorsal or ventral root involvement.

The H wave is thought to be due to a spinal reflex, with electrical stimulation of afferent fibers in the mixed nerve to the muscle and activation of motor neurons to the muscle, accomplished through a monosynaptic connection in the spinal cord. The reflex and wave are named in honor of Hoffmann who had observed in 1918 that the CMAP associated with ankle and knee jerks were comparable in latency and configuration to those evoked by submaximal stimulation of tibial and femoral nerves and reasoned that abolition of the late response with supramaximal stimulation and brief latency (30 msec in the calf) must be a result of fast conducting nerve fibers and a short central delay. (Adapted from the 1987 Report of the Nomenclature Committee of the American Association of Electromyography and Electrodiagnosis. AAEE glossary of terms in clinical electromyography. *Muscle Nerve* 1987;**10S**:G5–G23. Copyright 1987. By John Wiley and Sons, Inc. Reprinted by permission of John Wiley and Sons, Inc.) cf. **F wave, A wave.**

Normal Values of H-Reflex Latency According to Height

147–160 cm	163–175 cm	178–193 cm
28.46 ± 1.8	29.9 ± 2.12	31.5 ± 1.2

The upper limit of normal is 35 msec and the normal side-to-side latency difference is <1.1 msec.

The reflex is hardly obtainable elsewhere, with the exception of the flexor carpi radialis.[2766]

Haab, Otto (1851–1931) Swiss ophthalmologist, in Zurich.

Haab reflex Bilateral pupillary constriction when one eye is confronted with a bright light; the consensual pupillary reaction.

HAART **H**ighly **A**ctive **A**nti**R**etroviral **T**herapy—combinations of three or more anti-HIV drugs including nucleoside and non-nucleoside reverse transcriptase inhibitors and protease inhibitors.

Haas sex-linked disease with copper metabolism defect A syndrome characterized by psychomotor retardation, seizures, low serum copper and ceruloplasmin levels, and impaired absorption of copper from the gut, but differing from **Menkes disease** in the virtual absence of pili torti, absence of hypothermia, normal birth weight at term, and later demise.[2352]

Habel syndrome A congenital dysmorphic syndrome manifesting also generalized hirsutism, skeletal maldevelopments, seizures, spasticity, hydrocephalus, and mental and developmental delay.[337]

habenula (Lat, a bridle or strap) A thalamic nucleus situated above the pineal where it was considered by the ancients to drive and control the seat of the soul.

habituation Decrease in size of a reflex motor response to an afferent stimulus when the latter is repeated, especially at regular and recurring short intervals. (From the 2001 Report of the Nomenclature Committee of the American Association of Electromyography and Electrodiagnosis.[10] Used by permission, copyright © 2001, AAEM.)

habromania (Gr, graceful + madness) A form of insanity in which the patient is abnormally merry.

Hachinski dementia score A brief scale rating decline in the performance of everyday activities (an 8-point score) and in personal habits (up to 20 points). Although innovative in its use of a patient's easily assessed functional abilities as the basis for scoring, it has been little utilized in comparison with other similar diagnostic scales, and far less than its sibling, the ischemia score (see next entry).

Hachinski Ischemia score A validated instrument (Chart H–1) designed to differentiate the demented patient with multiple infarcts from the patient with **Alzheimer disease;** it does this successfully, not so much on the basis of any difference in mental state but on the basis of other clinical temporal and historical data.

Chart H–1. The Hachinski Ischemic Score

Feature	Score
Abrupt onset	
Stepwise deterioration	1
Fluctuating course	2
Nocturnal confusion	1
Relative preservation of personality	1
Depression	1
Somatic complaints	1
Emotional incontinence	1
History of hypertension	1
History of strokes	2

Evidence of associated atherosclerosis	1
Focal neurological symptoms	2
Focal neurological signs	2

From Hachinski VC, Iloff L, Zilkha K, et al. Multi-Infarct Dementia. Arch Neurol 1975;32:632–7. © American Medical Association 1975. Reproduced by kind permission.

A score of 4 or more suggests that the patient does not have pure **Alzheimer disease,** and that a vascular component is a cause of or contributing to the clinical syndrome.[2356]

A revised and reduced *variation* of the scale has been proposed by Rosen et al.,[4779] in which the assessment is limited to the following clinical features: abrupt onset, stepwise deterioration, history of stroke, focal neurological signs, emotional incontinence, and somatic complaints.

Haenel, H. (1874–1942) German neurologist who studied at Freiburg, Munich, and Berlin and graduated at Heidelberg University. He practiced in Halle and Dresden.

Haenel sign Lack of pain in the eye when it is pressed by the examiner. The sign is positive in the presence of tertiary neurosyphilis.

Bradycardia and hypotension, the normal responses to this maneuver, are also absent.[2364]

Haenel variant A form of muscular dystrophy affecting only the arms.

Haff disease An inflammatory myopathy resulting in **myoglobinuria** and due to the ingestion of eels or fish contaminated by industrial toxins, probably arsenic. The first report was from the Kurische Haff (harbor) area of Königsberg, Germany.[248]

Hornet stings may produce a similar syndrome.

hag (the old hag) An evil spirit in female form, believed in some cultures to oppress the chest in subjects with **sleep paralysis.**

Hagberg disease A *variant* of **Krabbe leukodystrophy.**

Hagberg lipofuscinosis See **neuronal ceroid lipofuscinosis.**

Hagenbach-Bing myopathy See **myopathica rachitica.**

Hague Seizure Severity Scale A 13-item self-administered scale based on the reports by parents of their child's seizures.[913]

Hahn sign Persistent rotation of the head from side to side in cerebellar disease.

hair-brain syndrome A congenital, recessively inherited syndrome characterized by cataract, sexual infantilism, dwarfism, nail dystrophy, brittle hair, and physical and mental delay.[2773]

Hajdu-Cheney syndrome A congenital, sporadic, or dominantly inherited dysmorphic syndrome character-

ized by basilar impression, craniofacial and peripheral dysostoses, spinal osteoporosis, and chondrodystrophy.[2373] See **osteopetrosis.**

Hakim-Adams syndrome See **normal pressure hydrocephalus.**

Halal syndrome A congenital dysmorphic syndrome manifesting also pigmentary retinopathy, goiter, microcephaly, and mental and developmental delay.[337]

Hall disease See **Wilson disease.**

Hall, Marshall (1790–1857) English physician who trained in Edinburgh and after making a grand tour of European centers, settled to practice in Nottingham and later in London, but was never appointed to any London hospital.

He was a comparative anatomist and neurophysiologist who discovered and interpreted the role of the spinal cord in reflex activity,[2381] introducing the terms **reflex arc** and **spinal shock** (1850) and demonstrating conclusively the dualistic nature of neural functioning, both volitional and reflex.

He also suggested an association between epilepsy and anemia of the medulla oblongata and was the first to describe the **grasp reflex** and **spinal shock.** He published at least 15 major books, collections of lectures, and tracts on neurology or neurophysiology, and over 150 papers. His advocacy of the establishment of a hospital for epileptics in 1852 (now the **National Hospital**) speeded its foundation.

Marshall Hall

Hall syndrome 1. (hydrencephaloid, spurious hydrocephalus) A syndrome thought by Marshall Hall to suggest hydrocephalus in infants or children with anemia, gastrointestinal complaints, and tachycardia. He published his comments in a volume of essays in 1825; from the descriptions given, however, dehydration following gastroenteritis seems a most likely etiology. 2. (Pallister-Hall syndrome) A sporadic, lethal, congenital dysmorphic syndrome characterized by features of **Turner syndrome** with synostosis of the coronal suture, imperforate anus, various visceral, endocrine and skeletal abnormalities, and a tendency for hypothalamic hamartoblastomas to develop.[2379]

Haller, Albrecht von   (1708–1777) Swiss anatomist, botanist, and professor of medicine at Göttingen University. He was for a time physician to the English King George II.

Haller was reputed to have had 1300 publications, among which were his demonstrations that all CSF eventually drains into the venous system, that nerves are irritable structures, and that peripheral stimulation causes impulses to be sent to the brain. He was also the first to describe the foramen of Luschka.

Hallerman-Streiff-François syndrome   (oculomandibulardyscephaly with hypotrichosis) A rare oculoauriculocephalic anomaly comprising short stature, brachycephaly with prominent frontal and parietal bones, long beaked nose, thin sparse hair, thin skin, microphthalmia and micrognathia, congenital cataracts, dental anomalies, nystagmus, optic atrophy, and mental delay.

The dysmorphism leads to an appearance of "bird-headedness" and unilateral proptosis is also described.[2382]

Julius Hallervorden

Hallervorden, Julius   (1882–1965) German neuropathologist who trained at Königsberg and worked as a psychiatrist in Landsberg. He described the syndrome named for him and his mentor Hugo Spatz while working in Munich in 1922. He later joined Spatz at the Kaiser Wilhelm Institute in Berlin and, after World War II, in Frankfurt.

Hallervorden (not himself a member of the National Socialist party, but dependent upon it in wartime Germany and thus himself brutalized) participated actively in the Nazi-inspired euthanasia programs, thus collecting extensive data on the pathologies leading to mental illness or retardation.[5124]

Hallervorden-Spatz disease   (Martha-Alma disease, progressive pallidal degeneration, adult amaurotic idiocy) A rare, recessively inherited condition with onset in childhood, marked by the deposition of iron and other pigments in the globus pallidus and substantia nigra, and by glial proliferation, cerebral demyelination, and the presence of spheroids in the axons and dendrites or neuronal cell bodies of the basal ganglia and thalamus. Linkage to 20p12–3t has been established.

Clinically, optic atrophy, pigmentary retinal degeneration, progressive dystonia, chorea, dysarthria, mental deterioration, parkinsonism, and pyramidal signs occur.[2383] In some cases there is also evidence of a motor neuropathy. The condition ends in death after 5–20 years. When this condition occurs in early childhood, it and **infantile neuroaxonal dystrophy** are identical.[5962] See also **neuroaxonal dystrophies.**

Diagnostic criteria have been suggested by Swaiman[5432] and are presented in Chart H–2.

Chart H–2. Diagnostic Criteria for Hallervorden-Spatz Disease

Obligatory features:
  Onset before the age of 20
  Progressive course
  Presence of extrapyramidal signs
Corroborative features:
  Presence of pyramidal signs, progressive dementia, pigmentary retinopathy, optic atrophy, and/or seizures
  Autosomal recessive transmission
  Hypodensities on MRI scanning
  Presence of sea-blue histiocytes
Excluding features:
  Abnormal copper, ceruloplasmin, hexosaminidase or GM_1 levels
  Neuronal ceroid lipofuscinosis
  Severe retinal abnormality
  Dominant inheritance
  Caudate atrophy
  Absence of extrapyramidal features

From Swaiman K. Hallervorden-Spatz syndrome and brain iron metabolism. Arch Neurol 1991;**48**:1285–1293. © *American Medical Association 1991. Reproduced by kind permission.*

Variants are a *late-onset* form with dysarthria, dementia, extrapyramidal rigidity, tremor, and incontinence accompanying the cerebral atrophy and striatal gliotic changes,[2809] and an *infantile* form with features similar to those of the late-onset form.

Hallgren syndrome   See **von Graefe–Sjögren syndrome.**

Hallipré sign   Dorsiflexion of the wrist during attempted grip on the side of a radial nerve lesion.

Hallpike, Charles Skinner   (1900–1979) British neuro-otologist who trained at Guy's Hospital in London. His early clinical and research interests in diseases of the ear led to his appointment to the National Hospital, Queen Square, after he defined the pathology of Ménière syndrome (endolymphatic hydrops), where he founded and directed the neuro-otology unit, which he led until his retirement. He is best remembered for his precise definition of methods and norms for **caloric tests** and for his clinical analysis of the more common causes of vertigo which led to his original description of **vestibular neuronitis** and to the modern characterizations of **Ménière syndrome** and **benign paroxysmal positional vertigo.**[312]

hallucinations   (from Lat, to wander mentally) Subjective perceptions without objective stimuli.

hallux   (from Lat, the big toe) The great toe.

Halpern syndrome   See **dysequilibrium syndrome.**

Halstead aphasia screening test   A part of the **Halstead-Reitan battery.**[4655] An abbreviated and amended form is also available.[2521]

Halstead-Reitan battery   An evaluative tool for a wide range of psychological activities, including parts of the **Wechsler Adult Intelligence Scale,** the category test, the Reitan **trail-making test,** an aphasia screening examination, and the **finger tapping test.** By these means, abstract thought, motor performance, rhythm and perception, gnosis, trail-making, sensory functions, grip strength, auditory perception, time perception, verbal and nonverbal memory, perceptual motor speed, spatial relations, finger gnosis, double simultaneous stimulation, and personality are all assessed.[4655] An impairment score is derived from the patient's overall performance on this complex battery.

Haltia-Santavuori syndrome   See **neuronal ceroid lipofuscinosis.**

HAM   Acronym for **HTLV-1-associated myelopathy.** See **tropical spastic paraparesis.**

hamartoma   (from Gr, to miss the goal) A collection of cells that are misplaced within the CNS as a result of faulty migration during embryonal development. They consist typically of masses of neurons, glia, and fiber bundles and may contain neurosecretory granules.

While commonly asymptomatic, hamartomas may act as a focus for seizure discharges in certain sites, such as the temporal lobes or the hypothalamus. In the latter site they may be manifest by **gelastic seizures.**

Hamilton Rating Scale   (HRS) An interviewer- and observer-rated measure of psychological and somatic symptoms determining the severity of depressive illness.[2405]

One of the earliest-published and still probably the most widely used of the depression scales, this was not designed as a diagnostic instrument but rather as a tool for assessing change in depressed patients under treatment. This instrument scores more of the somatic symptoms of depression than do others.[2404]

hammer palsy   Unilateral shoulder girdle weakness, once thought to be due to excessive use of the hammer but more probably a form of **brachial plexopathy.**

Hammersmith Motor Ability score   A scale for scoring muscle power, of particular value in the assessment of children with muscular dystrophies[5035] (see Chart H-3).

Chart H–3. The Hammersmith Motor Ability Score

1. Lifts head	11. Standing on toes
2. Supine to prone over right	12. Standing on right leg
3. Supine to prone over left	13. Standing on left leg
4. Prone to supine over right	14. Hops on right leg
5. Prone to supine over left	15. Hops on left leg
6. Gets to sitting	16. Gets off chair
7. Sitting	17. Climbing step right leg
8. Gets to standing	18. Descending step right leg
9. Standing	19. Climbing step left leg
10. Standing on heels	20. Descending step left leg

All movements are attempted and scored as follows: 2, for every completed movement; 1, for help and/or reinforcement; 0, if unable to achieve the movement. (From Scott, OM, Goddard C, Dubovitz V. Quantitation of muscle function in children; a prospective study in Duchenne muscular dystrophy. Muscle Nerve *1982;**5**:291–301. Reproduced by permission. © 1982, John Wiley & Sons, Inc.)*

Hammond syndrome   See **athetosis.**

Hammond, William Alexander   (1828–1900) American neurologist, professor of anatomy and physiology at Maryland, and later Surgeon-General of the Army. It was he who recognized the importance of the study of neurological disorders arising from the injuries sustained during the American Civil War, appointing Dr. S. **Weir Mitchell** to head a neurological unit in Philadelphia established for this purpose. Court-martialled on trumped-up charges precipitated by his peremptory and dictatorial manner, he was dismissed after 2 years as surgeon-general, but was later reinstated when Congress quashed the verdict. Meanwhile, he had returned to private practice in New York, where he was shortly afterwards appointed professor of neurology at the City University, and later at Bellvue.

His *Treatise on Diseases of the Nervous System* (New York, 1871) was the first American textbook of neurology and went to nine editions. It preceded that of **Gowers** by 10 years. His description of athetosis, contained within it,[3759] led to the eponymous labeling of that condition for over half a century. Hammond was a distinguished lecturer who also wrote novels and plays, and was a founder of the **American Neurological Association** (of which both he and his son were to be presidents) and of the Army Medical Museum, now the Walter Reed Army Institute of Research.

Hand, A. (1868–1949) American pediatrician. He thought that the osteolytic bone lesions that he detected in his patient were tuberculous. See **Hand-Schüller-Christian disease.**

hand cramps Focal dystonias of the hands precipitated by various skilled activities such as writing or playing musical instruments.[1084]

hand flexor reflex Flexion of the wrist in response to tapping of the flexor tendons at the wrist or the palmar surface of the fingers when the fingers are loosely supported by the examiner. The contraction is enhanced in cases of pyramidal lesions above C6, but also in states of emotional tension.

A similar extensor reflex can also be obtained.

hand washing Persistent intertwining and rotation of the hands, a characteristic motor automatism in **Rett syndrome.**

hand–arm vibration syndrome An acquired progressive disease comprising vasospasm with blanching of the fingers; neuropathy with paresthesias, numbness, impaired finger coordination and hand dexterity; and musculoskeletal involvement. It is due to prolonged occupational exposure to high-amplitude vibrations.[3755,4396,5514] See **vibration white-finger.**

handcuff neuropathy Numbness of the thumb and index finger as a result of compression damage to the superficial radial nerve resulting from the too-tight application of handcuffs (or even wristwatches). Damage to the ulnar and to the median nerve from the same cause have also been recorded.[5038] See also **Wartenberg syndromes.**

handedness The preferential use of one hand (or foot) for motor tasks such as writing (or kicking). Such a preference is usually seen after the age of 2 years, and if present before that age suggests the presence of impairment of motor control in the opposite hand. The perception of "correctness" in using the right hand is suggested by the positive connotations of the words *right* and *dextrous* and by the pejorative *sinister*, although the Book of Judges records the exploits of 700 left-handed slingers, who allegedly never missed their targets.

The dominant hemisphere for speech may be inferred from handedness, all right-handers (but only *most* left-handers) having speech dominance in the left hemisphere. See also **Wada test.**

handicap 1. A disability affecting a person's social or professional activities, requiring adoption of a change in lifestyle. 2. A disadvantage resulting from an impairment or disability, limiting or preventing the fulfilment of a role for a person. However, age and social and cultural factors must be considered when assessing a handicap. See also **disability, impairment.**

HaNDL **H**e**a**d**a**che with **N**eurologic **D**eficits and CSF **L**ymphocytosis, a self-limited syndrome that otherwise resembles migraine with aura. Conventional cerebral angiography can provoke a similar condition. (HJM)[489]

hand–mouth reflex See **Babkin reflex.**

Hand-Schüller-Christian disease (generalized xanthomatosis, histiocytosis X, lipoid granulomatosis, craniohypophysial xanthomatosis) A disease marked by the widespread deposition of masses of cholesterol-laden histiocytes, leading to the classic triad of exophthalmos, diabetes insipidus, and osteolytic bone lesions in the orbit or in the base of the skull.

Other signs may include papilledema; extraocular palsies and nystagmus; involvement of lower cranial nerves, cerebellum, and pyramidal tracts; increased intracranial pressure; hepatosplenomegaly; pulmonary infiltration; skin eruptions; xanthelasmas and xanthomas; and lymphadenopathy.[2410] The neurological complications are variable and nonspecific, depending on the sites of accumulation of the abnormal cells.

This represents one of those conditions to which none of the usually accepted eponyms should apply, the condition having been recognized in 1865 by the English pathologist Thomas Smith (1833–1909), whereas Hand published a description of it in 1893; Schuller, in 1915; and Christian, in 1919.

A. Schuller (1874–1957) was an Austrian radiologist, who first suggested the trans-sphenoidal approach for operations on the pituitary. His description of the abnormalities to be found on skull X-ray studies was unparalleled and he was appointed professor in Vienna but fled the city, leaving his sons, when threatened by Nazism. He emigrated to Australia where his opinions were widely sought.

H.A. Christian (1876–1951) was an American physician who was head of the medical service at Peter Bent Brigham Hospital in Boston. His report covered all the important points of the disease.[1829]

Hane whistle-smile sign The failure of patients with **Parkinson disease** to smile when they are asked to whistle.[2412]

hanging sensory loss (suspended sensory loss) Altered sensation and weakness in the arms but not in the legs, occurring as a result of a central cord lesion. The pathology affects the medial portion of the descending lateral corticospinal tract, the anterior horn cells at that level, and both the crossing fibers and the more central fibers in the spinothalamic tract; these latter fibers carry impulses from the arms and upper trunk.

hangman fracture A fracture of the neural arch of the second cervical vertebra bilaterally with associated rupture of the anterior longitudinal ligament and C2–3 spondylolisthesis. The odontoid process is not displaced.

This fracture may occur as the result of a severe extension injury; the use of a submental knot in judicial hanging is intended to induce it, with immediate effective transection of the cervical cord at that level. Less severe cord injury (or occasionally none at all) may result when the fracture occurs in other traumatic conditions such as motor vehicle accidents.[704]

Hanhart disease Recessively inherited **hereditary spastic paraparesis** associated with mental deficiency.[5047]

Hansen disease See **leprosy.**

Hansen, Gerhardt Henrik Armauer (1841–1912) Norwegian physician who correctly related the presence of *Mycobacterium leprae* to clinical **leprosy** in 1871.

happy feet See **burning feet syndrome.**

happy puppet syndrome A congenital dysmorphic syndrome manifesting also jerky, puppet-like movements, and frequent spontaneous paroxysms of laughter in retarded, often microcephalic infants or children with infantile spasms, optic atrophy, cerebellar signs, and generalized seizures.[691] See **Angelman syndrome.**

haptic (Gr, touching) The tactile and proprioceptive image of one's own body and the recognition of external objects using touch alone. An older use of the word, now defunct, indicated mental alienation (Hippocrates).

Harada syndrome (uveomeningoencephalitic syndrome, Harada-Vogt-Koyanagi syndrome, Vogt-Koyanagi syndrome) A syndrome of bilateral uveitis, exudative choroiditis and retinal detachment, vitiligo, depigmentation and loss of the hair, and signs of meningoencephalitis, invariably with CSF pleocytosis, seen mainly in people living in the Far East and occurring most commonly in adults.[2429]

Harada-Vogt-Koyanagi syndrome See **Harada disease.**

Harboyan syndrome A recessively inherited syndrome characterized by nerve deafness and congenital corneal dystrophy.[3713]

hard exudates Small, glistening knobs seen on the retina in patients with chronic papilledema. They are considered to be composed of axoplasmic protein, extruded with continuing damage to the retinal nerve fibers.

hard palate reflex (Hennebert sign) Protrusion of the lips with stimulation of the hard palate; a sign of diffuse cortical dysfunction.

HARD+E syndrome See **hydrocephalus, agyria, retinal dysplasia, and encephalocele syndrome, Walker-Warburg syndrome.**

Hardy-Wilson system A grading scale for pituitary tumors with suprasellar extension.[859]

Hare syndrome See **Pancoast syndrome.**

harelip A congenital failure of fusion producing a fissure in the upper lip, resembling that normally seen in the hare and similar animals.

harlequin syndrome The happy nomination of a condition marked by the sudden onset of loss of thermoregulatory flushing and sweating on one side of the face without associated miosis, due to local autonomic dysfunction resulting from a cervical sympathetic deficit located at the pre- or postganglionic level on the non-flushing side.

That this deficit sometimes represents a lesion of the second sympathetic neuron is suggested by the increased gustatory sweating on that side, but the syndrome may also follow damage to the sympathetic pathway in the brainstem. Possibly this is due to sprouting of preganglionic sympathetic fibers originally destined for the salivary glands. Impairment of sympathetic activity on one side of the face without ptosis and miosis indicates a lesion of T2,3 in the cord at the intermediolateral column or white rami, as T3 carries most vasomotor and sudomotor fibers for the head and neck. Ocular sympathetic fibres leave in T1.

The lesion is usualy located at the level of postganglionic sympathetic fibers, probably because of transsynaptic postganglionic neuronal degeneration at the level of the stellate ganglion The finding of cholinergic supersensitivity in the iris muscles of patients with this syndrome indicates a relationship with **Holmes-Adie syndrome, Ross syndrome,** and the persistent autonomic deficit occasionally associated with acute inflammatory polyneuropathy.[1520,3243,3960]

Harlow, J.W. American physician who looked after Phineas **Gage** and reported his findings in 1848.[2454]

harmonic A wave appearing at a frequency that is a multiple of some given fundamental frequency; an example would be alpha activity at 16 Hz.

harmonious hypersomnia See **idiopathic CNS hypersomnolence.**[4021]

harmonious oxycephaly See **oxycephaly.**

HARP syndrome See **hypoprebetalipoproteinemia, acanthocytosis, retinitis pigmentosa, and pallidal degeneration.**

Harris neuralgia See **cluster headache.**

Harris, Sir Wilfred John (1869–1960) English neurologist, educated at Cambridge and the University of London, who later trained under Hughlings-**Jackson** and Sir William **Gowers** at the **National Hospital,** Queen Square. His consultant appointments were at the Maida Vale Hospital (linked with the National) and at St. Mary's, where he organized the first department of neurology in any British teaching hospital. He was also the first president of the Association of British Neurologists.

He is best remembered for his studies on the trigeminal nerve, for his delineation of the features of cluster headache (the "periodic migrainous neuralgia of Wilfred Harris"), and for his successful introduction of percutaneous alcohol injection of the gasserian ganglion in the treatment of intractable trigeminal neuralgia, on one occasion injecting the second and third division fibers before an audience of neurologists at Queen Square.

Cluster headache has been labeled with his name, on account of the full description which he provided; he later changed his name for it to *ciliary neuralgia*.[2463]

Harris syndrome (functional hypoglycemia) Weakness, hunger, anxiety, and mild confusion with signs of excessive sympathetic activity due to hypoglycemia. See **Whipple triad.**

Harrod syndrome A congenital dysmorphic syndrome manifesting visceral, genital, and skeletal malformations, dolichocephaly, and mental and developmental delay.[337]

Hart syndrome   See **Hartnup disease.**

Hartmann apraxia   Apraxias resulting from tumors of the frontal lobe described by Fritz Hartmann (1871–1937), an Austrian neurologist and professor at Graz.[2471,5047]

Hartnup disease (Hart syndrome) A recessively transmitted cerebellar syndrome of childhood due to a defect in the renal tubular resorption and intestinal transport of amino acids, and characterized by a skin rash resembling that of pellagra, optic atrophy, pyramidal signs, dystonia, tremors, episodic ataxia, and episodes of delirium. Biochemical abnormalities include severe neutral and basic aminoaciduria and the urinary excretion of indican and glycinuria, but normal ammonium levels.

The intestinal absorption of tryptophan and thus the synthesis of nicotinamide are reduced, so some of the features of the disease are not surprisingly also those of **pellagra** and treatment with nicotinamide is of some value.

The condition was named for the family in which it was first detected by Dr. Charles Dent at the Middlesex Hospital in London.[368,5468] See also **cerebellar ataxias** (*variants*).

Hartsfield syndrome   A congenital dysmorphic syndrome manifesting also skeletal maldevelopments and craniosynostosis, encephalocele, holoprosencephaly, and callosal abnormalities.[337]

Harvey syndrome   A dominantly inherited syndrome of recent description, characterized by athetosis, hypotonia, areflexia, pyramidal signs, mental retardation, and periodic attacks of fever with unconsciousness, the neurological dysfunctions having their onset in early childhood in most cases.[2472]

Harvey, William   (1578–1657) English physician and physiologist. He is remembered in neurology for his descriptions of the venous drainage from the brain, the distinctions he made between motor and sensory nerves, and for his descriptions of patients with epilepsy and syringomyelia.

Hashimoto encephalopathy   A subacute condition affecting euthyroid subjects, mainly women. It is associated with autoimmune thyroiditis and presents with acute, stroke-like focal neurologic deficits with mild cognitive impairment or with dementia, focal or generalized seizures including myoclonus, psychoses, and altered consciousness.

Unlike the encephalopathy associated with hypothyroidism, this type responds to steroid therapy but not to thyroxine replacement. High levels of antithyroid autoantibodies are characteristric, and elevated protein levels or intrathecal IgG synthesis may be present in cerebrospinal fluid without pleocytosis. The EEG may show rhythmic delta activity. See also **hyperthyroidism.**[995,5106]

A *variant* presentation is *Hashimoto-associated ataxia*, an acute-onset cerebellar syndrome associated with abnormal behavior and high-intensity T2 signals in the cerebellum, responding remarkably to steroids and thyroid hormone therapy.[3599]

Haspeslagh syndrome   A congenital dysmorphic syndrome manifesting also short stature; cardiac, thyroid, and skeletal anomalies; microcephaly; pyramidal signs; nystagmus; and mental and developmental delay.[337]

Hassin sign   (Langley-Sherrington sign, ear-wagging) Protrusion of the pinna of the ear on the side of a **Horner syndrome,** of which this is an additional feature. Contraction of the anterior and posterior auricularis muscles (supplied by the posterior auricular branch of the seventh cranial nerve) is responsible, but the reason for this is unknown.[3267,3268] See also **ear-wiggling.**

hatters' shakes   (paralysis agitans mercurialis) A coarse distal tremor seen in those exposed on a longtern basis to organic mercury such as the sublimate, which was used in the raising of the nap on felt hats in the 19th century. See also **mad as a hatter.**

Hauptmann, Alfred   (1881–19??) German neurologist who introduced phenobarbitone (luminal) for the treatment of epilepsy in 1907.

Hauptmann-Thannhauser   muscular   dystrophy See **Emery-Dreifuss muscular dystrophy.**

Hauser ambulation index   An assessment instrument designed to determine changes in the ability of patients with **multiple sclerosis** to ambulate.[2479] The 10 levels are described in Chart H–4. See also **Rivermead mobility index.**

Chart H–4. The Hauser Ambulation Index

0. Asymptomatic; fully active
1. Walks normally, but reports fatigue that interferes with athletic or other demanding activities
2. Abnormal gait or episodic imbalance; gait disorder is noticed by family and friends; able to walk 25 feet (7.5 meters) in 10 seconds or less
3. Walks independently; able to walk 25 feet (7.5 meters) in 20 seconds or less

4. Requires unilateral support (cane or single crutch) to walk; walks 25 feet (7.5 meters) in 20 seconds or less

5. Requires bilateral support (canes, crutches, or walker) and walks 25 feet (7.5 meters) in 25 seconds, or requires unilateral support but needs more than 20 seconds to walk 25 feet. (7.5 meters)

6. Requires bilateral support and more than 20 seconds to walk 25 feet (7.5 meters); may use wheelchair occasionally

7. Walking limited to several steps with bilateral support; unable to walk 25 feet (7.5 meters); in wheelchair for most activities

8. Restricted to wheelchair; able to transfer self independently

9. Restricted to wheelchair; unable to transfer self independently

From Hauser SL, Dawson DM, Lehrich JR, et al. Intensive immunosuppression in progressive multiple sclerosis. N Engl Med J 1983;308:173–180. Reproduced by kind permission.

haut mal (Fr, high + illness) An old term for major epilepsy (generalized tonic-clonic seizures).

Haven syndrome Pain in the wrist progressing proximally, pallor of the hand and wrist, and loss of the radial pulse, ascribed by Haven to compression of the subclavian artery by the scaleni. Perhaps it is a form of vasogenic **thoracic outlet syndrome**.[2482]

Haver, Clopton English anatomist of the 18th century who described the vascular channels within bone now named for him (Haversian canals).

haypitcher's palsy Suprascapular neuropathy. This is also an occupational hazard of baseball pitchers.

head 1. The uppermost or anterior part of the body, including the cranium and face in vertebrates. 2. The upper end of a long bone. 3. The origin of a muscle.

head banging (jactitatio capitis nocturna) A syndrome occurring in some babies or young children during the lightest stages of non–rapid eye movement sleep, characterized by rhythmic, repetitive, to-and-fro rocking movements or by banging of the head on the pillow or crib side[1716] (see also the ASDA Diagnostic Classification,[234] and Chart J–1).

head circumference The greatest circumference of the head measured with the tape lying on the occiput and the frontal bones.

Graphs for the normal values in males and females at different ages have been published.[4088] See **occipitofrontal circumference.**

head extension vertigo The physiological occurrence of vertigo or postural imbalance induced when the head is maximally extended and terminating when it returns to the normal position, considered to be due to the inefficiency of otolith function in this position.[727]

head flexion test (Hyndham sign) Pain in the leg experienced with passive head flexion, as a result of irritation of the lumbar roots in patients with prolapsed intervertebral disks.

head heave maneuver A test of utricular function in which the examiner places his palms over the ears of the seated patient and makes a fast lateral translation of 1–2 inches. The appearance of corrective saccades indicates the presence of a hypometric slow-phase response, and when this is present asymmetrically, the labyrinthine lesion is likely to be on the side to which the head was pushed.[4575]

head injury See **craniocerebral trauma.**

head lag Passive extension of the neck with backward drooping of the head, occurring when the supine infant is raised toward the sitting position by the examiner pulling on the infant's arms; a sign of weakness of the neck flexors.

The normal reaction is for the head to be maintained in the line of the body or even slightly flexed. In a small infant the head may initially be supported by one hand.

In the Dubowitz neurological criteria, score 0 for complete lag; 1 for partial head control; 2 for ability to maintain the head in line with the body; and 3 if the infant brings the head anterior to the body.[1528]

head nodding See **spasmus nutans.**

head retraction reflex Brief extension of the neck in response to a tap on the maxilla when the patient's head is slightly flexed. The reflex was described by **Wartenberg**[5858] as a sign of bilateral supracervical lesions of the pyramidal tract.

head rolling See **jactitatio capitis nocturna.**

Sir Henry Head

Head, Sir Henry (1861–1940) English neurologist and neurophysiologist. He was educated at Charterhouse and Trinity College, Cambridge, worked with Hering in

Prague on respiratory physiology, and continued studies in Cambridge and London leading to graduation in medicine in 1890. His earlier posts were held at University College Hospital and at the National Hospital; and he eventually was appointed physician to the London and University College Hospitals. He was fluent in French and German (which was then essential for the editorship of *Brain*, which he held from 1910 to 1925, during which time he consolidated the prestige of that journal).

Although publishing in many fields of neurology, he wrote over 20 papers on sensation between 1905 and 1918, which comprised perhaps one of his most lasting legacies. These papers were collected together in his *Studies in Neurology* (London, 1920). He mapped the dermatomes, in one experiment having his own superficial radial nerve sectioned in order to define the resulting area of sensory loss, and described the anatomy and variations of all of the major peripheral nerves and of the brachial plexus.[2500,4713]

The studies performed on his own nerves led to his differentiation of forms of sensation between deep sensibility (pressure and proprioception); sharp, bright, localized **epicritic** pain; and deep, persistent, unlocalized, more vivid, less acute skin pain and more extreme heat and cold (**protopathic pain**)[2498] after nerve injury. Head also postulated the existence of epicritic and protopathic systems, the functions of which are now thought to be mediated in the central rather than in the peripheral nervous system.[2540]

Many of his other studies were made possible by his post as consultant to a hospital for officers in London during and after World War I. In 1900 he localized the site of herpetic inflammation to the dorsal root ganglia.[2497] During the later years of his career, he resigned his hospital appointments on developing the earliest evidence of **Parkinson disease** and devoted the greater party of his activities to the study of aphasia. This culminated in the publication of his book, *Aphasia and Kindred Disorders of Speech* (1926), in which he divided the forms of aphasia among *verbal* (inability to form words internally or externally), *syntactical* (loss of balance and rhythm of speech with retained comprehension), *semantic* (failure to recognize the intention and significance of words), and *nominal* (loss of the use of names), a scheme found difficult to employ by others.

He has been described as erudite, obsessional, critical, original, and energetic, full of enthusiasm and possessed of a vivid scientific imagination. He had a wide and devoted following as a teacher, published a volume of poetry (*Destroyers and Other Verses*, Oxford, 1919), and had the capacity to discourse with wit and profound knowledge on a range of subjects, any one of which would mark the speaker as expert.[2540,2541]

Headache The official journal of the *American Headache Society* publishing original articles dealing with headache and all aspects of pain (clinical and basic science). Web site: http://ahsnet.org/journal/.

headache (cephalalgia) Pain in the head, of numerous varieties. The International Headache Society has published a comprehensive classification of headache[1051] (Chart H–5), supplanting that suggested in 1978 by an *ad hoc* committee.[4140] The numbers placed before the various headache types in this newer classification are omitted elsewhere in this book.

Chart H–5. International Headache Society Classification of Headache Syndromes

1. **Migraine**
   1.1 Migraine without aura
   1.2 Migraine with aura
       1.2.1 Migraine with typical aura
       1.2.2 Migraine with prolonged aura
       1.2.3 **Familial hemiplegic migraine**
       1.2.4 **Basilar migraine**
       1.2.5 Migraine aura without headache
       1.2.6 Migraine with acute onset aura
   1.3 **Ophthalmoplegic migraine**
   1.4 **Retinal migraine**
   1.5 Childhood **periodic syndrome**s that may be precursors to or associated with migraine
       1.5.1 **Benign paroxysmal vertigo of childhood**
       1.5.2 **Alternating hemiplegia of childhood**
   1.6 Complications of migraine
       1.6.1 **Status migrainosus**
       1.6.2 Migrainous infarction
   1.7 Migrainous disorder not fulfilling above criteria
2. **Tension-type headache**
   2.1 Episodic tension-type headache
       2.1.1 Episodic tension-type headache associated with disorder of pericranial muscles
       2.1.2 Episodic tension-type headache unassociated with disorder of pericranial muscles
   2.2 Chronic tension-type headache
       2.2.1 Chronic tension-type headache associated with disorder of pericranial muscles
       2.2.2 Chronic tension-type headache unassociated with disorder of pericranial muscles
   2.3 Headache of the tension type not fulfilling above criteria
3. Cluster headache and chronic paroxysmal hemicrania
   3.1 **Cluster headache**
       3.1.1 Cluster headache, periodicity undetermined
       3.1.2 Episodic cluster headache
       3.1.3. **Chronic cluster headache**
           3.1.3.1. Unremitting from onset
           3.1.3.2 Evolved from episodic
   3.2 **Chronic paroxysmal hemicrania**
   3.3 Cluster headache-like disorder not fulfilling above criteria
4. Miscellaneous headaches unassociated with structural lesions
   4.1 **Idiopathic stabbing headache**
   4.2 **External compression headache**
   4.3 **Cold stimulus headache**
       4.3.1 External application of a cold stimulus
       4.3.2 Ingestion of a cold stimulus
   4.4 **Benign cough headache**
   4.5 **Benign exertional headache**

4.6 **Headache associated with sexual activity**
    4.6.1 Dull type
    4.6.2 Explosive type
    4.6.3 Postural type
5. Headache associated with head trauma
  5.1 Acute post-traumatic headache
    5.1.1 With significant head trauma and/or confirmatory signs
    5.1.2 With minor head trauma and no confirmatory signs
  5.2 Chronic post-traumatic headache
    5.2.1 With significant head trauma and/or confirmatory signs
    5.2.2 With minor head trauma and no confirmatory signs
6. Headache associated with vascular disorders
  6.1 Acute ischemic cerebrovascular disease
    6.1.1 Transient ischemic attack
    6.1.2 Thromboembolic stroke
  6.2 Intracranial hematoma
    6.2.1 Intracerebral hematoma
    6.2.2 Subdural hematoma
    6.2.3 Epidural hematoma
  6.3 **Subarachnoid hemorrhage**
  6.4 Unruptured vascular malformation
    6.4.1 **Arteriovenous malformation**
    6.4.2 Saccular aneurysm
  6.5 Arteritis
    6.5.1 **Giant cell arteritis**
    6.5.2 Other systemic arteritides
    6.5.3 Primary intracranial arteritis
  6.6 Carotid or vertebral artery pain
    6.6.1 Carotid or vertebral dissection
    6.6.2 **Carotidynia** (idiopathic)
    6.6.3 Post-endarterectomy headache
  6.7 Venous thrombosis
  6.8 Arterial hypertension
    6.8.1 Acute pressor response to exogenous agent
    6.8.2 **Pheochromocytoma**
    6.8.3 Malignant (accelerated) hypertension
    6.8.4 Pre-eclampsia and eclampsia
  6.9 Headache associated with other vascular disorder
7. Headache associated with nonvascular intracranial disorder
  7.1 High cerebrospinal fluid pressure
    7.1.1 **Benign intracranial hypertension**
    7.1.2 High-pressure hydrocephalus
  7.2 Low cerebrospinal fluid pressure
    7.2.1 **Post–lumbar puncture headache**
    7.2.2 Cerebrospinal fluid fistula headache
  7.3 Intracranial infection
  7.4 Intracranial **sarcoidosis** and other noninfectious inflammatory diseases
  7.5 **Headache related to intrathecal injections**
    7.5.1 Direct effect
    7.5.2 Due to chemical meningitis
  7.6 Intracranial neoplasm
  7.7 Headache associated with other intracranial disorder
8. Headache associated with substances or their withdrawal
  8.1 Headache induced by acute substance use or exposure
    8.1.1 Nitrate/nitrite-induced headache
    8.1.2 Monosodium glutamate–induced headache
    8.1.3 Carbon monoxide–induced headache

    8.1.4 Alcohol-induced headache
    8.1.5 Other substances
  8.2 Headache induced by chronic substance use or exposure
    8.2.1 Ergotamine-induced headache
    8.2.2 **Medication-induced headache**
    8.2.3 Other substances
  8.3 **Headache from substance withdrawal (acute use)**
    8.3.1 Alcohol withdrawal headache (hangover)
    8.3.2 Other substances
  8.4 **Headache from substance withdrawal (chronic use)**
    8.4.1 **Ergotamine withdrawal headache**
    8.4.2 **Caffeine withdrawal headache (rebound headache)**
    8.4.3 Narcotic abstinence headache
    8.4.4 Other substances
  8.5 Headache associated with substances but with uncertain mechanism
    8.5.1 Birth control pills or estrogens
    8.5.2 Other substances
9. **Headache associated with noncephalic infection**
  9.1 Viral infection
    9.1.1 Focal noncephalic
    9.1.2 Systemic
  9.2 Bacterial infection
    9.2.1 Focal noncephalic
    9.2.2 Systemic (septicemia)
  9.3 Headache related to other infection
10. Headache associated with metabolic disorder
  10.1. Hypoxia
    10.1.1 **High-altitude headache**
    10.1.2 **Hypoxic headache**
    10.1.3 Sleep apnea headache
  10.2 Hypercapnia
  10.3 Mixed hypoxia and hypercapnia
  10.4 Hypoglycemia
  10.5 Dialysis
  10.6 Headache related to other metabolic abnormality
11. Headache or facial pain associated with disorder of cranium, neck, eyes, ears, nose, sinuses, teeth, mouth, or other facial or cranial structures
  11.1 Cranial bone
  11.2 Neck
    11.2.1 Cervical spine
    11.2.2 Retropharyngeal tendinitis
  11.3 Eyes
    11.3.1 Acute glaucoma
    11.3.2 Refractive errors
    11.3.3 Heterophoria or heterotropia
  11.4 Ears
  11.5 Nose and sinuses
    11.5.1 Acute sinus headache
    11.5.2 Other diseases of nose or sinuses
  11.6 Teeth, jaws, and related structures
  11.7 Temporomandibular joint disease
12. Cranial neuralgias See **trigeminal neuralgia, glossopharyngel neuralgia, nervus intermedius neuralgia, superior laryngeal neuralgia, occipital neuralgia.**
13. Headache not classifiable

From: Classification Committee of the International Headache Society. Classification of headache disorders, cranial neuralgias and facial pains; and diagnostic criteria for primary headache disorders. Cephalalgia 1988;8(suppl):1–96. Reproduced by kind permission of Elsevier Science.

headache associated with intrathecal injections
The following diagnostic criteria are suggested by the Headache Classification Committee of the International Headache Society[1051] and are reproduced by kind permission of Elsevier Science.

A. Headache follows intrathecal injection within 4 hours.
B. Headache is diffuse and present also in the recumbent position.
C. Headache clears completely within 14 days. (If it persists consider **low CSF–pressure headache**; see **idiopathic intracranial hypotension**.)

headache associated with noncephalic infection
This definition and the following diagnostic criteria are suggested by the Headache Classification Committee of the International Headache Society.[1051] (from: Classification of headache disorders, cranial neuralgias and facial pains; and diagnostic criteria for primary headache disorders. *Cephalalgia* 1988;**8** [suppl]:1–96, reproduced by kind permission of Elsevier Science).

A. Symptoms and/or signs of noncephalic infection.
B. Laboratory diagnosis of systemic or focal noncephalic infection.
C. Headache as a new symptom or of a new type occurs concomitantly with infection.
D. Headache disappears less than 1 month after successful treatment or spontaneous remission of infection.

Viral infection, *bacterial infection*, and *headache related to other infection* are also included here.

headache associated with sexual activity   (benign sex headache, coital cephalalgia) Headache precipitated by masturbation or coitus, usually starting as a dull bilateral ache while sexual excitement increases and suddenly becoming intense at orgasm, in the absence of any intracranial disorder. Dull, explosive, and postural types are defined (see **headache**). This definition and the following diagnostic criteria are suggested by the Headache Classification Committee of the International Headache Society[1051] (from: Classification of headache disorders, cranial neuralgias and facial pains; and diagnostic criteria for primary headache disorders. *Cephalalgia* 1988;**8** [suppl]:1–96, reproduced by kind permission of Elsevier Science.)

A. Headache is precipitated by sexual excitement.
B. Headache is bilateral at onset.
C. Headache is prevented or eased by ceasing sexual activity before orgasm.
D. Headache is not associated with any intracranial disorder such as aneurysm.

headache associated with substances but with uncertain mechanism   This category would include headache in association with ingestion of estrogens and other substances.

Headache Disability Inventory   A validated 25–item scale assessing the effects of daily living in terms of disability suffered by people with recurrent headaches.[2785] See also **Headache Impact Test, MIDAS.**

headache due to chemical meningitis   The following diagnostic criteria are suggested by the Headache Clas-

sification Committee of the International Headache Society[1051] (from: Classification of headache disorders, cranial neuralgias and facial pains; and diagnostic criteria for primary headache disorders. *Cephalalgia* 1988;**8** [suppl]:1–96, reproduced by kind permission of Elsevier Science).

A. Headache follows intrathecal injection within 5–72 hours.
B. Headache is diffuse and present also in the recumbent position.
C. Cerebrospinal fluid pleocytosis with negative culture is evident.

headache from substance withdrawal   (*acute use*)
The following diagnostic criteria are suggested by the Headache Classification Committee of the International Headache Society[1051] (from: Classification of headache disorders, cranial neuralgias and facial pains; and diagnostic criteria for primary headache disorders. *Cephalalgia* 1988;**8**[suppl]:1–96, reproduced by kind permission of Elsevier Science).

A. Headache follows acute use of a substance.
B. A certain required minimum dose should be indicated.
C. Headache occurs when the substance is largely or completely eliminated, but may last longer.
D. Headache is relieved or improved by renewed intake of the substance.

Alcohol withdrawal headache is an example.

headache from substance withdrawal   (*chronic use*)
The following diagnostic criteria are suggested by the Headache Classification Committee of the International Headache Society[1051] (from: Classification of headache disorders, cranial neuralgias and facial pains; and diagnostic criteria for primary headache disorders. *Cephalalgia* 1988;**8**[suppl]:1–96, reproduced by kind permission of Elsevier Science).

A. Headache occurs after use of a high daily dose (specified when possible under each substance) of a substance for ≥3 months.
B. Headache occurs within hours after elimination of the substance.
C. Headache is relieved by renewed intake of the substance.
D. Headache disappears within 14 days after withdrawal of the substance.

Headache Impact Test   A validated tool assessing the burden of disability suffered by people with migraine, either in a 6-question paper-based form or by accessing it on the internet (http://www.headachetest.com/). See also **Headache Disability Inventory, MIDAS.**

headache induced by acute substance use or exposure   The following diagnostic criteria are suggested by the Headache Classification Committee of the International Headache Society.[1051] (from: Classification of headache disorders, cranial neuralgias and facial pains; and diagnostic criteria for primary headache disorders. *Cephalalgia* 1988;**8**[suppl]:1–96, reproduced by kind permission of Elsevier Science).

A. Headache occurs within a specified time after substance intake.

B. A certain required minimum dose should be indicated.

C. Headache has occurred in at least $^1/_2$ of exposures and at least 3 times.

D. Headache disappears when substance is eliminated or within a specified time thereafter.

headache induced by chronic substance use or exposure   The following diagnostic criteria are suggested by the Headache Classification Committee of the International Headache Society.[1051] (from: Classification of headache disorders, cranial neuralgias and facial pains; and diagnostic criteria for primary headache disorders. *Cephalalgia* 1988;**8** [suppl]:1–96, reproduced by kind permission of Elsevier Science).

A. Headache occurs after daily doses of a substance for ≥3 months.

B. A certain required minimum dose should be indicated.

C. Headache is chronic (15 days or more per month).

D. Headache disappears within 1 month after withdrawal of the substance.

headache not classifiable   The following diagnostic criterion is suggested by the Headache Classification Committee of the International Headache Society.[1051] (from: Classification of headache disorders, cranial neuralgias and facial pains; and diagnostic criteria for primary headache disorders. *Cephalalgia* 1988;**8**[suppl]:1–96, reproduced by kind permission of Elsevier Science).

Any type of headache which does not fulfil criteria for one of the disorders described in the remainder of the classification.

headache of the tension type not fulfilling criteria for episodic or chronic tension-type headache   Headache believed to be a form of tension-type headache which does not quite meet the operational diagnostic criteria for any of the forms of tension-type headache. The following diagnostic criteria are suggested by the Headache Classification Committee of the International Headache Society.[1051] (from: Classification of headache disorders, cranial neuralgias and facial pains; and diagnostic criteria for primary headache disorders. *Cephalalgia* 1988;**8**[suppl]:1–96, reproduced by kind permission of Elsevier Science).

A. Fulfils all but one criterion for one or more forms of tension-type headache (specify type/s).

B. Does not fulfil criteria for migraine without aura.

headache scale   A list of 30 adjectives (pulling, tight, tiring, dull, splitting, sharp, stabbing, throbbing, etc.) used to describe pain by headache sufferers.[2797]

Using such a list, clusters of headache descriptions have been defined, but different analyses have identified 2, 5, or 7 clusters, and the purpose of the scale appears to assist in the qualitative determination of the characteristics of head pains rather than in diagnosis or management.

headache with neurologic deficits and CSF lymphocytosis   A benign and transient syndrome with these manifestations. Characteristic features include the pres-

ence of severe headaches, neurological deficits lasting for less than 3 days on each occcasion, CSF lymphocytosis of 16–350 cells/mm^3, and limitation of the condition to less than 3 months. Additional featues include a modest rise in CSF protein and pressure, transient focal nonepileptiform EEG changes, and sometimes a viral prodrome or fever.[489]

Mollaret cells are absent from the CSF but the condition otherwise resembles **Mollaret meningitis.**

Head-Holmes syndrome   The sensory deficits resulting from cortical lesions.[2498] The utility of retaining this eponymous syndrome may now be expended, but the original paper is a treasure.

headphone neuralgia   A syndrome resembling glossopharyngeal neuralgia and thought to be caused by compression of the aural branches of that nerve by the hard earpieces of, e.g., personal entertainment devices, stethescopes, or hearing aids, or by idiopathic craniofacial polyneuritis.[5203]

Head-Riddoch syndrome   (autonomic hyperreflexia syndrome) Sweating, flushing, pilomotor erection, nasal stuffiness, blurred vision, headache, and occasionally generalized seizures occurring as a result of excessive autonomic activity following extrinsic or intrinsic stimulation of quadriplegic patients below the level of their high spinal lesions.[2499]

Head's areas   (Head's zones) The dermatomes, precisely delineated by Henry Head as his graduation thesis at Cambridge and published in *Brain* in 1893.[2492]

The term has also been applied to the areas of hyperalgesia occurring in association with disease of the underlying viscera, but, in effect, these are also the dermatomes.

Head's principles   1. "When any level of activity is attacked, the most complex functions, and those that have appeared most recently are the first to suffer; they are also disturbed to a greater degree and to a wider extent than those which are simpler or more inevitable in their expression."

2. "The negative manifestations of a lesion appear in terms of the affected level." (Thus, lesions of the speech area produce disturbances of speech.)

3. "A negative lesion produces positive effects by releasing activities normally held under control by the functions of the affected level." The mass reflex and thalamic pain are examples.

4. "The functions of the nervous system have been slowly evolved by a continuous process of development. The methods by which this gradual process from lower to higher efficiency have been reached are still manifest in the phenomena of its normal activity . . . [thus] what at lower levels appeared a variable response became with the progress of evolution, voluntary control."

5. "Integration of function within the nervous system is based on a struggle for expression between many

potentially different physiological activities." (Thus, a warm stimulus may be perceived as warm, cold, or painful according to its position on the skin and the state of the receptors.)[2495]

Head's zones   See **Head's areas.**

head-shaking nystagmus   A horizontal jerk nystagmus appearing after vigorous head-shaking for 15 seconds, thus suggesting the presence of **dynamic vestibular imbalance.** See **vestibular nystagmus.**

head-thrust response   A baby is held in the sitting position with the body leaning slightly forward. When a hand placed against the back of the head thrusts the head forward, the normal infant opposes the movement.[6064]

head-tilt test   See **Bielschowsky test.**

head-turning sign   The action of patients with dementing diseases, who repeatedly turn to ask their spouse the answers to questions put by the examiner (Dr. Rémi Bouchard, personal communication).

health   1. The ability of all parts of the body to perform their respective functions without giving rise to awareness of incapacity or discomfort. 2. The absence of disease. 3. A state of mental, physical, and emotional well-being.

heat hematoma   An artifactual extradural hematoma subjacent to a fissure fracture of the skull, found in some victims of death in extreme heat.[6]

heat stroke   (coup de la chaleur) Hyperpyrexia following exposure to unusually high temperatures, and associated with pupillary constriction, complex automatisms, and raised serum creatine kinase values.

heat-flow disc   A method of assessing changes in skin blood flow by measuring the rate of heat loss from a disk placed on the skin.[1573]

Heart and Stroke Foundation of Canada   A charitable organization. Address: 222 Queen St., Ste. 1402, Ottawa, Ontario K1P5V9, Canada. Tel: 613-569-4361. Web site: www.heartandstroke.ca/.

heautognosis   (Gr, of oneself + knowledge). Self-knowledge.

heautoscopy   A multimodal reduplicative hallucination of one's own person; a combination of autoscopy and an out-of-body experience, resulting in the perception of a **doppelgänger;** a primary somesthetic illusion of being separated from, and outside, one's own body. It most commonly is a manifestation of complex partial seizures arising from parietal or deep temporal foci.[812]

heaviness   Not itself a primary sensory mode, but rather the sense of the movement required to lift a mass, or the discrimination of relative pressures (depending on whether the limb is allowed to move). Gordon

Holmes stated, "Every paretic limb exaggerates the load it carries, if sensation be normal"—that is, objects feel heavy when lifted by paretic muscles, a "sense of effort" being used to estimate the weight of a lifted object.[2017]

Hebb, Donald   (1904–1985) Preeminent Canadian psychologist at McGill University. He is remembered in particular for his postulate, building on the work of William James, that when the axon of a neuron is close enough to excite a particular cell and does so repeatedly, the threshold for further such excitations is reduced. Thus synapses are modified by pre- and postsynaptic activity.

hebephrenia   (from Gr, puberty + the mind) A variety of schizophrenia, occurring mainly in young people and unaccompanied by major paranoid ideation. The affect is changeable and "silly," the thought disorder and hallucinations exuberant.

Heberden, William   (1710–1801) English physician and classical scholar who trained at Cambridge and practiced in London. His clinical skills and his writings on rheumatism, angina, and varicella placed him in the forefront of the profession and he was elected to fellowship of both the Royal College of Physicians and the Royal Society. He also described night blindness (nyctalopia).

His son, William Heberden, Jr., published in 1804 a book on pediatrics said "to have been of such superlative excellence that it might well be attributed to the father"—which must be the most backhanded compliment that any medical author has received.

hebetude   (from Lat, to make blunt) Dullness of intellect as with a slight reduction in conscious level.

Hebold syndrome   See **encephalotrigeminal angiomatosis.**

Hecáen, Henri   (1912–1983) French neurologist, psychiatrist, and neuropsychologist, a founding father of behavioral neurology and neuropsychology. His medical training was at the University of Bordeaux and he later studied with Jean Lhermitte and Henri Ey before joining the French Centre National de la Récherche Medicale. He was in turn director of the language pathology laboratory and of the research laboratory for neuropsychological studies at the Institut National de la Santé.

Hecáen's important clinical research on brain–behavior relationships complemented his political organization of the discipline, through the foundation of the journal *Neuropsychologia* (of which he was founding editor-in-chief) and indirectly of the International Neuropsychological Society. His best-known studies were of apractagnosia, aphasia, visual agnosia, and cerebral lateralization.[81]

heel reflex   Plantar flexion or spreading out of the toes in response to a tap in the heel, seen in patients with pyramidal lesions. In babies, this normally leads to extension of the leg.[6064]

heel-(knee)-shin test   A test of coordination in which the subject is required to run one heel smoothly down the other shin.

Miller **Fisher**[1841] suggested a modification (shin-tapping) whereby the subject also taps the heel repetitively on the shin before continuing to slide it down toward the foot.

heel-to-ear maneuver   A test forming part of the battery used in **gestational assessment.** The heel of the supine baby is gently drawn up toward the head, and the distance between them is measured. Normally the foot will get as far as the chest, but any further flexion is a sign of immaturity or hypotonia.[1527,1528]

Heerfordt syndrome   (uveoparotid fever) Bilateral facial paralysis (and occasional pareses of the fifth, eighth, and bulbar cranial nerves) with bilateral uveitis, fever, and parotid enlargement occurring as a manifestation of **sarcoidosis.**[2510] Both optic and peripheral neuropathies have also been reported.

C.F. Heerfordt (b. 1871), a Danish ophthalmologist, described the syndrome in 1909.

Heide syndrome   A congenital dysmorphic syndrome manifesting also macrocephaly, frontal bossing, osteoporosis, acral defects, optic atrophy with blindness, and mental and developmental delay.[337]

Heidenhain, Adolf   (b. 1893) German neuropsychiatrist and pathologist.

Heidenhain disease   An insidiously progressive spongy degeneration of the adult cortex with neuronal loss and gliosis, leading to severe dementia, cortical blindness, rigidity, athetosis, ataxia, dysarthria, cerebellar signs, and myoclonus and leading to death within months of the onset of the illness.[2515,3858]

Heidenhain noted that the condition strongly resembles **Creutzfeldt-Jakob disease** but that the latter manifests a slower course with more pyramidal and extrapyramidal features; his patients showed mainly involvement of the occipital lobes, the frontal lobes being relatively spared. See **Creutzfeldt-Jakob disease.**

height vertigo   A visually induced physiological syndrome of subjective instability in postural balance and locomotion, coupled with a fear of falling and with vegetative symptoms, which occurs when the distance between the observer and visible stationary objects becomes critically large.[727]

Heilbronner sign   Flattening of the thigh on the side of a pyramidal lesion.

Heimann-Bielschowsky phenomenon   Instability of gaze in a blind eye, with uni- or bidirectional drifting or nystagmus occurring in that eye during fixation of an object by the other eye.[5234]

Heine, Jacob von   (1800–1879) German physician who trained at Wurzburg and, as a result of family connections, was asked to found an orthopedic institute near Stuttgart. He published his report on **poliomyelitis** (infantile paralysis) in 1840,[2522] noticing almost all the clinical features of the disease, localizing the pathology correctly to the anterior horn cells, demonstrating its epidemic nature, showing that a single infectious agent could produce different syndromes in different people, and dealing at length with methods of management and rehabilitation.

Oskar Medin (1874–1928) studied the epidemic form of the disease.

Heine-Medin disease   See **poliomyelitis.**

helicopodia   (Gr, circling + leg) Circumduction of the leg during walking, as is seen in hemiparetic patients.

heliotrope rash   The mauve discoloration of the eyelids in some patients with dermatomyositis. A memorable term, but not as memorable as the alternative Victorian phrase "violaceous hue," which for some reason (certainly not accuracy) has been retained in this context where neither word is used from year to year in any other.

helix   (Gr, a spiral) The outer border of the pinna, the external ear.

Heller disease   (dementia infantilis, childhood schizophrenia, Heller-Zappert syndrome) A disease of unknown cause in which, after normal infancy, behavioral disturbances with overactivity, tics, immature behavior, and stereotypic movements lead to progressive dementia with eventual speech regression and mutism, withdrawn helplessness ("separated from his surroundings by a glass wall"), and incontinence in the second or third year of life, despite a lack of focal neurological findings. No pathology was described by Heller in his major paper,[2523] nor in a briefer report in 1909.

It is uncertain that this is a single condition. Julius Zappert[6105] described further cases of dementia infantilis and proposed the eponym now used. The condition is probably akin to, if not identical to, infantile autism,[2523] but it is also possible that the cause is a subacute encephalitis.

Heller, Theodor   (1869–1938) Austrian psychiatrist. Born in Vienna into a family with a tradition of service to the blind, he also began training appropriately for that task, diverting to the study of the problems affecting all handicapped children. His life was largely spent in training the mentally handicapped, but he also wrote on a wider field of child psychiatry.

Heller-Zappert syndrome   See **Heller disease.**

Hellsing syndrome   See **hereditary facial spasm.**

Helmholtz, Hermann Ludwig Ferdinand von (1821–1894) German physicist and physiologist, professor of anatomy and physiology variously at Konigsberg, Bonn, Heidelberg, and Berlin. Of interest to neurologists were his studies on the speed of neural transmission (1850), his pioneering books on optics and acoustics,[2995] and his invention of the ophthalmoscope in 1851.[2529] The English mathematician Charles Babbage had produced a similar instrument 4 years previously, but no report of it was published until 1854.

He put forward the resonance theory of hearing, stating (1862) that vibrations in the stapes are transmitted to the perilymph and thus to the basilar membrane, each basilar fiber responding at its own particular frequency.

Helweg-Larsen disease A dominantly inherited hereditary cochleovestibular atrophy manifesting progressive hearing loss from early adult life and anhidrosis as a result of the nondevelopment of sweat glands.[2530]

hem- Greek prefix indicating blood.

hemangiectatic hypertrophy See **Klippel-Trenauny-Weber syndrome.**

hemangioblastoma A benign, circumscribed, cystic tumor of blood vessels usually occurring in adults and arising in the cerebellum or spinal cord from unknown cell origins.

Histologically, it is characterized by cells with uniform nuclei and foamy cytoplasm containing lipid, surrounded by a fine reticulin network and many thin-walled blood vessels. Some produce erythropoietin, leading to polycythemia. In the cerebellum, the tumors eventually cause signs of posterior fossa compression and obstructive hydrocephalus.[2825]

The tumors are familial in **von Hippel–Lindau disease,** in which condition the gene maps to the short arm of chromosome 3.

hemangioma calcificans Slowly growing calcified hemangiomas usually found within one temporal lobe close to the fissure of Sylvius and frequently associated with complex partial seizures. Tuberculomas, hemangiomas, and hematomas are other calcified lesions found in this region.[4404]

hemangiomas Vascular tumors of bone that may occur in the spinal column, leading to compression of the spinal cord. See **cavernous angioma.**

hemangiopericytic meningioma (hemangiopericytoma) A rare, primary, potentially malignant tumor of the nervous system with histological similarities to angioblastic meningiomas. See **meningioma.**

hemangiopericytoma See **hemangiopericytic meningioma.**

hematoencephalon Intracranial bleeding.

hematoma A mass of blood; a blood clot.

hematomyelia Hemorrhage into the spinal cord, with a tendency to spread longitudinally over several segments, particularly within the gray matter, and usu-

ally due to trauma or (when spontaneous) to rupture of an occult arteriovenous malformation. The name was first applied by Ollivier d'Angers in 1827.

hematorrachis Hemorrhage into the spinal canal.

hematosidosis (anabolic GM_3 gangliosidosis) A polioencephalopathy. See **GM_3 gangliosidosis.**

hemeralopia (Gr, day + obscure + vision) Impaired vision in bright illumination.

hemi- (Gr, half) The Latin equivalent word is **semi-,** the French, **demi-.**

hemi-3 syndrome (**h**emihypertrophy, **h**emiparesthesias, **h**emiareflexia) A sporadic, developmental syndrome consisting of hemihypertrophy, hemihypesthesia, hemiareflexia, and progressive scoliosis, perhaps due to a defect of the dorsal lip of the neural tube or neural crest. The hemihypertrophy may be quadrantal and it spares the face; the muscles are large and strong. The hypesthesia affects the modalities of pain and temperature. An increased prevalence of neural tube defects in the family is notable.[4178] Mental retardation and seizures are further complications.[4708]

hemiachromatopsia Loss of color vision in one half-field, all colors appearing as gray, while perception of white objects is unaffected.

hemiagnosia for pain A rare manifestation of a right hemisphere lesion described by Pierre **Marie.** Although patients are hyperpathic on the left, they are unable to localize the source or to define the nature of the severe discomfort.

hemiakinesia See **inattention.**

hemianhidrosis (from Gr, half + derivative + sweating) Lack of sweating on one side of the body, usually due to a lesion of the sympathetic fibers within the CNS.

hemianopia (hemiopia, hemianopsia) Loss of vision in one half of the field of each eye. Such a loss is usually to one or the other side. The various tpes of hemianopia are lested in Chart H–6.

Chart H–6. Types of Hemianopia

Homonymous hemianopia The deficits are of the corresponding right or left fields in each of the two eyes.

Bitemporal hemianopia The loss is in the right half-field in the right eye and in the left half-field in the left eye, as is characteristically associated with a midline lesion compressing the optic chiasm.

Altitudinal hemianopia The visual field defect may also be of the upper or the lower half if the deficit is demarcated by the equator.

Sectoral hemianopia: a homonymous altitudinal field defect with a linear horizontal edge, produced by lesions of the nonstriatal visual pathways.[2663]

Binasal hemianopia The nasal fields are lost, in each eye. Because the field defect is a mirror image in the two eyes, such forms of hemianopia may be known as *heteronymous hemianopias.*

Complicated hemianopias The hemianopia is complicated by the presence of an oculomotor palsy.

Quadrantic hemianopias Those in which the deficit is of one quarter of the field only; these may be bitemporal or binasal, and above or below the equator.

Functional hemianopia Hemianopia in the absence of organic disease of the visual pathways. This form has been reviewed by Gittinger.[2129]

See also **congruence.**

hemianopic color blindness Residual color blindness (shown by inability to match colors) in a field that was formerly hemianopic.

hemianopic hallucinations Pure visual hallucinations within a hemianopic half-field (or in the area of a lesser visual field defect), the lesion involving the visual cortex. Migrainous visual hallucinations are an example.[1862,3119]

hemianopsia See **hemianopia.**

hemiasomatognosia See **Anton-Babinski syndrome.**

hemiataxia See **hemiataxy.**

hemiataxia-hypesthesia An unusual lateral thalamic stroke syndrome due to infarction in the territory of the thalamogeniculate artery and characterized clinically by isolated hemiataxia and ipsilateral sensory loss involving any modalities.[3822]

hemiataxy (hemiataxia) Unilateral motor incoordination.

hemiathetosis Athetosis occurring on one side of the body only.

hemiatrophia cerebri Severe acquired atrophy of one cerebral hemisphere in children, following an initial acute insult and associated partial seizures. See also **HHE syndrome.**[5480]

hemiatrophy Unilateral shrinkage of a body part due to various degrees of involvement of skin, subcutaneous tissue, fat, and/or bone.

Though classically the sequel to infantile cortical lesions, it is also described in association with acquired neurological diseases and it occurs idiopathically.[4790]

hemiballism(us) (Gr, half + jumping) (hemichorea) An uncommon hyperkinetic disorder characterized by sudden, violent, persistent, unilateral, proximal flinging movements of an arm or leg due to a lesion (usually a **lacunar infarct**) involving the contralateral subthalamic nucleus of Luys.[1871] The term was applied first by **von Economo.** See **ballism.**

In a *variant form,* the condition is inherited as a recessive trait.

hemibasal syndrome See **Garcin syndrome.**

hemibulbar syndrome See **Babinski-Nageotte syndrome.**

hemichorea See **hemiballism(us).**

hemiconvulsions, hemiplegia, epilepsy syndrome See **HHE syndrome.**

hemicrania (Gr, half + the head) (megrim) Headache affecting one side only; classic migraine. *Hemicrania alternans* affects the two sides alternately; *angioparalytic (or neuroparalytic) hemicrania* is **complicated or hemiplegic migraine.**

hemicrania alternans See **hemicrania.**

hemicrania continua A rare, benign, unilateral headache of continuous type and moderate severity, for which no precipitants are identified and which is absolutely responsive to indomethacin. It is more common in females. The pain may or may not pulsate but tends to fluctuate in intensity, with severe exacerbations (stabbing headaches) sometimes superimposed on background pain of moderate severity. The side on which it is felt seldom changes between attacks. Cycles persist over weeks to years.[4114] There are few accompanying autonomic signs compared to those occurring in **chronic paroxysmal hemicrania,** which this headache otherwise resembles[664,4113,5200] but ipsilateral lacrimation, ptosis, rhinorrhea, and nasal congestion and conjunctival injection are occasional accompaniments.

A much-amended fusion of the diagnostic criteria suggested by Goadsby and Lipton[2142] and by Pareja et al.[4329] is given here; the latter authors' perceived subdivisions of the clinical syndrome (*H. vera, H. generis incerti*)[4328] is not.

A. Head pain has persisted for over 1 month.
B. Obligatory features:
   1. Strict unilaterality without side shift, usually in anterior/auricular regions
   2. Absolute and protracted effect of indomethacin
   3. Long-lasting, repetitive attacks lasting up to weeks at a time, tending towards a fluctuating pattern
   4. Continuous pain ranges from mild to severe but is never excruciating
   5. No identifiable precipitants
C. Associated features with unusually severe pain attacks:
   1. Conjunctival injection
   2. Lacrimation
   3. Nasal congestion and rhinorrhoea
   4. Ptosis and eyelid edema
D. Nonobligatory features:
   1. Female gender
   2. Few autonomic accompaniments
   3. Few typical migraine or cervicogenic headache features
   4. Inefficacy of serotonin agonist therapy

hemicranianosis See **Brissaud-Lereboullet syndrome.**

hemidystonia Involuntary sustained posturing of the arm, leg, and face of one side.

In most cases, the responsible lesion is situated in the contralateral putamen, caudate, or thalamus, disconnecting the thalamus from the striatum. The corticospinal pathways are essentially preserved. The possible etiologies are many.[3644,4426]

hemifacial atrophy   See **Parry-Romberg syndrome.**

hemifacial microsomia (first arch syndrome, mandibular dysostosis) A congenital anomaly of unknown cause, manifesting unilateral hypoplasia of the facial soft tissues and underlying bones, with failure of formation of the mandibular ramus and condyle and ipsilateral microtia.[2218]

The condition may be a *variant* of **oculoauriculovertebral dysplasia.** See also **Goldenhar syndrome.**

hemifacial spasm (Brissaud-Meige syndrome) An acquired, progressive syndrome characterized by frequent, repetitive, unilateral, involuntary tonic or tonic-clonic of the facial muscles.

There are two forms. In the first, brief twitches occur simultaneously in several facial muscles, often with blinking and accompanied by isolated bursts of 20 to 40 repetitive motor unit discharges on the EMG at up to 400 Hz and lasting for about 0.5 second. In the second form, prolonged spasms occur erratically with electrical discharges at a slower rate.[2591]

Both ephaptic transmission after nerve injury and the appearance of a new trigger in the nerve trunk which would give rise to a locally generated electrical discharge have been postulated to be the cause. Some consider the basis to be a form of segmental myoclonus, while others believe that impingement of local dilated or redundant arteries upon the facial nerve exit zone is responsible, which has led to the institution of surgical procedures designed to achieve separation. Though criticized as simplistic, the theory of electrical cross-talk or chatter between artery and nerve has electrical validity,[2458] and the procedure, though potentially hazardous, has at least the merit of cure in numerous instances.[2812]

The theory of vascular compression of the nerve is not new; it was propounded also by Brissaud in 1895.

In a *variant form,* autosomal dominant inheritance has been reported.[5361]

hemifield slide Diplopia with deviation of images either horizontally or vertically as an effect of bitemporal hemianopia, which prevents binocular fixation and suppression of the false image which is necessary in the presence of slight imbalance of motor input to the eyes.[3060]

hemihypertrophy-hemianesthesia-hemiareflexia-scoliosis   See **hemi-3 syndrome.**

hemihypertrophy-nevi-hamartoma   See **proteus syndrome.**

hemimasticatory spasm A rare facial movement disorder characterized by isolated, involuntary, unilateral, painful contractions of the masticatory muscles (masseter, temporalis, and pterygoid) which tend to hypertrophy.

This paroxysmal cranial neuropathy is considered to be due to irritation leading to ectopic activity in the proximal trigeminal motor nerve root, perhaps by vascular structures; the EMG findings are similar to those observed in **hemifacial spasm.**[5568]

In a *variant form,* the syndrome accompanies facial hemiatrophy.[2962]

hemimegalencephaly A congenital dysmorphic syndrome manifesting also macrocrania, hemipareses, hemianopia, refractory grand mal and myoclonic seizures in the neonatal period, infantile spasms with hypsarrhythmia, nystagmus, heterotopias, diffuse gliosis, and high-output cardiac failure in infants. The affected hemisphere is enlarged and may show agyria or pachygyria.[354,4391]

hemiopia (Gr, half + the eye) Half of the (normal) visual field. The term is, however, often used erroneously in place of **hemianopia.**

hemiparalexia An unusual dyslexic syndrome due to lesions in the left posterior callosum and characterized clinically by substitutions of left-sided (initial, beginning-of-word) letter substitutions during oral reading of words.[571]

hemiparesis (Gr, half + want of strength) Reduction of muscle strength on one side of the body. The word is colloquially used for weakness as opposed to paralysis (**hemiplegia**).

hemiparetic cerebral palsy Congenitally derived hemparesis, appearing in two main forms: arm-dominant, which is associated with relatively large cortical or subcortical lesions and clinically with epilepsy and cognitive deficits, and leg-dominant, in which the lesions are of the subcortical white matter and are less often asociated with these problems.[2698]

hemiparetic seizures (focal inhibitory seizures, local or unilateral atonic seizures, status hemiparalyticus, partial seizures with subsequent hemigeneralization) Epileptic equivalents in which unilateral paresis is accompanied by paroxysmal epileptiform discharges.

This uncommon form of focal seizure is due to discharges arising from the contralateral hemisphere without disturbance of consciousness, as shown by EEG abnormalities and radionucleotide uptake in the contralateral hemisphere. Treatment of the seizures clears both the paralysis and the abnormal brain scan. The episodes represent an ictal rather than postictal event and are neither migrainous nor due to demonstrable focal pathology.[2421] See also **Todd paralysis.**[2421]

hemiparkinsonism-(somatic) hemiatrophy syndrome The association of early life hemispheric injury with contralateral focal hemiatrophy and pyramidal signs, with the late development on that side of slowly progressive parkinsonism unresponsive to L-dopa, and with early dystonia, appearing before the ingestion of medications.[3077] The condition is a rare form of secondary **parkinsonism.**

hemiplegia   (Gr, half + striking) Severe weakness, as due to a stroke, affecting any part of the upper motor neuron pathway, on one side of the body.

In **alternating** or *crossed hemiplegia* the weakness affects the ocular movements or face on one side and the trunk and limbs on the other. See **Weber syndrome, Millard-Gubler syndrome, Foville syndrome, Jackson syndrome.**

hemiplegia alternans superior peduncularis   See **Weber syndrome.**

hemiplegia cruciata   (crossed hemiplegia, syndrome of the decussation) Corticospinal tract damage leading to a pyramidal syndrome affecting the arm on the same side and the leg on the other.

The lesion must be at the cervicomedullary junction on the side of the arm weakness, at which site the fibers destined to cross to the corticospinal tract on the other side of the cord controlling the leg have not yet crossed (unlike those destined for the arm, which have).

hemiplegic amyotrophy   (hemiplegic atrophy) Wasting of muscles in a limb affected by an upper motor neuron lesion.

Such wasting is considered due to a combination of disuse, transsynaptic degeneration, and loss of central trophic influences on the lower motor neuron.[1018]

hemiplegic atrophy   See **hemiplegic amyotrophy.**

hemiplegic epilepsy   The term of Hughlings-**Jackson** for **partial seizures.**

hemiplegic gait   Characteristically that gait requiring exaggeration of upward pelvic tilt with rolling circumduction of the affected leg during the phase of weight-bearing on the opposite leg, in order to compensate for the lengthening effect of the paretic leg's posture. This is held extended at the hip and knee, the ankle being plantar flexed. The adducted, pronated, and flexed posture of the arm is a further diagnostic clue.

hemiplegic migraine   See **familial hemiplegic migraine.**

hemipontine syndrome   Hemorrhage into the lateral part of the pons; it is an unusual occurrence, most hemorrhages being central and bilateral. The major signs include alternating hemiparesis and thermoanalgesia, as well as **skew deviation** of the eyes. Consciousness is preserved, and many patients make reasonable functional recoveries. See also **dorsal tegmental syndrome.**

hemi-see-saw nystagmus   A rare variant of **see-saw nystagmus** in which one half-cycle of see-saw nystagmus alternates with a quick phase in the other direction.[2390]

hemisensory syndrome   A **lacunar syndrome.** See **pure sensory stroke.**

hemisomatic spasms   A syndrome of unilateral spasms affecting the face and ipsilateral arm, resulting from a lesion at the ipsilateral cerebellopontine angle.[118] Only the extension of movements to the arm differentiates this condition from **hemifacial spasm.**

hemispasm   A dystonic or convulsive movement affecting one side of the body only.

hemispatial agnosia   See **neglect.**

hemispatial neglect   (inattention) An abnormal relationship between the patient and the environment on the side opposite a hemispheric lesion (usually the right hemisphere) in which objects and events on that side, including that half of the patient himself, are ignored to a greater or lesser extent.

hemisphere   (Gr, half + a ball or sphere) Half a sphere—thus the cerebral and cerebellar hemispheres, because of their shape.

hemispherectomy   Surgical removal of most or all of one cerebral hemisphere, rarely performed but of value in children with intractable epilepsy.[34]

hemispheric epilepsy   A syndrome of childhood or adolescence manifesting an intractable seizure disorder (tonic-clonic, myoclonic, tonic, atonic, or absence-like) with generalized ictal features that are focal in most cases, without demonstrable etiology or related structural abnormality of the CNS. Diffuse unilateral spike–waves are seen on EEG consistently appearing over the same hemisphere. The etiology is seldom determined.[611]

hemispheric stroke scale   An instrument for assessing and quantitating deficits following ischemic stroke, under the headings *level of consciousness* (derived from the **Glasgow Coma scale**); *language; other cortical functions and cranial nerves; motor examination and gait;* and *sensory function.*[39] See also **stroke scales.**

hemivertebra   A congenital anomaly characterized by the failure of normal development of one half-side of a vertebra. While the condition may be symptomless, some degree of scoliosis is the usual result.

hemodilution   A technique for lowering the hematocrit, usually by about 30%, in order to increase cerebral blood flow and maximize tissue oxygenation, as following stroke. Methods may either increase blood volume (hypervolemic) or, by bloodletting at the same time as cell-free fluids are administered, allow it to remain normal (isovolemic). The method is of unproven value in the treatment of stroke.

hemoglobinopathy encephalopathy   A diffuse encephalopathy occurring in children having hemoglobin H, and who present with mental retardation. The responsible gene maps to 16pter–p13.5.

hemophilic encephalopathy   A diffuse encephalopathy.[1586]

Hemophilus influenzae **meningitis**   A dangerous form of meningitis most commonly affecting children less than 5 years old and immunocompromised adults.

hemorrhagic leukoencephalitis   See **acute disseminated encephalomyelitis.**

Henneberg, Richard   (1868–1962) German neurologist who gave early accounts of **metachromatic leukodystrophy.**

Henneberg sign   1. Induction of vertigo and nystagmus in subjects with a fistula of a semicircular canal by the examiner's fingertip pressure over a patient's external auditory meatus.[2538] 2. See **hard palate reflex.**

Henneberg syndrome   (luetic otitic-nystagmus syndrome) The occurrence of nystagmus and vertigo with alterations of pressure within the external auditory meatus; a feature of congenital syphilis, often accompanied by interstitial keratitis and chorioretinitis.[2537] The phenomenon was described by Camille Henneberg (1867–1962), a Belgian otologist.

Increased vertigo and/or nystagmus also occur when the pressure in the external auditory meatus is increased, as by manual pressure on the tragus, in patients with a fistula between the perilymph and the middle ear resulting from any cause.

Henoch, Eduard Heinrich   (1820–1910) German physician.

Henoch syndrome   The disease was called "electrical chorea" by Henoch, who noted it in children with asymmetrical and variable lightning-like twitches in the shoulder and neck muscles which disappear in sleep but later become generalized and chronic. The term was later appropriated for that syndrome described by **Dubini,** which is probably quite different. See **paramyoclonus multiplex.**

Henoch-Schönlein purpura   A hypersensitivity vasculitis of children in which both stroke and subarachnoid hemorrhage may occur apart from the gastrointestinal and renal manifestations.

Henzschell syndrome   See **Apert syndrome.**

hepatic carnitine palmityl transferase deficiency   A syndrome with onset in infancy, characterized by fasting hypoglycemia. As a result of lack of carnitine palmityl transferase activity, long-chain fatty acid oxidation, ketogenesis, and gluconeogenesis are all impaired. No muscle disorder is associated.[677]

hepatic encephalopathy   A severe neuropsychiatric syndrome characterized by abnormal mental and other neurological status, occurring in patients with severe acute or chronic hepatic insufficiency or primary biliary cirrhosis. The clinical features range from mild cognitive impairment to coma, and may include **aster-**

ixis, tremor, ataxia, ophthalmoplegia, myelopathy, neuropathy, and autonomic insufficiency, usually in the presence of high levels of blood ammonia.[1318,1936] **Triphasic waves** are commonly found on the EEG in each of the two forms described:

1. That due to acute hepatic insufficiency causing rapidly raised intracranial pressure with deepening drowsiness up to coma as a result of cytotoxic brain edema; death may ensue.
2. *Portosystemic encephalopathy,* in which the clinical development is slower, passing from personality change and altered sleep patterns through ataxia and asterixis to stupor and coma.

hepatic neuropathy   A mild, demyelinating, sensorimotor peripheral neuropathy due either to the metabolic disorder that induced hepatic insufficiency, or the metabolic consequences of the organ failure.[1318]

Acute inflammatory demyelinating polyneuropathy may complicate viral hepatitis[3360] and a mild but painful sensory neuropathy is described in biliary cirrhosis.[5551]

hepatocerebral degeneration   A condition resembling **Wilson disease,** described 2 years later. The clinical features are those of cortical and basal ganglion disturbance. See **acquired hepatocerebral degeneration, Alpers disease.**

hepatocerebral syndrome   See **acquired hepatocerebral degeneration.**

hepatolenticular degeneration   See **Wilson disease.**

hepatorenal glycogenosis   See **glycogen storage diseases.**

hepatosplenomegaly and adrenocortical deficiency   A rare, recessive, congenital, musculoskeletal disorder manifesting diarrhea and vomiting during the first year of life, followed by sensorineural hearing loss and pigmentary retinopathy, subnormal mentality, distal progressive muscular atrophy, hepatosplenomegaly, and adrenal insufficiency. There are reduced levels of tissue arachidonic and other polyunsaturated fatty acids, prostanate and phosphate are identified in the plasma.

The condition may be a disorder of phytanic acid metabolism distinct from Refsum disease.[1581]

Heracles   A Greek god (Hercules in Latin), whose name was applied to epilepsy by Hippocrates, because of the strength and violence of the motor movements of the seizures.

herald hemiparesis   The occurrence of mild hemiparesis when brainstem signs may be absent or few, prior to the massive deficit produced by a succeeding basilar artery occlusion. There is nothing about the hemiparesis, however, which allows the subsequent events to be predicted.[1859]

hereditary acrolabial telangiectasia   A dominantly inherited syndrome characterized by blue discoloration of the lips, nails, and nipples, widespread telangiectasias of the skin, and migraine headaches.[3893]

hereditary adult-onset leukodystrophy A dominantly inherited, chronic, progressive neurological disorder of unknown nature characterized by the appearance of cerebellar, pyramidal, and autonomic symptoms and signs in mid-adult life, clinically and radiologically similar to X-linked a**drenoleukodystrophy** but with a different pattern of transmission, and to **multiple sclerosis** except for the symmetry of radiological findings.[1632]

hereditary amyloid neuropathy   See **Andrade neuropathy.**

hereditary anhidrotic sensory neuropathy   See **hereditary sensory and autonomic neuropathy** (recessive).

hereditary areflexic dystasia   See **Roussy-Levy syndrome.**

hereditary arthro-ophthalmopathy   See **Stickler syndrome.**

hereditary ataxia   See **cerebellar ataxias, Friedreich ataxia.**

hereditary benign chorea   See **hereditary nonprogressive chorea.**[3197]

hereditary brachial plexopathy (familial recurrent brachial plexus neuropathy) A dominantly inherited syndrome of young adult life, characterized by unusual sensitivity of fibers of the brachial plexus to intercurrent stretch or pressure, probably as a result of a subclinical polyneuropathy, and leading to temporary but still prolonged conduction block.[5513] Clinically, it presents with attacks of pain and weakness with atrophy of the muscles of the shoulder girdle and proximal arm. See also **neuralgic amyotrophy.**

Cranial mononeuropathies and **Horner syndrome** are also occasionally found in such patients.[702]

hereditary branchial myoclonus with spastic paraplegia A dominantly inherited condition with adult onset, manifesting rhythmic, myoclonus-like movements of the palate, pharynx, larynx, and face; truncal ataxia; and pyramidal signs, and leading to death in 5–10 years.[1429] See also **branchial myoclonus.**

hereditary bulbar atrophy (Fazio-Londe atrophy) See **juvenile motor neuron disease.**

hereditary carnitine deficiency   See **carnitine deficiency.**

hereditary cerebellar ataxia   See **cerebellar ataxias.**

hereditary cerebellar ataxia with mental deficiency See **cerebellar ataxias** (*variants*).

hereditary cerebral hemorrhage with amyloidosis–Dutch type   See **Dutch cerebral hemorrhage.**

hereditary cerebral vasculopathy A dominantly inherited leukoencephalopathy appearing first in the third decade, characterized by dysarthria, progressive visual loss, dementia, and gait disturbance, thus resembling **multiple sclerosis,** except that there is also visible retinal vasculopathy.[2255]

hereditary ceruloplasmin deficiency (hereditary ferroxidase deficiency) An autosomal recessive disorder characterized by subcortical dementia, involuntary movements, retinal degeneration, and diabetes mellitus in association with onset in adult life. Low serum levels of ceruloplasmin and iron overload, especially in the brain, pancreas, and liver, are characteristics. Serum ceruloplasmin is very low or absent, while ferritin levels are high. The mutation is mapped to chromosome 3q.[3990]

hereditary chin trembling   See **hereditary quivering of the chin.**

hereditary continuous motor neuron discharges with neuropathy A familial syndrome of distal weakness and atrophy with myokymia or fasciculations and delayed relaxation after voluntary contraction.[3242]

hereditary coproporphyria An uncommon, dominantly inherited form of **porphyria.** The neurological features complicate some acute attacks and include the occurrence of proximal motor neuropathy affecting the arms more than the legs (often asymmetrically) and also the face and autonomic system, in the setting of other features of the disease, including photosensitivity, abdominal pain, vomiting, tachycardia, hypertension, and often seizures and delirium.[4756]

hereditary demyelinating neuropathy of infancy A demyelinating peripheral neuropathy with onset in infancy, clinically resembling type III **hereditary motor and sensory neuropathy** (Déjèrine-Sottas disease) some-times with bulbar and diaphragmatic involvement. Four point mutations in the peripheral myelin protein 22 (*PMP22*) gene have been found, but the disease is genetically heterogeneous.[5676]

hereditary dentatorubropallidoluysian atrophy (familial myoclonic epilepsy and choreoathetosis, progressive pallidal atrophy, dentatorubral atrophy, dyssynergia cerebellaris myoclonica) A combined systemic degeneration of the dentatofugal and pallidofugal pathways, clinically manifesting chorea, dystonia, athetosis, ballism, and/or ataxia.[5470]

Criteria for diagnosis are the presence of a dominantly inherited myoclonic epilepsy syndrome with or without cerebellar signs or choreoathetosis with MRI evidence of dentatorubralpallidoluysian atrophy.

Hereditary Disease Foundation A charitable organization maintaining grant programs to support scientific projects in major medical and basic science laboratories, and disseminating information to organizations and individuals. Address: 1303 Pico Blvd., Santa Monica, CA 90405-1553. Tel: 310-450-9913. Web site: http://www.hdfoundation.org/.

hereditary distal muscle dystrophy   See **Gowers syndromes.**

hereditary distal myopathy   Genetically determined syndromes of distal muscle weakness and wasting, first described by **Gowers.**[2241]

Two forms are recognized: (*1*) the autosomal dominant *distal late hereditary myopathy* of Welander[5908] with onset after the age of 20 years, and with slow progression of symptoms starting in the hands and wrist extensors in both sexes; and (*2*) another dominantly inherited form, characterized by the infantile onset of bilateral foot drop, weakness later affecting the hands and wrists, but with no further progression after the age of 18 years.[3563]

hereditary distal spinal muscular atrophy   A syndrome of progressive symmetrical wasting and weakness presenting in childhood or adolescence. It resembles a form of peroneal muscular atrophy (types 1 or 2 **hereditary motor and sensory neuropathy** but there is less arm weakness, relative preservation of the muscle stretch reflexes, and normal clinical sensory examination and motor and sensory conduction study findings.

Other *variants* are *scapuloperoneal, facioscapulohumeral,* and *generalized* forms.[2445]

hereditary dysphasic dementia   A dominantly inherited dementing disorder of later adult life with prominent nonfluent dysphasia and parkinsonism.

Pathologically, features of **Pick, Alzheimer,** or **Parkinson diseases** are found in association with spongy degeneration of the cortex.[3996] See also **primary progressive aphasia.**

hereditary dysphasic disinhibition dementia   See **frontotemporal dementia.**

hereditary dystonia with contractures and abnormal muscle   A congenital syndrome characterized by joint contractures, chorea, dystonia, and muscle fiber hypotrophy with ring fibers.[337]

hereditary dystonia with lightning jerks, responsive to alcohol   See **hereditary myoclonic dystonia.**

hereditary dystonia-parkinsonism syndrome of juvenile onset   See **dopa-responsive dystonia.**

hereditary dystonic lipidosis   See **Fabry disease.**

hereditary endotheliopathy with retinopathy, nephropathy, and stroke   A dominantly inherited disorder manifesting these features, presenting clinically with visual impairment, migraine-like headaches, dysarthria, hemiparesis, and apraxias in young adult life. The presence of contrast-enhancing subcortical lesions indicates that this is a multi-infarct syndrome, though separate from **CADASIL.**[2833]

hereditary essential myoclonus   A dominantly inherited myoclonic disorder with onset before the age of 20 years, characterized by involuntary contractions of single muscles or groups of synergic muscles, resulting in jerks of various amplitudes. The movements involve the arms, legs, trunk, and neck (particularly the arms and neck) and are most frequent and intense proximally. Movements are always rapid and brief and are sometimes asynchronous; accompanying EMG activity lasts less than 500 msec. The movements are increased by activities requiring fine coordination, such as writing, and by conscious attempts to inhibit them. No other neurological deficits are found, the course is benign, and the condition does not decrease life span.[3571]

Distinction from paramyoclonus multiplex is made mainly on the basis of the family history and exacerbation with activity.[1299]

See also **paramyoclonus multiplex, myoclonus, essential myoclonus, hereditary myoclonic dystonia.**

hereditary facial spasm   (Hellsing syndrome) A slowly progressive, complicated polyneuropathy, dominantly inherited and manifesting uni- or bilateral hemifacial spasm, with facial weakness, **Argyll Robertson pupils,** gaze disturbances, reduced caloric reactions, optic atrophy, hyporeflexia, and mild lower motor neuron paresis in the legs with pes cavus and trophic foot ulcers but normal distal sensation. To date, the condition seems to have been reported only from Sweden.[3519] The syndrome is probably a form of hereditary hypertrophic neuropathy, resembling Déjèrine-Sottas neuropathy (**hereditary motor and sensory neuropathy type 3**).

hereditary ferroxidase deficiency   See **hereditary ceruloplasmin deficiency.**

hereditary fructose intolerance   A congenital dysmetabolic state due to the absence of fructose-1-phosphate aldolase B, the enzyme responsible for the assimilation of dietary fructose, and characterized in infancy by failure to thrive, vomiting, and hypoglycemia. In adults, the symptoms are those of hypoglycemia, including convulsions after fructose ingestion.[1152]

In a *variant* form, fructose 1:6–diphosphatase activity is deficient. The clinical features are similar.

hereditary hemorrhagic telangiectasia   (Rendu-Osler-Weber hemangiomatosis) A dominantly inherited disorder characterized by the presence of multiple dermal, mucosal, and visceral telangiectasias that bleed recurrently.

Neurologically, emboli resulting from pulmonary arteriovenous fistulas, intracranial aneurysms with hemorrhage, and telangiectasias within the CNS are the major complications.[4749]

Hereditary Hemorrhagic Telangiectasia Foundation International, Inc.   A charitable organization concerned with this condition. Address: PO Box 8087, New

Haven, CT 06530. Tel: 1–800–HHT-NETW (USA) or 313–561–2537 (Canada).

hereditary hypertrophic neuropathy, trigeminal neuralgia, and deafness   See **hereditary motor and sensory neuropathy, type 1.**

hereditary hypertrophic neuropathy with paraproteinemia   See **gammopathic neuropathy.**

hereditary kinesthetic reflex epilepsy   See **paroxysmal kinesigenic choreoathetosis.**

hereditary late-onset chorea   A variant of **Huntington disease** with onset over the age of 50 years.[759]

hereditary leukoencephalopathy and palmoplantar keratoderma   A recessively inherited neurocutaneous syndrome with childhood onset, manifesting spastic quadriparesis and cognitive impairment in adult life.[3476]

hereditary liability to pressure palsies   See **hereditary pressure-sensitive neuropathy.**

hereditary macular dystrophies with encephalopathy (cerebroretinal degeneration)   Those **sphingolipidoses** or **mucolipidoses,** usually recessively inherited, associated with cone or rod-cone dystrophies or with pigmentary retinopathy. See also **neuronal ceroid lipofuscinosis.**

hereditary mirror movements   A dominantly inherited syndrome with childhood onset, characterized by the performance of movements with one limb mirroring those voluntarily performed in the other, and by mental and developmental delay.[4999] See **mirror movements.**

hereditary motor and sensory neuropathies (HMSN) A heterogeneous group of familial disorders characterized by the onset in childhood of denervation affecting the feet and legs well before the hands and arms, and leading to slowly progressive weakness and muscle atrophy. The prototype was described by **Charcot** and **Marie**[981] and independently by **Tooth** in the same year. The responsible gene lies on chromosome 1, but at two sites, with and without linkage to the Duffy locus. Many *variant forms* have been identified (see Chart H–7).

Some order was brought to the classification of the hereditary mixed neuropathies when nerve conduction studies showed that, in most families, the motor conduction velocity was grossly reduced but in others it was reduced only to a figure still greater than 70% of the normal or 38 m/s. Both this syndrome and the next (HMSN 1 and HMSN 2) are also known by the names of Charcot, Marie, and Tooth (CMT), and as *peroneal muscular atrophy.*[2446] Despite the advances of recent years, the classifications below are best regarded as *work in progress.*

Dyck[1567] classified the whole group; Chart H–7 is based on this work. The organization of the many entities is difficult today, however, because variant classifications are also extant.[2441,4958,5711] There follows an abbreviated listing of the conditions that are further defined below.

CMT 1   Dominant, demyelinating, with low motor nerve conduction velocity (MNCV) (the same as HMSN 1)

Types A (17p11.2), B (1q22–q23), C, and D (10q21) are differentiated, on the basis of their genetic loci.

This grouping includes Déjèrine-Sottas neuropathy (HMSN 3), with very slow MNCV; although most cases are sporadic the genetic forms map to the same loci. A defect of peripheral myelin protein (PMP-22) is responsible.

CMT 2   Dominant, axonal, with normal or low normal MNCV (this may be the same as HMSN 2)

Types A (1p35–p36), B (3q13–q22), C, D (7p14), and E (1q22) are differentiated, on the basis of their genetic loci.

CMTX   X-linked, demyelinating, mapped to Xq13,1; and CMTX2 to Xq24. A defect of connexin 32 is responsible.

Hereditary neuropathy with liability to pressure palsies (perhaps a variant of HMSN 1)

Dominant or sporadic; types A and B are differentiated. One form is linked to Xp11.2. and another to 17p.11.2. A defect of peripheral myelin protein (PMP-22) is responsible.

CMT 3   A recessive, axonal form.

Congenital hypomyelination neuropathy. Both dominant and recessive forms are described.

Linkages to 1q22 and 10q21 have been established.

CMT 4   Recessive, demyelinating (also known as AR-CMT 2)

Types A (8q13–q21), B (11q13), C (5q23–q33), and L (8q24) have been differentiated.

CMT 5   Dominant; axonal loss, with pyramidal signs.

CMT 6   Dominant; axonal loss, with optic atrophy.

Chart H–7. Classification of the Hereditary Motor and Sensory Neuropathies

Hereditary motor and sensory neuropathy type 1 (Charcot-Marie-Tooth disease, demyelinating form; peroneal muscular atrophy, CMT 1; HMSN 1, Hoffmann disease, Roussy-Lévy syndrome): A relatively common, dominantly (sometimes recessively) inherited, slowly progressive, hypertrophic motor and sensory neuropathy due to a duplication of DNA on the short arm of chromosome 17 (type 1A at 17p11.2–p.12), or due to a mutation on chromosome 1 at 1q22 (type 1B).[2326] A 1C genotype is also described. CMTX may also be classified here. Mutations in the early growth response gene have been found here and in subjects with congenital hypomyeliniating neuropathy (see below).

The usual clinical onset is in childhood; widespread segmental demyelination of the peripheral nerves is found and the motor nerve conduction velocities in the median nerves are below 38 m/s. Distal weakness and wasting, especially in the legs, areflexia, nerve thickening, and reduction of all forms of sensation distally are commonly detected and pes cavus, scoliosis, essential tremor (*Roussy-Lévy syndrome*), or ataxia may be present.

Charcot-Marie-Tooth disease X-linked (CMTX) comprises X-linked and X-linked dominant *variants* of HMSN 1, for which, in some kinships, the responsible gene maps to Xq11–q13.[2748,4837]

Other variant forms include the following:

HMSN with optic atrophy The latter feature may be of the **Leber** type.[3775] See also *HMSN 6,* below.

HMSN with spasticity The association of typical type 1 HMSN with pyramidal signs and abnormal auditory brainstem evoked responses. See *HMSN 5,* below.

HMSN with ataxia The association of congenital, dominantly inherited type 1 HMSN with cerebellar signs and sometimes choreoathetosis.[5279] This probably is the Roussy-Levy syndrome, wrongly placed.

Hereditary hypertrophic neuropathy, trigeminal neuralgia, and deafness A demyelinating sensorimotor neuropathy with onset in infancy or childhood, manifesting also sensorineural deafness and facial pain.[337]

HMSN with continuous motor unit activity A rare, dominantly inherited *variant* form of type 1 HMSN with associated fasciculations, myotonia, myokymia, and cramps.[5744]

HMSN with corneal dystrophy A congenital demyelinating sensorimotor peripheral neuropathy manifesting also cloudy corneas, hypotonia, multiple fractures, and cutaneous ulcers.[337]

Hypertrophic neuropathy with facial involvement A sensorimotor axonal and demyelinating neuropathy with onset in childhood or youth, manifesting also kyphoscoliosis, trigeminal neuralgia, facial spasm, and dysmyelination with onion bulb formation in the peripheral nerves.[337]

HMSN with nephropathy A syndrome of progressive muscle wasting in a distribution characteristic of peroneal muscular atrophy with severe nephritis and neural deafness. This may be a variant of **Alport syndrome.**[2422]

HMSN with excessive myelin outfolding A recessively inherited, hypomyelinating but hypertrophic sensorimotor peripheral neuropathy with onset in youth, with this unusual pathological finding.[343] Confusingly (because the standard classification of Dyck is now in the process of amendment), this is known also as CMT 4B. Juvenile-onset glaucoma has been associated with this form.[3072]

HMSN with features of Noonan syndrome Typical HMSN type 1a with giant proximal nerve hypertrophy, not linked to neurofibromatosis.[5158]

HMSN-Lom A recessively inherited demyelinating neuropathy associated with sensorineural deafness and mapped to chromosome 8q24.[5547]

Congenital cataracts–facial dysmorphism–neuropathy syndrome There are added microcornae, mental retardation, small stature, and a predominantly motor neuropathy, sometimes[965] pyramidal signs and mild chorea. It maps to chromosome 18qter.

HMSN Russe A recessively inherited syndrome characterized by severe leg and distal arm weakness, distal pansensory loss, foot and hand deformities, and Charcot joints, mapped to chromosome 10q.[5547]

Hereditary motor and sensory neuropathy type 2 (Charcot-Marie-Tooth disease, neuronal form; peroneal muscular atrophy, HMSN 2; CMT 2; CMT 4; AR-CMT 2) is a slowly progressive, usually dominantly inherited motor and sensory neuropathy with onset at any age but mainly during the second decade. Its clinical features resemble those of type 1 but tend to be less severe and involve the hands less often. The

nerves are not thickened, tremor and ataxia are uncommon accompaniments, the motor nerve conduction velocities in the median nerves are above 38 m/s, and nerve biopsy specimens show neuronal atrophy.[4330]

Three autosomal dominant loci have been identified: 1p35–p36 (CMT 2A), 3q13–q22 (CMT 2B), and 7p14 (CMT 2D). Type 2B is a distal sensorimotor axopathy associated with juvenile onset of distal motor weakness and sensory loss, with preserved ankle reflexes. Type 2C is remarkable for the vocal cord pareses and diaphragmatic paralysis occurring.[1578]

Recessive forms (disorders classified under the alternative terminology as CMT 4) have been mapped to 8q13.q21.1 (CMT 4A); 11q23 (CMT 4B); 5q23.q33 (CMT 4C); 8q24 (CMT 4D); and 19q13.1–13.3 (CMT 4F).[469]

Variants include the following:

Benign HMSN type 2 with ptosis, parkinsonism, and dementia The combination of **multiple system atrophy** (ptosis, parkinsonism, orthostatic hypotension, hyperreflexia, and mild dementia) with HMSN 2, dominantly inherited, and carrying a benign prognosis for life.[5484]

HMSN type 2 with neurofilamentous accumulations A dominantly inherited sensorimotor axonal and demyelinating neuropathy with onset in childhood or youth, also characterized by pes cavus and cardiomyopathy, but without kinky hair. Nerve biopsy specimens show the presence of neurofilamentous accumulations and axonal swellings.[5774]

HMSN type 2 with deafness (CMT 4D) A sensorimotor axonal and demyelinating neuropathy with congenital or childhood onset, manifesting also sensorineural deafness.[335]

HMSN type 2 with acrodystrophy and severe limb weakness[5546]

HMSN type 2 with parkinsonism A rare familial variant with adult onset.[860]

HMSN type 2 with optic atrophy and deafness A sensorimotor axonal and demyelinating neuropathy with congenital or childhood onset manifesting also sensorineural deafness, optic atrophy, and nystagmus.[4791]

HMSN type 2 with mental retardation, optic atrophy, and pyramidal signs A recessively inherited, severe, but slowly progressive sensorimotor axonal neuropathy with onset in childhood, manifesting the above signs and retinal colloid bodies.[3543]

HMSN with myopathy Typical HMSN with the added histological features of myopathy, presumably as the result of repeated de- and reinnervation.

HMSN with dementia and dysautonomia A dominantly inherited syndrome consisting of slowly progressive limb weakness due to sensorimotor axonal neuropathy, attacks of vomiting, labile blood pressure, attacks of altered consciousness, mental retardation, and cerebral atrophy.[4286]

Parkinsonism with cerebellar ataxia and peripheral neuropathy A rare variant form with adult onset.

Charcot-Marie-Tooth disease related to spinal muscular atrophy, distal type

Charcot-Marie-Tooth peroneal muscular atrophy and **Friedreich ataxia.** An X-linked variety

Hereditary motor and sensory neuropathy type 3 (Déjèrine-Sottas syndrome, progressive hypertrophic interstitial neuropathy, onion bulb neuropathy) is a severe, congenital, axonal and demyelinating motor and sensory neuropathy with abnormal motor development and gross slowing of MNCV.

In some cases, this may be no more than the homozygous expression of a dominant gene for HMSN 1,[3529] but in most, the condition is transmitted as a recessive characteristic[4279] or occurs sporadically. The mutiple genotypes (1q22–q23; 17p11.2; 10q21.q22; 8q23.q24) indicate the heterogeneity of the disorder.

Pupillary changes, optic atrophy, deafness and pigmentary retinal degeneration, hoarse voice, hypotonia, and bulbar weakness have been variously described in some kinships with HMSN 3.[2446] The condition has been subdivided according to the presence of hypomyelination and onion bulbs, the absence of myelin, and a congenital neuronal form.[335,1345]

The first postmortem examination in this condition was performed by **Déjèrine** on a patient of his who had died and had been buried for 4 days before he arranged her exhumation; the weather at the time being extremely cold, he found the body in a perfect state of preservation, allowing him to confirm the nerve enlargement.[4928]

Clinical variants include the following:

Congenital hypomyelination neuropathy A form with congenital onset, severe hypomyelination and the presence of atypical onion bulbs.[2346] Clinically, hypotonia, arthrogryposis, and severe weakness are seen. In yet other cases, neither myelin nor onion bulbs are present.

Hypertrophic neuropathy with facial weakness and kyphoscoliosis A form with onset in early adult life, presenting with trigeminal neuralgia, facial spasm, and palsy in addition to the usual findings.

Hereditary auditory, motor, vestibular, and sensory neuropathy In this complex condition with these features, linkage to 8q24 has been achieved.[855]

Hereditary motor and sensory neuropathy type 4 (Refsum disease, heredoataxic hemeralopic polyneuritis, heredopathia atactica polyneuritiformis, phytanic acid storage disease) A recessively transmitted inborn error of metabolism marked by the accumulation of exogenous phytanic acid due to a defect of the alpha oxidation mechanism of β-methyl-substituted fatty acids.

Clinically, the onset is in childhood with hypertrophic sensorimotor neuropathy, pigmentary retinal degeneration with concentric constriction of the visual fields and night blindness, cerebellar ataxia, ichthyosis, and increased CSF protein and blood phytanic acid levels. Pupillary abnormalities, cataract, anosmia, nerve deafness, epiphyseal abnormalities, and electrocardiographic abnormalities are sometimes associated.[4631]

Variants include the following:

Hypertrophic interstitial neuropathy with cataracts A congenital sensorimotor demyelinating hypertrophic neuropathy with cataract and kyphosis.

Adult Refsum disease variant with impaired pipecolic acid oxidation A rare syndrome with the Refsum disease phenotype but with evidence of both mitochondrial and peroxisomal disorders, such as raised levels of pipecolic as well as of phytanic acid.[5622]

Hereditary motor and sensory neuropathy type 5 (HMSN with spasticity) is a dominantly inherited sensorimotor demyelinating hypertrophic neuropathy with onset in infancy, childhood, or youth, also characterized by spasticity and pes cavus.[1576,1965,2447]

Hereditary motor and sensory neuropathy type 6 (HMSN with optic atrophy) is a recessively inherited sensorimotor axonal or demyelinating hypertrophic neuropathy with onset in early childhood, complicated by deafness, nystagmus, and optic atrophy.[3873] Features of HMSN 5 and 6 may coexist.[1447] In a *variant* form, the neuropathic element is minimal and lancinating pains suggest the presence of a sensory neuropathy.[959]

Hereditary motor and sensory neuropathy type 7 (HMSN with pigmentary retinopathy) is a syndrome of HMSN with onset in childhood or adult life and with the added features of ataxia, pigmentary retinopathy, and sometimes sensorineural deafness and radiological evidence of cerebellar atrophy.

The cases reported thus resemble *HMSN type 4* (Refsum disease) but lack a detectable biochemical abnormality and peripheral nerve hypertrophy. Biopsy specimens show a reduction in the numbers of myelinated fibers without onion bulb formation.[5660]

To this classification may be added other *variant* forms:

A form mapping to Xq13 (*X-linked HMSN type 2 with deafness and mental retardation*) The onset is in infancy or childhood and sensorineural deafness and mental and developmental delay are present.[337]

HMSN with peripheral neurofibromatosis A hypertrophic, demyelinating, sensorimotor neuropathy with onset in infancy or childhood, manifesting also sensorineural deafness, seizures, café-au-lait spots, and neurofibromas.[337]

HMSN with epilepsy A form of HMSN with congenital onset, manifesting developmental delay, cerebellar ataxia, chorea, athetosis, and seizures.[337]

HMSN with arthrogryposis A rare *variant* form of HMSN with congenital onset.[6097]

HMSN with heart block A rare *variant* form of HMSN complicated by cardiomyopathy.[3283]

See also **scapuloperoneal syndrome, hereditary neuropathy with liability to pressure palsies.**

hereditary motor and sensory neuropathy with corneal dystrophy   See **hereditary motor and sensory neuropathy, type 1.**

hereditary motor and sensory neuropathy with continuous motor unit activity   See **hereditary motor and sensory neuropathy, type 1.**

hereditary motor and sensory neuropathy with dementia and dysautonomia   See **hereditary motor and sensory neuropathy, type 2.**

hereditary motor and sensory neuropathy with myopathy   See **hereditary motor and sensory neuropathy, type 2.**

hereditary motor and sensory neuropathy with optic atrophy   See **hereditary motor and sensory neuropathy, type 6.**

hereditary motor and sensory neuropathy with pigmentary retinopathy   See **hereditary motor and sensory neuropathy, type 7.**

hereditary motor and sensory neuropathy with spasticity   See **hereditary motor and sensory neuropathy, type 5.**

hereditary motor neuropathies (HMN; distal hereditary motor neuronopathies) Recessively inherited disorders, characterized by weakness and wasting due to selective degeneration of the motor neurons. The first four major forms defined were all thought to be allelic on chromosome 5q (5q11.2–13.3.), but with many variants. New forms continue to be detected.

The term *spinal muscular atrophy* has been applied to many of these conditions, as shown in Chart H–8, but in this book that term will be used with reference to the acquired rather than to the inherited forms. The following classification is after Harding and Thomas.[2446]

Chart H–8. Classification of the Hereditary Motor Neuropathies

Hereditary motor neuropathy type 1 (severe/acute Werdnig-Hoffman disease, acute infantile spinal muscular atrophy type 1, infantile neuronal degeneration, amyotonia congenita, hereditary poliodystrophy) is a recessively inherited, fatal degenerative disease affecting bulbar and spinal motor nuclei with onset at birth or in the first 6 months of life, and manifesting generalized symmetrical weakness and fasciculations but with sparing of type 1 fibers in muscle biopsy specimens using ATPase stains. The responsible gene maps to chromosome 5 (5q11.2).

The disease was first described by Werdnig in 1891; Hoffmann later reported its familial nature.[2601,5918] Instances of adult-onset **amyotrophic lateral sclerosis** have been recorded in the same families.

The following criteria for the diagnosis of *spinal muscular atrophy, type 1* have been suggested:[1063]

1. Clinical symptoms of anterior horn cell disease: areflexia or hyporeflexia, muscle atrophy, fasciculations
2. Early onset and progressive course: age at onset, $<1/2$ year; age at death, <4 years; never able to sit unsupported
3. Creatine kinase normal: <10 times higher than reference value
4. Electromyographic study shows signs of anterior horn cell involvement
5. Muscle biopsy findings are compatible with those of anterior horn cell disease.
6. Exclusion criteria:
   No symptoms of other neurological systems: no sensory loss, no central motor neuron symptoms, no mental retardation
   No arthrogryposis
   No evident facial involvement
   No other major organ involvement

Variant forms include the following:

1. A form with atrial and ventricular septal defects and joint contractures.[3914]
2. A form with pathological evidence of sensory fiber involvement.[4531]
3. *Cervical spinal muscular atrophy* A variant considered to be due to a restricted form of hereditary motor neuropathy resulting in progressive muscle wasting of the arms but generalized hyporeflexia and EMG evidence of widespread denervation.[2235]
4. A nonprogressive congenital variant considered to be due to an infarct or malformation of the lower cervical spinal cord, resulting in muscle wasting and contractures of the arms.[1294]
5. *Congenital Werdnig-Hoffman disease with glial bundles in the spinal roots* Whether this is a distinct variant is uncertain, since any form of HMN 1 may be associated with these glial bundles, but the bundles are not necessarily the cause of the disease, which is an anterior horn cell degeneration.[3914]
6. *Infantile neuronal degeneration* A recessively inherited form clinically resembling HMN 1, in which there is additional widespread neuronal loss and gliosis in both the gray and white matter in the thalamus, pons, cerebellum, and spinal cord and segmental demyelination in the peripheral nerves,[5331] as in **infantile neuroaxonal dystrophy.**
7. *Dominant congenital benign spinal musular atrophy* A nonprogressive form of neurogenic weakness with leg contractures.[1962]

Hereditary motor neuropathy type 2 (early-onset spinal muscular atrophy, chronic or arrested Werdnig-Hoffmann disease, intermediate spinal muscular atrophy, infantile spinal muscular atrophy, arrested; chronic infantile form) is a recessively inherited, degenerative disease affecting bulbar and spinal motor nuclei with onset at or after 6 months of age and manifesting progressive, symmetrical, mainly proximal weakness and fasciculations, mild distal tremor, pes cavus, kyphoscoliosis, and contractures leading to crippling but with survival at least to 3 years of age and sometimes even into adult life.[2327] Mapping to 12q24 has been achieved in a distal form.

In *variant* forms[335] (*1*) there is dominant inheritance of a slowly progressive chronic motor neuropathy with more pelvic than shoulder girdle involvement;[6119] (*2*) *infantile spinal muscular atrophy, arrested*, a nonprogressive form, is complicated by contractures.[1887]

Hereditary motor neuropathy type 3 (juvenile or pseudomyopathic spinal muscular atrophy, [Wohlfart-] Kugelberg-Welander disease, chronic juvenile amyotrophic lateral sclerosis) is a slowly progressive degenerative disease affecting spinal more than bulbar motor nuclei with usual onset between the ages of 5 and 15 years and manifesting progressive symmetrical, mainly proximal weakness with fasciculations, ophthalmoplegia and eventually kyphoscoliosis, cardiomyopathy, and contractures, but with survival into middle age or later, and without sensory signs.[3183,6015] The responsible gene maps to chromosome 5 (5q11.2).

When the disease is purely of the lower motor neuron type and has its onset before 24 months, the transmission is usually dominant; after that age, transmission is usually recessive. When the disease shows both upper and lower motor neuron features, inheritance is recessive.

Variant forms include the following:

1. *Juvenile spinal muscular atrophy with hexosaminidase A deficiency* (*GM_2 ganglioside*) A recessively inherited form with the particular features of onset in youth, cognitive dysfunction, postural tremor, muscle pain or cramps, and neuronal inclusions.[3916,6119]
2. A form in which the signs involve both proximal and distal muscles, and the course is rapid. This has only been reported from Papua, New Guinea.[5041]
3. *Juvenile spinal proximal muscular atrophy* Usually recessively inherited, but both dominant[4383] and X-linked forms[5658] have been reported.
4. A form in which progressive external ophthalmoplegia is associated.
5. Further variants include the **monomelic** form, which is usually sporadic;[5250] spinal muscular atrophy with **fa-**

cioscapulohumeral distribution,[1782] of which there is an X-linked variety (Skre syndrome);[5206] and Hirayama-type juvenile muscular atrophy, characterized by the rapid appearance of self-limited distal amyotrophy of one arm in young men.[2585]

Hereditary motor neuropathy type 4 (juvenile onset) is an uncommon, dominantly inherited variant in which the onset occurs between the ages of 6 months and 15 years, the course is slow, and the outcome benign.[4383]

Hereditary motor neuropathy type 5 (adult spinal muscular atrophy) includes forms of HMN with autosomal recessive (seldom dominant) inheritance and onset in early adult life, presenting with cramps, atrophy, and neurogenic weakness complicated variously by such features as truncal ataxia, myotonia, hydrocephalus ex vacuo, or external hydrocephalus. Mapping to 7p has been achieved.

Variants are the following:

A *proximal spinal muscular atrophy* which may have dominant, recessive, or X-linked inheritance,[4677] and another form presenting in the context of **GM₂ gangliosidosis.**[4082]

Motor neuronopathy affecting predominantly the hands A dominantly inherited condition mapped to gene 7p (but heterogeneous) with onset in youth of asymmetric distal weakness and wasting of the hands more than of the feet in the absence of sensory disturbances or pyramidal signs.

Other *variants* of the above syndromes include the following:

1. Forms with associated lesions of the nervous system

Anterior horn cell disease with cerebellar hypoplasia in infants A syndrome consisting of severe mental retardation, cortical blindness, and extensive peripheral paralysis of the lower motor neuron type and representing a combination of HMN 1 with extreme hypoplasia and atrophy of the cerebellum and of the ventral part of the pons.[2234]

Anterior horn cell disease with pontocerebellar hypoplasia A congenital form with the particular features of contractures; facial, bulbar, trunk, and limb weakness; abnormal motor conduction speeds with segmental demyelination; and pathological changes in the cerebellum, pons, medulla, and basal ganglia.

Amyotrophic dystonic paraplegia[2121]

Amyotrophic lateral sclerosis and *variants*

Amyotrophic lateral sclerosis–parkinsonism–dementia complex of Guam

Amyotrophic lateral sclerosis with dementia[4454]

Amyotrophic lateral sclerosis with autosomal dominant familial parkinsonism[713]

Amyotrophic lateral sclerosis with Pick disease[1382]

Arthrogryposis multiplex congenita 1. The neurogenic form with distal involvement.[2380] The neurogenic form with pulmonary hypoplasia. 2. A recessive form with renal and hepatic abnormalities and rarefaction of the anterior horns.[4125] 3. A distal, X-linked form including one type with anterior horn cell disease;[2380] other forms are attributed to nonprogressive intrauterine myopathy or connective tissue disease.

Bulbar spinal muscular atrophy of childhood (see **Fazio-Londe syndrome**)

Bulbar palsy with deafness (see **Vialetto–van Laere syndrome**)

Bulbar palsy with deafness and pigmentary retinopathy.

Bulbar palsy with olivopontocerebellar atrophy, (see **cerebellar ataxias**)

Chronic asymmetrical spinal muscular atrophy A form with onset in young adult life and with the particular features of asymmetrical muscle atrophy, muscle pain or cramps, fasciculations, and neurogenic weakness.[2442]

Chronic spinal muscular atrophy with pallidonigral degeneration A recessively (occasionally dominantly) inherited form with the addition of resting tremor, akinesia, and cogwheel rigidity without myoclonus or dementia, with severe degenerative lesions in the pallidum and substantia nigra.

Clinically, there are fasciculations, proximal limb weakness, hyporeflexia or areflexia, and extrapyramidal syndromes including resting tremor, akinesia, and cogwheel rigidity. Evidence of neurogenic atrophy is obtained from EMG and from muscle biopsy specpcimens. Neurofibrillary degeneration is not present and there is no pathology resembling that of **amyotrophic lateral sclerosis.** The condition is regarded as a chronic spinopallidonigral degeneration because of the neuronal loss in the anterior horns, the globus pallidus, and the substantia nigra without **Lewy bodies** or neurofibrillary degeneration.[5075]

Congenital lower motor neuron disease with arthrogryposis A form with the particular features of lordosis, scoliosis, club foot, varus joint contractures, and neurogenic trunk and limb weakness.

Adult proximal spinal muscular atrophy (Finkel late-onset type of spinal muscular atrophy included) Clinically, this is not different from recessive and X-linked forms.

Hereditary muscular atrophy with ataxia, retinitis pigmentosa, and diabetes mellitus A syndrome inherited as a dominant characteristic, with onset in adolescence and a slowly progressive course.[1999] See also **NARP.**

Hereditary motor and sensory neuropathy, type 2 (neurogenic form)

Kuskokwim disease

Progressive spinal muscular atrophy with chorea and deafness

Progressive muscular atrophy with chorea and optic atrophy

Spinal muscular atrophy with amyotrophic lateral sclerosis Both recessive[2447] and dominant forms are described, the latter malignant, progressive, and resembling typical severe **amyotrophic lateral sclerosis.**[3597]

Spinocerebellar ataxia and deafness

Spinal muscular atrophy, optic atrophy, and deafness

Spinal muscular atrophy with deafness

Distal spinal muscular atrophy with vocal cord paralysis[6092]

Spinal muscular atrophy with Joseph disease (Azorean ataxia, **Joseph disease,** spinopontine atrophy, nigrospinodentatal degeneration)[4789]

Spinal muscular atrophy with **olivopontocerebellar atrophy,** type 4[3252]

Spinal muscular atrophy with bulbar palsy[1476]

Spinal muscular atrophy with ophthalmoplegia

Spinal muscular atrophy with retinitis pigmentosa

Spinal muscular atrophy with retinitis pigmentosa and hereditary spastic paraplegia

Spinal muscular atrophy with microcephaly and mental retardation A form with the particular features of microcephaly, deafness, mental and developmental delay, and onset in infancy.[5293]

Spinal muscular atrophy with mental retardation

Spinal muscular atrophy, mental retardation, seizures, and orofacial dysplasia

Spinal muscular atrophy with myoclonus A slowly progressive form of spinal muscular atrophy also manifesting stimulus-sensitive myoclonus.[2811]

Spinal muscular atrophy with oculopharyngeal muscular atrophy A form with onset in young adult life and with the particular features of ptosis, ophthalmoplegias, bulbar weakness, myopathic face, fasciculations, neurogenic muscle weakness, and raised creatine kinase levels, and with variable fiber diameter and increased endomysial connective tissue on muscle biopsy.

Spinal muscular atrophy with recessive spinocerebellar degeneration (**Friedreich ataxia**)[5707] The condition may be due to peripheral neuropathy (**hereditary motor and sensory neuropathy, type 2**) rather than to anterior horn cell disease.

Spinocerebellar ataxia with rigidity and peripheral neuropathy A variant form with fasciculations and parkinsonism as well as signs of peripheral motor neuropathy.[6126] See also **hereditary motor and sensory neuropathy, type 2 with parkinsonism.**

Troyer syndrome See **hereditary spastic paraplegia.**

Neuronal intranuclear hyaline inclusion disease A single sporadic case, manifest by amyotrophy, dementia, seizures, choreoathetosis, and sphincter disorder.

Spastic paraplegia with amyotrophy of hands (Silver disease) A rare, dominantly or recessively inherited variant with childhood or early adult onset manifesting pyramidal signs in the legs and global wasting of the small hand muscles. Other neurological signs have also been recorded.[5159]

Distal spinal muscular atrophy Sporadic or recessive forms that may be confined to the hands.[4198]

Spinal muscular atrophy in **xeroderma pigmentosum**

Spinal muscular atrophy in **infantile neuroaxonal dystrophy** (Seitelberger disease)

Spinal muscular atrophy in amyotrophic choreoacanthocytosis (see **neuroacanthocytosis**) Both autosomal recessive and autosomal dominant inheritance patterns are described.

Spinal muscular atrophy with **Huntington disease**[1916]

Spinal muscular atrophy with lysosomal enzyme deficiencies A recessively inherited syndrome.[2230]

Spinal muscular atrophy with **phenylketonuria** A recessively inherited syndrome.[3811]

Spinal muscular atrophy with hydroxyisovaleric aciduria A recessively inherited syndrome.[1631]

Amyotrophic lateral sclerosis *with luysopallidonigral atrophy*[2261]

Spinal muscular atrophy with pallidonigral degeneration[5075]

2. Forms with distinct regional involvement:

Hereditary motor neuropathy affecting the arms A slowly progressive demyelinating motor neuropathy affecting only the distal motor nerves of the arms.[3249]

Chronic neurogenic quadriceps amyotrophy

Distal and segmental muscular atrophy of upper extremities A form with the particular features of fasciculations, muscle atrophy, neurogenic weakness, and sensory neuropathy with paresthesia and without any typical inheritance pattern.[4384]

Distal spinal muscular atrophy A form with onset at any age, from infancy to adult life, and with the particular features of high arches of the feet, bulbar as well as distal involvement, retention of muscle stretch reflexes, and resting tremor. Both dominant and recessive inheritance have been described. Motor nerve conduction velocities suggest primary neuronal involvement.[2445] See **hereditary motor and sensory neuropathy, type 2.**

Distal spinal muscular atrophy with a hoarse voice A form with the particular features of onset in childhood, youth, or young adult life and presentation with hoarseness as a result of recurrent laryngeal nerve involvement.[6092] In this syndrome, ragged red fibers have been detected.[335]

Facioscapulohumeral atrophy A dominantly inherited neurogenic form resembling facioscapulohumeral dystrophy, with onset in childhood or youth.[1782]

Familial **amyotrophic lateral sclerosis**

Fazio-Londe syndrome[1753]

Focal cervical poliopathy of distal arm (*juvenile muscular atrophy of unilateral upper extremity*) A condition with a benign course, usually reported from Japan, in which the anterior horns of the spinal cord between C5 and T1 show shrinkage and necrosis of large and small nerve cells and mild gliosis. A circulatory disorder is considered the likely cause.[2584]

Infantile spinal muscular atrophy in **incontinentia pigmenti** An X-Linked dominant form, lethal in males.[3281]

Juvenile bulbar spinal muscular atrophy See **Fazio-Londe syndrome.**

Monomelic spinal muscular atrophy

Multiple contracture syndrome See **Pena-Shokeir phenotype.**

Neuropathy–motor neuron disease with visual pathway disorder

Oculopharyngeal spinal muscular atrophy A rare, dominantly inherited variant manifesting external ophthalmoplegia, bulbar signs, and distal weakness and wasting, manifesting first in early adult life.[3702]

Progressive ophthalmoplegia in Kugelberg-Welander disease A form with the particular features of ptosis, ophthalmoplegias, and bulbar weakness, with onset in early childhood.[26]

Scapuloperoneal atrophy (Stark-Kaeser syndrome) A dominant, recessive, or X-linked syndrome characterized by slowly progressive neurogenic weakness and wasting in this distribution.[2900] The phenotypes have been reviewed by Baraitser.[335]

Scapuloperoneal atrophy, cardiopathy, and inflammatory myopathy The neurogenic status of this form is not certain, as there is a definite myopathic component.[2839] See also **Emery-Dreifuss syndrome** (autosomal dominant form).[3886]

Spinal muscular atrophy and pallidonigral degeneration A form with the particular added features of pyramidal signs, rigidity, and rest or postural tremor, with onset in mature adult life.

Spinal muscular atrophy, **Ryukyuan type.**

Spinal muscular atrophy (HMSN) with calf hypertrophy A form with the particular features of onset in young adult life, muscle hypertrophy, pain and cramp, raised creatine kinase levels, and slow progression.[688] Duplication of 17p.11.2 has been reported in this condition.

Forms with limb girdle, **scapuloperoneal,** *or peroneal distribution*

X-linked variety (Kennedy disease, spinobulbar muscular atrophy): A form mapping to Xq21.3–q12, presenting clinically in young adult life with bulbospinal weakness and atrophy, and testicular failure. See **X-linked bulbospinal muscular atrophy.**

Spinal muscular atrophy due to mitochondrial disease A form in which the picture of spinal muscular atrophy is accompanied by cardiomyopathy and cytochrome oxidase (COX) deficiency.[4843]

A recessively inherited form with weakness and atrophy of the legs and pyramidal features, with onset in childhood and linked to a mutation at chromosome 9p21.1–p12.[1029]

See also **Vialetto–van Laere syndrome, Fazio-Londe disease.** Other, acquired forms are noted under **spinal muscular atrophy.**

hereditary motor neuronopathy affecting the arms See **hereditary motor neuropathy** (*variants*).

hereditary motor system disease (chronic juvenile amyotrophic lateral sclerosis) A recessively inherited, slowly progressive syndrome with the onset in childhood or youth of bilateral pyramidal and lower motor neuron signs affecting bulbar and spinal muscles and without sensory loss.[2403]

hereditary multi-infarct dementia See **familial subcortical dementia with arteriosclerotic leukoencephalopathy.**[5259]

hereditary multiple exostoses A dyschondroplasia, usually dominantly inherited, characterized clinically by the development of multiple osteogenic exostoses from the metaphyses of long bones more often than from other bones. Neurological involvement may include paraparesis resulting from cord compression.[1795] The condition was first described by Stanley in 1894.

hereditary muscular atrophy with ataxia, retinitis pigmentosa, and diabetes mellitus See **hereditary motor neuropathy** (*variants*).

hereditary myoclonic dystonia (hereditary dystonia with lightning jerks responsive to alcohol) A dominantly inherited syndrome with childhood onset, characterized by dystonia and myoclonus affecting mainly the neck and arms. Both kinds of abnormal movement respond dramatically to alcohol ingestion.[4563]

A similar syndrome (but with onset in adult life) was reported by Davidenkow in 1926.

hereditary myoclonic encephalopathy A recessively inherited **mitochondrial encephalomyelopathy.** See **Unverricht-Lundborg-Lafora syndrome.**

hereditary myoclonus and progressive distal muscular atrophy A dominantly inherited multifocal neuronal degeneration of adult life characterized by **stimulus-sensitive myoclonus** and slowly progressive distal neurogenic muscle atrophy.

Bulbar weakness, extrapyramidal signs, myoclonus, neurogenic muscle atrophy and weakness, raised serum creatine kinase levels, and paroxysmal EEG discharges are other features described.[2811]

hereditary myokymia (normocalcemic tetany) A dominantly inherited syndrome of generalized myokymia and muscle cramping without evidence of peripheral neuropathy, typically with spontaneous, regularly recurring bursts of motor unit potentials arising distally in the nerve fibers.[260,5108]

hereditary myokymia and muscle stiffness A syndrome of continuous involuntary quivering of muscles causing movements in the eye, face, and limbs. In cases of generalized muscle stiffness and delayed relaxation, the term **neuromyotonia** has been applied (see **idiopathic neuromyotonia, myokymia**).[260,2015,2343,3500]

Most cases are without familial occurrence; familial cases usually have an associated peripheral neuropathy.

hereditary myokymia with periodic (episodic) ataxia (Van Dyke Hanson syndrome) A rare, dominantly inherited syndrome of childhood onset paroxysmal ataxia lasting 1–2 minutes and induced by vestibular stimulation, movement or shock; the movements probably represent an epileptic manifestation.

Other features include persistent widespread myokymia which supervenes in youth and affects the face, hands, arms, and legs: truncal shaking or jerking movements of the head, arms, and legs; carpopedal spasms; and lower motor neuron disease without overt peripheral neuropathy. The condition is considered to represent a form of motor neuropathy on the basis of muscle biopsy findings.[5725]

hereditary myopathy limited to females A slowly progressive dominantly inherited limb-girdle type of muscular dystrophy with onset in childhood or early adult life and expression limited to females, in which muscle biopsy specimens reveal isolated muscle fiber necrosis and phagocytosis.[2546]

hereditary nephritis and nerve deafness (distal muscle wasting, nephritis and deafness) A syndrome featuring evidence of both **hereditary motor and sensory neuropathy** and **Alport syndrome.**[2422]

hereditary neuralgic amyotrophy See **neuralgic amyotrophy.**

hereditary neurocutaneous vascular malformation The association of intracranial arteriovenous malformations with cutaneous hemangiomas, in the absence of retinal lesions. The condition has been reviewed by Baraitser.[335]

hereditary neuromyotonia See **neuromyotonia.**

hereditary neuropathy with liability to pressure palsies See **hereditary pressure-sensitive neuropathy.**

hereditary nonprogressive athetotic hemiplegia A congenital syndrome, dominantly inherited and nonprogressive after childhood, characterized by congenital left-sided hemihypoplasia, hemiparesis, and hypertonicity; left hand athetosis after the age of 8 years; and right-sided cerebral atrophy or hypoplasia.[2349]

hereditary nonprogressive chorea (hereditary benign chorea, benign familial chorea; OMIM 118700) A rare, dominantly inherited, nonprogressive and eventually self-limiting syndrome characterized by the appearance in childhood or adult life of chorea, athetosis, and gait and limb ataxia without current or subsequent intellectual or neurological impairment. It is linked to chromosome 14q.[1793]

The condition is associated with striatal hypometabolism,[2366] but no abnormality is detected on cerebral imaging.[1731] In *variant forms*, **essential tremor** or some intellectual deficits do occur.[3337] See **chorea, Huntington disease.**

hereditary nystagmus   See **congenital nystagmus.**

hereditary parkinsonism and neuropathy   See **hereditary motor neuropathy** (*spinocerebellar ataxia with rigidity and peripheral neuropathy*), **hereditary motor and sensory neuropathy, type 2** with parkinsonism, **parkinsonism-plus.**

hereditary parkinsonism-dystonia   See **dopa-responsive dystonia.**

hereditary paroxysmal ataxia   A dominantly inherited syndrome characterized by the onset in childhood of paroxysmal bouts of ataxia, dysarthria, and nystagmus, lasting 1–6 hours on a weekly basis and responsive to acetazolamide.[2284]

hereditary persistent distal cramps   A dominantly inherited syndrome of muscle cramps involving distal muscle groups with accompanying continuous muscle discharges that wax and wane. Clinically, the condition is marked by intermittent painful stiffness of the intrinsic hand muscles and of the calves. The cause is unknown.[2896]

hereditary photomyoclonus   A dominantly inherited syndrome consisting of deafness, diabetes mellitus, nephropathy, and light-sensitive seizures with dementia. The pathological features resemble those of **subacute spongiform encephalopathy.**[2551]

hereditary piebaldness and congenital deafness   An autosomal or sex-linked recessive disorder manifesting depigmentation of the head and arms with pigmented spots, congenital neural deafness, and normal vestibular function.[6035]

hereditary poliodystrophy   See **hereditary motor neuropathy.**

hereditary polycystic osteodysplasia with progressive dementia   A rare, recessively inherited syndrome characterized by the onset in young adult life of bone pain, ankle and wrist swelling, pyramidal signs, myoclonic and other seizures, and dementia.[44]

hereditary polyneuropathy, oligophrenia, premature menopause, and acromicria   A syndrome of slowly progressive paresis in the hands and feet, starting in childhood and leading to moderate incapacity; areflexia; reduced motor nerve conduction velocity; oligophrenia; premature menopause without hypophyseal failure; and disproportionate smallness, with short arms and legs and acromicria.[3518]

hereditary pressure-sensitive neuropathy   (hereditary recurrent pressure palsies, hereditary neuropathy with liability to pressure palsies [HNPP], tomaculous neuropathy, familial recurrent pressure palsy, familial recurrent polyneuropathy)[4395,5075] A dominantly inherited syndrome of young adult life characterized by unusual sensitivity of the peripheral nerves to intercurrent pressure (probably as a result of subclinical polyneuropathy), leading to painless, temporary, but still prolonged conduction block.[1595,3561,5513] A deletion at 17p11.2–12 has been detected, the same site as that involved in HMSN 1A, but the condition is genetically heterogeneous.

There may be associated electrophysiological evidence of a generalized neuropathy as well as local conduction block at the site of nerve compression. A wide range of symptoms is described, from numbness, paresthesias, or absent reflexes to paralysis and objective sensory loss. The ulnar, median, radial, and common peroneal nerves are those most commonly affected, but any nerve is at risk, including the fifth and eighth cranial nerves. Even such trivial compressive traumas as using scissors, knitting, squatting, plaster casts, and wearing tight shoes have been incriminated.

Biopsy specimens show a **tomaculous neuropathy** with axonal loss. The syndrome of **familial (or hereditary) neuralgic amyotrophy** may be associated but is not the same condition.[1347,2232]

In variant forms, the syndrome is manifest as recurrent brachial plexus palsies,[5362] or is sporadic.[4650]

hereditary proximal spinal muscular atrophy   See **hereditary motor neuropathy.**

hereditary putaminal necrosis   A dominantly inherited degenerative syndrome characterized by bilateral isolated necrosis of the putamen and globus pallidus with vascular proliferation and gliovascular lesions in the thalamus.

Clinically, the syndrome is first expressed in infancy, the major findings being psychomotor retardation and increasing apathy with seizures, inability to lift the head from the pillow, difficulties with swallowing and eating, and apparent blindness. Various movement disorders are described in some kinships, including pyramidal syndromes, athetosis, and ataxia.

The disorder has also been described with onset in later life.[1521] See also **infantile bilateral striatal necrosis.**

hereditary quivering of the chin   (geniospasm, hereditary chin trembling, trembling chin) A congenital, dominantly inherited syndrome (chromosome 9q) characterized by transient fine tremors of the mentalis muscles occurring during emotional stimulation; they disappear in calmness and sleep and go away with increasing age.[1952,4786]

In *variant forms*, nystagmus and nocturnal myoclonus have also been described.[2219] In fact, the disorder may be a form of localized myoclonus.[1421]

hereditary recurrent focal neuropathy See **hereditary pressure-sensitive neuropathy.**

hereditary recurrent pressure palsies See **hereditary pressure-sensitive neuropathy.**

hereditary sensory and autonomic neuropathy (HSAN) A group of similar sensory neuropathies which may be classified as shown in Chart H–9 (compiled after Dyck[1567] and Donaghy et al.[1488]).

Chart H–9. Classification of the Hereditary Sensory and Autonomic Neuropathies

Autosomal Dominant Inheritance

Dominantly inherited sensory neuropathy (Denny Brown or Hicks neuropathy, HSAN 1 of Dyck, hereditary sensory radicular neuropathy, hereditary perforating ulcers of the feet, familial mutilating ulcerative acropathy, hereditary lumbosacral syringomyelia, familial neurogenic osteoacrolysis, hereditary sensory neuropathy with peroneal muscular atrophy, acrodystrophic neuronopathy)[1391,2564] is a dominantly inherited sensory more than motor neuropathy with onset in childhood, youth, or early adult life, also manifesting autonomic signs, and sometimes sensorineural deafness, neurogenic muscle atrophy, particular loss of pain and temperature sensations, spontaneous lancinating pains, multiple fractures, and mutilating acropathy.[1392,1682] Genetic linkage to 9q22.1–q22.3 has been established.

Personal observations of kinships in Newfoundland (as in France[1526]) indicate that there may also be notable lower motor neuron involvement.

Variants include the following:

HSAN 1 with spastic paraplegia A dominantly inherited sensory neuropathy with congenital or childhood onset of loss of pain, temperature and touch sensations leading to mutilating acropathy, neurogenic bladder, spasticity, and both myelinated and unmyelinated fiber loss.[942]

Hereditary sensory neuropathy with deafness A form with sensorineural deafness. Dementia[2656] and ataxia have also been recorded as complications but in such cases, widespread cell loss and gliosis in other areas suggest that this may represent a form of **familial multisystem atrophy.** In a related form, loss of gastric motility is also described.

Ulcerative mutilating acropathy with abnormal CSF amino acids An inherited sensory neuropathy with onset in youth, manifesting also loss of pain, temperature, and touch sensations; incontinence; and generalized skin atrophy.

Hereditary sensorimotor neuropathy with ulceromutilation A form similar to the prototype above but without genetic linkage to it (see www.neuro.wustl.edu/neuromuscular/sensory-large+small.html).

Autosomal Recessive Inheritance

Congenital sensory neuropathy (HSAN type 2 of Dyck, lumbosacral syringomyelia, congenital insensitivity/indiffer-

ence to pain) A slowly progressive form of HSAN in which all modes of sensation are affected from the earliest years and in which lancinating pains are frequent.[4049,4225] Both progressive and nonprogressive forms have been described.

The phenomenon of *congenital insensitivity to pain* (CIP) resembles this neuropathy in its manifestations but a central origin seems more likely,[1910] especially because the sensory nerve action potentials are missing in this form but not in CIP, spontaneous pains are common, and there is in HSAN 2 a graded reduction of sensation centrifugally in the limbs, the trunk remaining sensitive.

Variants with **tonic pupils** or with dominant inheritance have also been described.

Familial dysautonomia (Riley-Day syndrome, HSAN type 3 of Dyck, congenital insensitivity to pain with dysautonomia) An inherited sensory and autonomic axonal neuropathy with congenital onset. The major clinical features include short stature, sparse and depigmented hair, absent or sparse tears, optic atrophy, nerve deafness, smooth tongue with loss of the fungiform papillae, kyphoscoliosis, hyporeflexia, loss of pain and temperature sensations, impaired temperature control, hyperhidrosis, orthostatic hypotension, and loss of the histamine flare in the skin. Nerve biopsy specimens show both myelinated and unmyelinated fiber loss.[53,4695] Mapping to 9q31–q33 has been achieved.

A *variant dominant form* with onset in the fifth decade manifesting ataxia as well is also described (www.wustl.edu/neuromuscular/sensory-small.html).

Congenital insensitivity to pain with anhidrosis (HSAN 4 of Dyck, hereditary anhidrotic sensory neuropathy, syndrome of the neural crest, familial dysautonomia type 2): A sensory neuropathy (or a developmental disorder?) with congenital or early childhood onset. The major clinical features are loss of pain, temperature, and touch sensation with self-mutilation, poor temperature control, multiple fractures, hypohidrosis, cutaneous ulcers, and intellectual impairment. Nerve biopsy specimens show loss of both small myelinated and unmyelinated fibers.[5436] Mapping to 1q21–q22 has been achieved.

Variants are described with dominant inheritance, or with a nonprogressive course.[4155]

HSAN with spastic paraplegia: (Cavanagh variant) A recessively inherited sensory neuropathy with congenital or childhood onset of loss of pain, temperature and touch sensations, neurogenic bladder, spasticity, and both myelinated and unmyelinated fiber loss. This condition resembles the dominantly inherited variety but is more severe.[942]

HSAN with neurotrophic keratitis A congenital syndrome of loss of pain and temperature sensations with mutilating acropathy, corneal ulceration and opacification, and anhidrosis.[1488]

HSAN with predominant loss of small myelinated fibers

X-linked Inheritance Pattern

HSAN, X-linked An otherwise typical form of sensory neuropathy with onset in infancy, childhood, or youth of loss of pain, touch, and temperature sensations, complicated by neuropathic deformity and ulceration of the feet, joint stiffness and arthritis, abnormal sensory conductions, and pathologically a loss of myelinated fibers. The condition is marked by minimal involvement of the muscle stretch reflexes and absence of autonomic involvement.[2856] The gene lies in the dxys 1–p58–1 region of the X chromosome.[4837]

Other Forms

Sensory neuropathy with hereditary ataxia (congenital sensory neuropathy with selective loss of small myelinated fibers, congenital insensitivity to pain, HSAN type 5 of Dyck) A congenital, dominantly inherited sensory neuropathy with loss of pain and temperature sensations and acropathy, manifesting also cloudy corneas, pupillary abnormalities, hyperactivity, self-mutilation, paroxysmal headache, paresthesias, and flushing, and both myelinated and unmyelinated fiber loss in peripheral nerves.[3484]

Congenital insensitivity to pain A dominantly inherited congenital syndrome consisting of cloudy corneae, hyperactivity, and self-mutilation. Paroxysmal headaches, loss of pain and temperature sensations, paresthesia, and flushing are the other features.[400,2858]

HSAN with dysautonomia and corneal insensitivity A congenital syndrome comprising loss of pain sensation, poor temperature control, absent or sparse tears, flushing, corneal ulceration, and myelinated fiber loss. See **hereditary sensory and autonomic neuropathy** (recessive).

HSAN with tonic pupils A sensory neuropathy with childhood onset in which there is loss of pain and temperature sensations associated with features of the **Holmes-Adie syndrome**.[3887]

Congenital pain asymbolia with auditory imperception A congenital syndrome consisting of auditory agnosia, loss of pain sensation, and speech delay.

In yet other *variant forms*, motor neuropathy, mental retardation, **Friedreich ataxia,** cerebellar degeneration, hypotonia, skeletal dysplasias, and dysmorphism are variously associated. See also **congenital asymbolia, Fabry disease, Tangier disease.**

hereditary sensory and autonomic neuropathy with deafness   See **hereditary sensory and autonomic neuropathy** (dominant).

hereditary sensory and autonomic neuropathy with dysautonomia and corneal insensitivity   See **hereditary sensory and autonomic neuropathy** (other).

hereditary sensory and autonomic neuropathy with neurotrophic keratitis   See **hereditary sensory and autonomic neuropathy** (recessive).

hereditary sensory and autonomic neuropathy with spastic paraplegia   See **hereditary sensory and autonomic neuropathy.**

hereditary sensory and autonomic neuropathy with tonic pupils   See **hereditary sensory and autonomic neuropathy** (other).

hereditary sensory radicular neuropathy   See **hereditary sensory and autonomic neuropathy, type 1**

hereditary spastic ataxia   A dominantly inherited hereditary cerebellar ataxic syndrome of adult life with added pyramidal signs and sometimes retinal degeneration and vestibular impairment.[500] See also **familial spastic ataxia, cerebellar ataxias.**

hereditary spastic dystonia   An inherited dystonic syndrome manifesting also optic atrophy, dystonias and rigidity with evidence of putaminal necrosis on MRI or CT scans. The condition may be a form of **mitochondrial encephalopathy.**[825]

hereditary spastic paraparesis   See **hereditary spastic paraplegia.**

hereditary spastic paraparesis with wasting and growth retardation   See **Troyer syndrome.**

hereditary spastic paraplegia   (HSP; hereditary spastic paraparesis, familial spastic paraplegia, Strümpell-Lorrain syndrome) Inherited degenerative diseases, usually dominantly inherited, with particular effects on the pyramidal tracts and occurring in pure and in complicated forms. The condition was first described by Strümpell in 1880.[5386]

The *"pure" form* (in which there are no other neurological findings) has been mapped variously to chromosomes 2p22–p21 (SPG4; OMIM 182601); 14q11.2q–24.3 (SPG3, OMIM 182600); 15q11.1 (SPG6, OMIM 600363); 8q232–q24 (SPG8, OMIM 603563); 10q23–q24.1 (SPG9, OMIM 601162); 12p13 (SPG10, OMIM 604187); 19q13 (SPG12, OMIM 604805); and 2q24 (SPG13, OMIM 605280). Autosomal dominant is far more common (70%) than autosomal recessive transmission (8p12–q13, SPG5, OMIM 270800; 16q24.3, SPG7, OMIM 602783; 15q13–15, SPG11, OMIM 604360; 3q27–q28, SPG14, OMIM 605229; AR symmetrical spastic cerebral palsy, 2q24–25, OMIM 603513; AR Charlevoix-Saguenay spastic ataxia, 13q12 OMIM 270550) or X-linked (Xq22). In all, about 18 loci have been mapped to date (2001).[5475]

Clinically, the onset is at any age; children show delay in the development of motor skills while adults complain of easy tiring, tripping, and stiffness. In all, typical pyramidal signs are found (mainly in the legs), except that spasticity is especially marked in comparison to the relative preservation of strength. Pes cavus is seen in about a quarter of affected subjects. Sensory complaints are generally lacking, but autopsy findings show posterior column degeneration in some cases.[687,1564] Cognitive decline appears to be associated with the 2p and 8q mutations. The gene responsible for at least SPG4 is spastin.

Dominant forms are SPG 3A, SPG 4, SPG 6, SPG 8, SPG 9, SPG 10, SPG 12, SPG 13, SPG 17 and SPG 19. Most are uncomplicated, though SPG 9 is associated with cataracts, neuropathy, and gastro-esophageal reflux.

The *recessive forms* have numerous phenotypes, including pure HSP with early onset; pure HSP with late onset; HSP with mental retardation; HSP with both mental retardation and peripheral neuropathy; and

HSP with cerebellar ataxia; other CNS and PNS disturbances have also been reported.[1148,5475] The first gene identified for the recessive forms was paraplegin.

X-linked forms (SPG1, Xq28, OMIM 308840; SPG2, Xq22, OMIM 312920; SPG16, Xq11 m2, OMIM 300266) also have numerous additional clinical features.[5475]

The best initial description of this form was that of **Strümpell**[5386] in 1880. A complete review has been published.[3741]

Numerous kinships with clear additional features complicating hereditary spastic paraplegia have been described. In these *"complicated" forms*, amyotrophy resembling that of **hereditary motor and sensory neuropathy;** distal involvement; mental retardation; deafness; optic atrophy; pigmentary retinal degeneration; extrapyramidal features; ataxia and dysarthria; sensory neuropathy; and skin lesions have been detected variously. The compilation in Chart H–10 is based upon Harding's[2439] and Baraitser's[335] reviews of the major *variants*. See also the Web site of the Spastic Paraplegia Foundation (http://www.hspinfo.org/) for further information.

Diagnostic criteria for family members in pure HSP have been suggested, as follows.

Suggested Diagnostic Criteria for Family Members from Families with Pure Hereditary Spastic Paraplegia

Status	Criteria
Definitely affected	Progressive gait disturbance + frank corticospinal tract involvement of lower limbs, including grade 4 hyperreflexia and extensor plantar reflexes
Probably affected	Individuals lacking history of progressive gait disturbance, or asymptomatic individuals with signs of spastic paraparesis. Examined only once and so not proven to have a progressive gait disturbance + frank corticospinal tract involvement of lower limbs, including grade 4 hyperreflexia and extensor plantar reflexes. (Serial examinations may allow recategorization as definitely affected.)
Possibly affected	Asymptomatic + normal gait + questionably abnormal corticospinal tract signs, e.g., mild hyperreflexia, unsustained clonus, but downgoing plantar reflexes
Definitely unaffected	Asymptomatic + normal neurological examination + age greater than maximal age of symptoms in family
Probably unaffected	Asymptomatic + normal neurological examination + age younger than maximal age of symptoms in family

Alternative diagnoses should first be excluded, and the family history should be consistent with autosomal dominant, autosomal recessive, or X-linked recessive inheritance. These criteria are perhaps most useful for standardization in a research setting and are open to criticism. Many definitely affected individuals lack grade 4 hyperreflexia. The criteria for the definitely unaffected category are insufficiently rigorous in view of the wide range in age at onset that may occur in some families

Chart H–10. Variant (Not "Pure") Forms of Hereditary Spastic Paraplegia

Charlevoix-Saguenay syndrome A form that is slowly progressive and recessively inherited with its onset in childhood, characterized by dysarthria, nystagmus, ataxia, pyramidal and posterior column signs, impaired vertical pursuit movements of the eye, and sphincter involvement, reported from Quebec.[676] It is mapped to 13q.11.

Familial spastic paraparesis and deafness A rare X-linked syndrome characterized by short stature, hypogonadism, elevated CSF protein levels, and, in some cases, pigmentary retinopathy and lens opacities.[1126]

Familial spastic paraparesis and dementia Forms that are usually dominantly inherited. See **familial multi-infarct dementia, Worster-Drought syndrome.**

Familial spastic paraplegia with amyotrophy of the hands (Silver disease, hereditary spastic paraparesis with amyotrophy) A rare dominantly or recessively transmitted variant with childhood or early adult onset, manifesting pyramidal signs in the legs and global wasting of the small hand muscles. Various other neurological features have also been described in this condition.[2034,5159] In a further variant, the onset is in childhood, and leukodystrophy, cerebellar deficits, and mild mental retardation are other features.[2002]

Hereditary spastic paraparesis with ataxia A dominantly inherited form appearing in adult life, in which the spastic syndrome is accompanied by pathological evidence of degeneration of the pyramidal and spinocerebellar tracts and of the posterior columns, with the expected clinical features.[4989] In still other forms, extrapyramidal features are also found.[1788] See also **hereditary spastic ataxia, familial spastic ataxia, cerebellar ataxias.**

Hereditary spastic paraparesis with deafness An X-linked degenerative disorder with onset in late childhood, manifesting nerve deafness, spastic paraparesis, tremor, ophthalmic abnormalities, sensory deficits, short stature, cataract, hypogonadotrophic hypogonadism, elevated CSF protein levels, and absent or delayed somatosensory evoked potentials. Except for the normal levels of very long–chain fatty acids, the condition resembles **adrenomyeloneuropathy.**[5913]

Hereditary spastic paraparesis with brachydactyly and cone-shaped epiphyses A congenital or childhood variant with brachydactyly and epiphyseal dysplasia, reported once.

Hereditary spastic paraparesis with dementia A dominantly inherited adult *variant* characterized by the occurrence of dementia late in the course of the disease.[6043] The 2p and 8q mutations appear most liable to induce this syndrome.

Hereditary spastic paraparesis with optic atrophy, dementia, and cardiac involvement Forms in which any of these features complicate the spastic paraparesis.[5424] Further variants are reviewed by Baraitser.[335] Inheritance patterns vary.

Hereditary spastic paraparesis with seizures A dominantly inherited form with a tendency toward seizures and with familial associations with multiple sclerosis. It is due to a frame shift in the spastic (SPG4) gene.[3793]

Hereditary spastic paraparesis, mental retardation, and precocious puberty A childhood variant with dysarthria, early puberty, paraparesis, and mental and developmental delay.

Hereditary spastic paraparesis with oligophrenia (X-linked) A congenital *variant* with added mental retardation, facial palsy, athetosis and ataxia.[279]

Hereditary spastic paraparesis with dysarthria and cutaneous lesions An infantile variant with dysarthria, pigmentary disturbances, and abnormal EEG.

Hereditary spastic paraparesis with extrapyramidal features A childhood variant, usually dominantly inherited, characterized by athetosis or dystonia, rigidity, and hyperreflexia.[1434]

Hereditary spastic paraparesis and macular degeneration (Kjellin syndrome) A variant form presenting in youth with pigmentary retinal degeneration, distal motor neuropathy, spasticity, and mental and developmental delay. Another recessive form that is typical but with severe dysarthria has been linked to the SPG15 locus on 14q.[2690]

Hereditary spastic paraparesis with peroneal neuropathy and crural hypopigmentation A dominantly inherited childhood **neurocutaneous syndrome** with high palate, dysarthria, lordosis, pes cavus, patchy depigmentation of the skin, and peroneal motor neuropathy.[5356]

Hereditary spastic paraparesis with peripheral retinal degeneration A recessively inherited *variant* occurring in young adult life, manifesting pigmentary retinopathy, spasticity, and mental impairment.[5206] Forms with dominant inheritance or with sensory losses have also been reported.[335]

Hereditary spastic paraparesis with sensory neuropathy A dominantly or recessively inherited *variant* with onset in childhood or early youth, characterized by the addition of a neuropathy resembling **hereditary sensory and autonomic neuropathy, type 2.**[3030,4941]

Hereditary spastic paraparesis with mental impairment and thin corpus callosum A recessively inherited *variant* characterized by these features and mapped to 15q13–15.[5131]

Hereditary spastic paraparesis with syndactyly A *variant* with onset in youth or early adult life, characterized by sensorineural deafness, osseous syndactyly of the fingers, spasticity, and incontinence.

Kjellin syndrome

MASA syndrome An X-linked recessive *variant* with onset in youth, characterized by **M**ental retardation, **A**dducted thumbs, **S**huffling gait (due to paraparesis), and **A**phasia.[546]

Mast syndrome A static form with onset in young adult life, characterized by spastic paraparesis, athetosis, dysarthria, and dementia, described in the Pennsylvanian Amish people.[1195]

A form with features of peroneal muscular atrophy

A form resembling **amyotrophic lateral sclerosis**

Spinal muscular atrophy with spastic paraplegia, mental retardation, and ichthyosis See **Sjögren-Larsson syndrome.**

Spastic paraparesis, ataxia, mental retardation (SPAR) A dominantly inherited disorder manifesting these features, with marked atrophy of the spinal cord.[2381]

Spinal muscular atrophy with retinitis pigmentosa and **hereditary spastic paraplegia**

Troyer syndrome (hereditary spastic paraparesis with wasting and growth retardation) A static form with onset in childhood, characterized by pseudobulbar palsy, athetosis, short stature, speech defect, and mental and developmental delay, described in some Pennsylvanian Amish people.[1196]

Yet other variants with added **cerebellar signs, dystonia** or **choreoathetosis,** sensory neuropathy, abnormal skin pigmentation, or **hyperekplexia** or with seizures are also described.[4636]

hereditary spastic paraparesis with cognitive loss An autosomal dominant form of hereditary spastic paraparesis (HSP), manifesting late-onset cognitive impairment (subcortical dementia) and with genetic linkage to the SPG4 locus on chromosome 2p as reported in pure HSP.[5882] See also the entries above.

hereditary spinal arachnoid cyst, distichiasis, lymphedema syndrome A congenital dysmorphic syndrome manifesting also vertebral abnormalities, kyphosis, spinal tumors, congenital cardiac malformations, pyramidal signs, and thick fiber sensory neuropathy.[337]

hereditary stiff baby syndrome The earliest, infantile expression of **hyperekplexia.** See **startle epilepsy.**

hereditary striatal degeneration (holotopistic striatal degeneration) A dominantly inherited syndrome characterized by apathy and psychomotor retardation appearing in infancy or childhood. Dysarthria, rigidity, and chorea are the main features in older individuals.[3922]

hereditary thermosensitive neuropathy A dominantly inherited dremyelinating neuropathic syndrome characterized by reversible episodes of ascending muscle weakness, paresthesias, and areflexia triggered by elevations of body temperature above 38.5°C.[3567]

hereditary torsion dystonia See **dystonia.**

hereditary transcobalamin II deficiency A congenital dysmorphic syndrome characterized also by red blood cell abnormalities, hypotonia, microcephaly, seizures, cerebellar and pyramidal signs, cerebral atrophy, and neurodegenerative regression.[337]

hereditary tyrosinemia A recessively inherited deficiency of fumarylacetoacetate, an enzyme required in the final step of tyrosine metabolism.

The disorder is manifest in infancy. The clinical features largely reflect the presence of slowly progressive hepatic failure and of a renal Fanconi syndrome; abrupt episodes of vomiting, painful peripheral neuropathy, muscle weakness, and self-mutilation are also described.[3907]

hereditary vertical nystagmus A dominantly inherited syndrome with congenital onset characterized by vertical nystagmus which may be associated with mild ataxia and titubation.[1913]

hereditary whispering dysphonia A dominantly inherited condition characterized by inability to speak above a whisper except under strong emotion, and often accompanied by involuntary movements.[4336]

heredity (from Lat, inheritance) The laws whereby the characteristics of humans tend to repeat themselves in their descendants.

hérédoakinesie paroxystique douloureuse A rare familial disease characterized by paroxysmal attacks of paralysis with severe limb pains.

The condition was described by Koulkov in the early 1900s but seems to have disappeared.[574]

heredoataxic hemeralopic polyneuritis See **hereditary motor and sensory neuropathy, type 4.**

heredofamilial mononeuritis multiplex with brachial predilection A dominantly inherited condition in which there are recurrent episodes of painful, acute brachial plexus neuritis, although cranial and other spinal nerves have also been described as affected.[5513]

hérédofamilial optic atrophy See **Leber optic atrophy, optic atrophy, Behr disease.**

heredofamilial tremor See **essential tremor.** This variant is dominantly inherited. The tremor is symmetric and affects the hands and arms first.

heredopathia atactica polyneuritiformis See **Refsum disease** (**hereditary motor and sensory neuropathy, type 4**).

Hering, Heinrich Ewald (1866–1948) Austrian physiologist at Cologne who is remembered for his identification of the nerve of the carotid sinus and his studies of respiratory reflexes. Henry **Head** and **Bielschowsky** were his pupils.

Hering nerve A branch of the ninth cranial nerve, afferent from the carotid sinus, described by Hering in 1923.

Hering's Law Each member of a yoked pair of ocular motor muscles must receive equal innervation, so that they move in parallel. While this is true in the normal state, small differences in innervation can occur in the presence of unilateral ocular muscle weakness.

Herman Pallister Opitz syndrome A congenital syndrome characterized by scynostosis of the coronal suture, hypertelerism, severe mental retardation, facial dysmorphism, and skeletal deformities.[2553]

hernia A swelling produced by the protrusion of a viscus through an aperture in the walls of the cavity that contains it.

herniation 1. Abnormal protrusion of part of the brain (or of other structures such as intervertebral disks) outside their normal boundaries. Herniation of the cingulate gyrus across the midline below the falx,

of the brainstem vertically down through the tentorial opening, of the uncus down over the tentorial free edge, of the cerebellum upward, and of the cerebellar tonsils down through the foramen magnum are examples of the reaction of the brain as a whole to major increases in intracranial pressure. The **central syndrome** and the **uncal syndrome** are the most clinically important results. Lateral shift of the brainstem, however, is likely to be the factor causing most of the clinical signs.[1863]

2. Protrusion, displacement, or extrusion of a fragment of disk material independent of its relationship to the spinal ligaments or nerve roots. That degree of disk herniation in which there is the extrusion of a fragment from the disk space. See also **disk prolapse, disk protrusion.**

Herophilus of Chaldecon (335–280 B.C.) A Greek physician, a teacher at the Ptolemaic school in Alexandria. Although he is credited with the first recorded descriptions of the brain, its membranes, and sinuses, and noted the origin of motor and sensory nerves from the spinal cord, as well as many other anatomical and physiological facts, none of his works actually survive.[1478]

He considered that the brain was the organ of intelligence and the fourth ventricle was the seat of the soul (300 B.C.). The *torcular Herophili* (Gr, cellar) is the name given to the confluence of the superior sagittal, straight, and both transverse cerebral venous sinuses at the posterior edge of the tentorium, regarded by Herophilus as a reservoir of blood.

herpes (Gr, creeping) Hippocrates used this word for a spreading skin eruption, especially one which runs around the body. The word was subsequently used for many other forms of dermatosis.

herpes simplex encephalitis A necrotizing encephalitis with a particular predilection for the medial temporal and inferior frontal lobes. It is the most common cause of severe sporadic encephalitis in the Western world, affecting subjects at any age. Subjects presenting with behavioral and personality changes, evidence of raised intracranial pressure, and meningism and focal neurological signs, occurring subacutely or acutely, are usually treated with acyclovir without resorting to brain biopsy, the former standard for diagnosis.[2769] Focal EEG changes and MRI demonstration of uni- or bilateral edema deep in the temporal lobes are, in this context, strongly suggestive markers for the disease.

herpes viruses Viruses of the class include herpes simplex and zoster, the Epstein-Barr virus, and cytomegalovirus.

herpes zoster (Gr, creeping + a girdle) The clinical expression of infection with the herpes zoster virus. Infection may have no consequence or may lead, after a period of latency, to inflammation of the dorsal root ganglia or the ganglia on the afferent cranial nerves, as described by Sir Henry **Head** in 1900. This is most commonly manifest as pain, an erythematous vesicular rash next appearing within 3–4 days and leaving with either no residua or with skin atrophy and further long-lasting pain. In some cases, the virus attacks the anterior horn cell pool at the same levels as it affects the posterior roots, causing wasting, weakness, and reflex loss at those segmental levels.

Herpes was first described as an infectious condition by **Landouzy** in 1884. The term *shingles* derives from the Latin *cingulum*, a belt, presumably referring to the distribution of the rash even though it is unilateral.

herpes zoster cranialgia   Facial pain caused by acute herpes zoster. This definition and the following diagnostic criteria are suggested by the Headache Classification Committee of the International Headache Society[1051] (Reproduced from: Classification of headache disorders, cranial neuralgias and facial pains; and diagnostic criteria for primary headache disorders. *Cephalalgia* 1988;**8** [suppl]:1–96 by kind permission of Elsevier Science.)
   A. Pain is followed by a herpetic eruption in the distribution of the nerve affected within 1 week of onset.
   B. Pain subsides within 6 months after onset of the rash.

herpes zoster myelopathy   The rare occurrence of transverse myelitis at the level of a herpetic infection of the dorsal root ganglia, causing motor and sensory long tract signs below that level and due to direct infection of the cord.[2606]

herpetic neuralgia   Continuous aching, burning, or itching pains experienced during the eruption of the herpetic rash, sometimes with superimposed lancinating pains.[4494] See also **postherpetic neuralgia.**

Herrick syndrome   1. A congenital dysmorphic syndrome manifesting also skeletal maldevelopments, microcephaly, seizures, spasticity, cerebral and cerebellar atrophy, hydrocephalus, and skin telangiectasia.[2550] 2. (Dresbach disease, sickle cell anemia) Chorioretinal disease, retinal venous thrombosis, and secondary glaucoma, occurring in patients with sickle cell disease.[2550]

Herrmann disease   A dominantly inherited syndrome characterized by photomyoclonus, deafness, diabetes, and nephropathy, and, in some cases, progressive cerebral neuronal degeneration with periodic acid-Schiff–positive glycolipid storage.[2551] Seizures, dementia, nystagmus, and pyramidal and cerebellar signs are also described in such cases.

Herrmann-Opitz syndrome   See **craniosynostosis.**

Hermann-Pallister-Opitz syndrome   See **craniosynostosis.**

Hers disease   A condition in which glycogen accumulates in tissues because of a lack of hepatic phosphorylase; hepatosplenomegaly, hypoglycemic attacks, mild ketosis, and retardation of growth are the main clinical features.[2554] See **glycogen storage disease,** type 6.
   Dr. H.G. Hers is a Belgian biochemist.

Hersh syndrome   A congenital dysmorphic syndrome manifesting also sensorineural deafness, retinitis pigmentosa with visual impairment, strabismus, nystagmus, and mental and developmental delay.

Hertwig-Magendie syndrome   See **skew deviation.**

Hertz   (Hz) Units of frequency, equivalent to cycles per second.

Heschl gyri   (transverse temporal gyri) The gyri immediately behind the insula on the mesial and superior aspect of the superior temporal gyrus, thought to be concerned with the elaboration of auditory sensation.

Heschl, Richard L.   (1824–1881) Austrian physician who became, in succession, professor of anatomy at Olmutz, of pathology at Krakau, and of clinical medicine at Graz University.

Hess, Walter Rudolf   (1881–1973) Swiss physiologist who studied the control of autonomic system functioning. For this work he was awarded the Nobel prize in 1949.

hetero-   (Gr, different; the other one of two) Prefix denoting different.

heterochromia iridis   (Gr, different + color + irises) (heteroglaucos) An alteration in the color and structure of the iris, in which the color of all or a part of one iris differs from that of the other, associated with hypo- or hyperplasia of the iris. The color change may be complete or partial and uni- or bilateral.
   Simple heterochromia is thought to be due to genetic mosaicism; *complicated heterochromia*, due to ocular disease, and *sympathetic heterochromia*, due to damage to the superior cervical ganglion at birth. Although many other diseases have been reported as occurring in association (Gladstone[2132] references 77 diseases), the condition itself is of no pathological significance and the simple form is by far the most common; anxious parents may be reassured that it was manifested by Alexander the Great. However, deafness has been described in association.[337]
   See also **Waardenburg syndrome, Horner syndrome.**

heterogeneous system degeneration   See **Steele-Richardson-Olszewski syndrome.**

heteromodal (polymodal) association areas   Cortical regions which are not devoted to any single modality and which receive convergent input from several sensory association areas and from limbic–paralimbic areas. The prefrontal cortex, posterior parietal cortex, and inferior temporal lobe are examples.[3851]

heteronymous hemianopia   Binasal or bitemporal hemianopia. cf. **homonymous hemianopia.**

heteronymous reflexes   Reflex contractions of muscles not supplied directly by the nerve stimulated (on the same or the opposite side) as a result of facilitation of transmission in interneuronal pathways coactivated by group I and group II afferents, and due to alterations in suprasegmental control. An example is contraction of the biceps brachii in response to stimulation of the median nerve in the cubital fossa. The phenomenon is relevant in the control of posture and balance.[3890]

heterophoria   That condition in which both globes are directed normally during fixation upon near or far objects, but one or both deviate when one eye is occluded and the other eye fixates. Thus, there is a latent tendency for deviation of the eyes. See **cover test, phoria.**

heterotopia   (Gr, different + position) (ectopia) Misplacement of a part of the body during development. Within the nervous system, cortical cells land in places other than the cortex as a consequence of arrest of normal neuronal migration during embryogenesis; thus malformations due to abnormal neuronal migration occur. Subependymal, subcortical, and band heterotopia (double cortex) are distinguished. In all cases, the diagnosis is best made with MRI.[4612] Most commonly, islands of gray matter are found in the subcortical white matter.

With subependymal (periventricular) heterotopias, the presentation is likely to be with temporal or occipital lobe–type seizures in the first two decades of life. *Bilateral nodular periventricular heterotopia* (subependymal heterotopia) is an error of neuronal migration in which subependymal clumps of gray matter protrude into the lumen of the ventricles; it is sometimes associated with cerebellar hypoplasia or with other disorders of CNS development such as the Chiari malformation and with frontonasal dysplasia and with gastrointestinal and renal anomalies. Mental retardation is common but seizures are the main manifestation. The condition appears to be lethal in males, so is seen in females almost exclusively. It is mapped to Xq28, but autosomal linkage is also described.

In a variant form, also mapped to Xq28, these features are accompanied by seizures, mental retardation, and partial syndactyly in the hands and feet. See also **Zellweger syndrome.**

Band heterotopia (double cortex syndrome) is characterized by the presence of a demarcated layer of neurons in the white matter, where they arrested during migration to their cortical sites. Mutations at 17p13.3, Xq22.3–q23 are sometimes found. Mental and developmental delay and partial or generalized seizures are the usual clinical accompaniments, with other seizure types appearing in due course.[356]

A major review has been published,[358] and a classification of heterotopia proposed:

Heterotopia
1. Subependymal (periventricular) heterotopia
   a. Periventricular nodular heterotopia (PNH)
      i. Bilateral PNH with FLN1 mutations
      ii. Other PNH
      iii. PNH with abnormal overlying cortex
   b. Periventricular laminar/ribbon heterotopia
2. Subcortical heterotopia (other than band heterotopia)
   a. Large subcortical heterotopia with abnormal cortex and hypogenetic corpus callosum
   b. Single subcortical heterotopic nodule
   c. Excessive single neurons in white matter
3. Marginal glioneuronal heterotopia

From Barkovich AJ, Kuzniecky R, Jackson GG, et al. Classification system for malformations of cortical development. Neurology 2001;57:2168–78. *Reproduced by kind permission.*

See also **microcephaly, megalencephaly, lissencephaly, cobblestone complex, poilymicrogyria.**

heterotropia   (tropia) Eye deviations manifest during binocular vision. *Esotropia* indicates the adduction and *exotropia*, the abduction of one eye. See **strabismus, cover test, heterophoria.**

heterotypic granular cortex   Those regions of visual, auditory, or general sensory neocortex where the usual six layers are ill defined because small stellate cells overflow into the second and fifth layers.

Heubner arteritis   See **Heubner disease.**

Heubner disease   (Heubner arteritis) Syphilitic arteritis of the cerebral vessels, described by Heubner in 1874.

Heubner endarteritis   See **endarteritis obliterans.**

Heubner, Otto Johann Leonhard   (1843–1926) German pediatrician, professor of medicine at Leipzig. He demonstrated the presence of a leptomeningeal anastomotic circulation in 1874.

Heubner recurrent artery   An early branch of the anterior cerebral artery, supplying the superior and anterior part of the internal capsule.

Heubner-Möbius syndrome   See **Möbius syndrome.**

hexosaminidase deficiency   Inherited deficiencies of β D-*N*-acetylhexosaminidase, leading to the abnormal accumulation of gangliosides and related substances within neurones. See **GM$_2$ gangliosidosis.**

The hexosaminidase isoenzymes (A, B, and S) are part of a complex system metabolizing GM$_2$ gangliosides and related substances; when they fail, the gangliosides accumulate within the nervous system. The B form of the enzyme is coded for on chromosome 5.

The numerous phenotypes have been defined by Johnson[2871] and are given in Chart H–11.

Chart H–11. Hexosaminidase Deficiency Phentotypes

Infantile Encephalopathies

Alpha locus	Tay-Sachs disease and variant
Beta locus	Sandhoff disease and variants
Activator locus	AB variant

Late Infantile/Juvenile

Alpha locus	Juvenile Tay-Sachs disease and variant
Beta locus	Juvenile Sandhoff disease

Cerebellar Ataxia

Alpha locus	Atypical spinocerebellar ataxia
Beta locus	Juvenile ataxia (Ramsay Hunt phenocopy)

Motor Neuron Diseases

Alpha locus	Amyotrophic lateral sclerosis phenocopy
	Hereditary motor neuropathy, type 3 phenocopy

Adult-onset Encephalopathy

Activator locus	Adult GM$_2$ gangliosidosis

Asymptomatic or Presymptomatic Adults

Alpha locus	Total or near-total hexosaminidase deficiency
Beta locus	Hexosaminidase A and B or B deficiency

Adapted from Johnson WG. The clinical spectrum of hexosaminidase deficiency diseases. Neurology 1981;31:1453–1456, by kind permission.

Ataxia, excessive startle responses, dementia, seizures, involuntary movements, pyramidal signs, and cherry-red spots on the retina are recorded variously in these conditions, and phenotypes resembling **amyotrophic lateral sclerosis** or **hereditary motor neuropathy type 3** also represent expressions of hexosaminidase deficiency.[2871] See also **cerebellar ataxias.**

Chronic hexosaminidase A and B deficiency is a *variant* condition in which progressive dystonia and pyramidal and cerebellar signs occur during childhood.[2170]

HHE syndrome (**H**emiconvulsions, **H**emiplegia, **E**pilepsy **S**yndrome, acute acquired postconvulsive hemiplegia, Gastaut syndrome) An epileptic syndrome characterized by persistent, unilateral, clonic motor seizures accompanied by high-voltage delta activity and spikes on the EEG and followed by flaccid hemiplegia lasting over a week with suppression of EEG activity on the appropriate side. In three-quarters of all cases, complex partial clonic or other seizures begin, usually within 2 years. Most affected children have evidence of intellectual failure.

The syndrome is uncommon, but is described in children following acute unilateral cerebral lesions.[2048]

HHH syndrome 1. (**H**yperornithemia, **H**yperammonemia, **H**omocitrullinemia syndrome) See **ornithinemia.** 2. (*hemiparesis, hemiatrophy and hemiathetosis*) A dominantly inherited nonprogressive athetotic hemiplegic syndrome.[2349]

HHHO syndrome (**H**ypotonia, **H**ypomentia, **H**ypogonadism, **O**besity syndrome) See **Prader-Willi syndrome.**

hiccoughs (hiccups, singultus) Intermittent, rhythmic, chronic, spasmodic contractions of the diaphragm accompanied by similar contractions of the accessory muscles of respiration. The sudden inspiration is terminated almost immediately by abrupt closure of the glottis, producing the audible sound. The cause may lie in structural or functional disorders of the medulla affecting the region of the vagal nuclei and the nucleus tractus solitarius, or in damage to the vagi or to the afferent or efferent nerves of the respiratory muscles.

The functional utility of this involuntary respiratory reflex has not been determined. In 1883 Short was the first to recognize the relationship between hiccoughs and phrenic nerve irritation. The condition is usually self-limiting but in protracted cases, Hippocrates advised apnea, which is sound, because an increase in the arterial carbon dioxide tension does have an inhibitory effect. Over 100 other therapies have been suggested, including digital or chemical stimulation of the pharynx, ocular compression, prayers to St. Jude, and drugs such as phenothiazines, demerol, metoclopramide, carbamazepine, nifedipine, meperidine, quinidine, orphenadrine, and digital rectal massage, recalling the comment of Dr. Charles Mayo; "The amount of knowledge on any subject such as this can be considered as being in inverse proportion to the number of different treatments suggested and tried for it."[3752]

hiccups See **hiccoughs.**

Hicks disease See **hereditary sensory and autonomic neuropathy, type 1.**

hidden figures test (Gollin test) A figure-matching task testing visuoperceptual functions, in which the stimuli to be matched are embedded in more complex figures. Like other similar tests, it is sensitive to damage localized to the parietal cortex.[2231]

hidrotic ectodermal dysplasia A familial syndrome comprising cataract, hyperpigmentation of the skin with telangiectasias, hyperkeratosis, and nail dystrophy. See also **neurocutaneous syndromes, Clouston disease.**

high-altitude cerebral edema A vasogenic encephalopathy presenting with headache and cognitive impairments due to low ambient partial pressures of oxygen and characterized by intense T2 signal in white matter areas, especially the splenium of the corpus callosum, and reversible white matter edema. The condition is considered to be due to movement of fluid and protein out of the vascular compartment.[2360]

high-altitude headache See **hypoxic headache.**

high-density lipoprotein deficiency See **Tangier disease.**

high-frequency filter A circuit that reduces the sensitivity of the EEG channel to relatively high frequencies. For each position of the high-frequency filter control, this attenuation is expressed as a percent reduction in output pen deflection at a given frequency, relative to frequencies unaffected by the filter, i.e., in the mid-frequency band of the channel.

At present, high-frequency filter designations and their significance are not standardized for instruments of different manufacture. For instance, for a given instrument, a position of the high-frequency filter control designated at 35 Hz may indicate a 30% (3 Db) or other stated percentage reduction, in sensitivity at 35 Hz compared to the sensitivity, for example at 10 Hz. (Adapted from the 1974 report of the Committee on Terminology, IFCN. In: Chatrian GE, Bergamini L, Dondey M, *et al.* A glossary of terms most commonly used by clinical electroencephalographers. *EEG Clin Neurophysiol* 1974;37:538–548.[989])

high-frequency response The sensitivity of an EEG channel to relatively high frequencies, determined by the high-frequency responses of the amplifier-writer combination and of the filter used and expressed as a percentage reduction in the output pen deflection at certain specific high frequencies, relative to other frequencies in the mid-frequency band of the channel. (Adapted from the report of the Committee on Terminology, IFCN,[989] © 1974, with permission from Elsevier Science.)

high median neuropathy See **pronator syndrome.**

high-pressure hydrocephalus headache (including post-traumatic high-pressure hydrocephalus) The following diagnostic criteria are suggested by the Headache Classification Committee of the International Headache Society[1051] (Classification of headache disorders, cranial neuralgias and facial pains; and diagnostic criteria for primary headache disorders. *Cephalalgia* 1988;**8** [suppl]:1–96).

  A. Patient fulfils the following criteria for high pressure hydrocephalus: ventricular enlargement on neuroimaging, and intracranial pressure >200 mm of water.
  B. Headache occurs with increased intracranial pressure, and is alleviated or abolished by reduction of intracranial pressure with a time lag of less than 24 hours.

Hilger syndrome See **carotidynia.**

hill of vision A three-dimensional representation of visual acuity in which the horizontal and vertical parameters representing the dimensions of visual space are joined by another representing the differential sensitivity to light of different parts of the retina. The fovea is most sensitive, and would be shown as forming the summit of the hill, slightly removed from the bottomless crater, which is the optic nerve head/blind spot.

Hillig syndrome A congenital dysmorphic syndrome manifesting also hepatosplenomegaly, skeletal maldevelopments, macrocephaly, and mental and developmental delay.[337]

Hill-Lowenberg syndrome See **Pelizaeus-Merzbacher disease.**

Hilton, John (1804–1878) English anatomist, surgeon to Guy's Hospital, London, and sometime president of the Royal College of Surgeons. He described his law in his famous book, *Rest and Pain* (London: Bell, 1863).

Hilton's Law "The same trunks of nerves whose branches supply the groups of muscles moving a joint, furnish also a distribution of nerves to the skin over the insertions of the same muscles . . . and the interior of the joint."

hindbrain That part of the developing brain which separates into the medulla oblongata and the cerebellum and which contains the fourth ventricle.

Hines, Edgar Alphonso, Jr. (b.1906) Physician at the Mayo Clinic, the originator (with Dr. G.E. Brown) of the **cold pressor test** in 1932.

Hippel, Eugen von (1867–1939) German ophthalmologist who trained in Heidelberg and Göttingen and who studied further with Leber and later became professor at Halle and then Göttingen University.

Apart from describing the syndrome named for him, he published on numerous eye deformities, cataract, optic nerve lesions, and sympathetic ophthalmia.

Eugen von Hippel

hippocampal sclerosis Severe neuronal loss and gliosis of the hippocampal CA1 sector and subiculum, uni-or bilaterally; a major cause of partial seizures, arising as a developmental defect or due to febrile seizures in childhood or in association with various forms of dementia in adult life.

hippocampal theta activity Regular, high-amplitude waves recorded by subcortical electrodes during rapid eye movement sleep and wakefulness in animals and occasionally in people.[2005]

hippocampus (Gr, a horse, and Lat, a field or race-track) A curved cell mass with distinct zones lying in the inferomesial part of the temporal lobe and covered by the gyrus of the same name.

hip-pocket sciatica Irritation of the sciatic nerve as a result of carrying a wallet in the back pocket of the trousers.

The condition is likely to be more prevalent during times of high inflation.

Hippocrates (460–370 B.C.) Greek physician from the island of Cos in the Aegean; the father of medicine. The Hippocratic writings are almost certainly a collection of manuscripts by a number of authors, though presumably based on his books. It is said that Hippocrates taught beneath the sycamore tree (*Plantanus orientalis*) that stands to this day on Cos; scions of this tree populate many medical campuses. (HJM)

Hippocrates described numerous neurological conditions as well as some neuroanatomy, based in part upon dissections performed on goats as well as humans. He identified thought, intelligence, and dreams as functions of the brain, but also considered that it changed pneuma into animal spirits and excreted the residua.

Diseases identified by him included both focal and generalized tonic-clonic seizures, pupillary inequality, nerve palsies, ophthalmoplegia, myelopathy, apoplexy (including both subarachnoid and intracerebral hemorrhages), mental disorders, and aphasia. His comment that epilepsy was not any more sacred than other diseases seems to have been forgotten for the next 2000 years.

Hippocrates phrenitis An acute, febrile, fatal syndrome consisting of severe nausea and vomiting, acute cachexia, profound mental confusion, and intense generalized motor agitation. Hippocrates also included under *phrenitis* other causes such as malaria, typhoid, and alcoholic crises.

The term was derived from the belief that the diaphragm was the organ of mind, so in delirium (which is what Hippocrates was describing in the cases he reported with the diagnosis of phrenitis) there must be irritation of the diaphragm.[5631]

hippus (from Gr, hippos—continual winking) Physiological oscillation of the size of the pupils. The irregular pupillary constriction and dilatation occur continuously in dim, diffuse lighting with a cycle time of 660 msec. or longer, and is of variable amplitude. The finding is within normal limits, but its cause is not known.

Hirano bodies Eosinophilic cylindrical structures up to 30 μm long, containing filaments derived from cytoskeletal proteins and found within the cytoplasm of hippocampal neurons in relation to advancing age, but with increased frequency in patients with numerous dementing and degenerative diseases, including **Alzheimer** and **Pick diseases, kuru,** and **amyotrophic lateral sclerosis.**

Dr. Asao Hirano is a contemporary American neuropathologist.

Hirano parkinsonism-dementia See **Lytico-Bodig.**

Hirano-Kurland-Sayre combined neurological degeneration A dominantly inherited disease resembling **amyotrophic lateral sclerosis** but with the added features of degeneration of the posterior columns, spinocerebellar tracts, and Clarke's column, and the presence of intracytoplasmic argyrophilic inclusions (**Lewy bodies**) in the anterior horn cells.[2581]

Hirano–Lewy body disease See **amyotrophic lateral sclerosis, Hirano-Kurland-Sayre combined neurological degeneration.**

Hirayama disease (*juvenile muscular atrophy of the upper limbs*) A rare cervical myelopathy described in young Japanese males who present with asymmetric distal weaksss and wasting of one arm, initially progressive and then static after years. The precise cause is unknown.[2585] See **hereditary motor neuropathy, type 3.**

Hirayama juvenile muscular atrophy See **hereditary motor neuropathy.**

Hirschberg sign See **adductor reflex of the foot.**

Hirschsprung disease A disorder characterized by absence of ganglion cells in the intestine. The condition is most commonly seen in males and usually presents with constipation in the first 3 months of life. In three-quarters of cases the involvement is limited to the rectosigmoid region. The condition is sometimes associated with **Down syndrome, neurofibromatosis,** or **neuroblastoma.**[1616] Harald Hirschprung (1830–1916) was a Danish pediatrician at Copenhagen.

A *variant* is *Hirschsprung (cleft palate, mental retardation) syndrome*, a congenital dysmorphic syndrome manifesting also speech delay, Hirschprung syndrome, microcephaly, cerebellar signs, and mental and developmental delay.[337]

His, Wilhelm (1831–1904) Swiss anatomist from Basel, a student of Remak. He originated the terms *dendrite, neuropil, neuroblast,* and *spongioblast*. His main interest was the embryogenesis of the nervous system.

histamine flare test The subcutaneous injection of 0.1 ml of a 1:1000 solution of histamine acid phosphate, with assessment of the area of erythema (the flare) produced through local axon reflexes.

Once used for localization of the site of a sensory nerve lesion (normal flare size with proximal radicular lesions; reduced flare size with distal plexus or other lesions), it has been largely supplanted by nerve conduction studies.

histaminic cephalgia See **cluster headache.** Horton incriminated histamine in the pathogenesis of this condition in part because of the provocative role of histamine in precipitation of the attack. He has still not been proved right or wrong.

histidinemia A recessively inherited syndrome resulting from a deficiency of l-histidase and characterized clinically by motor and behavioral delay in some cases.[5042]

histiocytosis (systemic histiocytosis, Erdheim-Chester disease) A rare systemic disorder seen mainly in males with onset in later adult life, characterized by fever, cardiovascular and dermal features, metaphyseal cortical thickening of the long bones, and hypothalamic or orbital infiltration, the former associated with diabetes insipidus.[5236]

histiocytosis X See **generalized xanthomatosis.**

histoplamosis Infection by this dimorphic fungus, usually presenting as pulmonary infiltrations but able to disseminate in immunocompromised people, in which case meningoencephalitis is a potential complication.

histrionic palsy A synonym for **Bell palsy,** so known in the nineteenth century on account of the resultant loss of the power of facial expression.

Hittner syndrome A congenital dysmorphic syndrome manifesting also deafness, microphthalmia, retinal and iris colobomas, and mental and developmental delay.[337]

Hitselberg sign Hypoesthesia of the posterior wall of the external auditory meatus as a result of a proximal lesion affecting the seventh cranial nerve (which is not purely a motor nerve).

Eduard Hitzig

Hitzig, Eduard (1838–1907) German neuropsychiatrist, eventually professor of psychiatry at Zurich and then Halle University. He described girdle zones and, by animal experiments performed in his home during 1870–1874 in conjunction with Fritsch, a zoologist, defined the extent of the motor areas in primates using electrical stimulation of the cortex.

Hitzig girdle (zone) Analgesia in the T3–T6 regions in early **tabes dorsalis.**[5047]

HIV encephalopathy See **HIV-1–associated nervous system diseases.**

HIV meningoencephalitis (giant cell encephalitis, multinucleated cell encephalitis, subacute encephalitis) The *acute form* is an uncommon complication occurring early in the course of HIV infection and characterized by altered consciousness, seizures, mental dysfunction, evidence of inflammation in the CSF, and diffuse changes on the EEG, leading to ultimate recovery from the acute illness.

The *chronic form* (chronic HIV meningitis) is a frequent complication of HIV infection, occurring often prior to the appearance of AIDS and (if symptomatic at all) characterized by headache and mild meningeal signs, cranial neuropathies, and chronic inflammatory changes in the CSF.[1834]

HIV myelopathy See **HIV-associated myelopathy.**

HIV myopathy A proximal myopathy complicating HIV type 1 infection or (less often) its treatment with zidovudine and characterized by weakness, elevated serum CK, and muscle biopsy appearances of myofiber degeneration, variable inflammatory infiltrates, inclusion bodies, and mitochondrial abnormalities.[6051]

HIV neuropathy See **HIV-associated multiple mononeuropathy, HIV-associated progressive polyneuropathy, HIV-associated autonomic neuropathy, HIV-associated predominantly sensory neuropathy, HIV-associated acute inflammatory demyelinating polyneuropathy, HIV-associated lumbosacral polyradiculopathy.**

Radiculopathies (cytomegalovirus, herpes zoster), vasculitic neuropathy, lymphomatous neuropathy, and forms associated with drug therapy are also described in patients with HIV infections.

HIV wasting disease See **HIV-associated myopathy.**

HIV-associated acute inflammatory demyelinating polyneuropathy (HIV-1–associated Guillain-Barré syndrome) A neuropathic syndrome resembling **acute inflammatory demyelinating polyneuropathy** complicating HIV infection. The following diagnostic criteria have been suggested (from American Academy of Neurology AIDS task force. Nomenclature and case definitions for neurological manifestations of HIV type 1 infection. *Neurology* 43:625–627), reproduced by kind permission.

Probable (must have):

1. Guillain-Barré Syndrome by previously published criteria except that the CSF cell count can be as high as 50 cells/mm³.

Possible (must have one of the following):

1. Other potential etiology present (must have each of the following):
   a. As above No. 1
   b. Other potential etiology is present and the cause of No. 1 is uncertain.
2. Incomplete clinical evaluation (patients must have each of the following):
   a. As above No. 1
   b. Etiology cannot be determined (appropriate laboratory investigations not performed).

HIV-associated aseptic meningitis An acute aseptic meningitis with headache, meningism, cranial neuropathies, and fever occurring at the time of seroconversion (AIDS-related complex), reflecting the initial response of the nervous system to the infection. The CSF shows a monocytic pleocytosis.[3728]

HIV-associated autonomic neuropathy The occurrence of such autonomic symptoms as fainting due to orthostatic hypotension, cardiac irregularities, hypohidrosis, impotence, diarrhea, and urinary dysfunction occurring in patients suffering the later stages of HIV infection.

Whether it is the disease or its treatment that is responsible is not yet determined.[5178]

HIV-associated cognitive/motor complex (chronic AIDS encephalopathy, AIDS–dementia complex, AIDS-related dementia, subacute encephalitis) A group of dementing or motor system disorders due to primary infection of the nervous system by the HIV; the most common neurological manifestation of AIDS, present in up to 75% of those affected with the disease.[1834]

Clinically, it presents with insidious mental slowing with impaired concentration, memory loss, depression, loss of libido, social withdrawal and mild motor deficits (unsteady gait, leg weakness, tremor) with frontal release signs, advancing to a state of apathy, abulia, mutism, and profound mental failure.[3728] All of the following diagnoses require laboratory evidence for confirmation of systemic HIV-1 infection (enzyme-linked immunosorbent assay confirmed by Western blot, by polymerase chain reaction, or by culture). Diagnostic criteria have been suggested;[4524] those in the following entries include minor adaptations. (Reproduced from the American Academy of Neurology AIDS task force. Nomenclature and case definitions for neurological manifestations of HIV type 1 infection. *Neurology* 1991;**43**:625–627, by kind permission.)

Operational Definition of HIV-1 Dementia

Probable (must have each of the following four criteria):

1. A. Acquired abnormalities, for at least 1 month, in at least two of the following cognitive domains: attention/concentration, information-processing speed, abstraction/reasoning, visuospatial skills, memory/learning, and speech/language.
   B. Cognitive dysfunction affecting work performance or activities of daily living. This impairment should not be explainable just by systemic illness.
2. At least one of the following:
   A. Acquired abnormality in motor function or performance, as documented on clinical examination, such as slowing of ability to perform rapid movements, abnormal gait, limb incoordination, hyperreflexia, hypertonia, weakness; or as recorded during neuropsychological testing, fine motor speed manual dexterity, and perceptual motor skills.
   B. Decline in motivation or emotional control or change in social behavior. This may include alteration in personality with apathy, inertia, irritability, emotionality, newly developing impairment of judgement, and socially inappropriate behavior or disinhibition.
3. Absence of clouding of consciousness during a period sufficient to establish criterion 1 above.
4. Exclusion of another etiology as causal of the symptoms, including CNS opportunistic infection or neoplasm, and psychiatric disorder, by history, clinical examination, laboratory (for example, blood tests and lumbar puncture) and neuroimaging.

Possible (must have one of the following):

1. Criteria 1, 2, and 3 above in *probable* are present but an alternative potential cause is present.
2. Criteria 1, 2, and 3 above in *probable* are present but there was incomplete clinical evaluation.

HIV-associated leukoencephalopathy (progressive diffuse encephalopathy) A syndrome characterized by diffuse damage to the cerebral white matter with loss of myelin and reactive astrogliosis, and presenting in the same way as **progressive multifocal leukoencephalopathy** but with a particular tendency to cause dementia.[3727]

HIV-associated lumbosacral polyradiculopathy (cytomegalovirus polyradiculitis, myeloradiculitis) A severe but reversible cauda equina syndrome manifesting bilateral leg weakness, areflexia, and loss of sphincter function with rapid progression of the paraplegia over days. A mononuclear pleocytosis is notable in the CSF.

Although cytomegalovirus infection is a common cause, lymphoma, toxoplasmosis, and syphilis can produce the same syndrome.[5249]

HIV-associated multiple mononeuropathy A multifocal sensory axonal inflammatory neuropathy presenting rarely with multiple sensory complaints, often in association with fever, cachexia, and cytomegalovirus retinopathy, within the context of HIV infection.[5178]

HIV-associated myelopathy (vacuolar myelopathy, HIV myelopathy) A vacuolar myelopathy presenting with a syndrome of motor and sensory deficits characteristic of spinal cord disease and due to direct infection of the cord with HIV. It is found to occur in a quarter of all patients dying from AIDS.[1835,4425] Gait disturbance, leg weakness, and urinary incontinence are the major clinical features. Diagnostic criteria have been suggested by the American Academy of Neurology AIDS Task Force and are given in Chart H–12.

Chart H–12. Diagnostic Criteria for HIV-Associated Myelopathy

Probable (must have each of the following):

1. Acquired abnormality in lower extremity neurological function disproportionate to upper extremity abnormality, verified by reliable history of lower extremity weakness, incoordination and/or urinary incontinence, and neurological examination (paraparesis, lower extremity spasticity, hyperreflexia or the presence of Babinski sings, with or without sensory loss).
2. Disturbance in No. 1 is severe enough to require constant unilateral support for walking.
3. Although mild cognitive impairment may be present, criteria for HIV-1–associated dementia complex are not fulfilled.
4. Evidence of another etiology, including neoplasm, compressive lesion, or multiple sclerosis, must be sought from history, physical examination, and appropriate laboratory and radiological investigation (e.g., lumbar puncture, neuroimaging, myelography). If another potential etiology is present, it is not the cause of the myelopathy. This diagnosis cannot be made in a patient infected with both HIV-1 and HTLV-1; such a patient should be classified as having possible HIV-1–associated myelopathy.

Possible (must have one of the following):

1. Other potential etiology present (must have each of the following):
   a. As above Nos. 1, 2, and 3
2. Incomplete clinical evaluation (must have each of the following):
   a. As above Nos. 1, 2, and 3
   b. Etiology cannot be determined (appropriate laboratory or radiological investigations not performed.

Reproduced from the American Academy of Neurology AIDS task force. Nomenclature and case definitions for neurological manifestations of HIV type 1 infection. Neurology 1993;43:625–627, by kind permission.

HIV-associated myopathy (HIV wasting disease) A myopathic syndrome complicating HIV infection.[5177] Diagnostic criteria have been suggested and are given in Chart H–13.

Chart H–13. Diagnostic Criteria for HIV-Associated Myopathy

Probable (must have each of the following):

1. Symptoms of proximal lower and/or upper extremity weakness, documented by physical examination.
2. No other etiology (including toxic exposure to zidovudine). EMG and muscle biopsy may be necessary to rule out certain other etiologies.

Possible (must have one of the following):

1. Other potential etiology present (must have each of the following):
   a. As above No. 1.
   b. Other potential etiology is present and the cause is uncertain.
2. Incomplete clinical evaluation (must have each of the following):
   a. As above No. 1.
   b. Etiology cannot be determined (appropriate laboratory investigations not performed).

Reproduced from the American Academy of Neurology AIDS task force. Nomenclature and case definitions for neurological manifestations of HIV type 1 infection. Neurology 1991;43:625–627, by kind permission.

HIV-associated nervous system diseases The complex of disorders affecting the nervous system in patients with clinical expression of HIV infection. The conditions are listed in Chart H–14.

Chart H–14. The HIV-Associated Nervous System Diseases

HIV-associated cognitive motor complex
1. *Severe manifestations*
   HIV-associated dementia complex
   Acute **HIV meningoencephalitis**
   HIV-associated myelopathy
   HIV-associated leukoencephalopathy
   Opportunistic infections (toxoplasmosis, cryptococcosis, cytomegalovirus encephalitis, primary CNS lymphoma, progressive multifocal leukoencephalopathy, mycobacterial infections)
2. *Mild manifestations*
   HIV-1-associated minor cognitive-motor disorder
   HIV-1-associated neurocognitive disorder
   HIV-1-associated neurobehavioral abnormalities
HIV-associated acute inflammatory demyelinating polyneuropathy
HIV-associated autonomic neuropathy
HIV-associated multiple mononeuropathy
HIV-associated myopathy
HIV-associated predominantly sensory neuropathy
HIV-associated progressive encephalopathy of childhood
HIV-associated progressive polyneuropathy

The syndromes of **amyotrophic lateral sclerosis** and of pure sensory neuropathy may also be related to HIV infection. Malignancies of the CNS (primary CNS lymphoma, Kaposi sarcoma) and opportunistic infections (*toxoplasma*, viruses, fungi, bacteria) are other complications.[1834]

HIV-associated predominantly sensory neuropathy (distal symmetrical polyneuropathy). A painful axonal neuropathy, the most common peripheral neuropathy in patients with HIV infection. Diagnostic criteria are listed in Chart H–15. A similar neuropathy occurs in this context as a result of exposure to neurotoxins or Vitamin B_{12} deficiency.

Chart H–15. Diagnostic Criteria for HIV-Associated Predominantly Sensory Neuropathy

Probable (must have each of the following):

1. Distal limb sensory symptoms (feet > hands) of a peripheral nature, with numbness, burning, or pain.
2. Neurological examination confirming a distal, relatively symmetrical polyneuropathy in which sensory abnormalities predominate.
3. Electrodiagnostic studies indicative of a polyneuropathy with features of both axonal loss and demyelination.
4. Normal CSF cell count and only minimal, if any, elevation of protein level, with negative VDRL.
5. No other etiology (including toxic exposure to dideoxyi-

nosine). Nerve biopsy may be indicated to rule out certain etiologies such as amyloid, but is not a requirement.

Possible (must have each of the following):

1. Other potential etiology present (must have each of the following):
   a. As above Nos. 1, 2 and 3
   b. Other potential etiology is present and the cause is uncertain.
2. Incomplete clinical evaluation (must have each of the following):
   a. As above Nos. 1 and 2
   b. Etiology cannot be determined (appropriate laboratory investigations not performed).

*Reproduced from the American Academy of Neurology AIDS task force. Nomenclature and case definitions for neurological manifestations of HIV type 1 infection. Neurology 1991;**43**:625–627, by kind permission.*

HIV-associated progressive encephalopathy of childhood   A dementing syndrome complicating HIV infection in children. The major clinical features include loss of developmental attainments or failure to achieve them, and acquired symmetrical motor deficits such as pareses, hypertonia, hyperreflexia, ataxia, and gait disturbance.

Diagnostic criteria have been suggested and are given in Chart H–16.

Chart H–16. Diagnostic Criteria for HIV-Associated Progressive Encephalopathy of Childhood

Probable (must have each of the following):

1. Evidence for systemic HIV-1 infection
   a. Infants and children <15 months
      i. Virus in blood or tissues, or
      ii. Presence of HIV-1 antibody and evidence of cellular and humoral deficiency or other conditions meeting Center for Disease Control case definition for AIDS.
2. At least one of the following progressive findings present for at least 2 months:
   a. Failure to attain or loss of developmental milestones or loss of intellectual ability, verified by standard development scale or neuropsychological tests.
   b. Impaired brain growth (acquired microcephaly or brain atrophy demonstrated on serial CT or MRI scans).
3. Evidence of another etiology, including active CNS opportunistic infection or malignancy, must be sought from history, physical examination, and appropriate laboratory and radiological investigation (e.g., lumbar puncture, neuroimaging). If another potential etiology is present, it is not thought to be the cause of the above cognitive/motor/behavioral/developmental symptoms and signs.

Possible (must have one of the following):

1. Other potential etiology present (must have each of the following):
   a. As above, Nos. 1 and 2
   b. Other potential etiology is present but the cause of No. 2 is uncertain.
2. Incomplete clinical evaluation (must have each of the following):
   a. As above, Nos. 1 and 2
   b. Etiology cannot be determined (appropriate laboratory or radiologic investigations not performed).

*Reproduced from the American Academy of Neurology AIDS task force. Nomenclature and case definitions for neurological manifestations of HIV type 1 infection. Neurology 1991;**43**:625–627, by kind permission.*

HIV-associated progressive polyneuropathy   (HIV-associated polyradiculomyelitis) A rapidly progressive, painful syndrome of leg and sacral paresthesias, moving on to areflexic paraparesis with ascending sensory loss producing saddle anesthesia and both peripheral muscle and bladder denervation, in the context of severe immunosuppression and occurring in patients suffering the later stages of HIV infection.[1618] The usual causative organism is cytomegalovirus.

An alternative system of classification based on the underlying pathology has been suggested[831] and is given in Chart H–17.

Chart H–17. Proposed Neuropathology-Based Terminology of HIV-Associated Disease of the Nervous System, Recommended in a Consensus Report

Central Nervous System

HIV encephalitis
HIV leukoencephalopathy
Vacuolar myelopathy and vacuolar leukoencephalopathy
Lymphocytic meningitis
Diffuse poliodystrophy
Cerebral vasculitis, including granulomatous angiitis

Peripheral Nervous System

(HIV-1-associated) acute inflammatory demyelinating (polyradiculo-) neuropathy
Chronic inflammatory demyelinating (polyradiculo-)neuropathy
(HIV-1-associated) predominantly sensory axonal neuropathy
Ganglionitis, ganglioradiculitis, (polyradiculo-)neuritis
Necrotizing vasculitis, vasculitic neuropathy

Myopathies

(Poly)myositis
Necrotizing myopathy
Nemaline rod myopathy
Vesicular myopathy, mitochondrial myopathy
Necrotizing vasculitis

*Reproduced from Budka H. Cerebral pathology in AIDS. Curr Opin Neurol Neurosurg 1992;**5**:917–923 by kind permission.*

HIV-1-associated dementia complex   (AIDS–dementia complex, HIV-associated neurocognitive disorders, subacute AIDS encephalitis, chronic AIDS encephalopathy) The most common neurological complication in patients with AIDS, affecting at least half of them. HIV, *toxoplasma* or cytomegalovirus infection, or lymphoma may variously be responsible.[4524] The diagnostic criteria are given in Chart H–18.[1269]

Chart H–18. HIV-1-Associated Dementia Complex (ADC) Modified American Academy of Neurology Algorithm

Criteria for 1 and 2 must be met:

1. Scores 1 SD below age- and education-adjusted norms on two of eight neuropsychological tests or 2 SDs below the norms on one of eight tests

2. Patient requires assistance or has difficulty (due to either physical or cognitive deficit) in one of the following instrumental activities of daily living (IADL):

Using the telephone
Handling money
Taking medication
Performing light housekeeping
Doing laundry
Preparing meals
Shopping for groceries
Getting to places out of walking distance and must meet either 1 or 2 of the following:

1. Any impairment in the following: lower extremity strength, coordination, finger tapping, alternating hand movements, leg agility, or performance on grooved pegboard 2 SDs below mean (dominant hand)

2. Self-reported frequent depression that interferes with function, loss of interest in usual activities, or emotional lability, or irritability

Staging of HIV-1-Associated Dementia Complex

Mild: must attribute IADL to a cognitive source
Moderate: satisfies neurologic and psychiatric criteria for mild ADC plus functional impairment in either telephone use, medication taking, or money handling plus two or three other lADLs or ADLs (indoor mobility, eating, dressing, grooming, toileting, getting in and out of bed, bathing) attributed to a cognitive source
Severe: satisfies neurologic and psychiatric criteria for moderate ADC and has in addition to impairment in telephone use, medication taking, or money handling at least four lADLs or ADLs attributed to a cognitive source

A further description of this state is provided by Fischer and Enzensberger:[1834]

Possible (must have one of the following):

1. Other potential etiology present (must have each of the following):
   a. As in Nos. 1, 2, and 3 in Chart H–18
   b. Other potential etiology is present but the cause of No. 1 is uncertain.

2. Incomplete clinical evaluation (must have each of the following):
   a. As in Nos. 1, 2, and 3 in Chart H–18
   b. Etiology cannot be determined (appropriate laboratory or radiological investigations were not performed).

See also **HIV-1 associated minor cognitive-motor disorder.**

Children also develop an HIV-associated neurodevelopmental disorder, characterized by developmental delay, hypertonia, microcephaly, and basal ganglia calcification. The neurological involvement most often occurs in the absence of opportunistic infections and neoplasms, which is not the case for adults.

HIV dementia generally, but not invariably, progresses quickly (over weeks or months) to severe global dementia, mutism, and death.[150] (Reproduced from the American Academy of Neurology AIDS task force. Nomenclature and case definitions for neurological manifestations of HIV type 1 infection. *Neurology* 1991;**43**:625–627, by kind permission.)

HIV-1-associated distal symmetrical polyneuropathy See **HIV-associated predominantly sensory neuropathy.**

HIV-1-associated Guillain-Barré syndrome See **HIV-associated acute inflammatory demyelinating neuropathy.**

HIV-1-associated Guillain-Barré syndrome See **HIV-associated acute inflammatory demyelinating neuropathy.**

HIV-1-associated minor cognitive-motor disorder Cognitive changes such as impaired concentration, inattention, mild memory loss, slowed verbal responses, and blunted affect accompanying HIV infection but not alone diagnostic of AIDS. Diagnostic criteria have been suggested and are given in Chart H–19.

Chart H–19. Diagnostic Criteria for HIV-Associated Minor Cognitive-Motor Disorder

Does not meet criteria for H1V-l-associated cognitive/motor disorder and meets 1 and 2 of the following:

1. Deficit in at least two of the following:
   Mental slowing: digit symbol at least 1 SD below age- and education-adjusted norms
   Memory: Rey Auditory Verbal Learning Test (total) at least 1 SD below norms
   Motor dysfunction: any impairment in finger tapping or pronation/supination
   Incoordination: mild impairment in gait or clumsiness
   Emotional lability or apathy/withdrawal

and

2. Deficit in at least one of the role function measures attributed in part to cognitive function:
   Need for frequent rests
   Cuts down on amount of time in activities
   Accomplishes less than desired
   Cannot perform activities as carefully as one would like
   Limited in work or activities
   Difficulty performing activities
   Requires special assistance to perform activities.

*Adapted from American Academy of Neurology AIDS task force. Nomenclature and case definitions for neurological manifestations of HIV type 1 infection. Neurology **43**:625–627. Reprinted by kind permission.*

HIV-1-associated neurocognitive disorder See **HIV-1–associated dementia complex.**

HIV-1–associated peripheral nervous system disorders See **HIV-associated myopathy, HIV-associated predominantly sensory neuropathy, HIV-associated acute inflammatory demyelinating polyneuropathy.** All of these diagnoses require laboratory evidence for systemic HIV-1 infection (enzyme-linked immunosorbent assay confirmed by Western blot, by polymerase chain reaction, or by culture).

Hobson-McCarley model A model system of the neural basis of sleep which hypothesizes an aminergic, rapid eye movement–off state controlled by the locus ceruleus and raphé nuclei, and a cholinergic rapid eye movement–on system in opposition controlled by the giganticocellular field of the pons.

Hochsinger sign   Closure of the fist in response to pressure exerted on the inner side of the biceps brachii in tetany,[5047] presumably as a result of ischemia induced distally by compression of the brachial artery proximally.

The sign was described by Carl Hochsinger (1869–1942), an Austrian pediatrician.[2595]

hocquet diabolique   Intractable hiccups, recorded as a complication of numerous central (CNS) and peripheral (chest, abdomen) causes. The most prolonged case of hiccups was one lasting 8 years, during which time the patient was estimated to have "hic'ed" 100 million times. He sought assistance from any source and received, it is said, 60,000 suggestions for cure but only one of these (prayer to St. Jude) succeeded.[3752] See **hiccoughs.**

Hodgkin disease   A localized or systemic lymphoma. Neurological complications include epidural compression of the spinal cord, cranial nerve palsies, progressive multifocal leukoencephalopathy, and parenchymal sarcomas.

Hoehn and Yahr scale   A rating scale for the overall level of impairment in Parkinson disease.[2598] See Chart H–20.

Chart H–20. Hoehn and Yahr Scale for Parkinson Disease (modified)

0.	No signs of disease
1.	Unilateral disease, usually with minimal or no functional impairment
1.5.	Unilateral disease + axial involvement
2.	Bilateral or midline disease without impairment of balance
2.5.	Mild bilateral disease with recovery on pull test
3.	Mild to moderate bilateral disease; some postural instability; physically independent. [The first sign of impaired righting reflexes, here made evident by unsteadiness when the patient turns or when is pushed from standing equilibrium with the feet together and eyes closed; it indicates mild to moderate disability.]
4.	Severe disability. Still able to stand and walk unassisted, but markedly incapacitated.
5.	Wheelchair-bound or bedridden unless aided

From Hoehn MH, Yahr MD. Parkinsonism: onset, progression and mortality. Neurology 1967;17:427–442. Reprinted by kind permission.

Hoffmann disease   See **hereditary motor neuropathy, type 1.**

Hoffmann, Johann   (1857–1919) German neurologist, who graduated from Heidelberg with a thesis on acute ascending paralysis. There he worked at first under **Friedreich** and then, **Erb.** In 1910 he was elected full professor of medicine and, shortly before his death, professor of neuropathology.

His many clinical contributions include those following, his differentiation of **myotonic dystrophy** and **myotonia congenita,** the **H reflex,** and an accurate description of **hereditary motor neuropathy, type 1,** acknowledging the previous report of **Werdnig.**

Hoffmann, Paul   (1884–1962) German physician who described the following sign independently of Tinel.

Hoffman reflex   1. (Hoffmann-Tromner reflex, digital reflex) Sudden release of the flexed distal phalanx of the second, third, or fourth digits leads to flexion of the terminal phalanx of the thumb and of the last two interphalangeal joints of other fingers of that hand in the case of pyramidal tract disease affecting that limb.[1226]

The phenomenon has the same significance as the **finger flexion reflex,** of which it is a variant. The first account of it was actually published by Curschmann (one of Hoffmann's students) in 1911, 10 years after he had described it orally.

2. See **H reflex.**

Hoffmann sign   Increased irritability of regenerating sensory nerves in response to mechanical stimuli. See also **Tinel sign.**

Hoffman syndrome   (hypothyroid myopathy) Stiffness, slowed contraction and relaxation, and persistent painful muscle contractions following effort, made worse by exertion and associated with muscle hypertrophy in adult hypothyroid patients.[2602,2603] See **pseudomyotonia.**

Kocher-Debré-Sémélaigne syndrome is only different by virtue of the lesser amount of pain felt, and its original description in cretinoid patients. See **hypothyroid myopathy, pseudomyotonia.**

Hoffmann-Charcot-Marie-Tooth   syndrome See **hereditary motor and sensory neuropathy, types 1 and 2.**

Hoffmann-Tromner reflex   See **Hoffman reflex.**

Hollenhorst plaque   A visible cholesterol embolism in the retinal arterioles accompanied sometimes by **amaurosis fugax.** It suggests the presence of atherosclerosis in the carotid system.

Hollenhorst syndrome   Permanent or temporary blindness as a result of chorioretinal infarction that results from persistently increased ocular pressure. This might be caused by malpositioning of a patient lying face down during surgery with the head supported in a head rest.

Ophthalmoplegias, proptosis, chemosis, corneal edema, and retinal detachment are other features reported.[2617]

hollow hand sign   (of Garcin) Adduction and flexion of the thumb when the fingers are extended voluntarily. This is a sensitive sign indicating a pyramidal lesion affecting the upper limb.

Holmes cerebellar ataxia   An **autosomal dominant cerebellar ataxia.** See **Holmes disease.**

Holmes disease   1. (cerebelloolivary degeneration, Holmes cerebellar ataxia) Originally described as a recessively inherited cerebellar ataxia with hypogonadism,[2619] the appellation has been given to various forms of ataxias, including some dominantly inherited, on the basis of similar pathology. The condition is now classified as an **autosomal dominant cerebellar ataxia**.[2438] 2. (visual disorientation) Disorders in the perception of space, with inability to recognize the position, distance, or size of objects seen, accompanied by disorders of accommodation and of convergence, impairment of visual fixation, and absence of the blink reflex.[2621]

Holmes, Oliver Wendell (1809–1894) American literary figure and physician, practicing in Boston. In the latter role, he introduced the terms *anesthesia* and *anesthetic* to medicine.

Holmes rebound sign See **rebound**.[5357] The rebound is normally present, exaggerated in spastic limbs, and lost in cerebellar disease.

Holmes, Sir Gordon Morgan (1876–1965) Irish neurologist who trained in Dublin and in Germany (with Weigert and Edinger) before taking up junior positions at, and then becoming physician to, the **National Hospital,** Queen Square, between 1909 and 1941. He was elected a Fellow of the Royal Society in 1933.[732]

Gordon Holmes, as much as Hughlings-**Jackson,** could be called the father of British neurology and has been described as "the outstanding neurological exponent of the World." Well-grounded in neuroanatomy and neurophysiology after his extensive training in Germany, his life's work reflected his preoccupation with the pathophysiology of disease; the huge advances that he made were the result of close clinical observation and accurate reporting, as in the case of the seminal paper on sensation that he wrote with **Head** in 1911, and his papers on signs of spinal cord injury in 1915, on cerebellar disease in 1922, and on neuro-ophthalmology in 1919.[2627]

His most triumphant work was performed in field hospitals on the battlefields of northern France, where, despite appalling conditions, he and Sir Percy Sargent, his neurosurgical colleague, made painstaking observations that led to numerous papers on neurological localization—studies only made possible by the ambient carnage. They showed, for example, that the upper retina was represented in the upper part of the visual area and the macular area at the pole, and then wrote a landmark paper on cerebellar injuries.[2620,2628] Holmes' collected papers have been published.[2627]

A precise and exacting man, he expected from others the standards of observation of which he himself was a master. In the opinion of this author, his book *An Introduction to Clinical Neurology* (Edinburgh, 1946) remains the finest introductory text in neurology yet written.

Holmes syndrome 1. A congenital dysmorphic syndrome of modern description, characterized by pes cavus, microcephaly, delayed closure of the fontanelles, and mental and developmental delay.[337] 2. See **visual disorientation.**

Holmes tremor See **rubral tremor.**

Holmes-Adie syndrome (Adie syndrome, Kehrer-Adie syndrome, Markus syndrome, Markus-Adie syndrome, Weill-Reys syndrome) The combination of **Adie pupil** and loss of the muscle stretch reflexes, either in the legs or universally, and usually occurring in young women.[2623]

Adie had also noted the association in his 1931 paper in the *British Medical Journal.*[41]

A *variant* is *Holmes-Adie syndrome with segmental hypohidrosis* (**Ross syndrome**).

Holmes-Logan infantile CNS degeneration A hereditary dysmorphic syndrome of infancy, characterized also by growth failure, optic atrophy, ophthalmoplegia, areflexia, choreoathetosis, and severe mental and motor retardation, noted over the first 3 years of life.[2630]

Holmes-Stewart syndrome See **Jackson cerebellar "fits"**

Holmgren, Alarik Frithiof (1831–1897) Norwegian ophthalmologist and professor of physiology at Uppsala who introduced the wool-skein sorting test for the diagnosis of color-blindness in 1874.

holocarboxylase deficiency 1. (Biotin-responsive multiple carboxylase deficiency) A neonatal disorder due to a deficiency in three biotin-dependent mitochondrial carboxylase enzymes. Onset of symptoms occurs in the neonatal or infantile periods, with metabolic (lactic) acidosis, tachypnea, hypertonia, irritability, lethargy, and coma, responsive to biotin therapy.[4290]

2. Juvenile- or late-onset form. See **biotin-responsive encephalopathy.**

holokinetic movements Extensive jerky, abrupt, rapid, and awkward movements of extensive parts of the body, as may occur in some dystonic and dyskinetic states.[4180]

holoprosencephaly (Gr, whole + front + brain) (holotelencephaly, arhinencephaly, telencephalosynapsis) A congenital, heterogeneous, but sometimes dominantly inherited dysmorphic anomaly in which the forebrain is not divided by a midline fissure. The basal ganglia and thalami may be fused, and the pyramidal tracts are absent in some forms. Clinical manifestations also include hypotelorism, microcephaly, and mental and developmental delay. At least four separate gene mutations are known to be associated.

The condition is subdivided according to the degree of completeness of the fusion of the two frontal lobes. In the *alobar* form there is a small cerebrum with but a single ventricle, and there are no lobes nor fissures. In the *semilobar* form, there is an incomplete midline fissure but the cerebral cortex is in continuity across the midline, at least anteriorly. In the *lobar* form, the hemispheres are joined by a band of neocortex at the frontal pole or the orbital surface or over the corpus callosum (**cingulosynapsis**), or are separated; but the corpus callosum is absent.

The terminological difficulties of this classification have been discussed.[3108] Various chromosomal syndromes may be associated with this anomaly.[2219]

holoprosencephaly and limb defects   See **Steinfeld syndrome.**

holoprosencephaly with congenital heart disease and polydactyly   A congenital dysmorphic syndrome characterized by skeletal, genital and cardiac abnormalities, hydrocephalus, and holoprosencephaly.

holoprosencephaly with endocrine dysgenesis   A congenital dysmorphic syndrome characterized by adrenal hypoplasia, hypopituitarism, small sella turcica, and holoprosencephaly.

holotelencephaly   See **holoprosencephaly.**

holotopistic striatal degeneration   See **hereditary striatal degeneration, infantile symmetrical necrosis of the neostriatum.**

Holter valve   A pair of stainless steel valves connected by tubing and used in procedures to reduce intracranial pressure by drainage into another body part such as the peritoneum.

Holtermüller syndrome   See **cloverleaf skull.**

Holtermüller-Weidermann syndrome   See **cloverleaf skull.**

Holzer stain   A glial stain using phosphomolybdic acid and crystal violet, useful for showing fibrous astrocytic processes.

Homen, Erst Alexander (1851–1926)   Finnish pathologist, professor at Helsingör. His major interest was the pathological anatomy of neurological infections and inherited diseases.

Homen syndrome   Generalized rigidity, vertigo, amnesia, apraxia, speech disorders, and progressive dementia occurring with lesions of the lenticular nucleus.[2635]

Homeric laughter   A literary allusion to Homer: "Where unextinguished laughter shakes the skies . . ." referring here to episodic outbursts of irrepressible hearty laughter not provoked by any merry ideas, occurring with pseudobulbar palsy resulting from any cause (such as multiple sclerosis or kuru), and occasionally after prefrontal lobotomy or as an epileptic manifestation. Such **emotionalism** is, however, more usually seen as weeping.[595] See **spasmodic laughter.**

homocarnosinosis   A recessively inherited syndrome with onset in childhood or adult life and characterized by hepatosplenomegaly, spastic paraplegia, mental deterioration, and markedly elevated levels of homocarnosine in the CSF.[5196]

homocysteine   An essential amino acid, high blood levels of which have been implicated as risk factors for silent brain infarcts and white matter lesions.[5753a]

homocystinuria   (cystiathionine beta-synthetase deficiency, Field syndrome, Carson syndrome) A recessively inherited dysmorphic syndrome with infantile onset, the responsible gene (for cystathionine l:I-synthase) mapping to 21q22.3.

Clinical characteristics include fine fair hair, pale skin with facial flushing, myopia, cataract, dislocation of the lens, optic atrophy, and a tendency for multiple cerebrovascular, coronary, and renal arterial occlusions to develop. Mental retardation, various psychiatric disorders including schizophreniform psychosis, seizures, pyramidal signs, dystonias, hepatomegaly, and osteoporosis are also described. Excessive amounts of homocystine are present in the blood and urine.[5941]

Variants include the following:
N-methylene-tetrahydrofolate methyltransferase deficiency type In this disorder, decreased blood methionine levels occur and megaloblastic anemia is reported, each due to deficiency of this enzyme required for the metabolism of homocysteine and for activation of vitamin B_{12}. Clinically, the phenotypes are diverse, but mental retardation, impaired memory, hallucinations, features of **Marfan syndrome,** nystagmus, and ataxia may occur.[1248]
N-methylene-tetrahydrofolate reductase type There is a failure of homocysteine metabolism in childhood, associated clinically with any combination of pyramidal signs, seizures, myopathy, chorea, and psychosis.[1944]
Homocystinuria with methylmalonic aciduria A combinations of the two defects, leading to a syndrome of dystonia with associated megaloblastoc anemia.

homolateral ataxia and crural paresis   Originally considered to be a **lacunar syndrome** manifesting cerebellar ataxia, weakness, and pyramidal signs involving the limbs of the same side, the leg more than the arm, due to a supratentorial lesion in the capsular-corona radiata region or in the paracentral area supplied by the anterior cerebral artery.[629,1866] (See **ataxic hemiparesis.**) The condition may actually be a crossed cerebral–cerebellar **diaschisis.**[2126]

homologous   (Gr, agreeing) The same in value, structure, or position.

homonomous   (Gr, subject to the same law) The same on the two sides of the body; similarly constituted.

homonymous   (Gr, the same + name) Having the same name, but possibly a different meaning.

homonymous diplopia   See **diplopia.**

homonymous hemianopia   Loss of vision in the same half-field in each eye due to a lesion at a point in the visual pathway in or behind the lateral geniculate bodies. See also **bitemporal hemianopia, binasal hemianopia.**

homonymous hemianoptic paracentral scotoma   A syndrome characterized clinically by difficulty in reading and fixation of objects located close to the central field on the side of the defect, normal visual acuity, and a homonymous scotoma that does not include the macula. There is maintenance of the peripheral field so that vision is retained in that portion of the field that lies between the periphery and the scotoma. The condition usually has a sudden onset and may be due to vascular lesions in or near the lateral geniculate bodies.[112]

homunculus   (diminutive of Lat, man) A caricature representing the cortical regions for the various body parts overlying the motor and sensory cortices.

The name was adopted despite the ancient assertion of the disciples of **Paracelsus** that a figure so named was produced by digesting semen in a glass, incubated within a dunghill.

Hooft syndrome   A recessively inherited disorder of tryptophan metabolism characterized by tapetoretinal degeneration, physical and mental retardation, erythematous skin rashes, hypoglycemia and hypolipidemia, and abnormalities of the nails and teeth.[2638]

Hooke, Robert   (1635–1703) English scientist who in his *Micrographia* wrote of seeing "little boxes or cells, distinct from one another" under the microscope, thus introducing the concept of the cellular structure of the body.

Hooper, Robert   (1773–1835) English physician, practicing in London. Spillane[5280] relates that he performed over 4000 autopsies, gathering his observations into a book, *The Morbid Anatomy of the Human Brain,* in 1828, which was the first atlas of neuropathology.

Hooper Visual Organization test   A complex, modern, nonverbal test of perceptual processing, in which the subject is required to assemble mentally the separated parts of a line drawing and to name the object depicted; right hemisphere functions are thus examined.[2639]

Hootnick-Holmes syndrome   See **acrocephalopolysyndactyly.**

Hoover, Charles Franklin   (1865–1927) American neurologist who was diverted to medicine after training for the Methodist ministry. On graduation from Ohio Wesleyan University, he trained in Europe and on his return to America was quickly appointed as a teacher of physical diagnosis and physician at Cleveland City Hospital, and later professor of medicine at Case Western Reserve University. Most of his publications were on cardiorespiratory medicine. He described his sign in 1908.

Hoover sign   A test of feigned weakness in the legs. It can be elicited in two ways.[214]

1. When a normal subject is asked to *raise*, for example, the right leg off the bed, the left foot will be felt to press down with a similar force as is required to raise the right one. In simulated hemiparesis, when the "normal" leg is raised the "paralyzed" leg will show this downward pressure but, in the setting of organic hemiparesis, it will not. In hysterical weakness of one leg, the lack of downward pressure by the other (normal) leg suggests that no effort is being made to elevate the affected one. See **Grasset sign.**

2. A patient's firm voluntary pressure of the sound leg *downward* upon the bed leads to a slight lifting of the other one in normal and also in hemiparetic patients, but such elevation does not occur in patients with hysterical or simulated weakness.[214]

The sign has some validity, but is not always reliable, although Hoover claimed to prefer it to the **Babinski sign,** which he found "unsatisfactory."[2642]

Hopf syndrome   See **acrodermatitis chronica atrophicans.**

Hopkins Symptom check list   An assessment tool assessing symptoms in a 57-item questionnaire and providing data on both mental and physical health.

Hopkins syndrome   The occurrence of acute flaccid paralysis, resembling poliomyelitis, following an attack of asthma. This is a rare condition, more commonly described in children. Flaccid paralysis, atrophy, and fasciculations of one limb, without pain or sensory change, are the typical findings.[1323]

An enterovirus other than poliovirus is presumably responsible for both the lower motor neuron lesions and the lower respiratory tract infection that triggered the asthma attack, but the combination of muscle relaxants and steroids is also under scrutiny as a cause.[2649]

The occurrence of **acute myopathy** following treatment of acute asthma with steroids and/or pancuronium has also been reported.[3218] See also **critical care neuropathy, postventilatory paretic syndrome.**

Hopkins Verbal Learning test   A simple, recently developed test of learning and recent memory with six alternate forms, allowing assessment of free recall, recognition, discrimination, and semantic versus serial clustering.[720]

hopping nystagmus   See **square-wave jerks.**

horizontal gaze palsy   Inability to turn the eyes conjugately to one side, due to a lesion of the pons and the peripontine reticular formation on the same side, or to a lesion of the frontal eye field on the other. See also **Vulpian sign.**

horizontal insomnia   Back pain made worse by recumbency and requiring that the patient sit up to sleep. The usual cause is the presence of a mobile cauda equina neoplasm that causes complete myelographic block in the supine position.

horizontal nystagmus   Nystagmus in which the abnormal eye deviations occur in the horizontal plane.

horn players palsy   An **overuse syndrome** presenting with mononeuropathy in the arm.

Horner, Johann Friedrich   (1831–1886) Swiss ophthalmologist who trained with von **Graefe** and was professor in Zurich. In 1869 he gave the first complete description of the ocular changes that occur with sympathetic denervation[2654] (though Claude Bernard had described the same changes in animals 7 years before). He also demonstrated that color-blindness was a sex-linked characteristic.[1829]

Johann Friedrich Horner

Horner syndrome   (Bernard-Horner syndrome, oculosympathetic palsy) Reduction in the size of the pupil, both in light and in dark, with narrowing of the palpebral fissure due to ptosis of the upper lid and elevation of the lower lid, due to a lesion at any point along the homolateral sympathetic pathway. Acute lesions affecting the third neuron in the wall of the common carotid artery may also produce temporary flushing and anhidrosis of the same side of the face. Enophthalmos is an associated clinical sign encumbered by subjectivity.

Pharmacological testing assists in localizing the site of the lesion; thus, a brisk constriction with 4% cocaine drops is seen because of denervation hypersensitivity when the lesion affects the third (postganglionic) neuron.

The syndrome was described in animals by Francois Pourfoir du Petit in 1727. E.S. Hare[2451] in England (in 1838) and later Claude Bernard[518] in France gave precise accounts of the changes before Horner's report of 1869.[2451] An American origination by **Weir Mitchell** is also claimed.[3062]

A *variant* is *dominant congenital Horner syndrome*, in which the lesion is partial and is thought to lie in the middle fossa.[2369]

hornet-sting myopathy   An acute myopathy with myoglobinuria due to the venom from the bite of this insect.[5134] See also **Haff disease.**

horopter   A set of points in space which pass through the fixation point in a semicircle, concave toward the observer.

Sir Victor Horsley

Horsley, Sir Victor   (1857–1916). Pioneering British neurosurgeon who trained at, and later was on the staff of, University College Hospital and the **National Hospital,** Queen Square, starting in 1886. He performed experiments using brain stimulation in humans[2658] and, in his first year on the staff of the National Hospital, became the first ever to attack an epileptogenic lesion surgically (in a Scottish man of 22 with scarring after a local infection had complicated a depressed skull fracture. It was on this occasion that Dr. Hughlings-**Jackson** remarked that Horsley had missed the opportunity of putting a joke into a Scotsman's head).

Horsley also introduced bone wax to seal off the edges of a craniotomy and pioneered other methods of ensuring antisepsis; he attempted to relieve trigeminal neuralgia by posterior fossa exploration, was the first to remove a pinealoma and to operate in the region of the pituitary, and he was co-inventor of a prototype stereotactic frame for intracranial surgery.[2660]

The procedure in 1886 was a spectacular success, as was another he performed in the following year when he successfully removed a spinal fibromyxoma clinically localized by Jackson, but, after another few dozen operations (including one performed on his son, who had also developed seizures), Horsley appeared to lose interest in such surgery and turned to medical politics. It was much due to his pressure that regulations were adopted which led to the elimination of **rabies** in England, and he made devoted efforts to improve the regulation of the medical profession, to encourage female suffrage, and to stop vivisection. He was a founder member of the Neurological Society of London and was elected a Fellow of the Royal Society. He volunteered (and was accepted) for military service at the age of 57 and died in Mesopotamia, probably of typhoid or heat stroke, in 1916.[3535,3536,5508]

Hortega, Pio del Rio (1882–1945) Spanish neuroanatomist who trained with **Cajal,** in whose laboratory he identified microglial cells and oligodendroglia as a result of improvements that he had made to Cajal's staining techniques. Rio Hortega delayed publication of his findings because this information contradicted Cajal's opinions, and, when he did publish, he was dismissed. For the remainder of his career he worked elsewhere in Madrid, and (having taken the Republican side in the Spanish Civil War) he went on to work in Paris, Oxford, and Buenos Aires.[1829]

Horton arteritis See **giant cell arteritis.**

Horton, Bayard Taylor (b. 1895) American neurologist at the Mayo Clinic. Apart from his description of **cluster headache,** he is remembered for his identification of the syndrome of **giant cell arteritis.**

Horton headache (syndrome) See **cluster headache.**

hospital addiction See **Munchausen syndrome.**

hot cross bun skull (Parrot sign) Bossing of the frontal bones in congenital syphilis.

hot feet See **burning feet syndrome.**

hot (and dry) foot sign Erythema of the lateral part of the sole of the foot in association with an S1 radiculopathy, which is commonly due to neoplastic lumbosacral plexopathy.

hot water epilepsy (immersion epilepsy) The occurrence of seizures (usually of complex partial type) after the head of children aged 6 months to 10 years has been bathed in very hot water. Water at colder temperatures or hot water applied to other parts of the body has also been recorded as initiating seizures.[4762] The condition has usually been reported from India.

hot-bath sign See **Uhthoff symptom.**

hour glass tumors See **dumbbell tumors.**

Houssay syndrome Relief from the signs of diabetes mellitus by naturally occurring extirpation of the anterior pituitary, as by a pituitary adenoma.

The name follows the demonstration that hypophysectomy relieves the hyperglycemia, ketonuria, and fluctuating blood sugar levels and allows survival without insulin for months in pancreatectomized animals.[876]

Howship, J. (1781–1841) English surgeon.

Howship syndrome See **obturator neuralgia.**

Howship-Romberg syndrome Pain referred to the inside of the knee resulting from irritation of the obturator nerve at the hip, as by a hernia. See **obturator neuralgia.**

Hozay–van Bogaert syndrome See **van Bogaert syndrome.**

HRS See **Hamilton rating scale.**

HSAN See **hereditary sensory and autonomic neuropathy.**

HTLV See **human T-cell lymphotropic virus.**

HTLV-1–associated myelopathy See **tropical spastic paraparesis.**

Huber, Johann Jacob (1707–1778) Swiss professor of anatomy and botany in Göttingen and later at Kassel.

Huber's ganglion A ganglion in the posterior root of C1, not always present.

Huc-Alajouanine-Gopcevitch syndrome See **Alajouanine syndrome.**

Huchard ataxia Forms of gait disturbance seen in in hysterical patients.[2681]

Hughes, C.H. (1839–1916) American neurologist and psychiatrist, professor in St. Louis.

Hughes reflex Downward movement of the penis when the prepuce is pulled upward. The significance of this phenomenon is unclear.

Hughes scale A rating scale allowing the determination of improvement in patients with acute polyneuropathy, devised by Prof. R.A.C. Hughes, a contemporary English neurologist.[2696]

Hughlings-Jackson, J. See **Jackson,** J.H-. Jackson adopted the hyphen and preferred its use.

Huguenin edema Acute congestive cerebral edema.

human pincushion A Bohemian from Prague who had some form of congenital insensitivity to pain and who, in the 19th century, staged performances in which objects were thrust through parts of his anatomy to his complete indifference. His performances were temporarily halted by decree when many members of his American audience were cast into a swoon, unable to tolerate his faithful re-enaction of the Crucifixion. See **congenital indifference to pain.**

human T-cell lymphotropic virus (HTLV) A RNA retrovirus with at least three types, capable of inducing human "slow-virus" neurological disease. Visna, AIDS, and HTLV-1–associated myelopathy (**tropical spastic paraparesis**) are representative disorders.

humeroperoneal myopathy A dominantly inherited form of proximal myopathy which in every other way resembles the **Emery-Dreifuss muscular dystrophy.**[2113]

humeroradial synostosis plus   See **Keutel syndrome.**

Humes melanosis and hydrocephalus syndrome   A congenital dysmorphic syndrome manifesting also macrocephaly, hydrocephalus, and patchy skin pigmentation.[337]

humors   The four fluids, yellow and black bile, phlegma and blood, which were thought in Galenical medicine to produce disease when present in abnormal proportions or when themselves abnormal.

Humpty-Dumpty syndrome   A form of disability neurosis, the subject appearing unable to believe in his recovery.[1909]

hung-up reflexes   Persistent contraction of a muscle stimulated by a tap on its tendon; this is seen both in chorea when involuntary contraction of the muscle interrupts the relaxation phase and in hypothyroidism.

hunkering   A test of virility in parts of the southern United States, the competitors trying to remain longest in the squatting position. See **sciatic neuropathy.**

Hunt epilepsy   Pyridoxine-dependent seizures, described by Dr. A.D. Hunt and others in 1954.[2700]

Hunt, James Ramsay   See **Ramsay Hunt, J.** Hunt did not assume a hyphen and it would be reasonable to place entries concerning him here, except that the compound name is so universally employed.

Hunt juvenile paralysis agitans   See **parkinsonism plus, juvenile parkinsonism syndromes.**

Hunt paralysis   See **juvenile parkinsonism syndromes.**

Hunter, C.H.   (1872–1955) Scottish-Canadian physician, professor of medicine at University of Manitoba. His single description of two Canadian brothers with the disease named for him was published in 1917 while he was in England, 2 years before the report of Gertrud Hurler from Munich.

Hunter oculoencephalohepatorenal syndrome   A congenital dysmorphic syndrome or recent description, characterized by retinal colobomas, strabismus, cerebellar and extrapyramidal signs, and mental and developmental delay.[337]

Hunter syndrome   Deficiency of iduronate sulfatase, inherited as a sex-linked recessive trait. Severe and mild forms are distinguished, with optic atrophy, pigmentary retinal degeneration, deafness, and nodular skin lesions; mental retardation, spinal flexion deformities, and cataracts are not seen until later, if at all.[2709] See **mucopolysaccharidoses.**

Hunter-McAlpine syndrome   A congenital dysmorphic syndrome manifesting also short stature, ptosis, skeletal malformations, microcephaly, craniosynostosis affecting the coronal sutures, and mental and developmental delay.[2708]

Hunt-Hess Scale   A scale in common use for recording the status of patients with **subarachnoid hemorrhage,** published in 1968.[2706]

Chart H–21. Status of Patients with Intracranial Aneurysm with and without Subarachnoid Hemorrhage (Hunt-Hess Scale)

Grade	Symptoms and signs
0.	Unruptured aneurysm; no history nor other manifestation of subarachnoid hemorrhage
1.	Asymptomatic or minimal headache and slight nuchal rigidity
1a.	No acute meningeal or brain reaction, but fixed neurological deficit
2.	Moderate to severe headache, nuchal rigidity, no neurological deficit other than cranial nerve palsy
3.	Drowsiness, confusion, or mild focal neurological deficit
4.	Stupor, moderate to severe hemiparesis; may also include early decerebrate rigidity and vegetative disturbances
5.	Deep coma, decerebrate rigidity, moribund appearance

From Hunt HE, Hess RM. Surgical risks as related to time of intervention in the repair of intracranial aneurysms. J Neurosurg 1968;28:14–20. Reproduced by kind permission.

Huntington Association (International)   A charitable organization. Address: c/o Gerritt Dommerholt, Callunahof 8, 7217 ST Harsfen, The Netherlands. Tel: 31-573-341-595.

Huntington disease   A progressive, autosomal dominantly inherited neurodegenerative disorder due to expansion of a CAG trinucleotide repeat in exon 1 of the gene coding for the hungtintin gene on chromosome 4p16.3, while another Huntington-like syndrome is mapped to 20p.[3611] Mutations are rare and penetrance is complete. ("Unstable and whimsical as the disease may be in other respects, in this it is firm, it never skips a generation to again manifest itself in another; once having yielded its claims, it never regains them."[2710])

Symptoms are usually manifest in the third to fifth decades; they include abnormal movements (chorea), deterioration in personality and in cognitive abilities, and psychiatric disturbances. Neuropsychological deficits include slowness of thought, learning failures, and inability to shift mental set or attention, traditionally regarded as cortical functions but now shown to correlate better with atrophy of the caudate nucleus. Pathologically, there is loss of neurons from the neostriatum and cortex, especially the frontal cortex.

The disease had been known to many generations of the family that Huntington described, and was known as "magrums" or "megrims" to the people of colonial New England; many affected subjects were burnt as witches, as it was popularly believed in those days that the families in which the disease appeared were cursed because they had dared to pantomime Christ's sufferings on the cross in this derisory manner. Thilenius reported a case in 1816, Rufs another in 1834, and Waters yet another, published in Robley Dunglison's *Practice of Medicine* in 1842 (Vol 2, p. 312). It formed the subject of an inaugural thesis (now lost) by Charles Rollin Gorman of Lucerne, Pennsylvania in 1848 and was again reported by Irving Lyon in the *American Medical Times* of 1863. References to Huntington disease appeared in the German literature in 1885 and 1887, since that time the eponym has been firmly established.[5935] The disease was imported to America from Bures in Suffolk, U.K., by the wife of a young Englishman in 1630; the match being disapproved of by his family (her father was choreic), he married her and emigrated.

The following diagnostic criteria have been defined:[1907]

Definite Huntington disease 1. Chorea or the characteristic impairment of voluntary movement that was not present at birth, was insidious in onset, and had become gradually worse; and 2. A family history of at least one other member with these typical symptoms of the disease. Dementia and emotional symptoms are usually present but are not required and are not alone sufficient for the diagnosis.

Probable Huntington disease The clinical features as above, but with a family history that is unobtainable because of adoption or unknown parentage.

In early cases, impairment of movements requiring rhythm and speed, slow voluntary (saccadic) eye movements, mild speech abnormalities, impaired balance on tandem walking, and bradykinesia occur. In advanced cases, severe slowing or absence of both saccades and pursuit eye movements, severe dysarthria or mutism, inability to walk, long tract motor signs, and extreme slowing of all movements are evident.

Variants are listed in Chart H–22.

Chart H–22. Variants of Huntington Disease

Hereditary nonprogressive chorea (*hereditary nonprogressive chorea without dementia*) A dominantly inherited syndrome characterized by the onset in childhood of chorea in the face and arms, with the later appearance of dysarthria and axial dystonia and without dementia, rigidity, seizures, or cerebellar ataxia.[2366,3197] In a further subgroup, progression does occur.[4940]

Familial essential benign chorea A dominantly inherited syndrome of nonprogressive chorea, sometimes with added **essential tremor.**[584,4451] This and the last condition are not clearly distinguished.

Huntington chorea, myoclonic variant A cause of very atypical progressive myoclonic epilepsy.

Juvenile Huntington disease (rigid or Westphal variant) A form characterized by the onset in youth of a rigid-akinetic syndrome, the clinical course afterward resembling that of the later-onset form. This form is more likely to occur in cases with paternal transmission.[2150]

*Spinal muscular atrophy with **Huntington disease*** See **motor neuronal diseases.**

A Huntington-like syndrome mapped to 20p

Huntington, George Sumner (1851–1916) A general practitioner who was born into a family tradition of care for the people of East Hampton, Long Island. After receiving a classical education and medical training at the New York College of Physicians and Surgeons, he described the familial dementia now named for him, briefly but completely[2710] within a year of graduation, while practicing in Ohio. Here, apart from 2 years spent in North Carolina (for the good of his health), he remained for the rest of his professional life without making any further notable contributions to the medical literature.

Huntington sign When a patient is asked to cough forcibly when lying supine with the legs over the side of the bed, the hip will flex and the knee extend on the side of a pyramidal lesion.

Huntington's Disease Association (UK) A charitable organization. Address: 108 Battersea High Street, London SW11 3HP, UK. Tel: 020 7223 7000. Web site: www.hda.org.uk/.

Huntington's Disease Society of America A charitable organization. Address: 140 West 29th St., 7th Floor, New York, NY 10001-5300. Tel: 212-242-1968, 1-800-345-HDSA. Website: http://www.hdsa.org/.

Huntington Society of Canada A charitable organization. Address: 151 Frederick St., Suite 400, Kitchener, Ontario N2H 2M2, Canada. Tel: 519-749-7063. Web site: http://www.hsc-ca.org/.

Hunt–van Bogaert syndrome See **pure pallidal atrophy.**

Hurler, Gertrud (1889–1965) German pediatrician who trained at Munich and worked in Neuhauser.

Hurler syndrome See **mucopolysaccharidoses.**

Hurler syndrome variant See **neurovisceral lipidosis.**

Hurler-Scheie syndrome See **mucopolysaccharidoses.**

Hurst disease (hemorrhagic leukoencephalitis) See **acute disseminated encephalomyelitis.**

Hutchinson facies Extension of the neck and contraction of the frontalis muscles in an attempt to compensate for the ptosis of **tabes dorsalis.**

Hutchinson pupil Unilateral dilatation of a pupil with impaired light and accommodation reactions due to compression of the parasympathetic fibers in the third cranial nerve, as caused by a swollen herniating temporal lobe. Initially the affected pupil may constrict because of irritation of the nerve, dilating later and finally becoming fixed.

The same pattern of events may occur with a time lag in the other eye as a result of the stretching of its third nerve as the brainstem also herniates downward.

Hutchinson, Sir Jonathan   (1828–1913) English surgeon, dermatologist, and ophthalmologist at the London Hospital and professor at the Royal College of Surgeons. He was elected a fellow of the Royal Society in 1882 and was knighted 5 years before his death. His interests were legion, as may be deduced from the following entries, but he was especially interested in syphilis and was said to have gained experience from a million patients with that disorder;[1829] but assuming 40 years in practice, 50 weeks a year and 5 days a week, this translates into 100 patients per day, which is ridiculous.

Sir Jonathan Hutchinson

Hutchinson, Sir Robert   (1871–1943) Scottish radiologist, who investigated the use of radium implants in the management of bladder cancers.

Hutchinson teeth   Notching of the permanent incisors in congenital syphilis.[2716] With interstitial keratitis and bilateral nerve deafness, this constitutes the **Hutchinson triad.**

Hutchinson triad   Interstitial keratitis, notching of the central incisors, and nerve deafness, occurring in congenital syphilis.[2715]

Hutchinson tumor   Neuroblastoma of the left adrenal gland with a secondary deposit in the orbit, less often in other cranial areas, occurring in infants and young children who present with proptosis, papilledema, or optic atrophy and frequently extraocular palsies.

The right-sided tumor metastasizes to the liver.[2718]

Hutchinson-Gilford syndrome   See **progeria.**

hyaline body myopathy   A dominantly inherited, slowly progressive, scapuloperoneal myopathic syndrome characterized by the presence of subsarcolemmal hyaline aggregates in type 1 fibers of skeletal muscles.[3691]

hyalinosis cutis et mucosae   See **Urbach-Wiethe disease.**

hyaloid remnants   Residua of the embryonic vascular channels in the eye which may overlie the optic disk, causing apparent blurring on ophthalmoscopy.

Hyams cerebral palsy and glaucoma syndrome   A congenital syndrome manifesting short stature, buphthalmos, spasticity, and mental and developmental delay.[337]

hydranencephaly   (hydroanencephaly) An uncommon congenital abnormality consisting of more or less complete replacement of the cerebral hemispheres by fluid, contained within a thin-walled capsule composed of glial tissue and meninges. The normally sized skull thus transilluminates brilliantly.

It occurs as the result of a severe ischemic cerebral lesion, usually of the carotid territory, and during the fifth month of intrauterine development. **Cruvheilier** gave the first description in 1829.[1207]

hydrargyria   Mercury poisoning.

hydrencephaloid   See **Hall syndrome.**

hydroanencephaly   See **hydranencephaly.**

hydrocephalus   (Gr, water + brain) (hydrocrania) Dilatation of the cerebral ventricles, first described by Vesalius in 1550 but known to the Hippocratic authors.

In *internal hydrocephalus*, there is an obstruction to the flow of CSF somewhere between its site of production in the ventricles and the subarachnoid space in the posterior fossa. In *external hydrocephalus*, the obstruction is between the roof foramina of the fourth ventricle and the arachnoid granulations in the dural venous sinuses.

Although grossly but accurately described by Vesalius, it was Morgagni (1682–1771) who noted in 1769 it's occurrence in young children, with cranial enlargement, separation of the sutures, thinning of the skull, dilatation of the lateral ventricles, and a normal cerebellum and brainstem. One of his patients undoubtedly had a **Chiari malformation.**[5609]

In a *variant X-linked form*, the responsible gene maps to Xq28.

hydrocephalus, agyria, retinal dysplasia, and encephalocele syndrome   (HARD+E syndrome, Warburg syndrome) See **Walker-Warburg syndrome.**

hydrocephalus ex vacuo   (external hydrocephalus) An increase in the volume of CSF resulting solely from independent atrophy of brain tissue. See **normal pressure hydrocephalus.**

hydrocephalus with polydactyly   (Biemond syndrome, definition 2) A syndrome of hydrocephalus, iris colobomata, hypogenitalism, polydactyly, mental retardation, and obesity.[562]

hydrocephalus-costovertebral dysplasia with Sprengel deformity   See **Waaler anomaly.**

hydrocrania   See **hydrocephalus.**

hydrolethalus syndrome   A recessively inherited dysmorphic syndrome characterized also by hydrocephalus; cardiac, renal, genital, and skeletal malformations; and a tendency to die *in utero* or shortly after birth.[4889]

hydromyelia   (Gr, water + marrow) The term applied by Olliver d'Angers in 1827 to cystic dilatation of the central canal of the spinal cord.

The condition is usually congenital and results from increased pressure of CSF in the fourth ventricle and hypertrophic arachnoiditis of its roof, as with a **Chiari malformation.**

hydrophobia   (Gr, water + fear) The repulsion of water or any fluid to drink, manifest by those about to die from **rabies,** owing to the violent paroxysms of muscle contraction that the sufferer now knows will follow any attempt to swallow.

hydrops   (Lat, dropsy) See **idiopathic intracranial hypertension.**

hydrostatic cerebral edema   Excessive water content of the brain extracellular space, usually as a result of increased intravascular pressure, as in hypertensive encephalopathy.

hydroxyamphetamine test   (paredrine test) One drop of 1% hydroxyamphetamine solution is instilled into the eye. A normal pupil will not respond by dilating, but the pupil on the side of a lesion of the first- or second-order sympathetic neuron will.

The drug releases vesicles of stored norepinephrine from the healthy nerve terminals of the long ciliary nerves, resulting in dilatation of the pupil in normal subjects and those with a first-order sympathetic neuron lesion, but this effect is not seen in those with a lesion of the third-order neuron in the sympathetic pathway to the eye. See also **cocaine test.**

hydroxyisovaleric aciduria   A disorder of branched-chain amino acid metabolism considered due to deficiency of dimethylacrylyl coenzyme A-carboxylase, characterized clinically by the features of hereditary motor neuropathy, and notable for the infant's strong odor of cat urine.[5364]

hydroxykynureninemia   A rare syndrome in infancy characterized by mental retardation, hemolytic anemia, and hepatosplenomegaly in the presence of excessive urinary excretion of xanthenuric acid and hydroxykynurenine.[1248]

3–hydroxy-3–methyl coenzyme A lysase deficiency   A rare disorder resulting from a failure of leucine catabolism, and characterized clinically by acidosis, hypoglycemia, hypotonia, seizures, and progressive reduction of consciousness in infancy or childhood.[1752]

hygroma   A fluid-filled cavity. Those in the subdural space have usually followed trauma or meningitis.

Hyndham sign   See **head flexion test.**

hyp-   (Gr, a diminution) Prefix denoting diminution.

hypacusis   Diminution in hearing.

hypalgesia   (Gr, under + sense of pain) (hypalgia) A diminution in the perception of pain.

hypalgia   See **hypalgesia.**

hyper-   (Gr, over, in excess of) Prefix denoting excess.

hyperabduction syndrome   See **thoracic outlet syndrome.**

hyperacusis   Abnormal perception of sounds as being loud. Increased keenness of hearing for quiet sound stimuli is not associated. This is a common symptom in patients with migraine attacks and with any disease causing cerebral irritability such as meningitis.

hyperaldosteronism   Increased production of aldosterone, usually due to an adenoma of the adrenal cortex in adults. A neurological complication is a myasthenia-like syndrome appearing as intermittent severe weakness or paralysis, associated with tetany, paresthesias, and hypertension. Raised sodium and reduced potassium and magnesium serum levels are also present and a vacuolar myopathy may also be associated.[1714]

hyperalgesia   (hyperalgia) An abnormally increased response to a stimulus that normally is indeed painful.

hyperalgia   See **hyperalgesia.**

hyperammonemia-orthinemia-homocitrullinuria (HHH) syndrome   (OMIM 238970) A recessively inherited inborn error of metabolism in which there is impairment of transport of ornithine across the inner mitochondrial membrane. Clinically, it is expressed in childhood and characterized by vomiting, irritability, seizures, and ataxia in the first year of life and by hyperammomnemia, homocitrullinuria, and gyrate atrophy of the choroid and retina with visual field constriction, myopia, pyramidal signs, ataxia, myoclonic seizures, episodic disturbances of consciousness due to intermittent hyperammonemia, and mental retardation.[335,5133] The responsible affected *ORNT1* gene maps to chromosome 13q14.[5656] See also **ornithinemia.**

hyperammonemias   A group of inherited disorders involving any of the five enzymes of the urea cycle and presenting as intermittent ataxic syndromes associated with elevated serum ammonia levels and leading to diffuse encephalopathies. **Arginase deficiency, argininosuccinuria, citrullinemia, carbamyl-phosphate synthetase deficiency, hyperornithinemia,** and **ornithine transcarbamoylamase deficiency** are described.[390,5247] Levels of ammonia are also raised in **pyruvate carboxylase deficiency.**

The usual presentation is of a catastrophic illness in the first week of life with poor suck, hypotonia, vomiting, lethargy, and hyperventilation, progressing to seizures and eventually to coma. The EEG shows low voltage with theta and delta activity. Imaging suggests the presence of cerebral edema.

Individuals with partial syndromes present later; children present with anorexia, ataxia, behavioral disturbances, and hyperactivity, and adults present with migrainous headaches, nausea, ataxia, dysarthria confucion, hallucinatioins and visual impairment, clinical signs including pyramidal signs, papilledema, decerebrate/decorticate posturing, and coma. Hyperammonemic episodes tend to be precipitated by high-protein meals, infections, surgery, and pregnancy or delivery.[390] In children, valproic acid has also been associated with hyperammonemic encephalopathy.

hyperammonemic syndromes   See also **cerebellar ataxias** (*variants*).

hyperaphia   Increased sensibility to touch.

hyper-beta-alaninemia   An aminoaciduria due to deficiency of β-alanine α-ketoglutarate transaminase, characterized by infantile seizures and by elevations in the plasma and urine levels of β-alanine and β-immunoisobutyric acid.[5043]

hypercapnic headache   (mixed hypoxia and hypercapnia) A metabolic cause of headache resembling **migraine** included in that category of the International Headache Society's Classification (see Chart H–5) as are **hypoglycemic** and **dialysis headaches.**

hypercolumn   The alternating arrangements of the columns of cells in the cortex, each column having a specific receptivity to inputs at different orientations.

hyperconvergence   Spasm of the muscles producing convergence.[1847]

hyperdense MCA sign   Unusual density of the middle cerebral artery on neuroimaging, highly suggestive of embolic or atherothrombotic MCA occlusion in the appropriate clinical context but not specific when present in isolation. It is likely due to calcium or to the hemorrhagic components of the acute plaque. False-positive hyperdensity may be seen in asymptomatic patients with a high hematocrit or calcific atherosclerotic disease.

hyperdense sylvian fissure branch sign   Hyperdensity on CT scans of the more distal branches of the middle cerebral artery in the sylvian fissure within hours of their embolic occlusion.

hyperdynamia   Abnormally increased strength.

hyperekplexia   (stiff baby syndrome) A rare dominantly (seldom recessively) inherited syndrome with in-

complete penetrance which in its major form comprises an excessive **startle response** to unheralded sensory stimuli and generalized stiffness and transient hypertonia from early infancy; falling attacks ("falling like a log") without unconsciousness, often leading to injuries such as concussion; nocturnal leg jerking; episodic generalized shaking resembling generalized spontaneous clonus or repetitive myoclonus; generalized hyperreflexia; and an insecure and hesitating or puppet-like gait due to fear of falling, all in the absence of gross brain pathology. The episodes are maximal at night. Seizures and mental retardation are inconstant features.[2450] There is an increased incidence of associated neurologic and electroencephalographic abnormalities

The pattern of muscle recruitment suggests that the condition represents a widespread elevated gain of the vestigial withdrawal reflexes in the brainstem and spinal cord due to increased excitability of the reticular neurons.[3700] The condition has been mapped to 5q33–q35, involving the glycine receptor, α_1 subunit, binding strychnine.

Excessive startle was identified as leading to seizures by Alajouanine and Gastaut but it was later recognized that a nonepileptic surprise reaction also exists.

In *variant* minor forms, an inconstant excessive startle response brought out by a febrile illness and in adults by emotional stress and improving with time is the only feature,[167] or the clinical manifestations first appear in youth.

hyperemesis gravidarum   A syndrome of recurrent vomiting occurring in the first trimester of pregnancy, but occasionally persisting thereafter and liable to be complicated by vitamin deficiency and **Wernicke-Korsakoff syndrome.**

hyperendorphin syndrome of necrotizing encephalopathy   A *variant* of **subacute necrotizing encephalomyelopathy** characterized by attacks resembling acute morphine poisoning with prolonged apnea and unconsciousness, temporarily reversible with nalorphine. The postmortem brain changes are the same as those of the parent syndrome.[723]

hyperesthesia   1. The term of Henry **Head** for a most unpleasant prolonged stinging sensation felt in areas sensitive to pinprick but not to light touch; it follows peripheral nerve injury and is due to a loss of the normal inhibitory effects of local touch receptors. An increased sensitivity to sensory stimuli, often with an added unpleasant quality. **Hyperpathia** has the same meaning. 2. Increased sensitivity (decreased threshold) to a stimulus.

hyperflexion-hyperextension syndrome   See **acceleration injury syndrome.**

hypergeusia   A morbid sensitivity to taste sensations—more a disorder of reaction than one of sensation, as taste thresholds are not necessarily affected.

hyperglycinemia An inborn error of metabolism causing both a primary organic acidemia and a secondary defect in the metabolism of glycine. The *non-ketotic* form is due to a primary error in the metabolism of glycine; the *ketotic* form (see **proprionic acidemia**) is due to an error in proprionic acid metabolism, but their features are similar.

Microencephaly, severe hypomyelination of those systems that myelinate only after birth, and spongy degeneration of the brain are the pathological characteristics; lethargy, myoclonus and epileptic seizures, and progression to decerebration and death after only 1 or 2 days of normal development after birth are the usual findings.[5145] The condition may also occur as a response to therapy with sodium valproate.

In a *variant* form, the hyperglycinuria is paroxysmal and associated with paroxysmal kinesigenic dystonia.

hypergraphia (echographia, graphomania, anosognosic graphomimia, graphoreé, phonographie) 1. A disturbance of writing seen in patients with right hemisphere lesions, characterized by writing on the right side of the paper only, inability to maintain a straight line, and the repetition of letters.[5736,6062] This syndrome is known as *multiple loop agraphia*. 2. Unusually detailed and copious but graphically normal writing observed as a compulsive phenomenon in patients with complex partial seizures[5878] or with frontal lobe dementia.[2970]

A distinction between hypergraphia as defined here and "automatic writing behavior" has been suggested,[5740] although the value of this remains unproven.

hyperhidrosis Morbidly increased sweating. See also **episodic hyperhidrosis.**

hyperhomocystinemia A monogenic disorder with genetic heterogeneity, mapped to 1p36.3, predisposing the subject to stroke.[2363]

hyperinsulin neuronopathy A motor axonal neuropathy associated with excessive insulin production.[4033]

hyperkalemic periodic paralysis See **familial periodic paralysis.**

hyperkalemic periodic paralysis with dysrhythmias (Andersen syndrome) See **familial periodic paralysis.**

hyperkeratosis-syringomyelia See **Fischer syndrome.**

hyperkinesia (Gr, above + movement) A condition in which a subject makes excessive and even continuous movements, these themselves not necessarily being abnormal.

hyperkinetic state A condition of childhood in which the patient manifests stimulus-oriented behavior, distractibility, shortened attention span, lack of tolerance of frustration, and lack of fear. See **attention-deficit hyperactivity disorder.**

hyperkinetic tremor See **cerebellar tremors.**

hyperlexia 1. The presence of outstanding reading ability in brain-damaged children who otherwise manifest retardation in the normal development of language, with failure of spontaneous speech, dysarthria, echolalia, and evidence of a hyperkinetic syndrome. An associated to-and-fro rocking movement during reading is nearly invariable. The children's drive to examine and read written material is at times compulsive.[3806] 2. The acquisition of reading skills at an unusually early age.[9]

hyperlysinemia A hyperammonemic syndrome characterized by failure to thrive, hypotonia due to lax ligaments, and seizures occurring in infancy.[2088] Mental retardation is common but not invariable, and a few normal children with this condition have been reported.

hypermetamorphosis The tendency to change behaviors unusually quickly; a feature of the **Kluver-Bucy syndrome.**

hypermethioninemia A rare, fatal, diffuse encephalopathy occurring in infancy, probably a variant of **hereditary tyrosinemia.** It is characterized clinically by irritability, lethargy, and intracranial hemorrhage.[1248]

hypermetria An excessive range of movement of a limb due to delays in starting and in completing the arrest of a limb in its trajectory toward a target.[2625] It appears to be based on misjudgment of the required point of arrest of a limb during extension (overshoot), which is a sign of cerebellar disease affecting the lateral lobes.

hypermetric saccades A normal single saccade that only stops past the point of fixation of the desired target (overshooting), requiring thus a further small corrective saccade in order to place the image of the target back on the fovea (a refixation eye movement). See also **hypometric saccades, pulse dysmetria.**

hypermnesia The rare condition of abnormally enhanced memory, met with occasionally in *idiots savants.*

hypernormal CT scans CT scan images in which the sulci are narrow and the ventricles are small, not because the brain is normal but because of the presence of chronic, bilateral, isodense subdural hematomas.[2786]

hyperopia (Gr, above + the eye) Far-sightedness (in the ophthalmological sense), in which the entering rays are focused behind the retina because of inadequate refraction by the media.

hyperopsia Abnormally acute vision.

hyperornithinemia A rare hyperammonemic syndrome of childhood presenting with irritability, ataxia, constriction of the visual fields, and myoclonus. The precise biochemical abnormality is unknown.[2439] See **HHH syndrome.**

In a *variant* form, there is associated gyrate atrophy of the retina with optic atrophy.

hyperornithinemia, hyperammonemia, homocitrullinemia syndrome   See **HHH syndrome.**

hyperosmia   1. Abnormal sensitivity in the realm of odor detection. 2. Increased sensitivity to the qualities of odors without any decrease in the threshold for their detection. This latter definition represents the current usage of the word.

hyperostosis   1. Bony overgrowths or excrescences. 2. Thickening of normal bone as in **hyperostosis frontalis interna.**

hyperostosis corticalis generalisata congenita (dominant osteosclerosis, Caffey Silverman syndrome) The milder, dominantly inherited form of **endosteal hyperostosis** characterized by hyperostosis and osteosclerosis of the skull, mandible, and other parts of the skeleton, and commonly complicated by seventh and eighth cranial nerve deficits.[6044] See also **hyperostosis corticalis generalisata familiaris.**

hyperostosis corticalis generalisata familiaris   (van Buchem syndrome, Buchem syndrome, chronic hyperphosphatemia tarda) The severe autosomal recessive form of **endosteal hyperostosis** characterized by hyperostosis and osteosclerosis of the skull, mandible, and other parts of the skeleton, commonly complicated by seventh and eighth cranial nerve deficits, and occasionally with increased intracranial pressure and optic nerve involvement.[5710]

hyperostosis cranialis interna   A dominantly inherited hyperostotic and osteosclerotic disease with onset in youth, manifesting intracranial hyperostosis, osteosclerosis of the calvaria and skull base only, recurrent facial palsy, and variable involvement of cranial nerves I, II, and VIII.[3593]

hyperostosis frontalis interna   (Morgagni-Stewart-Morel syndrome, calvarial hyperostosis) Thickening and condensation of the frontal bones, seen almost exclusively in females. Obesity and hypertrichosis but no neurological deficits accompany this phenomenon, although all manner of troubles were ascribed to it by Morgagni (1769).[3974]

A *variant* is *hyperostosis frontalis interna with cataracts*, which is a congenital dysmorphic syndrome characterized also by skeletal deformities, cataract, strabismus, short neck, thick calvarium, fasciculations, and mental and developmental delay.[337]

hyperoxaluria type 1   (glycolic aciduria) A recessively inherited **peroxisomal disorder** resulting from a deficiency of alanine glyoxalate aminotransferase and characterized by hyperoxaluria, hyperglycolic aciduria, the formation of calcium oxalate stones in the urine, and nephrocalcinosis.[1277]

Combined axonal and demyelinating polyneuropathy, causing painful paresthesias or weakness, is a noted complication.[2377] Renal failure usually leads to death before the end of the second decade.

hyperparathyroid myopathy   A syndrome consisting of fatigue, wasting, quadriceps weakness with intact reflexes, and skeletal pain, occurring in the presence of a parathyroid adenoma.[1021]

hyperparathyroidism   Overactivity of the parathyroid glands, leading to proximal and bulbar muscle weakness, wasting, aching, and fatigue with hyperactive muscle stretch reflexes. The findings in osteomalacia are similar.[5239]

More severe neurological disturbances, including ataxia, internuclear ophthalmoplegia, and pyramidal signs, have also been reported.[4363]

hyperpathia   (Gr, excessive + pain) 1. Great torment of mind. 2. Delay in the perception of a stimulus with an after-sensation and overreaction to the painful stimulus, as frequently occurs in association with **causalgia. Hyperesthesia** has the same meaning and represents the current usage of the term. 3. A painful syndrome of increased reaction to a stimulus in association with a raised threshold for perception of that stimulus.

hyperphagia   Pathological overeating, as may result from some hypothalamic lesions. See **bulimia.**

hyperphenylalaninemia   Diffuse encephalopathies occurring in a number of conditions, such as **phenylketonuria, dihydropteridine** and **dihydrobiopterin synthetase deficiency, persistent hyperphenylalaninemia,** and **phenylalanine transferase deficiency,** in all of which there is an abnormality of the phenylalanine hydroxylase enzymic system.[1248]

hyperphoria   A latent tendency for one eye to deviate to a position above that assumed by the other.

hyperpipecolic acidemia   A recessively inherited peroxisomal disorder with onset in infancy, characterized clinically by hypotonia, hepatomegaly, and nystagmus; thereafter, progressive quadriparesis and mental retardation occur as a result of demyelination in the CNS. Elevated serum pipecolate levels are found.[2060] See **Zellweger disease, neonatal adrenoleukodystrophy.**

hyperpolarization   A change in the existing membrane potential to a more negative value. See also **polarization.**

hyperpraxia   Excessive activity, as in manic conditions.

hyperprolinemia   A metabolic error characterized by a deficiency of proline oxidase or of a related dehydrogenase. The syndrome is regarded as a diffuse encephalopathy which in some cases causes renal and ocular disease, seizures, mental retardation, and various CNS disorders, but which may be asymptomatic.[3945]

hyperpyrexia associated with muscle contraction
See **diencephalic autonomic seizures.**

hypersensitivity raking Unusual responsiveness to
the visual environment, considered to be a manifestation of **Parkinson disease** and a factor leading to **freezing** of gait.[3848]

hypersensitivity vasculitis A group of vasculitis syndromes resulting from abnormal responses to foreign
antigens. In **serum sickness** and **Henoch-Schönlein
purpura,** neurological complications are reported.

hypersexuality Abnormally increased sexual drive
and activity. In neurology, it may indicate the presence
of bilateral frontal lobe damage or the **Kluver-Bucy
syndrome.**

hypersomnia (somnolence) A climate of sleepiness;
enhanced proclivity toward sleep punctuated by spells
in which awareness of environmental stimuli is actually
lost. It is a feature of the **Kleine-Levin, Pickwickian,**
and various psychiatric syndromes.[653] See **idiopathic
hypersomnia.**

hypersomnia with increased 5–HIAA in the CSF A
syndrome characterized by a high normal sleep time of
12–14 hours/day over several consecutive days, the
raised serotonin levels presumably reflecting hyperactivity of serotonergic mechanisms.

hypersomnia-bulimia See **Klein-Levin syndrome.**

hypersomnolence (excessive daytime drowsiness)
The condition of experiencing prolonged nocturnal
sleep and long periods of gradual and resistible non–
rapid eye movement stage 1–2 sleep (subwakefulness)
during waking hours, especially in the morning. *Essential hypersomnolence* is defined as "chronic persistent
daytime drowsiness without obvious organic cause."[4337]
   Variants include the following:
   Secondary hypersomnolence resulting from some metabolic
      or neurological disorder of the nervous system
   Neurotic hypersomnolence A condition consisting of life-
      long fatigue, hypersomnia, and sometimes sleep reversal
      as a complication of neurotic or depressive disease.
   Nocturnal hyperkinesis with daytime hypersomnolence Is the
      occurrence of severe myoclonus, restlessness, bruxism,
      and frequent arousals during the night, with daytime
      drowsiness.
   Sleep apnea
   Long-cycle hypersomnia A condition of recurrent hyper-
      somnolence occurring at intervals longer than a day. It is
      also seen in the **Kleine-Levin syndrome;** it is secondary
      to drug or alcohol abuse, and occurs in shift workers.

hypertelorism (orbital hypertelorism, ocular hypertelorism, teleorbitism) A craniofacial anomaly in which
there is unusual widening of the space between the eyes,
and thus increased interorbital and interpupillary distances, due to maldevelopment of the lesser wings of the
sphenoid bones. Mental retardation is sometimes associated even when the condition is present in isolation,[2277]

but it is also a feature of numerous other developmental
syndromes. The condition is usually sporadic but may be
inherited as a dominant or recessive trait.[4,1026,2219]
   In adults, the normal distance between the inner canthi is 30–33 mm, and between the pupils it is more than
64 mm.
   Orbital hypertelorism exists when there is true lateralization, (i.e., out-turning) of the orbits; *interorbital
hypertelorism* is the term used when there is no such
lateralization, as is commonly the case in **craniosynostosis.**[4] The term was originally coined by Dr. David
Greig, conservator of the Edinburgh museum, in 1924.
See also **Greig syndrome.**

hypertelorism-hypospadias syndrome (BBB syndrome, Elsahy-Waters syndrome) A dominantly inherited developmental syndrome with incomplete penetrance and variable expressivity, so that males are
mainly affected.
   Clinically, it is characterized by wide-spaced inner
canthi (telecanthus), hypospadias, cryptorchidism,
mental retardation, cranial asymmetry, and strabismus.[1026] Coarctation of the aorta, cleft lip and palate,
and micrognathia may also be associated.

hypertensive headache The popular perception of
high blood pressure as a cause of headache, for which
there is no good evidence except in association with hypertensive encephalopathy.

hypertensive encephalopathy An acute syndrome
due to a rapid rise in blood pressure, occurring primarily in patients with chronic, poorly controlled hypertension.
   Clinically, headache, obtundation, seizures, and
sometimes transient neurological deficits are common,
nausea, vomiting, seizures, focal signs, and visual disturbances less so. The level of consciousness is relatively
more depressed than the severity of the neurological
signs, and papilledema, flame-shaped hemorrhages,
and retinal exudates are almost invariable. The diastolic
blood pressure is usually >130 mmHg, and there is no
gross bleeding into or around the brain on imaging or
as detected by lumbar puncture. The CSF pressure is
usually increased.[1464]
   Neuropathologic changes consist of fibrinoid necrosis of arterioles, thrombosis of arterioles and capillaries, and parenchymal lesions such as microinfarcts and
petechial hemorrhages secondary to the vascular lesions, which are not confined to the brain but affect
also the eyes, kidneys, and other organs. In the CNS the
brainstem was most severely affected. Cerebral edema
is not observed, even in patients with increased CSF
pressure and papilledema.[1003]
   See also **eclampsia.**

hyperthyroid myopathy A syndrome of proximal
muscle weakness with atrophy and myopathic EMG abnormalities complicating nearly all cases of hyperthy-

roidism. See also **acute thyrotoxic myopathy, familial periodic paralysis.**

hyperthyroid neuropathy   (Basedow paraplegia) An acute flaccid proximal neuropathy or plexopathy complicating hyperthyroidism.[1762]

hyperthyroidism   See **amyotrophic lateral sclerosis, endocrine exophthalmos, myasthenia gravis, familial periodic paralysis.**

hypertonia   (Gr, excessive + tone) Increased muscle resistance to passive stretching, as occurs with upper motor neuron lesions.

hypertonia of opposition   1. Rigidity in neurodegenerative diseases associated with a general attitude of flexion, particularly of the neck muscles, and with a positive limb placement sign.[5673,5674] The association of hypertonia in the upper limbs with dyspraxia. See also **arteriosclerotic rigidity.**

hypertonic bladder   See **Bors Comarr classification.**

hypertrichosis and gingival fibromatosis   A congenital dysmorphic syndrome manifesting also generalized hirsutism, seizures, and mental and developmental delay.[337]

hypertrichosis–mental   retardation–seizures   A congenital dysmorphic syndrome characterized by generalized hirsutism, coarse facial features, gum hypertrophy, seizures, and mental and developmental delay.

hypertrophia   (hypertrophy) (Gr, above + nourishment) See **hypertrophy.**

hypertrophia musculorum vera   A dominantly inherited syndrome with the onset in youth or adult life of muscle hypertrophy with muscle pain, cramps, and often paresthesias, but without weakness.[4469]

A *variant* is *hypertrophia musculorum vera and ataxia*, which is a congenital syndrome characterized by painful muscle hypertrophy, fasciculations, and neurogenic weakness, cerebellar ataxia, raised serum creatine kinase levels, and sensory neuropathy.[4200]

hypertrophic brachial plexus neuritis   A dominantly inherited disorder linked to 17q24, possibly a form of **neuralgic amyotrophy** or a painless manifestation of hereditary pressure-sensitive neuropathy. In yet other cases it appears to be due to localized chronic autoallergic or viral inflammation, producing marked hypertrophy of the nerves of the plexus.[1234,5712] See **multifocal inflammatory demyelinating neuropathy.**

hypertrophic branchial myopathy   A syndrome of isolated enlargement of the masseter and/or temporalis muscles, either sporadically or in association with hypothyroidism.[3406] See **branchial myopathy.**

hypertrophic cervical pachymeningitis   Chronic inflammation of the spinal meninges, including the lep-

tomeninges, producing compression of the spinal cord and nerve roots.[972] Whether this is due to infections or to autoimmune disease is not certain.

hypertrophic granulomatous cranial pachymeningitis   Inflammatory swelling of the intracranial dura mater as a result of **Wegener granulomatosis** or infection.[1790]

hypertrophic inflammatory neuropathy involving bilateral brachial plexus   See **multifocal inflammatory demyelinating neuropathy.**

hypertrophic interstitial neuritis   (Déjèrine-Sottas syndrome) See **hereditary motor and sensory neuropathy, type 3.**

hypertrophic interstitial neuropathy with cataracts   See **hereditary motor and sensory neuropathy, type 1.**

hypertrophic mononeuritis, focal upper limb demyelinating neuropathy   See **multifocal inflammatory demyelinating neuropathy.**

hypertrophic myelomalacia   See **Foix-Alajouanine syndrome.**

hypertrophic myopathy   Generalized enlargement of muscles that are strong.[1959] When not physiologically induced, this is probably **Thomsen disease.** See **hypertrophia musculorum vera.**

hypertrophic neuropathy   Neuropathies in which there is visible or palpable thickening of the cutaneous (anterior tibial, supraclavicular, greater superficial petrosal, radial sensory) or other superficial nerves such as the ulnar or peroneal. This occurs, for example, in **hereditary motor and sensory neuropathies types 1, 3, and 4; amyloid** and **diabetic neuropathies; neurofibromatosis; Roussy-Cornil syndrome;** and **Marie syndrome.**

hypertrophic neuropathy with facial involvement   See **hereditary motor and sensory neuropathy, type 1.**

hypertrophic neuropathy with facial weakness and kyphoscoliosis   See **hereditary motor and sensory neuropathy, type 3.**

hypertrophic spinal meningitis   (Charcot-Joffroy syndrome, epidural ascending spinal paralysis) A syndrome clinically resembling **syringomyelia** or **amyotrophic lateral sclerosis** but with pain in the neck and back and often sphincter disturbances and vasomotor changes in the limbs, and associated with chronic granulomatous inflammation of the cervical spinal meninges.[980] See **Spiller syndrome.**

hypertrophy   (hypertrophia) Abnormal enlargement of a tissue or organ.

hypertropia   Vertical strabismus, one eye being elevated with respect to the other.

hypertryptophanemia   An aminoacidopathy characterized by elevated serum tryptophan levels with the massive urinary excretion of indoleacetic, lactic, and pyruvic acids and characterized clinically by ataxia, spasticity, mental retardation and pellagrinoid skin rash. The responsible enzymatic defect might be of tryptophan transaminase.[5243]

hyperuricemia, deafness, and ataxia   A rare syndrome of elevated blood uric acid levels appearing in late childhood with progressive spinocerebellar ataxia, sensorineural deafness, weakness, and renal insufficiency occurring after puberty. The condition is probably dominantly inherited but the biochemical lesion is unknown.[4783]

hypervalinemia   A diffuse encephalopathy characterized by vomiting, nystagmus, hyperkinesias, ataxia, and failure to thrive in infancy. The EEG shows a pattern of sharp waves and spikes.[5465]

hyperventilation syndrome   (Da Costa syndrome, overbreathing) The state in which the ventilatory activity is greater than what is physiologically required, leading to a lowering of P_aCO_2 and consequent cerebral vasoconstriction. This then causes a variety of symptoms (paresthesias, weakness, tetany) that are often accompanied by other symptoms of anxiety. Psychogenic causes are the most common.[3721]

hyperventilation-epilepsy syndrome   The occurrence of epilepsy as a result of hyperventilation was described by Rosett in 1924, and, in the following year, Foerster showed that seizures could be induced thus in many epileptic patients. If overbreathing leads to seizures, surely underbreathing should stop them; and Durham recounts the use of artificial pneumothorax as a treatment modality, noting that between the two World Wars it was recorded that patients with tuberculosis treated thus had far fewer "seizures."[1563]

hyperviscosity syndrome   See **Waldenstrom macroglobulinemia.**

hypesthesia   Decreased sensitivity to sensory stimuli, usually applied to common sensory modes. **Hypoesthesia** has the same meaning.

hyphema   The presence of red blood in the anterior chamber of the eye due to infection or hemorrhage.

hypnagogic hallucinations   The occurrence of vivid waking auditory or visual perceptions incorporated into dream-like periods during the lightest stages of non–rapid eye movement sleep (or immediately upon awakening, hypnopompic hallucinations) in normals and in the rapid eye movement sleep periods of narcoleptics. They represent the sleep dream imagery of rapid eye movement sleep occurring inappropriately, and include a recall of scenes from recent waking experience. They may be accompanied by visual, auditory, or somesthetic sensory illusions. When combined with sleep paralysis, the subject experiences a true nightmare.

See also **hypnopompic hallucinations, narcolepsy,** and Chart S–6.

hypnagogic imagery   Vivid sensory images occurring at the onset of sleep, both in rapid eye movement sleep–onset periods[249] and with non-rapid eye movement sleep awakenings, when they are briefer and less affectively charged.

hypnagogic jerks   (fron Gr, sleep + leading) See **sleep starts.**

hypnagogic startle   A sudden bodily jerk observed commonly at the onset of sleep and resulting in at least momentary awakening.[249]

hypnic headache   A rare, benign, regularly occurring, diffuse, and self-limited nocturnal headache affecting patients usually over the age of 60 years during rapid eye movement sleep and lasting up to an hour. The head pain lasts from 15 to 60 minutes and is typically generalized, although it may be unilateral and is not accompanied by photophobia or phonophobia.[4602]

It is distinct from **cluster headache** by virtue of its diffuse site and relative lack of severity and by the absence of ocular and nasal symptoms.

hypnic jerks   (sudden bodily jerks on falling asleep) Shock-like starts, affecting the whole body, occurring in non–rapid eye movement sleep stages 1 and 2 and thus at sleep onset in normal people. See **sleep starts.**

hypnogenic paroxysmal dystonia   Episodes characterized by coarse, violent movements of the limbs with tonic spasms, vocalization, or laughter, occurring mainly or only at night. A familial form is recognized.[3511] See **nocturnal paroxysmal dystonia.**

hypnopompic hallucinations   The occurrence of vivid waking auditory or visual perceptions incorporated into dream-like periods immediately upon awakening.

hypnosis   A state of altered awareness induced by suggestion and associated with further abnormal suggestibility, focused awareness, loss of critical judgment, amnesia and possibly anesthesia, time regression, and ability to maintain fixed postures.

The condition can be induced at least to some extent in all humans, and in some animals.[4337]

hypnotic-dependent sleep disorder   Insomnia or excessive sleepiness associated with tolerance of or withdrawal from hypnotic medications.[234]

hypo-   (Gr, below, under, less than).

hypobaropathy   See **altitude insomnia.**

hypobetalipoproteinemia   A dominantly inherited syndrome manifest in youth or young adult life by low levels of cholesterol, β-lipoproteins and triglycerides, sometimes with **acanthocytosis.** The responsible gene maps to 2p24–p23.

The neurological features are extremely variable, if any occur at all; seizures, multifocal lesions of white matter, myelopathy, sensorimotor neuropathy, and ataxia have all been reported in different kinships. The most common symptom complexes are spinocerebellar degeneration or peripheral neuropathy.[2439,3638] See also **cerebellar ataxias** (*variants*).

hypoceruloplasminemia   A dominantly inherited syndrome characterized by low-serum ceruloplasmin levels in the absence of other evidence of **Wilson disease**.[1149]

hypochondriasis   A morbid concern with one's health, generally manifested as a belief that one is or is about to be affected by a disease. The problem may be a manifestation of chronic anxiety or of depression.

hypocretins   Hypothalamic peptides concerned with feeding and with sleep. See **orexins.**

hypoesthesia   Decreased sensitivity to sensory stimuli, usually applied to common sensory modes. **Hypesthesia** has the same meaning.

hypogastric reflex of Bekhterev   See **abdominal reflexes.**

hypogenic dystonia   See **familial paroxysmal dystonic choreoathetosis** (*familial paroxysmal hypogenic dystonia*).[3511]

hypoglossal nerve   (Gr, beneath + the tongue) The twelfth cranial nerve, containing purely motor fibers, all of which pass to the tongue muscles.

hypoglossal–alternating hemiplegia syndrome   A vascular syndrome of the medulla due to a paramedian lesion that damages the pyramid and the fasciculus of the twelfth cranial nerve on one side to produce the **alternating hemiplegia.** See also **Jackson syndrome.**

hypoglossal-facial anastomosis   An operation performed to normalize facial movement in people with hemifacial spasm or in those who have lost facial nerve function as a result of surgery for the treatment of cerebellopontine angle tumors.

Autogenous nerve grafts may produce better results because functional reinnervation from the stump of the divided seventh cranial nerve leads too often to synkinetic mass action of the facial muscles during attempts to move the tongue.

hypoglycemic amyotrophy   A syndrome of distal muscle wasting associated with hypoglycemia, probably due to damage to the anterior horn cells or motor roots. Recovery occurs clinically with evidence of reinnervation accomplished by axonal sprouting.[2464]

hypoglycorrachia   An unnecessary term meaning low glucose levels in the CSF.

hypokalemic myopathy   Muscle membrane damage with resulting weakness and myoglobinuria, complicating chronic potassium depletion.

hypokalemic periodic paralysis   A familial syndrome of attacks of flaccid weakness of the trunk and limbs, precipitated by food and sometimes relieved by exercise. See **familial periodic paralysis.**

hypokinesia   Poverty of willed movement. See **akinesia.**

hypomagnesemia   Tremors, twitches, and seizures, often with mental confusion, agitation, and hallucinations and a positive **Chvostek sign,** as a result of magnesium deficiency.[1888]

hypomania   A state judged to be more intense than simple euphoria (or unwonted cheerfulness) but less intense than mania, the etiologies of which it shares.

hypomelanosis of Ito   (incontinentia pigmenti achromicans, systemic achromic nevus) An uncommon, sporadic or dominantly inherited congenital neuroectodermal disorder described by Ito in Japan in 1952. The responsible gene maps to 9q33–qter. It is characterized by the presence of a whorled or swirling pattern of skin hypopigmentation, shown up by viewing the skin under a Wood light. Heterotopias of the white matter lead to mental retardation, convulsions, disturbances of language, and hypotonia or pyramidal signs in most affected children.[207,4847]

Short stature, skeletal abnormalities, cloudy corneas, microphthalmia, myopia, retinitis pigmentosa, strabismus, nystagmus, macrocephaly, alopecia, and low densities in the white matter on CT scans may also be associated.

hypometria   A reduction in the amplitude of limb movements that are otherwise normally formed. A lesion of the contralateral **supplementary motor area** has been incriminated.[3795]

hypometric saccades   A normal single saccade that stops before fixation of the desired target is achieved (undershooting), requiring thus a further small corrective saccade to place the image of the target on the fovea (a refixation eye movement). See also **hypermetric saccades, pulse dysmetria, postsaccadic drift.**

hypomimia   Reduced facial expressivity, as seen in parkinsonism or depressive states.

hyponatremic encephalopathy   A combination of brain swelling and increased intracranial pressure, leading to increased pressure on the brain, decreased cerebral blood flow, and sometimes cerebral herniation, due to the retention of free water and an osmotic imbalance between the extracellular fluid and neural tissues. **Central pontine myelinolysis** is not necessarily a feature.[5582]

hypo-osmotic brain edema   Excessive water content of the brain's extracellular space as a result of hypo-osmolality of the blood, as seen in patients with the **syndrome of inappropriate ADH secretion** or after the massive replacement of blood with hypotonic fluids.

hypoparathyroidism Impaired activity of the parathyroid glands, leading to the neurological complications of increased intracranial pressure, seizures, and tetany in a few cases.

Other complications occasionally reported include the features of Addison disease, ptosis, blepharospasm, increased intracranial pressure, superficial moniliasis, proximal myopathy, seizures, and tetany.[2043,3528,5091]

hypophosphatasia (phosphoethanolaminuria) A fatal, recessively inherited, neonatal syndrome characterized by craniostenosis, skeletal deformities, and hypercalcemia.

Variants include forms occurring in later years with a syndrome resembling rickets, and the occurrence of low levels of serum alkaline phosphatase without symptoms.[1738]

hypophosphatemia A condition of reduced serum phosphate levels below 2 mmol/L, as may occur in diabetes mellitus, alcoholism, renal tubular acidosis, hepatic disease, excessive alkali ingestion, etc.

Profound hypophosphatemia can produce severe proximal and respiratory flaccid weakness resembling that in **acute inflammatory demyelinating polyneuropathy.** The condition may be due to the decreased absorption of phosphate or its increased renal excretion cellular uptake. It also occurs in association with abnormalities of vitamin D metabolism.

Clinically, the condition is marked by anorexia, proximal muscle weakness and waddling gait, irritable paresthesias, dysarthria, and seizures,[4998] while, with extreme reduction of phosphate levels (<0.5 mg/dl), an encephalopathy ensues with irritability, dysarthria, confusion, seizures, and coma. Acute rhabdomyolysis is a further complication.

hypophysial nanism See **Burnier syndrome.**

hypophysitis (*lymphocytic hypophysitis*) A rare destructive autoimmune inflammatory disease of the pituitary often causing severe hypopituitarism.[1881]

It occurs mainly in females, usually during or after a pregnancy and is thus difficult to differentiate from **Sheehan syndrome.**

Granulomatous hypophysitis is a similarly presenting condition characterized clinically by pituitary enlargement, hypopituitarism, and diabetes insipidus. Various granulomatous diseases may be responsible and the condition may also be idiopathic.

hypoplasia of the cerebellum and pons See **Paine syndrome.**

hypoplasia of the thenar eminence A congenital condition characterized only by thenar muscle hypoplasia and with malformation of the underlying bones.[943] See also **Souques syndrome.**

hypoprebetalipoproteinemia, acanthocytosis, retinitis pigmentosa, and pallidal degeneration (HARP

syndrome) A variant form of **Hallervorden-Spatz disease,** characterized by the onset in childhood of orofacial dyskinesias, dystonia, pigmentary retinopathy, progressive dementia, prominent facial dyskinesias, and dystonias with associated hypo-pre-β-lipoproteinemia, abundant acanthocytosis, and evidence of iron deposition in the basal ganglia.[2570] The condition is allelic with pantothenate kinase-associated neurodegeneration.

hypopyon The presence of pus in the anterior chamber of the eye as a result of anterior uveitis.

hypospadias-dysphagia syndrome See **G syndrome.**

hypothalamic crossroads syndrome See **hypothalamique carrefour syndrome.**

hypothalamic ganglionic hamartoma A developmental defect consisting of a mass of redundant gray matter, usually attached to the mamillary bodies.

Compression of the hypothalamus may lead to excessive gonadotropin production, resulting in precocious puberty. The condition is more common in males.

hypothalamic hamartoma See **hamartoma.**

hypothalamic hypophysiotrophic hormones Synaptically active peptide molecules released from the hypothalamus with effects upon the release of other hormones.

hypothalamic syndrome The clinical syndromes resulting from various hypothalamic disorders. They include disturbances of appetite, sleep, water metabolism, sexual function, thermoregulation, and behavior. See **syndrome of inappropriate ADH secretion, Fröhlich syndrome, Kleine-Levin syndrome,**[4467] **diabetes insipidus.**

hypothalamic-midbrain dysregulation syndrome See **diencephalic autonomic seizures.**

hypothalamique carrefour syndrome (hypothalamic crossroads syndrome) A stroke syndrome characterized by the association of sudden visual loss, hemiplegia, hemianesthesia, apraxia, astereognosis, and asynergias.[4577]

hypothermia A state in which the core body temperature is below 34°C. As temperatures fall to 32.2°C, there is a linear depression of cerebral metabolism, with shivering, ataxia, apathy, dysarthria, impaired judgement, and maladaptive behavior. Between 32.2°C and 28°C there is a progressive depression of the level of consciousness with EEG slowing, reduction in shivering, and muscle rigidity. Hallucinations may occur and there is mydriasis. Below 28°C there is no movement, a loss of cerebral autoregulation, reduction in cerebral blood flow, loss of ocular and muscle stretch reflexes, and progressive attenuation of the EEG.[1280]

hypothyroid encephalopathy See **myxedema coma.**

hypothyroid myopathy 1. (Hoffmann syndrome) A syndrome of stiffness, slowed contraction, and relaxation (**pseudomyotonia**), and persistent painful muscle contractions following effort, made worse by exertion and occurring in hypothyroid patients.[2602] See also **Kocher-Debré-Semelaigne syndrome**. 2. Girdle muscle hypertrophy with weakness.[4165]

hypothyroid neuropathy   A symmetrical, distal, sensorimotor, demyelinating polyneuropathy complicating primary hypothyroidism, and presenting with cramps, hyporeflexia, distal pain, and paresthesias. The symptoms remit slowly with thyroid replacement.[1577] The same condition may occur because of thyrotropin deficiency.[2246] Axonal polyneuropathy is also described.[4098]

Mononeuropathies such as the **carpal tunnel syndrome** due to mucinous compression of the nerve were also described, but are now uncommon because of earlier diagnosis of the thyroid disorder.

hypotonia   1. Decreased resistance to the passive stretching of a limb muscle, as interpreted by an observer from the feel of the limb manipulated by the examiner or from an increase in the to-and-fro movements of the leg when the knee jerk is tested with the patient in the sitting position and the legs hanging freely (pendular knee jerk).

It occurs in association with lesions of the extrapyramidal pathways, the cerebellar system, or of the reflex arc. If " . . . the outstretched arms rest lightly on a bar, the normal limb keeps its position or sags a little when the bar is suddenly removed, but the hypotonic arm falls through a greater angle and may fail to maintain its new posture. This is more striking if the hand carries even a moderate weight. . . . When the arms are extended horizontally, the affected limb is more easily displaced by a tap on the wrist. . . . When shaken, the distal segments of the limbs swing more passively and through a greater range" (Sir Gordon **Holmes**[2627]).

Determination of the existence of hypotonia is difficult and comprises part of the artistic quality of this discipline. Holmes described increased drooping (flexion) of the wrist when the flexed elbows are placed on a level surface as a characteristic sign of hypotonia; in the case of the upper limb, this is perhaps one of the easiest signs to interpret.

The traditional view that hypotonia is due to a reduction in stretch reflexes now appears incorrect, reduction in tone being the result of weakness preventing voluntary activity.[5719a]

2. The resistance to stretch of a muscle forming part of a damaged reflex arc or of muscles on the side of a lesion of the cerebellum or its connections.

hypotonia-hypomentia-hypogonadism-obesity syndrome   See **Prader-Willi syndrome**.

hypotonic cerebral palsy   A form of cerebral palsy mimicking generalized lower motor neuron disease, recognized by Otfried **Foerster** in 1909. See **cerebral palsy.**

hypotrophy   Failure of growth to a normal size.

hypotropia   Manifest vertical deviation of an eye.

hypovolemia   Reduction in the volume of the intravascular compartment.

hypoxanthine   The oxidation of hypoxanthine forms superoxide radicals which may cause postischemic damage.

hypoxic degenerative polioencephalopathy   A diffuse encephalopathy. See **hypoxic-ischemic encephalopathy.**

hypoxic headache   Hypoxia is associated with three headache varieties:

> *High-altitude headache* The following diagnostic criteria are suggested by the Headache Classification Committee of the International Headache Society[1051] Classification of headache disorders, cranial neuralgias and facial pains; and diagnostic criteria for primary headache disorders. *Cephalalgia* 1988;**8**[suppl]:1–96) and are reproduced by kind permission.
> A. Occurs within 24 hours after sudden ascent to altitudes above 3000 meters.
> B. Is associated with at least one other symptom typical of high altitude: Cheyne-Stokes respiration at night; desire to overbreathe; exertional dyspnea.
> *Hypoxic headache* (low-pressure environment, pulmonary disease causing hypoxia) Occurs within 24 hours after acute onset of hypoxia with arterial oxygen tension of ≤70 mgHg, or in chronic hypoxic patients with arterial oxygen tension persistently at or below this level.
> *Sleep apnea headache*

Headaches resulting from hypercapnia, mixed hypoxia and hypercapnia, hypoglycemia, **dialysis**, and other metabolic disorders are also included in this category of the International Headache Society's Classification.

hypoxic neuropathy   Focal or multifocal central fascicular or sector axonal fiber degeneration, leading to endoneurial hypoxia; the basis of most diabetic and some other neuropathies.[1569]

hypoxic-ischemic encephalopathy   (hypoxic degenerative polioencephalopathy) A syndrome of diffuse neuronal destruction involving primarily the cerebral cortex, basal ganglia, and thalamus. It is most commonly seen in neonates after complicated deliveries, and is characterized clinically by reduced Apgar scores, hypotonia, seizures, or coma initially, with mental and motor delay, seizures (including **infantile spasms**), and spastic or athetotic cerebral palsy developing in those infants who survive.[6]

hypoxic-ischemic injury   Changes in the CNS following trauma or a severe reduction in cerebral blood flow, usually after cardiac arrest. The condition is characterized by widespread cortical neuronal loss, small areas of patchy infarction in the watershed interarterial zones, cerebral infarction in the territory of a major vessel, or any combination of these.

Clinically, patients suffering such injury frequently show evidence of increased intracranial pressure and episodes of systemic hypotension, often secondary to severe systemic injury as a result of the initial trauma. The territory of the posterior cerebral artery is that most frequently involved.

hypsarrhythmia (from Gr, high + lack of + rhythm) An age-related EEG pattern consisting of high-voltage, arrhythmic, chaotic slow waves at 1–3 Hz interspersed with multifocal spike discharges, without consistent synchrony between the two sides of the head or between different areas on the same side during wakefulness and between seizures. (Adapted from the report of the Committee on Terminology, IFCN,[989] © 1974, with permission from Elsevier Science.) Many variations are also described.[612]

These findings are usually associated with infantile spasms (**West syndrome**) but may also be noted in neurofibromatosis and in certain metabolic diseases of the nervous system.

Hyrtl's loop Small, recurrent branches between the two hypoglossal nerves in the geniohyoid muscle recorded by Joseph Hyrtl (1810–1894), the Hungarian anatomist, in 1842.[4979]

hyster- (Gr, uterus) Hysteria was considered from ancient times to be a condition of the womb because it was only recognized in females; it was supposed that the womb (considered as an animal endowed with the faculties of sensation and motion) wandered indignantly through the body when dissatisfied in its ardent desire to bear children. Pregnancy was determined to be the most effective remedy. The author exhorts his readers to suggest a better explanation.

hysteria (psychogenic disease, conversion syndrome, abnormal illness behaviour, somatoform disorder) A condition in which the mental mechanism of **dissociation** is used as if to protect the subject from the awareness of painful mental content. Within neurology, it is manifest as symptoms and signs that can be ascribed to abnormal function or loss of function in any parts of the nervous system, for which no chemical, electrical or structural cause can be determined; but because perhaps half of the patients so diagnosed do in fact turn out to have such "organic" disease after prolonged follow-up, it might be best to make the diagnosis only in retrospect after 5 years or more. There is no hysterical symptom that cannot be produced by well-defined nonhysterical causes.

The first two of these alternative terms for the condition are those usually employed;[3545] others are modified newspeak. It will have been noticed that neither this author nor any other[5207,5827] can frame a satisfactory definition of hysteria, although classic descriptions were given by Thomas **Willis** in 1671 and by Henry **Head** in 1922. However, according to Buzzard, "the figure of Hysteria shrinks in proportion as the various forms of organic disease acquire greater solidity and sharper definition."[858] The word was introduced by William Cullen in 1766.

Eames[1594] classifies the presentations as follows: *hysterical personality disorder*,[1055] *Briquet syndrome* (the sta-

ble syndrome of hysteria); *conversion hysteria* (focal presentations); and *Charcot syndrome* ("gross hysteria," seen also in patients with prior diffuse brain insults such as hypoglycemia or hypoxia). See also **functional disease.**

hysterical flutter   See **psychogenic flutter.**

hysterical gait   No single abnormality is here subsumed, but characteristic findings are the variability of the deficits with time and circumstance, their unphysiological nature, and the absence of physical findings of neurological examination in the bed, although none of these is unique to this gait disorder.

hysterical neurosis   See **somatization disorder.**

hysterical nystagmus   See **psychogenic flutter.**

hysterical personality   (psychopathy) A set of traits described as including the following clinical points listed in Chart H–23.[1055]

Chart H–23. Traits Associated with the Hysterical Personality

1. Superficial charm and "intelligence"
2. Absence of delusions and other signs of irrational thinking
3. Absence of nervousness or psychoneurotic manifestations
4. Unreliability
5. Untruthfulness and insincerity
6. Lack of remorse and shame
7. Inadequately motivated antisocial behaviour
8. Poor judgement and failure to learn by experience
9. Pathologic incapacity to love
10. General poverty in major adjective reactions
11. Specific loss of insight
12. General unresponsiveness in interpersonal relations
13. Fantastic and uninviting behavior with drinking, sometimes without
14. Suicide threats are seldom carried out.
15. Sex life is impersonal, trivial, and poorly integrated.
16. Failure to follow any life plan

From Cleckley H. The Mask of Sanity. St. Louis, Mosby, 1964.

hysterical pseudodementia   See **Ganser syndrome.**

hysterical seizures   Attacks resembling epileptic seizures in which there is a wide range of events, including bizarre behavior; the EEG is normal during and after the attack, and there is no relationship to medication.

The attacks may start gradually. Tongue biting, incontinence, abnormal neurological signs, and nocturnal occurrence are rare, and post-seizure drowsiness and confusion are absent. The patient frequently retains vivid recollections of the attack[1416,3680] and of one or more episodes of sexual abuse during childhood.

hysterical sensory loss   Subjective abnormalities of sensation, seldom conforming to the anatomical distribution of a nerve or a root, commonly involving all modes of sensation, and considered to reflect the use of the mental mechanism of dissociation. See also **Waddell signs, hysteria.**

"hysterical" signs Clinical signs suggestive of nonorganic pathology. There follows a clinically derived compendium; no single one of these signs is itself sufficient to make the diagnosis with any confidence.

Sensory

1. Vibration is felt when the tuning fork is placed on one side of the sternum, forehead, or incisor teeth but not when it is placed across the midline on the other side, which is unphysiological.

2. During sensory testing, the patient may be asked to say "yes" if she or he feels the touch, pin, etc. and "no" if not.

3. Distal arm anesthesia ends precisely at the shoulder line, as if it were the top of the sleeve.

4. Psychogenic hemiparesis is often complicated by hemianesthesia that extends to the midline, affects all modalities of sensation, and may be accompanied by an ipsilateral decrease or loss of vision, hearing, taste, and smell. Anesthesia of the affected half of the body is rare in organic hemiparesis. If present, the cause is usually a cerebral lesion. In both psychogenic and organic paralyses secondary contractures and vasomotor changes occur.

Formal Motor Testing

5. Collapse during toe walking, always toward the "good" side.

6. Give-way weakness on testing the abductor digiti quinti and palpating the tendon of the flexor carpi ulnaris.

7. See the **forearm rolling test.**

8. In organic hemiparesis there is sparing only of the upper portion of the face; in psychogenic paralysis there is also sparing of the face, tongue, platysma, and sternocleidomastoid muscles. In organic hemiparesis the muscle stretch reflexes are exaggerated, the abdominal reflexes are diminished or absent, the Babinski and other corticospinal tract responses are present, and there may be clonus; in psychogenic paresis the muscle stretch reflexes are normal or increased in range but have normal speed, the abdominal reflexes are normal or increased, there are no corticospinal tract responses, and there is no persistent clonus. In organic hemiparesis the gait is of the unilateral spastic variety with circumduction of the leg; in psychogenic paralysis the gait is bizarre and there may be dragging of the foot.

9. See **Hoover sign, Babinski** trunk-thigh **sign, Neri sign** of combined flexion of the thigh and leg, **Bechterew sign, Raimiste** arm and leg **signs.**

10. Asynchronous leg and arm movements occur in tonic clonic seizures (although bilateral asynchronous movements without loss of consciousness may be accompanied by EEG findings of 6 per second spike and wave).

11. Any hyperactivity of the muscle stretch reflexes is characterized by an increase in the range of movement rather than in the speed of response.

12. Pseudoclonus at the knee or ankle is irregular and poorly sustained and is not stopped by plantar flexion of the foot.

13. Subjects with nonorganic weakness of one lower extremity may use a cane on the wrong side.

14. Cutaneous reflexes are not affected in psychogenic paralyses, but the abdominal reflexes may be increased.

15. The Babinski sign and the related dorsiflexor and fanning responses are only seen in organic conditions.

16. Tests for power, tone, and coordination may be normal if carried out while the patient is lying down.

Gait

17. On testing stance, any body swaying occurs from the hips rather than from the ankles; trembling and shaking occur without signs of fear or pain. The truly ataxic patient makes every effort to maintain the erect posture and to avoid falling, whereas the simulator or hysteric usually reels from side to side or falls *en masse* without trying to maintain equilibrium. Patients may appear to be about to fall to the floor, but either catch themselves or, if they do fall, do so in a theatrical manner, without injury.

18. If subjects with either hysteria or malingering are asked to carry out various commands, such as touching a finger to the nose or alternately pronating and supinating the hands while standing with their feet together, they may cease to sway and fall.

19. Patients with organic ataxia can usually maintain an upright position with very slight support from a wall or table, or by lightly touching the examiner's hand, by watching the floor, or by placing the feet a short distance apart; the patient with psychogenic ataxia is not aided by these measures.

20. In hysterical astasia-abasia, although subjects seem unable to stand or walk, they may be able to move the limbs for other purposes, and may skip, jump, run or walk backwards without difficulty.

21. Locomotion is accompanied by superfluous movements of other parts of the body.

Cranial Nerves

22. A large mirror moved in front of the face of patients who claim to be blind leads to eye movements when the mirror is moved since the subjects can't avoid moving their eyes. (However, patients with cortical blindness perceive the objects but make no sense of them and will also move their eyes when confronted with a moving mirror.)

23. The complaint of restriction of the visual fields turns out to be tunnel vision rather than restricted funnel vision on bedside testing and on perimetry.

24. Subjects may be unable to find their own hand in the peripheral field, but this is a function of proprioception rather than vision.

25. Subjects simulating deafness may react to the sound of coins thrown to the floor after saying goodbye.

General

26. Pelvic/coital rocking in pseudoseizures, especially if the subject grabs a bed rail to obtain more effective rocking.

27. Puffed-up cheeks with breath-holding.

28. Events occurring just after the change of nursing shifts.

29. The presence of wrist scars from previous suicidal gestures.

30. Detection of a Medic-Alert or similar bracelet stating "see wallet card."

hysterical twilight state See **Ganser syndrome.**

hysteroepilepsy The simulation of epileptic seizures by those who do not suffer from them. The differentiation has been aided by video monitoring, but in the 19th century, **Charcot** considered that in hysteroepilepsy the onset of the seizure was preceded by a peculiar mental state and gradual flexion of one limb; violent limb movements preceded the tonic spasm; attacks were brought on or arrested by compression of the ovaries or other "hysterogenic areas"; and standard treatment failed to stop the attacks.[3680] See also **hysterical seizures.**

iatros (Gr, physician) As iatro-, a prefix signifying a relationship with physicians or with the art of medicine.

ice-cream headache See **cold stimulus headache.**

ice-cream cone sign A sign seen in subjects with a sterile abscess in the gluteal muscles as a result of receiving multiple injections at that site. The swelling is visible and palpable as a conical, fluctuant mass with a line of needle marks leading to it. (Dr. Asa Wilbourn, personal communication, 1993).

Iceland amyloid angiopathy A form of **familial amyloidosis** with involvement of the cerebral vessels, as in **cerebral amyloid angiopathy.**

Icelandic disease See **chronic fatigue syndrome, postinfection fatigue syndrome.**

I-cell disease (inclusion cell disease, **mucolipidosis, type 2**) An inherited condition of deficiency of intracellular lysosomal hydrolases in which large cytoplasmic inclusions are detectable in cultured skin fibroblasts.

The clinical manifestations are seen in infancy and include gingival hyperplasia and both psychomotor and growth retardation, as well as facial telangiectasias, kyphosis, skeletal and vertebral abnormalities, arthritis, and seizures, with the slow development of corneal opacities; abnormal excretion of mucopolysaccharides is not a feature. The condition resembles both **Hurler** and **pseudo-Hurler syndromes.** A major review is that of Kolodny and Cable.[3121]

ice-pack test A bedside diagnostic maneuver in **myasthenia gravis** in which a small bag of crushed ice is held over one eye while the myasthenic patient who is currently experiencing diplopia looks upward. The ice pack is removed when the patient indicates that it hurts and the degree of diplopia and speed of opening of the eyelid are assessed. A lack of fatigability in the cooled eye relative to the other eye and faster opening of that eyelid suggests the diagnosis.[5079]

ice-pick pains Recurrent twinges of sharp, needle-like pains in the head, lasting for a second or so and occurring mainly in patients with migraine.[4604] See **idiopathic stabbing headache.**

It is a puzzle that something so characteristic and common should not have been recognized until the last decade.

ice water test Introduction of 100 ml of ice cold water into the bladder leads to its immediate contraction if the bladder is uninhibited, with detrusor instability. With the patient in the supine position, 100 ml of sterile saline water at 4–8° C is injected manually. If cystometric capacity was <200 ml, a volume of about half the individual cystometric bladder capacity is used. The

fluid is left inside the bladder for 3 minutes. The test is considered positive if an involuntary bladder contraction ≥15 cm H_2O is registered. Autonomic hyperreflexia, manifested as systolic blood pressure increase ≥50 mmHg within 3 minutes of ice water instillation, occurs commonly.[964]

ichthyosis (Gr, fishiness) Scaliness of the skin (reptilian skin); a feature in **Rud** and **Refsum syndromes** and **Sjögren-Larsson syndrome.**

Variants of the latter are an ichthyotic condition appearing in adult life that is associated with progressive spastic paraparesis but without mental impairment; and a neurocutaneous syndrome resembling **myotonic dystrophy** but inherited as an X-linked characteristic.[3787]

ichthyosis and neutral lipid storage disease A congenital dysmorphic syndrome manifesting also sensorineural deafness, cataract, retinal dysplasia, myopathic weakness, and mental and developmental delay.[337]

ichthyosis linearis neuropathica See **nevus unis lateralis.**

ichthyosis-alopecia-photophobia See **Eramo syndrome.**

ichthyosis–Little disease See **Sjögren-Larsson syndrome.**

ictal amaurosis A rare **inhibitory seizure** disorder of childhood, in which temporary blindness is associated with occipital EEG paroxysms and succeeded by headaches and nausea.[2120]

ictal catatonia A syndrome of nonconvulsive status epilepticus characterized by catalepsy, waxy flexibility, mutism, muscle rigidity, psychotic negativism, stereotypies, and **verbigeration,** associated with concurrent abnormal discharges on the EEG.[3411]

ictal deafness A rare **inhibitory seizure** disorder associated with a left posterior temporal focus.[2091]

ictal nystagmus See **epileptic nystagmus.**

ictal paralysis (inhibitory seizure paralysis, somatic inhibitory seizure) A form of nonconvulsive seizure presenting as transient paralytic attacks involving the face, hand and/or leg, usually lasting from 2 minutes to a day. Serious structural pathology is commonly absent.

ictus (Lat, a blow or stroke) A sudden neurological happening, such as a cerebrovascular event or a seizure.

ictus emeticus Paroxysmal vomiting as an epileptic event. The causative lesion was right-sided in most but not all of the cases described. Two features suggesting that the symptom is in fact ictal are the patient's unawareness of the act of vomiting and the association of this with other ictal events.[3152]

Idaho syndrome   A craniofacial malformation characterized by scaphocephaly, strabismus, skeletal abnormalities such as ulnar deviation of the fingers, congenital heart malformations, and physical and mental delay.[4]

ideation   Thoughts and feelings generated spontaneously, in the absence of obvious extrinsic stimuli.

ideational agraphia   A selective inability to write letters or words in the absence of any difficulty in copying them.[399]

ideational apraxia   A defect in the actual handling of common objects or a loss of conceptual knowledge relating to the use of tools, on account of spatiotemporal errors; however, the subject retains the correct intent and the gross motor power and coordination required for these purposes. The error patterns include perseveration, omission, or incorrect ordering of those acts that are components of multistage complex actions requiring the manipulation of objects, along with a loss of pantomime ability in response to command or imitation.

The diagnostic clue is that patients can do things spontaneously that they cannot manage when they are asked to do them, although they understand the command itself. Usually the phenomenon is seen in the left limbs in association with left sided deep parietofrontal and occipitofrontal and anterior callosal lesions, so dysphasia and a right hemiparesis coexist in most cases. The condition may be considered a **disconnection syndrome.**

The causative lesion, in dextrals, is in the dominant parietal lobe, but in **callosal apraxia,** there is disconnection of the engrams for skilled movement in the right hemisphere from the speech centers on the left.[5873] See **apraxia.**

idioglossia   1. Severe retardation of articulatory development, often accompanied by congenital auditory imperception or retardation of language development, and leading to a form of abnormal speech in which the subject uses individual words for objects, persons and affective states.[109] 2. A private language developed by two or more people, particularly twins, which is unintelligible to others.

ideomotor apraxia   See **apraxia.**

ideomotor prosodic apraxia   A condition in which spontaneous everyday speech has normal prosody, but the subject cannot produce the same acoustical features underlying prosody to command, described in the context of **Alzheimer disease.**[2906]

idiomuscular   Peculiar to muscle.

idiomuscular contraction   See **myotatic irritability.**

idiopathic   (Gr, of itself, individual + disease) Now used to refer to disease arising spontaneously, with no known cause.

idiopathic acute lethal catatonia   See **acute lethal catatonia.**

idiopathic adult hydrocephalus   See **normal pressure hydrocephalus**

idiopathic brachial plexopathy   See **neuralgic amyotrophy.**

idiopathic calcification of the basal ganglia   A syndrome inherited in either dominant or recessive modes, with the onset in childhood or adult life of spasticity, rigidity, bradykinesia, tremor, dystonia, chorea, and dementia,[3494] accompanied by evidence of basal ganglion calcification on MRI or CT scans. In a few cases, there are no clinical features of the calcification at all.

In a *variant* form, familial ataxia and pigmentary macular degeneration are found.[5380] The differences from so-called **Fahr disease** are subtle at best. See **striatopallidal calcification.**

idiopathic CNS hypersomnolence   (NREM narcolepsy, harmonious hypersomnia) A syndrome characterized by excessive daytime sleepiness without sleep attacks, unresponsive to cerebral stimulants, and with a tendency for affected subjects to exhibit automatic behavior due to microsleeps.

Subjects are more able to resist sleep than those with **narcolepsy,** but still need frequent daytime naps and experience abnormally heavy and prolonged nocturnal sleep, sometimes with **sleep drunkenness** on awakening[4810] (see also Chart S–6, **idiopathic recurring stupor, subwakefulness syndrome**).

idiopathic cranial polyneuropathy   The association of self-limited facial pain and involvement of (mainly motor) cranial nerves such as the III, V, and VII and the bulbar nerves (or either of these features in isolation) with diverse etiologies. The condition was first recognized by **Gowers** and is hardly separable from the **superior orbital fissure syndrome** or the **Tolosa-Hunt syndrome** (which themselves may be identical).[2893]

idiopathic dementia/autism   See **infantile autism.**

idiopathic enuresis   See **sleep-related enuresis.**

idiopathic familial intracerebral arterial calcification   See **striatopallidal calcification.**

idiopathic generalized epilepsies   (age related) (OMIN 600669) Forms of generalized epilepsy in which all seizures are initially generalized, with an EEG expression that is a generalized, bilateral, synchronous and symmetrical discharge (such as that described in the seizure classification of the corresponding type). The patient usually has a normal interictal state, without neurological or neuroradiological signs. In general, interictal EEGs show normal background activity and generalized discharges, such as spikes, polyspikes, spike–waves, and polyspike waves of >3 Hz. The discharges are increased by slow wave sleep. The term *id-*

iopathic as defined by the ILAE is reserved for certain partial or generalized epileptic syndromes with particular clinical characteristics and with specific EEG findings, and should not be used to refer to epilepsy or seizures without obvious cause.[1115]

The various syndromes of idiopathic generalized epilepsies comprise (either alone or in combination) absence, generalized tonic-clonic, or myoclonic seizure disorders but otherwise differ mainly in the age of onset. (Adapted from Commission for Classification and Terminology, ILAE. Proposal for Revised Classifications of Epilepsies and Epileptic syndromes. *Epilepsia* 1989; 30:389–399.) By permission from Blackwell Science. In some cases, mapping to 8q24 has been achieved.

See also **benign neonatal familial convulsions, benign neonatal convulsions, benign myoclonic epilepsy in infants, childhood absence epilepsy, juvenile absence epilpsy, juvenile myoclonic epilepsy, epilepsy with tonic-clonic seizures on awakcning, eyelid myoclonia with typical absences.**

idiopathic generalized glycogenosis See **glycogen storage diseases.**

idiopathic headache See **episodic tension-type headache.**

idiopathic hypercalcemia See **Williams syndrome.**

idiopathic hyperCKemia A common presentation of dystrophinopathy, seen mainly in males in a minority of whom clinical and/or histopathologic evidence of a neuromuscular disorder develop between 1 and 7 years after detection of hyperCKemia. Such conditions include distal myopathy, **myoadenylate deaminase deficiency,** subclinical hypothyroidism, **polymyositis,** mitochondrial myopathy, sarcoid myopathy, McArdle disease, **central core disease, multicore disease, inclusion body myopathy,** and **Duchenne muscular dystrophy** carrier status. The frequency of diagnosis of the condition has diminished since the development of knowledge regarding the variable presentations of dystrophinopathies and recognition that beta-blockers, antipsychotics, and cholesterol-lowering drugs may also be responsible.[52] Unexplained persistently increased CK levels in an otherwise healthy patient should alert the anesthesiologist to the possibility of **malignant hyperthemia** syndrome and/or myopathy.

idiopathic hypersomnia A disorder of presumed CNS cause that is associated with normal or prolonged major sleep episodes and excessive sleepiness, consisting of prolonged sleep episodes composed of non–rapid eye movement sleep and lasting 1 to 2 hours. The following diagnostic criteria have been suggested (Chart I–1).[234]

Chart I–1. Diagnostic Criteria for Idiopathic Hypersomnia

A. A complaint of prolonged sleep episodes, excessive sleepiness, or excessively deep sleep.

B. Presence of a prolonged nocturnal sleep period or frequent daily sleep episodes.

C. The onset is insidious, and typically before age 25 years.

D. The complaint is present for at least 6 months.

E. The onset does not occur within 18 months of trauma.

F. Polysomnography demonstrates one or more of the following:
   1. A sleep period that is normal or prolonged in duration
   2. Sleep latency less than 10 minutes
   3. Normal REM sleep latency
   4. A multiple sleep latency test that demonstrates a sleep latency less than 10 minutes
   5. Less than two sleep-onset REM periods

G. Absence of any medical or psychiatric disorder that could account for the symptom.

H. Does not meet the diagnostic criteria of any other sleep disorder causing excessive sleepiness, e.g., narcolepsy, obstructive sleep apnea syndrome, or post-traumatic hypersomnia.

From ASDA Diagnostic Classification Steering Committee. The International Classification of Sleep Disorders Diagnostic and Coding Manual. *Rochester, MN. American Sleep Disorders Association, 1990. Reproduced by kind permission of the American Academy of Sleep Medicine.*

idiopathic hypertrophic cranial pachymeningitis A rare, chronic, fibrotic, granulomatous, inflammatory condition of the dura mater, presenting usually with headache, papilledema, cranial nerve palsies, seizures, confusion, and hydrocephalus, more commonly occurring in the Far East. The CSF may or may not show evidence of chronic inflammation with raised protein and white cell counts. The MRI and CT images show the thickening of the basal dura. No organism has been implicated as responsible in the cases reported to date. The signs usually dissipate after the institution of steroid therapy. See also **Tolosa Hunt syndrome.**

idiopathic inflammatory myopathies A heterogeneous group of inflammatory muscle diseases from which no infectious agent can be isolated but sharing the features of the presence of inflammatory infiltrates within skeletal muscles and muscle fiber destruction. Disturbances of the immune system are considered responsible in many cases.

The conditions have been classified[3687] as follows (see Chart I–2). See also **eosinophilic fasciitis.**

Chart I–2. Classification of the Idiopathic Inflammatory Myopathies

Generalized

Polymyositis (further subclassified)
Dermatomyositis (further subclassified)
Inclusion body myositis
Granulomatous myositis Sterile muscle inflammation with giant cells, indistinguishable from sarcoidosis except for the absence of sarcoid granulomas elsewhere.
Eosinophilic polymyositis The presence of an inflammatory myopathy as a complication of a systemic hypereosinophilic syndrome characterized by eosinophilia, anemia, hypergammaglobulinemia, cardiac and pulmonary involvement, skin changes, peripheral neuropathy, and encephalopathy.[3304]

Eosinophilic perimyositis[5073]
Interstitial myositis
Angiopathic myositis An inflammatory myopathy associated with **Churg-Strauss syndrome, Wegener Granulomatosis**, or **polyarteritis nodosa**.[3688]

Localized

Focal (localized) nodular myositis[1212]
Monomelic myositis (Gr, single + limb)
Proliferative myositis
Orbital myositis
Myositis associated with linear scleroderma
Myositis associated with panniculitis

From Mastaglia FL, Ojeda V. Inflammatory myopathies. Ann Neurol 1985;17:215–227; 317–323. Reported by kind permission.

idiopathic insomnia A lifelong inability to obtain adequate sleep, presumably due to an abnormality of the neurological control of the sleep–wake mechanism. The suggested American Sleep Disorders Association diagnostic criteria are given in Chart I–3.

Chart I–3. Diagnostic Criteria for Idiopathic Insomnia

A. There is a complaint of insomnia, along with a complaint of decreased functioning during wakefulness.
B. The insomnia is long-standing, typically beginning in early childhood, if not at birth.
C. The insomnia is relentless, unvaried through periods of both poor and good emotional adaptation.
D. Polysomnography demonstrates one or more of the following:
   1. An increased sleep latency
   2. Reduced sleep efficiency
   3. An increased number and duration of awakenings
   4. Often a reversed first night effect
E. No medical or psychiatric disease can explain the early onset of insomnia.
F. Other sleep disorders producing insomnia can occur simultaneously, e.g., adjustment sleep disorder.

From ASDA Diagnostic Classification Steering Committee. The International Classification of Sleep Disorders Diagnostic and Coding Manual. Rochester, MN: American Sleep Disorders Association, 1990. Reproduced by kind permission of the American Academy of Sleep Medicine.

idiopathic intracerebral vascular calcification A rare, probably dominantly inherited disorder characterized by pigmentary retinal degeneration, calcification of the basal ganglia, thumb deformities, pectoralis muscle hypoplasia, and peroneal muscular atrophy with mental retardation.[4449]

idiopathic intracranial hypertension (pseudotumor cerebri, serous meningitis; toxic, minor, or pseudomeningitis; meningismus; Julien-Marie-See syndrome; increased intracranial pressure without localizing signs; Dupré syndrome) First described by Quincke (an originator of lumbar puncture) in 1891,[4559] this condition is characterized by a rise in intracranial pressure (>200 mm CSF) in the absence of an intracranial mass lesion or of hydrocephalus. It represents a disorder of CSF dy-

namics resulting from increased intraabdominal and intrapleural pressure, leading to increased cardiac filling and jugular venous pressures.[5406,5811]

Clinically, it presents with papilledema, visual obscurations, and occasionally a sixth cranial nerve palsy without other clinical signs, most often in female subjects. Over 120 disorders have been described as being associated with it, the most common being obesity, but in 30% of the cases in which such clinical features are noted, a different pathology is finally detected.[5898] See also **otitic hydrocephalus**

Diagnostic criteria[5230] (modified from those originally suggested by **Dandy**) include the following:

1. Clinical features of increased intracranial pressure (e.g., headache, papilledema)
2. Increased intracranial pressure at lumbar puncture (>250 mm CSF)
3. Absence of localizing findings on CNS examination. False localizing signs may be present.
4. Normal neurodiagnostic studies (apart from CSF pressure > 220 mm CSF in the nonobese and >250 mm CSF in the obese). There is no evidence of venous obstructive disease.
5. No disturbance of consciousness
6. Normal CSF constituents
7. Benign course apart from visual deterioration
8. No other cause of increased intracranial pressure is found.

Reproduced from: Smith JL. Whence pseudotumor cerebri? *J. Clin. Neuro-Opthalmol.* 1985;**5**;55–6 by kind permission.

idiopathic intracranial hypotension See **spontaneous intracranial hypotension**.

idiopathic late-onset cerebellar ataxias A heterogeneous group of ataxic syndromes that were generally reported as *olivopontocerebellar atrophies* (OPCAs) by Déjèrine and Thomas in 1900 but first described by Menzel in 1891.

Clinically, the onset is usually around 40 years of age with gait ataxia, cerebellar and spastic speech, some arm incoordination, impassive facies, and hypertonia. The stretch reflexes are brisk and the plantar responses upgoing. Dementia and nystagmus are more marked in the OPCAs than in the cortical cerebellar atrophies (see below), but pursuit movements and optokinetic nystagmus are much affected in both forms.

Numerous *variant* forms of OPCA are recognized, usually with dominant inheritance and associated with various other problems. Linkage to chromosome 6 has been found in some kinships but not in others. These conditions closely resemble *parenchymatous or cortical cerebellar atrophy* (CCA), but, in the latter, the olivary and pontine changes are less marked and optic atrophy, pigmentary retinal degeneration, and ophthalmoplegia do not occur. See **cerebellar ataxias.**

idiopathic leg pain Chronic, deep, mild muscular pain felt especially during rest after exercise. Both the cause and the cure are unknown.

idiopathic Lewy body disease   See **Lewy body disease.**

idiopathic localization-related epilepsies   Childhood epilepsies with partial seizures and focal EEG abnormalities. They are age related, without demonstrable anatomical lesions, and are subject to spontaneous remission.

Clinically, patients have neither a neurological nor an intellectual deficit, nor a history of antecedent illness, but frequently have a family history of benign epilepsy. The seizures are usually brief and rare, but may be frequent early in the course of the disorder. The seizure patterns may vary from case to case, but usually remain constant in the same child. The EEG is characterized by normal background activity and localized, high-voltage repetitive spikes, which are sometimes independently multifocal. Brief bursts of generalized spike–waves can occur. Focal abnormalities are increased by sleep and are without change in morphology. (Reproduced from the Commission for Classification and Terminology, ILAE. Proposal for Revised Classifications of Epilepsies and Epileptic syndromes. *Epilepsia* 1989;**30**:389–399,[1114] by kind permission of Blackwell Science.)

idiopathic lumbosacral plexitis   See **lumbosacral plexitis.**

idiopathic neonatal convulsions   Focal clonic or multifocal clonic seizures, and minimal seizures including tonic deviation, eyelid blinking, lip smacking, sucking or swallowing, or alterations in muscle tone with assumption of bizarre postures occurring in the neonatal period, and most commonly due to **hypoxic-ischemic encephalopathy.** Myoclonic seizures also occur, but less commonly.

idiopathic neurogenic anorectal incontinence   A syndrome of adult life, characterized by weakness of the anal sphincter with loss of the anal reflex, usually occurring in women. It is often due to denervation of the puborectalis muscle resulting from prolonged constipation or from the process of childbirth.[4340]

idiopathic neuromyotonia   (continuous muscle fiber activity, neurogenic benign fasciculations, pseudomyotonia and pseudotetany, chronic or sporadic tetany, acquired myotonia, pseudomyotonia, generalized myokymia, quantal squander, Isaacs syndrome, Isaacs-Mertens syndrome) A sporadic, probably autoimmune syndrome of abnormal, spontaneous distal motor unit activity of neural origin (**neuromyotonia**) manifesting benign fasciculations, generalized myokymia, delayed muscular relaxation (pseudomyotonia), pseudotetany, hyperhidrosis, painful spasms, cramps, and stiffness at rest and in sleep (but exacerbated by exercise); muscle hypertrophy; and abnormal motor nerve conduction velocities. The face and branchial muscles may be affected. The condition is heterogeneous in nature and causation; most cases are sporadic, a few are paraneoplastic or autoallergic.[3242,5826]

The condition may be of any degree of severity and in some cases is permanent; in others, the symptoms are worsened by voluntary muscle contraction but abate after repetitive effort. The lesion is localized to the distal part of the motor unit and may represent motor axonal hyperexcitability, but its nature is obscure.[1066]

Variant forms are **neurogenic Isaacs syndrome,** characterized by onset in youth, pes cavus, myotonia, pseudohypertrophy, myokymia, fasciculation, neurogenic weakness, and loss of pain sensation with neural myelinated fiber loss; an inherited form; and forms associated with **hereditary motor and sensory neuropathy,**[3242] *chronic inflammatory polyneuropathy, squamous cell carcinoma of the lung,*[5826] and *exposure to 2,4-D or to penicillamine.*

idiopathic ophthalmoplegia   (Collier syndrome) A syndrome reported from the Far East resembling the superior orbital fissure syndrome with involvement of the third, fourth, sixth, and the first two divisions of the fifth cranial nerves. The optic nerve may also be involved. The erythrocyte sedimentation rate is typically raised.

Clinically, diplopia, ptosis, giddiness, headache, facial numbness , chemosis, retro-orbital pain, proptosis, conjunctivitis, and/or progressive blindness are the usual features. The signs clear within 2 months, in some cases requiring steroids to do so.[5502] See **superior orbital fissure syndrome.**

idiopathic orofacial dystonia   See **cranial dystonia.**

idiopathic orthostatic hypotension   See **progressive autonomic failure.**

idiopathic painless brachial plexopathy   A syndrome resembling neuralgic amyotrophy with neurogenic muscle weakness and atrophy but without pain. See **neuralgic amyotrophy.**

idiopathic parkinsonism   A syndrome characterized by resting tremor, rigidity, bradykinesia, and impairment of postural reflexes. See **Parkinson disease.**

idiopathic postural orthostatic tachycardia syndrome   A form of autonomic neuropathy seen mainly following a viral illness in women, who complain of the acute onset of fatigue and light-headedness, postprandial bloating or vomiting, and tachycardia, exaggerated with tilting. The condition is considered to be possibly due to decreased plasma volume or red blood cell mass, or to adrenergic hypersensitivity resulting from postganglionic sympathetic denervation.[4991] See also **pandysautonomia.**

idiopathic recurrent myoglobinuria   See **myoglobinuria** (*variant*).

idiopathic recurring stupor   A rare syndrome characterized by the occurrence of transient episodes of stupor or coma in the absence of toxic or structural brain disease and with accompanying 14-Hz activity on the EEG, as a result of a disturbance of the gamma aminobutyric acidergic systems.[5592,5593]

idiopathic sensory neuronopathy   An acute, subacute, or chronic asymmetrical sensory neuropathy affecting large rather than small fibers in the extremities, face, and trunk, occurring mainly in females aged between 40 and 60 years. Patchy areflexia is notable but there is no motor weakness. All sensory modes may be affected and the Romberg test is usually positive. Progression is variable but usually slow. Antineuronal antibodies are not detected. The condition is not associated with distant carcinoma, nor with abnormalities of the CNS or of the CSF, and the cause is unknown.[2963] See also **cryptogenic sensory polyneuropathy.**

idiopathic stabbing headache   (likely to be renamed "primary stabbing headache" in a future revision of the IHS criteria) Transient stabs of pain in the head that occur spontaneously in the absence of organic disease of underlying structures or of the cranial nerves. (See **ice-pick pains**) Similar pains can occur with tumors at the base of the brain and in the third ventricle, with disorders at the cranio-cervical junction such as the **Chiari malformation,** with **subdural hematoma** and with **pheochromocytoma.**

The following diagnostic criteria are suggested by the Headache Classification Committee of the International Headache Society. (from: Classification of headache disorders, cranial neuralgias and facial pains; and diagnostic criteria for primary headache disorders. *Cephalalgia* 1988;**8**[suppl]:1–96) reproduced by kind permission.

A. Pain confined to the head and exclusively or predominantly felt in the distribution of the first division of the trigeminal nerve (orbit, temple, and parietal area).
B. Pain is stabbing in nature and lasts for a fraction of a second. Occurs as single stabs or series of stabs.
C. It recurs at irregular intervals (hours to days).
D. Diagnosis depends upon the exclusion of structural changes at the site of pain and in the distribution of the affected cranial nerve.

idiopathic steroid-responsive chronic lymphocytic meningitis   A steroid-responsive, chronic meningitis for which an etiological cause is seldom found. Leptomeningeal biopsy and long-term follow-up seldom identify the underlying cause.[982]

idiopathic stimulus-sensitive myoclonus   See **stimulus-sensitive myoclonus.**

idiopathic subcortical degeneration   See **pallidonigral degenerations.**

idiopathic torsion dystonia   See **dystonia.**

idiopathic vertebral sclerosis   Narrowing of a disk space with diffuse sclerosis of the anterior inferior part of the vertebral body, usually of L4. The condition can only be diagnosed radiographically. The condition

mainly affects women and is a cause of severe low back pain.[5938]

idiospasm   Cramp or spasm occurring only in one area.

idiosyncrasy   (Gr, one's own + mixing together) The special or peculiar temperament or body habit of a person whereby one differs from the ordinary. This peculiarity extends to susceptibility to certain diseases and to the actions of different drugs.[4512]

idiotic aphasia   See **Worster-Drought-Allen syndrome.**

iduronate sulfatase   The enzyme deficient in mucopolysaccaridosis type 2 (Hunter disease), leading to the accumulation of dermatan and heparan sulfate.

iduronidase   The enzyme deficient in mucopolysaccaridoses types 1 and 1A (Hurler disease) and leading to the accumulation of dermatan and heparan sulfate.

Ilheus encephalitis   A rare form of encephalitis due to a flavivirus member of the togavirus group of arboviruses, occurring in South America.

iliac reflex   Contraction of the lower abdominal muscles in response to a tap on the iliac crest, seen occasionally in patients with pyramidal lesions above T10.

iliohypogastric neuralgia   Continuous burning or lancinating pain felt in the distribution of this nerve, usually following partial injury to it.

The pain is felt in the midline above the pubis but may also radiate to the hip; hypoesthesia may be noted in the same region.

ilioinguinal neuralgia   Continuous burning or lancinating pain felt in the distribution of this nerve, usually following its partial injury. The pain is felt in the groin and pudenda and hypoesthesia may be noted in the same region. The pain of **genitofemoral neuropathy** is practically indistinguishable from this condition.[3129]

Illinois Test of Psycholinguistic Abilities   A test profile designed to delineate communication deficits in children and to suggest remedial programs. Tests of **cognitive closure,** visual memory, and visual and auditory reception are also of value in adults. The test is reviewed by Lezak.[3392]

Illness Severity score   A modified form of the **disability status scale** for **multiple sclerosis** with weighting added to stress pyramidal and cerebellar dysfunction and incorporating additional areas of disease activity and a further factor reflecting the phase of illness. The score is proposed as a useful method for evaluating progression in clinical trials of multiple sclerosis therapy.[3867]

illusions   Misperceptions of objective environmental stimuli, affecting any sensory modality.

illusory splitting   Fragmentation of visual perception, such that the parts of an object or person seen appear to be fractured and displaced from one another. It has been described as a feature of migraine auras.[4470]

illusory visual spread   A form of visual perseveration in the spatial sense, in which the object appears to extend beyond its normal boundaries; or its colors may similarly extend such that the colors of a dress may appear to expand onto the face or arms of the wearer. This is unusual manifestation of disease of the visual cortex.[1170,1175]

iminoglycinuria   A benign inborn metabolic disorder presenting with nerve deafness and sometimes mental retardation, in which there is increased urinary excretion of proline, hydroxyproline, and glycine.[4784]

imitation behavior   A disturbance in motor response in which patients imitate the gestures and behavior of the examiner despite the fact that they have not been asked to do so, and continue with such imitations although asked to stop. It represents an early stage of **utilization behavior** and is interpreted as demonstrating impairment of the frontal lobe's normal function of inhibiting parietal lobe function.[3393]

imitation synkinesis   Involuntary symmetrical movements tending to reproduce on one side of the body those movements executed by the other. The condition is usually associated with thalamic or parietal lesions and sometimes with lesions of the posterior columns or the peripheral nervous system, and thus is seen in body regions where lemniscal sensation is lost or diminished but motor function is at least relatively intact.[877] A *cerebellar* form is also distinguished.[5647]

immediate memory   See **short-term memory.**

immersion epilepsy   See **hot water epilepsy.**

immersion foot   Cold-induced **Wallerian degeneration** of peripheral nerves.

immune-mediated neuropathies   Those neuropathies associated with high titers of autoantibodies directed against a specific neural antigen. These are listed in Chart I–4. See also **acute inflammatory and demyelinating polyneuropathy, gammopathic neuropathies.**

Chart I–4. The Immune-Mediated Neuropathies

Multifocal motor neuropathy with persistent conduction block

Anti-MAG-associated neuropathy A syndrome of paresthesias in the legs progressing slowly to a distal symmetrical demyelinating sensorimotor peripheral neuropathy, accompanied by high levels of anti-MAG (myelin-associated glycoprotein) IgM antibodies.[3290]

Paraneoplastic sensory neuronopathy associated with small cell lung cancer and anti-Hu antibodies: A subacute, progressive, paraneoplastic syndrome characterized by paresthesias and painful distal dysesthesias, sensory deficits affecting all modalities, and asymmetrical proximal sensory signs accompanied by high levels of IgG anti-Hu antibodies that bind to neuronal nuclei. In some cases, **lim-**

bic encephalitis, seizures, diplopia, bulbar signs, and autonomic dysfunction are also found.[1391,2260]

Acute axonal motor neuropathy with anti-GM1 antibodies and campylobacter infection (Chinese paralytic disease): An acute, life-threatening axonal motor neuropathy resembling **acute inflammatory demyelinating polyneuropathy** but with early and severe axonal damage, associated with infection by *Campylobacter jejuni*, and accompanied by high titers of anti-GM_1 antibodies.

Painful sensory neuropathy with antisulfatide antibodies, A syndrome characterized by slowly progressive distal sensory loss involving both large and small fibers, accompanied by pain and paresthesias and with detectable IgM and IgG antibodies to sulfatide.[4417]

---

immunoblastic sarcoma   See **primary CNS lymphoma.**

immunodeficiency syndromes with encephalopathy   Microcephaly, encephalopathy, developmental delay, incoordination, and basal ganglion calcification in infants with AIDS.[445]

immunophilins   A family of proteins that act as receptors for the immunosuppressant drugs CsA and FK506 in immune tissue, and are highly enriched in the nervous system. They regulate the mitochondrial permeability transition pore, modulate the stability and function of ion channels, and act as molecular chaperones for a variety of proteins. CsA and FK506 and their derivatives inhibit the function of the immunophilins and provide neuroprotective and neuroregenerative actions in experimental models of stroke, Parkinson disease, neuropathies, etc.

impaired sleep-related penile tumescence   The inability to attain or sustain a penile erection during sleep as a result of organic disease affecting the central autonomic nervous system. Such impairment in penile expansibility is a marker for the presence of organic impotence.[5844]

impairment   1. A failure of function due to musculoskeletal or cerebral injury. 2. The disturbance of a specific function at the level of the organ, for instance, the elements of the neurological examination that make up stroke scales, which are typical examples of impairment scales.

impersistence   The inability to maintain a particular activity. This can be considered abnormal only with reference to the concept of the "reasonable person," but does resemble that lack of attention and concentration commonly found in the confused and demented as well as the interruption of static postures by such abnormal movements as chorea. Impersistence of eyelid closure is also a feature of acute hemispheric disease.[1411]

The tests include examination of the ability of the patient to maintain the tongue protruded, the eyes closed, or the arms outstretched; and those in the **Dartmouth battery,** particularly with regard to gaze. See also **perseveration.**

implicit memory   Knowledge without awareness of the possession of that knowledge; the unconscious retention of learned material; memory where retention is implicit in the performance of tests, although it is not explicitly requested. Frontal and temporal cortices (rather than the hippocampi and perirhinal areas) appear essential for this capacity.[1542]

Tests are usually administered as an evaluation of some function other than memory (such as reading or the learning of motor skills) and memory is assessed indirectly from changes in the performance of the task in question. See also **explicit memory tests, working memory.**

impotence   (Gr, want of power) Inability to generate or sustain a satisfactory penile erection; sexual incapacity.

impulse   (from Lat, to push against) A force communicated suddenly, such as the passage of a wave of depolarization through tissues.

impulse blocking   See **blocking.**

impulsive petit mal   See **benign juvenile myoclonic epilepsy.**

imubacco   See **Tourette syndrome,** for which this is the Japanese term.

inactivity, record of electrocerebral   The absence over all regions of the head of identifiable electrical activity of cerebral origin, whether spontaneous or induced by physiological stimuli or pharmacological agents.

The determination of electrocerebral inactivity requires advanced instrumentation and stringent technical precautions. Tracings of electrocerebral inactivity should be held in clear contradistinction to low-voltage EEGs and records displaying low-amplitude delta activity. (Adapted from the report of the Committee on Terminology, IFCN,[989] © 1974, with permission from Elsevier Science.)

inadequate sleep hygiene   A sleep disorder due to the performance of daily living activities that are inconsistent with the maintenance of good quality sleep and full daytime alertness. These include practices that produce arousal, and those that are inconsistent with the principles of sleep organization.[234]

Diagnostic criteria have been suggested and are given in Chart I–5.

Chart I–5. Diagnostic Criteria for Inadequate Sleep Hygiene

A. Complaints of either insomnia or excessive sleepiness
B. Presence of at least one of the following:
  1. Daytime napping at least two times each week
  2. Variable wake-up times or bedtimes
  3. Frequent periods (two to three times per week) of extended amounts of time spent in bed
  4. Routine use of products containing alcohol, tobacco, or caffeine in the period preceding bedtime
  5. Scheduling exercise too close to bedtime
  6. Engaging in exciting or emotionally upsetting activities too close to bedtime
  7. Frequent use of the bed for nonrelated activities (e.g., television watching, reading, studying, snacking, etc.)
  8. Sleeping on an uncomfortable bed (poor mattress, inadequate blankets, etc.)
  9. Allowing the bedroom to be too bright, too stuffy, too cluttered, too hot, too cold, or in some other way not conducive to sleep
  10. Performing activities demanding high levels of concentration shortly before bed
  11. Allowing to occur in bed such mental activities as thinking, planning, reminiscing, etc.
C. Polysomnography demonstrates one or more of the following:
  1. Increased sleep latency
  2. Reduced sleep efficiency
  3. Frequent arousals
  4. Early morning awakening, or
  5. A multiple sleep latency test that shows excessive sleepiness
D. No evidence of psychiatric or medical disorder that accounts for the sleep disturbance
E. Absence of other sleep disorder either producing difficulty in initiating or maintaining sleep or excessive sleepiness

Adapted from The International Classification of Sleep Disorders Diagnostic and Coding Manual. *Rochester, MN: American Sleep Disorders Association, © 1990. Reproduced by kind permission of the American Academy of Sleep Medicine.*

inapperceptive agnosia   That form of **agnosia** in which the subject is unable to copy objects visualized.

inappropriate ADH syndrome   See **syndrome of inappropriate ADH secretion.**

inappropriate crying   See **emotionalism.**

inattention   Lack of response to stimuli for which the primary perceptive mechanism and pathways are intact.

This is usually a phenomenon detected unilaterally (**neglect**), when the subject fails to perceive a stimulus in the presence of competing stimuli from the opposite side (normally within the same sensory modality, *sensory inattention*). Many or all sense channels may be involved in this way, or the condition may affect one (e.g., vision or touch) selectively. With unimodal inattention, the responsible lesion is of the right inferior parietal lobe, while with multimodal inattention, lesions of the centrum semiovale may also be responsible.[1804]

Motor inattention (hemiakinesia) is the term used to describe a disinclination for direct motor activity, or using the limbs on one side, in the absence of any detectable motor deficit; in such cases, normal power can be demonstrated, at least briefly, with encouragement. Premotor cortical and thalamic lesions are considered to be responsible. See also **hemispatial neglect.**

Global inattention is synonymous with **motor impersistence.**

incapacity status scale   See **Kurtzke scales.**

inching   A technique used in sensory nerve conduction studies, whereby the median nerve is stimulated at points separated by 1–2 cm along its course in the palm. A record of the sensory nerve action potential is made from the finger distally, or from the wrist proximally, in an attempt to define precisely the site of compression of the nerve in **carpal tunnel syndrome.**[804]

incidentaloma An asymptomatic pituitary adenoma shown on CT or MRI scans, to the surprise of the physician and the likely consternation of the patient when informed.

incisura (from Lat, to cut into) A cleft. The term formerly applied to the cerebral or cerebellar fissures.

incisura scapulae syndrome Atrophy and weakness of the infraspinatus muscle as a result of compression of the distal extension of the suprascapular nerve at the level of the scapular notch.

incisural sclerosis The term of **Penfield** for the mesial temporal lobe gliosis occurring as a remote effect of temporal lobe ischemia resulting from difficulties during parturition. [RMS]

inclusion body encephalitis See **subacute sclerosing panencephalitis.**

inclusion body myopathy (*myopathy with congenital joint contractures, ophthalmoplegia and rimmed vacuoles*) A dominantly inherited proximal syndrome with these features, the contractures normalizing in later childhood.[1283]

inclusion body myositis (myopathy) (IBM) A benign, usually sporadic, slowly progressive inflammatory myopathy resembling chronic polymyositis but more common in adult males, who present with painless asymmetrical proximal and distal weakness occasionally with dysphagia; skin or ocular, facial or respiratory muscle involvement; fatigue; or arthralgias. The weakness does not respond to steroid therapy.[2892,4704] Both dominant and recessive forms are described.

Other features of diagnostic value are the tendency for loss of the knee jerks and predominant involvement of the wrist and finger flexors, the quadriceps, and the tibialis anterior muscles. Serum creatine kinase levels are normal or slightly raised.[2037]

Three distinct subsets of IBM have been recognized: *(a) sporadic IBM*, an inflammatory vacuolar myositis with the distinct clinical phenotype described below; *(b) familial inflammatory IBM*, an inflammatory vacuolar myositis occurring in several family members of the same generation with clinical and histological phenotype identical to that of the sporadic form; and *(c) hereditary inclusion body myopathy*, a group of noninflammatory vacuolar myopathies of recessive or dominant inheritance. The recessive disease is characterized by quadriceps sparing and is linked to chromosome 9p. The dominant form comprises a heterogenous group of vacuolar myopathies not yet genetically identified.[1241]

The diagnostic criteria are microscopic; biopsy specimens show the presence of ragged red fibers, rimmed vacuoles, and intranuclear filaments, as well as many of the usual changes of myositis.[2936] Both myopathic and neurogenic EMG patterns may be found. The condition is unresponsive to current treatments. Adenovirus has been isolated from a few cases.

The entity has been reviewed[5603a] and diagnostic criteria[2283] have been proposed:

Proposed Diagnostic Criteria for Inclusion Body Myositis

I. *Characteristic features and inclusion criteria*
   A. Clinical features
      1. Duration of illness >6 months
      2. Age of onset >30 years old
      3. Muscle weakness
         Must affect proximal and distal muscles of arms and legs *and*
         Patient must exhibit at least one of the following features:
         a. Finger flexor weakness
         b. Wrist flexor more than wrist extensor weakness
         c. Quadriceps muscle weakness (≤grade 4 MRC)
   B. Laboratory features
      1. Serum creatine kinase <12 times normal level
      2. Muscle biopsy
         a. Inflammatory myopathy characterized by mononuclear cell invasion of non-necrotic muscle fibers
         b. Vacuolated muscle fibers
         c. Either (*i*) Intracellular amyloid deposits (must use fluorescent method of identification before excluding the presence of amyloid) *or* (*ii*) 15 to 18-nm tubulofilaments by electron microscopy
      3. Electromyography must be consistent with features of an inflammatory myopathy (however, long-duration potentials are commonly observed and do not exclude diagnosis of sporadic inclusion body myositis).
   C. Family history
      Rarely, inclusion body *myositis* may be observed in families. This condition is different from hereditary inclusion body *myopathy* without inflammation. The diagnosis of familial inclusion body *myositis* requires specific documentation of the inflammatory component by muscle biopsy in addition to vacuolated muscle fibers, intracellular (within muscle fibers) amyloid, and 15 to 18-nm tubulofilaments.
II. *Associated disorders*
   Inclusion body myositis occurs with a variety of other, especially immune-mediated conditions. An associated condition does not preclude a diagnosis of inclusion body myositis if diagnostic criteria (below) are fulfilled.
III. Diagnostic criteria
   A. *Definite* inclusion body myositis
      Patients must exhibit all muscle biopsy features including invasion of non-necrotic fibers by mononuclear cells, vacuolated muscle fibers, and intracellular (within muscle fibers) amyloid deposits or 15 to 18-nm tubulofilaments. None of the other clinical or laboratory features are mandatory if muscle biopsy features are diagnostic.
   B. *Possible* inclusion body myositis
      If the muscle shows only inflammation (invasion of non-necrotic muscle fibers by mononuclear cells)

without other pathological features of inclusion body myositis, *then* a diagnosis of possible inclusion body myositis can be given if the patient exhibits the characteristic clinical (A.1, 2, 3) and laboratory (B.1, 3) features. From Griggs RC, Askanas V, DiMauro S, et al. Inclusion body myositis and myopathies. *Ann.Neurol.* 1995;**38**:705–13, reproduced by kind permission. Alternative diagnostic criteria are presented at http://www.enmc.org/pdf/emery81.pdf.

Variant forms include *familial inclusion body myositis*, a dominantly inherited form of the disease,[4107] and a form presenting with dysphagia.[4700]

inclusion cell disease   See **I-cell disease.**

incomplete activation   Motor unit action potentials firing, on requested maximal effort, in decreased numbers at their normal physiological rates, within the basal firing range of 5 to 10 Hz. Causes include upper motor neuron syndrome, pain on muscle contraction, hysteria/conversion reaction, and malingering. Contrast with reduced recruitment. (From the 2001 Report of the Nomenclature Committee of the American Association of Electromyography and Electrodiagnosis.[10] Used by permission, copyright © 2001, AAEM.)

incontinence   Inability to contain the natural evacuations, leading to the inadvertent or uncontrolled passage of urine or feces or both.

incontinentia pigmenti   (Bloch-Sulzberger syndrome, cutaneous meningeal melanosis) An X-linked (or autosomal) dominant mesodermal and ectodermal dysplastic condition causing a variety of pigmented skin lesions, including vesical and bullous eruptions, hyperkeratosis, warts, dermal atrophy, and alopecia, with additional problems such as microphthalmia, cataract, dental and retinal dysplasia, blue sclerae, hemivertebrae with scoliosis and other skeletal malformations; and, in a third of the cases, neurological disorders, including optic atrophy, chorioretinitis, nystagmus, mental retardation, microcephaly, cerebellar atrophy, hydrocephalus, spastic pareses, and seizures, rarely with anterior horn cell degeneration.[909,3280,3281] The condition is lethal *in utero* for hemizygous males, and so is seen to excess in female infants.

The differentiation between the syndromes of Naegeli and of Bloch is based on the appearance of the disease in both sexes in the former, but only in females in the latter.[605]

Variants are *incontinentia pigmenti achromicans* (see **hypomelanosis of Ito**) and *infantile spinal muscular atrophy* with incontinentia pigmenti.[3281]

incontinentia pigmenti achromicans   See **hypomelanosis of Ito.**

increased intracranial pressure without localizing signs   See **idiopathic intracranial hypertension.**

increment   Increase in the size of a compound motor action potential during repetitive motor nerve stimulation, due to an increase in the number of muscle fibers responding to the stimuli. See also **decrement, potentiation, pseudofacilitation.**

incremental exercise test   A procedure whereby the force of muscular contraction required to perform motor tasks is correlated with the force expended by the patient at different levels of required exertion. There should be a precise correlation between the force demanded and that expended; when this is not the case, the presence of "strength withheld" or other forms of noncompliance is likely. *Incremental ergonometry* is a further development of the same principle.

incrementing response   A reproducible increase in amplitude and/or area of successive M waves to repetitive nerve stimulation. The rate of stimulation and the number of stimuli should be specified. It is commonly seen in two situations. In normal subjects the configuration of the M wave may change in response to repetitive nerve stimulation so that the amplitude progressively increases as the duration decreases, leaving the area of the M wave unchanged. This phenomenon is termed **pseudofacilitation.** Also, in neuromuscular transmission disorders, the configuration of the M wave may change with repetitive nerve stimulation so that the amplitude and the area of the M wave progressively increase. This phenomenon is termed "facilitation." cf. **decrementing response.** (From the 2001 Report of the Nomenclature Committee of the American Association of Electromyography and Electrodiagnosis.[10] Used by permission, copyright © 2001, AAEM.)

incubus   (from Lat, to lie down upon) A male devil, thought in the Middle Ages to be seeking sexual intercourse with women during their sleep. The word is now used occasionally for the sense of extreme pressure on the chest. See **night terror, sleep terrors;** also **succubus.**

incurvation reflex   With the infant held in ventral suspension, the examiner runs her finger along the paravertebral area, close to the spine. This normally induces a firm swinging of the baby's pelvis toward the stimulation.[6064]

incycloduction   See **duction.**

indeterminate leprosy   An early stage in the development of leprosy, manifest by no more than the presence of an anesthetic, depigmented macule that has the potential for resolution or for progression to either the tuberculoid or the lepromatous forms of the disease.

indeterminate tremor syndrome   Bilateral postural or kinetic tremor of the hands and forearms, or isolated head tremor associated with equivocal neurological signs or concomitant neurological signs of doubtful significance (such as a slightly unsteady gait, mild dementia in an elderly person, hypomimia, reduced arm swing, or mild bradykinesia).[1422,1630] See **essential tremor,** of which this is likely to be a *variant.*

index   (from Lat, to point out) 1. A pointer; the second digit, next to the thumb. 2. Numerous measurements and ratios of measurements between the points of the body and especially of the head, used mainly by anthropologists but not of great value in medicine. See **cephalic index.**

index of suspicion   The clinician's awareness of the relative likelihood of one pathological condition as opposed to another within the context of his or her work.

indifferent electrode   (reference electrode) See **reference electrode, recording electrode.**

induced nystagmus   (flash-induced, drug-induced nystagmus, provoked nystagmus) Forms of **vestibular nystagmus** appearing in normal subjects only in response to some exciting external event. See **arthrokinetic nystagmus, audiokinetic nystagmus, vestibular nystagmus** (caloric nystagmus), **optokinetic nystagmus, pseudo-caloric nystagmus, anticipatory nystagmus.**

infant Hercules syndrome   See **Kocher-Debré-Semelaigne syndrome.**

infantile adrenoleukodystrophy   A recessively inherited, rapidly progressive syndrome characterized by severe neuropathy from birth, seizures, and hepatomegaly.[2135] See **adrenoleukodystrophy.**

infantile amaurotic familial idiocy   See **gangliosidosis** (Tay-Sachs disease).

infantile autism   (idiopathic autism) A syndrome characterized by failure to establish communication with others, an obsession to continue "sameness," failure of language communication, aloofness, preoccupation with handling small objects, and an inability to anticipate with appropriate body positioning the likelihood of being picked up.[2916]

Clinically, the condition usually presents toward the end of the first year of life with diminution in crying, motor activity, feeding, language, and response, although motor milestones are normal. Stereotypic movements and gestures are common. The condition is likely to be multifactorial; no single biochemical or structural abnormality is typically associated and there is no characteristic abnormality on laboratory examination. See also **Heller disease.**

infantile bilateral striatal necrosis   See **familial bilateral striatal necrosis**

infantile botulism   A syndrome consisting of constipation, cranial nerve deficits, pupillary involvement (dilation), and hypotonic weakness with an EMG pattern of brief, small, abundant (for power exerted) motor unit potentials, considered to be due to damage to the motor end-plate resulting from botulinus toxin.[1054] See **botulism.**

infantile cerebellar ataxia   See **acute cerebellar ataxia.**

infantile CNS degeneration   A syndrome characterized by optic atrophy, ophthalmoplegia, areflexia, hypotonia, dysmorphic facies, and severe mental and motor retardation. Microcephaly and seizures may also occur. The course is slowly progressive, but the full-blown syndrome appears within the first 3 years of life. The cause is unknown.[2630]

infantile CNS spongy degeneration   See **Canavan leukodystrophy.**

infantile cortical hyperostosis   (Caffey-Silverman syndrome) A dominantly inherited infantile syndrome characterized by facial swelling due to the formation of new bone (especially of the mandible), excessive bone formation in long bones with pain and pseudoparalysis, fever, and irritability. The condition resolves slowly within a year or two.[867]

infantile facioscapulohumeral dystrophy   A more malignant variant of **facioscapulohumeral dystrophy,** also dominantly inherited, with onset in infancy and death in adolescence.[296]

infantile hexosaminidase deficiency   A cause of very atypical progressive myoclonus epilepsy. See **GM$_2$ gangliosidoses.**

infantile lactic acidosis with failure to thrive   A form of **mitochondrial encephalomyopathy.**

infantile metachromatic leukodystrophy   See **metachromatic leukodystrophy.**

infantile muscular atrophy   See **hereditary motor neuropathy.**

infantile myasthenia   See **myasthenia gravis.**

infantile myoclonic petit mal   See **centrencephalic myoclonic-astatic epilepsy.**

infantile neuroaxonal dystrophy   (Seitelberger disease) A recessively inherited, fatal, primary axonopathy of infancy affecting multiple tracts in the CNS. It is characterized by extrapyramidal dysfunction and often by the involvement of optic, cerebellar, and spinal systems. Failure of mental and motor growth, dystonia, dementia, spasticity, areflexia, generalized analgesia, optic atrophy, pendular nystagmus, deafness, and other cranial nerve palsies and peripheral neuropathy result, and the children never walk or talk, eventually dying decerebrate before the age of 10 years.[2719] The following diagnostic criteria have been suggested:[4074]

1. Unequivocal histologic evidence in the form of axonal swellings and spheroid bodies in skin biopsies
2. Onset of symptoms before the age of 3 years
3. Clinically, psychomotor deterioration, with increasing pyramidal tract signs and with marked truncal hypotonia
4. Relentlessly progressive course leading to spastic tetraplegia, blindness, and dementia by the age of 4 years

Reproduced from Nardocci N, Zorzi G, Farina L, et al. Infantile neuroaxonal dystrophy. *Neurology* 1999;*52:* 1472–8, by kind permission.

Pathologically, the presence of dystrophic axons containing spheroid bodies is notable throughout the CNS and in peripheral tissues. The condition was first reported by Seitelberger.[5054] It runs a shorter course and starts at an earlier age than **Hallervorden-Spatz disease,** which it otherwise resembles and from which distinction may be impossible. The question is reviewed by Baraitser.[335]

Variants include the following:

Neuroaxonal dystrophy with tubular acidosis A rare, congenital, dysmetabolic syndrome characterized by renal tubular acidosis, axonal neuropathy, cerebral and cerebellar atrophy with ataxia and pyramidal signs, resting tremor, and mental and developmental delay.[3539]

Juvenile neuroaxonal dystrophy A rare dementing illness in children, with axonal spheroids.[1499]

Forms with *neonatal onset* or *X-linked inheritance*

Spinal muscular atrophy in infantile neuroaxonal dystrophy

infantile neuronal ceroid lipofuscinosis A recessively inherited form of neuronal ceroid lipofuscinosis, characterized by psychomotor retardation, hypotonia, trunk and limb ataxia, severe visual deficits due to retinal dystrophy and optic atrophy, myoclonic jerks, and microcephaly, with onset in infancy.[4912] See **neuronal ceroid lipofuscinosis.**

infantile neuronal degeneration A variant form of **hereditary motor neuropathy type 1** (which it resembles clinically). It is recessively inherited and there is additional widespread neuronal loss and gliosis in both the gray and white matter in the thalamus, pons, cerebellum, and spinal cord as well as segmental demyelination in the peripheral nerves.[5331]

infantile Niemann-Pick disease See **sphingomyelin storage diseases.**

infantile osteopetrosis and neuronal storage disease A recessively inherited congenital neuroaxonal storage disease characterized by osteopetrosis, osteosclerosis with multiple fractures, enlarged liver and spleen, anemia, cerebral atrophy and macrocephaly, optic atrophy, pyramidal signs, mental and developmental delay, and neuronal inclusions.[138]

infantile paralysis (infantile palsy) See **poliomyelitis.**

infantile phytanic acid storage disease A recessively inherited peroxisomal disease characterized by elevated plasma phytanic acid levels with minor facial dysmorphism, sensorineural deafness, cataract, pigmentary retinopathy with visual failure, ichthyosis, electrocardiographic abnormality, enlarged liver, myoclonus, nystagmus, cerebellar ataxia, painful sensorimotor peripheral neuropathy, and developmental delay.[5911] See also **hereditary motor and sensory neuropathy, type 4.**

infantile polymyoclonia See **myoclinic encrephalopathy of infancy.**

infantile Refsum disease See **infantile phytanic acid storage disease.**

infantile sleep apnea See **sleep apnea.**

infantile spasms See **West syndrome.**

infantile spasms, hemimegalencephaly and hemi-hypsarrhythmia See **West syndrome.**

infantile spasms, X-linked See **West syndrome.**

infantile spinal muscular atrophy, arrested See **hereditary motor neuropathy, type 2.**

infantile striatonigral degeneration A progressive, familial neurodegenerative disorder characterized by degeneration of the cerebellum, dentate nucleus, substantia nigra, globus pallidus, inferior olives, and intermediolateral columns of the spinal cord, and clinically associated with mental and motor regression starting from the latter part of the first year of life, seizures and myoclonus, ataxia, pyramidal signs, and neuropathy, all progressing to death within the first 5 years of life.[2509]

infantile subacute necrotizing encephalopathy See **Leigh disease.**

infantile sudanophilic leukodystrophy See **adrenoleukodystrophy.**

infantile symmetrical necrosis of the neostriatum See **infantile bilateral striatal necrosis.**

infantile tremor syndrome A syndrome described in India comprising the abrupt onset in summer of a rapid, high-intensity tremor, apathy, and hypokinesia in children between the ages of 6 months and 2 years. The tremors affect the face and arms mainly, the latter being abducted at the shoulders and flexed more distally, like a bird drying its wings. The illness is self-limiting over a few weeks, but the children may then show developmental retardation. Anemia is the only constant pathological finding.

The cause is unknown,[4475] but it is thought to be a meningoencephalitis, as about half the affected children have fever. Apart from the tremor and an expressionless pallid facies, there are no accompanying physical signs.[5485]

infantile X-linked ataxia and deafness A familial syndrome comprising progressive cerebellar dysfunction, dementia, deafness, hypotonia, optic atrophy, esotropia and later vomiting, dysphagia with choking, increasing weakness, lethargy, and death. Pathologically, the maximum neuronal loss is in the dentate and olivary nuclei.[4975]

infantile-onset spinocerebellar ataxia with sensory neuropathy A recessively inherited ataxic syndrome, presenting with ataxia, hypotonia, athetosis, and areflexia between the ages of 9 and 18 months, with later-developing ophthalmoplegia and sensorineural hearing loss.[3139]

infarct Ischemic coagulative necrosis of tissue resulting from obstruction of the lumen of the artery supplying the infarcted area. The concept was formulated initially by **Virchow.**

infectious chorea   See **Sydenham chorea.**

infectious hepatitis   A systemic viral infection with a particular tendency to damage the liver. Neurological complications such as meningitis, encephalitis, and polyneuropathy occasionally occur.[3360]

infectious mononucleosis   A disease due to the Epstein-Barr virus, preferentially affecting children and young adults and causing fever, lymphadenopathy, pharyngitis and splenomegaly. Neurological complications include lymphocytic meningitis, encephalomyelitis, facial palsy, polyneuropathy, and mononeuropathy, but occur in less than 10% of the cases.[2063] In the context of CNS involvement, however, the classic features of mononucleosis listed above need not be present.[1416]

infectious polyneuritis   See **acute inflammatory demyelinating polyneuropathy.**

infective endocarditis   Bacterial infection of the cardiac valves with an incidence of neurologic complications of 30%, almost all occurring in patients with left-sided valvular disease and when the endocarditis is caused by virulent organisms such as *S. aureus* and the *Enterobacteriaceae.* The clinical presentation is dependent on the area of the central nervous system involved by infected (micro)emboli. A complication is intracranial mycotic aneurysm.[5667]

inferior calcaneal neuropathy   Compression of this nerve, presenting usually with heel pain. The associated weakness/wasting of the abductor digiti quinti is seldom clinically apparent.[4335]

inflammatory myopathy   See **dermatomyositis, polymyositis, inclusion body myositis.**

inflammatory myopathy, scapuloileoperoneal atrophy, and cardiomyopathy   A dominantly inherited syndrome with onset in the second to fifth decades, characterized by slowly progressive muscle weakness in the scapuloileoperoneal distribution and cardiopathy. Muscle biopsy specimens show both neurogenic and myopathic changes with inflammatory cell reactions and perivascular cuffing, the latter considered to be a manifestation of a secondary polymyositis.[2839]

inflammatory sensory polyganglionopathies   Disorders affecting primarily the spinal sensory ganglion cells, posterior roots and peripheral nerves and leading to prominent sensory deficits. Both **paraneoplastic** and nonmalignant inflammatory disorders are responsible.

In the *malignant form*, ataxic and/or hyperalgesic syndromes occur with or without accompanying dysautonomia. Progression is usually subacute. The most striking clinical features are paresthesias, dysesthesias, and eventually anesthesia, loss of reflexes with retained strength, and constipation. Antineuronal nuclear antibodies are present in the serum. Small-cell carcinoma of the lung is the most common association.

In the *nonmalignant form*, ataxic and/or hyperalgesic syndromes occur, usually with subacute or chronic progression. The clinical features resemble those of the other form, but autonomic signs are not detectable. Extractable nuclear antigen is present in the serum. Other dysimmune conditions such as **Sjörgren syndrome,** connective tissue disease, HIV, or other viral infections[5217] are commonly associated. This form may thus be regarded as a variant of **acute inflammatory demyelinating polyneuropathy.**

information-memory-concentration test   The forerunner of most of today's scales for diagnosing or rating dementia, it was originally combined with pathological measurements. The test items concern orientation, recall of significant dates and personal factors, and tests of counting and reversed sets (20 to 1, months of the year; see Chart I–6). Though validated in the original papers, this test appears to have been superseded by those of more recent origin.[603] See **Blessed Roth Dementia Scale, Modified Mini-Mental State.**

Chart I–6. The Information-Memory-Concentration Test

Information

Name.
Age.
Time (hour), time of day, day of week, date, month, season, year.
Place: Name, street, town.
Type of place (e.g., home, hospital, etc.).
Recognition of two persons (one point for each).

Memory

Personal: Date of birth, place of birth, school attended, occupation, name of siblings/name of spouse, name of any town where patient worked/lived, name of employers.
Non-Personal: Date of first World War (1/2 if within 3 years), date of second World War (1/2 if within 3 years), monarch, prime minister.
Five-minute recall (score 0–5 points): Mr. John Brown, 42 West Street, Gateshead.

Concentration

Months of year backwards, counting 1-20, counting 20-1.

*From Blessed G, Tomlinson BE, Roth M. The association between quantitative measures of dementia and of senile changes in the cerebral grey matter of elderly subjects. Br J Psychiatry 1968;**114**:797. Reproduced by kind permission.*

infra-   (Gr, beneath). Prefix denoting beneath.

infraorbital neuralgia   Pain felt in the distribution of that nerve with a persistent quality, unlike the stabbing pain of **trigeminal neuralgia,** although the same treatments may give relief. The cause is seldom determined.

infraspinatus reflex   Exaggerated contraction of the infraspinatus when it is tapped. A sign of minimal clinical value even with lesions of the corticospinal pathway above the C5 level.

ingravescent apoplexy   The slow, rather than the abrupt, onset of a stroke syndrome. This is usually due to thrombosis of a major artery or of a dural venous sinus as opposed to embolism or hemorrhage.

inherited prion disease   See **Jakob-Creutzfeldt disease.**

inherited tendency to pressure palsies   See **hereditary pressure-sensitive neuropathy**

inhibition   (from Lat, to hold in) The arrest of functional activity of an organ or structure as an effect of a restraining influence exerted by a neuronal system.

inhibitional palsy of Chavasse   Apparent paresis of the contralateral yoke muscle (*a*) in response to hypoactivity of that muscle (*b*) which is normally antagonistic to the action of a paretic muscle (*c*).

Thus with a right lateral rectus palsy (*c*), there will be overaction of the left medial rectus (the yoke muscle) and contracture of the ipsilateral antagonist (the right medial rectus). This latter muscle (*b*) is now hypoactive, which leads to the paresis of its contralateral yoke muscle, the left lateral rectus (*a*), especially if the paretic eye is used for fixation.[2133]

inhibitory epilepsy   Rare seizure type in which it is surmised that inhibitory impulses originating from higher centers act on the upper motor neuron itself, leaving the anterior horn cell, and possibly the upper motor neuron input to the gamma efferents is switched off. Differentiation from postepileptic paralysis is difficult because both may have associated seizures.[5190] Inhibitory simple partial (nonconvulsive) seizures also occur, presenting as focal neurological deficits with EEG evidence of appropriate focal seizure activity, for example, after neurosurgical procedures.[218]

Epileptic aphasic seizures, ictal deafness, ictal amaurosis, epileptic **negative myoclonus, Todd paresis,** and *brief focal atonia* are other forms described. See also **chalastic fits.**

inhibitory nerve   A nerve capable of slowing, restraining, or preventing secretion or contraction of the gland or muscle that it innervates.

inhibitory phenomenon   A rare form of seizure disorder in which attacks of paralysis are not preceded by convulsive movements in the same territory.[2421] See also **Todd paralysis.**

inhibitory postsynaptic potential   (IPSP) A local graded hyperpolarization of a neuron in response to activation at a synapse by a nerve terminal. cf. **excitatory postsynaptic potential.** (From the 2001 Report of the Nomenclature Committee of the American Association of Electromyography and Electrodiagnosis.[10] Used by permission, copyright © 2001, AAEM.)

inion   The apex of the external occipital protuberance. The name is the Greek word for the tendon at the back of the neck.

injection myopathy   Local inflammation following needling of a muscle, especially when antibiotics, digoxin, penicillin, or narcotic analgesics are injected into it. If such inflammation is widespread, it may induce a transient rise in the serum creatine kinase levels.[3301]

injection paralysis   Poliomyelitis in a single limb into which an injection had been given for any reason in the last 2 to 3 weeks.[6053]

injury potential   1. The potential difference between a normal region of the surface of a nerve or muscle and a membrane region that has been injured; also called a "demarcation," or "killed end" potential. Approximates the potential across the membrane because the injured surface has nearly the same potential as the interior of the cell. 2. In electrodiagnostic medicine, the term is also used to refer to the electrical activity associated with needle electrode insertion into muscle. (From the 2001 Report of the Nomenclature Committee of the American Association of Electromyography and Electrodiagnosis.[10] Reproduced by permission of the Association and of John Wiley and Sons, Inc.) See also **fibrillation, insertion activity, positive sharp wave.**

inner cerebral trauma   See **diffuse axonal injury.**

inner speech   (endophasy) Goldstein defines this as follows: "The totality of processes and experiences which occur when we are going to express our thoughts, etc. in external speech and when we perceive heard sounds such as language. Inner speech is, on the one hand, in relation to the non-language mental processes; on the other hand, to the external instrumentalities (external speech)."[2174]

Thus, there is a central language process coming between nonverbal thought and expressed speech or, in short, silent processes of thought.[1179]

innervation   The nerve supply of a structure.

Innsbruck coma scale   An assessment instrument with excellent predictive value with regard to poor outcome in patients with severe head injuries (see Chart I–7).[478]

Chart I–7. The Innsbruck Coma Scale

Neurological assessment	Score
Reaction to acoustic stimuli	
Turning towards stimuli	3
Better-than-extension movements	2
Extension movements	1
None	0
Reaction to pain	
Defensive movements	3
Better than extension movements	2
Extension movements	1
None	0

Body posture

Normal	3
Better-than-extension movements	2
Extension movements	1
Flaccid.	0

Eye opening

Spontaneous	3
To acoustic stimuli	2
To pain stimuli	1
None	0

Pupil size

Normal	3
Narrow	2
Dilated	1
Completely dilated	0

Pupil response to light

Sufficient	3
Reduced	2
Minimum	1
No response	0

Position and movements of eyeballs

Fixing with eyes	3
Sway of eyeballs	2
Divergent	1
Divergent fixed	0

Oral automatisms

Spontaneous	2
To external stimuli	1
None	0

From Benzer A, Mitterschliffthaler G, Marosi M, et al. *Prediction of non-survival after trauma: Innsbruck coma scale.* Lancet 1991;**338**:977–978. Reproduced by kind permission of Elsevier Science.

input circuit   A system consisting of the EEG electrodes and intervening tissues, the electrode leads, jack box, input cable, and electrode selectors. (Adapted from the report of the Committee on Terminology, IFCN,[989] © 1974, with permission from Elsevier Science.)

input impedance   The impedance that exists between the two inputs of an EEG amplifier, measured in ohms (generally megohms), with or without the additional specification of input shunt capacitance (measured in pico-farads [pF]). This is not a synonym for **electrode impedance.**

input terminal 1   (recording electrode) The input terminal of a differential amplifier at which negativity, relative to the other input terminal, produces an upward deflection. Synonymous with active or exploring electrode. (From the 2001 Report of the Nomenclature Committee of the American Association of Electro-

myography and Electrodiagnosis.[10] Used by permission, copyright © 2001, AAEM.)

input terminal 2   (reference electrode) The input of a differential amplifier at which negativity, relative to the other input terminal, produces a downward deflection. (From the 2001 Report of the Nomenclature Committee of the American Association of Electromyography and Electrodiagnosis.[10] Used by permission, copyright © 2001, AAEM.) See **active electrode.**

input voltage   The potential difference between the two input terminals of a differential EEG amplifier.

insensitivity to pain   See **pain asymbolia, hereditary sensory and autonomic neuropathy.**

insertion activity   Electrical activity from myofibrils caused by insertion or movement of a needle electrode within a muscle. See also **fibrillation** potential and **positive sharp wave.**

insertions   The appearance in speech of material related to thoughts at a remote time past—a form of perseveration, but with excessive delay. A sign in dementia, patients sometimes making inapposite use of words that would have been in context half an hour before.[1858]

Inside MS   A neurological journal devoted to multiple sclerosis, and the official publication of the National Multiple Sclerosis Society. Address: National Multiple Sclerosis Society, 733 Third Avenue, New York, NY 10017. Web site: http://www.nationalmssociety.org/InsideMS.asp.

insistence   A useful term suggested by Miller Fisher for stubborn ideational perseveration along a train of thought from which the demented patient's mind is not to be derailed. The patient ignores all inducements to change the subject or to desist from the repeated utterance, and may become overtly hostile if pressed to do so or if ignored.[1858]

insomnia   The subjective impression of inadequacy in the quantity or quality of sleep. The condition may be transient or chronic and is due to nonpsychiatric factors in perhaps one case in four. The varieties of insomnia have been listed by Parkes,[4337] as follows;

> **Sleep-onset insomnia**
> Sleep maintenance insomnia
> Early morning waking
> Phase-shift disorders
> Cyclical insomnia

In *persistent, psychophysiological insomnia*, the lack of sleep represents a learned pattern.[2478]

Total absence of sleep (*agrypnia*) in a man with Morvan fibrillary chorea and **vesperal hallucinations** has been reported.[1831]

inspiratory gasp   A clinical test of autonomic vasomotor control in which brief, dermal vasoconstriction is sought when a subject takes a sudden inspiratory gasp.

inspiratory speech   See **spasmodic dysphonia.**

instinctive grasp reaction   See **groping.**

instructional deficit   Inability to perform a test satisfactorily or at all because of inability to comprehend the instructions.

Instrumental Activities of Daily Living Scale   An assessment instrument by which eight functions (telephoning, shopping, preparing food, housekeeping, doing laundry, traveling, taking medication, and handling finances) are evaluated on 3- to 5-point rating scales completed by family members on the basis of the capacity of a family member living with them to cope unaided with such activities.[3299] See **activities of daily living.**

instrumental phase reversal   Simultaneous pen deflections in opposite directions caused by a single wave recorded in two bipolar derivations. This inversion is purely instrumental in nature, i.e., due to the same signal being simultaneously applied to the input terminal 1 of the other amplifier.

When observed in two linked bipolar derivations, phase reversal indicates that the potential field is maximal or less frequently minimal at or near the electrode common to such derivations, so the phenomenon can be used to localize EEG activities, whether normal or abnormal. See also **true phase reversal, bipolar montage, differential amplifier.** (Adapted from the report of the Committee on Terminology, IFCN,[989] © 1974, with permission from Elsevier Science.)

insufficient sleep syndrome   A disorder occurring in an individual who persistently fails to obtain sufficient nocturnal sleep required to support normal alert wakefulness. Diagnostic criteria have been suggested and are given in Chart I–8:[234]

Chart I–8. Diagnostic Criteria for Insufficient Sleep Syndrome

A. The patient complains of excessive sleepiness or (in prepubertal children) of difficulty in initiating sleep.
B. Habitual sleep episodes are shorter in duration than expected for the age of the individual.
C. When the habitual sleep schedule is not maintained (e.g., on weekends or in vacation time), patients will have a sleep episode that is greater in duration than the habitual sleep episode and will awaken spontaneously.
D. The abnormal sleep pattern is present for at least 3 months.
E. A therapeutic trial of a longer sleep episode eliminates the symptoms.
F. Polysomnographic monitoring performed over the patient's habitual sleep period demonstrates:
1. Sleep latency less than 15 minutes longer, a sleep efficiency >85% and a final awakening of less than 10 minutes
2. A multiple sleep latency test that demonstrates excessive sleepiness
G. There is no evidence of significant underlying medical or psychiatric disorder to account for the symptoms.
H. The disorder does not meet the criteria for any other sleep disorder producing either insomnia or excessive sleepiness.

From ASDA Diagnostic Classification Steering Committee. The International Classification of Sleep Disorders Diagnostic and Coding Manual. Rochester, MN: American Sleep Disorders Association, 1990. Reproduced by kind permission of the American Academy of Sleep Medicine.

insula   (Lat, island) (Island of Reil) That area of cortex lying deep in the sylvian fissure, covered by the opercula of the frontal and parietal lobes.

insular sclerosis   The first name applied to **multiple sclerosis** by Moxon, who first described the condition in England.

integrated EMG   Mathematical integration of the full wave rectified EMG signal. It reflects the cumulative EMG activity of a muscle over time. (From the 2001 Report of the Nomenclature Committee of the American Association of Electromyography and Electrodiagnosis.[10] Used by permission, copyright © 2001, AAEM.)

integrative action of the nervous system   The term of **Sherrington** for the coordination of movements as a response to sensory stimuli, the coordination being regarded as the simultaneous and successive compounding of simple reflexes; the cooperation of reflexes with allied or harmonious tendencies and the prevention of simultaneous activity in reflex arcs that have antagonistic functions.[5119]

integrator nystagmus   See **gaze-paretic nystagmus.**

integument   (Lat, upon + to cover) A covering, such as the skin.

intellect   (from Lat, perceiving or choosing between) The power or reasoning and of understanding.

intellectual aura   See **dreamy state.**

intelligence   1. The faculty of using means to attain ends, with understanding. 2. A set of (cognitive) abilities comprising the senses, gnosis, and reflection.[2503] 3. That set of abilities measured by intelligence tests.

At least two forms of intelligence are recognized: *fluid intelligence* is that required for the solution of new problems, while *crystallized intelligence* refers to the manipulation of previously learned information.[2653]

intention   An end which a subject decides to attain.

intention myoclonus   See **action myoclonus.**

intention rigidity   The occurrence of "freezing," often leading to falling, when a patient with **myotonia congenita** has to do something suddenly.

intention spasm   The simultaneous contraction of agonists and antagonists during performance of a precise voluntary movement, rendering correct execution of the movement impossible. A form of dystonia.

intention tremor   A form of kinetic tremor due to an oscillation of a limb during the performance of a voluntary goal-directed movement that requires precision in the final placement of part of that limb on a distant target. Such to-and-fro movements, increasing in amplitude as the limb approaches the distant target, are taken as a sign of cerebellar disease on the same side. See also **cerebellar tremors, tremor.**

inter-   (Lat, between). Prefix denoting between.

intercalated nodes Nodes of Ranvier with an unusually short internodal distance, occurring in the course of remyelination after previous segmental demyelination of peripheral nerves.

intercostal neuralgia (segmental neuralgia) Paroxysmal, sharp pain in the distribution of an intercostal nerve, precipitated by spinal movements, usually with cutaneous tenderness.

The primary form is rare, and local spinal or generalized (infectious or metabolic) causes are more often incriminated as causal agents, although the mechanism is usually unclear.

interdigital neuralgia See **Morton metatarsalgia.**

interdigital neuropathy See **Morton metatarsalgia.**

interdischarge interval The time between corresponding points upon consecutive discharges of the same potential. (Adapted from the 2001 Report of the Nomenclature Committee of the American Association of Electromyography and Electrodiagnosis.[10] Used by permission, copyright © 2001, AAEM.)

interdose withdrawal headache See **analgesic rebound headache.**

interelectrode distance The spacing between pairs of electrodes. The distances between adjacent EEG electrodes placed according to the standard 10-20 system or more closely spaced electrodes are frequently referred to as *short* or *small inter-electrode distances.* Larger distances such as the double or triple distance between standard electrode placements are often termed *long* or *large inter-electrode distances.* (Adapted from the report of the Committee on Terminology, IFCN,[989] © 1974, with permission from Elsevier Science.)

interference Unwanted electric activity recorded from the surrounding environment.

interference pattern Electric activity recorded from a muscle with a needle electrode during maximal voluntary effort. A full interference pattern implies that no individual motor unit action potentials can be clearly identified. A reduced interference pattern (intermediate pattern) is one in which some of the individual motor unit action potentials may be identified while others cannot, owing to superimposition of waveforms. The term discrete activity is used to describe the electric activity recorded when each of several different motor unit action potentials can be identified in an ongoing recording because of limited superimposition of waveforms. The term *single unit pattern* is used to describe a single motor unit action potential, firing at a rapid rate (should be specified) during maximum voluntary effort. The force of contraction associated with the interference pattern should be specified. See also **recruitment, recruitment pattern.** (From the 2001 Re-

port of the Nomenclature Committee of the American Association of Electromyography and Electrodiagnosis.[10] Used by permission, copyright © 2001, AAEM.)

interference pattern analysis Quantitative analysis of the interference pattern. This can be done either in the frequency domain using fast Fourier transformation (FFT) or in the time domain. It can be done using a fixed load (e.g. 2 kg), at a given proportional strength (e.g., 30 of maximum), or at random strengths. The following are measured in the time domain: (*a*) the number of turns per second and (*b*) the amplitude, defined as the mean amplitude between peaks. (From the 2001 Report of the Nomenclature Committee of the American Association of Electromyography and Electrodiagnosis.[10] Used by permission, copyright © 2001, AAEM.)

interictal That period intervening between acute events affecting the nervous system - for example, the time after one seizure and before the next.

intermanual conflict A state in which one hand performs an action that is undone by the other hand. See **alien hand syndrome**

intermediary coup contusions Single- or multiple-contusion hemorrhages in the deeper structures of the brain.[6]

intermediary nerve of Wrisberg The small sensory component of the seventh cranial nerve, conveying common sensation from the anterior wall of the external auditory meatus.

intermediary sleep stage Non–rapid eye movement sleep stage 2.[249]

intermediate filaments Fibrous proteins that mediate cell type–specific features of cytoarchitecture, including α-internexin, cytokeratins, desmin, lilensin, glial fibrillary acidic protein (GFAP), lamins, nestin, neurofilaments, paranemin, peripherins, phakinin, synemin, and vimentin. Intermediate filament-associated proteins responsible for other disorders include αB-crystallin, desmoplakin, emerin, gigaxonin, and plectin. (This entry is abstracted from the Neuromuscular Web site at Washington University, St. Louis, (http://www.neuro.wustl.edu/neuromuscular/maltbrain.html) by courtesy of Dr. Alan Pestronk.)

intermediate interference pattern See **interference pattern.**

intermediate petit mal seizures An epileptic syndrome characterized by features of both classic typical absence attacks and the **Lennox-Gastaut syndrome.** The clinical seizure patterns include typical absences and tonic-atonic seizures, but motor phenomena including automatisms and change in muscle tone may occur, as may generalized tonic-clonic seizures, or tonic seizures during sleep. The attacks can be precipitated by hyperventilation. The patients frequently show a degree of mental impairment. EEG discharges consist of slow spike–wave complexes, but the frequency of the complexes varies during short periods of time.[3515]

intermediate spinal muscular atrophy   See **hereditary motor neuropathy, type 2.**

intermittent ataxias   Cerebellar syndromes, usually recessively inherited and with an early age of onset. Most are associated with a metabolic deficit.[2439]

intermittent branched-chain ketoaciduria   A recessively inherited, intermittent ataxic syndrome, a variant of **maple syrup urine disease.** Various stresses such as infections and surgery may lead to attacks of lethargy, hyporeflexia, ataxia, vomiting, coma, and possibly death. In such attacks, the urinary levels of ketoacids are high.[2439] See also **cerebellar ataxias.**

intermittent claudication of the cord   The occurrence of pain, leg weakness, and ascending sensory deficits during exercise, relieved by rest and lumbar spinal flexion, and resulting either from steal of the blood supply from the lower cord segments and cauda equina or from compression of lumbosacral roots at many levels as a result of extension during activity in the setting of spinal stenosis.

The term was introduced by **Déjèrine,** as his patients had pyramidal signs on walking and thus their gait was disturbed. Verbiest detected radicular symptoms on exercise and the condition was subsequently called *intermittent claudication of the cauda equina* or *neurogenic claudication.* Since the term is derived from the Latin word for limping, and it is the patient rather than the cord that limps, it is an obvious misnomer. See **lumbar spinal stenosis.**

intermittent oculosympathetic paresis   See **periodic miosis.**

intermittent painful ophthalmoplegia   See **superior orbital fissure syndrome.**

internal anal sphincter reflex   Contraction of the sphincter in response to dilatation, as from a gloved finger. The reflex is mediated by the presacral (sympathetic) nerves. See also **external anal sphincter reflex.**

internal arousal insomnia   See **persistent DIMS.**

internal auditory artery occlusion   An arterial occlusion leading to labyrinthine infarction and to the syndrome of acute vertigo and unilateral hearing loss.[3043]

internal border-zone (subcortical junctional infarcts)   Small infarcts in paraventricular regions or high in the internal capsule resulting from distal middle cerebral artery occlusion beyond the takeoff of the perforating vessels but before the bifurcation of the artery, or from severe extracranial carotid occlusive disease. Clinically, hemiparesis with hemisphere specific neuropsychological dysfunction are the usual findings.

internal carotid artery web   A linear filling defect in the proximal part of the internal carotid artery, seen in the arteriogram of some patients with **fibromuscular dysplasia.**[3986]

internal hamstring reflex   (semitendinosus reflex, semimembranosus reflex, posterior tibiofemoral reflex) Contraction of the hamstrings in response to a tap on the tendons of these muscles, on the medial aspect of the popliteal fossa. The reflex informs on the state of the L4–5 and S1–2 reflex arcs.

internal hydrocephalus   Expansion of the ventricles, assumed to be due to increased intracranial pressure. This term and **noncommunicating hydrocephalus** are interchangeable.

internal purulent pachymeningitis   See **subdural empyema.**

International Academy for Child Brain Development   A professional society, based at 8801 Stenton Ave, Philadelphia, PA 19118.

International Association for the Study of Pain   A charitable association in this field. Address: 909 NE 43rd St., Ste. 306, Seattle, WA 98105. Tel: 206-547-6409.

International Brain Research Organization   A professional society founded by H.H. Jasper in 1960 to promote international cooperation in research on the nervous system. Address: 51. Boul. de Montmorency, F-75016, Paris, France. Web site: http://www.ibro.org/.

International Continence Society Classification   A system of classifying neurogenic bladder disorders.[2745]

Detrusor:	Normal, overactive, underactive
Urethra:	Normal, overactive, incompetent
Sensation:	Normal, hypersensitive, hyposensitive

See also **Bors-Komarr classification, Krane-Siroky classification.**

International Federation of Clinical Neurophysiology   Formerly the International Federation of Societies for Electroencephalography and Clinical Neurophysiology, IFCN. A professional organization concerned with the practice of clinical neurophysiology, teaching, and research worldwide, equal representation being accorded to EEG and EMG. National societies from 36 countries are affiliated. The journal *Clinical Neurophysiology* is the official publication of the Federation.

International Federation of Multiple Sclerosis Societies   A professional organization to which all national societies are affiliated, concerned with cooperation in multiple sclerosis research, the publicizing of research information, and the standardization of materials and methodologies in multiple sclerosis research. It is based at 3rd Floor Skyline House, 200 Union Street, London SE1 OLX, UK.

International Huntington Association   A charitable organization. Address: c/o Gerritt Dommerholt, Callunahof 8, 7217 St. Harsfen, The Netherlands. Tel: 31-573-431-595.

International Joseph Disease Foundation   A charitable organization, based at P.O. Box 2550, Livermore, CA 94550. Tel: 925-449-2060.

International Polio Network   A charitable organization providing support and information on this condition. Gazette International Networking Institute, 4207 Lindell Blvd., #110, St. Louis, MO 63108-2915. Tel: 314-534-0475. Web site: http://www.post-polio.org/.

International Research Council of Neuromuscular Disorders   A professional society, the members of which are active in research into diseases of nerve and muscle. Address: P.O. Box 41, New Bremen, OH 45869.

International Rett Syndrome Association   A nonprofit organization for parents of children with **Rett syndrome,** interested professionals, and others. It offers an information and referral service and support groups, and assists research. Address: 9121 Piscataway Rd, Ste. 2-B, Clinton, MD 20735. Tel: 301-856-3334, 1-800-818-7388.

International Society of Neuropathology   A professional organization for members of national societies of neuropathology. It is based at Dept. of Pathology, Richardson Laboratory, Queen's University, Kingston, Ontario, Canada K7L 3N6. Brain Pathology Editorial Office, UCLA Medical Center, Neuropathology CHS 18-126, Los Angeles, CA 90095.

international 10-20 system   A system of electrode placement on the scalp in which EEG electrodes are placed either 10 or 20% of the total distance on a line on the scalp between the nasion and inion in the sagittal plane and between the right and left preauricular points in the coronal plane. Notes on the derivation of the system, a fuller descriptin of it and a self-test protocol can be accessed at the Web site: http//members.aol.com/aduial/1020sys.html.

International Tremor Foundation   A charitable organization publishing information for patients with essential tremor or Parkinson disease or both, as well as for physicians involved in their care. Address: 7046 W. 105th St., Overland Park, KS 66212-1803. Tel: 913-341-3880.

Internet Handbook of Neurology   A comprehensive information source based at the University of Debrecen, Hungary, with superb illustrations of the neuroanatomy and neuropathology of many neurological diseases as well as links to other resources. Sites include www.neuropat.dote.hu/movement.htm and www.neuropat.dote.hu/dementia.htm.

Internet Journal of Neurology   A free, on-line journal publishing reviews and original material. Web site: http://www.ispub.com/ostia/index.php?xmlFilePath=journals/ijn/front.xml.

internodes   The portions of nerve fibers between nodes of Ranvier.

internuclear ophthalmoplegia   (ataxic nystagmus, Bielschowsky-Lutz-Cogan syndrome) A term introduced by **Lhermitte** to describe the clinical phenomenon of horizontal jerk nystagmus in the abducting eye and impaired adduction of the other eye on lateral gaze, the lesion being in the medial longitudinal fasciculus on the side of the adduction failure. Lutz (a Cuban ophthalmologist in Havana) defined two varieties. In his *anterior form*, the lateral rectus functions normally but the medial rectus is paralyzed on movement toward the side of the lesion, though it supports convergence. In his *posterior form* the lateral rectus is paralyzed, but the medial rectus functions normally. The validity of this definition is questioned, and the absence of convergence in the affected medial rectus would suggest that the lesion is higher—that is, more anterior. Dissociated optokinetic nystagmus and ocular dysmetria are also commonly present.[5231]

The syndrome may be bilateral,[5381] in which case multiple sclerosis is the most common cause, but any brainstem pathology and even myasthenia gravis can be responsible.[560,4818]

internuncial cells/fibers   Those which relay impulses between major tracts, such as the corticospinal, and target neuronal cell bodies, such as the anterior horn cells.

interossei phenomenon   When the arm is stretched out, the fingers abduct in the presence of a pyramidal lesion. See **fifth finger sign.**

interparietal sulcus   A horizontal sulcus separating the superior and inferior parietal lobules.

interpeak interval   Difference between the peak latencies of two components of a waveform.

interpotential interval   Time between two different potentials. Measurement should be made between the corresponding parts of each waveform. (From the 2001 Report of the Nomenclature Committee of the American Association of Electromyography and Electrodiagnosis.[10] Used by permission, copyright © 2001, AAEM.)

interpretative cortex   The term of **Penfield** for those parts of the temporal cortex which, when stimulated spontaneously or exogenously, lead to the occurrence of experiential hallucinations or illusions or interpretative responses.[4403]

interpretative illusions   The term of **Penfield** for illusions of things formerly seen or heard or experienced, occurring as manifestations of spontaneous epileptic seizures. Such phenomena include auditory and visual illusions, illusions of recognition (déjà vu), and illusional emotions.[4403]

interscapular reflex (scapular reflex) Contraction of the periscapular muscles in response to a tap on the spine between the scapulae, described as present in the case of a lesion of the corticospinal tracts above C5.

Intersocietal Commission for the Accreditation of Vascular Laboratories A nonprofit organization established with the support of 11 medical organizations to provide a mechanism for the accreditation of facilities that perform comprehensive testing for vascular disease using noninvasive modalities. Address: 8840 Stanford Blvd., Ste 4900, Columbia, MD 21045. Tel: 410-872-0100.

interstitial brain edema Increase in the amount of water in the extracellular space adjacent to the ventricles, as a result of increased intraventricular pressure, as occurs with acute obstructive hydrocephalus.

interstitial cells As classified by Cajal, astrocytes and oligodendroglia of epiblastic origin and microglia of mesoblastic origin.

interstitial radiotherapy (brachytherapy) A technique for the focusing and collimation of intense beams of gamma radiation in the treatment of deep-seated, inoperable brain lesions.

interventional neurology The subspecialty comprising the performance of therapeutic maneuvers for neurological conditions that rely on technical procedures (such as CT or MRI, arteriography or electromyography) for the proper direction of the intervention. Nerve blocks, biopsy, angioplasty, thrombolysis, local delivery of chemotherapy, botulinus toxin injection, and trigger-point injection are examples. Most such procedures are not commonly performed by neurologists.[3133]

intestinal neuronal dysplasia A condition characterized pathologically by hyperganglionosis in the myenteric and submucosal plexuses of the colon or small bowel with giant ganglia, isolated heterotopic ganglion cells in the lamina propria, and increased acetylcholinesterase activity in the parasympathetic fibers of the lamina propria and circular muscle. The clinical condition presents in infancy with obstinate constipation resembling that of **Hirschsprung disease,** megacolon, or rectal bleeding.[2536]

Multiple endocrine neoplasia syndrome type 2b, **Hirschsprung disease,** or **neurofibromatosis** are sometimes associated.

intestinal pseudo-obstruction The occurrence of repeated episodes of small bowel dilatation, the clinical picture suggesting obstruction but without any lesion detectable at operation. The causes include both neuropathic and myopathic disorders. See **intestinal neuronal dysplasia, familial visceral neuropathy, megacystis-microcolon-intestinal hypoperistalsis syndrome, Hirschsprung disease.**

intra- (Lat, inside). Prefix denoting inside.

intracerebral hemorrhage (intraparenchymal hemorrhage) Bleeding into the substance of the brain or its ventricles. Depending on the cause, this may be in the putamen, thalamus, pons, cerebellum or elsewhere in the subcortical white matter, as is most usual in patients with hypertension; or in the cortex or subcortical regions, as in those with arterial diseases such as **cerebral amyloid angiopathy,** etc. Arteriovenous malformations, aneurysms, cavernous and venous angiomas, tumors, dural sinus thromboses, coagulopathy, and vasculitis are other causes.[4565]

The clinical diagnosis is suggested by (1) the demonstration of an intracerebral hematoma by CT or MRI scan, *and* (2) at least one of the following: depression of conscious level; unilateral or bilateral paresis; unilateral or bilateral sensory deficit; visual field deficit; impairment of speech or dysphagia or ataxia; or the occurrence of sudden severe headache, in the context of acute stroke.

intracerebral steal When there is diminution of response to metabolic factors, for example CO_2, a rise in P_aCO_2 may lead to a fall in regional cerebral blood flow (rCBF). Here, blood is directed away from the diseased brain with abnormal reactivity to the normally reactive brain which can dilate with CO_2. Or RCBF may be increased in areas of hypocarbia, termed *intracerebral countersteal.*

intracranial arteritis with spontaneous benign outcome See **isolated benign cerebral vasculitis.**

intracranial hypotension Positional headache due to intracranial hypotension is one of the low CSF pressure symptoms that include vertigo, nausea, vomiting, visual symptoms, auditory symptoms, and rarely, cognitive changes. The mechanism of low CSF pressure after craniectomy is likely related to loss of hydrostatic pressure following removal of the skull vault.[1640]

intracranial pressure The pressure inside the cranial cavity, normally 0–10 mm Hg and always <15 mmHg.

intracranial pressure monitoring Constant assessment of the intraventricular pressure by means of a catheter introduced into the frontal horn of a lateral ventricle and connected to an external transducer, thus requiring puncture of the brain; or by inserting a hollow metal screw subdurally through a burrhole. The normal intraventricular pressure ranges between 0 and 15mmHg (lower in children). Continuous monitoring, although an invasive procedure with some hazards, is the only reliable way of ascertaining intracranial pressure and thus assists in the management of patients with increased pressures, such as that due to **Reye syndrome,** coma following subarachnoid hemorrhage or intracerebral hematoma, hypoxia, encephalitis, and head injury, with the aim of preventing brain death, which is the typical result of a great increase in such pressure.[3880,4123,4767]

intracranial pressure waves   Three principal varieties are described:

A waves (plateau waves) are sustained increases in intracranial pressure lasting from 5 to 20 minutes, followed by a fall to normal levels and are due to episodes of cerebral vasodilation without an increase in blood flow, as during rapid eye movement sleep periods. They indicate poor compliance (or "venting") in response to slight increases in pressure.

B waves are much briefer and occur every 1–3 minutes, in association with phasic changes in respiration.

C waves correspond with spontaneous alterations in arterial perfusion pressure and indicate decreased cerebral vascular resistance.[3517]

intradural enterogenous cyst   A spinal malformation leading to a myelopathic syndrome of spasticity and loss of pain and touch sensations in infancy or childhood. See **neurenteric cyst.**

intradural meningeal cyst   See **arachnoid diverticula.**

intramedullary   (Lat, within + marrow) Situated within the brainstem or spinal cord. Even though the lesion may thus be far from the medulla oblongata, the word is still often used in this confusing manner. **Intrinsic** is preferable, however.

intraoperative monitoring   The use of electrophysiological stimulating and recording techniques in an operating room setting. The term is usually applied to techniques used to detect injury to nervous tissue during surgery or to guide the surgical procedure. (From the 2001 Report of the Nomenclature Committee of the American Association of Electromyography land Electrodiagnosis.[10] Used by permission, copyright © 2001, AAEM.)

intraparenchymal hemorrhage   See **intracerebral hemorrhage.**

intrasellar arachnoid diverticulum   See **empty sella syndrome.**

intrasellar cistern   See **empty sella syndrome.**

intrasellar cyst   The presence of an arachnoid cyst within the sella turcica causing focal erosion of bone, unlike the situation in **empty sella syndrome,** which does not lead to this finding.

intrauterine seizures   Abnormal movements assumed to be a form of epilepsy occurring toward the end of pregnancy, in that the fetus is suffering from pyridoxine dependency or any form of brain dysplasia.[434]

intravascular lymphoma   A multifocal malignant lymphoma that may be either systemic or confined to the CNS (including the lower spinal cord). Typical presenting syndromes are of multiple subcortical infarcts; paraparesis, pain, and incontinence; subacute encephalopathy; or cranial and/or peripheral neuropathy, all accompanied by nonspecific constitutional symptoms. Pathologically, the intravascular collections of large lymphoid B cells are instrumental in causing the multiple microinfarcts.[2136] **See malignant angioendotheliomatosis.**

intravenous digital subtraction angiography   An invasive radiological test in which a large volume of contrast material is injected rapidly, so that the dye travels as a bolus through the pulmonary system, the left heart, and the aorta to the brachiocephalic vessels.

Such studies are successful only if the cardiac output is normal, so that the dye travels as a dense bolus. The injection of large volumes of dye may precipitate congestive heart failure or renal failure, and the technique is being supplanted by intraarterial digital arteriography[4141] or magnetic resonance angiography.

intrinsic   (from Lat, on the inside) Within, inherent, special to.

intrinsic sleep disorders   Sleep disorders that either originate or develop within the body or arise from causes within the body. They were classified by the **American Sleep Disorders Association** (now the American Academy of Sleep Disorders) as follows:[234]

1. **Psychophysiological insomnia**
2. **Sleep state misperception**
3. **Idiopathic insomnia**
4. **Narcolepsy**
5. **Recurrent hypersomnia**
6. **Idiopathic hypersomnia**
7. **Post-traumatic hypersomnia**
8. Obstructive **sleep apnea**
9. Central **sleep apnea** syndrome
10. **Central alveolar hypoventilation syndrome**
11. **Periodic limb movement disorder**
12. **Restless legs syndrome**
13. Intrinsic sleep disorder not otherwise specified

intron   A segment of a gene.

intrusions   The inappropriate recurrence of a response or of a type of response following a preceding test item or procedure due to proactive inhibition; or the recall of information learned previous to that which was most recently learned and which is now requested.

The resemblance to **perseveration** is close; the difference lies in the fact that the intrusion error occurs not immediately following the first response but even minutes later. In each case, diffuse organic brain disease is likely.[1989] In speech, these are known as **insertions.**

inv dup (15) syndrome   A chromosomal disorder resulting in tetrasomy or partial tetrasomy of 15q. The phenotypes are variable but multiple types of seizure, motor delay, hypotonia, facial dysmorphism, and lack of social interaction are common and mental retardation is always present. See also **Prader-Willi syndrome.**[391]

inverse bobbing   See **ocular dipping.**

inverse cerebellum   (ventral cerebellum) Grossly abnormal development of the cerebellum such that the folia project ventrally, covering the basilar artery, as a result of inability of the cerebellum to grow in the appropriate direction because of the presence of an occipital encephalocele. The malformation is usually accompanied by other anomalies.[5237]

inverse jaw-winking   See **Amin-Amat syndrome.**

inverse latent macro square wave jerks   An unusual variety of **square-wave jerks** which are present with binocular vision at a distance but which cease with monocular fixation (i.e., when one eye is closed).

inverse Marcus Gunn pupil   See **Amin-Amat syndrome, Wartenberg winking-jaw phenomenon.**

inverse myasthenia   See **Lambert-Eaton myasthenic syndrome.**

inverse Uhthoff symptom   See **Uhthoff symptom.**

inversion of the radial reflex   (inverted supinator reflex) A phenomenon described first by **Babínski** in 1910, comprising the replacement of the brachioradialis reflex by finger flexion. This is taken to indicate the presence of a cord lesion at the 5-level. An increase in the triceps jerk is usually detectable as well.[1706]

inversion recovery   (IR) An MRI pulse sequence that begins by inverting the magnetization of the nucleus with a 180° pulse and then, after a time (T1), measures the recovery of the magnetization to equilibrium.[4009] This sequence provides an image with twice the T1-weighting discrimination of the spin-echo sequence, at the expense of a longer imaging time.

inverted ocular bobbing   See **reverse ocular bobbing.**

inverted optokinetic nystagmus   (inverted pursuit) A variant of the normal pattern, in which the fast component of the optokinetic nystagmus is in the direction of the movement of the visual stimulus. This may be seen in some patients with **congenital nystagmus.**

inverted pursuit   See **inverted optokinetic nystagmus.**

inverted reflexes   Occasional variant forms of the usual muscle stretch reflexes, modified in certain conditions by the underlying pathology and the method of elicitation.[5858] Contraction of the muscles is supplied by an adjacent segment below that stimulated by the hammer when a reflex is sought in the normal way.

Thus, tapping the biceps tendon (C5) leads to contraction of the brachioradialis muscle (C6) when there is a cord lesion at C5 which produces signs of a lower motor neuron lesion at that level but of an upper motor neuron lesion as seen from C6 (Babínski's inversion of the radial reflex), or tapping the quadriceps tendon (L3,4) leads to contraction of the hamstrings (L5–S1) with a lesion at L3–4.

Despite the inherent logical confusion, the former is known as the *inverted supinator reflex,* the latter as the *inverted knee jerk.*[696]

inverted supinator reflex   See **inversion of the radial reflex.**

involuntary crying   See **emotionalism.**

involuntary (EMG) activity   Motor unit action potentials that are not under volitional control. The condition under which they occur should be described, e.g.. spontaneous or reflex potentials. If elicited by a stimulus, its nature should be described. cf. **spontaneous activity.** (From the 2001 Report of the Nomenclature Committee of the American Association of Electromyography and Electrodiagnosis.[10] Used by permission, copyright © 2001, AAEM.)

inward fits   The term of Dr. J. Hughlings-**Jackson** for laryngismus stridulus (stridor due to tetany in rickets).

ion channel diseases   (channelopathies) A group of disorders caused by mutations in genes encoding ion (sodium, potassium, calcium, chloride) or ligand (glutamate, GABA, glycine, acetylcholine) channels and with clinical expression in any tissue, but predominantly skeletal muscle or the central nervous system. "Channels" are macromolecular protein complexes within the lipid membrane forming functional pores in the cell membrane through which ions flow to depolarize or hyperpolarize the cell.

Skeletal muscle sodium channelopathies include **hyperkalemic periodic paralysis, paramyotonia congenita,** and potassium-aggravated **myotonia.** Skeletal muscle calcium channelopathies include **hypokalemic periodic paralysis, malignant hyperthermia,** and **central core disease.** Skeletal muscle chloride channelopathies include **Thomsen** and **Becker myotonia.**

A neuronal sodium channelopathy underlies the generalized epilepsy–febrile seizures plus syndrome and familial generalized epilepsy with febrile seizures plus. Neuronal potassium channelopathies include **familial benign neonatal convulsions** and **episodic ataxia** type 1. Neuronal calcium channelopathies include episodic ataxia type 2; familial hemiplegic migraine; and **cerebellar ataxia** type 6. A neuronal glycine receptor channelopathy is **hyperekplexia.**

Muscle acetylcholine receptor channelopathies underly the congenital **myasthenic syndromes.**

Some forms of epilepsy (e.g., autosomal dominant frontal lobe nocturnal epilepsy), the Lambert-Eaton **myasthenic syndrome, Alzheimer disease, Parkinson disease,** and schizophrenia may result from dysfunction of voltage-gated sodium, potassium, and calcium channels, or acetylcholine- and glycine-gated channels. Vision disorders, e.g., **congenital stationary night blindness,** and total color-blindness may also be linked to mutations in ion channels.[946,5421]

ipsilesional neglect   The unusual situation in which there is impairment of processing of stimulus data originating from the side ipsilateral rather than contralateral to a hemispheric lesion. An example is that of patients with a right hemispheric lesion who deviate their responses *to the left* in a **line bisection** task.[3209]

ipsipulsion   See **saccadic lateropulsion.**

IPSP   See **inhibitory postpsynaptic potential.**

IR   See **inversion recovery.**

iridoplegia   Paralysis or immobility of the iris; thus, loss of all pupillary reflexes.

iridoplegia interna   See **Adie syndrome.**

iris   (Gr, a bright-colored circle) The pigmented contractile organ demarcating the pupil of the eye.

irregular generalized spike–wave activity   (atypical or rapid spike–wave activity) The occurrence of generalized bursts of spike and spike–wave complexes, occurring irregularly at about 3.5 to 6 Hz, commonly found in patients with idiopathic generalized epilepsy.

irregular potential   See **serrated action potential.**

irregular sleep–wake pattern   A condition characterized by variable temporal disorganization of sleep and waking behavior which occur at irregular intervals for irregular durations. Nocturnal sleep is interrupted and total sleep time is maintained at a normal level only by the individual taking irregular naps by day. The following diagnostic criteria have been suggested (Chart I–9).[234]

Chart I–9. Diagnostic Criteria for Irregular
Sleep–Wake Pattern

A. A complaint of either insomnia or excessive sleepiness
B. Irregular pattern of at least three sleep episodes during a 24-hour period
C. Presence of the sleep pattern for at least 3 months
D. Total average sleep time per 24 hour period is normal for age
E. Evidence of disturbed chronobiological rhythmicity by either
    1. Demonstration of loss of the normal sleep–wake pattern by continuous polysomnographic monitoring for at least 24 hours, or
    2. Demonstration of loss of the normal temperature pattern by continuous temperature monitoring for at least 24 hours.
F. Absence of any medical or psychiatric disorder that would account for the symptom
G. Does not meet criteria for any other sleep disorder causing insomnia or excessive sleepiness

From ASDA Diagnostic Classification Steering Committee. The International Classification of Sleep Disorders Diagnostic and Coding Manual. Rochester, MN: American Sleep Disorders Association, 1990. Reproduced by kind permission of the American Acedemy of Sleep Medicine.

irritability   (from Lat, to provoke) 1. Abnormal excitability. 2. The property of movement in response to a stimulus, possessed by muscles only. (Robert **Whytt**).

irritable legs   See **Ekbom syndrome.**

Isaacs syndrome   See **idiopathic neuromyotonia.**

Isaacs-Mertens syndrome   See **idiopathic neuromyotonia.**

ischemia   (Gr, staunching of blood) Local anemia due to reduction of its blood supply. The term was introduced by **Virchow.**

ischemia test   A method of increasing the sensitivity of repetitive nerve stimulation in the diagnosis of **myasthenia gravis,** in which the ulnar nerve is stimulated supramaximally at 3 Hz for 4 minutes, after which the nerve is again stimulated at 3 Hz for brief periods every 30 seconds. The decrement in the ulnar-supplied muscles is assessed; if none occurs, the arm is made ischemic by a blood pressure cuff inflated above the systolic pressure at a point above the site of stimulation, and the procedure is repeated.

In even mild generalized myasthenia, the first part of the procedure usually induces a marked decrement in the amplitude of the muscle action potential and even if it does not, such a decrement is highly likely under ischemic conditions.[3045] See also **regional curare test, single fiber electromyography.**

ischemic cerebrovascular disease   Cerebral ischemia or infarction resulting from reduction of blood flow to part or all of the brain, as opposed to hemorrhage into the brain or its coverings.

ischemic chiasmal syndrome   Binasal field defects due to ischemia of the optic chiasm, as a result of atheroma of the cervical or intracranial carotid artery or of the anterior cerebral arteries.[5565]

ischemic conduction resistance   Hypoxia may lead to the down-regulation of enzymes, decreased Na-K-adenine triphosphatase activity, and consequently reduced oxygen requirements. This may explain the phenomenon in which damaged nerves (in diabetes) continue to conduct despite induced ischemia.

ischemic forearm exercise test   A standardized test of muscle glycogenolysis in which the forearm is made ischemic by occlusion of the brachial artery and blood is sampled from the draining veins before, during, and after work is done with the forearm muscles, sometimes measured by ergometry. In normal subjects, peak lactate levels (3–5 times the resting levels) are found at 3 minutes after cessation of work; both decreases in lactate production (in the **glycogen storage diseases**) and increases in production (in certain metabolic myopathies) may be found in abnormal cases.[4045] See also **myoadenylate deaminase deficiency.**

A nonischemic form of the test in which the isometric exercise is performed at 70% of the maximal voluntary contraction for 30 seconds. has also been proposed.[2609]

ischemic monomelic neuropathy   The occurrence of multiple axonal neuropathies in a single limb, occurring abruptly, simultaneously, and without evidence of muscle necrosis, as a result of acute occlusion of, or shunt placement within, a major limb artery.[5966]

ischemic muscular necrosis syndrome   See **Bywaters syndrome.**

ischemic myopathy   A syndrome characterized by changes in muscle which histologically resemble those of **Duchenne muscular dystrophy,** but which are due to peripheral vascular disease.[1680]

ischemic neuropathy   Any injury of peripheral nerves caused by compromise of their blood supply.

ischemic oculopathy   A syndrome of periorbital pain and transient or persistent visual loss resulting from chronic ocular ischemia, as may occur with acute or chronic carotid artery occlusion.

Clinically, the major features include tenderness of the globe, episcleral vascular congestion, conjunctival injection, hyperemia and cellular deposits in the anterior chamber, neovascularization of the iris (rubeosis iridis), a mid-dilated sluggish pupil, increased intraocular pressure, attenuated or dilated retinal vessels, and **venous stasis retinopathy.**[3102]

ischemic optic neuropathy   A condition of older people who develop sudden segmental monocular visual field defects (**scotomas**) as a result of infarction of the anterior, retrolaminar part of the optic nerve, in the absence of inflammation, nerve compression, demyelination, or generalized hypoperfusion. **Crowding** of the disk is said to predispose to the condition.

In most cases the cause is not apparent, but, in a few, **cranial arteritis,** hypertension, diabetes, or atherosclerosis are diagnosed. The other eye may be affected subsequently.[624]

In *variant* forms, the condition follows cataract extraction[921] or complicates collagen vascular disease, migraine, uremia, or severe ocular ischemia.

ischemic papillopathy   Swelling of the optic disk in association with **ischemic optic neuropathy.**

ischemic penumbra   A marginal zone of tissue surrounding a brain infarct within which the cells are functionally impaired since they are perfused at a level between the thresholds of functional impairment and of morphological integrity. Such metabolically challenged cells are, however, still viable and able to survive and recover function if perfusion improves.[251]

ischemic vascular dementia   Dementia resulting from cerebrovascular disease. See **vascular dementia.**

ischuria paradoxa   Dribbling incontinence in **tabes dorsalis.**

Ishihara plates   See **pseudoisochromatic plates.**

Ishihara, Shinobu   (1879–1959) Japanese professor of ophthalmology at Tokyo University, who in 1917 developed isochromatic plates for the detection of various forms of color-blindness.[2754]

island of vision   The term of **Traquair** for the variable sensitivities of different parts of the retina to light and contrast, the use of different illuminations of the stimuli yielding a set of values that chart these sensitivities over a large area of the retinal surface. The resultant chart is thus drawn in three dimensions—two for area and one for sensitivity.[1636] See also **hill of vision.**

-ismus   A suffix indicating spasm—thus pharyngismus, laryngismus, esophagismus, etc.

isocortex   The greater part of the six-layered cortex, consisting of two kinds of cortical structure: (1) the *idiotypic* cortex (**koniocortex**) of the primary motor and primary sensory areas, which represents the most highly developed part of the cortical mantle: and (2) the *homotypical* cortex, which is the **association cortex,** some of which is *unimodal* and some, *heteromodal* (polymodal, multimodal, supramodal, polysensory or high-order association cortex) in its response to differing kinds of stimulation.

isoelectric focusing   A technique used to separate IgG on the basis of different charges or isoelectric points. It is the most sensitive test for detecting humoral immune responses, and when followed by IgG-specific antibody staining, is employed in the detection of oligoclonal bands in the CSF.[173]

isoelectric line   In electrophysiologic recordings, the display of zero potential difference between the two input terminals of the recording apparatus. See **baseline.** (From the 2001 Report of the Nomenclature Committee of the American Association of Electromyography and Electrodiagnosis.[10] Used by permission, copyright © 2001, AAEM.)

isokinetic dynamometry   A method of quantitating muscle power which requires subjects to exert their maximum force against that of a hydraulic or motor-driven instrument, which then measures the torque produced at the anatomical joint tested.[1366]

isolated angiitis of the nervous system   (primary angiitis of the central nervous system, granulomatous angiitis) A relapsing, focal, necrotizing, giant cell angiitis of young or middle-aged adults, characterized by sterile inflammation of the small and medium-sized intracranial, intraspinal, or intraocular vessels exclusively.

Clinically, severe headache, lethargy and malaise, confusion, nausea, vomiting, or myelopathic signs appear first, followed by multifocal neurological symptoms and signs. Fever, myalgia, and arthralgia are uncommon, as is presentation as subarachnoid hemorrhage. Abnormal cell and protein levels in the (sterile) CSF, the arteriographic finding of alternating areas of dilatation or constriction in any of the cerebral arteries, and the proliferation of mesenchymal cells in the intima and adventitia or in all layers of the vessel wall, with giant cells seen on leptomeningeal and cortical biopsy specimens, allow the diagnosis.[871,5194] The disease is unlikely to be homogeneous; numerous etiologies may be responsible.[1158,2414]

The following diagnostic criteria have been suggested.[102]

1. The appropriate clinical presentation of multifocal strokes or encephalopathy in association with headaches
2. Cerebral angiography showing changes consistent with vasculitis (such as segmental stenosis, irregularity of small of medium-sized vessels' lumina, beading, and an aneurysmal appearance)
3. Exclusion of systemic infection, neoplasm, or toxic exposure
4. Leptomeningeal or cortical biopsy demonstrating vascular inflammation and exluding other (such as infectious or malignant) causes of the vascular inflammation

In *variant forms*, the spinal cord is involved rather than the brain; or children are affected.[3274]

See also **isolated benign cerebral vasculitis, microangiopathic syndrome of enephalopathy, hearing loss and retinal arteriolar occlusions.**

isolated benign cerebral vasculitis (benign distal cranial arteritis, intracranial arteritis with spontaneous benign outcome) A disease of intracranial vessels unassociated with other primary pathological processes and demonstrating segmental narrowing on angiography.

Clinically, the condition typically affects young adults who present with headache, nausea, and focal deficits. Whether this is truly an inflammatory disease or a manifestation of arteriospasm is uncertain.[5068]

isolated disk reabsorption   See **disk reabsorption.**

isolated finger flexion   A rare syndrome due to **neuromyotonia** of the flexor digitorum sublimies muscles, causing progressive, painless, involuntary flexion of the fourth and fifth fingers and eventually to contractures. The cause is unknown, but may be related to chronic pulmonary obstructive disease or its treatment.[3928]

isolated gait ignition failure   (gait apraxia, magnetic gait, slipping clutch gait, lower-half parkinsonism, arteriosclerotic parkinsonism, trepidant abasia, Petren gait) A gait pattern characterized by marked difficulty with initiating gait (*start hesitation*) and maintaining locomotion (*turn hesitation*, **freezing**) in the absence of impairment of equilibrium, cognition, limb praxis, or parkinsonism. Once locomotion is initiated, steps are short and barely clear the ground, giving the gait a shuffling appearance. However, with continued stepping the stride lengthens, foot clearance becomes normal, and the arms swing as they should.

Diversion of the patient's attention, negotiating narrow passages, or turning may precipitate freezing and a resumption of shuffling. Certain tricks (such as kicking the bottom of a cane) may be employed by the patient to maintain progress. Postural responses and stance base are normal, and falls are rare.

The pattern is associated with lesions of the basal ganglia or of the frontal lobes or their connections.

(Adapted from Nutt JG, Marsden CD, Thompson PD. Human walking and high-level gait disorders, particularly in the elderly. *Neurology* 1993;**43**:268–279 by kind permission.)

isolated hemihypertrophy   A congenital dysmorphic syndrome characterized by multiple renal cysts and tumors, asymmetrical limb hypertrophy, and mental and developmental delay.[337]

isolated lissencephaly sequence   A developmental anomaly characterized by type 1 **lissencephaly** of variable severity, bitemporal hollowing with a prominent occiput, severe or profound mental retardation with minimal developmental progress, early hypotonia and subsequent hypertonia, decreased spontaneous movements, feeding difficulties, and seizures, including **infantile spasms.**

Numerous other anomalies may accompany the above, which represent minimal diagnostic criteria.[1480]

isolated polymyositis   See **primary idiopathic polymyositis.**

isolated speech deafness   See **pure word deafness.**

isolated trigeminal neuropathy   Chronic, persistent sensory disturbance of the face, usually numbness in one or more divisions of the trigeminal nerve, affecting pain, temperature, and light touch rather than other sensory modes, but sparing motor functions and without demonstrable pathology or evidence of any lesion compressing the trigeminal nerve fibers.[5284]

isolated voice tremor   Tremulousness of the voice in the absence of tremor in any other body part. Both dystonia of the vocal cords and essential tremor appear to be capable of causing this.[1422]

isolation aphasia   A form of aphasia in which the subject can repeat but cannot speak spontaneously, nor comprehend. See **transcortical aphasias** (*mixed form*).

isometric contraction   Muscle contraction that occurs without any change in the length of the muscle fibers (and thus without movement at a joint), as when pushing against an immovable object.

isometric tremor   That form of tremor occurring normally when muscle activity is exerted at maximal force against an unyielding object, or against the antagonists of the muscle in question. See also **tremor.**

isopter   1. The extent of the visual field that is plotted with a given stimulus. 2. Retinal zones of equal visual sensitivity.

isothermagnosia   The perception of thermal stimuli at all temperatures as being warm; an occasional finding in patients with high spinal cord lesions.

isotonic contraction   Muscle contraction that occurs with shortening of the muscle fibers but without any further increase in the tension within them after the initial contraction has occurred, as is the case when an object is lifted from off the ground.

isotope cisternography   A diagnostic technique for studying the flow of the CSF, useful in the diagnosis of **normal-pressure hydrocephalus** and in identifying the site of a CSF leak. Radioactive-iodine labeled albumin is injected into the lumbar subarachnoid space and the patient is scanned repeatedly over the next 72 hours. Normally, the isotope will be seen to ascend to the basal cisterns in 4–6 hours, collecting around the superior sagittal sinus in 24 hours, after which it is reabsorbed.

isovaleric acidemia   A rare organic aciduria due to deficiency of isovaleryl-coenzyme A dehydrogenase, leading to a block in the pathway of leucine catabolism. The condition is characterized clinically by an intermittent ataxic syndrome in infants, who present with vomiting, ketosis, ataxia, hyperreflexia and coma, and in whom cardiomyopathy, congenital heart disease, simple partial seizures, intracerebral hemorrhage, and mild mental and motor delay may also be found.

Most affected infants die before they are a year old. Aminoaciduria, hyperammonemia, and gliosis and spongy changes in the CNS are characteristic pathological findings. The condition is notable for the odor of stale sweat given off by the child, especially during the acute attacks.[830,2439]

itch   An unpleasant sensation that provokes the desire to scratch. Although relief of itch by contralateral ventrolateral cordotomy suggests that the spinothalamic tract is involved in the transmission of itch-related information, there is persuasive evidence that itch and pain are independent sensory modalities. (HJM)[4817] The subject has been reviewed by Tuckett.[5663a]

See also **mitempfindungen.**

iter cerebelli   (Lat, a passage + cerebellum) The cerebral aqueduct (of Sylvius).

iterative discharge   See **repetitive discharge.**

ivory osteomas   Slowly growing solid tumors that arise within the nasal sinuses and may extrude into the orbit or the anterior cranial fossa.

Iwashita syndrome   A syndrome comprising polyneuropathy, skin hyperpigmentation, edema, hepatosplenomegaly, and hypertrichosis complicating myelomatosis.[2762] See **POEMS.**

J receptors   Receptors lying in the walls of pulmonary capillaries, which when excited cause apnea, hypotension, and bradycardia through vagal activity.

jabs and jolts syndrome   A syndrome of head pain in which brief, stabbing pains lasting a second or a few seconds appear in various locations, or sometimes in a single localized area. The jabs may occur in isolation or in association with other headaches such as migraine or cluster headaches. The phenomenon is probably the same as a prolonged **ice-pick pain.**[5195]

jack-in-the-box phenomenon   The appearance as though objects were jumping about; a distortion of vision due to aberrations produced by wearing strong positive lenses.

jack-knife convulsions   See **jack-knife spasms.**

jack knife spasms   (jack-knife convulsions, infantile spasms, salaam attacks) Massive myoclonic jerks with trunk flexion as seen in **West syndrome.** See **flexor spasms.**

Jackson cerebellar "fits"   (Stewart-Holmes syndrome, Holmes-Stewart syndrome) A form of movement disorder in which the head is drawn back, the spine extended, the forearms and hands flexed with the arms kept to the sides, and the legs extended. A persistent hyperextended posture remains present between the attacks.

Originally described by Jackson in 1871 as resembling seizures, the invariable presence of posterior fossa pathology causing raised intracranial pressure suggests that this rather resembles tonic decerebrate posturing.[2778] Wurffbain had described the same entity in 1671.

Holmes' name is also applied to this entity, but in his paper he made it plain that he had never seen what Jackson had described.[5357]

Jackson, John Hughlings- (1835–1911)   One of the greatest figures in the history of neurology, he was born in Yorkshire and apprenticed to a physician in York, training further at St. Bartholomew's Hospital in London before working in a Poor-Hospital in York and then at the London Hospital and Moorfields Eye Hospital. **Brown-Séquard** helped to secure his appointment as assistant physician to the **National Hospital** in 1862 and he joined the staff of the London Hospital in the following year. He was elected a Fellow of the Royal Society in 1878, the same year in which he, with others, founded the journal **Brain.** He retired from practice at the London Hospital in 1894 and from the National Hospital in 1906. It was by his work at these hospitals that Hughlings-Jackson, out of the chaos of speculative and descriptive medicine, organized and laid the foundations of modern neurology and became

himself, without doubt, the greatest living neurologist and scientific clinician of the 19th century in England.

Jackson defined the intellectual "aura" (he disliked the term), or dreamy state—smell and taste, hallucinations of reminiscences (déjà vu) and epigastric sensations with chewing movements, and a defect (not a loss) of consciousness—which he had first described in 1876. He applied the term *uncinate fits* in 1899. His best-studied patient was a physician, Dr. Z., who lived close by Jackson's house[5509] and who later died from an overdose of chloral; at autopsy a small patch of softening was found in the left uncinate region.

He introduced the routine use of the ophthalmoscope; described a patient with Tourette syndrome in 1865; expounded his system of **levels of organization** in *Brain* (1887); and divided speech into the propositional and emotional, regarding aphasia as a loss of propositional speech. His studies of epilepsy, aphasia, apraxia, stroke, functional localization, and levels of organization within the nervous system were made without his ever performing a laboratory experiment.[5439] Jackson's contributions in the area of speech were summarized by Head[2493] as the differentiation between speechlessness and plentiful words wrongly used, between *internal* and *external speech*, and between *intellectual* and *propositional* speech; the statement of the principle that the loss of power of performance varies with the complexity of the act; the recognition of the power of intellectual expression by movements of any kind; and the characterization of agnosia as nonlanguage aphasia.

His contributions in ophthalmology were summarized by Taylor in 1915,[5511] who noted Jackson's recognition of the importance of the use of the ophthalmoscope, the nature of optic neuritis and atrophy, the occurrence of headache as a result of refractive errors, ocular vertigo, and the anatomical innervation of levator palpebrae superioris by the fifth as well as the third cranial nerve in the Marcus **Gunn syndrome.**

Walshe[5832] considered that the areas in which Jackson exerted the most influence (1) the nature of the relationship between mind and brain, noting that Jackson adopted the doctrine of psychophysical parallelism—mental states arose during but not from the activities of the brain; (2) movements and their organization; (3) speech and loss of speech; (4) the duality of symptoms, positive and negative; (5) the hierarchy of levels in the nervous system; (6) the meaning of the term *representation*; and (7) evolution and dissolution in the nervous system

Broadbent[761] published a full review of Jackson's work during his lifetime.

Jackson's laws   1. Those neural functions that are most lately developed are also the first to be lost. This is restated in a variation as Jackson's rule: after epileptic attacks, simple nervous processes are more quickly regained than are complex ones. 2. "The study of the causes of things must be preceded by the study of things caused."

Jackson syndrome (Jackson-MacKenzie syndrome, alternating hypoglossal hemiplegia) A brainstem disorder, the main clinical features being homolateral ninth, tenth, and twelfth cranial nerve palsies, producing anesthesia of the pharynx and larynx, paresis of the soft palate, sternomastoid and trapezius muscles and of the tongue, and contralateral hemiparesis, usually occurring as a result of a medullary tegmental stroke or tumor.[2775,5431]

Some indicate that the eleventh nerve is also affected, but the condition of the trapezius and sternomastoid muscles was only mentioned by Jackson in an earlier report of his case, a patient who also had syphilis or tuberculosis and who had suffered a number of prior vascular events as a result of severe and generalized atheroma.

This is thus another type of **alternating hemiplegia.** The syndromes of **Tapia** and of **Schmid** are variants.

Sir Stephen Mackenzie (1844–1909) trained at the London Hospital and in Berlin, returning to join the staff of the London Hospital where he worked as a pathologist and dermatologist. He reported two cases of unilateral bulbar paresis in 1886.[3554] The two syndromes are considered sufficiently alike to allow their fusion.

Jacksonian epilepsy   See **Jacksonian march.**

Jacksonian march (Jacksonian epilepsy, Bravais-Jackson epilepsy) The spread of tonic-clonic epileptic movements through contiguous body parts on one side of the body as the causative epileptic discharge successively excites adjacent cortical regions.[2774]

Dr. L. Bravais had described the same events in his graduation thesis of 1827 for the University of Paris, but contributed no analysis of their cause.

Jackson-MacKenzie syndrome   See **Jackson syndrome.**

Jackson-Weiss syndrome A dominantly inherited form of craniosynostosis characterized also by large, broad toes and fusions of the tarsal bones. It has been mapped to chromosome 10q.

Jacob disease (spastic pseudosclerosis) See **Wilson disease.**

Jacobsen, Ludwig Levin (1783–1843) Danish physician and anatomist. His name is appended to the tympanic plexus and canal as well as to the nerve.

Jacobsen nerve The tympanic branch of the ninth cranial nerve.

Jacobsohn reflex Flexion of the fingers in response to a tap on the lower end of the radius. When enhanced,

this may be evidence of a pyramidal tract lesion or of heightened emotional tone, or it may be normal.[5858]

Dr. L. Jacobsohn was a German neurologist in Berlin.

Jacod syndrome (triad) (Negro-Jacod syndrome, petrosphenoidal space syndrome) Dysfunction of cranial nerves II, III, IV, V, and VI in the retrosphenoidal space, due to compression or infiltration by tumors of the middle cranial fossa such as nasopharyngeal carcinomas. Unilateral visual loss, progressive ophthalmoplegia, and trigeminal pain and numbness are the presenting features.[2788]

Negro described the syndrome from Italy in 1921, and Jacod described it from France in the same year.

Jacod-Rollet syndrome Dysfunction of the optic nerve with exophthalmos, due to optic gliomas or other tumors at the orbital apex or to aneurysm of the internal carotid artery.

jactitatio capitis nocturna (head rolling, body rocking, body rolling, rhythmie du sommeil) A form of **ritualistic movement** performed by some infants and young children and consisting of rhythmic movements of the head, frequently persisting through the night. A group of stereotyped, repetitive movements involving large muscles, usually of the head and neck, typically occurring immediately prior to sleep onset and sustained into light sleep. See also **head banging.**

Diagnostic criteria have been suggested and are given in Chart J–1.[234]

Chart J–1. Diagnostic Criteria for Jactitatio Capitis Nocturna

A. Rhythmic body movements occur during drowsiness or sleep.
B. At least one of the following types of disorder is present:
   1. The head is forcibly moved in an anterior–posterior direction— *head-banging type.*
   2. The head is moved laterally while in a supine position— *head-rolling type.*
   3. The whole body is rocked while on the hands and knees—*body-rocking type.*
   4. The whole body is moved laterally while in a supine position—*body-rolling type.*
C. Onset typically occurs within the first 2 years of life.
D. Polysomnographic monitoring during an episode demonstrates:
   1. Rhythmic movements during any stage of sleep or in wakefulness; and
   2. Absence of seizure activity in association with the disorder.
E. Absence of any other medical or psychiatric disorder that causes the symptom, e.g., epilepsy.
F. The disorder does not meet the diagnostic criteria for other sleep disorders producing abnormal movements during sleep, e.g., sleep bruxism.

From ASDA Diagnostic Classification Steering Committee. The International Classification of Sleep Disorders Diagnostic and Coding Manual. Rochester, MN. American Sleep Disorders Association, 1990. Reproduced by kind permission of the American Academy of Sleep Medicine.)

jactitation   (Lat, to pour forth frequently) Originally a restless tossing of parts of the body; but now the word is used for repetitive movements resembling myoclonus.

Jadassohn nevus phakomatosis   See **epidermal nevus syndrome.**[2793]

Jaeger, Eduard Ritter von Jaztthal   (1818–1884) Austrian ophthalmologist who, in 1860, introduced the test types still in occasional use today.

Jaeger test types   A visual test card using the printers' designation of type sizes. Jaeger 1+ is equivalent to 20/20 vision.

Jaffe-Lichtenstein syndrome   See **fibrous dysplasia.**[2796]

Jahnke syndrome   A variant of **Sturge-Weber syndrome** in which glaucoma does not occur. See **encephalofacial angiomatosis.**

jake paralysis   (Jamaica ginger paralysis) A clinical syndrome due to poisoning by triorthocresyl phosphate, a chemical introduced as a contaminant by American makers into an (illicit) alcoholic extract of ginger sold in the southern United States around 1929, and later by others into cooking oil sold in Algeria and Vietnam. At least three notorious outbreaks resulted.

Symptoms include cramping leg pains and weakness proceeding to quadriparesis due to a severe motor neuropathy and later due to an upper motor neuron syndrome, which improves only minimally.[3977]

Jakob, Alfons Maria   (1884–1931) German neuropathologist. He studied medicine at Munich, Hamburg and Berlin, graduating at Strasbourg University in 1908 and later worked with Kraepelin, Nissl, and Alzheimer. After World War I he returned to Hamburg where he practiced academic and private neuropsychiatry and was also head of the anatomical laboratory of the university psychiatric clinic until his early death.

His most important contributions concerned cerebral trauma, demyelination, neurosyphilis, extrapyramidal diseases, and brain anatomy and histology. **Alpers** described the disease bearing Jakob's name, having worked on the case with him in his laboratory. The paper on three patients with this form of dementia was received 9 months after that of **Creutzfeldt** and was published in the following year.[2798]

Jakob-Creutzfeldt disease   See **Creutzfeldt-Jakob disease.**

Jamaican ginger paralysis   See **Jake paralysis.**

Jamaican neuritis   See **Strachan syndrome.**

Jamaican neuropathy   A form of tropical myeloneuropathy of unknown cause(s), manifesting spastic and ataxic variants.

Clinically, the disease has its onset in adult life and leads to weakness, sensory ataxic gait, numbness or dysesthesias in the legs, distal loss of proprioception and vibration, and decreased muscle stretch reflexes (*ataxic form*) or to a radicular back pain, spastic gait, bladder disturbances, increased muscle stretch reflexes, and upgoing plantar responses with few sensory complaints (*spastic form*). (See also **tropical spastic paraparesis.**) Optic atrophy, deafness, and an axonal peripheral neuropathy may occur in either form.[352]

Jamaican optic neuropathy   A rapidly progressive bilateral optic neuropathy of unknown cause, resulting in dense central scotomas, reported so far only in West Indian and West African people.[1749]

Jamaican vomiting sickness   A severe metabolic encephalopathy due to poisoning with hypoglycine A (present in unripe akee fruit) and characterized by anorexia, vomiting, progressive encephalopathy, and elevation of serum ammonia levels, thus resembling **Reye syndrome.**[3956,5463] or **glutaric acidemia type 2.**

jamais vécu   (Fr, never + lived) The sensation that, although the current situational experience is in fact well known, it appears strange, as if it were completely unfamiliar. This is occasionally a normal percept but is typically considered to be a feature of complex partial seizures arising from a lesion in the mesial temporal neocortex.[4403]

See also **jamais vu.**

jamais vu   An awareness that although the visual percepts are well known, they appear strange as if they were completely unfamiliar. This is occasionally normal, but it is typically considered also to be a feature of complex partial seizures arising from a lesion in the mesial temporal neocortex.[4403]

See also **déjà vu, jamais vécu.**

James-Lange theory   The hypothesis that emotion merely represents the perception of the autonomic changes induced by exciting causes. "Anger, fear, love, hate, joy, grief, shame, pride and their varieties, may be called the coarser emotions, being coupled, as they are, with relatively strong bodily reverberations.

Our natural way of thinking about these coarser emotions is that the mental perception of some fact excites the mental affection called the emotion, and that this latter state of mind gives rise to the bodily expression. My theory, on the contrary, is that the bodily changes follow directly the perception of the exciting fact, and that our feeling of the same changes as they occur is the emotion."[2802]

Janin tetanus   See **Rose disease.**

Jansky-Bielschowsky lipofuscinosis   See **neuronal ceroid lipofuscinosis.**

Janz syndrome   See **juvenile myoclonic epilepsy of Janz.**

Japanese encephalitis   Direct infection of the brain with a flavivirus member of the togavirus group of arboviruses, occurring in India, China, and adjacent countries of the Far East and borne by mosquitos.

Clinically, the condition is most likely to cause disease in children and the elderly, in whom a syndrome of aseptic meningitis with headache, malaise, fever, headache and added confusion, muscle weakness, extrapyramidal and other focal signs, and sometimes convulsions occur, progressing in severity. Acute flaccid paralysis is a variant presentation. The disease carries a mortality of up to 40%.[6030]

Other neurotropic flavivirus encephalitides include St. Louis, West Nile, Murray Valley, Russian spring-summer, Western and Far-Eastern tick-borne, and Louping ill.[5257]

Jarcho-Levin syndrome   A recessively inherited congenital developmental disorder characterized by facial dysmorphisms, short stature, hemivertebrae, block vertebrae, missing vertebrae, and spina bifida.[2068]

In a *variant* form, the condition is dominantly inherited.

jargon   1. (undifferentiated jargon) Recurrent, stereotypical utterances that are out of context with the current subject of conversation. 2. A form of speech containing many neologisms but with a preserved syntactical framework, the use of some grammatical words, phonemic variability, and the preservation of appropriate intonation and stress.

jargon aphasia   Fluent, paraphasic speech that is grammatical and profuse but so distorted by phonetic and phonemic errors as to be incomprehensible. The phenomenon is usually evidence of a posterior dominant hemispheric lesion.

Jarisch syndrome   See **Gorlin-Goltz syndrome.**

Jasper, Herbert Henri   (1906–1999) American-born neurologist, electroencephalographer, and experimental neurophysiologist who worked with **Penfield** at the Montreal Neurological Institute in Canada in the investigation of brain function, using electrical clues. His pioneering work on brain stimulation in the conscious patient contributed hugely to our understanding of cerebral localization and to the successes of Penfield in epilepsy surgery. He was Penfield's co-author in their landmark book, *Epilepsy and the Functional Anatomy of the Human Brain.* From 1960 he was executive secretary of the International Brain Research Organization.[1766]

jaw jerk   See **jaw reflex.**

jaw reflex   (masseter reflex, mandibular reflex, jaw jerk) Contraction of the masseter and temporalis muscles in response to a brisk downward tap on the lower teeth or on a finger placed on the mental region.

Usually invisible, the movement of the jaw can be seen and felt in cases of bilateral suprapontine disease (spastic bulbar palsy). The reflex was first described by de Watteville in 1886.[2643, 5858]

A brief tap downward on the examiner's finger resting just below the patient's lower lip, the mouth relaxed and open, normally leads to no visible or palpable response, but with bilateral upper motor neuron lesions above the level of the pons and in states of marked anxiety, reflex contraction of the masseters results and the mouth closes smartly.

jaw winking   see **Gunn phenomenon.**

jaw-closing spasm   Involuntary paroxysmal contractions of the masseter muscles causing sudden opening, deviation, or closing of the jaw, and probably representing an unusual focal dystonia.

Jeanne sign   Hyperextension of the metacarpophalangeal joint of the thumb in patients with partial paralysis of the flexor pollicis longus muscle due to an ulnar nerve lesion, this nerve often assisting the median nerve in supplying that muscle.

Jefferson, Sir Geoffrey   (1886–1961) English neurosurgeon at Manchester. He described the syndromes resulting from aneurysms of the internal carotid artery in the cavernous sinus, pointing out that the trigeminal nerve is variably involved, anterior aneurysms involving the first division only, those in the middle of the sinus affecting the first and second divisions, and posterior aneurysms affecting all three divisions.[2822,2823] See **cavernous sinus syndrome.**

Jefferson syndrome   See **cavernous sinus syndrome.**

Jendrassik, E.   (1858–1921) Hungarian neurologist in Budapest.

Jendrassik maneuver   The induction of sustained voluntary contraction of distant muscle groups in order to enhance the muscle stretch reflex responses, described by Jendrassik in 1883.[2834]

Jennings syndrome   (endocardial fibroelastosis with neurological dysfunction) A congenital dysmorphic syndrome manifesting also genital maldevelopments, cardiomyopathy, hypoglycemia, seizures, plagiocephaly, and mental and developmental delay.

jerk nystagmus   That form of nystagmus in which the speed of the deviations of the eyes differs in the two directions, and in which the speed of eye deviation in one direction (drift) is slower than that of the restitution phase (correction).

jerking stiff-man syndrome   A syndrome with onset in young adult life; characterized by progressive scoliosis, cerebral atrophy, cerebellar and pyramidal signs, downbeat nystagmus, axial rigidity, leg rigidity, stimulus-sensitive myoclonus, and muscle cramps.[75] See also **stiff man syndrome.**

jerk-locked averaging   A technique for back-averaging the EEG with respect to a myoclonic discharge recorded on the simultaneously recorded EMG. It is used to study the scalp distribution of myoclonus-related spikes or the time interval separating an EEG spike and a myoclonic discharge, and for the detection of myoclonus-related EEG spikes that may be undetectable on the usual polygraphic record.[5127] Time-locking is seen with cortical but not with reticular reflex **myoclonus.**

jerk-locked evoked potentials A technique for studying cortical excitability following a myoclonic jerk. The stimulus is presented at varying times in relation to a myoclonic discharge and the EEG and EMG are back-averaged using the EMG pulse as a trigger. In cortical reflex myoclonus, cortical excitability can be demonstrated thus.

Jervell-Lange-Nielson syndrome A recessive disorder characterized by sensorineural deafness, mutism, heart block (prolonged Q-T interval), recurrent syncope, and a tendency to sudden death.[1829]

Jervis syndrome A congenital familial syndrome of inconspicuous and nonprogressive cerebellar signs and mental deficiency, occurring in both sexes but leading to death in the first year of life in the more severe cases. Degeneration of the granular layer and Purkinje cells of the cerebellum and of the inferior olives is noted.[2855]

jet lag See **rapid time zone change.**

Jeune asphyxiating thoracic dystrophy See **Jeune syndrome.**

Jeune syndrome 1. (Jeune-Tommasi syndrome) A recessively inherited disorder of childhood, characterized by the presence of pigmented spots on the skin, polydactyly, short limbs and ribs, severe nerve deafness, optic atrophy, hypotonia and ataxia, and mental retardation. The condition is progressive to death due to myocardial sclerosis or renal failure.[2857]

2. (Jeune asphyxiating thoracic dystrophy, thoracic-pelvic-phalangeal dystrophy) A recessively inherited syndrome characterized by cone-shaped phalangeal epiphyses, pigmentary retinopathy, pelvic bony changes, and small, shortened ribs, which may cause death from respiratory insufficiency during infancy as a result of thoracic constriction.[4184]

Hepatic or renal failure is the cause of death in childhood in those who escaped that fate earlier.

Jeune-Tommasi syndrome See **Jeune syndrome.**

jiggle Shape variability of motor unit action potentials recorded with a conventional EMG needle electrode. A small amount occurs normally. In conditions of disturbed neuromuscular transmission, including early reinnervation and myasthenic disorders, the variability can be sufficiently large to be easily detectable by eye. Quantitative methods for estimating this variability are not yet widely available. (From the 2001 Report of the Nomenclature Committee of the American Association of Electromyography and Electrodiagnosis.[10] Used by permission, copyright © 2001, AAEM.)

jimpy mice A strain of mouse affected by a mutation of the X chromosome affecting the proteolipid gene and leading to a form of demyelination, which provides an animal model for **Pelizaeus-Merzbacher disease.**

jimson weed *Datura stramonium*, a plant whose pods, stems and leaves contain atropine and scopolamine. Ingestion leads to an acute anticholinergic syndrome with pupillary dilatation, psychosis, hyperpyrexia, and hallucinosis.

jitter The variability of consecutive discharges of the interpotential interval between two muscle fiber action potentials belonging to the same motor unit. Usually expressed quantitatively as the mean value of the difference between the interpotential intervals of successive discharges (the mean consecutive difference, A/CD). Under certain conditions, it is expressed as the mean value of the difference between interpotential intervals arranged in the order of decreasing interdischarge intervals (the mean sorted difference, MSD). See **single fiber electromyography.** (From the 2001 Report of the Nomenclature Committee of the American Association of Electromyography and Electrodiagnosis.[10] Used by permission, copyright © 2001, AAEM.)

jittery legs See **burning feet syndrome.**

Joffroy, Alexis (1844–1908) French physician, practicing in Paris.

Joffroy reflex Contraction of the glutei with pressure on the buttocks, seen in patients with paraparesis.

Joffroy signs 1. Failure of the forehead to wrinkle on upward gaze in dysthyroid ophthalmopathy.[2861] 2. Impairment in tests of simple arithmetic as an early sign of **general paresis of the insane.**[4723]

jogger's foot See **medial plantar neuropathy.**

Johnson, Dr. Samuel (1709–1784) English lexicographer and author. Boswell's invaluable biography and other descriptions have made it clear that he suffered from **Tourette syndrome;** his mannerisms, vocal utterances, and habits were recognized by himself as abnormal and by others as bizarre or frightening, but the brilliance of his intellect and the wit of his conversation diminished, within the minds of his companions, the relevance of such eccentricities. He described poignantly the effects upon his speech of the left hemispheric stroke which he suffered in the last year of his life.

Johnson syndrome (adherence syndrome, oculomotor pseudoparalysis) Fibrosis of any of the oculomotor muscles in early childhood (but usually the lateral or superior recti), leading to the appearance of palsy but distinguished by the results of **forced duction tests,** which are abnormal. **Duane syndrome** is similar but affects both lateral recti.[2866]

joint position sense (conscious and unconscious proprioception) The faculty of being able to localize the position of body parts without the aid of vision. The pathways ascend to the thalamus in the posterior columns of the spinal cord.

Jolliffe syndrome   The encephalopathy of **pellagra.**

Jolly, Friedrich   (1844–1904) German neurologist.

Jolly sign   The position of abduction of the shoulder and flexion of the elbow adopted by people with C7 root lesions. When bilateral, the sign is also known by the names of Bradburne or Thorburn.

Jolly test   A technique described by Dr. Friedrich Jolly,[2878] who applied an electric current to excite a motor nerve while recording the force of muscle contraction. The method was later refined by recording the M waves evoked by repetitive supramaximal nerve stimulation (at 2–50 Hz) to detect a defect of neuromuscular transmission. (Adapted from the 1987 Report of the Nomenclature Committee of the American Association of Electromyography and Electrodiagnosis. AAEE glossary of terms in clinical electromyography. *Muscle Nerve* 1987;**10S:**G5–G23. Copyright 1987 by John Wiley and Sons. Inc. Reprinted by permission of John Wiley and Sons. Inc.) The term was formerly used for repetitive nerve stimulation.

jolt accentuation   Worsening of a headache when the patient's head is rotated to-and-fro by the examiner 2–3 times each second. The phenomenon is commonly present in patients with intracranial pathology of many kinds, including migraine, and in those conditions causing CSF pleocytosis.[5677]

Jones syndrome   A congenital dysmorphic syndrome characterized by short trunk and neck, lordosis, scoliosis, skeletal deformities, platyspondyly, dolichocephaly, J shaped sella turcica, and mental and developmental delay.[337]

Joplin 'neuroma'   Interdigital neuropathy of the foot comprising isolated compression of the medial plantar nerve, causing pain and numbness of the medial aspect of the hallux. Though called a neuroma, the tissue expanding and compressing the nerve is actually fibrous.[2880]

Jorgenson syndrome   A congenital X-linked or autosomal dominant dysmorphic syndrome manifesting also short stature, strabismus, ptosis, blepharophimosis, xerophthalmia and often resulting blindness, various skeletal maldevelopments, microcephaly, cortical hyperostosis, and mental and developmental delay.[2883]

Joseph disease   1. (SCA 3, Machado-Joseph disease, Azorean neuropathy, nigrospinodentatal degeneration, ataxia plus, autosomal dominant cerebellar atrophy with optic atrophy, dementia, extrapyramidal signs and lower motor neuron lesions, Azorean ataxia, nigrospinodentatal degeneration, dominant striatonigral degeneration; OMIN 109150) A dominantly inherited multisystem disorder with differing phenotypes, manifesting variously progressive cerebellar ataxia, dystonia, progressive external ophthalmoplegia, and peripheral neuropathy, and mapped to 14q24–q32, where there is expansion of an unstable trinucleotide CAG repeat.

The disease is seen in descendants of William Machado, once a resident of Sao Miguel in the Portuguese Azores Islands. The name *Joseph* is the surname of the Portuguese-Californian family with this disease described in 1976.[4793,5289]

The condition is best classified with the progressive, late-onset cerebellar ataxias of unknown cause until the underlying biochemical defect is ascertained. Three overlapping phenotypes have been described.[1147] All three have been recorded in each of the separate families affected; the major clinical features are as follows:[4067]

1. *Nigrospinodentatal degeneration with nuclear ophthalmoplegia* (Joseph phenotype): A form with onset in the second or third decade, with ophthalmoplegia, pyramidal and extrapyramidal signs (chorea, dystonia, rigidity), facial myoclonus, face and tongue fasciculations, prominent eyes due to lid retraction, and death by the age of 45 years.
2. *Dominant striatonigral degeneration* A form with onset in adult life (20–45 years) and characterized by the same ophthalmoplegia, face and tongue fasciculations, pyramidal and extrapyramidal signs, and marked ataxia.
3. *Machado disease* A late-onset variant, beginning after the third decade and characterized by progressive cerebellar gait ataxia, hyporeflexia, hypotonia, distal atrophy, and distal sensory loss.

Eventually, peripheral neuropathy is common to all types, but initially the presentations tend to be with ataxia, progressing to ataxia with peripheral neuropathy and eventually to ataxia with peripheral neuropathy and striatal signs.[1922] Rapid eye movement sleep disturbance is a common problem, especially in patients with the Joseph phenotype.

Variants include forms with pigmentary retinal degeneration, myoclonus and deafness, essential tremor, late onset (usually over 50 years), periodic expression, and features of spinal muscular atrophy. See **motor neuronal diseases.**

2. A recessively inherited congenital syndrome consisting of mental retardation, renal disease, urogenital malformations, sensorineural deafness, and convulsions with hyperprolinemia and the increased urinary excretion of proline, hydroxyproline, and glycine.[2884]

Joubert syndrome   A rare, recessively inherited congenital syndrome, characterized by episodic tachypnea and apnea, colobomas of the iris and retina, pigmentary retinopathy with blindness, ptosis due to congenital ocular fibrosis, torsional nystagmus, skew deviation of the eyes, renal lesions, syndactyly, microcephaly, cerebellar vermis aplasia with ataxia, **Dandy-Walker malformation,** cranial meningocele, and mental retardation. Linkage to chromosome 9q has been achieved but the condition is genetically heterogeneous.

Although the disease is nonprogressive, most affected children die at an early age as the result of these neurological problems.[2885]

Joubert syndrome with orofaciodigital anomalies
See **Egger syndrome.**

Journal of Child Neurology   An interdisciplinary subspecialty journal examining aspects of nervous system disorders in children and adolescents. Web site: http://bcdecker.yy.net/cgibin/tangocgi.exe/tango/decker/journals/journal.qry?function=view&ID=10&_User Reference=5950453235/.

Journal of Clinical Neuromuscular Disease   A subspecialty journal published by Lippincott, Williams and Wilkins. Web site: http://www.jcnmd.com/.

Journal of Clinical Neuroscience   The official journal of the Neurosurgical Society of Australasia, the Australian Association of Neurologists, the Australian and New Zealand Society for Neuropathology, the **Taiwan Neurosurgical Society** and the **Asian/ Australian Society of Neurological Surgeons,** published by Harcourt Brace. Web site: http://www.harcourt-international.com/journals/jocn/.

Journal of Cognitive Neuroscience   (*J. Cogn. Neurosci.*) A neurological subspecialty journal. Address: Massachusetts Institute of Technology, 55 Hayward St., Cambridge, MA 02142.

Journal of Communication Disorders   (*J. Commun. Disord.*) Address: Elsevier Science Publishing Company Inc., Madison Square Station, P.O. Box 882, New York NY 10159-0882. A neurological subspecialty journal.

Journal of Comparative Neurology   A basic neuroscience journal. Web site: http://www.interscience.wiley.com/jpages/0021-9967/.

Journal of Geriatric Psychiatry and Neurology   (*J. Geriatr. Psychiatry Neurol.*) The official journal of the **Alzheimer Foundation.** Address: 8177 South Harvard, M/C-114, Tulsa, OK 74137.

Journal of Headache and Pain   A subspecialty journal, published by Springer. Web site: http://link.springer.de/link/service/journals/10194/index.htm.

Journal of Nervous and Mental Disease   (*J. Nerv. Ment. Dis.*) A private publication founded by James S. Jewell of Chicago in 1874 and owned at one time by Dr. Bernard **Sachs** of New York. The journal emphasized psychiatric rather than neurological articles, though this was due in part to the relative numbers of articles submitted, and in 1919 turned further towards psychiatry with the founding of the rival *Archives of Neurology and Psychiatry.* Web site: http://www.jonmd.com/.

Journal of Neuroimmunology   The official Journal of the International Society for Neuroimmunology. Web site: http://www.elsevier.com/locate/jneuroim.

Journal of Neural Transmission   A subspecialty neuroscience journal published by Springer. Web site: http://link.springer.de/link/service/journals/00702/about.htm.

Journal of Neurology   (*J. Neurol.*) The official journal of the European Neurological Society and organ of the Deutsche Gesellschaft für Neurologie. Address: Springer-Verlag GmbH & Co. KG, Heidelberger Platz 3, D-100 Berlin 33 Germany. Web site: http://link.springer.de/link/service/journals/00415/.

Journal of Neurology, Neurosurgery and Psychiatry   (*J. Neurol. Neurosurg. Psychiatry*) A British journal of the neurosciences, published monthly, which was founded in 1920 by Alexander Bruce as the *Review of Neurology and Psychopathology* (1903–1918), and which became the *Journal of Neurology and Psychopathology* (edited first by Ninian Bruce and then by Kinnier **Wilson** until his death). It was published by the British Medical Association after 1926. A new series began in 1938, as the *Journal of Neurology and Psychiatry*. The present name was taken in 1944. Web site: http://jnnp.bmjjournals.com/.

Journal of Neuro-Ophthalmology   The official journal of the North American Neuro-Ophthalmology Society, published by Lippincott, Williams and Wilkins. Web site: http://www.jneuro-ophthalmology.com/.

Journal of Neurosurgery   (*J. Neurosurg.*) A neurosurgical journal. Address: 1224 W. Main St., Ste. 450, Charlottesville, VA 22902. Web site: http://www.thejns-net.org/jns/issues/current/toc_fs.html.

Journal of Neurotrauma   The official journal of the National Neurotrauma Society. Web site: http://www.liebertpub.com/NEU/default1.asp.

Journal of Sleep Research   The official Journal of the European Sleep Research Society, published by Blackwell Synergy. Web site: http://www.blackwell-science.com/~cgilib/jnlpage.asp?Journal=JSR&File=JSR&Page=aims.

Journal of Speech, Language, Hearing Research   (*J. Speech Lang. Hear. Res.*) A neurological subspecialty journal. Address: American Speech-Language-Hearing Association, 10801 Rockville Pike, Rockville, MD 20852.

Journal of Stroke and Cerebrovascular Diseases   (*J. Stroke Cerebrovasc Dis.*) A neurological subspecialty journal. Address: National Stroke Association, 300 East Hampden Avenue, Suite 240, Englewood, CO 80110. Web site: http://www.strokejournal.org/scripts/om.dll/serve?action=searchDB&searchDBfor=home&id=jscd.

Journal of the History of the Neurosciences   (J. Hist. Neurosci.) A quarterly publication sponsored by the World Federation of Neurology History of Neurosciences Research Group, containing contributions relating to the development of basic neuroscience and clinical neurology from the remote and more recent past. Address: Swets and Zeitlinger Publishers, P.O. Box 825, 2160 SZ Lisse, The Netherlands.

Journal of the Neurological Sciences   (*J. Neurol. Sci.*) The official journal of the World Federation of Neurology. Address: Elsevier Science Publishers B V, P.O.

Box 211, 1000 AE Amsterdam, The Netherlands. Web site: http://www.elsevier.nl/locate/jns.

Journal of Tropical and Geographical Neurology (*J. Trop. Geogr. Neurol.*) The official journal of the World Federation of Neurology Research Group on Tropical Neurology, founded in 1991. Address: Neurological Unit, Harvard Medical School, Beth Israel Hospital, 330, Brookline Ave., Boston, MA 02215.

J-shaped sella   The appearance seen when the tuberculum sella and the anterior clinoids are eroded. This is a typical feature in patients with gliomas of the optic nerve but is also found in **Down syndrome,** in gangliosidoses, and occasionally in normal subjects.[2618]

Juberg-Hayward syndrome   A recessively inherited congenital dysmorphic syndrome manifesting also short stature, hypoplastic or absent radii, clinodactyly, microcephaly, cleft palate, and mental and developmental delay.[2888]

Judgement of Line Orientation test   A test for perceptual disturbances involving the posterior part of the right hemisphere, in which the subject is required to match the orientation of a line drawn on a paper with a standard set of other lines arranged like spokes on a protractor.[474]

jugular   (from Lat, the throat) So translated by the Benedictine monk who made the first medieval translations of Galen's works, Galen having called it the "sacrificial vein."

jugular foramen syndrome   Involvement of various combinations of cranial nerves IX, X, and XI by a lesion at the jugular foramen. If the twelfth nerve is also involved, the condition is known as the **Collet-Sicard** or posterior lacerocondylar syndrome. See **Vernet syndrome.**

Variant syndromes described and separately named (with the cranial nerves involved)[5431] include the following:

Avellis	(X; some have contralateral spinothalamic loss)
Collet-Sicard	(IX, X, XI, XII)
Jackson	(Complete X, XI, XII; no comment on taste)
Lannois-Jouty	(IX, X, XI, XII)
Mackenzie	(IX, X, XI XII)
Schmidt	(X, XI)
Tapia	(XI, XII)
Vernet	(VII, IX, X, XI, XII)
Villaret	(Collet-Sicard syndrome with cervical sympathetic palsy)

Cervical sympathetic palsy, hemiparesis and other signs may, however, accompany any of these.

Julien-Marie-See syndrome   See **idiopathic intracranial hypertension.**

jumpers   See **dancing mania.**

jumping Frenchmen of Maine (goosey)   A familial syndrome seen mainly in males, characterized by brief involuntary movements occurring from infancy, precipitated by startle without alteration in consciousness, and sometimes accompanied by echolalia, echopraxia, and automatic obedience. It was described in 1878 by George Beard among French-Canadian workers in Maine, and is still present in their descendants living in Quebec.[407]

Tourette translated the article and compared this condition to **tics** in 1881. **Latah** and **myriachit** are similar conditions to jumping and were described first in English by **Hammond** in 1884.[5349]

jumpy stump   Involuntary twitching of an amputation stump, usually associated with lancinating pain, persisting for up to years after the amputation. Voluntary movements and local cutaneous stimuli may act as precipitants.

junctional infarct   Infarction in the border zone between the territories of the superficial (pial) perforating medullary branches of the middle cerebral artery (MCA) and the deep perforators from the MCA trunk, carotid siphon, anterior choroidal artery, anterior cerebral artery trunk, Heubner's artery, and posterior communicating artery. More plainly, they are for the most part infarcts in between superficial and deep territories supplied by the MCA.

junctional scotoma   (junctional visual field loss) That visual field defect due to a lesion present at the point where the optic nerve runs back into the chiasm, compressing both and leading to total visual loss or field constriction in the homolateral eye and an upper quadrantic temporal field defect in the other, the latter being due to compression of those optic nerve fibers from the contralateral inferior nasal retina looping forward in von Willebrand's knee. See **Traquair scotoma.**

junctional visual field loss   See **junctional scotoma.**

juster reflex   Finger flexion with stimulation or irritation of the palm. The normal response is extension.[4723]

juvenile absence epilepsy   (OMIM 600131) A seizure disorder in which the absences are the same as those occurring in pyknolepsy, those accompanied by retropulsive movements being less common. The first manifestations are evident around puberty. The seizure frequency is less than that in pyknolepsy, with absences occurring less frequently than every day, mostly sporadically. Association with generalized tonic-clonic seizures is frequent, such seizures preceding the absence manifestations more often than they do in childhood absence epilepsy, often occurring on awakening. Not infrequently, the patients also have myoclonic seizures. Sex distribution is equal. The spike waves are often >3 Hz. Response to therapy is excellent. (From the Commission for Classification and Terminology, ILAE. Proposal for revised classifications of epilepsies and epileptic syndromes. *Epilepsia* 1989;**30:**389–399 and reproduced by kind permission of Blackwell Science.)

Onset in adult life is also described.[1548]

juvenile Alzheimer disease See **congophilic angiopathy.**

juvenile amaurotic familial idiocy See **GM$_2$ gangliosidoses.**

juvenile amyotrophic lateral sclerosis See **amyotrophic lateral sclerosis.**

juvenile amyotrophy of distal upper extremity See **monomelic amyotrophy.**

juvenile bulbar palsy 1. See **Fazio-Londe syndrome.** 2. See **Vialetto–van Laere syndrome.** 3. See **amyotrophic lateral sclerosis.**

juvenile bulbar spinal muscular atrophy See **Fazio-Londe syndrome.**

juvenile cerebromacular degeneration A clinical syndrome of dementia and visual loss, with diverse causes.

juvenile Creutzfeldt-Jakob disease See **Creutzfeldt-Jakob disease.**

juvenile dermatomyositis See **childhood dermatomyositis or polymyositis associated with vasculitis.**

juvenile distal and segmental atrophy of upper extremities See **monomelic amyotrophy.**

juvenile distal (nonprogressive) muscular atrophy A syndrome of insidiously progressive asymmetrical muscle atrophy in the hands and forearms with a self-limiting clinical course, usually reported in males from the Orient. A neurogenic etiology is probable.[5186]

Of clinical interest is the usual sparing of the brachioradialis muscle. Bladder, pyramidal, and sensory signs are absent, and the EMG shows evidence of both myopathic and neurogenic disease.

juvenile distal spinal muscular atrophy of upper extremities See **monomelic amyotrophy.**

juvenile dystonic lipidosis A juvenile variant of Niemann-Pick disease type C, itself a heterogeneous group of disorders generally manifesting dementia, epilepsy, and vertical gaze pareses in infancy or adult life, and in which sea-blue histiocytes and foam cells are found in the bone marrow. The nature of the primary biochemical defect remains unknown. See **sphingomyelin storage disorders.**[2940]

juvenile epilepsy See **juvenile myoclonic epilepsy of Janz.**

juvenile galactosialidosis (type 2 juvenile sialidosis) A lysosomal storage disease in which sialyloligosaccharides are stored. The onset is in youth or young adult life and the condition is characterized by mental retardation, coarse facies, corneal clouding, a macular cherry-red spot, deafness, seizures, and myoclonus. See **sialidosis.**

juvenile global tremor A slow tremor at 1–1.5 Hz seen throughout the body, reportedly associated with bilateral olivary disease and with a likely metabolic basis.

juvenile GM$_2$ gangliosidosis with hexosaminidase A deficiency A recessively inherited syndrome characterized by ataxia, loss of speech, spasticity, athetosis, and minor motor seizures in early childhood, with death by age 15. Late pigmentary retinopathy is also described.[4189] See **GM$_2$ gangliosidosis.**

juvenile head trauma syndrome See **traumatic spreading depression syndrome.**

juvenile Leigh disease See **infantile bilateral striatal necrosis.**

juvenile lipofuscinosis See **neuronal ceroid lipofuscinosis.**

juvenile motor neuron disease (hereditary bulbar atrophy) A sporadic variant of **amyotrophic lateral sclerosis** most commonly seen in the pople of southern India. It is characterized by slower progress than the classical form; the lower motor neuron lesions of the limbs and bulbar muscles are accompanied by fasciculations and hearing loss; and the stretch reflexes are increased asymmetrically. The highest cerebral functions are spared.[5794]

juvenile muscular atrophy of the upper extremity See **monomelic amyotrophy**

juvenile muscular atrophy of unilateral upper extremity (distal chronic spinal muscular atrophy affecting the hands) A benign syndrome of distal, segmental muscular atrophy of the upper limb with juvenile onset, affecting mainly the intrinsic hand muscles and those of the forearms.[2585]

It usually occurs sporadically, but familial cases have also been recorded. See **hereditary motor neuropathy** (*variants*), **monomelic amyotrophy.**

juvenile muscular atrophy simulating muscular dystrophy Forms of **hereditary motor neuropathy** in which the neurogenic nature of the disorder is not initially apparent.[773]

juvenile myasthenia Clinically, electrophysiologically, and immunologically, typical **myasthenia gravis** occurring in childhood.

It always has its onset after the age of 1 year and usually after 10 years. All degrees of severity occur, as with adults, including an acute fulminating form.[1780]

juvenile myoclonic epilepsy of Janz (impulsive petit mal, Janz syndrome, myoclonic epilepsy of adolescents, benign myoclonic juvenile epilepsy; OMIM 254770) A generalized, idiopathic, and age-related convulsive syndrome with onset around puberty, characterized by clusters of seizures with bilateral single or repetitive, arrhythmic, irregular myoclonic jerks, predominantly affecting the arms.

The jerks may cause some patients to fall suddenly

without noticeable disturbance of consciousness (but the intensity of the jerks is usually so mild that only the patient can perceive them). Generalized seizures also occur often, absences less frequently. The seizures usually occur shortly after awakening and are often precipitated by sleep deprivation, fatigue, and photic stimulation. Interictal and ictal EEG have rapid, generalized, often irregular spike–waves and polyspike–waves; there is no close phase correlation between the EEG spikes and the jerks. The response to appropriate drugs is good. (Adapted from Commission for Classification and Terminology, ILAE. Proposal for revised classifications of epilepsies and epileptic syndromes. *Epilepsia* 1989;**30**:389–399.) The condition is mapped to 6p21.2–p11 and to 15q.14; both dominant and recessive transmissions are described. Generalized tonic-clonic seizures, myoclonus, and absences may all occur.[1548,2814]

In summary, this is a rather benign form of seizure disorder, in which nocturnal or early morning tonic-clonic epileptic seizures and repetitive attacks of myoclonus on awakening begin in adolescence but remain as a lifelong trait, and in which the neurological and mental state of those affected is normal.

juvenile neuroaxonal dystrophy   A rare variant of **neuroaxonal dystrophy,** characterized by the onset in childhood or young adult life of progressive myoclonic epilepsy, cerebellar ataxia, and intellectual deterioration.

Dysarthria, pyramidal and extrapyramidal signs, resting tremor, incontinence, and axonal neuropathy are other features.[1499] See also **infantile neuroaxonal dystrophy.**

juvenile neurogenic muscle atrophy with lysosomal enzyme deficiencies   A syndrome of childhood onset, characterized by mental retardation, features of Marfan syndrome, neurogenic muscle atrophy and hyporeflexia, multiple epithelial dysplasia, increased urinary secretion of dermatan sulphate and decreased lysosomal enzyme activities (β-galactosidase, β-glucuronidase and N-acetyl β-D-glucose amylidase).[2230]

juvenile nonprogressive muscular atrophy localized in hand and forearm   See **monomelic amyotrophy.**

juvenile parkinsonism syndromes   (corpus striatum syndrome, Hunt paralysis, pallidopyramidal disease) A pure **system disease** of unknown cause, causing parkinsonian syndromes of bilateral rigidity and tremor with diurnal variation, and paralysis of certain

automatic and associated movements. The disease has its onset in the first two decades of life and is associated with lesions of the efferent motor neurons of the globus pallidus. The response to L-dopa is gratifying.[6081]

There tends to be a high familial incidence in these varieties and Lewy bodies are absent in patients examined before the age of 20 years. The condition was first noted by Ramsay **Hunt** in 1917.

A *variant* is *juvenile-onset parkinsonism with dystonia*, an uncommon dominantly inherited disease characterized by the onset in the first two decades of life of L-dopa–responsive parkinsonism with prominent dyskinesias, such as equinovarus posturing of the feet, on–off oscillations, and slow progression of symptoms.

The presence of motor fluctuations distinguishes this from **Segawa disease,** which it otherwise closely resembles.[2094,2703]

juvenile progressive spinal muscular atrophy   See **hereditary motor neuropathy.**

juvenile Sandhoff disease   A syndrome of progressive cerebellar disorder and mental and motor delay with onset in childhood, associated with total deficiency of hexosaminidase.[3558] See **GM$_2$ gangliosidosis.**

Other *variant* forms include partial deficiency of the enzyme producing the same clinical picture, and a syndrome of tremor, cherry-red spots, and mild truncal ataxia without dementia, associated with total deficiency of hexosaminidase B.[2871]

juvenile segmental muscular atrophy   See **monomelic amyotrophy.**

juvenile spinal muscular atrophy   See **hereditary motor neuropathy, type 3.**

juvenile spinal muscular atrophy with hexosaminidase A deficiency (GM$_2$)   See **hereditary motor neuropathy** (*variants*).

juvenile type of distal and segmental atrophy of upper extremities   See **monomelic amyotrophy**

Juvenile Unknown Mitochondrial Problems (J.U.M.P. Foundation) A charitable organization. Address: 2232 South Main St., Suite 130, Ann Arbor, MI 48103. Tel: 313-327-5070. See also http://www.umdf.org/ (**United Mitochondrial Disease Foundation**).

juvenile-onset parkinsonism with dystonia   See **juvenile parkinsonism syndromes, young-onset Parkinson disease.**

K complex A burst of waves on the EEG of variable appearance, consisting most commonly of a high-voltage diphasic slow wave frequently associated with a **sleep spindle.** Its amplitude is generally maximal in proximity to the vertex.

K complexes occur during sleep, apparently spontaneously or in response to sudden sensory stimuli and are not specific for any individual sensory modality. See also **vertex sharp transients.** (Adapted from the report of the Committee on Terminology, IFCN,[989] ©1974, with permission from Elsevier Science.)

Such EEG waveforms are recorded from all head regions during non–rapid eye movement sleep stages 2–4 at 2–3/minute, and are characterized by an initial slow negative wave followed 700 msec later by a positive wave. They may represent nonspecific evoked potentials since they are sometimes induced by external stimuli. [2865]

Kabuki make-up syndrome A dominantly inherited congenital dysmorphic syndrome characterized by depression of the tip of the nose, short stature, ectropion, congenital cardiac anomalies, brachydactyly, recurrent infections, and mental and developmental delay, seen mainly in Japan.[4138]

The name derives from the supposed resemblance of the affected subjects' faces to those of a class of Japanese traditional actors.

Kaeser syndrome See **scapuloperoneal syndrome** (*scapuloperoneal muscular atrophy without sensory disturbance*). Kaeser's name is sometimes given to this condition but his description came 25 years after that of Davidenkow.

kainic acid An excitotoxic amino acid.

kakke The Japanese name for **beriberi.**

Kahlbaum, Karl Ludwig German psychiatrist who described **catatonia** in 1868.

Kahlbaum syndrome (catatonia) The association of at least one motor sign of catatonia (catalepsy, posturing or waxy flexibility) and at least one sign of psychosocial withdrawal or excitement and/or bizarre repetitions (mutism, negativism, impulsiveness, grimacing, stereotypies, mannerisms, command automatism, echopraxia or echolalia, verbigeration).

The syndrome was first described by Kahlbaum in 1868, but catatonia itself is nonspecific with a range of psychiatric and organic neurological causes.[364]

Kallmann syndrome (olfactogenital dysplasia) A syndrome of (usually) X-linked dominant hypogonadotrophic hypogonadism with olfactory agenesis and consequent hyposmia, sometimes associated with color blindness.[2910] The responsible gene maps to Xp22.3.

Other features found have included mental retardation, hypotelorism, scoliosis, renal agenesis, pes cavus, spasticity, and sensory neuropathy. The disease has also been reported in females.

kappa rhythm A rhythm consisting of bursts of alpha or theta frequency occurring over the temporal areas of the scalp of subjects engaged in mental activity.

The cerebral origin of this rhythm is unproven. It is best recorded between electrodes located lateral to the outer canthus of each eye. (Adapted from the report of the Committee on Terminology, IFCN,[988] © 1974, with permission from Elsevier Science.)

Karnofsky scale See **quality of life.**

Karsch syndrome A rare, recessively inherited, congenital syndrome consisting of nystagmus, strabismus, pigmentary retinal degeneration, and splitting of the hands and/or feet.[2943]

Kashida sign The appearance of muscle spasms and tingling in response to warming or cooling the skin, reported to occur in tetany.[374]

Katsantoni syndrome (Coté-Katsantoni syndrome) A congenital dysmorphic syndrome manifesting also sparse, brittle hair and nails, ptosis, torticollis, nystagmus, osteosclerosis, atrial septal defect, abnormal immunoglobulins, and mental and developmental delay.[601]

Katz activities of daily living scale A well-known and reliable instrument for evaluating a patient's ability to perform six activities in the realm of basic self-care (*bathing, dressing, toileting, transferring, continence, and feeding*) independently, requiring some assistance, or requiring total assistance, and thus of value in the assessment and management of elderly demented people.[2955–2957]

Kaufman Assessment Battery for Children A diagnostic test for cognitive impairment in children.[3]

Kaufman syndrome (oculocerebrofacial syndrome) A congenital dysmorphic syndrome manifesting also fusion of vertebrae with scoliosis, myopia, pendular nystagmus, strabismus, ptosis, brachycephaly, microcephaly, intracranial calcifications, and mental and developmental delay.[2964]

Kawasaki disease (mucocutaneous lymph node syndrome) An acute febrile illness of unknown cause, usually affecting young children and manifest by cervical and hilar adenopathy, thrombocytosis, and coronary artery aneurysms. Encephalopathy and aseptic meningitis with increased intracranial pressure, muscle tenderness and weakness, and elevated creatine kinase level[3144]have also been described.

Kayser, Bernard (1869–1954) German ophthalmologist practicing in Stuttgart.

Kayser-Fleischer ring An orange, gold, or greenish deposit, about 2 mm wide, around the limbus of the cornea and due to copper deposition within the Descemet membrane. It is found in cases of **Wilson disease,** for which it is pathognomonic, but it may not be visible to the naked eye (it was not described by Wilson), requiring the use of a slit lamp to exclude its presence.[2974]

Kearns-Sayre syndrome (Kearns-Shy syndrome, Kearns-Sayre-Daroff syndrome, oculocraniosomatic neuromuscular disease with ragged red fibers) A laudable coalescence of two conditions (progressive external ophthalmoplegia and the Kearns-Sayre syndrome) through the demonstration that a deficiency of cytochrome-c oxidase and the presence of mitochondrial abnormalities in muscle and sweat glands are factors common to patients with various combinations of progressive ophthalmoplegia, pendular nystagmus, heart block, pigmentary retinal degeneration, cerebellar ataxia, pyramidal signs, mild facial and somatic muscle weakness, retarded somatic growth, and raised CSF protein levels.

The syndrome as initially described has its onset in youth and is characterized by choroidal atrophy and retinal changes resembling **retinitis pigmentosa,** external ophthalmoplegia, small stature, deafness, an elevated CSF protein level, and cardiac conduction block,[2986] with which proximal and distal lipid storage myopathy, cerebellar ataxia, dementia, hypoparathyroidism, and basal ganglion calcification may be associated. Familial factors play an undefined role in its genesis.[2939]

Kearns-Sayre-Daroff syndrome See **Kearns-Sayre syndrome.**

Kearns-Shy syndrome See **Kearns-Sayre syndrome.**

Keating syndrome See **glycogen storage disease** *type 9, phosphoglycerate kinase deficiency.*

Kehrer, Ferdinand Adalbert (1883–1966) German neurologist. He described the auriculopalpebral reflex (closure of the eyes in response to various stimuli such as sudden noise, in the presence of increased intracranial pressure).

Kehrer-Adie syndrome See **Adie pupil, Holmes-Adie syndrome.**

Keipert syndrome An X-linked or autosomal, recessively inherited dysmorphic syndrome characterized also by digital anomalies (broad terminal phalanges), hydrocephalus, mental retardation, and deafness.[2990]

A classification of hypertensive retinopathy developed by Keith, Wagener and Barker.[2990a] It combines the clinical findings of atherosclerosis and hypertension and is that most generally employed. The four levels comprise:

1. Mild-to-moderate narrowing or sclerosis of the arterioles
2. Moderate-to-marked arteriolar narrowing, local and/or generalized, with exaggeration of the light reflex and compression of the venules at arteriovenous crossings
3. The same retinal arteriolar narrowing with focal constriction, retinal edema showing as 'cotton-wool patches', and/or hemorrhages into the retina
4. The changes listed in # 3 with added papilledema.

Other schemes for classification (Schie, Leishman) are presented at the following web site: http://www.medal.org/ch19.html.

Keith-Wagener scale

Kemp sign Reduction in back pain with flexion of the lumbar spine, seen in patients with prolapsed intervertebral disks.

Kennedy, Robert Foster See **Foster Kennedy, Robert.**

Kennedy syndrome 1. (Foster Kennedy sign) See **Foster Kennedy syndrome.** 2. See **bulbospinal muscular neuronopathy.**

Kenney-Alter-Sung syndrome See **progressive proximal spinal and bulbar muscular atrophy of late onset.**

Kenny self-care scale An instrument for the assessment of a patient's abilities in self-care and ambulation, of particular value in the elderly.[716]

keratan sulfate One of the glycosaminoglycans, forming part of the mucopolysaccharide that accumulates and is excreted in the **mucopolysaccharidoses.**

keratic precipitates Deposits of inflammatory and epithelioid cells on the posterior surface of the cornea.

keratoconjunctivitis sicca See **Sjögren syndrome.**

keratoconus A conical forward-projection of the cornea due to corneal dystrophy as occurs in **Marfan syndrome,** trisomy 21 syndrome, **Leber amaurosis,** and other keratopathies.

The condition may also occur in isolation as a dominantly or recessively inherited malformation. See also **Munson sign.**

keratosis follicularis A dominantly inherited diffuse encephalopathy characterized by dwarfism, alopecia, and hyperkeratosis.[5942]

Microcephaly, cerebral atrophy, seizures, and mental and developmental delay have also been described in association.

kernicterus (bilirubin encephalopathy, nuclear jaundice) A syndrome of hypotonia, lethargy, and poor sucking response, leading to spasticity, opisthotonos, seizures, and eventually mental retardation, deafness, choreoathetosis, dystonia, ataxia, and a pyramidal syndrome as a toxic effect of unconjugated bilirubin that crosses the immature blood–brain barrier unimpeded in children with hemolytic disease of the newborn or other hyperbilirubinemic syndromes.[5738]

The condition was first described by Johannes Orth (1847–1923), a German physician, in 1875.

Kernig sign   The classic test for meningeal irritation, as in meningitis, described by Kernig in 1882 but a full description of it was only published 23 years later.[3010] To elicit the sign, the hip is flexed on the pelvis and the knee flexed also; the knee is then gradually extended by the examiner. Resistance due to involuntary hamstring contraction suggests irritation of the L5 and S1,2 roots.

The test is now almost invariably done with the patient supine, but in his original paper, Kernig described its elicitation in the sitting position as well.

See also **attitude en chien de fusi, Brudzinski signs, Edelmann great toe phenomenon (toe reflex), neck rigidity.**

Kernig, Vladimir Mikhailovich   (1840–1917) Russian neurologist, born in Latvia, who became director of the Obohovsk Hospital in St. Petersburg until his retirement in 1911.

Kernohan, J.W.   (b. 1897) Irish neuropathologist who emigrated to America and worked at the Mayo Clinic. He introduced a grading system for gliomas as well as describing the following syndrome.

James Watson Kernohan

Kernohan notch syndrome   (clivus edge syndrome) Unilateral or bilateral pyramidal signs resulting from direct compression of a cerebral peduncle in the **uncal syndrome,** and further indirect compression of the contralateral peduncle as a result of its displacement across the midline to abut the contralateral tentorial free edge, indenting ("notching") the peduncle.[3012]

The name of H.W. Woltman, a colleague of Kernohan at the Mayo Clinic, has also been applied to this syndrome.

Kerr syndrome   Stiffness and dryness of the skin for a few segments below a spinal cord lesion.

Kestenbaum number   A rough measure of the relative afferent pupillary defect, obtained by comparing the size of each pupil while the other one is in darkness.

Kestenbaum also counted the vessels crossing the edge of the optic disk and believed that a substantial reduction was an indication of optic neuropathy, though this has not been confirmed as a valid marker for that condition.

Kestenbaum syndrome   See **Sylvian aqueduct syndrome.**

ketogenic diet   A high-fat, high-protein diet used in the management of intractable generalized or partial seizure disorders in children and adults. As over three-quarters of the calories are derived from fats, chronic kctoacidosis results and this appears to have anticonvulsant activity.

3-ketothiolase deficiency   (beta-ketothiolase deficiency) A congenital metabolic aminoaciduric syndrome manifesting an abnormality in consciousness, neonatal respiratory distress, and mental and developmental delay.[337]

ketotic hyperglycinemia   A recessively inherited primary organic acidemia presenting in infancy with failure to thrive, seizures, hypertonia, cerebellar ataxia, and mental and motor delay, induced by the ingestion of milk protein (casein).[1011] See **proprionic acidemia, cerebellar ataxias** (*variants*).

ketotifen   A drug that blocks the secretion of mast cells, which are thought to contribute to the origin and growth of neurofibromas.

Keutel syndrome   (humeroradial synostosis plus) A recessively inherited congenital dysmorphic syndrome manifesting also skeletal and genital abnormalities, microcephaly, meningocele, deafness, and mental and developmental delay.[3027]

keyhole aqueduct syndrome   (pure **syringobulbia**) The occurrence of a syrinx in the midbrain and upper pons communicating with the aqueduct and fourth ventricle without associated syringomyelia. The condition is associated with gliosis of the cerebellum, and presents clinically with signs and symptoms of cerebellar and brainstem dysfunction with dysarthria, nystagmus, deafness, and internuclear ophthalmoplegia.

The syrinx may be a centimeter or more in its widest diameter, and is in the shape of an old-fashioned keyhole.[1353]

Kienbock disease   Post-traumatic **syringomyelia.**[3035] See also **hematomyelia.**

Kienbock, Robert   (1871–1953) Austrian radiologist, professor at Vienna University, who described both the following condition and that of osteochondritis of the semilunate bone.

Killian-Pallister mosaic syndrome   (chromosome 12p tetrasomy) A congenital dysmorphic syndrome characterized by facial dysmorphism and skeletal abnormalities, brachycephaly, strabismus, ptosis, hypotonia, cerebral atrophy, seizures, and mental and developmental delay.[4308]

Kiloh-Nevin syndromes   1. **anterior interosseous syndrome.**[3038] 2. **ocular myopathy** A syndrome of dominantly inherited progressive weakness of the external ocular muscles with adult onset. The difficulty of distinguishing myopathic from neuropathic changes in these muscles has led to uncertainty as to the actual pathology, but, in many cases, further spread of the weakness to the facial and bulbar and ultimately to the girdle muscles, coupled with the frequent finding of **ragged red fibers** on muscle biopsy specimens, has swung the balance in favor of a myopathy (probably mitochondrial), as originally described.[3037]

This condition and **Kearns-Shy syndrome** are presumably the same.

kindling   The progressive and permanent reduction in seizure threshold that occurs when certain brain regions are stimulated repeatedly. Initially stimulus-bound, the seizures later occur spontaneously and eventually become intractable.[3786]

kinesia paradoxica   The remarkable ability of some patients with akinetic parkinsonism to regain normal motor freedom for a short time, usually when under acute emotional stress (as when their hospital ward catches fire, and they are capable of short-lived but useful movement, such as running out of the building).

kinesics   1. The complex of all an individuals' gestural activity, conscious or unconscious, replacing or embellishing speech.[1179]

2. The study of limb, body, and facial movements associated with nonverbal communication.

kinesigenic choreoathetosis   An uncommon paroxysmal movement disorder characterized by the onset in childhood or youth of dystonic spasms, chorea, and athetosis precipitated by walking or other muscle activity, and seizures but without succeeding dementia.[3017]

Whether this is a form of reflex epilepsy or a movement disorder with basal ganglion origin is undetermined. See **paroxysmal kinesigenic choreoathetosis, familial kinesigenic choreoathetosis.**

kinesin   One of a family of proteins found within axons, which are able to translocate axoplasmic vesicles along the microtubules, and thus are responsible for axoplasmic transport.

kinesiologic EMG   (dynamic EMG) The muscle electrical activity recorded during movement. This gives information about the timing of muscle activity and its relative intensity. Either surface electrodes or intramuscular fine wire electrodes are used. (From the 2001 Report of the Nomenclature Committee of the American Association of Electromyography and Electrodiagnosis.[10] Used by permission, copyright © 2001, AAEM.)

kinesiology   The study of movement.

kinesiometer   An instrument for measuring the range of motion of a joint.

kinesthesis   (Gr, to move + perception) The sense of movement determined by conscious and unconscious awareness of the current state of extension (and thus the length) of the muscles, so in turn of the varying positions of a limb. The afferent impulses actually come from tendon organs and the older term muscular sense for the senses both of movement and of static position is not therefore appropriate.

This, the sixth, or "muscular," sense or sense of movement, was known to Aristotle but was described precisely by Sir Charles **Bell** in 1826 and assigned by him to the posterior columns. Bastian introduced the term in its current usage.

kinetics   The internal and external forces affecting the moving body.

kinetic cerebellar tremor   See **cerebellar tremors.**

kinetic deviation   See **past pointing.**

kinetic nystagmus   See **optokinetic nystagmus.**

kinetic perimetry   That (conventional) form of perimetry in which a test spot of given size and contrast is moved from the periphery into the center of the subject's visual field,[1636] the points of first perception being charted.

kinetic tremor   Tremor occurring during a voluntary movement.[1422] When the amplitude of the tremulous movements is increased at the end of the movement of a limb toward a target, the terms *intention or terminal tremor* may be used. When a kinetic tremor occurs only during certain activities, such as writing, it is also known as **task-specific kinetic tremor.** See **tremor.**

King-Denborough syndrome   A congenital myopathy complicated by malignant hyperthermia occurring in children with short stature, generalized muscle weakness, dysmorphism with anti-Mongolian slant to the eyes, and multiple congenital skeletal abnormalities.[3048] See **malignant hyperthermia.**

kinking   Acute-angle tortuosity of an artery, such as the carotid. The pathological significance of such a directional change is disputed, unless it is associated with stenosis.

kinky hair syndrome   See **Menkes disease.**

kinky hair–photosensitivity–mental retardation See **Calderon syndrome.**

Kinsbourne-Warrington syndrome   See **opsoclonic meningoencephalitis.**

kippdeviationen/kippnystagmus   Horizontal, conjugate, large-amplitude oscillations of the eyes which are suppressed by visual fixation at a rate of 2.5 Hz. [1290] See also **square-wave pulses.**

Kisch, B   (b. 1890) German physiologist who, like **Kehrer,** described the **auriculopalpebral reflex.**

Kit test   Upward movement of the umbilicus of the supine patient with a cord lesion at T10, on saying the word *kit* loudly. This is due to the retained activity of the upper but not of the lower fibers of the rectus abdominis muscle which contract during the expiration required to say the word.

See also **Beevor sign,** in which the same movement is produced (rather more reliably) by neck flexion.

Kitamura syndrome   See **thyrotoxic periodic paralysis.**

Kjellin syndrome   A recessive form of **hereditary spastic paraplegia** complicated by muscular atrophy, mental retardation, and pigmentary retinal degeneration.[3073]

kleeblattschädel anomaly   (cloverleaf skull) A combination of anomalies based upon the presence of craniosynostosis, leading to a trilobar skull with associated hydrocephalus. Retraction of the upper lids and proptosis lead to the **sunset sign,** and both strabismus and visual failure due to optic nerve compression are common.

Associated features include bony ankylosis of the limbs, hydrocephalus, EEG abnormalities, motor and mental retardation, cerebellar deformities, and polymicrogyria, while numerous other developmental defects have been reported less commonly.[2633]

Klein syndrome   A dominantly inherited dysmorphic syndrome, characterized also by hypertelorism, blepharophimosis, partial albinism, deafness, syndactyly, and bone dysplasias.[3078] See **mandibulofacial dysostosis.**

Klein-Lisak syndrome   See **Andersen syndrome.**

Kleine, Willi   German neuropsychiatrist who published a series of five cases of periodic somnolence, two of which also showed morbid hunger, in 1925. He considered hypothalamic pathology as a possible basis for it. Four years later, Max Levin, an American neurologist, reported a further case and in 1936 he summarized the features of seven cases reported as a new syndrome of periodic somnolence and morbid hunger. See **Kleine-Levin syndrome.**

Kleine-Levin syndrome   (hypersomnia-bulimia) A syndrome characterized by recurrent periods of excessively prolonged sleep in adolescent males, intermixed with periods of normal sleep architecture lasting for a few days or weeks, occurring every few months, and eventually ending with recovery. During the abnormal sleep phases, apathy, irritability, confusion, hyperphagia (compulsive eating), and sexual disinhibition may occur (See also Chart S–6).

A confusional state, hallucinosis, irritability, or a schizophreniform state may occur around the time of the attacks. Thalamic rather than hypothalamic disease was detected in the only case so far to come to postmortem examination. The syndrome was reported by Antimoff in 1898, more fully (in German) by Kleine in 1925[3080] and in English by Levin.[337a] Critchley provided a further review.[1174]

Variants of the syndrome include forms due to hypothalamic pathology, **menstruation-related hypersomnia,** and cyclical depression, and a form characterized by insomnia rather than by hypersomnia.[4337] See also **recurrent hypersomnia.**

Klemm tetanus   See **Rose disease.**

Klippel, Maurice   (1858–1942) French neurologist at the **Salpêtrière.** He described the following two conditions as well as a familial form of frontal cranial hypertrophy resembling that seen in craniocleidodysostosis.[3088]

Klippel-Feil anomaly   (congenital cervical synostosis, congenital webbed neck, congenital brevicollis) Fusion of two or more cervical vertebrae, with or without occipitalization of the atlas, and basilar impression.

Three types are described: (*1*) complete fusion of the cervical vertebrae; (*2*) a decreased number of cervical vertebrae, and (*3*) Subtotal fusion of some cervical vertebrae.

In all cases, the neck is short, the hairline low, and neck movements are limited.

The major neurological complications are myelopathy and radiculopathy, resulting from the bony or associated neural malformations[5282] but synkineses, pyramidal signs, and a syringomyelic syndrome have also been described.[4006]

Some patients have other skeletal abnormalities, including **dysraphism** with hydrocephalus, scapular winging, cleft palate, micrognathia, deafness, and spinal tumors.[2219,3087]

A *variant* is **Wildervanck syndrome.**

Klippel-Trenaunay-Weber syndrome   (Parkes-Weber syndrome, hemangiectatic hypertrophy) A congenital **neurocutaneous syndrome,** characterized by spinal vascular malformations with dermal hemangiomas of the trunk and limbs, telangiectasias, arteriovenous communications, varices and nevi at the same segmental levels, and asymmetrically hypertrophic limbs.[3089,3481] Irregular dominant inheritance is suggested.

Macrocephaly, hypertrophy of other areas, subcutaneous calcification, syndactyly, malabsorption, seizures, glaucoma, and other ocular abnormalities are other features described. Weber's paper in 1907 referred to the account of the condition by Kallischer in 1899 but not to that of Klippel and Trenaunay, which had been published in 1900.[3089]

Manifestations of other neurocutaneous disorders such as **tuberous sclerosis** and **neurofibromatosis** have been described in association.[335]

Klippel-Weil sign   When the contracted fingers of the patient are quickly extended by the examiner, flexion and adduction of the patient's thumb indicate the presence of pyramidal disease.[3086]

Kloepfer syndrome   A recessively inherited syndrome with onset in infancy, characterized by amentia, cortical blindness, deafness, infantilism, and a photosensitive erythematous skin rash.

Pathologically, there is subcortical demyelination and marked loss of cortical neurons. The biochemical basis for the condition is not known.[3091]

Klumpke, Augusta Déjèrine-   (1859–1927) Parisian neurologist, the wife of Dr. Jules Déjèrine. She was born in San Francisco and studied medicine in Paris, becoming the first woman Interne des Hôpitaux in Paris (in the face of substantial opposition on the grounds of her gender, as might be expected).

Klumpke palsy   (Déjèrine-Klumpke palsy) Lower brachial plexus injury, with consequent weakness and wasting of the C8–T1 musculature. When due to violent physical abduction/stretch injury, the sympathetic fibers may also be damaged, with consequent **Horner syndrome.** The syndrome usually follows birth injury (traction of the after-coming arm with breech delivery), arrest of a fall by grabbing on to a projection, or motor vehicle accidents.[2556]

Klüver-Bucy syndrome   A disconnection syndrome of the temporal lobes from midline structures. Clinically, this is characterized by hyperphagia, loss of the ability to make correct choices under visual control (visual agnosia, "psychic blindness"), restlessness, excessive oral exploratory behavior and appetite, overattentiveness to visual stimuli (hypermetamorphosis), sexual libertarianism, and loss of the ability to learn new skills. The syndrome was first described in monkeys following lesions of both hippocampi.[3093]

In humans, bilateral temporal lobe damage (usually in the context of head trauma, encephalitis, or dementia, or with dysfunction of one remaining temporal lobe) may lead to a blunted, affectless, apathetic state with inability to learn new data; occasional arousing to hypersexuality; bulimia; and a tendency toward hypermetamorphosis.[3410]

Knapp streaks   Angioid streaks on the retina, as seen in pseudoxanthoma elasticum. See **angioid streaks, Grondblad-Strandberg syndrome.** Dr. Herman Knapp (1932–1911) was an American ophthalmologist.

knapsack palsy   Brachial plexopathy as a result of compression by the straps of a knapsack or a hod.[4687] See also **Rieder paralysis, upper brachial plexus palsy.**

knee flexor reflex   Contraction of the flexor muscles of the knee and of others in the leg in response to a tap behind the calcaneum, either as part of a generalized (increased) flexor response or as the result of vibrations set up by the tap.

knee jerk   (patellar reflex, quadriceps reflex) Contraction of the quadriceps muscle when its tendon is percussed; like other muscle stretch reflexes, it is augmented in pyramidal tract disease affecting that level and reduced with damage to the reflex arc, in this case at the L3–4 level.

The *contralateral quadriceps reflex* (tapping one patellar tendon leads to extension of the other knee as well) is part of a generalized mass movement (a crossed-extensor response) in patients with severe pyramidal disease.

knee-bending sign   Slight flexion of one knee occurring while the subject is standing. The sign indicates root irritation at L5 or S1.[1150] See **Neri sign** No. 1.

Knobloch-layer syndrome   A recessively inherited congenital syndrome consisting of cataract, macular degeneration, detached retina, myopia, cardiac situs inversus, lung hypoplasia, pendular nystagmus, and occipital encephalocele.[1087]

knock-knees   See **genu valgum.**

Kny disease   See **paramyoclonus multiplex.**[3104]

Kocher, E.T.   (1841–1917) Swiss surgeon who became professor of surgery at Berne University and advanced the techniques of thyroidectomy (an operation commonly required in those days in the goitrous regions of Switzerland). He was awarded the Nobel prize in 1909 for his contributions to the understanding of thyroid disease.[1829]

Kocher reflex   Contraction of the abdominal wall when the patient's testicles are squeezed by the examiner.

Kocher sign   (globe lag) The delay in ascent of the eyeball relative to the upper eyelid on looking upwards in dysthyroid ophthalmopathy.

Kocher-Debré-Sémelaigne syndrome   (muscular hypertrophy in cretins, infant Hercules syndrome, hypothyroid myopathy) The association of general enlargement of muscles with slow muscle contraction and relaxation and **myoedema** in patients with cretinism or adult hypothyroidism.[1324] Painful muscle spasms are not a feature but aching pain, stiffness, and slow muscle contractions, with "hung-up" reflexes and a stiff gait, dysarthria, and paramyotonia, are other features.[3109] The only differences between this and **hy-**

pothyroid myopathy (Hoffmann syndrome) appear to be the absence of pseudomyotonia and the amount of pain felt, as both states may occur in the same patient at different times.

The condition was described first by Kocher in 1892.[3109] The contribution of Debré and Sémelaigne was to demonstrate the response of the symptoms to treatment with thyroid extract, in 1935. The underlying mechanism is uncertain, but possibly an increased intracellular potassium concentration makes the endplate less sensitive to acetylcholine and the cell less excitable; or it may reflect the failure of myosin heavy-chain switching from the neonatal to the adult IIb form of myosin as a result of the absence of thyroxine.

Koenen tumor   Periungual or subungual fibromas occurring after puberty and diagnostic of tuberous sclerosis.[2179]

Koerber-Salus-Elschnig syndrome   Retraction nystagmus and failure of up-gaze, described in patients with a pineal tumor or a cysticercus cyst in the region of the sylvian aqueduct.

The best of the original descriptions was that of Salus,[4891] a pupil of Eleshnig. See **dorsal midbrain syndrome.**

Kofferath syndrome   A combination of **Duchenne-Erb palsy** (upper brachial plexus palsy) and phrenic nerve paresis following birth injury.[6135]

Koh blocks   A set of cubes bearing designs in four colors which the subject is asked to arrange to match a printed pattern. The test was used to assess posterior right parietal function but because of its complexity has now been superseded by the block design test on the **Wechsler Adult Intelligence scale.**

Kohler syndrome   A congenital dysmorphic syndrome manifesting also cataract; congenital heart disease; pulmonary, renal, genital, and endocrine abnormalities; and cerebellar atrophy.[337]

Kohlmeier-Degos disease   See **malignant atrophic papulosis.**

Kohlschutter syndrome   A congenital X-linked or autosomal recessive inherited dysmorphic syndrome, manifesting also hypohidrosis, myopia, abnormality of the dental enamel, intractable seizures, pyramidal signs, and mental and developmental delay.[3114]

Kojewnikow A.   See **Kozhevnikoff.**

koniocortex   (Gr, dust + Lat, bark) The primary receptive areas of the cortex; the granular primary sensory cortex. It includes the primary visual cortex, the primary auditory cortex on Heschl's gyrus, the primary somatosensory cortex on the postcentral gyrus, and the primary motor cortex on the precentral gyrus.

Konzo   An abrupt-onset, nonprogressive, epidemic upper motor neuron disease (tropical myelopathy) presenting as spastic paraparesis. It occurs in children and young adults in central African countries such as Zaire. The cause is considered to be cyanide intoxication due to excessive consumption of improperly processed cassava.[2672]

Kopf tetanus   Cephalic tetanus, the wound often being cranial and the onset occurring with trismus.

Kornzweig, Abraham Leon   (b. 1900) American ophthalmologist who practiced at the Mt. Sinai Hospital in New York. See **abetalipoproteinemia.**

Koro   (Indonesian; shrinking tortoise) An acute anxiety reaction occurring in Oriental males who fear that their penis is receding into the abdomen and insist that it be grasped firmly, by themselves or others.[1829] One cause of such a fear, in some cultures, is the belief that ghosts (who, of course, lack penises) disguise themselves in order to steal those of the living.

Korsakoff psychosis   See **Wernicke-Korsakoff encephalopathy.**

Korsakoff, Sergei Sergeyovich   (1854–1900) Russian neuropsychiatrist who studied at the University of Moscow, receiving his MD degree with a thesis on alcoholic paralysis in 1887. He later took charge of the university psychiatric clinic. His contributions, apart from summarizing findings on the syndrome named after him and which he described as an entity between 1887 and 1889, included a classification of mental diseases and works on paranoia and memory disturbances. He also wrote a major textbook of psychiatric disease.

While Korsakoff noted that the syndrome often follows an episode of **delirium tremens,** he also reported 16 cases of nonalcoholic origin.

Sergei Sergeyovich Korsakoff

Korsakoff syndrome (Korsakoff psychosis) See **Wernicke-Korsakoff encephalopathy.**

Kousseff syndrome A recessively inherited, congenital dysmorphic syndrome characterized also by short stature, facial hemangiomas, webbed neck, sacral meningomyelocele, arthropathy, congenital cardiac disease, and distal weakness.[3143]

Kozhevnikoff, Aleksei Yakovlyevich (Kojewnikow, A.Y.) (1836–1902) Russian neuropsychiatrist who graduated from Moscow University and studied further in Paris, London, and Germany before returning to Moscow. He was eventually elected professor of nervous and mental disease there. He described the form of epilepsy described in the next entry,[3146] as well as **lathyrism,** the microanatomy of the cerebral and cerebellar cortices, the neuropathology of myasthenia and bulbar paralyses, **amyotrophic lateral sclerosis,** and familial spastic diplegia (reported when studying with **Charcot** in Paris). He was the author of a successful textbook of neurology. In Moscow, **Korsakoff** was at one time his pupil and later his assistant.

Kozhevnikoff syndrome 1. (*partial continuous epilepsy*) A particular form of rolandic partial epilepsy occurring in both adults and children and related to a variable lesion of the motor cortex.

Its principal features are (*a*) motor partial seizures, always well localized; (*b*) often late appearance of myoclonus in the same site were somatomotor seizures occur; (*c*). an EEG with normal background activity and a focal paroxysmal abnormality (spikes and slow waves); (*d*) occurrence at any age in childhood and adulthood; (*e*) frequently demonstrable etiology (tumor, vascular); and (*f*) no progressive evolution of the syndrome (clinical, electroencephalographic, or psychological, except in relation to the evolution of the causal lesion).

The condition may also result from mitochondrial encephalopathy (MELAS). (From Commission for Classification and Terminology, ILAE. Proposal for revised classifications of epilepsies and epileptic syndromes. *Epilepsia* 1989;**30**:389–399 With permission from Blockwell Science.)

See **epilepsia partialis continua.**

2. Atrophy of the neck and shoulder muscles and later of the muscles of mastication, attributed to a lesion in the region of the mesencephalon (Osler, 1928 quoted by Durham[1563]).

Kozlowski syndrome A recessively inherited dysmorphic syndrome, characterized by generalized skin atrophy with excessive wrinkling, short stature, dislocation of the hips, microcephaly, seizures, and mental and developmental delay.[3147]

Krabbe, Knud Haraldsen (1885–1961) Danish neurologist who trained at the University of Copenhagen and studied in London and with **Marie** in Paris, where he developed an interest in the pineal gland. He became head of the neurology department in Copenhagen. His full account of the following condition was published in 1916; other major contributions were his complete description of **Sturge-Weber syndrome** in 1934[3148a] and his description of **congenital universal muscular hypoplasia** in 1947. The journal *Acta Neurologica et Psychiatrica Scandinavica* was founded in 1926, largely at his instigation.

His colleague Viggo Christensen was professor of neurology at Copenhagen University.

Krabbe leukodystrophy (globoid cell leukodystrophy, Christensen-Krabbe syndrome, galactosylceramide lipidosis; OMIM 245200) A recessively inherited, lysosomal degenerative disorder of myelin (leukodystrophy) occurring in infancy or later childhood with a fatal course, characterized by a deficiency of galactosylceramide β-galactosidase, the deposition of galactocerebroside, and the presence of **globoid cells.** The responsible gene for galactosylceramidase maps to chromosome 14q31.

Clinically, *early and late infantile* and *juvenile* forms are distinguished; the former is characterized by fevers, psychomotor regression, irritability, optic atrophy, tonic seizures, opisthotonos, deafness, cortical blindness, basal ganglion and pyramidal signs, demyelinating sensorimotor peripheral neuropathy, and a raised CSF protein level with onset after 4 months of age. The disease progresses to decerebration and death within 2 years.

The *late infantile* type is characterized by optic atrophy, dysarthria, dementia, hypotonia, cerebellar signs, spasticity, myoclonus, and motor neuropathy with onset after 6 months of age.[3148]

A *juvenile or adult* presentation with dementia, cortical blindness, optic atrophy, pyramidal signs, and often peripheral neuropathy is also recognized.[1189]

The diagnosis is made by finding the characteristic multinucleated globoid cells with severe astrocytic gliosis in an almost totally demyelinated brain and in nerve biopsy specimens.[3148]

Other *variants* are *Hagberg disease* (prolonged floppy infant syndrome), which is characterized by the late onset of the usual clinical features,[335] and a form with added *congenital fiber type disproportion.*[1336]

Krabbe syndrome See **Sturge-Weber syndrome.**

Krabbe universal muscular hypoplasia A wasting disease of infancy, probably a form of **hereditary motor neuropathy.**

Kraepelin dementia A dementing syndrome with onset in early adult life, manifesting behavioral disturbances, extrapyramidal rigidity, and cerebral atrophy with gliosis and spongy changes.

Kraepelin, Ernst (1856–1926) German psychiatrist, professor at Dorpat, Heidelberg, and later Munich University. His major contributions were in the classification of mental symptoms and diseases, the descriptions of schizophrenia, and the provision of an academic milieu in which assistants such as **Nissl,** Jakob, **Barany,** and Spatz flourished.

Krane-Siroky classification   A system for classifying disorders of micturition based on urodynamic data.[3154]

Detrusor Hyperreflexia
    Coordinated sphincters
    Striated sphincter dyssynergia
    Smooth sphincter dyssynergia
    Nonrelaxing smooth sphincter
Detrusor Areflexia
    Coordinated sphincters
    Nonrelaxing striated sphincter
    Denervated striated sphincter
    Nonrelaxing smooth sphincter

    See also **Bors-Komarr classification, International Continence Society classification.**

Kratschmer reflex   Inhibition of breathing when a baby encounters a bad smell. The reflex appears to persist, however.

Krause corpuscles   Rounded end-bulbs on sensory nerves in such sensitive areas as the lips and glans penis.

Krause syndrome   (retinal dysplasia, congenital encephalo-ophthalmic dysplasia, encephalo-ophthalmic syndrome) The combination of retinal and cerebral dysplasia with microphthalmos, malformations of the retina, choroid and optic nerve, persistent remains of the hyaloid artery, and microcephaly. Affected children, who are usually born prematurely, show failure of mental development and hydrocephalus and are blind. Oxycephaly and encephalocele may also be found.[3157]

    The condition was described by Dr. A.C. Krause, an American ophthalmologist, in 1946. Trisomy 13–15 may be responsible for the syndrome.

Krause, Wilhelm Johann Friedrich   (1833–1910) German professor of anatomy at Göttingen University and later at Berlin.

Kraus-Ruppert syndrome   A congenital dysmorphic syndrome, characterized by hypogonadotrophic hypogonadism, small testes, microcephaly, syndactyly, and mental and developmental delay.[337]

Kretschmer, Ernst   (1888–1964) German neuropsychiatrist.

Kretschmer syndrome   See **apallic syndrome.**

Krishaber disease   See **depersonalization.**

Krishaber, Maurice   (1836–1883) Hungarian-French physician who studied medicine at Vienna, Prague and Paris Universities, graduating from the last in 1864. He settled and practiced in Paris. His original publication on depersonalization recorded 38 cases, representing a huge range of mental and neurological symptoms, but linked by the common thread of, at some time, loss of the sense of personal identity. Krishaber considered this

to be a neurological condition due to focal pathology, but this view is currently not held.[5140]

Kristiansen syndrome   Progressive dissociated anesthesia, hyperpathia, spontaneous pain, hemiballismus, diplopia, seizures, and behavioral changes leading on to bulbar palsies, as a result of an intrinsic thalamic/brainstem lesion.[4723]

Kubisagari   See **vertige paralysant, Gerlier disease.**

Kufs disease   (late or adult amaurotic familial idiocy, adult ganglioside lipidosis) The dominantly inherited adult form of **neuronal ceroid lipofuscinosis,** in which there is deposition in neurons and other cells of an abnormal lipoprotein with characteristic ultrastructural patterns.

    Clinically, it presents with photosensitive progressive myoclonic epilepsy or with progressive mental deterioration, seizures, and facial dyskinesias, but without pigmentary retinal degeneration.[504,3180]

Kufs, Hugo Frederick   (1871–1955) German neuropathologist, who practiced in Leipzig.

Kugelberg-Welander disease   See **hereditary motor neuropathy, type 3.**

Kulenkampff-Tarnow syndrome   (cervicolingumasticatory syndrome) A drug-induced dyskinesic syndrome. See **tardive dyskinesia, cervicolinguomasticatory syndrome.**[3185]

Kurtzke, John F.   Contemporary American neurologist.

Kurtzke scales   (Expanded Disability Status Scale, EDSS; Disability Status Scale, Incapacity Status Scale) Clinical rating scales for evaluating the disabilities of patients with multiple sclerosis. The Expanded Disability Status Scale[3198] extends the older (1955) scale, which had been widely adopted in clinical and research settings. The EDSS is now half of a bifid rating system, assessing overall disability, while the remainder (the functional scale) represents "a series of grades in each of eight functional groupings . . . In each portion there is a numerical rating which is mutually exclusive in its category, and the higher the number, the greater is the dysfunction. Only objectively verifiable defects due to multiple sclerosis as elicited upon neurological examination are included. Symptoms are discarded." The Kurtzke[3198] Scale is given in Chart K–1 and the EDSS in Chart K–2.

Chart K–1. The Kurtzke Scale

A. Functional Systems

Pyramidal functions

  0. Normal
  1. Abnormal signs without disability
  2. Minimal disability
  3. Mild or moderate paraparesis or hemiparesis; severe monoparesis

4. Marked paraparesis or hemiparesis, moderate quadriparesis, or monoplegia
5. Paraplegia, hemiplegia, or marked quadriparesis
6. Quadriplegia
V. Unknown

Cerebellar functions

0. Normal
1. Abnormal signs without disability
2. Mild ataxia
3. Moderate truncal or limb ataxia
4. Severe ataxia, all limbs
5. Unable to perform coordinated movements due to ataxia
V. Unknown
X. Used throughout after each number when weakness (grade 3 or more on pyramidal) interferes with testing

Brainstem functions

0. Normal
1. Signs only
2. Moderate nystagmus or other mild disability
3. Severe nystagmus, marked extraocular weakness, or moderate disability of other cranial nerves
4. Marked dysarthria or other marked disability
5. Inability to swallow or speak
6. Unknown

Sensory functions (revised 1982)

0. Normal
1. Vibration or figure-writing decrease only, in one or two limbs
2. Mild decrease in touch or pain or position sense, and/or moderate decrease in vibration in one or two limbs; or vibratory (with or without figure writing) decrease alone in three or four limbs
3. Moderate decrease in touch or pain or position sense, and/or essentially lost vibration in one or two limbs; or mild decrease in touch or pain and/or moderate decrease in all proprioceptive tests in three or four limbs
4. Marked decrease in touch or pain or loss of proprioception, alone or combined, in one or two limbs; or moderate decrease in touch or pain and/or severe proprioceptive decrease in more than two limbs
5. Loss (essentially) of sensation in one or two limbs; or moderate decrease in touch or pain and/or loss of proprioception for most of the body below the head
6. Sensation essentially lost below the head
V. Unknown

Bowel and bladder functions (revised 1982)

0. Normal
1. Mild urinary hesitancy, urgency, or retention
2. Moderate hesitancy, urgency, retention of bowel or bladder, or rare urinary incontinence
3. Frequent urinary incontinence
4. In need of almost constant catheterization
5. Loss of bladder function
6. Loss of bowel and bladder function
V. Unknown

Visual (or optic) functions

0. Normal
1. Scotoma with visual acuity (corrected) better than 20/30
2. Worse eye with scotoma with maximal visual acuity (corrected) of 20/30 to 20/59
3. Worse eye with large scotoma, or moderate decrease in fields, but with maximal visual acuity (corrected) of 20/60 to 20/99
4. Worse eye with marked decrease of fields and maximal visual acuity (corrected) of 20/100 to 20/200; grade 3 plus maximal acuity of better eye of 20/60 or less
5. Worse eye with maximal visual acuity (corrected) less than 20/200; grade 4 plus maximal acuity of better eye of 20/60 or less
6. Grade 5 plus maximal visual acuity of better eye of 20/60 or less
V. Unknown
X. Added to grades 0 to 6 for presence of temporal pallor

Cerebral (or mental) functions

0. Normal
1. Mood alteration only (does not affect disability status scale score)
2. Mild decrease in mentation
3. Moderate decrease in mentation
4. Marked decrease in mentation (chronic brain syndrome—moderate)
5. Dementia or chronic brain syndrome—severe or incompetent
V. Unknown

Other functions

0. None
1. Any other neurological findings attributed to muoltiple sclerosis (specify)
V. Unknown

From Kurtzke JF. Rating neurological impairment in multiple sclerosis: an expanded disability scale (EDSS). Neurology 1983;33:1444–1452. Reproduced by kind permission.

Chart K–2. Expanded Disability Status Scale (EDSS)

0. Normal neurological examination (all grade 0 in FS; cerebral grade 1 acceptable)
1.0. No disability, minimal signs in one FS (i.e., grade 1 excluding cerebral grade 1)
1.5. No disability, minimal signs in more than one FS; disability, minimal signs in more than one FS (more than one grade 1 excluding cerebral grade 1)
2.0. Minimal disability in one FS (one FS grade 2, others 0 or 1)
2.5. Minimal disability in two FS (two FS grade 2, other 0 or 1)
3.0. Moderate disability in one FS (one FS grade 3, others 0 or 1), or mild disability in three or four FS (three/four FS grade 2, others 0 or 1), though fully ambulatory
3.5. Fully ambulatory but with moderate disability in one FS (one grade 3) and one or two FS grade 2; or two FS grade 3; or five FS grade 2 (others 0 or 1)
4.0. Fully ambulatory without aid, self-sufficient, up and about some 12 hours a day despite relatively severe disability consisting of one FS grade 4 (others 0 or 1),

or combinations of lesser grades exceeding limits of previous steps. Able to walk without aid or rest some 500 meters

4.5. Fully ambulatory without aid, up and about much of the day, able to work a full day, may otherwise have some limitation of full activity or require minimal assistance; characterized by relatively severe disability, usually consisting of one FS grade 4 (others 0 or 1) or combinations of lesser grades exceeding limits of previous steps. Able to walk without aid or rest for some 300 meters

5.0. Ambulatory without aid or rest for about 200 meters; disability severe enough to impair full daily activities (e.g., to work full day without special provisions). (Usual FS equivalents are one grade 5 alone, others 0 or 1; or combinations of lesser grades usually exceeding specifications for step 4.0.)

5.5. Ambulatory without aid or rest for about 100 meters; disability severe enough to preclude full daily activities. (Usual FS equivalents are one grade 5 alone, others 0 or 1; or combinations of lesser grades usually exceeding those for step 4.0.)

6.0. Intermittent or unilateral constant assistance (cane, crutch, or brace required to walk about 100 meters with or without resting). (Usual FS equivalents are combinations with more than two FS grade 3+.)

6.5. Constant bilateral assistance (canes, crutches, or braces) required to walk about 20 meters without resting. (Usual FS equivalents are combinations with more than two FS grade 3+.)

7.0. Unable to walk beyond about 5 meters even with aid, essentially restricted to wheelchair; wheels self in standard wheelchair and transfers alone; up and about in wheelchair some 12 hours a day. (Usual FS equivalents are combinations with more than one FS grade 4+; very rarely, pyramidal grade 5 alone.)

7.5. Unable to take more than a few steps; restricted to wheelchair; may need aid in transfer; wheels self but cannot carry on in standard wheelchair a full day; may require motorized wheelchair. (Usual FS equivalents are combinations with more than one FS grade 4+.)

8.0. Essentially restricted to bed or chair or perambulated in wheelchair, but may be out of bed itself much of the day; retains many self-care functions; generally has effective use of arms. (Usual FS equivalents are combinations, generally grade 4+ in several systems.)

8.5. Essentially restricted to bed much of the day; has some effective use of arm(s); retains some self-care functions. (Usual FS equivalents are combinations, generally 4+ in several systems.)

9.0. Helpless bed patient; can communicate and eat. (Usual FS equivalents are combinations, mostly grade 4+.)

9.5. Totally helpless bed patient; unable to communicate effectively or eat/swallow. (Usual FS equivalents are combinations, almost all grade 4+.)

10.0. Death due to multiple sclerosis.

FS, functional systems. (From Kurtzke JF. Rating neurological impairment in multiple sclerosis: an expanded disability scale (EDSS). Neurology 1983;33:1444–1452. Reproduced by kind permission.)

kuru (laughing death syndrome) See **Lytico-Bodig.** The term is derived from the local word meaning "to shiver."

Kushtha See **leprosy.**

Kuskokwim syndrome A recessively inherited congenital syndrome characterized by multiple joint contractures, mainly affecting the knees and ankles, hypoplasia of the lumbar vertebrae with spondylolisthesis, and atrophy (less often hypertrophy) of local muscles.[4421]

Kussmaul, Adolf (1822–1902) Peripatetic German physician, sometime professor or professor emeritus of medicine at Heidelberg University. He made advances in a number of areas of medicine, including the invention of the stomach pump, and he was the first to describe the following; polyarteritis nodosa (1866); progressive bulbar paralysis (1873); diabetic coma with the respiratory pattern now bearing his name (1874); and pulsus paradoxus, thoracentesis, gastroscopy, and mesenteric thrombosis. He was the first to use the term *poliomyelitis.*

Kussmaul aphasia (aphrasia paranoica) Voluntary mutism, simulating aphasia, in cases of paranoia; a clinical syndrome of stupor followed by overtalkativeness, described by Kussmaul in 1877. ("The insane often remain for months and years in absolute silence; they would be taken for aphasics if they did not begin to speak unexpectedly at a given moment.")[3202]

Kussmaul respirations Deep and rapid breathing in acidotic states, such as diabetic ketosis or uremia.

Kwashiorkor (M'Bwaki, red boy, plurideficiency or malignant malnutrition syndrome) Depigmentation of hair and skin, edema, growth failure, lassitude, apathy, photophobia, and fatty infiltration of the liver with hypoalbuminuria as a result of starvation in children, who develop the signs after weaning in countries afflicted by family, regional, or national famine.[5649]

Kwok quease Poisoning by monosodium glutamate. See **Chinese restaurant syndrome.**

kyphosis (from Gr, bent) Flexion curvature of the spine, either *regular* over a large number of segments, or *angular*, affecting one or two levels only.

L

L nystagmus A form of nystagmus that occurs during prolonged linear (or translational, not rotational) movements of the head. The receptors for such movements are the otolithic organs.[5205] See **vestibular nystagmus.**

L-2-hydroxyglutaric acidemia A rare, recessively inherited, chronic metabolic error characterized by mental retardation, pyramidal and extrapyramidal signs, ataxia, organic acidemia and hyperlysinemia, subcortical leukoencephalopathy, and cerebellar atrophy.[380]

la belle indifférence The lack of emotional expression in the presence of an overt bodily disorder, shown by patients with hysterical conversion syndromes (when it is regarded as culpable) and by Stoics (when it is regarded as laudable). Physicians who can tell the difference are called *psychiatrists*; those who cannot, *cynics.*

Brave, ignorant, agnosic, parkinsonian, and depressed patients may also decline to wear their emotions on the sleeves of their hospital gowns, but the tempting phrase will nevertheless often lead to their inclusion with the hysterics until an experienced physician examines them.

la crampe des écrivains See **writer's cramp.**

La Crosse encephalitis A mosquito-borne arboviral cause of potentially severe encephalitis or aseptic meningitis, characterized often by hyponatremia, seizures, focal neurological signs, and increased intracranial pressure.[3762]

la main étrangère See **alien hand (limb) syndromes.**

la rage See **rabies.**

Labbé, Charles (1852–1889) French anatomist at the medical faculty in Paris.

Labbé's vein The posterior anastomotic vein, crossing the temporal lobe about 5 cm behind its tip.

labials (Lat, pertaining to the lips) Those consonants such as *B*, *M*, and *P* requiring use of the lips for articulation. See also **articulated labials, modified labials,** and **dentolabials.**

laboratory-supported multiple sclerosis Diagnostic categories of **multiple sclerosis** in which two previous attacks are separated both in time and in the location of the lesions; one clinical or one paraclinical feature is present; and the results of CSF oligoclonal banding are positive (*laboratory-supported definite*). Other categories are also defined.

In the *laboratory-supported probable* category, there have been two prior attacks and the results of CSF oligoclonal banding are positive.[4504] See **Poser criteria.**

labyrinth (from Gr, a place with many turnings) The internal ear, composed of the cochlea, vestibule, and the semicircular canals, both osseous and membranous.

labyrinthine apoplexy Acute vertigo and vomiting with succeeding permanent vestibuloparesis, probably resulting from occlusion of a branch of the artery of the internal auditory meatus.

labyrinthine nystagmus See **vestibular nystagmus.**

labyrinthine reflex The sign is most easily elicited in infancy; the child is held up by, and facing, the examiner, who then rotates about his own axis for several turns to the right, then to the left. The baby will look ahead in the direction of the rotation and, after stopping, will look back in the opposite direction.[6064] See **vestibulo-oculogyric reflex.**

labyrinthine righting reflex See **righting reflexes.**

labyrinthine Romberg sign When subjects with unilateral labyrinthine disease stand with their feet together and their eyes closed, they feel a sensation of being drawn to one side and there is slow lateral flexion of their neck to that side.

labyrinthitis See **acute peripheral vestibulopathy.**

Lacheretz-Allain syndrome A congenital dysmorphic syndrome characterized by female pseudohermaphroditism, nephropathy, multiple synostoses, acrocephaly, and craniosynostosis.[3217]

lacrimal (Lat, a tear) Pertaining to lacrimation; weeping.

lactate dehydrogenase deficiency A rare, recessively inherited, metabolic myopathy in which this muscle isoenzyme is missing, thus causing incomplete block of glycolysis. The responsible gene maps to chromosome 11p15.

Clinically, the condition is marked by fatigue, exercise intolerance, muscle cramps and myoglobinuria following heavy exercise, without detrimental storage of excess glycogen.[1452,2917]

lactate stress testing Estimation of serum lactate levels following exercise rather than at rest used in the diagnosis of mitochondrial diseases. Abnormally increased levels reflect impairment of function of respiratory chain enzymes in muscle so that anaerobic replaces aerobic metabolism and shifts the pyruvate/lactate equation towards lactate. The addition of exercise enhances the diagnostic yield of the test.[1823]

lactic acidemia A metabolic acidosis due to a failure in pyruvate catabolism, in which lactate levels exceed 2.2 mmol/L. The causes include many inborn errors of metabolism, mitochondrial disorders, systemic diseases, and intoxications. An idiopathic congenital form also exists.[2758] See **pyruvate dehydrogenase deficiency, pyruvate carboxylase deficiency, Leigh disease, mitochondrial diseases, carnitine deficiency.**

lactosylceramidosis   A rare, neurovisceral, glycolipid storage polioencephalopathy characterized by the intracellular accumulation of lactosylceramide and clinically by the appearance in infancy of cerebellar and pyramidal signs and optic atrophy with a progressive course to death in the vegetative state.[1315]

lacunar dementia   That form of dementia associated with multiple small infarcts in the subcortical brain regions as a result of occlusive hyalinosis of the small penetrating vessels.[66] See **Binswanger disease.**

lacunar infarcts   Infarcts in the deep white matter or the brain, presumed to be due to occlusion of single perforating arteries supplying the internal capsule, striatum, thalamus, pons, or cerebellum. The classic syndromes are pure motor hemiparesis, sensorimotor stroke, pure sensory stroke, dysarthria–clumsy hand syndrome, and ataxic hemiparesis. See also **striatocapsular infarcts, thalamic infarcts, white-matter medullary infarcts, extended large subcortical infarcts.**

lacunar skull   (Lükenschädel) The "soap-bubble" radiological apearance of the inner table of the skull seen in some newborn infants with spina bifida and other developmental anomalies. Although this resembles copper-beating, it is not associated with increased intracranial pressure and it tends to go away within the first 6 months of life.

lacunar state   The presence of multiple, small, cavitating infarcts in the white matter, due to multiple **lacunes.** The term was introduced by Déchambre in 1838[1325] and amplified by Durand-Fardel 4 years later, but the clinical correlations were made with greatest effect by Pierre **Marie** in 1901 and by Dr. C. Miller **Fisher** between 1953 and 1982.

lacunar syndromes   Constellations of more or less constant clinical signs considered to arise from the presence of **lacunes** in certain areas of the cerebral white matter.[3453] The syndromes defined at present are listed in Chart L–1.[1853]

Chart L–1. Lacunar Syndromes

1. **Pure sensory stroke**
2. **Pure motor hemiparesis**
3. **Ataxic hemiparesis** (homolateral ataxia and crural paresis, however, is an example of crossed cerebral-cerebellar **diaschisis**)
4. **Dysarthria-clumsy hand syndrome**
5. *Modified pure motor hemiparesis with aphasia*, characterized by pyramidal signs mainly in the face and hand, with initial dysarthria and due to a lesion of the genu and anterior limb of the internal capsule
6. *Pure motor hemiparesis sparing the face*, in which unilateral pyramidal signs in the limbs with initial nystag-

mus and vertigo are due to an infarct of the medullary pyramid
7. *Mesoencephalothalamic syndrome* characterized by third cranial nerve palsy, impairment of upward gaze and abulia, and due to bilateral paramedian infarcts of the subthalamic and thalamic region or of the midbrain. See also **top of the basilar syndrome**
8. **Thalamic dementia**
9. *Pure motor hemiparesis with horizontal gaze palsy* in which a transient **one-and-a-half syndrome** is associated with hemiparesis; this is due to a paramedian pontine infarct[1853]
10. *Pure motor hemiparesis with crossed third nerve palsy* (**Weber syndrome**)
11. *Pure motor hemiparesis with crossed sixth nerve palsy* in which these findings are due to a low paramedian pontine infarct[1853]
12. *Pure motor hemiparesis with confusion*, a rare syndrome due to a small deep infarct interrupting the thalamofrontal connections, in which the hemiparesis is associated with acute confusion and a memory deficit
13. Cerebellar ataxia with crossed third nerve palsy (**Claude syndrome**)
14. **Sensorimotor stroke** (thalamocapsular)
15. **Hemiballism** or hemichorea
16. **Lower basilar branch syndrome**
17. **Lateral medullary syndrome**
18. **Lateral pontomedullary syndrome**
19. *Acute loss of memory* due to an infarct of the corpus callosum
20. **Locked-in syndrome**
21. Miscellaneous:
    Weakness of one leg with ease of falling
    Pure dysarthria, a presumed **lacunar syndrome** characterized by the sudden onset of dysarthria without any angiographic or CT abnormality
    Acute dystonia of thalamic origin, a presumed **lacunar syndrome**

Adapted from Fisher CM. Lacunar strokes and infarcts; a review. Neurology 1982;32:871–876, by kind permission.

Other lacunar syndromes identified[4259] besides those in Chart L–1, include third nerve palsy, nuclear and prenuclear syndromes of the third nerve, vertical gaze palsy, **internuclear ophthalmoplegia, one-and-a-half syndrome,** focal **dystonia** of the arm, and unilateral **asterixis.**

Hachinski[2355] has suggested the following diagnostic criteria, given in Chart L–2.

Chart L–2. Diagnostic Criteria for Lacunar Syndromes

Component	Diagnostic Criteria	Exclusions
Etiology	Hypertension (present on past history or prescribed for)	Seizures, severe unusual headache, vomiting, loss of consciousness
Deficit	Pure motor hemiplegia in face, arms or leg	Abnormal higher function (aphasia, neglect apraxia, agnosia)
	Pure sensory stroke in face, arms, or leg	

	Motor sensory stroke in face, arms, or leg	Hemianopia
	Ataxic hemiparesis	
	Dysarthria clumsy hand syndrome	
CT	Compatible with a small, deep infarct or normal (or normal isotope brain scan)	Superficial CT lesion Deep lesion >1 cm Focal abnormality
EEG	Normal or symmetrically abnormal	
Angiography	No tight stenosis of the internal carotid, middle, cerebral, vertebral, or basilar arteries	

Adapted from Hachinski VC. Classification of stroke for clinical trials. Stroke 1990;21:(Suppl II)27–29, by kind permission.

Lacunar transient ischemic attacks are also described, in which isolated motor or sensory symptoms involve at least two of the three areas face, arm, and leg.[3250]

lacune   (from Lat, a pond, or Fr, a small lake) The term used by Pierre **Marie** in 1901 and reintroduced by Miller Fisher in 1965 to describe small (<1 cm), deep cystic cavities in the white matter of the cerebrum, brainstem, and cerebellum, representing healed infarcts resulting from occlusion of deep penetrating cerebral arterioles.[1837] For larger lesions he suggested the term *giant lacune*; others prefer *lagoon*.

Three forms have been described: *type 1*, with small areas of cerebral infarction; *type 2*, with cystic scars which are the residue of small hemorrhages; and *type 3*, in which areas of perivascular dilation are not associated with infarction.[3702]

Lacunes are associated with a prior history of hypertension, with atherosclerosis of the cerebral vessels and cerebral hemorrhages. When numerous, they produce the **état criblé.** Over 20 clinical syndromes have been identified as resulting from lacunes in various sites (see Chart-L-1 above), but most are probably asymptomatic.[1853] In some cases the clinical diagnosis is plain, but, in more, the differentiation from other stroke pathologies is impossible.

The underlying lesion is said to be ischemic infarction resulting from lipohyalinosis, or occlusion of the mouth of the branching vessel, but the sites of the lacunes (exactly the same as the sites of primary intracerebral hemorrhage), the presence of hematin-laden macrophages around them, the absence of pathological reports of recent acute lacunes, and the occasional CT image of small, deep hemorrhages in the appropriate areas suggest that incriminating ischemic infarction in every case is not warranted.

The wholesale ascription of clinical presentations to the collection of lacunar states has been criticized.[3245]

The following criteria for *possible lacunar stroke* have been suggested:[3891]

All of the following must be met:

1. Clinical presentation of lacunar syndrome, these being pure motor hemiparesis, pure sensory stroke, ataxic-hemiparesis, or the dysarthria-clumsy hand syndrome
2. Age ≥ 0 years or a history of hypertension or diabetes
3. CT or MRI performed ≥72 hours after stroke shows appropriate subcortical lesion <2 cm in diameter or demonstrates no lesion appropriate to the stroke
4. No obvious other cause of small vessel disease (e.g., vasculitis)
5. Arterial imaging shows no evidence of significant occlusive disease

Laehr reflex   (Laehr-Henneberg reflex, hard palate reflex) Contraction of the orbicularis oculi and lowering of the upper lip when the hard palate is tickled. This sign may be found in cases of pseudobulbar palsy.

Laehr-Henneberg reflex   See **Laehr reflex.**

Lafora bodies   (amyloid bodies, myoclonus bodies, polyglucosan bodies) Rounded periodic acid-Schiff–positive, argyophilic, intracytoplasmic inclusion bodies with a dense central basophilic core and a rim that takes up less stain, found in the larger neurons of the thalamus, dentate nuclei, and substantia nigra, in progressive myoclonic epilepsy (**Lafora body disease**) and less abundantly in normal-aged brains.

Lafora body disease   (progressive myoclonic epilepsy with Lafora bodies; OMIM 254780) A recessively inherited polioencephalomyelopathy of late childhood or early adult life, characterized clinically by progressive dementia, dysarthria, visual loss, pyramidal and cerebellar signs, and focal occipital, photoconvulsive progressive myoclonic, and other seizure types, leading to death in 2–10 years from the onset of symptoms. It is mapped to 6q24.

The EEG shows both generalized and focal or multifocal posterior discharges, photoconvulsive responses, and slowing of the background rhythms. The diagnostic pathological finding of basophilic intracytoplasmic PAS-positive inclusions in cells of the dentate nucleus, thalamus, and brainstem was described by Lafora in 1911,[3224] 20 years after Unverricht's original identification of progressive myoclonic epilepsy.[5689] The diagnosis is made by detecting **Lafora bodies** within neuronal processes in the central nervous system. Similar accumulations occur in the liver, heart, skin, and skeletal muscles. In practice, the method of choice for confirming the diagnosis is axillary skin biopsy.[1098]

Lafora body disease differs from **Unverricht-Lundborg-Lafora syndrome** in its slightly later mean age of onset, less severe myoclonus, and earlier and relentless cognitive decline; but this does not mean to say that the underlying abnormality is not the same. See also **adult polysaccharidosis.**

The following *variants* are described:

Progressive myoclonic epilepsy without Lafora Bodies A precisely similar clinical condition in which the Lafora bodies are not detected.[3709]

Juvenile neuronopathic Gaucher disease type 3 A cause of progressive myoclonus epilepsy, with the added clinical features of horizontal and vertical supranuclear gaze palsies, hepatosplenomegaly, and cerebellar signs.[4142]

Lafora, Gonzalo Rodriguez (1886–1971) Spanish neurologist, neuropathologist, and psychiatrist, who graduated from Madrid, taking further training there with **Cajal** and in a number of German centers. While working in Washington D.C., he described the amyloid bodies known by his name. After a further period as an exile in Mexico during the Spanish Civil War, he returned to Cajal's laboratory in Madrid for the remainder of his career.

laforin   A protein with unknown function, seemingly relevant in the pathogenesis of **Lafora body disease.**

lag-in-pulse sign   Delay in the re-establishment of the radial pulse after manual compression of the radial artery proximally, seen in the vasogenic form of the **thoracic outlet syndrome.**

lagophthalmos   (from Gr, a hare + the eye) Inability to close one or both eyes fully while at rest, as may occur with bilateral seventh cranial nerve palsies or myopathy affecting the facial muscles.

The name derives from the ancient belief that hares sleep with their eyes open. Iritis and corneal nodules are predictable complications.

lalling   (from Lat, to sing a lullaby) 1. The earliest speech sounds made by infants, varying between cooing and the repetitive utterance of consonants. The name was formerly used for that mode of speech in which the *R* sound is replaced by that of *L* 2. The imperfect pronunciation of letters or words as by small children or by the inebriated. It includes slurring, **mogilalia,** and **paralalia.**

lambda   The Greek letter *L*, written as an inverted *V* and thus appropriately applied to the cranial posterior suture separating the parietal and occipital bones—hence also *lambdoid* (of this shape).

lambda wave   A sharp transient on the EEG, mainly electropositive relative to other areas and occurring over the occipital regions of the head of waking subjects during visual exploration. It is time-locked to saccadic eye movement and its amplitude varies but is generally below 50 uV. (Adapted from the 1974 report of the of the Committee on Terminology, IFCN,[989] by permission of Elsevier Science.)

These bi- or triphasic waves are recorded in parieto-occipital regions with intermittent stimulation and are absent in darkness or with a neutral visual field.

lambdoid wave   See **positive occipital sharp transient of sleep.**

Lambert-Brody syndrome   An X-linked disorder of childhood characterized by electrically silent muscle contractions with impairment of relaxation, similar to myotonia clinically but without percussion myotonia and electrically silent. It is due to impairment of calcium reuptake by the sarcoplasmic reticulum as a result of calcium-adenosine triphosphatase deficiency in type 2 myofibrils.[266,2942]

Lambert-Eaton myasthenic syndrome   (Eaton-Lambert syndrome, inverse myasthenia; LEMS) An autoimmune disorder of presynaptic neuromuscular transmission affecting the P/Q Ca^{2+} channels, resulting from impaired release of acetylcholine from the motor endplate due to blockade of functional calcium channels in the presynaptic membrane by autoantibodies; a **paraneoplastic syndrome** associated with carcinoma (usually small cell carcinoma of the lung) occurs in at least 60% of all cases. Thus, the classification recognizes the syndrome with and without malignant disease. See also **neuromuscular transmission disorders.**

Clinically, the condition is manifested by mild girdle weakness, especially of the hips and thighs, transiently improving with brief sustained exercise; fatigability; muscle aching; cramps; paresthesias; and hyporeflexia. The extraocular, facial, and bulbar muscles tend to be spared but impotence, ptosis, and dryness of the mouth and eyes are common features of autonomic involvement and hypometric saccades may be recorded. Both the weakness and the depression of reflexes abate with repeated effort because of the augmented mobilization of acetylcholine quanta, as seen by the post-tetanic potentiation recorded with repetitive electrical stimulation studies[3231,3232,4243] and by the paradoxical lid elevation with sustained upward gaze.

The same condition had been described by Anderson and others in England 3 years before the report of Lambert and Eaton, but they did not perform repetitive stimulation and probably did not understand the nature of the defect in full.

lamellated cytoplasmic inclusion disease   A neuronal storage disease characterized by the childhood onset of cerebral atrophy with spasticity, rigidity, chorea, and mental and developmental delay with sensorimotor neuropathy. Nerve or rectal biopsy specimens show inclusions and cytoplasmic bodies.[337]

laminin   A major structural protein in vertebrate muscle.

Lamy-Maroteaux syndrome   (diastrophic dwarfism, cherub dwarfism) A recessively inherited dysmorphic syndrome characterized by extreme short stature due to shortness of the limbs, kyphoscoliosis, joint contractures, hand deformities, and bilateral club foot.[3636]

The neurological Maroteaux-Lamy syndrome is a **mucopolysaccharidosis.**

Lancaster red-green test   A quantitative test measuring the degree of diplopia, in which red and green filters are placed successively over the subject's eyes, and the subject and the examiner each project a light (one red, one green) onto a screen in the nine cardinal positions of gaze. The separation of the images as seen by the subject is measured in each case.[4668]

The test has been found valuable in demonstrating even small improvements of ocular motility in myasthenic patients given edrophonium.

Lance-Adams syndrome (chronic posthypoxic myoclonus) Multifocal cortical **action myoclonus** with cerebellar ataxia and some mental slowing, due to subcortical ischemic anoxia[3240] as after cardiorespiratory arrest. It presents with multifocal cortical action myoclonus, often stimulus-sensitive, and with mild cognitive derficits. An exaggerated startle response and brainstem reticular reflex myoclonus are also described. [5919]

Dr. James Lance and Dr. Raymond Adams are contemporary Australian and American neurologists.

Lancet One of the longest established medical journals, publishing also neurological papers. Web site: http://www.lancetneuronet.com/.

lancinating pain Pain of a sharpness resembling that of a stab with a needle or scalpel. The pain of **trigeminal neuralgia** is typically described thus.

Landau reflex Extension of the neck, spine, and legs when the normal infant is held in ventral suspension, but flexion of the legs and trunk when the head is flexed by the examiner.

The reflex normally appears between the third and sixth month, and is lost at the end of the first year. Children with spastic states may show exaggeration of the reflex while those with neuromuscular disease may not exhibit it at all, and instead droop listlessly from the examiner's hands.[3908] See also **developmental reflexes.**

Landau syndrome A syndrome of retarded mental development with psychomotor seizures, dysplastic facial changes resembling acromegaly, and later generalized amyotrophy, slowly progressing and leading to early death. The pathogenesis is unknown.[3248]

Landau-Kleffner syndrome (acquired verbal auditory agnosia with convulsive disorder, acquired epileptic aphasia, Andermann syndrome) A childhood syndrome, characterized by the acute or subacute appearance of regression of previously acquired language skills, leading eventually to mutism in young children whose former language development was proceeding normally. Verbal auditory agnosia and a rapid reduction in spontaneous speech are typical. Often associated are auditory agnosia and behavioral disorders, without intellectual deterioration. Nonverbal skills are unaffected. Epileptic seizures (usually generalized tonic-clonic or partial motor) and behavioral and psychomotor disturbances occur in two-thirds of the patients; the EEG findings include spike–wave discharges, especially during slow-wave sleep. Both the seizures and the EEG abnormalities are likely to remit before the age of 15 years. (Modified from Commission for Classification and Terminology, ILAE. Proposal for revised classifications of epilepsies and epileptic syndromes. *Epilepsia* 1989;30:389–399. Reproduced by kind permission of Blackwell Science.)

The condition responds poorly to anticonvulsant drugs, but steroids lastingly correct both the regression in higher functions and the EEG abnormalities.[3247]

In a *variant* form there is associated selective gait disorder and paroxysmal dystonia.[4106]

Landing syndrome See **GM₁ gangliosidosis.**

Landing-Oppenheimer disease See **neuronal ceroid lipofuscinosis.**

Landouzy camptodactyly Irreducible contractures at the interphalangeal joints of the fingers (especially the fifth) due to fibrosis of the tendon sheaths.[3256]

Landouzy, Louis-Théophile-Joseph (1845–1917) French physician, professor of therapeutics, and later dean of the faculty of medicine in Paris. His description of **facioscapulohumeral muscular dystrophy**[3255] was his only important contribution to neurology, most of his work being on tuberculosis. However, he did also describe muscle atrophy in association with sciatica, which some have called *Landouzy syndrome* or *Landouzy sciatica.*[3253]

Louis-Théophile-Joseph Landouzy

Landouzy-Déjèrine syndrome See **facioscapulohumeral dystrophy.**

Landouzy-Grasset law When a unilateral cerebral lesion produces hemiplegia, the head is turned to the side of the lesion if the paralysis is flaccid and to the side of the affected limbs if it is spastic.[3254] See also **Vulpian sign, Prevost sign.**

Landry de Thezillat, Jean-Baptiste-Octave (1826–1865) French neurologist, born in Limoges, whose description of acute infectious polyneuropathy in 1859[3258] (making most of the important clinical points and leading to the names *acute ascending* or *Landry paralysis*) preceded that of Guillain, Barré, and Strohl by nearly 60 years, although **Kussmaul** also described two cases in the same year.

His original account emphasized the sensory as well as the motor findings, but obviously omitted reference to the CSF, as lumbar puncture had not then been introduced. Following this report he left Paris for financial reasons and devoted the remainder of his professional life to the management of patients at the Auteuil spa. He returned to Paris in 1865 to help in the care of patients during a cholera epidemic, and died from the disease despite the attention of **Charcot**.[1829]

Jean-Baptiste-Octave Landry de Thezillat

Landry-Guillain-Barré (-Strohl) syndrome See **acute inflammatory demyelinating polyneuropathy.**

Langdon-Down, J.L.H.   See **Down, J.L.H.L.**

de Lange, Cornelia Catherina   (1871–1950) Dutch pediatrician who graduated from Amsterdam University and worked in Zurich before returning, eventually becoming professor of pediatrics.

Langer-Gierdon syndrome   (thoracic-pelvic-phalangeal dystrophy) A dysmorphic syndrome characterized by microcephaly, polydactyly, hypotonia, deafness, an unusually bulbous nose, redundant folds of skin in cervical regions, and both physical and mental retardation, due to a chromosomal deletion at 8q24.[4046]

Langerhans cell histiocytosis   A rare granulomatous disease with predilection for the pituitary gland and hy-pothalamus, typically presenting with skull lesions, proptosis, and diabetes insipidus. See also **hypophysitis.**

Langley, John Newport   (1852–1925) English physiologist, professor of physiology at Cambridge. He devoted most of his research to a study of the autonomic nervous system, differentiating the sympathetic and parasympathetic systems by 1894. Both these names and *orthosympathetic* were suggested by him, and he also differentiated and named the pre- and postganglionic fibers.[3267]

John Newport Langley

Langley nerves   Pilomotor nerves.

Langley-Sherrington sign   Protrusion of the pinna of the ear on the side of a **Horner syndrome**. See **Hassin sign.**

language   1. An essentially human method of expressing ideas and feelings by way of a system of visual or auditory symbols; the expression and reception of ideas and feelings.

2. Expression of mental content through muscular activity with the intention of communicating it to another person. It is the symbolic representation of many forms of sensory experience, the symbols taking the form of written or spoken words and of gestures (including *body language*) used for the expression and communication of thoughts or feelings.[2174,4641]

language disorder   Disturbances of reading, writing, spelling, calculation, and verbal memory or learning as well as dysphasia.

language-induced epilepsy   A reflex seizure disorder in which the seizures are triggered by multiple language-related functions, including reading, speaking, and writing.[2084]

Lannois-Jouty syndrome   A syndrome of paresis of cranial nerves IX, X, XI, and XII, indicating a lesion of the skull base. See **Avellis syndrome.**

Lantermann A.J.   German anatomist whose paper reporting what are now known as **Schmidt-Lantermann clefts** in myelin followed that of Schmidt by 3 years.

lardaceous hegemony   The term of Dr. H.L. Parker for the fatty imperatives of the antiepileptic **ketogenic diet.**

Larrey, D-J.   (Baron) (1766–1842) French surgeon who headed the medical services in Napoleon's armies. His experiences gained from the military carnage he witnessed led to numerous original descriptions of diseases or of methods for their management and (apart from surgical topics) included accounts of **Jacksonian seizures,** of contralateral paresis with cerebral injury, homolateral paresis with cerebellar injury, and aphasia with cerebral lesions.[1829]

Larsen disease   A congenital dysmorphic syndrome manifesting also sensorineural deafness, optic atrophy, retinal cone dystrophy with night blindness, hepatic disorder, hypertension, diabetes, hypothyroidism, and a large sella turcica.[337]

larval discharges   Runs of abnormal activity on the EEG, such as those frequently associated with clinical seizure activity, but which in these cases are unaccompanied by seizures.

larval epilepsy   (Lat, a mask + seizures) An antique name for **complex partial seizures,** in which the evidence for epilepsy is masked by the atypical nature of its manifestations.

laryngeal abductor paralysis   An X-linked congenital syndrome of dysphonia with stridor and mental retardation, due to agenesis of the nucleus of the nerve in the medulla. A sixth cranial nerve palsy may be associated. [576]

laryngeal adductor paralysis is also described as a dominantly inherited abnormality.[3546]

laryngeal dystonia   Dystonic spasms of the vocal cords which adduct on phonation, resulting in **spastic dysphonia**. The cause is not known.[157] See also **Meige syndrome.**

laryngeal epilepsy   See **cough syncope.**

laryngeal nystagmus   See **ocular myoclonus.**

laryngeal vertigo   See **cough syncope.**

laryngisimus stridulus   Laryngeal spasm in children with hypocalcemia (usually as a result of rickets), which causes arrest in inspiration followed by relaxation of the vocal cord adduction and results in a crowing inspiratory sound.

Laségue, Ernest-Charles   (1816–1883) Parisian neuropsychiatrist, who had already held a chair of rhetoric when he entered the University of Paris. He graduated in 1846, became a student of **Trousseau,** and eventually became physician at the **Salpêtrière** and later at the Pitié Hospital. It was his student, J-J. Forst, who published Laségue's 1864 observations on straight-leg raising (in his doctoral thesis in 1881), although the same sign had already been described by Lazarevic in 1880.

Laségue also gave a superb description of paranoid dementia praecox (schizophrenia) in 1852 and of anorexia nervosa (hysterical anorexia) in 1878,[3286] just after the first note by **Gull** in the *Lancet* of 1868. On the two descriptions Seckersen remarks: "It is interesting to note the extraordinary differences in the descriptions of the same condition by the two men. While Gull's comments are as direct and precise as a pathological report, Laségue conveys a sense of the spirit and feeling of these people, the nuances of their disturbed relationships and the subtleties of their psychiatric upheaval."[5047]

Laségue's acquaintance with such cases sprang from his appointment as physician to the Paris prefecture in 1849, where all persons arrested on a charge of lunacy were brought. Under Trousseau, whose favorite pupil he was, he acted as chef de clinique from 1852 to 1854. In the remainder of his career, he published over 115 papers on subjects as diverse as cretinism, hysteria, alcoholism, migraine, vertigo, typhoid, rheumatism, and syphilis.[5047]

Ernest-Charles Laségue

Laségue signs   1. (straight-leg raising) A sign of lumbosacral root irritation. Pain and limitation of further movement occur when the patient's hip is slowly, passively flexed with the knee extended, but not when the hip is flexed with the knee also flexed. The test can be augmented by passive dorsiflexion of the ankle, which causes more pain in the back in positive cases.

Laségue originally likened the stretching of the sciatic nerve over the ischium when the leg is elevated to the tuning of a violin string by his son-in-law, but thought that the pain came from compression of the nerve by muscles.[3284] **Wartenberg**[5863] noted that the sign (and a more correct interpretation of its genesis) was described by Lazarevic, a physician in Belgrade in 1880, a year before the thesis of Forst.

2. **Laségue syndrome** In hysterical anesthesia, the patient will be unable to move the limb when the eyes are closed, but can do so when they are opened.[3285,3286]

Lashley, Karl (1890–1958) American neurophysiologist and psychologist. He defined the law of mass action, noting that the degree of impairment in maze learning by rats was proportional to the volume of brain removed but was not dependent on the site of the ablation, thus giving support to those who believed in the functional equivalence of the cortex. He later modified his view, considering such equipotentiality to exist only within regions.[3287]

Lassa fever An acute arenavirus illness endemic in central Africa, characterized by an insidious onset of influenza-like symptoms followed, in severe cases, by a generalized bleeding diathesis, encephalopathy, and death. Early diagnosis may be possible using polymerase chain reaction technology. The Junin and Machupo arenaviruses are responsible for the similar conditions of Argentine and Bolivian hemorrhagic fever, respectively.

lata See **latah.**

latah (lata) A chronic condition manifest by excessive startle responses to noise or touch with involuntary mimicry, tics, striking out, coprolalia, and automatic obedience to commands, occurring mainly in adult females in Africa and the Far East.[5174]

It was recorded first in the sixteenth century, but in modern times was described in 1883 by Beard among Malaysians.[6066] See also **jumping Frenchmen of Maine.**

late amaurotic familial idiocy See **GM₂ gangliosidoses, neuronal ceroid lipofuscinosis.**

late component (of a motor unit action potential) See **satellite potential.**

late cortical cerebellar atrophy See **olivopontocerebellar atrophy, autosomal dominant cerebellar ataxias, Marie-Foix-Alajouanine syndrome.**

late distal myopathy A form of muscular dystrophy appearing in mature adult life, affecting first the hands but later also the feet.[5908] See **distal myopathy.**

late hereditary myopathy See **distal muscular dystrophy.**

late infantile amaurotic familial idiocy See **GM₂ gangliosidoses, neuronal ceroid lipofuscinosis.**

late infantile metachromatic leukodystrophy See **metachromatic leukodystrophy.**

late post-traumatic epilepsy Seizures occurring more than a week after craniocerebral trauma. They are more likely to recur than those occurring within the first week.

late response A general term used to describe an evoked potential in motor nerve conduction studies having a longer latency than the M wave. Examples include **A wave, F wave,** and **H wave.** (From the 2001 Report of the Nomenclature Committee of the American Association of Electromyography and Electrodiagnosis.[10] Used by permission, copyright © 2001, AAEM.)

late-life muscular dystrophy See **chronic polymyositis.**

latency The interval between a stimulus and a response. The onset latency is the interval between the onset of a stimulus and the onset of the evoked potential. The peak latency is the interval between the onset of a stimulus and a specified peak of the evoked potential. (From the 2001 Report of the Nomenclature Committee of the American Association of Electromyography and Electrodiagnosis.[10] Used by permission, copyright © 2001, AAEM.)

latency of activation The time required for an electric stimulus to depolarize a nerve fiber (or bundle of fibers as in a nerve trunk) beyond threshold and to initiate an action potential in the fiber(s). This time is usually of the order of 0.1 msec or less. (From the 2001 Report of the Nomenclature Committee of the American Association of Electromyography and Electrodiagnosis.[10] Used by permission, copyright © 2001, AAEM.)

latent Concealed, not yet manifest.

latent convergent strabismus See **esophoria.**

latent nystagmus (monocular "fixation" nystagmus, unimacular nystagmus) A congenital form of jerk nystagmus which appears (in both eyes) only when one eye is occluded, and in which the slow phase has a decreasing-velocity exponential curve. The fast phase is in the direction of gaze of the viewing eye. Strabismus is always present as well.

The condition is a disorder of tonic innervation which is precipitated by an inability to adjust properly to the differences between monocular and binocular perceptual domains.[1369]

Manifest latent nystagmus is similar, occurring in both eyes of subjects with image suppression due to squint or amblyopia, who for this reason are actually viewing with one eye only, even though both are open.[1369]

latent period   See **latency.**

latent tetany   See **spasmophilia.**

late-onset ataxia, rigidity, and peripheral neuropathy   A dominantly inherited degenerative disease of late onset, characterized by cerebellar ataxia, muscular rigidity, bradykinesia, dysarthria, muscle atrophy, and spasticity in various combinations in affected individuals.[6126] See also **cerebellar ataxias** (*variants*).

late-onset cerebellar ataxias   See **cerebellar ataxias** (*variants*).

late-onset proximal myopathy with diabetes mellitus   A syndrome with onset in later adult life, comprising muscle pain and cramp, cataract, diabetes, and proximal myopathic weakness.[337]

late-onset proximal riboflavine-responsive myopathy with combined multiple acyl CoA dehydrogenase and respiratory chain deficiency   A rare syndrome resulting from the impaired oxidation of fatty acids with onset in later adult life, and comprising lipid storage myopathy with severe proximal weakness.[190]

An *infantile variant* in which the presentation is with nonketotic hypoglycemia, hypotonia, failure to thrive, and acute attacks resembling **Reye syndrome,** and a *juvenile* form with progressive limb-girdle and axial myopathy and secondary carnitine deficiency are also described.

lateral   (Lat, belonging to the side).

lateral antebrachial cutaneous neuropathy   Compression of the terminal cutaneous branch of the musculocutaneous nerve at its point of exit beside the biceps tendon, resulting in pain and sensory deficit in the territory of that nerve.[2763]

lateral bulbar syndrome   See **lateral medullary syndrome.**

lateral cervical puncture   Percutaneous insertion of a needle into the spinal cord through the C1–2 interspace under fluoroscopic control, performed to interrupt the spinothalamic tracts as a method of pain control.

In an adaptation, the needle is advanced only into the subarachnoid space for the collection of CSF.[6132]

lateral epicondylitis   (tennis elbow) A common syndrome of adults characterized by pain in the region of the lateral epicondyle, which is exacerbated by gripping with the hand (and perhaps caused by overuse of that function in the arm), and associated with tenderness over the origin of the extensor carpi radialis brevis at the lateral humeral epicondyle.

The **forced elbow extension test** result is usually positive.[5799]

lateral femoral cutaneous nerve   An independent branch of the lumbar plexus, this long nerve runs into the thigh, passing beneath the lateral part of the inguinal ligament. There, it may be entrapped by the ligament itself or by a pad of fat beneath it, leading to complaints of pain and numbness in its distribution, which is equivalent to an area about the size of a hand located on the lateral part of the thigh. The precise diagnosis is occasionally aided by nerve conduction studies. Decompression of the nerve may relieve symptoms in such cases.

lateral femoral cutaneous neuropathy   See **meralgia paresthetica.**

lateral foot reflex   (von Monakow reflex) Eversion of the foot in response to light stroking of the lateral edge of the sole, seen in patients with pyramidal lesions.

lateral hamstring reflex   See **external hamstring reflex.**

lateral hypothalamic syndrome   A rare syndrome characterized by loss of appetite amounting to aphagia, resulting from lesions of the lateral hypothalamus.

lateral inferior pontine syndrome   Deafness, facial palsy, homolateral facial numbness, and cerebellar ataxia, usually due to a small pontine vascular lesion.

lateral medullary nystagmus   See **Bruns nystagmus.**

lateral medullary syndrome   (Wallenberg syndrome, lateral bulbar syndrome, syndrome of the posterior inferior cerebellar artery) The syndrome resulting from occlusion of the vertebral artery or of its branch, the posterior inferior cerebellar artery, and manifested by acute vertigo, vomiting, hiccups, dysarthria, dysphagia and dysphonia, homolateral cerebellar ataxia, Horner syndrome, and alternating thermoanalgesia (loss of temperature and pinprick sensation on the same side of the face and on the trunk and limbs on the opposite side).

The syndrome was described in full detail by **Wallenberg** in 1895,[5816] who encountered it in a young man who perhaps had herpetic angiitis when he was first seen but whose arteries were severely and generally diseased when Wallenberg performed the autopsy 4 years later, at which time the stenoses of the posterior inferior cerebellar arteries confirmed his predictions.

The classic syndrome is of inestimable value to teachers of neurology because of the precise clinicopathological correlations which it allows,[1225] but it may also occur as a **lacunar syndrome.**[1853,1867] Further downward extension results in the **Opalski syndrome.**

In a variant form, *face-arm-trunk-leg sensory loss* occurs on the contralateral side.[5788]

lateral plantar neuropathy   Damage to this nerve within or just distal to the tarsal tunnel, producing pain and numbness of the lateral plantar surface of the foot. See also **tarsal tunnel syndrome.**[4216]

lateral pontomedullary syndrome   A lacunar syndrome with features resembling the **lateral medullary** or **Foville syndromes.** Clinically, it is characterized by vertigo, vomiting, facial weakness, dysarthria, dysphagia, tinnitus, ataxia, nystagmus, **Horner syndrome,** and **alternating thermoanalgesia.**[1853,4381,4434]

The usual pathology is a small occlusion of one of the short circumferential branches of the vertebral artery, but the same features may also occur as a result of local compression or infiltration. See also **lower basilar branch occlusion.**

lateral temporal seizures   Simple seizures characterized by auditory hallucinations or illusions or dreamy states, visual misperceptions, or language disorders in the case of a language-dominant hemisphere focus. These may progress to complex partial seizures if propagation to mesial temporal or extratemporal structures occurs. The scalp EEG shows unilateral or bilateral midtemporal or posterior temporal spikes that are most prominent in the lateral derivations.[1114]

An autosomal dominantly inherited form is described with onset in youth or young adult life of visual and auditory hallucinations and a benign course. Linkage to chromosome 10q has been shown.[4513]

lateral transtentorial herniation   See **uncal herniation.**

lateralization   1. Specialization of cerebral function within one or other hemisphere. 2. Localization of disease to one or other part of the neuraxis.

The concept that there was specialization in the function of one hemisphere was introduced by Dax in 1836, countering the older idea of organic duality with functional unity, but it was Broca who developed the idea to the point of effective proof, leading to his dictum that we speak with the left hemisphere. **Hughlings-Jackson** took the hypothesis on to the next stage; if the left hemisphere is specialized for speech, what is the special function of the right hemisphere?

Geschwind and Galaburda showed that cerebral dominance is founded on asymmetries of structure for speech, particularly of the posterior part of the superior temporal gyrus—the planum temporale.[2083]

A test for determining the side of a brain lesion was suggested by Heimburger and Reitan;[2521] the subject is asked to copy a square, a Greek cross and a triangle, to name each of the figures, to spell each name, and to repeat the phrase "He shouted the warning".

lateralized   Involving mainly the right or the left side of the body.

laterocollis   A focal dystonia characterized by sustained involuntary contractions of the neck muscles, which result in abnormal lateral flexion of the head on the neck. See **cervical dystonia.**

lateropulsion   (Lat, to the side + to push) Involuntary drawing of the body or veering of the gait toward one side; a characteristic sign after cerebellar or lateral medullary infarction.[1441]

Latham-Munro disease   A recessively inherited syndrome consisting of congenital deafness and both myoclonic and grand mal epilepsy.[3289]

lathyrism   (from Gr, the vetch) An ancient neurodegenerative syndrome seen mostly in males on the Indian subcontinent, who develop subacutely progressing muscle cramps, paresthesias, urgency and frequency of micturition, and nocturnal erections and ejaculations proceeding to pyramidal weakness and spasticity following chronic consumption of the seeds of the chickling or grass pea (*Lathyrus sativus*) in times of war, famine, or pestilence. This substance contains an excitotoxic amino acid (B(n)oxalyl aminoalanine) that may be responsible for causing this **central-distal axonopathy.**[3506,3900] Little or no recovery occurs. See also **epidemic spastic paraplegia.**

latissimus dorsi reflex   A tap on the examiner's finger placed on the tendon of the muscle (which forms the posterior wall of the axilla) leads to its contraction, causing adduction and internal rotation of the shoulder. The maneuver informs (a little) about the status of the C6, 7, 8 reflex arcs.

laughing death   (kuru) See **Lytico-Bodig.**

Launois syndrome   See **pituitary gigantism.**

Launois-Bensaude syndrome   See **familial multiple symmetrical lipomatosis with peripheral neuropathy.**

Laurence, John Zachary   (1828–1870) English ophthalmologist who was a founder of the Royal Eye Hospital and editor of the first journal of ophthalmology published in English.

Laurence-Moon-Biedl syndrome   A recessively inherited diffuse encephalopathy, characterized by the combination of obesity, spastic paraparesis, mental deficiency, pigmentary retinal degeneration with severe rod degeneration leading to blindness, and renal anomalies suggesting abnormal maturation.[3291] Polydactyly is unusual in this form of the disorder, but is common in the variant **Bardet-Biedl syndrome.**[2456]

The first description (by Laurence and Moon) was in 1866,[3291] Bardet's report appearing in 1920.[346] R.C. Moon (1844–1914) was an American ophthalmologist and A. Biedl (1869–1933), a Czech physician.

law of denervation   See **Cannon's law.**

law of dynamic polarity   The observation (of Ramon y **Cajal**) that the nerve impulse passes from the dendrite through the cell body to the axon.

law of motor correspondence   See **Hering law.**

law of reciprocal innervation   Agonist and antagonist muscles do not normally contract against each other (Sir Charles **Sherrington**).

law of regression   see **Ribot law.**

law of specific nerve energies The concept of Johannes Müller (1838) that there is an intrinsic difference between the nervous mechanisms subserving the five senses, such that the same stimulus applied to different nerves would evoke different sensations. Thus, different nerve fibers subserving, for example, touch, cold, and tickle would exist. This "specific fiber" theory has now given way to the "pattern" theory.

Lawford syndrome A variant of **Sturge-Weber syndrome** in which glaucoma occurs without any increase in the volume of the globe.[3297]

Laxova syndrome A lethal, congenital, recessively-inherited dysmorphic syndrome manifesting also strabismus, seizures, microcephaly, lissencephaly, muscle atrophy, tremor, syndactyly, and mental and developmental delay. Agenesis of the corpus callosum may also be present.[3300] See **Neu-Laxova syndrome.**

lazaroids Cytoprotective steroid derivatives, of possible value in patients with cerebral ischemia or with physical or chemical injury of the brain.

Lazarus complex A term applied by Thomas Hackett in 1972 to those symptoms affecting the survivors of cardiac arrest who have, as it were, been "raised from the dead." These include anxiety, depression, nightmares, insomnia, a sense of alienation, and occasionally a delusional state.

Such symptoms usually occur as a result of anoxic brain damage, but are nevertheless based on the normal mental mechanisms of denial and isolation (inhibition) of the affective response, projection, and displacement.

Lazarus movements (Lazarus sign) A Moro-like automatism comprising spontaneous flexion of the arms, occurring (rarely) in brain-dead people, perhaps as a result of spontaneous discharge of cervical motor neurons.[4766]

le main en griffe See **claw hand.**

le pied en griffe See **claw foot.**

lead colic Cramping abdominal pains as a result of lead poisoning, best described by George Baker (1722–1809), who realized that the lead was coming from the glaze inside the cider presses used in his Devonshire village.

lead encephalopathy A syndrome of headache, irritability, tremulousness, and giddiness, progressing to seizures, raised intracranial pressure, stupor, and coma, and due to lead poisoning.

lead hyperesthesia Excessive hyperexcitability of the sensory nerves giving rise to paroxysmal pain, as a result of lead poisoning. *Lead neuralgia* has the same meaning.

lead neuralgia See **lead hyperesthesia.**

lead palsy A focal motor neuropathy most prone to affect the radial nerve, first described by Thomas Cadwalader (1708–1779), an American physician. Benjamin Franklin later showed that the lead had come from the pipes leading off the distillate (Jamaica rum), a favored beverage of New Englanders at that time. Mild sensory and autonomic symptoms may also occur. The pathophysiology may involve the precipitation of lead-induced porphyria.[4838] See also **Remak paralysis.**

lead pipe rigidity A type of increase in muscle tone in which the resistance of the patient's limb is constant in magnitude throughout the range of passive excursion. In keeping with modern advances in plumbing technology, the term *plastic rigidity* is nowadays often substituted.

lean spastic dwarfism See **Coffin syndrome.**

Leao, Aristide A contemporary Brazilian neurophysiologist.

leaping ague See **dancing mania.**

learning 1. The modification of thought, feeling, or action as a result of experience. 2. The body of (usually considered exceptional) knowledge possessed by an individual.

Learning Disabilities Association of America A charitable association in this field. Address: 4156 Library Rd., Pittsburgh, PA 15234. Tel: 412-341-1515.

Learning Disabilities Association of Canada A charitable organization. Address: 323 Chapel St., Ottawa, Ontario K1N 7Z2, Canada.

Leber congenital amaurosis (hereditary retinal aplasia, retinal abiotrophy) A recessively inherited congenital syndrome of near-blindness due to abnormalities of the retinal photoreceptors, with absent electroretinographic potentials.

The clinical features include pendular nystagmus, photophobia, pigmentary retinal degeneration, optic atrophy, chorioretinitis, keratoconus, and cataract. Multiple renal cysts, intellectual failure, seizures, hypotonia, morphological abnormalities of muscle, and deafness have been recorded in some cases.[3312,4029] These features resemble those of **neuronal ceroid lipofuscinosis.**[4450]

In a *variant* form, diffuse CNS demyelination is associated and the affected individuals show psychomotor retardation.[1221]

Leber disease, dystonia, and basal ganglia low densities See **hereditary spastic dystonia.**

Leber miliary aneurysms Telangiectasia and varicosity of the retinal capillaries, which become unusually permeable as a result. This may represent the pathological basis of **Coats disease.**

Leber optic atrophy (Leber hereditary optic neuropathy) An acute, sequentially bilateral optic neuropathy causing painless permanent visual loss and occurring mainly in young males (>80%) over the age of

10; women are affected much less frequently. The condition affects the second eye within 3 months. Pseudoedema of the retinal nerve fiber layer, peripapillary microangiopathy, and tortuosity of the retinal vessels are characteristic signs. There is an absence of peripapillary staining on fluorescein retinal angiography.

Though familial and following a transmission pattern resembling that of X-linked recessive disorders, being maternally transmitted, this transmission does not follow the usual Mendelian principles[3304,3310] and it is a **mitochondrial encephalopathy,** usually resulting from point mutations at 11778, 3460, or 14484 in the mitochondrial genome.[4709] It is considered to reflect both this abnormality of respiratory chain enzymes and also the operation of an exogenous factor. The diagnosis is proven by mtDNA analysis. In the typical form, the triad listed above is present.

In *variant* forms the clinical presentation is compatible with Leber disease but the microangiopathy is not seen in the subject (although it may be present in family members).[3470] Other evidence of neurological disease (such as headaches, emotional instability, myoclonic and other seizures, mental retardation, tremor, dystonia, hypotonia, peripheral neuropathy, or pyramidal signs), cardiac arrhythmias, or **broad band** disease may also be present (*Leber-plus syndrome).*[4028,4139] Similar but mitochondrial damage is likely to be responsible for **Cuban optic neuropathy, tobacco-alcohol amblyopia,** and certain toxic optic neuropathies.

Theodor Leber

Leber, Theodor Karl Gustav von   (1840–1917) German ophthalmologist, who graduated from Heidelberg University and trained further in France and Germany. He was elected professor of ophthalmology at Göttingen and then Heidelberg University where he remained for the rest of his life, describing the hereditary optic neuropathy named for him in 1871. He first proposed the term *tapetoretinal degenerations.*

Leeuwenhoek, Antonius van   (1632–1723) Dutch draper and biologist, the first to describe the striations in muscle and the sarcolemma as well as spermatozoa and many other structures, based on his observations made with the microscope,[5735a] for which he was elected a corresponding Fellow of the Royal Society.

He also described respiratory myoclonus (**diaphragmatic flutter**) as the cause of paroxysms of epigastric pulsation and dyspnea in himself, differentiating the problem from one of cardiac origin, as his diaphragmatic contractions were not in time with his pulse.

left-handedness   (sinistrality) A preference for using the left side of the body for performing fine motor tasks such as writing, using scissors, a knife, or a sporting implement. It occurs in some 10% of the population, and more often in males. Left-eyedness also occurs.

Except for the nuisance value of being left-handed in a world run mainly by and for right-handers, there is little that is negative about the preference, although there is a statistical excess of subjects with autism, stuttering, dyslexia, migraine, allergies, and immune diseases in a population of strong sinistrals.

A major review of cerebral lateralization and hypotheses about its nature was presented in the last paper of Norman **Geschwind.**[2083]

left-right confusion   Impairment of the ability to differentiate the two sides, usually as a result of right parietal lobe disease. See **Gerstmann syndrome.**

left-sided syndrome   1. Weakness of the left arm and leg (but of the right side of the face), left optic atrophy, loss of auscultatory blood pressure in the left arm, and staggering gait with a tendency to fall to the left, all occurring in the presence of renal failure and generalized atherosclerosis.[5880]

2. The complaint of both positive and negative painless sensory symptoms, felt on the left side of the body (face, neck, and arm more than leg) mainly by females, in whom no objective physical signs can be found and no underlying structural pathology demonstrated.[5325] In some cases, anxiety with hyperventilation appears relevant in causation, but the phenomenon of unilateral *right*-sided symptoms being nearly 10 times less likely to occur than those on the left is unexplained.[4820]

leg jerks   See **periodic limb movement disorder.**

leg phenomenon   See **Pool-Schlesinger sign.**

leg sign   (Barré sign) With the patient prone, the knees are flexed so that the lower leg is vertical. Return of a leg to the extended position (on the bed) suggests the presence of a pyramidal lesion (but also argues in favor of gravity).

Legallois, Julien-Jean-César   (1770–1814) French physiologist, notable for his isolation of the medullary respiratory center and for demonstrating neurogenic influences on the heart.

Legionnaire disease   A widespread infection by organisms of the class *Legionnairaceae*, most commonly occurring in epidemics and producing mainly respiratory tract disease. The latter is associated with weakness, headache and myalgia, cough, and high fever. Gastrointestinal symptoms are also common. Neurological signs, including emotional lability, confusion, delirium, or CNS depression, occur in about one-third of the cases.

leg-straightening reflex   The legs and body normally straighten when the sole of an infant's foot is pressed onto the surface of the examining table. See also **developmental reflexes.**

Leichtenstern, Otto Michael Ludwig   (1845–1900) German physician in Cologne. He had a particular interest in infectious diseases, but also gave a good account of subacute combined degeneration of the cord in 1884.

Leichtenstern phenomenon   Hyperalgesia when any bone is pressed, found in patients with meningitis.[325]

Leigh disease   (subacute necrotizing encephalomyelopathy) A fatal, recessively inherited mitochondrial disease of infancy or childhood (rarely occurring in adults, in whom the disease may be relatively mild), of unknown cause but with a major biochemical defect in the deficiency of cytochrome-*c* oxidase and thus in the oxidation of pyruvate.[3326] Serum lactate and pyruvate levels may be raised. Abnormalities of the pyruvate dehydrogenase complex and (rarely) of the NADH-Co-Q reductase system have also been described.

Clinically, it is characterized by psychomotor retardation, weakness, hypotonia, feeding difficulties with failure to thrive, and dystonias, seizures, myoclonus, visual deterioration due to optic atrophy, metabolic acidosis with vomiting, tachypnea, apneic spells, reduced consciousness, nystagmus and other ocular signs, pyramidal and cerebellar signs, and hepatomegaly. The eye signs and the histological appearances are similar but not identical to those of **Wernicke disease** and, as in that condition, abnormalities of liver function and of cardiac and skeletal muscle may also be found.[2149,5726] However, the response to vitamin B therapy is usually disappointing.

Dr. A. Denis Leigh (1915–1998) was a consultant psychiatrist at Bethlem-Maudsley Hospital in London. The following *variants* have been identified:

See **Alpers disease.** The differentiation of this condition from Leigh disease is uncertain.

Acute neonatal Leigh disease A fatal recessively inherited syndrome with rapid progression, characterized by hypotonia, acidosis, and cardiomyopathy with sudanophilic leukoencephalopathy.[5056]

Juvenile Leigh disease A sporadic syndrome of adolescence characterized by weakness, exercise intolerance with dys-

pnea, parkinsonism, pyramidal and cerebellar signs, and dementia. [5726]

Adult Leigh disease A sporadic pleomorphic condition, usually diagnosed initially as multiple sclerosis but with no MRI abnormalities in the initial stages, despite clinical evidence of brainstem involvement (respiratory failure, nystagmus, oculomotor palsies, palatal myoclonus, reticular myoclonus, etc.), visual failure, ataxia, and spasticity. Coma and paroxysmal brainstem failure with apnea may occur.[2262]

leiodystonia   A chronic but intermittent disturbance of regulation of the autonomic nervous system manifesting as hypotension, pallor, dilated pupils, perspiration, and impotence, described in the 1930s in Europeans living in the tropics and probably representing a combination of dehydration and depression.[4314,4314a]

leiomyoma   (Gr, smooth + muscle + tumor) A benign tumor of unstriated muscle, as in the uterus or prostate gland.

Leishmaniasis   (kala-azar) Infection with *Leishmania donovani*, resulting from the bite of a sandfly and causing a parasitic reticuloendotheliosis. Peripheral neuropathy is a complication, perhaps reflecting the nutritional deficiency that results from anorexia in this condition.[5067]

Leiter International Scale   (Arthur adaptation) A nonverbal test of cognitive ability, used in children and young people.

leitungaphasie   See **conduction aphasia.**

Lejeune disease   See **cri du chat syndrome.**

Lejonne-Lhermitte disease   (olivo-rubro-cerebellar atrophy) A syndrome of adult onset, characterized by atrophy and gliosis of the olives, cerebellar cortex, dentate nucleus, and both superior and inferior cerebellar peduncles.[3336]

Lemierre, André-Alfred   (1875–1956) French physician in Paris, who specialized in infectious diseases.

Lemierre-Boltanski-Justin-Besançon syndrome   (tuberculous alcoholic polyneuritis) Regarded by the original authors as a specific variety of polyneuropathy with twin etiologies, it seems likely that this condition represents the occurrence of both polyneuropathy and tuberculosis as complications of alcoholic malnutrition, although it is singular that the cases reported initially were all in relatively young women with marked cachexia, cirrhosis, and miliary tuberculosis. The condition is not now reported from the Western world.[3339]

Lemieux-Neemeh syndrome   A congenital syndrome, perhaps recessively transmitted, manifesting sensorineural deafness, nephropathy, and sensorimotor neuropathy, resembling **hereditary motor and sensory neuropathy.**[3340]

lemniscal system   (from Gr, bandage or woolen strand) One of two somatosensory systems (the other is the **spinothalamic**) comprising the ascending fiber pathway, which transmits tactile and kinesthetic impulses from the large myelinated fibers in the peripheral nerves and posterior columns to the medullary gracile and cuneate nuclei, from which second-order afferents arise that decussate and pass to the ventrobasal thalamic nuclei. Nerve cells from here project to the primary somatosensory area of the postcentral cortex.

The system is highly adaptive, rapidly conducting, and mode- and place-specific, and appears to provide the anatomical base for the discriminative and localizing functions of the nervous system.

LEMS See **Lambert-Eaton myasthenic syndrome.**

lengthening reaction 1. When a tonic muscle is stretched, it assumes, by virtue of its proprioceptive arc, a new tonic length which is approximately that to which it has been stretched.[5120]

2. **Sherrington** later wrote that in trying to bend the knee of a decerebrate animal, "the attempt causes further accentuation of the stretch reflex in muscles which are already highly responsive to stretching. If the attempt to flex the joint is maintained, there comes a point and time at which the muscle suddenly gives way and allows any degree of flexion to be imposed on it (the **clasp-knife** reaction). This is the lengthening reaction and it marks the partial or total abolition of the stretch reflex."[4567]

Lennox disease See **Lennox-Gastaut syndrome.**

Lennox, William Gordon (1884–1960) American humanitarian, clinical neurophysiologist, and epileptologist who trained at Harvard and, after a period spent in China, at the Rockefeller Medical School. After satisfying in part his missionary zeal, he returned to Harvard and began his lifelong studies of the cerebral circulation and later, the nature and treatment of the epilepsies.

He collaborated during the long period of his research output with Stanley Cobb, H.G. Wolff, F.A. and E.L. Gibbs, and others. Prominent among the studies completed and published as a long series of papers was his investigation of the electrical activity of the brain, using the newly introduced EEG. His major book *Epilepsy and Related Disorders* (written with his daughter, Dr. Margaret Lennox-Buchthal) was immediately hailed as a classic.

In addition to his important laboratory studies, he built up a major epilepsy service and taught widely on all aspects of epilepsy, not the least being the importance of education of the patient, the family, and the community.

Lennox-Gastaut syndrome (severe myokinetic epilepsy of childhood with slow spike and wave, childhood encephalopathy with diffuse slow spike–waves, Lennox syndrome, minor motor seizures, myoclonic-astatic seizures)[1] A polioencephalopathy characterized by the association of slow spike–wave activity in the EEG, mental retardation, and various types of intractable seizure (including tonic-axial, absence, atonic, myoclonic, and generalized tonic-clonic seizures) in children aged 1–8 years. The seizure frequency is high, and status epilepticus is frequent (stuporous states with myoclonic, tonic, and atonic seizures).[3345]

The EEG usually shows abnormal background activity, slow spike–waves (1–2.5 Hz), and often multifocal abnormalities. During sleep, bursts of fast rhythms appear. Seizures are difficult to control, and their development is mostly unfavorable. In 60% of the cases, the syndrome occurs in children suffering from a previous encephalopathy, but is primary in other cases. (From the revised ILAE Classification,[1114] reproduced by kind permission of Blackwell Science.)

Known causes are metabolic and dysgenetic, and many peri- or postnatal acquired disorders can also precipitate the syndrome.[1236]

The term is widely used to refer to a number of conditions, indicating that the precise delineation of the syndrome has not yet been achieved.

1. A syndrome of epilepsy in childhood accompanied by diffuse, slow spike-wave patterns on the EEG (see above). In this childhood epileptic encephalopathy there are diffuse, interictal, slow spike–wave complexes and multiple seizures including tonic seizures as well as atonic and myoclonic attacks, atypical absences, and even absence, tonic, or myoclonic status. The classic EEG feature is a diffuse, slow spike–wave pattern originally described as a "petit mal variant." Secondary or symptomatic forms of the syndrome are common. Aicardi defines the syndrome as one limited to those cases characterized clinically by brief tonic and atonic seizures and atypical absences as the predominant types of attacks and from the EEG viewpoint by at least some 2-Hz (slow) diffuse spike–wave activity. Myoclonic seizures may also occur, as may 3-Hz (fast) spike–wave activity.[56] 2. **Myoclonic epilepsies.** 3. An epileptic syndrome secondary to diffuse or mild focal brain damage and characterized by astatic and myoclonic seizures, mental retardation, the presence of neurological signs, and, in most cases, neuroradiological abnormalities.

In the *myoclonic variant*, the frequency and intensity of the myoclonic jerks are both unusually high. The EEG is typical except that it is activated by overbreathing.[56]

Lenoble-Aubineau syndrome (nystagmus-myoclonus syndrome) An X-linked, congenital, nonprogressive syndrome of nystagmus with myoclonic contractions of the extraocular and limb muscles occurring in response to cold and muscle percussion. Pigmentary retinopathy, tremor of the head and arms, muscle fasciculations, hyperactive reflexes, and vasomotor disturbances made worse by cold are also described.

The syndrome was described first in 1898 in the residents of Brittany[3346] and appears to be confined to Breton and British Celts.

lenticular, lenticulate   (from Lat, a lens or a lentil)

lentiginosis-deafness-cardiopathy syndrome   See **LEOPARD syndrome.**

Lenz micropthalmia syndrome   An X-linked recessive or autosomal dominant syndrome characterized by micropthalmia; skeletal abnormalities of the hands; renal, genital, and dental abnormalities; and mental retardation with microcephaly.[3347]

Lenz-Majewski syndrome   (hyperostotic dwarfism) A congenital dysmorphic syndrome manifesting also short stature, polysyndactyly, dental and dermal abnormalities, delayed closure of the fontanelles, a thick calvarium, sclerosis of the skull, osteoporosis, and spasticity.[3582]

Leonardo da Vinci   (1452–1519) Italian artist, anatomist, and scientist. A brilliant contributor in many areas of science, art, and medicine. He himself dissected corpses and was probably the illustrator for Vesalius. In these pictures, he published many structures that others proclaimed in prose only centuries later.

There is dispute as to his handedness, some suggesting that he was left-handed, others that he only used the left hand after he suffered a right hemiparesis.

Leonhard syndrome   An acquired syndrome characterized by a disturbance in the sense of time, constructional apraxia, dysgraphia, and dyscalculia.[1177,3350]

leontiasis ossea   Bilateral hypertrophy of the bones of the cranial vault, leading to a lion-like appearance; first described by Marcello Malpighi (1628–1694), an Italian anatomist.

LEOPARD syndrome   (dominant lentigines and congenital deafness, lentiginosis-deafness-cardiomyopathy syndrome) A dominantly inherited neurocutaneous syndrome consisting of multiple **L**entigines over the entire body, **E**lectrocardiographic conduction defects (due to hypertrophic cardiomyopathy), **O**cular hypertelorism giving a triangular shape to the face, **P**ulmonary stenosis, **A**bnormal genitalia, growth **R**etardation, and severe congenital neural **D**eafness with normal vestibular function.[2217] Scoliosis, spina bifida, dwarfism, and scapular winging are also described inconsistently. See **multiple lentigenes syndrome.**

leprechaunism   See **Donohue syndrome.**

lepromatous leprosy   (nodular leprosy, cutaneous leprosy) That form of the disease in which the bacterial proliferation in the skin and peripheral nervous system proceed unabated, leading to multiple mononeuropathies, the nerve territories involved being those in the distal, cooler parts of the body, where the skin nodules and macules are most abundant.

The clinical features include those of a predominantly thin-fiber hypertrophic neuropathy with patchy sensory loss that eventually becomes confluent; mutilating acropathy; Charcot joints, and autonomic involvement.[4863]

leprosy   (from Gr, scaly) (Hansen disease, elephantiasis anesthetica, Kustha) A mildly contagious disease with a long incubation period, caused by infection with the *Mycobacterium leprae* (Hansen bacillus), which has an affinity for cells originating from the neural crest. **Tuberculoid, lepromatous, dimorphous,** and **indeterminate** forms are described.

Leprosy was Hippocrates' name for psoriasis; later what we know today as leprosy was called *leontiasis* by Arateus of Cappadocia, while Lucretius and Celsus called it *elephantiasis*.[5204] *Kushtha* (in the Indian Vedas manuscripts of 1300 B.C.) was probably the same disease, but English biblical translators, using Arabian medical texts as well as Hebrew sources, rendered the Hebrew word *tsara'ath* ("zaraath"), meaning any variety of skin disease requiring separation from the tribe, as *leprosy*, which led to use of the term for **Hansen disease,**[2417] the leprosy we recognize. There is good evidence that syphilis, not leprosy, was a more likely cause of the contagions referred to in Mosaic texts. [EWM]

This age-old condition was known in India at least 2500 years ago but was also found throughout Europe at least since the return to the Mediterranean shores of Alexander the Great. While it was taught that this was the most common cause of neuropathy worldwide, limited control of the disease has meant that diabetes is now likely to be more prevalent as a cause. The various forms of leprosy are listed in Chart L–3.

Chart L–3. The Forms of Leprosy

The *tuberculoid* form indicates the presence of increased resistance, as is seen mainly in African patients, in whom classically there are a few asymmetrical lesions, the skin is dry, scaly, and anesthetic in places, and there is evidence of a thin-fiber neuropathy in such areas. The lepromin test result is strongly positive, and the nerves are enlarged and granulomatous. Acid-fast bacilli are not found.

In an *intermediate form (BT type)*, the clinical features are the same, but the number of lesions is markedly increased and there is more scaling induration of the skin and less evidence of neuropathy and sensory loss.

In the second major form (*borderline, intermediate dimorphic, or BB type*), the skin lesions consist of rounded red papules that are not anesthetic. Intermediate between this and the third major form is a type characterized by the presence of macular, papular, or nodular lesions that are asymmetrical (BL type), and which contain substantial numbers of acid-fast bacilli.

In the third major *lepromatous* form (LL type), there is decreased resistance or even no resistance to the acid-fast bacilli. The lepromin test result is negative and mycobacteria are abundant.

In a diffuse *variant*, the whole skin is thickened; this has given rise to the name *pretty leprosy* as facial wrinkles are abolished; and in a nodular lepromatous form, nodules form plaques in the skin in all regions, although less on the scalp and in the axillae and groins. A late finding in this form is the presence of generalized symmetrical polyneuropathy.

In a variant form (*neural leprosy*) only the nerves are involved and the skin is unaffected; however, anesthetic patches are detected, mainly distally and in the colder acral parts. Dementia is a rare complication. See also **mutilating acropathy, ocular leprosy.**

leptocephaly (from Gr, thin + head) A malformation due to premature fusion of the anterior fontanelle and the metopic suture, leading to elongation of the skull and narrowing of the forehead.[4]

leptomeningeal cyst See **arachnoid diverticula.**

leptomeningeal glioneuronal heterotopias Irregular nodules of glial tissue, sometimes containing neurons, budding from the pial surface, or forming nests within the leptomeninges.[417]

leptomeninges (Gr, thin + membrane) The pia and arachnoid—the delicate as opposed to the coarse (dural) meninges.

leptomeningitis Inflammation of the arachnoid and pia mater. Although the term was originally used to refer to inflammation of these thinner meninges, it has now been replaced by the simpler **meningitis** to embrace all forms of infection of the meninges.

Léri, André (1875–1930) French physician who trained in Paris and took further training with **Charcot** and **Marie** at the **Salpêtrière.** He practiced in Paris, writing mainly on rheumatic and neurological topics.

André Léri

Léri reflex See **Léri sign.**

Léri sign (Léri reflex) Flexion of the elbow of the patient's relaxed arm in response to forceful and painful passive flexion of the fingers and hand on that side; it is said to be increased in subjects with lesions of the pyramidal tracts or of the frontal lobes.[3353] The difference between this and the **bending reflex** is not easy to appreciate.

Léri syndrome (pleonosteosis) A dominantly inherited congenital osteodystrophy with premature ossification of the epiphyses, leading to dwarfism, corneal opacities, and cataract, and often compression of the median nerve in the carpal tunnel.[5139]

Lériche syndrome Occlusion of the aorta or iliac arteries causing ischemic pain in the buttocks and legs, as well as, variably, either **impotence** or **priapism.**[3354]

Lermoyez, M. (1858–1929) French otolaryngologist.

Lermoyez syndrome Tinnitus, nausea, vomiting, and deafness with temporary improvement in hearing after the onset of vertigo. The attacks complicate a condition of gradually increasing deafness, as in **Ménière syndrome,** but generally occur in younger adults.[3357]

Leroy, Raoul (b. 1868) French psychiatrist.

Leroy syndrome (lilliputian hallucinosis) The perception of hallucinations of small people, animals, etc., against a background of normal size. The phenomenon thus differs from **micropsia,** in which everything is seen in miniature.

The occurrence of such hallucinations was recorded by Macarius in *The Lives of the Saints* (fourth century A.D.), who dismissed them with the words, "Arise, Oh Lord, that your enemies might be dispersed, that they may flee before Thy face; for our soul is full of illusions."[5047] From then on they were usually documented in religious mystics or in those suffering from systemic infections or toxic exposure such as to ether, hashish, cocaine, hyoscine, or caffeine. Organic brain diseases held responsible have been many and various—**general paralysis of the insane,** seizures, temporoparietal tumors, and lobar hematomas, for example—and these hallucinations have also been reported in dementing states and in schizophrenia.

Finally, they have also been recorded in healthy people, including Ben Jonson (the playwright), who regarded them as products of his "overheated imagination."

Les Turner ALS Foundation, Ltd. A charitable organization. Address: 8142 N. Lawndale Ave., 60076–3322. Tel: 847–679–3311, 888–ALS-1107.

Lesch-Nyhan syndrome A congenital X-linked recessive syndrome with the abnormal locus situated at chromosome Xq26, characterized clinically by choreic, dystonic, and athetoid movements, pyramidal signs, hyperuricemia with urinary stone formation, mental retardation, and compulsive self-destructive behavior such as biting the lips, cheeks, and fingers. Deficiency of hypoxanthine-guanine phosphoribosyl-transferase[3359] and low levels of immunoglobulin E are commonly found.[3447]

lethal catatonia   A rare syndrome resembling the **neuroleptic malignant syndrome,** characterized by prolonged mental and physical excitement and agitation leading on to stupor and hypotension with muscle rigidity, hyperpyrexia, increased serum creatine kinase levels, and death.

The autonomic features and abnormal movements characteristic of the neuroleptic malignant syndrome are not seen in this condition.[3592]

lethal multiple pterygium syndrome   A congenital, recessively inherited dysmorphic syndrome characterized by low birth weight, dwarfism, hypertelorism, cleft upper lip and palate, webbed neck often with a cystic hygroma, fusion of vertebrae, hydranencephaly, congenital hernia of the diaphragm, congenital cardiac anomalies, lung hypoplasia, webbing of the elbows and knees, radioulnar synostosis, symphalangism of the fingers, and neurogenic muscle weakness.[3723]

lethargic encephalitis   See **encephalitis lethargica.**

lethargy   (Gr, forgetful) The ancient meaning has given way to that of a state of drowsy inertia.

letter fluency test   A test of language in which subjects are asked to name verbally as many words beginning with the letters *F*, *A*, and *S* as they can within 1 minute, proper names and different forms of the same word being disallowed.[2418] See also **category fluency test.**

Letterer-Siwe histiocytosis   A diffuse encephalopathy of infants, who also manifest osteolytic bone lesions, hepatosplenomegaly, a reduction in all blood cell types with hemorrhage, and skin infiltration. The condition is a disseminated form of histiocytosis.

Lettsom, John Coakley   (1744–1815) A popular and successful English Quaker physician working in the Virgin Islands, where he was the first to describe alcoholic peripheral neuropathy.[2995] He later returned to practice in London, where he also probably became aware of **delirium tremens** and of the **Wernicke-Korsakoff** syndrome.

leucine encephalin   An opioid peptide in the brain with a role in the mediation of pain perception.

leukemia   A systemic hematological malignancy with neurological complications including intracerebral hemorrhages, the accumulation of leukemic cells within the brain, **progressive multifocal leukoencephalopathy,** and infiltration of the meninges.

leukoaraiosis   (from Gr, white + rarefied) A modern descriptive term for the presence of lucencies (patchy diffuse areas of low attenuation) in the deep white matter surrounding the frontal and occipital horns and in the centrum semiovale, as seen on CT scans.[2358]

It is clinically associated with advancing age, a history of hypertension, motor weakness, upgoing plantar responses, and signs of the multi-infarct rather than of the Alzheimer type of dementia.

leukocytoclastic angiitis   See **Churg-Strauss syndrome.**

leukodystrophies   A group of genetically determined degenerative disorders selectively affecting the myelin of the cerebral or peripheral nervous system. At least 10 separate disorders and their subgroups were classified by Baraitser.[335] Some additions are made in Chart L–4.

Chart L–4. The Leukodystrophies

Aicardi-Goutières syndrome
Alexander disease

X-linked Forms

Adrenoleukodystrophies
   Adrenoleukomyeloneuropathies
   Infantile sudanophilic leukodystrophy
Cerebrotendinous xanthomatosis
Cockayne syndrome
18q syndrome

Glial or Glioneuronal Degenerations

Alpers disease
Canavan disease
Glioneuronal degeneration
Globoid-cell leukodystrophy   (Krabbe disease)
Infantile neuroaxonal dystrophy
Leigh disease
Martha-Alma (Hallervorden-Spatz) disease
Menkes disease
Metachromatic leukodystrophy
Multiple sulfatidase deficiency   (Austin disease)
Pelizaeus-Merzbacher disease
Polycystic lipomembranous osteodysplasia with sclerosing leukoencephalopathy
Reye syndrome
Sjogren-Larsson syndrome

Orphan Genetic Leukodystrophies

Adult-onset autosomal dominant leukodystrophy
Vacuolating megalencephalic leukodystrophy
Fatal infantile leukoencephalopathy (CACN, vanishing white matter disease)
Dominantly inherited leukodystrophy with cerebellar deficits and spastic paraparesis

Modified from Baraitser 1990[335] and Berger et al. (2001).[493]

leukodystrophy, cerebellar deficits, and spastic paraparesis   A dominantly inherited disorder with onset in early childhood characterized by progressive spastic paraparesis, cerebellar deficits, and mild mental deterioration, resulting in severe disability in the third to fourth decades of life. Brain MRI shows diffuse white matter involvement but no biochemical or genetic deficits have been determined.[1981]

leukoencephalopathy   Any disease primarily affecting the white matter of the brain. See also **posterior leukoencephalopathy, toxic leukoencephalopathy, hereditary adult-onset leukoencephalopathy.**

leukoencephalopathy with neuroaxonal spheroids A rare, dominantly inherited, progressive, diffuse white matter disorder with onset in adult life, characterized by seizures, evidence of frontal lobe dysfunction, pyramidal signs, ataxia, and mild extrapyramidal signs. The MRI shows cortical atrophy and multifocal white matter changes especially in frontal regions. Biopsy reveals the presence of axonal spheroids in the white matter.[5718]

leukoencephalopathy with ragged red fibers   See **MERRF.**

leukoencephalopathy with vanishing white matter (CACH) A chronic-progressive and episodic disease of childhood and youth, probably recessively-inherited, manifesting episodes of deterioration following infections and minor head traumas that result in unexplained coma. MRI signals from the white matter resemble those of CSF as a result of extensive cystic degeneration of the cerebral white matter, the cortex being preserved.[5719] See **fatal infantile leukoencephalopathy.**

leukoma   A corneal scar.

levator   (from Lat, to lift up) The first name of those muscles elevating, for example, the eyelids, the pelvic floor, and the scapula.

levator dehiscence-disinsertion syndrome   Separation of the levator palpebrae superioris muscle from its origin as a result of inflammation, also described after local surgical procedures and in the elderly; a cause of ptosis.

levels of organization   A concept of Hughlings-**Jackson** whereby he postulated the existence of separate hierarchically ordered brain regions that function together to produce a motor effect. The *highest level* is made up of centers of the prefrontal lobes and governs the most complex movements of all parts of the body from the eyes to the perineum. ("The central nervous system knows nothing of muscles, it only knows movements. . . . There are, shall we say, thirty muscles in the hand, these are represented in the nervous system in thousands of combinations—that is, as very many movements. It is just as many chords, musical expressions and tunes, can be made out of a few notes.") The *second level* is composed of centers of the rolandic region (so-called motor regions of the cerebral cortex) and possibly of the ganglia of the corpus striatum as well. It is responsible for mediating complex movements of all parts of the body from the eyes to the perineum. The *lowest level*, corresponding to the pons, medulla, spinal cord, and motor units, represents the simplest movements of all parts of the body mediated

by a series of lower motor centers.[47,708] In fact, at this last level the CNS structures mainly function as lines of communication.

The analogy of an army is appropriate; at the highest level, the general determines the strategy, namely what is to be accomplished by military means; the staff determine the mechanisms whereby that goal is to be accomplished; and, at the lowest level of organization (corresponding to the motor unit), the soldiers try to do it.

Levic syndrome   See **progressive nuclear ophthalmoplegia syndrome.**

Levin, Max   (b.1901) American neuropsychiatrist, born in Latvia, who graduated from Johns Hopkins University and worked in neurology and psychiatry in Philadelphia and Pittsburg before returning to Johns Hopkins and eventually becoming clinical professor of neurology at the New York Medical College.

He is best remembered for his description of the **Kline-Levin syndrome** in 1936;[3373a] his other publications chiefly focused on toxic psychoses and delirium.

Levine syndrome   See **neuroacanthocytosis.**

Lévy, Gabrielle   (1886–1935) French neurologist who collaborated with Roussy in describing the **Roussy-Lévy syndrome.**

Lewis-Besant dystrophy   A rare congenital muscular dystrophy localized to the diaphragm and pectoralis muscles and leading to early death.[3384]

Lewis-Sumner syndrome   (multifocal acquired demyelinating sensory and motor neuropathy; MADSAM) An immune-mediated form of neuropathy with slow progression presenting with asymmetrical weakness and atrophy and impaired sensation in the distribution of specific peripheral nerves, with evidence of persistent multifocal conduction block over short segments of the affected nerves. Muscle cramps and fasciculations are common complaints.

Whether this condition is the same as or distinct from **multifocal motor neuropathy with conduction block** or **chronic inflammatory demyelinating polyneuropathy** is not resolved.[4347,4917] See also **multifocal inflammatory demyelinating neuropathy.**

Lewy, (Lewey) Fritz Heinrich   (1885–1950) German neuropathologist, neurologist, and psychiatrist who left Germany urgently in 1934 to live in the United States, where he held academic appointments at the University of Pennsylvania.

Lewy bodies   Intracytoplasmic eosinophilic hyaline inclusions staining for ubiquitin, signifying the presence of neuronal injury and found in the cortex, substantia nigra, autonomic nervous system, basal nucleus of Meynert, and brainstem nuclei in patients with **Parkinson disease, Hallervorden-Spatz disease, dopa-responsive dystonia,** idiopathic **diffuse Lewy body disease,** and some other disorders affecting the basal ganglia.[3389]

They are also found in the anterior horn cells in **amyotrophic lateral sclerosis** and have been found in asymptomatic elderly people. The most consistent association is with dementia in patients with Parkinson disease.[2097] Lewy bodies are detected more frequently with increasing age.[2094]

Lewy-body disease   See **diffuse Lewy-body disease.**

lexical agraphia   A form of agraphia marked by the impairment of writing of words but not of speech, of spelling without impairment of phoneme–grapheme conversion, nor of reading. There is thus a specific difficulty in spelling words with irregular phoneme–grapheme transformations. The condition has been reported in the context of a left parieto-occipital lesion.[412]

lexical system   One of two reading method systems (the other being the **phonological system**) in which reading is considered to be performed by lexical or semantic processing. This system is affected when *surface dyslexia* occurs, in which subjects can read pronounceable nonsense words but not orthographically irregular words.

lexicon   The words contained in a language and their semantic definitions.[3505]

Leyden ataxia   See **acute cerebellar ataxia.**

Leyden, Ernst Victor von   (1832–1910) German physician who became professor of medicine at Berlin University after **Frerichs.** He was most successful in his practice, in which he concentrated on tuberculosis and neurological diseases, especially poliomyelitis, tabes, and muscular dystrophy. He also described a form of ataxia (pseudotabes), periodic vomiting, and the following disorders.

Leyden neuritis   (lipomatous neuritis) Neuropathy with fatty replacement of the degenerating nerve fibers. Leyden's paper[3390a] was entitled "On Poliomyelitis and Neuritis" (in German) and this condition may be a variant of that viral motor neuropathy.

Leyden paralysis   1. See **Weber syndrome.** 2. Quadriplegia associated with pontine hemorrhage, described by Leyden in 1875.

Leyden syndrome   (cerebral peduncle syndrome) See **Weber syndrome.**

Leyden-Möbius muscular dystrophy   A recessively inherited muscular dystrophy affecting the pelvic girdle initially and beginning in adult life.[3390] The classification of this among similar syndromes is in flux. See **limb girdle muscular dystrophy.** See also **scapulohumeral dystrophy.**

Lhermitte, Jean-Jacques   (1877–1959) French neurologist who trained in Paris and after graduation became chef de clinique under Raymond at the Salpêtrière. He later emphasized psychiatry in his practice and held the Chair of Mental Diseases at the Hôpi-

tal Ste. Anne. He coined the term **internuclear ophthalmoplegia** (sometimes known as *Lhermitte syndrome*), described the sign described in the next entry and **peduncular hallucinosis,** and made significant contributions to the study of **narcolepsy,**[3395] **encephalitis lethargica,** herpes, neuropathies, **Huntington disease,** sleep, phantom limb, and disturbances of the body image.[1053,5047]

Lhermitte sign   (barber's chair sign) Described in 1924 by Lhermitte (but before him by **Babiński**), this is more properly a symptom, comprising a sensation as of an electric shock or paresthesia that shoots down the back and/or into the limbs when the neck is flexed or with coughing or neck rotation.[3401]

Although Lhermitte regarded the sign as diagnostic of multiple sclerosis, any cervical cord lesion, intrinsic or extrinsic, is capable of inducing it.

Lhermitte syndrome   1. See **peduncular hallucinosis.**[3399] 2. See **internuclear ophthalomoplegia.**

Lhermitte-Cornil-Quesnel syndrome   (progressive pyramidopallidal degeneration) A rare syndrome of slowly progressive degeneration of the pyramidal and pallidal systems, manifest as pathological emotionality, generalized muscle rigidity, pseudobulbar palsy, and parkinsonian signs and chorea. Pathologically, there is cell loss in the basal ganglia and dentate nucleus with calcium deposition.[3397,3400]

Dr. Lucien Cornil (1888–1952) was a French physician who trained in Paris and worked with Roussy and Lhermitte during World War I on spinal cord injuries. He later became professor of experimental medicine at Marseille.

Lhermitte-Duclos disease   (granular cell hypertrophy, cerebrellar hamartoma, dysplastic gangliocytoma of the cerebellum, Purkinjeoma, Cowden disease, diffuse cerebellar cortical hypertrophy) A sporadic or dominantly inherited hamartomatous condition of cerebellar hypertrophy with onset in childhood or adult life, characterized by hypertrophy of the ganglion cells in the granular and molecular layers and excessive myelination of axons in the molecular layer. The gyri are coarse. Whether the condition represents a neoplasm, a malformation, or a hamartoma remains undetermined.

Clinical manifestations include macrocephaly, increased intracranial pressure, and mental and developmental delay.[4291,5769] See also **Cowden disease,** which may indeed be a variant of this condition.

Lhermitte-McAlpine syndrome   A syndrome of gradual onset and slow progression affecting adults and characterized by parkinsonism and choreic movements of the face and bulbar muscles with pseudobulbar and pyramidal signs and marked hypertonia, with only slight weakness. Pathological examination shows lesions in the putamen, globus pallidus, and pyramidal tracts.[3400]

Lichtenstein-Knorr syndrome   A rare, congenital, recessively inherited ataxic syndrome characterized also by progressive deafness and skeletal anomalies.[3403]

Lichtheim aphasia   (subcortical sensory aphasia) A form of expressive dysphasia in which the patient is mute but able to indicate with the fingers the number of syllables in the word the patient would like to utter.[3404]

Lichtheim, Ludwig   (1845–1928) German pathologist and neurologist who graduated from Zurich University and eventually succeeded **Quincke** as professor of medicine at Berne. He later moved to Königsberg.

Lichtheim made important contributions to the study of aphasia, describing subcortical aphasia in 1885, and wrote also on the topics of pseudobulbar palsy, brain tumors, meningitis, the spinal cord in pernicious anemia (once known as *Lichtheim syndrome*), and oculomotor palsies, as well as on general pathology.[5047]

Lichtheim syndrome   See **subacute combined degeneration of the cord**.[3607]

lid apraxia   See **apraxia of eyelid opening**.

lid lag   Abnormal delay in descent of the eyelid when the globe of the eye rotates downwards. This classic sign was described by von **Graefe** in hyperthyroidism. See **Graefe sign**.

lid nystagmus   *Type 1.* Jerky vertical movements of the eyelids, mimicking (but exceeding the amplitude of) an underlying vertical nystagmus.[246] *Type 2.* Rapid, phasic twitches of the eyelids occurring with lateral deviation of the eyes in patients with horizontal jerk nystagmus, as in the **lateral medullary syndrome**. *Type 3.* Similar movements to the last, occurring on convergence in the presence of cerebellar or medullary lesions.[1291,4905] *Type 4.* The association of type 3 lid nystagmus with neck extension movements during attempts at upward gaze.[2133] This is described in the **Miller Fisher syndrome**.

lid retraction   Elevation of the upper lid, giving rise to a staring gaze and occurring in association with the **dorsal midbrain syndrome**. See **Collier sign**.

lid twitch sign   See **Cogan twitch sign**.

Liepmann disease   Motor apraxia; the inability to perform skilled acts in the presence of normal motor power and coordination, differentiated by Liepmann into three varieties: ideational, ideomotor, and limb-kinetic.[3409] See **apraxia**.

Liepmann, Hugo Karl   (1863–1925) German psychiatrist and humanitarian who graduated in philosophy and then in medicine from Berlin University and who then studied further under **Weigert** and **Wernicke**. He directed a mental hospital for some years, then entered private practice, since he was excluded from a chair in psychiatry because of his Jewish heritage.

He showed in 1904 that the left hemisphere is dominant for praxis in right-handed people; other topics on which he contributed were alcoholic delirium, agnosias, and the effects of callosal lesions.

During the final blockade of Germany in 1918, he refused to eat any better than did his patients and as a result lost 60 pounds in weight, but it was his **Parkinson disease** that led him to suicide in 1925.

light blindness   Episodic binocular visual impairment related exclusively to exposure to light. The cause is usually bilateral stenosis or occlusion of the internal carotid arteries that produces a delay in the regeneration of visual pigment in the pigment epithelial layer of the retina.[5960]

light reflex   Constriction of the pupil stimulated by light, the first modern description being that of **Robert Whytt** in 1751.

light sleep stage   Non–rapid eye movement sleep stages 1 and 2.[249]

light stress test   (photostress test) A method of assessing the degree of macular disease as opposed to optic nerve disease, based on the impairment of photochemical processes in the retina as a result of local disease. The function tested is the delay in the regeneration of visual pigment after retinal "bleaching" with the light; optic nerve disease is not associated with any delay in the return of visual acuity in this test.[2134]

The best-corrected vision is assessed in each eye, and then bright light is directed into one eye for 10 sec. The amount of time elapsing before the patient can read one line larger than he could prior to the light stimulation is recorded, and the process is then repeated in the opposite eye. Normally, the recovery takes less than 1 minute (and usually less than 30 seconds) but in the presence of macular disease, recovery takes longer than a minute, while in the presence of optic nerve disease, the recovery time should be normal.[2134]

light-near dissociation   Pupillary constriction occurring when a person focuses on a close object, but not in response to light stimulation. The mechanism is more likely to be found in the much more extensive innervation of the ciliary muscle than of the sphincter; after infection or other injury to the ciliary ganglion, some of the nerves passing to the ciliary muscle sprout into channels destined for the sphincter muscle instead.

lightning encephalopathy   Syndromes exhibited by victims of lightning strikes. In the acute stage, these include immediate but transient unconsciousness, amnesia, and pareses, due most likely to circulatory arrest with hypoxic encephalopathy, less commonly due to stroke. Delayed syndromes can also occur; these are progressive and include parkinsonism, myelopathy, and a syndrome resembling **amyotrophic lateral sclerosis**.[1001]

lightning eye movements   Uncommon, fast, horizontal ocular dyskinesias of small amplitude which represent disordered saccadic deviations and which may be seen with lesions of the parapontine reticular formation.[253] See also **square-wave jerks, opsoclonus, ocular myoclonus.**

lightning eyes   See **opsoclonus.**

lightning pains   Sudden lancinating pains occurring chiefly in the legs but also in the trunk, arms, or even head. They are paroxysmal, lasting some hours or a day or two, and represent irritation of the dorsal roots, typically seen in **tabes dorsalis.**[979] Similar pains occur in **trigeminal neuralgia.**

lightning polyneuropathy   An acute polyneuropathy resulting from extensive peripheral nerve damage as a result of being struck by lightning.

Apart from death, cataract, autonomic dysfunction, renal failure, **rhabdomyolysis,** and respiratory distress syndrome are also documented complications of this mishap.[2483]

lightning streaks   (Moore lightning streaks) Brief, alarming, but benign luminous visual impressions arising as a result of separation of the vitreous from the surface of the retina.[3964]

lightning stroke   A syndrome of subtle cognitive impairment described in survivors of a lightning strike, manifest as loss of consciousness with subsequent amnesia, fatigue, loss of energy, irritability and emotional lability with associated impairments in attention, memory, and visual reaction times.[5742] The similarity to **chronic fatigue syndrome** is obvious.

Lihastautiliitto R. Y.   A member society of the European Alliance of Muscular Dystrophy Societies, based at De Muskelhandikappades Forbund RF, Lantinen Pitkakatu 35, SF-0100 Turku, Finland.

lilliputian hallucinations   The hallucinated perception of small people, alone or with small animals. The beings are mobile, colored, and generally multiple and are seen by the subject within real external space (which itself is of normal size). The lilliputian people occasionally speak, not surprisingly in small voices. The phenomenon occurs in toxic encephalopathies such as those due to alcohol, cocaine, or marijuana abuse and (rarely) as an aura in migraine.[3358] See also **Leroy syndrome.**

limb apraxia   See **apraxia.**

limb placement reaction   When a healthy baby is supported and the anterior aspect of the tibia or the ulna is brought into contact with the edge of a table, the leg or the arm is lifted and placed on the surface of the table. See **placing reaction.**

limb shaking   The occurrence of brief, irregular, coarse, wavering movements of an arm or leg, or both; it is evidence of a transient ischemic attack in the carotid territory[1842] and occurs as a result of **cerebrovascular insufficiency.**[332]

limb-girdle muscular dystrophy   (Erb-Landouzy syndrome, Erb dystrophy, dystrophia muscularis progressiva) A heterogeneous group of diseases, sporadic or variously inherited, which share the common characteristic of slowly progressive girdle and proximal limb weakness (often sparing the deltoid muscles at first) with later spread to the pelvic girdle and limbs.[1692] Heel-cord contractures are commonly found, myopathic features are notable on muscle biopsy specimens, and serum CK levels are very high. The condition starts at variable ages between birth and later adult life, and it is unlikely that it represents a single entity, a number of conditions formerly so diagnosed now being classified as, for example, **congenital myopathies.** Genetic analysis suggest that at least three dominant and seven recessive forms exist, with similar but variable phenotypes.[6107]

LGMD1 is autosomal dominantly inherited, mapped to 5q22; the LGMD2 group, recessively, but in the case of the latter numerous chromosomal mutation sites have been identified, including 15–q15.1 (LGMD2A); 2pter–p12 (LGMD2B); 3q12 (LGMD2C); 17q12–q21.33 (LGMD2D); 4q12 (LGMD2E); 5q33–q34 (LGMD2F); 17q11–q12 (LGMD2G); and 9q31–q33 (LGMD2H). These variously encode for calpain-3, dysferlin, sarcoglycans, and telethonin.[1460,1530]

Variants include the following:
Bethlem myopathy
Quadriceps myopathy
A recessive or sporadic form with pelvic-femoral involvement[5393]
Limb-girdle muscular dystrophy and Wolff-Parkinson-White syndrome A myopathic syndrome with onset in adult life, characterized by proximal myopathic weakness and cardiomyopathy.[5906]
Late-onset limb-girdle muscular dystrophy with diabetes A myopathic syndrome with onset in adult life, characterized by proximal myopathic weakness with cataract and diabetes.[5441]
Other *variants with* earlier onset, or of later onset with dominant inheritance[773,1036] The dominant form maps to chromosome 5q22.3–31.3.

limb-girdle myasthenia   A rare syndrome of abrupt onset manifesting proximal weakness and fatigability without involvement of the bulbar or extraocular muscles, occurring in childhood or adult life. It is likely that this is a heterogeneous group of conditions.[1780]

limbic   (Lat) Edged, a border or fringe—hence "limbo," the suburbs of hell.[5204]

limbic dementia   A rare amnestic syndrome with cognitive and behavioral changes including marked confabulation, denial of illness, distractibility, and change of affect, resulting from complete, selective **limbic lobe** destruction in a previously normal nervous system.

The functions primarily lost, however, are not those cognitive abilities usually associated with intelligence, but those which add an affective quality to all perceptions.

Clinically, the presentations resemble both the **Wernicke-Korsakoff** and the **Klüver-Bucy** syndromes. Herpes simplex encephalitis is a typical cause.[2040]

limbic encephalitis   A **paraneoplastic syndrome** of the CNS occurring in adult life and due to sterile inflammatory or degenerative changes in the temporal parts of the limbic system gray matter, resembling those of a viral encephalitis and complicating small cell lung carcinoma in most cases.

The clinical manifestations include personality changes, irritability, depression, seizures, and sometimes dementia, followed within weeks by an abrupt permanent impairment of recent memory, variable focal neurological signs stemming from medullary, spinal, or peripheral nerve disease, and subsequently dementia and altered consciousness.[1136,2040]

The diagnosis requires neuropathological examination or the presence of the four following criteria: (1) a compatible clinical picture; (2) an interval of <4 years between the development of neurological symptoms and tumour diagnosis; (3) exclusion of other neuro-oncological complications; and (4) at least one of the following: CSF with inflammatory changes but negative cytology; MRI demonstrating temporal lobe abnormalities; or EEG showing epileptic activity in the temporal lobes.[2332]

Commonly associated neoplasms are small cell carcinoma of the lung (50%), and carcinomas of the testis and breast. Neurological symptoms precede the cancer diagnosis in most patients by a median of 3 months or so. Antineuronal antibodies (e.g., anti-Hu, anti-Ta, anti-Ma) are present in most cases. Pathologically, perivascular inflammatory infiltrates, microglial nodules, neuronal loss, and gliosis are the major features, seen especially in Ammon's horn and the amygdala but also in the hypothalamus, orbitofrontal cortex, and cingulate gyri.

limbic epilepsy   Epileptic syndromes in which complex partial seizures involving the medial aspect of the temporal lobe are associated with behavioral disturbances and evidence of psychopathology, such as the **schizophrenia-like psychoses.**[5627,5900]

limbic lobe   Also known as the *gyrus fornicatus* (Lat, arched gyrus), the lobe on the medial aspect of the cerebral hemispheres was named this by **Thomas Willis,** who noted that the structures comprising it encircle the gray matter of the thalamus and basal ganglia.

These structures include the cingulate and parahippocampal gyri, the hippocampal formation, fornix, amygdala, mammillary bodies, mamillothalamic tract, and the dorsomedial and other thalamic nuclei.

limbic P3 potentials   Event-related potentials normally recorded with depth electrodes placed in limbic structures. The absence of such potentials predicts with high sensitivity the presence of a local epileptogenic focus.[4543]

limbic system   A C-shaped circuit defined first by James **Papez** in 1939, comprising the hippocampus, fornix, mammillary bodies, bundle of Vicq d'Azir, anterior thalamic nucleus, cingulate gyrus, and cingulum. Its cortex is of the four-layered variety and it is younger in phylogeny than the archicortex of the temporal lobe. The complete role of the system is not confidently defined, but the functions of smell, emotion, and memory are almost certainly dependent upon this region.

limb-kinetic apraxia   See **apraxia.**

limit dextrinosis   See **glycogen storage diseases.**

limit-setting sleep disorder   A childhood disorder characterized by the inadequate enforcement of bedtimes by a caretaker, with resultant stalling or refusal to go to bed at an appropriate time.[234]

limp man syndrome   A rare syndrome characterized by intermittent attacks of hypotonia with failure to maintain posture as a result of continuous, partial, fluctuating **cataplexy.**[5310]

Lindau, Arvid   (1892–1958) Swedish pathologist who trained at Lund and in Europe and America before returning to Lund, where he was eventually appointed professor of pathology.

Lindau disease   Cavitating myelopathy due to spinal hemangioblastoma.

Lindenov-Hallgren syndrome   A syndrome of infancy characterized by the combination of pigmentary retinal degeneration, congenital deafness, and vestibulocerebellar ataxia, often with mental retardation.[3416]

Lindstrom syndrome   A congenital dysmorphic syndrome, characterized also by low birth weight, short stature, short neck, skeletal malformations, nevi, cryptorchidism, cerebral atrophy, seizures, hydrocephalus, and pyramidal signs.[337]

line bisection test   A diagnostic maneuver to detect evidence of visual **neglect,** in which the subject is asked to draw vertical lines bisecting each of several horizontal lines randomly printed on the right- or the left-hand side of a sheet of paper. In the presence of neglect, the point marked will veer towards the damaged, nondominant hemisphere, and thus away from the neglected side. The lines on the right-hand side of the paper may also be ignored. By using multiple lines, the test discriminates between right and left hemisphere lesions, whereas to ask a patient to bisect a single line is unlikely to yield such information.[4957]

linear envelope   EMG Moving average of the full wave–rectified EMG, obtained by low pass filtering. See also **integrated EMG.**

linear scleroderma *"en coup de sabre"*   A rare, sporadic disorder characterized by an atrophic band-like region of induration as a result of collagen depositon in the forehead and scalp, extending deeply to involve also the underlying muscles and bone, leading to local atrophy as in the **Parry-Romberg syndrome** of idiopathic progressive facial hemiatrophy. Neurologically, complex partial seizures, cerebral atrophy, ventricular enlargement, parenchymal calcifications, and white matter changes are the main features. Although the condition overlaps with some collagen vascular diseases, it is more likely to be a developmental disorder.[1032]

linear sebaceous nevus syndrome of Jadassohn See **epidermal nevus syndrome.**

lingual dystonia Dystonia affecting the tongue. See **dystonia.**

lingual seizures A rare form of stimulus-sensitive epilepsy, characterized by the occurrence of painful involuntary tongue movements, with head turning and clonic movements of the corner of the mouth; the EEG shows a centrofrontal spike discharge.[4103]

lingual syndrome See **benign childhood epilepsy with centrotemporal spikes.**

linguals Speech sounds formed with the aid of the tongue. "D", "L", "N", "R", "T", and "Th" are also known as *tongue-point* or *alveolar sounds;* "S", "Sh", "Z", "Zh", "Ch", and "J" are also known as *dentals, tongueblade,* or *palatoalveolar sounds.* "K", "G", and "Ng" are articulated between the back of the tongue and the palate; they are also known as *velars, gutturals,* or *tongue-back sounds.*

linkage The connection of a pair of electrodes to the two respective input terminals of a differential EEG amplifier (Adapted from the 1974 report of the of the Committee on Terminology, IFCN,[989] by permission of Elsevier Science.)

linked potential See **satellite potential.**

Linnaeus, Carolus (Charles Linné) (1707–1778) Swedish physician and botanist practicing in Stockholm, where he was professor of medicine and physician to the Swedish court and later professor of botany. He was the first to give a full description of aphasia.

lipid myopathies (lipid storage myopathies) Inherited disorders of muscle leading to a syndrome of proximal and distal myopathic fatigue, weakness, pain, and cramping after prolonged exercise, usually in muscled adult men who cannot run (but, paradoxically, who *can* lift weights).

In some cases, true myotonic discharges are recorded on the EMG. The muscle free carnitine levels are normal or depressed. Muscle biopsy specimens show evidence of lipid storage, mainly in the type 1 muscle fibers, brought about by failure of the enzyme systems responsible for the metabolism of free fatty acids within the muscle. Borderline delayed ketosis is found with fasting.[1211]

The prototype is **carnitine palmityl transferase deficiency;**[1459] other conditions await delineation[773] and

are likely to be genetically diverse with multiple etiologies.[5246] These include **glycogen storage disease, mitochondrial myopathy, arthrogryposis, multisystem triglyceride storage disorder, and pyruvate decarboxylase deficiency.** See also **carnitine deficiency.**

Variants are listed in Chart L–5.

Chart L–5. Variant Forms of Lipid Myopathy

Congenital ichthyosis with lipid storage myopathy (Chanarin-Miranda syndrome) A lipid storage myopathy characterized by proximal limb weakness, congenital ichthyosis, ectropion, and steatorrhea. Abnormal lipid accumulations are found in muscle, skin, leukocytes, and liver.[963] The subject has been reviewed by DiMauro et al.[1459]

Lipid (storage) myopathy with joint contractures A congenital recessively inherited syndrome, characterized by proximal myopathic weakness, hypotonia and fatigability, muscle pain and cramps, myotonia, cleft palate, scoliosis, clubfoot, joint contractures, abnormal levels of plasma lactate, and normal or mildly depressed muscle free carnitine levels, with borderline delayed ketosis accompanied by neutral lipid storage in muscle biopsy specimens.[5246]

Lipid (storage) myopathy with congenital onset A syndrome of generalized hypotonia with the development of nonprogressive proximal muscle weakness with easy fatigability. Muscle biopsy specimens show a lipid storage myopathy. Serum carnitine levels are normal.[2853]

Alpha-glycerophosphate dehydrogenase deficiency A mitochondrial disorder presenting as a glycogen storage disease with progressive ophthalmoplegia.[1458]

Riboflavine-responsive lipid myopathy with carnitine deficiency [394]

For further information, access the Washington University Web site http://www.neuro.wustl.edu/neuromuscular/html.

lipid neuromyopathy A dominantly inherited mitochondrial myopathic syndrome, characterized by proximal weakness, loss of vibration sensation, myelinated fiber loss, and excess lipid in muscle fibers, and due to a systemic defect in fat metabolism.[244]

lipid storage diseases See **lipidoses.**

lipid storage myopathies See **lipid myopathies.**

lipidoses (lipid storage diseases) Lysosomal storage diseases characterized by the accumulation of abnormal amounts of lipid within neurons and macrophages within the nervous system. Those involving myelin in the white matter are termed **leukodystrophies.** Those in which the nature of the material stored is known are known as **sphingolipidoses.** Representative disorders are **Gaucher** and **Nieman-Pick** diseases, **Krabbe** globoid leukodystrophy, **metachromatic leukodystrophy, Fabry** disease, **Tay-Sachs** disease and its variants, and **GM₁ gangliosidosis.**

lipodystrophic muscular hypertrophy with encephalopathy (Beradinelli syndrome) A rare condition of childhood, characterized by a deficiency of fatty tissue; hirsutism; muscular hypertrophy and excessive linear growth; enlarged hands, feet, and liver; and hyperpigmentation without endocrine dysfunction. Diabetes and hyperlipidemia are also occasionally found.[479]

lipodystrophy   Atrophy of the subcutaneous fat; when occurring on one side of the face only, this is known as **Parry-Romberg syndrome.**

lipofibromatous hamartoma   Extensive fatty infiltration of a nerve (usually the median nerve at the wrist and seen most often in children) causing a compression mononeuropathy.[2868]

lipofuscin   (ceroid, wear-and-tear pigment) A pale yellow-brown, periodic acid-Schiff–positive sudanophilic pigment, accumulating in the cytoplasm of nerve and muscle cells with increasing age and acting as a marker of the wear and tear of life. The substance is particularly notable in the thalamus and the hippocampus; and more diffusely in aged brains in parkinsonism, Alzheimer disease, and certain lysosomal diseases.

lipofuscinosis   (juvenile cerebroretinal degeneration) A chronic lipid storage disease resembling Tay-Sachs disease in its clinical manifestations, but not biochemically. See **neuronal ceroid lipofuscinosis.**

lipogranulomatosis   See **Farber disease.**

lipohyalinosis   The characteristic pathological change in the intracerebral arterioles of patients with hypertensive vascular disease, consisting of segmental arterial disorganization associated with the presence of macrophages laden with hemosiderin, and indicating that some extravasation of erythrocytes has occurred.

lipohyalinotic aneurysm   See **microaneurysm.**

lipoid granulomatosis   See **Hand-Schüller-Christian disease, generalized xanthomatosis.**

lipoid proteinosis   (hyalosis cutis et mucosae) A congenital dysmorphic syndrome manifesting also alopecia; hyperkeratosis; nasal, facial, and other skin tumors; leukoplakia; hoarse voice; intracranial calcification; and seizures. See **Urbach-Wiethe disease.**

lipomas   Intracranial or intraspinal midline developmental abnormalities consisting of masses of adipose tissue, usually sited above the corpus callosum, in relation to the cerebellum, within the spinal canal (see **spinal epidural lipomatosis**), or extrinsically at the level of the cauda equina.

lipomatosis with proximal myopathy   A rare lipid storage myopathy, sometimes with a mitochondrial 8344 mutation. See **multiple symmetric lipomatosis.**

lipomatous neuritis   See **Leyden neuritis.**

lipomembranous osteocystic osteodysplasia   (brain, bone, and fat disease) An unusual recessively inherited cystic disease of bone characterized by pathological

fractures, progressive dementia, seizures, calcifications of the basal ganglia, and death in the fourth to sixth decades.[585]

lipomeningomyelocele   A subcutaneous lipoma that extends intradurally through a defect in the posterior vertebral arch, extending thus down as far as the conus medullaris.

The lesion is large and may compress the lowest spinal nerve roots. Cutaneous manifestations such as an angioma, a patch of hair, or an open sinus tract may be notable. See also **dysraphism.**

lipopigments   Autofluorescent materials which stain with Sudan black, but which are insoluble in conventional lipid solvents. They are found in various types of juvenile cerebromacular degeneration, but also represent normal aging pigment (lipofuscin) and include the material known as *ceroid.*

Lisch nodules   Melanocytic hamartomas that appear as well-defined, dome-shaped elevations projecting from the surface of the iris and are clear, yellow, or brown. They are found in **neurofibromatosis type 1.**[3501]

Lissauer atrophy   See **Lissauer paralysis.**

Lissauer dementia   See **Lissauer paralysis.**

Lissauer, Heinrich   (1861–1891) German neuropsychiatrist who trained in Heidelberg, Berlin, and Leipzig and practiced as a psychiatrist in Breslau,[1478] publishing on the topics of **general paralysis of the insane,** pharmacology, and pathological anatomy (Lissauer tract, 1885) before his early death.

Lissauer paralysis   (Lissauer atrophy, Lissauer dementia) A variety of **general paralysis of the insane** marked by diffuse atrophy of the cerebral cortex, leading to seizures, strokes, and prominent focal neurological syndromes.

The condition was described in a note edited posthumously, by a pupil. Although diffuse cortical loss and subcortical demyelination were detected, the major lesion appears to be that caused by a widespread vasculopathy.[5369]

Lissauer tract   (dorsolateral tract, marginal tract) A fiber pathway in the root entry zone of the spinal cord containing mainly unmyelinated fibers running in both directions. The fibers terminate within one or two segments of their entry level within the root entry zone or cross the midline to ascend in the contralateral spinothalamic tract. Lissauer published his description of this tract in 1885.[3429a]

lissencephaly   (Gr, smooth + brain) (agyria) A rare developmental disorder of neuronal migration, characterized by the complete or partial failure of gyral formation in the cerebral hemispheres and by increased thickness of the cortical gray matter. In some cases, the responsible gene maps to 17p13.3, indicating a mutation in the doublecortin gene. The diagnosis is best made using MRI. The types, subtypes and diagnostic criteria for lissencephaly are summarized in Chart L–6.

Chart L–6. Types of Lissencephaly and Their Diagnostic Criteria

Classic or *type 1 lissencephaly* (OMIM 601545) is recessively inherited (17p.13.3) and characterized by agyric and macrogyric regions composed of four layers and resulting from failure of neuronal migration at 10 to 14 weeks gestation.

Subtypes include the following:

X-linked lissencephaly with subcortical band heterotopia in carrier females. Infantile spasms and mixed seizure types, mental retardation, and facial dysmorphisms are typical features.

Miller-Dieker syndrome (OMIM 247200) In this disorder the agyric and pachygyric regions of the cortex have only four layers. Clinical features include congenital cardiac anomalies, craniofacial anomalies, enlarged liver, seizures, hypotonia, microcephaly, and camptodactyly. Abnormalities at chromosome 17p13.3 are usually detectable.

X-linked lissencephaly with absent corpus callosum and ambiguous genitalia (XLAG) with trilayered cortex, dysplastic basal ganglia, spongy white matter, intractable seizures, hypotonia and early death. Mental retardation and seizures are common among related females.[653a]

Minimal diagnostic criteria have been suggested:

A. Type 1 lissencephaly
B. Bitemporal hollowing, midface hypoplasia, short nose with upturned lip, and micrognathia
C. Profound mental retardation, feeding problems, decreased spontaneous movements, early hypotonia with later hypertonia, and seizures, including **infantile spasms**

Isolated lissencephaly sequence This form is characterized by lissencephaly, microcephaly, enlarged ventricles, and heterotopias, presenting clinically as mental retardation, spasticity, and seizures but with minimal facial dysmorphism.[1484]

Type 2 lissencephaly is characterized by a thick and disordered cortex with fibroglial proliferation and without obvious cell layers. Clinically, this form is associated with hydrocephalus and other major malformations.

Type 3 lissencephaly is characterized by a thick and disordered cortex with fibroglial proliferation and without obvious cell layers. Clinically, this form is associated with hydrocephalus and other major malformations. See **cobblestone complex.**

Type 4 lissencephaly is characterized by the association with extreme microcephaly.

In *Walker lissencephaly* (Walker-Warburg syndrome, **HARD+E syndrome**), there is also hydrocephalus due to an arachnoid cyst of the posterior fossa, obliteration of the subarachnoid space, cerebellar hypoplasia and unilateral microphthalmia. This condition is thought to result from an intrauterine infection.[355,961]

Minimal diagnostic criteria have been suggested:[1480]

A. Type 2 lissencephaly
B. Cerebellar dysplasia with vermis hypoplasia
C. Retinal malformations, with hypoplastic ganglion cells, nerve fiber layer, and optic nerves
D. Congenital muscular dystrophy
E. Profound mental retardation, feeding problems, decreased spontaneous movements, early hypotonia with later hypertonia, and seizures, including **infantile spasms**

An alternative classification is that of Aicardi (1994).[59]

Lissencephalies/Subcortical Band Heterotopia (SBH) Spectrum

1. Classical lissencephaly (LIS; agyria-pachygyria) and subcortical band heterotopia (SBH)
   a. Miller-Diecker syndrome with deletions of LIS1 and telomeric genes
   b. Lissencephaly or SBH with LIS1 mutations
   c. Lissencephaly or SBH with DCX (XLIS) mutations (an X-linked dominant form, OMIM 300067, linked to Xq22,3–q22 with multiple seizure types and mental retardation)
   d. Baraitser-Winter syndrome
   e. Other lissencephaly and SBH loci
2. Lissencephaly with agenesis of the corpus callosum (LACC)
   a. LACC with neonatal death
   b. LACC
   c. X-linked LACC with abnormal genitalia (XLAG)
3. Lissencephaly with cerebellar hypoplasia (LCH)
   a. LCH identical to classical LIS except moderate vermis hypoplasia
   b. LCH with AP gradient, malformed hippocampus, and globular cerebellum
      i. LCH with RELN mutations
      ii. Other loci
   c. LCH with severe brainstem and cerebellar hypoplasia, and neonatal death
   d. LCH with brainstem and cerebellar hypoplasia
   e. LCH with abrupt AP gradient
   f. LCH with agenesis of the corpus callosum, brainstem and cerebellar hypoplasia
4. Lissencephaly, not otherwise classified
   a. Lissencephaly with T-cell deficiency
   b. Winter-Tsukahara syndrome (WTS)

Other conditions which lissencephaly may accompany are listed by Dobyns.[1480]

List syndrome   See **Chiari malformation.**

Listings law   Under normal conditions there are no torsional eye movements during voluntary saccades (up/down, right/left) when the head is stationary. This not always true, however.[2526]

literal alexia   An inability to recognize written letters,[673] as seen in patients with lesions of the dominant angular gyrus.

literal paraphasia   The selection of wrong words by patients with dysphasias.

little Broca aphasia   See **Broca aphasia.**

Little club   A group of pediatric neurologists and others constituting a medical advisory board for the British Spastics Society, holding annual conferences and publishing occasional studies on cerebral palsy over the last 40 years. The name of the club honors Dr. W.J. **Little.**

Little disease   Congenital spastic paraparesis, a form of **cerebral palsy,** which Little recognized to be the result of birth injury and most likely to occur in children who had convulsions in the postpartum stage.[3436] He acknowledged the recognition of asphyxia neonatorum, infantile hemiplegia, and infantile apoplexy by others such as Duges and Cruveilher, but emphasised the types of abnormal labor (unnatural presentations, delayed labor, cord around the neck, breech presentations, instrumentation, etc.) and postpartum injuries that could produce cerebral injury. His second paper contained descriptions of spasticity, hemiparesis, torticollis, mental retardation, and cranial deformities, all resulting from perinatal injury.[3437]

little toe reflex of Puusepp   See **toe reflex.**

Little, William John   (1810–1894) English general practitioner and later orthopedic surgeon who trained in London and later practiced at the London Hospital and at the orthopedic institution which he helped to found. He himself was afflicted with an equinus deformity of the left foot as a result of infantile paralysis, for which he obtained some surgical relief while in training in Germany with Stromeyer. It is perhaps ironic that spastic diplegia, the disease that he described in his book *Treatment of Deformities in the Human Frame* (1853), is associated with a similar foot deformity.

His major interest was the diagnosis and management of cerebral palsies, the types of which he classified as generalized rigidity, paraplegia (cerebral diplegia, Little disease), hemiplegic rigidity, and a form with abnormal movements (1861), later called *athetosis* by **Hammond.** Nicholas André in France had reported on cerebral diplegia in 1741.

Little was the first to demonstrate the importance of perinatal injury in the causation of the conditions. Other contributions included his advocacy of saline injections or transfusions in cases of cholera and the performance of tenotomy of the Achilles tendon for contractures, he himself having obtained relief from surgery.

Liveing, Edward   English physician, migraineur, and migrainologist. His book *On Megrim, Sick-Headache and some Allied Disorders* (London, 1873) established the unique nature of migraine headaches and gave a very complete account of their manifestations.

liver flap   See **asterixis.**

liver-lover's headache   The headache of increased intracranial pressure resulting from **idiopathic intracranial hypertension** and due to excess consumption of liver. The liver is supposed to contain large amounts of vitamin A, a known precipitant of idiopathic intracranial hypertension, but this is mainly so in polar bears.

Liverpool Seizure Severity scale   A tool to assess seizure severity (not frequency) through the comments of the patient rather than family or attendants.[302] See also **VA scale, Chalfont scale, Hague scale.**

Livingston, Samuel   (1908–1984) American neurologist and epileptologist who graduated in medicine from Vanderbilt University. He practiced privately but also directed the epilepsy clinic at Johns Hopkins University from which he published a stream of important papers on the social and pharmacological management of seizures. His popular book *Living with Epileptic Seizures* (1963) made him a household name in nearly 2% of the Western world.

livresse du sommeil   See **confusional arousals.**

loa-loa   A filarial nematode whose larvae are transmitted to the human host by the bite of a fly of genus *Chrysops*. These larvae mature to the adult parasites which migrate through subcutaneous tissue including the conjunctivas—whence the popular name "eyeworm." Fertile adult females release microfilaria into the bloodstream diurnally, and biting flies then become infected to complete the life cycle. Loiasis is endemic in central and western Africa, but most residents are asymptomatic in spite of high microfilarial burdens. Eosinophilia is prominent. Visitors are prone to develop symptoms including itching, urticaria, and a fugitive form of angioedema known as the Calabar swelling that occasionally causes compressive neuropathy. The most serious complication of loa-loa infection is encephalitis, which may occur following attempted treatment with antihelminthic agents such as diethylcarbamazine. As this is likely to be a reaction to the destruction of the parasites, pretreatment with steroids is advisable. (HJM)

lobar atrophy   Acquired focal cortical atrophy, leading to such syndromes as **primary progressive aphasia** and **posterior cortical atrophy.**

lobar cerebral hemorrhage   Bleeding into the cerebrum outside the basal ganglia and thalamus, not due to arteriovenous malformation or to trauma.

This is less common than hypertensive hemorrhage into the ganglionic-thalamic region, the brainstem, and cerebellum and has a better prognosis. The clinical features of the hemorrhages in different lobes have been summarized. [4770] Hypertension, cerebral amyloid angiopathy, and fibrinolytic therapy are important antecedents.[3941]

lobar holoproscencephaly   A developmental forebrain disorder in which the cerebral hemispheres are only partially separated by a fissure, which is deepest posteriorly.

Mental and developmental delay without hydrocephalus are the usual results.[1385] See also **holoproscencephaly.**

lobar sclerosis   See **Pick disease.** The term was employed because of the massive astroglial proliferation within the cortex sometimes seen in that condition.

Lobstein, Jean Georges Chretien Martin   (1777–1835) French neurologist who gave an early description of **Apert syndrome** in 1833.[3449]

Lobstein syndrome   See **Apert syndrome.**

lobular sclerosis   See **multiple sclerosis.**

local atonic seizures   See **hemiparetic seizures.**

local epilepsy   See **localization-related epilepsies and syndromes.**

local tetanus   That form of **tetanus** in which the symptoms appear first in a single limb, from which they may or may not spread to other areas.

localization   A cortical function relating the site of a stimulus to the entire remainder of the body schema; there is no pathway in the cord for this purpose.

The localization of functions within the nervous system was remarked indirectly by Hippocrates, but this insight gave way to error, in the idea that the whole brain was considered equipotential with regard to sensation and activity, forming altogether the seat for overall sensation—the **sensus communis.** The concept of functional localization was further supported in 1809 when **Rolando** stimulated animal brains and produced lateralized responses, but the flowering of the concept only came when **Gall** and **Spurzheim** published their studies in **phrenology**[2009a] and claimed that certain faculties of the mind resided in particular areas of gray matter.

These studies led them to generate maps of ridiculous complexity, but for a time their concepts held sway, untempered by persisting criticism and, in time, apparent experimental disproof; thus, **Flourens** and others failed to elicit motor activity by stimulation of the hemispheres of animals, although **Todd** had done so successfully before, and Bouillaud also earlier in the nineteenth century had shown that speech disorders followed lesions of the frontal lobe.

It was the work of Hughlings-**Jackson** in the field of focal seizures, however, that established a degree of cerebral localization, especially his demonstration that cortical discharging lesions lead to focal motor seizures. By this, he contradicted the opinion then held that motor activity originated only from the brainstem and basal ganglia. Further studies by **Hitzig, Ferrier, Horsley,** and others, using electrical stimulation of the cortex, confirmed the existence of localization of function.

localization-related epilepsies and syndromes   (focal, local or partial epilepsy) Disorders in which semiologic studies or findings at investigation disclose a localized origin of the seizures. This includes not only patients with small, circumscribed, constant epileptogenic lesions (anatomical or functional), i.e., true focal epilepsies, but also those with less well-defined lesions, whose seizures may originate from variable loci. In most symptomatic localization-related epilepsies, the epileptogenic lesions can be traced to one part of one cerebral hemisphere, but in idiopathic age-related epilepsies with focal seizures, corresponding regions of both hemispheres may be functionally involved. (From Commission for Classification and Terminology, ILAE. Proposal for revised classifications of epilepsies and epileptic syndromes. *Epilepsia* 1989;**30**:389–399 by kind permission of Blackwell Science.)

localized adhesive spinal arachnoiditis   See **arachnoid diverticula.**

localized hypertrophic neuropathy   A focal sensorimotor neuropathy with many characteristics of **hereditary motor and sensory neuropathy, type 3,** except that it is localized to one or more peripheral nerves, such as the radial.[200] The nerves are enlarged with the formation of perineuronal whorls, despite a loss of myelinated axons. The condition is sustained usually as the result of trauma. See also **perineurinoma.**

localized nodular myositis   (focal nodular myositis) A condition of slowly increasing, painful, localized inflammatory swelling, initially of the thigh or calf muscles but sometimes extending to other sites or becoming generalized, in the presence of elevations in the serum creatine kinase levels and the erythrocyte sedimentation rate.[3687]

The disease affects young and middle-aged adults, sometimes evolving into a diffuse proximal myopathy accompanied by dysphagia and resembling the "facioscapulohumeral syndrome," but sometimes with eosinophilic infiltration. Recurrence is rare after excision, but in a few cases polymyositis develops.

Muscle biopsy specimens show intense interstitial polymorphic infiltration of muscle with scattered foci of fiber destruction and regeneration. The condition is considered to be an unusual presentation of polymyositis.[1217] See also **proliferative myositis,**[2513] **eosinophilic perimyositis.**

localized scleroderma   See **morphea.**

locked-in syndrome   (pseudocoma, the de-efferented state, ventral pontine syndrome [or state], ventral brainstem syndrome, Monte Cristo syndrome, cerebromedullary disconnection, pontopseudocoma, akinetic mutism, pontine locked-in syndrome, pontine disconnection syndrome) A term proposed by Plum and Posner[4466] for the near-total motor paralysis resulting from lesions of both cerebral peduncles or of the ventral pons at or above the abducens nuclei, with retained though inexpressible consciousness. Only eye opening, vertical (not lateral) eye movements, and convergence remain in the full form of the syndrome; the patients are truly mute and akinetic. The EEG shows the pattern of wakefulness. The **Glasgow Coma scale** scores will be 4–2–1 or less.

Major pontine lesions sparing the ascending reticular activating system are the most common causes, but any condition that deprives the patient of motility—myasthenia gravis, poliomyelitis, **acute inflammatory demyelinating neuropathy,** and muscle relaxant administration, for example—can do the same thing. The syndrome may also occur as a **lacunar syndrome** (bilateral **pure motor hemiparesis**).[1853,1867]

Darolles first described the syndrome in 1875, in a patient who had sustained a basilar artery occlusion. In 1941, Cairns[870] described **akinetic mutism** in a patient with an epidermoid cyst in the third ventricle, who neither spoke nor moved but who followed the observer with her eyes, could be made to carry out simple commands, and would withdraw from painful stimuli. This suggests a different condition, perhaps **abulia,** as the patient could move, but did not do so. A full review of the syndrome and the etiologies encountered has been published.[4365] In Alexandre Dumas' novel, *The Count of Monte Cristo*, the elderly M. Noirtier communicated only by eye blinks signifying yes or no, but retained perfect understanding.

lockjaw Tonic spasm of the masseter muscles, classically seen in **tetanus,** for which this was an alternative name.

Locock, Sir Charles (1799–1875) English obstetrician who, noting in 1857 that impotence had been reported as a side effect of bromide treatment and believing that seizures were a manifestation of abnormal sexual tendencies, including masturbation, suggested the use of bromides as treatment for epilepsy.[3451] Serendipitously, it worked.

locomotor ataxia (ataxy) An antique term for **tabes dorsalis.**

locus ceruleus (Lat, place + dark or sky blue) Medullary adrenergic nuclei situated bilaterally in the floor of the fourth ventricle, involved in sensory, autonomic, and perhaps motor functions, arousal, and attention.

Loewi, Otto (1873–1961) German-American physiologist who detected the presence of cholinesterase in motor end-plate regions and demonstrated that it was inhibited by eserine (1924–1926), and who proved the role of chemical substances in neural transmission.

He demonstrated that the vagus nerves liberate acetylcholine, establishing the theory of chemical transmission in the nervous system, and he isolated both cholinesterase and physostigmine, an anticholinesterase.

logical memory A form of verbal memory tested by getting the patient to recall details of a trite story, each successful recollection (either immediately or after a filled interval) adding to the subject's score. The model is used in the **Wechsler Memory Scale.** Typical examples are the story of the donkey and the salt, and of the Boston woman who lost her purse.

logopathy (Gr, word + disease) A morbid affection of speech.

logorrhea (Gr, word + flow) Uninhibited speech output, occurring in schizophrenia and in confusional states.

logospasmus choreiformis The pathological insertion of the same word into sentences, when it is out of context with regard to the patient's otherwise normal speech.

lollipop sign The appearance on CT scans of swelling of the inferior rectus muscle in **dysthyroid ophthalmopathy.**

Lombard sign Elevation of the pitch of the voice when normal subjects read with their normal ear subjected to white noise, compared to its pitch when they read without such stimulation. The test is of value in the detection of feigned unilateral deafness.

Lomtadse sign Dorsiflexion of the hallux when the examiner's knuckles are pressed upon and run distally down the tibial spine. Lomtadse believed that the sign indicated the presence of both a cortical and a capsular lesion causing hemiparesis, but it can equally well be interpreted as yet another form of stimulation leading to the Babinski response. The **Soederbergh phenomenon** is very similar.

London Dysmorphology Database 3.0 A database of over 3000 non-chromosomal multiple congenital anomaly syndromes, useful in diagnosis and in providing genetic counselling for rare syndromes associated with mental retardation and congenital anomalies, with over 28,000 references. Web site: http://www.oup.co.uk/isbn/0-19-268738-7. The database was conceived and compiled by Dr. Michael Baraitser and Dr. Robin Winter, and is published by Oxford University Press, Walton St., Oxford, UK OX2 6DP. A dysmorphology photographic library of over 7500 images is also available. See also **London Neurogenetics Database.**

London Handicap scale A validated six-question health outcome measure designed to assess disadvantage as a result of ill health. The questions concern the items contributing to handicap as defined by the World Health Organization; namely, mobility, physical independence, occupation, social integration, orientation, and economic self-sufficiency.[2474]

London Neurogenetics Database A comprehensive, computerized, menu-driven database assisting in the recognition of over 2400 defined neurogenetic syndromes by means of a listing of selected features; allowing a search for a differential diagnosis of specific clinical features; reviewing the clinical manifestations of named disorders; and providing references to recent or seminal papers.

The database was conceived and written by Dr. Michael Baraitser and Dr. Robin Winter, and is published by Oxford University Press, Walton St., Oxford, UK OX2 6DP. See also **London Dysmorphology Database.**

lone status epilepticus Abrupt presentation of status epilepticus in a previously healthy adult with no past history of neurological disease. There is good recovery from the attack, but it is nevertheless most likely to have been caused by a cerebral tumor.[4284]

long Q-T syndrome   Syncope or cardiac arrest following unexpected stimuli and resulting from prolongation of cardiac cell repolarization due to dysfunction of ion channels. Sudden, alerting adrenergic stimuli such as an unexpected loud noise cause tachycardia and new depolarization that occurs prior to the complete repolarization of the cardiac myocyte. The resultant reduction in cerebral blood flow may trigger syncope, seizures or even sudden death. The arrhythmia classically associated is the torsade des pointes. A gene mutation affecting a potassium channel expressed in cardiac muscle is the likely cause. ECG shows a QTc >460 msec (normal <420 msec).

long sleeper   A variant of the normal sleep patterns, characterized by a perceived need to sleep for longer than is usual in a subject's age group and accommodation of this perception. The sleep architecture is normal. [2470] See also the American Sleep Disorders Association Diagnostic Classification, **sleep disorders** (Chart S–6)[234] and **short sleeper.**

long thoracic nerve of Bell   The nerve supply to the serratus anterior muscle, arising from C 5, 6, 7. It was identified by Sir Charles **Bell** in 1821 as the "external respiratory" nerve.[438]

Palsy resulting from damage to the nerve is usually the result of neuralgic amyotrophy or direct trauma but may be familial.[4436]

long-chain acyl-coenzyme A dehydrogenase deficiency   A rare, genetically determined enzyme defect resulting in episodic juvenile-onset recurrent myoglobinuria, hypoketotic hypoglycemic coma, and hypertrophic cardiomyopathy, triggered by fasting.[5516]

long-cycle hypersomnia   See **hypersomnolence.**

longitudinal bipolar montage   An EEG montage consisting of derivations from pairs of electrodes along longitudinal, usually anteroposterior arrays. (Adapted from the 1974 report of the of the Committee on Terminology, IFCN,[989] by permission of Elsevier Science.)

long-latency reflex   A reflex with many synapses (polysynaptic) or a long pathway (long-loop) so that the time to its occurrence is greater than the time of occurrence of short-latency reflexes. See also **long-loop reflex.** (From the 2001 Report of the Nomenclature Committee of the American Association of Electromyography and Electrodiagnosis.[10] Used by permission, copyright © 2001, AAEM.)

long-latency somatosensory evoked potential   That portion of a somatosensory evoked potential normally occurring more than 100 msec after stimulation of a nerve in the upper extremity at the wrist, or the lower extremity at the knee or ankle.[146]

long-loop reflex   A reflex thought to have a circuit that extends above the spinal segment of the sensory input and motor output. It may involve the cerebral cortex. It should be differentiated from reflexes arising from stimulation and recording within a single or adjacent spinal segments (i.e., a segmental reflex). See also **long-latency reflex.** (From the 2001 Report of the Nomenclature Committee of the American Association of Electromyography and Electrodiagnosis.[10] Used by permission, copyright © 2001, AAEM.)

look nystagmus   A wide-amplitude, slow variety of **optokinetic nystagmus** induced by having a patient follow a succession of moving vertical stripes presented before him.

The nystagmus is faster and of smaller amplitude when the subject stares through the striped stimulus (*stare nystagmus*).[3330]

Looser syndrome   See **Apert syndrome.**

Lopez-Hernandez syndrome   A congenital dysmorphic syndrome characterized by fusion of the vermis and pons with resulting cerebellar ataxia and trigeminal anesthesia, and manifesting also short stature, parietal alopecia, cloudy corneas, craniosynostosis, and mental and developmental delay.[3471]

lordosis   (Gr, bent backward) An extended posture of the spine, usually as an exaggeration of the normal lumbar curve, so that the small of the back is hollowed and the chest prominent.

Lorente de No, Rafael   American neurobiologist who described the role of the internuncial pool in reflex sympathetic dystrophy and the CA 1, 2, 3, 4 regions of the hippocampus.

Lorenzo's oil   A 4:1 combination of glycerol trioleate and glycerol trierucate, formerly used with uncertain success in the treatment of **adrenoleukodystrophy.**[5023]

loss of memory   Isolated amnesia occurring as a **lacunar syndrome.**[1853,1867]

lotus footdrop   Sciatic neuropathy in the thigh, sustained as a result of prolonged meditation in the customary yoga position.[5773] See also **yoga footdrop.**

Lou Gehrig disease   See **amyotrophic lateral sclerosis.** Gehrig (1903–1941) was an acclaimed American baseball player (New York Yankees) whose eventual, originally inexplicable, decline in performance on the field was the result of this disease.

loudness recruitment   A sign of cochlear or brainstem disease, characterized by the perception of a great increase in the loudness of sounds, which are actually only slightly more intense than sounds previously presented below that threshold. See **Equal Loudness Balance test.**

Louis-Bar, Denise   A Belgian neuropathologist who described the syndrome named for her (see next entry) in 1941,[3478] although there had been a report of the same condition in 1926.

Boder and Sedgwick published a more detailed account in 1958[616a] and noted the frequent infections; selective deficiency of IgA was found in one patient 3 years later.

Louis-Bar syndrome (ataxia-telangiectasia, Boder-Sedgwick syndrome) A rare, recessively inherited syndrome of neurological deterioration and failure of DNA repair in which there are breaks on chromosome 11 at 11q22–q23. See **ataxia-telangiectasia.**

louping Ill An encephalitic illness due to direct infection by a flavivirus member of the togavirus group of arboviruses, occurring in Scotland and Northern Ireland and responsible for a form of ataxia in sheep, but only occasionally affecting humans.[6030]

low-affinity fast channel syndrome A variant metabolic disorder underlying the clinical phenotype of congenital myasthenia gravis.

Lowe oculocerebrorenal syndrome See **oculocerebrorenal syndrome.**

Lowenberg-Hill syndrome A dominantly inherited syndrome of tremor associated with patchy demyelination of the cerebral white matter; a variant of the **Pelizaeus-Merzbacher** form of leukodystrophy.[3491]

Lowenthal sclerosis A hereditary syndrome of congenital generalized muscle hypotonia, joint hyperextensibility, kyphoscoliosis, blepharoptosis, hyperhidrosis, and skeletal deformities in which biopsy specimens show firm adhesion of the muscles to the overlying subcutaneous adipose tissues.[3493]

lower basilar branch syndrome A **lacunar syndrome** characterized clinically by dizziness, diplopia, gaze palsy, dysarthria, cerebellar ataxia, and numbness of the face.[1853,1867] See also **lateral pontomedullary syndrome.**

lower body parkinsonism See **frontal gait disorder.**

lower brainstem (bulbar) encephalitis A chronic, progressive **paraneoplastic syndrome** most likely associated with carcinoma of the prostate and characterized by loss of voluntary horizontal gaze and later by spasms of the bulbar muscles.

Notable pathological features are the presence of perivascular round-cell infiltrates and microglial nodules in the brain stem.[316]

lower motor neuron lesion Any pathology that affects the cell body of the motor neuron, its axon and branches, or the motor end-plate. Diseases of the muscle are sometimes included, mainly because they may also lead to hypotonia, wasting, weakness, and depressed muscle stretch reflexes, although the muscles can hardly be regarded as neurons.

lower-half headache Another term for **cluster headache.** It certainly draws attention to the site of the pain, but by no means are all headaches affecting the lower part of the face due to that condition, and the term is now seldom employed.

lower-half parkinsonism A gait disturbance resembling that of Parkinson disease but with few or no other signs of the full syndrome. Whether this is due to that disease or is merely associated with periventricular ischemia in older people is uncertain. See **isolated gait ignition failure, frontal gait disorder.**

lower-level seizures (pontobulbar seizures) Positive electrical events arising from lesions of the brainstem or spinal cord. The modern concept that this could occur was that of Hughlings-**Jackson,** based on his delineation of a hierarchy of functional levels within the brain, although others such as **Galen, Rolando,** and **Flourens** had considered this same possibility before him.[3168]

low-frequency filter (high-pass filter) A circuit that reduces the sensitivity of the EEG channel to relatively low frequencies. For each position of the low-frequency filter control, this attenuation is expressed as a percentage reduction of the output pen deflection at a given stated frequency relative to frequencies unaffected by the filter, i.e., in the mid-frequency band of the channel.

Low-frequency filter designations and their significance are not standardized for instruments of different manufacture. For instance, in a given instrument, a position of the low-frequency filter control, designated *0.5 Hz*, may indicate a 30% (or 3 decibel) or other stated percentage reduction in sensitivity at 0.5 Hz, compared to the sensitivity, for example, at 10 Hz. The same position of the low-frequency filter control may also be designated by the time constant. See also **time constant.** (Adapted from the 1974 report of the of the Committee on Terminology, IFCN,[989] by permission of Elsevier Science.)

low-frequency response The sensitivity of an EEG channel to relatively low frequencies, determined by the low-frequency response of the amplifier and by the low-frequency filter (time constant) used, and expressed as the percentage reduction in the output pen deflection at certain stated low frequencies relative to other frequencies in the midfrequency band of the channel. See also **low frequency filter, time constant.** (Adapted from the 1974 report of the of the Committee on Terminology, IFCN,[989] by permission of Elsevier Science.)

low-pressure headache See **post–lumbar puncture headache.**

low-pressure hydrocephalus See **normal-pressure hydrocephalus.**

Lowry syndrome (Lowry-MacLean syndrome, cranial synostosis and fibular aplasia) A recessively inherited congenital craniofacial malformation syndrome characterized by short stature, beaked nose, bilateral fibular aplasia, proptosis, glaucoma, **Brushfield spots,** atrial septal defect, intestinal malrotation, seizures, microcephaly, callosal abnormalities, hydrocephalus, craniosynostosis affecting all sutures, and mental and developmental delay.[3495] See also **craniosynostosis.**

Lowry-MacLean syndrome   See **Lowry syndrome.**

low-voltage EEG   A waking EEG record characterized by activity with an amplitude not greater than 20 uV over all head regions. With appropriate instrumental sensitivities, this activity can be shown to be composed primarily of beta and theta (and to a lesser degree delta) waves, with or without alpha activity over the posterior area.

Low-voltage EEGs are susceptible to change under the influence of certain physiological stimuli, sleep, pharmacological agents and pathological processes. They should be held in clear contradistinction to the tracings of **electrocerebral inactivity** (which are records consisting primarily of delta waves of relatively low voltage) and to tracings which display low voltages over limited regions of the head. (Adapted from the 1974 report of the of the Committee on Terminology, IFCN,[989] by permission of Elsevier Science.)

lubag   An X-linked recessive syndrome characterized by dystonia and parkinsonism, described only in Filipinos.[5971]

Lubarsch-Pick disease   See **amyloidosis.**

Luciani, Luigi   (1842–1919) Italian neurophysiologist and rector of the University of Rome who performed ablation experiments on the cerebellum and was the first to conclude that it serves as the regulatory center for tonic, static, and voluntary movement functions.

Luciani triad   Asthenia, atonia and ataxia, three major manifestations of cerebellar disease. See also **Charcot triad** of nystagmus, ataxia, and slurred speech.

lucid dreaming   The awareness of dreaming while it is occurring, coupled with a limited ability to control the script.[3576]

lucid interval   That period commencing with the awakening of a patient following concussion and the onset of coma due to brain compression by a resulting intracranial (usually extradural) hemorrhage.

The patient who awakens following concussion from severe head trauma, and whose conscious level shortly thereafter declines again, probably has a fracture of the squamous temporal bone with laceration of the middle meningeal artery, causing an epidural hematoma. This latter is the cause of the delayed coma, through rapid brain compression. In this interval, the patient is likely to be fully conscious, and her thinking may be lucid.

The phenomenon was first described by H-F. le Dran in 1731.

lückenschädel   See **lacunar skull.**

Lucky syndrome   A congenital dysmorphic syndrome manifesting also tall, thin stature, skeletal deformities including arachnodactyly, erythema, strabismus, ptosis, facial telangiectasia, hypotonia, muscle atrophy, and mental and developmental delay.[4360]

lucubration   (from Lat, to work by the light of a lamp) Insomnia.

lues   (Lat, a pestilence or a criminal) See **syphilis.** The word was used in previous centuries meaning an expiation, such as epilepsy; an epidemic, such as dysentery; and as a contagion, such as syphilis.[4512] Only the latter survives.

luetic otitic-nystagmus syndrome   See **Hennebert syndrome.**

Luft disease   (nonthyroidal hypermetabolism) A rare hypermetabolic **mitochondrial myopathy** due to the uncoupling of oxidative phosphorylation in the mitochondria of skeletal muscles. Patients complain of fever, heat intolerance, sweating, dyspnea at rest, polyphagia, polydipsia, and polyuria without weight gain, and sometimes with slight muscle weakness. Muscle biopsy specimens demonstrate a profusion of ragged red fibers.[3509]

Dr. Rolf Luft introduced the concept of mitochondrial myopathies in 1962.[3509]

Lujan syndrome   A congenital, X-linked dysmorphic syndrome manifesting also tall stature, atrial septum defect, arachnodactyly, macrocephaly, joint laxity, callosal malformations, and mental and developmental delay.[337]

lumbago   (Lat, pain in the loins) Etymologically, a very proper word for back pain, but it has lost its respectability because of popular usage, and is no longer commonly employed in medicine.

lumbar   (from Lat, the loins) Of or belonging to the loins or low back.

lumbar puncture   An invasive procedure (insertion of a needle between the lumbar vertebra into the subarachnoid space for the purpose of obtaining cerebrospinal fluid), introduced in the living with great bravery by **Quincke** in Germany and Walter Essex **Wynter** in England,[6056] both in 1891.

Cotugno had obtained CSF from the dead a century before, and **Corning,** a physician in New York, put a needle into the spinal column in 1889, but there is evidence that he did not attempt to withdraw spinal fluid.[2210] Despite the introduction of the procedure in England, it was not performed at the **National Hospital** until after the retirement of Sir William **Gowers,** who disapproved of it, perhaps because all four of Wynter's meningitic patients died.

Practice parameters regarding the indications, contraindications, and methodology of lumbar puncture (diagnostic, therapeutic, and incidental and in adults and children) have been reviewed by the American Academy of Neurology.[144]

lumbar spinal stenosis   (Verbierst syndrome, pseudoclaudication syndrome) Narrowing of the lumbar spinal canal over several segments as a result of multiple disk protrusions or other pathology; pain, weakness, and ascending numbness in the legs as a result of exercise, relieved by rest and by flexion of the spine, are typical symptoms.[5748]

This syndrome is sometimes improperly called *intermittent claudication of the cord*, but it is probably the spinal nerve roots that are ischemic and, anyway, the spinal cord cannot limp.[2968]

lumbarization   The fusion of the S1 vertebra with that at L5, effectively producing a state of having six lumbar vertebrae separated from the remainder of the sacrum by a disc and joint capsule.

Low back pain can result, but there may be no clinical effects at all.[1974]

lumbosacral plexopathy   (lumbosacral plexus neuritis) An acutely or subacutely evolving monophasic syndrome of painful neurogenic muscle weakness in the legs with areflexia, atrophy, and sensory disturbances such as paresthesias in the distribution of the spinal nerves and the plexus at and below L1, usually unilaterally. The numerous causes include microvasculitis and, less often, compression, malignant infiltration, and diabetes; often no cause is ascertainable, in which case there is a tendency for slow recovery.[4898,5752] The criteria for diagnosis resemble those for **neuralgic amyotrophy,** except that it is the lumbosacral rather than the brachial plexus which is involved.

A *variant* syndrome of *painful lumbosacral plexopathy* has been described, which presents with acute pain, weakness, hyporeflexia, and muscle atrophy in the legs with slow recovery, occurring as a manifestation of ischemic axonal neuropathy in the absence of evidence of cancer, vasculitis, or other autoimmune disease (although an autoimmune etiology is assumed and the erythrocyte sedimentation rate is high).[699] In other variant forms, *lower lumbosacral plexopathy* occurs postpartum, producing perineal sensory disturbances and sphincter failure without leg weakness; or an upper plexopathy occurs as a rare obstetric complication in the third trimester or in the intra- or postpartum periods, and is associated with upper (L2–S1) lesions causing obturator, femoral, or sciatic nerve palsies.[2756]

lumbosacral plexus neuritis   See **lumbosacral plexopathy.**

lumbosacral radiculoplexus neuropathy   (LSRPN) (nondiabetic) A subacute lumbosacral plexopathy associated with weight loss, beginning focally or asymmetrically in the thigh or leg but usually extending to local regions and to the other side. Morbidity is prolonged because of pain, paralysis, autonomic involvement, and sensory loss and recovery is usually delayed and incomplete. In biopsied distal nerves, changes are found similar to those found in the diabetic form and are typical of ischemic injury and of microvasculitis.

This disorder mirrors the diabetic variety in its clinical features, course, pathological findings (ischaemic injury from microvasculitis), and long-term outcome.[1579]

lumbosacral syringomyelia   See **hereditary sensory and autonomic neuropathy** (recessive).

lumbrical   (Lat, like a worm) Small intrinsic hand muscles, named in the seventeenth century for their resemblance to (rather fat) worms.

Lundberg syndrome   1. (hereditary neurological disease with facial spasm, myopathy-oligophrenia-cataract) The occurrence of slowly progressive peripheral paresis in the hands and feet, starting in childhood with areflexia and reduced conduction velocities; moderate oligophrenia; multiple cranial nerve lesions (optic atrophy, pupillary abnormalities, facial spasms or palsy, cataract, speech delay); ataxia; premature menopause; and disproportionate smallness of the limbs. The condition is considered to be related to **hereditary motor and sensory neuropathy.**[3518]

2. *acromicria, mental retardation, polyneuropathy* A congenital recessively inherited syndrome characterized by short stature, hypogonadotrophic hypogonadism with premature menopause at 20 to 25 years of age, small hands and feet, ophthalmoplegias, nystagmus, oculomotor apraxias, bulbar palsies, a slowly progressive motor peripheral neuropathy resembling hereditary motor and sensory neuropathy type 1, and mental and developmental delay.[3518]

3. **benign acute childhood myositis** (myalgia cruris epidemica) A syndrome of transient pain and tenderness in the calves and elevated serum creatine kinase levels occurring in children within a week of an upper respiratory infection.[3516]

lupus anticoagulant   A circulating immunoglobulin (IgG, IgM, or both) autoantibody directed against phospholipids which interferes with the in vitro phospholipid-dependent tests of coagulation, such as the activated partial thromboplastin time, producing an anticoagulant effect; but, paradoxically, its presence is associated clinically with thrombocytopenia, prothrombin deficiency, pulmonary emboli, deep vein thromboses (type 1), arterial thromboses (type 2), cerebrovascular thrombotic disease leading to ocular or focal cerebral deficits, mainly in younger women (type 3), or any combination of these (type 4).

Although initially detected in subjects with **systemic lupus erythematosus,** it is also sometimes found in normal subjects and those with complicated migraine, seizures, or chorea; those with viral infections including HIV infection; those with malignancy or lymphoproliferative disorders; or those taking chlorpromazine, procainamide, etc. Suspicion of its presence is aroused by finding an increased partial thromboplastin time or elevated levels of anticardiolipin antibodies.[3377]

lupus cerebritis   See **systemic lupus erythematosus.**

Luria, Aleksander Romanovich   (1902–1977) Russian aphasiologist who distinguished six aphasic syndromes: efferent (Broca aphasia), afferent apraxic, amnesic, sensory, semantic, and dynamic.

Luria-Nebraska Battery   A complex timed instrument for the assessment (by neuropsychologists) of perseveration and other functions that may be affected in states of cognitive decline. The battery is derived from the techniques used by **Luria,** but is itself a North American creation,[2162] and its validity and reliability are not unquestioned.[3392]

Luschka foramen   The paired lateral foramina in the meningeal roof of the fourth ventricle.

Luschka, Hubert von   (1820–1875) German, professor of anatomy at Tübingen University.

Luschka joints   Originally described as narrow joint cavities between a small bony eminence on the posterior rim of the superior surface of the bodies of the C3, 4, 5, 6, 7, and T1 vertebrae (the uncus), forming part of the medial wall of the adjacent intervertebral foramen, and the inferior facet of the superjacent vertebra—the lateral intervertebral joints. These "joints," however, probably represent nothing more than fissures in the lateral part of the cervical disks.[4375]

Luschka syndrome   See **Sturge-Weber disease.**

Lust phenomenon   (peroneal sign) Eversion and dorsiflexion of the ankle in response to tapping the common peroneal nerve; a sign of **tetany.**

luxury perfusion   Abundant cerebral blood flow in a region with impaired ability to extract oxygen, as a result of ischemic or other damage.[3288] This localized reactive hyperemia is due to a local chemical effect of lactic acidosis in and around ischemic tissue, and also occurs following trauma and seizures.

A reduction in oxygen and glucose uptake larger than the drop in perfusion is known as *relative luxury perfusion.*

Luys, Jules-Bernard   (1828–1897) French neurologist who became chief of the neurology service of the **Salpêtrière** and the Charité Hospitals. He first described the subthalamic nucleus in 1865, but is also remembered for his demonstration of the degeneration of the anterior horn cells in progressive muscular atrophy.

luysopallidonigral atrophy and amyotrophic lateral sclerosis   A rare variant, characterized by anterior horn cell loss and corticospinal tract degeneration in association with dystonias, rigidity, and hyperkinesias.[2261]

In a further *variant* form, signs of spinal muscular atrophy are also found. See **motor neuronal diseases.**

Lyle syndrome   1. See **cortical blindness.** 2. See **syndrome of the mesencephalic gray matter.**

Lyme disease   (Garin-Bujadoux-Bannwarth syndrome, Bannwarth syndrome; neuroborreliosis) A tickborne, seasonal, spirochetal disease endemic in North America, Europe, and Australia with cutaneous manifestations such as spreading red papules and erythema chronicum migrans, occurring initially at the site of a tick bite. Later, neurological and finally arthropathic symptoms and signs may appear.[5329] In addition, atrioventricular conduction defects are described.

The neurological features of note are nonspecific chronic malaise, headache, and pains, progressing over perhaps 6 months in about 15% of the cases to become a chronic meningoencephalopathy accompanied by painful polyradiculopathies and neuropathies, both cranial and peripheral. The seventh cranial nerve is that most often affected. A lymphocytic pleocytosis and raised protein levels are found in the CSF.[885,3598,4639] The spirochaete *Borrelia burgdorferi* was first isolated from patients living in Lyme, Connecticut, but the first reports of the disease were from southern France in 1922 and from Germany by Bannwarth in 1941.[331]

Criteria for the diagnosis of definite nervous system Lyme disease have been suggested[2396] and the place of the polymerase chain reaction (PCR) defined.[4288]

1. Possible exposure to appropriate ticks in an area where Lyme disease occurs.
2. One or more of the following;
   i. Erythema migrans, the pathognomic rash, or histologically proven borrelia lymphocytoma or acrodermatitis
   ii. Immunologic evidewnce of exposure to *B. burgdorferi* (e.g., positive serologic test)
   iii. Culture, histologic, or PCR proof of the presence of *B. burgdorferi*
3. Occurrence of one or more of the (typical) neurological disorders (such as lymphocytic meningitis with or without cranial neuritis or painful radiculoneuritis, encephalomyelitis, peripheral neuropathy, or encephalopathy) after exclusion of other potential etiologies. Additional testing is indicated, based on the likelihood that a given neurological disorder is causally related to Lyme borreliosis. If CNS disease is suspected, CSF should be examined for intrathecal antibody production, culture, or PCR.

Lympho-   (Gr, water)

lymphocytic choriomeningitis   See aseptic meningitis The condition was first described by Arvid Johan Wallgren in 1924.

lymphocytic meningoradiculitis   See **Bannwarth syndrome.**

lymphogranuloma inguinale   See **lymphogranuloma venereum.**

lymphogranuloma venereum (lymphogranuloma inguinale) A chlamydial infection that occasionally progresses to cause aseptic meningitis or encephalitis.[1558]

lymphoma A generic term for Hodgkin disease, lymphosarcoma, reticulum cell sarcoma, and follicular lymphoma. Neurologic complications include the effects of local deposits on the brain, spinal cord, and the cranial (oculomotor, fifth and seventh cranial nerves) and peripheral nerves, **progressive multifocal leukoencephalopathy,** peripheral neuropathy, cauda equina compression, **polymyositis,** and such infections as **herpes zoster** and **cryptococcosis.** See also **primary CNS lymphoma.**[3779]

lymphomatoid granulomatosis A lymphoreticular proliferative and granulomatous disorder with polymorphic cellular infiltrates, mainly affecting the lungs and skin, but also capable of causing central or peripheral nervous system abnormalities, the former usually presenting as a neoplasm or multifocal disease, the latter as a sensorimotor neuropathy.[2607,3407]

lymphomatous leptomeningitis See **neurolymphomatosis.**

lymphomatous neuropathy See **neurolymphomatosis.**

lypemania (Gr, grief + madness) Esquirol's term for depressive illness.

lypothymia (Gr, grief + the spirit) Great sadness.

lysine cystinurnia with benign myopathy A rare congenital familial disorder presenting with severe muscular hypotonia, respiratory failure, and feeding difficulties, but with eventual improvement in most cases. The condition is accompanied by dwarfism but there is no mental defect. Aminoaciduria and mild renal acidosis are also present.[1043]

lysine intolerance A rare, diffuse encephalopathy due to a failure in the intestinal transport of dibasic amino acids and a resulting deficiency of available arginine, ornithine, and lysine.

Clinically, the condition is characterized by cataract, short stature, hepatosplenomegaly, and weakness, with aminoaciduria.[4411]

lysinuric protein intolerance See **familial protein intolerance.**

lysis The destruction of an object; in medicine, usually a cell or a chemical substance such as an enzyme.

lysis of myofibrils in type 1 fibers A rare, congenital myopathy presenting with severe weakness and hypotonia, with lumbar lordosis, and characterized pathologically by small type 1 myofibrils, within which oxidative activity is absent but adenosine triphosphatase activity is increased in some peripheral zones.[4877]

lysosomal enzyme defects See **lysosomal storage diseases.**

lysosomal glycogen storage disease A dominantly inherited disease that presents with vacuolar myopathy, cardiomyopathy, and weakness in infants and proximal limb weakness and diaphragmatic paralysis but no cardiac involvement in adults. A deficiency of lysosomal α-1,4 amylo-glucosidase is usually detected at all ages. See **Pompe disease.**

lysosomal storage diseases (lysosomal enzyme defects) Genetically determined disorders in which the intracytoplasmic enzymes that normally metabolize peptide and glycosidic linkages are deficient, so that the substances normally degraded accumulate within and cause swelling of the lysosomes that contain undigested metabolic products in various types of cells.[1248] Their overall frequency may be 1 in 5000 live births. Confident diagnosis requires skin biopsy.[4515]

Disorders affecting the nervous system include the **sphingolipidoses, mucopolysaccharidoses, mucolipidoses, glycoproteinoses, cystinosis,** and some **glycogenoses.** In all, over 40 such diseases are known. See **GM$_1$ gangliosidosis, GM$_2$ gangliosidosis** (Tay-Sachs and Sandhoff disease, AB variant), **sulfatidoses, metachromatic leukodystrophy** and *variants*, and **mucosulfatidosis, Gaucher disease** types 1, 2, and 3, **Krabbe disease, sphingomyelin storage disorders, Fabry disease, Jansky-Bielschowsky disease** (types A, B, C, D), **Spielmeyer-Vogt disease, mucopolysaccharidoses** (Hurler; Hunter; Sanfilippo types A, B, C, and D; Morquio; Maroteaux-Lamy; and β-glucuronidase deficiency), **glycogen storage disease type 2,** oligosaccharidoses (**fucosidoses, mannosidosis,** and **aspartylglucosaminuria**), **Wolman disease, sialidosis type 1, adrenoleukodystrophy, neuronal ceroid lipofuscinosis** and **acid phosphatase deficiency.**[2138,3121] In most of these, the clinical features include progressive psychomotor retardation and abnormal facial appearances.

lysosomes Membrane-bound intracytoplasmic bodies containing the hydrolytic enzymes required for the degradation of lipids, proteins, and nuclides, which form an integral part of the structure of normal cells.[2138]

lyssa See **rabies.**

lyssophobia (Gr, rage or canine madness + fear) Pseudohydrophobia. A condition resembling **rabies** without true respiratory muscle spasm.

Lytico-Bodig (Hirano parkinsonism-dementia, laughing death) The vernacular term for the amyotrophic lateral sclerosis-parkinsonism-dementia complex occurring in the Chamorro people of Guam and Rota in the Western Pacific.[2007,5271] See **amyotrophic lateral sclerosis.**

M

M wave   A compound muscle action potential evoked from a muscle by an electric stimulus to its motor nerve. By convention, the M wave elicited by a supramaximal stimulus is used for motor nerve conduction studies. Ideally, the recording electrodes should be placed so that the initial deflection of the evoked potential from the baseline is negative. Common measurements include latency, amplitude, and duration. It is also referred to as the motor response. Normally, the configuration is biphasic and stable with repeated stimuli at slow rates (1 to 5 Hz). See **repetitive nerve stimulation.** (From the 2001 Report of the Nomenclature Committee of the American Association of Electromyography and Electrodiagnosis.[10] Used by permission, copyright © 2001, AAEM.)

MAAP Services   (for Autism, Asperger Syndrome, and PDD) A charitable organization in this field. Address: P.O. Box 524, Crown Point, IN 46308. Tel: 219-662-1311. E-mail: chart@netnitco.net Web site: http://www.maapservices.org/index.html.

Mabry muscular dystrophy   An X-linked muscular dystrophy with incomplete penetrance, in which muscle weakness and wasting appear between the ages of 5 and 35 years, the pelvic muscles being affected first.

Later clinical features include calf pseudohypertrophy, ECG abnormalities, and very slow progression, such that ambulation is still possible until mature adult life, and survival to late middle age is usual.[3537]

See **X-linked muscular dystrophy.**

MacCormack reflex   Adduction of the contralateral thigh after tapping the patellar tendon, due to reflex disinhibition in patients with bilateral pyramidal tract disease.

MacCormack, W   (1836–1901) Irish surgeon practicing in Belfast.

MacEwen pupil   See **MacEwen signs.**

MacEwen signs   1. Increased resonance on combined percussion and auscultation of the head. When the parietal region is tapped with the finger, a short, high-pitched note can be heard with the stethoscope placed over the frontal region in children with increased intracranial pressure, so long as the fontanelles are closed. The sound becomes quieter when the tapping finger approaches the stethoscope.[3548,4723] This is a form of auscultatory percussion and is not the same as the **cracked-pot note** heard without a stethoscope in similar conditions. 2. (MacEwen pupil) The pupil of a patient comatose from alcohol intoxication dilates briefly when the patient is stimulated but not awakened, while that of a patient comatose from structural disease does not dilate with such mild stimulation.[3547]

MacEwen, Sir William   (1848–1924) Scottish surgeon who trained with Lord Lister in Glasgow. He became Regius Professor of Surgery in Glasgow, was elected a Fellow of the Royal Society in 1895, and was knighted in 1902. Even before this honor was bestowed, however, he used to speak of himself in the first person plural.

His 1879 paper in the *Glasgow Medical Journal,* "Tumour of the Dura Mater—Convulsions—Removal of Tumor by Trephining—Recovery", was not only an account of a spectacular surgical *tour de force* but combined within the title the introduction, patient and methods, results, and conclusions sections, while the discussion seems superfluous. His later publications concerned above all his treatment of cerebral abscesses and sinus thrombosis, summarized in his book *Pyogenic Diseases of the Brain and Spinal Cord* (1893).

MacEwen triangle   (suprameatal triangle) A space bounded by the lower part of the posterior end of the zygoma, the superior posterior edge of the external auditory meatus, and the mastoid process, a landmark for identifying the position of the underlying middle meningeal artery.

Machado-Joseph Azorean disease   See **Joseph disease.**

Mackenzie syndrome   Dysfunction of cranial nerves IX, X, XI, and XII with a Horner syndrome, resulting from infiltration by a tumor of the retroparotid space below the base of the skull.[3554]

macro-   (Gr, long or large). Prefix denoting long or large.

macrocephaly   (macrocrania) Enlarged head circumference, greater than 2 standard deviations above the mean for the person's age and sex.

Although this is a frequent feature of numerous named clinical syndromes, macrocrania may also exist in isolation, when it is a factor increasing the risk of perinatal brain damage but is otherwise harmless.

macrocephaly and callosal agenesis   See **Young syndrome.**

macrocephaly with angiomatosis   A congenital syndrome comprising asymmetrical limbs, macrocephaly, and capillary and cavernous hemangiomas with papilledema,[337] presumably due to raised intracranial pressure with obstructive hydrocephalus.

macrocrania   See **macrocephaly.**

macro–creatine kinase   Variant forms of creatine kinase, including CK-BB with immunoglobulin, and aggregates of mitochondrial creatine kinase.[3265]

macrodactyly   (Gr, macros, long + dactylos, finger) Enlargement of a digit, as may occur rarely in **neu-**

rofibromatosis, with arteriovenous malformations, with **localized hypertrophic neuropathy,**[200] or in the syndrome described in the next entry.

macrodactyly with connective tissue nevi and hemi-hypertrophy A congenital neurocutaneous syndrome, characterized by scoliosis, asymmetrical limbs, macrodactyly, calcification of muscle and subcutaneous tissues, and patchy depigmentation of the skin.[337]

macrodystrophia lipomatosa A condition occurring in young people, characterized by hypertrophy of the finger or part of the hand as a result of infiltration of the soft tissues (including the nerves traversing the region) by fat.

The disorder may be a form of **neurofibromatosis,** but there is very little disturbance in the function of the nerves affected.

macroelectromyography (macro-EMG) General term referring to the technique and conditions that approximate recording of all muscle fiber action potentials arising from the same motor unit. See **macro–motor unit action potential.** (From the 2001 Report of the Nomenclature Committee of the American Association of Electromyography and Electrodiagnosis.[10] Used by permission, copyright © 2001, AAEM.)

macro-EMG See **macroelectromyography.**

macro-EMG needle electrode A modified single-fiber electromyography electrode insulated to within 15 mm from the tip and with a small recording surface (25 urn in diameter) 7.5 mm from the tip. (From the 2001 Report of the Nomenclature Committee of the American Association of Electromyography and Electrodiagnosis.[10] Used by permission, copyright © 2001, AAEM.)

macroglobulinemia A group of conditions characterized by a marked increase in the amount of IgM in the blood. This may occur as an isolated condition, or may complicate lymphomas, collagen vascular diseases, or some hemolytic anemias.

Clinically, malaise, fatigue, weakness, and the usual features of a demyelinating sensorimotor peripheral neuropathy are the most prominent features; this last disorder may present acutely, thus the overall condition resembles **acute inflammatory demyelinating polyneuropathy.**[2228] See **Bing-Neel syndrome.**

macroglossia (Gr, long + tongue) Enlargement of the tongue to the extent that it protrudes beyond the teeth or alveolar ridge at rest. It occurs with hypothyroidism, lymphangioma, hemangioma, and muscle dystrophies (primary form) and as a result of infiltrations such as amyloid and benign and malignant masses (secondary form).

macrogyria A rare neuronal migration disorder consisting of an increase in the width (and therefore a decrease in the number) of the cerebral cortical gyri. This is sometimes combined with **microgyria.**

In its most extreme form, it is associated with complete absence of the gyri.[5324]

macro–motor unit action potential (macro-MUAP) The average electric activity of that part of an anatomic motor unit that is within the recording range of a macro-EMG electrode. It is characterized by consistent appearance when the small recording surface of the macro-EMG electrode is positioned to record action potentials from one muscle fiber. The following characteristics can be specified quantitatively: (1) maximal peak-to-peak amplitude, (2) area contained under the waveform, and (3) number of phases. (From the 2001 Report of the Nomenclature Committee of the American Association of Electromyography and Electrodiagnosis.[10] Used by permission, copyright © 2001, AAEM.)

macro-MUAP See **macro–motor unit action potential.**

macroprolactinoma A prolactin-secreting pituitary adenoma >10 mm in diameter and liable to compress local structures such as the optic chiasm.

macropsia The apparent magnification of objects seen—a perceptual distortion in which objects appear too large to the subject. Both retinal lesions and complex partial seizures may be responsible.

macrosaccadic oscillations Sequences of large- or small-amplitude square wave saccadic jerks (1°–30°) which oscillate with increasing and decreasing amplitude, bypassing the fixation point with each reversal. They are absent in darkness. Such oscillations reflect excessive gain within the saccadic system and typically occur in patients with lesions of the deep midline cerebellar structures.[5059]

Adaptive changes made to muscle activation during periods of weakness may become maladaptive, with return of strength as when edrophonium chloride is given to patients with myasthenia gravis, in which condition these oscillations may also be found.

macro–square-wave jerks (kippdeviationen/kippnystagmus) Unwanted saccadic movements (saccadic intrusions) appearing as large-amplitude square-wave jerks (10°–40°), followed by corrective saccades after an interval.

These bursts of square-wave jerks of large amplitude occur at about 2 Hz during fixation. Both eyes suddenly and conjugately move off the target with a saccade, but after a latent period of about 80 msec a nonvisually evoked reflex saccade returns them to the target. They may, however, be present in darkness. They have been described in patients with acute cerebellar lesions and with chronic ataxic syndromes, including **multiple sclerosis.**[1370] See also **square-wave pulses.**

macrotia (Gr, macros, long + otos, ear) Enlargement of the ears, occasionally dominantly inherited.

macula lutea   (Lat, a small spot + yellow) The portion of the retina to the temporal side of the optic disk, about 1 mm in diameter, which contains the greatest concentration of cone receptors and where the blood vessels are all of capillary size. At its center is the fovea, where even capillaries are absent.

macular degeneration   Hereditary or acquired absence or degeneration of the cone cells of the retina (**pigmentary retinopathy**) or of both cones and rods. The former presents with bilaterally diminished visual acuity, impaired color vision, and photophobia by day (**hemeralopia**). Various degenerative or metabolic neurological disorders are frequently associated.

macular dystrophy-deaf-muteness syndrome   See **Amalric syndrome.**

macular ischemia   Focal ischemia of the macula, resulting usually from presumed embolism or hematological disorders such as sickle cell disease, and manifest clinically by the presence of a central scotoma.[5604]

macular sparing   That condition in which the macular representation on the involved side is wholly or partly unaffected despite the presence of homonymous visual field defects, leaving an island of central vision within a sea of blindness. It occurs probably as a result of the large area of the visual cortex devoted to the representation of the macula. See also **sparing of fixation.**

macular star   The glistening sheen upon the retina radiating around the fovea or between the fovea and the optic disk, indicating the presence of retinal edema.

maculoanesthetic leprosy   See **tuberculoid leprosy.**

maculopapillary fibers   The bundle of nerve fibers running from the macula to the optic nerve head. These are especially, but not selectively, susceptible to damage from demyelination; in such cases, a striped appearance (*retinal slits*) is sometimes seen when they are viewed with red-free (i.e., green) light through the ophthalmoscope.

mad as a hatter   An opprobrious term popularized by the fiction of Lewis Carroll, but with a root in truth, in that sublimate of mercury was once used to rub up the nap on the felt used in making hats; the resultant encephalopathy (with visual field constriction, neuropathy, depression, and tremor) suffered by the hatters led to the name.

mad cow disease   See **bovine spongiform encephalopathy.** The Web site http://www.mad-cow.org/ provides data on mad cow disease, Creutzfeldt-Jacob disease (CJD), prions, spongiform encephalopathies, scrapie, BSE, CWD, TME, and TSE.

madarosis   Loss of the outer part of the eyebrow as occurs in **leprosy** and hypothyroidism.

MADD   See **myoadenylate deaminase deficiency syndrome.**

Maddox rod   A test instrument comprising a disk composed of parallel red glass cylinders which can be employed in estimating the degree of diplopia in the nine cardinal positions of gaze. The presence of the rod placed before one eye prevents fusional vergence.

When the disk is placed over one eye (by convention, the right), a bright white light source is seen as a red line with that eye, and its position and orientation can be compared with the white image seen by the unoccluded eye.[3330] See also **red glass test, Lancaster red-green test.**

Madelung disease   See **familial multiple symmetrical lipomatosis with peripheral neuropathy.**

Madras neuropathy   A variant of **amyotrophic lateral sclerosis** in which eighth cranial nerve involvement and bulbar palsy, with slowing of motor nerve conduction velocities, are commonly found. The condition, reported from Madras, India, may be dominantly or recessively inherited.[215]

Maffucci syndrome   A rare, sporadic, neurocutaneous syndrome of unknown cause characterized by multiple enchondromas, visceral and cutaneous hemangiomas, bony malformations, and phlebolithiasis. It was described by Dr. Angelo Maffucci, an Italian physician, in 1881. Primary brain tumors and syndromes consequent upon compression of the CNS by the bony abnormalities are the usual neurological complications.[3] This condition and **Ollier disease** may be the same.[3821]

Magendie, François   (1783–1855) French professor of physiology and pathology at the Collège de France and physician at the Hôtel-Dieu. He confirmed the report of **Bell** (published in 1811) that the anterior spinal roots were motor, but was the first to show that the posterior roots were sensory (the Bell–Magendie law) in 1822, although his report was somewhat hesitant. He described the cerebrospinal fluid in 1825,[3565] and in 1842 described the **foramen** in the fourth ventricular roof that bears his name. He was also the first to describe **decerebrate rigidity.**

His claim to have discovered CSF (which he thought was secreted by the pia-arachnoid membrane at the surface of the brain and flowed into the ventricles through the midline foramen which he had described in 1828) was false. Key and Retzius restored a correct understanding of the formation, direction of flow, and absorption of CSF in 1876, Luschka redescribed the lateral foramina, and Magendie's errors were forgotten; but the name lives on.[5608]

magnet reaction   See **grasp response.**

magnet reflex   When the examiner's finger pushes the sole of a baby's foot so that the knee and the hip flex, and then slowly withdraws her finger, the baby's leg normally extends so that the foot remains in contact with it.

magnetic apraxia   Bimanual grasping of objects seen or felt, occurring in patients with orbital frontal lobe lesions, perhaps through release of parietal lobe activity.[3393]

magnetic foot   See **tonic foot response.**

magnetic gait   See **isolated gait ignition failure.**

magnetic gait apraxia   See **frontal gait disorder.**

magnetic gaze attraction   Persistence of a subject's gaze upon one object among a number presented, especially within the remaining normal homonymous half-field, seen in subjects with right hemispheric lesions. The phenomenon is commonly associated with unilateral spatial neglect.[1093]

magnetic resonance angiography   (MRA) A development of MRI scanning, allowing accurate visualization of arterial anatomy.

magnetic resonance imaging   (MRI, nuclear magnetic resonance) A technique adapted for neuroimaging that measures the absorption or emission of electromagnetic energy by nuclei in a static magnetic field after excitation by a suitable radiofrequency stimulus.[779]

The method uses the principles of nuclear magnetic resonance and the same computer techniques used for CT scanning to produce a map of the body's soft (water-containing) tissues. This requires high-strength magnetic fields, in which the magnetic properties of hydrogen atoms (protons) and the sensitivity of the spin of those nuclei to radiofrequency signals are studied. There are no known side effects, and the technique complements and often replaces CT scanning as a means of imaging inaccessible structures. Thus, it has been estimated that MRI has 10 times the power of CT in the resolution of the lesions of multiple sclerosis.[6028] A review of its nature and diagnostic value has been published.[1601]

Diffusion-weighted imaging is a refinement of MR technique that measures the Brownian motion of water; it is of value in the diagnosis of ischemic disease, producing increased signals in ischemic tissue. *Perfusion-weighted imaging* measures the relative blood flow in tissues using the patient's own blood or injected contrast agents such as gadolinium.

magnetic resonance spectroscopy   (MRS) A technique based on the principles of **magnetic resonance imaging,** but which also examines the concentration and distribution of elements other than the hydrogen proton, such as P^{31}, thus providing information on the metabolism of tissues without such intervention as biopsy. Such examinations have yielded information of the greatest value in primary muscle diseases and in cerebral ischemic states.

magnetization transfer ratio   (MTR) The magnitude of the exchange of magnetization between free water (which is normally visible on conventional T1- and T2-weighted MRI images) and bound water (which, being fixed within lipid membranes and proteins, is normally invisible on conventional MRI scans) following selective saturation of the bound water pool. The ratio gives an indication of the amount of macromolecular material present in a unit of brain.

Myelin is the most prevalent complex macromolecule present in the brain and MTR may this indicate the extent of demyelination.[2042]

magnetoencephalography   (MEG) The measurement, recording, and display of magnetic fields mainly perpendicular to the skull (and thus emanating from the sulci) produced by ionic flow across active neuronal membranes, which are the same ionic currents as produce EEG signals. This is a technique still in its infancy with regard to clinical diagnosis, but currently under scrutiny as to its ability, usually in combination with EEG, to localize abnormal electrical discharges within the brain.[145,1080]

magnetometer   A device capable of measuring the smallest magnetic fields of the brain, and which is thus able to detect the location, depth, orientation, and polarity of intracerebral spike discharges.

Magnus, Rudolf   (1873–1927) Dutch professor of pharmacology at Utrecht and a neurophysiologist. He demonstrated the existence of the antidiuretic factor in pituitary extracts, but is best known for his studies of postural, tonic labyrinthine, righting, and neck reflexes in the decerebrate animal, which led to huge advances in understanding of the activity of the vestibular apparatus.

The *Magnus-de Kleijn reflex* consists of extension of the limbs and rigidity on the side to which the head is turned passively, with flexion of the limbs with decreased tone on the other side; it is seen in subjects with decerebration.

Magoun, H.W.   Neurophysiologist who with **Moruzzi** delineated the reticular activating system.

Maida Vale Hospital for Nervous Diseases   Formerly the London Hospital for the Paralysed and Epileptic. A division of the **National Hospital,** Queen Square, London.

main d'accoucheur   (Fr, osteTRIcian's hand) See **carpopedal spasm.**

main de fakir   (Fr, Fakir's hand) A minor **dystonia,** not uncommon in the elderly, in whom this may be the first or only sign of a basal ganglion disorder. Flexion at the metacarpophalangeal joints, extension of the interphalangeal joints, and adduction of the thumb are the movements producing this appearance.

main en griffe   (Fr, hand in the shape of a claw) The manual posture seen in the setting of most lower motor neuron lesions chronically affecting the C8–T1 roots, and thus those fibers destined for the median and ulnar nerves. In this posture, the metacarpophalangeal joints are extended and the interphalangeal joints flexed; contractures of the long flexors also play a part in causing this. **Duchenne** first used the term in describing the appearance of the hands in **amyotrophic lateral sclerosis,** but it is more commonly seen with severe ulnar nerve pareses.

main en pince   (Fr, hand + claw) Partial flexion of the first two digits and full flexion of the remaining fingers, the posture of the hand thus slightly resembling a crab's claws; seen in some patients with severe motor neuropathies or syringomyelia.

The name was applied by Pierre **Marie** and **Guillain.**

main en poing fermée   (Fr, hand with the fist clenched) Clenching of the fist, as the first or only sign of a minor **dystonia,** as is not uncommon in the elderly. See also **fisting.**

main succulente   (Marinesco hand sign) The term applied by **Marinesco** to the cold, edematous, shiny, and livid appearance of the hand in some cases of syringomyelia.

Maintenance of Wakefulness test   A variation of **polysomnography,** in which subjects with complaints of excessive sleepiness are assessed.[3912]

Mainzer-Saldino syndrome   A congenital dysmorphic syndrome characterized by short stature, retinitis pigmentosa, hepatic and renal insufficiency, broad hands with arachnodactyly and cone-shaped phalangeal epiphyses, cerebellar signs, and mental and developmental delay.[337]

Majewski syndrome   See **short rib–polydactyly, type 2.**

major causalgia   See **reflex sympathetic dystrophy.**

major motor seizure   See **generalized tonic-clonic seizure.**

Major Problems in Neurology   (*Major Probl. Neurol.*) A neurological review book series. Address: W.B. Saunders Co., The Curtis Center, Independence Square West, Philadelphia, PA 19106-3399.

make/break test   An extension of the technique of hand-held dynamometry, in which the patient's power is tested isometrically (power being generated against immovable resistance—"make") and compared with that generated isotonically (power generated up to a maximum against increasing resistance—"break"). An increase of more than 20% in the force exerted can be generated by patients with functional weakness tested with the "break" rather than the "make" technic.[5720]

mal   French for evil, pain, or sickness—hence *mal a tête* for headache; *mal d'amour* for toothache (married mans toothache, part of the **Couvade syndrome**); *mal de mer* for seasickness; *mal de montagne* for mountain sickness; *grand and petit mal* epilepsies; *mal Saint, mal sacre, mal de terre, mal de St. Jean,* and *and mal haut* for forms of epilepsy; and many other secular (*mal francais, mal des allemands, mal Neapolitain, mal espagnol mal de Brunn, mal de chien*) or saintly (e.g., *mal divin, mal de SSt. Mervuis, Sement, Homme, Job, or Euphemie*) attributions for syphilis.[4512]

mal perforant   Painless perforating ulcers of the digits, most commonly seen in patients with **hereditary sensory and autonomic neuropathy** but also in **tabes dorsalis** or **syringomyelia.**

malabsorption encephalopathy   Fatigue, weakness, and physical and mental retardation, usually with evidence of subacute combined degeneration of the spinal cord and polyneuropathy, resulting from chronic malnutrition with steatorrhea.[5065]

maladie des tics compulsifs/impulsifs   See **Tourette syndrome.**

malaise   The subjective awareness that one is not perfectly well. In its mildest form, Miller Fisher[1860] notes typical symptoms being tiredness, a wish to sleep longer, disinclination for activity, loss of enthusiasm and cheerfulness, diminished appetite, and a disinclination to clear thinking. In more severe degrees of affliction, lack of strength, energy, initiative, appetite, alertness, and intellectual effort may be disabling. These symptoms are a part of the effort syndrome, and also of depression, but they are not usually accompanied by notable affective change and are closely linked temporally with organic diseases, both serious and trivial. Their neural substrate remains elusive and, in fact, no pathology may exist.

malar   (Lat) Of the cheek bone.

malaria   Infection with *Plasmodium vivax, malariae, falciparum,* or *ovale,* as a result of transfer of the sporozoites of the organism resulting from a mosquito bite. Congestion of cerebral capillaries with *P. falciparum*–laden red blood cells is the cause of the multifocal encephalopathy, perhaps the most common nontraumatic encephalopathy in the world, presenting with fever, seizures, and focal cerebral signs and known as *cerebral malaria.*[1289]

Diagnostic criteria for cerebral malaria have been suggested[4120] and include a deep level of unconsciousness (such that a painful stimulus is not localized) in the presence of a *P. falciparum* asexual parasitemia, after the correction of hypoglycemia and exclusion of other encephalopathies, especially bacterial meningitis and locally prevalent viral encephalitides. Other neurological complications include mononeuropathy and perhaps radiculopathy.

malformation   A defective part of an organ or of a region of the body resulting from an abnormality of development.

malignant   (from Lat, to act spitefully) Disposed to harm.

malignant angioendotheliomatosis (malignant intravascular lymphoma, malignant systematized angioendotheliomatosis, neoplastic angioendotheliomatosis) A rare, rapidly fatal disorder of adult life, characterized by the intravascular proliferation of atypical mononuclear cells, leading to ischemic damage to many organs, but especially the CNS.

Clinically, a subacute progressive dementing syndrome is the most typical presentation; cortical blindness; disturbances of gait, the special senses, and speech; and motor and sensory deficits progress to cause death within a year.[403,3098]

The same term is applied to a condition of intravascular malignant metastasis or lymphomatous spread occurring in adults.

malignant atrophic papulosis (Kohlmeier-Degos disease, Degos syndrome, fatal cutaneointestinal syndrome) A rare, fatal, cutaneous and systemic vaso-occlusive disease of unknown cause. The numerous painless skin lesions (the effects of the vasculopathy) are papular or atrophic and are scattered all over the trunk, while small infarcts also occur in the gastrointestinal tract and conjunctivae, and occasionally in the CNS.[1329]

The condition occurs mainly in adult males; occasional involvement of the CNS has been reported, with nonspecific signs of disseminated disease (ptosis, ophthalmoplegias, dysarthria, bleeding diatheses, seizures, and hemipareses) resulting from vascular thrombosis.[3749]

malignant brain edema Increased cerebral blood flow as a result of a failure of autoregulation. This is typically seen in children after severe head injury.[4350]

malignant fasciculation Large, polyphasic fasciculation potentials firing at a slow rate. This pattern has been seen in progressive motor neuron disease, but the relationship is not exclusive. (From the 2001 Report of the Nomenclature Committee of the American Association of Electromyography and Electrodiagnosis.[10] Used by permission, copyright © 2001, AAEM.)

malignant hyperpyrexia See **malignant hyperthermia.**

malignant hypertensive headache (accelerated hypertensive headache, including hypertensive encephalopathy). The following diagnostic criteria are suggested by the Headache Classification Committee of the International Headache Society[1051] (from: Classification of headache disorders, cranial neuralgias and facial pains; and diagnostic criteria for primary headache disorders. *Cephalalgia* 1988;**8**[suppl]:1–96. Reprinted by kind permission of Blackwell Science.)

A. Headache associated with grade 3 or 4 retinopathy (Keith-Wegener classification)
B. Diastolic blood pressure persistently above 120 mmHg
C. Appropriate investigations rule out vasopressor toxins, medication, or pheochromocytoma as causative factors.
D. Headache is temporally related to rise in blood pressure and disappears within 2 days after reduction of blood

pressure. If hypertensive encephalopathy is present, headache may persist up to 7 days after reduction of blood pressure.

malignant hyperthermia (malignant hyperpyrexia, King-Denborough syndrome, and in animals, capture myopathy) A dominantly inherited defect in the transmembrane transport of calcium, which may lead to muscle rigidity, hyperthermia, tachycardia, tachypnea and hypertonicity with acidosis, raised serum creatine kinase levels hypercapnea, hypoxemia, and **rhabdomyolysis** with myoglobinuria and potentially renal failure. The condition occurs in the presence of depolarizing muscle relaxants, inhalational anesthetics, or tricyclic drugs.[3261] In cases with ryanodine receptor disturbance, the responsible gene maps to chromosome 19q12–q13.2.

Screening is possible in those with a suspected family history (usually of death related to anesthesia), as baseline serum creatine kinase levels are usually elevated, but a firmer diagnosis can be achieved by an in vitro test on a muscle biopsy specimen activated with caffeine.[1712]

The original syndrome was characterized by short stature, mandibular hypoplasia, ptosis, spinal deformity, and pectus carinatum,[3048] but the condition also complicates various other subclinical, dominantly inherited, or myotonic myopathies[2461] and **Noonan syndrome.** See also **neuroleptic malignant syndrome** (which is clinically similar but pharmacologically distinct), **ecstasy.**

Malignant Hyperthermia Association A charitable organization. Canada: Address: 200 Elizabeth Street, EC 11-307, Toronto, Ontario, M2N 2A5, Canada. Tel: 416-340-3238. U.S.: Address: P.O. Box 1069, 39 E. State Street, Sherburne, NY 13460. Tel: 800-644-9737.

malignant inflammatory sensory polyganglionopathies (See also **nonmalignant inflammatory sensory polyganglionopathies**) A group of dysimmune disorders of dorsal root ganglia and autonomic and CNS structures affecting adults usually with small-cell carcinoma of the lung and presenting with ataxic and/or hyperalgesic syndromes, with or without autonomic dysfunction and cerebral, cerebellar, or other CNS involvement. Women may be more prone to these conditions than men. The presence of antineuronal nuclear antibodies (ANNA or anti-Hu) strongly suggests the presence of the small-cell carcinoma. The condition was originally described by **Denny-Brown** in the 1940s.[1391] See also **inflammatory sensory polyganglionopathies.**

malignant intravascular lymphoma See **malignant angioendotheliomatosis.**

malignant malnutritional syndrome See **kwashiorkor.**

malignant melanoma See **melanoma.**

malignant meningioma See **meningeal sarcoma, meningioma.**

malignant monophasic multiple sclerosis (Marburg disease) A fulminant monophasic demyelinating disease of unknown cause usually affecting young adults and leading to severe disability (blindness, paraplegia, etc.) and early death; and with pathological features characteristic of multiple sclerosis but with unusually extensive axonal loss.[3603]

malignant neurofibroma   See **neurofibromas.**

malignant schwannoma   See **schwannoma.**

malignant sensory neuropathy   See **subacute sensory neuronopathy**

malignant systematized angioendotheliomatsis See **malignant angioendotheliomatsis.**

malignant tumors   Tumors that are rapidly growing and often invasive, and that histologically show frequent mitoses, necrosis, vascular proliferation, and endothelial hyperplasia.

malignant vasovagal syncope   See **neurocardiogenic syncope.**

malingering   The conscious, motivated simulation of disease.

Mallory body myopathy   See **myofibrillar (desmin-storage) myopathy.**

Mallory stain   (PTAH stain) A method of demonstrating glial fibers histologically, using mercuric chloride, phosphotungstic acid, and alcohol. Muscle fibers, myelin, and astroglia stain blue; collagen stains brown.

malnutrition syndrome   A syndrome described in black African infants in the month or two following treatment of severe malnutrition. Clinically, the findings include parkinsonian tremor and rigidity with hyperreflexia, and sometimes myoclonus, opisthotonos, and insomnia. The author suggests that the condition results from relative deficiency of some essential dietary factor such as a trace element or vitamin in the context of sudden replenishment of protein stores.[2902]

maltase deficiency myopathy   See **glycogen storage diseases.**

malum vertebrale suboccipitale   Tuberculous caries of the atlanto-occipital region.

mandibular dysostosis   See **hemifacial microsomia.**

mandibular reflex   Tapping the chin causes elevation of the mandible in the normal newborn.[6064] See also **jaw jerk.**

mandibulofacial dysostosis   (Franchescetti syndrome, Franchescetti-Zwahlen-Klein syndrome, Treacher Collins syndrome) A dominantly (or X-linked recessively) inherited congenital dysmorphic syndrome, characterized by antimongolian slant of the eyes, malar and mandibular hypoplasia, colobomas of the lower lids, ocular malformations, prominent low-set ears with deformed pinnas, absent auditory canals, a flat malar region, cleft palate, webbed neck, pulmonary stenosis, cryptorchidism, microcephaly, dwarfism, and mental and developmental delay. Cervical vertebral anomalies and various other systemic abnormalities may also occur.[1106]

The condition was well described by Dr. E. Treacher-Collins,[1106] an English ophthalmologist at Moorfields Eye Hospital, but the very first account was that of Allen Thompson, professor of physiology at Edinburgh University in 1847. Franchescetti and Klein analyzed 65 cases in 1949 and integrated many unrelated observations into one logical clinical complex.

mandibulofacial syndromes   A group of genetically determined malformations in which abnormal formations of the facial bones represent a common factor.

mandrake   (*Atropa mandragora*) A plant whose root has anesthetic properties, used in ancient days to alleviate pain before amputations, and also as an enchantment, since it was considered capable of rendering a person invisible.

mands   Self-limiting statements concerning the needs of the speaker.[1179] See also **tacts.**

manganism   Chronic manganese intoxication, presenting as a syndrome resembling **Parkinson disease** and with progression of gait disturbance, rigidity, and speed of distal movements even after cessation of exposure.[2676]

mania   (Gr, violent madness) (delirium furiosum) A psychosis characterized by both mental and physical excitement. The term is still employed to refer to one aspect of bipolar depressive illness, and occasionally dipsomania (morbid alcoholic ingestion), but is seldom used in other contexts in modern medical parlance. The dancing mania (tarantism) came and went in 1374. Many other descriptive Latinisms to do with mania are also no longer current.

mania à potu   (mania inebriosa) Alcoholic delirium. See **delirium tremens.**

mania inebriosa   See **mania à potu.**

manifest latent nystagmus   See **latent nystagmus.**

man-in-the-barrel syndrome   The association of weakness of the arms with intact leg power, as though the patient were constrained within a barrel. Brainstem functions are retained. The usual cause of this unusual syndrome is cerebral hypoperfusion, such as may occur after myocardial infarction. Bilateral infarction of the motor cortices, in the "watershed" areas, is also a cause.[3934]

Mann syndrome   The association of a positive Romberg sign, diminution of the corneal reflex, past pointing, and loss of arm swing on the same side as a contusion of the brain, with restricted movement of the eyes to that side.

The syndrome, which has uncertain validity and which does not permit localization of the responsible lesion to a single site, was described by Dr. Ludwig Mann (1866–1936), a German neuropathologist and professor of neurology in Breslau.[3590]

Mannkopf sign   Pressure over a painful area usually causes an increase in the pulse rate of 10–30/min, but this increase does not occur in subjects with feigned pain, though it may do so in those in hysterical states.[1349a]

mannosidase deficiency   A rare, inherited, lysosomal storage disease of glycoprotein catabolism, characterized by facial dysmorphism, deafness, mental retardation, impairment of speech, and sometimes peripheral neuropathy or encephalopathic signs with spasticity; the clinical features are, however, very variable.

The diagnosis is made by finding severe reduction in β-mannosidase activity and elevation of urinary disaccharides.[3295]

mannosidosis   1. A rare, congenital lysosomal storage disease due to deficiency of α-mannosidase, leading to the deposition of excessive amounts of glycoprotein (mannosyl-oligosaccharides). The responsible gene maps to chromosome 19p13.2–q12.

The clinical features, particularly the dysmorphism, resemble those of **Hurler syndrome** and include mental retardation, corneal opacities, nerve deafness, hepatosplenomegaly, osteoporosis, vertebral anomalies, short stature, sensorineural deafness, cataract, umbilical hernia, jaundice, mucopolysacchariduria, immunoglobulin deficiency, thickening of the calvarium, pyramidal signs, and mental and developmental delay.

As *variants*, both rapidly progressive infantile and more lenient juvenile forms occur.[3065]

2. Beta-mannosidosis (OMIM 25841) is a rare congenital lysosomal storage disease of glycoprotein catabolism due to deficiency of β-mannosidase. Deafness and other neurological signs and facial dysmorphisms are the usual features; peripheral neuropathy has also been described.

Manta syndrome   A rapidly progressive asymmetrical tetraparesis, ending fatally from denervation as a result of rapidly progressive anterior horn cell disease without any involvement of the upper motor neuron.[3597] The cause is not determined.

mantakassa   A form of acquired spastic paraplegia due to cyanide toxicity from cassava consumption in the residents of Mozambique.

Manto syndrome   The unusual association of **spasmodic torticollis** and **thoracic outlet syndrome**.[1473]

manual muscle testing   Clinical techniques for evaluating the strength of muscle contractions semiquantitatively, using the subjective judgments of the examiner, who provides the resistance to the patient's limb movement. The modified **Medical Research Council scale** represents one such system.[3829]

maple syrup urine disease   A recessively inherited leukoencephalopathy due to a block in the oxidative decarboxylation of leucine, isoleucine, and valine.[3837] The responsible gene maps to chromosome 19p13.1–q13.2. See also **branched-chain ketoaciduria.**

Clinically, vomiting, seizures, and spasticity with intermittent opisthotonos are the usual signs, occurring first when protein is introduced into the infant's diet. Most infants die within a month of birth after rapid cerebral deterioration. The serum leucine levels are raised and hypoglycemia is common. Boiled urine assumes a yellow cast in the DPNH test.[3835]

A *variant* is *thiamine-dependent maple syrup urine disease*, which is characterized by similar but milder symptoms in the presence of some residual branched-chain ketoacid dehydrogenase activity and is responsive to thiamine treatment.[1557]

marasmus   (Gr, wasting) Emaciation of the body with stunting of growth, as in **protein-calorie malnutrition** and the **diencephalic syndrome**.[2032]

marble bone disease   See **Albers-Schönberg disease, osteopetrosis.**

marble brain disease   See **carbonic anhydrase II deficiency.**

Marburg disease   See **malignant monophasic multiple sclerosis.**

March of Dimes Birth Defects Foundation   A charitable organization. Address: 1275 Mamaroneck Ave., White Plains, NY 10605. Tel: 888-663-4637. Web site: http://www.modimes.org/.

march syndrome   See **anterior tibial syndrome.**

marche à petits pas   (Fr, gait with little steps) A feature of parkinsonism and also of diffuse cerebral dysfunction, as in **Alzheimer disease.** See **frontal gait disorder.**

Marchi stain   A method of staining a block of neural tissue, achieved by immersing it in a mixture of osmium tetroxide, and an oxidizing agent; degenerating myelin products stain black.

Marchi, Vittorio   (1851–1908) Italian physician and anatomist. After graduation at Modena, he was assistant to **Golgi** for a time, and later worked in Florence and Modena. His name is occasionally given to the spinothalamic tract, but he is best remembered for the staining technique that he described in 1886.

Marchiafava, Ettore   (1847–1935) Italian physician who graduated from the University of Rome, where he eventually became professor of pathology and of clinical medicine. He published important work on malaria, vasculitis, and pathological anatomy as well as on the following condition.

Ettore Marchiafava

Marchiafava-Bignami disease   (corpus callosum degeneration, progressive alcoholic dementia) Degeneration of the middle layer of the corpus callosum throughout its extent, occurring classically in male Italian drinkers of red wine, but also described among alcoholics in other lands. The anterior and hippocampal commissures, cerebellar peduncles, optic chiasm, and deep white matter pathways may also be affected.

Clinically, confusion, seizures, dementia, aphasia, apraxias, pyramidal signs, rigidity, disconnection syndromes, mutism, and coma result; death follows shortly.[3605]

The mellifluous names of the original describers have fixed this syndrome in the minds of neurologists, almost none of whom will ever see it.

Marchiafava-Micheli syndrome   Paroxysmal nocturnal hemoglobinuria, a potential cause of cerebral venous thrombosis and more often of back pain.[2870]

Marcus Gunn, Robert   (1850–1909) Scottish ophthalmologist who trained in Vienna and at Moorfields Eye Hospital in London. See **Gunn, R. M.**

Marcus Gunn phenomenon   See **Gunn phenomenon.**

Marcus Gunn pupil   See **Gunn pupil.**

Marden-Walker syndrome   A recessively inherited dysmorphic syndrome characterized by blepharophimosis, kyphoscoliosis, arachnodactyly, micrognathia, cleft palate, multiple joint contractures present during the first year of life, and cataract.[3606]

Cleft palate, pectus carinatum, congenital cardiac anomalies, camptodactyly, clubfoot, joint contractures, neurogenic muscle atrophy with hypotonia and hyporeflexia, agenesis of the corpus callosum, and mental and developmental delay are also occasionally described.

Marden-Walker–like syndrome   See **Suliman syndrome.**

Marek disease   A demyelinating neuropathy of poultry caused by a herpes virus with pathological similarities to **acute inflammatory polyneuropathy**

Marfan, Antonin-Bernard-Jean   (1858–1942) French pediatrician who trained in Toulouse and Paris, working for most of his life in Paris as professor of therapeutics in one or another of the children's hospitals. The topics he published on most often were tuberculosis, diphtheria, and nutrition, but he is best remembered for describing the following syndrome.

Marfan syndrome   A polygenic, dominantly inherited disorder of connective tissue, the responsible gene mapping to 15q21.1, where the gene *FBN1* codes for fibrillin, a component of extracellular microfibrils. Its variable manifestations affect the eyes and the cardiovascular and skeletal systems.

The major clinical features include displacement of the lens, myopia, blue sclerae, dolichocephaly, high arched palate, scoliosis with chest deformity, pectus carinatum or excavatum, inguinal hernia, flat arches of the feet, abnormally long limbs (the span of the body being greater than its height), arachnodactyly, laxity of joints, aortic and mitral valve lesions, and aortic dissecting aneurysm.[3608,4552] The lower-segment (pubis to sole) measurement is greater than that of the upper segment (vertex to pubis), the ratio averaging 0.85 (normal, 0.93).[2219] A brief but comprehensive handbook has been published for the National Marfan Foundation of New York.[4551]

In a *variant* form (*Marfan myopathic syndrome*), a slowly progressive myopathy is associated with early weakness in girdle distribution.[2152]

marginal gliosis   See **Chaslin gliosis.**

marginal tract   See **Lissauer tract.**

Marie, Pierre   (1853–1940) French neurologist who trained in law before entering medicine. After his internship, he became a pupil of **Charcot** and eventually chef de clinique when aged 65, after many years at the Bicêtre.

He gave original descriptions of hypertrophic pulmonary osteoarthropathy, achondroplasia, and **craniocleidodysostosis** and, in 1886, with Charcot, described what is now known as **hereditary motor and sensory neuropathy** (peroneal muscular atrophy or Charcot-Marie-Tooth disease). In 1885, he had described acromegaly, and noted its association with a pituitary tumor. In 1893, he identified the hereditary ataxia now named for him (see next entry) and later described ankylosing spondylitis. His classification of the aphasias in 1906[3616] was notable for his vehement contradiction of **Broca** in its denial of any special role for the left third frontal convolution in speech.[712] He also questioned the existence of Aran-Duchenne progressive muscular atrophy in a paper in 1897.[3615]

Marie was a founder of the *Revue Neurologique* with Brissaud in 1893. He did not succeed **Charcot** as professor of diseases of the nervous system on the latter's death, but only in 1917 after the deaths of **Raymond** and then **Déjèrine.** Within 6 years, his closest family having died, he resigned and retired to the south of France.[7]

Marie ataxia (Nonne-Marie syndrome) A dominantly inherited spastic-ataxic syndrome with gaze palsies, which is probably not different from the olivopontocerebellar atrophy type 1 of Menzel, but may not comprise a single entity. Marie distinguished the condition from **Friedreich ataxia** on the grounds of later age of onset and the presence of hyperreflexia and pyramidal signs; oculomotor pareses; a reduction in visual acuity and of the visual fields and color vision; and the absence of Rombergism, pes cavus and scoliosis.[3614] Optic atrophy and, in some cases, mental deterioration may occur late in the course of the disease.

One may remark a tendency to put most non–Friedreich ataxic patients into this category, which is what Marie seems to have done. However, a modern classification places this condition with the late-onset autosomal dominant **cerebellar ataxias.**[2438]

Marie syndrome   See **pituitary gigantism.**

Marie-Foix retraction sign   In patients with pyramidal lesions, pressure on the toes or vigorous plantar flexion at the ankle leads to flexion at the hip and knee and to attempts to dorsiflex the ankle.

Marie-Foix sclerosis   Nonprogressive lesions of the white matter with sclerosis following perinatal encephalopathy or associated with acquired multifocal cerebrovascular disease.[3617]

The condition has been mistaken for a form of **Schilder disease** and the eponym *Schilder-Foix disease* has been coined as a result.

Marie-Foix syndrome   Unilateral cerebellar ataxia with contralateral hemiparesis and thermoanalgesia, resulting from a rostral lateral pontine lesion. See **lateral pontomedullary syndrome,** which is almost if not exactly the same thing.

Marie-Foix-Alajouanine syndrome (late cortical cerebellar atrophy) A sporadic, adult-onset cerebellar syndrome with atrophic changes limited to the cerebellum and inferior olives, resembling Holmes cerebellar atrophy, except that the latter is inherited in an autosomal dominant manner. It is occasionally accompanied by dementia, pyramidal signs, or absent ankle jerks. See **autosomal dominant cerebellar ataxias, olivopontocerebellar atrophy.**

Marie-Léri syndrome   Acromegaly, described by Marie in 1886, by von Recklinghausen in 1890, and by Leri in 1913.[3353]

Marie-Sée syndrome   The occurrence of **idiopathic intracranial hypertension** in children, here due to vitamin A intoxication. The condition was originally described in 1951[3613] by Dr. J. Marie.

Marin-Amat syndrome (inverted Marcus Gunn phenomenon) Abnormal synkinetic movements following facial nerve paresis and manifesting as eye closure when the jaw is opened wide.

The condition has been described as the opposite of the **Gunn phenomenon** (jaw-winking)[3619,4581] but probably represents a normal associated movement rather than the manifestation of any abnormal trigeminofacial anastomosis. It may be noted in passing that, when the mouth is opened unusually wide, as in yawning, the eyes close anyway.

Dr. Marin-Amat was a Spanish ophthalmologist.

Marinesco bodies   Eosinophilic intranuclear inclusions found in the pigmented brainstem nuclei and substantia nigra, in numbers proportional to the subject's age; also found mainly in the substantia nigra in elderly people and in those with hepatic encaphalopathy.

Georges Marinesco

Marinesco, Georges (Marinescu, Georghe) (1863–1938) Romanian neurologist who trained under **Charcot** and Weigert and later became professor of neurology at Bucharest. He identified and named **chroma-tolysis,** the lesions of the substantia nigra in **Parkinson disease,** and neuronophagia. He also wrote on salvarsan therapy for syphilis, painful amputation neuromas, pathological anatomy, diseases of muscle, and conditioned reflexes, and published a number of books on neurology and pathology.

Marinesco hand sign (*main succulente*) The cold, livid, and edematous hand in syringomyelia, resulting from sympathetic irritation. This was the subject of Marinesco's graduation thesis.[3622]

Marinescu-Radovici reflex See **palmomental reflex.**

Marinesco-Sjörgen(-Garland) syndrome A rare, recessively inherited, congenital degenerative disorder, characterized clinically by progressive cerebellar ataxia, nystagmus, cataract occurring at any age but usually in early childhood, and a variable degree of mental retardation.

Skeletal anomalies such as dwarfism, kyphoscoliosis, and pes cavus; pigmentary retinopathy; hypertension; hypergonadotropic hypogonadism; delayed motor development; dysarthria; myopathy;[385] pyramidal signs; and peripheral neuropathy with inclusions seen on nerve biopsy specimens have also been described in this condition.[5076]

The first report of the syndrome was in 1904. Marinesco published a description in 1931 and Sjögren emphasized the genetic nature of the disease in 1950.[3623] See also **Gillespie syndrome,** in which aniridia is present rather than cataract but is otherwise identical.

Mariotte spot The **blind spot.**

Markus syndrome See **Adie pupil, Holmes-Adie syndrome.**

Markus-Adie syndrome See **Holmes-Adie syndrome.**

Maroteaux-Lamy syndrome 1. (mucopolysaccharidosis type 6) See **mucopolysaccharidoses.** 2. (pyknodysostosis; from Gr, dense + bone + condition) A recessive syndrome of mental retardation, dwarfism, delayed closure of the fontanelles, skull and spinal dysplasia with deformity, a double row of teeth, and blue sclerae.[3635]

Marsden, C. David (1938–1998) Preeminent British neurologist and neurophysiologist, professor and chairman of neurology at the National Hospital, Queen Square, and prolific contributor to knowledge, especially in the fields of movement disorders and genetics. He described such syndromes as **painful legs and moving toes, reticular reflex, cortical** and **propriospinal myoclonus,** and **abdominal dyskinesias,** and in the words of Stanley Fahn, "brought order into the spectrum of dystonia." He was elected a Fellow of the Royal Society in 1983.

Marshall syndrome See **dominant saddle nose, myopia, cataract, and hearing loss.**

Martha-Alma disease See **Hallervorden-Spatz disease.**

Martin-Albright syndrome See **pseudohypoparathyroidism.**

Martin-Bell syndrome See **fragile X syndrome.**

Martin-Gruber anastomosis A common anomalous connection between the median and ulnar nerves, usually in the upper forearm. In the most common form, fibers of the median nerve leave the trunk of that nerve and run with the ulnar nerve to the hand where they innervate the thenar muscles as usual. The anomaly occurs in between 10% and 30% of humans and may be dominantly inherited.

Variants on the common pattern have been identified[5306] and electrical criteria for anomalous innervation have been suggested, as follows:[161]
A. Median to ulnar
1. The compound muscle action potential (CMAP) is higher over the abductor pollicis brevis (APB) with elbow than with wrist stimulation of the median nerve.
2. The CMAP over the first dorsal interosseous is higher with elbow than with wrist stimulation of the median nerve.
3. Recording of a negative potential over the abductor digiti minimi (ADM) on stimulation of the median nerve at the elbow.
B. Ulnar to median
1. The CMAP over the APB is higher on stimulation of the median nerve at the wrist than at the elbow.
2. The CMAP over the ADM is lower on stimulation of the ulnar nerve at the wrist than at the elbow, and there may be an additional recording of a CMAP from the ADM with stimulation of the median nerve at the wrist (the Riche-Cannieu anastomosis, leading fibers from the median to the hypothenar muscles). A proximal Martin-Gruber anastomosis may mimic ulnar neuropathy at the elbow.

Martsolf syndrome See **cataract–spasticity–mental retardation syndrome.**

MASA syndrome (**M**ental retardation, **A**phasia, **S**huffling gait, **A**dducted thumbs) A congenital syndrome inherited as an X-linked trait and characterized by short stature, aphasia, adducted thumbs, spasticity, and psychomotor retardation.[546] See **hereditary spastic paraplegia.**

masked epilepsy A nineteenth century term for what are now known as **complex partial seizures.**

masking The stimulation of one ear with white noise or with a band of sound at frequencies close to the test frequency, while the acuity in the other ear is tested; a technique designed to prevent the perception of the test sound by the ear not being studied.

mass lesions (space-occupying lesions) Pathological collections of abnormal material that are (but should not be) inside the cranium, where they act to increase intracranial pressure. The alternative term is rejected, as the author cannot think of any lesions apart from psychiatric disorders and amputations which do not occupy space.

mass reflex   (Riddoch mass reflex) Diffuse activity of the disinhibited spinal cord below the level of a complete or near-complete lesion of the descending motor pathways, appearing after the period of **spinal shock.** The clinical manifestations include flexor spasms and autonomic discharge, the latter leading to detrusor contraction, hypertension, bradycardia, sweating, and piloerection. The reflex occurs in response to external (painful or tactile) or internal (infections, full bladder) stimuli below the level of the lesion.[2499,4683]

masseter inhibitory reflex   Inhibition of contraction of the muscle bilaterally resulting from unilateral trigeminal sensory stimulation, especially of the mental n. Electrophysiologically, the reflex has both early and late phases.[2643]

masseter reflex   See **jaw reflex.**

masseteric hypertrophy   (masticatory muscle hypertrophy) Uni- or bilateral hypertrophy of the masseters, usually in subjects prone to grinding their teeth (**bruxism**).[2340] Such enlargement of the temporalis and masseter muscles is due to reactive muscle fiber hypertrophy with type 1 fiber predominance. The condition may also occur as a familial condition,[3657] as a manifestation of **branchial myopathy,** or from unknown causes.[2459]

massive infantile spasms   See **West syndrome.**

Masson stain   A trichrome connective tissue stain that colors astrocytes, myofibrils, and myelin red-brown and collagen blue-green.

MAST syndrome   1. A recessive form of hereditary spastic paraparesis with extrapyramidal features, dementia, and pyramidal signs found in an Old Order Amish kinship in Pennsylvania.[1195] See **hereditary spastic paraplegia.** 2. A compression mononeuropathy resulting from the wearing of **M**edical **A**nti**S**hock **T**rousers.

mastication reflex   See **Wolfing reflex.**

masticatory dysfunction   Persistent or repeated clenching of the masseter muscles, usually seen in patients under stress and causing pain felt diffusely over the side of the face, usually unilaterally, extending from the temple down to the jaw.

masticatory muscle hypertrophy   See **masseteric hypertrophy.**

masticatory palsy   Weakness of the muscles supplied by the fifth cranial nerve.

mastocytosis   (systemic mastocytosis) A syndrome characterized by urticaria pigmentosa, spinal anomalies, platyspondyly, malabsorption, dizziness, seizures, recurrent migraine-like headaches with hypotension,

osteoporosis, osteosclerosis or osteopetrosis, and distal myopathic weakness. Intracerebral hemorrhage has also been reported. Hives, flushing, lacrimation, and anaphylaxis are the more visible features; hepatosplenomegaly and anemia, abdominal cramps, and respiratory distress are the main systemic manifestations. The benign localized form affects the skin only (urticaria pigmentosa).[3131,3203]

Mastroiacovo syndrome   A congenital dysmorphic syndrome characterized by thinness, micrognathia with an open-mouth appearance, scoliosis, cryptorchidism, arachnodactyly, joint contractures, hypotonia, seizures, muscle atrophy, strabismus, and mental and developmental delay.[337]

masturbation   (from Lat, the hand + licentious conduct) Stimulation of erogenous zones by means other than contact with the erogenous zones of another person.

This solitary activity was widely regarded as a cause of neurological disease during the nineteenth century, but is not now considered to have any such long-term effects. Ladame (1890) wrote that is was likely to "favour the evolution of . . . disease by exhausting an already enfeebled spinal cord."[3222] *Autres temps, autres moeurs.*

Matas test   See **carotid compression test.**

maternal rubella syndrome   See **Gregg syndrome.**

Mathew scale   A popular neurological scoring system designed for the evaluation of stroke patients[3694] (see Chart M–1).

Chart M–1. The Mathew Scale: Neurological Evaluation in Patients with Acute Stroke

Factor	Score
Mentation	
Level of Consciousness	
Fully conscious	8
Lethargic but mentally intact	6
Obtunded	4
Stuporous	2
Comatose	0
Orientation	
Orientated × 3 modalities	6
Orientated × 2	4
Orientated × 1	2
Disorientated	0
Speech	
Reitan test	0–23
Cranial Nerves	
Homonymous hemianopsia	
Intact fields	3
Mild	2
Moderate	1
Severe impairment	0

Conjugate Deviation of Eyes

Intact	3
Mild	2
Moderate	1
Severe impairment	0

Facial Weakness

Intact	3
Mild	2
Moderate	1
Severe impairment	0

Motor Power (Each Limb Separately)

Normal strength	5
Contracts vs. resistance	4
Elevates against gravity	3
Gravity eliminated	2
Flicker	1
No movements	0

Performance on Disability Status Scale

Normal	28
Mild impairment	21
Moderate impairment	14
Severe impairment	7
Death	0

Reflexes

Normal	3
Asymmetrical/pathological	2
Clonus	1
No reflexes elicited	0

Sensation

Normal	3
Mild sensory abnormality	2
Severe sensory abnormality	1
No response to pain	0

Adapted from Mathew NT, Meyer JS, Rivera VM, et al. Double blind evaluation of glycerol tretment in acute cerebral infarction. Lancet 1972;2:1327–1329, by permission of Elsevier Science.

Mattis Dementia Rating Scale A screening instrument designed to detect the presence of brain pathology in impaired geriatric patients.

Consciousness, insight, affective tone, attention, memory, verbal and motor perseveration, constructional ability, conceptual ability, and naming are examined.[3711] See also **Extended Scale for Dementia.**

matutinal vertigo That common form of vertigo in which symptoms are commonly precipitated, *inter alia*, by arising from bed in the morning. It occurs with both central and peripheral causes of the vertigo and it has no localizing value, but is seldom present in **Ménière disease.**[508] See **benign positional vertigo.**

Maurois syndrome See **pituitary gigantism.**

Mauthner, Ludwig Wilhelm Hungarian pediatrician who trained and worked in Vienna, where he founded and ran a hospital for sick children; in 1844 he published the first textbook of pediatric neurology.[7]

maximum volumetric isometric contraction A valid technique for evaluating the strength of muscle contractions against unyielding resistances, and thus a method of estimating motor unit loss.[178] See also **Tufts Quantitative Neuromuscular examination.**

Mayer disease See **neuronal ceroid lipofuscinosis.**

Mayer finger-thumb reflex (Mayer sign) Adduction of the thumb, with extension at the interphalangeal joint and flexion of the metacarpophalangeal joint, in response to forcible flexion of D2, 3, 4 when the patient's hand is in full supination. Normally present, it disappears with a pyramidal lesion.[3716]

Mayer, K. (1862–1931) Austrian neurologist.

Mayer sign 1. (See **Mayer finger-thumb reflex**). 2. See **Wartenberg sign.**

Mayer-Gross apraxia See **constructional apraxia.**[3718]

Mayer-Gross sign See **closing-in phenomenon.**

Mayer-Gross, Willi (b. 1889) German psychiatrist.

Mayo Clinic Scale for Reflex Assessment A scheme enumerating the activity of muscle stretch reflexes, with 9 points ranging from absent (−4) through normal (0) to continuous clonus (+4) but not improving interrater agreement.[3595] See also **MRC scale; NINDS scale.**

Mayou, Marmaduke Stephen (b. 1876) English ophthalmologist who described familial cerebromacular degeneration (Batten-Mayou disease) in 1904. See **gangliosidoses.**

May-White syndrome (autosomal dominant cerebellar ataxia, ataxia with myoclonus and deafness) A dominantly inherited multisystem degeneration causing progressive myoclonic epilepsy, sensorineural deafness, ataxia, sensorimotor peripheral neuropathy, and muscle atrophy, beginning in adolescence.[3715] In some cases, changes typical of mitochondrial disease have been reported.

M'Bwaki See **Kwashiorkor.**

McArdle disease See **glycogen storage diseases.**

McArdle sign Increase in weakness produced by neck flexion and relieved by extension, probably due to conduction block in demyelinated segments of the cervical cord.

The mechanism for this is likely to be ischemia induced by the flexion when the spinal canal is narrowed by degenerative joint disease.

McCarthy, D.J. (1874–1965) American neurologist who published two papers on the supraorbital reflex in 1901 (in German).

McCarthy reflex (McCarthy sign) Percussion of the superior orbital region causes blinking of the homolateral eyelid; a normal finding in infants.[6064] See **orbicularis oculi reflex.**

McCarthy sign   See **orbicularis oculi reflex.**

McCrae syndrome   A syndrome consisting of X-linked mental retardation and deafness with mental and developmental delay.[337]

McCune-Albright syndrome   (polyostotic fibrous dysplasia) A sporadic congenital syndrome of progressive fibrous dysplasia of the long bones and skull, leading to complaints of bone pain, fractures, and cranial nerve palsies; irregular brown-pigmented patches are found on the skin, their outline said to resemble that of the coast of Maine; and various endocrine disturbances occur, especially precocious puberty in girls.

The syndrome was first reported by McCune in 1936 but a fuller paper[3739] and an extensive review by Albright[91] both appeared in the following year.

Jaffé-Lichtenstein syndrome is similar, but the endocrine and dermal abnormalities are not present.

McDonald-Halliday criteria   A system of criteria for the diagnosis of multiple sclerosis, published in 1977 and introducing the concept of isolated spinal involvement[3744] (see Chart M–2).

Chart M–2. McDonald-Halliday Criteria for the Diagnosis of Multiple Sclerosis

Proved

Diagnosis established at necropsy

Clinically Definite

Some physical disability
Remitting or relapsing course
History of two or more episodes, and
Evidence of lesions at two or more necessarily separate sites in the CNS, and
Lesions predominantly in the white matter, and
Age at onset of symptoms 15–50 years, and
History of signs or symptoms for 1 year or longer, and
No better explanation.

Early Probable or Latent

Slight or no disability
Single episode suggestive of multiple sclerosis, and
Evidence of lesions at two or more sites in the CNS, *or*
Remitting and relapsing course, and
Evidence of one or more lesions associated with multiple sclerosis.

Progressive Probable

Progressive history of paraplegia, and
Evidence of lesions at two or necessarily separate sites in the CNS, and
Other causes excluded.

Progressive Possible

Progressive history of paraplegia, and
Evidence of only one lesion, and
Other causes excluded.

Suspected

Single episode suggestive of multiple sclerosis without evidence of any lesion or with evidence of a single lesion only, *or*
Recurrent optic neuritis (unilateral or bilateral) with one additional episode not involving the optic nerve but without evidence of lesions outside the eye.

McDonald WI, Halliday AM. Diagnosis and classification of multiple sclerosis. Br. Med. Bull. 1977;33:4–9. Reproduced by kind permission.

A recent revision of these criteria is reproduced under **multiple sclerosis.** See also **Schumacher panel criteria, Poser criteria.**

McGill Pain Inventory   A questionnaire consisting primarily of three classes of word descriptors—sensory, affective, and evaluative—that are used by patients who describe the pains from which they suffer, and containing a scale of the intensity of the pain. A background history also forms part of the questionnaire, as do enquiries about accompanying symptoms, the timing and geography of the pain, the pain modifying activities used, and the effect of the pain upon sleep and sexual activity.[3824]

McGregor's line   The line drawn from the upper surface of the posterior edge of the hard palate to the most caudal point of the occipital curve in the true lateral X-ray of the skull.

Though originally thought to be of value in the diagnosis of **basilar impression,** CT scanning or anteroposterior tomography of the foramen magnum are now preferred.[5282]

McHenry, Lawrence Chester   (1929–1985) American neurologist, born in Oklahoma, where he later trained in medicine, afterwards receiving his neurological training in Boston. During his army service, he became interested in cerebral blood flow and published extensively in that field over many years, from the Army Institute of Research and from Jefferson Medical College Hospital, Philadelphia; but his abiding interest was medical—specifically neurological—history. He entitled his magnum opus *Garrison's History of Neurology,* even though he was revising what was originally a book chapter into a whole book, some 5 times as long as the original.

In 1972 he became professor of neurology at the Bowman Gray School of Medicine and for the remainder of his life continued in the teaching and practice of his specialty and the encouragement of further historical research into its past, an area in which he had become internationally preeminent.

McLellan classification   A system for the classification of voiding dysfunction. Spastic and atonic forms were defined, the latter reclassified by Lapides into motor paralytic and sensory paralytic forms.

McLeod syndrome   (benign X-linked myopathy with acanthocytes, Xp21 myopathy) A rare, X-linked, recessive, multisystem disorder characterized by acanthocytosis, anisocytosis, and weakened blood cell antigenicity in the Kell blood group system, due to a mutation of the *XK* gene.[5444] Clinically, psychiatric disturbances are common presenting signs;[2895] subclinical myopathy with areflexia and raised serum creatine kinase levels, chorea, peripheral neuropathy, cardiomyopathy, and caudate atrophy seen on MRI scans are less commonly found.[1273]

The name comes from that of the blood donor in whom the disorder was first detected. The responsible gene maps to Xp21.2–p21-1 on the short arm of the chromosome, close to that of **Duchenne dystrophy.**

McQuarrie syndrome (idiopathic infantile or neonatal hypoglycemia) Hypoglycemia causing convulsions and nonlocalizing signs in small children in whom no pathological abnormality is consistently detected.[3789]

MCTD Abbreviation for medium-chain triglyceride disease.

mean consecutive difference See jitter.

mean sorted difference See **jitter.**

measles inclusion body encephalitis A fatal encephalitic illness seen in some immunocompromised patients exposed to measles virus. It is characterized clinically by obtunded delirium and myoclonus, and pathologically by the finding of measles antigen within neurons and by the presence of eosinophilic intranuclear inclusions.

MEB disease See **muscle, eye, brain disease.**

mechanical hyperalgesia A decrease in the threshold but an increase in the suprathreshold magnitude of pain induced by mechanical stimulation of the skin. A *static form* (tested by gentle skin pressure and mediated by unmyelinated fibers) and a *dynamic form* (tested by light skin stroking and mediated by myelinated fibers) have been defined.[4194]

Meckel cave The dural sac overlying the medial tip of the petrous portion of the temporal bone, in which lies the Gasserian ganglion of the fifth cranial nerve.

Meckel, Johann Freidrich (the elder; 1724–1774) German anatomist who described the sphenopalatine ganglion (Meckel ganglion) and the dural space lodging the Gasserian ganglion (Meckel cave) in 1748.[4000] He also defined the syndrome named for him in 1822.

Meckel syndrome See **dysencephalia splanchocystica.**

Meckel-Gruber syndrome See **dysencephalia splanch-nocystica.**

medial brachial fascial compartment syndrome A potential complication of axillary artery angiography, the result of hematoma formation with damage to the lower brachial plexus.[5241]

medial epicondylitis (golfers' elbow) A syndrome of pain on the medial aspect of the elbow, radiating distally. It results from tendinitis of the long wrist and finger flexors occasioned by excessive use of those muscles.

medial forebrain bundle A complex collection of ascending and descending fibers running through the lateral hypothalamus, including noradrenergic fibers from the medulla and dopaminergic fibers of the nigrostriatal pathway.

medial medullary syndrome See **Déjèrine syndromes.**

medial pectoral neuropathy An entrapment syndrome in which the nerve is compressed as it passes through the pectoralis minor, leading to wasting of the inferior sternal part of the pectoralis major muscle.[4804]

medial plantar neuropathy (jogger's foot) A focal neuropathy resulting from compression of this nerve in the tarsal tunnel, giving rise to local tenderness and distal sensory loss.[4218]

medial pterygoid reflex A stretch reflex elicited in the EMG laboratory with needle electrodes in the muscle and stimulation given by performing the jaw jerk. The reflex may be useful in the localization of brainstem or peripheral trigeminal nerve lesions.[2643]

medial tegmental paralysis See **Babinski-Nageotte syndrome.**

median cleft face syndrome See **frontonasal dysplasia.**

median facial cleft syndrome See **frontonasal dysplasia.**

median longitudinal bundle (fasciculus) A fiber bundle running between the oculomotor nuclei in the medulla and mesencephalon, first described by Benedict Stilling in 1846, but named by His in 1895.

median pubic reflex Tapping the symphysis pubis leads to contraction of the muscles of the abdominal wall and adduction of the leg in patients with hyperexcitability of the spinal cord resulting from lesions of the corticospinal tracts above T11.

Medical Outcomes Study 20-item scale An instrument for measuring aspects of **quality of life.**

Medical Research Council scale A popular nonlinear scale for the clinical grading of the strength of individual muscles. The defined grades (in a modified form) are given in Chart M–3.

Chart M–3. Modified Medical Research Council Scale

5	Normal strength
5−	Barely detectable weakness
4+	Same as 4, but stronger
4	Muscle is weak but moves the joint against a combination of gravity and some resistance.
4−	Same as 4, but weaker

3+ The muscle is capable of transient resistance but collapses abruptly.

3 Muscle cannot move against resistance but moves the joint fully against gravity. With the exception of knee extensors, the joint must be moved through the full mechanical range against gravity. If a patient has contractures that limit movement of the joint, the mechanical range will be to the point at which the contractures cause a significant resistance to the movement.

3− Muscle moves the joint against gravity but not through the full extent of the mechanical range of the joint.

2 Muscle moves the joint when gravity is eliminated.

1 A flicker of movement is seen or felt in the muscle.

0 No movement[3829]

From Mendell JR, Florence J. Manual muscle testing. Muscle Nerve 1990;13:S16–S20. © 1990. Reprinted by permission of John Wiley and Sons, Inc.

Despite the increase of the number of steps from 5 to 10 through the expansion of the fifth, fourth and third grades, the scale is still bottom-heavy, grades 4 and 5 representing over 90% of the potential strength of a muscle. See also **Mayo Clinic scale, NINDS scale.**

medication-induced headache (analgesic rebound headache) A form of **chronic daily headache** occurring in those with preexisting migraine or tension-type headaches for which they have taken analgesics, aspirin, acetaminophen, opioids, benzodiazepines, ergot preparations, or triptans on a regular basis for their headaches (usually 3 days/week or more). The new headache usually has characteristics of the previous ones, but occurs characteristically on waking and is partially relieved (but not removed) by further ingestion of the usual remedy. A re-setting of the tolerances of pain receptors in the brain is supposed to underlie the problem. Treatment demands abstention from the causative drug, but the "rebound" headaches resulting may last up to 2 weeks.

Medin, Oskar (1874–1928) Swedish physician in Stockholm. He described in great detail the Stockholm poliomyelitis epidemic of 1887, and the disease was accordingly known for some time by the name of Medin and of **Heine.**

medioplantar reflex (of Guillain and Barré) Tapping the heel or the middle of the sole elicits plantar flexion of the ankle in patients with pyramidal lesions. This represents merely an alternative method of eliciting the ankle jerk.

medium-chain acyl CoA dehydrogenase deficiency See **acyl CoA dehydrogenase deficiency.**

Medscape A commercial internet site covering many areas of medicine, including neurology: http://www.medscape.com/neurologyhome.

medulla oblongata (Lat, marrow + oblong shape) That part of the brainstem between the pons and the spinal cord. Formerly, according to **Willis** and others, the word signified the entire brainstem, but it has been restricted to its present extent since Haller's text was published in 1750.[5204]

medullary respiratory centers Dorsal and ventral nuclear masses (the solitary nucleus and tract, and the nucleus ambiguus) which act as pattern generators for respiratory activity.

medullary satiety Diminution in appetite and early satiety, thought to be due to a lesion of the area postrema in the medulla.[3670]

medullary sheath The Schwann cell layer of peripheral nerves; the investment of myelin-containing Schwann cells surrounding the axons.

medullary tegmental paralysis See **Babinski-Nageotte syndrome.**

medullary tube The tube formed by the closure and union of the laminae dorsales in the embryo, and from which the brain and spinal cord develop. Its walls constrict to become the forebrain or proscencephalon, the interbrain or thalamencephalon, the midbrain or mesencephalon, the hindbrain or epencephalon, and the afterbrain or metencephalon. The tube itself becomes the cerebral ventricles of the brain and the central canal of the spinal cord.

medullated (myelinated) nerve fibers (myelinated nerve fibers) Those nerve fibers which are individually surrounded by myelin-containing Schwann cells and which are thus greater in diameter, visibility, and conductive ability than the nonmedullated fibers which are invaginated into nonmyelin-containing Schwann cells.

medulloblastoma (Cushing tumor, medullomyoblastoma) A malignant **primitive neuroectodermal tumor** arising from the cerebellum (in children, from the vermis or medullary velum) and composed of sheets of small, round cells with oval hyperchromatic nuclei and small amounts of fibrillary cytoplasm, frequently arranged in rosettes with the nuclei at the periphery of the cells. Local invasion of the cerebellum and brainstem is usual, and the tumor seeds throughout the spinal subarachnoid space in many cases. This is the most common primary brain tumor in childhood. Unbalanced translocations, with loss of chromosome 17q and changes in chromosome 1, are the most common karyotypic abnormalities described.

Clinically it presents with signs of midline cerebellar and medullary dysfunction and ultimately leads to signs of raised intracranial pressure.[1205]

Variants include *desmoplastic medulloblastoma*, in which local invasion of the meninges leads to the occurrence of an intense fibrous reaction; *medullomyoblastoma*, in which striated muscle and epithelial cells appear; and *medulloepithelioma*, characterized by the tubular arrangements of cells resembling the "epithelial" cell pattern in the primitive neural tube.[6]

medulloepithelioma   A primitive malignant tumor of the cerebral hemispheres containing a columnar epithelial layer resembling that of the primitive neural tube,[2932] lacking cellular differentiation and frequently hemorrhage and necrotic. They occur in the first 5 years of life and are highly malignant. See **medulloblastoma.**

medullomyoblastoma   See **medulloblastoma.**

meeting badge neuropathy   Superficial radial (sensory) nerve injury as a result of compression against this personal label when the arms were crossed for a prolonged period. See also **cheiralgia paresthetica.**

MEG   See **magnetoencephalography.**

megaconial myopathy   A familial muscular disorder presenting with slowly progressive weakness from infancy and associated with an excess of giant mitochondria and morphological inclusions within such organelles.[5151]

This is a member of the group of benign, nonprogressive, congenital myopathies presenting in infancy with weakness and hypotonia which result in significant motor delay.

megacystis-microcolon–intestinal hypoperistalsis syndrome   (Berdon syndrome) A congenital visceral myopathy with two variant types: *type 1* is dominantly inherited and is characterized by esophageal dilation, megaduodenum, redundant colon, and megacystis; *type 2* is recessively inherited and is characterized by dilation of the stomach and small intestine with external ophthalmoplegia and ptosis.[572]

megadolichobasilar anomaly   (S aneurysm) A rare condition consisting of the abnormal elongation and widening of the basilar arteries, usually in adult males, first described by **Dandy** in 1947. The distortion may be so great that aqueductal and cranial nerve compression syndromes result.[620]

megalencephaly   (Gr, big + brain) (macrocephaly) Enlargement of the brain with or without histological abnormalities, as shown by a rapid increase in the occipitofrontal circumference of the head above the 98th percentile during the first year of life.

This occurs with such infiltrative or storage diseases as **GM₂** gangliosidosis, Niemann-Pick disease, sulfatidosis, **tuberous sclerosis,** and **glioblastomatosis** and also as a familial characteristic without associated disease. The primary form is developmental or it can be associated with other inherited disease. In the secondary form, the brain enlargement results from the accumulation of excessive lipid. See also **macrocephaly, megalobarencephaly, megalocephaly, microcephaly.**

Anatomic and *metabolic* forms are recognized. In the former, the brain is enlarged because of an increase in the number or size of its cells. In the latter, the enlargement reflects the accumulation of a metabolic product without any increase in the number of cells. Diagnostic criteria are given in Chart M–4.[1384]

Chart M–4. Diagnostic Criteria for Asymptomatic (Benign) Familial Anatomic Megalencephaly

1. Occipitofrontal circumference more than two standard deviations above the mean or above the 98th percentile
2. No clinical evidence of increased intracranial pressure in the form of bulging fontanelles, palpably split sutures, or persistent vomiting
3. Normal developmental and neurological examination findings
4. Absence of any neurocutaneous signs, or craniofacial or somatic anomalies that may identify a specific syndrome
5. One or more of the parents or siblings has a large occipitofrontal circumference but is neurologically normal, or the increased occipitofrontal circumference can be traced through several generations.
6. Follow-up visits establish the normality of the patient's developmental course, and the occipitofrontal circumference curve levels off and, although it remains high, begins to parallel the normal curve.
7. Radiographic demonstration of normal or only slightly enlarged ventricles in one of the family members with an enlarged occipitofrontal circumference, establishing that the condition is megalencephhaly, not arrested hydrocephalus or some other lesion
8. Negative chemical screening test results for metabolic disorders or lysosomal enzyme deficits in those patients lacking some of the other criteria

From DeMyer W. Megalencephaly; types, clinical syndromes and management. Pediatr Neurol 1986;2:321, by kind permission.

In a *variant* form, megalencephaly is associated with polymicrogyria and hydrocephalus.[358]

megalobarencephaly   An abnormal increase in the weight of the brain. This is a more accurate term than megalencephaly, in that a brain may be enlarged as a result of hydrocephalus, but it remains susceptible to misinterpretation in the presence of brain edema.

megaloblastic madness   Cognitive and emotional symptoms resulting from deficiency of vitamin B₁₂.

megalocephaly   The word usually employed to indicate enlargement of the head, although the derivation suggests rather enlargement of the brain. See also **megalencephaly.**

megalocornea with skeletal abnormalities   A congenital dysmorphic syndrome characterized by frontal bossing, low-set posteriorly rotated ears, hypertelorism, macrocornea, micrognathia, open-mouth appearance, gibbus, kyphoscoliosis, camptodactyly, clubfoot, acrocephaly, and mental and developmental delay.[337]

megalocornea–mental retardation   See **Neuhauser syndrome.**

megalopapilla   Congenital enlargement of the optic disk, sometimes associated with midline cranial defects, dysmorphism, and midline clefting.[2169]

megalopsia   Exaggerated **macropsia,** a condition in which everything looks abnormally big. A word generated by neologismophiles for neologismophiles.

megaphagia   Excessive ingestion of food without inducing hunger; often a compulsion. The condition should be distinguished from morbid hunger. The word was suggested by Critchley as more precisely derived than *hyperphagia* in the context of the **Kleine-Levin syndrome.**

megaseme   The term of **Charcot** for a skull with an orbital index >90, but this measurement is not now considered to be of practical usefulness.

megasthenic   Possessed of great muscular power. The necessity for the word must be limited, but it is reassuring to come across an exaltation of the normal in a work otherwise devoted to the abnormal.

megrim   (from Middle English and Fr, a headache; derived from Gr, a pain on one side of the face) An obsolete term for **migraine,** but applied still to a staggering disease in horses.

Meige, Henri   (1866–1940) French neurologist who trained in Paris and studied with **Charcot.** He gave the first good description of the symmetrical dystonic spasms of the facial muscles occurring in oromandibular dystonia, and of **Munchausen syndrome.** He was cofounder of the *Revue Neurologique* and of the Société de Neurologie in Paris.

Because some paintings by Pieter Brueghel the Elder (1525–1569) depict faces in similar dystonic postures, the name of Brueghel has been added to that of Meige (see next entry), but unaccountably those of Stanley Spencer and William Blake (British artists of the distortive school) have not.[3814]

Meige syndrome   (idiopathic orofacial dystonia, Brueghel syndrome) A segmental cranial dystonia of adult onset characterized by blepharospasm, oromandibular dystonia, apathy, depression, tics, bulbar weakness, rigidity, chorea, and tremor at rest. See **cranial dystonia.**

Meinecke syndrome   A congenital dysmorphic syndrome characterized by brachydactyly (short, broad thumbs), wide-spaced teeth, speech delay, patchy pigmentation of the skin, seizures, and mental and developmental delay.[337]

Meissner, Georg   (1829–1905) German anatomist, professor of physiology and anatomy at Basel, later at Freiburg and Göttingen Universities.

Meissner's corpuscles   Expansions of sensory nerve endings sensitive to touch.

Meissner's plexus   The submucous plexus of the intestine, described in 1853.

melancholy   See **chronic fatigue syndrome.**

melanocytoma   (cellular blue nevus) A rare, relatively benign pigmented nevoid tumor of the meninges or elsewhere, presenting as an intradural, extrinsic mass lesion. The histological patterns resemble those of schwannoma, dermal nevi, and neuroblastomas, and the tumor shows positive immunochemical reactions for the S-100 protein.[3216]

melanodermic leukodystrophy   See **adrenoleukodystrophy.**

melanoma   A tumor usually arising from neural crest tissues and skin, commonly malignant, and with likely autosomal dominant inheritance, mapped in some cases to 9p. In familial cases, other family members may have at least multiple dysplastic nevi of skin. Cerebral or optic gliomas appear to be associated. Multiple secondary metastases to the brain are common.[2961]

MELAS   (**M**itochondrial **E**ncephalopathy, **L**actic **A**cidosis, and **S**troke; OMIM 540000) A maternally transmitted mitochondrial disease with onset in infancy or childhood, characterized by recurrent migraine-like headaches, vomiting, hemiplegia ("stroke-like episodes" not conforming to known vascular territories) and hemianopia.

Other features include dementia, partial seizures, cortical blindness, ataxia, deafness, short stature, intracranial calcification, and cardiomyopathy. Increased lactate levels in the blood and CSF, ragged red fibers/abnormal mitochondria in muscle biopsy specimens, and spongy degeneration of the cortex with basal ganglion calcification are the laboratory abnormalities usually detected.[1448,4372] Non–insulin-dependent diabetes mellitus may also develop. Myoclonus, cerebellar lesions, retinal pigmentary changes, and heart block are not present.

The following diagnostic criteria have been suggested:[2583]

1. Stroke before the age of 40
2. An encephalopathy charaterized by seizures, dementia, or both
3. Blood lactic acidosis or ragged red fibers in skeletal muscle, or both

See also **MERRF, mitochondrial diseases.**

Melkersson-Rosenthal syndrome   The unusual combination of recurrent facial palsies with facial edema, migraine headaches, and fissuring of the tongue (lingua plicata).[3819] Ocular complications are also described. *Miescher cheilitis* is considered to be the same thing.[2764]

The syndrome is usually sporadic, but dominant inheritance has been recorded. Hubschmann described it in 1894; Melkersson, in 1928;[3819] and Rosenthal, in 1931.

melodic intonation therapy   The utilization of the retained capacity of some aphasic patients to sing when they cannot speak, whereby short phrases are incorporated first into a musical recitative and thereafter into progressively less and less intonational speech. One recalls the epigram of Dr. Samuel Johnson: "That which is too silly to be said may yet be sung," but that was in the context of opera.

The success of the method is thought to indicate the recruitment of the undamaged right hemisphere into the process of language production.[15,84]

membrane instability   The tendency of a cell membrane to depolarize spontaneously, with mechanical irritation or after voluntary activation.[146]

It may be used to describe the occurrence of spontaneous single muscle fiber action potentials such as fibrillation potentials during needle electrode examination. (From the 2001 Report of the Nomenclature Committee of the American Association of Electromyography and Electrodiagnosis.[10] Used by permission, copyright © 2001, AAEM.)

memory   (from Lat, memoria, memory) The ability to retain and recall experiences; a physical system by which a record or representation of organized spatiotemporal events is made which thus can be carried forward in time. One mechanism (explicit memory) deals with those memories for which there is conscious awareness and is dependent on frontotemporal cortex, hippocampal, and perirhinal function. In the other form (**implicit memory**) the memory is acquired without intention, is maintained without awareness, and does not depend on hippocampal function.[1542]

Memory Assessment Clinics Test Battery   A complex memory test instrument assessing also attention and psychomotor speed, and designed to assess memory function in normal elderly subjects and patients with **age-associated memory impairment** or **Alzheimer disease.**[3279]

Memory for Designs Test   An instrument for assessing visual recall and reproduction,[2252] and thus right hemisphere function.

Memory Impairment Screen   A validated, sensitive, and specific 4-minute, four-item delayed free- and cued-recall trest of memory impairment, usable as a screening test for dementias.[854]

Memory Loss Scale   An abbreviated test of mental status emphasizing orientation, but also assessing attention, abstraction, mental tracking, language, memory, and praxis.[3631]

memory tests   See **Computerized Everyday Memory Battery, Wechsler Memory Scale,**[5887] **Memory Assessment Clinics Test Battery, Memory for Designs Test, Memory Impairment Screen, Modified Mini-Mental State Examination, Recognition Memory Test, Buschke selective reminding tests**, **Babcock sentence, Rey tests**. Lezak[3392] has provided a critique and compendium of the tests available.

menace reflex   See **palpebral reflex.**

Mendel, Kurt   (b. 1874) German neurologist.

Mendel-Bekhterev sign   1. (dorsocuboidal reflex, tarsophalangeal reflex, dorsal foot response) Percussion over the dorsal aspect of the cuboid bone leads to plantar flexion of the toes in patients with pyramidal lesions. The normal response is dorsiflexion.[3828] See **dorsal foot response.** 2. (carpometacarpal reflex, carpophalangeal reflex) In the hand, percussion over the carpal bones causes flexion of the wrist and fingers in patients with pyramidal lesions.

Mengel syndrome   A recessively inherited syndrome characterized by early-onset severe neural hearing loss, leading to complete deafness after the age of 6 years, but normal vestibular responses.[3833]

Ménière disease   Idiopathic, symptomatic, endolymphatic hydrops leading to a syndrome of intermittent aural vertigo with nausea, vomiting, progressive tinnitus, and low-tone deafness with increased endolymphatic pressure.

This relatively common syndrome was first described in 1861,[3834] and Ménière followed this with a further series of papers on the same subject. Hallpike and Cairns showed in 1938 that dilatation of the membranous labyrinth was commonly associated.[4323]

The name was once applied to suppurative or hemorrhagic labyrinthitis as well.

Prosper Ménière

Ménière, Prosper   (1799–1862) French otologist who trained in Angers and Paris and initially was assistant to Baron Dupuytren at the Hôtel Dieu. He failed in his attempt to become professor of medicine in Paris, but instead directed the Institute for Deaf-mutes, which provided him greater experience in the diagnosis and management of otological problems, and also more time to devote to the study of literature, of which he was passionately fond.

The syndrome that he described was certainly that known today by his name, but the only evidence which he adduced for his belief that the lesion affected the inner ear was a brief mention of vertigo in patients who died suddenly and had had a blood-tinged or grayish exudate in the semicircular canals; the cause of this was not given, but Ménière considered tuberculosis to be the likely cause in one patient.[5373]

meningeal angiomatosis See **Sturge-Weber syndrome** (*van Bogaert–Divry* form).

meningeal apoplexy An ancient term for **subarachnoid hemorrhage.**

meningeal carcinomatosis See **carcinomatous meningitis.**

meningeal gliomatosis Diffuse or multifocal invasion of the cranial and/or spinal leptomeninges by malignant glioma. The condition was considered rare before more recent studies showed otherwise.[6099]

meningeal hemorrhage An old term for **extradural hemorrhage.**

meningeal hydrops See **idiopathic intracranial hypertension, arachnoid diverticula.**

meningeal sarcoma An uncommon malignant tumor arising from the arachnoid and resembling a fibrosarcoma or malignant fibrous histiocytoma histologically, and liable to recur, invade, and metastasize.

meninges (from Gr, a membrane) The membranous coverings of the CNS, comprising the dura mater, arachnoid, and pia mater.

meningioangiomatosis without neurofibromatosis An uncommon cerebral dysplasia characterized by the localized proliferation of fibrous tissue in the arachnoid membrane and by perivascular fibrous tissue infiltration of the subjacent cortex. Clinically, the condition presents with seizures.[3189]

meningioblastoma See *anaplastic meningiomas* in Chart M–5.

meningioma (dural endothelioma, fungus durae matris) The most common benign and slow-growing brain tumor of adult life arising from the meningoepithelial arachnoid cells of the arachnoid membrane or from the choroid plexus. Multiple deletions of chromosome 22 (22q12.3–qter) are frequently found in its rare familial forms, almost all these patients having neurofibromatosis (NF2). An extracranial origin is rare and metastasis quite exceptional, but recurrence is not uncommon. They represent about 20% of all intracranial tumors. Their slow growth leads to late detection in most cases; although headache, visual disturbances, loss of intellectual functions, and memory disturbances are common presentations, certain features are typical at different sites. *Olfactory groove meningiomas* sometimes cause uni- or bilateral anosmia.

The histological appearances vary and numerous variant subtypes are differentiated (see Chart M–5).

Chart M–5. Varieties of Meningioma Pathology

Meningoepithelial (syncytial) meningiomas are characterized histologically by the uniformity of nuclei with prominent nucleoli, the formation of whorls of cells, the presence of desmosomes between adjacent cells and of fibrous collagenous bands within the tumors, and by the absence of reticulin in most forms.

Fibroblastic meningiomas are characterized by the presence of sheets of elongated spindle cells with arachnoid cell nuclei; they contain **psammoma bodies.**

Transitional meningiomas combine features of both fibroblastic and meningoepithelial meningiomas.

Psammomatous meningiomas contain numerous **psammoma bodies.**

Angiomatous meningiomas resemble syncytial or transitional forms but contain many blood vessels, around which reticulin is prominent.

Angioblastic meningiomas comprise *hemangioblastic* forms that resemble **hemangioblastomas** located elsewhere in the body, and the *hemangiopericytic* variety, which contains numerous thin-walled blood vessels and has a strong tendency to invade locally and to recur after removal.

Papillary meningiomas contain collagenous cores of papillae comprised of sheets of uniform cells; pseudorosettes are common. These tumors are aggressive in their growth.

Anaplastic meningiomas are malignant tumors with the usual histological features of malignancy, and may invade locally, recur, and metastasize.[6] See also **meningeal sarcoma.**

There are other forms in which bone, fatty tissue, cartilage cells, or melanin are present.

The tumor was first described by Felix Platter in his book *Observationem in Hominis Affectibus* (1614) but was first fully documented by Cushing,[1230] who noted their origin from cell rests in the arachnoid; their appearance as solid masses or *en plaque*; the associated cranial hyperostosis; and the particular sites where they arise, which he listed as intraspinal, foraminal, suprasellar, olfactory groove, sphenoidal ridge, sylvian cleft, convexity (including parasagittal, falx, and true convexity tumors), transverse sinus, and cerebellopontine angle. They may also occur (rarely) in the lateral ventricles.

meningioma en plaque The appearance of a **meningioma** that forms a flattened mass, usually adjacent to the dura mater at the skull base or over the convexity.

meningiomatosis The presence of multiple meningiomas arising due to continuous spread through the CSF to other locations. This happens in less than 10% of the population with meningiomas.

meningism (meningismus) A clinical syndrome resembling mild meningitis, and due to irritation without direct infection of the meninges. See **serous meningitis.**

meningismus See **meningism.**

méningite de voisinage   See **parameningeal infections.**

meningitis   Inflammation of the meninges by bacterial, viral, fungal, or other infectious agents or as a result of chemical irritation or malignant invasion. **Leptomeningitis** is the usual alternative term, indicating that the finer meninges are affected. **Pachymeningitis** indicates inflammation of the dura. **Basal meningitis** is that form in which the meninges of the skull base are maximally affected; **chronic lymphocytic** and **carcinomatous** (malignant) meningitis and **spinal arachnoiditis** are entered elsewhere.

meningitis circumscripta spinalis   See **chronic spinal meningitis.**

meningitis serosa circumscripta   Nonpurulent meningitis with focal signs, resulting either from subjacent cortical infarcts or from the presence of loculated arachnoid, forming cysts and giving rise to signs appropriate to an expanding mass lesion.

For the spinal form *meningitis serosa circumscripta spinalis*, see **spinal arachnoiditis.**

meningitis tuberculosa chronica circumscripta   A subacute or chronic variety of tuberculous meningitis in which the tubercles elicit a jelly-like exudate upon the meninges, in which there is but a limited mesodermal reaction.[6000]

meningocele   A defect of neural tube closure at any level of the neuraxis, leading to the exposure of meninges, which do not contain nervous tissue. There is no associated neural deficit.[3874]

meningocerebral angiodysplasia   A developmental anomaly of the cerebral vasculature, characterized by the presence of multiple tortuous and dilated vessels on the surface of the cerebral cortex, with subjacent infarcts and calcification.

meningococcal meningitis   (cerebrospinal fever) An acute meningitis seen mainly in youth, resulting from infection with *Neisseria meningitidis*, a gram-positive diplococcus.

The condition was described first by Thomas **Willis** in his book *The London Practice of Physick* (1684), and next by Gaspard Vieusseux (1746–1814), a Geneva physician in 1805.[4979] The organism was first discovered by Anton Weichselbaum, a German pathologist (1845–1920), in 1887.

meningoencephalitis   Inflammation of the meninges and of the underlying substance of the brain.

meningoencephalocele   (hernia cerebri) A developmental anomaly (a **craniofacial malformation**), characterized by the presence of a sessile or pedunculated swelling in the glabellar region, composed of glial tissue and fibrous tissue, protruding through a skull defect. Telecanthus and elongation of the nose are invariably present, and hydrocephalus due to atresia of the foramen of Monro, agenesis of the corpus callosum, cortical atrophy, seizures strabismus, and mental retardation are common accompaniments.[4]

meningoencephalomyelitis   Inflammation of the meninges, brain tissue, and spinal cord.

meningoepithelial meningioma   See **meningioma.**

meningomyelitis   Inflammation of the meninges and of the underlying substance of the spinal cord.

meningomyelocele   A severe defect of neural tube closure occurring at any level of the neuraxis, leading to the exposure of both the meninges and the neural contents of the spinal canal to the outside. These represent the most common physically disabling birth defects in humans. The relative roles of genetic and environmental causes have not yet been determined.

The condition is associated with severe motor and sensory deficits in the legs, and frequently with the **Chiari malformation** and resulting **hydrocephalus.** The presence of the disorder is suggested antenatally by the finding of high levels of α-fetoprotein in the amniotic fluid and in maternal blood.

meningovascular syphilis   A form of tertiary **syphilis,** characterized by cerebral arteritis and by lymphocytic infiltration of the meninges with or without **gummas.** The clinical effects result from a basal meningitis with optic and lower cranial nerve involvement, and from multiple small cerebral infarcts resulting from obliterative endarteritis.

Pachymeningitis cervicalis hypertrophicans is a variant in which the cervical meninges are matted together, leading to compressive and vascular myelopathy.

Menkes disease   1. (trichopoliodystrophy, kinky-hair disease, steely-hair disease) An X-linked, recessive, degenerative disorder due to a deficiency of copper as a result of its impaired absorption, leading to failure of function of copper-dependent enzymes such as cytochrome-*c* oxidase. The responsible gene maps to chromosome Xq12–q13.

The main clinical features are failure to thrive, with seizures in infancy, severe mental retardation, dysmorphism, ivory-white and brittle hair that feels like steel wool (pili torti), short stature, bony changes, poikilothermia, poor feeding, abnormal temperature control, and arterial tortuosity from the age of 2 months. Generalized seizures, cerebral atrophy, callosal dysgenesis, and demyelination accompany these features. The disorder leads eventually to decerebration and death within 2 years. It was first defined by Dr. Milton Alter[3836] while he was a junior resident.

In a *variant* form, chorea, athetosis, hypotonia, seizures, and psychomotor retardation are associated with low copper and ceruloplasmin levels, and intestinal copper absorption is reduced.[2352] 2. See **branched-chain ketoaciduria.**[3837]

menopausal muscular dystrophy See **chronic polymyositis.**

menstrual migraine Attacks of migraine that occur on days −2 to +3 of the menstrual cycle and at no other time. The headache is associated with increased circulating prostaglandin levels.[419]

A *variant* is *menstrually associated migraine*, in which the attacks occur at any time of the cycle but with increased frequency at period times.

menstrual-associated syndrome A syndrome characterized by marked hypersomnolence in association with menstruation.[569]

mental 1. (from Lat, the mind) Relating to the mind. 2. Relating to the chin.

mental coprolalia The unwanted intrusion of obscene words into the thoughts of patients with **Tourette syndrome.**

Mental Health Inventory A 31-question, multiple-choice self-assessment instrument designed to survey experience of anxiety, depression, behavior/emotional control, general positive affect, and emotional ties in response to life events experienced by the subject.[5746]

mental neuropathy Numbness of the chin, most commonly due to malignant infiltration of the mental nerve.[3681]

mental retardation A state of abnormal development manifested by impaired intelligence and inadequate ability to learn. Nonspecific X-linked forms without other distinguishing neurological features have been mapped to chromosome Xq11–q12 or Xp22.

mental retardation, aphasia, shuffling gait, adducted thumbs See **MASA syndrome.**

mental retardation, diabetes mellitus, hypogonadism, and nerve deafness A rare recessive syndrome characterized by these features, in which pigmentary retinal degeneration has also been described.[1606]

Mental Status Questionnaire (MSQ) A widely used, formalized bedside screening test of cognitive function. Like the many others developed in the last quarter-century, it is brief (requiring only 5 minutes or so to put the 10 questions on orientation, memory, and general knowledge to the patient); focuses on cognitive factors rather than on affect, thought disorder, or behavioral features; and is valid, reliable, and simple to both give and score. However, it is rather insensitive.[2903]

See also **Modified Mini-Mental Status Examination.**

mentation Use of the mind or intellect.

Menzel disease A dominantly inherited form of **cerebellar ataxia** causing pyramidal, cerebellar, and posterior column dysfunction.[1590,3839] See **olivopontocerebellar atrophy, autosomal dominant cerebellar ataxia.**

MEPP See **miniature end-plate potentials.**

meralgia paresthetica (Gr, the thigh + pain) (lateral femoral cutaneous neuralgia, Roth-Bernhardt disease, Bernhardt-Roth [Rot] paresthesia) Paresthesias, hypoesthesias, numbness, and often burning pain in the distribution of the lateral cutaneous nerve of the thigh, supposedly often caused by compression of the nerve by a fat pad under the lateral part of the inguinal ligament and most commonly seen in middle-aged men.[519,4809] Lumbar plexus or L2, 3 lesions can cause the same picture.

Despite the usual eponyms, the condition was first described by Remak.

A *familial form* has been described.[3675]

meranesthesia (Gr, part + deprivative + feeling) Partial anesthesia.

mercuric encephalopathy See **pink disease, Minamata disease.**

mercuric neuropathy A syndrome resembling **amyotrophic lateral sclerosis** resulting from the ingestion of organic mercury. Weakness, wasting, fasciculations, hyperreflexia, and up-going plantar responses are found, and a blue line on the gum margins is noted in some patients.[2919]

Meretoja syndrome Dominantly inherited generalized **amyloidosis** with lattice dystrophy of the cornea, progressive cranial neuropathies, and late peripheral neuropathy.[3842]

merged gyri A cortical dysplasia, characterized by fusion of the gyral surfaces of the brain; a forme fruste of **polymicrogyria.**[417]

meridrosis Localized sweating.

Merkel disks A form of sensory nerve ending, sensitive to touch.

Merkel, Karl Ludwig (1812–1876) German anatomist.

mermaid syndrome See **caudal regression syndrome.**

meropia Partial dullness or obscuration of vision.

MERRF (**M**yoclonic **E**pilepsy with **R**agged **R**ed **F**ibers, Fukuhara syndrome, leukoencephalopathy with ragged red fibers; OMIM 545000) A maternally transmitted mitochondrial disorder with onset in infancy, childhood, or early adult life, characterized by short stature, myoclonus, nerve deafness, generalized tonic-clonic seizures, ataxia, myopathy with ptosis, and mental and developmental delay, with lactic acidosis, spongiform encephalopathy, and the presence of ragged red fibers in muscle biopsy specimens.[1983,3348,3348a]

Optic atrophy, deafness, pyramidal signs, peripheral neuropathy resembling hereditary motor and sensory neuropathy, migraine, and hypoventilation are other inconstant features described. See also **MELAS, mitochondrial myopathies.**

Merrill Palmer scales of mental development   A composite nonverbal test of perceptual and motor skills designed for children under the age of 5 years.

Merritt, H. Houston   (1902–1979) A leading American neurologist who was educated at Chapel Hill and at Vanderbilt and Johns Hopkins Universities, then at the Boston City Hospital and in Munich. His professional life was spent first at Harvard (where with Tracy Putnam he was first to complete clinical studies of diphenylhydantoin in 1937),[3845] and then in New York at Columbia University where he was professor and chairman of the department of neurology and established model departments of neurology at Montefiore and the New York Neurological Institute. He was also sometime dean of the medical school and vice-president for medical affairs.

Merritt was an outstanding clinician, a superb teacher (his *Textbook of Neurology* passed through six editions before his death), and a productive researcher, but he also was active on the boards of charitable organizations in the neurological field, and of the National Institute of Neurological Diseases.

As one of the most influential neurologists in the United States, he promoted neurology as an independent clinical discipline and fostered the organization of dedicated neurological training programs with a strong basic science component. His residency program trained a remarkable proportion of those physicians who today are most influential in American neurology. Merritt was also instrumental in the foundation of the National Institute of Neurological and Communicative Disorders and Stroke and as a research worker himself, published over 200 papers, particularly on the topics of epilepsy, syphilis, cerebrovascular disease, and nutritional disease.

Merwarth syndrome   See **rolandic vein occlusion.**

Merzbacher, Ludwig   (1875–1942) German physician who trained in Strasbourg and practiced mainly in Argentina. In 1910 he added to the 1885 description by Friedrich **Pelizaeus** of the syndrome now known by both of their names, having re-studied members of the same family.

mesaticephalic   **Broca**'s term for a skull with a **cephalic index** between 75 and 80. The significance of the shape is not known.

mesencephalic artery syndrome   See **top of the basilar syndrome.**

mesencephalitis and rhombencephalitis   A syndrome of subacute progression, manifesting drowsiness; oculomotor, facial, and bulbar palsies; anarthria; and cerebellar ataxia without limb weakness. There may be mild pyrexia. The CSF contains increased numbers of mononuclear cells.

Despite severe bulbar failure occurring at some time during the course of the disease, eventual recovery may be complete.[553] See **Bickerstaff brainstem encephalitis.**

mesencephalon   (Gr, the middle brain) (mesocephalon) That part of the brain derived from the middle cerebral vesicle and comprising the brainstem structures below the hypothalamus and above the pons.

mesial temporal lobe epilepsy syndrome   See **temporal lobe epilepsy.**

mesial temporal sclerosis   (Ammon's horn sclerosis, hippocampal sclerosis, incisural sclerosis, pararhinal sclerosis) Loss of nerve cells with gliosis in Sommer's sector of the hippocampus, usually with additional abnormality elsewhere in the temporal lobe.

After many years of uncertainty as to whether such changes were the cause or the effect of complex partial seizures, Falconer concluded that they signified prior anoxia due to repetitive seizures in infancy, were themselves epileptogenic, and were the most common lesions found in tissue specimens removed after anterior temporal lobectomy for the management of drug-resistant epilepsy,[1735,1736] but the issue remains unsettled and the seizures may in some cases be the result rather than the cause of the sclerosis.[5735]

mesiobasal limbic seizures   See **amygdalohippocampal seizures.**

Mesmer, Franz Anton   (1734–1815) Austrian physician and metaphysician who trained originally for the priesthood and then for law before changing to medicine, the subject in which he graduated from Vienna University in 1765. He was interested in the effect of the planets on the human body, which he considered similar to their effects on each other; this formed the subject of his dissertation and led to his proposition of the existence of animal magnetism (*gravitas animalis*), a mysterious fluid permeating all organic and inorganic substances. Mesmer thought that obstruction to the flow of this fluid was the basis of disease, and that such obstructions could be relieved by putting the patients into a trance and then inducing a convulsion.

His ideas were rejected by orthodox physicians in Vienna, and he left for Paris, where his success was phenomenal, thanks to adept stage management, the innocuous nature of the treatments, and the high prevalence of naïveté and ignorance. By 1784, these had diminished enough to allow the creation of a commission of inquiry into the basis of Mesmer's system, of which Benjamin Franklin, Antoine Lavoisier, and Dr. Armand Guillotin were members. Their conclusions that mesmeric fluid did not exist and that the effects of Mesmer's treatments were but the result of imagination led to his departure from Paris and to his further demonstrations being given in a traveling format.

Mesmer considered that he was dealing with physical rather than with mental forces. It was James **Braid** who introduced the term *hypnotism* for the trance-like state induced in his subjects by Mesmer, and who regarded this as a mental state of heightened suggestibility.

mesocephalon   See **mesencephalon.**

mesoencephalothalamic syndrome   Isolated bilateral internal and external ophthalmoplegias; the oculomotor palsies, vertical gaze paresis, and **abulia** result from a vascular lesion in thalamic and high brainstem regions. This may occur as a **lacunar syndrome.**[1853,1867] See **syndrome of the mesencephalic gray matter.**

mesolimbocortical dementia   A rare, insidiously progressive, dementing syndrome of unknown cause, characterized pathologically by nonspecific neuronal loss and gliosis in the limbic system and also in the mesencephalic dopaminergic fields, their terminal fields in the cortex and the caudate nuclei, substantia nigra, and inferior olive.

Clinically, late-onset, slowly progressive personality changes; loss of memory, insight, judgement, and self-care skills; behavioral disturbances such as those in the **Klüver-Bucy syndrome;** and sometimes **parkinsonism,** all giving rise to features of a **subcortical dementia,** are the most prominent features.[5611,5751]

mesomelia and nephritis syndrome   See **Funderbunk syndrome.**

meta-   Greek prefix, signifying "beyond."

metabasis   The changing over from one thing to another, as suggested by its derivative *metabolism.* However, a change in the appearance of symptoms of disease is also an acceptable, if somewhat archaic, meaning.

metabolic craniopathy   See **Morel-Stewart-Morgagni syndrome.**

metabolic headache   (headache associated with metabolic disorder) The following diagnostic criteria are suggested by the Headache Classification Committee of the International Headache Society[1051] (from Classification of headache disorders, cranial neuralgias and facial pains; and diagnostic criteria for primary headache disorders. *Cephalalgia* 1988;**8**[suppl]:1–96).

A. Symptoms and/or signs of a metabolic disorder
B. Confirmation by laboratory investigations when specified under the subform
C. Headache intensity and/or frequency related to variations in the metabolic disorder with a specified time lag
D. Headache disappears within 7 days after normalization of the metabolic state.

metabolic myopathy   See **lipid myopathies; carnitine deficiency, riboflavin responsive; acid maltase deficiency; glycogen storage disease; myopathy.**

metabolic poliodystrophy   Anterior horn cell disease due to chemical disorders, such as hypoglycemia or lead poisoning.

metachromasia   A change in color.

metachromatic leukodystrophy   (Greenfield disease, Scholtz syndrome, van Bogaert–Nijssen-Pfeiffer disease, sulfatide lipidosis; OMIM 250100). A group of recessively inherited lysosomal storage diseases caused by deficiency of arylsulfatase A and leading to intralysosomal storage of cerebroside sulfate in the white matter of the CNS and peripheral nerves. The resulting progressive demyelination causes a variety of neurological symptoms. The responsible gene maps to chromosome 22q13.13–qter or, when there is a lack of sphingolipid activator protein, to 10q21–q22.

Symmetrical and severe demyelination of the cerebral and cerebellar hemispheres occurs as a result of damage to oligodendroglia, and leads to axonal damage, pyramidal degeneration with isomorphic gliosis, and loss of myelin in the peripheral nerves, with sparing of the subcortical U fibers. Sulfatide (a cerebroside sulfuric acid ester, which is a metachromatic material causing a brown stain in the presence of acidic cresyl violet) is deposited in white matter, nerves, neurons such as the anterior horn cells; in the dentate and other nuclei;[2268] and in the liver, kidney, testes, and pituitary. CT scanning shows bilateral white matter lucencies in the cerebrum and cerebellum, with cortical atrophy.

There are three types of arylsulfatase: A and B are lysosomal; C is microsomal. The A form is deficient in the late infantile, juvenile, and adult forms of metachromatic leukodystrophy. Some allelic types of the disease are recognized. Clinically, the disease is heterogeneous, and different forms are classified according to the age at onset of symptoms (late infantile, juvenile, and adult; see Chart M–6).

Chart M–6. Allelic Forms of Metachromatic Leukodystrophy

The *late infantile* form is most common. Clinically, it presents at the age of 1–2 years with irritability, poor eating, gait disorder, floppy posture, loss of motor skills, optic atrophy, squint, and nystagmus. With further decline, spasticity takes over, despite evidence of a peripheral neuropathy, and seizures, myoclonus, cortical blindness, mental deterioration, decerebration, and opisthotonos lead to death.

In the *juvenile* form, the onset is between 3 and 16 years of age with gait disturbance and behavioral change. The neuropathy is less prominent, but mental changes, dystonia, and incontinence may be severe.[2401]

The *adult* form is rare; clinical features include insidious dementia, psychoses, optic atrophy, ataxia, pyramidal and extrapyramidal signs, and neuropathy with onset after the age of 16 years.[5840] The neuropathy has been reported as occurring in isolation.

Other *variants* include the following:

Metachromatic leukodystrophy due to cerebroside sulfatase activator defect A phenotype resembling the juvenile form, in which the enzyme activity is reduced but not absent.[5094]

The *Austin variant* (O variant, multiple sulfatase deficiency) A recessively inherited mucosulfatidosis—a nonallelic variant. The features are similar to those of the *late infantile* variety, with progressive motor and intellectual deterioration, ichthyosis, and hepatosplenomegaly, progressing to blindness, deafness, decerebrate rigidity, and dementia; but the biochemistry resembles that of some of the gangliosidoses and mucopolysaccharidoses, with storage of gangliosides in the cortical neurons.[268]

Adult-onset form of metachromatic leukodystrophy with nor-aryl sulfatase A form characterized by the onset in adult life of dementia, ataxia, spasticity, orthostatic hypotension, diffuse demyelination, and low-density lesions in the white matter on CT scans.

Metachromatic leukodystrophy with heterozygous compound allele (pseudodeficiency) A form characterized by the onset in infancy of gaze palsy, dysarthria, ataxia, spasticity, psychomotor arrest, cerebral atrophy, and diffuse gliosis and demyelination. The same apparent deficiency may also occur in healthy people.

Metachromatic leukodystrophy with early juvenile onset A form characterized by the onset in childhood of optic atrophy, seizures, ataxia, pyramidal and extrapyramidal signs, sensorimotor peripheral neuropathy, and dementia.

Metachromatic leukodystrophy without arylsulfatase deficiency A form characterized by dementia, pyramidal signs, hypertrophic demyelinating sensorimotor peripheral neuropathy, neurogenic bladder, and developmental delay.

Metachromatic leukodystrophy with retinitis pigmentosa A form characterized by the onset in infancy of pigmentary retinal degeneration, dysarthria, dysphagia, dystonia, ataxia, pyramidal signs, demyelinating sensorimotor peripheral neuropathy, diffuse demyelination with low-density lesions in the white matter on CT scanning, and mental and developmental delay.

metamorphopsia Distortion (alteration of size, shape, or angulation) of objects seen. When persistent, it is usually due to ocular disease or to bilateral occipital or occipitotemporal lesions.

In some cases, the distortion affects only one or two quadrants of the visual field, making the environment grotesque.

metamorphosis The change of an object from one form or structure to another.

metaphyseal dysplasia A **craniotubular dysplasia** with cranial bone sclerosis, associated sometimes with muscle weakness, scoliosis, or optic atrophy.[5521] See **Pyle disease.**

metastatic Shifting of disease from one place in the body to another.

metencephalon That part of the brain derived from the posterior part of the third cerebral vesicle during embryonic development and comprising the medulla oblongata, the eighth cranial nerve, and the fourth ventricle.

methacholine test Instillation of one drop of 2.5% methacholine into the conjunctival sac normally has no effect, but produces miosis within 15 minutes, lasting for up to 2 hours, in states of parasympathetic denervation with denervation hypersensitivity, as with the **Adie pupil.** See also **pilocarpine test.**

methionine malabsorption syndrome See **oasthouse disease.**

methioninemic myopathy A rare inborn metabolic error manifest in infants by high circulating levels of methionine; it presents as a proximal myopathic syndrome with hyporeflexia and mental retardation.[2062]

methyl crotonyl-coenzyme A–carboxylase deficiency A congenital metabolic disorder characterized by neonatal seizures, hypotonia, spinal muscular atrophy, alopecia, patchy skin abnormalities, neurodegenerative regression, and organic aciduria with metabolic acidosis.[337]

5-10-methylenetetrahydrofolate reductase deficiency A rare, inherited error in the pathway for synthesis of methionine, presenting as an infantile dysmorphic syndrome of pyramidal signs with spasticity, cognitive deterioration, myoclonic seizures, microcephaly, sensory ataxia, rigidity, tremor, motor neuropathy, neurogenic bladder, cerebral atrophy, and diffuse cerebral demyelination with aminoaciduria.[5808]

3-methylglutaconic aciduria A rare, congenital, dominantly inherited syndrome characterized by chorea, truncal and limb ataxia, optic atrophy, retinal aplasia, sensorineural deafness, severe hypotonia giving way to spasticity by the age of 6 years, and mild mental retardation, with excessive excretion of 3-methylglutaconic acid (MGA) in the urine. The clinical features closely resemble those of **Behr syndrome.**

Three syndromes are differentiated according to the amounts of MGA excreted, in which the same features, and also macrocephaly, seizures, pigmentary retinal degeneration, and cataracts, are seen in varying combinations.[1139]

methylmalonic acidemia A group of rare, congenital, inborn metabolic errors, usually manifesting neonatal seizures, dystonias, feeding problems, apneic attacks, and mental and developmental delay, but occasionally with minor signs only. Organic aciduria, hyperammonemia, and raised plasma lactate levels are characteristically found.[3132]

methylmercuric encephalopathy See **Minamata disease.**

metopic (Gr, between the eyes) Relating to the forehead. An antique term for the frontal bone. A *metopic suture* is a persistent sagittal suture between the right and left sides of the frontal bone.

metopion (Gr, the forehead) An alternative term for the glabella or interorbital region.

metrizamide encephalopathy A syndrome of asterixis, sometimes with generalized seizures, and with severe stuttering speech, occurring as a toxic manifestation of metrizamide myelography. Impaired brain glucose metabolism may be responsible for some of these effects.

Metrizamide is a nonionic contrast agent derived from glucose and metrazoic acid, widely used for imaging of the CSF spaces.[526]

Meyer, Adolf (1866–1950) Swiss-American neurologist and psychiatrist born in Zurich, who became professor of psychiatry at Cornell after emigration and later went to Johns Hopkins University. Although outstanding as a psychiatrist, his early neurological and pathological studies led to his identification of the following anatomical fact.

Meyer loop (Fleschig loop) The lowermost fibers of the geniculocalcarine (optic) radiation, which pass through the temporal lobe and loop around the tip of the temporal horn on their way to the calcarine cortex. These carry impulses from the inferior nasal quadrant of the retina, and thus lesions of the temporal lobe may produce a superior quadrantanopia.[1073]

Meyer phenomenon Mydriasis in response to abdominal pressure; described in psychiatric patients. For a sign so trite the word *phenomenon* seems overstated; perhaps *happening* would be more appropriate?

Meyer-Betz disease Paroxysmal myoglobinuria, unassociated with other evidence of muscle disease, but occurring after heavy exertion or during infections, with associated muscle pain and swelling. The myoglobinuria is liable to lead to renal impairment.[3130,3861]

Meynert amentia An acute confusional psychosis. See **Wernicke-Korsakoff encephalopathy.**

Meynert decussation The decussation of the dorsal tegmental tract.

Meynert fasciculus (habenulopeduncular tract) A small bundle passing from the habenula of the thalamus to the interpeduncular region, described by Meynert in 1867.[3862a]

Meynert, Theodor Hermann (1833–1892) German professor of psychiatry and later of neurology in Vienna, where he combined neurological science with psychiatric research, convinced that diseases of the mind must reflect disease of its substrate, the brain. His anatomical studies revealed the central projections of the sensory fields onto the cortex, the functional topography of which he mapped out, differentiating between the association fields and the primary receptive areas. He also studied the morphology of the brainstem in detail.

MGUS See **monoclonal gammopathy of uncertain significance.**

Michel defect A developmental defect comprising the absence of the otic capsule and the eighth cranial nerve.

Michel syndrome (clefting with ocular anomalies) A congenital dysmorphic syndrome characterized by sensorineural deafness, telecanthus, hypertelorism, iris adhesions, corneal opacities, strabismus, impairment of upward gaze, ptosis, blepharophimosis, epicanthic folds, cleft upper lip and palate, and mental and developmental delay.[4]

Mickey illness severity score A weighting system providing an overall score of functional disability in patients with **multiple sclerosis,** based on **Kurtzke**'s functional systems score and his disability status scale.[3867]

micrencephaly Reduction in brain weight to a value less than 2 standard deviations below the mean for a given age, with any size of cranium. **Broca** considered that brain weights below 1049 g in males and below 907 g in females were abnormal. **Microcephaly** is also commonly present.

micro- Greek prefix signifying smallness.

micro border-zone infarct The distribution of lesions occurring after arterial occlusion.

micro syndrome Microphthalmia and cerebellar and callosal hypoplasia, usually with X-linked inheritance.[4374]

microadenoma A functioning adenoma within the pituitary gland which has caused no detectable expansion of the gland by virtue of its size, arbitrarily defined as <10 mm in diameter.

microaneurysm 1. (lipohyalinotic aneurysm) Focal bulging of the wall of an arteriole damaged by **lipohyalinosis** and arteriolosclerosis with an increase in the diameter of the vessel's lumen. This is seen mainly in the putamen, caudate, and thalamus, and to a lesser extent in the cerebral cortex. 2. (saccular miliary aneurysm) Focal bulging of the wall of an arteriole, its new wall being composed of fibrin thrombus and organized red blood cells, resulting from prior bleeding from the arteriole. **Charcot-Bouchard aneurysms** are considered to include both of these forms.

microangiopathic encephalopathy and hearing loss A syndrome with onset in young adult life, characterized by sensorineural deafness, vascular abnormalities of the retina, dysarthria, dementia, aggressive behavior, cerebellar ataxia, and spasticity. See **RED-M syndrome.**

microcephalic primordial dwarfism A congenital dysmorphic syndrome characterized by low birth weight, dwarfism with short (or absent) limbs and metacarpal bones, alopecia, beaked nose, micrognathia, short neck, rhizomelia of the upper limbs, dislocation of the elbows and hips, Perthes disease, delayed skeletal maturation, hyperkeratosis, microcephaly due to early closure of the fontanelles, and mental and developmental delay.[337]

microcephaly A reduction in the circumference of the head, the occipitofrontal circumference measuring less than 2 standard deviations below the mean for the person's **gestational age,** gender, and race.

This may be due to failure of development of the underlying brain or of the skull bones themselves during the first 4 months of gestation, or may result from premature fusion of the cranial sutures. The result is usually severe psychomotor delay. In familial cases, recessive, dominant, and X-linked inheritance have all been described. In such cases, the cerebrum is small and contains evidence of multiple neuronal migration defects, but the cerebellum is usually of normal size. Sporadic cases are also common.[3770]

In *primary microcephaly*, anomalies of induction and migration have occurred during the first 7 months of intrauterine life; in the secondary form, the reduction in brain size is due to infectious, traumatic, metabolic, or anoxic lesions incurred in the last 2 months of gestation or in the perinatal period.[3835]

A classification of the congenital microcephalies has been suggested.[358]

1. Microcephaly with normal to thin cortex
   a. Primary microcephaly (microcephaly vera)
   b. Extreme microcephaly with simplified gyral pattern
2. Microlissencephaly (MLIS: extreme microcephaly with thick cortex)
   a. MLIS with thick cortex (**Norman-Roberts syndrome**)
   b. MLIS with thick cortex, severe brainstem, and cerebellar hypoplasia (Barth MLIS syndrome)
   c. MLIS with intermediate cortex, abrupt AP gradient
   d. MLIS with mildly to moderately thick (6–8 mm) cortex
3. Microcephaly with polymicrogyria or other cortical dysplasias
   a. Extreme microcephaly with diffuse or asymmetric polymicrogyria
   b. Extreme microcephaly with agenesis of the corpus callosum and cortical dysplasia

From Barkovich AJ, Kuzniecky R, Jackson GG, et al. Classification system for malformations of cortical development. Neurology 2001;57:2168–78, by kind permission.

Variant forms are listed in Chart M–7.

Chart M–7. Variant Forms of Microcephaly

Microcephaly and chorioretinal dysplasia A dominantly inherited anomaly characterized by microphthalmia, dysplasia of the optic nerve and retina, detached retina, pigmentary retinopathy with blindness, strabismus, early closure of the fontanelles, microcephaly, and psychomotor retardation.[5523]

Microcephaly-chorioretinopathy A recessively inherited syndrome of dwarfism, microphthalmia, optic atrophy, aplasia or dysplasia of the retina, pigmentary retinopathy, microcephaly, and cutis marmorata.[890]

Microcephaly, motor neuron disease, and nigral degeneration A congenital dysmorphic syndrome characterized by the onset in early childhood of dysarthria, dementia, microcephaly, tremor at rest, dystonias, fasciculations, neurogenic muscle atrophy and cerebral atrophy.[337]

Multiple epiphyseal dysplasia–microcephaly-nystagmus A congenital syndrome characterized by short stature, small pelvis, epiphyseal dysplasia, microcephaly, nystagmus, and mental and developmental delay.[3496]

Microcephaly with spasticity and seizures A congenital dysmorphic syndrome characterized by tonic-clonic and myoclonic seizures, microcephaly, spasticity, and cerebral atrophy.[835] See **Paine syndrome.**

In other *variant* forms, lymphedema, retinopathy, cervical spine anomalies, intracranial calcification, and/or pyramidal signs are associated. These and a summary of syndromes in which microcephaly also occurs are reviewed by Baraitser.[335]

See also **COFS** and the syndromes of **Aicardi, Cockayne, Coffin and Siris, de Lange, dysencephalia splanchnocystica, Dubowitz, Hallermann-Streiff-Francois, Meckel, Pen-Shokeir phenotypes, Rett, Rubinstein and Taybi, Seckel,** and **Smith, Lemli, and Opitz.**

microcephaly with basal ganglion calcification   See **Aicardi-Goutières syndrome.**

microcephaly–absent phalanges–short stature–retardation syndrome   See **Drayer syndrome.**

microcephaly-albinism–limb defects   See **Castro-Gago syndrome.**

microcephaly-syndactyly syndrome   See **Filippi syndrome.**

microcompression   An operative technique in which a small balloon is inflated in a position where it will compress a nerve, such as the fifth cranial nerve in Meckel's cave, in cases of trigeminal neuralgia resistant to medical treatment.

microcoria   A synonym for **miosis.**

microdeletion syndromes   Inherited conditions caused by the deletion of small segments of chromosomes at a variable number of contiguous loci.

microdiskectomy   Microsurgical excision of prolapsed intervertebral disks, of value in patients with segmental signs who have not responded to conservative treatment, including **chemonucleolysis,** and in those with osseous **spinal stenosis.**

microdrift   Dysconjugate slow eye movements of $<1°$ in amplitude, occurring during fixation of an object. They are of no known pathological significance.

microdysgenesis   The presence of nests of ectopic neurons and glia in the first layer of the cerebral cortex. This is often associated with focal dysplasia of adjacent cortical layers, including focal microgyria, and with superficial excrescences known as *brain warts.*

This abnormality may be asymptomatic or else associated with dyslexia or seizures.[2967]

microflutter   See **ocular flutter, microsaccadic flutter.**

microglia   (Gr, small + glue) The smaller supporting neuroglial cells in the CNS; interstitial cells of mesoblastic origin representing the reticuloendothelial system in the CNS, having both the morphology and staining characteristics of macrophages. They were first described by Rio **Hortega** in 1921. See **primary CNS lymphoma.**

microglial stars Clusters of activated microglia around damaged or dead neurons.

microglioma (microgliomatosis, reticulum cell sarcoma) A form of reticulosis affecting the brain and producing clinical signs of a fast-advancing intracranial tumor.[4853] See **primary CNS lymphoma.**

microgliomatosis See **microglioma.**

microglossia Smallness of the tongue, congenital or acquired.

micrognathia Congenital smallness of the jaw.

micrographia Smallness of the handwriting; a classic sign in bradykinesia, as in parkinsonism.

microgyria (hemiatrophy of the brain) A developmental abnormality of prenatal origin, characterized by a decrease in the cell population of the middle cerebral cortical layer leading to decreased width and therefore an increased number of cerebral cortical gyri focally. It is sometimes combined with **macrogyria.** Such laminar destruction of the middle layer only is considered evidence of an acquired injury rather than of a neuronal migration defect.[3]

Clinically, seizures and a degree of mental impairment are commonly present.[5218,5222]

micromelia Small limbs.

microneurography The technique of recording peripheral nerve action potentials in humans by means of intraneural electrodes.

micropapilla See **optic nerve hypoplasia.**

microphthalmia A congenital ocular malformation in which the presence of some ocular development can be determined by clinical means. Microcephaly and other brain malformations are occasionally associated. See **Walker-Warburg, Meckel,** and **Neu-Laxova syndrome.**

micropsia The illusion of reduction in the size of objects seen, as in some forms of complex partial seizure.

microsaccades Small-amplitude, rapid saccadic oscillations of the eyes contributing to ocular "noise" in normal subjects and suppressed during the performance of close work.[3330]

microsaccadic flicks See **microsaccadic flutter.**

microsaccadic flutter (microflutter, microsaccadic flicks) The rare phenomenon of conjugate saccadic horizontal ocular oscillations at 15–30 Hz, invisible to the naked eye and inconsistently associated with neurological disease, although considered to reflect abnormal function of the brainstem omnipause neurons.[236]

The perplexed lexicographer notes the high validity but the slight importance of this phenomenon but recalls with relief that

> A symbol said "I represent
> The meaning someone else has meant.
> I personally have no leanings
> Toward any of the many meanings."

microsleeps Brief periods in which the EEG activity is that of stage 1 or 2 non–rapid eye movement sleep activity but lasting less than 10 seconds, interrupting wakefulness and impairing sustained attention. They occur in normal people after sleep deprivation and may be associated with **excessive daytime sleepiness** and with automatic behavior.[249]

microsomia Smallness of the whole body—head, trunk, and limbs.

MICROSTROKE A computer-based system designed to use the clinical features of a patient's case to diagnose the type of stroke suffered.[5297] See also **TOPOSCOUT.**

microsurgery Surgical procedures utilizing the operating microscope and small instruments for meticulous operations within a confined space. Microvascular decompression of the fifth cranial nerve in the cerebellopontine angle for relief of **trigeminal neuralgia** is an example.

microtia Small ears. A sporadic congenital syndrome of middle ear anomalies, ear atresia, and conductive hearing loss.[3]

microtremor Dysconjugate, low-amplitude, high-frequency ocular vibrations, of no known pathological significance.

microtropia Divergence of the ocular axes, leading to a manifest deviation so small that the **alternate cover test** fails to reveal it. A degree of diplopia may yet result.[2133]

microtubules Cytoskeletal structures within axons synthesized within the cell body, consisting of polymerized dimers of tubulin protein forming a hollow tube, about 20 nm in diameter and 1 mm long. They are longitudinally oriented and are linked by crossbridges to neurofilaments, and move centrifugally within the axoplasm at up to 3 mm/day.

miction (from Lat, to pass water) The act of passing water. The word is hardly used now, but it appears to be the better derivation to describe normal urinary functioning.

micturition (Lat, a desire to pass water) 1. A constant inclination to urinate. 2. The act of passing water—the modern, but slightly incorrect meaning. See also **miction.**

micturition syncope Syncope that occurs during or after voiding, usually in the case of elderly men who rise from their beds at night for this purpose, and thus are at risk by virtue of attaining the upright posture when peripherally vasodilated, and also because of the Valsalva maneuver required to overcome the effects of prostatism.[1079]

MIDAS (**MI**graine **D**isability **A**ssessment **S**cale) A tool for the evaluation of the effects of headaches on those who suffer from them. A pediatric version is also available. Web site: http://www.migraine-disability.net/.

See also **Headache Impact test.**

midbrain   The **mesencephalon.**

midbrain corectopia   A shift in the geometric center of a pupil, which becomes oval, in association with disease of the brainstem.

midbrain deafness   Total deafness as a result of degeneration of the lateral lemnisci and inferior colliculi, described following a head injury.[2669]

midbrain infarction   Localized posterior circulation infarctions, usually in the territories of paramedian branches of the basilar artery supplying the midbrain and presenting with overt eye movement disorders such as those due to III n. palsies, vertical gaze palsies, pure motor hemiparesis, and/or four-limb ataxia but with few other localizing findings. Infarcts in the territories of the mesencephalic branches of the posterior cerebrla artery and the superior cerebellar artery are distinctly less common.[628]

midbrain "myasthenia"   The occurrence of some ocular signs of myasthenia (fatigable ptosis, lid twitch, ophthalmoparesis) as a result of a midbrain tumor.[4570]

midbrain pseudo-sixth   Impairment of ocular abduction as a result of **convergence spasm** without any lesion of the sixth cranial nerve.[896]

midbrain tremor   (cerebellar outflow tremor, red and black tremor) A predominantly unilateral tremor at 1.5–3 Hz, involving both proximal and distal muscles, present at rest but successively increased by maintenance of a posture and by volitional movement. Occasional large-amplitude tremor bursts may induce a quasi-myoclonic component.[1819] See **rubral tremor.**

midcervical central cord syndrome   Numbness of the fingertips and clumsiness of the hands with tightness felt at midthoracic levels resulting from midline cervical disk protrusions at C3–4.[4066]

middle cranial fossa syndrome   See **Raeder paratrigeminal syndrome.**

middle finger test   The patient extends the elbow, wrist, and middle finger and holds them against resistance. Increase of pain in the region of the lateral part of the elbow indicates pressure on the posterior interosseous nerve, as with compression underneath the arcade of Frohse.[3432]

midfacial hypoplasia   Dominantly inherited or sporadic malformations (dysmorphisms) occurring in holoproscencephaly, or in **Apert** or **Crouzon syndromes,** characterized by maldevelopment of the parts derived from the frontonasal process.

Deafness and facial dysmorphisms (hypotelorism, flattening of the nose, **cebocephaly, ethmocephaly, cyclopia,** an indistinct philtrum, palatal deformity, mandibular hypoplasia, malformations of the temporomandibular joints and tongue, fusion of the jaws, and other anomalies of the cranial bones) may be associated.

midlatency SEP   That portion of the waveforms of a somatosensory evoked potential normally occurring within 25–100 msec after stimulation of a nerve at the wrist, within 40–100 msec after stimulation of a nerve at the knee, and within 50–100 msec after stimulation of a nerve at the ankle. (Adapted from the 1987 Report of the Nomenclature Committee of the American Association of Electromyography and Electrodiagnosis. AAEE glossary of terms in clinical electromyography. *Muscle Nerve* 1987;**10S:**G5-G23. Copyright 1987 by John Wiley and Sons, Inc. Reprinted by permission of John Wiley and Sons, Inc.)

midline fusion defect syndrome   See **Wolf-Hirschorn syndrome.**

midline hyperplasia with malformation of the fornical system   A congenital dysmorphic syndrome characterized by meningocele, hydrocephalus, and cerebellar atrophy.

midline nevus flammeus with intracranial vascular disease   See **Sturge-Weber syndrome.**

midline spikes   An encephalographic finding during interictal periods, consisting of the appearance of spikes with maximal amplitude at the Fz, Pz, and Cz positions, with phase reversals in the waking or sleeping states. They correlate well with the presence of various forms of epilepsy, including generalized tonic-clonic and focal motor seizures and less commonly myoclonic or atonic attacks.[1613]

midwinter insomnia   A seasonal form of the **delayed sleep phase syndrome** encountered in the "Land of the Midnight Sun."[3421]

Mietens syndrome   A recessively inherited, congenital dysmorphic syndrome manifesting also strabismus, corneal clouding, horizontal and rotary nystagmus, short limbs with flexion contractures, and mental retardation.[3870]

migraine   (from Gr, half + skull, through Lat, hemicrania to Fr; migraine) A familial systemic syndrome encompassing various forms of head pain or evidence of focal disturbance of the nervous system. The condition was known to Hippocrates, Celsus, Arateus, and Galen, but the first modern account was that of Thomas **Willis** and a more formal description was provided by John **Fothergill** in a pamphlet *Remarks on that com-*

plaint commonly known under the name of sick headach, published in 1777.[4001] The history of the development of thought in the area has been recounted by Pearce,[4377] who quotes Liveing's definition of 1873: "A form of centrencephalic seizure, the activity of which is projected rostrally upon the cerebral hemispheres and peripherally via the autonomic nervous system," and notes that we are little wiser now. The classification of the International Headache Society[1051] is reproduced in Chart M–8.

Chart M–8. Classification of Migraine

1.1 Migraine without aura
1.2 Migraine with aura
   1.2.1 **Migraine with typical aura**
   1.2.2 Migraine with prolonged aura
   1.2.3 Familial hemiplegic migraine
   1.2.4 Basilar migraine
   1.2.5 **Migraine aura without headache**
   1.2.6 **Migraine with acute onset aura**
1.3 Ophthalmoplegic migraine
1.4 Retinal migraine
1.5 Childhood periodic syndromes that may be precursors to or associated with migraine
   1.5.1 Benign paroxysmal vertigo of childhood
   1.5.2 Alternating hemiplegia of childhood
1.6 Complications of migraine
   1.6.1 Status migrainosus
   1.6.2 **Migrainous infarction**
1.7 **Migrainous disorder not fulfilling above criteria**

From The Classification Committee of the International Headache Society. Classification of headache disorders, cranial neuralgias and facial pains; and diagnostic criteria for primary headache disorders. Cephalalgia 1988;8(suppl):1–96. Reprinted by kind permission of Blackwell Science.

Knowledge of the pathophysiology of migraine has advanced far since the first edition of this book, though not far enough to allow confident mapping of the underlying chain of events. Cortical hyperexcitability, evidenced by laboratory techniques and by the persistence of the afterimage following fundoscopy,[1419] and the activity of a brainstem generator of impulses activating the trigeminovascular complex and thus leading to the liberation of vasoactive peptides in the extra- and intracranial arterial walls, in turn causing progressive pain perception through other brainstem mechanisms appear to be the major elements of the process.

migraine accompagnée See **migrainous accompaniments.**

migraine accompaniments (migraine accompagnée) Transient and reversible neurological deficits occurring in the absence of a current headache and of any other detectable cause, supposed to be occurring on the same basis as the rest of the migrainous syndrome, whatever that may be. Not all patients who have such problems have migraine headaches as well.

Clinically, scintillating scotomas, blindness, blurred vision, numbness, paresthesias, aphasia, dysarthria and motor weakness are the more common symptoms.

Clues to the migrainous nature of the syndrome are as follows:

A. The presence of visual symptoms
B. A gradual buildup and migration of any scintillating display
C. A march of paresthesias
D. The serial progression of symptoms
E. The occurrence of two or more identical spells
F. Accompanying headache
G. A duration of 15–25 minutes
H. The occurrence of a flurry of accompaniments
I. Recurrence of similar spells over a period of years
J. The exclusion of cerebral thrombosis, subclavian steal, epilepsy, thrombocythemia, polycythemia, hyperviscosity, and lupus anticoagulant
K. Normal cerebral arteriographic findings[1856]

migraine aura without headache (migraine equivalents, acephalgic migraine) Migrainous aura unaccompanied by headache. The following diagnostic criteria are suggested by the Headache Classification Committee of the International Headache Society[1051] (from Classification of headache disorders, cranial neuralgias and facial pains; and diagnostic criteria for primary headache disorders. *Cephalalgia* 1988;**8**[suppl]:1–96) and are reproduced by kind permission.

A. Fulfils criteria for **migraine with aura**
B. No headache

Perhaps more usefully, the condition has been diagnosed when the focal neurological symptoms come on gradually, and spread or intensify over a period of minutes; positive visual symptoms occur as classically in migraine; headache is absent or mild if present; and the patient did not have simiar symptoms previously in the context of classical migraine or in association with a more severe headache.[1390]

migraine coma (meningitic migraine) A repetitively occurring, self-limited, generalized encephalopathy with delirium, rarely reported in patients with prior classic or familial migraine, but sometimes following head trauma.[1129]

The attacks are preceded by severe headache and vomiting and lead to clouding of consciousness to pyramidal signs, often accompanied by fever and further reduction in consciousness, with recovery in about 2 days. Despite the alternative title, the CSF is usually normal, although pleocytosis may occur some days after admission.

migraine equivalents See **migraine aura without headache.**

Migraine Foundation A Canadian charitable association. Address: 120 Carlton St. Ste. 210, Toronto, Ontario M5A 4K2. Canada. Tel: 416-920-4916.

migraine madness Psychosis occurring in temporal association with migraine in subjects known to have that condition in the past without such mental abnormality.

The state may last days or weeks, and recur over many years. Delusions, both paranoid and other, visual hallucinations, **reduplicative paramnesia,** and speech disturbances are described. Migraine-induced ischemia of the nondominant hemisphere is considered to be responsible.[1990] See also **dysphrenic migraine.**

migraine stroke   See **migrainous infarction.**

migraine with acute-onset aura   Migraine with aura developing fully in less than 5 minutes. The following diagnostic criteria are suggested by the Headache Classification Committee of the International Headache Society[1051] (from Classification of headache disorders, cranial neuralgias and facial pains; and diagnostic criteria for primary headache disorders. *Cephalalgia* 1988;**8**[suppl]:1–96). Reprinted by kind permission of Blackwell Science.

A. Fulfils criteria for **migraine with aura**
B. Neurological symptoms develop within 4 minutes
C. Headache lasts 4–72 hours (untreated or unsuccessfully treated)
D. Headache has at least two of the following characteristics: unilateral location; pulsating quality; moderate or severe intensity (inhibits or prohibits daily activities); aggravation by walking stairs or similar routine physical activity
E. During headache at least one of the following occurs: nausea and/or vomiting; photophobia and phonophobia
F. Thromboembolic transient ischemic attack and other intracranial lesions are ruled out by appropriate investigations.

migraine with aura   (classic migraine, classical migraine, ophthalmic migraine, hemiparesthetic migraine, hemiplegic migraine, aphasic migraine, migraine accompangneé, complicated migraine) An idiopathic, recurring disorder manifesting with attacks of neurological symptoms unequivocally localizable to the cerebral cortex or brainstem, usually gradually developed over 5–20 minutes and usually lasting less than 60 minutes.

Headache, nausea, and/or photophobia usually follow neurological aura symptoms directly, or after a free interval of less than an hour. The headache usually lasts 4–72 hours, but may be completely absent (Code 1.2.5 in Chart M–8). This definition and the following diagnostic criteria are suggested by the Headache Classification Committee of the International Headache Society[1051] (see Chart M–9).

Chart M–9. Diagnostic Criteria for Migraine with Aura

A. At least two attacks fulfilling B
B. At least three of the following characteristics:
1. One or more fully reversible aura symptoms indicates focal cerebral cortical and/or brainstem dysfunction.
2. At least one aura symptom develops gradually over more than 4 minutes.
3. Two or more symptoms occur in succession.
4. Headache follows aura with a free interval of less than 60 minutes. It may also begin before or simultaneously with the aura.
C. At least one of the following:
1. History, and physical and neurological examination

findings do not suggest one of the disorders listed in groups 5 to 11 (see **headache**).
2. History and physical and neurological examination findings do suggest such a disorder, but it is ruled out by appropriate investigations.
3. Such a disorder is present, but migraine attacks do not occur for the first time in close temporal relation to the disorder.

From Classification of headache disorders, cranial neuralgias and facial pains; and diagnostic criteria for primary headache disorders. Cephalalgia 1988;**8**(suppl):1–96. Reprinted by kind permission of Blackwell Science.

A *variant* is *migraine with aura, fluishing spells, myalgias, asthma and advanced sleep phase syndrome.*

migraine with interparoxysmal headache   A condition in which occasional but increasingly frequent episodes of migraine headache are separated by periods during which further headaches occur, similar to but not identical to the patient's usual migraine and which occur daily and chronically. The condition has been considered a "transformational syndrome" between migraine and chronic daily headache.[4915] See **rebound headache.**

migraine with prolonged aura   Migraine with one or more aura symptoms lasting more than 60 minutes and less than a week. Neuroimaging findings are normal. Following are the diagnostic criteria suggested by the Headache Classification Committee of the International Headache Society[1051] (from Classification of headache disorders, cranial neuralgias and facial pains; and diagnostic criteria for primary headache disorders. *Cephalalgia* 1988;**8**[suppl]:1–96. Reprinted by kind permission of Blackwell Science.)

A. Fulfils criteria for code 1.2 (see Chart M–8), but at least one symptom lasts between 60 minutes and 7 days. If neuroimaging reveals relevant ischemic lesion, code as 1.6.2 migrainous infarction (see Chart M–8) regardless of symptom duration.

migraine with typical aura   (ophthalmic, hemiparesthetic, hemiparetic, hemiplegic, or aphasic migraine, migraine accompagnée) Migraine with an aura consisting of homonymous visual disturbances, hemisensory symptoms, hemiparesis or dysphasia, or combinations thereof. Gradual development, duration under 1 hour, and complete reversibility characterize the aura associated with headache.

Following are the diagnostic criteria suggested by the Headache Classification Committee of the International Headache Society[1051] (from: Classification of headache disorders, cranial neuralgias and facial pains; and diagnostic criteria for primary headache disorders. *Cephalalgia* 1988;**8**[suppl]:1–96. Reprinted by kind permission of Blackwell Science):

A. Fulfils criteria for **migraine with aura** including all four criteria under B.
B. One or more aura symptoms of the following types: homonymous visual disturbance; unilateral paresthesias and/or numbness; unilateral weakness; aphasia and unclassifiable speech difficulty.

migraine without aura (common migraine, hemicrania simplex) Idiopathic, recurring headache disorder manifesting in attacks lasting 4–72 hours. Typical characteristics of headache are unilateral location, pulsating quality, moderate or severe intensity, aggravation by routine physical activity, and association with nausea, photophobia, and phonophobia. This definition and the diagnostic criteria in Chart M–10 are suggested by the Headache Classification Committee of the International Headache Society.[1051]

Chart M–10. Diagnostic Criteria for Migraine without Aura

A. At least five attacks fulfilling B–D below
B. Headache attacks lasting 4–72 hours, untreated or unsuccessfully treated. (In the case of children, the IHS criteria suggest 2–48 hours.)
C. Headache has at least two of the following characteristics:
  1. Unilateral location
  2. Pulsating quality
  3. Moderate or severe intensity (inhibits or prohibits daily activities)
  4. Aggravation by walking stairs or similar routine physical activity
D. During headache at least one of the following occurs:
  1. Nausea and/or vomiting
  2. Photophobia and phonophobia
E. At least one of the following occurs:
  1. History, physical and neurological examination findings do not suggest one of the disorders listed in groups 5–11 under **headache.**
  2. History and/or physical and/or neurological examination findings do suggest such a disorder, but it is ruled out by appropriate investigations.
  3. Such a disorder is present, but migraine attacks do not occur for the first time in close temporal relation to the disorder. See also **symptomatic migraine.**

From Classification of headache disorders, cranial neuralgias and facial pains; and diagnostic criteria for primary headache disorders. Cephalalgia 1988;8(suppl):1–96. Reprinted by kind permission of Blackwell Science.

A *variant* is **familial migraine with vertigo and essential tremor.**[313]

migraine–cluster headache syndrome The occurrence of headaches that are predominantly of one of these types, but with at least one major timing factor (random vs. clustering, frequency, duration, hour of onset) or three other major features of the other (prodrome; aura; nausea, vomiting; incapacitation leading to bed, etc., with migraine; and with eye redness and tearing; Horner syndrome; rhinorrhea; and physical mobility with cluster headache).[5256]

migrainous disorder not fulfilling criteria Headache attacks believed to be a form of **migraine,** but which do not quite meet the operational diagnostic criteria for any of the forms of migraine. This definition and the following diagnostic criteria are suggested by the Headache Classification Committee of the International Headache Society (from Classification of headache disorders, cranial neuralgias and facial pains; and diagnos-

tic criteria for primary headache disorders. *Cephalalgia* 1988;**8**[suppl]:1–96. Reprinted by kind permission of Blackwell Science.)
  A. Fulfils all criteria but one, for one or more forms of migraine
  B. Does not fulfil criteria for tension-type headache

migrainous infarction (complicated migraine; migraine stroke) One or more migrainous aura symptoms not fully reversible within 7 days and/or associated with neuroimaging confirmation of ischemic infarction. This definition and the following diagnostic criteria are suggested by the Headache Classification Committee of the International Headache Society[1051] (from Classification of headache disorders, cranial neuralgias and facial pains; and diagnostic criteria for primary headache disorders. *Cephalalgia* 1988;**8**[suppl]:1–96). Reprinted by kind permission of Blackwell Science.
  A. Patient has previously fulfilled criteria for migraine with aura
  B. The present attack is typical of previous attacks, but neurological deficits are not completely reversible within 7 days and/or neuroimaging demonstrates ischemic infarction in the relevant area.
  C. Other causes of infarction are ruled out by appropriate investigations.

The condition is considered to be due to prolongation of the migrainous process beyond its usual temporal limits.[634] The occipital lobe is most commonly affected.

migrainous neuralgia   See **cluster headaches.**

migrainous vertigo The occurrence of vertigo or dysequilibrium as a manifestation of an underlying migraine attack. Diagnostic criteria have been suggested, as follows:[866]
  1. Recurrent vestibular symptoms (rotatory/positional vertigo, other or illusory self or object motion, head motion intolerance)
  2. Migraine according to International Headache Society criteria
  3. At least one of the following symptoms during two vertiginous attacks;
    a. Migrainous headache
    b. Photophobia
    c. Phonophobia
    d. Visual or other auras
  4. Other causes are excluded by appropriate investigations.

migralepsy The association of features of migraine and epilepsy in the same attack. The term was suggested by Sir William **Gowers.**

migrant sensory neuritis (of Wartenberg) A self-limiting condition characterized by the repetitive brief occurrences of a sudden, searing pain in the territory of a sensory nerve, precipitated by movement of a limb and leading sometimes to sensory deficits.

It has been considered that this may occur because of stretching resulting from movements of a limb,[3708] but **multiple sclerosis** is sometimes a more acceptable explanation.

migration abnormalities   See **heterotopias, lissencephaly.**

Main Pathological Types of Migration Abnormality[59,1481]

Major Abnormalities

1. *Type 1* **lissencephaly**-*agyria* Smooth brain, four-layer cortex with thick layer of arrested heterotopic neurons, resembling a fetal brain at 13 weeks of gestation.
2. *Type 2 lissencephaly* (Walker-Warburg syndrome) Totally disorganized cortex divided by gliomesenchymal trabeculae into glomeruli with disoriented cells.
3. Pachygyria Few, thick gyri, similar to lissencephaly with less numerous heterotopic neurons.
4. Polymicrogyria Multiple small gyri with "cauliflower" appearance; four-layer cortex without heterotopic neurons but paucicellular layer in continuity with normal layers 4–5. Other types include unlayered microgyria.
5. Localized cortical dysplasia (The term *dysplasia* is used in a general sense to designate all developmental cortical abnormalities or in the restricted sense of focalized defect of cortical organization.) Absent lamination and anarchic distribution of neurons and glial cells are typical. In one type, balloon cells similar to those in tuberous sclerosis are found.

Minor Abnormalities That May Exist Alone or in Association with Major Anomalies

6. Glioneuronal heterotopias Verrucous cortex, excess cell migration into the molecular layer, and meninges.
7. Microdysgenesis Excess number of neurons in molecular layer, irregular thickness of neuronal layers, heterotopic neurons in the outer white matter.

migratory recurrent cranial neuritis   A syndrome of repetitive cranial nerve palsies lasting a few weeks and affecting the same or different nerves (usually the cranial nerves II to VI), with headache.[5502] See also **acute painful ophthalmoplegia.**

migratory seizures   See **fragmentary seizures.**

Mikulicz-Gougerot-Sjörgren syndrome   See **Sjögren syndrome.**[3978]

Milan Overall Dementia assessment   A composite tool for the assessment of cognitive impairment, composed of an autonomy scale measuring everyday coping skills; four items concerning orientation; and nine neuropsychological tests assessing attention, intelligence, memory, language, space cognition, and visual perception.[1008]

mild Broca aphasia   See **Broca aphasia.**

mild head injury   (mild traumatic brain injury) A traumatic incident resulting in loss of consciousness for less than 30 minutes, or in dazing without loss of consciousness at all; an initial **Glasgow Coma scale** score of 13 to 15 without subsequent deterioration; and an absence of focal neurological deficits, depressed skull fracture, intracranial bleeding, or other pathology.[1718]

Symptoms such as headache; dizziness; fatigue; irritability; impaired concentration, memory, and the ability to perform mental tasks; insomnia; depression; and reduction in tolerance to stress, alcohol, and excitement are, however, common, and remarkable for their transience in the presence of verbal motivation.[2992]

mild postural cerebellar tremor   See **cerebellar tremors.**

mild traumatic brain injury   See **mild head injury.**

milestones   The motor skills acquired, in order, by the developing infant. These are listed in Chart M–11.

Chart M–11. Developmental Milestones

Months*	Motor Skills
1	Watches mother
1–2	Smiles
1	Extends neck in prone position, raising head briefly
2	Vocalizes, apart from crying
3	Lifts head prone when held in ventral suspension
4	Laughs; turns head towards meaningful sound
5	Grasps with whole; hands come together in play; rolls over alone
6	Head held erect while sitting; raises upper body on arms in prone position; transfers objects between hands; drinks from a cup (held); looks at own hands; stretches arms out to mother
7	Simple sounds (ba, da, goo, etc.)
8	Double-syllable words (dada, mama, etc.)
9	Sits supported
10	Responds to own name
11	Crawls; pulls up to standing; walks while holding on
12	Pincer (finger-thumb) grasp
14	Says at least one meaningful word
15	Builds a tower of two cubes; walks unsupported
16	Picks up and drinks from a cup
24	Builds a tower of 6 cubes; uses pronouns (I, me, you)
36	Builds a tower of 9 cubes; copies a circle
48	Copies a cross
60	Copies a triangle
60–96	Dry at night

The latest date by which the milestones are normally first attained.

See also **Denver Developmental Screening test.**

Milgram test   When the supine patient raises both legs a few inches off the bed for 30 seconds, back pain suggests the presence of radiculopathy, caused by the increased intrathecal pressue induced by the maneuver.

miliary aneurysms   (from Lat, millet seeds) The term of **Charcot** (1866) and of Bouchard (1872) for the tiny dilatations of arterioles now known by the names of both. See **Charcot-Bouchard aneurysm.**

milk-alkali syndrome   See **Burnett syndrome.**

milkmaid sign   Variability in the isometric force exerted by the wrist and by individual fingers during attempts to grasp an object. The sign is positive in choreic states.[5976]

Millard, Auguste   (1830–1915) French physician who graduated from the University of Paris where he practiced and published extensively in the areas of pediatrics and internal medicine.

Millard-Gubler syndrome   (Gubler paralysis) A pontine lesion affecting the seventh cranial nerve nucleus and the descending pyramidal fibers on one side of the ventral pons, causing homolateral facial paresis and contralateral hemiplegia.[2304] The syndrome may also include a sixth cranial nerve palsy.

Credit for localization of the syndrome belongs to Gubler. Millard had his anecdotal contribution (a letter) published immediately after it in the same issue of the *Gazette Hebdomadaire Médicine et Chiurgerie*, although he had previously described the same condition, but without any useful analysis.[3875]

Miller, Henry   (1913–1976) English neurologist. After completing medical studies at the University of Newcastle-upon-Tyne, he trained in psychiatry and neurology in Newcastle and London, returning to northern England for the rest of his clinical career, except for wartime service.

His teaching and almost prescient clinical skills were legendary. The clinical research topics he explored included multiple sclerosis, accident neurosis, and numerous other topics in neurology and psychiatry, not all of the latter being welcomed by colleagues in psychiatry, perhaps in part because in his writing he displayed readability, irreverence, individuality, courage, and common sense. Some of his *obiter dicta* are not to be forgotten: "the best instrument for obtaining the plantar response is the ignition key of a Bentley" and "hemiplegic multiple sclerosis is a rarity and only to be diagnosed by me" are classic examples.

He was variously professor of neurology, dean of the medical school, and, later, vice-chancellor of his university; Secretary-General of the World Federation of Neurology; and visiting professor at numerous universities. He also held many other positions in national or international neurology by election or acclamation. The book *Remembering Henry* was compiled within a decade of his death by those who knew him and displays a true renaissance figure who contributed to the form as well as to the substance of neurology.

Miller Fisher syndrome   (Fisher syndrome, ophthalmoplegia-ataxia-areflexia syndrome, acute oropharyngeal palsy, brainstem "encephalitis") A self-limited syndrome in which truncal and limb ataxia, ptosis, and conjugate gaze palsies leading to ophthalmoplegia, the involvement of other cranial nerves, and hyporeflexia without significant motor or sensory deficits in the limbs are the leading signs. Other features include acellular CSF with high protein levels and occasionally internal ophthalmoplegia.[1838] IgG antibodies to GQ1b and GT1a have been detected.[5990] Sensory loss is unusual.

Long considered to be a variant of the **acute inflammatory demyelinating polyneuropathy** syndrome, it has been suggested that this syndrome is ac-

tually a manifestation of brainstem encephalitis;[67] whether this represents a central or a peripheral lesion (or both) is debated. Anti-GQ1b IgG antibodies have been found in both of these conditions and in acute ophthalmoparesis. A similar condition was reported by Collier in 1932. See also **multiple cranial nerve palsies syndrome, mesencephalitis, rhombencephalitis.**

Variants include the absence of the ophthalmoplegia; a syndrome of bilateral ptosis, ataxia, and areflexia;[6080] and an ataxic form of **acute inflammatory polyneuropathy.**

Diagnostic criteria in Chart M–12 have been suggested by Ropper et al.[4772]

Chart M–12. Diagnostic Criteria for Miller Fisher Syndrome

Clinical Features

A. Bilateral, relatively symmetrical weakness of several extraocular muscles, and ptosis
B. Limb and gait ataxia with cerebellar tremor
C. Areflexia in all limbs by 1 week
D. Progression of the above three features over several days to 3 weeks
E. Minimal or no limb, facial, or oropharyngeal weakness, or paresthesias
F. Normal alertness, no cerebellar dysarthria except as a result of the previous feature; no Babinski signs

Laboratory Abnormalities that Confirm the Diagnosis

A. Variable, usually slight, elevation of CSF protein concentration
B. Abnormal motor nerve conduction and late responses in the legs

From Ropper AH, Wijdicks EFM, Truax BT. Guillain-Barré Syndrome. Philadelphia: F.A. Davis, 1991, by permission.

Miller-Dieker syndrome   (OMIM 247200) The association of lissencephaly with facial dysmorphism, hypertelorism, cloudy corneae, congenital cardiac and renal anomalies, enlarged liver, polydactyly, syndactyly, seizures (infantile spasms), decerebrate posturing, and microcephaly, described by Dr. J.Q. Miller.[3881] The responsible chromosomal deletion is of a band on 17p13.3. See **lissencephaly.**

Milles syndrome   A variant of the **Sturge-Weber syndrome** in which an angioma of the choroid occurs without glaucoma.

Millikan-Siekert syndrome   See **vertebrobasilar insufficiency.**

Mills, Charles Karsner   (1845–1931) American neurologist, the first professor of neurology in the United States, who operated the first neurological ward, at Philadelphia General Hospital. (Later neurological wards were created at Bellvue in 1898 for Dana, at Mount Sinai in 1900, and at Boston City Hospital in 1909. By 1923, eight independent neurological departments existed in the United States.)

Mills described ascending and descending forms of progressive paralysis, alcoholic polyneuropathy, and geniculate ganglion neuralgia. His classic and highly popular textbook, *The Nervous System and Its Diseases—A Practical Treatise on Neurology* (Philadelphia), was published in 1898 and was notable for its inclusion of sections on the neurological examination and on functional localization.

Mills disease Chronic, unilateral, progressive ascending paralysis with wasting but also hyperreflexia, starting in the leg and later affecting the arm and eventually the other side as well; this is an entity of uncertain nature, but probably a form of **amyotrophic lateral sclerosis,**[3894] though some have considered it to represent **acute inflammatory demyelinating polyneuropathy.**

mimetic (Gr, imitative) Apt to imitate. 1. Applied to diseases that resemble others in their manifestations, such as syphilis, AIDS, and systemic lupus erythematosus. 2. Human actions that copy those of others.

mimetic palsy See **emotional facial palsy.**

mimetic smile Retained ability to contract the lower facial muscles on the hemiparetic side during the spontaneous act of smiling or laughing, while voluntary contraction of these muscles is impossible on command, because of an upper motor neuron lesion above the pons.

The disparity results from the anatomical situation; while the coorticobulbar tract mediates the volitional "smile," the mimetic smile depends on the functional integrity of fibers from the central tegmental tract derived from the hypothalamus, thalamus, and globus pallidus. Thus the subject with a high supranuclear lesion may laugh symmetrically even though the lower facial quadrant is paretic when attempting voluntary, nonemotional movements.

mimic palsy Facial palsy. See **Bell palsy.**

mimic spasm Facial muscle spasm, probably due to **dystonia.**

mimo-causalgia See **reflex sympathetic dystrophy.**

Minamata disease A toxic encephalomyeloneuropathy due to chronic mercury poisoning, which occurred between 1953 and 1956 in people living by a bay in southern Japan, methyl mercury having been concentrated in fish caught and eaten by them. Salivation, cerebellar signs, numbness due to sensory neuropathy, deafness, concentric constriction of the visual fields, and delirium or dementia were the major signs recorded.[3725] Low-level exposure is under investigation as a factor reducing motor skills and auditory and visual functions in the young.

mind (Middle English, from Saxon; to remember) 1. The power of human intelligence. 2. The sum total of the phenomena of the functional activity of the brain, subdivided into feeling, will or volition, and thought, through which all subjective and objective experience is derived.

miner's nystagmus A form of pendular nystagmus accompanied by light intolerance and oscillations of the head in people who have worked for years in darkness. Whether this entity really exists is questionable.

miniature end-plate potential (MEPP) The postsynaptic muscle fiber potentials produced through the spontaneous release of individual acetylcholine quanta from the presynaptic axon terminal. As recorded with monopolar or concentric needle electrodes inserted in the end-plate region, MEPPs are monophasic, negative, of short duration (<5 msec), and generally less than 20 uV in amplitude. (From the 2001 Report of the Nomenclature Committee of the American Association of Electromyography and Electrodiagnosis.[10] Used by permission, copyright © 2001, AAEM.)

minicore-multicore myopathy (MMM) A benign, congenital, nonprogressive myopathy in which the muscle fibers have histochemical defects of both oxidative and myofibrillar adenosine-triphosphatase enzymes and show disorganization of myofilaments.[1666]

minimal brain damage See **minimal brain dysfunction.**

minimal brain dysfunction (minimal brain damage, Struwwelpeter syndrome, hyperkinetic syndrome) A syndrome of incoordination, overactivity, impulsivity and emotional lability, reduced attention span, and often specific learning deficits, apparent when the child first attends school.[1058] See **attention-deficit hyperactivity disorder.**

minimal change myopathy Weakness of presumably congenital origin associated with normal or near-normal muscle biopsy.[1744] See **benign congenital myopathy.**

minimal ice water caloric test A test of labyrinthine function using 0.2 ml of ice-cold water with the head elevated 30° and tilted toward the opposite side for the first 10 seconds. The patient should wear +20D lenses.

The standard test popularized by **Bárány** used 10–20 ml, which induces nystagmus, past-pointing, and drift, but also nausea and vomiting in many cases. This modification results in nystagmus for a shorter period, but without the unpleasant associations.[4093]

minimal record of disability (MRD) A rating scale published by the National Multiple Sclerosis Society of the United States, designed to quantitate the effects of **multiple sclerosis.** It was last modified in 1984.[2746]

The record was designed to follow the three-tier classification of dysfunction developed by the World Health Organization. As applied to neurological disorders these are the following:

1. *Impairment* Clinical signs and symptoms produced by damage to the nervous system.

2. *Disability* The personal limitations imposed upon the activities of daily living by the neurologic impairment.

3. *Handicap* The social and environmental effects of the disability.

minimal seizures (subtle seizures) An epileptic seizure pattern in newborns, characterized by tonic deviation; jerking of the eyes or eyelids; lip smacking, sucking, or swallowing; abnormal limb movements; and brief alterations of muscle tone with assumption of bizarre postures. Seizures presenting as autonomic dysfunction only also fall into this category. Clonic jerks of the eyelids or limbs are occasionally seen in the later stages.[56]

minimally conscious state A state of reduced consciousness characterized by inconsistent but discernible sustained and reproducible evidence of consciousness, retention of sleep–wake cycles, and ability to localize sound and noxious stimuli and to fixate visually, with some ability to vocalize and show emotional facial movement.[2092]

The major purpose of defining this condition appears to be its differentiation from the **persistent vegetative state.**

Mini-Mental State Examination (MMSE) A standardized and formal 11-item examination of certain mental functions, including orientation, concentration, data retention, registration, calculation ability, recall, language, visuospatial functions, and praxis. It is used as a screening test for dementia and for the serial assessment of geriatric patients. The original test[1905] has been expanded (See **Modified Mini-Mental State Examination**[5524]) by the addition of items, including date and place of birth, some abstract thought items, and more memory and naming tasks so that the maximum score is now 100.

minimum conduction velocity The nerve conduction velocity measured from slowly conducting nerve fibers. Special techniques are needed to produce this measurement in motor or sensory nerves.

minipolymyoclonus Subtle, small-amplitude, multifocal movements, once considered to represent myoclonic jerks but more likely due to fasciculations of enlarged motor units causing twitching predominantly in the fingers and hands, and preceded by a synchronous, frontocentrally predominant negative slow wave in the condition of **primary generalized epileptic myoclonus.**[5972]

The movements resemble small-amplitude coarse tremors, and may also be seen in patients with anterior horn cell disease.[2726,5292] See also **cortical tremor.** (From the 2001 Report of the Nomenclature Committee of the American Association of Electromyography and Electrodiagnosis.[146] Used by permission, copyright © 2001, AAEM.)

Minnesota Child Development Inventory A questionnaire for parents, used to assess general development, gross and fine motor activity, language, comprehension, and personal and social skills, etc. in their infants.

Minnesota Multiphasic Personality Inventory A comprehensive self-administered inventory allowing an assessment of personality factors.[2475]

Minnesota Test for the Differential Diagnosis of Aphasia An aphasia battery.[5006] See also **Western Aphasia Battery, Boston Diagnostic Aphasia Examination, Porch Index.**

Minnesota thermal disks A set of mounted disks made of copper, stainless steel, glass, and polyvinyl chloride, respectively, which are placed upon prepared areas of skin and which, because of the different rates of heat transfer between such materials and the skin, will feel relatively warmer or cooler than one another to the normal subject.

The disks have been used for the semiquantitative assessment of temperature sensation.[1573]

Minor causalgia See **reflex sympathetic dystrophy, causalgia.**

Minor disease A syndrome resembling **syringomyelia,** occurring after blunt stretching or compressive trauma to the spinal cord, usually at cervical levels.[3901] See **central hematomyelia.**

minor epileptic status See **status epilepticus.**

minor head injury A cranial trauma producing an initial loss of consciousness limited to 20 minutes or less, a **Glasgow Coma scale** score of over 13–15 on admission, and requiring hospitalization for less than 48 hours.[4699]

minor hemisphere syndrome See **apractagnosia.**

minor intervertebral disorder Mechanical lesions of the **mobile segment** of the spine (particularly of the facet joints) without demonstrable pathology, but leading to pain referred to the appropriate dermatomal territory.[3578]

minor ischemic stroke An acute ischemic disturbance of focal neurological function with symptoms lasting more than 24 hours and less than 1 week.

Minor, Lazar Salomavitch (1855–1942) Russian neurologist and neuropathologist, professor in Moscow, who described hematomyelia (**Minor disease**) in 1892 and thereafter **serous meningitis** (Minor pseudomeningitis), the **Minor method,** the **Minor sign,** and **Minor tremor.**

minor meningitis See **idiopathic intracranial hypertension.**

Minor method The use of an iodine-alcohol–castor oil application to demonstrate areas of sweat production, invented by Dr. L. **Minor.**

minor motor epilepsy   See **Lennox Gastaut syndrome.**

minor motor seizures   Myoclonic, astatic, or brief atonic seizures, or any type of seizure of limited expression regardless of clinical and EEG features.[56] The term is honored more in the breach than in the observance. See **absence seizures.**

Minor pseudomeningitis   See **serous meningitis.**

Minor sign   The patient with sciatica arises by putting weight on the healthy leg, bending the other one, placing one hand on the back, and flexing the spine.[4723]

minor status   See **absence status.**

Minor tremor   A familial tremor with childhood onset, described by Dr. L. **Minor** in 1925; it is increased by stress, is unassociated with other neurological problems, and is properly known as **essential tremor.**

miosis   (Gr; lessening) Constriction of the pupil to a diameter of 3 mm or less as a result of accommodation (physiological), decreased sympathetic or increased parasympathetic activity, or the effects of drug administration.

miotics   Agents that produce pupillary constriction, many also causing contraction of the ciliary muscle and thus disturbing accommodation. Eserine (physostigmine), pilocarpine, and opioids are examples.

mirror agnosia   See **Ramachandran sign.**

mirror focus   Excessive electrical activity arising in a contralateral homologous site to a primary epileptic focus as a result of repetitive transmissions across the corpus callosum.

mirror movements   Symmetrical involuntary movements of the opposite side of the body involving the use of the homologous contralateral muscles, very commonly seen in childhood but thereafter generally suppressed except in some left-handers; hemiparetics (see **Leonardo da Vinci**), especially if congenital; and dyslexic children. Reports of increased left-handedness and mirror writing among children in institutions for the mentally retarded are of uncertain merit. The basis is likely to be abnormal branching of crossed fast-conducting fibers from the undamaged primary motor cortex to homologous motor neuron pools.[1039] See also **alien hand syndrome.**

In a *variant* form, *hereditary mirror movements,* an anatomical variation of the corticospinal tracts has been considered to be the basis of the phenomenon.[2365,2918,3153]

mirror test   If a large mirror is moved to and fro in front of the face of a subject who claims blindness, movements of the eyes indicate that vision is in fact retained.

mirror writing   (spiegelschrift) Reversed writing, sometimes performed by mentally retarded people and more easily performed in normal subjects by those who are left handed. **Da Vinci,** paretic in his right hand, wrote with the left in this manner.

miscellaneous headaches unassociated with structural lesion   A category of headache recognized by the International Headache Society,[1051] provided below (from Classification of headache disorders, cranial neuralgias and facial pains; and diagnostic criteria for primary headache disorders. *Cephalalgia* 1988;**8**[suppl]: 1–96). Reprinted by kind permission of Blackwell Science.

4.1 **Idiopathic stabbing headache**
4.2 **External compression headache**
4.3 **Cold stimulus headache**
    4.3.1 External application of a cold stimulus
    4.3.2 Ingestion of a cold stimulus
4.4 **Benign cough headache**
4.5 Benign exertional headache
4.6 **Headache associated with sexual activity**
    4.6.1 Dull type
    4.6.2 Explosive type (benign sex headache)
    4.6.3 Postural type

misdirection syndrome   Adduction and depression of the eye on attempted vertical gaze, elevation of the eyelid, and miosis due to abnormal mass discharges in aberrant regenerating fibers of the third cranial nerve after injury. These features, occurring periodically, thus resemble those of **cyclic oculomotor paralysis.**[5822]

misery perfusion   Locally increased oxygen extraction occurring in an area of chronic reduction of cerebral blood flow. It may follow a small focal infarct or may itself lead to symptoms of **transient ischemic attacks.**

miso-   Greek prefix denoting hatred of something.

misoplegia   (Gr, hate + stroke) Behavior suggesting hatred of a paralyzed limb, as seen occasionally in patients with a left hemiplegia due to a right hemispheric infarct, who reject, push away, or curse their offending members.

misplaced objects task   A visuospatial recall task in which the subject places cardboard cutouts of household items into the rooms of a two-dimensional representation of a seven-room house, and after a delay is asked to recall which rooms of the house the objects are in.[1192]

Mitchell, Silas Weir   See **Weir Mitchell, S.W.**

Mitchell's treatment   A method for the treatment of neurasthenia, introduced by **Weir Mitchell.** As it consisted of removal from the responsibilities of home, rest in bed, massage, electrical stimulation of the limbs twice daily, and somewhat excessive feeding, it proved most popular and it was deemed successful in many cases.

mitempfindungen   (Ger, with sympathy) See **referred itch.**

mitochondrial cytopathy   A heterogeneous group of multisystem disorders mainly affecting cardiac and skeletal muscle and the CNS, many with added features. Some examples are the following:

1. (Fanconi-Toni-Debré form, cystinosis) A rare, recessively inherited, congenital syndrome comprising short stature, sensorineural deafness, cloudy corneas, cataract, retinitis pigmentosa, cardiomyopathy, renal tubular acidosis, glycosuria, aminoaciduria, cystinuria, and mental and developmental delay or dementia with widespread excessive storage of cystine. Seizures, ophthalmoplegia, intermittent ataxia, pyramidal and extrapyramidal signs, sensorimotor peripheral neuropathy and proximal myopathic weakness are other clinical features recorded. Raised levels of lactate and the presence of ragged red fibers and abnormal mitochondria in muscle biopsy specimens are markers indicating this to be a mitochondrial disease.

2. *Late-onset optic atrophy, ataxia, and myopathy* is associated with a mutation of a complex 2 gene.[581]

3. In other *variant* forms, onset occurs in childhood or youth; or the features are predominantly or exclusively those of a muscle disease,[4427] or those of disorder of the CNS.

mitochondrial diseases (mitochondriopathies) A heterogeneous group of disorders in which an impairment in mitochondrial functions due to single- or multiple-point deletions of mtDNA or nDNA are considered to be the basic defects.[3057] Aside from the clinical presentations, diagnosis may be assisted by the results of a **lactate stress test,** rather more than resting serum lactate levels.[1823] See also http://www.neuro.wustl.edu/ neuromuscular/mitosyn.html for further analysis.

Two main groupings of the phenotypes can be made (see Chart M–13).

Chart M–13. Mitochondrial Diseases Affecting the Nervous System

Presentation as Myopathy

Carnitine palmitoyl transferase deficiency
Chronic progressive myopathy
Fatal myopathy
Kearns-Sayre syndrome (Kearns-Shy syndrome)
Lethal infantile cardiomyopathy
Luft disease
Malignant hyperthermia
MNGIE
Progressive external ophthalmoplegia
Transient neonatal myopathy

Presentation as Encephalopathy

Subacute necrotizing encephalopathy
Alpers disease (subacute poliodystrophy)
Acute encephalopathy of infancy
MERFF
MELAS
Mitochondrial cytopathy
Leber optic atrophy
Leigh disease
Aminoglycoside-associated deafness
Glutaric aciduria 2
Diabetes with deafness
Fumarase deficiency
Pyruvate dehydrogenase deficiency
Pyruvate decarboxylase deficiency
NARP syndrome

Accompanying these disorders, or in isolation, there may be cardiomyopathy, growth retardation, endocrinopathy, a malabsorption syndrome, and abnormal liver function test results. Pathological abnormalities suspicious for these conditions include an increase in the CSF pyruvate/lactate ratios, systemic lactic acidosis, and the presence of abnormal mitochondria, with or without inclusions, in biopsy specimens.

mitochondrial disease, X-linked A congenital syndrome comprising cardiomyopathy, respiratory difficulties, abnormality in consciousness, proximal myopathic weakness and hypotonia, and the usual biochemical and muscle biopsy hallmarks of mitochondrial disease.[337] See also **United Mitochondrial Disease Foundation.**

mitochondrial electron transport chain A composite set of energy-producing metabolic pathways in the body comprising the following enzymes:

Complex I	NADH:CoQ oxide reductase
Complex II	Succinate CoQ reductase DHO-QO
Complex III	CoQ cytochrome idoreductase
Complex IV	Cytochrome-*c* oxidase
Complex V	ATP synthase

Clinical Features Useful in Identifying Patients with Respiratory Chain Disease

Rank 1	Rank 2	Rank 3
PEO	Myoclonic epilepsy	Failure to thrive
Elevated lactate in blood/CSF	Ataxia	Small stature
Maternal inheritance	Myopathy	Dementia
Low density in putamen on CT scan	Stroke-like episodes after seizures	Metabolic acidosis
SSAM in muscle biopsy	Deafness	Developmental regression
		Retinal pigmentation
		Cardiomyopathy
		Optic atrophy

Rank 1, features that alone are highly suggestive of respiratory chain disease; rank 2, features that in combination are suggestive of respiratory chain disease; rank 3, features which are commonly associated with respiratory chain disease but not suggestive of it unless associated with category 1 (or possibly 2) features. CT, computed tomography; progressive external ophthalmoplegia. From Jackson MJ, Schaefer JA, Johnson MA et al. Presentation and clinical investigation of mitochondrial respiratory chain disease. Brain 1995;118:339–57, by kind permission.

mitochondrial encephalomyopathies Members of a clinically and biochemically heterogeneous group of complex sporadic inborn errors of metabolism, affecting the energy pathways of mitochondrial metabolism in many systems, in particular defects of the respiratory chain and other enzyme systems involving the citric acid cycle or electron transport systems, and due to abnormal structure or function of mitochondria.[1448] These are inherited through the maternal line. In such cases, both muscle and the CNS at least are affected.

Failure to thrive, seizures, ataxias, psychomotor regression, hypotonia, and organ failure, including visual failure, are typical effects when the condition presents in infancy; they are usually due to cytochrome-*c* oxidase deficiency, and are often fatal.

Three main symptom complexes are reported (Chart M–14).

Chart M–14. The Mitochondrial Encephalomyopathies

1. Muscle weakness with severe exercise intolerance, including the hypermetabolic state **Luft disease** and *mitochondrial myopathy with nonsense mutation of the COX1 gene*[2931]
2. The same as No 1, complicated by chronic progressive external ophthalmoplegia, etc. The best-studied of these are the following:
   A. Congenital/neonatal onset
      Alpers disease
      Canavan disease
      Familial myoclonic epilepsy with ragged red fibers
      Fatal infantile myopathy with cytochrome-*c* oxidase deficiency
      Leigh disease
      Menkes disease (trichopoliodystrophy)
      Methylmalonic acidemia
      NARP (**N**europathy, **A**taxia, and **R**etinitis **P**igmentosa)
      Myopathy with multiple deletions of mitochondrial DNA
      Ramsay Hunt syndrome (dyssynergia cerebellaris myoclonica)
      Zellweger syndrome
   B. Onset in childhood, youth, or adult life
      Kearns-Sayre syndrome
      Adult-onset mitochondrial myopathy with progressive external ophthalmoplegia, presenting usually with fatigue and mild muscle weakness with elevated serum lactate levels[1385]
      MELAS
      MERRF
      Mitochondrial neurogastrointestinal encephalomyopathy (MNGIE)
3. Various combinations of CNS syndromes, such as seizures, dementia, deafness, headache, somnolence, vomiting, pigmentary retinopathy, optic atrophy, ataxia, myoclonus and/or involuntary movements, short stature, and psychomotor retardation, often with myopathy or neuropathy,[3978] and sometimes with involvement of other organ systems.[1724,4427]

Certain syndromes such as **MERRF, MELAS, maternally inherited myopathy and cardiopathy,** and **Leber hereditary optic neuropathy** are maternally transmitted and due to point mutations in mitochondrial DNA. In all of these conditions, the hallmark is the presence of **ragged red fibers** in muscle biopsy specimens stained with Gomori trichrome, a marker suggesting that the primary abnormality is of the mitochondria, although the finding is not always present and is not specific for any primary mitochondrial disease.[4943]

Described syndromes include the following:
1. Ataxia, intellectual impairment, myoclonic jerks, seizures, and small stature accompanied by muscle biopsy findings of abnormal accumulations of mitochondria and lipid droplets, with decreased cytochrome-*c* reductase activity in the mitochondrial respiratory chain[4693]

2. Hepatic failure, hypotonia, and failure to thrive in infancy with early death[5638]
3. Progressive dementia, chorea, cerebellar ataxia, deafness, and peripheral neuropathy without myopathy[4092]
4. Parkinsonism, deafness, and peripheral neuropathy[5577]

mitochondrial encephalopathy, lactic acidosis, and stroke   See **MELAS.**

mitochondrial myelomyopathy   (3-M syndrome) A progressive myelopathy described in adult males, with associated myopathy and the usual evidence of excessive storage of mitochondria, lipids, and glycogen in muscle biopsy specimens.[4209]

mitochondrial myopathies   Neurological diseases with maternal inheritance (Chart M–15) in which 4% or more of the fibers in a muscle biopsy specimen show peripheral mitochondrial accumulations (using the Gomori trichrome and succinate dehydrogenase stains),[3979] and with deficiencies in oxidative phosphorylation enzymes, mutations in mitochomndrial DNA, elevated resting serum lactate levels, abnormal ^{31}P magnetic resonance spectra of resting muscle, and a lowered anaerobic threshold. At least three of these features should be present for the diagnosis to be made.

Three overlapping syndromes have been identified, encompassing the conditions listed in the entries for **mitochondrial-lipid-glycogen disease of muscle, mitochondrial myelomyopathy,** and **mitochondrial peripheral neuropathy:**

1. Ophthalmoplegia and limb weakness (**Kearns-Sayre syndrome**)
2. Proximal weakness and fatigability
3. **Mitochondrial cytopathy**

Chart M–15. The Mitochondrial Myopathies

Mitochondrial myopathy—complex I deficiency A syndrome comprising optic atrophy, neurodegenerative regression, ophthalmoplegia, rigidity, dystonia, proximal and distal myopathic weakness, muscle pain and cramps, fatigability and cardiomyopathy, and the usual biochemical and biopsy hallmarks of mitochondrial disease. In this category is included **fatal infantile encephalomyopathy,** which is a similar encephalopathy of later onset. **MELAS** and **Alpers disease** are other manifestations of complex I deficiency.[3983]

Respiratory chain complex I deficiency An underdiagnosed energy generation disorder.[3057]

Mitochondrial myopathy—complex III deficiency A syndrome with onset in childhood or adolescence, comprising myoclonus, pigmentary retinopathy, ptosis, progressive external ophthalmoplegia, nerve deafness, ataxia, pyramidal signs, proximal and distal myopathic weakness, muscle pain and cramps, fatigability and cardiomyopathy, with the usual biochemical and biopsy hallmarks of mitochondrial disease.[3983]

Mitochondrial myopathy—complex IV deficiency See **fatal infantile mitochondrial myopathy.**

Benign reversible infantile myopathy—cytochrome oxidase deficiency (complex IV deficiency) A syndrome with onset in infancy, comprising proximal hypotonia and weakness also affecting the face, macroglossia, and severe lactic acidosis, remitting within the first 2 years of life.

Mitochondrial myopathy, encephalopathy, lactic acidosis, and stroke The most common mitochondrial encephalomyopathy. See **MELAS.**

Mitochondrial myopathy, myoclonic epilepsy, and ragged-red fibers See **MERRF.**

Mitochondrial myopathy with myotonia A syndrome with onset in childhood, comprising dwarfism, kyphoscoliosis, high arches of feet, ophthalmoplegia, myopathic muscle atrophy or hypertrophy, myotonia, hypertrophic motor neuropathy, glycogen storage, basal ganglia calcification, and the usual biochemical and biopsy hallmarks of mitochondrial disease.[337]

Mitochondrial myopathy with multiple deletions of mitochondrial DNA A dominantly inherited form, characterized by progressive external ophthalmoplegia, dysphagia, cataract, lactic acidosis, exercise intolerance, and early death. Ragged red fibers are found on muscle biopsy specimens; muscles also contain diminished amounts of mitochondrial enzymes, and mitochondrial deletions are detected in muscle cells only.[5078]

Further *variant* forms are described:

A form associated with a mild axonal or demyelinating *sensorimotor peripheral neuropathy*[5079] The onset may be in youth or adult life; the sensory peripheral neuropathy is associated variously with cerebral atrophy, optic atrophy, ophthalmoplegia, proximal neurogenic and myopathic weakness and atrophy, and the usual biochemical and biopsy hallmarks of mitochondrial disease.

A form associated with *cardioskeletal myopathy* and chronic magnesium-losing nephropathy.[4692]

A rare metabolic myopathy presenting in young adult life with *exercise-induced muscle pain*, myoglobinuria, and elevated serum creatine kinase levels, due to a failure of oxidative metabolism involving mitochondrial transport systems.

A form with onset in late adult life, presenting with insidious progressive muscle weakness, often axial and accompanied by fatigability.[2876]

---

mitochondrial neurogastrointestinal encephalomyopathy (MNGIE) A recessively inherited mitochondrial syndrome with early childhood onset, due to multiple deletions of mitochondrial DNA (thymidine phosphorylase mutations). Clinically, it is characterized by ophthalmoparesis, ptosis, peripheral neuropathy, leukoencephalopathy, recurrent nausea, vomiting or diarrhea with resultant cachexia, intestinal dysmotility, peripheral neuropathy, and histologically abnormal mitochondria in muscle. Serum lactate levels are raised.[5686]

mitochondrial peripheral neuropathy A syndrome with onset in youth or adult life, comprising optic atrophy, ophthalmoplegia, proximal neurogenic and myopathic weakness and atrophy, sensory peripheral neuropathy, cerebral atrophy, and the usual biochemical and biopsy hallmarks of mitochondrial disease.[337]

mitochondrial-lipid-glycogen disease of muscle A spontaneously reversible syndrome of muscle weakness, hypotonia, and hyporeflexia, with hepatomegaly and macroglossia, in infants with evidence of excessive storage of mitochondria, lipids, and glycogen in muscle biopsy specimens.[2850] See **benign infantile mitochondrial myopathy.**

mitochondrion An intracellular organelle concerned with the synthesis of ATP from ADP and phosphate by oxidative phosphorylation, the pathway using reducing potential generated by several oxidative systems, in particular the citric acid cycle; and possessing its own DNA.[2488]

mitral valve prolapse with ophthalmoplegia A progressive mitochondrial disease characterized by ataxia, ophthalmoplegia, ptosis, and myopathy, including cardiomyopathy manifested as heart block or mitral valve prolapse with regurgitation. Muscle biopsy specimens show the usual ragged red fibers, or congenital fiber type disproportion.[1293]

The condition is likely to represent a *variant* of **Kearns-Sayre disease.**

mitten hand A hand affected by **syndactyly** of the second through fifth digits.

mixed connective tissue disease An overlap syndrome, with features of **systemic lupus erythematosus, progressive systemic sclerosis,** and **polymyositis,** and characterized by the presence of high titers of speckled-pattern fluorescent antinuclear antibody.

Neurological complications occur in half of all cases, and include **aseptic meningitis,** paranoid psychosis, trigeminal neuropathy, peripheral neuropathy, and seizures.[458]

mixed dementia Dementing illnesses for which more than one etiology can be adduced. A diagnosis of mixed dementia should be made when one or more other systemic or brain disorders are present and are thought to be causally related to the dementia. The degree of confidence in the diagnosis of **ischemic vascular dementia** (IVD) should be specified as possible, probable, or definite, and the other disorder(s) contributing to the dementia should be listed—for example, mixed dementia due to probable IVD and possible Alzheimer disease, or mixed dementia due to definite IVD and hypothyroidism.

mixed headache (chronic daily headache) Headache with the characteristics of both **migraine** and **muscle contraction headaches** and which tend to occur on a near-daily basis in patients with added symptoms of sleep disturbance, depression, or anxiety, and a tendency to ingest excessive quantities of analgesic medications.[4914] See also **rebound headache.**

mixed hypoxia and hypercapnia See **hypercapnic headaches.**

mixed nerve A nerve containing both motor and sensory axons.

Miyoshi myopathy   See **distal muscular dystrophy.**

MMM   See **minicore-multicore myopathy.**

MNCV   Abbreviation for motor nerve conduction velocity.

mnemonist   One possessed of an extraordinary capacity for the memorization of facts.[3522]

mobile segment   The segment between two vertebrae including the intervertebral disk, the articular facets, and all the muscles and ligaments related to them, believed by Maigne to act as a unit so that any pathology affecting one also affects the others.[3578]

mobile spasm   Gowers defined this as follows: "Tonic spasm, slowly varying in relative degree in different muscles, causing slow, irregular movements, chiefly conspicuous in the hand, and slow irregular incoordination. . . . A disorder of movement seen after hemiplegia."[2240]

Möbius, Paul Julius   (Moebius) (1853–1907) German neurologist who graduated in philosophy and then in medicine from Leipzig University, and became assistant to Strümpell in Heidelberg. He described ophthalmoplegic migraine in 1884[3926] and the syndrome named for him 4 years later.[3927] Möbius is also remembered for his differentiation of exogenous and endogenous disease states, but not for his publications on the weak-mindedness of women.[1829]

Paul Julius Möbius

Möbius sign   The inability to maintain ocular convergence in hyperthyroidism.

Möbius syndrome   1. **ophthalmoplegic migraine.** 2. (congenital facial diplegia, oculofacial paralysis, congenital oculofacial paresis, nuclear agenesis, congenital facial-abducens paralysis, congenital nuclear agenesis/aplasia, congenital facial palsy, congenital bulbar palsy, agenesis of cranial nerve nuclei) Congenital aplasia of the sixth and seventh nerve nuclei, leading to the inability to abduct the eyes from the midline, loss of facial movements with dysarthria and drooling, poor eye closure, and exposure keratopathy. The strabismus may also arise as a result of third or of fourth nerve palsy. Malformations of the skeleton or limbs may occur in association.

Atrophy of the tongue, micrognathia, weakness of the muscles of mastication and of the soft palate, clubfoot, syndactyly or absence of fingers or toes, aplasia of the sternomastoid and pectoral muscles, and congenital dislocation of the hips may also be found in association,[3927] as may developmental delay. Denervation of the spinal musculature due to anterior horn cell lesions and cerebellar and hypothalamic anomalies are also described. The MRI may show medullary hypoplasia and flattening of the floor of the fourth ventricle.[4389]

Möbius first described his syndrome in a 50-year-old man, though the condition is congenital and static in nature. Despite the eponym, the first description was by von **Graefe** in 1880. While the sixth nerve palsy is the main cause of the oculomotor disorder, supranuclear influences are also responsible.[5699]

In a progressive *myopathy resembling* **facioscapulohumeral dystrophy**, congenital facial diplegia may be a presenting sign, giving rise to diagnostic confusion.[2425]

Variant forms[3885] include *Möbius syndrome with hypogonadotrophic hypogonadism;*[4235] a form with *hypogonadism* of hypothalamic/pituitary origin and an acute peripheral neuropathy;[27] a form with *absence of the pectoral muscles* (see **Souques syndrome**); and *Levic syndrome* (**progressive nuclear ophthalmoplegia**).[3367]

3. See **akinesia algera.**

modality   A type of sensation. It was considered by Sinclair (1955) that for every sensation there exists a specific nervous apparatus terminating in a specific type of nerve ending, rather in keeping with Müller's doctrine of the specific irritability of nerves, but today the synthesis of pattern theory and specific irritability has left acceptable only the concept that there is a degree of functional specificity of the receptors.

It is supposed that impulse patterns arising peripherally enable central cells to define the stimulus; the significant characteristics of these patterns depend on such factors as the specificity, adaptation, threshold, and location of the various receptors called into action.[874]

modality-specific anomia   See **anomia.**

modified labials   Those vowels (primarily *O* and *U*) which depend for their utterance upon intact lip function. See also **articulated labials, dentolabials.**

Modified Mini-Mental State Examination

Chart M–16. Modified Mini-Mental State Examination

1. When and where were you born? (5):
   Year 0 1 State 0 1 Town 0 1 Day 0 1 Month 0 1
2. Recall of three words (score no. of presentations) (3):
   Shirt 0 1 Brown 0 1 Honesty 0 1
3. Counting 5 to 1 (write the answers) (2): 5 4 3 2 1 0
   Spell "WORLD" backwards   (5): 5 4 3 2 1 0
4. First delayed recall (9):
   Shirt 3; Cue—something to wear 2; Multiple—shoes, socks, shirt 1; Missed completely 0
   Brown 3; Cue—a color; 2; Multiple—blue, black, brown 1; Missed 0
   Honesty 3; Cue—a good personal quality 2; Multiple—honesty, charity, modesty 1; Missed 0
5. Today's date (15):
   Date: Accurate 3; Missed by 1 or 2 days 2; Missed by 3–5 days 1; Missed by >1 week 0
   Month: Accurate/within 5 days 2; Missed by 1 month 1; Missed by >1 month 0
   Day of week: Accurate 1; Missed 0
   Season: Accurate/within 1 month 1; Missed 0
   Year: Accurate 8; Missed by 1 year 4; Missed by 2–5 years 2; Missed by >5 years 0
6. Spatial orientation (5):
   Hospital/office/home 0 1; City town 0 1;
   Province/state 0 2; Country 0 1
7. Naming (5):
   Forehead 0 1; Shoulder 0 1; Knuckle 0 1; Chin 0 1; Elbow 0 1
8. Four legged animals (write down the animals named in 30 seconds) (10):
9. Similarities (6):

   Arm-leg

   Limbs, extremities 2; Body parts, bend, move, joint 1; Very weak or no similarity 0

   Laughing-crying

   Feeling, emotion 2; Expressions, sounds, relieve tension 1; Very weak or no similarity 0

   Eating-sleeping

   Necessary bodily functions 2; Bodily functions, relaxing, good for you 1; Very weak or no similarity 0
10. Repetition: "I would like to go home." (5):
    Correct 2; 1 or 2 missed words 1; More than 2 missed words 0.
    "No ifs (1 0) ands (1 0) or buts" (1 0)
11. Read and obey "CLOSE YOUR EYES" (3):
    Obeys without prompting 3; Obeys after prompting 2; Reads aloud only 1; None of the above 0
12. Writing "(I) would like to go home." (1 minute) (5):
    0 1 2 3 4 5
13. Copying two pentagons (1 minute) (10):

Each pentagon		Intersections	
5 approximately = sides	4 4	4 corners	2
5 unequal (>2:1) sides	3 3	Not 4-corner	1
Other enclosed figures	2 2	enclosure	
2 or more lines	1 1	No intersection/	0
Less than 2 lines	0 0	no closure	

14. Three-stage command (3): "Take this paper with your "Left/right hand" 1 0 "Fold it in half" 1 0 "Hand it back to me" 1 0
15. Second delayed recall (9): Scored as above #4.

The maximum scores on each subtest are shown in parentheses.
(From Teng EL, Chui HC. The modified mini-mental state (3MS) examination. J Clin Psychiatr 1987;48:314–318. Copyright 1987. Physicians Postgraduate Press. Reprinted by permission.)

modified motor assessment scale A system for measuring the recovery occurring in patients with stroke, in the areas of movement from the supine position to side-lying or to sitting on the side of the bed; balanced sitting; movement from a sitting to a standing position; walking; upper arm function; hand movements; and advanced hand activities.[3455] See also **Barthel Index of Activities of Daily Living.**

modified pure motor hemiparesis with "aphasia" A **lacunar syndrome** with these features, resulting from a thalamic-parathalamic lacune.[1853,1867]

modified radius reflex Flexion of the fingers in response to a tap on the radius, occurring in patients with a pyramidal lesion. If the normal elbow flexion response to brachioradialis stretch is also not seen, the presence of a lesion at C5 in the cord is likely (inversion of the radial reflex).

Moebius See **Möbius.**

Moebius Syndrome Foundation A charitable organization in this field. Address: P.O. Box 147, Pilot Grove, MO 65276. E-mail: vmccarrell@mid-mo.net. Web site: http://www.moebiussyndrome/.

Moerman syndrome A lethal congenital dysmorphic syndrome, characterized by dwarfism; kyphoscoliosis; vertebral and limb anomalies; skeletal, cardiac, pulmonary, and renal anomalies; **Dandy-Walker malformation;** and callosal agenesis.[337]

Moersch-Woltman syndrome A condition of progressive fluctuating muscular rigidity and spasm described in 1956.[3926] See **stiff man syndrome.**

mogigraphia (Gr, with painful effort + to write) An old name for **writers cramp.**

mogilalia The imperfect pronunciation of a single letter such as *G, K, L, R,* or *S.*

Mohr syndrome 1. See **orofaciodigital syndrome II.** 2. Circumscribed left posterior cerebral artery infarction with right hemianopia and deficits in color perception and memory.[3936]

Mohr-Tranebjaerg syndrome An X-linked condition mapped to Xq21.3–Xq22, manifesting deafness and dystonia.[5623]

Mollaret meningitis A recurrent form of aseptic lymphocytic meningitis characterized by marked pleocytosis of the CSF and lasting for a few days. The condition occurs abruptly usually in adults with fever and meningism, who return to normal over a few days but suffer recurrences over years. It was described by Dr. Pierre Mollaret, a French physician, in 1944.[3944] Herpes simplex type 2 has been incriminated as the causal organism.

The following diagnostic criteria have been suggested:

1. Recurrent attacks of fever occur with clinical evidence of meningeal irritation.
2. The attacks last several days, are accompanied by myalgias, and are separated by symptom-free intervals lasting weeks or months.
3. During the attacks, there is CSF pleocytosis, including the presence of numerous polymorphonuclear cells and large mononuclear endothelial cells (Mollaret cells) with irregular nuclear and cytoplasmic membranes; these disappear after 24 hours, leaving a CSF picture of lymphocytic meningitis.
4. The disease remits spontaneously.
5. No causative microorganisms have been found (this may now be incorrect, as herpes simplex virus type 1 has been isolated in some cases).[824]

molluscum fibrosum   The subcutaneous papular, nonplexiform neurofibromas in **neurofibromatosis.**

molybd-   Latin prefix signifying the metal lead. Thus the terms Molybd-amaurosis, -amblyopia, -epilepsia, -ocolic, -oparesis, -spasmus, etc. to refer to various symptoms complicating lead poisoning. The name was perhaps bestowed before the discovery of molybdenum, an essential trace element in the human.

molybdenum cofactor deficiency   (OMIM 252150) A rare, recessively inherited, progressive neurodegenerative disorder caused by a deficiency in sulfite oxidase, which induces severe neuronal loss, astrogliosis, and spongiform encephalopathy.[4888]

Mona Lisa syndrome   Contracture of the facial muscles after **Bell palsy,** leaving an enigmatic (half-) smile on the patient's face.[46]

Monakow, Konstantin von   (1853–1930) Russian-German neurologist whose noble family emigrated from Russia for political reasons. He trained in Zurich, where he was later appointed professor. He is remembered best for his definition of **diaschisis,** but also showed the connections between the lateral geniculate nuclei and the occipital cortex and isolated two anatomical parts: **Monakow's bundle,** the rubrospinal tract (1909), and **Monakow's nucleus,** the external cuneate fasciculus.

Something of an eccentric, he left instructions in his will that his spinal cord be examined to determine the cause of his chronic **thenar hypoplasia,** but this was not done.[1829]

Monakow syndromes   1. Hemiplegia, hemianesthesia, and hemianopia due to occlusion of the contralateral anterior choroidal artery; Monakow showed that the artery supplies part of the lateral geniculate body and gave some clinical details.[3947] Further descriptions

Konstantin von Monakow

of the anatomy and clinical significance of the artery have been published.[19]

2. Dysmorphic microcephaly, the very large nose and ears being the main facial characteristics. The brain weighed 25 g in the original case, the cerebral and cerebellar hemispheres being almost absent and the pons, thalamus, and hypothalamus also being small.[3948]

Monbrun-Benisty syndrome   Severe unilateral orbital and cranial pain radiating to the occiput and accompanied by facial vasodilatation, sweating, and hyperesthesia and by lacrimation, without the pathology of sympathetic ophthalmia.

The condition follows ocular injury or removal, and the eye pain is considered to be a form of **causalgia.**[3949]

Mondini defect   A developmental disorder characterized by deafness, due to aplasia of the bony and membranous labyrinths of the inner ear. It was first described by Dr. C. Mondini, an Italian anatomist, in 1791 but more fully in 1792.[4324]

Mondonesi reflex   See **bulbomimic reflex.**

Monge disease   See **mountain sickness, high-altitude headache.**

mongolism   See **Down syndrome.**

Moniz, Antonio Caetano de Egas   (1874–1955) Portuguese neurosurgeon and diplomat, professor of neurosurgery at Lisbon, who introduced prefrontal leucotomy in 1936[1612] and arteriography in 1927, using 25% sodium iodide.[1611] He won the Nobel prize in 1949, oddly enough for the less useful of the two procedures.

Moniz reflex   A variant method of eliciting the Babinski response, the stimulus being passive ankle plantar flexion.

monoamine oxidase inhibitors Drugs that inhibit the enzymes responsible for breaking down serotonin, monoamines, and norepinephrine in the body. See also **serotonin syndrome.**

monochromatopsia The tinting of all perceptions with a specific color—yellow in digitalis poisoning, for example; perhaps rose in euphoria.

monoclonal gammopathy of uncertain significance (MGUS) A generally benign monoclonal gammopathy (IgG, IgA, IgD, IgM) frequently associated with sensory or motor neuropathy.[2128,2996] The IgG-MGUS and IgM-MGUS conditions differ, in that an insidious course, raised CSF protein level, more sensory loss, slower nerve conduction velocities, and anti-myelin-associated glycoprotein (anti-MAG) antibodies are found in the latter, which is also the more common of the two. In the IgG form, weakness is the predominant feature.

In the motor form, the weakness is predominantly distal, asymmetric, and slowly progressive. Conduction block is not present.[4418]

The following criteria for the diagnosis of MGUS (as opposed to multiple myeloma) have been suggested:[3210]

A. Monoclonal serum protein, <2 g/L
B. Normal serum albumin levels
C. Marrow plasma cells, <5%
D. Absence of bone lesions, anemia, and monoclonal urine protein
E. Observation shows no change over 3 years.

Chart M–17. Criteria for the Diagnosis of Demyelinating Polyneuropathy Associated with MGUS[4170]

A causal relation between demyelinating polyneuropathy and MGUS should be considered in a patient with

1. Demyelinating polyneuropathy according to the electro-diagnostic criteria for idiopathic chronic inflammatory demyelinating polyradioneuropathy
2. Presence of an M protein (IgM, IgG, or IgA), without evidence of malignant plasma cell dyscrasias such as multiple myeloma, lymphoma, Waldenstrom macroglobulinemia, or amyloidosis
3. Family history negative for neuropathy
4. Age >30 years

The relation is *definite* when the following is present:

1. IgM M protein with anti-MAG antibodies

The relation is *probable* when at least three of the following are present in a patient without anti-MAG antibodies:

1. Time to peak of the neuropathy >2 years
2. Chronic slowly progressive course without relapsing or remitting periods
3. Symmetrical distal polyneuropathy
4. Sensory symptoms and signs predominate over motor features.

A causal relation is *unlikely* when at least three of the following are present in a patient without anti-MAG antibodies:

1. Median time to peak of the neuropathy is within 1 year.
2. Clinical course is relapsing and remitting or monophasic.
3. Cranial nerves are involved.

4. Neuropathy is asymmetrical.
5. Motor symptoms and signs predominate.
6. History of preceding infection.
7. Presence of abnormal median sensory nerve action potential (SNAP) in combination with normal sural SNAP

After Notermans NC, Franssen H, Eurelings M, et al. Diagnostic criteria for demyelinating polyneuropathy associated with monoclonal gammopathy. Muscle Nerve 2000;23:73–9. © 2000. Reprinted by permission of John Wiley and Sons, Inc.

See also **multiple myeloma, POEMS syndrome.**

monocular (from Lat, relating to one eye)

monocular diplopia(uniocular diplopia) See **diplopia.**

monocular elevation failure A deficit in up-gaze in one eye, despite the supranuclear level of the causative lesion.[3361]

monocular "fixation" nystagmus See **latent nystagmus.**

monocular nystagmus An unusual dissociated motor ocular sign in which involuntary oscillations of only one eye in any direction(s) are present in the primary position of gaze. In the presence of visual loss, the nystagmus is pendular in the affected eye.

It has been reported in numerous neurological conditions and is not a localizing sign.[2791]

monomania A form of mental illness in which the subject is irrational on one subject only, appearing quite normal in other areas of mental activity.

monomelic amyotrophy (benign focal amyotrophy; benign focal atrophy; benign juvenile focal muscular atrophy of upper extremities; benign monomelic amyotrophy; distal amyotrophy of predominantly the upper limbs; focal cervical poliopathy of distal upper extremity causing juvenile muscular atrophy; juvenile amyotrophy of distal upper extremity; juvenile distal spinal muscular atrophy of upper extremities; juvenile muscular atrophy of the upper extremity; juvenile nonprogressive muscular atrophy localized in hand and forearm; juvenile segmental muscular atrophy; juvenile type of distal and segmental atrophy of upper extremities; monomelic atrophy; monomelic spinal muscular atrophy; nonfamilial juvenile central neurogenic muscular atrophy; nonfamilial juvenile distal spinal muscular atrophy of upper extremity; nonfamilial spinal segmental muscular atrophy in juvenile and young subjects; spinal monomelic amyotrophy; unilateral juvenile muscular atrophy of upper limbs) A rare sporadic form of **amyotrophic lateral sclerosis** presenting as asymmetric, painless atrophy and weakness of the distal upper limbs of young adults, seldom accompanied by pyramidal signs.[1493] The occurrence of this condition and monomelic atrophy mainly in Oriental males suggests that they may be identical.

monomelic atrophy (benign focal amyotrophy, monomelic spinal muscular atrophy) A sporadic syndrome of progressive wasting of a limb, usually the arm, with evidence of spinal cord atrophy at the appropriate levels and with clinical and electrical evidence of chronic anterior horn cell disease. Most often reported from the Orient, the condition usually affects young men and is benign and, after a year or two, nonprogressive.[2233] See also **monomelic amyotrophy.**

monomelic myopathy   A rare congenital syndrome characterized by hypertrophy of muscle and bone, confined to a single extremity.[947] Percussion myotonia may also be detectable.

monomelic myositis   A form of **polymyositis** in which the weakness and atrophy are confined to a single limb.

monomelic spinal muscular atrophy   See **monomelic amyotrophy.**

monomyositis   Eosinophilic infiltration and painful inflammation of one muscle or a part of one muscle.

mononeuritis multiplex   See **multiple mononeuropathy.**

monophasia   An extreme degree of loss of expressive language due to localized brain disease, whereby the patient is unable to emit anything more than extremely few stereotyped utterances, either verbal or nonverbal, despite insight into the occurrence of the problem.[1178] See **stereotypy.**

monophasic wave   An EEG waveform developed on one side of the baseline only.

monoplegia   (Gr, one + a stroke) 1. Paralysis of one muscle or of a group of muscles only. 2. Paralysis of a single limb. The latter is the preferred usage today.

Brachial (arm), crural (leg) and faciolingual forms are seen and are "more common in disease of the cortex" (Sir William **Gowers**).[2240] Crural monoplegia also occurs with thoracic or lumbar cord disease, but any peripheral lesion can cause monoplegia.

monoplegia anesthetica   See **Morvan disease.**

monoplegia masticatoria   Unilateral weakness of the muscles supplied by the trigeminal nerve, usually without accompanying sensory changes.[5282]

monopolar needle recording electrode   A solid wire, usually stainless steel, and usually coated, except at its tip, with an insulating material. Variations in the voltage between the tip of the needle (active or exploring electrode) positioned in a muscle and a conductive plate on the skin surface or a bare needle in subcutaneous tissue (reference electrode) are measured.

By convention, this recording condition is referred to as a *monopolar needle electrode recording*. It should be emphasized, however, that potential differences are always recorded between two electrodes. (Adapted from the 1987 Report of the Nomenclature Committee of the American Association of Electromyography and Electrodiagnosis. AAEE glossary of terms in clinical electromyography. *Muscle Nerve* 1987;**10S:**G5–G23.

Copyright 1987 by John Wiley and Sons, Inc. Reprinted by permission of John Wiley and Sons, Inc.)

monopolar recording   An inaccurate term, but commonly used to describe (*1*) the use of an intramuscular needle exploring electrode in combination with a surface disk or subcutaneous needle reference electrode, and (*2*) a similar combination of needle electrodes used to record nerve activity.[146]

monotherapy   The philosophy that one medication is better than two for treating a single complaint. Though not always achievable, this is accepted as desirable in the management of epilepsy, but not necessarily in that of other conditions.

Monrad-Krohn, Georg Herman   (1884–1964) Norwegian neurologist from Bergen who trained in Oslo and thereafter at the National Hospital and the Salpêtrière before returning to Oslo as physician at the Oslo Neurological Clinic and then professor of neurology. His book *Clinical Examination of the Nervous System* (London, 1921) quickly became the classic in many translations, by which he is better remembered even than his clinical research publications on leprosy, facial palsies, and aphasia.

Monrad-Krohn sign   Paradoxical emotional hypermimia occurring in bilateral upper motor neuron facial weakness, regarded as a release from some normal suppression—phenomenon of liberation—by Monrad-Krohn in 1924.

Monro, Alexander   (*primum*; 1697–1767) Professor of anatomy at Edinburgh University. He first noted that the nerves of the body were "composed of small parallel threads."

Monro, Alexander   (*secundum*; 1733–1817) Scottish anatomist, holding the chair of the department of anatomy at Edinburgh University in succession to his father of the same name. He first described the interventricular foramen in 1753; his son (also Alexander, and thus known as *tertius*, and also professor of anatomy at Edinburgh) wrote in his *Elements of the Anatomy of the Human Body*, "Hence at this place the lateral ventricles of the brain communicate with each other, and with the third ventricle. This aperture has been very particularly described by my Father in his work in the Nervous System" (Vol. 2, p. 363).

Of this Monro, the third of the line (1773–1859), it is said[5204] that he contributed little that was new himself, but relied extensively upon the notes of his grandfather, even including such statements as "When I was a student at Leyden in 1719."

Monro-Kellie hypothesis   Since the brain is incompressible and the cranial cavity inelastic, compensation for an increase in the volume of any of one of the intracranial contents must be attained through diminution in the volume of the others.

This insight was first expressed in 1783 but was repeated by Kellie in 1824.

monstrocellular sarcoma   (giant cell fibrosarcoma) See **glioma.**

montage   The particular arrangement or pattern of placement of electrodes on the scalp, allowing the simultaneous display of potential changes at numerous sites on the EEG record.

Monte Cristo syndrome   See **locked-in syndrome.**

Montgomery-Asberg Depression Rating Scale   A 10-item rating scale assessing the features of depression, shown to have high validity and an ability to demonstrate changes in depressive symptomatology.[3957]

Mood Assessment scale   See **geriatric depression scale.**

Mood Scales—Elderly   A set of 50 adjectives referring to five factors (tense-irritable, considerate, cognitive disturbance, inept helpless, depressed) to be rated by the caregivers of elderly subjects.[4601]

Moon molars   Mulberry-like molar teeth seen in patients with congenital syphilis, described by H. Moon (1845–1892), a dental surgeon at Guy's Hospital in London.

Moore lightning streaks   Flashes of light (phosphenes) perceived by normal patients with eye closure when brief pressure is exerted on the globe, and occasionally perceived by those with intraocular pathology. They are named for R.F. **Moore.** See **lightning streaks.**

Moore, M. T.   (b. 1901) American neuropsychiatrist, professor at the University of Pennsylvania.

Moore, Robert Foster   (b. 1878) London ophthalmologist who described the **pseudo–Argyll Robertson pupil** in 1924.[3963]

Moore syndrome   Abdominal pain as a manifestation of a seizure. The recurrent attacks of abdominal pain occur in children and young adults and are associated with abnormal EEG changes and occasionally are followed by generalized tonic-clonic convulsions.[3961] They are named for M.T. **Moore.** See **abdominal epilepsy.**

morbid   (Lat, sickly) Of or belonging to disease; unhealthy.

morbid hunger   (bulimia) Excessive appetite with decreased satiety after eating.

morbidity   Predisposition to disease.

morbific   Causing disease.

morbus   (Lat, disease) A sickness. Hence a large number of alternative names for certain diseases such as *morbus celsi* for catalepsy; *M. aphrodisius, gallicus, hispanicus,* and *indicus* for syphilis; *M. astralis, attonitus, caducus, comitialis, convivialis, daemonicus, deificus, divinus, foedus, herculeus, infantilis, insputatus, interlunis, lunaticus, magnus, major, mensalis, popularis, puerilis, sacer, sancti johannes* or *valentini, sclestus, seleniacus, viridellus,* and *vitriolatus* for epilepsy; *M. cerebralis whytii* for meningitis; and *M. gesticulatorius, lascicus,* and *saltatorius* for chorea.

Such names allow a measure of understanding of ancient views of the disease in question. In the case of epilepsy, one may understand from the above that it is a frightful disease, has major and minor forms, occurs in children and in company, leads to stunning of the mind, to falling to the ground with strong movements, is influenced by God, the gods, or devils and, by that lesser light, the moon (at least when it recurs regularly on a monthly cycle); breaks up a meeting by its occurrence, and leads others to spit upon the sufferer.

morbus gallicorum   (Lat, the French disease) Syphilis. This term was used by those other than the French, who regarded it as an English disease.

morbus medicorum   The disease of patients who "seek advice from many physicians, trusting those who pander to their apprehensions. . . .[2240] For the best chance of recovery, [they] should keep away from doctors" (Gowers). The dangers of the condition include susceptibility to **Ulysses syndrome.**

morbus sacer   (Lat, disease + holy) The term of Linnaeus for a disorder involving continuous distortion of the limbs without affection of the mind. It is probably the same as the mobile spasms described by **Hammond,** and thus **athetosis.**

Morel, Benedict Augustin   (1809–1873) Austrian-French psychiatrist who trained at the **Salpêtrière** and practiced in northeastern France. He introduced the terms *dementia praecox* (which was later popularized by Kraepelin), and *obsession,* and published widely on psychiatric disorders and their history and on forensic psychiatry.[5653]

Morel disease   (alcoholic laminar cortical sclerosis) Symmetrical neuroglial proliferation in the third cortical layer occurring in alcoholics, mainly in the frontal regions, and combined with generalized astrocytic hyperplasia. Clinically, the syndrome comprises dementia, dysarthria, weakness, gait disturbance, and tremor.[3971]

Morel, Ferdinand   (1868–1957) Swiss psychiatrist, born in Geneva, who trained in medicine in Paris after early studies in philosophy. He trained under **Charcot** and returned to graduate in Geneva, where he remained for most of the rest of his life, becoming professor of psychiatry and director of Bel Air Psychiatric Hospital in 1938.

Morel-Stewart-Morgagni syndrome   (metabolic craniopathy) Frontal hyperostosis, obesity, hirsutism, hypertension, amenorrhea, diabetes mellitus and insipidus, headache, vertigo, lethargy, somnolence, seizures, and psychiatric manifestations, occurring in adult women.[3970]

The condition was originally considered to be due to a diencephalic lesion, but its identity is now in question, the association of any endocrinopathy with the skull changes being at best suspect. See **hyperostosis frontalis interna.**

Morel-Wildi syndrome   Asymptomatic disseminated nodular dysgenesis of the frontal cortex, manifest as small, pearl-like prominences.[3972]

Moreno syndrome   A congenital dysmorphic syndrome characterized also by gigantism, high birth weight, tall stature, advanced skeletal maturation, epiphyseal dysplasia, micrognathia, scoliosis, brachydactyly, joint contractures, macrocephaly, early closure of the fontanelles, ridged cranial sutures, ossification defects of the skull, umbilical hernia, spasticity, wide metaphysis, and cutis laxa.[337]

Morgagni, Giovanni Battista   (1682–1771) Italian physician and pathological anatomist, and professor at Padua. His book *De Sedibus et Causis Morborum Peranatomen Indagatis Libri Quinique* was published in 1769.[3975] He was the first to give an account of **subarachnoid hemorrhage** and to note that hydrocephalus in children (but not in adults) caused enlargement of the head.

Morgagni syndrome   See **hyperostosis frontalis interna.**

moria   (Gr, silliness) Naïve, childish excitement, a behavioral pattern sometimes seen with prefrontal lobe lesions.

Morgagni-Stewart-Morel syndrome   See **hyperostosis frontalis interna.**

Morin's pathway   An ascending pathway in the dorsomedial portion of the lateral funiculus of the cat, relaying in the dorsal horn and lateral cervical nucleus before crossing to join the medial lemniscus. Ascending fibers probably take a similar route in humans and may have a role in the perception of vibratory stimuli.[874]

morning glory syndrome   A dysmorphism of the optic disk, characterized by a deep, funnel-shaped pit surrounded by heaped-up glial tissue, the retinal vessels radiating out in all directions. The anomaly is associated with enlargement of the blind spot, but other visual disturbances may not be present.[3046] The name springs from a fanciful resemblance to the shape of the flower.

morning paralysis   See **poliomyelitis.**

morning sleepiness   See **delayed sleep phase syndrome.**

morning/evening comparison test   A simple test for the diagnosis of **myasthenia gravis** which involves measuring the difference in the width of the palpebral fissures between morning and night.[4977]

Moro, E.   (1874–1951) Austrian pediatrician who described the reflex named for him in 1918.

Moro reflex   (embrace reflex, body startle reflex) Abduction and extension of the arms and opening of the hands followed by adduction of the arms, in response to sudden withdrawal of support from the head of the normal baby (aged less than 3–4 months) held up at 45°, the head being allowed to fall back for an inch or two. This is also elicited by any sudden stimulus, such as a loud noise, sudden displacement of the body of the infant, or a blow to the bed on which the infant lies.[6064] The reflex can be elicited after 30 weeks of gestation and is lost by 5 months of age.

The reflex is inhibited in hypertonic states and is asymmetrical in hemiplegia and with local disease of the arms.[4341] See also **developmental reflexes.**

moron   (from Gr, sluggish) A term selected by **Binet** for that class of the intellectually deprived with a mental age of 0–2 years.

morphea   (localized scleroderma) A slowly progressive atrophic inflammatory process, pathologically resembling **eosinophilic fasciitis** but without the eosinophils and involving a localized area of skin and subjacent tissues. Such focal scleroderma may rarely affect the brain, resulting in focal deficits and perhaps partial seizures.

In some cases, it leads to facial, limb, or generalized hemiatrophy.[5028]

morpheme   The smallest meaningful unit of language, which occurs either as a word or part of a word.

Thus, *troubleshooting* contains three morphemes: *trouble-*, *shoot-*, and *-ing*. The acceptable use of words depends on the morphemes they contain. Morphemes may be appended to words—for example, verb endings, *-ed*, *-ing*; noun modifiers, *-es*, *-s*; adverb endings, *-ly*; and adjective modifiers, *-er*, *-est*.[3505]

morphology   The morphemes contained in a language and the system of rules followed by speakers when combining morphemes into phrases.[3505]

morphosynthesis   The physiological process underlying the perception of both visual and tactile form, making possible accurate localization in space.

Morquio disease   See **mucopolysaccharidosis type 4.**

Morquio, Luis   (1867–1935) Uruguayan professor of pediatrics at Montevideo, who also trained in Paris in neurology with **Charcot.**

Morquio-Brailsford syndrome   See **mucopolysaccharidosis type 4.**

Morton metatarsalgia   (interdigital neuralgia) A syndrome of constant aching pain with lancinations felt in the sole of the foot and due to compression of a digital neuroma by the heads of the second to third or the third to fourth metatarsals.

The syndrome usually occurs in older women, mainly while standing or walking, and can be relieved surgically.[4002]

Morton, Thomas   (1835–1903) American surgeon who trained at the University of Pennsylvania and, after further training there, became a member of its staff as well as of other hospitals in the region, some of which he had helped to found. He was the first to ligate the common carotid artery (for the treatment of orbital aneurysm) in 1864.

Morvan, Augustin-Marie (1819–1897) French physician in Brittany, whose writings were praised by **Charcot.** He is remembered for the two conditions named for him, but produced nothing else in medicine, although as a fervid republican his life was greatly occupied in the management of current political and social problems.

Morvan chorea (fibrillary chorea, chorea fibrillaris) A disorder of very uncertain provenance, first described by Morvan in 1890 as the combination of fibrillary chorea of the calf and other leg muscles (myokymia or neuromyotonia) with shooting pains, hyperhidrosis, albuminuria, and encephalopathy with delirium, terminating fatally in one patient with severe insomnia that later led to delirium and coma.[4004] Cramps, weakness, and pruritis have also been recorded as part of the syndrome. Most patients have an underlying thymoma.

S.A.K. **Wilson** was confident that it was "neither chorea nor myoclonus" and regarded it as "a meaningless term except as synonymous for flickering contractures of muscles." The condition went unremarked for 40 years after Morvan's publication until Mollaret described another case in 1930. Where it stands now is uncertain, but it may represent generalized myokymia as a toxic effect of gold therapy; or simply benign calf fasciculations. See also **myokymia.**

In *variant* forms, the condition exists in association with a rare brain disease (**agrypnia**) which is characterized by total abolition of the ability to sleep,[1830,1831] or is associated with a myasthenia-like syndrome as a paraneoplastic manifestation of thymoma.[3315]

Morvan disease (monoplegia anesthetica) Dissociated analgesia with severe trophic changes and paralysis of the limbs (usually the arms). The sense of touch may be retained but pain and temperature sensations are much affected and may be entirely lost.

Regarded as synonymous with **syringomyelia** during the first half of this century, this disease could equally well have been a form of **hereditary sensory and autonomic neuropathy,** perhaps type 2, as the losses of pain and of common sensation distally (mutilating acropathy) occur in both conditions.[4004]

Moschowitz disease (thrombotic thrombocytopenic purpura, thrombotic microangiopathy). A rare, acute, and often lethal systemic autoimmune vasculopathy with widespread effects, such as fever, purpura, thrombocytopenia, and hemolytic anemia. In the nervous system, the main features are delirium, various focal neurological signs, and seizures.[4007]

MOSES See **Multidimensional Observation Scale for Elderly Subjects.**

Moskowskij sign Right-sided mydriasis in patients with acute appendicitis or other abdominal sepsis. Why this should occur (if it is indeed confirmed) is not known.

Mosso, Angelo (1846–1910) Italian physiologist.

Mosso's ergometer An early device for measuring muscle force in fatigable and other states. Mosso also remarked in 1884 on a patient whose symptoms suggest **paroxysmal choreoathetosis.**

moth-eaten fibers The biopsy appearance of myofibrils (especially those of type 1) in which the normally regular myofibrillary network seen in the oxidative enzyme preparation is disturbed, giving rise to a whorled appearance and lack of reactivity to NADH as a result of a loss of mitochondria. The change is not specific but is most common in inflammatory myopathies. The significance of this finding is that of **cores,** of which it may represent a stage in development.[5442]

motility (from Lat, movement) The power of movement or of contractility.

motion sickness Nausea and vomiting induced by unfamiliar bodily accelerations or intersensory mismatch during passive locomotion in vehicles, and reduced or inhibited by visual perception of a static environment.[727]

motivation A force based on personality, reflexes, and the totality of individual experience, inclining one towards a course of action.

motor (Lat, a mover) giving, imparting or producing movement.

motor agrammatism The term of Goldstein for the speech in motor aphasia, with suppression of the "little tools of language" such as articles, pronouns, and connectors, such that speech is ultimately reduced to nouns, infinitives, and names.

motor and sensory demyelinating mononeuropathy multiplex See **multifocal inflammatory demyelinating neuropathy.**

motor and sensory neuropathy, dementia, and dysautonomia A rare autosomal recessive syndrome with adult onset, also marked by pigmentary retinal degeneration, described in a single family.[4286]

motor aphasia See **aphasia.**

motor apraxia See **apraxia.**

motor aprosodia A condition characterized by the loss of melody in vocal output with an associated decrease in the use of gesture. The monotonous verbal output lacks emotional quality. The underlying lesion is of the right inferior motor cortex. See **aprosodia.**

motor area See **motor cortex.**

motor asynergy (Lat, motor + Gr, not affording assistance) Ataxia.

motor block See **freezing.**

motor centers Those areas of the cortex which, when stimulated, produce coordinated movement of a limb.

motor cortex (motor area, precentral area, Brodman's area 4, area gigantopyramidalis) An arbitrary term for that part of the precentral convolution lying adjacent to the fissure of Rolando, in which the giant cells of Betz are found. The anterior border is ill defined, and its functions and those of the **premotor cortex** overlap or may even be the same except that damage to this area leads to contralateral hemiparesis and later to hyperreflexia and hypertonia.

motor cortex seizures Epilepsies mainly characterized by simple partial seizures, their localization depending on the side and topography of the area involved. In the case of seizures involving the lower prerolandic area, there may be speech arrest, vocalization or dysphasia, tonic-clonic movements of the face on the contralateral side, or swallowing. Generalization of the seizure frequently occurs.

In the rolandic area, partial motor seizures without march or Jacksonian seizures occur, particularly beginning in the contralateral upper extremities. In the case of seizures involving the paracentral lobule, tonic movements of the ipsilateral foot may occur as well as the expected contralateral leg movements. Postictal or **Todd paralysis** is frequent. (From the Commission for Classification and Terminology, ILAE. Proposal for revised classifications of epilepsies and epileptic syndromes. *Epilepsia* 1989;**30:**389–399.[1114] Reprinted by kind permission of Blackwell Science.)

motor end plate A specialized area on the surface of the myofibril where it is unusually responsive to depolarization by packets of acetylcholine arriving from the motor nerve terminal.

motor end point (motor point) The site where a motor nerve enters a muscle, which is also the point over a muscle where its contraction may be elicited by a minimal-intensity, short-duration electric stimulus. These sites were first noted and defined by **Remak** and have recently regained prominence because they are the regions where injections of botulinum toxin are most effectively placed to alleviate unwanted muscle contractions.

motor evoked potentials The electrical events accompanying muscle contraction recorded by electrodes placed over or within the muscle in question and best assessed following magnetic stimulation of the motor cortex.

The magnetic stimulation technique may one day be found useful in monitoring spinal cord function in the awake patient, but the potentials are lost during anesthesia.

motor extinction Inhibition of activity in one limb during voluntary movement in the other.[5874]

motor hyperactivity Excessive involuntary muscle contraction as a result of lesions of the central or peripheral nervous systems.

The causes include **spasticity; stiff man syndrome,** which is probably an autoimmune syndrome due to the presence of antibodies to α-glutamic acid dehydrogenase, leading to a decrease in the amount of γ-aminobutyric acid present; **tetanus,** in which the toxin reduces levels of glycine/γ-aminobutyric acid; **segmental myoclonus;** and increased motor neuron excitability, as with **fasciculations, myokymia,** and **neuromyotonia.**

motor impersistence (global inattention) A term introduced by Miller Fisher[1839] to describe an inability to sustain simple acts such as conjugate gaze, tongue protrusion, mouth opening, or the exertion of steady manual grip pressure, all in the absence of a detectable motor deficit. The sign suggests right hemispheric damage.[3023] Compare with **perseveration.**

motor inattention See **inattention.**

motor latency The interval between the onset of a stimulus and the onset of the resultant compound muscle action potential (M wave). The term may be qualified as either *proximal* or *distal,* depending on the relative position of the stimulus.[146]

motor negativism A consistent increase in resistance to the passive stretch of a muscle, occurring bilaterally as a sign of diffuse cerebral dysfunction and unilaterally as a result of a focal lesion of the contralateral hemisphere. See **paratonia.**

motor nerve conduction velocity The speed of conduction of the nerve impulse down a motor nerve (varying normally in different nerves between 45 and 55 m/s), first measured by von **Helmholtz** in 1850.

motor nerve involvement syndrome A congenital storage disorder manifesting osteoporosis, lytic lesions of bone, demyelinating motor neuropathy, and inclusions on nerve or rectal biopsy specimens.[337]

motor neuron A neuron with its cell body in the anterior horn of the spinal cord, its single axon passing out in the anterior root to inervate the myofibrils within that **motor unit.**

motor neuron disease See **amyotrophic lateral sclerosis.**

motor neuronal diseases Disorders primarily affecting the anterior horn cells, the motor roots or the motor nerves of the body, cranial or spinal. The classification in Chart M–18 is closely based on that of the World Federation of Neurology.[6039] See also **radiculopathy** (*disorders of motor nerve roots),* **neuropathy** (*disorders of peripheral nerve),* **neuromuscular transmission disorders,** and **myopathy** (*disorders of muscle).* The term has also been used to include disorders with upper motor neuron involvement.[1487]

Chart M–18. Spinal Muscular Atrophies and Other Disorders of Motor Neurons

A1. Autosomal recessive, biochemical abnormality unknown
1. Spinal muscular atrophy, type 1; **hereditary motor neuropathy, type 1** (Werdnig-Hoffman)

2. Spinal muscular atrophy, type 2; **hereditary motor neuropathy, type 2** (Kugelberg-Welander)

3. Spinal muscular atrophy, type 3; **hereditary motor neuropathy, type 3** (Kugelberg-Welander)

4. Proximal spinal muscular atrophy of adults, indistinguishable from recessive and X-linked forms, **hereditary motor neuropathy, type 4.**

5. Scapuloperoneal muscular atrophy. See **hereditary motor neuropathy.**

6. (Distal) spinal muscular atrophy of childhood. See **hereditary motor and sensory neuropathy, type 2.**

7. **(Distal) spinal muscular atrophy** (of adults). See **hereditary motor neuropathy** (*variants*).

8. Spinal muscular atrophy with microcephaly and mental retardation

9. Spinal muscular atrophy, **Ryukyuan** type

10. Progressive muscular atrophy with chorea and optic atrophy

11. **Arthrogryposis multiplex congenita,** neurogenic type

12. **Arthrogryposis multiplex congenita** with pulmonary hypoplasia

13. Multiple contracture syndrome, Finnish type; see **Pena-Shokier phenotypes.**

14. **Kuskokwim disease** (arthrogryposis-like disorder)

15. Charcot-Marie-Tooth disease, progressive ataxia, and tremor. See **hereditary motor and sensory neuropathy, type 2.**

16. Charcot-Marie-Tooth disease (same as 15?)

17. Progressive bulbar palsy of childhood. See **Fazio-Londe disease.**

18. Progressive bulbar palsy with deafness. See **progressive bulbar palsy** (*Vialetto–van Laere syndrome*).

19. Bulbar palsy, with deafness and retinitis pigmentosa

20. Bulbar palsy with olivopontocerebellar atrophy. See **cerebellar ataxias** (unknown etiology, late onset).

21. Spinal muscular atrophy with amyotrophic lateral sclerosis, spinocerebellar ataxia, and deafness. See **amyotrophic lateral sclerosis.**

22. Spinal muscular atrophy with optic atrophy and deafness

23. Spinal muscular atrophy with deafness

24. Spinal muscular atrophy with ophthalmoplegia

25. Spinal muscular atrophy with retinitis pigmentosa

26. Spinal muscular atrophy with retinitis pigmentosa and **hereditary spastic paraplegia**

27. Troyer syndrome. See **hereditary spastic paraplegia.**

28. Spinal muscular atrophy and mental retardation. See **hereditary motor neuropathy** (*variants*).

29. Spinal muscular atrophy, mental retardation, seizures, and orofacial dysplasia

30. Spinal muscular atrophy, restricted forms (e.g., one or both hands or quadriceps)

31. Spinal muscular atrophy with recessive spinocerebellar degeneration or **Friedreich ataxia**

32. Spinal muscular atrophy with spastic paraplegia, mental retardation, and ichthyosis. See **Sjögren-Larsson syndrome.**

33. **Neuronal intranuclear hyaline inclusion disease** (single sporadic case, manifest by amyotrophy, dementia, choreoathetosis, seizures, and sphincter disorder)

34. Spinal muscular atrophy or axonal neuropathy in **xeroderma pigmentosum** (spinal cord may be found abnormal at utopsy)

35. Spinal muscular atrophy in **infantile neuroaxonal dystrophy**

36. Spinal muscular atrophy in **Hallervorden-Spatz disease**

37. Spinal muscular atrophy in amyotrophic **choreoacanthocytosis**

A2. *Autosomal recessive, biochemical abnormality known*

1. Spinal muscular atrophy with hexosaminidase deficiency. See **GM₂ gangliosidosis.**

2. Spinal muscular atrophy with lysosomal enzyme deficiencies

3. Spinal muscular atrophy with **phenylketonuria**

4. Spinal muscular atrophy with **hydroxyisovaleric aciduria**

A3. *Autosomal dominant, biochemical abnormality unknown*

1. Spinal muscular atrophy, ataxia, retinitis pigmentosa, and diabetes mellitus

2. Spinal muscular atrophy, juvenile, proximal type (usually autosomal recessive, but dominant forms are reported) (Tsukagoshi). *Variants* include the **monomelic** form, which is usually sporadic and spinal muscular atrophy of **facioscapulohumeral distribution.**

3. **Progressive muscular atrophy with malignant course,** a form which is fatal within 1 year, but which is not clearly different from autosomal dominant **amyotrophic lateral sclerosis.**

4. Progressive muscular atrophy with amyotrophic lateral sclerosis. See **amyotrophic lateral sclerosis.** This entity is not clearly different from peroneal muscular atrophy with pyramidal features.

5. **Amyotrophic dystonic paraplegia**

6. **Madras** type

7. **Amyotrophic lateral sclerosis–parkinsonism–dementia complex of Guam**

8. Spinal muscular atrophy with olivopontocerebellar atrophy. See **cerebellar ataxias** (unknown etiology, late onset).

9. Amyotrophic lateral sclerosis with dementia. See **amyotrophic lateral sclerosis.**

10. Distal spinal muscular atrophy with vocal cord paralysis

11. Spinal muscular atrophy with bulbar palsy. See **amyotrophic lateral sclerosis.**

12. **Arthrogryposis multiplex congenita,** distal, type 1 (neurogenic or myopathic)

13. Charcot-Marie-Tooth disease, neuronal type. See **hereditary motor and sensory neuropathy, type 2.**

14. Scapuloperoneal atrophy with cardiopathy. See **Emery-Dreifuss syndrome.**

15. Scapuloperoneal amyotrophy. See **Kaeser syndrome.**

16. Spastic paraplegia with amyotrophy of hands. See **amyotrophic lateral sclerosis.**

17. **Distal spinal muscular atrophy** confined to the hands (see **hereditary motor neuropathy,** *hereditary motor neuropathy affecting the arms*)

18. Spinal muscular atrophy, facioscapulohumeral type (see **hereditary motor neuropathy**)

19. Proximal spinal muscular atrophy, adult type (Finkel late-onset type). See **hereditary motor neuropathy, type 5.**

20. Spinocerebellar ataxia with parkinsonian rigidity and peripheral neuropathy and fasciculations

21. Spinal muscular atrophy with myoclonus. See **hereditary motor neuropathy.**

22. Spinal muscular atrophy with **Joseph disease**
23. Scapuloperoneal atrophy with cardiopathy and inflammatory myopathy. See **hereditary motor neuropathy.**
24. Amyotrophic lateral sclerosis with **Pick disease**
25. Amyotrophic lateral sclerosis with autosomal dominant familial **parkinsonism.** See **amyotrophic lateral sclerosis.**
26. Spinal muscular atrophy with **Huntington disease**
27. Amyotrophic lateral sclerosis with **pallidonigroluysian atrophy**
28. Spinal muscular atrophy with **pallidonigral degeneration**
29. **Motor neuronopathy predominantly affecting the hands**

A4. *X-linked recessive, biochemical abnormality unknown*
1. Spinal and bulbar muscular atrophy (**Kennedy disease**)
2. X-linked proximal juvenile spinal muscular atrophy. See **Kennedy syndrome.**
3. X-linked scapuloperoneal muscular atrophy with cardiomyopathy. See **Emery-Dreifuss syndrome.**
4. Charcot-Marie-Tooth peroneal muscular atrophy and **Friedreich ataxia.** See **hereditary motor and sensory neuropathy, type 2.**
5. X-linked spinal muscular atrophy with facioscapulohumeral distribution. See **hereditary motor neuropathy.**
6. **Arthrogryposis multiplex congenita** with renal and hepatic abnormality
7. **Arthrogryposis multiplex congenita,** distal, X-linked

A5. *X-linked dominant, lethal in males*
1. Infantile spinal muscular atrophy in **incontinentia pigmenti**

B. *Congenital and developmental abnormalities*
1. **Möbius syndrome**
2. Congenital absence of muscles. See **David anomaly.**
3. Amyotrophy with developmental anomalies of the spinal cord or nerve roots: **hydromyelia, syringomyelia,** or **syringobulbia** (often with **Chiari malformation**); **spinal dysraphism; meningomyelocele;** aplasia of spinal cord (amyelia)
4. Spinal muscular atrophy with **pontocerebellar hypoplasia**[2234]
5. **Arthrogryposis multiplex congenita** of non-neural, nonmyopathic origin

C. *Motor neuron disorders attributed to physical causes*
1. Trauma: direct injury of spinal cord (birth injury, spinal fracture); traumatic **hematomyelia**
2. Amyotrophy due to destruction, compression, or compressive ischemia of anterior horn cells
3. **Progressive vascular myelopathy** (amyotrophy due to ischemia of anterior horns)[2830]
4. Amyotrophy after electrical injury[1748]
5. Amyotrophy after radiotherapy[3226]

D. *Motor neuron disorders attributed to toxins, chemicals, or heavy metals*
The following agents have been incriminated: tetanus toxin, strychnine, **botulinum toxin** (adult and infantile forms),[1054] lead,[881] **mercury,** organic phosphates (triorthocresyl phosphate, **jake paralysis**), saxitoxin and related marine toxins, dapsone,[2634] and phenytoin.[1466]

E. *Motor neuron disorders attributed to viral infection*
E1. *Acute disorders*
1. Paralytic acute anterior **poliomyelitis,** due to poliomyelitis or to other enteroviruses

2. Amyotrophy in **Russian spring-summer encephalitis**
3. **Herpes zoster**[5538]
4. Amyotrophy with acute hemorrhagic conjunctivitis[3126]
5. Amyotrophy with asthma.[421] See **Hopkins syndrome.**
6. Amyotrophy in acute transverse myelitis, cause undetermined

E2. *Subacute or chronic disorders*
1. Amyotrophy in **Creutzfeldt-Jakob** disease[110]
2. Amyotrophy due to human immunodeficiency virus.[2599] See **HIV infection.**
3. Persistent infection by poliovirus in agammaglobulinemia
4. Late **post-poliomyelitis muscular atrophy (post-polio syndrome)**[1244]
5. Syndrome of benign fasciculation and cramps in survivors of paralytic poliomyelitis or other forms of acute myelitis[1805]
6. Amyotrophy after **encephalitis lethargica**[2271]
7. **Delayed cramps and fasciculation after poliomyelitis or myelitis**

F. *Disorders of motor neurons with immunological abnormality*
1. Motor neuron diseases with monoclonal paraproteinemia (including Waldenstrom macroglobulinemia, multiple myeloma, chronic lymphatic leukemia)[5153]
2. Amyotrophy with Hodgkin disease[4987] or non-Hodgkin lymphoma
3. Carcinomatous motor neuron disease.[3906] See **amyotrophic lateral sclerosis** (paraneoplastic ALS).

G. *Disorders of motor neurons of undetermined etiology*
1. **Amyotrophic lateral sclerosis,** including **monomelic** and the sporadic and both adult- and childhood-onset inherited forms[2473,3201]
2. Juvenile **amyotrophic lateral sclerosis**[4094]
3. Amyotrophy in **Shy-Drager syndrome**
4. Amyotrophy in sporadic **Pick disease**[3899]
5. **Quadriceps amyotrophy** (sporadic, neurogenic)[1998]
6. Muscle pain–fasciculation syndrome

H. *Disorders of motor neurons in endocrine disorders*
1. **Tetany** (hypocalcemia, hypomagnesemia, alkalosis)
2. Amyotrophy in hypoglycemic hyperinsulinism
3. Amyotrophy, fasciculation, and upper motor neuron signs (amyotrophic lateral sclerosis) in **hyperthyroidism**[1869]
4. Amyotrophy in **hyperparathyroidism**[4363]

I. *Disorders of motor neurons manifest by hyperactivity*
1. **Ordinary muscle cramps**
2. **Benign fasciculation-cramp syndrome** (syndrome of Foley and Denny-Brown)
3. **Occupational cramps** and writer's cramp
4. **Isaacs syndrome**[5826]
5. **Tetanus**
6. Strychnine intoxication
7. **Stiff man syndrome**
8. **Satoyoshi syndrome**[4927]
9. Myelopathy with rigidity, spasm, or continuous motor unit activity
10. Myokymia with hyperhidrosis and impaired muscle relaxation[2015]
11. Black widow spider bite
12. **Tetany**
13. **Spinal myoclonus**
14. **Facial myokymia**
15. **Hemifacial spasm**

16. **Painful legs and moving toes**[5281]
17. **Ekbom syndrome.** See **restless legs syndrome**[2460]

This classification is amended from that of the World Federation of Neurology (World Federation of Neurology Classification Subcommittee. Classification of neuromuscular diseases. J Neurol Sci 1988;*86:333–360) and is reproduced by kind permission of Prof. P.K. Thomas, Lord Walton, and the World Federation of Neurology.*

motor neuronopathy   A disorder of the anterior horn cells and/or of the cranial nerve motor nuclei, as in **amyotrophic lateral sclerosis,** some dysimmune polyneuropathies, **diabetic amyotrophy, porphyria,** postradiation neuropathies, and **lead poisoning.** cf. **multifocal motor neuropathy with conduction block.**

motor neuronopathy predominantly affecting the hands   A dominantly inherited condition mapped to gene 7p (but heterogeneous) with onset in youth of asymmetric distal weakness and wasting of the hands more than of the feet in the absence of sensory disturbances or of pyramidal signs.

motor neuropathy predominantly affecting the arms   A neuropathy with onset in childhood, characterized by neurogenic brachial muscle atrophy and weakness. See also **hereditary motor neuropathy, amyotrophic lateral sclerosis.**

Either a *variant* or the same condition is *motor neuronopathy predominantly affecting the hands*, a dominantly inherited condition mapped to gene 7p (but heterogeneous) with onset in youth of asymmetric distal weakness and wasting of the hands more than of the feet in the absence of sensory disturbances or of pyramidal signs.

motor paralytic bladder   A dilated and flaccid bladder resulting from detrusor weakness and lack of tone due to damage to its motor nerve supply, as in lesions of the conus medullaris or severe autonomic neuropathy. As a result, the bladder stretch reflex fails and it becomes a large urine-containing sac with dribbling incontinence resulting.

motor persistence   The ability to sustain motor activity, diminished in patients with an attention deficit-hyperactivity disorder.

motor point   See **motor end point.**

motor response   1. The compound muscle action potential (M wave) recorded over a muscle with stimulation of the nerve to that muscle. 2. The muscle twitch or contraction elicited by stimulation of the nerve to a muscle. 3. The muscle twitch elicited in the muscle stretch reflex. (From the 1987 Report of the Nomenclature Committee of the American Association of Electromyography and Electrodiagnosis. AAEE glossary of terms in clinical electromyography. *Muscle Nerve* 1987;**10S:**G5–G23. Copyright 1987 by John Wiley and Sons, Inc. Reprinted by permission of John Wiley and Sons, Inc.)

motor system degeneration   A dominantly inherited syndrome resembling **Azorean neuropathy,** but occurring in people without Portuguese ancestry.[2501]

motor system diseases   See **amyotrophic lateral sclerosis.**

motor tics   Irregularly repetitive, involuntary, abrupt, rapid, purposeless, coordinated movements of multiple muscle groups, occurring in stereotyped sequences, preceded often by a conscious urge to perform the movement but persisting in sleep; they can be suppressed for a period by an effort of will. Those involving an isolated body part, such as shrugging or eye-blinking, are known as *simple tics*; those comprising a more coordinated movement pattern such as jumping or touching are known as *complex tics. Phonic tics* (vocalizations) may also be simple or complex, the latter comprising perceptible words or phrases. Brief, jerky movements merit the label *clonic tics,* but slower, prolonged forms occur as well (**tonic** or **dystonic tics**). See also **sensory tics.**

motor unit   The anatomical unit of an anterior horn cell, its axon, the neuromuscular junctions, and all of the muscle fibers innervated by the axon.

motor unit action potential   (MUAP) An action potential reflecting the electrical activity of a single anatomical motor unit; the compound action potential of those muscle fibers within the recording range of an electrode.

With voluntary muscle contraction, the MUAP is characterized by its consistent appearance with, and relationship to, the force of contraction. The parameters listed in Chart M–19 should be specified, quantitatively if possible, after the recording electrode is placed so as to minimize the rise time (which by convention should be <0.5 msec).

Chart M–19. Parameters of the Motor Unit Action Potential

1. *Configuration*
   A. Amplitude, peak-to-peak (uV and mV)
   B. Duration, total (msec)
   C. Number of phases (monophasic, biphasic, triphasic, tetraphasic, polyphasic)
   D. Sign of each phase (negative, positive)
   E. Number of turns
   F. Variation of shape, if any, with consecutive discharges
   G. Presence of satellite (linked) potentials, if any
2. *Recruitment characteristics*
   A. Threshold of activation (first recruited, low threshold, high threshold)
   B. Onset frequency (Hz)
   C. Recruitment frequency (Hz) or recruitment interval (msec) of individual potentials

Adapted from the 1987 Report of the Nomenclature Committee of the American Association of Electromyography and Electrodiagnosis. AAEE glossary of terms in clinical electromyography. Muscle Nerve 1987;10S: *G5–G23. (Reprinted by permission of John Wiley and Sons, Inc. © 1987)*

motor unit estimation   An electrophysiological technique in which threshold and then increasing electrical stimuli are given to a motor nerve, the sizes of the muscle evoked potentials being measured and the average divided into the size of the evoked potential recorded with maximal stimulation to provide an estimate of the number of functioning motor units in that muscle.[3732]

motor unit territory   The area in a muscle over which the muscle fibers belonging to an individual motor unit are distributed.[146]

motricity index   A scoring system for the power of selected movements which can be derived for the upper and lower limbs or for one side of the body after the motor evaluation of patients with vascular hemiplegia.[1396]

The first group of tests is performed with the patient sitting. It includes measures of *arm function* (pinch grip, elbow flexion, shoulder abduction) and of *leg function* (hip flexion, knee extension, and ankle dorsiflexion).

A *trunk control test* may be added, in which the subject is assessed on the ability to roll over to the weak or to the strong side, to sit up from the supine position, and to maintain balance while sitting on the side of a bed. Scores for the arms, for the legs, and for one side may be derived.

Mott, Sir Frederick Walker   (1853–1916) English physician and pathologist, who proved conclusively the relationship between syphilis and general paresis by finding spirochetes in the brain of paretic patients. He also described the pathology of neuronal degeneration in the Royal College of Physicians Croonian lectures of 1900.

Mouchet syndrome   Ulnar nerve paresis resulting from a distal fracture of the humerus. This is worthy of note only because the description was of a fracture of the *condyle externe*, suggesting the lateral epicondyle rather than the medial, as was actually the case.

Dr. Albert Mouchet was a French physician, born in 1869.

mounding phenomenon   A focal contracture of a skeletal muscle in response to a direct tap on the muscle. It was first observed (in recently dead animals) by Schiff in 1858; its genesis has been determined to be calcium liberation from the sarcoplasmic reticulum.[3925]

Mount Fuji sign   The CT scan appearance in the supine patient in the presence of a large amount of subdural air that compresses both frontal lobes.[4869] The dark, conical frontal lobes are capped by white, from the air present.

Mount-Reback syndrome   See **paroxysmal kinesiogenic choreoathetosis.**

mountain sickness   1. (acute mountain sickness) Cerebral edema and pulmonary symptoms developing within hours of arriving at altitudes above 2500 m. Headache, anorexia, nausea, vomiting; and dyspnea at rest, cough, pink frothy sputum, and audible rales are typical clinical features. Retinal hemorrhages may accompany these findings. See also **high-altitude headache.** The pulmonary problems at least are responsive to steroids. 2. (Monge disease, chronic moun-

tain sickness) The occurrence of polycythemia and pulmonary hypertension in subjects living at high altitudes for long periods (years), the clinical effects consisting of fatigue and mental slowing.[5428]

mouthing   Repetitive chewing and licking throughout wakefulness with tongue protrusions, seen in edentulous elderly patients and inhibited briefly by eye closure or by a touch on the face. Midline cerebellar lesions are considered responsible.[198] See also **oromandibular dystonia.**

Movement Disorder Society   A professional organization dedicated to disseminating information on recent advances in both clinical and basic sciences related to movement disorders, and to the education of physicians and the public. Tel: 414-276-2145. Web site: http://www.movementdisorders.org/.

movement disorders   Those neurological conditions in which the major clinical expressions involve reduced normal movements or excessive or abnormal involuntary movements of the limbs, face, or trunk and which in most instances are considered to reflect disease of the extrapyramidal system.

Movement Disorders   (Mov. Disord.) The official journal of the **Movement Disorder Society.** Address: John Wiley and Sons, 111 River Street, Hoboken, NJ 07030. Web site: http://www.intrascience.wiley.com/. movementdisorders.

movement phosphenes   Phosphenes induced by movement of the eyes; an occasional accompaniment of **optic neuritis.**[1313]

movement-induced seizures   A questionable variety of seizure in which the actual voluntary movement of a limb induces a motor response resembling that in **startle-induced seizures,** but which may actually be a movement-induced paroxysmal dyskinesia.

Moving Forward   A charitable organization in the field of myoclonus. Address: 2934 Glenmore Ave., Kettering, OH 45409. Tel: 937-293-0409.

Moxon, William   Eighteenth-century physician to Guy's Hospital, London, who gave the first account of **multiple sclerosis** ("insular sclerosis") in the English literature.

moyamoya disease   (Jpn, hazy, like a puff of smoke) (Nishimoto-Takeuchi-Kudo disease) A form of large-vessel occlusion affecting the intracranial supraclinoid carotid artery, in which a secondary network of proliferating collateral arterioles is seen to arise from the carotid artery proximal to the occlusion.[5430]

Children or young adults with such an abnormality usually present with hemiplegia; adults present with subarachnoid hemorrhage, although dementia, dysphasia, pyramidal or extrapyramidal signs, and cerebral atrophy have all been recorded.[3176] The angiographic appearances (described first by Takeuchi[5473a] in 1961) resemble a mist or puff of smoke arising from the floor of the skull; a similar appearance can occur in disease of the posterior circulation.

The clinical picture is that of bilateral basal vascular occlusive disease with telangiectasia involving the basal ganglia as a result of occlusion of the internal carotid artery.[5423]

In a *variant* condition, *moyamoya disease and Ollier disease*, there is associated enchondromatosis and lytic lesions of bone, skeletal cysts, or tumors leading to multiple fractures.

Moynahan syndrome   A recessively inherited syndrome characterized by alopecia, hypohidrosis, seizures and mental retardation.[4024]

Dr. E.J. Moynahan was a British dermatologist at Guy's Hospital.

Mozart effect   Slight and transient improvement in spational reasoning skills detected in normal subjects as a result of exposure to the music of Mozart, specifically his sonata for two pianos (K448). Such music (also that of J.S. Bach and of his son, J.C. Bach) has been shown to contain long-lasting periodicities and repetition of melodic lines, considered somehow responsible for the effect.[2836]

A decrease in the manifestations of neurological disease such as seizure activity has also been described as an extension of the effect; the fact that some patients showing it are in coma indicates that an emotional reaction to the beauty of the music is not itself the relevant mechanism.

MPTP   (methyl-phenyl-tetrohydropyridine) A substance synthesized in the illicit, nonprofessional, but highly commercial production of heroin, and which is intensely toxic to the nigrostriatal pathways in humans and some monkeys to the extent that ingestion leads inexorably and quickly to a **parkinsonian** syndrome.

MRA   See **magnetic resonance angiography.**

MRD   See **minimal record of disability.**

MRI   See **magnetic resonance imaging.**

MSLT   See **minimal sleep latency test.**

MSQ   See **Mental Status Questionnaire.**

mu rhythm   (arceau rhythm, wicket rhythm, comb rhythm) An EEG rhythm at 7–11 Hz composed of arch-shaped waves occurring over the centroparietal regions of the scalp during wakefulness. Its amplitude varies but is mostly below 50 uV. It is blocked or attenuated most clearly by contralateral movement, the thought of movement, readiness to move, or tactile stimulation. (Adapted from the 1974 report of the Committee on Terminology, IFCN[989] by permission of Elsevier Science.)

The rhythm is seen in rolandic regions and is of no known pathological significance.

MUAP   See **motor unit action potential.**

Muckle-Wells syndrome   (dominant urticaria, amyloidosis, nephritis and hearing loss) A dominantly inherited cochleovestibular syndrome of childhood, characterized by progressive renal impairment due to amyloidosis, recurrent urticarial rashes, fever, and neural deafness.[4032]

mucocele   Benign cysts composed of mucus-secreting epithelium situated within the nasal sinuses, but capable of eroding into the orbit or cranial cavity.

mucocutaneous   lymph   node   syndrome   See **Kawasaki disease.**

mucolipidoses   Sphingolipid and mucopolysaccharide lysosomal storage diseases in which lipid-like and polysaccharide-like material is deposited in the tissues. See **sialidosis.**

mucopolysaccharidoses   (Ellis gargoylism, Pfaundler-Hurler syndrome) A group of lysosomal disorders of mucopolysaccharide metabolism resulting from deficient activity of the enzymes that degrade mucopolysaccharides; they are usually autosomal recessively inherited, and involve the storage of glycos-aminoglycans (mucopolysaccharides) in the lysosomes of various tissues. The catabolism of dermatan sulfate, heparan sulfate, and/or ketaran sulfate is thus blocked, and in some cases, that of chondroitin sulfate as well. The types are listed in Chart M–20.

Chart M–20. Types of Mucopolysaccharidosis

Hurler syndrome (type 1-H) A lethal, recessively inherited, systemic disease appearing within the first year of life, due to α-L-iduronidase deficiency, which leads to the deposition of dermatan and heparan sulfate in the joints, liver, spleen, and skin. Clinically, the syndrome is characterized by short stature, gargoyle-like facies, prominent lips and tongue, cataract, hypertelorism, psychomotor retardation, macrocephaly, thickened skin, hepatospleno-megaly and cardiomegaly, arthropathy, kyphoscoliosis, and sometimes spastic quadriparesis due to C1–2 subluxation.[2712] Entrapment neuropathies are also often found. The children usually die of respiratory or cardiac failure.

Hurler-Scheie syndrome (type 1-H/S) A recessively inherited syndrome in which deficiency of α-L-iduronidase leads to the accumulation of dermatan and heparan sulfate and in which the clinical features resemble those of both of the syndromes suggested by its name. The responsible gene lies on chromosome 22.

Scheie syndrome (type 1-S or 5) A recessively inherited systemic mucopolysaccharidosis due to deficiency of the enzyme α-L-iduronidase, in which dermatan sulfate and heparan sulfate are deposited. Diffuse congenital corneal haziness and the later development of pigmentary retinopathy, cataract, dwarfism, joint ankylosis, mild dysmorphism, skeletal defects, carpal tunnel syndrome, coarctation of the aorta, and hepatosplenomegaly are the main clinical features. Urinary levels of chondroitin sulfate B are high.[4949] The condition differs from most other mucopolysaccharidoses in that the physical and mental statures of the patients are not diminished. It is allelic with Hurler syndrome.

Although the term *Hunter-Hurler syndrome* is also applied, these and **Hunter** diseases are separate, though similar, mucopolysaccharidoses.

Hunter syndrome (type 2) An X-linked form due to deficiency of iduronate 2-sulfate sulfatase appearing in childhood and characterized by short stature, enlarged nose with a depressed nasal bridge, coarse facial features, delayed tooth eruption, kyphosis, beaked vertebrae, platyspondyly, pectus carinatum, thick ribs, inguinal and umbilical hernias, enlarged liver, joint stiffness, mucopolysacchariduria, oligosacchariduria, macrocephaly, J-shaped sella turcica, epiphyseal dysplasia, and psychomotor retardation. Mild and severe forms are distinguished on the basis of the degree of mental impairment and on the course of the disease. The responsible gene maps to chromosome Xq27.3.

Sanfilippo syndrome (types 3 A, B, C) Recessively inherited systemic mucopolysaccharidoses of young children due to the absence of any one of three sulfamidase enzymes that are responsible for the degradation of heparan sulfate, which is therefore accumulated; thus, the A, B, and C forms are differentiated. *N*-sulfatase (sulfaminidase) is deficient in type A; *N*-acetylglucosaminidase, in type B; and *N*-acetyl transferase, in type C, in which heparan sulfate is deposited.

Clinically the conditions are similar and are marked by severe mental deterioration with aggressive behavior, coarse facial features, cataract, dwarfism, joint ankylosis, skeletal defects, hepatosplenomegaly, vertebral abnormalities, joint stiffness, seizures, ataxia, mucopolysacchariduria, and abnormal lysosomal enzymes. In the B form, there is striking visceral involvement. Urinary levels of heparan sulfate are high.[4910]

In a *variant* form, the disorder presents as a dementing disease in early adult life.

Morquio disease (type 4A and 4B, Morquio-Brailsford syndrome) An autosomal recessive metabolic disease presenting in early childhood, due to deficiency of *N*-acetyl-galactosamine-6-sulfate sulfatase (type A) or *β*-galactosidase (type B), in which keratan sulfate and chondroitin-6-sulfate are deposited in tissues and excreted in the urine. The clinical manifestations include coarse facial features, corneal opacities, deafness without mental deterioration, dwarfism, hyperextensible joints, aortic valve anomalies, epiphyseal dysplasia, platyspondyly, and osteoporosis, the latter leading to widespread skeletal deformities. In the case of the spine, these may cause vertebral subluxation such as atlanto-axial dislocation and cord compression.[3095,3992,3993] The responsible gene for Morquio syndrome B maps to chromosome 3p21–p14.2. J.F. Brailsford (1888–1961) was an English radiologist practicing in Birmingham.

In related *variant forms*, neuronal storage or corneal opacities occur as well.

Maroteaux-Lamy syndrome (type 6) A recessively inherited lysosomal storage disease (mucopolysaccharidosis type 6) with deficiency of arylsulfatase B and accumulation of dermatan sulfate. It exists in severe, intermediate, and mild forms, the latter appearing in adult life.

The main clinical features are dwarfism, facial dysmorphism with prominent lips and tongue, severe skeletal deformity, deafness, corneal opacities, hepatosplenomegaly and car-diomegaly, kyphoscoliosis, and sometimes spastic quadriparesis due to C1–2 subluxation. Hydrocephalus and carpal tunnel syndrome are the other main neurological complications. The urine contains large amounts of chondroitin sulfate B.[3636] Mental retardation is not a feature.

A milder *variant* is also described.

Beta-glucuronidase deficiency (type 7, Sly disease) A rare, recessively inherited disorder of mucopolysaccharide metabolism due to a defect on chromosome 7 with deficiency of *β*-glucuronidase and the accumulation of dermatan and heparan sulfate.

Clinically, it presents with short stature, mental retardation, macrocephaly, corneal clouding, hepatosplenomegaly, and polymorphic skeletal malformations.[5211]

Di Ferrante syndrome (type 8) A rare, recessively inherited disorder of mucopolysaccharide metabolism due to a defect on chromosome 7 with deficiency of glucosamine-6-sulfate sulfatase. Clinically, it presents in childhood with psychomotor delay, hepatomegaly, coarse hair, and odontoid anomalies.[2124]

Other *variant* conditions are *O'Brien mucopolysaccharidosis*, characterized by short stature, gibbus, mucopolysacchariduria, rhizomelia of the upper limbs, bowed radius and ulna, skeletal and joint anomalies, and mental and developmental delay,[337] as well as a form presenting with multiple nerve entrapments.[2937] See also **National Mucopolysaccharidosis Society.**

mucormycosis A severe infection with the fungus *Phycomycetes* which may be manifested in pulmonary, disseminated, intestinal, and rhinocerebral forms. Debilitated subjects with systemic illnesses such as diabetes, leukemia, organ failure, renal acidosis, etc. are the most susceptible.

The rhinocerebral manifestations include the orbital apex syndrome, cavernous sinus syndrome, and carotid occlusion. A nasopharyngeal form that includes multiple cranial nerve palsies is also described. Depression of consciousness may occur in association with any of these.[4587]

mucosulfatidosis A diffuse encephalopathy with onset in infancy and due to deficiency of arylsulfatases and other enzymes, leading to the accumulation of sulfatide, heparan, and dermatan sulfate, etc. The condition is regarded as a variant form of **metachromatic leukodystrophy.**

Muenchmeyer syndrome See **myositis ossificans.**

mulibrey syndrome A rare, recessively inherited dysmorphic syndrome characterized by **Mu**scle, **Li**ver, **Br**ain and **Ey**e anomalies. **Nanism,** hypotonia, hypertelorism, hepatomegaly, pigmentary retinopathy, cerebral ventricular enlargement, pericarditis, and skeletal malformations are the most constant clinical features.[4410]

Müller, Eduard (1876–1928) German neuropsychiatrist in Breslau.

Müller, Heinrich (1820–1864) German, professor of anatomy at Wurzburg.

Müller, Johannes (1801–1858) German professor of physiology at Berlin who in 1826 propounded the law of specific nerve energies, which states that each sense organ responds to any stimulus with impulses giving rise to its particular sensation and is supplied by nerves sensitive only to that one form of stimulation. Thus, specific sense organs are responsible for specific modalities of sensation.

In 1831, Müller published accounts of his stimulation experiments on frogs and finally demonstrated without doubt the sensory functions of the posterior roots and the motor functions of the anterior roots, thus sealing the observations of **Bell** and of **Magendie** in this area.

Müller sign Early loss of the abdominal reflexes in **multiple sclerosis,**[4037] named after **Eduard Müller.**

Müller's Law (law of specific nerve energies) Every nerve fiber subserves one modality of sensation, whatever stimulation its end-organ receives, propounded by Johannes Müller in 1826.

Müller's muscle Smooth muscle fibers in the upper eyelid, weakly assisting the levator palpebrae superioris. It is named after **Heinrich Müller.**

multicore myopathy (myopathy with multicore and central nuclei, congenital myopathy with multifocal degeneration of muscle fibers) A benign, congenital, and nonprogressive myopathy characterized by the presence of multiple, small, randomly distributed areas of myofibrillar disorganization with a local decrease in mitochondrial oxidative enzyme activity. Multicores, a focal loss of cross-striations, and a failure of fiber-type differentiation are also noted, as in **central core disease,** but they occur only patchily within the muscle biopsy specimens.[1663,1666,5442]

Clinically, lifelong (proximal more than distal) limb and facial weakness, delayed motor development, ptosis, dolichocephaly, ophthalmoplegias, and slightly raised creatine kinase levels are the only constant associations.[1666] The respiratory muscles and myocardium are rarely affected. A case has been reported with onset in adult life.[658]

multicystic encephalopathy (polyporencephaly) Multiple areas of cavitation in the cerebral cortex and in the subcortical white matter, found in infants following **hypoxic-ischemic encephalopathy,** usually in the territory of the anterior or middle cerebral arteries. See also **porencephaly, encephalomalacia.**

Multidimensional Observation Scale for Elderly Subjects (MOSES) A scale designed for observers to evaluate aspects of functioning in elderly residential patients in five areas of functioning, including self-care, disoriented behavior, depressed or anxious mood, irritable behavior, and withdrawn behavior. These factors are determined after rating the subject on 40 areas of function.[2527]

Multidimensional Pain inventory An instrument for assessing cognitive, behavioral, and affective aspects of pain, yielding scores for pain severity; interference; life control; affective distress; support; punishing, solicitous, and distracting responses; household chores; outdoor work; activities away from home; and social activities.[3013]

multifidus syndrome A myofascial pain syndrome with the trigger point below the posterior superior iliac spine.[3443]

multifocal acquired demyelinating sensory and motor neuropathy (MADSAN) See **multifocal inflammatory demyelinating neuropathy.**

multifocal demyelinating CIDP (**multifocal CIDP, Lewis-Sumner syndrome**) A slowly progressive, or relapsing distal asymmetrical neuropathy of adult life, the weakness affecting mainly the arms. A proximal syndrome is also described, affecting mainly the phrenic and suprascapular nerves. Any sensory loss is mild and distal. Electrophysiology shows multifocal conduction block, variably slow nerve conduction velocities, and long distal latencies. The CSF protein is raised, usually to <100 mg/dl, and MRI shows swollen nerves in brachial plexus. The pathology is patchy nerve demyelination with some axonal loss.

multifocal demyelinating neuropathy with persistent conduction block See **multifocal inflammatory demyelinating neuropathy.**

multifocal giant-cell encephalitis A chronic encephalitis associated with HIV infection, characterized by the perivascular accumulation of microglia, monocytes, and macrophages, with virus-containing multinucleated giant cells.[6]

multifocal inflammatory demyelinating neuropathy (MIDN) An asymmetric sensory or sensorimotor demyelinating neuropathy not fulfilling criteria for **multifocal motor neuropathy with persistent conduction block** or **chronic inflammatory demyelinating polyneuropathy.** Clinically, the disorder starts in one limb, slowly progressing asymmetrically. Electrically, there is evidence of multifocal demyelination and conduction block in motor and sensory nerves. MRI may show swelling of nerves in the brachial plexus and biopsy shows inflammatory changes.[5714]

The condition known as **multifocal motor sensory demyelinating neuropathy** is possibly the same condition, as may be **idiopathic sensory neuropathy.**

multifocal interstitial myositis with localized lipoatrophy An inherited myopathy characterized by the young adult onset of proximal and distal myopathic weakness with inflammatory cells in muscle.[337]

multifocal motor and sensory demyelinating neuropathy See **multifocal inflammatory demyelinating neuropathy.**

multifocal motor neuropathy with persistent conduction block An acquired, chronic, progressive, asymmetrical, sensorimotor or pure motor demyelinating neuropathy occurring in young adult life, clinically resembling **amyotrophic lateral sclerosis** or **multiple mononeuropathy,** but most pronounced distally in the arms, in which at least two nerves show persistent, asymmetrical and multifocal, persistent, partial motor **conduction block** away from the usual sites. Atrophy is relatively mild, fasciculations and cramps are common, and myokymia is occasional. Sensory symptoms are not to be expected and there is relative preservation of the muscle stretch reflexes. Optic neuritis is associated in some cases, but other cranial nerves and the pyramidal system are seldom involved. Electrophysiology shows the presence of focal segmental distal nerve conduction block, evidenced by >50% reduction of compound motor action potential amplitudes; axonal loss is a late finding.

In sural nerve biopsy specimens the pathological findings include both demyelination and remyelination, and there is a variable degree of fiber loss. Anti-GM_1 or NP-9 lipid antigen IgM antibodies are detected in over 90% of cases.[3388] Diagnostic criteria have been suggested;[5713]

The condition may considered a variant of **chronic inflammatory demyelinating polyneuropathy,** differing in its distal and asymmetric presentation, the rarity of sensory symptoms, localized electrophysiological findings, and lack of the inflammatory signs and onion bulbs seen in the widespread peripheral nerve demyelination of that condition.

In *variant* forms, the condition presents with ophthalmoplegia,[4528] or no conduction block is found.[4301] Definitions of this and most other neuromuscular syndromes are superbly presented at http://www.neuro.wustl.edu/neuromuscular.

multifocal pseudohypertrophic neuropathy See **multifocal inflammatory demyelinating neuropathy.**

multifocal sensorimotor demyelinating neuropathy A likely variant of **multifocal motor neuropathy with persistent conduction block** in which there are also sensory complaints, raised CSF protein levels, a shorter course, a better steroid response, and sensory nerve conduction abnormalities.[4210]

multifocal sensory demyelinating neuropathy Yet another likely variant of **multifocal motor neuropathy with persistent conduction block,** here presenting with sensory complaints, raised CSF protein levels, a response to IvIg and evidence of demyelinating sensory neuropathy on near-nerve conduction studies only.[4211]

multi-infarct dementia A relatively common and partially reversible form of dementia due to multiple focal cortical infarctions.[2357] The **Hachinski Ischemic scale** was devised to reflect the clinical features of this and other **vascular dementias.** The presence of brainstem and pyramidal signs, gait disorder, and depression are features not specifically rated on the Hachinski scale which suggest multi-infarct dementia rather than **Alzheimer disease.**

Dementia occurring as a result of multiple cerebral emboli or following cardiac arrest or cardiac surgery might also be included under this heading. See **vascular dementia.**

APA Diagnostic Criteria for Vascular Dementia
A. The development of multiple cognitive deficits manifested by both;
   1. Memory impairment
   2. One (or more) of the following cognitive disturbances:
      a. aphasia
      b. apraxia
      c. agnosia
      d. disturbance in executive functioning (i.e., planning, organizing, sequencing, abstracting)
B. The cognitive deficits in Criteria A1 and A2 each cause significant impairment in social or occupational functioning and represent a significant decline from a previous level of functioning.
C. Focal neurological signs and symptoms . . . or laboratory evidence indicative of cerebrovascular disease . . . that are judged to be etiologically related to the disturbance.
D. The deficits do not occur exclusively during the course of a delirium.

(Adapted from American Psychiatric Association. APA Diagnostic and Statistical Manual of Mental Disorders. Fourth Edition, Text Revision. Copyright 2000, American Psychiatric Association.)

A *variant* is *multi-infarct dementia, familial type* (familial vascular encephalopathy, Worster-Drought syndrome), which is a syndrome of adult onset characterized by cerebral atrophy with dementia, facial palsy, pyramidal signs, and arteriopathy.

multilead electrode Three or more insulated wires inserted through apertures in a common metal cannula with their bared tips flush with the cannula's outer circumference. The arrangement of the bare tips relative to the axis of the cannula and the distance between each tip should be specified. See **electrode.** (From the 2001 Report of the Nomenclature Committee of the American Association of Electromyography and Electrodiagnosis.[10] Used by permission, copyright © 2001, AAEM.)

multi-minicore disease A recessively inherited benign congenital myopathy associated with multifocal zones of degeneation of sarcomeres, with lack of oxidative activity.[1677] Weakness is axially predominant and severe respiratory difficulty and scoliosis are common features, but the phenotype is variable.[1799]

multi-MUP analysis A template-matching, decomposition EMG method used for motor unit action potential analysis. (From the 2001 Report of the Nomenclature Committee of the American Association of Electromyography and Electrodiagnosis.[10] Used by permission, copyright © 2001, AAEM.)

multiple acyl coA dehydrogenase–deficient myopathy A carnitine-deficient lipid storage myopathy with organic aciduria due to an inborn error of the enzymes catalyzing the oxidation of straight- and branched-chain acyl coenzyme A and glutaryl coenzyme A. Muscle weakness with recurrent episodes of hypoglycemia and an odor of sweaty feet are the leading features. Both mild and severe (lethal) forms occur.

In some cases, the condition, a mitochondrial disorder, is remarkably responsive to large doses of thiamine.[1440] See also **glutaric aciduria type 2.**

multiple acylcoenzyme A dehydrogenation disorders Mitochondrial disorders including **glutaric aciduria type 2,** characterized by a deficiency in the electron transfer flavoprotein or its dehydrogenase. In the *severe* (MAD: S) form, infants present with seizures and are found to have nonketotic hypoglycemia and metabolic acidosis. In the *mild* form (MAD: M) the **sudden infant death syndrome,** an illness resembling **Reye syndrome,** or a lipid storage myopathy (see next entry) may occur; such conditions may respond to riboflavine.[5637]

Multiple Affect Adjective Checklist A self-report questionnaire appropriate for the repeated assessment of disturbed mood states.[6137]

multiple basal cell nevi syndrome See **Gorlin-Golz syndrome.**

multiple carboxylase deficiency A neonatal metabolic syndrome due to a deficiency in biotin holocarboxylase synthetase,[4290] and characterized clinically by alopecia, sensorineural deafness, conjunctivitis, hypotonia, seizures, cerebellar ataxia, tremor, eczema, erythema, psychomotor delay, and eventually death in coma. High plasma ammonia and lactate levels and organic aciduria are found.[5576]

In the *neonatal* form the deficiency is of numerous carboxylase enzymes including pyruvate carboxylase and holocarboxylase synthetase, while in the *late-onset* form, biotinidase is deficient.

multiple cerebral/retinal arteriovenous malformations See **Wyburn-Mason syndrome.**

multiple congenital articular rigidities See **arthrogryposis multiplex congenita.**

multiple congenital contractures (multiple-contracture syndrome) A lethal autosomal recessive syndrome characterized by intrauterine growth retardation with multiple contractures and facial abnormalities.

The condition is a variant of the **Pena-Shokeir phenotype,** differentiated by the presence of severe fetal hydrops and the increased severity in this condition. See also **multiple pterygium syndrome.**[2560]

multiple cranial nerve palsies syndrome 1. A variant of **acute inflammatory demyelinating polyneuropathy,** described first by Guillain in 1937, in which a number of cranial nerves (usually at least four, including the oculomotor nerve) are affected bilaterally. The CSF protein level is elevated and ataxia or areflexia may also be found, but limb strength and sensation are typically unaffected. The prognosis for recovery is excellent.[5141]

See also **Miller Fisher syndrome; facial diplegia; ataxia, areflexia, and facial diplegia.**

2. Painful ophthalmoplegia related to a granulomatous inflammatory process in the cavernous sinus, preceded by facial palsy; an extended form of **Tolosa-Hunt syndrome.**[5528]

multiple discharge Four or more motor unit action potentials of the same form and nearly the same amplitude occurring consistently in the same relationship to one another and generated by the same axon. See **double** and **triple discharge, multiple discharge.** (From the 2001 Report of the Nomenclature Committee of the American Association of Electromyography and Electrodiagnosis.[10] Used by permission, copyright © 2001, AAEM.)

multiple endocrine neoplasia Type 1 is a dominantly inherited syndrome characterized by pituitary, pancreatic, adrenal, and/or parathyroid hyperplasia or adenomatosis. Chromophobe, basophil, or eosinophil pituitary adenomas may also complicate the syndrome.[5920]

Type 2 (Sipple syndrome) is a dominantly inherited disorder characterized by carcinoma and/or hyperplasia of the adrenal or thyroid glands; parathyroid hyperplasia uncommonly; a physique resembling that of **Marfan syndrome;** neuromas of the tongue, lips, and eyelids; autonomic symptoms due to ganglioneuromatosis in the alimentary tract; pheochromocytoma; and signs of **hereditary motor and sensory neuropathy.**[1571]

Type 2b is a rare autosomal dominant condition linked to chromosome 10q.11.2, in which medullary carcinoma of the thyroid, pheochromocytoma, ganglioneuromatosis, or various skeletal disorders are associated with pes cavus, atrophy of the peroneal muscles, lingual tumor-like excrescences, and thickened lips.[906]

multiple epiphyseal dysplasia with mild myopathy A dominantly inherited myopathy mapped to 20q13.3 and presenting with knee pain in childhood, mild symmetric weakness of neck flexion, shoulder abduction, and elbow extension and with pelvic girdle weakness. Evidence of osteoarthritis with joint space narrowing, osteophytes, and and femoral condylar bony flattening appears in mid-adult life. The serum CK is mildly elevated and muscle biopsy shows mild myopathic changes.

multiple epiphyseal dysplasia–microcephaly–nystagmus See **Conradi-Hünermann syndrome.**

Multiple Errands test A test of frontal lobe planning function, in which the subject has to complete a number of errands, such as shopping in an unfamiliar mall, according to a set of prelearned guidelines.[5089]

multiple evanescent white spot syndrome The presence of small, white dots deep to the retina and causing transient visual impairment. This may be a variant of the **big blind spot syndrome;** it is considered likely to be due to a virus infection.[1486]

multiple exercise-related mononeuropathies with colic   A dominantly inherited syndrome characterized by painful motor neuropathies with abdominal pain, occurring after strenuous exercise.[5640]

multiple exostosis   A rare, sporadic or dominantly inherited syndrome characterized by cartilaginous and bony protuberances, most often involving the metaphyseal regions of tubular long bones and capable of causing pressure on local nerves or myelopathy.[1797]

multiple lentigenes syndrome   See **LEOPARD syndrome.**

multiple lipomatosis with chronic encephalopathy
1. The presence of benign intracranial lipomas in the corpus callosum or elsewhere. The symptoms in such patients are frequently the result of other brain malformations rather than of the lipomas.[301] 2. See **encephalocraniocutaneous lipomatosis.**

multiple mononeuropathy   (mononeuritis multiplex) Acute haphazard infarction of various nerves, usually occurring asymmetrically, with resultant rapid motor and reflex loss, pain, and some sensory deficits adopting the sensory and/or motor topography of the nerves involved.

The sequential involvement of several nerves may, over the course of development, yield a clinical picture that gives a false appearance of symmetrical polyneuritis. The causes comprise any of numerous systemic diseases, particularly the systemic vasculitides,[1570] Lyme disease, AIDS, and leprosy; diabetes; and multiple schwannomas, and they also develop following dialysis.[1760] Each of these pathologies causes **persistent conduction block** at the usual sites of nerve compression.

multiple myeloma   A gammopathy frequently complicated by slowly progressive neuropathies of various types. These include a mainly distal amyloid deposition with sensory and autonomic neuropathy; a distal axonal polyneuropathy; a sensory neuronopathy; or a neuropathy resembling **chronic inflammatory demyelinating polyneuropathy.**

See also **POEMS, monoclonal gammopathy of uncertain significance.**

multiple nevoid basal cell carcinoma syndrome   A dominantly inherited syndrome characterized by frontal and temporal skull bossing, the presence of multiple nevoid basal cell carcinomas in childhood or early adult life, and skeletal malformations including kyphoscoliosis.[2222]

Hydrocephalus, blindness due to corneal cataract, glaucoma, coloboma of the choroid and optic nerve, strabismus, a marfanoid build, and numerous other endocrine, oral, and muscular abnormalities may be associated.[2219]

multiple peripheral nerve entrapments   A syndrome that represents an unusual phenotypical variant of the Hunter syndrome (**mucopolysaccharidosis** type 2), in which multiple peripheral entrapments occur, particularly of the median and ulnar nerves.[2937]

multiple pterygium syndrome   A rare, recessively inherited dysmorphic syndrome, characterized also by microcephaly, ptosis, vertebral fusion defects, scoliosis, and mental retardation.[1702]

multiple sclerosis   (insular sclerosis, lobular sclerosis, polysclerosis, sclérose en plaques) A common demyelinating disease of unknown cause, most frequently affecting young adults and characterized by the presence of islands of perivascular demyelination anywhere in the central nervous system which give rise to intermittent or progressive neurological signs.

Various defining diagnostic criteria have been drawn up (see **Schumacher panel criteria, McDonald-Halliday criteria,** and **Poser criteria**).[4504] **Charcot**'s criteria were published in 1868.[969] The first descriptions of the disease were by Jean Cruveilhier in 1835, Carswell in 1838, and **Frerichs** in 1849. A checklist of symptoms in multiple sclerosis[2328] and an **Illness Severity score**[3867] have been created. See also **primary progressive multiple sclerosis, relapse.**

Various sets of MRI criteria have also been suggested and are presented below.

Offenbacher et al.[4205] proposed that there be at least three areas of increased signal, with two of the following characteristics in addition:
1. Abutting the body of the lateral ventricles
2. Infratentorial lesion location
3. Size >5 mm

McDonald et al.[3743] suggest that three of the following features should be present:
1. One gadolinium-enhancing lesion or nine T2-weighted hyperintense lesions if there is no gadolinium-enhancing lesion
2. At least one infratentorial lesion
3. At least one juxtatentorial lesion
4. At least three periventricular lesions

Magnetic Resonance Imaging Criteria for Dissemination of Lesions in Time
1. If a first scan occurs 3 months or more after the onset of the clinical event, the presence of a gadolinium-enhancing lesion is sufficient to demonstrate dissemination in time, provided that it is not at the site implicated in the original clinical event. If there is no enhancing lesion at this time, a follow-up scan is required. The timing of this follow-up scan is not crucial, but 3 months is recommended. A new T2- or gadolinium-enhancing lesion at this time then fulfills the criterion for dissemination in time.
2. If the first scan is performed less than 3 months after the onset of the clinical event, a second scan done 3 months or more after the clinical event showing a new gadolinium-enhancing lesion provides sufficient evidence for dissemination in time. However, if no enhancing lesion is seen at this second scan, a further scan not less than 3 months after the first scan that shows a new T2 lesion or an enhancing lesion will suffice.

Clinical diagnostic criteria were suggested first by Schumacher et al.,[5011] later by **Poser** et al.,[4504] and more recently by McDonald and colleagues[3743] (see Chart M–21), whose suggestions are reproduced here by kind permission.

Chart M–21. Diagnostic Criteria for Multiple Sclerosis (MS)[3743]

Clinical Presentation	Additional Data Needed for MS Diagnosis
Two or more attacks; objective clinical evidence of 2 or more lesions	None.*
Two or more attacks; objective clinical evidence of 1 lesion	Dissemination in space, demonstrated by MRI† or 2 or more MRI-detected lesions consistent with MS *plus* positive CSF‡ or await further clinical attack implicating a different site.
One attack; objective clinical evidence of 2 or more lesions	Dissemination in time, demonstrated by MRI† or second clinical attack.
One attack; objective clinical evidence of 1 lesion (mono-symptomatic presentation; clinically isolated syndrome)	Dissemination in space, demosntrated by MRI† or 2 or more MRI-detected lesions consistent with MS *plus* positive CSF‡ *and* dissemination in time, demonstrated by MRI§ or second clinical attack.
Insidious neurological progression suggestive of MS	Positive CSF‡ *and* dissemination in space, demonstrated by 1. 9 or more T2 lesions in brain *or* 2. 2 or more lesions in spinal cord, or 3. 4–8 brain *plus* 1 spinal cord lesion *or* abnormal VEP‖ associated with 4–8 brain lesions, *or* with fewer than 4 brain lesions *plus* 1 spinal cord lesion demonstrated by MRI and dissemination in time, demonstrated by MRI§ *or* continued progression for 1 year.

If criteria indicated are fulfilled, the diagnosis is MS; if the criteria are not completely met, the diagnosis is possible MS, if the criteria are fully explored and not met, the diagnosis is not MS.

*No additional tests are required; however, if tests MRI, CSF are undertaken and are negative, extreme caution should be taken before making a diagnosis of MS. Alternative diagnoses must be considered. There must be no better explanation for the clinical picture.

†MRI demonstration of space dissemination must fulfill the criteria derived from Barkhof et al.[352A] and Tintore et al.[5591a]

‡Positive CSF determined by oligoclonal bands detected by established methods (preferably isoelectric focusing) different from any such bands in serum or by a raised IgG index.

§MRI demonstration of time dissemination must fulfill the criteria listed above.

‖Abnormal visual evoked potential of the type seen in MS (delay with a well-preserved wave form).

From McDonald WI, Compston DAS, Edan G, et al. Recommended Diagnostic Criteria for Multiple Sclerosis: Guidelines from the International Panel on the Diagnosis of Multiple Sclerosis. Ann. Neurol. 2001;50:121–7. © 2001. John Wiley and Sons, Inc. Reprinted by permission of John Wiley and Sons, Inc.

Primary progressive multiple sclerosis is the term for those forms of the disease that are progressive from their onset.[5560] *Secondary progressive multiple sclerosis*

indicates that the condition has become progressive after an initial relapsing-remitting course. The pathogenesis and eventual prognosis of these two forms is not known to differ, but they do exhibit differences in their MRI appearances, the former group developing fewer new lesions with less gadolinium enhancement over an observed period.

A possible variant is *transitional progressive multiple sclerosis* with an unusual presentation and course of disease.[1815] See also **benign multiple sclerosis; chronic progressive multiple sclerosis.**

Multiple Sclerosis Functional Composite   A test battery comprising three timed tests of neurologic function: a 25-foot walk, the nine-hole peg test, and a 3-second version of the **PASAT.** The battery correlates with the **EDSS,** MRI lesion load, and self-reported quality of life.[4846]

Multiple Sclerosis Rating scale   A system for quantitating the findings noted on physical evaluation of patients with **multiple sclerosis.**[5191]

Multiple Sclerosis Association of America   A nation wide nonprofit health agency providing patient and educational services and research support. Address: 706 Haddonfield Rd., Cherry Hill, NJ 08002. Tel: 856-488-4500 800-532-7667; E-mail: msaa@msaa.com. Web site: http://www.msaa.com/.

Multiple Sclerosis Clinical and Laboratory Research A subspecialty journal published by Arnold. Web site: http://www.arnoldpublishers.com/journals/pages/mul_scl/13524585.htm.

Multiple Sclerosis Foundation   A charitable organization in this field. Address: 6350 North Andrews Ave., Ft. Lauderdale, FL 33309. Tel: 954-776-6805; 888-673-6287. E-mail: support@msfocus.org. Web site: http://www.msfocus.org/.

Multiple Sclerosis Society of Canada   A charitable organization dedicated to enhancing the quality of life of people coping with multiple sclerosis. Address: 2550 Argentia Rd., Suite 230, Mississauga, ON, Canada, L59 7N8. Tel: 1-888-CMSA; 905 812-3511. Web site: http://www.mssociety.ca/.

multiple sclerosis stages   Arbitrary gradings of multiple sclerosis according to the temporal pattern of the disease.

1. Stable multiple sclerosis
2A. Infrequent relapses (less than 1/year)
2B. Slowly progressive (deterioration in expanded disability status scale of <0.5/year)
3A. Frequent clinical relapses (more than one attack/year)
3B. Rapidly progressive (deterioration in expanded disability status scale of >0.5/year)

multiple sensory neuritis   See **Wartenberg sensory neuritis.**

Multiple Sleep Latency Test   (MSLT) A standardized test of sleepiness carried out in a sleep laboratory by day, in which the subject is allowed to fall asleep but is awakened shortly after each successful attempt; the latency to the onset of sleep is measured on each occasion while the usual parameters assessed during **polysomnography** are recorded. The test is of value in determining the premature onset of rapid eye movement sleep in patients with narcolepsy.[927] See also **maintenance of wakefulness test.**

multiple sulfatase deficiency (Austin disease) A rare, recessively inherited metabolic disorder (a *variant* of **metachromatic leukodystrophy**), due to the deficiency of expression of at least seven distinct lysosomal sulfatases. Deficiency of arylsulfatases A, B, and C, as well as of other enzymes, leads to the accumulation of sulfatides, sphingolipids, glycolipids, and other substances in the tissues and body fluids.

Clinical phenotypes resemble either **mucopolysaccharidoses** with the addition of ichthyosis, hypotonia and later hypertonia, minor ataxia, myoclonus, sensorineural deafness, pigmentary abnormality of the macula, optic atrophy, cerebellar and pyramidal signs, and mental and developmental delay; or they resemble **metachromatic leukodystrophy** (late infantile form).[267]

multiple symmetric lipomatosis (Madelung disease) A rare sporadic or inherited mitochrondriopathy presenting in adult life, characterized by the development of multiple lipomas of the neck and shoulder regions, frequently associated with peripheral neuropathy, proximal myopathy, and/or deafness.[4044] See **familial multiple symmetrical lipomatosis with peripheral neuropathy.**

multiple system atrophy A term introduced by Graham and Oppenheimer in 1969 to include all of the adult-onset degenerative conditions of unknown cause showing selective involvement of various combinations of defined nuclei and long tracts within the CNS, as first described by Déjèrine and Thomas in 1900. Such structures have included the retinas; the optic, thalamic, and pyramidal pathways; the cerebellar cortex and deep nuclei; the inferior olives; the vestibular nuclei; the posterior columns; the spinocerebellar and spinothalamic tracts; and the anterior horn cells.

Clinically, any combination of extrapyramidal, pyramidal, cerebellar, and autonomic features may occur, and both gaze palsies and other disturbances of eye movements are described, as has the phenotype of **amyotrophic lateral sclerosis.**[5165] Onset is usually after the age of 45 years. The response to L-dopa is transient and incomplete.

Pathologically, the hallmarks of the conditions are the distribution of the lesions in the olivopontocerebellar, pyramidal, and striatonigral systems and in the nuclei of Onuf, innervating the external sphincter muscles; the presence of argyrophilic intracellular cytoplasmic and nuclear inclusions in oligodendrocytes, neuronal cell bodies, and axons; and the absence of

neurofibrillary tangles and (usually) of Lewy bodies. The cellular pathology has been reviewed.[3275]

The **olivopontocerebellar atrophies,**[1346] **striatonigral degeneration,**[37] and the **Shy-Drager syndrome**[5148] are all subsumed under this general heading. The characteristics of the two major forms have been summarized as follows:[4560]

Striatonigral degeneration type (predominant parkinsonism) Sporadic, adult-onset parkinsonism, nonresponsive or poorly responsive to L-dopa, without dementia, but manifesting down-gaze progressive supranuclear palsy with severe symptomatic autonomic failure, with or without cerebellar or pyramidal signs and areflexia. The features distinguishing this from other causes of the parkinsonian syndrome include the presence of autonomic symptoms, the occurrence of falls, a poor response to levadopa, the presence of speech or bulbar dysfunction and the absence of dementia and of levadopa-induced confusion.[5917]

Olivopontocerebellar atrophy type (predominantly cerebellar) A sporadic, adult-onset cerebellar and/or pyramidal syndrome with severe symptomatic autonomic failure and/or parkinsonism, manifest by mild bradykinesia or rigidity.

Diagnostic criteria for these two types have been suggested.[4560]

Striatonigral Degeneration	Degree	Olivopontocerebellar Atrophy
Sporadic onset, non-poorly responsive parkinsonism	Possible	—
The above + severe symptomatic autonomic failure ± cerebellar ± autonomic signs	Probable	Sporadic adult-onset cerebellar ± pyramidal syndrome with severe symptomatic autonomic failure and/or parkinsonism
Postmortem confirmation	Definite	Postmortem confirmation

In each case, autonomic failure is defined as postural syncope or presyncope and/or marked urinary incontinence or retention not due to other causes.

(From Quinn N. Multiple system atrophy—the nature of the beast. J. Neurol. Neurosurg. Psychiatry 1989; supplement:78–89, by kind permission.)

More recently, consensus criteria for the diagnosis of multiple system atrophy (MSA) have been defined (see Chart M–22).[2123]

Chart M–22. Criteria for the Diagnosis of Multiple System Atrophy

In this outline of clinical domains, features, and criteria used in the diagnosis of MSA, a feature (A) is a characteristic of the disease and a criterion (B) is a defining feature or composite of features required for diagnosis.

  I. *Autonomic and urinary dysfunction*
    A. Autonomic and urinary features
      1. Orthostatic hypotension (by 20 mmHg systolic or 10 mmHg diastolic)
      2. Urinary incontinence or incomplete bladder emptying
    B. Criterion for autonomic failure or urinary dysfunction in MSA

Orthostatic fall in blood pressure (by 30 mmHg systolic or 15mm Hg diastolic) *or* urinary incontinence (persistent, involuntary partial, or total bladder emptying, accompanied by erectile dysfunction in men) *or* both

II. *Parkinsonism*
   A. Parkinsonian features
      1. Bradykinesia (slowness of voluntary movement with progressive reduction in speed and amplitude during repetitive actions)
      2. Rigidity
      3. Postural instability (not caused by primary visual, vestibular, cerebellar, or proprioceptive dysfunction)
      4. Tremor (postural, resting, or both)
   B. Criterion for parkinsonism in MSA
      Bradykinesia plus at least one of items 2 to 4

III. *Cerebellar dysfunction*
   A. Cerebellar features
      1. Gait ataxia (wide-based stance with steps of irregular length and direction)
      2. Ataxic dysarthria
      3. Limb ataxia
      4. Sustained gaze-evoked nystagmus
   B. Criterion for cerebellar dysfunction in MSA
      Gait ataxia plus at least one of items 2 to 4

IV. *Corticospinal tract dysfunction*
   A. Corticospinal tract features
      1. Extensor plantar responses with hyperreflexia
   B. Corticospinal tract dysfunction in MSA: no corticospinal tract features are used in defining the diagnosis of MSA

Diagnostic Categories of Multiple System Atrophy

   I. *Possible MSA*: one criterion plus two features from separate other domains. When the criterion is parkinsonism, a poor levodopa response qualifies as one feature (hence only one additional feature is required).
   II. *Probable MSA*: criterion for autonomic failure/urinary dysfunction plus poorly levodopa responsive parkinsonism or cerebellar dysfunction.
   III. *Definite MSA*: pathologically confirmed by the presence of a high density of glial cytoplasmic inclusions in association with a combination of degenerative changes in the nigrostriatal and olivopontocerebellar pathways.

Exclusion Criteria for the Diagnosis of Multiple System Atrophy

   I. *History*
      Symptomatic onset under 30 years of age
      Family history of a similar disorder
      Systemic diseases or other identifiable causes for features listed in Chart M–21
      Hallucinations unrelated to medication
   II. *Physical examination*
      DSM criteria for dementia
      Prominent slowing of vertical saccades or vertical supranuclear gaze palsy
      Evidence of focal cortical dysfunction such as aphasia, alien limb syndrome, and parietal dysfunction

   III. *Laboratory investigation*
      Metabolic, molecular genetic, and imaging evidence of an alternative cause of features.

In a further *variant* form, the progression of the disease to death is rapid.[5165]

Adapted from Gilman S, Low PA, Quinn N, et al. Consensus statement on the diagnosis of multiple system atrophy. J. Aut. Nerv. Syst. 1998;74:189–92, with permission from Elsevier Science.

multiple-contracture syndrome.   See **multiple congenital contractures.**

multiple-spike complex   (polyspike complex) A sequence of two or more spikes recorded on the EEG.

multiple-step hypometric saccades   Refixations of the eye upon a target requiring more than two saccadic steps. This is occasionally present in normal subjects when fatigued but is always abnormal if dominantly present in one or other direction. In such cases, pyramidal or cerebellar disease may be the cause.

multiple-step saccadic refixations   Eye movements composed of multiple dynamic steps and pulses (**saccades**).

multiple-tic syndrome   See **Tourette syndrome.**

multiplex   (Lat, plaited or folded many times) A derivation ill employed within the term *mononeuritis multiplex*, in which nothing of the sort happens.

multisensory syndrome   The effect of a mismatch between the visual, vestibular, and proprioceptive inputs informing subjects about their orientation in space, occurring as a result of disease affecting any two or all of them; thus a form of physiological vertigo.

Clinically, it is a condition characterized by the sensation of severe imbalance occurring as a result of deficits in conscious or unconscious proprioception, visual acuity, peripheral vision, dark adaptation, contrast sensitivity, and accommodative capacity, usually seen in elderly people.[1511]

multisystem atrophies   A heterogeneous group of diseases characterized by cell loss and variable amounts of gliosis occurring in one or more neuronal groups.[2950,4249] See **system degenerations.**

multisystem disorder with cerebellar atrophy   A recessively inherited syndrome with adult onset, characterized by ophthalmoplegias, cerebellar and pyramidal signs, athetosis, anterior horn cell involvement, and sensory and autonomic neuropathy. See **multi-system atrophies.**

multisystem mitochondrial cytopathy   A rare syndrome consisting of ophthalmoplegia, pigmentary retinal degeneration, cardiac lesions, and dystonias.[272]

multisystem neuronal degeneration   A syndrome of infancy characterized by pigmentary retinal degeneration, optic atrophy, failure to thrive, nerve deafness, progressive distal muscular atrophy with adrenal cortical hormone deficiency, hepatosplenomegaly, and mental and developmental retardation. Tissues show a consistent reduction in the contents of arachnidonic acid and other polyunsaturated fatty acids, but not of phytanic acid.

The syndrome resembles **adrenoleukodystrophy,** but that condition is not apparent at birth, tends to have a defined subacute onset, and is unassociated with retinitis pigmentosa, deafness, or hepatosplenomegaly. Generalized **gangliosidosis** is ruled out by finding an absence of deposited gangliosides, and phytanic acid levels are normal, thus excluding **Refsum disease.**[1581]

multisystem triglyceride storage disorder   A recessively inherited congenital dysmorphic syndrome due to a defect in the degradation of endocellularly synthesized triglycerides; a neutral lipid storage disorder.

Clinically it is characterized by microcephaly, short stature, lordosis, enlarged liver and spleen, vacuolated granulocytes, ichthyosis, diffuse depigmentation of the skin, proximal lipid storage myopathy, neurogenic atrophy, and mental and motor delay.[1439]

Nystagmus, retinopathy, opacities of the lens and corneas, and nerve deafness are other features described. The underlying biochemical deficit is not yet determined.

Mulvihill progeria-like syndrome   A congenital dysmorphic syndrome characterized by thinness, short stature, sparse fine hair, metopic ridges, sensorineural deafness, myopia, premature aging, micrognathia, dental anomalies, wide-spaced nipples, hypospadias and small penis, diabetes, deficient adipose tissue, hypohidrosis, skin atrophy and telangiectasia, microcephaly, bulbar weakness, and mental and developmental delay.[337]

Munchausen syndrome   (hospital addiction, peregrinating problem patient syndrome, chronic factitious disorder with physical symptoms). The repetitive, factitious simulation of severe organic disease leading to numerous hospital consultations, admissions, and unnecessary operations. The patients also give false names, addresses, occupations, and histories. When recognized, or when apparently bored with their hospital experience, they discharge themselves, usually against forceful medical advice if their operation was recent. Their underlying motives have been listed as a desire to be the center of interest, a grudge against physicians and hospitals which is satisfied by such deceptions, a desire for drugs, a desire to escape from the police, and a need for board and lodging.

The title has literary allusions. Henri **Meige** was actually the first to describe the syndrome, in his graduation thesis (University of Paris, 1893) but it was Dr. Richard Asher[238] who defined the condition recently and dedicated the syndrome to Karl Friedreich Hieronymous, Baron Munchhausen (1720–1797), whose dramatic accounts of his exploits as an army captain serving with the Russian army against the Turks in the 1763–1772 war were similarly fabulous; it was thought that, at times, he seemed to lie merely for the sake of lying, according to the German writer and geologist Rudolph Erich Raspe in his fictional work, *Baron Munchausen's Narrative of his Marvellous Travels and Campaigns in Russia* (London, 1785), published without the consent of the (real) Baron Munchhausen (sic).

Asher defined three varieties of the syndrome: the acute abdominal type (*laparotomophilia migrans*), which is the most common; the hemorrhagic type; and the neurological type, this last type presenting with complaints of paroxysmal headache, loss of consciousness, or peculiar fits. He noted the consistent pattern of behavior, with no obvious motive nor gain from it, but found no consistent psychiatric abnormality. The syndrome can also occur by proxy, as when a parent claims that a child has symptoms and may go on to contaminate samples collected and repeatedly presents the child for medical attention, while there is recovery when the child is separated from that parent ot guardian.[3797]

Munchmeyer, Ernst   (1846–1880) German physician who first described **myositis ossificans,**[4042] although "a woman who has become as hard as wood" was mentioned by a Dr. Patin in a letter to Dr. Falret, a physician in Troyes, in 1648.[5047]

Munchmeyer syndrome   See **myositis ossificans.**

Munch-Petersen encephalomyelitis   See **Redlich encephalitis.** Dr. Carl Julius Munch-Petersen was a Danish physician who described this form of encephalomyelitis in 1932.

Munich Coma scale   A tool for the assessment of behavioral arousal (or depth of coma) using two additive scales that measure *susceptibility to stimulation* by electrical, tactile, acoustic and optical stimuli, and *reactivity*, for which motor, mimic, orienting, and communicative movements are assessed. Verbal responses are not examined.[749]

Despite the sensitivity of this instrument, the **Glasgow Coma scale** has been utilized more widely.

Munk, Hermann   German anatomist who suggested the presence of a postrolandic sensory cortex in 1868.

Munson sign.   Protrusion of the lower lid on downward gaze as a result of pressure from **keratoconus.**

Munzer-Rosenthal syndrome   See **Rosenthal syndrome.**

Muratov syndrome   Hemichorea following a cerebrovascular episode, the lesions being in the mesencephalon and thalamus.[4047]

Murdoch syndrome   A congenital dysmorphic syndrome characterized by sensorineural deafness, telecanthus, hypertelorism, colobomas and atrophy of the iris, detached retina, myopia, antimongolian slant, dental enamel abnormalities, inguinal hernia, recurrent infections, seizures, and mental and developmental delay.[337]

Murray valley encephalitis (Australian X disease) Direct infection of the brain (polioencephalitis) by a flavivirus member of the togavirus class of arboviruses occurring endemically in Victoria (Australia) and New Guinea. The clinical features resemble those of Japanese encephalitis.[460,1056]

Murri, Augusto (1841–1932) Italian physician.

Murri syndrome A generalized parenchymatous cerebellar atrophy of late adult onset, presenting with slowly progressive signs of vermis involvement and probably caused by chronic alcohol abuse in the original cases reported.[4050]

muscae volitantes Vitreous floaters, composed of collagen fibrils and leading to the perception of specks drifting around in the visual field, lagging behind but restituting in position after a voluntary eye movement.

Unlike some other phenomena pertinent to aging, these are benign. See **floaters.**

muscle (dim. of Lat, a little mouse) The contractile organ of the body.

Muscle & Nerve (Muscle Nerve) A specialist scientific journal published monthly since 1977 by John Wiley and Sons. The journal has been adopted as the official organ of the **American Association of Electrodiagnostic Medicine** and publishes original contributions in the field of neuromuscular disease with an emphasis on electrodiagnosis. Address: John Wiley and Sons, 111 River Street, Hoboken, NJ 07030. Web site: http://www.interscience.wiley.muscleandnerve/.

muscle action potential See **compound muscle action potential.**

muscle aplasia The congenital absence of certain muscles or groups of muscles. Syndromes include the absence of the glutei, the thenar muscles, the trapezii, and the pectoralis major, either alone (**Poland anomaly**) or with the absence of the serratus and latissimus dorsi (a dominantly inherited syndrome).[335] See **Souques syndrome, thenar hypoplasia.**

muscle atrophy Reduction in the size or number of the myofibrils, and thus of the fascicles within muscles, as a result of disuse or disease.

muscle carnitine palmitoyl transferase deficiency (CPTase deficiency) A myopathy characterized by cramps and myoglobinuria, usually related to exercise but also induced by fasting or a high-fat diet, and due to a defect in the utilization of the long-chain fatty acids by skeletal muscle resulting from a deficiency of muscle CPTase.[1451]

muscle cramps Painful involuntary contractions of muscles, usually associated with electrical activity (cramp discharge). Muscle cramps may be accompanied by other types of repetitive discharges, and, in some metabolic myopathies such as McArdle disease (a glycogen storage disease), the painful contracted muscle may show **electrical silence.**[146]

muscle cramp syndrome A dominantly inherited syndrome charcaterized by neurogenic muscle cramps at rest, in sleep, and with exertion.[1010]

muscle disease See **myopathies** for general classification.

muscle, eye, brain disease (MEB disease, Santavuori syndrome) A congenital, recessively inherited dysmorphic syndrome characterized by anterior chamber and lens abnormalities, glaucoma, optic atrophy, choroidal and retinal hypoplasia with colobomas, myopia, seizures, pendular nystagmus, distal myopathic weakness, cerebral atrophy, and hydrocephalus. The mutant gene is mapped to 1p32–p34.

See also **Fukuyama congenital muscular dystrophy**[4913] and **Walker-Warburg syndrome,** both of which are also characterized by congenital muscle dystrophy and cerebral malformations based on migration disorders with differing genetic locations.[1133]

muscle fiber action potential Action potential recorded from a single muscle fiber.

muscle fiber conduction velocity The speed of propagation of a single muscle fiber action potential, usually expressed in meters per second. It is usually less than most nerve conduction velocities, varies with the rate of discharge of the muscle fiber, and requires special techniques for measurement. (From the 2001 Report of the Nomenclature Committee of the American Association of Electromyography and Electrodiagnosis.[10] Used by permission, copyright © 2001, AAEM.)

muscle hypertrophy Enlargement of a muscle due either to an increase in the size of its myofibrils or (pseudohypertrophy) replacement or displacement of the myofibrils by material such as fat or amyloid. Myofibrils increase in size physiologically in response to repetitive, strong voluntary contraction or pathologically as the result of abnormal electrical activity, such as **myotonic** or **complex repetitive discharges.**

muscle pain–fasciculation syndrome See **cramp-fasciculation syndrome.**

muscle phosphofructokinase deficiency See **glycogen storage diseases.**

muscle phosphorylase b kinase deficiency See **glycogen storage diseases.**

muscle quantitation Methods for determining the power of muscle on a prospective basis. These have included the **Medical Research Council scale,** muscle strength myometry using an instrument to measure the voluntary strength of muscle groups, and assessments of motor ability (**Hammersmith Motor Ability score**).[5035] See also **quantitative neuromuscular examination.**

muscle sense The term of Sir Charles **Bell** for *position sense* (proprioception) or *sense of movement* (kinesthesis). These are, however, derived from information transmitted from tendon and joint receptors and not from any receptors within muscles themselves.

muscle stretch reflexes   Reflex muscle contraction in response to a sudden lengthening stimulus. An oblique early description of the phenomenon was provided by Robert **Whytt**. These reflexes were called *tendon reflexes* by Erb in 1875,[1688] who published his paper in a journal edited by Westphal, whose own observations on the knee phenomenon were printed in a paper adjacent to that of Erb. **Gowers** revised this term to *knee jerk*, which is prosaic and restricted but memorable.

The term *deep tendon reflex* is rejected, both because the tendons struck are actually superficial and because the response to afferent discharges emanating from the Golgi tendon organs is actually an inhibition of contraction.

Scales for reflex activity have been designed; see **NINDS myotatic reflex scale.**

muscle tone   (tonus) The constant, slight tension characteristic of healthy muscle which offers a steadily maintained resistance to passive stretching, thus the amount of resistance to passive stretch supplied by muscles. It is recognized by the resistance experienced when the limbs are moved or displaced by the examiner.[2627]

In the case of postural muscles, it is also defined as "the steady contraction of muscles dependent on the activity of spinal reflexes but modifiable by supra-segmental mechanisms, the function of which is the maintenance of posture or postural adaptation" (Sir Charles **Sherrington**).[5120]

In healthy states, tone is related to the inherent elasticity of the muscles, but in disease states it reflects a reduction in supraspinal influences on the reflex arc or is due to damage to the reflex arc itself.

muscle-contraction headache   See **episodic tension-type headache.**

muscle-paretic nystagmus   (myasthenic nystagmus) A form of gaze-evoked nystagmus resulting from abnormal fatigability of the extraocular muscles (as in **myasthenia gravis**), in which a slow drift of the tiring, deviated eyes towards the primary position is corrected by brief saccadic movements resembling genuine nystagmus.[4978]

muscles of fixation   Muscles that stabilize neighboring joints and thus assist in the efficient performance of the contraction of other muscles. See also **agonists, antagonists, synergists.**

muscular atrophy, diabetes mellitus, and ataxia   A rare, dominantly inherited syndrome characterized by the onset in childhood or adolescence of the features listed in the title, together with pigmentary retinal degeneration. The intellect is unaffected and the phytanic acid levels are normal.[4286]

muscular atrophy in cretins   See **Debré-Sémélaigne syndrome.**

muscular dystrophy   Inherited progressive disorders of muscle. Those that are assigned to this heading[6039] are listed in Chart M–25 (Disorders of Muscle; A. Heritable myopathies; 1. Muscular dystrophies).

Unlisted *variants* include *muscular dystrophy (Manitoba) variant*, a recessively inherited muscular dystrophy with onset in early childhood of proximal muscle atrophy and weakness, and **benign X-linked muscular dystrophy** (Waida). See **Becker muscular dystrophy.**

Muscular Dystrophy Association   A charitable organization providing support and information on these conditions. Address: 3300 East Sunrise Dr., Tucson, AZ 85718-3208. Tel: 520-529-2000; 800-572-1717. E-mail: mda@mdausa.org. Web site: http://www.mdausa.org/.

Muscular Dystrophy Association of Canada   A Canadian charitable association in this field. Address: 2345 Yonge St., Ste. 900, Toronto, Ontario, M4P 2E5, Canada. Tel: 416-488-7523. Web site: http://www.mdac.ca/.

Muscular Dystrophy Family Foundation   A charitable organization in this field. Address: 2330 North Meridien St., Indianapolis, IN 46208. Tel: 317-923-6333; 800-544-1213. E-mail: mdff@mdff.org. Web site: http://www.mdff.org/.

Muscular Dystrophy Campaign   Formerly **Muscular Dystrophy Group of Great Britain and Northern Ireland,** a charitable organization and member society of the European Alliance of Muscular Dystrophy Societies. Address: 7-11 Prescott Place, London SW4 6BS, UK.

muscular infarction   A rare complication of diabetes, in which thrombotic occlusive disease of the small muscular arteries of the quadriceps leads to infarction of that muscle.[327]

muscular pain–fasciculation syndrome   A chronic neuromuscular syndrome characterized by muscle aching and burning pain, fasciculations, cramps, fatigue, and occasional paresthesias affecting the legs more than the trunk, girdle muscles, and arms, worsened by physical activity and due to a mild axonal motor neuropathy.[2686]

Musella Foundation for Brain Tumor Research and Information   A charitable organization in this field. Address: 1100 Peninsula Blvd. Hewlett, NY 11557. Tel: 516-295-4740. E-mail: musella@virtualtrials.com. Web site: http://www.virtualtrials.com/.

mushroom myopathy   A subacute syndrome of myopathy caused by mushroom ingestion.[2186]

music   The art or science of arranging sounds in notes and rhythms to give a desired pattern or effect (Jacobs, 1967, quoted by Brust[821]). See also the definitions of Critchley and Henson.[1182]

musical alexia and agraphia Inability to comprehend or reproduce musical notation (as opposed to verbal language); a function still unlateralized as well as inexactly localized, despite the popular belief that receptive amusia follows damage to the language-dominant side and expressive amusia follows nondominant frontal lobe damage.[821]

musical hallucinations Hallucinated music occurring in association with deafness, or with lesions of the brainstem, or of the frontal or temporal regions.[3813]

musician overuse syndrome Painless focal dystonia of the hand occurring as an occupational dystonia.[1972] Strict union regulations prevent overuse of the musicians themselves.

musicogenic epilepsy (musicolepsy, musicolepsia, sonogenic reflex epilepsy, audiogenic epilepsy) A form of reflex epilepsy occurring in young adults who suffer simple or complex partial seizures, more rarely secondary generalized atonic-clonic seizures precipitated by certain musical airs or sometimes by music played by certain combinations of instruments. However, thinking about, remembering, or playing music may also act as precipitant.[1167] The first description has been attributed to Merzjejeuvski, who presented a case in St. Petersburg in 1884.

The seizure may be on either side in this condition (even though music function is considered to be lateralized to the right hemisphere, at least in nonmusicians) and the stimulus may be exquisitely specific; for example, in Sutherling's patient,[5426] the seizures were triggered only by playing a specific hymn on the organ ("Now Thank We All Our God"). Critchley and Henson[1182] reviewed the reports to 1977.

musicolepsia See **musicogenic epilepsy.**

musicolepsy See **musicogenic epilepsy.**

Muskelsvindfonden A member society of the European Alliance of Muscular Dystrophy Societies based at Kongsvang Allé 23, 8000 Aarhus C, Denmark.

Musset sign A rhythmic nodding of the head as a consequence of ballistic (vascular) forces resulting from severe aortic incompetence. The name remembers the French novelist and poet Alfred de Musset (1810–1857), who was thus affected as a result of a syphilitic aortic aneurysm.

Mutchinick syndrome A congenital dysmorphic syndrome characterized by dwarfism, fine hair, hypertelorism, blepharophimosis, antimongolian slant, higharched palate, brachycephaly, microcephaly, spasticity, and mental and developmental delay.[337]

mutilating acropathy See **ulceromutilating acropathy, hereditary sensory and autonomic neuropathy.**

mutism 1. Loss of the power of making sounds with the larynx. 2. Loss of the power of making articulate sounds or speech; absence of verbal output.

mutism and subsequent dysarthria See **cerebellar mutism.**

myalgia Pain arising from muscles, especially following exertion. Pathologies such as tumor, infection, ischemia, or infarction are important causes, but for neurologists, **polymyositis** and other inflammatory diseases of muscle such as **polymyalgia rheumatica,** and almost all metabolic muscle diseases such as **cramps, chronic fatigue syndrome, lipid myopathy, myalgia cruris epidemica, myoadenylate deaminase deficiency, glycogen storage disease, mitochondrial encephalomyopathy,** and **hypothyroid myopathy** are of particular interest.

A *variant* is *exercise-induced pain, stiffness, and tubular aggregations in skeletal muscle* with a persistent elevation of the serum creatine kinase levels but normal EMG and forearm ischemic exercise test results. A muscle biopsy specimen shows aggregations of tubular structures in most fibers.[813]

myalgia cruris epidemica See **benign acute childhood myositis.**

myalgic encephalomyelitis See **postinfection fatigue syndrome, chronic fatigue syndrome.**

myasthenia (Lat, muscle + debility). Muscle fatigability.

myasthenia gravis (Erb-Goldflam syndrome) An autoimmune disorder, more common in women, in which antibodies to the acetylcholine motor end-plate receptors (AChR) lead to their loss of structure and function. The pathogenic effects on neuromuscular transmission are mediated by antibody-induced antigenic modulation of end-plate AChR, end-plate membrane destruction through complement fixation and recruitment of inflammatory cells, and antibody-induced blockade of the function of the remaining AChR molecules.

Clinically, it is characterized by impairment of neuromuscular transmission, leading to fluctuating weakness and fatigability of, in order of severity, the ocular, bulbar and limb muscles. The deficit is lessened by cooling and increased with warmth,[665] which may be of value during electrical testing. See also **ice-pack test.**

The generalized *adult* form is that generally recognized; it was described in an Amerindian in 1644 and by Thomas **Willis** in 1672,[5988] but the first modern descriptions were those of **Erb**[1690,1691] and of Sir Samuel Wilks (1824–1911), who described the manifestations as part of a treatise on bulbar paralysis in 1877.[5975]

Two subgroups are differentiated: a *severe* (or even *acute fulminating*) type, most common among young women, is associated with the HLA8 antigen; and another form, occurring mainly among older patients, is associated with thymoma and with the presence of the HLA2 or A3 antigens.

Physostigmine, the first effective treatment, was introduced by Dr. Mary Walker, an intern at St. Alfege's

Hospital, Greenwich, who tried it in a 56-year-old woman with myasthenia, having discussed the similarity of myasthenia and curare poisoning with the visiting neurologist, Dr. **Denny Brown.** She published the result as a letter in *Lancet*[5810] (cited by Keynes[3028]).[4678]

A classification of the types of acquired autoimmune myasthenia gravis has been suggested[5753] and is reproduced with adaptation in Chart M–23. It may be noted, however, that different forms may occur in the same family.

Chart M–23. Classification of Acquired Autoimmune Myasthenia Gravis

Adult form as above

Familial myasthenia gravis (recessive form) A form characterized by strabismus; ptosis; enlarged thymus; ophthalmoplegias; and facial, distal, and proximal myopathic weakness and fatigability with onset before the age of 2 years. In a similar form with later onset (2–20 years) there is no recognizable pattern of inheritance.[834]

Myasthenia gravis and dystonia with diurnal fluctuation A form characterized by congenital ptosis, ophthalmoplegias, dystonia, tremor, and muscle fatigability.

Chronic limb-girdle myasthenia gravis An uncommon form presenting in adult life with limb-girdle weakness and fatigability without ocular or bulbar involvement and in patients without a positive family history.[4215]

Other variants of the syndrome include the following:

A. *Heritable varieties*

1. *Familial infantile myasthenia gravis* A presynaptic syndrome of myasthenia, inherited as a dominant or recessive trait, and characterized by fluctuating ptosis and ophthalmoplegia; feeding difficulties in infancy; facial, distal, and proximal myopathic weakness and fatigability after exercise; and attacks of apnea precipitated by crying, vomiting, or fever. Enlargement of the thymus and unusually small synaptic vesicles in the nerve terminals are found.[3964,4070] The condition responds to anticholinesterases and may remit in time.

Other presynaptic syndromes include *familial infantile myasthenia with tetanic facilitation* and *congenital Lambert-Eaton syndrome*.[3671]

2. *Congenital myasthenia gravis* A recessively inherited group of myasthenic syndromes occurring in infants, in which antibodies to AChR motor end-plate receptors are absent. Thymectomy, immunosuppression, and plasmapheresis are ineffective and spontaneous remissions do not occur. Presynaptic (impaired resynthesis or packaging of ACh); synaptic (absence of acetylcholinesterase from the end-plate), and postsynaptic (abnormal receptor) varieties are defined. Various mutations are responsible for each. The clinical patterns described include the following (adapted from Beeson et al., 1997).[423]

In the *typical form*, infants are born to nonmyasthenic mothers. The disease resembles the typical postsynaptic form, except that antibodies to ACh motor end plate receptors are absent, the external ocular muscles are prominently involved, and the usual forms of treatment are ineffective. At least three subgroupings are described in this category.[834]

3. *End-plate acetylcholinesterase deficiency* is a postsynaptic form in which acetylcholinesterase is absent or markedly deficient at the neuromuscular junction. It presents in adult life with severe fatigue, weakness, episodes of respiratory distress, refractoriness of anticholinesterases, and repetitive compound motor action potentials in response to a single stimulus.[4224]

In another form, the ophthalmoplegia is mild and nonprogressive, and there is proximal, distal and facial myopathic atrophy and weakness with fatigability. Muscle biopsy specimens show small-group atrophy and fiber-type predominance. Antibodies to ACh motor end-plate receptors are absent and immunosuppressants are ineffective.[1780]

Congenital myasthenia with ptosis, ophthalmoplegia, proximal weakness, and fatigability unresponsive to anticholinesterase agents is yet another clinical pattern.[5635]

In a recessively transmitted *variant*, facial malformations such as prognathism are associated with a postsynaptic neuromuscular transmission defect.[4870]

4. *Juvenile myasthenia gravis* An acquired autoimmune disorder in which circulating antibodies to ACh receptors and complement together reduce the number of functioning ACh receptors available on the motor end-plate, and thus interfere with normal neuromuscular transmission.[180] The clinical features are the same as those in No. 1 above, but with slightly earlier onset.

5. *Myasthenia with familial limb-girdle myopathy (familial limb girdle myasthenia)* A recessively inherited variant presenting in childhood with fatigability and proximal weakness, occasionally complicated by cardiomyopathy.[3790]

6. *Myasthenia gravis with myotonic dystrophy* A form characterized by the presence of myotonia complicating otherwise typical adult myasthenia.

7. **Pseudocholinesterase deficiency** (suxamethonium paralysis)

8. **Congenital end-plate ACh receptor deficiency** A postsynaptic syndrome of myasthenia in which there is a deficiency of ACh receptors because of their abnormal synthesis, reactivity, or degradation.[5767]

9. *Myasthenia with (congenital) end-plate acetylcholinesterase deficiency* A rare, recessively transmitted, postsynaptic disorder characterized by congenital ptosis, kyphoscoliosis, lordosis, and neonatal myopathic distal and proximal weakness, atrophy, and fatigability.[1662,1168,1669] Decrementing responses can be found in all voluntary muscles and, because of the prolonged interactions of ACh and its receptors, a single supramaximal stimulus to a motor nerve eliciting more than one compound muscle action potential.[422]

10. **Slow-channel congenital myasthenic syndrome** A dominantly inherited or sporadic post-synaptic disorder presenting in childhood or young adult life with selective weakness, fatigability, and atrophy of the muscles of the neck, shoulder girdle, and forearms, with variable involvement of the extraocular and other muscles, due to abnormally slow closure of the ACh receptor ion channel.[1670] An acquired form, presenting in adult life, is also described.[6009]

11. *Decrease of the amplitude of the miniature end-plate potential without ACh receptor deficiency* A putative defect in ACh synthesis or packaging.[1662]

12. *Abnormality of synaptic vesicles* with reduction in quantal release.[3961] See *familial infantile myasthenia gravis*, above.

13. *Congenital persistent (neonatal persistent) myasthenia* A syndrome characterized by congenital ptosis, ophthalmoplegia, and distal and proximal myopathic weakness and fatigability.

14. *Infantile myasthenia* A form characterized by ptosis and respiratory distress in the neonate, with muscle fatigability.

15. *ACh receptor channel fast closure* A congenital myasthenic syndrome characterized by ocular and limb weakness and fatigability from birth, with later improvement. High conductance and fast closure of the ACh receptor channel are demonstrable.[1671]

16. *Abnormal interaction between ACh and the ACh receptor*[5678]

17. *Acetylcholine receptor deficiency*[1671] A postsynaptic, recessively inherited form occurring in the neonatal period or in infancy.

18. Presynaptic disorders involving the resynthesis or packaging of Ach.[3966]

19. *High-conductance fast-channel syndrome*[1671] A form recessively inherited and characterized by neonatal onset.

20. *Acetylcholinesterase deficiency* A recessively inherited, neonatal synaptic form in which acetylcholinesterase is absent or markedly deficient at the neuromuscular junction. These forms have been reviewed.[423]

B. *Toxic*
   1. **Botulism**
   2. **Tick paralysis**
   3. **Puffer-fish paralysis** (tetrodotoxin)
   4. Magnesium intoxication
   5. Kanamycin and other antibiotics[3791]
   6. *Myasthenia due to penicillamine* A disorder mimicking idiopathic myasthenia gravis, even to the detection of anti-ACh receptor antibodies, occurring in subjects taking penicillamine.[2036] Anticonvulsants and quinidine have also been implicated as causing the same problem.

C. *Autoimmune*
   1. **Myasthenia gravis** (see above)
      a. *Transient neonatal myasthenia* A form in which the affected infant is born of a woman with myasthenia; within 72 hours of birth, feeding difficulties, generalized weakness, respiratory difficulties, and facial weakness with ptosis are seen, lasting a few days. Pharmacological tests are frequently positive and the condition responds to anticholinesterase medication and respiratory support.[4069]
      b. Ocular myasthenia with peripheral neuropathy and spastic paraparesis[823]
      c. Generalized myasthenia
         i. Severe, especially in young women, correlated with HLA-8
         ii. In older patients, often with thymoma and with HLA-2 or 3
      d. Myasthenia with thyrotoxicosis
      e. Myasthenia with hypothyroidism[5472]
      f. Myasthenia with other autoimmune diseases
      g. Myasthenia combined with **Lambert-Eaton myasthenic syndrome**[4213]
      h. Myasthenia with the **Satoyoshi syndrome**[4922]
D. **Lambert-Eaton syndrome**

ACh, acetylcholine; HLA, human lymphocyte antigen. (After Verma P, Oger J. Treatment of Acquired Autoimmune Myasthenia Gravis. Can. J. Neurol. Sci. 1992;19:360–75,[5753] reproduced by kind permission.

A scale for rating the severity of myasthenia gravis, based on that of Osserman, used five degrees of severity, but a more modern scale has been devised by Jaretzki et al.[2815] These authors also provide a classification of disease severity, based on assessment of 13 single functions.

Myasthenia Gravis Clinical Severity Classification

Class I Any ocular muscle weakness; may have weakness of eye closure but all other muscle strength is normal.

Class II Mild weakness affecting other than ocular muscles. May also have ocular muscle weakness of any severity.

Class IIa Predominantly affecting limb, axial muscles, or both; may also have lesser involvement of oropharyngeal muscles

Class IIb Predominantly affecting oropharyngeal, respiratory muscles, or both. May also have lesser or equal involvement of limb, axial muscles, or both.

Class III Moderate weakness affecting muscles other than ocular muscles; may also have ocular muscle weakness of any severity.

Class IIIa Predominantly affecting limb, axial muscles, or both; may also have lesser involvement of oropharyngeal muscles.

Class IIIb Predominantly affecting oropharyngeal, respiratory muscles, or both; may also have lesser or equal involvement of limb, axial muscles, or both.

Class IV Severe weakness affecting muscles other than ocular muscles; may also have ocular muscle weakness of any severity.

Class IVa Predominantly affecting limb and/or axial muscles; may also have lesser involvement of oropharyngeal muscles.

Class IVb Predominantly affecting oropharyngeal, respiratory muscles, or both; may also have lesser or equal involvement of limb, axial muscles, or both.

Class V Defined by intubation, with or without mechanical ventilation, except when employed during routine postoperative management. The use of a feeding tube without intubation places the patient in class IVb.

From Jaretzki AI, Barohn RJ, Ernstoff RM, et al. Myasthenia Gravis: Recommendations for Clinical Research Standards. *Ann. Thoracic Surg.* 2000;**70**:327–34, reproduced by kind permission.

See also **midbrain myasthenia.**

Myasthenia Gravis Association A charitable organization. Address: Keynes House, Chester Park, Alfreton Road, Derby DE21 4AS, UK. Tel: 01332-290219. Web site: http://www.mgauk.org/.

Myasthenia Gravis Foundation of America, Inc. A voluntary organization dedicated to the conquest of myasthenia through programs of research, education, and information and patient services, including support, diagnostic, and therapeutic services. Address: 5841 Cedar Lake Road, Ste. 204, Minneapolis, MN. Tel: 952-545-9438, 1-800-541-5454. Web site: http://www.myasthenia.org/.

Myasthenia Severity scale A scale for assessing impairment in myasthenic crisis.[4564]

Dyspnea   1 = intubated; 2 = dyspnea at rest;
           3 = dyspnea on exertion; 4 = no dyspnea

Cough   1 = intubated; 2 = weak; 3 = normal

Ocular   1 = weakness at rest; 2 = weakness on fatigue; 3 = none

Bulbar   1 = weakness at rest; 2 = weakness on fatigue; 3 = none

Extremities   1 = worst affected muscle 3/5 or less; 2 = worst affected muscle 4/5 motor strength or weakness on fatigue; 3 = no detectable weakness

myasthenic crisis Abrupt deterioration in strength in a myasthenic patient, due to exacerbation of the defect in neuromuscular transmission, either as a result of the natural progression of the disease or because of the effects of drugs that further reduce the availability of acetylcholine to the end-plate.

myasthenic myopathy 1. The occurrence of fatigability in patients with primary myopathic diseases; the symptoms may be partially responsive to anticholinesterase medication. 2. Persistent proximal weakness and wasting complicating long-standing **myasthenia gravis.**

myasthenic nystagmus An asymmetric gaze-evoked nystagmus that may be in any direction and that is relieved by intravenous edrophonium chloride. See **muscle-paretic nystagmus.**

myasthenic syndrome See **Lambert-Eaton myasthenic syndrome.**

myasthenic syndrome in hypothyroidism A *variant* that may resemble the **Lambert-Eaton myasthenic syndrome** but is considered to be due to conduction block in the fine terminals of the motor axons.[5472]

mycotic aneurysm (septic aneurysm) An aneurysm developing because of weakening of an arterial wall as the result of infection. Bleeding into the substance of the brain or into the subarachnoid space may result. See **aneurysm.**

mydriasis Pupillary dilatation, usually accepted as being >6 mm in diameter. It is due to paresis of the iris by drugs (mydriatics) or disease or is due to emotion.

This use of the word is attributed to Galen, but Areteus used it to refer to pupillary constriction and Hippocrates is said to have used the word *mydros* for the cautery tool that he employed—an instrument likely to produce fear and its attendant sympathetic manifestations. See also **Pourfour du Petit syndrome.**

mydriatic A drug that paralyzes the iris and causes pupillary dilation. Atropinic derivatives, ephedrine, cocaine, and some synthetic agents are examples.

myelencephalon The term of Huxley for **metencephalon.**

myelin (from Gr, marrow) The insulating fatty substance ensheathing axons, so named by Virchow in 1854.

myelin basic protein An immunogenic structural component of myelin; it forms about 40% of the total protein. When injected with Freund's adjuvant into animals, it induces experimental allergic encephalomyelitis, a paralytic disease. There is evidence that it appears in a higher concentration in the blood of multiple sclerosis patients during an exacerbation.

myelin stains Histological enhancement methods that preferentially stain myelin. They include the Weigert-Pal, Spielmeyer, Weil, and Marchi methods, variously employing hematoxylin, osmium tetroxide, Luxol fast blue (a copper-containing dye staining myelin bright blue), and metallic salts with borax ferricyanide, iron alum, lithium, and/or alcohol. See also **axon stains.**

myelin-associated glycoprotein (MAG) A component of myelin, metabolites of which can be detected in the CSF but which cannot be linked to active demyelination. Patients with high serum IgM antibody levels to MAG may present with gait ataxia and polyneuropathy.

myelinated nerve fibers Fibers bearing myelin and also nonmyelinated and demyelinated fibers, the diameter of which is in the range of the normal population of myelinated fibers.[2346] See **medullated (myelinated) nerve fibers.**

myelination The process of myelin accumulation around axons during pre- and postnatal development, and following demyelination.

myelinoclastic disease Conditions in which normally formed myelin is damaged, as opposed to **dysmyelinating** diseases, in which the myelin itself is abnormally constituted.[4500]

myelinopathia centralis diffusa See **vanishing white matter disease.**

myelinopathy A pathological process affecting peripheral nerves in which there is paranodal or segmental demyelination. cf. **neuronopathy, axonopathy.**

myelinosclerosis centralis diffusa See **fatal infantile leukodystrophy.**

myelitis Originally this was defined as "inflammation of the central nervous system with particular effects upon the myelin" (Marshall Hall), but this definition has been discarded in favor of one which regards myelitis as inflammation of the spinal cord only, inflammation of the brain being called **encephalitis** and both together, **encephalomyelitis.**

Classifications have consisted of the following categories: *topical* (transverse, ascending or descending, central, marginal, or funicular), *structural* (poliomyelitis, leukomyelitis), or *etiological*. **Neuromyelitis** indicates the combined involvement of the spinal cord and cranial or peripheral nerves. See **acute intrinsic myelopathy.**

myelitis with predilection or anterior horn cells resembling motor neuron disease A **paraneoplastic syndrome** associated with carcinoma, usually of the lung, breast, or stomach, and manifesting muscle weakness and atrophy with fasciculations and pyramidal signs affecting the bulbar and/or spinal muscles and resembling typical **amyotrophic lateral sclerosis** in everything but a slower course to death.[711]

myelocele   (Gr, marrow + a cavity) A form of failure of closure of the neural tube in which the protruding sac contains meninges and CSF, but no nervous tissue.

myelodysplasia   Developmental abnormalities of the spine and spinal cord. These include **diplomyelia, myeloschisis, hydromyelia, syringomyelia,** and **diastematomyelia.**

myelography   The introduction of a solution of iodinated substances into the subarachnoid space at lumbar levels to outline the extent of the space by radiography as a diagnostic test for intrinsic or extrinsic spinal cord or root disease. This is a useful but unpleasant test, now giving way to MRI scanning where it is available.

myeloma   See **multiple myeloma.**

myelomalacia   Noninflammatory softening of the spinal cord.

myelomeningitis   Inflammation of the spinal cord and the meninges surrounding it.

myelomeningocele   See **meningomyelocele.**

myeloneuropathy   A disorder affecting both the spinal cord and the peripheral nerves or nerve roots. **Tabes dorsalis** was a classic example but other conditions are probably (in aggregate) more prevalent today. See **Cuban** and **Tanzanian epidemic neuropathy, recurrent optic neuromyelitis with endocrinopathy, HTLV-1 myelopathy. Vernant disease,** tuberculous neuropathy, and hemorrhagic fevers are other listed causes.

myelopathic muscular atrophy   See **amyotrophic lateral sclerosis.**

myelopathy   Disease of the spinal cord. See also **progressive necrotic myelopathy; myelitis; myeloneuropathy, pseudocervical cord syndrome.**

myelopathy complicating diabetes mellitus.   See **diabetic myelopathy.**[2107]

myelopathy with optic neuritis   See **neuromyelitis optica.**

myeloplegia   Paralysis resulting from a lesion of the spinal cord.

myeloradiculitis   See **HIV-associated lumbosacral polyradiculopathy.**

myelotomy   See **cordotomy.**

myenteric   (Gr, muscle + the intestines) The smooth muscle in the wall of the intestines.

myenteric plexus   (Gr, myenteric + weaving) Auerbach's plexus of autonomic nerve fibers within the muscular wall of the intestines.

Myerson, Abraham   (1881–1948) Lithuanian-American psychiatrist and neurologist who trained at Tufts University and became professor of neurology and of psychiatry at Harvard. Most of his major publications were on psychiatric topics but he is remembered for the following signs.

Myerson reflex   Contraction of the biceps and pectoralis on both sides or only on the opposite side, when the clavicle is tapped. The reflex is present in patients with pyramidal lesions.[4052]

Myerson sign   See **orbicularis oculi reflex.**

myesthesia   Muscle sense; the sense of the position of the parts of the body as a result of afferent impulses from muscle receptors and thus a form of proprioception.

Myhre syndrome   (growth deficiency–clefting–retardation) A congenital dysmorphic syndrome characterized by muscular build, high birth weight, short stature, cleft upper lip, cleft palate, platyspondyly, constrictive pericarditis, thick ribs, duodenal ulcers, hypoplastic iliae, hypospadias, cryptorchidism, arthropathy, deafness, hypermetropia, spina bifida occulta, thick calvarium, muscle hypertrophy, facial weakness, and mental and developmental delay.[337]

myo-   Greek prefix signifying relationship with muscle.

myoadenylate deaminase   (MADA) A muscle enzyme responsible for catalyzing the deamination of adenosine monophosphate, producing energy and ammonia.

myoadenylate deaminase deficiency syndrome (MADD) A common familial or acquired metabolic myopathy resulting from myoadenylate deaminase deficiency. It is often asymptomatic, but in some cases is expressed clinically as a syndrome of muscle pain, cramp, and fatigue induced by exercise, sometimes with fixed proximal weakness and wasting, hyporeflexia, paresthesia, and repeated infections in childhood or young adult life.[773] Using the ishemic forearm test, serum ammonia levels increase absolutely by 100 μg/dl in normals, and by less than this amount in those with MADD. The lactate/ammonia ratio is high in this condition but low in the glycogenoses.

The *acquired form* is associated with a range of other muscle disorders. Adenosine monophosphate deaminase activity is undetectable in the muscle biopsy specimens of such patients.[1456]

myoatrophy   Muscle atrophy; a more proper but less euphonious term than amyotrophy.

myoclonia   (Gr, muscle + confused motion) Intermittent convulsive jerks of muscles. See **myoclonus.**

myoclonic absence attacks   (clonic absence attacks) An epileptic syndrome characterized by rhythmic jerks occurring at 3 Hz throughout the body, but most obviously seen in the shoulder girdle, frequently leading to elevation of the arms and backward tilting of the head. The attacks occur in infancy, childhood, or youth, and are accompanied by 3-Hz spike-and-wave discharges on the EEG. Mental deterioration is a feature in some patients. See **myoclonus.**

myoclonic astatic seizures (akinetic seizures, static seizures, minor motor epilepsy, propulsive petit mal, akinetic petit mal, severe myokinetic epilepsy of childhood with slow spike-and-wave) A syndrome of the first 3 years of life, characterized by refractory atonic or akinetic (minor motor) seizures that are increased in the drowsy state by myoclonus and by mental and developmental delay. The last may be due to static encephalopathy. The EEG typically records background theta activity and slow (2–4 Hz) spike–wave activity between seizures, and generalized multiple spike–wave bursts during them.[4207] See **Lennox-Gastaut syndrome.** See also **myoclonus, myoclonic epilepsies, absence seizures.**

myoclonic dystonia Unusual irregular, tremor-like dystonic movements of subcortical origin, lasting 50–200 msec, often superimposed upon sustained dystonic contractions. Time-locked EEG discharges do not precede the movements.[4187] See also **hereditary myoclonic dystonia, dystonia.**

myoclonic encephalopathy A collection of cerebral diseases in which myoclonus occurs. Mitochondrial encephalopathies, malabsorption syndromes, multiplesystem atrophy, and the various causes of the **Ramsay-Hunt syndrome** are examples.

myoclonic encephalopathy of infancy (infantile polymyoclonia, dancing eyes syndrome, dancing eyes–dancing feet, opsoclonus, ataxic conjugate movements of the eyes, Kinsbourne-Warrington syndrome) A generalized, recurrent but nonprogressive, self-limiting, and benign myoclonic disorder of late infancy. Clinical features of diagnostic value include the acute onset of opsoclonus and somatic myoclonus (especially of the trunk and head) in a previously normal infant, often following a minor infection or complicating aseptic meningitis. The condition runs a fluctuating but protracted course, but may remit with steroid therapy.[1585,3052] No laboratory abnormalities are found. See **opsoclonus.**

In *variant* forms, the condition is associated with **neuroblastoma**[5845] or with progressive cranial nerve palsies.

myoclonic encephalopathy with progressive cranial nerve palsies See **Unverricht-Lundborg-Lafora syndrome.**

myoclonic epilepsies (myoclonic astatic epilepsy) Seizure syndromes of infancy and childhood characterized by various types of tonic, atonic, and myoclonic seizures, leading to repeated falls. The condition is resistant to therapy. See **early myoclonic epilepsy, benign myoclonic epilepsy in infants, severe myoclonic epilepsy in infants, myoclonic absences,**[5495] **juvenile**

myoclonic epilepsy of Janz, Unverricht-Lundberg-Lafora syndrome.

The term is considered by some to be interchangeable with **Lennox-Gastaut syndrome.**

myoclonic epilepsy of adolescents See **juvenile myoclonic epilepsy.**

myoclonus epilepsy with Lafora bodies See **myoclonus.**

myoclonic epilepsy with ragged-red fibers (Fukuhara syndrome)[1984] See **MERRF,** and also **mitochondrial diseases.**

myoclonic epilepsy with supranuclear ophthalmoplegia See **myoclonus.**

myoclonic ocular jerks See **ocular myoclonus.**

myoclonic seizures A seizure state in which EMG records during the attacks show biphasic or polyphasic potentials, lasting between 20 and 100 msec, followed by a tonic contraction of the affected muscles or by a transient suppression of normal tonic activity lasting up to 350 msec; EEG findings include generalized burst or polyspike-and-waves or spike–wave activity.[56]

myoclonic status epilepticus See **status epilepticus.**

myoclonic triangle That part of the brainstem bounded by the inferior olivary nuclei, the cerebellar dentate nucleus, and the red nucleus, with their interconnection in the central tegmental tract and the superior and inferior cerebellar peduncles. The term recognizes that lesions of any of these structures may give rise to ocular (and sometimes to reticular) **myoclonus.**[2318] See **Guillain-Mollaret triangle.**

myoclonic variant of Lennox-Gastaut syndrome A form of the syndrome in which the frequency and intensity of the myoclonic jerks are both unusually high. The EEG is typical, except that it is activated by overbreathing.[56] See **Lennox-Gastaut syndrome.**

myoclonic writer's cramp The occurrence of repetitive myoclonic jerks precipitated by writing.[4611]

myoclonique de la calotte See **palatal myoclonus.**

myoclonus Sudden regular or irregular brief, jerky, or shock-like involuntary contractions of muscle fibers, muscles, or muscle groups, as a manifestation of hyperexcitability in the nervous system at any level between the cerebral cortex and the spinal cord, and unassociated with alteration in consciousness.

The term derives from **Friedreich** in 1881, who called such movements "paramyoklonus multiplex." Two major subdivisions of myoclonus are defined, according to whether or not the movements are fragments of an epileptic syndrome. *Epileptic myoclonus* is said to be focal, elicited by stimuli, accompanied by large somatosensory evoked potentials and enhancement of long-loop reflexes, and responsive to anticonvulsants. *Cortical reflex myoclonus* is considered to represent a fragment of partial epilepsy; *reticular reflex myoclonus* and *primary generalized epileptic myoclonus* are fragments of types of **generalized epilepsy.** *Nonepileptic myoclonus* consists of massive spontaneous bodily jerks, with normal somatosensory evoked potentials and long-loop reflexes and with a poor response to anticonvulsants.[3773]

Using an anatomical basis for classification, **spinal/propriospinal, segmental, brainstem-reticular,** and **cortical** forms are defined. *Essential myoclonus* is the term used when none of the above appear appropriate. The existence of *psychogenic myoclonus* attests to the astounding variety of responses of the stressed human.

Positive myoclonus refers to abnormal involuntary movements produced by single motor units or groups of motor units discharging synchronously but not rhythmically for about 100 msec in many or all of the muscles of a limb. *Negative myoclonus* (**asterixis**) is also described. The electrical characteristics of myoclonus have been reviewed.[5128]

Myoclonus may also be classified according to whether it is triggered by stimuli (**stimulus-sensitive [reflex] myoclonus**) or is spontaneous (**on-stimulus–sensitive myoclonus**)[2385] or again by whether it is *rhythmic* (see **palatal** and **ocular myoclonus**), *oscillatory* (see **ballistic movement overflow myoclonus**), or *arrhythmic* (most forms). The palatal form, characterized by fast-recurring, small-amplitude movements of the palate, probably represents **myokymia.** See also **photomyogenic response.**

A listing of forms of myoclonus is presented in Chart M–24.

Chart M–24. Causes of Myoclonus

1. *Epileptic myoclonus* Myoclonic syndromes in which rapid bursts of action potentials occur as neurons discharge synchronously, detectable as spikes on the EEG. The EMG burst length associated with the muscle jerk is usually <50 msec; muscles active in the same jerk are activated synchronously and an EEG correlate can be identified.[2384] Such epileptic myoclonic syndromes include the following:
   a. *Fragments of epilepsy*
      Isolated epileptic myoclonic jerks
      Epilepsia partialis continua
      Idiopathic stimulus-sensitive myoclonus
      Photosensitive myoclonus and myoclonic absences in petit mal
      Cortical reflex myoclonus
      Reticular reflex myoclonus
      Photic reflex myoclonus
      Primary generalized epileptic myoclonus
      Unverricht-Lundborg-Lafora syndrome
   b. *Childhood myoclonic epilepsies*
      Benign myoclonus of infancy (cryptogenic myoclonic epilepsy[56]) An idiopathic syndrome characterized by the onset in the first year or two of life of myoclonic and generalized tonic-clonic seizures that disappear in adolescence. The affected children are otherwise neurologically unimpaired; but the EEG shows spike/polyspike-and-wave activity.[4740]

Severe myoclonus of infancy An idiopathic syndrome characterized by the onset in the first year of life of myoclonic and clonic seizures with progressive neurological deterioration. The EEG shows spike/polyspike-and-wave activity.[4740] See also **neonatal myoclonic encephalopathy.**
      West syndrome (Infantile spasms)
      Myoclonic astatic epilepsy (**Lennox-Gastaut syndrome**)
      Myoclonic astatic epilepsy of early childhood An idiopathic syndrome characterized by the onset in the first 5 years of life with myoclonic, astatic, absence, and generalized tonic-clonic seizures. The affected children are neurologically unimpaired at onset, but the prognosis is variable. The EEG shows spike/polyspike-and-wave activity.[1496]
      Early myoclonic encephalopathy An idiopathic, probably recessively inherited syndrome characterized by the onset in the first month of life with massive myoclonic seizures, progressing to infantile spasms during the first 6 months of life.[56]
      Myoclonic absences A syndrome with onset in childhood or youth, characterized by absence attacks with myoclonus, associated in some cases with progressive intellectual decline. The EEG shows 3-Hz spike-and-wave discharges.[5495]
      juvenile myoclonic epilepsy (of Janz) A syndrome with onset in youth, characterized by myoclonic and generalized tonic or tonic-clonic seizures, especially upon waking from sleep. The EEG typically shows polyspike and wave discharges.
   c. **Benign familial myoclonic epilepsy** (Rabot)
   Other *variant forms* include the following:
   Myoclonus and chorea A syndrome of infancy or childhood characterized by myoclonic seizures, cerebellar ataxia and chorea.[3197]
   Myoclonus, deafness, and cerebellar ataxia A syndrome of childhood characterized by sensorineural deafness, cerebellar ataxia, and myoclonus. See **May-White syndrome.**[3715]
   Myoclonus-dystonia A dominantly inherited syndrome characterized by myoclonic and dystonic muscle contractions, mainly of the neck and arms, in the absence of other signs of neurological disease and with a relatively benign course. The movements are often responsive to alcohol. The condition has been mapped to 7q21–q31.[4182] Obsessive-compulsive disorder and alcohol dependence may also be associated.[4930]
   Familial chorea with myoclonic epilepsy An apparent association of these two syndromes.[5471]
   Myoclonus epilepsy with Lafora bodies A degenerative disease with onset in childhood or youth, manifesting dysarthria, dementia, seizures and myoclonus, cerebellar ataxia and spasticity, and neuronal inclusions (Lafora bodies).
   Myoclonus epilepsy with supranuclear ophthalmoplegia A rare, recessively inherited syndrome of ataxia followed years later by epilepsy, myoclonus, mild dementia, and supranuclear ophthalmoplegia. Pigmentary retinopathy has also occurred in this condition.[3458]
   Myoclonic epilepsy with signs of spinal muscular atrophy
2. *Nonepileptic myoclonus* Myoclonic syndromes in which the underlying disorder is not characterized as epileptic on the basis of the EEG and in view of the lack of accompanying clinical events. The EMG burst length associated with the muscle jerk is usually 50–300 msec, muscles active in the

same jerk are usually activated asynchronously and may be alternating, and no EEG correlate can be identified.[2384] This form includes the following disorders:

Physiological myoclonus Sleep jerks (**hypnic jerks**), sneezing, hiccough, and myoclonus induced in otherwise normal subjects by anxiety or exercise.

Essential myoclonus A sporadic or familial syndrome characterized by the occasional occurrence of isolated myoclonic jerks in the absence of other neurological deficits. This syndrome also includes **periodic movements of sleep** or nocturnal myoclonus.

Ballistic movement overflow myoclonus

Exaggerated **startle**

Segmental myoclonus See **spinal myoclonus; propriospinal myoclonus; palatal myoclonus**

Symptomatic myoclonus Syndromes in which a progressive or static encephalopathy dominates the clinical picture, and in which myoclonus is a characteristic clinical feature. Classes of disease associated include storage diseases; spinocerebellar degenerations; basal ganglion degenerations; dementing diseases; viral, metabolic, toxic, and physical encephalopathies; and other conditions involving focal CNS damage. See **Lafora body disease, dyssynergia cerebellaris myoclonica, lipidoses, MELAS, MERFF.**

See also **paramyoclonus multiplex, photomyogenic response, palatal myoclonus, myoclonic dystonia, opsoclonus.**

myoclonus bodies   See **Lafora bodies.**

myoclonus, deafness, and cerebellar ataxia   See **myoclonus.**

Myoclonus Research Foundation, Inc.   A public charity supporting research in myoclonus, investigating its basic mechanisms, and developing new therapies. Address: 200 Old Palisade Road, Suite 17D. Fort Lee, NJ 07024. Tel: 201-585-0770. Web site: http://www.myoclonus.com/.

myodynamometer   An instrument for measuring muscle power.

myodynia   Muscle pain. The term has now been replaced by **myalgia.**

myodysplasia fibrosa multiplex   See **familial myosclerosis.**

myodystrophia fetalis deformans   See **arthrogryposis multiplex congenita.**

myoedema   Slow dimpling and then elevation of a muscle due to localized contraction following percussion, the contraction spreading across the muscle surface. It resembles myotonia except that it is electrically silent, but is classically seen in some hypothyroid patients and also in **cachexia.**[4128]

myofascial pain dysfunction   See **Costen syndrome.**

myofascial pain syndromes   (fibromyalgia, fibromyositis, myofibrositis, fibrositis, myofascial pain, myospasm; "fibrositis" was Gowers' term in 1904) Syndromes of enduring localized muscle aching or pain,

stiffness, fatigue, and local tenderness without definite pathology, muscle biopsy or EMG abnormalities, known cause, or cure. Weakness of muscle is, however, a real feature.[4162] The condition is a common cause of prolonged pain and disability.

Certain muscles are particularly vulnerable—such as the upper fibers of the trapezius, gluteus medius, piriformis, spinati, deltoid, and sartorius. Prolonged stress, spinal degenerative disease, irritable bowel disturbances, a sensation of joint swelling, anxiety, paresthesias, skinfold tenderness, and certain features of somatic dysthymia such as nonrestorative sleep are all associated.

The condition is commonly and appropriately diagnosed by those who believe in it, but is ignored or derided by others.[6101] The criteria of the American College of Rheumatology require symptoms of generalized pain for at least 3 months and pain by palpation at 4 kg at more than 11 of 18 specified tender point locations, ignoring the usual systemic symptoms.[6020]

myofibrillar (desmin-storage) myopathy   (desmin storage myopathy, familial desminopathy, spheroid body myopathy, cytoplasmic body myopathy, Mallory body myopathy, familial cardiomyopathy with subsarcolemmal vermiform deposits, myopathy with intrasarcoplasmic accumulation of dense granulofilamentous material) Hereditary myopathies presenting with proximal, distal, and respiratory muscle weakness; a scapuloperoneal syndrome and/or cardiomyopathy; and a myopathic EMG and normal or elevated serum CK levels. Pathologically, focal degradation primarily affects the myofibrils, which may contain hyaline spheroid cytoplasmic inclusions reacting intensely for actin, and in which numerous proteins such as desmin, lamin-B, gelsolin, ubiquitin, dystrophin, *g*-sarcoglycan, and α1-antichymotrypsin as well as amyloid may accumulate.[137] See also **inclusion body myositis, intermediate filament disorders, myopathy.**

The following entries are in part abstracted from the Neuromuscular Web site at Washington University, St. Louis (http://www.neuro.wustl.edu/neuromuscular/maltbrain.html), by courtesy of Dr. Alan Pestronk.

Myofibrillar myopathy with desmin mutations (OMIM 601419) Dominant or recessively inherited myopathies mapped to chromosome 2q35 and resulting from a mutation in the desmin gene. The *dominant form* produces early distal progressing to proximal weakness and wasting leading eventually to wheelchair use in most cases. Cardiac involvement is common with right bundle branch block, ST segment depression, and syncopal episodes, sometimes requiring a pacemaker. The serum CK levels are normal or mildly elevated, and the EMG and biopsy findings are myopathic.

A variant is *familial hypertrophic cardiomyopathy*, also dominantly inherited and characterized by a desmin point mutation causing cardiomyopathy. This form has also been mapped to chromosome 10q.[3816]

In the *recessive form*, the syndrome is dominated by cardiomyopathy with onset in early childhood, progressing to facial, girdle, and respiratory muscle weakness within a decade or two. High arched palate and scoliosis are associated features. Biopsy shows hyaline/desmin plaques resembling Mallory bodies and amorphous subsarcolemmal material, immunoreactive for desmin and dystrophin.

Myofibrillar myopathy; αB-crystallin mutations (type 1) A dominantly inherited condition due to a missense mutation at 11q22.3–q23.1. Clinically, the onset is in early adult life with slowly progressing proximal and distal, facial, and bulbar weakness, but cardiac death can occur as a result of cardiac arrhythmias, conduction block, or congestive failure. Associated signs include lens opacities and intestinal malabsorption. Serum CK levels are somewhat elevated, and the EMG and muscle biopsy findings are myopathic with loss of the intermyofibrillar network in type 1 fibers, accumulations of granulofilamentous material containing phosphorylated desmin, and autophagocytosis.

Myofibrillar myopathy with arrhythmogenic right ventricular cardiomyopathy (ARVC) A dominantly inherited condition due to a mutation at 10q22.3. Clinically, the onset is in adult life of mild axial, distal, or generalized muscle weakness with cardiomyopathy and rhythm disturbances. The EMG is myopathic and biopsy findings include myofibrillar disorganization, rimmed vacuoles, and accumulation of desmin.

In a *variant* form, also dominantly inherited, the onset of proximal and distal weakness with dysphagia occurs at any time, and cardiac findings are less common. Muscle biopsy shows the presence of cytoplasmic or spheroid bodies associated with desmin.

myofibrositis   See **myofascial pain syndromes.**

myogelosis   See **myofascial pain syndromes.**

myoglobin   A respiratory pigment with a low renal threshold, found in muscles; it is capable of binding oxygen, which it releases only under conditions of low partial pressure of oxygen, as with sustained exertion and in certain diseases, as mentioned under **myoglobinuria.**

myoglobinuria   The excretion of myoglobin into the urine as a result of necrosis of muscle membranes, with the subsequent liberation of all of their contents into the circulation. Clinically, the affected muscles are weak, swollen, and tender during attacks and the urine may be pink, red, or black, depending on the degree of myoglobinemia. The condition results from impairment of fuel usage by skeletal muscle in numerous conditions.

Hereditary and acquired causes of the syndrome are numerous;[4825,4829] metabolic disorders such as the **glycogen storage diseases, malignant hyperthermia, lipid myopathies,** and others with an unknown metabolic basis are in the former group; overexertion, muscle ischemia, electric shock, crush injury, **polymyositis,** and metabolic and toxic causes (e.g., drugs, *hornet venom*[457] and **quail myopathy**) account for most of the latter. Renal failure is a well-recognized complication of myoglobinuria from any cause.

Variant forms include *idiopathic recurrent myoglobinuria*, in which limb weakness and elevated creatine kinase levels persist between the attacks, the EMG shows a myopathic pattern, and neither an enzyme deficiency nor a biochemical abnormality is ascertainable.[516]

Familial myoglobinuria is a severe intermittent myoglobinuria in which attacks are precipitated by exercise or by infection.[4932]

myograph   An instrument for recording the attributes of muscular contraction. See **electromyogram.**

myohypertrophia kymoparalytica   A syndrome of muscular hypertrophy, cramps, wave-like muscular contractions, and pareses of unknown nature. It was described by Oppenheim,[4251] but is not now reported; possibly the condition represents a form of dystonia.

myoid cell   A thymic cell somewhat resembling a myofibril that may express acetylcholine receptors on its surface.

***myo*-inositol**   Disturbed metabolism of *myo*-inositol is associated with a reduction in nerve conduction velocities, presumably through an effect on the Na-K-ATPase system. Impaired axonal conduction results and axonopathy follows, from which it has been considered that the disturbance of *myo*-inositol in diabetes mellitus is a cause of the peripheral neuropathy. This is as yet unproven.

myokinetic epilepsy   See **absence seizures.**

myokymia   (from Gr, muscle + wave) (fibrillary contractions) Involuntary, localized, writhing, undulating, persistent quivering contractions of a muscle due to a process arising in the peripheral portion of its motor nerve and leading to spontaneous, synchronous, repetitive discharges of motor unit potentials.

Electromyographically, continuous, repetitive, brief discharges of groups of two to six motor unit potentials, firing at 5–60 Hz, are recorded. The differential diagnosis has been considered.[260,2343] See **neuromyotonia, myokymic discharge, fasciculations, fasciculation potential.** Neuromyotonia and myokymia appear to represent loci on a spectrum of abnormal activity in muscle due to aberrant neural input.[2344]

Myokymia often accompanies motor nerve lesions of any type, but can also occur without demonstrable pathology; in such cases, the most common site is the orbicularis oculi muscles of people who are tired or anxious. Irritation of the fasciculus of the seventh cranial nerve within the brainstem by a plaque of **multiple sclerosis** or a brainstem neoplasm are rare causes. The condition may also be hereditary[5108] or toxic.[3917] The review of Albers et al. remains current and complete.[76]

Superior oblique myokymia is a misnomer, as the condition is really a microtremor. See also **Isaacs syndrome (neuromyotona), cramp-fasciculation syndrome, episodic ataxia, Morvan disease.**

Variant forms are listed in Chart M–25.

Chart M–25. Variant Forms of Myokymia

Myokymia and impaired muscle relaxation with continuous muscle discharge A disorder of peripheral nerves characterized by generalized muscle twitching, weakness, stiffness, cramping, and hyperhidrosis, persistent during sleep, and initial fatigue, followed by increasing strength with continued effort. Nerve conduction velocities are reduced.[3500]

Hereditary myokymia and paroxysmal ataxia A dominantly inherited syndrome mapped to chromosome 12p with a missense mutation in the *KCNA1* gene. The attacks of ataxia with slowed movements and tremor last up to 15 min, are precipitated by kinesigenic stimuli, exertion, and startle, and are responsive to acetazolamide. The myokymia may lead to generalized stiffness or be simply minimal contractions of distal muscles.[3497] See also **cerebellar ataxia** (*variants*).

Idiopathic generalized myokymia See **neuromyotonia.**

Myokymia and ataxia with continuous muscle discharge A congenital degenerative disease characterized by clubfoot, joint contractures, cerebellar ataxia, tremor at rest, myokymia, and raised creatine kinase levels.[337]

Morvan fibrillary chorea A form of generalized myokymia, probably occurring as a toxic effect of gold therapy.

Generalized myokymia and muscle cramping without peripheral neuropathy EMG findings are of spontaneously recurring regular bursts of motor unit potentials, termed **myokymic discharges,** with normal motor and sensory nerve conduction velocities. Repetitive discharges follow each motor nerve stimulus.[261]

---

myokymic discharge   A form of involuntary activity in which motor unit action potentials fire repetitively and may be associated with clinical **myokymia.** Two firing patterns have been described: 1. Commonly, the discharge is a brief, repetitive firing of single motor unit action potentials for a short period (up to a few seconds) at a uniform rate (2 to 60 Hz) followed by a short period (up to a few seconds) of silence, with repetition of the same sequence for a particular potential at regular intervals. 2. Rarely, the potential recurs continuously at a fairly uniform firing rate (1 to 5 Hz). Myokymic discharges are a subclass of grouped discharges and repetitive discharges. See also **ephapse** and **ephaptic transmission.** (From the 2001 Report of the Nomenclature Committee of the American Association of Electromyography and Electrodiagnosis.[10] Used by permission, copyright © 2001, AAEM.)

myolemma   (sarcolemma) The connective tissue layer investing myofibrils.

myoleukoencephalopathy   a mitochondrial disease presenting with features overlapping those of MERRF and MELAS, with in addition severe myopathy and seizures.[1330]

myology   The study of the nature, structure, function, and pathology of muscles.

myoma   A tumor consisting of muscle fibers. If these are striated, the name **rhabdomyoma** is applied; if they are unstriated, it is known as a **leiomyoma.**

myomesin   The major structural protein of the M line in vertebrate muscle.

myonecrosis   (gas gangrene) Infection and subsequent decomposition of muscle, usually by *Clostridium perfringens or welchii,* the exotoxin of which causes large areas of muscle necrosis with marked systemic reaction. *S. pyogenes* and *group B Streptococcus* may do the same.

Clinically, pain out of proportion to the appearance of the wound, extensive edema of the overlying skin, watery or purulent exudates, fever, and skin necrosis are in succession the main findings, leading to hypovolemic shock, intravascular hemolysis, and organ failure.

myoneural junction   The structures comprising the mechanism for the transmission of nerve impulses from nerve to muscle. These include the axon terminal, the synaptic cleft, and the **motor end plate.**

myoneurogastrointestinal encephalopathy   (MNGIE) A rare mitochondrial disorder comprising external ophthalmoplegia, muscle atrophy, polyneuropathy, and hyperdensities of the cerebral white matter, associated with acidosis. The condition is a mitochondrial multisystem disorder considered due to a partial defect of the cytochrome-*c* complex of the respiratory chain.[347]

myopalmus   (Gr, muscle + swinging) Twitching of muscle.

myopathic carnitine deficiency   See **carnitine deficiency.**

myopathic motor unit potential   Low-amplitude, short-duration, polyphasic motor unit action potentials. Use of the term is discouraged. It incorrectly implies specific diagnostic significance of a motor unit action potential configuration. See **motor unit action potential.** (From the 2001 Report of the Nomenclature Committee of the American Association of Electromyography and Electrodiagnosis.[10] Used by permission, copyright © 2001, AAEM.)

myopathic recruitment   An increase in the number and firing rate of motor unit action potentials compared with normal for the strength of muscle contraction. (From the 2001 Report of the Nomenclature Committee of the American Association of Electromyography and Electrodiagnosis.[10] Used by permission, copyright © 2001, AAEM.)

myopathica rachitica   (Hagenbach-Bing myopathy) A severe hypotonic myopathy occurring in infants with rickets.

myopathies   Diseases in which the structure or function of muscles is compromised. Many (but not all) of those that are inherited are subsumed under the heading of **muscular dystrophies,** but the term myopathy is all-encompassing and all dystrophies are myopathies, though not all myopathies are dystrophies. Some of them are considered under the heading **congenital myopathy,** others under, e.g., **mitochondrial myopathies,** or by name when listed in bold print; the remainder are dealt with as shown in Chart M–26. See also **distal myopathy.**

Chart M–26. A Listing of the Myopathies

A. *Heritable myopathies*
  1. *Muscular dystrophies*
    a. X-linked types
      1. X-linked recessive (severe) **Duchenne muscular dystrophy**
      2. Myopathy in manifesting Duchenne carriers
      3. X-linked Duchenne dystrophy due to chromosomal translocation in females or to Turner syndrome[694]
      4. X-linked recessive form. See **Becker muscle dystrophy.**
      5. X-linked recessive myopathy (Xp21) with **glycerol kinase deficiency**
      6. X-linked myopathy (Xp21) with **McLeod syndrome**
      7. X-linked recessive dystrophy with contractures and cardiomyopathy
      8. X-linked recessive congenital muscle fiber hypotrophy with central nuclei
      9. X-linked dominant lethal myopathy in hemizygous boys
      10. X-linked **myotubular myopathy,** lethal in neonates
      11. X-linked **scapuloperoneal muscular dystrophy** with lethal cardiomyopathy
      12. X-linked vacuolated myopathy[5765]
    b. **Facioscapulohumeral muscular dystrophy**
      1. Autosomal dominant involving face, scapulohumeral and anterior tibial muscles
      2. Severe infantile form
      3. Childhood form with **Möbius syndrome**
      4. With sensorineural deafness alone, or with **Coats disease** of the retina or tortuosity of retinal vessels
    c. **Scapuloperoneal muscular dystrophy**
      1. Autosomal dominant
      2. X-linked (may be Emery-Dreifuss type) (see A.11 above)
      3. With inflammatory changes and cardiopathy
    d. **Limb-girdle muscular dystrophy**
      1. See **quadriceps myopathy**
      2. Limb-girdle muscular dystrophy with Wolff-Parkinson-White syndrome
      3. Late-onset proximal myopathy with diabetes mellitus
    e. *Autosomal recessive dystrophy of childhood,* resembling **Duchenne dystrophy,** but more benign and affecting both sexes. The condition is more common in Tunisia and in parts of the Middle East.[457]
    f. **Distal muscular dystrophy**
      1. **Welander distal myopathy** on 2p13[55]
      2. Autosomal dominant with tibialis anterior weakness on 2q31 (tibial muscular dystrophy)[2430]
      3. Autosomal dominant with infantile onset
      4. Autosomal recessive variety with rimmed vacuole formation and lamellar (myeloid) bodies
      5. Hereditary distal myopathy with sarcoplasmic bodies and intermediate (skeletin) filaments
      6. Autosomal recessive, with high creatine kinase
      7. Autosomal dominant variety of late onset with desmin storage[5696]
      8. Distal myopathy with proximal weakness and early respiratory failure[1012,4129]
      9. Autosomal recessive inclusion body myopathy on 9p1–q1[2991]
      10. Distal myopathy on chromosome 14[3227]
      11. Autosomal dominant inclusion body myopathy with rimmed vacuoles, ophthalmoplegia, and variable joint contractures on 17p13.1[3660]
    g. *Autosomal dominant dystrophy with humeropelvic distribution and cardiomyopathy*[1784]
    h. **Emery-Dreifuss dystrophy** with dominant inheritance
    i. Benign muscular dystrophy with contractures but without cardiomyopathy[295]
    j. **Myositis ossificans** (autosomal dominant fibrodysplasia ossificans progressiva)
    k. **Ocular myopathies** (progressive external ophthalmoplegias)
      1. Isolated (autosomal dominant) with or without ragged red fibers
      2. With pigmentary retinal degeneration (dominant or sporadic)
      3. **Kearns-Sayre syndrome** (with retinal degeneration, short stature, heart block, ataxia, and high CSF protein content)
      4. With curare sensitivity
      5. **Oculopharyngeal muscular dystrophy,** usually autosomal dominant, sometimes recessive
      6. Oculopharyngeal myopathy with distal myopathy and cardiomyopathy, and other varieties of **oculopharyngodistal myopathy**
      7. **Familial multicore disease** with ophthalmoplegia
      8. Progressive ophthalmoplegia with mental retardation
      9. Congenital ophthalmoplegia in the **Goldenhar-Gorlin syndrome**
      10. X-linked recessive ophthalmoplegia and myopia
      11. **Neonatal ophthalmoplegia with microfibers**
      12. **Nemaline myopathy** with ophthalmoplegia and mitochondrial abnormalities
      13. **Nemaline myopathy** with cardiomyopathy
      14. **Familial paralysis of horizontal gaze**
      15. Late-onset **oculogastrointestinal muscular dystrophy**
      16. **Familial static ophthalmoplegia**
See also **myofibrillar (desmin-storage) myopathy.**
  2. *Myopathies of unknown etiology, usually congenital*
    a. **Congenital muscular dystrophy,** including some cases of **arthrogryposis multiplex congenita** with infantile cataract
    b. Congenital muscular dystrophy with severe mental retardation

c. **Benign congenital myopathy** without specific features

d. **Benign congenital or infantile hypotonia**

e. Central core disease

f. **Nemaline** (rod-body) myopathy

g. Myotubular (**centronuclear**) myopathy and variants

h. **Familia! myosclerosis** (myodysplasia fibrosa multiplex)

i. Myopathy in **Marfan syndrome** and variants: centronuclear myopathy with type 1 fiber hypotrophy, and "fingerprint" inclusions with Marfan syndrome

j. **Marinesco-Sjögren syndrome** (familial congenital myopathy with cataract, gonadal dysgenesis, and oligophrenia)

k. Myopathies with characteristic histochemical abnormalities
   1. **Type 1 fiber hypotrophy**
   2. **Congenital fiber-type disproportion**
   3. **Congenital myopathy with uniform fiber type** (type 1)
   4. Congenital fiber type disproportion in **Krabbe disease**
   5. **Reducing body myopathy**
   6. **Congenital myopathy with trilaminar muscle fibers**
   7. **Congenital myopathy with multifocal degeneration of muscle fibers**

l. Rigid spine syndrome[4474]

m. Myopathy with features of both centronuclear myopathy and multicores See **myofibrillar myopathy.**

n. Myopathies with cytoplasmic[3317] or with "fingerprint" inclusions[1661] See **myofibrillar myopathy.**

o. **Multicore disease**

p. **Sarcotubular myopathy**

q. **Tubular aggregate myopathy**

r. Familial neuromuscular disease with type 1 fiber hypoplasia, tubular aggregates, cardiomyopathy, and myasthenic features[1477]

s. Congenital myopathy with type 2 fiber hypoplasia[776]

t. Myopathy with crystalline intranuclear inclusions[2835] See **myofibrillar myopathy.**

u. Autosomal dominant "spheroid body" myopathy See **myofibrillar myopathy.**

v. **Hypertrophic branchial myopathy**

w. **Monomelic hypertrophic myopathy**

x. **Cytoplasmic body neuromyopathy** with respiratory failure and weight loss See **myofibrillar myopathy.**

y. **Zebra body myopathy**

z. Myopathy with absence of muscle glycogen and neutral lipid in the **neuroleptic malignant syndrome**

aa. **Benign myopathy**

bb. **Myopathy with merosin-deficient fibers** See **myofibrillar myopathy**

cc. *Vocal cord and pharyngeal muscular dystrophy* on 5q31[1768]

dd. **Late-onset riboflavin-responsive myopathy with multiple acyl CoA dehydrogenase deficiency** A lipid-storage myopathy presenting with weakness and wasting of the trunk and limbs in late adult life.[190] See also **lipid myopathy.**

ee. *Fatal infantile hypertonic muscular dystrophy* A progressive myopathy appearing soon after birth with continuous muscle activity and progressive weakness to death before the age of 18 months, described in Canadian Aboriginal infants. The pathology shows fibrosis, necrosis, and regeneration.[3221]

ff. *Myopathy with intrasarcoplasmic accumulation of dense granulofilamentous material* See **myofibrillar (desmin-storage) myopathy.**

gg. **Myopathy with cardiomyopathy** A dominantly inherited condition similar to limb-girdle muscular dystrophy 1B with the onset in childhood or young adult life of proximal symmetrical weakness affecting mainly the pelvic girdle and with the occurrence of dysrhythmias and conduction disturbances potentially leading to sudden death. Serum CK levels are somewhat elevated and the EMG and muscle biopsy are myopathic. See http://www.neuro.wustl.edu/neuromuscular/maltbrain.html.

hh. *Dominant myopathy with ankle contractures and high CK* A dominantly inherited condition characterized by proximal symmetric weakness with onset in youth or young adult life and joint contractures. Serum CK levels are very high and muscle biopsy findings are typically myopathic. See http://www.neuro.wustl.edu/neuromuscular/maltbrain.html.

ii. *Myopathy with abnormal merosin* (laminin-2) 4 A progressive form with likely autosomal recessive inheritance characterized by onset in youth or adult life, female preponderance, facial, neck, and shoulder girdle weakness without scapular winging, weakness of the hamstrings and hip adductors and flexors, and ventilatory impairment. Hypertrophy of the calves and brachioradialis is reported. Serum CK levels are greatly increased and the EMG and biopsy findings are myopathic. See http://www.neuro.wustl.edu/neuromuscular/maltbrain.html.

3. *Myotonic disorders*
   a. **Myotonic dystrophy**
   b. **Myotonia congenita** (autosomal dominant form, Thomsen disease)
   c. **Myotonia congenita** (autosomal recessive form)
   d. **Schwartz-Jampel syndrome:** myotonia, dwarfism, facial dysmorphism and diffuse bone disease
   e. **Paramyotonia congenita** (Eulenburg)
   f. **Paramyotonia** without paralysis on exposure to cold
   g. *Familial granulovacuolar lobular myopathy with electrical myotonia* See **myotonia congenita.**
   h. *Myotonia with painful cramps* See Chart M–26.

B. *Trauma to muscle by external agents*
   B1. *Physical*
      1 **Crush syndrome**
      2. Ischemic infarction or atrophy
      3. **Volkmann contracture**
      4. **Compartment syndromes**
         a. Anterior tibial syndrome
         b. Posterior compartment (tibial) syndrome
         c. Lateral (peroneal) compartment syndrome
         d. Triceps surae compartment syndrome
         e. Extensor compartment syndrome of the forearm
         f. Rectus abdominis compartment syndrome
      5. Congenital or idiopathic **torticollis**

B2. *Toxic*
  1. **Haff disease**
  2. Snake-bite by *Enhydrina schistosa*
  3. Saxitoxin poisoning
  4. **Myoglobinuria** caused by hornet venom
  5. **Quail myopathy**
B3. *Drugs*
C. *Inflammatory*
  C1. *Infections of muscle*
    1. **Viral myositis**
      a. **Benign acute myositis**
      b. Acute myopathy with **rhabdomyolysis**
      c. **Epidemic pleurodynia** due to coxsackie B5 (also B1, B3, and B4)
      d. **Postviral fatigue syndrome** (benign postinfection "myositis")
    2. **Bacterial**
    3. Fungal myositis (e.g., disseminated candidiasis)
    4. Protozoal myositis
    5. Cestode myositis
    6. Nematode myositis
  C2. *Other inflammatory disorders of muscle*
    1. **Dermatomyositis**
    2. **Polymyositis** (possibly an organ-specific autoimmune disease)
      a. Acute polymyositis with myoglobinuria
      b. Subacute polymyositis
      c. Chronic polymyositis (including chronic myositis fibrosa)
    3. **Polymyositis** with autoimmune disease, including systemic lupus erythematosus, rheumatic fever, rheumatoid arthritis, systemic sclerosis, scleroderma (morphoea), polyarteritis nodosa or giant cell arteritis, Sjögren disease, Werner disease, localized nodular myositis, chronic graft-versus-host disease, benign acute childhood myositis, and acne fulminans with inflammatory myopathy.
    4. **Polymyositis** or dermatomyositis with malignant disease
    5. **Polymyositis** with associated virus particles
    6. Acute fulminant myoglobinuric **polymyositis** with picornavirus-like particles
    7. **Eosinophilic polymyositis**
    8. Cyclic eosinophilic **polymyositis** and hyperimmunoglobulin E
    9. **Inclusion body myositis** and variants
    10. Orbital myositis (**pseudotumour orbiti**)
    11. Polymyositis with **HIV** infection
  C3. *Inflammatory disorders of muscle of unknown etiology*
    1. **Sarcoidosis** with myopathy
    2. **Granulomatous polymyositis** and giant cell myositis
    3. **Polymyalgia rheumatica**
    4. Localized **myositis ossificans**
    5. **Fibrositis** and nodular fasciitis; myositis proliferans or pseudotumor
    6. Myopathy in relapsing panniculitis (**Weber-Christian syndrome**)
    7. Myositis with **necrotizing fasciitis**
    8. **Psoriatic myopathy**
    9. Myopathy in **Reye syndrome**
D. *Metabolic myopathies*
  D1. *Muscle disorder associated with endocrine disease*
    1. Hyperthyroidism (see **acute thyrotoxic myopathy**)

2. Hypothyroidism (girdle myopathy, **Debré-Sémélaigne syndrome, Hoffmann syndrome, pseudomyotonia,** neuromyopathy following iodine[131] therapy)
3. **Hypopituitarism** with myopathy
4. **Acromegaly** with muscle hypertrophy or myopathy
5. **Exophthalmic ophthalmoplegia** (infiltrative ophthalmopathy or ophthalmic Graves disease)
6. **Cushing disease** myopathy (and iatrogenic corticosteroid myopathy)
7. ACTH myopathy in **Nelson syndrome**
8. **Addison disease** with myopathy
9. **Primary aldosteronism** (with hypokalemic periodic paralysis)
10. **Hyperparathyroidism** with myopathy
11. **Hypoparathyroidism** with myopathy
12. Myopathy in other forms of metabolic bone disease such as **osteomalacia**
13. Myopathy with calcitonin-secreting medullary carcinoma of the thyroid
D2. *Heritable myopathies, biochemical abnormality known*
  1. **Glycogen storage disease** involving muscle
    a. **Glycogenosis** type 1 (von Gierke disease)
    b. Glycogenosis type 2 (Pompe disease)
      1. Infantile form
      2. Adult or late-onset variety
    c. Glycogenosis type 3 (Cori-Forbes disease)
    d. Glycogenosis type 4 (Andersen disease, adult polyglucosan body myopathy)
    e. Glycogenosis type 5 (McArdle disease)
      1. Usual form, with onset in childhood or adolescence
      2. Infantile form
      3. Late-onset **myophosphorylase deficiency**
    f. Glycogenosis type 7 (Tarui disease) due to phosphofructokinase deficiency
      1. Typical form, lack of M subunit
      2. Hemolysis with myopathy, lack of L subunit Infantile myopathy
    g. **Phosphoglycerate kinase deficiency**
    h. **Phosphoglycerate mutase deficiency**
    i. Lactate dehydrogenase deficiency
    j. Lysosomal glycogen storage disease without acid maltase deficiency
    k. Mixed enzyme deficiencies (e.g., phosphofructokinase and phosphorylase kinase)
  2. Other inherited disorders of carbohydrate metabolism
    a. Muscle fructose 1,6-diphosphatase deficiency with atypical **central core disease**
    b. Myopathy due to glycolytic abnormality involving phosphohexoisomerase
  3. **Myoadenylate deaminase deficiency** (with cramps and exertional myalgia)
  4. **Familial periodic paralysis** and related syndromes
    a. Hypokalemic periodic paralysis
    b. Hyperkalemic periodic paralysis (adynamia episodica hereditaria), sometimes with cardiac arrhythmia
    c. Normokalemic periodic paralysis
    d. Myotonic periodic paralysis (paramyotonia congenita), possibly a variant of b. above
    e. Thyrotoxic periodic paralysis

5. **Mitochondrial myopathies** and **lipid storage myopathies**
   a. Lipid storage myopathies of uncertain origin
      1. Lipid storage myopathy and congenital ichthyosis (Chanarin-Miranda syndrome)
      2. Congenital myopathies with lipid storage
      3. Associated with recognized disease (glycogenosis type 1, hyper β-lipoproteinemia, pyruvate decarboxylase deficiency, arthrogryposis)
      4. Autosomal recessive lipid storage myopathy with electrical myotonia, lipid in leukocytes, and defect in long-chain fatty acid utilisation
      5. Autosomal dominant lipid storage neuromyopathy with systemic abnormality of fat metabolism
      6. Idiopathic lipid storage myopathies with glycogen storage, and structurally abnormal mitochondria
   b. Alpha-glycerophosphate dehydrogenase deficiency See **lipid myopathy.**
   c. Deficiencies involving the carnitine acyl-carnitine carrier system
      1. Muscle **carnitine deficiency**
      2. **Systemic carnitine deficiency** with cardiomyopathy
      3. Partial muscle carnitine deficiencies
      4. **Carnitine palmitoyl transferase deficiency;** CPT 2 deficiency with normal CPT 1, CPT deficiency with myoglobinuria and respiratory failure
      5. Combined carnitine and CPT deficiencies
   d. Defects of mitochondrial substrate utilization
      1. Pyruvate decarboxylase deficiency
      2. Dihydrolipoyl transacetylase deficiency
      3. Dihydrolipoyl dehydrogenase deficiency
      4. Pyruvate dehydrogenase phosphatase deficiency
      5. Pyruvate carboxylase deficiency
      6. Carnitine acetyltransferase deficiency

Many mitochondrial disorders cause myopathy but the clinical picture is often dominated by progressive encephalopathy, hypotonia, lactic acidosis, and respiratory insufficiency.

   e. Defects of the respiratory chain
      1. Defects of NADH oxidation
      2. Cytochrome-*b* deficiency
      3. Cytochrome-*c* oxidase deficiency
      4. Combined cytochrome deficiencies.
      5. Encephalomyopathy with decreased succinate-cytochrome-*c* reductase deficiency
   f. Defects of energy conservation and transduction
      1. Hypermetabolic mitochondrial myopathy (**Luft disease**)
      2. Other **mitochondrial myopathies** with "loose coupling"
      3. Mitochondrial ATPase deficiency
      4. Myopathy due to a malate-aspartate shuttle defect[2489]

The mitochondrial myopathies in e. and f. are associated with diverse clinical syndromes that include ophthalmoplegia, severe hypotonia, cramps, myoglobinuria, exercise-induced myalgia, and limb weakness, occurring at different stages of life. **Fukuhara syndrome** comprises myoclonic epilepsy and ragged red fibers (MERRF). The controversies about the delineation of specific disorders have been reviewed by Petty et al.[4427]

   6. **Malignant hyperpyrexia** (halothane, suxamethonium, ketamine, psychotropic agents, etc.)
   7. Progressive muscle spasm, alopecia, diarrhea, and malabsorption (**Satoyoshi syndrome**)
   8. Myopathy in **lysine-cystinuria**
   9. **Xanthenuric myopathy**
   10. Myopathy in **Lafora disease**
   11. **Tubular aggregate myopathy** often associated with myalgia
   12. **Cytoplasmic body myopathy**
   13. Benign **reducing body myopathy**
D3. *Other metabolic myopathies*
   1. **Alcoholic myopathy**
      a. Acute, with myoglobinuria
      b. Subacute or chronic proximal
      c. Hypokalemic
   2. **Nutritional myopathy**
      a. Protein deficiency; malnutrition due to anorexia nervosa or malabsorption
      b. Human myopathy due to vitamin E deficiency
      c. Chronic myopathy with hypocalcemia and hypophosphatemia
   3. Myopathy in chronic renal failure (see **uremic myopathy**)
   4. **Acute polymyopathy** during total parenteral nutrition
   5. Potassium depletion myopathy
   6. **Carnitine deficiency** induced during hemodialysis
   7. Riboflavin-responsive **lipid myopathy** with carnitine deficiency
   8. **Myoglobinuria** (other than that due to glycogen storage disease, mitochondrial or lipid storage myopathies, and CPT deficiency)
      a. Exertion (including military training, running, skiing, compartment syndromes, status epilepticus, electric shock, myoclonus, and severe dystonia)
      b. Crush or ischemic injury to muscle (see above)
      c. Metabolic depression or distortion (including carbon monoxide or drug intoxication, diabetic ketoacidosis, hyperosmolar states, renal tubular acidosis, hyper- and hyponatremia, hypokalemia, and hypophosphatemia)
      d. Myoglobinuria due to drugs and toxins (see above), including the ingestion of **quail**
      e. Abnormalities of body temperature (including hypothermia due to cold or hypothyroidism, or fever due to toxins, vaccines, heat stroke, malignant hyperpyrexia, or the malignant neuroleptic syndrome)
      f. Infections (including viral, bacterial, and *Mycoplasma* infections, and the toxic shock syndrome)
      g. Autoimmune muscle disease (polymyositis and dermatomyositis)
      h. Idiopathic recurrent myoglobinuria, sometimes leading to myopathy with persistent weakness
      i. Chronic myopathy due to drugs (chloroquine, emetine, steroids, penicillin, vincristine, colchicine; repeated intramuscular injections of meperidine or pentazocine)
      j. Proximal myopathy in diabetes mellitus[5445]

E. *Myopathy associated with malignant disease*
   1. **Carcinomatous myopathy** (other than polymyositis)
   2. **Lambert-Eaton syndrome**
   3. **Carcinomatous embolic myopathy**
   4. Proximal myopathy due to discrete carcinomatous metastases in muscle
   5. Myopathy in the **carcinoid** syndrome
F. *Myopathy associated with myasthenia gravis*
G. *Myopathy in **thalassemia***
H. *Other disorders of muscle of unknown or uncertain etiology*
   1. Acute muscle necrosis of unknown cause, or complicating chronic alcoholism, carcinoma, or intensive care treatment See **acute quadriplegic myopathy.**
   2. **Amyloid myopathy**
      a. Primary familial
      b. Primary sporadic (sometimes causing pseudohypertrophy of muscle)
      c. In myelomatosis
      d. With angiopathy
   3. **Disuse atrophy**
   4. Muscle **cachexia** (in wasting diseases and in the elderly)
   5. Muscle wasting in contralateral cerebral lesions (particularly of parietal lobe)
   6. **Granular nuclear inclusion body disease** affecting skeletal muscle and the nervous system
I. *Tumors of muscle*
   1. **Rhabdomyoma**
   2. **Rhabdomyosarcoma**
      a. Adult pleomorphic type
      b. Embryonal botryoid type
      c. Embryonal alveolar type
   3. **Desmoid fibroma**
   4. **Alveolar sarcoma**
   5. Angioma
   6. Other connective tissue tumors occasionally occurring in muscle

Unclassified Myopathies

Familial myopathy with thrombocytopenia
Myopathy complicating methioninemia
Myopathy complicating **mucolipidosis** type 4

CPT, carnitine palmityl transferase. See also the continuously updated Web site from Washington University: http://www.neuro.wustl.edu/ neuromuscular/maltbrain.html.

*(Adapted from World Federation of Neurology Classification Subcommittee. Classification of neuromuscular diseases. J Neurol Sci 1988;**86:** 333–360.) The classification used here is closely based on that of the World Federation of Neurology.[6039] It is adapted by kind permission of Prof. P.K. Thomas, Lord Walton, and the World Federation of Neurology. It uses basically the same ennumeration.*

myopathy and chronic renal failure   Proximal weakness and wasting of myopathic type in association with severe osteomalacia secondary to renal disease, mainly affecting the flexors and other proximal leg muscles, commonly asymmetrical and partially responsive to vitamin D therapy.[1890]

myopathy (Bender type)   A congenital myopathic syndrome, comprising proximal and facial muscle atrophy, weakness and hypotonia, ptosis, ophthalmoplegia, kyphoscoliosis, feeding problems in infants, and the presence of fiber hypotrophy, central nuclei, fiber-type predominance, and central core-like lesions in muscle biopsy specimens.[337]

myopathy following adrenalectomy   A condition of proximal weakness and wasting with unusual pigmentation in patients prescribed steroid hormones following adrenalectomy for Cushing disease.[4527]

myopathy with characteristic sarcoplasmic bodies and skeletin (desmin) filaments   See **myofibrillar myopathy.**

myopathy with cylindrical spiral inclusions   A myopathic syndrome with onset in childhood, comprising proximal weakness and atrophy, lordosis, myotonia, and muscle pain and cramps.[337]

myopathy with exercise intolerance and weakness   A limb-girdle myopathic syndrome presenting at any time of life, sometimes with ophthalmoplegia.[3983]

myopathy with focal loss of cross-striations and multicores   A congenital myopathic syndrome, comprising proximal and facial muscle atrophy, weakness and hypotonia, ptosis, ophthalmoplegia and lordosis, and central nuclei with the finding of central core-like lesions on muscle biopsy specimens.

myopathy with inclusion bodies   See **myofibrillar myopathy.**

myopathy with lysis of myofibrils in type 1 fibers   See **type 1 fiber hypotrophy with central nuclei.**

myopathy with Mallory body–like inclusions   See **myofibrillar myopathy.**

myopathy with merosin-deficient fibers   A syndrome of rapidly evolving and severe weakness leading to incapacity and respiratory insufficiency, reported in subjects following severe illness and steroid administration. Serum CK levels are normal or mildly elevated and the EMG is myopathic. Pathology shows lack of myosin-ATPase staining in many small, angular fibers with marked loss of myosin. Slow recovery is usual.[117]

myopathy with mucolipidosis type 4   A congenital myopathic syndrome, a *variant* of mucolipidosis type 4, characterized by cloudy corneas, optic atrophy, retinitis pigmentosa, joint contractures, spasticity, athetosis, proximal and distal weakness and hypotonia, and mental and developmental delay.[337]

myopathy with multicore and central nuclei   See **multicore disease.**

myopathy with tubular aggregates   Proximal myopathic syndromes characterized by the presence of cytoplasmic aggregates of membranous tubules derived from the sarcoplasmic reticulum, mainly in type 2 fibers. Three variants are described:

1. *Autosomal dominant (or recessive)*, presenting with slowly progressive proximal weakness in childhood or early adult life, sometimes with extraocular muscle weakness or ankle contractures and with normal serum CK levels.
2. *Autosomal dominant*, a slowly progressive form with onset in adult life of proximal and sometimes distal weakness, muscle pain, cramps, and exertional stiffness. Serum CK levels are normal or slightly raised. Muscle biopsy shows the presence of tubular aggregates in type 2 muscle fibers and type 2 muscle fiber atrophy.
3. *Sporadic*, a slowly progressive form with onset in adolescence of proximal weakness. The serum CK levels are normal or mildly elevated. Muscle biopsy reveals the presence of tubular aggregates in type 1 and 2 muscle fibers.

The above entries were abstracted from the Neuromuscular Web site at Washington University, St. Louis, http://www.neuro.wustl.edu/neuromuscular/maltbrain.html, by courtesy of Dr. Alan Pestronk.

myopathy with tubulomembranous inclusions   An inherited myopathic syndrome with onset in youth, characterized by high-arched palate and facial, proximal, and distal myopathic weakness. See **tubular aggregate myopathy.**

myopathy-oligophrenia-cataract   See **Lundberg syndrome.**

myophosphorylase deficiency   The biochemical cause of McArdle disease (type 5 glycogenosis), leading to a metabolic myopathy characterized by the deposition of subsarcolemmal glycogen in skeletal muscles and occasionally in endothelial cells. See **glycogen storage diseases.**

myopia   (from Gr, to close + eye; thus to close the eye) Shortsightedness; the condition in which rays of light entering the eye are brought to focus anterior to the retina, within the vitreous humor. The eye is thus adapted for near-vision.

myopic crescent   A pale crescent surrounding part of the optic disk in myopes, due to choroidal atrophy in this region.

myorhythmia   (skeletal myoclonus) A coarse, rhythmic, irregular, alternating tremor of small amplitude which may be intermittent or continuous and present at rest, but is intensified by posture and voluntary activity, occurring at 1–4 Hz (usually about 2 Hz) in the limbs ipsilateral to a dentate or superior cerebellar peduncle lesion or contralateral to a lesion of the inferior olive.[3690] It disappears in sleep.

Muscles such as the superior oblique or those of the palate may also be involved; this phenomenon is variously regarded as myoclonic (implying a central origin) or myokymic (when the origin is presumed to be peripheral). The phenomenon is sometimes associated with **branchial myoclonus.**[3690] See also **midbrain tremor.**

myosclerosis   (fibrosing myositis) A heterogeneous condition, in which the consistency of muscles is increased to a woody hardness. Dystrophic, neurogenic, and inflammatory causes are recognized.[701]

myosin   A major muscle protein, selectively absent in certain myopathies as above and in critical illness myopathy.

myosis   See **miosis.**

myositis   (polymyositis) Inflammatory myopathies due to infection by viruses, bacteria, fungi, or parasites or occurring as manifestations of autoallergic disease (**idiopathic inflammatory myopathies**).

Viral infections may produce the syndromes of **benign acute myositis, acute rhabdomyolysis** or **epidemic pleurodynia,** and possibly **chronic myopathy.** Bacterial infections lead to **acute suppurative myositis. Fungal myositis** is considered separately. Protozoa, cestodes, and nematodes are the agents leading to **parasitic myositis.**[3687] Numerous other forms of inflammatory myopathy are considered under **polymyositis.** See also **focal steroid responsive myositis.**

Myositis Association of America   A charitable organization providing information and support. Address: 755-C Cantrell Ave., Harrrisonburg, VA 22801. Tel: 540-433-7686. Web site: http://www.myositis.org/.

myositis of chronic graft-versus-host disease   A rare complication of bone marrow transplantation presenting with severe proximal weakness. Muscle biopsy specimens show necrotic fibers with anti-IgG deposits and interstitial inflammation.[4673]

myositis ossificans   (Munchmeyer syndrome, fibrodysplasia ossificans progressiva, myositis ossificans progressiva, Patin syndrome) A rare, dominantly inherited, severe, disabling disorder of childhood characterized by painful swelling due to fibrosis and ossification of affected muscles and of local fascia and other fibrous tissues. The proximal limb muscles are most affected, but the heart and intercostal muscles may also be involved, a situation eventually incompatible with life in some cases.[4042] Spinal anomalies and malformations of the hallux may be associated.[4456] Radiologically, the mass is encircled by a rim of calcification and is separated from underlying bone.

The same condition was probably that described by Guy Patin in 1648 and again by John Freke (1688–1756), an English physician, in 1740 as "a case of extraordinary exostoses on the back of a boy."[1951,4979] *Variants* include the following:[2455]

Myositis ossificans traumatica A condition of localized calcification in muscle damaged in the remote past and the most common form, in which the lesions arise following trauma.

Pseudomalignant nontraumatic myositis ossificans A form of **proliferative myositis**[3225] occurring in reponse to repeated minor muscle traumata even if no major injury is recalled.

A familial form in which the mass is located within the paravertebral muscles[2455]

Heterotopic bone formation occurring within muscles in patients with prior poliomyelitis, polymyositis, burns, paraplegia, infections, etc., without obvious cause. [2455]

myositis ossificans progressiva   See **myositis ossificans.**

myositis proliferans   See **nodular fasciitis.**

myospasm   See **myofascial pain syndromes.**

myospasm gravis   See **Satoyoshi syndrome.**

myospasmus   (Gr, muscle + contraction) Muscle cramp or spasm.

myotalgia senilis   An uncommon syndrome occurring in elderly people who suffer darting or aching pains, undiagnosable neuralgias, dysesthesias, and painful cramps in the legs associated with movement. The underlying pathology is not elucidated.

myotatic   (Gr, muscle + a stretching). Resulting from muscle stretching.

myotatic irritability   1. (goggia) Mounding or dimpling of a muscle tapped by the finger or tendon hammer, common in chronic debilitated states but classically evidence of **myotonia.** 2. Excessive reactivity of the muscle stretch reflexes (Sir William **Gowers**).

myotatic reflexes   The term of **Gowers** for the muscle stretch reflexes. The myotatic unit comprises muscle stretch receptors and their afferents, the intraspinal connections that these make with the alpha motor neuron, the motor neurons themselves, and the muscle fibers of that motor unit.[3405]

myotatic reflex scale   Adopted by the American National Institute of Neurological Disorders and Stroke (NINDS), this five-point scale rates the activity of muscle stretch reflex responses as follows:[2386]

0   Reflex absent
1   Reduced reflex response, including a trace response or one only evident with reinforcement
2   Response in lower lalf of normal range
3   Response in upper half of normal range
4   Response enhanced, maybe including clonus

The scale is thus bottom heavy; the need for two gradings for normal responses and only one to include all levels of hyperreflexia is not easily comprehensible, but reliability has been claimed.[3440]

myotatic unit   The reflex arc—all of the neural and muscular structures required for the occurrence of a muscle stretch reflex; thus, the muscle receptors and their afferent fibers, the segmental spinal pathways, the alpha motor neuron, and the muscle.

myotome   1. (metamere) A segment of the muscular system of the vertebrate embryo. The word dates from Goodsir's use of it in 1857. The muscles comprising a particular myotome are all those which are innervated by one spinal nerve root. 2. An instrument for cutting muscle sections.

myotomy   The division of a muscle to release contractures.

myotonia   1. Repetitive discharges of muscle fiber action potentials, at 20–80 Hz, resembling fibrillations or positive sharp waves and occurring with decreasing frequency and amplitude, each run having a duration of between 0.1 and 30 seconds. The runs are initiated by needle insertion, needle movement, muscle contraction, or muscle percussion. The phenomenon of prolonged after-contraction of a muscle after voluntary effort has ceased, usually diminishing with continuing muscle activity. The basis for this is abnormal muscle fiber contraction associated with abnormal and continued sarcolemmal membrane excitation and with a reduction in the potential difference across the membrane, the precise mechanism of which is still uncertain. 2. Muscle tension (obsolete). 3. The clinical observation of delayed relaxation of a muscle after voluntary contraction or percussion. Such delayed relaxation may be electrically silent, or may be accompanied by propagated electrical activity such as **myotonic discharge, complex repetitive discharge,** or **neuromyotonic discharge.**

Paradoxical myotonia (in paramyotonia) worsens with repeated activity. *Delayed myotonia* appears after a period of muscle contraction; see **myotonia fluctuans.**

A historical review is that of Thomasen.[5557]

The following genetic classification of the myotonias has been suggested:[4542]

1. Sodium channel diseases
   Hyperkalemic periodic paralysis
   Paramyotonia congenita
   Myotonia fluctuans
2. Protein kinase–related disease
   Myotonic dystrophy
   Proximal myotonic myopathy
3. Chloride-channel diseases
   Myotonia congenita (autosomal dominant)
   Myotonia congenita (autosomal recessive)
4. Unknown cause
   Schwarz-Jampel syndrome (chondrodystrophic myotonia)
   Hyperkalemic periodic paralysis with dysrhythmias
   Dominantly inherited painful myotonia[3474]

Adapted from Ptacek LJ, Johnson KJ, Griggs RC. Genetics and physiology of the myotonic muscle disorders. *N Engl J Med* 1993;**328**:482–489, by permission.

myotonia acquisita   Transient **myotonia,** which is not of genetic origin and is precipitated by exercise, or as a result of trauma, infectious or metabolic disease (such as poisoning with diazocholesterol or 2.4-D), or polyneuropathy.[5476] See **pseudomyotonia, Talma disease.**

myotonia atrophica   See **myotonic dystrophy.**

myotonia congenita   (Thomsen disease) A nonprogressive, nondystrophic myopathy with infantile or childhood onset, marked by abnormal electrical afterdischarges in muscles subjected to voluntary contraction and leading to a failure of relaxation which is made worse by rest and cold. The resultant cell membrane hyperexcitability results in reduction in sarcolemmal chloride conductance. Both dominant, (mapped to 7q35) and (less commonly in North America) recessive inheritance (*Becker myotonia)* are recorded, the former having an earlier onset but lesser severity, the latter sometimes associated with muscle dystrophic changes and periodic paralysis.

Clinically, painful, electrically silent muscle contractions, action and percussion myotonia, paradoxical myotonia in the cold, and severe cold insensitivity affecting especially the face are other notable symptoms. The EMG findings that repetitive muscular contractions do not alter the recruitment pattern and that, after cooling of the hand, the myotonic activity increases differentiate this condition from **paramyotonia congenita.**[4132]

Dr. Thomsen himself was thus affected and there was a strong family history of it (affecting at least four generations), but he was stirred to publish on the subject only because his affected son was being accused of malingering in an attempt to escape military service.[5569] Ernst von Leyden (1832–1910) gave an account of the disease in the same year.[3390]

Variant myotonic syndromes in this class are described,[5378] as listed in Chart M–27.

Chart M–27. Variant Myotonic Syndromes

Becker variant A recessively inherited disorder of the muscle chloride channel (CLCN1) at chromosome 7q35. Clinically, the symptoms are more severe than in the dominant form. The onset is in childhood, presenting with myotonia of the leg muscles, improving with continuing activity (the "warm-up" phenomenon). Muscle hypertrophy may be seen in the leg and gluteal muscles. Initially strength is normal but with brief exercise there is rapid occurrence of weakness, returning to normal with further activity. Some permanent distal weakness may be apparent. EMG findings include distal more than proximal myotonia, reduced with maximal contraction, and other features of mild myopathy. A decremental response occurs, especially at 30 Hz stimulation frequency.

Myotonia congenita and painful muscle contraction (type 2) (myotonia with painful cramps) A congenital syndrome of hypothyroidism, myotonia, and muscle pain.[4900]

Myotonia congenita with severe cold sensitivity (type 3) A dominantly inherited syndrome in which the abnormal muscle contractions are markedly increased at low temperatures.

Myotonia with centronuclear myopathy An inherited syndrome characterized by cataract, ptosis, ophthalmoplegia, torticollis, pes cavus, joint contractures, and proximal and distal myopathy with myotonia.

Recessive generalized myotonia A progressive myotonic syndrome characterized by childhood onset with marked muscle stiffness, especially in the legs, and only mild proximal muscle weakness.

Paramyotonia congenita A rare, dominantly inherited, nonprogressive syndrome with onset in childhood and

characterized by muscle stiffness worsened in cold temperatures, with increased and prolonged weakness after exercise (especially of the hand, facial, and bulbar muscles).[1710] Delayed eye opening after tight closure is characteristic. Independent attacks of paralysis also occur in some cases, precipitated, for example, by potassium loading.

Myotonia, myokymia, hyperhidrosis, and muscle wasting A benign syndrome of young men, manifesting these features. The EMG and muscle biopsy findings are generally normal.[2273]

Familial hyperkalemic periodic paralysis with myotonia

Familial granulovacuolar lobular myopathy with electrical myotonia[2890]

Recessive myotonia congenita with dystrophic features[4061]

Acetazolamide-responsive myotonia A dominantly inherited disorder of the sodium channel mapped to 7q35 and characterized by muscle hypertrophy without weakness, "paradoxical" myotonia made worse by repeated activity, muscle pain and stiffness, aggravation by potassium, and response to acetazolamide. See the Washington University, St. Louis, Neurology Web site: http://www.neuro.wustl.edu/neuromuscular/maltbrain.html.

The above chart is based on but modified from the classification of Streib (1987).[5378]

See also **paramyotonia congenita, myotonic dystrophy.**

myotonia congenita and painful muscle contraction See **myotonia congenita.**

myotonia congenita with severe cold sensitivity See **myotonia congenita.**

myotonia fluctuans (sodium-sensitive myotonia) A rare skeletal muscle sodium channel disease (SCN4A sodium channel α-subunit) presenting as a variant form of **myotonia** and characterized by dominant inheritance, exercise-induced, delayed-onset myotonia variable from day to day, and the absence of weakness. Symptoms are made worse with potassium loading but are minimally affected by cold.[4680] The responsible gene is mapped to 17q23.

A *variant* is *acetazolamide-responsive myotonia* (see above).

myotonia, myokymia, hyperhidrosis, and muscle wasting See **myotonia congenita.**

myotonia permanens A syndrome of continuous myokymia with marked muscle hypertrophy and superimposed attacks of marked muscle stiffness as a result of sodium channel impairment.[3323]

myotonia with centronuclear myopathy See **myotonia congenita.**

myotonia with dwarfism and bone disease A rare dysmorphic syndrome with these characteristics.[25]

myotonic chondrodystrophy See **Schwartz-Jampel syndrome.**

myotonic discharge   Repetitive discharge which occurs at rates of 20 to 80 Hz. There are two types: 1. Biphasic (positive–negative) spike potentials less than 5 msec in duration resembling fibrillation potentials. 2. Positive waves of 5 to 20 msec duration resembling positive sharp waves. Both potential forms are recorded after needle electrode insertion, after voluntary muscle contraction, or after muscle percussion, and are due to independent, repetitive discharges of single muscle fibers. The amplitude and frequency of the potentials must both wax and wane. This change produces a characteristic musical sound in the audio output of the electromyogram due to the corresponding change in pitch, which has been likened to the sound of a dive bomber (but that is incorrect as the sound of a dive bomber is characterized by increasing pitch, while myotonic discharges sound more like the whine of a rapidly departing motor cyclist). cf. **waning discharge.** (After the 2001 Report of the Nomenclature Committee of the American Association of Electromyography and Electrodiagnosis.[10] Used by permission, copyright © 2001, AAEM.)

myotonic dystrophy   (DM1, Batten-Gibb disease, Batten-Steinert-Curschmann disease, Steinert disease, Deleage disease, dystrophia myotonica, myotonica atrophica, OMIM 160900) A multisystem disease inherited in an autosomal dominant manner, the gene having been localized to 19q13.3 on chromosome 19 and considered due to an expansion of an unstable cytosine-thiamine-guanine trinucleotide repeat. The mutation is identified by the p5B1.4 probe.

The main features of the full syndrome include distal, centripetal, and cranial muscular atrophy with weakness, including respiratory muscle weakness; myotonia, shown best in the distal hand and faciobulbar muscles; cardiomyopathy; endocrinopathy with frontal balding, diabetes, and hypogonadism; and posterior polar cataract, reduced intraocular pressure, and slow pupillary reactions as well as diminished insight into the gravity of the condition. Fragments of the syndrome may occur alone.[4539]

An *infantile* form, occurring in the children of affected mothers (not of affected fathers) is unusually severe in the neonatal period, seems to modify the degree of affliction during childhood, and reappears in serious form in youth.

This is the most prevalent genetic dystrophy in the Western world, although **Duchenne dystrophy** has a higher incidence. The first descriptions were those of C.L. **Dana** in 1888 and of Francisque Deleage (b. 1862) in his 1890 graduation thesis for the University of Paris (although he thought that it was a variety of Thomsen disease). Hoffmann gave a partial description in 1900, and Steinert gave a fuller one in 1904.

The condition was the first disease in which the phenomenon of anticipation was reliably demonstrated. It is also of interest because the Ypsilante brothers, leaders of the Greek revolution of 1821 in which Greece was successfully wrested from the control of the Ottoman Empire, suffered from it.[2457]

Defined *variants* of the syndrome are expanding in number, but all multisystem myotonic disorders are subsumed under the heading of myotonic dystrophies. They include the following:

Myotonic dystrophy with hypersomnia and alveolar hypoventilation The typical signs of myotonic dystrophy are accompanied by excessive somnolence and alveolar hypoventilation.

Myotonic dystrophy and hypertrophic neuropathy A form characterized by neurogenic muscular atrophy and demyelinating sensorimotor neuropathy in addition to the usual signs of the disease.[337]

Myotonic dystrophy and axonal-demyelinating polyneuropathy A form characterized by the presence of a severe sensorimotor polyneuropathy in addition to the usual signs of the disease.[5783]

Unclassified familial myopathy resembling Steinert disease A proximal myopathy with the usual non-neurological findings of myotonic dystrophy but without clinical or electrical evidence of myotonia.[5518]

See also **proximal myotonic myopathy** (and its subvariants), **action nyotonia, percussion myotonia, paradoxical myotonia.**

Myotonic Dystrophy Association   See **Muscular Dystrophy Association.**

myotonic periodic paralysis   See **paramyotonia congenita.**

myotonic (Adie) pupil   See **Holmes-Adie syndrome.**

myotonic pupillary reaction   See **Adie pupil.**

myotonica atrophica   See **myotonic dystrophy.**

myotubes   Multinucleated cell structures seen early in fetal development (7 weeks) and composed of fused myoblasts. In postnatal life, myotube-like structures are found in one form of congenital myopathy.

myotubular myopathy   See **centronuclear myopathies.**

myriachit   A familial tic-like disorder affecting both sexes, occurring epidemically in Siberia, the movements precipitated by startle and lasting hours, sometimes accompanied by echolalia. See also **Tourette syndrome.**

myxedema   (Gull disease, hypothyroidism)[2330] The painless, nonpitting edema of the shin described in hypothyroidism. Such edema was considered so specific that its name was also used for the whole syndrome of hypothyroidism.

myxedema cerebellar syndrome   Ataxia and incoordination complicating hypothyroidism, remitting with successful treatment of that condition.[2828]

myxedema coma   (hypothyroid encephalopathy) A recurrent acute encephalopathy with confusion leading to coma with pyramidal signs and seizures or myoclonus, and a low-voltage EEG marked by generalized slow-wave activity. It is seen in myxedema with Hashimoto disease and results from a marked depression of the hypoxic respiratory drive, leading to further hypoxia, hypercapnia, and coma resulting from CO_2 narcosis. Hyponatremia due to inappropriate antidiuretic hormone secretion, hypothermia, and hypoglycemia may also contribute, and pituitary and adrenal insufficiencies are incriminated. The mortality rate may range up to 30%.[3338]

The illness is usually precipitated by cold, chest infections, stroke, congestive heart failure, or use of sedative drugs, typically in patients with a history of thyroid disease, and often with evidence of dementia or **myxedematous madness.** The condition was first recognized in 1879 by William Ord.

myxedematous madness　The colorful term used by Richard Asher in 1949[237] for a syndrome (also well described by A.J. Cronin in *The Citadel*, 1937) comprising disturbances in mentation often accompanying severe hypothyroidism. These include delirium, melancholia, paranoid psychoses and sometimes restless violence, hallucinations, depression, dementia, extreme somnolence, and sometimes hypothermia. No one of these manifestations is predominant. There are no focal signs except for localized EEG changes. See **myxedema coma.**[237]

N

N-acetylaspartic aciduria A congenital syndrome resulting from aspartoacyalase deficiency and manifesting spasticity, macrocephaly, tremor, diffuse cerebral demyelination, and mental and developmental delay with organic aciduria.[337]

NADH–coenzyme Q reductase deficiency An inherited mitochondrial myopathy characterized by complex 1 defects that lead to exercise-induced fatigue, acute attacks of weakness provoked by exercise, alcohol, or fasting, and lactic acidosis.[3981]

Naegeli syndrome See **incontinentia pigmenti.**

Naffziger, Howard Christian (1884–1961) American neurosurgeon who trained and saw war service with **Cushing.** He was later professor at the University of California, San Francisco.

Naffziger signs 1. Compression of both jugular veins increases CSF pressure which, being transmitted to the lumbar theca, stretches both the meninges and the attached nerve roots and causes (or increases) pain in patients with root irritation at those levels.[4196] 2. Pressure on the scalenus anterior muscle above the clavicle leads to paresthesias of the hand in patients with **thoracic outlet syndrome.** 3. Shift of the pineal gland (visible on skull x-ray when calcified) as a sign of an expanding intracranial mass, such as a subdural hematoma.

Naffziger syndrome (scalenus syndrome) See **thoracic outlet syndrome.**

Nagel anomaloscope A device for detecting defects in color vision, in which the subject has to match the appearance of a monochromatic yellow field to one of a number of mixtures of red and green lights.[4381]

Nageotte, Jean (1866–1948) French neurologist, born in Dijon. He graduated from the University of Paris, and was later appointed physician at the Bicetre hospital and then at the **Salpêtrière.** He succeeded Ranvier as professor of comparative histology at the Collège de France.

Nageotte was a friend of **Babiński**, with whom he collaborated in studies of the CSF and in describing medullary tegmental paralysis, and he was also the first correctly to ascribe the lesion in **tabes dorsalis** to the dorsal roots.

Naidu variant See **adrenoleukodystrophy.**

naked axons Nonmyelinated nerve fibers or demyelinated fibers of usually myelinated axons; the axons of the Remak fibers.

NAME syndrome (**N**evi, **A**trial myxoma, **M**yxoid neurofibromata, **E**piphelides) A congenital dysmorphic syndrome characterized also by gynecomastia; tumors of the breast, testes, and heart; abnormal genital pigmentation; adrenal hyperplasia; large sella turcica; osteoporosis; acanthosis nigricans; nevi; cavernous hemangioma; skin cysts; and neurofibromas.[4629]

Name–Face test A test of visual verbal associations in which names appear with photographs.[1802]

Nance-Sweeney dwarfism A recessively inherited congenital chondrodystrophy characterized by dysmorphism; short stature; calcification of the ear cartilage, subcutaneous tissue, and muscle; macrocephaly; conductive and sensorineural deafness; brachydactyly; scoliosis; and other skeletal anomalies.[4072]

nanism Dwarfism.

nanocephaly (from Gr, a dwarf + the head) Abnormal smallness of the head; the same as microcephaly.

narcolepsy (from Gr, numbness + a seizure) A disorder of excessive sleepiness often associated with the occurrence of manifestations of rapid eye movement (REM) sleep such as **hypnagogic hallucinations, cataplexy,** and **sleep paralysis** during waking periods.

Clinically, in its fullest expression, the syndrome is characterized by excessive daytime sleepiness, **hypnagogic hallucinations, cataplexy, sleep paralysis,** microsleep lapses, amnesic automatisms, memory blackouts, diplopia, and disturbed nocturnal sleep. In early cases, the disorder may be monosymptomatic. The onset is generally in youth or young adult life. The symptoms additional to the sleep attacks make up a tetrad of narcoleptic symptoms occurring more often in association with **REM-onset sleep patterns** as seen on the EEG, whereas patients who have **idiopathic CNS hypersomnolence** have sleep attacks with non–rapid eye movement sleep (**NREM**) onset. **Sleep apnea** may also complicate the syndrome, which characteristically begins in youth. A positive family history is common, and tight linkage to HLA DQB1 0602 has been demonstrated, but the responsible gene maps to chromosome 6p21.3. The pathophysiology appears to involve acquired damage to hypothalamic cells secreting the peptide hypocretin.

While Gélineau[2067] gave the first modern account of the syndrome in 1880 (his patient had sleep attacks and cataplexy), he acknowledged Caffé's earlier identification of the disorder in 1862, but not that by H.B. Schindler, an ophthalmologist in Breslau, in 1829. In fact, Thomas **Willis** had recounted his treatment of patients with excessive sleepiness 200 years before in *De Anima Brutorum* and **Westphal** described it 3 years before Gélineau, but the latter named it. The American general "Stonewall" Jackson probably suffered from this condition, but it did not seem to diminish his military effectiveness.

See also Chart S–6, **sleep disorders.**[234,2320]

Diagnostic criteria were first suggested by Yoss and Daly,[6085] but newer ones have been suggested and are listed in Chart N–1.[234]

Chart N–1. Diagnostic Criteria for Narcolepsy

A. A complaint of excessive sleepiness or sudden muscle weakness

B. Recurrent daytime naps or lapses into sleep that occur almost daily for at least 3 months

C. Sudden bilateral loss of postural muscle tone in association with intense emotion (cataplexy)

D. Associated features include the following:
1. Sleep paralysis
2. Hypnagogic hallucinations
3. Automatic behaviors
4. Disrupted major sleep episode

E. Polysomnography demonstrates one or more of the following:
1. Sleep latency less than 5 minutes
2. REM sleep latency less than 20 minutes and
3. A multiple sleep latency test that demonstrates a mean sleep latency of less than 5 minutes
4. Two or more sleep-onset REM periods

F. HLA typing demonstrates DR2 positivity

G. Absence of any medical or psychiatric disorder that could account of the symptoms

H. Other sleep disorders may be present, but are not the primary cause of the symptoms, e.g., periodic limb movement disorder or central sleep apnea syndrome.

From ASDA Diagnostic Classification Steering Committee. The International Classification of Sleep Disorders Diagnostic and Coding Manual. Rochester, MN: American Sleep Disorders Association, 1990. Reproduced by kind permission of the American Academy of Sleep Medicine.

Variants include the following:
Secondary narcolepsy (symptomatic), in which some symptoms of the condition appear in patients with various diseases affecting the brainstem
Narcolepsy with congenital oculomotor pareses
Narcolepsy with congenital cataract
Narcolepsy with diplopia and strabismus[4337]
See also *idiopathic hypersomnia.*

Narcolepsy Network   A charitable organization providing support and information on this condition. Address: 10921 Reed Hartman Highway, Cincinnati, OH 45242. Tel: 513-891-3522. Web site: http://narcolepsynetwork.org/.

narcosis   (from Gr, benumbing) The condition of those under the influence of sedative agents.

narcotic abstinence headache   See **rebound headache** in which headaches on withdrawal from other substances are included.

NARP syndrome   A sporadic, X-linked or autosomal recessive syndrome characterized by sensory peripheral Neuropathy resembling Refsum syndrome (**hereditary motor and sensory neuropathy, type 4**) but with normal serum phytanic acid levels, and including Ataxia and Retinitis Pigmentosa with normal lipoprotein levels. The biochemical abnormality is not known and the condition may be a mitochondrial disorder. Sen-

sorineural deafness and evidence of cerebellar atrophy have also been detected in such patients.[3683,5660] It has been reported in a single sibship.

See also **Cockayne syndrome, Hallgren syndrome, von Graefe–Sjörgren syndrome, lipidoses, cerebellar ataxias.**

nasal reflex   1. (sternutatory reflex, sneeze reflex) Sneezing in response to nasal tickle. 2. (nasal reflex of Bechterew) Contraction of the ipsilateral facial muscles in response to nasal tickle. An abrogation of No. 1.

nasal reflex of Bechterew   See **nasal reflex.**

nascent   (from Lat, to be born) In the process of being born.

nascent motor unit potentials   Very low–amplitude, short-duration, highly polyphasic motor unit action potentials observed during the early stages of reinnervation. The use of the term is discouraged, as it incorrectly implies diagnostic significance of a motor unit action potential configuration. See also **motor unit action potential.** (After the 2001 Report of the Nomenclature Committee of the American Association of Electromyography and Electrodiagnosis.[10] Used by permission, copyright © 2001, AAEM.)

nasion   The median point of the junction between the two frontal and the two nasal bones; thus, the center point above the bridge of the nose.

nasolacrimal reflex   The secretion of tears in response to chemical stimulation of the nasal mucosa.

nasomental reflex   See **buccal reflex, orbicularis oris reflex.**

nasopalpebral reflex   (glabellar tap, orbicularis oculi reflex) Blinking in response to tapping on the bridge of the nose.[6064] See **McCarthy reflex.**

nasopharyngeal electrode   An electrode introduced through the nasal passages to lie against the nasopharyngeal wall, its tip thus close to the body of the sphenoid bone.

nasopharyngeal torticollis   See **Grisel syndrome.**

Nasu-Hakola lipodystrophy   (polycystic lipomembranous osteodysplasia with sclerosing leukoencephalopathy; OMIM 221770) A dysmorphic syndrome with juvenile or young adult onset, characterized by bony cysts and multiple fractures, progressive early dementia with dyspraxia, agnosia and dysphasia, seizures, myoclonus, pyramidal signs, frontal lobe atrophy, and calcifications of the basal ganglia.[4313]

nates   (Lat, the rump) The buttocks. The nates cerebri are the corpora quadragemini, from their supposed resemblance to the foregoing.

Nathalie syndrome   A congenital syndrome characterized by short stature, sensorineural deafness, cataract, absent or hypoplastic breasts, ECG abnormality, and axonal motor neuropathy.[337]

National AIDS Network   A charitable association. Address: 1012 14th Street N.W., Suite 601, Washington, D.C. 20005. Tel: 202-347-0390.

National Aphasia Association   A charitable organization. Address: 29 John Street, Suite 1103, (NAA) New York, NY 10038. Tel: 212-267-2814. Web site: http://www.aphasia.org/.

National Association for Down Syndrome   A charitable organization. Web site: http://www.nads.org/.

National Ataxia Foundation   A charitable association in this field. Address: 2600 Fernbrook Lane, Suite 119, Minneapolis, MN 55391. Tel: 763-553-0020. Web site: http://www.ataxia.org/.

National Brachial Plexus/Erb's Palsy Association, Inc.   A charitable organization in this field. Address: P.O. Box 23, Larsen, WI 54947. E-mail: erbspalsy@usa.net. Web site: http://www.nbpepa/.

National Brain Tumor Foundation   A charitable organization. Address: 414 Thirteenth St., Suite 700, Oakland, CA 94612-2603. Tel: 1-800-934-CURE. Web site: http://www.braintumor.org/.

National Chronic Pain Outreach Association   A charitable organization in this field. Address: PO. Box 274, Millboro, VA 24460. Tel: 540-862-9437. E-mail: ncpoa@cfw.com. Web site: http://www.ijdf.net/.

National Disability Sports Alliance   A charitable organization in this field. Address: 25 West Independence Way, Kingston, RI 02881. Tel: 401-792-7130. E-mail: info@ndsaonline.org. Web site: http://www.ndsaonline.org/.

National Down Syndrome Congress   A charitable association in this field. Address: 1370 Center Drive, Ste. 102, Atlanta, GA 30338. Tel: 770-604-9500, 800-232-NDSC. Web site: http://www.ndsccenter.org/.

National Down Syndrome Society   A charitable association in this field. Web site: http://www.ndss.org/.

National Dysautonomia Research Foundation   A charitable organization in this field. Address: 421 W. Fourth Street, Suite 9, Red Wing, MN 55066-2555. Phone: 651-267-0525, Web site: http://www.ndrf.org/.

National Easter Seal Society   A charitable organization. Address: 230 West Monroe Street, Suite 1800. Chicago, IL 60606. Web site: http://www.easter-seals.org/.

National Epilepsy Library   See **Epilepsy Foundation of America.** Web site: http://www.efa.org/services/library/html.

National Eye Institute   A government health research organization. Address: National Institutes of Health, Bldg. 31, Rm. 6A32, Bethesda, MD 20892-2510. Tel: 301-496-5248; Professionals: 800-869-2020. E-mail: 2020@b31.nei.nih.gov. Web site: http://www.nei.nih.gov/.

National Foundation for Jewish Genetic Diseases   A charitable association in this field. Address: 250 Park Ave., Ste. 1000, New York, NY 10177. Tel: 212-371-1030. Web site: http://www.nfjgd.org/.

National Gaucher Foundation   A charitable organization in this field providing information and support. Address: 5410 Edson Lane, Suite 260, Rockville, MD 20852-3130. Tel: 301-816-1515: 800-428-2437. E-mail: ngf@gaucherdisease.org. Web site: http://www.gaucherdisease.org/.

National Head Injury Foundation   See **Brain Injury Association.**

National Headache Foundation   A charitable organization. Address: 428 W. St. James Place, 2nd Floor, Chicago, IL 60614-2750. Tel: 1-888-NHF-5552, 312-878-7715. Web site: http://www.headaches.org/.

National Hospital, Queen Square   The first hospital dedicated to the care and cure of patients suffering from neurological diseases, it was opened in Queen Square, London, England, in 1860, largely through the efforts of Miss Joanna Chandler, who saw the great need for such an institution and determined to devote her life to supply such a place for the treatment of the paralyzed and epileptic. The stated object of the hospital was to "give relief to such persons as are disqualified for the duties of life by either paralysis or epilepsy and are proper objects of charity. Those who need only partial relief . . . will be treated as outdoor patients." The appointment to its staff of some of the best-known London practitioners saved the hospital from the hostility of the medical profession, and it flourished although existing almost totally upon the proceeds of charitable appeals. New buildings were added, the Rockefeller Foundation contributing funds for the erection of research laboratories in 1934, and for over 100 years, the hospital, with the Institute of Neurology built later, was preeminently the center for the study of neurological disorders in Great Britain, receiving referrals from all parts of the United Kingdom.

Dr. J. Hughlings-**Jackson,** Sir William **Gowers,** Dr. **Brown-Sequard,** Sir David **Ferrier,** Sir Gordon **Holmes,** Sir Victor **Horsley,** Dr. Marcus **Gunn,** Dr. S.A.K. **Wilson,** Sir Francis **Walshe,** Sir Charles **Symonds,** and Dr. W.J. **Adie,** among others, were members of the staff of the hospital during its first hundred years of operation.[2626]

National Hydrocephalus Foundation   A charitable organization. Address: 12413 Centralia Road, Lakewood, CA 90715-1623. Web site: http://nhfonline.org/.

National Institute of Aging   A U.S. government organization. Address: Building 31, Room 5C27, 31 Center Dr., MSC 2292, Bethesda, MD 20892. Tel: 301-496-1752. Web site: http://www.nia.nih.gov/.

National Institute of Child Health and Human Development   A government health research organization.

Address: National Institutes of Health, Bldg. 31, Rm. 2A32, Bethesda, MD 20892-2425. Tel: 301-496-5133; 800-370-2943. E-mail: NICHDClearinghouse@mail.nih. gov. Web site: http://www.nichd.nih.gov/.

National Institute of Deafness and Other Communication Disorders   A government health research organization. Address: National Institutes of Health, Bldg. 31, Rm. 3C35, Bethesda, MD 20892-2320. E-mail: nidcdinfo@nidcd.nih.gov. Tel: 301-496-7243. Web site: http://www.nidcd.nih.gov/.

National Institute of Mental Health   A government health research organization. Address: 6001 Executive Blvd., Rm. 8184, MSC 9663, Bethesda, MD 20892-9663. Tel: 301-443-4513. Tel: (Depression Info) 800-421-4211; (Anxiety Info) 888-ANXIETY (269-4389); (Panic Info) 888-64-PANIC (64-72642). E-mail: nimhinfo@nih.gov. Web site: http://www.nimh.nih.gov/.

National Institute of Neurological and Communicative Disorders and Stroke   See **National Institute of Neurological Disorders and Stroke.**

National Institute of Neurological Disorders and Stroke   (National Institute of Neurological Disease and Blindness, National Institute of Neurological and Communicative Disorders and Stroke) A U.S. government organization established in 1951 with a $1.9 million budget as an institute for research in neurological diseases. The institute functioned to increase study in basic sciences; to initiate research in targeted areas, such as neonatal brain damage, stroke, and neurogenetics; and to provide research and training fellowships in the neurological disciplines.

Its name was changed to the National Institute of Neurological and Communicative Disorders and Stroke in 1968 and subsequently to the current one. Address: NIH Neurological Institute, P.O. Box 5801, Bethesda, MD 20824. Tel: 800-352-9424. Web site: http://www.ninds.nih.gov/.

National Institute of Neurological Disorder and Stroke myotatic reflex scale   A standardized scale adopted in that center for the assessment of muscle stretch reflexes.

0. Absence of the reflex
1. Reduced responsiveness, or presence only with reinforcement
2. Responsiveness assessed as in the lower half of the normal range
3. Responsiveness assessed as in the upper half of the normal range
4. Hyperflexia, including clonus

Adapted from Hallet M. NINDs myotatic reflex scale. Neurology 1993; 43:2723.

The scale is bottom heavy, and any level of reflex activity, from 1 to 4, may actually be present in a normal subject.

National Institutes of Health   The premier U.S. governmental health organization and the home of

PubMed. Web site: http://www.nih.gov/ or http://www.nbi.nlm.nih.gov/entrez/query.fcgi.

National Institutes of Health Office of Rare Diseases   A U.S. governmental agency. Tel: 301-402-4336. Web site: http://rarediseases.info.nih.gov/.

National Library of Medicine   The foremost United States medical library, providing asscess to Medline/ PubMed. Web site: http://www.nlm.nih.gov/.

National Mental Health Association   A charitable organization. Address: 2001 N. Beauregard St., 13th Fl., Tel: 703-684-7722, 1-800-969-NMHA. Web site: http://www.nmha.org/.

National Migraine Foundation   See **National Headache Foundation.**

National Mucopolysaccharidosis (MPS) Society   A charitable association in this field. Address: 102 Aspen Dr., Downingtown, PA 19335. E-mail: info@mpssociety.org. Web site: http://www.mpssociety.org/.

National Multiple Sclerosis Society   An American charitable organization devoted to supporting research into the causes and treatment of multiple sclerosis, and to providing support for those affected by the disease through the formation of chapters for education, counseling, referral, and advocacy. Address: 733 Third Ave., New York, NY, 10017-3288. Tel: 212-986-3240 or 1-800-FIGHT MS (344-4867). Web site: http://www.nmss.org/.

National Neurofibromatosis Foundation, Inc.   A charitable organization devoted to supporting research into the causes and treatment of neurofibromatosis, promoting the development of diagnostic protocols and clinical centers, publishing educational materials, and supporting those affected by the disease through the formation of chapters for education, counseling, referral, and advocacy. Address: 95 Pine Street, 16th Fl., New York, NY 10005. Tel: 212-344-NNFF, 1-800-323-7938. Web site: http://www.nf.org/.

National Neurological Research Specimen Bank   A research organization. Address: Human Brain and Spinal Fluid Resource Center, W. Los Angeles Healthcare Center, 11301 Wilshire Blvd., Los Angeles, CA 90073. Tel: 310-268-3536. Web site: http://www.loni.ucla.edu/~nnrsb/NNRSB/.

National Niemann-Pick Disease Foundation, Inc.   A charitable organization in this field. Address: P.O. Box 49, Ft. Atkinson, WI 53538. Tel: 920-563-0930; 877-287-3672. E-mail: nnpdf@idcnet.com. Web site: http://www.nnpdf.org/.

National Organization for Rare Disorders, Inc.   A charitable association in this field. Address: 55 Kenosia Ave., P.O. Box 1968, Danbury, CT 06813-1968. Tel: 203-744-0100. 800-999-6673. Web site: http://www.rarediseases.org/.

National Parkinson Foundation, Inc. A charitable association in this field. Address: 1501 N.W. 9th Avenue, Miami, FL 33136-1494. 1-800-327-4545. Web site: www.parkinson.org/.

National Rehabilitation Information Center A health research and support organization. Address: 4200 Forbes Blvd. Suite 202, Lanham, MD 20706. Tel: 800-346-2742; 301-459-5900. E-mail: naricinfo@ heitechservices.com. Web site: http://www.naric.com/.

National Reye's Syndrome Foundation A charitable organization providing support and information on this condition. Address: 426 North Lewis St., Bryan, OH 43506. Tel: 419-636-2679, 1-800-233-7393. Web site: http://www.reyessyndrome.org/.

National Sleep Foundation A charitable organization providing support and information on sleep disorders. Address: 1522 K Street, NW, Suite 500, Washington, DC 20005. Tel: 202-347-3471. Web site: http://www.sleepfoundation.org/.

National Society to Prevent Blindness See **Prevent Blindness America.**

National Spasmodic Dysphonia Association A charitable association providing support and information on this condition. Address: One E. Wacker Drive, Ste. 2430, Chicago, IL 60601-1905. Tel: 800-795-NSDA. Web site: http://www.dysphonia.org/nsda/.

National Spasmodic Torticollis Association A charitable organization providing support and information on this condition. Address: 9920 Talbert Ave., #233, Fountain Valley, CA 92708. Tel: 1-800-487-8385. Web site: http://www.torticollis.org/.

National Spinal Cord Injury Association A charitable organization providing support and information on this condition. Address: 6701 Democracy Blvd., Bethesda, MD 20817. Tel: 301-588-6959, 1-800-962-9629. Web site: http://www.spinalcord.org/.

National Stroke Association A charitable organization committed solely to stroke prevention, treatment, rehabilitation, and community reintegration. It provides packaged training programs; on-site assistance; and physician, patient, and family education materials to acute care and rehabilitation hospitals; organizes workshops; operates the Stroke Information and Referral Center; and produces professional publications (*Stroke: Clinical Updates* and *Journal of Stroke and Cerebrovascular Disease*). Address: 9707 E. Easter Lane, Englewood, CO 80112. Tel: 303-649-9299, 1-800-STROKES. Web sites: www.strokejournal.org/. www.stroke.org/.

National Tay-Sachs and Allied Diseases Association A charitable organization providing support and information on this condition. Address: 2001 Beacon Street, Ste. 204, Boston, MA 02135. Tel: 800-906-8723. Web site: http://www.ntsad.org/.

National Tremor Foundation A charitable organization. Address: Harold Wood Hospital (DSC), Gubbins Lane, Romford, Essex, RM3 OBE UK. Tel: 01708 386 399. Web site: http://www.tremor.org.uk/.

National Tuberous Sclerosis Association A charitable organization providing support and information on this condition. Address: 8000 Corporate Drive, Ste. 120, Landover, MD 20785. Tel: 301-459-9888; 1-800-225-NTSA (6872). Web site: http://tsalliance.org/redirect.asp.

natural killer neuropathy A widespread multifocal, axonal, inflammatory neuropathy attacking roots and peripheral nerves, in association with CSF pleocytosis, in the context of natural killer cell leukemia.[616]

Nature Neuroscience A basic science journal. Web site: http://www.nature.com/neurosci/.

nausea The desire or urge to vomit, unaccomplished.

NCS See **nerve conduction studies.**

near point The closest place in front of the eyes at which an object is still in focus.

near reflex See **near triad.**

near response Pupillary constriction (accommodation) with vergence of the eyes during gaze upon an object near to the face. See **near triad.**

near synkinesis See **near triad.**

near triad (near response, near reflex, near synkinesis) The three mechanisms whereby the eye disposes itself to allow focused close vision. They comprise **convergence, miosis,** and pupillary constriction (**accommodation**).

near-constant-frequency trains See **complex repetitive discharge.**

near-field A region of electrical activity where the isopotential voltage lines associated with a current source change rapidly over a short distance. The terms *near-field* and *far-field* are arbitrary designations, as there are no agreed-upon criteria defining where the near-field ends and the far-field begins. cf. **far-field.** (From the 2001 Report of the Nomenclature Committee of the American Association of Electromyography and Electrodiagnosis.[10] Used by permission, copyright © 2001, AAEM.)

near-field potential Electrical activity of biological origin generated near the recording electrodes.

Use of the terms *near-field potential* and *far-field potential* is discouraged because all potentials in clinical neurophysiology are recorded at some distance from the generator and there is no consistent distinction between the two terms. (Adapted from the 1987 Report of the Nomenclature Committee of the American Association of Electromyography and Electrodiagnosis. AAEE glossary of terms in clinical electromyography. *Muscle Nerve* 1987;**10S:**G5-G23. Copyright 1987 by John Wiley and Sons, Inc. Reprinted by permission of John Wiley and Sons, Inc.)

neck   All that part of the body which lies between and connects the head and the thorax.

neck phenomenon   See **Brudzinski signs.**

neck rigidity   Active reflex resistance to passive flexion of the neck. A sign of meningeal irritation from any cause, and of increased intracranial pressure.

Increased tone of the neck extensors is also a feature of **progressive supranuclear palsy,** and increased resistance to flexion occurs in subjects with cervical spinal disease, but in such cases other signs of meningeal irritation (**Kernig sign, Brudzinski sign**) should be absent.

neck torsion nystagmus   See **cervical nystagmus.**

neck-eye loop   See **cervico-ocular reflex.**

neck-righting reflex   See **righting reflex.**

neck-righting response   A variation of the **tonic neck reflex,** seen in the first 10 months of life, in which rotation of the infant's head to one side induces rotation of the shoulder and pelvis and eventually of the whole body to that side.

The reflex may be induced clinically in order to compare motor activity on the two sides of the body.

neck-tongue syndrome   The occurrence of pain in the neck and numbness on one side of the tongue induced by turning the head and likely to be due to irritation of the C2–3 cervical roots as they course between the axis and atlas. The following diagnostic criteria are suggested by the Headache Classification Committee of the International Headache Society[1051] (from Classification of headache disorders, cranial neuralgias and facial pains; and diagnostic criteria for primary headache disorders. *Cephalalgia* 1988;8[suppl]:1–96 and are reproduced by kind permission of Blackwell Science.)

   A. Pain and numbness in area of distribution of the lingual nerve and second cervical root

   B. Precipitation by sudden turning of the head

Repeated minor subluxations of the C1–2 articulatory process with compression and stretch injury of adjacent nerves such as the C2 ramus may be responsible. Afferent fibers from the lingual nerve join the hypoglossal nerve and then enter the upper cervical rami, which accounts for the tongue symptoms. The pain is thought to be due to stretching of the joint capsule of the lateral articulating process.[3241]

A recent review has been published.[4261]

necrosis   (from Gr, a state of death) Irreversible destruction of some or all of the cellular elements of a tissue.

necrotizing fasciitis   An uncommon, severe, and potentially lethal condition manifesting gross swelling of an affected part with severe fever and necrosis of the overlying skin, fever, shock, and multisystem involvement resulting from bacterial infection.[3817]

Type 1 is caused by mixed anaerobes, enterococci, and gram-negative aerobes and tends to destroy fat and fascia, while type 2 is caused by *Streptococcus* group A and is characterized by severe local pain, systemic toxicity and shock, organ failure and extending necrosis of skin and subcutaneous tissues.[590]

In a *variant* form, *necrotizing fasciitis with polymyositis,* the infection is considered secondary to the immunosuppression associated with the polymyositis.[926]

See also **myonecrosis.**

necrotizing granulomatous angiitis with a predilection for the CNS   See **allergic angiitis and granulomatosis.**

necrotizing leukoencephalopathy   Rapidly progressive necrosis of the white matter of the brain as a complication of the combined treatment of leukemia with methotrexate and cranial irradiation.

Clinically, confusion, ataxia, and quadriparesis lead to seizures, stupor, and eventual death. See also **somnolence syndrome.**

necrotizing leukoencephalopathy with CNS vasculitis   A fatal dysimmune condition, a rare complication of celiac disease, presenting with progressive cerebellar ataxia, epilepsy, myoclonus, peripheral neuropathy, pyramidal tract signs, tremor, and evidence of brainstem involvement. Pathologically, there is extensive gliosis and neuronal loss in the cortex, cerebellum, brainstem, and deep gray matter.[4849]

necrotizing myelopathy   A rare **paraneoplastic syndrome** occurring in patients with a variety of malignancies and characterized by the subacute onset of painless motor, sensory, and sphincter dysfunction with evidence of a transverse cord lesion at a defined level, with accelerating progression. Pathologically, there is massive transverse cord necrosis at that level.[2411]

necrotizing myopathy   Moderate and scattered necrosis of muscle fibers occurring as a toxic effect of drugs such as clofibrate, lovastatin, and epsilon-aminocaproic acid.

Clinically, myalgia, muscle tenderness, and weakness are the main complaints. The serum creatine kinase levels are raised and the electrical and pathological findings are those of nonspecific degeneration of myofibrils.[3301,3188]

Nederlandse Vereniging voor Neurologie   A professional organization based at P.O. Box 20050, 3502 LB Utrecht, The Netherlands.

needle electrode   An electrical device used for recording or stimulating that is positioned near the tissue of interest by penetration of the skin. Types include: bifilar (bipolar) needle recording electrode, **concentric needle electrode, macro-EMG** needle electrode, **monopolar needle recording electrode, multilead electrode, single fiber needle electrode,** and **stimulating electrode.** (From the 2001 Report of the Nomenclature Committee of the American Association of Electromyography and Electrodiagnosis.[10] Used by permission, copyright © 2001, AAEM.)

needle-in-the-eye syndrome The occurrence of repetitive, sudden, brief, lancinating pains felt in one eye. No pathology is known to be associated and the condition is benign.[4376]

See also **ice-pick pains, benign paroxysmal cranial neuralgia, exploding head syndrome.**

needle-like occipital spikes Innocuous, unusually brief spikes recorded over the occipital regions in congenitally blind children. The spikes disappear during adolescence and are considered to reflect only functional deafferentation.[3228] See also **benign occipital spikes.**

Neftel disease (hysterical astasia-abasia) Inability to walk, although all appropriate leg movements can be made in the supine position.

Neftel, W.B. (1830–1906) Russian-American physician who trained in Moscow and, after service in the Crimean War, emigrated to New York.

negative afterimages The ephemeral complementary image of a bright object which remains for a while when darkness supervenes, as with eye closure, so that what was bright is now seen as dark and *vice versa.*

negative delta sign See **empty delta sign.**

negative myoclonus Silent periods of between 35 and 200 msec duration that interrupt voluntary background EMG activity and result in jerky myoclonic movements such as asterixis.[6093] See also **myoclonus, asterixis.**

A *variant* is *epileptic negative myoclonus* in which brief postural lapses of a body segment are time-locked with EEG spike activity in contralateral central areas, where almost continuous paroxysmal activity is recordable. The syndrome occurs in subjects with partial epilepsies or various etiologies, who complain of action-activated jerks of an arm, each jerk being related to a silent period on the EMG lasting 100–400 msec. Motor neglect and impaired awareness of the disorder are commonly associated.[2311]

negative symptoms Those clinical features (such as paresis or sensory loss) which appear due to the removal of a normal state of tonic activation of part of the nervous system. They may be compared with **positive symptoms** (such as epileptic events) which occur from abnormal activation within the nervous system. The distinction was made first by Hughlings-**Jackson.**

neglect 1. (hemispatial agnosia) The phenomenon whereby objects or occurrences in one half-field are perceived but to which responses are inhibited. This has been interpreted as a defect in the orienting response, due either to hemispatial hypokinesia restricted to acts that have to be performed on the side of the inattention or to a hemispatial memory defect.[2519] See also **paralexia, paragraphia.**

2. Inability to direct the focus of awareness toward behaviorally relevant sensory events in one direction of extrapersonal space.[3851] The phenomenon is most often found with right hemisphere lesions, sensory events occurring within the left extrapersonal hemispace having a diminished or no impact upon awareness. See **extinction.** The processes preventing neglect in healthy subjects are mediated by the posterior parietal cortex, prefrontal cortex, and the cingulate gyrus; damage to any of these may give rise to the syndrome of unilateral neglect. See also **visual neglect.**

3. (*representational neglect*) Neglect of space that is not actually seen but only imagined. Neglect of the space that is seen is known as *perceptual neglect.* The phenomenon is seldom considered in daily neurological practice.

neglect syndrome A disorder characterized by hemi-inattention, extinction of double simultaneous stimuli, hemiakinesia, allesthesia, hemispatial neglect, anosognosia, and anisodiaphoria.[5367]

It is probably due to impairment of attention-arousal systems induced by dysfunction of those neuronal networks that form the basis of corticolimbic-reticular interaction.[2520]

Negri, Adelchi (1876–1912) Italian physician and pathologist who trained at Pavia University and was assistant to **Golgi.** He became professor of microbiology at Pavia and wrote mainly on hematology, dysentery, malaria, and rabies.[1829]

Negri bodies Eosinophilic intracytoplasmic inclusions composed of virus particles, seen in the Purkinje cells of the cerebellum and in the hippocampal pyramidal cells in **rabies,** described by Negri in 1905 (although he thought that they were parasitic protozoa).[4723]

Structures which are similar but without the core are known as **Lyssa bodies** and are not specific for rabies.[3876]

Negro, Camillo (1861–1927) Italian neurologist in Turin.

Camillo Negro

Negro sign (phenomenon)   1. (toothed trochlea phenomenon) Cogwheel rigidity, described by Camillo Negro in 1901 in his parkinsonian patients. In **Gowers'** words; "The least degree of tremor is felt during passive movement of a rigid part." 2. Apparent decrease in the upward excursion of the globe on the affected side when the patient with a lower motor neuron lesion of the facial nerve attempts to look up.[4086]

Negro-Jacod syndrome   See **Jacod syndrome.**

Neill-Dingwall syndrome   A recessively inherited syndrome manifesting signs similar to those of **Cockayne syndrome** (dwarfism, microcephaly, pigmented chorioretinitis, cerebellar signs and short trunk), but with the absence of cataract and the presence of hepatomegaly and intracranial calcifications.[4087]

Nelson syndrome   1. The excessive secretion of ACTH and MSH by a chromophobe pituitary adenoma, developing after adrenalectomy and leading to hyperpigmentation and features of Cushing syndrome. Myopathy is a complication.[4090] 2. See **acrocallosal syndrome.**

nema   Greek for a "thread."

nemaline myopathy   (rod body myopathy, congenital rod disease) A dominantly or recessively inherited or sporadic congenital myopathy characterized by the presence of **rod bodies** composed of actin and α-actinin in muscle biopsy specimens. The responsible dominant gene maps to chromosome 1q21–q23. Mutations in five separate genes (*TPM3, NEB, ACTA1, TPM2,* and *TNNT1*) have been described; all encode for protein components of muscle thin filaments.

   The clinical pictures vary. In the *recessive* form, infants with the severe form have progressive hypotonia, weakness, and atrophy in proximal muscles with feeding and respiratory difficulties and the condition is sometimes fatal; in milder forms, this is a mild, progressive myopathy with hypotonia, small muscles, feeding problems, genealized weakness, and some face, trunk, and limb dysmorphisms. A *dominant* form is nonprogressive when presenting in early childhood. In adults the course can resemble either of the progressive or nonprogressive forms.[5149] The greatest involvement is found in the facial, trunk flexor, ankle dorsiflexor, and toe extensor muscles.

   The diagnosis is suggested when this clinical picture is encountered in a subject with features resembling **Marfan syndrome** (high-arched palate, arachnodactyly, and span greater than height) and it is confirmed by light and electron microscopy of a muscle biopsy specimen that shows characteristic rod-bodies within the myofibrils (mainly of type 1).[3659]

   Diagnostic criteria have been suggested.[4861]

   Variants include the following:

   An *adult onset* form, characterized by cardiomyopathy and proximal and distal myopathic weakness with the typical microscopic findings just described.[3812]

A *severe* form, characterized by congenital presentation with high-arched palate, feeding problems, joint contractures, and severe facial and proximal myopathic weakness.

Forms with *ophthalmoplegia and mitochondrial abnormalities* are described, in some cases, as well as the myopathy affecting the face, neck, limbs, and trunk.[1985]

See also **central core disease,** with which this condition may overlap.

A clinical classification has been proposed.[5819]

Inclusion Criteria	Exclusion Criteria
Severe congenital NM	No spontaneous movements neonatally
	Cardiomyopathy or ophthalmoplegia
	No spontaneous respiration neonatally
	Contractures at birth
	Fractures at birth
Intermediate congenital NM	Infantile onset
	Cardiomyopathy or ophthalmoplegia
	Contractures developing in early childhood
	Breathing and moving at birth
	Inability to maintain respiratory independence after early childhood
	Failure to sit or walk independently
	Use of wheelchair before 11 years
Typical congenital NM	Onset in infancy or early childhood
	Contractures or fractures at birth
	Weakness most pronounced in facial, bulbar, and respiratory muscles and neck flexors
	Failure to sit or walk independently
	Weakness initially primarily proximal
	Use of wheelchair before 11 years
	Late distal involvement
	Cardiomyopathy or ophthalmoplegia
	Milestones delayed but reached
	Unusual distribution of weakness
	Slowly progressive/nonprogressive course
Childhood-onset NM	Childhood or juvenile onset
	Cardiomyopathy or ophthalmoplegia
	No facial weakness
Adult-onset NM	Adult onset
Other forms	Cardiomyopathy or ophthalmoplegia

NM, nemaline myopathy. See also http://www.neuro.wustl.edu/neuromuscular/maltbrain.html.

From Wallgren-Pattersson C, Laing, NG. Report of the 70th ENMC International workshop: Nemaline Myopathy. 1999, Naarden, The Netherlands. Neuromusc. Disorders. 2000;10(4–5):299–306, with kind permission from Elsevier Science.

nemaline rods   Intramyofibrillar material found in the foregoing myopathy, but scattered reports have recorded them in many other conditions, mainly involving neurogenic muscle disease.

nematodes   Worms of the class **nemathelminths,** including the hairworms and threadworms, with a body cavity. Examples of neurological relevance are *Ascaris, Trichina,* and *Filaria.*

neo-   Greek prefix denoting new.

neocortical death   See **persistent vegetative state.**

neocortical temporal lobe epilepsies   Seizures characterized by elementary or complex hallucinations, complex psychic phenomenon such as hallucinations and delusions, dreamy states, emotional manifestation, and visceral sensory disturbances. They include primary rhinencephalic, frontal, opercular, frontobasal cingulate, temporal pole, and posterior neocortical seizures.[56] See **temporal lobe epilepsy.**

neologism   1. A word newly created, either in response to a communicative need within a category of intellectual activity or as a result of disease of the brain. In the latter case, the word cannot be defined by the inventor and represents a failure of production of normal speech. 2. The replacement of a desired word with an articulate sound devoid of conventional meaning.

neologistic jargon   A form of **jargon aphasia** in which more than 80% of the words enunciated are unintelligible. The causative disease is usually in the left superior temporal and inferior parietal regions.[3019]

neonatal adrenoleukodystrophy   See **adrenoleukodystrophy.**

neonatal cerebellar atrophy with retinal dystrophy   A rare and fatal congenital syndrome of retinal dystrophy, arthrogryposis, vomiting and generalized edema with postmortem evidence of cerebellar atrophy.[2449] See **cerebellar ataxias** (1. *congenital cerebellar ataxias*).

neonatal endotoxin encephalopathy   A form of **periventricular leukomalacia** occurring in the perinatal period, considered to be due to the effect of endotoxins.[2117]

neonatal familial hyperparathyroidism   A congenital dysmetabolic syndrome manifesting also constipation, hepatosplenomegaly, hypercalcemia, hypotonia, seizures, osteoporosis, and multiple fractures.[337]

neonatal herpes simplex infection   Infection by herpes simplex virus (type 2), usually acquired by the infant during passage through the maternal genital tract.

Clinically, a disseminated form of the disease damages the liver and adrenal glands, while neurological symptoms and signs include seizures, cranial nerve palsies, lethargy, and coma due to a diffuse encephalitis as a result of direct infection of the brain by the virus. The disease is often fatal, but in those who survive, the long-term consequences include seizures, microcephaly, blindness, and pyramidal signs.[5950]

neonatal myasthenia   The occurrence of the features of **myasthenia gravis** in the infants of mothers with that condition.[5360] Immunosuppressants and plasma exchange are effective therapies, if required at all, although they are not effective in **congenital myasthenia.**

neonatal myoclonic encephalopathy   (early myoclonic encephalopathy) A syndrome characterized clinically by the occurrence of erratic fragmentary myoclonus of early onset usually in association with other seizure types and with the EEG finding of a suppression–burst pattern. Associated seizures include partial motor seizures, massive myoclonus, and atonic spasms.

All affected infants have severe neurological impairment and the disease is frequently fatal before the age of 6 months. In some cases, recessive inheritance is considered likely.[56]

neonatal ophthalmoplegia with microfibers   A congenital myopathy characterized by nonprogressive hypotonia, weakness, and hoarseness; permanent external ophthalmoplegia; and, on muscle biopsy, marked variation in fiber size, some being less than 3 μm in diameter.[2423]

neonatal persistent myasthenia   See **myasthenia gravis** (*congenital or developmental*).

neonatal seizures   An **epileptic seizure** occurring in the first 4 weeks of life.[1115] Such forms of seizure differ from those of older children and adults. The most frequent neonatal seizures are described as subtle, because the clinical manifestations are frequently overlooked. These include tonic, horizontal deviation of the eyes with or without jerking, eyelid blinking or fluttering; sucking, smacking, or other buccal-lingual oral movements; swimming or pedaling movements; and occasionally apneic spells.

Other neonatal seizures occur in the form of tonic extension of the limbs, mimicking decerebrate or decorticate posturing. These occur particularly in premature infants. Multifocal clonic seizures characterized by clonic movements of a limb, which may migrate to other body parts or other limbs, or focal clonic seizures, which are much more localized, are also described. In the latter, the infant is usually not unconscious. Rarely, myoclonic seizures occur, when the EEG pattern is frequently that of suppression–burst activity.[3720] The tonic seizures have a poor prognosis because they frequently accompany intraventricular hemorrhage. The myoclonic seizures also have a poor prognosis because they are frequently a part of the early myoclonic encephalopathy syndrome. (From Commission for Classification and Terminology, ILAE. Proposal for revised classifications of epilepsies and epileptic syndromes. *Epilepsia* 1989;**30**:389–399,[1114] with kind permission from Blackwell Science.

neoplasm   (Gr, new + to form) An abnormal, independent proliferation of cells characterized by histological diversity from the matrix from which it takes its origin (Bland-Sutton); a tumor.

neoplastic angioendotheliosis   See **malignant angioendotheliomatosis.**

neovascularization   The formation of a new system of blood vessels within a tissue, such as the retina in diabetes.

nephrolithiasis-mitochondrial cytopathy   See **Donaldson syndrome.**

nephropathy with retinitis pigmentosa, cerebellar ataxia, and skeletal abnormalities   A recessively inherited syndrome reported once; juvenile nephronophthisis is a feature.[3580]

nephrosialidosis (Gr, kidney + saliva) (severe infantile sialidosis) A congenital lysosomal storage disease due to deficiency of β-galactosidase, leading to storage of sialo-oligosaccharides and presenting with a nephrotic syndrome, coarse facies, corneal clouding, multiple dysostoses, a cherry-red spot at the macula, seizures, and mental and developmental delay. See also **sialidosis.**

Neri signs 1. Flexion of the knee with forward bending of the trunk indicates lumbar root irritation on that side. The same knee flexion occurs in patients with a pyramidal tract lesion on the affected side. 2. (pronation sign) In hemiparesis or monoparesis, flexion of the sound arm lying pronated and extended leads to supination of the contralateral paretic arm. 3. In organic hemiparesis, with the patient lying supine, spontaneous bending of the knee occurs when the leg is passively lifted.[4101]

Neri, Vincenzo (b. 1882) Italian neurologist who trained at the **Salpêtrière.**

nerve (Middle English, from Lat, a tendon) Anatomical collections of bundles of nerve fibers and their supporting connective tissue and vascular and lymphatic elements, with their origin in nuclei situated within or beside the brainstem or spinal cord. Over 250 have been named.

The early Greeks did not distinguish between nerves and tendons (hence the word *aponeurosis*) until this was achieved at Alexandria by **Eristratus** and **Herophilus.**

nerve action potential (NAP) Strictly defined, refers to an action potential recorded from a single nerve fiber. The term is commonly used to refer to the compound nerve action potential. See **compound nerve action potential.** (From the 2001 Report of the Nomenclature Committee of the American Association of Electromyography and Electrodiagnosis.[10] Used by permission, copyright © 2001, AAEM.)

nerve agents Organic esters of phosphoric acid derivatives capable of inactivating acetylcholinesterase by permanent binding, and thus leading to syndromes of cholinergic excess, both nicotinic and muscarinic. Centrally, weakness, circulatory and respiratory depression, seizures, and coma occur at the time of exposure; delayed effects include anxiety symptoms, giddiness, memory disturbances, headaches, insomnia, confusion, and ataxia.[2334]

nerve compression syndromes Combinations of motor and sensory deficits, often with positive **Tinel signs** during the recovery phase, caused by compression and thus ischemia of peripheral nerves.

The median, ulnar, radial, suprascapular, axillary, femoral, sciatic, common peroneal, and posterior tibial nerves and their cutaneous branches are those most often affected.

nerve conduction study (NCS, electroneurography) Recording and analysis of electric waveforms of biologic origin elicited in response to electric or physiologic stimuli. The waveforms are compound sensory nerve action potentials, compound muscle action potentials, or mixed nerve action potentials. The compound muscle action potentials are generally referred to by letters that have historical origin: M wave, F wave, H wave. T wave, A wave, and Rl, R2 waves. It is possible under standardized conditions to establish normal ranges for amplitude, duration, and latency of the waveforms and to calculate the maximum conduction velocity of sensory and motor nerves. The term generally refers to studies of waveforms generated in the peripheral nervous system, whereas evoked potential studies refers to studies of waveforms generated in both the peripheral and central nervous systems. (From the 2001 Report of the Nomenclature Committee of the American Association of Electromyography and Electrodiagnosis.[10] Used by permission, copyright © 2001, AAEM.)

nerve conduction velocity (NCV) The speed of action potential propagation along a nerve fiber or nerve trunk. Generally assumed to refer to the maximum speed of propagation unless otherwise specified. See **conduction velocity.** (From the 2001 Report of the Nomenclature Committee of the American Association of Electromyography and Electrodiagnosis.[10] Used by permission, copyright © 2001, AAEM.)

The speed of conduction of nerve impulses (normally as a result of saltatory conduction), in both motor and sensory nerves at normal temperatures in adults, ranges between 45 and 65 m/sec. These values apply to the fastest-conducting, most heavily myelinated, A or alpha fibers, which also have the largest axons; B and C fibers conduct at substantially slower rates but cannot normally be measured in the clinical laboratory because the action potentials they induce are overshadowed by those produced by the faster-conducting fibers. In the newborn the rates are about one-third of the values cited above, rising to adult values by about the age of 8 years.

The velocity of nerve conduction was first measured by Helmholtz in 1850.

nerve deafness–optic atrophy–dementia syndrome An X-linked syndrome manifesting sensorineural deafness, optic atrophy, and neurodegenerative regression with onset in early adult life.[2847]

nerve fiber The axon and its sheath, its outer limit being the endoneurial membrane; the Schwann cells investing the fiber may be myelinated or not.

nerve fiber action potential Action potential recorded from a single axon.

nerve fiber–bundle defect A visual field defect occurring with either a retinal or optic nerve lesion which follows the pattern of loss of retinal nerve fibers. Examples are altitudinal defects, temporal sector defects, steps, and nasal scotomas.

nerve growth factor   A substance synthesized in the Schwann cells of the peripheral nervous system, and transported retrogradely to the perikaryon.

nerve injury   The three-heading classification of Seddon[5048] was criticized by Sunderland[5416] who defined five forms, given in Chart N–2; the Seddon schema, however (**neurapraxia, axonotmesis, neurotmesis**), has found so much favour by clinicians that it is more generally used.

Chart N–2. Sunderland's Five Groups of Nerve Injury

First degree (interruption of conduction with preservation of anatomical continuity) Conduction is blocked at the site of injury, but the continuity of all components comprising the nerve trunk, including the axon, is preserved. There is no wallerian degeneration and the disturbance which is responsible for blocking the conduction is fully reversible, so that function is rapidly and completely restored.

Second degree (disintegration with regeneration of axons) Disintegration of the axon occurs with distal wallerian degeneration, but the general arrangement of the axon sheath and the other neural structures is retained, so that regeneration of the axons is down the appropriate endoneurial tube in all cases.

Third degree (disorganization of the contents of the funiculi, with loss of continuity of the endoneurial tubes) The bundles of funiculi remain in continuity, but there is disorganization of their internal structure, such that the continuity of the endoneurial tubes is lost and there is distal axonal disintegration and wallerian degeneration. As a result of interfunicular fibrosis, the regenerating axons do not sprout down their original endoneurial tubes.

Fourth degree (complete disorganization of the internal structure of the nerve) Breaching and disorganization of the funiculi occur with retained continuity of the anatomical nerve trunk. The involved segment becomes a tangle of connective tissue, Schwann cells, fibrosis, and axon sprouts, and the chance that an axon will grow back down its own endoneurial tube is remote.

Fifth degree Severance of the nerve trunk[5416]

From Sunderland S. A clasification of peripheral nerve injuries producing loss of function. Brain 1951;74:491–516, by kind permission.

nerve potential   Equivalent to **nerve action potential.** Also commonly, but inaccurately, used to refer to the biphasic form of end-plate activity observed during needle electrode examination of muscle. The latter use is incorrect, because muscle fibers, not nerve fibers, are the source of these potentials.

nerve trunk action potential   See **compound nerve action potential.**

nerve roots   The nerve fiber bundles entering and leaving the spinal cord and brainstem. The motor function of the anterior roots and the sensory function of the posterior roots were detected by Georg Prochaska in 1779, but the first (but partial) account in English was that of Sir Charles **Bell** in 1811,[437a] published 10 years later, while Magendie completed the differentiation in the following year.

nerve sheath myxoma   See **pseudocyt.**

Nervenzart   A German neurological journal. Web site: http://link.springer.de/link/service/journals/00115/index.htm.

nervi erigentes   The pelvic parasympathetic nerves leaving the cord at S2–4, described by Carl Ludwig in 1866.

nervous system   The compilation of the whole of the central and peripheral nervous systems, thus comprising in humans the cerebral hemispheres and their ascending, descending, and commissural connections, the thalamus, basal ganglia, and limbic system, the brain stem and cerebellum, the cranial nerves, the spinal cord with its spinal nerves, and the autonomic nervous system.

The differentiation between the central and peripheral nervous systems is made on the basis of the type of cells investing the axons; these are oligodendroglia in the former and Schwann cells in the latter.

nervus intermedius   The name given by **Wrisberg** to that part of the seventh cranial nerve which runs as a separate bundle, lying between the remainder of the seventh and the eighth nerves.

nervus intermedius neuralgia   A rare disorder characterized by brief paroxysms of pain felt deeply in the auditory canal. This definition and the following diagnostic criteria are suggested by the Headache Classification Committee of the International Headache Society[1051] and are reproduced by kind permission.
  A. Pain paroxysms felt in the depth of the ear, lasting for seconds or minutes, of intermittent occurrence
  B. Presence of a trigger zone in the posterior wall of the auditory canal
  C. Exclusion of a structural lesion

Neuhauser syndrome   (megalocornea-mental retardation) A congenital dysmorphic syndrome characterized also by abnormalities of the cornea and iris, seizures, hypotonia, and mental and developmental delay.[337]

Neu-Laxova syndrome   A lethal congenital dysmorphic syndrome characterized also by microphthalmia, cataract, ascites, edema of hands, syndactyly, joint contractures, microcephaly, intracranial calcification, lissencephaly, and cerebellar and callosal anomalies.[4102]

neural   Of or belonging to a nerve or the nervous system.

neural amyotrophy with familial retinitis pigmentosa See **NARP syndrome.**

neural crest A line of epiblastic cells situated on the dorsal lips of the neural tube, from which cells migrate to form some cranial nerves (III, V, VII, VIII, IX, and X), peripheral sensory ganglia and satellite cells, autonomic ganglia and plexuses, the Schwann cells, some endocrine glands or parts of them (e.g., thyroid, parathyroid and thymus), much of the meninges, the skin and bones of the face, the tooth-enamel organs, and almost all pigmented cells in the body, though not those of the retina.[3313]

A *syndrome of the neural crest* arising from a failure in its differentiation has been proposed to consist of loss of superficial or deep pain sensibility, autonomic dysfunction, dysplasia of dental enamel, meningeal thickening and cystic change, mild mental retardation, hyporeflexia, blond hair, blue-green eyes, and a pale complexion.[795]

neural induction The process of the formation of primitive neural elements as the first part of the process of organogenesis, leading to differentiation of the neural plate and then to formation of the neural tube.

neural myxedema bodies Round, granular, glycogen-containing bodies in the dorsal root entry zone of the spinal cord and in the cerebellar vermis of patients with myxedema.[4525]

neural tube The infolding of the dorsal ectoderm forming a tube from which the brain and spinal cord develop. It was first noted by Remak and confirmed by Huxley.[5204]

neural tube defects A group of developmental disorders occurring from failure of normal closure of the neural tube between 22 and 29 days after conception. The most severe forms are **anencephaly** and **meningomyelocele** (spina bifida).

neuralgia (Gr, nerve + pain) Pain felt in the distribution of a nerve or nerve root, due usually to a proximal lesion of that nerve. The characteristics of such pains tend toward constancy in their intermittency, brevity, severity, and explosive onset and in the usual finding of normal function in the territory supplied by the nerve in between attacks, but these criteria do not hold for **postherpetic neuralgia.** The pain may be sharp, even lancinating, when affected by **ephaptic transmission,** but is burning and constant in inflammatory conditions.

Further comments are entered for the particular varieties of neuralgia—**trigeminal, geniculate, glossopharyngeal, occipital, vagal,** and **superior laryngeal** forms are described. While **tabetic crises** could also be considered to be neuralgias, using the preceding criteria, they are not usually so classified.

The history of the term has been reviewed.[71]

neuralgic amyotrophy (Spillane syndrome, Parsonage-Turner syndrome, shoulder-girdle syndrome, shoulder-girdle neuritis, brachial neuritis, [idiopathic] brachial plexopathy, brachial plexus neuropathy, acute brachial plexitis/plexopathy/neuritis/neuropathy, hereditary peripheral neuropathy predominantly affecting the arms) A syndrome characterized by the acute onset of pain in the shoulder and arm followed by variable weakness and atrophy of muscles, usually unilaterally and most often in the C5–6 (upper trunk of the brachial plexus) distribution, but any upper limb muscles can be affected, as can the diaphragm. The cause is unknown.[4348]

Sensory functions are much less affected. Sometimes a single nerve (usually the long thoracic) or multiple unrelated nerves (e.g., the phrenic, axillary, anterior interosseous, and/or suprascapular) are involved. The syndrome is more common in males in early adult life, and is often preceded by a variety of infectious, traumatic, or immunological events. Laboratory studies other than EMG are unhelpful in diagnosis. The prognosis for eventual recovery is good.

Spillane actually described the entity 5 years before Parsonage and Turner.[4348]

The following diagnostic criteria have been reviewed:[4899]

A. Acute onset over the course of hours or days
B. Pain in the shoulder girdle and arm, often severe
C. Subsequent weakness and atrophy in the territory of individual nerves arising from the brachial plexus
D. Little or no sensory loss
E. Eventual recovery
F. EMG findings consistent with axonal neuropathy
G. Normal CSF
H. Frequent antecedent viral infection, vaccination, or serum sickness

From Sander JE, Sharp FR. Lumbosacral plexus neuritis. *Neurology* 1981;**31**:470–3, by kind permission.

Variants include the following:

A *dominantly inherited* form with predilection for the brachial plexus (OMIM162100) described in 1887, presenting with recurrent attacks of pain and weakness lasting for a few days and leading to muscle atrophy. It is mapped to 17q24–qter. This condition is nearly identical with the classic picture in affecting the brachial plexus most often, but the lesions are more extensive and may involve the recurrent laryngeal nerves, isolated limb nerves, or the lumbosacral plexus.[223,426,2066] Dysmorphic features such as hypotelorism, syndactyly, short stature, and epicanthic folds may accompany the neural problems.

A chronic painless form has been described[4995] as well as another occurring postpartum.

In rare cases, a multifocal relapsing sensory neuropathy occurs, resembling **sensory perineuritis.**[5548]

See also **hereditary pressure-sensitive neuropathy, multiple exercise-related neuropathy with colic, carpal tunnel syndrome** (familial variant), **meralgia paresthetica, giant axonal neuropathy, lumbosacral plexopathy.**

neuralgic osteopathy   See **Camera syndrome.**

neurapraxia   (Gr, nerve + lack of + action) (transient block) A minimal lesion of a peripheral nerve usually due to compression or stretch injuries, producing paralysis that is usually incomplete, unaccompanied by peripheral axonal degeneration and with rapid, spontaneous, and complete recovery. This is one of three types of nerve injury described by Seddon.[5048] See **conduction block.** See also **axonotmesis, neurotmesis.**

neurasthenia   (Gr, nerve + weakness) Nervous exhaustion, a fashionable diagnosis by any of its many names. It is polite to regard this condition as possibly organic, but without demonstrable pathology—a refuge for physicians and patients.

First described by Jean-Antoine-Eugène Bouchat (1818–1891) in a monograph entitled "De l'état nerveux aigu et chronique ou nervosisme" (Paris, 1860), it was more fully detailed by George **Beard** in 1869[406,408] and described as a "want of nervous force . . . most frequently met with in civilized, intellectual communities. They are part of the compensation for our progress and refinement." Symptoms identified included "general malaise, debility of all the functions, poor appetite, abiding weakness in the back and spine, fugitive neuralgic pains, hysteria, insomnia, hypochondriasis, disinclination for consecutive manual labour, severe and weakening attacks of sick headache . . . and other analogous symptoms and at the same time gives no evidence of anemia or of other organic disease. We have reason to suspect that the central nervous system is mainly at fault and that we are dealing with a typical case of neurasthenia."

Beard treated the condition with general electrization, the patient's feet being placed on a sheet of copper to which the "negation pole" was attached; the positive pole was a large sponge applied to the (moistened) head. Violent muscular contractions were produced. He also used hypnotism and "air, sunlight, water, food, rest, diversion, muscular exercise and . . . strychnine, phosphorus, arsenic, etc. which directly affect the nervous system." Beard's practice flourished and the diagnosis and treatment were each so convenient that alternatives seldom required consideration. The treatment employed by Weir **Mitchell** was similar and produced results as good. See also **chronic fatigue syndrome.**

neurasthenic nystagmus   See **gaze-evoked nystagmus.**

neurectasy   (Gr, nerve + stretch) Manual traction on a nerve exposed at operation in an attempt to relieve pain and numerous other neurological symptoms. Early scepticism in the late eighteenth century gave way to later incredulity and the procedure has now been abandoned.[2982]

neurenteric   Relating to the nerves and to the intestines.

neurenteric cyst   (dorsal enteric cyst, archenteric cyst or enterogenous cyst) A congenital defect due to herniation of the ventral yolk sac and its adherence to the dorsal ectoderm, resulting in the presence of an intraspinal cystic mass with an endodermal epithelial lining. Secondary spinal cord or nerve root compression may occur at any age.

A classification of such developmental disorders has been achieved by Smith.[5227] See also **intradural enterogenous cyst.**

neurilemma   (Gr, nerve + covering) Described originally by **Schwann** and named for him, thus indicating the Schwann cell sheath, although the intent was to label the connective tissue covering of nerve fibers, the epi- and the perineurium.

neurites   (nerve sprouts) Small axon sprouts, regenerating from the tip of a severed axon at a node of Ranvier.

neuritic plaques   (senile plaques) Spherical argyrophilic structures, 5–200 μm in diameter, comprising a dense central core of amyloid fibrils surrounded by a clear halo, outside which is a ring of neurofilamentous and mitochondrial material derived from degenerating dendritic and axonal nerve terminals.

They are found in the cerebral cortex, hippocampal regions, and gray matter, and relate in number to the age of the subject, although they are not always present even in the brains of very elderly people.[6] Such plaques are also characteristic findings in Alzheimer disease.

neuritis   Inflammation of nerves from any cause. However, the word has been used in a far less specific way in the past century to include almost any nerve disorder other than tumor. It should be retained for inflammatory disease, unsullied by association with noninflammatory diseases that affect nerve conduction.

neuroacanthocytosis   (choreoacanthosis, Levine-Critchley syndrome, familial neuroacanthocytosis, familial amyotrophic chorea with acanthocytosis, familial chorea with acanthocytosis) A heterogeneous (recessively or dominantly inherited or sporadic) multisystem degenerative disorder seen in children or young adults, and characterized by movement disorders (chorea, motor and phonic tics, dystonias, and orofacial dyskinesias causing dysphagia and dysarthria with lip and tongue biting, followed by orolingual ["eating"] dystonia), proximal or distal muscle weakness and atrophy, and personality changes or cognitive impairment. The chorea is slowly progressive and involves the bulbar muscles first and most. Psychoses, behavioral disorders with tongue biting, parkinsonism, vertical ophthalmoparesis, self-mutilation, seizures, and occasionally cardiac involvement have also been recorded.

The clinical picture and pathological findings of striatal degeneration with caudate atrophy may resemble those of **Huntington disease**,[155] but to this are added neuropathy and myopathy, and the serum creatine kinase levels are high.[3376] Wet blood or Wright-stained fast dry smears usually reveal that over 15% of red blood cells are acanthocytes.

Other features recorded include evidence of a sensorimotor axonal neuropathy affecting the larger myelinated fibers, the occurrence of cerebellar or pyramidal signs, and CT evidence of cortical atrophy.[2435] Bulbar involvement and sphincter disturbances are additional but inconstant features.[2805,2808] Caudate atrophy and hypometabolism have been seen. Neuronal loss and gliosis is particularly prominent in the striatum and pallidum but also may affect the thalamus, substantia nigra, and anterior horns of the spinal cord.

Two forms are distinguished, according to whether the serum β-lipoproteins are normal or absent; the presence of a malabsorption syndrome is a marker for the second of these possibilities. The multiple phenotypes have been reviewed by Baraitser.[335] See also **McLeod syndrome.**[6014]

Variants are *spinal muscular atrophy in choreoacanthocytosis,* **hypobetalipoproteinemia,** and *hypoprebetalipoproteinemia,* each of which may present similarly.[5350]

The multisystem neurological involvement in this disorder has been reviewed.[2435]

neuroanatomy   A basis of sound neurological practice. Various entries in this book allude to neuroanatomical structures, since it is supposed that the reader has already the basic knowledge. For illustrations of neuroanatomy, the following Web sites are recommended:

http://anatomy.yonsei.ac.kr/neurolink.htm
http://www.bcm.tmc.edu/oto/studs/fn.html
http://www.anatomy.wisc.edu/
http://www.neuropat.dote.hu/anatomy.htm
http://info.med.yale.edu/caim/cnerves/contents_detailed.html
http://anatome.ncl.ac.uk/tutorials/brain1/text/index.html
http://www.med.harvard.edu/AANLIB/cases/java/case.html

neuroaxonal dystrophies   A group of sporadic or recessively inherited conditions characterized by neuronal degeneration and fragmentation of the axon with the formation of homogenous round eosinophilic bodies, at first in the distal part of the nerve, in which numerous spheroids are present in distal axons and throughout nerve cell processes. These conditions include **Martha-Alma (Hallervorden-Spatz) disease,** nutritional disorders, old age, and **infantile neuroaxonal dystrophy.**

Clinically, affected children show rigidity, chorea, dystonia, tremor, seizures, dementia, and pigmentary retinopathy; in adults, the inheritance pattern is dominant and there is evidence of parkinsonism with dementia and dystonias.[5962]

Neurobehavioral Rating Scale (revised)   A tool based on a structured 20-minute interview, of use in the assessment of patients after head injury. It provides rating scores for agitation, anxiety, articulation, blunting of affect, calculation, conceptual thought, comprehension, depression, disinhibition, emotional withdrawal, excitement, guilt, hallucinatory behavior, hostility, attention, difficulties in mental flexibility, irritability, reduced alertness, insight, judgement, memory, mood lability, orientation, planning, repetition of speech, retardation, somatic concern, suspicion, thought content, and word-finding/naming.[3370,3731]

neuro-Behçet disease   The occurrence of predominantly neurological features in Behçet disease, an idiopathic multisystem inflammatory disease of young adults.

Diagnostic criteria are the presence of recurrent aphthous stomatitis with at least two of the following:[2557] (*1*) genital aphthous ulcers, (*2*) uveitis, (*3*) cutaneous or large-vessel vasculitis, (*4*) synovitis, and (*5*) meningoencephalitis.

neuroblastoma   An uncommon malignant, solid, soft tumor of the central or peripheral nervous system, arising from undifferentiated sympathetic neuroblasts of the adrenal medulla, or from sympathetic ganglia (neural crest cells); a type of **primitive neuroectodermal tumor.** Such tumors are dominantly inherited in a fifth of the cases, and usually occur in infants or children in either location,[2661] in which population they are the most common solid tumor found.

Apart from the usual focal neurological signs of a mass lesion and of raised intracranial pressure, such tumors are remarkable for the **opsoclonus** that is often present.[724]

Cerebral neuroblastomas occur mainly in children within the cerebral hemispheres. Histologically, they are characterized by sheets of cells with small and hyperchromatic nuclei with little cytoplasm, and occasionally they show focal glial or neuronal differentiation and rosette formation. *Olfactory neuroblastomas* (**esthesioneuroblastomas**) are rare *variants* arising in the anterior cranial fossa and consist of small cells with fibrillary cytoplasm containing cytokeratin and staining positively for protein S-100. *Abdominal neuroblastomas* arise from the chromaffin cells of the adrenal gland or from the sympathetic chain. *Differentiated neuroblastomas* (central neurocytomas) are rare *variants* of the above, usually occurring in young adults and with a good prognosis. They are characterized by the presence of vesicles or of synaptic structures. See also **ganglioneuroblastoma.**

neuroborreliosis   See **Lyme disease.**

neurobrucellosis   The occurrence of predominantly neurological features in patients suffering from brucellosis.

Clinically, headache, fatigue and myalgia are the usual early features and transient ischemic attacks, strokes, acute confusional states, myelopathy, anterior horn cell disease, multisystem degenerations, polyradiculopathy, sciatica, neuralgic amyotrophy, mononeuritis, and cauda equina syndromes at later stages are the more common presentations.[89,5087]

neurocardiogenic syncope (neurally mediated syncope, ventricular syncope) Bradycardia, hypotension due to profound generalized vasodilatation, decreased cerebral blood flow, and often reduction in consciousness resulting from a failure of the normal compensatory responses to the assumption of the upright posture, in the absence of serious cardiac disease. A paradoxical withdrawal of sympathetic activity (and increased parasympathetic activity) occurs, probably resulting from excessive activation of cardiac mechanoreceptors. Norepinephrine levels are high, accounting for the presence of pallor and sweating.[20]

Tilt-table testing suggests four categories of hypotension, only the first represeing true neurocardiogenic syncope:

1. Malignant vasovagal syncope in which there is an abrupt drop in systolic blood pressure (mean drop over 100 mmHg) with severe bradycardia and maybe loss of consciousness after a mean of 18 minutes
2. Orthostatic hypotension with a drop of systolic pressure of more than 20 mmHg within a minute of tilting
3. Delayed orthostatic hypotension, with a mean drop of 40 mmHg after 20 minutes
4. Psychogenic or other causes (Dr. Brad Hiner, personal commnication, 1995)

The Neurology and Neurosurgery Forum provides an explanation for lay people at http://www.medhelp.org. Harvard maintains a site on the topic at http://neuromancer.mgh.harvard.edu/cgi-bin/Ultimate.cgi.

The National Dysautonomia Research Foundation (NDRF), a foundation for this type of disease, is at http://www.ndrf.org/. A patient support network can be found at http://www.medhelp.org/network.htm.

Neurocase A journal of the Oxford University Press dealing with single case studies and reviews of brain–behavior relationships. Web site: http://neucas.oupjournals.org/.

neurocentral (Gr, nerve + the center of a circle) Relating to the centrum and the neural arch of a vertebra.

neurocirculatory asthenia See **chronic fatigue syndrome.**

neurocristopathy A neurological disorder due to abnormal development of structures arising from the **neural crest. Neurofibromatosis** is an example.[641]

neurocutaneous angiomatosis See **Sturge-Weber syndrome.**

neurocutaneous melanosis A rare, sporadic, congenital neurocutaneous syndrome characterized by numerous benign pigmented nevi (giant hairy nevus) mainly in the cycle-shorts area of the skin, with widespread deposits of pigmented cells in the leptomeninges and in the cerebral and cerebellar white matter. For the diagnosis to be made, no malignant melanoma may be present in other organs.

The affected children have seizures, hydrocephalus, and brain hamartomas; they are also mentally retarded and show a variety of neurological deficits.[5704]

neurocutaneous syndromes (choristomas) A group of heterogeneous disorders involving both the skin and the nervous system and marked by a tendency to neoplasia. See also **phakomatoses.**

In all, over 35 different forms are known,[1931] and these are listed in Chart N–3.

Chart N–3. A Listing of Neurocutaneous Syndromes

Dominantly inherited **Hypomelanosis of Ito; lentiginosis-deafness-cardiopathy; neurofibromatosis; nevoid basal-cell carcinoma syndrome; Sturge-Weber syndrome; tuberous sclerosis; von Hippel-Lindau syndrome; Waardenburg syndrome.**

Recessively inherited **argininosuccinic aciduria; ataxia-telangiectasia (Louis-Bar syndrome); biotin-responsive multiple carboxylase deficiency; Chediak-Higashi disease; citrullinuria; Cockayne syndrome; fucosidosis; homocystinuria; giant axonal neuropathy; hereditary motor and sensory neuropathy type 4** (Refsum disease); **hereditary sensory neuropathy, type 3** (familial dysautonomia); **neuroichthyosis; phenylketonuria; Sjörgen-Larsson syndrome; Werner syndrome** (progeria) and **xeroderma pigmentosum.**

Uncertain transmission **Albright syndrome; Cobb syndrome; Divry-van Bogaert syndrome; focal dermal hypoplasia; hereditary hemorrhagic telangiectasia; linear nevus sebaceous; Meckel-Gruber syndrome; neurocutaneous melanosis, peroneal neuropathy with crural hypopigmentation; poikilodermia congenitale; progeria; Rud syndrome; Sturge-Weber syndrome.**

X-*Linked Inheritance:* **adrenoleukodystrophy; Fabry disease; incontinentia pigmenti and Menkes kinky-hair disease.**

neurocysticercosis Infestation of the CNS by the encysted larvae of *Taenia solium,* the pork tapeworm, representing the most common cause of cystic lesions in the brain worldwide and probably the most common cause of acquired seizures. Cysts in the brain parenchyma and subarachnoid space lead to psychiatric symptoms, variably raised intracranial pressure, and focal signs, but the first clinical manifestation is usually intractable epilepsy.[5725]

In a spinal form, the cysts may be extra- or intramedullary and lead to an increase in the CSF protein content, pressure, and cell count, with eosinophilia. Laboratory (CT and pathology) results in acute, transitional, and inactive stages have been described.[916]

The following criteria for diagnosis have been suggested:[1357]

Diagnostic Criteria for Neurocysticercosis

Absolute

1. Histologic demonstration of the parasite from biopsy of a brain or spinal cord lesion

2. Cystic lesions showing the scolex on CT or MRI
3. Direct visualization of subretinal parasites by funduscopic examination

Major

1. Lesions highly suggestive of neurocysticercosis on neuroimaging studies[*]
2. Positive serum EITB[†] for the detection of anticysticercal antibodies
3. Resolution of intracranial cystic lesions after therapy with albendazole or praziquantel
4. Spontaneous resolution of small, single enhancing lesions[‡]

Minor

1. Lesions compatible with neurocysticercosis on neuroimaging studies[§]
2. Clinical manifestations suggestive of neurocysticercosis[**]
3. Positive CSF ELISA for detection of anticysticercal antibodies or cysticercal antigens
4. Cysticercosis outside the CNS[***]

Epidemiologic

1. Evidence of a household contact with *Taenia solium* infection
2. Individuals coming from or living in an area where cysticercosis is endemic
3. History of frequent travel to disease-endemic areas

ELISA, enzyme-linked immunosorbent assay.

[*]CT or MRI showing cystic lesions without scolex, enhancing lesions, or typical parenchymal brain calcifications.

[†]Enzyme-linked immunoelectrotransfer blot assay using purified extracts of Taenia solium antigens, as developed by the Centers for Disease Control and Prevention (Atlanta, GA).

[‡]Solitary ring-enhancing lesions measuring <20 mm in diameter in patients presenting with seizures, a normal neurologic examination, and no evidence of an active systemic disease.

[§]CT or MRI showing hydrocephalus or abnormal enhancement of the leptomeninges, and myelograms showing multiple filling defects in the column of contrast medium.

[**]Seizures, focal neurologic signs, intracranial hypertension, and dementia.

[***]Histologically confirmed subcutaneous or muscular cysticercosis, plain X-ray films showing "cigar-shaped" soft tissue calcifications, or direct visualization of cysticerci in the anterior chamber of the eye.

Reprinted from Del Brutto OH, Rajshekhar V, White AC, et al. Proposed diagnostic criteria for neurocysticercosis. Neurology 2001;**57**:177–83. Copyright (2001), with permission from Elsevier Science.

neurocytoma A tumor derived from neuronal cells, usually presenting in young adults, and usually found in the lateral ventricles. The very vascular mass contains neurotubules, neurosecretory granules, clear vesicles, and well-developed intercellular junctions; it resembles neuroblastoma, but is better differentiated. It may cause sudden death, acute hydrocephalus, or a frontal lobe syndrome.[6069]

Neurodegeneration A journal devoted to neurodegenerative disorders, neuroprotection, and neuroregeneration, incorporated into *Experimental Neurology*. Address: Academic Press, 525 B Street, Suite 1900, San Diego, CA 92101–4495. Web site: http://www.academicpress.com/en.

neurodegenerative disease A collective term for the numerous atrophic symmetrical diseases of unknown etiology and pathogenesis which progressively damage specific systems within the nervous system following at least some period of apparently normal functioning. See also **tauopathies, synucleinopathies, amyloidopathies.**

neurodynia An obsolete term signifying pain from nerve disease. See **causalgia.**

neuroectodermal dysplasia A disorder of the development of structures of ectodermal origin; **incontinentia pigmenti, hypomelanosis of Ito,** and **basal cell nevus syndrome** are examples.

neuroectodermal melanolysosomal disease (Elejalde syndrome) A congenital dysmorphic syndrome manifesting also short stature, depigmentation of skin and hair, myopia, seizures, and mental and developmental delay.[337]

neuroectodermal tumors Primary intracranial tumors which arise from neuroectoderm. They include **astrocytomas, glioblastoma multiforme, oligodendrogliomas, ependymomas, choroid plexus papillomas, primitive neuroectodermal tumors,** and **neuronal tumors.**

neuroectomesodermoses See **phakomatoses.**

Neuroendocrinology A subspecialty medical journal. Web site: http://www.karger.ch/journals/nen/nen_jh.htm.

neuroepidemiology The study of the natural history of neurological disease, including its frequency of occurrence, severity and course; the context in which it occurs; and the characteristics of those who suffer from it.[3199]

Neuroepidemiology A subspecialty medical journal. Web site: http://www.karger.com/journals/ned/ned_jh.htm.

neuroepithelial cyst (colloid cyst) A congenital cyst originating from neuroepithelial folds, including those in ectopic, endothelium-lined structures, or originating from the cleft of Rathke's pouch, and found in or beside the third ventricle or intraspinally.

Their clinical expression occurs through the obstruction of CSF flow or compression of local structures.

neuroepithelioma See **dysembryoma.**

neuroepithelium The epithelial layer of the sense organs that contain the endings of the nerves of special sense, such as the second and the eighth cranial nerves.

neurofaciodigitorenal syndrome A recessively inherited congenital dysmorphic syndrome, characterized also by short stature, renal agenesis, digital anomalies, megalencephaly, hypotonia, and mental and developmental delay.[1950]

neurofibrillary degeneration (tangles) Intraneuronal basophilic masses composed of paired helical filaments in tangles that displace the nucleus. They are found in the hippocampal regions, the frontotemporal cortex, and the pigmented nuclei of the brainstem in relation to advancing age. They were described first by **Alzheimer.** Their presence is described after cerebral trauma; in **Alzheimer disease, postencephalitic parkinsonism,** the **ALS-parkinsonism-dementia complex of Guam,** in **subacute sclerosing panencephalitis,** in adults with **Down syndrome,** and in normal aged brains.

Variant (straight) filaments are seen in **progressive supranuclear palsy** and in sporadic motor neuron disease.[6]

neurofibromas Benign, unencapsulated tumors of the nerve sheath of mixed composition, containing fibroblasts, Schwann cells, and other cells, which infiltrate the nerve from which they arise, as well as local tissues; and thus are frequently multiple, as in **neurofibromatosis.**

Histologically, they are characterized by the presence of loosely packed spindle cells seen separating the axons of a nerve, with collagen bands and mucoprotein located interstitially. Malignant change is rarely described.[6]

neurofibromatosis (von Recklinghausen syndrome, central neurofibromatosis) A dominantly inherited or sporadic neurocutaneous syndrome manifesting genetic heterogeneity. Both types, NF-1 and NF-2, may occur in mosaic forms.

Neurofibromatosis 1 is a dominantly inherited neurocutaneous syndrome due to a genetic abnormality at 17q11.2, the site of a gene coding for neurofibromin. It is characterized by scoliosis; bifid ribs; early puberty in males; renal artery stenosis; renal tumors; absent or hypoplastic patella; adrenal tumors; mental and developmental delay; seizures; macrocephaly; arterial disorders in the CNS; brain tumors; pseudoarthrosis; patchy depigmentation of skin; café-au-lait spots and axillary, groin, or submammary freckles; dermal fibromas; and nodules in the iris (**Lisch nodules**). Lipomas and other pedunculated skin lesions are also found.

Complications include plexiform neurofibromas, cerebral tumors such as cerebral and optic gliomas and meningiomas, vestibular schwannomas, spinal neurofibromas, neurofibrosarcomas, aqueduct stenosis, learning disabilities, and scoliosis. Visceral and endocrine tumors are also associated.[4621]

Neurofibromatosis 2, or central (bilateral acoustic) neurofibromatosis, is due to a genetic abnormality on chromosome 22 (at 22q11.21–q13.1). It is characterized clinically by sensorineural deafness; facial weakness; cerebellar signs; cerebral, brainstem, and optic nerve gliomas; meningiomas, sarcomas, or neurofibromas; and café-au-lait spots. The bilateral acoustic schwan-

nomas may be the only features, however. The excessive frequency of benign and malignant neuroectodermal tumors in neurofibromatosis is likely due to the defective production of neurofibromatin, an antioncogene.

The condition was first described by Robert Smith, an Irish physician in 1849, 33 years before von Recklinghausen's account.[4621]

Criteria for the diagnoses have been suggested[3663] and are given in Chart N–4.

Chart N–4. Diagnostic Criteria for Neurofibromatosis

Neurofibromatosis 1 may be diagnosed when two or more of the following are present:
  A. Six or more café-au-lait macules whose greatest diameter is >5 mm in prepubertal patients and >15 mm in postpubertal patients
  B. Two or more neurofibromas of any type, or one plexiform neurofibroma
  C. Freckling in the axilla or inguinal region
  D. Optic glioma
  E. Two or more Lisch nodules (iris hamartomas)
  F. A distinctive osseous lesion such as sphenoid dysplasia or thinning of long bone cortex, with or without pseudoarthrosis
  G. A parent, sibling, or child with neurofibromatosis 1, according to the above criteria

Neurofibromatosis 2 may be diagnosed when one of the following is present:
  A. Bilateral eighth cranial nerve masses are seen with appropriate imaging techniques (CT or MRI)
  B. A parent, sibling, or child with neurofibromatosis 2 *and* either a unilateral eighth nerve mass or any two of the following: neurofibroma, meningioma, glioma, schwannoma, or juvenile posterior subcapsular lenticular opacity

*From Martuza, RL, Eldridge R. Neurofibromatosis 2. N Engl J Med 1988;**318:**684–688. Copyright 1988, Massachusetts Medical Society. All rights reserved.*

Variant conditions are the following:
  Noonan features with neurofibromatosis A dominantly inherited congenital dysmorphic syndrome, characterized also by short stature; ptosis; short webbed neck; vertebral and other skeletal, dermal, and congenital cardiac anomalies; seizures; macrocephaly; mental and developmental delay; and the usual features of neurofibromatosis.[4797]
  Segmental neurofibromatosis A form with restriction of the cutaneous and neoplastic features to a few adjacent segments of the body.[3888]
  Spinal and cutaneous neurofibromatosis The occurrence of multiple schwannomas has been described as sporadic but probably represents a variant of NF-2.[1715]
  Godfried-Prick-Carol-Prakken syndrome Dermal atrophy, mongoloid facies, mental deficiency, and cardiac conduction disturbances are added features.[910]

Neurofibromatosis, Inc. A charitable organization providing support and information on this condition. Address: 9320 Annapolis Road, Suite 300, Lanham, Maryland 20706-3123. Tel: 301-918-4600, 1-800-942-6825. Web site: http://www.nfinc.org/.

neurofilaments Small (10-nm) organelles which exist within the axoplasm, determining its diameter. The filaments are especially notable in larger axons, and move centripetally at up to 3 mm/day.

Neurogastroenterology and Motility A subspecialty medical journal. Web site: http://www.blacksci.co.uk/~cgilib/jnlpage.asp?Journal=ngem&File=ngem.

Neurogenetics A subspecialty medical journal. Web site: http://link.springer-ny.com/link/service/journals/10048/index.htm.

neurogenic acro-osteolysis See **ulceromutilating acropathy.**

neurogenic arthropathy (Charcot joints) A clinical syndrome of painless joint enlargement with crepitus, effusions, laxity of ligaments, and excessive mobility leading to dissolution of the joint, and associated with a loss of nociceptive sensation, as in **hereditary sensory neuropathy, tabes dorsalis, diabetic or amyloid neuropathies,** and **leprosy.**

neurogenic benign fasciculations See **idiopathic neuromyotonia.**

neurogenic bladder The condition of the bladder after interruption of its motor or sensory nerve supply. See **reflex neurogenic bladder, autonomous neurogenic bladder, motor paralytic bladder, deafferented bladder.**

neurogenic claudication The complaint of ascending numbness and weakness of the legs which occurs in association with postural extension of the lumbar spine, as during shaving, and both with standing and exercise in patients with lumbar **spinal stenosis.** The similarities with vasogenic claudication are many but, in the neurogenic form, the absence of cramps and of paresthesias and the procurement of relief by the adoption of the flexed posture are differentiating points.

The term *claudication* is derived from the Latin *claudicare,* to limp; perhaps deriving also from that deficit of the Roman Emperor Claudius. The word is poorly applied here, because, when patients with lumbar spinal stenosis become symptomatic, they do not limp but rather stop walking and bend forward, a maneuver that enlarges the internal dimensions of the spinal canal. Such people should rely on bicycles for local transport.

neurogenic diabetes insipidus Transient reduction in the secretion of antidiuretic hormone following head injury or cranial surgery.

neurogenic fever See **neurogenic hyperthermia.**

neurogenic hyperthermia ("neurogenic fever") Fever reflects the action of a pyrogen upon an intact hypothalamus. Lesions of the anterior hypothalamus may impair the body's ability to dissipate heat, leading to hyperthermia, but do not change the hypothalamic set point. The hypothalamus contains two areas maintaining temperature homeostasis—one located anteriorly, concerned with heat dissipation and containing the "hypothalamic thermostat," and a posterior area involved in heat generation. Electrical stimulation of the posterior area produces shivering, piloerection, peripheral vasoconstriction, and behaviors raising body temperature. Lesions of this area prevent the normal response to cold.

In true fever, pyrogens such as interleukin 1 act on anterior hypothalamic neurons to raise the set point of the hypothalamic "thermostat" through a prostaglandin E2-mediated system. Sensing a difference between the current and desired temperatures, these neurons stimulate activity in the posterior thalamic center to increase thermogenic activities. Once body temperature has reached the new set point, these activities normally subside. In patients with neurogenic hyperthermia, antipyretics are ineffective in lowering the elevated temperature but external cooling is effective unless rigidity produces a large internal heat load; heat-generating activities such as shivering are not increased with cooling back to a normal body temperature; there is a history of trauma, infarct, or tumor in the hypothalamus, spinal cord injury, familial dysautonomia, or autonomic neuropathies; and the syndrome may be seen in late stages of neurodegenerative disorders.

Subarachnoid blood, air, or iodinated contrast may cause a low-grade fever from an inflammatory response in the subarachnoid space, but there is accompanying evidence of inflammation in the CSF. Diencephalic epilepsy and complex partial status epilepticus may be associated with temperature elevations thought to be secondary to episodic hypothalamic dysfunction.[1461,1696,4401]

neurogenic inflammation An early response to tissue injury. In the context of migraine, the term applies to the vasodilatation and extravasation of plasma that occur following stimulation of the unmyelinated afferent C-fibers supplying dural and scalp blood vessels.

neurogenic pulmonary edema The occurrence of pulmonary edema as a complication of generalized tonic-clonic seizures, first reported by Shanahan in 1908. The precise mechanism of this effect remains uncertain.[5525]

neurogenic sarcoma An uncommon malignant tumor of the peripheral nerve sheath.

neurogenic thoracic outlet compression syndrome An uncommon lower trunk brachial plexopathy predominantly damaging the T1 fibers in the median motor nerve fibers to the thenar muscles and in the the medial antebrachial cutaneous nerve fibers.[3372] See **thoracic outlet syndrome.**

neuroglia (Gr, nerve + glue) The name applied by Virchow (1846) to the supporting cells (as opposed to the neurons) of the CNS; the differentiation was achieved without benefit of special stains, which had not then been invented.

neuroglioma See **glioma.**

neuroichthyoses Genetically determined diffuse encephalopathies, including **Sjögren-Larsson syndrome, Rud syndrome,** keratitis-ichthyosis-deafness syndrome, ichthyosis with neutral lipid storage, and **Refsum syndrome.**

Neuroimmunomodulation A subspecialty medical journal. Web site: http://www.karger.com/journals/nim/nim_jh.htm.

neuroimmunophilins A family of proteins expressed in the nervous system that act as receptors for some immunosuppressant agents and with a likely role in neuroprotection and regeneration.[1897]

neurokinin A peptide substance discovered by Wolff, with a possible role in the genesis of **migraine.**

neurolabyrinthitis See **acute peripheral vestibulopathy.**

Neuroland A valuable free website, www.neuroland.com/, maintained by Dr. Charles Tuen, containing current data on numerous neurological diseases, including multiple sclerosis, headache, pain, stroke, polyneuropathy, seizures, anticonvulsants, low back pain, Parkinson disease, and infectious diseases, and on internal medicine.

neuroleptic malignant syndrome (lethal catatonia) An uncommon, fulminant, life-threatening, and unpredictable idiosyncratic reaction to neuroleptic medications (dopamine-receptor blocking agents) in adults, described by Delay and Deniker in 1968 and due to imbalance of 5-HT and dopamine, causing a relatively hypodopaminergic state.

The clinical features that develop over 1–3 days and last for up to 10 days include hyperthermia, autonomic instability (labile blood pressure, sweating, tachycardia, or bradykinesia), intense plastic muscular rigidity, altered consciousness with delirium, and elevated muscle enzyme levels in almost all cases. Mutism, tremor, choreic or dystonic movements, and incontinence occur in a majority and oculogyric crises, opisthotonos, seizures, and trismus are seen in a few patients. Shock, respiratory failure, and myoglobinuria can occur, with serious consequences.[3366] Dantrolene sodium, amantadine, and bromocriptine have all been found to have therapeutic benefit.[40]

The condition occurs at some time in 0.5% of subjects (especially young males) exposed to neuroleptic agents and is considered to have a central (presynaptic) origin.[2345] It is also described following withdrawal of L-dopa therapy in the treatment of idiopathic **Parkinson disease,** while an identical syndrome may be seen rarely in untreated catatonic schizophrenia.

Diagnostic signs have been defined: *major criteria* are fever, rigidity, and elevated serum creatine kinase levels; *minor criteria* are tachycardia, labile blood pressure,

tachypnea, altered consciousness, sweating, and leukocytosis. The presence of three major, or two major and four minor signs makes the diagnosis probable.[40]

In a *variant* form, an absence of muscle glycogen and neutral lipid is found on muscle biopsy specimens.[3654] See also **serotonin syndrome; malignant hyperthermia,** and the web site: http://www.neuro.wustl.edu/neuromuscular/index.html.

neurolipidoses Hereditary metabolic disorders in which abnormal lipid accumulations occur, such as in the **gangliosidoses.** Myoclonic epilepsy is often a prominent clinical feature.

Neurologic Clinics A quarterly periodical reviewing neurology topics, published by W.B. Saunders. Web site: http://www.us.elsevierhealth.com/fcgi-bin/displaypage.pl?isbn=07338619.

Neurological Disability score A semiquantitative method of assessing the disability produced by diseases of the *peripheral* nervous system, in which the degree of abnormality in clinical tests of the cranial nerves (6 items), muscle weakness (16 movements or muscles), muscle stretch reflexes (5), and sensation in the index finger and hallux (4 modalities in each site) on each side is scored between 0 (no deficit) and 4 (complete absence of function or severest deficit). The summed score is used to obtain a raw score whereby to evaluate progression of diabetic neuropathic symptoms.[1568,1580]

Deficits produced by lesions of the central nervous system are not considered in this scale.

Neurological Rating scale A simple assessment tool in **multiple sclerosis** in which dysfunction is scored in the categories of mentation and mood; cranial nerves (visual acuity, fields, discs and pupils, eye movements, and nystagmus); lower cranial nerves; motor and reflex functions in each limb; Babinski signs; sensory functions in each limb; cerebellar function in the upper and in the lower limbs; gait; and bladder/bowel/sexual dysfunction, the whole yielding a total impairment score. The maximum (normal) score is 100.[3867]

neurological examination A complex learned skill possessed by some physicians.

Neurological Institute of New York An institution founded in 1909 by Joseph Collins and Pearce Bailey, later attracting Ramsay **Hunt,** Charles **Dana,** Elsberg, and Sachs as members. It moved to Columbia Presbyterian Medical Center in 1929, and has expanded greatly since. Address: Columbia-Presbyterian Medial Center, 710 W. 168th St., New York, NY 10032-3784. Tel: 212-305-2700. Web site: http://cpmcnet.columbia.edu/dept/neurology/index.htm.

Neurological Society of London An institution founded in 1885 with Hughlings-**Jackson** as founding President, and Samuel Wilks, **Bastian,** Crighton-Browne, Broadbent, **Ferrier, Galton,** and Bucknill as councillors. Two years after its founding, it created the journal *Brain* as its organ.

neurologic web sites   A listing of the most respected Web sites in neurology can be found at http://www.neuroland.com/links/best_links.htm.

neurologist   (Gr, a nerve + a discourse) 1. One who is occupied with the study of the nerves and the nervous system. 2. A physician who is trained in the diagnosis and management of patients suffering from diseases of the nervous system, or their symptoms.

neurology   The study of the nervous system in health and disease. The term was originally that of Thomas **Willis,** who also described this labor as "The doctrine of the nerves." This phrase was taken by Spillane for his superb review of the history of the subject.[5280]

Neurology   A professional journal founded as the official publication of the **American Academy of Neurology** in 1951 with Dr. R. de Jong as the first editor. The journal has been published monthly since 1953. Web site: http://www.neurology.org/.

Neurology Alert   (*Neurol. Alert*) A neurological review/update publication. Address: American Health Consultants, 3525 Piedmont Road, Bldg. 6, Ste. 400, Atlanta, GA 30305. Web site: http://www.ahcpub.com/ahc_root_html/products/newsletters/na.html.

Neurology and Neurosurgery   An Excerpta Medica abstract journal providing a current awareness service, published by Elsevier . Web site: http://www.elsevier.com/inca/publications/store/5/0/5/9/7/7/.

neurolymphomatosis   (reticulosis of the nervous system, polyradiculitis with cellular infiltrates, lymphomatous neuropathy, lymphomatous leptomeningitis) Lymphomatous infiltration of the peripheral nerves producing various clinical pictures of sensorimotor peripheral and cranial neuropathies. These include those of acute inflammatory polyneuropathy, mononeuropathy, subacute or relapsing neuropathy, and cauda equina syndrome.

The condition is analogous to Marek disease, which afflicts Orpington roosters.[1431]

neuroma   (Gr, nerve + tumor) A benign tumor of nerves, first described by William Wood, a Scottish physician, in 1828.

neuroma sign   In patients with severe proximal brachial plexus lesions, if the side of the neck is tapped and paresthesias are felt in the distribution of a dermatome, the nerve root is likely to have been ruptured.

Neurometer   A commercial device for quantifying sensory thresholds, and thus potentially of use in the diagnosis and/or follow-up of patients with neuropathies.

neuromodulator   A substance altering the receptivity of a neuron to stimulation, as by altering the resting poten-

tial or changing synthesis in the cell for receptors, etc. Examples include secretin, bombesin, neuropeptide Y, substance P, vasoactive intestinal peptide, and glucagon.

neuromuscular blockade   Impairment of the passage of acetylcholine from the nerve ending, across the synapse to the motor end-plate, or reduction of the effect of acetylcholine at the latter site.

Neuromuscular Disease Center   (Washington University, St. Louis) A superb resource maintained by Dr. Alan Pestronk. It provides complete data for physicians on the clinical and laboratory aspects of all neuromuscular disorders and ataxias. Web site: http://www.neuro.wustl.edu/neuromuscular/index.html.

neuromuscular disorders   Diseases primarily affecting the nerve roots or peripheral nerves, the motor end-plates, or the muscles.

These have been listed and classified by the World Federation of Neurology. Chart N–5 contains a slightly adapted summary of this classification and uses similar ennumeration. Other entries in this book follow in general the order given here.

Chart N–5. Classification of Neuromuscular Disorders

1. *Spinal muscular atrophies and other disorders of motor neurons* (for further descriptions see **motor neuronal disorders** and specific diseases)
   A. Inherited muscle atrophies (**hereditary motor neuropathies)**
      A1. Autosomal recessive, biochemical abnormality unknown
      A2. Autosomal recessive, biochemical abnormality known
      A3. Autosomal dominant, biochemical abnormality unknown
      A4. X-linked recessive, biochemical disorder unknown
      A5. X-linked dominant, lethal in males
   B. Congenital and developmental abnormalities (see Chart M–17, **motor neuronal diseases,** for further consideration of groups B, C, D, E, F, G, H, and I)
   C. Disorders of motor neurons attributed to physical causes
   D. Disorders of motor neurons attributed to toxins, chemicals, or heavy metals
   E. Disorders of motor neurons attributed to viral infection
      E1. Acute disorders
      E2. Subacute or chronic disorders
   F. Disorders of motor neurons with immunological abnormality
   G. Disorders of motor neurons of undetermined etiology
   H. Disorders of motor neurons in endocrine disorders
   I. Disorders of motor neurons manifest by hyperactivity
2. *Disorders of motor nerve roots* (for further descriptions see **radiculopathy**)
   A. Congenital
   B. Acquired
3. *Disorders of peripheral nerve* (for further descriptions see **neuropathy** and entries for specific diseases)

A. Heritable, biochemical abnormality unknown
B. Congenital
C. Traumatic
D. Infections
E. Guillain-Barré syndrome (**acute inflammatory demyelinating polyneuropathy**) and related disorders
F. Neuropathy associated with connective tissue disorder
G. Metabolic neuropathy
H. Neuropathy in malignant disease
I. Neuropathy associated with other systemic or non-hereditary degenerative diseases
J. Chronic neuropathy with no known cause or association
K. Tumors of nerves

4. *Disorders of neuromuscular transmission* (for further descriptions see Chart N–6, **neuromuscular transmission disorders**)
   A. Heritable
   B. Congenital or developmental **myasthenia**
   C. Toxic
   D. Autoimmune
   E. **Lambert-Eaton syndrome**
   F. Cholinergic paralysis

5. *Disorders of muscle* (for further description and subclassification, see **myopathies**)
   A. Heritable myopathies
      A1. The muscular dystrophies
      A2. Congenital myopathies of unknown etiology
      A3. Myotonic disorders
   B. Trauma to muscle by external agents
      B1. Physical
      B2. Toxic
      B3. Drugs
   C. Inflammatory
      C1. Infections of muscle
      C2. Other inflammatory disorders of muscle
      C3. Inflammatory disorders of muscle of unknown etiology
   D. Metabolic myopathies
      D1. Muscle disorder associated with endocrine disease
      D2. Heritable myopathies, biochemical abnormality known
      D3. Other metabolic myopathies
   E. Myopathy associated with malignant disease
   F. Myopathy associated with **myasthenia gravis**
   G. Myopathy in thalassaemia
   H. Other disorders of muscle of unknown or uncertain etiology
   I. Tumors of muscle

6. *Disorders of supraspinal tonal regulation which may mimic neuromuscular disorders*

Adapted from the World Federation of Neurology Classification Subcommittee. Classification of neuromuscular diseases. J Neurol Sci 1988; 86:333–360, *by kind permission of the late Professor P.K. Thomas, Lord Walton, and the World Federation of Neurology. See also http://www. neuro.wustl.edu/neuromuscular/maltbrain.html.*

Neuromuscular Disorders   The official journal of the World Muscle Society covering all aspects of the neuromuscular disorders of childhood and adult life. The journal publishes original research, reviews, short communications, and book reviews. Web site: http://www. elsevier.com/inca/publications/store/9/7/3/.

neuromuscular transmission disorders   Diseases adversely influencing the process whereby depolarization of nerve leads to the depolarization of muscle. The classification in Chart N–6 is closely based on that of the World Federation of Neurology and uses the same ennumeration.

Chart N–6.   Disorders of Neuromuscular Transmission

A. *Heritable*
   1. Hereditary **myasthenia gravis**
      a. Congenital and juvenile[834]
      b. Myasthenia with myopathy[3790]
   2. **Pseudocholinesterase deficiency** (suxamethonium paralysis)
B. *Congenital or developmental myasthenia*
   1. Putative defect in acetylcholine synthesis or packaging
   2. **Congenital end-plate acetylcholinesterase deficiency**
   3. **Slow-channel syndrome**
   4. **Congenital end-plate acetylcholine receptor deficiency**
   5. Decrease of miniature end-plate potential amplitude without acetylcholine receptor deficiency
   6. Abnormality of synaptic vesicles[3964]
C. *Toxic*
   1. **Botulism**
   2. **Tick paralysis**
   3. **Puffer-fish paralysis** (tetrodotoxin)
   4. Magnesium intoxication
   5. Kanamycin and other antibiotics[3791]
   6. Penicillamine-induced myasthenia, also anticonvulsants, quinidine[2036]
D. *Autoimmune*
   1. **Myasthenia gravis**
      a. Transient neonatal myasthenia[2100]
      b. Ocular myasthenia, with peripheral neuropathy and spastic paraparesis[823]
      c. Generalized myasthenia
         i. Severe, especially in young women, correlated with HLA-8 antigen
         ii. In older patients, often with thymoma and with HLA-2 or A3 antigen
      d. Myasthenia with thyrotoxicosis
      e. Myasthenia with hypothyroidism[5472]
      f. Myasthenia with other autoimmune diseases
      g. Myasthenia combined with **Lambert-Eaton syndrome**[4213]
      h. Myasthenia with the **Satoyoshi syndrome** (muscle cramps, alopecia, and diarrhea)
E. ***Lambert-Eaton syndrome*** (a facilitating disorder of neuromuscular transmission)
   1. With malignant disease
   2. Without malignant disease
F. *Cholinergic paralysis* (e.g., due to poisoning with anticholinesterase compounds such as nerve gases, depolarizing drugs, or black widow spider venom)

Adapted from the World Federation of Neurology Classification Subcommittee. Classification of neuromuscular diseases. J Neurol Sci 1988;86: 333–360, *by kind permission of Professor P.K. Thomas, Lord Walton, and the World Federation of Neurology. See also http://www.neuro.wustl.edu/ neuromuscular/maltbrain.html.*

neuromyasthenia   See **chronic fatigue syndrome.**

neuromyelitis Originally signifying "inflammation of the nervous or medullary substance,"[4512] the word is now used to indicate the coexistence of inflammation of the spinal cord and a nerve, usually the optic nerve.

neuromyelitis optica (Devic disease, Devic-Gault syndrome, myelopathy with optic neuritis, optic myelitis, Schilder myelinoclastic diffuse sclerosis) A necrotizing and demyelinating disease with its attack targeted upon the spinal cord and both optic nerves, described from France by M.E. Devic in 1894[1424] and before him by Chisholm in England.

The disease, which may be a variant of **multiple sclerosis,**[2372] is uncommon in the Western world but not in Japan. Clinically, subacute visual failure is followed within days by signs of myelopathy, but brainstem, cerebellar, and cognitive disturbances do not occur.

Suggested diagnostic criteria, modified here, are as follows:

1. Clinically, acute involvement of the spinal cord and of one of both optic nerves, either coincidentally or separated by months or years, independent of the subsequent progression of the disease but without the development of brainstem, cerebellar, or cortical features at any time, without evidence of disease elsewhere in the CNS. The disease may be mono- or multiphasic.
2. The brain MRI appears normal, or shows deep white matter lesions, but there is enlargement of the spinal cord, sometimes with cavitation.
3. Oligoclonal bands are usually absent from the CSF and daily IgG synthesis is normal. There is a decrease in the serum/CSF albumin ratio.
4. Spinal cord necrosis and cavitation with thickened vessel walls are found; there is no inflammatory infiltration. Demyelination is found in the optic nerves but not elsewhere in the brain, brainstem, or cerebellum.[3587]

From Mandler RN, Davis LE, Jeffery DR, et al. Devic's neuromyelitis optica: A clinicopathological study of 8 patients. *Ann. Neurol.* 1993;**34:**168, by kind permission.

neuromyopathy Clinical disorders resulting from pathology affecting both nerve and muscle fibers. See **carcinomatous neuromyopathy, cachectic myopathy.**

neuromyositis (dermatoradiculoneuromyositis) The rare concomitant association of polyneuropathy and polymyositis, first described by Senator in 1888, and probably representing the chance concurrence of **acute inflammatory demyelinating polyneuropathy** and **polymyositis.**[3748]

neuromyotonia 1. (Isaacs syndrome, continuous muscle fiber activity, hereditary myotonia, continuous muscle fiber activity, continuous motor unit activity, idiopathic generalized myotonia, Isaacs-Mertens syndrome, quantal squander, generalized myokymia, normocalcemic tetany, neurotonia) A nonprogressive syndrome of continuous, generalized involuntary twitching or quivering in several muscles with impaired relaxation after contraction (**myokymia**) but without a true my-

otonic response. It is due to hyperexcitability of the peripheral motor axons, possibly as the result of autoimmune disease[2752;5846] mediated by IgG antibodies to voltage-gated potassium channels, although familial occurrence has been recorded.[3846] Electrically, there are irregular and abrupt spontaneous bursts of single motor unit potentials at a rate of between 2 and 300 Hz, prolonged over several seconds, associated with persistent muscle contraction The situation is complicated by the coexistence of **myotonia** in some cases.[2803] See also **pseudomyotonia, myokymia.**

Clinically, the condition presents at any age with continuing contraction of muscles at rest or following voluntary effort, leading to a delay in relaxation, and with muscle stiffness, cramps, weakness, and often twitching and increased warmth and sweating. The accompanying electrical activity may be intermittent or continuous.

The phenomenon resembles **myotonia** clinically, but, in this case, may be the result of many disorders of motor nerves which lead to ectopic or ephaptic neural discharges, as with myokymia following plexus irradiation. It responds to phenytoin and to carbamazepine. Lung and thymic neoplasms and myasthenia with antiacetylcholine receptor antibodies have been reported in association. See also **Schwartz-Jampel syndrome.**

2. A combination of subjective muscle stiffness and myokymia, sometimes with added muscle hypertrophy, supervening in some patients with **chronic inflammatory demyelinating polyneuropathy.**

3. (*ocular neuromyotonia*) Recurrent episodes of sustained contraction of the muscles supplied by a paretic third cranial nerve, both spontaneously and following eccentric gaze. The condition appears usually in the context of recent pituitary radiation therapy.[3362] Ephaptic neural transmission is the likely underlying mechanism.[5587]

Variants include the following:

A syndrome of muscle stiffness associated with a bronchial carcinoma, the stiffness precipitated by movement and accompanied by bizarre, high-frequency motor unit discharges appearing during and after voluntary contraction. The features are abolished by nerve block and reduced by phenytoin. HIV infection, thymus cancer, and Hodgkin disease are also associated. See also **stiff man syndrome.**[5826]

Morvan "chorea" (neuromyotonia, hyperhidrosis and encephalopathy)

Familial stiff man syndrome, manifesting hypertonia at birth, which regresses, only to return in adolescence.[4897] See also **limp man syndrome, idiopathic neuromyotonia.**

See also **continuous muscle fiber activity syndrome, Isaacs syndrome, Isaacs-Merten syndrome, quantal squander, generalized myokymia, pseudomyotonia, normocalcemic tetany, neurotonia,** and the Web site http://www.neuro.wustl.edu/neuromuscular/maltbrain.html.

neuromyotonic discharge Bursts of motor unit action potentials that fire at high rates (150 to 300 Hz) for a few seconds, often starting or stopping abruptly. The amplitude of the waveforms typically wanes. Discharges may occur spontaneously or be initiated by needle electrode movement, voluntary effort, ischemia, or percussion of a nerve. The activity originates in motor axons. It should be distinguished from myotonic discharges and complex repetitive discharges. This is one type of electrical activity recorded in patients who have clinical neuromyotonia. (From the 2001 Report of the Nomenclature Committee of the American Association of Electromyography and Electrodiagnosis.[10] Used by permission, copyright © 2001, AAEM.)

neuronal ceroid lipofuscinosis   (Gr, nerve + wax + fat) (cerebroretinal lipofuscinosis, Batten-Vogt disease, Batten-Mayou disease, Batten disease, Landing-Oppenheimer disease) A group of recessively inherited lysosomal storage diseases characterized by the accumulation of abnormal amounts of ceroid-lipofuscin, an autofluorescent lipopigment, in the lysosomes and by the presence of characteristic curvilinear or fingerprint inclusions in brain, skin, muscle, or rectal mucosa; an excessive accumulation of granular lipopigment in neuronal perikarya; and elevated levels of urinary sediment dolichols.

Clinically, all forms manifest progressive encephalopathy with psychomotor deterioration, visual failure, seizures, psychiatric disturbances, spasticity, ataxia and movement disorders, seizures, and death within about 10 years of the onset. Increased autofluorescent lipopigment is detectable in neuronal cells. For the many known mutations in neuronal ceroid lipofuscinosis, see http://www.ucl.ac.uk/ncl.

Five clinical varieties were described variously by Batten (1903)[392] Mayer (1904); Vogt (1904); Spielmeyer (1904); Jansky (1908); Bielschowsky (1913) and Sjögren (1931). Others have been added more recently by Wisniewski (2001)[6012] (See Chart N–7).

Chart N–7. Forms of Neuronal Ceroid Lipofuscinosis

1. *Infantile (Haltia-Santavuori, Hagberg, or Finnish type; OMIM 256730)* A form with onset at the end of the first year of life up to mid-adult life mapped to 1p32. Clinically, it is characterized by microcephaly, psychomotor deterioration, hypotonia and ataxia (giving way later to spasticity and rigidity), myoclonus and seizures, optic atrophy, and retinal dystrophy, accompanied by severe diffuse brain atrophy due to neuronal destruction and demyelination.[4912] Visual evoked responses are lost, and there is marked slowing on the EEG.

   In a *variant form,* onset is delayed for a few years.

2. *Late-infantile (Jansky-Bielschowsky, late amaurotic familial idiocy)* A recessive form mapped to 11p15 in which myoclonic and tonic-clonic seizures, atonic attacks, and atypical absences present at between 2 and 8 years of age, after which stimulus-sensitive myoclonus, ataxia, psychomotor failure, pigmentary retinopathy, and optic at-

rophy with visual failure occur. Intractable seizures and myoclonus, relentless dementia, and progressive ataxia and spasticity lead to death within 5 years.[505,561]

   A *Finnish variant* of this form maps to 13q22 and presents in childhood with cognitive and motor decline, seizures, and visual loss. It is distinguished from the typical form on the basis of pathological findings.

   A third (*Gypsy/Indian*) late infantile variant maps to 15q21 and presents in infancy or childhood with cognitive and motor decline, seizures, and visual loss.

3. *Juvenile (Batten, Mayer, Speilmeyer-Vogt, Spielmeyer-Sjögren)* A recessively inherited syndrome mapped to 16p11.2–12.1 and presenting with visual failure occurring between the ages of 4 and 10 years, sometimes with tonic-clonic and myoclonic seizures and followed by psychomotor regression, seizures, stuttering dysarthria, pyramidal signs, ataxia, and extrapyramidal dystonic rigidity. Optic atrophy, pigmentary macular degeneration, attenuation of the retinal vessels, and cardiac conduction defects[2207] are other typical findings.[392] The disease has no ethnic predilection.

   Earlier and more severe cases contrast with the slower course of those with later onset, known as the *chronic juvenile (Batten)* form, in which visual failure occurs in later childhood, sometimes with tonic-clonic and myoclonic seizures, followed by the slow development of psychomotor regression, seizures, stuttering dysarthria, pyramidal signs, ataxia, and extrapyramidal rigidity. Optic atrophy, pigmentary macular degeneration, and attenuation of the retinal vessels are characteristic findings.

4. *Adult (Kufs or Parry)* A recessively inherited (rarely dominant) variety in which hexosaminidase A is not absent but is severely decreased in content. The disease is characterized clinically by variable cerebellar, extrapyramidal (dystonic), cognitive, and psychiatric disturbances, lower motor neuron lesions, and often myoclonic or other seizures, usually with their onset in early adult life, with only minor if any dementia and without visual symptoms. The optic fundi are normal.[211,335,3180]

5. *Turkish variant* A form presenting in early childhood with motor decline, seizures, and visual loss, distinguished from other forms on the basis of pathological findings.

6. *Northern epilepsy (OMIM 600143)* A disorder presenting in childhood with cognitive decline and seizures and mapped to 8p23.[3264]

The following diagnostic criteria for type 4 have been suggested:[504]

1. Onset around the age of 30 years
2. Phenotypes of **progressive myoclonic epilepsy** or of behavioral change, dementia, and motor disturbances, there being visual failure in neither case
3. A clinical course of about 12 years to death with dementia
4. Elevated urinary sediment dolichol levels; a marked photoparoxysmal response on the EEG is seen in the first of the two phenotypes
5. Ultrastructural studies reveal fingerprint profiles or granular osmophilic deposits

From Berkovic S, Carpenter S, Andermann F, et al. Kufs' disease: a critical reappraisal. *Brain* 1988;**111**:27–62, by kind permission of Oxford University Press.

Other *variant forms* have been reported;

Early juvenile form A neuronal inclusion/storage disease with juvenile onset, characterized by dementia; seizures; cerebellar, pyramidal, and extrapyramidal signs; myoclonus; multifocal paroxysmal discharges; and abnormal electroretinogram.

Pigment form A neuronal inclusion/storage disease with dementia, ataxia, spasticity, resting tremor, and myoclonus.

Atypical form A form in which the features of retinal abnormalities or visual symptoms are not present.[2274]

Ceroid lipofuscinosis storage, sea-blue histiocytes, and posterior column dysfunction.[5433]

These conditions and the **gangliosidoses** were formerly classified together under the pejorative rubric "familial amaurotic idiocy." The subject has been reviewed by Zeman.[6121]

neuronal heterotopias   A form of dysplasia characterized by accumulations of clumps of neuronal cell bodies within the white matter of the brain.

neuronal intestinal dysplasia   A visceral neuropathy characterized by hyperganglionosis of the bowel with hyperplasia of the submucosal and myenteric plexus and the formation of giant ganglia; isolated heterotopic ganglion cells in the lamina propria and between the muscle fibers of the muscularis mucosae; and an increase in acetylcholine activity in the parasympathetic fibers of the laminar and circular muscle. The condition may be confined to the colon or may involve more diffuse regions of the small bowel.

Clinically, the disease presents with megacolon and pseudo-obstruction, resembling that seen in Hirschsprung disease. Associations with multiple endocrine neoplasia syndrome type 2b, **neurofibromatosis,** and **Hirschsprung disease** are well described.[4944]

neuronal intranuclear hyaline inclusion disease   A rare, slowly progressive, inherited neuronal storage disorder with onset in childhood, characterized pathologically by the presence of round, eosinophilic, antifluorescent inclusion bodies in neuronal nuclei in both the central and peripheral nervous systems.[2400,4043]

The variable phenotypes include cerebellar, extrapyramidal, and pyramidal signs; seizures; oculogyric spasms; lower motor neuron lesions; kyphoscoliosis; pes cavus; behavioral disturbance; tics; seizures; microcephaly; ophthalmoplegia; sensory and autonomic neuropathy; cerebral atrophy; and mental and developmental delay or (later) dementia.[4043]

In a *variant* form, the disorder presents in adult life with dementia, amyotrophy, choreoathetosis, seizures, and sphincter disorder.[5418]

neuronal migration disorders   Disorders that result from specific derangements in fetal neuronal development. Such developmental structural lesions are characterized by disorganization of the cortical architecture with an aberrant columnar and laminar neuronal arrangement. When severe, they present with severe seizure disorders, mental retardation, and incapacitating motor dysfunction, but minor formes frustes produce only syndromes of diluted severity.

The conditions encompassed by this term include **lissencephaly** (agyria), **Miller-Diecker syndrome, pachygyria** (macrogyria), **polymicrogyria, schizencephaly,** and other **heterotopias** of the gray matter.[168,3205] See also **focal neuronal migration disorders.**

neuronal storage diseases   Inherited conditions such as Tay-Sachs disease, **metachromatic leukodystrophy,** and the **gangliosidoses,** in which abnormal material accumulates within neuronal cell bodies.

neuronal tumors   Uncommon tumors showing histological features of neuronal differentiation to a variable extent and occurring mainly in the cerebral hemispheres of children and young adults or in the sympathetic system. **Gangliocytoma, ganglioglioma, ganglioneuroblastoma, neuroblastoma, paraganglioma-ganglioneuroma, anaplastic gangliocytoma,** and **esthesioneuroblastoma** are examples.

neuron(e)   A nerve cell and all of its processes; the unit structure of the nervous system.

The name was first applied by Heinrich Wilhelm Waldeyer (1837–1921), a German anatomist, who showed that all nerve fibers, axons, and dendrites are outgrowths of the neuronal cell bodies. The word was formerly used by Hippocrates to mean a tendon.

neuron doctrine   The cells in the cerebrum are linked by contact, not by continuity, and thus there is physiological autonomy of the nerve cell and its branches.

This point of view was supported by **Remak** against the **reticular theory,** which held that the cerebral gray matter formed a huge reticulum or nerve net, as was believed by **Gerlach, Golgi,** and **Weigert.** Using the Golgi silver stain, Ramon y Cajal showed that the neuron doctrine was correct, although Golgi was not converted even as they shared the Nobel prize in 1906.

Neuronet   An online resource center that addresses information needs in the fields of dementia, acute stroke, epilepsy, and multiple sclerosis. Access to NeuroNet is limited to physicians only and pre-registration is required. Web site: http://www.neuro-net.net/.

neuronopathy   1. A disease of the peripheral nervous system in which the primary neuropathological changes appear in the nerve cell body rather than the axon or the myelin sheath. 2. A motor neuropathy in which the anterior horn (or cranial nerve motor nucleus) cells, or a sensory neuropathy in which the dorsal root ganglion cells (or cranial nerve sensory nuclei), are the site of the pathology.[5337]

See **subacute motor neuronopathy.**

neuronophagia   (from Lat, nerve cell + to swallow) The ingestion and removal of dead neuronal tissue by phagocytic macrophages.

neuroparalytic hemicrania See **migraine with aura, familial hemiplegic migraine.**

neuroparalytic keratitis Corneal ulceration developing as a result of corneal anesthesia and consequent failure of the protective **blink reflex.**

neuropathic motor unit potential Abnormally high-amplitude, long-duration, polyphasic motor unit action potential. Use of the term is discouraged, as it incorrectly implies a specific diagnostic significance of a motor unit action potential configuration. See **motor unit action potential.** (From the 2001 Report of the Nomenclature Committee of the American Association of Electromyography and Electrodiagnosis.[10] Used by permission, copyright © 2001, AAEM.)

neuropathic pain Pain of neurological origin accompanied usually by allodynia, hyperalgesia to prick and temperature, summation, after-sensations, and unusual referral patterns.

Neuropathic Pain scale A five-question scale designed to assess distinct pain qualities associated with neuropathic pain.[2009]

neuropathic recruitment A recruitment pattern characterized by a decreased number of motor unit action potentials firing at a rapid rate. Use of the term is discouraged. See **reduced interference pattern, discrete activity, single unit pattern.** (From the 2001 Report of the Nomenclature Committee of the American Association of Electromyography and Electrodiagnosis.[10] Used by permission, copyright © 2001, AAEM.)

neuropathic tremor A form of coarse tremor at 3–6 Hz. with both postural and action components, usually affecting the arms and associated with the presence of thick-fiber peripheral sensory neuropathy.

See also *Roussy-Levy syndrome* (**hereditary motor and sensory neuropathy**).

neuropathy (Gr, nerve + disease) A disorder of one or more peripheral nerves, more correct than *neuritis* (the word more commonly used) because relatively few disorders of nerves are actually accompanied by inflammation. The word *neurosis* for this condition is obsolete. Disorders of the cell body are also known as neuronopathies; of the axon, axonopathies; and of the myelin sheath, demyelinating neuropathies. Motor, sensory, or autonomic nerves may be uniquely affected or the neuropathy may involve these elements in any combination. The classification in Chart N–8 is closely based on that of the World Federation of Neurology.[6039]

Further information about all neuropathies can be accessed at the Web site of Dr. Alan Pestronk: http://www.neuro.wustl.edu/neuromuscular/index.html.

Chart N–8. Classification of the Neuropathies

A. *Heritable, biochemical abnormality unknown*
   1. See **hereditary motor and sensory neuropathy.**
   2. See **hereditary sensory and autonomic neuropathy.**
   3. Hereditary neuropathies associated with specific biochemical abnormalities
      a. **Familial amyloid neuropathy**
         Type 1—Portuguese type (transthyretin abnormality)
         Type 2—Indiana type
         Type 3—Iowa type
         Type 4—Finnish type
         Type 5—Jewish type
         Type 6—Appalachian type
      b. **Porphyria**
      c. Analphalipoproteinemia See **Tangier disease.**
      d. **Abetalipoproteinemia**
      e. **Metachromatic leukodystrophy**
      f. Globoid cell leukodystrophy See **Krabbe leukodystrophy.**
      g. **Niemann-Pick disease**
      h. **Adrenoleukodystrophy** and **adrenomyeloneuropathy**
      i. **Fabry disease**
      j. **Refsum syndrome** See **hereditary motor and sensory neuropathy.**
      k. Glycogen storage diseases See **glycogen storage diseases** types 2 (Pompe) and 3 (Forbes-Cori) disease.
      l. **Primary hyperoxaluria**
   4. Miscellaneous hereditary neuropathies
      a. **Hereditary liability to pressure palsies**
      b. **Familial recurrent brachial plexus neuropathy**
      c. **Giant axonal neuropathy**
      d. **Ataxia-telangiectasia**
      e. **Cockayne syndrome**
      f. **Mitochondrial myopathies**
      g. **Neurofibromatosis** (von Recklinghausen disease)
      h. Hereditary hypertrophic neuropathy with paraproteinemia See **gammopathic neuropathy.**
      i. **Hereditary polyneuropathy with oligophrenia, premature menopause, and acromicria**
      j. Neuropathy in **neuroectodermal dysplasias**
      k. **Subacute necrotizing encephalomyelopathy**
      l. Peripheral neuropathy associated with **xeroderma pigmentosum**
      m. **Marinesco-Sjögren syndrome**
      n. Hereditary parkinsonism and neuropathy
      o. Neuropathy in spinocerebellar and cerebellar degenerations See **cerebellar ataxias**
      p. Neuropathy with **familial lipomatosis**
      q. **Distal hereditary upper limb muscular atrophy**
      r. **Hereditary thermosensitive neuropathy**
B. *Congenital*
   1. Congenital neuropathy with **arthrogryposis multiplex congenita**
   2. **Congenital neuropathy with absence of myelin** in the peripheral and central nervous systems
   3. **Congenital hypomyelination neuropathy**
C. *Traumatic*
C1. *Physical*
   1. Laceration, contusion, compression, or distraction of nerves or plexuses
   2. Birth trauma to brachial plexus See **upper brachial plexus palsy, Klumpke palsy**
   3. Compression neuropathies
      a. Of cranial nerves

i. **Bell palsy**
ii. **Clonic facial spasm**
iii. Recurrent familial facial palsy (**Melkersson syndrome**)
b. Of the upper extremity
    i. Cervical rib or **cervical band syndrome**
    ii. Median n. in the forearm (**pronator syndrome**)
    iii. Median n. under supracondylar process or **Struther's ligament**
    iv. Median n. in the forearm (**anterior interosseous syndrome**)
    v. Median n. at the wrist (**carpal tunnel syndrome**)
    vi. Ulnar n. at the elbow (**cubital tunnel syndrome**)
    vii. Ulnar n. at the elbow (the medial epicondyle)
    viii. Ulnar n. at the wrist or its deep branch in the palm
    ix. Radial n. in the spiral groove
    x. Radial n. in the forearm
    xi. Posterior interosseous n. in the forearm
    xii. Suprascapular n. at the shoulder
    xiii. Long thoracic n. at the shoulder
    xiv. Axillary n. at the shoulder
    xv. Musculocutaneous n. in the upper arm
c. Of the lower extremity
    i. Sciatic n. at the pelvic exit
    ii. Obturator n. in the obturator canal
    iii. Ilioinguinal n. at the groin
    iv. Genitofemoral nerve
    v. Femoral n. in the groin or upper thigh
    vi. Lateral cutaneous n. of the thigh (**meralgia paraesthetica**)
    vii. Common peroneal nerve
    viii. Deep peroneal n. (including compression terminally under the cruciate ligament on the dorsum of the foot)
    ix. Tibial nerve
    x. Posterior tibial n. in the tarsal tunnel
    xi. Medial plantar nerve
    xii. Digital n. (**Morton neuroma**)
d. Of the trunk
    i. Intercostal neuropathy
    ii. Lesions of dorsal branches or thoracic and lumbar spinal nerves (**notalgia paraesthetica**)
e. Multiple entrapments in **mucopolysaccharidosis**
4. Electric shock
5. Cold injury (**trench foot, immersion foot**)
6. Burns
7. Vibration injury (vibrating tools)
8. Radiation injury
9. Ischemic neuropathy
    a. Vasculitis[3032]
        i. Polyarteritis nodosa
        ii. Neuropathy in **systemic lupus erythematosus**
        iii. **Churg-Strauss syndrome**
        iv. **Diabetes mellitus**
        v. Giant cell arteritis
        vi. Cryoglobulinemia
        vii. Hypersensitivity angiitis
        viii. Neuropathy in **rheumatoid arthritis**
        ix. Neuropathy in **sarcoidosis**
        x. **Wegener granulomatosis**

        xi. Neuropathy in **Lyme disease**
    b. Arteriosclerotic occlusive disease
    c. Thromboangiitis obliterans (Buerger disease)
    d. Embolic infarction of nerve trunks
    e. Hemorrhage into nerve trunks
    f. Occlusion of large arteries by compression, e.g., tourniquet, trauma
    g. **Volkmann ischemic contracture**
    h. Anterior tibial **compartment syndrome**
    i. **Ischemic monomelic neuropathy**
    j. **Vasculitic neuropathy**
C2. *Toxic* (e.g., drugs, inorganic substances, organic substances, toxins derived from bacteria)
C3. *Of uncertain etiology* (? toxic, ? nutritional)
    1. Neuropathy and amyotrophy in
        a. **Jamaican** and other tropical neuropaties
        b. **South Indian paraplegia**
        c. Neuropathy in Nigerian **tropical ataxia** and **tropical spastic paraparesis**
    2. **Cryptogenic sensory polyneuropathy**
    3. Neuropathy in the **Spanish toxic oil syndrome**
D. *Infections*
    1. Direct infection of nerves:
        a. **Leprosy**
        b. **Herpes simplex**
        c. **Herpes zoster**
        d. Lymphoadenopathy-associated virus/HTLV III in AIDS
        e. Trypanosomiasis
        f. Nosematosis
    2. Neuropathies occurring in other infections
E. *Guillain-Barré syndrome and related disorders* (probably immunologically mediated)
    1. **Acute inflammatory demyelinating polyneuropathy**
    2. **Miller Fisher syndrome**
    3. **Chronic inflammatory demyelinating polyradiculoneuropathy**
    4. With CNS demyelination
F. *Neuropathy associated with connective tissue disorder*
G. *Metabolic neuropathy*
    1. Nutritional
        a. Specific deficiencies
        b. Of uncertain etiology (probably B_1, B_2, and B_6 vitamin deficiency)
    2. Neuropathies associated with endocrine disorder
        a. **Diabetes mellitus**
        b. Thyroid disorders
        c. Neuropathy in organic hyperinsulinism
        d. In **acromegaly**
    3. Neuropathy in blood dyscrasia
        a. Polycythemia vera
        b. Myelofibrosis
        c. Leukemia—acute and chronic
        d. Bleeding disorders—hemorrhage into nerves
        e. In sickle cell disease
    4. Neuropathy in renal failure
        a. Uremic polyneuropathy
        b. Mononeuritis multiplex following dialysis
        c. **Carpal tunnel syndrome** due to amyloid deposition
    5. Neuropathy in acute and chronic liver disease, including primary biliary cirrhosis

6. Neuropathy associated with paraproteinemia and dys-proteinemia (see **gammopathic neuropathy**)
   a. Multiple myeloma
   b. **Macroglobulinemia** (Waldenstrom)
   c. Cryoglobulinemia
   d. Benign monoclonal gammopathy—IgA, IgG, IgM
   e. Amyloidosis
   f. Paraproteinemia
   g. **Neuropathy with IgM binding to myelin-associated glycoprotein (MAG)**
   h. **Neuropathy with IgM binding to sulfatide**
H. *Neuropathy in malignant disease*
   1. **Carcinomatous neuropathy**
   2. Neuropathy in reticulosis—lymphoma, leukemia, myeloproliferative disorders See **subacute motor neuronopathy, subacute sensory neuronopathy.**
I. *Neuropathy associated with other systemic or nonhereditary degenerative diseases*
   1. Sarcoidosis
   2. Chronic obstructive pulmonary disease
   3. **Total lipodystrophy**
   4. **Acrodermatitis chronica atrophicans**
   5. **Critical illness polyneuropathy**
   6. Neuropathy with **retinitis pigmentosa and ataxia**
J. *Chronic neuropathy with no known cause or association*
   1. **Chronic sensorimotor neuropathy of undetermined cause**
   2. **Chronic idiopathic ataxic neuropathy**
K. *Tumors of nerves*
   1. Arising from supporting structures and/or axons
      a. **Plexiform neuroma**
      b. **Traumatic neuroma**
   2. Arising from supporting structures
      a. **Schwannoma** (neurinoma, neurofibroma), including acoustic neuroma
      b. Fibroma
      c. **Neurogenic sarcoma**
      d. Hemangioma
      e. Lipoma
      f. Neuroepithelioma (**dysembryoma**)

Adapted from the World Federation of Neurology Classification Subcommitee. Classification of neuromuscular diseases. J. Neurol. Sci. 1988;86: 333–360, by kind permission of the WFN, Lord Walton and Elsevier Science.

neuropathy associated with ataxia and retinitis pigmentosa See **NARP syndrome.**

Neuropathy Association Inc. An American charitable organization providing support and education and funding research into the causes and cure of peripheral neuropathies. Address: 60 East 42 St., Suite 942, New York, NY 10165-0999. Tel: 212-692-0662. Web site: http://www.neuropathy.org/.

neuropathy in acute and chronic liver disease A demyelinating neuropathy associated with acquired chronic hepatic insufficiency.[1318].

neuropathy in chronic obstructive pulmonary disease A chronic demyelinating sensorimotor peripheral neuropathy due either to malnutrition or to some unknown metabolic disorder affecting Schwann cells.[201]

neuropathy in hereditary Parkinson disease See **Parkinson disease.**[860]

neuropathy in Nigerian tropical ataxia. See **Nigerian neuropathy.**[5980]

neuropathy in spinocerebellar and cerebellar degenerations See **cerebellar ataxias.**

neuropathy of critical illness See **critical illness polyneuropathy.**

Neuropathy Screening Instrument A 15-item questionnaire and a brief structured examination protocol for use together in the diagnosis and follow-up of patieints with diabetic neuropathy.[1770]

Neuropathy Symptom profile A formal method of assessing the range and severity of symptoms of neuropathy, employing a true-or-false type of questionnaire that asks questions dealing with subjective weakness, functional weakness, cramps, abnormal sensation, prickling, deadness, burning, thermal insensitivity, pain on use of a limb, coldness, and aching. The profile gives rise to scores dealing in general with weakness, and with sensory and autonomic functions.

The instrument is thought suitable for screening a population at risk for neuropathy, for detecting and characterizing symptoms of neuropathy, and for controlled trials of therapy.[1568,1574]

Neuropathy Symptom score A formal method of assessing the range and severity of symptoms of neuropathy obtained by history, designed initially for use with patients suffering from diabetic neuropathies but also appropriate for use in patients suffering from neuropathies of other etiologies (see Chart N–9).[1575]

Chart N–9. Neuropathy Symptom Score

I. *Symptoms of muscular weakness*
   A. Bulbar
   B. Limbs
      1. Extraocular
      2. Facial
      3. Tongue
      4. Throat
      5. Shoulder girdle and upper arm
      6. Hand
      7. Glutei and thigh
      8. Legs
II. *Sensory disturbances*
   A. Negative symptoms
      9. Difficulty in identifying objects in the mouth
      10. Difficulty in identifying objects in the hands
      11. Unsteadiness in walking
   B. Positive symptoms
      12. "Numbness," "asleep feeling," "like novocain," "pricking" at any site
      13. Pain—burning, deep aching tenderness—at any location

III. *Autonomic symptoms*

    14. Postural fainting
    15. Impotence in male
    16. Loss of urinary control
    17. Night diarrhea[1580]

From Dyck PJ, Kratz KM, Lehman KA, et al. The Rochester Diabetic Neuropathy Study. Neurology 1991;41:799–807, by kind permission.

Other questions are added to assess completeness, reliability, and the presence of "neurasthenia." See also **Peripheral Neuropathy Symptom Questionnaire.**

neuropathy with IgM binding to GalNAc-GD$_{1a}$ and GM$_2$ gangliosides   A rare, distal, symmetrical sensorimotor **demyelinating** neuropathy of adult life presenting with gait disorder and distal pan-sensory loss, mild weakness, areflexia, and cerebellar signs. The course is slowly progressive over years.

Electrodiagnostic testing shows the demyelinating neuropathy. A serum M protein is detectable. See also http://www.neuro.wustl.edu/neuromuscular/index.html.

neuropathy with IgM binding to myelin-associated glycoprotein (MAG)   A rare, distal, symmetrical sensorimotor neuropathy of adult life presenting with weakness, gait disturbance, and tremor and slowly progressive over years. Electrophysiology shows evidence of a demyelinating neuropathy with prolonged distal latencies, slow nerve conduction velocity and temporal dispersion of compound motor action potentials, without conduction block. Evidence of axonal loss is eventually found. Serum IgM autoantibodies vs. MAG protein are detected, sometimes with anti-MAG titers >30,000. Waldenström's macroglobulinemia may coexist. Nerve pathology shows demyelination and subsequent axonal loss.

In a variant syndrome, the anti-MAG antibody titers are <10,000 and the clinical picture is dominated by sensory loss affecting small more than large fiber modalities, without motor involvement. See also http://www.neuro.wustl.edu/neuromuscular/index.html.

neuropathy with IgM binding to sulfatide   A rare, distal, symmetrical sensorimotor neuropathy of adult life presenting with distal paraesthesias and weakness, gait disorder, and tremor. Electrophysiology shows prolonged distal latencies and slowed nerve conduction velocity, with eventual evidence of axonal loss. A serum IgM autoantibody to sulfatide is detectable. See also http://www.neuro.wustl.edu/neuromuscular/index.html.

neuropathy with IgM paraproteinemia   See **gammopathic neuropathy.**

neuropathy–dementia–retinitis pigmentosa–dysautonomia syndrome   See **hereditary motor and sensory neuropathy, type 7.**

neuropathy–motor neuron disease with visual pathway disorder   A neuropathic syndrome characterized by the onset in childhood or youth of neurogenic muscle atrophy and weakness, demyelinating peripheral sensory neuropathy, hypohidrotic skin, and pyramidal signs. See **hereditary motor and sensory neuropathy** (*HMSN type 2 with mental retardation, optic atrophy, and pyramidal signs*).

Neuropediatrics   (formerly *Neuropediatrie*) The official journal of the Society for Neuropediatrics, founded in 1969. Address: Thieme Medical Publishers, 333 Seventh Avenue, New York, NY 10001. Tel: 212-760-0888. Web site: http://www.thieme.com/SID2060442868630/journals/pubid1432672485.html.

neuropeptide Y   A neurotransmitter found in the basal ganglia which has an effect upon appetite stimulation.

neurophysins   Precursors of vasopressin and oxytocin.

neuropil   The complex mesh of myelinated and unmyelinated axons and dendrites, and the processes of oligodendroglia, astrocytes, and microglia within the nervous system.

neuropore   (Gr, nerve + a passage) An opening from the neural tube in the developing nervous system. The *anterior* aspect connects the cavity of the brain with the epiblast; the *posterior* portion is the aperture of the neurenteric canal into the body cavity.

Neuropsychiatric Inventory   A validated tool evaluating the frequency and severity of 10 behaviors often found in patients with cognitive disturbance, aberrant motor behavior, agitation, anxiety, apathy, delusions, depression, disinhibition, euphoria, hallucinations, and irritability.[1215]

neuropsychiatry   1. An approach to the study of psychiatric disorders, whereby a neurological basis for them is presumed and sought; that aspect of psychiatry which seeks to advance the understanding of clinical problems through increased knowledge of brain structure and function.[3426] 2. A branch of psychiatry involving the study of organic psychosyndromes (such as the dementias, disorders resulting from toxic, traumatic, or developmental brain diseases, the psychological complications of the epilepsies, and memory disorders).

neuroptic myelitis   See **Devic disease.**

Neuroradiology   Springer-Verlag Berlin, Heidelberger Platz 3, 14197 Berlin, Germany. A neuroradiological journal. Web site: http://link.springer.de/link/service/journals/00234/.

neuroretinal rim   The edge of the optic cup.

neuroretinitis   1. The appearance of the retina when there has been leakage of edema fluid at the macula. The optic disk is swollen and a macular star figure is produced in the outer plexiform layer of the retina by the lipid-containing exudates derived from the capillaries at the disk head. The condition is not associated with multiple sclerosis.

Clinically, central visual loss occurs over hours and

is associated with a central scotoma and a macular star on ophthalmoscopy. Faster-progressing syndromes carry a worse prognosis. In some cases, evidence of vasculitis or infection (such as **Lyme disease**) may be found.

2. Inflammation of both the retina and the optic nerve.

neuroretinoangiomatosis   See **Bonnet syndrome.**

neurosarcoidosis   (disseminated sarcoid leukoencephalopathy) A rare disorder in which any part of the nervous system is affected with the lesions of sarcoidosis—comprising some 5% of all such cases. Meningeal, parameningeal, facial and other cranial nerve, hypothalamic, and pituitary infiltration; myelopathy; and many forms of peripheral neuropathy and plexopathy are characteristically described, and periventricular parenchymatous infiltration can also occur, leading to hydrocephalus.[5339] However, muscle biopsy findings suggest that muscle infiltration is even more common, though often subclinical.[5037]

In a *variant* form, evidence of angiitis is detected.[4099]

neuroschisis   A developmental abnormality characterized by splitting of the closed neural tube.

Neuroscience Links to Neurology and Neuroscience Journals   An Internet site (based in the United Kingdom) providing information about/access to neurological journals: http://www.uku.fi/neuro/links2.htm.

Neurosciences on the Internet   An Internet Web site providing an index of other sites concerned with (mainly basic) neuroscience: http://www.neuroguide.com/.

Neurosensory Center Comprehensive Examination for Aphasia   An aphasia battery.[5300,5301] See also **Boston Diagnostic Aphasia Examination, Western Aphasia Battery, Frenchay Aphasia Screening Test, Token Test, Reporters Test, Porch Index of Communicative Ability.**

neurosis   In the nineteenth century, a physical disease without apparent or discernible cause; now a pejorative term for disease without physical signs, for which the patient is usually blamed.

neurosonology   The study of the physical characteristics of the nervous system using high-frequency ultrasound.

Neurosurgery Clinics   A periodical reviewing neurosurgical topics, published by W.B. Saunders. Web site: http://www2.us.elsevierhealth.com/scripts/om.dll/serve?action=searchDB&searchDBfor=home&id=cnsu.

Neurosurgical Society of America   A professional association of young specialists in neurological surgery. Web site: www.neurosurgicalsociety.com/index.htm.

neuro-Sweet disease   The association of benign recurrent encephalitis with the features of Sweet syndrome, this latter characterized by malaise, fever, leukocytosis, mucosal ulceration, and symmetrical, tender, dull red skin plaques due to dermal cellular infiltrates that heal without scarring. The condition thus resembles **Behçet syndrome** but is associated with HLA B54, which is rare in the latter condition.[2589]

neurosyphilis   Those forms of secondary or tertiary syphilis in which there is involvement of the CNS, usually 2–18 months after the primary infection.[5172] The specific entities included are the following:
Meningovascular
   Asymptomatic neurosyphilis
   Acute syphilitic meningitis
   Cerebrovascular neurosyphilis
Parenchymatous
   Tabes dorsalis
   General paresis (of the insane)
   Optic neuritis
   Myelopathic
   Eighth cranial nerve involvement

neurotensin   An oligopeptide found in the hypothalamus and in the dorsal horn of the spinal cord, where it may act as a modulator in pain pathways.

neurothecoma   (dermal nerve sheath myxoma) A benign skin tumor consisting of nests of large stellate or spindle cells with a mucous matrix.

neurotic fatigue   A state of disinclination or incapacity to indulge in muscular exertion as a result of a generalized feeling of heaviness, tiredness, or stiffness of the muscles, for which no organic or biochemical reason can be detected. See **chronic fatigue syndrome.**

neurotic hypersomnolence   See **hypersomnolence.**

neurotmesis   (Gr, nerve + a cutting) Complete anatomical division of a peripheral nerve with disruption of the axons, their myelin sheaths, and the supporting connective tissue, resulting in wallerian degeneration of the axons distal to the injury site. This represents the most severe of the three types of nerve injury described by Seddon.[5048] cf. **axonotmesis, neurapraxia.**

neurotomy   Section or dissection of nerves.

neurotonia   (pseudomyotonia) Delay in the relaxation of a muscle following voluntary contraction, due to electrical hyperexcitability of its motor nerve.[5846] See **neuromyotonia.**

neurotonic discharges   Repetitive motor unit action potentials recorded from intramuscular electrodes during intraoperative monitoring. They are thought to arise from irritation or injury of nerves supplying the muscle from which the recording is made. (From the 2001 Report of the Nomenclature Committee of the American Association of Electromyography and Electrodiagnosis.[10] Used by permission, copyright © 2001, AAEM.)

neurotropic calcergy Selective calcification of the nerves of the autonomic nervous system, produced in rats by the injection of lead acetate and histamine.[5062]

neurotropism The theory of **Cajal** that neural growth is oriented by both generic and specific stimuli, the former from Schwann cells and the latter from motor end-plates and sensory receptors, all producing some factor attracting the axon.[6000]

neurotuberculosis Tuberculous infection of the nervous system, classified by Kinnier **Wilson**[6000] (Chart N–10).

Chart N–10. Classification of Neurotuberculosis

I. Tuberculosis of bone
  Skull (cranial osteitis)
  Spine
  Spinal caries
  Radicular compression
  Paraplegia
II. Tuberculosis of the meninges
  Pachymeningitis
  Leptomeningitis
  Tuberculous meningitis
    Acute, subacute, serous
  Meningeal tuberculosis
    Miliary
    Solitary pial tubercle
    Chronic meningeal tuberculosis
III. Tuberculosis of brain and cord
  Tuberculomas
  Encephalitis, myelitis
  Ocular
IV. Tuberculous neuritis
V. Psychoses of tuberculosis

From Wilson SAK Neurology. *London: Edward Arnold and Co., 1940.*

neuroviscerallipidosis See **GM₁ gangliosidosis.**

neurovisceral storage disease with vertical supranuclear ophthalmoplegia A genetic disorder of metabolism presenting between the ages of 1 and 15 years and characterized by vertical supranuclear ophthalmoplegia, limited convergence with normal pupillary functions, dementia, hearing loss, ataxia, rigidity, seizures, and hepatosplenomegaly. The bone marrow shows foamy histiocytes. See **sphingomyelin storage disorders,** type 3, **GM₁ gangliosidosis.**

neutral state syndrome A subwakefulness syndrome in which patients complain of excessive daytime sleepiness (hypersomnolence) without an increase in the total sleep time. The complaint is associated with a lack of nocturnal stages 3–4 non–rapid eye movement sleep, frequent daily microsleeps, and episodes of automatic behavior.[2324]

nevi-atrial myxomas, myxoid neurofibromata-epiphelides See **NAME syndrome.**

Nevin, Samuel (1905–1979) British neuropathologist, born in Belfast, where he took his medical training at Queen's University. After some years in junior positions at the **National Hospital,** he later became director of the research laboratory in the Institute of Psychiatry at the Maudsley Hospital and at Maida Vale, and professor of mental pathology at the University of London. A distinguished neuropathologist, most of his published work concerned the presenile dementias. His description with D.P. Jones of "progressive spongy encephalopathy" (**Creutzfeldt-Jakob disease**) defined that condition more clearly than any other report had done so to that date, although his conclusion favoring a vascular etiology was incorrect.[4110]

Nevin syndrome A progressive dementing illness with visual failure, pyramidal signs, speech disturbance, cerebellar signs, myoclonus, and accelerated death.

In the original papers, the authors considered that a vascular etiology underlay the rapidly progressive cerebral degeneration (a subacute spongiform encephalopathy) and that it was distinct from Creutzfeldt-Jakob disease, but that view is not now held.[4111] See **Creutzfeldt-Jakob disease.**

nevoid basal cell carcinoma syndrome (Gorlin-Goltz syndrome) A dominantly inherited **neurocutaneous syndrome** characterized by hypertelorism, frontal bossing, poly- and brachydactyly, kyphoscoliosis, and mental retardation. Pigmented papules appear between 12 and 35 years of age and undergo malignant transformation. There is also an increased incidence of **medulloblastoma,** squamous cell carcinoma, and odontogenic keratocysts.[2223]

nevus flammeus (Lat, a mole + fiery) (salmon patch, capillary nevus, capillary hemangioma) The port-wine stain that is characteristically present in the distribution of the trigeminal nerve in patients with **Sturge-Weber syndrome,** but also sometimes in the skin of the trunk or limbs; a dominantly inherited disorder without neurological features.[5113]

See also **midline nevus flammeus with intracranial vascular disease.**

nevus linearis sebaceous (of Jadassohn) See **epidermal nevus syndrome.**

nevus of Ito Pigmentation (melanoderma) of the lateral cervical area, shoulder, and thorax.[2760]

nevus of Ota (Ota syndrome) Localized periorbital pigmentation (melanoderma), which is especially marked on the eyelids, zygoma, and frontal regions, and sometimes extending to the lips, buccal cavity, and eyes. Heterochromia iridis is common. Ballooning of the posterior cranial fossa has also been described. The syndrome is more common in the black and the Asiatic races.

Neurological complications include malignant tumors of the nervous system, sensorineural deafness, the **Sturge-Weber syndrome,** spinocerebellar degenerations, and vascular malformations, including those located intracranially.[904,3678]

nevus unius lateris   (linear nevus, ichthyosis linearis neuropathica) A linear group of brown papules in the skin, usually present at birth and found in any part of the body. Cortical dysgenesis with epilepsy and mental retardation are commonly associated.[2614] See **epidermal nevus syndrome.**

new daily persistent headache   A benign headache syndrome of unknown etiology and pathophysiology occurring in adults without demonstrable structural lesions. Clinical criteria for diagnosis have been suggested by Silberstein et al.[5157] Reproduced by kind permission.

A. Average headache frequency >15 days/month for >1 month
B. Average headache duration >4 hours/day (untreated). Frequently constant without medication but may fluctuate
C. No history of tension-type headache or migraine that increases in frequency and decreases in severity in association with the onset of new daily persistent headache (over 3 months)
D. Acute onset (developing over <3 days) of constant unremitting headache
E. Headache is constant in location
F. Headache does not meet criteria for **hemicrania continua**
G. At least one of the following occurs:
  1. There is no suggestion of (any) disorder listed in International Headache Society diagnostic groups 5–11
  2. Such a disorder is suggested, but it is ruled out by appropriate investigations.
  3. Such a disorder is present, but first headache attacks did not occur in close temporal relation to the disorder.

The **Melkersson-Rosenthal syndrome** has been reported in association.

New England Journal of Medicine   A general medical journal publishing also numerous important papers on neurologic subjects. Web site: http://content.nejm.org/.

new variant Creutzfeldt-Jakob disease   A degenerative inflammatory disease of the nervous system resembling both Creutzfeldt-Jakob disease and bovine spongiform encephalopathy, of which it may itself be a variant. Suggested criteria are as follows:[5978]

1. A. Progressive neuropsychiatric disorder (depression, anxiety, apathy, withdrawal)
   B. Duration of illness >6 months
   C. Routine investigations do not suggest an alternative diagnosis
   D. No history of potential iatrogenic exposure
2. A. Early psychiatric symptoms
   B. Persistent painful sensory symptoms
   C. Ataxia
   D. Myoclonus or chorea or dystonia
   E. Dementia
3. A. EEG does not show the typical appearance of sporadic Creutzfeldt-Jakob disease (or no EEG performed)
   B. Bilateral pulvinar high signal on MRI scan

Definite: lA (progressive neuropsychiatric disorder) *and* neuropathological confirmation of NvCJD.
Probable: I *and* 4/5 of II *and* IlIA *and* IIIB.

Possible: I *and* 4/5 of II *and* IlIA.
Reproduced by kind permission.

New York Rating scale   An assessment instrument designed to provide a semiquantitative score of the impairments and disabilities suffered by patients with **Parkinson disease.**

As with many other similar scales, the battery provides a template for the neurological examination, including thus an appraisal of eye movements, blink rate, emotional and voluntary facial movements, swallowing, tongue movements, motor speech, neck rotation, shoulder and arm elevation, lying supine, writing, rising from a chair, normal and heel–toe walking, climbing stairs, sit-ups, trunk turning, straight-leg raising, foot movements, rigidity, general mobility, tremor, and contractures.[73]

New York University Computerized Test battery   A computerized evaluation designed to assess cognitive changes in normal elderly subjects and those with dementia or **age-associated memory impairment.**

The battery contains 12 subtests evaluating immediate and recent memory, language, concept formation, and psychomotor speed and attention. Use of the computer allows a simulated situation to be presented to the subject, whose reactions can then be directly assessed on the basis of their computer-interactive responses. The test is sensitive to drug effects and to changes in dementia.[1803]

Newcastle Dementia Scale   See **Blessed Roth Dementia Instrument.**

NGIE   A mitochondrial disease characterized by **Ne**uromyopathy with **G**astro**I**ntestinal symptoms and **En**cephalopathy.

N-hexane neuropathy   A subacute axonal sensorimotor peripheral neuropathy, with secondary demyelination, resulting from persistent exposure to *N*-hexane in the workplace. Optic neuropathy and involvement of the CNS are uncommon.[966]

nicotinic acid deficiency encephalopathy   An acutely evolving and often fatal syndrome of stupor or delirium with cogwheel rigidity of the limbs, sometimes with grasping and sucking reflexes, often with clinical evidence of pellagra, and in some cases with oculomotor and polyneuropathic features like those in **Wernicke-Korsakoff syndrome.**[2877]

Though commonly diagnosed (and apparently relieved by nicotinic acid) in the years after World War II, it is now seldom seen.

nictitating spasm   See **blepharospasm.**

nictitatio   See **spasmus nictitans.**

Nielsen syndrome   1. A condition of generalized weakness with fasciculations seen in states of terminal exhaustion.[4133] 2. (cingulate gyrus syndrome) Apathy, akinesia, mutism, and incontinence in the awake patient with bilateral damage to the cingulate gyri.[4130] Presumably the syndrome was described in patients in whom this damage was as a result of a tumor, which was also affecting other areas, because bilateral surgically created lesions of the cingulate gyri lead to similar but only minimal findings.

Niemann, Alfred   (1880–1921) He gave a short account of **Niemann-Pick disease** in 1914,[4134] but the account by Ludwig Pick (also a German pediatrician) 12 years later was more substantial.

Niemann-Pick cells   Foamy storage cells derived from macrophages, found in **sphingomyelin storage disorders.**

Niemann-Pick disease   See **sphingomyelin storage disorders.**

Nigerian neuropathy   (tropical ataxic neuropathy, tropical nutritional ataxia) A slowly progressive posterior column myelopathy and painful symmetrical demyelinating sensorimotor neuropathy (leading to severe proprioceptive loss) with bilateral optic atrophy and nerve deafness.

The condition is considered to be due to the ingestion of cyanide-containing foods such as cassava, and is conditioned by vitamin deficiency.[4272,5980] It is seen mainly in Central and West African countries.[2362]

A *variant* condition is *Nigerian acute seasonal ataxia* (encephalitis tremens), an acute cerebellar ataxic syndrome described in low-income Nigerians. The ataxia progresses in some cases to ophthalmoplegia and a reduction in consciousness, and may be due to acute thiamine deficiency resulting from the ingestion of thiamine-binding glycosides in certain foods consumed locally.[33]

night starts   See **periodic limb movement disorder.**

night terror   (pavor nocturnus, incubus, sleep terror) A **parasomnia** characterized by the sudden waking of the subject from non-rapid eye movement sleep (stage 3 or 4), screaming with terror, and violently mobile, with marked autonomic arousal, confusion, and great and inconsolable distress. Complete amnesia follows restoration of normal functioning.[3574] The condition is more common in children between the ages of 4 and 12 years but may also occur in young adult life[2054] (see also **dream anxiety attacks**).

The following diagnostic criteria have been suggested:
A. A sudden episode of intense terror occurs during sleep.
B. The episodes usually occur within the first third of the night.
C. Partial or total amnesia occurs for the events during the episode.
D. Polysomnographic monitoring demonstrates the onset of episodes during stage 3 and 4 sleep. Tachycardia usually occurs in association with the episodes.
E. Other medical disorders are not the cause of the episode, e.g., epilepsy.
F. Other sleep disorders can be present, e.g., nightmares.

From ASDA Diagnostic Classification Steering Committee.[234] *The International Classification of Sleep Disorders Diagnostic and Coding Manual.* Rochester, MN: American Academy of Sleep Medicine, 1990. Reproduced by kind permission.

nightmare   (Middle English, night + a crushing thing) (dream anxiety attack, REM nightmare) A vivid and frightening dream, often provoking a feeling of dread, oppression on the chest, or the conviction of paralysis, occurring during the middle third of the night during rapid eye movement sleep periods and leading to awakening with a normal sensorium. Diagnostic criteria have been suggested and are reproduced in Chart N–11.

Chart N–11. Diagnostic Criteria for Nightmares

A. At least one episode of sudden awakening from sleep with intense fear, anxiety, and feeling of impending harm
B. Immediate recall of frightening dream context
C. Alertness is full immediately upon awakening, with little confusion or disorientation
D. Associated features include at least one of the following:
    1. Return to sleep after the episode is delayed and not rapid
    2. The episode occurs during the later half of the habitual sleep period
E. Polysomnographic monitoring demonstrates the following:
    1. An abrupt awakening from at least 10 minutes of rapid eye movement sleep
    2. Mild tachycardia and tachypnea during the episode
    3. Absence of epileptic activity in association with the disorder
F. Other sleep disorders such as sleep terrors and sleepwalking can occur

From ASDA Diagnostic Classification Steering Committee. The International Classification of Sleep Disorders Diagnostic and Coding Manual. *Rochester, MN. By kind permission of the American Sleep Disorders Association, 1990.*

See also **hag, dream anxiety attack,** and cf. **night terror.**

nightwalkers   A name self-applied by those who suffer from **restless legs syndrome.**

nigrospinodentatal degenerations   (nigrostriatal degenerations) Hereditary disorders classifiable as progressive **cerebellar ataxias** (autosomal dominant forms of late onset) but not homogeneous in nature, in some cases the major extrapyramidal and/or cerebellar features being accompanied by, for example, nuclear ophthalmoplegia, pyramidal signs, sensory disturbances, muscle atrophy, or pes cavus.

Their final apportionment will have to await the detection of the underlying biochemical deficit.[6033] See also **Joseph disease.**

nigrostriatal degenerations   See **nigrospinodentatal degenerations.**

NIH stroke scale   A relatively short instrument for the semiquantitative assessment of deficits following stroke, used in numerous clinical trials[2175] (see Chart N–12).

Chart N–12. The NIH Stroke Scale

Each examination is assessed independently from previous examinations. A response must be checked for each item, using the following headings:

1a. Level of Consciousness
1b. Level of Consciousness—Questions
1c. Level of Consciousness—Commands
2. Gaze
3. Visual Fields
4. Facial Movement (Facial Paresis)
5. Motor Function—Arms (Left and Right)
6. Motor Function—Legs (Left and Right)
7. Limb Ataxia
8. Sensory
9. Best Language
10. Dysarthria
11. Neglect (Extinction and Inattention)

1a. Level of Consciousness

This global measure of responsiveness is assessed by the patient's interactions with the physician at the bedside when the patient is first examined. The physician should stimulate the patient (by patting or tapping the patient) to determine the best level of consciousness. On occasion, more noxious stimuli, such as pinching, may be required to check the level of consciousness.

0 = Alert. Patient is fully alert and keenly responsive.
1 = Drowsy. Patient is drowsy but can be aroused with minor stimulation. The patient obeys, answers, and responds to commands.
2 = Stuporous. Patient is lethargic but requires repeated stimulation to attend. The patient may need painful or strong stimuli to respond to or follow commands.
3 = Coma. Patient is comatose and responds only with reflexive motor or automatic responses. Otherwise, the patient is unresponsive.

1b. Level of Consciousness—Questions

Level of consciousness is checked by asking the patient to respond to two questions. The patient is asked the month of the year and his or her age. The answer must be correct—there is no partial credit for being close (for example, being off by 1 year in age). If the patient gives the wrong initial answer but then corrects it, the answer should still be scored as incorrect. Other measures of orientation such as time of day, location, etc. are not asked as part of this examination. If the patient has aphasia, the physician should judge the responses to questions in light of the language impairment.

0 = Answers BOTH correctly
1 = Answers ONE correctly
2 = BOTH incorrect

1c. Level of Consciousness—Commands

Here level of consciousness is checked by asking the patient to follow two commands. The patient is asked to open and close his or her eyes and then is asked to make a grip (close and open the hand). Only the initial response is scored. If a patient is aphasic and unable to follow verbal commands, the patient may imitate these movements (pantomime). For a patient who has hemiparesis, the response in the unaffected limb should be measured. For example, if the patient has a left hemiparesis, making a fist with the right hand is a normal response to the command. If a paralyzed patient does try to move the limb in response to a command but is unable to form a fist, it is counted as a normal response.

0 = Obeys BOTH correctly
1 = Obeys ONE correctly
2 = BOTH incorrect

2. Gaze

The position of the eyes at rest and movement of the eyes to command are tested. First look at the position of the eyes at rest. Spontaneous eye movements to the left or right should be noted. The patient is then asked to look to the left or right. Only horizontal eye movements are tested. Disorders of vertical gaze, nystagmus, or skew deviation are not measured. Reflexive eye movements (oculocephalic or oculovestibular) should be tested in patients who are unable to respond to commands. If a patient has ocular rotatory problems, such as a strabismus, but leaves the midline and attempts to look both right and left, he or she should be considered to have a normal response. If a patient has an isolated oculorotatory problem, such as an oculomotor (CN III) or abducens (CN IV) palsy, the score should be 1. If the patient has a conjugate deviation of the eyes that can be overcome by voluntary or reflexive activity, the score should be 1. If there is a conjugate lateral deviation that is NOT overcome with reflexive movements, the score should be 2.

0 = Normal. The patient has normal lateral eye movements.
1 = Partial gaze palsy. The patient is unable to move one or both eyes completely to both directions.
2 = Forced deviation. The patient has conjugate deviation of the eyes to the right or left, even with reflexive movements.

3. Visual Fields

Visual fields of both eyes are examined. In most cases, the physician asks the patient to count fingers in all four quadrants. Each eye is independently tested. If a patient is unable to respond verbally, the physician should check responses (attending) to visual stimuli in the quadrants or have the patient hold up the number of fingers seen. A quadrantic field cut should be scored 1. The entire half-field (both upper and lower quadrants) should be involved with a dense field loss to be scored 2. If a patient has severe monocular visual loss due to intrinsic eye disease and the visual fields in the other eye are normal, the physician should score the visual fields as normal. If the patient has monocular blindness due to primary eye disease and the visual fields in the other, "normal" eye demonstrate a partial or dense visual field defect, the visual loss should be scored as 1, 2, or 3 as appropriate.

0 = No visual loss
1 = Partial hemianopia. There is a partial visual field defect in both eyes. Included is a quadrantic field defect or sector field defect.
2 = Complete hemianopia. There is dense visual field defect in both eyes. A homonymous hemianopia is included.
3 = Bilateral hemianopia. There are bilateral visual field defects in both eyes. Cortical blindness is included.

4. Facial Movement (Facial Paresis)

The patient is examined by looking at the patient's face and noting any spontaneous facial movements. The facial movements in response to commands are also tested. Such commands may include asking the patient to grimace or smile, to puff out his or her cheeks, to pucker, and to close the eyes forcefully. If the patient is aphasic and is unable to follow commands, the physician should have the patient attempt imitative (pantomime) responses. The facial responses to painful stimuli (grimace) may substitute for responses to commands in a patient who has decreased levels of alertness.

   0 = Normal facial movements. There is no asymmetry.
   1 = Minor paresis. Asymmetrical facial movements or facial asymmetry occurs at rest. This response may be noted with a spontaneous smile but not with forced facial movements.
   2 = Partial paresis. There is unilateral "central" facial paresis. Decreased spontaneous and forced facial movements occur with changes most prominent at the mouth. Orbital and forehead musculature movements are normal.
   3 = Complete palsy. Dysfunction involves forehead, orbital, and circumoral muscles (the entire distribution of the facial nerve). Deficits may be unilateral or bilateral (facial diplegia) complete facial paresis.

5. Motor Function—Arms (Left and Right)

The patient is asked to extend his or her arm outstretched in front of the body at 90° (if sitting) or at 45° (if supine). The effort is made for a full 10 seconds. The physician should count to 10 aloud to encourage the patient to maintain the limb's position. If a limb is paralyzed, the physician may wish to test any "normal" limb first. If a patient is aphasic, directions may be achieved by nonverbal cues or pantomime. Patients may be "helped" by the physician by placing the limb in the desired position. If the patient has restricted limb function due to arthritis or non–stroke–related limitations, the physician should attempt to judge the "best" motor response. If the patient has decreased level of consciousness, an estimate of response to noxious stimuli should be measured. Volitional motor responses that are performed well should be graded as 0. If the patient has reflexive responses, such as flexor or extensor posturing, the response should be scored as 4. The only indication for scoring this item as 9, untestable, is if the limb is missing or amputated or if the shoulder joint is fused. A patient with a partial limb amputation should be tested.

   0 = No drift. The patient is able to hold the outstretched limb for 10 seconds.
   1 = Drift. The patient is able to hold the outstretched limb for 10 seconds but there is some fluttering or drift of the limb. If the limb falls to an intermediate position, the score is 1.
   2 = Some effort against gravity. The patient is not able to hold the outstretched limb for 10 seconds but there is some effort against gravity.
   3 = No effort against gravity. The patient is not able to bring the limb off the bed but there is some effort against gravity. If the limb is raised in the correct position by the examiner, the patient is unable to sustain the position.
   4 = No movement. The patient is unable to move the limb. There is no effort against gravity.
   9 = Untestable. May be used only if the limb is missing or amputated, or if the shoulder joint is fused.

6. Motor Function—Legs (Right and Left)

The supine patient is asked to hold the outstretched leg 30° above the bed. The limb should be held in this position for 5 seconds. The physician should count to 5 aloud to encourage the patient to maintain the limb's position. If the right leg is paralyzed, the examiner may wish to examine the "normal" left leg first. If a patient is unable to follow verbal commands, nonverbal cues may be used, or the limb may be placed in the desired position. If the patient has a decreased level of consciousness, an estimate of response to noxious stimuli should be measured. Volitional motor responses that are performed well should be scored 0. If the patient has reflexive responses, such as flexor or extensor posturing, the response should be scored 4. The only indication for scoring this item as 9, untestable, is if the limb is missing or if the hip joint is fused. Patients with artificial joints or partial limb amputations should be tested.

   0 = No drift. The patient is able to hold the outstretched limb for 5 seconds.
   1 = Drift. The patient is able to hold the outstretched limb for 5 seconds but there is unsteadiness, fluttering, or drift of the limb.
   2 = Some effort against gravity. The patient is unable to hold the outstretched limb for 5 seconds but there is some effort against gravity.
   3 = No effort against gravity. The patient is not able to bring the limb off the bed but there is effort against gravity. If the limb is placed in the correct position, the patient is unable to sustain the position.
   4 = No movement. The patient is unable to move the limb. There is no effort against gravity.
   9 = Untestable. May be used only if limb is missing or hip joint is fused.

7. Limb Ataxia

This item is aimed at examining the patient for evidence of a unilateral cerebellar lesion. It will also detect limb movement abnormalities related to sensory or motor dysfunction. Limb ataxia is checked by the finger-to-nose and heel-to-shin tests. The physician should test the "normal" side first. The movements should be well performed, smooth, accurate, and nonclumsy. There should not be any dysmetria or dyssynergia. Nonverbal cues may be given to the patient. If a patient has dysmetria or dyssynergia in one limb, the score should be 1. If a patient has dysmetria or dyssynergia in both the arm and leg on one side, or if there are bilateral signs, the score should be 2. If limb ataxia is present, the ataxia should be rated as present regardless of the possible etiology. This item may be scored 9, untestable, only if there is complete paralysis of the limbs (all Motor Function scores = 4), if the limb is missing, amputated, or fused, or if the patient is comatose (item 1a., Level of Consciousness = 3).

   0 = Absent. The patient is able to perform both the finger-to nose and heel-to-shin tasks well. The movements are smooth and accurate.
   1 = Present unilaterally in either arm or leg. The patient is able to perform one of the two required tasks well.
   2 = Present unilaterally in both arm and leg or bilaterally. The patient is unable to perform either task well. Movements are inaccurate, clumsy, or poorly done.

9 = Untestable. May be used only if all Motor Function scores = 4, if the limb is missing, amputated, or fused, or if item 1a., Level of Consciousness = 3.

8. Sensory

The patient is examined with a pin in the proximal portions of all four limbs and asked how the stimulus feels. The patient's eyes do not need to be closed. The patient is asked if the stimulus is sharp or dull and if there is any asymmetry between the right and left sides. Only sensory loss that can be attributed to stroke should be counted as abnormal—usually this will be a hemisensory loss. Sensory loss due to a non–stroke-related condition, such as a neuropathy, should not be graded as abnormal. If a patient has depressed level of consciousness, neglect, aphasia, or is unable to describe the sensory perception, the patient's nonverbal responses, such as a grimace or withdrawal, should be graded. If the patient responds to the stimulus, it should be scored 0. The response to the stimulus on the right and left sides should be compared. If the patient does not respond to a noxious stimulus on one side, the score should be 2. Patients with severe depression of consciousness should be examined.

0 = Normal. No sensory loss to pin is detected.

1 = Partial loss. Mild to moderate diminution in perception to pin stimulation is recognized. This may involve more than one limb.

2 = Dense loss. There is severe sensory loss so that the patient is not aware of being touched. The patient does not respond to noxious stimuli applied to that side of the body.

9. Best Language

The patient's language will be tested by having the patient identify standard groups of objects and by reading a series of sentences. Comprehension of language should be judged as the physician performs the entire neurologic examination. The physician should give the patient adequate time to identify the objects on the sheet of paper. Only the first response is measured. If the patient misidentifies the object and later corrects him- or herself, the response is still considered abnormal. The physician should then give the patient a sheet of paper with the series of sentences. The examiner should ask the patient to read at least three sentences. The first attempt to read the sentence is measured. If the patient misreads the sentence and later corrects him- or herself, the response is still considered abnormal. If the patient's visual loss precludes visual identification of objects or reading, the examiner should ask the patient to identify objects placed in his or her hand and the examiner should judge the patient's spontaneous speech and ability to repeat sentences. If the examiner judges these responses as normal, the score should be 0. If the patient is intubated or is unable to speak, the examiner should check the patient's writing.

0 = No aphasia. The patient is able to read the sentences well and is able to correctly name the objects on the sheet of paper.

1 = Mild to moderate aphasia. The patient has mild to moderate naming errors, word-finding errors, paraphasias, or mild impairment in comprehension or expression.

2 = Severe aphasia. The patient has severe aphasia with difficulty in reading as well as naming objects. Patients with either Broca's or Wernicke's aphasia are included here.

3 = Mute

10. Dysarthria

The primary method of examination is to ask the patient to read and pronounce a standard list of words from a sheet of paper. If the patient is unable to read the words because of visual loss, the physician may say the word and ask the patient to repeat it. If the patient has severe aphasia, the clarity of articulation of spontaneous speech should be rated. If the patient is mute or comatose (item 9; Best Language = 3) or has an endotracheal tube, this item can be rated as 9, untestable.

0 = Normal articulation. The patient is able to pronounce the words clearly and without any problem in articulation.

1 = Mild to moderate dysarthria. The patient has problems in articulation. Mild to moderate slurring of words is noted. The patient can be understood but with some difficulty.

2 = Near unintelligible or worse. The patient's speech is so slurred that it is unintelligible

9 = Untestable. May be used only if item 9; Best Language = 3, or if the patient has an endotracheal tube.

11. Neglect (Extinction and Inattention)

The presence of neglect is examined by the patient's ability to recognize simultaneous cutaneous sensory and visual stimuli from the right and left sides. The visual stimulus is a standard picture. The picture is shown to the patient and the patient is asked to describe it. The physician should encourage the patient to scan the picture and identify features on both the right and left sides of the picture. The physician should encourage the patient to compensate for any visual loss. If the patient does not identify parts of the picture on one side, the result should be considered abnormal. The physician then assesses the ability to recognize bilateral simultaneous touch to upper or lower limbs. The test is done by touching the patient with the patient's eyes closed. The test should be considered abnormal if the patient ignores sensory stimuli from one side of the body. If the patient has a severe visual loss and the cutaneous stimuli are normal, the score should be 0. If the patient has aphasia and is unable to describe the picture, but does attend to both sides, the score should be 0.

0 = No neglect. The patient is able to recognize bilateral simultaneous cutaneous stimuli on the right and left sides of the body and is able to identify images on the right and left sides of the picture.

1 = Partial neglect. The patient is able to recognize either cutaneous or visual stimuli on both the left and right, but is unable to do both successfully (unless severe visual loss or aphasia is present).

2 = Complete neglect. The patient is unable to recognize either bilateral cutaneous sensory or visual stimuli.

From Goldstein LB, Bertels C, Davis JN. Interrater reliability of the NIH stroke scale. Arch Neurol. 1989;46:660–2. Copyrighted 1989, American Medical Association, and reproduced by kind permission.

See also **Canadian Stroke scale, Orgogozo scale, stroke scales, Mathew scale, Nottingham 10-point Activities of Daily Living Index numbers item.**

NINCDS stroke data bank   A prospective observational study designed to provide a resource for research questions on the characteristics, clinical course, and outcome of patients hospitalized with acute stroke.

Within the study, a research classification scheme was developed to establish uniform diagnostic subgroups based on supporting data from angiography, from brain imaging using CT scanning, and from Doppler ultrasonography, and based on the nature of clinical syndromes and related medical conditions.

NINDS   See **National Institute of Neurological Disorders and Stroke.**

NINDS scale   A 5-point system for grading muscle stretch reflexes, ranging from absent (0) to a range of normal (+2 and +3) to clonus (+4). The scale does not seem to enhance interrater reliability.[3595] See also **Medical Research Council scale, Mayo Clinic scale.**

Nine-Hole Peg test   A simple and portable method for the evaluation of fine motor performance, sensitive in patients with slight but not severe disability.

The equipment required consists of nine wooden dowels (9 mm in diameter and 12 mm long) and a wooden base in which there are nine holes (10 mm in diameter and 15 mm deep) spaced 15 mm apart in three rows of three holes. The patient sits at a table and is asked to place the pegs in the holes, while the observer times the patient's performance from start to finish (but can stop at 50 seconds), recording the number of pegs correctly placed. The normal subject can place the pegs correctly within 18 seconds.[5415]

Nipah encephalitis   A form of encephalitis caused by a paramyxovirus and reported from Malaya. Clinically, severe encephalitis is accompanied by segmental myoclonus, areflexia, hypertension, and tachycardia and is fatal. See **encephalitis.**

Nishimoto disease   See **moyamoya disease.**

Nishimoto-Takeuchi-Kudo disease   See **moyamoya disease.**

N-methyl-D-aspartate   (NMDA) an excitatory amino acid, the receptors of which mediate relatively slow and long-lasting responses as compared to the non-NMDA receptors L-glutamate and L-aspartate. The amino acid is epileptogenic in animals by virtue of its power to depolarize neurons and to allow the generation of repetitive epileptiform discharges.[3160]

Nissl bodies   Blocks of intranuclear granular endoplasmic reticulin composed of protein, DNA, and RNA.

Nissl degeneration   Swelling of neuronal cell bodies with loss of chromophilic granules, occurring after nerve injury.

Nissl, Franz   (1860–1919) German neurologist and neuropathologist working in Frankfurt, Heidelberg, and finally in Munich. He noted that, within the swollen seventh cranial nerve neurons after section of the nerve, there was a loss of chromophilic granules that no longer stained with basic dyes such as methylene blue (an agent which he introduced for this purpose in 1858).

A clinician as well as laboratory-based physician, he enthusiastically adopted the technique of lumbar puncture and was known to his students as "punctator maximus."

Nissl granules   Described in 1894, these consist of granular basophilic material within the cytoplasm of perikarya. In chromatolysis, it breaks down to yield free ribosomes.

Nissl stains   Methods of enhancement of histological specimens, using thionine, toluidine blue, cresyl violet, or chrome-alum reagents with alcohol. The cresyl violet stains rough endoplasmic reticulum.

nitric oxide   (NO) An inorganic gas synthesized endogenously and derived from endothelial cells, capable of relaxing arterial walls. It thus has a function in cardiovascular control but also contributes to the role of macrophages as killers of pathogens, reducing platelet activation and acting as a diffusible messenger within the nervous system, where it modulates neuronal firing and regulates blood flow, among other functions. Excessive NO concentrations can destroy CNS neurons.[538]

nitroblue tetrazolium dye test   A laboratory test based on the ability of this dye to enter white blood cells in the presence of bacterial inflammatory products, where it is reduced and turns black.

It was used on CSF samples, where it was thought capable of differentiating aseptic from septic meningitis, but is now not much employed.

NMDA   See **N-methyl-D-aspartate.**

NMR   Acronym for **nuclear magnetic resonance,** generally euphemized to **magnetic resonance imaging** in order to quiet an excitable populace.

No to Hattatsu   (*Brain Dev.*) A Japanese journal of child neurology, founded in 1969. Address: Japan Publishing Co. Ltd., P.O. Box 5030, Tokyo International, Tokyo, Japan.

Noack syndrome   A form of mild acrocephaly (type 1) without neurological features. See **acrocephalopolysyndactyly.**

Nobile-Orazio ataxia scale   An observer-rated scale for gait ataxia.[4148]

0   Normal—stands on one foot with eyes closed
1   Stands/walks normally with eyes closed
2   Stands/walks normally with minor swaying with eyes closed, normally with eyes open
3   Stands/walks with some swaying with eyes open
4   Stands/walks on a wide base with eyes open
5   Standing/walking impossible without support

nocardiosis Infection with the fungus *Nocardia asteroides*, usually of the lungs in immunosuppressed people, with a tendency to spread to the brain as granulomatous meningitis or abscess.

The organism was first described by E.-I.-E. Nocard (1850–1903), a French veterinary pathologist.

nocioception (from Lat, to hurt or damage + perception) The awareness of pain.

nociceptive reflex (Lat, to hurt or damage + to take) (Riddoch reflex, Buzzard reflex) With pyramidal tract lesions, painful stimulation of the inner aspect of the arm or of the upper chest leads to abduction and external rotation of the shoulder with flexion at all joints of the arm. With quadriplegia, especially when due to high cervical cord lesions, the same stimuli induce adduction, internal rotation, and elevation of the shoulder; pronation of the elbow; extension of the elbow and wrists; and adduction and extension of the fingers and thumb.[1349a] This is considered to be an associated postural reaction in patients with loss of supraspinal inhibitory control of spinal reflex activity.

nociceptor A receptor that is activated by injury and that warns the subject by transmitting impulses leading to the sensation of pain. The term was introduced by **Sherrington** in 1906.

nocturnal arm dysesthesias See **Wartenberg cheiralgia paresthetica.** However, the symptom is usually due to **carpal tunnel syndrome.**

nocturnal eating (drinking) syndrome The condition characterized by recurrent wakening with the inability to return to sleep without eating or drinking. This is primarily a problem in infancy and early childhood but can also occur as a conditioned response in adult life.[5395]

nocturnal frontal lobe epilepsy See **autosomal dominant nocturnal frontal lobe epilepsy.**

nocturnal hemidystonia See **dystonia.**

nocturnal hemiplegia See **sleep paralysis.**

nocturnal hyperkinesis with daytime hypersomnolence See **hypersomnolence.**

nocturnal leg cramps Painful sensations of muscular tightness or tension usually felt in the calf but occasionally in the foot that occur during the sleep episode. The cramp frequently results in arousal from sleep and is accompanied by electrical evidence of muscle fiber contraction in the affected muscles.

Such cramps occur without other signs of peripheral neuropathy, usually in elderly people and in subjects of any age suffering from chronic renal failure or after vigorous treatment with diuretics. They represent a nightly curse to many aged people, but can often be prevented by oral calcium salts, quinine, or phenytoin.

nocturnal leg myoclonus See **periodic limb movement disorder.**

nocturnal myoclonus See **periodic limb movement disorder.**

nocturnal paroxysmal dystonia (hypnogenic paroxysmal dystonia, non-REM sleep–related dystonic dyskinetic episodes) A **parasomnia** characterized by repeated stereotyped dystonic or dyskinetic (choreoathetoid and ballistic) episodes during non-rapid eye movement sleep, lasting 15–60 seconds and preceded by EEG evidence of arousal. Severe sleep disruption may result. The following diagnostic criteria have been suggested (from ASDA Diagnostic Classification Steering Committee. *The International Classification of Sleep Disorders Diagnostic and Coding Manual.* Rochester, MN: by kind permission of the American Sleep Disorders Association, 1990).

A. Abnormal motor activity occurs during sleep.
B. Dystonic or dyskinetic episodes occur mainly during sleep.
C. Short-duration episodes typically last 15–60 seconds, and prolonged-duration episodes typically last 60 minutes.
D. Polysomnography demonstrates dystonic or dyskinetic movements occurring out of non–rapid eye movement sleep.
E. Episode is not associated with any medical or psychiatric disorder that can account for the symptom, e.g., frontal lobe epilepsy.
F. Episode does not meet the diagnostic criteria for other sleep disorders, such as rapid eye movement sleep behavior disorder or sleep terror.

The following *variant* forms have been described:
Typical attacks, but with dominant inheritance[3513]
Nocturnal paroxysmal dystonia with long-lasting attacks The attacks are similar but are more protracted, lasting between 2 minutes and an hour.[3510]
Nocturnal paroxysmal dystonia with intermediate duration attacks The attacks last between 2 and 5 minutes and consist of brief jerky movements affecting the limbs or trunk alternately, but are precipitated by arousal from sleep or by physical exercise-induced wakefulness.[3510]
Nocturnal paroxysmal dystonia with nocturnal wandering See **episodic nocturnal wandering.**
Behavioral arousals with abnormal motor pattern These present with complaints of sudden nocturnal awakenings that occur because of dystonic-dyskinetic movements following sudden awakening.[3510]
Atypical periodic movements in sleep A syndrome characterized by sudden, repetitive nocturnal awakenings from non–rapid eye movement sleep, occurring every 1–2 minutes, accompanied by fragmentary dystonic posturing or dyskinetic movements lasting 2–5 seconds.[3510]
Nocturnal paroxysmal hemidystonia See **dystonia.**

nocturnal psychogenic dissociative intrusion The occurrence of protracted, dissociative episodes including multiple-personality disorder occurring upon awakening from rapid eye movement sleep or non–rapid eye movement sleep. The condition is usually described in patients who have experienced childhood physical or sexual abuse and who in many cases have manifested sleepwalking or sleep terror.[4956]

nocturnal sleep epilepsy   Generalized seizures, restricted to, or predominantly occurring during, periods of sleep.

nocturnal start   See **periodic limb movement disorder.**

nocturnal tooth-grinding   See **bruxism.**

nocturnal vertigo   "The sensation of falling from a height when falling asleep or just after going to sleep" (Sir William **Gowers**).

nodes of Ranvier   Interruptions in the axonal sheath, places where the Schwann cell cytoplasm is in contact with the axon.

nodose ganglion   (Lat, a knot + Gr, a tumor) A relay station attached to the tenth cranial nerve just below the base of the skull, which contains the cell bodies of the afferent fibers from the pharynx, larynx, trachea, esophagus, and the thoracic and abdominal viscera.

nodular fasciitis   (myositis proliferans) A localized inflammatory pseudotumorous swelling in muscle resulting from local injury.[3009]

nodular leprosy   See **lepromatous leprosy.**

noise   1. Properly, artifactual potentials produced by electrodes, cables, the amplifier, or storage media, unrelated to the potentials of biological origin. 2. Colloquially in electromyography, physiological **end-plate activity.**
Noise refers thus to electric activity not related to the signal of interest. In electrodiagnostic medicine, this refers to waveforms generated by electrodes, cables, amplifier, or storage media and unrelated to potentials of biologic origin. The term has also been used loosely to refer to one form of end-plate activity. (Adapted from the 2001 Report of the Nomenclature Committee of the American Association of Electromyography and Electrodiagnosis.[10] Used by permission, copyright © 2001, AAEM.)

nominal aphasia   (nominal dysphasia) The term of Sir Henry **Head** for that form of speech disorder in which there is defective use of names and want of comprehension of words as names or indicators. Reading is difficult, writing affected, and copying is often impossible.[2496]
A graded naming diagnostic test has been described.[3765] See also **anomia.**

nominal dysphasia   See **nominal aphasia.**

nona   A form of sleeping sickness described by Gayet in 1875, in which mesencephalic and hypothalamic lesions were identified. Whether it was the same as **encephalitis lethargica** is impossible to tell.[4337]

noncommunicating hydrocephalus   That form of hydrocephalus in which there is obstruction to the circulation of CSF between the sites of its formation in the ventricles and brain, and the roof of the fourth ventricle. See **obstructive hydrocephalus.**

nonconcomitant deviation   Misalignment of the visual axes which varies with the position of gaze, changing according to which eye is fixating. In most cases, muscle paresis is responsible.

nonconvulsive seizure paralysis   Transient paralysis of one or more limbs due possibly to migraine, transient ischemic attacks, or inhibitory seizures. The syndrome has been analyzed superbly[1850] but a final conclusion is not always possible in a particular patient. See also **nonconvulsive status.**

nonconvulsive status   Abnormal variable seizure syndromes resembling dementia, delirium, sleepiness, or clouding of consciousness, with preserved motor and postural abilities and without clinical evidence of motor seizure activity, seen in patients of any age with a past history of generalized or partial seizures and persisting for hours, days, or even months, in association with EEG evidence of persistent seizure discharges. The condition is thus a form of absence status or complex partial status, and is usually precipitated by infection, low anticonvulsant levels, or withdrawal from benzodiazepines. The condition is underdiagnosed.
The more common clinical appearances include clouded consciousness with confusion, disorientation, and diminished responsiveness; myoclonic or clonic movements of the eyes, face, or jaw, and automatisms in absence status; and more severe but variable clouded consciousness, less frequent facial movements, and episodic adversive movements of head and eye movements. Slow recovery occurs after treatment but prolonged memory dysfunction may be a sequel.[1552]
Absence status (epilepsia minor continua, petit mal status, spike–wave stupor) is characterized by confusion or diminished responsiveness with occasional blinking or twitching, lasting hours to days, with generalized spike and slow-wave discharges on the EEG.
Complex partial status consists of prolonged or repetitive complex partial seizures (with a presumed focal onset) and produces an "epileptic twilight state" with fluctuating lack of responsiveness or confusion. In this group, the presence of some physical signs is more likely than in absence status.
Other confused, stuporous, or comatose patients with rapid, rhythmic, epileptiform discharges on the EEG may have "electrographic" status and should be considered in the same diagnostic category. While generalized convulsive status epilepticus (SE) produces lasting neuropathologic hippocampal damage, absence SE appears to cause no lasting effects. Complex partial SE is less uniform.[1517]
See also **absence status.**

nonepileptic myoclonus   Those forms of **myoclonus** which have no relationship to any **epileptic syndrome.**

These include **dystonic myoclonus; ballistic movement overflow myoclonus;** exaggerated startle; physiological phenomena such as hiccups, sneezing, and **sleep jerks; periodic movements of sleep;** and **segmental myoclonus** such as spinal and palatal myoclonus.

In such cases, the EMG burst length is between 50 and 300 msec, muscle jerking during the discharge may be asynchronous, and there is no correlated discharge recordable on the EEG.[2384] See also **epileptic myoclonus, myoclonus.**

nonepileptic seizures   1. A seizure of any type provoked by intercurrent disease (such as anoxia or head trauma) in a subject not formerly subject to recurrent seizures.

2. (pseudoseizures, functional, pseudoepileptic seizures, dissociative or psychogenic seizures, nonepileptic "attacks") Attacks resembling epileptic seizures but without a causal epileptic mechanism and considered to have a psychogenic basis. These clinical manifestations are presumed to be unrelated to an abnormal and excessive discharge of a set of neurons of the brain, including (a) disturbances in the brain function (vertigo or dizziness, syncope, sleep and movement disorders, transient global amnesia, migraine, enuresis), and (b) pseudoseizures (nonepileptic sudden behavioral episodes presumed to be of psychogenic origin; these may coexist with true epileptic seizures).[1115] Recent important commentaries have been published.[803,3167]

Unresponsiveness without motor manifestations may be the most common presentation, but partial seizure simulations are also common, in which any motor activity exhibited is usually coordinated. Side-to-side head movements, out-of-phase limb jerking, and pelvic thrusting are typical patterns, while bizarre and incongruous movement patterns are probably less common.[3333] Such attacks are rare in subjects who do not also suffer from true epileptic seizures as well. The EEG is nomal during the attacks.

nonfamilial juvenile central neurogenic muscular atrophy   See **monomelic amyotrophy.**

nonfamilial juvenile distal spinal muscular atrophy of upper extremity   See **monomelic amyotrophy.**

nonfamilial spinal segmental muscular atrophy in juvenile and young subjects   See **monomelic amyotrophy.**

nonfluency   Effortful, dysmelodic speech with impairment both of articulation and of grammar. Some call this *telegraphese.* **Dysprosody** (speech which lacks normal rhythm) is notable.

nonfluent aphasia   See **Broca aphasia, agrammatism.**

nonhypertrophic muscular dystrophy   See **Emery-Dreifuss syndrome.**

noninfantile Gaucher disease   A cause of Ramsay Hunt syndrome (cerebellar). See **glucosylceramide lipidosis.**

noninfections granulomatous angiitis with a predilection for the nervous system   See **isolated angiitis of the nervous system.**

nonketotic hyperglycinemia   (OMIM 238300) A recessively inherited (9p22) inborn error of the glycine cleavage system, causing ataxia and myoclonus and usually fatal within the first few weeks of life. See **cerebellar ataxias** (*variants*), **glycine encephalopathy.**

nonketotic hyperosmolar syndrome   Severe hyperosmolarity (>320 mOsm/L), hyperglycemia (>600 mg/100 ml), and dehydration occurring as the result of inability to drink enough fluid to keep pace with the osmotic diuresis caused by hyperglycemia, usually in elderly patients with mild or undiagnosed type 2 diabetes. The resultant impaired renal function reduces glucose loss, leading to elevations in blood glucose.

The onset is typically insidious with deterioration over weeks; severe acidosis and ketosis are not features. The level of consciousness generally correlates with the severity and duration of hyperosmolarity. Ten percent of patients present in coma, and an equal number have clear consciousness. Generalized or focal seizures, focal neurological signs, delirium, exacerbation of any pre-existing organic mental syndrome, and profound dehydration are the main features. The laboratory picture is of uncontrolled diabetes and dehydration, renal functional impairment, raised hemoglobin, abnormal liver function tests, and hypertriglyceridemia yielding a falsely low serum sodium ("pseudohyponatremia").

nonmalignant inflammatory sensory polyganglionopathies   (see also **malignant inflammatory sensory polyganglionopathies**) A group of uncommon dorsal root ganglion cell and autonomic neuronal disorders presenting as a sensory ataxic or hyperalgesic syndrome or both. Sensory nerve action potentials are small or absent. The CSF protein level is not raised. Sometimes positive tests for antinuclear antibodies, antibodies to extractable nuclear antigens, or rheumatoid factor suggest that connective tissue diseases are etiologically relevant.

non–Menkes-type copper deficiency with regression, lactic acidosis, and granulocytopenia   A rare syndrome of early childhood comprising low serum copper and ceruloplasmin levels, low granulocyte count, lactic acidosis, truncal ataxia, and neurodevelopmental regression, considered due to impaired copper transport across the intestinal wall and across the blood–brain barrier.[1978] See also Haas et al.[2352]

nonmetastatic syndromes   See **paraneoplastic syndromes.**

nonmigrainous vascular headaches   Headache with some characteristics of **migraine** but induced by specific circumstances, such as fever, hangover, or stroke (see **Willis headache**).

nonoptic aphasia   A form of aphasia due to malfunction of the semantic system in which there is impairment of spontaneous speech and of the generation of word lists, and reduction in semantic knowledge, but preservation of visual confrontation naming.[5147] The phenonenon is most often reported in Alzheimer disease.

nonprogressive congenital neuromuscular disease with uniform type 1 fibers   A congenital myopathy in which more than 99% of the muscle fibers belong to type 1. Clinically, the disease is characterized by delayed motor development, the early onset of mild proximal weakness, hyporeflexia, normal serum muscle enzyme levels, EMG changes of myopathy, and a nonprogressive course.[4212]

nonprogressive encephalopathy   The current term for cerebral palsy, also known as *infantile cerebral paralysis* by **Freud**. See **static encephalopathy.**

non–rapid eye movement sleep   (quiet sleep, synchronized sleep, deep sleep, delta sleep, NREM sleep) A slow, steady metabolic state characterized by low cardiac output, blood pressure, cerebral blood flow, and respiratory rate. Four stages are defined in Chart N–13.

Chart N–13. Stages of Non–Rapid Eye Movement Sleep

NREM stage 1 A stage of sleep following directly upon wakefulness and characterized by the EEG appearance of low-voltage activity with apha activity less than 50%, beta activity, and vertex spikes, and with slow rolling eye movements. This usually comprises some 5% of the total sleep time.

NREM stage 2 A stage of sleep characterized by the appearance of sleep spindles and K complexes on a low-voltage, mixed-frequency background and with delta activity comprising up to 20% of the stage. This stage usually comprises some 50% of the total sleep time.

NREM stage 3 A stage of sleep characterized by the appearance of high-amplitude delta waves (>75 uV, <2 Hz) for between 20% and 50% of the time, which occurs in the first third of the sleep period.

NREM stage 4 A stage of sleep characterized by the appearance of high-amplitude delta waves (>75 uV, <2 Hz) for more than 50% of the time and comprising, with NREM stage 3, slow-wave (SWS) or delta sleep.

See also **sleep stages, rapid eye movement sleep.**

non–rapid eye movement sleep–related dystonic dyskinetic episodes   See **nocturnal paroxysmal dystonia.**

nonspecific degeneration   See **frontal lobe dementia.**

nonspecific EEG abnormalities   Abnormal EEG activity, such as patterns of theta or delta activity occurring in bursts or rhythmic trains during wakefulness. Such activity may be produced by a wide variety of pathologies and alone has no diagnostic value.[4945]

nonspecific granuloma of the orbit   See **orbital pseudotumor syndrome.**

nonspecific lipid myopathy   A rare familial myopathy characterized by the deposition of lipid droplets in the muscle. Clinically, muscle weakness, abdominal cramps, and nausea following consumption of a fatty meal were described as the leading symptoms. Muscle carnitine levels are normal.[244]

nonspecific poliodystrophy and lactic acidosis   A **mitochondrial encephalomyelopathy** causing atypical **progressive myoclonic epilepsy.**

non–stimulus-sensitive myoclonus   Myoclonus occurring spontaneously at rest and periodic, rhythmic, or irregular in occurrence. See **myoclonus.**

nonsyndromic mental retardation   A recessively inherited developmental disability, mapped to 3p25–pter. Clinically, it is manifest as delay in the acquisition or maturation of language and social rather than of motor skills in children with no past history of hereditary or acquired disease known to be associated with mental retardation, no dysmorphism, normal vision and hearing, and no evidence of autism.[2571]

nonsystemic vasculitic neuropathy   A chronic multiple mononeuropathy (seldom a distal polyneuropathy) affecting only the peripheral nerves, without involvement of joints, skin, or viscera, lacking constitutional signs and due to an indolent necrotizing vasculitis.[1570]

nonthyroidal hypermetabolism   See **Luft disease.**

non–24-hour sleep–wake syndrome   A condition characterized by a chronic steady pattern comprising 1- to 2-hour daily delays in sleep onset and wake times in an individual living in society. As a result of these persistently incrementing delays in the times of sleep and of waking over successive days, the subject is at most times out of phase with the sleep–wake cycle of others in his environment. The most common pattern is of prolongation of the individual's sleep–wake cycle to 25 hours. The condition is seen particularly in males, often those with schizoid tendencies, and in the blind.[5883] Diagnostic criteria have been suggested[234] (see Chart N–14).

Chart N–14. Diagnostic Criteria for Non–24-Hour Sleep–Wake Syndrome

A. Primary complaint of either difficulty initiating sleep or difficulty in awakening

B. Progressive delays of sleep onset and offset with the inability to maintain stable entrainment to a 24-hour sleep–wake pattern

C. Presence of the sleep pattern for at least 6 weeks

D. Evidence of a progressive sequential delay of the sleep period revealed by:
   1. Polysomnography performed over several consecutive days on a fixed 24-hour bedtime and waketime schedule; or

2. Continuous 24-hour temperature monitoring over at least 5 days that shows a progressive delay of the temperature nadir.

E. Does not meet criteria for any other sleep disorder causing inability to initiate sleep or excessive sleepiness

From ASDA Diagnostic Classification Steering Committee. The International Classification of Sleep Disorders Diagnostic and Coding Manual. Rochester, MN. American Sleep Disorders Association, 1990, by kind permission.

nonvasculitic autoimmune inflammatory meningoencephalitis (NAIM) A syndrome of progressive cognitive decline, psychosis, and unsteady gait occurring in adults because of a steroid-responsive, nonvasculitic, autoimmune, inflammatory meningoencephalitic syndrome. The CSF shows elevated immunoglobulin (Ig)G index and IgG synthesis rates and the brain biopsy reveals perivascular lymphocytic infiltrates without vessel wall invasion.[932]

nonversive movements See **versive seizures.**

non-Wilsonian extrapyramidal disease with copper dysmetabolism A rare syndrome of hepatic copper metabolism characterized by hepatic copper accumulation, low levels of ceruloplasmin, and normal or low serum copper levels, but normal or raised urinary copper levels.

Clinically, extrapyramidal signs including dystonia and chorea occur in the absence of **Kayser-Fleischer rings** and without hepatic cirrhosis.[2507]

non-Wilsonian hepatocerebral degeneration See **acquired hepatocerebral encephalopathy.**

Nonne, Max (1861–1959) German neurologist, who trained with **Erb** in Hamburg, where he was later a colleague of Jakob.

Nonne reaction A qualitative test for excess globulin in the CSF.

Nonne syndrome See **Froin syndrome.**

Nonne-Marie syndrome Congenital cerebellar disease due to agenesis. See also **cerebellar ataxias, Marie ataxia.**

nonverbal auditory agnosia Difficulty in interpreting musical or nonlanguage environmental sounds, due to lesions of the auditory association cortex.

Noonan syndrome (Ullrich-Noonan syndrome, chromatin-positive Turner syndrome) A dominantly inherited or sporadic congenital dysmorphic syndrome seen mainly in girls, and characterized by ptosis, antimongolian slant of the eyes, broad nose, small jaw, hypertelorism, webbed neck, high-arched palate, low hairline, short stature, cubitus valgus, hypogonadism, seizures, sensorineural deafness, mild mental retardation, and congenital heart defects.[4154] The chromosome pattern XO is present. See also **neurofibromatosis.**

nootropic drugs A class of psychotropic drugs that raise levels of ATP in the brain, enhance the acquisition of new data, and reverse learning impairments in experimental animals with virtually no physiological effects in other bodily areas. The prototypical example was piracetam, a γ-aminobutyric acid analogue with diverse effects upon brain chemistry, facilitating performance on various learning and memory paradigms in humans and animals.[2131]

Nordic myoclonus See **Unverricht-Lundborg-Lafora syndrome, Baltic myoclonus.**

no-reflow Impairment of postischemic reperfusion of the brain, most often seen following transient arterial occlusion. It is mainly due to the accumulation of neutrophils within the lumen of the vessel.

normal pressure hydrocephalus (adult occult- or low-pressure hydrocephalus, hydrocephalus ex vacuo, cerebral enlargement, brain distension, Hakim-Adams syndrome, idiopathic adult hydrocephalus syndrome) An uncommon syndrome of adult life, characterized by the presence of grossly enlarged cerebral ventricles under normal pressure, urinary incontinence, gait apraxia, pyramidal signs, and mild "subcortical" dementia. The quality of the gait disorder suggests bifrontal damage. A fourth criterion should be perceptible behavioral decline over a period of weeks to months varying from mild apathy to severe psychomotor retardation.[38] It was probably identified by Riddoch in 1936.

The condition results from impairment of CSF flow and episodes of slightly raised CSF pressure with a pressure gradient between the ventricles and subarachnoid space, coupled with widespread reductuion in cerebral blood flow. The impairment of CSF flow is usually at the level of the basal cisterns.

Radioimmunosorbent assay scans may demonstrate reflux of the isotope into the ventricles after lumbar intrathecal injection and ventricular decompression sometimes leads to significant improvement in gait, but little in cognitive function. Neither the CSF tap test nor CSF conductance measurements provide information distinguishing patients whose conditions will or will not respond to shunting.[3584] However, a short history, any known cause of hydrocephalus, a predominance of the gait disorder, and CT or MRI evidence of hydrodynamic hydrocephalus are somewhat predictive of a good response to shunting, as is a positive response to external lumbar CSF drainage over a few days.[5737]

The disorder may also occur in children, who present with decreasing scholastic performance, delay in walking or frequent falls and impaired bladder control.[739a]

normal-volume hydrocephalus The occurrence of **slit ventricles** in children who formerly had suffered increased intracranial pressure and whose shunts had blocked.[1673]

Norman leukodystrophy (Norman-Tingey syndrome) A familial form of sudanophilic leukodystrophy with microcephaly, striate calcification, and pachygyria. Dwarfism, paraplegia, mental retardation, and the appearance of **progeria** are inconstant but notable features.[4158]

Norman Wood congenital amaurotic familial idiocy A congenital syndrome of extreme micrencephaly with gliosis and free neutral fat and the massive deposition of intracellular lipoid and cholesterol throughout the white matter of the brain.[4160]

Norman-Roberts lissencephaly A rare, recessively inherited, congenital dysmorphic syndrome, characterized also by microcephaly, heterotopias, **lissencephaly,** microcephaly, and ventricular dilatation.[4157]

Norman-Tingey syndrome See **Norman leukodystrophy.**

normocalcemic tetany See **hereditary myokymia, neuromyotonia.**

normokalemic familial periodic paralysis See **familial periodic paralysis.**

Norrbotten disease See **glucosylceramide lipidosis.**

Norrie disease (oculoacousticocerebral degeneration) A developmental disorder, inherited as an X-linked recessive trait, in which the eyes shrink and develop retrolental opacities, optic atrophy, and retinal phakomas in early childhood.

Other features include short digits, psychomotor regression, deafness, behavioral disturbances, and hallucinations.[4163] The responsible gene maps to chromosome Xp11.4.

North American Chronic Pain Association of Canada A charitable organization providing support and information on this condition. Address: 60 Lorne Ave., Partmouth, Nova Scotia B2Y 3E7, Canada. Tel: 902-465-5587, 1-866-470-7246. Web site: http://www.chronicpaincanada.org/.

northern epilepsy See **neuronal ceroid lipofuscinosis.**

Northwestern University Disability Scale One of the original instruments designed for the assessment of patients with **Parkinson disease** and providing scores in the categories of *walking, dressing, hygiene, eating and feeding, and speech.*[889] See also **Hoehn and Yahr Scale, Columbia Rating Scale, Unified Rating Scale for Parkinson Disease,** and **New York Rating Scale.**

nosocomial (Gr, hospital) Of or belonging to a hospital—for example, unusual infections acquired during hospitalization.

nosology (Gr, disease + a discourse) The practice of the naming and classification of diseases.

notalgia paresthetica A benign and self-limiting syndrome of burning paresthesia, pruritus, and hypoesthesia felt in the interscapular region, considered to be a consequence of dorsal spinal root compression at T2–6.[4461]

notch filter A filter that selectively attenuates a very narrow frequency band, thus producing a sharp notch in the frequency response curve of an EEG channel. A 60 (50) Hz notch filter is used in some EEG machines to provide attenuation of 60 (50) Hz interference under extremely unfavorable recording conditions. (Adapted from the 1974 report of the Committee on Terminology, IFCN,[989] by permission of Elsevier Science.)

Nothnagel, Carl Wilhelm Hermann (1841–1905) German internist, neurologist, and pathologist who trained with Virchow and Leyden. He became professor of medicine at Freyberg, Jena, and later Vienna University. He described the syndrome named for him in patients with tumors.

Carl Wilhelm Hermann Nothnagel

Nothnagel disease 1. "Vasomotor acroparesthesiae"; tingling, cyanosis, blanching, edema and even gangrene of the digits. A severe form of Raynaud phenomenon, described by Nothnagel in 1867.[4172] 2. Angina pectoris.

Nothnagel sign Loss of emotional but not voluntary facial movements with thalamic tumors.

Nothnagel syndrome (ophthalmoplegia-ataxia syndrome) Damage to the oculomotor nerves on one or both sides, and to the superior cerebellar peduncle, caused by a tumor in the mesencephalic tectum or by a mesencephalic vascular accident. Oculomotor nerve and vertical gaze palsies, depressed consciousness, and cerebellar ataxia are the clinical results.[4173]

The syndrome may be regarded as a variant of the **dorsal midbrain syndrome** or as **Benedikt syndrome** with an added paresis of vertical gaze.

notochord (Gr, back + string) The primitive skeletal axis of vertebrates, which forms a template for the differentiation of the vertebral column. It was discovered by Karl von Baer, a German embryologist (1792–1876).

Nottingham 10-point ADL Index A scale assessing the functional capacity of subjects after stroke or cerebral trauma.[1599] The items assessed are the patient's ability to do the following:

1. Drink from a cup
2. Eat
3. Wash face and hands
4. Transfer from bed to chair
5. Walk or use wheelchair indoors
6. Use the toilet
7. Undress
8. Dress
9. Make a hot drink
10. Get in and out of a bath

Nougaret night blindness A dominantly inherited syndrome of absence of the rod receptors of the retina. Dr. J. Nougaret (1637–1719) was a French physician.

Nova Scotia variant See **sphingomyelin storage disorders.**

NREM intrusion The interposition of non–rapid eye movement (NREM) sleep or of a component of NREM sleep such as increased EMG activity, or K-complexes, sleep spindles, or delta waves on the EEG, during rapid eye movement sleep periods.[249]

NREM narcolepsy See **idiopathic CNS hypersomnolence.**

NREM period The non–rapid eye movement sleep portion of the REM–NREM sleep cycle, consisting usually of stages 3 and 4 early in the night, and stage 2 later.[249]

NREM sleep See **non–rapid eye movement sleep.**

nuchal Of or belonging to the nape of the neck.

nuchocephalic reflex (Gr, neck + head) A sign of diffuse cortical dysfunction, elicited by rapidly turning the shoulders of a subject (standing with his eyes closed) to the right and left. The reflex is inhibited (normal) if the subject turns his head in the direction of the rotation, usually with a fraction of delay, and uninhibited if the original position of the head is maintained.[2838]

nuclear agenesis See **Möbius syndrome.**

nuclear jaundice See **kernicterus.**

nuclear magnetic resonance scanning (NMR) A variant of **magnetic resonance imaging,** allowing study of nuclei other than that of hydrogen (e.g., fluorine, carbon, sodium).

When magnetic nuclei such as ^{1}H, ^{31}P, ^{13}C, ^{23}Na, ^{19}F, or ^{15}N are placed in a strong magnetic field, they line up like tiny compass needles, even if they are incorpo-

rated in the molecules of a living organism. They precess about the flux lines of the field at characteristic resonant frequencies that vary with their chemical structure; such frequencies can be used to identify particular compounds.

NMR measurements are made by perturbing nuclear precession with radiofrequency energy, and then recording the similar radio waves the perturbed nuclei emit as they "relax" back to their equilibrium state. Magnetic nuclei in small molecules that tumble rapidly—water, lactate, and ATP, for instance—produce strong enough radio signals from within the brain to be detected.

Magnetic resonance spectroscopy (MRS) is the general term for the measurement of specific substances by detection of their characteristic resonant frequencies. MRI uses some strong signal—usually from water protons—to make pictures based on differences in the intensity and relaxation rates of the signal between different anatomical regions. The much weaker signals from sources such as ^{1}H in lactate, ^{31}P in ATP, and ^{13}C in glycogen can also be made into anatomical images that map the distribution of specific compounds. Of necessity, these are less detailed than water proton images, but they do provide chemically specific information.[4526]

nucleus A concentration of neuronal cell bodies within the brain or spinal cord. The term was first applied by J.C. **Riel** to the basal ganglia in 1808 but was first used by Benedict **Stilling** in 1846 in connection with the cells of origin of the cranial and spinal nerves.

nucleus basalis of Meynert A clump of neurons in the substantia innominata below the globus pallidus, the cells of which provide most of the cholinergic innervation of the cerebral cortex.

The nucleus suffers marked cell loss and a reduction in choline acetyltransferase activity in patients with **Alzheimer disease.**

nucleus of Perlia A median group of nerve cells situated between the oculomotor nuclei, the postulated center for ocular convergence. This hypothesized function, however, has been strongly criticized and, if the nucleus exists as a separate anatomical entity, it is more probably the origin of neurons innervating the inferior oblique and superior rectus muscles.[5864]

null point That position of the eyes in which a congenital nystagmus, present with gaze in some direction, disappears or shows the least amplitude.

numb cheek syndrome The occurrence of infraorbital neuropathy with numbness of the cheek and of the gums at the level of the upper incisor and canine teeth, usually as a result of malignant infiltration of the nerve.[882]

numb cheek–limp lower lid syndrome The association of the **numb cheek syndrome** with drooping of the homolateral lower eyelid, and also of the upper lip, due to damage to the infraorbital nerve and some distal branches of the facial nerve, and caused by the same processes that cause the following syndrome.[731]

numb chin syndrome   The occurrence of mental neuropathy with numbness in the distribution of the nerve, usually as a result of malignant infiltration of the nerve or atrophy of the mandible.

The condition was first reported by Sir Charles **Bell** in 1830.[1997]

numbness   The subjective awareness that stimuli applied to the skin or mucosae are not perceived. A positive feeling from the numb area, which cannot be verbalized, is also often present.

nurse's contracture   Tetany. This name was proposed by **Trousseau** because of the frequency of the condition in nursing mothers, suffering undoubtedly from hypocalcemia.

nutritional amblyopia   Slowly progressive visual failure with retro-ocular discomfort; optic atrophy and bilateral central or centrocecal scotomas are the usual findings.[4183] The condition may appear as a paraneoplastic nutritional deficiency state. See also **tobacco-alcohol amblyopia, Obal syndrome.**

nutritional deficiency with encephalopathy   Intellectual retardation resulting from specific or generalized nutritional deficits during gestation or infancy, and associated with a reduction in brain weight.

nutritional myopathy   1. Cachexia in association with starvation and protein malnutrition. 2. Myopathy in association with chronic deficiency of vitamin E,[4108] **hypocalcemia,** or **hypophosphatemia.**

nutritional neuropathy   A severe but reversible thick-fiber sensory neuropathy occurring in a state of general nutritional deprivation with minimal motor involvement, but with no evidence of a specific deficiency of vitamins or of other food factors.

Most cases have been recorded after gastric stapling for obesity; which nutrient or other substance is responsible for the syndrome through its deficiency is uncertain.[1767]   See **beri-beri, Strachan syndrome, Wernicke-Korsakoff encephalopathy, pellagra, alcoholic neuropathy, burning feet syndrome.**

nutritional optic neuropathy   See **tobacco-alcohol amblyopia.**

nyctalopia   (from Gr, night + sight) Impairment of twilight or night vision as occurs with deficiency of vitamin A, pigmentary retinal degeneration, or color blindness. The original Greek meaning was actually the opposite—the ability to see by night only, but it seems to have been reversed by Galen and the present meaning was that intended by Heberden (1768).[2504] Compare with **hemeralopia** (day-blindness).

Nylen-Bárány test   The patient who is seated on a table is quickly laid back into the supine position with the neck extended 45° over the end of the table and the head rotated 45° to one side, and is observed for vertigo, nausea, and nystagmus (onset, direction, and duration). After a period of restitution sitting up, the maneuver is repeated with the head rotated to the other side.

Lesions of the central and peripheral portions of the vestibular system induce the above physical signs, which are not seen in normal subjects.[1511] See also **central nystagmus, peripheral nystagmus.**

Nyssen–van Bogaert syndrome   See **metachromatic leukodystrophy,** also **opticocochleodentate degeneration.**

nystagmus   (from Gr, to nod in sleep) Involuntary rhythmic oscillations of the eyes; biphasic ocular oscillations with an initial slow component responsible for their genesis and continuation. **Vestibular nystagmus** was first described by Erasmus, the grandfather of Charles Darwin, in 1794. **Optokinetic nystagmus** was first noted by **Purkinje,** in people looking out of train windows.

Dell'Osso[1368] lists 47 types, with subgroups, and suggests a clinical classification, modified in Chart N–15.

Chart N–15. Listing of Forms of Nystagmus

Congenital, latent, manifest latent, spasmus nutans (infancy and childhood)
Acquired pendular
Acquired horizontal jerk (vestibular, gaze-evoked, gaze-paretic)
Special types **Cervical, circular/elliptical/oblique, convergence-evoked, dissociated, downbeat, lid, muscle-paretic** (myasthenic), **periodic/aperiodic alternating, physiological, rebound, rotary, see-saw, upbeat, voluntary**
Induced **Arthrokinetic, audiokinetic, caloric, drug-Induced, optokinetic, positional, rotational**

See also other terms referable to nystagmus: **anticipatory, arthrokinetic-induced, associated, ataxic, Bartel, bow-tie, Bruns, central, centripetal, convergence-retraction, direction-changing, direction-fixed, dissociated, divergence, downbeat, epileptic, flicker-induced, horizontal, induced, jerk, lateral medullary, miner's, optokinetic after-induced, pendular,** periodic downbeat, **peripheral, pursuit defect, rebound, reflex, retraction, somatosensory, spontaneous, torsional, uniocular,** upbeat, **vertical.** See also **oscillations.**

nystagmus retractorius   See **convergence-retraction nystagmus.**

nystagmus-blockage syndrome   (Ethan syndrome, compensation syndrome) The suppression of congenital nystagmus through the development of esotropia, and with head turning[2133,3330] or with forced convergence while fixating a distant object.

nystagmus-myoclonus syndrome   See **Lenoble-Aubineau syndrome.**

O

oasthouse disease (methionine malabsorption syndrome) A rare, recessively inherited, diffuse encephalopathy of infancy, characterized by malabsorption of amino acids, particularly methionine, and the excretion of α-hydroxybutyric acid, giving a smell of hops to the urine. The major clinical features are seizures, diarrhea and mental retardation.[5216]

ob- (Lat, against) A prefix indicating before, about, against, toward, or over.

Obal syndrome Relative central or ring scotomas, nyctalopia, impaired color vision (especially for green), and frequently evidence of peripheral sensorimotor polyneuropathy occurring in those starved for long periods, such as prisoners of war. See **nutritional amblyopia.**[4183]

obelion (Gr, sagittal) A cranial index marker point between the two parietal foramina, employed by **Charcot** but not now in common use.

Ober test A method of assessing the degree of tightness in the tensor fascia lata (TFL). With the patient lying in the lateral decubitus postion at the edge of the examination table, the superior thigh is flexed slightly and dropped off the edge of the table towards the floor with the knee extended. A tight TFL will not allow the thigh and leg to drop below the table edge. Comparison is made side to side.

Obersteiner, Heinrich (1847–1922) Austrian professor of neurology at the University of Vienna whose textbooks of neuroanatomy (1888) and neuropathology (1897) were regarded as classics in their day. His own neurological institute was opened in 1878, the first of its kind.

Obersteiner sign Perception of a stimulus given to one side of the body as if coming from the other side. See **allocheiria.** The phenomenon has been described in **tabes dorsalis, multiple sclerosis,** and **hysteria.**[4202]

obesity-polydactyly-iris coloboma See **Biemond syndrome.**

obfuscation (from Lat, to darken) A darkening or obscuration of vision, as in the case of **amaurosis.**

object agnosia The inability of a subject to name or recognize an object by sight, due to lesions in the visual association areas.

objective tinnitus See **tinnitus.**

obligate grasp reflex See **palmar grasp reflex.** This should diminish between 3 and 6 months of age and disappear after 6 months; its persistence suggests corticospinal tract dysfunction.

oblique nystagmus See **circular nystagmus.**

oblongata crises Episodes of apnea and coma occurring in tertiary syphilis and resembling gastric crises, although their pathophysiology is unknown.[3402] They were first described by Dusser de Barenne in 1913.

obmutescence Loss of speech.

obnubilation (Lat, clouding) Clouding of consciousness.

O'Brien mucopolysaccharidosis See **mucopolysaccharidoses.**

obscuration 1. Transient dimming or blacking-out of vision, typically experienced by patients with papilledema due to increased intracranial pressure, or in the case of preceding optic neuropathy. 2. Diminution (rather than extinction) of the perception of a stimulus applied to the side of the body or visual half-field opposite the side of a hemispheric lesion, such that the subject reports that the stimulus looks darker or feels weaker when presented at the same time as a similar stimulus given to the other side than when it is presented alone.[476]

obsessional slowness Significant slowness in preparation for executing a movement. This is commonly accmpanied by stooped posture and such signs as a positive **glabellar tap** in the absence of the other typical signs of Parkinson diseae. Cognitive difficulties, such as in shifting set and spatial orientation, may also be detected by neuropsychological testing.[2722]

obstetrical paralysis 1. Any nerve or spinal cord injury suffered by the fetus during delivery. Brachial plexopathy (**Erb palsy** or **Klumpke palsy**) (for a recent review see van Dijk et al., 2001)[5723] and spinal cord crush injury due to C3–4 fracture-dislocation sustained during breech delivery are examples. 2. Lumbosacral plexopathy suffered by the mother as a result of compression by the fetal head of the lumbosacral trunk (L4–5) and S1 root where they join and pass over the pelvic rim, or as a result of traction on the sciatic nerve or compression of the common peroneal nerve during a prolonged period in which the legs are held flexed in stirrups at the hip and knee. Small maternal size, a large fetus, midforceps rotation, and fetal malposition may place the mother at special risk of this nerve injury.[1755]

obstructive hydrocephalus Increased intracranial pressure with dilatation of the ventricles of the brain, as a result of obstruction to the flow of CSF anywhere between its site of origin in the ventricles and brain substance and the roof foramina of the fourth ventricle. See **noncommunicating hydrocephalus.** See also **communicating hydrocephalus.**

obstructive sleep apnea syndrome Cessation of airflow during sleep while thoraco-abdominal effort continues, as a consequence of narrowing and closure of the upper airway leading to (in order) oxygen desaturation, snorting, arousal, resaturation, and sleep again. Sleep fragmentation, hypoxemia, and cardiac and hemodynamic alterations such as bradycardia, increased pulmonary arterial pressures, and cardiac arrhythmias result.

The clinical features include daytime sleepiness and loud nocturnal snoring followed by periods of silence; enuresis; morning headaches; excessive movements in sleep; automatic behavior; poor memory; and intellectual deterioration. See also **polysomnogram.**[3044]

obtundation   (from Lat, blunting or dulling) A condition of mild to moderately reduced conciousness, the subject being rousable with verbal or slightly painful stimuli but tending to slip back into sleep after the stimuli cease.

obtundation status   A long-lasting decrease in the level of consciousness in the context of **severe myoclonic epilepsy of infancy** (a variety of complex partial status epilepticus).[679,5721,5803]

obturator   (from Lat, to stop up) The obturator foramen is more or less occluded by a fascial sheet; the obturator nerve derives its name by benefit of proximity.

obturator neuralgia   (Howship-Romberg syndrome, obturator neuropathy) Constant pain in the distribution of the obturator nerve, felt in the groin and the medial aspect of the thigh, often with hypoesthesia in that region and weakness of the adductors and rotators of the hip, due to a lesion of the nerve as after hip replacement or damage to the nerve during labor,[2673] or as a result of infiltration of the nerve by a pelvic tumor.

obturator neuropathy   See **obturator neuralgia.**

occasional seizure   A seizure occurring only in response to provocation by a definable external or internal event. **Febrile convulsions** represent a form of occasional seizure in which the attack is precipitated by a rapid rise in body temperature.

occipital apoplexy   Hemorrhage and hematoma formation in the occipital lobe as a result of bleeding from an **arteriovenous malformation.** Clinically, sudden intense headache and homonymous hemianopia are the major features.[5642]

occipital intermittent rhythmic delta activity   Fairly regular or approximately sinusoidal waves, mostly occurring in bursts at 2–3 Hz over the occipital areas of one or both sides of the head and frequently blocked or attenuated by opening the eyes. (From the revised ILAE Classification,[1114] reproduced by kind permission from Blackwell Science.)

occipital lobe   The paired posterior lobes of the brain, continuous with the parietal and temporal lobes anteriorly.

occipital lobe epilepsies   These syndromes are usually characterized by simple partial and secondarily generalized seizures. Complex partial seizures may also occur when the discharge spreads beyond the occipital lobe. The frequent association of occipital lobe seizures and migraine is complicated and controversial. The clinical seizure manifestations usually, but not always, include visual manifestations. Elementary visual seizures are characterized by fleeting visual manifestations, which may be either negative (scotoma, hemianopia, amaurosis) or, more commonly, positive (sparks or flashes, phosphenes). Such sensations appear in the visual field contralateral to the discharge in the specific visual cortex, but can spread to the entire visual field. Perceptive illusions, in which the objects appear to be distorted, may occur.

The following varieties can be distinguished: a change in size (macropsia or micropsia) or a change in distance, an inclination of objects in a given plane of space and distortion of objects, or a sudden change of shape (metamorphopsia). Visual hallucinatory seizures are occasionally characterized by complex visual perceptions (e.g., colorful scenes of varying complexity). In some cases, the scene is distorted or made smaller, and, in rare instances, the subject sees his or her own image (**heautoscopy**). Such illusional and hallucinatory visual seizures result from an epileptic discharge in the temporoparieto-occipital junction.

The initial signs may also include tonic and/or clonic contraversion of the eyes and head or the eyes only (oculoclonic or oculogyric deviation), palpebral jerks, and forced closure of the eyelids. Sensations of ocular oscillation or of oscillations of the whole body may occur. The discharge may spread to the temporal lobe, producing seizure manifestations of either lateral posterior temporal or hippocampal-amygdaloid seizures. When the primary focus is located in the supracalcarine area, the discharge can spread forward to the suprasylvian convexity or the mesial surface, mimicking those of parietal or frontal lobe seizures. Spread to the contralateral occipital lobe may be rapid. Occasionally, the seizure becomes secondarily generalized. (From the revised ILAE Classification,[1114] reproduced by kind permission from Blackwell Science.)

occipital lobe epilepsy and intercalated migraine (benign focal epilepsy with occipital lobe spike–waves, benign epilepsy with occipital paroxysms) A syndrome of childhood characterized by the sudden onset and resolution of visual disturbance accompanied by severe headache, nausea, and vomiting; the attacks are often followed by loss of consciousness, automatisms, or generalized seizure activity. The neurological examination and CT scan findings are normal but the EEG shows continuous occipital or posterior temporal high-voltage slow-and-sharp wave EEG activity that is suppressed by eye opening.[56]

The condition has also been regarded as a type of **basilar artery migraine.**

occipital lobe partial epilepsy, occipital cortical and subcortical calcification, and celiac disease   A recently described variant in which bilateral occipital calcification without physical signs, and in particular without evidence of **Sturge-Weber syndrome,** is associated with seizures and celiac disease.

occipital needle-sharp spikes   An EEG pattern consisting of brief occipital spikes in visually impaired children, having but a weak association with clinical epileptic seizures.[3075]

occipital neuralgia   A paroxysmal jabbing pain in the distribution of the greater or lesser occipital nerves, accompanied by diminished sensation or dysesthesia in the affected area. It is commonly associated with tenderness over the nerve concerned. This definition and the following diagnostic criteria are suggested by the Headache Classification Committee of the International Headache Society[1051] (from Classification of headache disorders, cranial neuralgias and facial pains; and diagnostic criteria for primary headache disorders. *Cephalalgia* 1988;8[suppl]:1–96), and reproduced by kind permission.
  A. Pain is felt in the distribution of the greater or lesser occipital nerves.
  B. Pain is stabbing in quality, although aching may persist between paroxysms.
  C. The affected nerve is tender to palpation.
  D. The condition is eased temporarily by local anesthetic block of the appropriate nerve.
The pain may mimic that of **thunderclap headache.**

occipital spikes   Repetitive spikes or sharp-and-slow wave EEG complexes recorded by occipital electrodes, mainly during eye closure.[4316]

occipitalization   Synostosis of the atlas to the occiput, affecting the anterior or posterior arches, or lateral masses, or any or all of them.[5282] The term *assimilation* is best used when all the bony elements of the atlas are fused.

occipitofrontal circumference   The circumference of the head when the tape measure lies upon the forehead and the occiput. A table of normal head circumferences for boys and girls has been prepared.[4088]

occiput   The posterior part of the head, lying behind the posterior fontanelle.

occlusion   (from Lat, to close up) Blockage of a hollow viscus; usually applied to pathological closure of an artery, but also to the eyes.

occult   Secret, hidden, unknown, and undiscoverable.

occupational cervicobrachial disorder   Functional and/or organic disturbances that result from neuromuscular fatigue due to work in a fixed position and/or to a repetitive movement of the upper extremities.[3562]

occupational cramp   (occupational dystonias, craft palsies) A nonprogressive, focal, activity-specific, dystonic syndrome presenting as muscle spasm or inability to execute a specific complex motor action by those who need to do so repetitively. Writers, pianists, bowlers (in cricket), telegraphists, violinists, and many others have been reported as afflicted.

Originally described by Kinnier Wilson[6000] and considered to be a central phenomenon, peripheral mechanisms may also be relevant.[4118]

occupational dystonias   See **occupational cramps.**

occupational nystagmus   See **miners' nystagmus.**

Ochsner, A.J.   (b. 1896) American surgeon, professor at Tulane University, who with Dr. M. DeBakey suggested a link between cigarette smoking and lung cancer in 1941. The proof of this link was obtained by Sir Richard Doll in England nearly 20 years later.

Ochsner sign   When the hands are clasped together, the index finger on the side of a median nerve injury does not flex.

O'Connell test   Straight-leg raising is performed, first in the sound leg, next in the affected leg, and finally in both together. An increase in the permissible flexion of the affected hip when both hips are flexed together, compared with the angle of flexion obtainable when the affected leg is flexed alone, suggests the presence of root irritation.

If both hips are flexed to a point short of that which induces pain, and the sound leg is lowered, pain felt on the side of the affected leg further indicates the presence of root irritation.[1349a]

ocular   (from Lat, oculus) To do with the eyes.

ocular agitation   See **restless eyes.**

ocular albinism   An inherited deficiency of retinal and ocular pigment, accompanied usually by abnormalities in smooth pursuit and by nystagmus of various types.[1739] See also **oculocutaneous albinism.**

ocular and visual reflex   The eyes of the newborn close under strong light.[6064] This observation appears somewhat trite. The author wonders whether the *failure* to close the eyes in strong light might be a more useful observation, as an indication of impaired vision or of facial power?

ocular angina   Periorbital pain due to ocular ischemia.

ocular apraxia   Congenital onset of dyspraxic eye movements with callosal abnormalities.[1070] See **Cogan syndrome.**

ocular bobbing   A form of saccadic oscillation characterized by fast, repetitive, irregular, nonrhythmic, downward movements of both eyes which return more slowly to the primary position. It is seen in patients with severe pontine dysfunction from any cause, who typically are unresponsive and also have paralysis of horizontal lateral gaze.

Typically, the initial phase of the eye movement is downward and fast, with a slower return to the primary position after a brief latent period. The condition was recognized and named by Fisher.[1843]

In *reverse ocular bobbing*, seen in pontine lesions and metabolic encephalopathy, the initial phase of the eyes' movement is fast upwards with a slow return to the mid-position. With *inverse bobbing* (*ocular dipping*), the primary eye movement is slow and downward, with a fast return to the midposition; anoxic encephalopathy is the usual cause.[1843,3809] *Converse ocular bobbing* leads to a slow upward eye movement with a fast return to the mid-position, and again is usually a result of pontine disease. Reports of *perverse* and *obverse bobbing* are eagerly awaited.

ocular counter-rolling   A slight compensatory movement made reflexly by the eyes when the head is persistently tilted to the side. The receptors are in the otolithic organs.

ocular dipping   (inverse ocular bobbing) Abnormal cyclic spontaneous eye movements along the vertical axis, usually seen in the course of coma due to anoxia or following seizures. The downward eye movement is slow and the upward return fast (the inverse appearance of ocular bobbing), and spontaneous, roving, horizontal eye movements are often noted. The responsible lesions are considered to be in the cortex and basal ganglia.[4764]

In *reversed ocular dipping*, the primary movement is upward and slow. In this condition, metabolic encephalopathy is a more likely cause. See also **ocular bobbing.**

ocular dysmetria   An inaccurate saccadic eye movement characterized by over- or undershooting at the end of a saccade which requires a correction to be made. The term is also employed to denote the presence of pathological ocular hypermetria.[1071] See also **dysmetric saccades, flutter dysmetria.**

ocular fibrillation   See **psychogenic flutter.**

ocular flutter   A brief run of spontaneous, intermittent, binocular, horizontal, ocular oscillations (repetitive saccadic oscillations) occurring during fixation on a point straight ahead or with re-fixation.[236,1071] Damage to the pause cells in the brainstem is considered to be responsible. Ocular flutter may present as the first sign of multiple sclerosis.[1929]

Microflutter represents the same, but the movements are of high frequency and low amplitude and are only seen during ophthalmoscopy. It may not indicate disease.

Ocular dysmetria   and other signs of cerebellar disease are usually associated. See also **oscillations.**

ocular hypertelorism   See **Greig syndrome, hypertelorism.**

ocular ischemic syndrome   (carotid artery syndrome) Acute ocular inflammation associated with decreased ocular perfusion as a result of carotid occlusive disease (usually atherosclerotic).

Clinically, corneal edema, neovascularization of the iris or disk, clouding of the lens, venous stasis retinopathy, and central retinal artery occlusion are the usual presenting signs.[2616]

ocular leprosy   Corneal ulceration (exposure keratitis) resulting from anesthesia caused by facial and trigeminal neuropathy in **leprosy.**

ocular microtremor   A high-frequency, low-amplitude, physiological tremor of the eyes at rest, due to excessive discharge of brainstem oculomotor mechanisms. The frequency of the microtremor is slowed with brainstem disease such as multiple sclerosis.[642]

ocular motor deviation   Drift of an eye from the primary position to take up another position so that the two visual axes are no longer aligned. These may occur when only one eye is viewing (**phorias**) or during binocular vision (**tropias**). They are shown well by the **cover test** or, in the case of vertical deviations, by the **Bielschowsky head tilt test.**

ocular myoclonus   (laryngeal nystagmus, lightning eye movements, pharyngeal nystagmus) A form of oscillation from the primary position of gaze, characterized by continuous, rhythmic, pendular, vertical oscillations of the eyes at 40–200 Hz, with dissociation between them, and unaffected by attempts to fixate, converge, or gaze.[5474] They are accompanied by slower (1–3 Hz) rhythmic movements of other branchial arch structures (**palatal myoclonus**) and of the trunk.

The condition is due to lesions of the dentatorubrothalamic pathway (Guillain-Mollaret triangle), especially the inferior olive, as after brainstem hemorrhage. See also **oscillations, square-wave jerks.**[3330]

Ocular myoclonus and **palatal myoclonus** can occur simultaneously, occasionally with similar myoclonus involving the pharyngeal and extraocular muscles, the diaphragm, neck, and (rarely) the shoulder muscles. The vascular, neoplastic, or inflammatory lesion is usually ipsilateral to the myoclonia, somewhere within the Guillain-Mollaret triangle. Unlike most other involuntary movements, this persists during sleep.

ocular myopathy   A muscular dystrophy inherited variously, with onset in youth or adult life and characterized by slowly progressive weakness of the external ocular muscles producing ptosis and external ophthalmoplegia, and slowly progressive weakness of the face. In some cases, weakness of the bulbar and eventually of the limb girdle muscles also ensues. Patients with this condition manifest extreme sensitivity to curare. The most common form is dominantly inherited. Ragged red fibers are frequently found on muscle biopsy specimens.

The condition was first reported by von **Graefe** in 1868.[5786] Further reports by **Gowers, Hutchinson, Möbius,** and others led to dispute as to whether the disease was primarily neurogenic or myopathic, but it has been concluded on balance that the latter is more often correct,[3037] although both positions may be, since mitochondrial diseases have multiple effects. Variant forms are listed in Chart O–1.

Chart O–1. Variant Forms of Ocular Myopathy

A sporadic form with added *pigmentary retinal degeneration*
Kearns-Sayre syndrome[2986]
Oculopharyngeal muscular dystrophy (usually autosomal dominant, sometimes recessive)[3434]
Oculopharyngeal myopathy with distal myopathy, cardiomyopathy, and other varieties of **oculopharyngopdistal myopathy**
Familial multicore disease with ophthalmoplegia[5442]
Progressive ophthalmoplegia with mental retardation
Goldenhar-Gorlin syndrome (oculoauriculovertebral dysplasia) with congenital ophthalmoplegia[95]
Ophthalmoplegia and myopia with X-linked recessive inheritance
Neonatal ophthalmoplegia with microfibers
Nemaline myopathy with ophthalmoplegia and mitochondrial abnormalities
Nemaline myopathy with cardiomyopathy[3812]
Familial paralysis of horizontal gaze
Oculogastrointestinal muscular dystrophy See **familial visceral myopathy.**[2747]
Familial static ophthalmoplegia

ocular neuromyotonia Intermittent spasm of some of the ocular muscles supplied by the third cranial nerve (rarely the fourth or sixth nerves), resulting in episodic diplopia due to noncomitant strabismus and **oscillopsia,** lasting up to half a minute, occurring either spontaneously or with sustained adduction of the affected eye, and sometimes painful. Almost all cases are unilateral.

The problem may occur following damage to the third nerve in the cavernous sinus,[4681] as after pituitary irradiation.

ocular oscillation and truncal myoclonus See **opsoclonus.**

ocular quiver See **dynamic overshoot.**

ocular retraction syndrome (Stilling syndrome) Congenital paresis or deficiency of convergence with impaired abduction and sometimes adduction, and with retraction of the affected eye(s) into the orbit on attempts to adduct.[2679] See also **Duane syndrome.**

ocular shuddering See **psychogenic flutter.**

ocular tilt reaction A transient postural abnormality following unilateral labyrinthine damage, consisting of the triad of ipsilateral head tilt, conjugate ocular tor-

sion, and skew deviation (ipsilateral eye lower) due to a unilateral otolithic lesion in the utricle or to a lesion of the mesencephalic tegmentum.[2391,5931]

ocular torsion (cyclorotation) Abnormal position of the eyes in the roll plane (about the line of sight), occurring as a feature of a peripheral or central **ocular tilt reaction.**[1442]

ocular torticollis An abnormal head posture, adopted to minimize the effect of congenital nystagmus (by attaining the **null-point**), or that of paresis of oculomotor muscles (by turning the head in the direction of action of the paretic muscle).[4841]

ocular vertigo That form of vertigo which occurs only as a result of diplopia.

oculoacousticocerebral degeneration See **Norrie disease.**

oculoauriculocutaneous syndrome (Burns syndrome) A rare congenital syndrome characterized by ichthyosis (erythroderma), deafness and keratitis.[848]

oculoauriculovertebral dysplasia (Goldenhar syndrome, Goldenhar-Gorlin syndrome, first and second branchial arch syndrome). Usually sporadic, but variably a dominant or a recessive syndrome, the main features include facial dysmorphism with auricular appendages and pretragal blind fistulas; hemivertebrae; visceral maldevelopments; epibulbar dermoid cysts, upper lid colobomas, microphthalmia, and strabismus; encephalocele; hydrocephalus; and macrostomia, microtia, and micrognathia due to asymmetrical cranial bone dysgenesis.

Cranial muscle hypoplasia (as may result from failure of development of the trigeminal nerve), conductive deafness, and cardiac defects may also occur, and many affected children are mentally retarded.[2165,2764] Incomplete manifestations are common.[2218] See also **hemifacial microsomia.**

In a *variant* form, paralysis of various extraocular eye movements are described, as a result of hypoplasia or agenesis of the extraocular muscles or nerves.[95]

oculobuccogenital syndrome See **Behçet syndrome.**

oculocardiac reflex (Aschner cardiac phenomenon) Compression of the eyeball leads to increased vagal tone, as detected by cardiac slowing, normally by 5–10 bpm. Painful stimulation of the skin of the neck may also induce this response as well as the **ciliospinal reflex.**

Bernard Aschner (b. 1883) was an Austrian gynecologist;[4979] his recognition of the sign is remarkable, unless he had become aware of the previous report by **Dagnini.**

oculocephalic reflex (doll's eye response, doll's head response, doll's eye movements, Puppenkopfphänomenon) Lateral deviation of the eyes (in parallel) in the direction opposite that of sudden passive rotation of the neck. The reflex is normally present but inhibited after a few hundred milliseconds, so that there is almost immediate restitution of the eyes to the primary position of gaze (straight ahead). In comatose patients, the restitution is seen late if the pathogenesis is diffuse cortical depression, not at all in cases of primary brainstem pathology, and asymmetrically if coma is due to, for example, a lesion producing an **uncal syndrome** and thus a third cranial nerve palsy. Reflex upward deviation of the eyes with sudden neck flexion represents the same reflex, turned 90°. These may be the only vertical movements possible in patients with supranuclear or collicular lesions preventing voluntary upward gaze, and indicate that the infranuclear mechanisms for vertical gaze are intact. Absence of the movements in a comatose patient suggests a severe degree of brainstem damage or depression of function stemming from toxic causes.

In most dolls marketed today, only vertical movements are present, and then only in the more expensive ones. Even these typically show movements of the eyelids rather than of the eyes. Bielschowsky introduced the term in 1939, dolls with lateral eye movements perhaps then being more populous than they are today.[4718] See also **vestibulocerebral response.**

oculocerebellar tegmental syndrome   A mesencephalic lacunar syndrome characterized by internuclear ophthalmoplegia, bilateral cerebellar ataxia, and contralateral hemiparesis.[4737]

oculocerebellomyoclonic syndrome   The occurrence of rapid, irregular movements of the eyes and limbs (**dancing eyes [dancing feet] syndrome**) in children with neuroblastoma.[4315]

oculocerebral hypopigmentation syndrome   See **Cross oculocerebral syndrome.**

oculocerebral malformative syndrome   See **Walker-Warburg syndrome.**

oculocerebrocutaneous syndrome   A rare, dominantly inherited, congenital dysmorphic syndrome, characterized by microphthalmia with orbital cysts, facial skin tags, cerebral atrophy, seizures, and mental delay.[1367]

oculocerebrofacial syndrome   See **Kaufman syndrome.**

oculocerebrofacial-skeletal syndrome   See **Pena-Shokeir phenotype.**

oculocerebrorenal syndrome   (Lowe oculocerebroretinal syndrome) An X-linked recessive metabolic disorder manifesting cataract, glaucoma, rickets and osteomalacia, retardation of physical and mental development, and eventually renal failure.[3489]

The main neurological features are craniosynostosis, pyramidal and lower motor neuron signs, nystagmus,

buphthalmos, and seizures. Periodic metabolic acidosis with urinary excretion of organic acids and variable aminoaciduria are the usual chemical findings. The responsible gene maps to chromosome Xq24–q26 or Xq25.

Defective renal and intestinal amino acid transport and disturbances in excretion of glycosaminoglycan may be the basis for the aminoaciduria and organic aciduria.

oculocraniosomatic dystrophy with ragged red fibers   See **Kearns-Sayre syndrome, mitochondrial myopathies.**

oculocutaneous albinism   1. Type 1a (tyrosinase-negative), the classic X-linked recessive syndrome characterized by nystagmus, sensorineural deafness, hypopigmentation of the fundus, and cutaneous albinism (piebaldness).[4628]

2. Tyrosinase-positive oculocutaneous albinism is a recessively inherited condition mapped to 15q11–q13, in which the biosynthesis of melanin is reduced in the skin, hair, and eyes. It may complicate the Prader-Willi and Angelman syndromes, each involving deletions of chromosome 15q.

A *variant* is *oculocutaneous albinism with deafness* (Woolf syndrome).

oculocutaneous syndrome   See **Harada disease.**

oculodento-osseous dysplasia   See **osteopetrosis.**

oculofacial paralysis   See **Möbius syndrome.**

oculogastrointestinal muscular dystrophy   See **familial visceral myopathy.**

oculogyric crises   Paroxysmal tonic or clonic contractions of the external ocular muscles deviating the eyes in any direction, but usually upward, and lasting seconds on each repeated occasion, preceded by an emotional upsurge and accompanied by an attentional disorder in which obsessive forced thinking occurs.

The episodes may be precipitated by psychical or sensory stimuli. They were first described in 1921 as complications of **encephalitis lethargica,** but now are more usually the result of poisoning by major tranquillizers.[3327]

oculogyric-auricular reflex   Retraction of the auricle and curling-back of the helix of the ear on far lateral gaze to the other side. Sometimes both auricles retract.

The reflex is a curiosity of no known pathological significance.

oculomandibular dyscephaly with hypotrichosis   See **Hallerman-Streiff-François syndrome.**

oculomandibulofacial syndrome   See **Hallermann-Streiff-François syndrome.**

oculomasticatory myorhythmia   The association of continuous, rhythmic, pendular vergence oscillations of the eyes with synchronous jaw movements, at about

1 Hz, reported only in **Whipple disease.**[5025] Ocular pareses may also occur.

oculomotor and facial palsy A syndrome of early adult life manifesting third, fourth, fifth, and sixth and/or seventh cranial nerve palsies; diabetes; and red blood cell abnormalities.[337]

The condition is probably a microangiopathy.

oculomotor apraxia See **Cogan syndrome.**

oculomotor nerve The third cranial nerve, which divides into two branches at the cavernous sinus. The superior branch supplies the superior rectus and levator palpebrae superioris, while the inferior branch supplies the medial and inferior recti and the inferior oblique muscles and carries the parasympathetic fibers to the pupil.

oculomotor psychoparalysis See **Johnson syndrome.**

oculomotor synkinesis Inappropriate elevation of the eyelid, movement of the eye, or changes in pupil size following remote damage to the third cranial nerve and presumed to be due to aberrant regeneration of its nerve fibers. The form occurring with slowly growing parasellar lesions is said to be *primary*; that occurring with acute acquired disorders of the nerve, such as trauma or aneurysmal compression, is termed *secondary.*

In *variant* forms, such synkineses occur without evidence of prior trauma, or in muscles innervated by both the superior and the inferior divisions of the nerve when only the former had been damaged, or bilaterally, or as a result of abnormal connections between the third and sixth cranial nerves.[5]

oculopalatal myoclonus The combination of **palatal myoclonus** with jerky oblique and rotatory nystagmoid movements and sometimes with pendular oscillations. This is known as the *lateral* form. A *mid-line* form is characterized by vertical to-and-fro pendular eye movements with symmetrical bilateral palatal myoclonus.[4064]

oculopalatocerebral syndrome A recessively inherited congenital dysmorphic syndrome, also characterized by short stature, microcephaly with cerebral atrophy, spasticity, mental retardation, conductive deafness, cleft palate, cloudy corneas, glaucoma, retinal phakomas, microphthalmia, and abnormalities of the vitreous.[1973] Cryptorchidism may be present.

oculopharyngeal muscular dystrophy (OMIM 164300) An unusual, dominantly inherited systemic myopathy affecting people of European descent in later life. Clinical features include ptosis, external ophthalmoplegia, upper facial weakness, dysphagia, and proximal lower leg weakness, but all voluntary muscles are affected eventually (although smooth and cardiac muscles are not). Muscle involvement is specific and symmetrical and involves, in order, the extraocular, tongue, diaphragm, pharynx, somatic, and limb muscles. The only characteristic diagnostic feature of the disease is the presence of rimmed vacuoles.[3434] The condition is mapped to chromosome 14q11–2.q13, where there is a stable trinucleotide repeat expansion in exon 1 of the poly(A) binding protein 2 gene (*PABP2*). It is a distinct disease entity, although it overlaps with oculopharyngodistal myopathy.

Morphological abnormalities of mitochondria are commonly detected on systemic muscle biopsy specimens, and the relationship of this condition to the **Kearns-Sayre syndrome** is close.[4048] Whether one regards this and **ocular myopathy** as the same or different conditions reflects more a frame of mind than a judgment based on scientific evidence.

Variants include a neurogenic form;[3702] a recessively inherited form; and *oculopharyngeal myopathy with distal myopathy and cardiomyopathy*, in which the usual features of slowly progressive ptosis, facial weakness, dysphagia, and atrophy are accompanied by distal weakness and cardiomyopathy with conduction system disorders. EMG suggests a myopathic disorder. Both familial and sporadic cases are described.[2229] Another *variant* is **oculopharyngodistal muscular dystrophy.**

oculopharyngeal spinal muscular atrophy A rare *variant* of **hereditary motor neuropathy, type 3**, in which the peripheral signs are accompanied by ophthalmoplegia and bulbar signs.[3702]

oculopharyngodistal muscular dystrophy (OMIM 164310) An unusual dominantly inherited systemic myopathy of adult life, characterized by progressive ptosis and extraocular palsy with eventual weakness of the facial and bulbar muscles and distal limb weakness.[4925] See **Satoyoshi syndrome, oculopharyngeal dystrophy.**

In *variant* forms, the muscle involvement progresses distally and cardiomyopathy and platybasia are associated,[2229] or intestinal pseudo-obstruction complicates the disorder.[136]

oculoplethysmography An investigational technique that indirectly assesses carotid blood flow (and thus the patency of the arterial lumen) by determining the amount of externally applied ocular pressure required to collapse the retinal arterioles and by recording the timing and amplitude of the pressure pulses in the eye occurring with each cardiac cycle.

With the advent of **magnetic resonance arteriography,** the test is threatened with redundancy.

oculorenalcerebellar syndrome A recessively inherited syndrome characterized by pigmentary retinal degeneration with optic atrophy, pyramidal and cerebellar signs, nephropathy, mental and developmental delay and progressive glomerulopathy.[2707,4360]

oculosensory reflex Dilation of the pupil in response to painful stimulation of the eye or of adjacent structures; a **pain reflex** mediated by the sympathetic pathways. See **ciliospinal reflex.**

oculosympathetic palsy   See **Horner syndrome.**

oculovestibular reflex   Deviation of the eyes towards the side of cold stimulation of a lateral semicircular canal, with a fast correcting saccade in the opposite direction in the conscious healthy subject. If such nystagmus is not elicited but only a tonic deviation of the eyes to the irrigated side occurs, the brain stem may be considered to be intact, but freed from suprabulbar control; a dysconjugate response (or none at all) indicates the presence of serious brainstem damage. See **caloric tests, vestibuloocular reflex.**

oculus   Latin for "eye." *Ocular* is thus derived.

odontoid   (Gr, like a tooth; the Latin form is *dens*) The peg-like odontoid process of the axis which projects superiorly and is retained by the transverse ligament; it does not resemble a tooth very closely in form.

odontotrichomelic-tetramelic ectodermal dysplasia A congenital dysmorphic syndrome characterized also by abnormalities of the hair, skin, teeth, and skeleton, as well as by aminoaciduria and seizures.[4360]

oenomania   (Gr, wine + madness) (oniomania) 1. Severe alcohol addiction; "a peculiar form of insanity excited by a drinking tendency" (Sir William **Gowers**). 2. A term for **delirium tremens.**

Oguchi syndrome   A recessively inherited syndrome characterized by night-blindness (hemeralopia), described in 1912 by Dr. C. Oguchi, a Japanese ophthalmologist, among others.

OHAHA syndrome   A rare, recessive form of ophthalmoplegic migraine occurring in infancy and characterized by **O**phthalmoplegia, **H**ypotonia, **A**taxia, **H**ypacusis, and **A**thetosis, as well as any of a selection of focal neurological deficits such as hemiparesis, athetosis, chorea, nystagmus, and strabismus.[6034]

ohmmeter   An instrument used to measure electrical resistance.

Ohtahara syndrome   A sporadic, primary, generalized seizure disorder occurring in infancy and characterized by burst–suppression on the EEG.[4226] See **early infantile epileptic encephalopathy with suppression burst.**

OKT3 encephalopathy   A syndrome of aseptic meningoencephalitis with obtundation, quadriparesis, and CT evidence of cerebral edema ascribed to the use of OKT3, a murine immunoglobulin monoclonal antibody (IgG2a) and immunosuppressant drug.[1097]

Oldendorf, William H.   (1925–1992) American neurologist, physicist, and physiologist who took the first conceptual and practical steps toward the realization of computerized tomographic scanning. For these insights, as well as for those regarding the nature of the blood–brain barrier, he was honored in the United States and abroad, though perhaps not to the extent that many thought appropriate. His book *A Quest for an Image of the Brain* is a classic in its time.

olecranon reflex   See **paradoxical triceps reflex.**

olfactogenital dysplasia   See **Kallmann syndrome, de Morsier syndromes.**

olfactory groove meningioma   See **meningioma.**

olfactory nerve   The first cranial nerve in today's classification, proposed by Soemerring, although it was not included as such by Galen (who was actually right because the first and second "nerves" are invested with oligodendroglia and not Schwann cells, and so are properly regarded as extensions of the central rather than as parts of the peripheral nervous system).

The function of the nerves was recognized by Alessando Achillini (1463–1512), the Italian anatomist. The derivation is from Latin or Greek roots with the expected meaning.

olfactory reference syndrome   The perception of (hallucinated) foul personal body odors by sensitive and obsessional depressed people, who thus exhibit secondary delusional states regarding the outraged reaction of others to their smell and whose contrite behavior includes excessive attention to self-cleanliness, self-isolation, and (in some cases) suicide.[4537]

oligoastrocytoma   See **oligodendroglioma.**

oligoclonal banding   A technique of protein immunoelectrophoresis, commonly used on CSF samples, whereby bands of immunogammaglobulin G with different migratory characteristics can be demonstrated using appropriate staining.

Normally, a single broad area is present, but the finding of such bands suggests the diagnosis of any chronic inflammatory disease of the nervous system; **multiple sclerosis** is the classic example. The technique is also applicable to serum, and when bands are found in serum as well as in CSF samples, the usefulness of the test as a diagnostic aid in neurological disease is compromised.[6120]

oligodendroglia   (Gr, few + branches + glue) Neuroglial cells of the supporting substance of the brain containing small oval nuclei and few fine processes. These are the myelin-forming cells of the CNS, and were first described by Rio del **Hortega** in 1921.

oligodendroglioma   A form of primary infiltrative intracranial glioma, first described by Bailey and **Cushing** in 1926, with defined histological criteria.[3507]

This usually well-differentiated malignant neuroectodermal tumor is composed of uniform small, round cells with few fibrillary processes. It usually arises in the cerebral hemispheres of adults and is normally slow growing, though, in less common anaplastic forms, it is capable of diffuse invasion through the cortex and white matter. Positive staining for **glial fibrillary acidic protein** is usual.[6] *Oligoastrocytomas* are mixed gliomas in which a prominent astrocytic component accompanies the features of oligodendrogliomas just mentioned. An *anaplastic oligodendroglioma* (showing necrosis, vascular proliferation, high cellularity, and obvious mitotic activity) is also recognized.

Clinically, the mean age at presentation is about 40 years, the sexes are equally affected, and the features such as headache, seizures, nausea, dementia, focal neurological signs, and increased intracranial pressure have often been present for some 5 years before the diagnosis is made. The tumor is most commonly located in the frontal lobe, and causes frontal ataxia in a high proportion of patients; intracranial bleeding, stroke syndromes, and meningismus due to leptomeningeal spread are other notable characteristics. In children, seizures are the most common presenting features.[3507,5973]

oligohydramnios syndrome   See **Potter syndrome.**

oligophrenia, epilepsy, and ichthyosis syndrome See **Rud syndrome.** Rud's description was, however, translated inexactly, and it is not certain that he described the condition known by his name.[857]

oligosaccharidoses Inherited storage diseases of childhood, including **fucosidosis, mannosidosis,** and **aspartylglucosaminuria.**

olivary hypertrophy Enlargement of the inferior olivary nuclei as a result of transsynaptic degeneration following ischemic or other damage to the central tegmental tract, its principal afferent pathway.[24]

The classic clinical accompaniment is **palatal myoclonus.**

olivopontocerebellar atrophies (Déjèrine-Thomas syndrome, parenchymatous cortical cerebellar atrophy, late cortical cerebellar atrophy, Marie-Foix-Alajouanine syndrome, Thomas atrophy) A collective term embracing a heterogeneous group of syndromes characterized by severe cerebellar ataxia and other complicating manifestations (dementia, parkinsonism, cramps, pigmentary retinal degeneration, optic atrophy, myoclonus, spasticity, posterior column dysfunction, musculoskeletal deformities, etc.), tenuously united by the common finding of neuronal loss in the basis pontis, inferior olives, and cerebellar cortex.[482]

The conditions are usually either dominantly inherited, as described by Menzel (1891),[3839] or sporadic (Déjèrine and Thomas, 1900).[1346,5536] A definitive synthesis and categorization was achieved by Konigsmark (1970),[3125] who defined five categories, but Harding[2438,2439] fitted them equally neatly into the group of **autosomal dominant cerebellar ataxias** of late onset.

The classic *Menzel type* is dominantly inherited with onset in youth or adult life and with a course of between 4 and 10 years to death. Gait ataxia, limb ataxia, dysarthria, dysphagia, and various abnormal movements such as tics, chorea, and parkinsonian features are sometimes recorded, as are the presence of bulbar palsies, internal and external ophthalmoplegias, py-

ramidal signs, and impairment of intellectual function.[1590] Posterior column dysfunction and demyelinating sensorimotor neuropathies have also been described. See also **autosomal dominant cerebellar ataxias, cerebellar ataxias.** Transition from typical sporadic olivopontocerebellar atrophy into **multiple system atrophy** with autonomic failure and parkinsonism has been recorded.[2122]

Variants are *olivopontocerebellar atrophy with velolaryngeal paralysis*, a cerebellar syndrome appearing in late life and complicated by bulbar palsy due to atrophy of the bulbar nuclei,[3276] and *olivopontocerebellar atrophy with liver cirrhosis and retinal dystrophy.*

olivorubrocerebellar atrophy   See **Lejonne-Lhermitte disease.**

Ollier disease (enchondromatosis, dyschondroplasia) A chondrodysplasia with maximal effects within the long bones, but also a potential cause of optic nerve compression and ophthalmoplegia.[1105,3821]

Dr. L.X.E.L. Ollier (1830–1900) was a French surgeon. See also **Maffucci syndrome.**

Ollivier d'Angers, Charles-Philippe (1796–1845) French neurologist. His book on the spinal cord and its maladies was the first in this area upon its publication in 1824, when he was 28 years old. In it he described spina bifida, **diastematomyelia,** and both compression and atrophy of the cord. In the third edition (1837), he coined the term **syringomyelia** but did not note the **dissociated anesthesia.** He also gave an account of the clinical features of cases of **multiple sclerosis** (recording the deterioration of function with heat) and **acute inflammatory demyelinating polyneuropathy** (reviewed by Spillane[5280]).

Ollivier disease Diffuse primary meningeal sarcomatosis.[530]

-oma The modern clinicopathological equivalent of the Galenic conception of "tumors against nature," a term introduced by Hooper in 1828.

Omenn syndrome   See **familial erythrophagocytic lymphohistiocytosis.**

omnipause neurons Neurons receiving impulses from the frontal cortex and superior colliculus, which exert inhibitory influences on saccadic mechanisms on those occasions when saccades are not required.[4686]

Onanoff, Jacques (b. 1859) Franco-Russian physician who studied at the University of Paris, graduating in 1892. He published papers with Paul **Blocq** on the diagnosis of neurological disease, but was then lost to history; presumably he returned to Russia.

Onanoff reflex   See **bulbocavernosus reflex.**[4239]

Onanism Strictly speaking, this refers to *coitus interruptus*, but the present meaning of the word is masturbation. "Judah commanded Onan, the son of Juda and the Canaanite Shua, to take Tamar, the widow of Er, in a leverite marriage. Onan withdrew during intercourse with Tamar and God slew him for this evil" (Genesis 38:8–10). The word was first employed by the anonymous author of a work entitled *Onania, or the heinous sin of self-pollution, and its frightful consequences, in both sexes* (ca. 1710). The author may have been a Dr. Bekkers, perhaps a clergyman turned quack but not an MD; he advertised secret pills (half-a-guinea a box) that were alleged to provide a remedy for masturbation, impotence, and sterility. The Swiss physician **Tissot** took up the name in his antimasturbatory diatribe *L'Onanisme* (Translated by Alexander Hume, 1781), their combined reputations coloring medical thought to the degree that the belief that masturbation leads to "debility of the brain and nervous system" only just now disappearing.[5047]

onchocerciasis   (river blindness) A metazoal infestation endemic in many parts of West Africa, leading to optic atrophy and blindness. See **Guinea worm infestation.**

onco-   (Gr, bulk) Prefix denoting bulk or mass.

oncocytoma   A nonfunctioning pituitary neoplasm.

oncogene   A group of genes with the power, when activated by unknown factors, to release cell systems from the ordinary constraints to multiplication and differentiation, thus stimulating normal cells to undergo malignant transformation.

oncosphere   Developed embryos of parasites such as **cysticercosis,** as may lodge in muscle and brain.

Ondine's curse   A rare congenital syndrome resulting from the primary failure of medullary automatic respiratory centers, leading to cessation of ventilation in sleep, almost permanent cyanosis, and eventually to hypoxic cerebral ischemia.

Bulimia, central diabetes insipidus, or other evidences of hypothalamic disturbance are associated in some cases. Insensitivity of the central chemoreceptors is held responsible for the failure in respiratory drive.[1873,3818]

Severinghaus coined the name with reference to the unlikely story of Ondine (a water nymph in a novel of that name by Giraudoux), who punished her unfaithful mortal husband (Hans, a knight) by depriving him of the ability to breathe while asleep.[5081]

In *variants* of the condition, Hirschsprung disease is associated; dysautonomic features are added; or it is acquired as a result of a medullary lesion in adults.

one-and-a-half syndrome   A clinical disorder of extraocular movements characterized by ipsilateral horizontal conjugate gaze palsy (the "one") associated with **internuclear ophthalmoplegia** on contralateral gaze (the "half").

The lesion is in the dorsal tegmentum of the pons, affecting the sixth cranial nerve nucleus or the parapontine reticular formation (the "center" for lateral

gaze) *and* the medial longitudinal fasciculus (leading to failure of adduction of the ipsilateral eye).[5813]

Brainstem infarction and **multiple sclerosis** are the more common causes. The condition was given its name by Miller Fisher in 1967.[1847]

oneirism   (from Gr, dreaminess) The positive aspects of disordered consciousness, including hallucinations, terrifying fantasies, and intense emotional experiences.

oneirodynia   (Gr, dream + pain) Unpleasant dreams.

oniomania   See **oenomania.**

onion bulbs   Superimposed reduplications of an axon's Schwann cell processes, with intermixed fibroblasts and collagen, leading to microscopical appearances that resemble the lamellations of an onion. This process occurs after repeated cycles of axonal swelling and regression with division of Schwann cells and the production of excessive amounts of myelin, which becomes redundant.

onion bulb neuropathy   See **hereditary motor and sensory neuropathy, type 3.**

onion-peel sensory loss   Facial anesthesia or hypoesthesia that is complete centrally, around the nose and mouth, but shades off peripherally, originally described by Déjèrine in 1914.[1341] It is seen in **tabes dorsalis** and with medullary lesions.

on–off effect   The rapid alteration in motility (improving or worsening) shown by patients with parkinson disease who are taking L-dopa, as a result of rapidly changing levels of the drug in the brain. The off periods are frequently accompanied by depressive mood swings.[2434]

onset frequency   The lowest stable firing rate for a single motor unit action potential that can be voluntarily maintained by a subject.

ontogenesis   (Gr, things which exist + origin) The process of development, from the ovum to the adult condition.

Opalski, Adam   (1897–1963) Polish neurologist.

Opalski cells   Large astrocytes with small, eccentric, pyknotic, densely staining nuclei displaced to the periphery, found in the cortical and subcortical regions of the brains of people with **Wilson disease** and **acquired hepatolenticular degeneration.**

Opalski syndrome   (submedullary syndrome) An extended form of the **lateral medullary syndrome,** in which there are also homolateral pyramidal signs due to downward extension of the ischemic lesion into the upper part of the cervical cord, there damaging the corticospinal tract, which at that level has crossed to the side of the medullary lesion.[4245]

open opercular sign   Bilateral, wide enlargement of the sylvian fissures, exposing the insulas, seen on CT scans of some children. A measurement of more than 3 mm between the caudal part of the frontal edge and the most rostral part of the temporal edge of the fissure is taken as abnormal.

The sign suggests that a patient's neurological impairment is due to arrested development,[5498] but it may also occur in other conditions and in normal infants.

open ring imaging sign   Contrast enhancement of a brain lesion shaped as an open ring or as a crescent circumscribed to the white matter on MRI or CT imaging. The sign is reported to be highly specific for demyelination.[3669]

opercular seizures   Seizures characterized by mastication, salivation, swallowing, laryngeal symptoms, speech arrest, epigastric aura, fear, and autonomic phenomena. Simple partial seizures, particularly partial clonic facial seizures, are common and may be ipsilateral. If secondary sensory changes occur, numbness may be a symptom, particularly in the hands. Gustatory hallucinations are particularly common in this area. (From the revised ILAE Classification,[1114] reproduced by kind permission from Blackwell Science.)

operculum   (Lat, a lid or cover) Those parts of the cortex of the frontal, parietal, and temporal lobes which cover the insula.

operculum syndrome   See **anterior operculum syndrome.**

ophthalmia   (Gr) Disease of the eyes.

ophthalmic migraine   See **migraine with aura.**

ophthalmodynamometry   1. The forerunner of oculoplethysmography, this test was designed to assess stenosis of the carotid artery by measuring blood pressure in the ophthalmic arteries by applying pressure to the globes using either a compression or suction apparatus; both diastolic and systolic blood pressures can be obtained. The technique is good at demonstrating but bad at excluding carotid disease.[4141] 2. Originally, the use of an instrument to measure the strength of ocular convergence.

ophthalmodynia   Pain in the eyes.

ophthalmopathic hallucinations   (syndrome of Charles **Bonnet**) Pure visual hallucinations associated with visual impairment resulting from disease of the ocular globes, optic nerves, or optic tracts.[1862]

ophthalmoplegia   (Gr, eye + stroke) Paresis of eye movements. The many causes have been summarized.[483]

ophthalmoplegia, demyelinating neuropathy, leukoencephalopathy, myopathy, and gastrointestinal dysfunction   See **mitochondrial encephalomyopathy.**

ophthalmoplegia, facial contraction, and progressive scoliosis   A rare syndrome characterized by the onset in infancy of ophthalmoplegias, scoliosis, and myokymia.[337]

ophthalmoplegia interna   Pupillary paralysis. The term was introduced by Jonathan Hutchinson in 1878. *Iridoplegia* is an alternative.

ophthalmoplegia-ataxia   See **Nothnagel syndrome.**

ophthalmoplegia-ataxia-areflexia syndrome   See **Miller Fisher syndrome.**

ophthalmoplegia-hypotonia-ataxia-hypacusis-athetosis syndrome   See **OHAHA syndrome.**

ophthalmoplegia-retinal degeneration   See **Barnard-Scholz syndrome.**

ophthalmoplegic migraine   Repeated attacks of headache associated with painful paresis of one or more ocular cranial nerves (usually the oculomotor nerve) in the absence of a demonstrable intracranial lesion. The duration of ophthalmoplegia varies from hours to months.

The following diagnostic criteria are suggested by the Headache Classification Committee of the International Headache Society[1051] (from Classification of headache disorders, cranial neuralgias and facial pains; and diagnostic criteria for primary headache disorders. *Cephalalgia* 1988;**8**[suppl]:1–96).

A. At least two attacks fulfilling B

B. Headache overlapping with paresis of one or more of cranial nerves III, IV, and VI

C. Parasellar lesion ruled out by appropriate investigations

Migraine headaches associated with total unilateral external ophthalmoplegia (with pupillary involvement) that outlasts the headache were first described by Paul **Möbius**[3926] in 1884. The criteria for the **superior orbital fissure syndrome**[2420] may be satisfied by the features of ophthalmoplegic migraine.

ophthalmoplegic neurolipidosis   A congenital syndrome characterized by strabismus, an enlarged liver and spleen, seizures, ataxia, and trigeminal nerve abnormalities.[4360]

ophthalmoplegia plus   The term of Drachman for cases of idiopathic progressive external ophthalmoplegia (PEO) occurring in association with any combination of retinal, brainstem, auditory system, vestibular system, hypothalamic, pyramidal, endocrine, cardiac, and/or muscular involvement.[1509]

In the same paper, Drachman noted reports of 14 different syndromes in which ophthalmoplegia had been described and the overlapping features in many; he therefore questioned the utility of designating disease entities merely on the basis of their clinical presentation, and discussed principles of nosology of relevance when this is done.

The syndrome of PEO is thus heterogeneous, although the **Kearns-Sayre syndrome** has been separated out as showing a more-or-less constant association of signs, and a common etiology in the presence of mitochondrial disease appears at least possible.

ophthalmoscope   A device for examining the interior of the eye, the observer's gaze running down the center of a beam of light angled by a mirror. The earliest instrument consisted merely of a tube that passed through a candle flame. It was invented by the English polymath Charles Babbage 4 years before Helmholtz in 1851[2529] described the machine that, adapted and refined, is still in use today. The concept was enthusiastically adopted by Hughlings-**Jackson** while working as an assistant to **Hutchinson** at Moorfields Eye Hospital in London.

opioid peptides   (Gr, poppy juice + digest) Endogenous morphine-like oligopeptides having a role as modulators in the transmission and processing of pain information.

opisthotonos   (Gr, stretched backward) Strong extensor muscular contractions leading to a bridge-like posture (Fr, *arc-en-cercle*) seen characteristically in the context of **rabies,** brainstem hemorrhage, posterior fossa tumor, meningitis, or encephalitis, but rather more commonly in dystonias or hysterical states.

The phenomenon was called *dolor inflexibilis* by Pliny.

Opitz trigonocephaly syndrome   See **C syndrome.**

Opitz-Frias syndrome   (hypospadias-dysphagia syndrome) A congenital dysmorphic syndrome manifesting also hoarse voice and stridor due to bulbar weakness; congenital gastrointestinal, cardiac, and lung anomalies; hypospadias; and mental and developmental delay.[4246]

Oppenheim disease   1. (amyotonia congenita) Congenital muscle weakness and hypotonia with the potential for recovery. Oppenheim's report contained no pathological data and the nature of the condition is uncertain;[4251] it was probably **hereditary motor neuropathy** or **benign congenital hypotonia,** or both. 2. Dystonia musculorum deformans (Oppenheim-Ziehen disease) See **dystonia.** 3. (pseudotabes, Sternberg-Cushing-Oppenheim syndrome) Optic atrophy, pupillary disturbances, impotence, and loss of the knee and ankle reflexes in association with a pituitary neoplasm but considered by Oppenheim and others to resemble **tabes dorsalis** with respect to these clinical features.[4084]

Oppenheim, Hermann   (1859–1919) German neurologist and psychiatrist, initially assistant to **Westphal** in Berlin but not succeeding him as professor of neurology for political reasons.[1829] Both his private practice and his 1894 two-volume textbook of neurology were extremely successful.

Oppenheim is credited with introducing the term **dystonia musculorum deformans** (1911),[4253] and with realizing that this is an organic rather than a neurotic disease.

Oppenheimer reflex   A variant of the **Babinski reflex** in which the hallux extends in response to a scratch on the inner side of the tibia or in response to firm finger pressure, sliding down the tibial spine.[4251]

Oppenheim-Ziehen disease   See **dystonia.**

opsoclonic meningoencephalitis   (Kinsbourne-Warrington syndrome) See **opsoclonus-myoclonus syndrome.**

opsoclonus   (lightning eye movements, ataxic conjugate movements, acute ocular oscillations, saccadomania, polymyoclonia, infantile polymyoclonia, ocular oscillations and truncal myoclonus, myoclonic encephalopathy of infancy). Ocular oscillations characterized by unpredictable, large-amplitude, irregular, rapid, involuntary, repetitive, multidirectional, and more or less conjugate saccades, which are increased by visual fixation but which occur both in the sleeping and waking states.

Opsoclonus is one feature of a syndrome complicating viral infections characterized by myoclonus, cerebellar signs, **hyperekplexia,** and vomiting.[3052,4315] The underlying lesion of the dentate nucleus may thus be postinfectious but it may also be associated with local or distant malignancies such as **neuroblastoma** or other malignancies with neural crest origin, and breast, lung, or uterine carcinoma. The anti-Ri antibody may be detectable in subjects with cancer, particularly cancer of the breast. See also **opsoclonus-myoclonus syndrome; oscillations.**

The word was introduced by Orzechowsky in 1913.[4265]

opsoclonus-myoclonus syndrome   (sporadic myoclonic encephalopathy, opsoclonic meningoencephalitis, dancing eyes, dancing feet syndrome) A self-limiting syndrome characterized by **opsoclonus** with oscillopsia and myoclonus, mainly of the legs with ataxia, dysarthria, learning and behavioral disorders, and mental retardation.[4514] When occurring in the setting of **neuroblastoma** or of small-cell or breast carcinoma in adults, it constitutes a **paraneoplastic syndrome,** but in as many cases the condition appears following a presumed viral infection and may be a postinfectious encephalopathy. See also **myoclonus.**

Opsoclonus Myoclonus Support Network, Inc.   A charitable organization in this field. Address: c/o 420 Montezuma Way, West Covina, CA 1791. E-mail: sandragreenberg@hotmail.com. Web site: http://www. geocities.com/opso-myoclonus/.

See also *Dancing Eye Syndrome Support Trust* (http://www.dancingeyes.org.uk/).

optacon   An electronic device measuring the sensation of vibration on the fingertips.[210]

optic   (Gr) Relating to sight.

optic ataxia   (misreaching) Severe impairment of visually guided movements, most evident when patients try to reach for an object and their manual groping resembles that of a normal person whose sight is distorted by a prism.[645]

The condition was originally described in 1909 by Balint[308] as occurring in the context of severe oculomotor impairment. The same problem resulting from parietal lobe disease was named *visual disorientation* by **Holmes.** The condition has been regarded as a disconnection syndrome between the visual and motor systems. See also **Balint syndrome.**

optic atrophy   Demyelination of the optic nerve as a result of hereditary or acquired disease. The prototypical dominantly inherited syndrome has its onset in childhood or youth. The mild reduction in visual acuity and blue-yellow dyschromatopsia are unaccompanied by other evidence of neurological impairment.

Variant syndromes are listed in Chart O–2.

Chart O–2. Variant Syndromes of Optic Atrophy

Leber optic atrophy, which is either an X-linked condition or a **mitochondrial cytopathy**

Adrenoleukodystrophy A *juvenile form* in which the visual defects are similar to those seen in patients with congenital tritan defects. The following diagnostic criteria have been suggested by Smith:[5220]

A. Autosomal dominant inheritance
B. Insidious onset between 4 and 8 years
C. Moderately reduced visual acuity to 6/20–6/60
D. Temporal pallor of the optic disks
E. Centrocecal enlargement of the blind spot
F. Full peripheral fields in response to white
G. Inverted peripheral fields in response to colors
H. Acquired blue-yellow dyschromatopsia

Conditions in which optic atrophy is part of a more widespread neurological disorder, including **Friedreich ataxia, late-onset cerebellar ataxias, hereditary motor and sensory neuropathy** (HMSN type 6), and conditions characterized by **osteopetrosis**[4791]

Early infantile recessive optic atrophy A rare recessive form characterized by severe but nonprogressive visual impairment with nystagmus and severe dyschromatopsia seldom discovered before the fourth year of life. The electroretinogram is normal. A similar *dominant form* is also described.[3074]

Optic atrophy, congenital cataract and ataxia A congenital syndrome characterized by cataract, optic atrophy, cerebellar ataxia, and extrapyramidal signs.[2020]

Optic atrophy, deafness, and sensory ataxia A syndrome with the onset in childhood of nerve deafness, optic atrophy, and cerebellar ataxia.[2848] Optic atrophy may also occur as a dominant trait in association with deafness alone.[3124]

Optic atrophy with spastic paraparesis An X-linked syndrome with the onset in childhood of optic atrophy, speech defects, scoliosis, pectus excavatum, ophthalmoplegias, seventh cranial nerve and bulbar palsies, pyramidal and cerebellar signs, athetosis, neurogenic muscle atrophy, and loss of pain and touch sensation.[3520]

Optic atrophy and tritanopia A rare association.[3162]

Familial bilateral optic nerve hypoplasia A rare association, reported both sporadically and with dominant or recessive inheritance.[335]

Optic atrophy-ataxia syndrome See **Behr syndrome.**

Optic atrophy also occurs incidentally in many other inherited disorders entered elsewhere, and due to e.g., **tabes dorsalis, multiple sclerosis,** vitamin B_{12} deficiency, ischemia, pressure on the optic nerve, and various toxins.

Secondary (consecutive) optic atrophy follows previous papilledema. In this case the appearance of the disc is not a "stark full moon in a deep red sky" but is yellower and irregular in outline.

optic chiasmal neuritis   Inflammation of the optic chiasm with swelling, well shown on MRI scans and usually due to demyelinating disease.[4115]

optic disk drusen   Hyaloid bodies situated in front of the lamina propria of the optic nerve head and sometimes visible within the optic disk, which appears swollen. Any associated field defects follow a nerve fiber–bundle pattern. Small hemorrhages on or beside the disk may be associated. Drusen become more prominent with age and may be inherited as an autosomal dominant characteristic.[3473] See **drusen.**

optic disk vasculitis   See **papillophlebitis.**

optic fixation reflex   Persistence of gaze directed upon an object despite passive rotation of the head; a sign suggesting the presence of a destructive frontal lobe lesion. Paresis of voluntary gaze may be associated.

optic myelitis   See **neuromyelitis optica.**

optic nerve aplasia   See **optic nerve hypoplasia.**

optic nerve dysplasia   See **coloboma, morning glory syndrome, optic pits, optic nerve hypoplasia.**

optic nerve gliomas   A heterogeneous collection of primary malignant tumors of the optic nerve. Their clinical expressions include visual failure, visual field defects, optic atrophy, papilledema, and evidence of hypothalamic or other local infiltration, including increased intracranial pressure.[132] The optic canal is characteristically enlarged.

The features of **neurofibromatosis** are present in half of the children affected. The tumors are substantially less common and more malignant (glioblastoma) in adults.

optic nerve hypoplasia   (micropapilla, partial optic aplasia, optic nerve aplasia, optic nerve dysplasia) A rare, sometimes dominantly inherited reduction in the number of axons in an optic nerve with a consequent reduction in the area of the optic nerve head, giving a horizontal optic disk diameter of less than 3.4 mm.

The causes of this abnormality are many and involve the eyes, the nervous system, or other systems; various malformations may be associated, especially when the hypoplasia is bilateral. The usual clinical presentation is of an **altitudinal field defect,** but visual acuity may be normal.[4096] Astigmatism and nystagmus may be associated.

optic neuritis   (optic neuropathy) Inflammation of the optic nerve as a result of any of numerous etiologies. Clinically, the syndrome presents most commonly with rapidly progressive loss of central vision revealed by perimetry, ocular pain on movement of the eyes, tender globes, and homolateral head pain. A central or centrocecal scotoma is demonstrable and acuity (especially to color and contrast) is almost always much decreased. Papillitis and flame hemorrhages are commonly seen when the inflammation is anterior, but the fundi appear normal with retrobulbar neuritis.

Bilateral involvement is etiologically and prognostically diverse, but children do not seem to develop **multiple sclerosis,** although some adults do at a rate which is not agreed upon by any two authors and which ranges between 13% and 85%, varying with the duration of follow-up. Whether optic neuritis not obviously due to another cause is a *forme fruste* of multiple sclerosis or is a separate entity is not agreed upon either.[1597, 3200] See also **ischemic optic neuropathy,**[501] **papilledema, relative afferent pupillary defect.**

optic neuropathy   Disease of the optic nerve(s). See **optic neuritis, Cuban optic neuropathy, Leber hereditary optic neuropathy, multiple sclerosis.**

optic nystagmus   See **optokinetic nystagmus.**

optic pits   A congenital optic disk dysplasia characterized by depression of the disk margin on the temporal side with nerve fiber loss, causing arcuate field defects and enlargement of the blind spot.[790]

optical apraxia   Impairment in performing saccadic eye movements on command.[3138] Impairment of hand–eye coordination results, although patients affected may perform such tasks as the finger–nose test better with the eyes closed than with them open. The condition is a feature of Balint syndrome. See **apraxia.**

opticocentral syndrome   See **opticocerebral syndrome.**

opticocerebral syndrome   (opticopyramidal syndrome) A syndrome of simultaneous optic nerve and watershed cerebral infarctions, usually with occlusion of the ipsilateral internal carotid artery and reversal of flow in the ophthalmic artery.[635,636]

opticocochleodentate degeneration   (Nyssen–van Bogaert syndrome) A congenital dysmorphic syndrome, characterized also by sensorineural deafness, optic atrophy, skeletal deformities, cerebral atrophy with seizures and pyramidal signs, and mental and developmental delay.[4038]

opticofacial reflex   See **orbicularis oculi reflex.**

opticopyramidal syndrome   See **opticocerebral syndrome.**

optokinetic after-induced nystagmus   (reverse postoptokinetic nystagmus). A physiological, brief reversal of the direction of nystagmus occurring after normal optokinetic nystagmus has been elicited.

optokinetic nystagmus   (railway nystagmus, elevator nystagmus, kinetic nystagmus, optomotor nystagmus, optic nystagmus, panoramic nystagmus, sigma nystagmus or train nystagmus, optokinetic after-induced nystagmus) A physiological form of reflex horizontal or vertical nystagmus induced by fixation on a series of moving visual targets in the environment.

The *subcortical* or *field* type requires stimulation of most of the visual field and is followed by an afternystagmus; it is impaired by brainstem or labyrinthine lesions. The *cortical* or *object* type resembles visual smooth-pursuit tracking, is not succeeded by an afternystagmus, and is impaired with posterior cortical lesions.

With routine clinical testing, employing a striped tape, the optokinetic response is normally symmetrical in both directions. In the presence of a frontal lobe lesion, the patient's eyes tend to drift slightly and slowly in the direction of tape movement. In the setting of parietal lesions, the response is lost when the object moves in the direction of the diseased lobe. There is a dissociated response in **internuclear ophthalmoplegia.**

The test was introduced as a clinical tool by Bárány in 1921, although the phenomenon was noted by **Purkinje** in onlookers during a cavalry parade in 1825. A recent very complete review is that of David.[1308]

optomotor nystagmus   See **optokinetic nystagmus.**

oral dysesthesias   See **burning mouth syndrome.**

oral reflex   See **buccal reflex, orbicularis oris reflex.**

oral-buccal apraxia   (pseudoplegia, aphemia, diplegia with dissociation) A term denoting the dissociation of voluntary and emotional movements, such as those of the face, jaws, throat, and larynx in the **anterior operculum syndrome.**[3601]

oral-facial-digital syndrome   (Mohr syndrome) See **orofaciodigital syndrome.**

orbi-   (Gr, a sphere).

orbicularis oculi reflex   (nasopalpebral reflex, blink reflex, McCarthy reflex, supraorbital reflex, frontal reflex, trigeminofacial rfeflex, glabellar reflex, Meyerson sign) Bilateral contraction of the orbicularis oculi and relaxation of the levator palpebrae superioris in response to visual, auditory, or tactile stimuli, the latter causing vibration in the muscle. It is tested clinically by tapping over the forehead as far back as the hairline (blink reflex), or by stretching the muscle itself by tapping the examiner's thumb which, with the index finger, is drawing back a fold of skin at the lateral angle of the patient's eye. Normally, a single blink is elicited in response to each of the first five or so repetitive taps, the reflex fatiguing thereafter. In patients with diffuse cerebral cortical dysfunction, either acute (delirium) or chronic (dementia), the blinking persists.

The reflex was first described by Overend in England in 1896 and described further by McCarthy 5 years later. It is unique by virtue of the number of types of stimuli that induce it, and its low threshold, enhancing thus its efficiency in protecting the cornea. It is enhanced in the presence of upper motor neuron facial weakness and postencephalitic parkinsonism.[5858]

orbicularis oris reflex (oral reflex, buccal reflex, nasomental reflex) Contraction of the levator muscles of the angle of the mouth when the upper lip or the side of the nose is percussed. The mentalis may also contract, adding wrinkling of the chin to the above signs.

The reflex is lost after the first year of life, but reappears in subjects with bilateral corticobulbar tract lesions and in those with parkinsonism.[5858] See **perioral reflex.**

orbicularis sign The patient is unable to close the eye on the paretic side without closing the other eye as well.[4723]

orbit (Lat, a track or circuit) Applied to the bony eye socket sometime in the Middle Ages.[5204]

orbital apex syndrome See **superior orbital fissure syndrome.**

orbital blowout fracture See **blowout fracture.**

orbital cysts and cerebral malformation See **Determan syndrome.**

orbital fibrositis See **orbital pseudotumor syndrome.**

orbital fissure syndromes See **orbital apex syndrome, superior orbital fissure syndrome, Foix syndrome, Jacod syndrome,** and **pseudotumor orbiti.**

orbital floor syndrome See **Dejean syndrome.**

orbital hypertelorism See **hypertelorism.**

orbital lipogranuloma See **orbital pseudotumor syndrome.**

orbital lymphomatosis See **orbital pseudotumor syndrome.**

orbital myositis Acute, persistent, painful focal inflammation of one or more extraocular muscles in adolescents or young adults, leading to ophthalmoplegias, redness of the eye, and chemosis without proptosis, but with a normal orbital CT image (thus differentiating the condition from the myositis of hyperthyroidism).[5299] See **orbital pseudotumor syndrome.**

orbital periostitis See **orbital pseudotumor syndrome.**

orbital pseudotumor syndrome (pseudotumor orbiti, orbital myositis, orbital periostitis, pseudoblastoma, orbital lymphomatosis, periostitis or fibrositis, granulome bizarre de l'orbite, chronic dacryo-adenitis, fibromatosis of the optic nerve sheath, superior orbital fissure syndrome, syndrome of Rochon-Duvigneau, or-

bital lipogranuloma, nonspecific granuloma of the orbit, Tolosa-Hunt syndrome, painful ophthalmoplegia) Space-occupying lesions of the orbit not due to common inflammations, specific granulomas, simple vascular lesions, hematomas, neoplasms, or lymphomas, nor to endocrine exophthalmos, but in which there is edema and cellular infiltration of the orbital contents.

The condition usually presents with malaise, unilateral ocular pain, visual loss, and proptosis, usually of one eye, and frequently there is evidence of a trigeminal sensory disturbance. The course is remitting, progressive, or chronic and the pathogenesis is autoimmune.[2827] See also **superior orbital fissure syndrome.**[3382]

orbital teratoma See **dermoid cyst.**

orbitofrontal seizures The seizure pattern is one of complex partial seizures with initial motor and gestural automatisms, olfactory hallucinations, and illusions and autonomic signs. (From the revised ILAE Classification,[1114] reproduced by kind permission from Blackwell Science.)

order of activation The sequence of appearance of different motor unit action potentials with increasing strength of voluntary contraction. See **recruitment.** (From the 2001 Report of the Nomenclature Committee of the American Association of Electromyography and Electrodiagnosis.[10] Used by permission, copyright © 2001, AAEM.)

ordinary headache See **episodic tension-type headache.**

orexins (hypocretins) Excitatory neuropeptide transmitters found only in the lateral hypothalamus. They are relevant in the control of sleep, arousal, and energy metabolism. Mutations of their genes are associated with narcolepsy in animal models and the ligand is likely to be defective in human **narcolepsy.**[4143]

organic acidemia (organic aciduria) Inborn errors of metabolism characterized by the presence of organic acids in the blood.

Clinically, the presentations are similar: failure to thrive in infancy, hypotonia, vomiting, hypoglycemia, seizures, and eventual coma are the common features. In some cases, psychomotor arrest occurs.[721]

Conditions of neurological importance are **proprionic acidemia, methylmalonic aciduria, isovaleric acidemia, betamethylcrotonylglycinuria, glutaric aciduria, glutathione synthetase deficiency, multiple carboxylase deficiency.** See also **maple syrup urine disease, hyperammonemias.**

Organic Acidemia Association A charitable organization. Address: 13210 35th Avenue, Plymouth, MN 55441. Tel: 763–559–1797. Web site: http://www.oaanews.orgl.

organic aciduria See **organic acidemia.**

organic brain syndrome A euphemism for a chemical or structural brain disease producing delirium or dementia. The only justification for its use is induced compliance with the dictates of expert professional committees.

organic dementias Those dementing illnesses associated with the presence of morphological alterations in the brain.

organic emotionalism See **emotionalism.**

organic mental syndromes Disorders affecting cognition or other aspects of mentation. They have been be grouped into six categories by the American Psychiatric Association (Chart O–3).

Chart O–3. Types of Organic Mental Syndrome

1. **Delirium**
2. **Dementia**
3. **Amnestic syndrome**
4. So-called *organic delusional syndrome, organic mood syndrome,* and *organic anxiety syndrome,* in which features both of schizophrenia and of mood and anxiety disorders can be identified
5. *Organic personality syndrome*
6. *Syndromes due to intoxication and withdrawal from psychoactive agents.* These are delirious states due either to the acute ingestion of psychoactive substances or to withdrawal from them after a period of regular ingestion. The terms *substance intoxication delirium* and *substance withdrawal delirium* are used to subsume such conditions in the APA DSM-IV (TR), © 2000 American Psychiatric Association.
7. *Organic mental syndrome not otherwise specified*

This scheme is based upon that of the American Psychiatric Association's Diagnostic and Statistical Manual of Mental Disorders (DSM-III-R). Washington, DC: American Psychiatric Association, 1994, now superseded by the APA DSM-IV (Text Revision), © 2000, American Psychiatric Associaton.

organic mercury cerebellar degeneration See **Minamata disease.**

organization The degree to which physiological EEG rhythms conform to certain hypothesized ideal characteristics displayed by a proportion of subjects in the same age group, free from a personal and family history of neurological and psychiatric diseases, and free also from other illnesses that might be associated with dysfunction of the brain.

The organization of physiological EEG rhythms progresses from birth to adulthood. Poor organization of such EEG rhythms as the alpha rhythm does not necessarily imply abnormality. (From Chatrian GE, Bergamini L, Dondey M, et al. A glossary of terms most commonly used by clinical electroencephalographers. *EEG Clin Neurophysiol* 1974;**37**:538–48,[989] with permission from Elsevier Science.)

organoid nevus syndrome A disorder of neuroectodermal proliferation characterized by unilateral facial linear sebaceous nevi and neurological manifestations such as asymmetrical macrocephaly, hemiparesis,

seizures, cognitive impairment, developmental delay, and focal or lateralized EEG abnormalities of the hypsarrhythmia or Lennox-Gastaut types, all appearing and progressing after birth.[1042]

orgasmic epilepsy Nocturnal somatosensory seizures arising from a central parietal focus and leading to complaints (?) of orgasm.[873]

orgasmic headache See **headache associated with sexual activity.**

Orgogozo scale A simple, brief, and rather reliable method of estimating the impairments suffered by patients with stroke (see Chart O–4).[4258] See also **stroke scales.**

Chart O–4. The Orgogozo Scale

Consciousness

15 Normal; awake and responsive to stimuli
10 Drowsiness; can be woken to remain awake through examination
5 Stupor; localizes and responds to painful stimuli
0 Coma; nonpurposeful response to painful stimuli

Verbal communication

10 Normal/not restricted; can sustain informative conversation
5 Difficult; limited to essential ideas, dysarthria included
0 Extremely difficult/impossible, for any reason

Eyes and headshift

10 Normal symmetrical horizontal eye movements
5 Gaze failure/unilateral neglect; gaze restricted on one side
0 Forced/tonic deviation; unable to gaze beyond midline

Facial movements

5 Normal/slight weakness; only minimal asymmetry at most
0 Paralysis, or marked paresis

Arm raising

10 Possible; can raise above horizontal against some resistance
5 Incomplete; only against gravity, not horizontally
0 Impossible; arm abduction impossible

Hand movements

15 Normal; no disability
10 Skilled; restriction of fine movements, slow/clumsy use
5 Useful; gross movements possible, can hold a walking stick
0 Useless; cannot hold or carry objects even if the hand moves

Arm tone

5 Normal/near normal
0 Severe spasticity or flaccidity

Leg raising

15 Normal; can be elevated from bed almost as other side
10 Possible against resistance; can be elevated, but weak
 5 Possible against gravity; not against resistance
 0 Impossible; cannot be lifted off bed

Foot dorsiflexion

10 Possible against resistance; even if weaker than normal
 5 Possible against gravity; can raise tip of foot off floor
 0 Foot drop; active dorsiflexion impossible

Leg tone

5 Normal/near normal
0 Overt spasticity or flaccidity
Total (out of 100)

From Orgogozo JM. Evaluation of treatments in ischemic stroke patients. In: Amery WK, Bousser MG, Rose FC, eds. Clinical Trial Methodology in Stroke, *pp 35–53. London: Baillière Tindall, 1989. Reproduced by kind permission of Elsevier Science.*

orientation   (Fr, to determine the east) Positioning oneself in space and, by extension, with relation to other people, places, structures or events.

ornithinemia   See **HHH syndrome.**

ornithine transcarbylamase deficiency   (OTC deficiency) A congenital intermittent ataxic syndrome inherited as an X-linked dominant trait and characterized by the accumulation of circulating neurotoxins, hyperammonemia, and low levels of citrulline and orotic aciduria, due to deficiency of OTC, a mitochondrial urea cycle enzyme. Urinary orotic acid levels are high; blood levels of glutamine and alanine are high, but those of citrulline, arginine, and argininosuccinic acid are normal.[390,880] The responsible gene maps to chromosome Xp21.1.

Clinically, lethargy, ataxia, vomiting, migraine-like headaches, ptosis, dysarthria, involuntary movements, seizures, and confusion occur from early infancy, with liver failure precipitated by dietary protein and fever. The children are mentally retarded. Cerebral atrophy and edema are noted terminally.

In a *variant* incomplete form, similar features present only in later childhood.

ornithosis   See **psittacosis.**

orobuccolingual dyskinesia   (orofacial dyskinesia) The occurrence of complex and often asymmetrical facial, oral, and lingual contortions including grimaces, tongue protrusion, licking movements, mouth opening, and vocalization.[2026]

The movements may represent a form of **tardive dyskinesia,** may occur spontaneously in the edentulous aged, and may be found in the context of various structural disorders of the basal ganglia.[130]

orofacial apraxia   Impairment in performing mouth or face actions on verbal command or imitation.[3138] See **apraxia, buccofacial apraxia.**

orofacial dyskinesia   See **orobuccolingual dyskinesia.**

orofaciodigital dysostosis   See **orofaciodigital syndrome** (1).

orofaciodigital syndrome   Inherited dysmorphic syndromes of three similar kinds (Chart O–5).

Chart O–5. The Orofaciodigital Syndromes

Orofaciodigital syndrome (orofaciodigital dysostosis) An X-linked dominant syndrome, lethal in males, characterized by high-arched palate and sometimes a hypoplastic mandible, polydactyly, syndactyly, brachydactyly, lobulation of the tongue, conductive deafness, facial and palatal clefts, lingual hamartomas, polycystic kidneys, alopecia, hydrocephalus, porencephaly, agenesis of the corpus callosum, and mental retardation.[334, 2220]

Orofaciodigital syndrome 2 (Mohr syndrome, Mohr-Majewski syndrome, acrofacial dysostosis) A recessively inherited dysmorphic syndrome characterized by high-arched palate, cleft lip, hypoplastic mandible, polydactyly, syndactyly, brachydactyly, lobulation and hamartomas of the tongue, conductive deafness, tibial hypoplasia, the **Dandy-Walker malformation, hydrocephalus,** and mental and developmental delay.[336,3938]

Orofaciodigital syndrome 3 A form characterized by facial dysmorphisms, lobulated tongue, mental retardation, myoclonus, skeletal abnormalities, and often abnormal eye movements.[5406]

orolingual tardive dyskinesia   A form of **tardive dyskinesia** in which there is involvement of the mouth and tongue.[2026]

oromandibular dysfunction   A collective term for abnormalities of dental occlusion and of the temporomandibular joints, which involves **bruxism.**

oromandibular dystonia   (Meige syndrome) A form of focal uni- or bilateral dystonia of unknown cause in which repetitive, strong, spasmodic contractions affect the masticatory muscles and thus the mouth, jaw, and tongue.[5478,5567] See **Brueghel syndrome.**

oropharyngeal palsy   See **Miller Fisher syndrome.**

Oroya fever   (Carrión disease, bartonellosis, verruga peruana, sitki) An infectious disease caused by *Bartonella bacilliformis* and transmitted by the bite of sandflies. Hemolytic anemia with vasculitis, disseminated hemorrhages, and meningoencephalitis are the major features. Clinically, these lead to acute fever, headache, and myalgias which are typically intense, and to vertigo, seizures, delirium, visual and auditory deficits, cranial and spinal nerve palsies, and frequently death.

The transmission and nature of the disease were determined by Carrión, a Peruvian medical student, who died as a direct result of his research.[5629]

orphan diseases   Rare conditions that are potentially susceptible to treatment, if economic factors allow the commercial search for it.

Orshansky sign   The knee-angle phenomenon in tabes.[4262]

ortho- (Gr, straight). Prefix denoting straight.

orthochromatic leukodystrophy (pigmented or-thochromatic leukodystrophy) A rare, sporadic or dominantly or recessively inherited dementing syndrome of adults presenting with initial depression, behavioral disorder, and inability to function prior to the appearance of severe dementia.

Pathologically, the findings include severe homologous demyelination, axonal loss, and gliosis in cerebral white matter, sparing the brainstem and cerebellum. Abundant lipofuscin granules are found in the microglia, macrophages, and astrocytes.[3101] See **leukodystrophy.**

orthodromic (Gr, straight + run) Propagation of an impulse in the direction which is the same as that of physiologic conduction—for example, conduction along sensory nerve fibers toward the spinal cord or of motor fibers away from it and toward the muscle innervated. cf. **antidromic.**

orthoses Devices for straightening limbs, preventing contractures, stabilizing joints (*static orthoses*), or assisting weak muscles to improve functional capacity (*dynamic orthoses*).

orthostatic headache Headache occurring on attaining the upright position, usually because of resultant intracranial hypotension (<6 mm water) in the presence of CSF hypovolemia.[1033] Spinal surgery including shunting, lumbar puncture, cranial trauma, dehydration, diabetic coma, uremia, infection, pseudo-Chiari malformations, skull-base tumors, and sexual intercourse have been noted as associated. See **idiopathic intracranial hypotension.**

orthostatic hypotension Reduction in arterial blood pressure on attaining the upright posture. Numerous criteria have been suggested.[4560] A typical example is a consistent and persistent fall of 30 mmHg or more in the systolic pressure and 15 mmHg or more in the diastolic pressure, accompanied by clinical symptoms (on attaining the upright position).

A fall of 30 mmHg systolic or of 20 mmHg mean blood pressure has also been considered sufficient for this diagnosis. See **progressive autonomic failure.**

orthostatic tremor (primary orthostatic tremor, shaky legs syndrome) A clinical syndrome seen in elderly people, characterized by a feeling of unsteadiness when standing (but not when walking, sitting, or lying) and rapid, regular, and asynchronous quiverings of the legs and trunk, especially when the subject is standing quietly. Patients often show evidence of essential tremor, of which this is considered by some to be a *forme fruste.* Other complaints include leg cramps and dystonia.[2516]

Electrophysiological findings are of rapid (frequency around 16 Hz), fast-firing burst discharges causing regular leg tremor in weight-bearing muscles, presumed to be generated by a central oscillator. It is not influenced by peripheral feedback and is synchronous between homologous leg muscles. The fast frequency of this muscle activity causes unsteadiness when standing (presumably due to partially fused muscle contraction), but only a fine ripple of muscle activity is visible. EMG studies show burst activity at 13–18 Hz in weight-bearing muscles. The major differences from essential tremor are the frequency of electromyographic burst firing, the invariable involvement of lower limb and paraspinal muscles, and the task-specific nature of the tremor in orthostatic tremor.[3781]

Ortner, N. (1865–1935) Austrian professor of medicine at Vienna.

Ortner syndrome (cardiovocal syndrome) Compression of the left recurrent laryngeal nerve by an enlarged left atrium, leading to dysphonia.[4264]

Orzechowski syndrome Opsoclonus, incapacitating postural tremor and fever, sometimes with signs suggesting encephalitis, complicating a recent viral upper respiratory infection.

This is probably a form of **postinfectious encephalomyelitis.**[1075]

OSAS (**O**bstructive **S**leep **A**pnea **S**yndrome) Collapse of the pharynx and cessation of airflow while the diaphragm continues the breathing effort. See **obstructive sleep apnea syndrome.**

oscillations (saccadic oscillations) Repetitive involuntary ocular **saccades** without intervening slow phases, thus differing from **nystagmus.**

Dell'Osso[1368] reviewed the following varieties: **convergence-retraction "nystagmus"; double saccadic pulses; dynamic overshoot; flutter dysmetria; macro-saccadic oscillations; macro-square-wave jerks; ocular bobbing; ocular dipping; ocular dysmetria; ocular flutter; ocular myoclonus; opsoclonus; psychogenic flutter; saccadic lateropulsion; saccadic double pulses; saccadic pulses; square-wave jerks; superior oblique myokymia;** and **voluntary "nystagmus."**

oscillopsia A subjective illusion of the rhythmic movement of the surrounding stationary world. This may be horizontal, vertical, or oblique and may vary.

It is the result of movement disorders affecting one or both eyes, stemming from lesions affecting the visual, oculomotor, or vestibular systems; but it can also occur with mechanical displacement of an eye (*chewing oscillopsia*). When unilateral, **superior oblique myokymia** and **palatal myoclonus** are likely associations.[449]

Osler, Sir William (1849–1919) Canadian physician who trained at the University of Toronto and in Montreal at McGill University and after graduation, spent some years in Europe. On his return to Canada at the age of 25, he was made professor of the "Institutes of

Medicine" (physiology) at McGill and lectured on pathology and physiology with such success that he moved to the University of Pennsylvania and then 5 years later became the first professor of medicine at Johns Hopkins University in Baltimore. Here he established an institution that revolutionized the teaching of medicine in North America by combining the British tradition of bedside teaching with the European tradition of the coordination of the wards and the laboratories. He accepted the Regius Chair of Medicine at Oxford in 1904, where he was also curator of the Bodleian Library.

From Johns Hopkins he published *On Chorea and Choreiform Affections* (Philadelphia, 1884) and *The Cerebral Palsies of Children* (1889) and the first editions of his classic textbook, *The Principles and Practice of Medicine* (1892), in which 300 pages were devoted to neurological topics. He contributed many chapters on neurology to the textbooks of internal medicine edited by others. He also published the first or the best current accounts of intracerebral hemorrhage, cerebral embolism, meningitis, and acute infectious polyneuropathy, noted the relationship of chorea and (rheumatic) heart disease, and recognized that jaundice may predispose to athetosis (1894). He also contributed many clinical reports on other neurological subjects. In later life, he published his reflective books, *Aequanimitas* and *A Way of Life*, each of which had wide appeal as a result of their depiction of his own philosophy of medicine. He was described as "the greatest personality in Medicine at the time of his death" at Oxford in 1919.

See Bliss, M. *William Osler: A Life in Medicine.* Toronto: University Toronto Press 1999.[604a]

osmotic demyelination syndrome Cellular edema due to an osmotic gradient caused by extracellular fluid dilution (for example, that due to hyponatremia); it leads to extrusion of intracellular cations as a corrective response. If the hyponatremia is quickly corrected, then the extracellular hyperosmolarity may lead to cell damage, as is thought to underlie the demyelination of the cells of the basis pontis in **central pontine myelinolysis.**

osteitis deformans See **Paget disease.**

osteochondromuscular dystrophy See **Schwartz-Jampel syndrome.**

osteogenesis imperfecta (van der Hoeve syndrome, Ekman syndrome, Spurway syndrome, Lobstein syndrome, Eddowes syndrome) A dominantly inherited disorder of collagen which leads to thin, brittle, osteoporotic, and easily fractured long bones, abnormal teeth, loose ligaments, and a tendency for the sclerotics to show a blue tinge.

Neurological complications include hydromyelia and communicating hydrocephalus; myelopathy due to

spinal deformity; macrocephaly; basilar invagination with brainstem compression; seizures; conductive deafness; spina bifida, platyspondyly, thin calvarium; and the consequences of accelerated atherosclerosis.[985] Arachnodactyly, syndactyly, keratoconus, cataracts, growth retardation, and osteopenia are other features described. The condition was first described in Sweden in 1788.[2219]

osteoglophonic dwarfism syndrome A congenital dysmorphic syndrome characterized by short stature, dental and metaphyseal deformities, craniosynostosis, and enlargement of the sella turcica.[432]

osteomalacic myopathy An acquired proximal myopathy characterized by muscle and bone pain, proximal muscle weakness without wasting, and normal serum creatine kinase levels but with typically myopathic muscle biopsy and EMG findings, occurring in patients with osteomalacia from any cause, except the X-linked form of type 1 hypophosphatemic rickets. Muscle biopsy and EMG findings are typically myopathic. The unusual finding in myopathy of retained brisk muscle stretch reflexes is characteristic here.[3301,3646]

osteopetrosis (Albers-Schönberg disease, marblebones) A rare recessively (rarely dominantly) transmitted condition manifesting generalized sclerosis of bone with thickening of cortical and spongy bone as well as increased fragility; hepatosplenomegaly, anemia, throbocytopenia, and susceptibility to infections; and thickening of the skull base, macrocephaly, and frontal bossing.

Neurological consequences may include optic atrophy with blindness, nystagmus, deafness, hydrocephalus, strabismus, facial palsy, intracranial hemorrhage, headache, mental retardation, seizures, basal ganglia calcification, and involvement of cranial nerves I and V.[3085,3124]

Variant forms are listed in Chart O–6.

Chart O–6. Variant Forms of Osteopetrosis

A type in which renal tubular acidosis and cerebral calcifications are associated[5210]

Osteoporosis, pseudoglioma, and mental retardation A congenital syndrome characterized by joint laxity, osteoporosis with multiple fractures, cloudy corneas, microphthalmia, pseudoglioma of the retina, blindness, and mental and developmental delay.

Acro-osteolysis with osteoporosis (Hajdu-Cheney syndrome) A congenital dysmorphic syndrome characterized by basilar impression, optic atrophy, and abnormal skull shape.[5910]

Oculodento-osseous dysplasia A congenital dysmorphic syndrome characterized by microphthalmia, syndactyly, and cranial hyperostosis with a tendency to cranial and spinal nerve palsy as a result of compression.[433]

osteophyte Ossified portions of the intervertebral disks which splay out posterolaterally, thus tending to impinge on the spinal nerves and the spinal cord.

osteoporosis   Low bone mass and microarchitectural deterioration of bone tissue, leading to enhanced bone fragility and consequent increase in fracture risk.[5953] Dual energy X-ray absorptiometry scanning is the best investigative tool allowing a confident diagnosis.

Steroid, phenobarbitone, and dilantin therapy and immobility resulting from any paretic disorder are the more important potential causes of interest to neurologists, and both bone pain and fractures as a result of falling are the more common consequences.[3448]

osteosclerosis fragilis   See **Albers-Schönberg disease.**

osteosclerosis-microcephaly-cataracts   A congenital syndrome characterized by cataract, congenital cardiac anomaly, microcephaly, and multiple fractures.[337]

osteosclerotic myeloma   See **POEMS.**

Österreichische Gesellschaft zur Bekämpfung der Muskelkrankheiten   A member society of the European Alliance of Muscular Dystrophy Societies. Address: Lazarettgasse 14, Postfach 23, A-097, Vienna, Austria.

Ostrum-Furst syndrome   The association of platybasia, congenital synostosis of the neck, and Sprengel deformity of the shoulder with mild facial weakness and some disturbances of the arm reflexes, reported in 1942.[1563,1996]

Osuntokun syndrome   Congenital asymbolia for pain (although the differentiation between sharp and dull sensations is retained) and auditory imperception of the significance of spoken words, without deafness.[4273]

Ota syndrome   See **nevus of Ota.**

otitic hydrocephalus   (sinus thrombosis causing intracranial hypertension) A syndrome of raised intracranial pressure with headache and often vomiting and diplopia, bilateral papilledema, normal ventricular size, and a normal neurological examination except for sixth nerve palsy, occurring as a result of thrombosis of the lateral dural venous sinuses following otitis media. The findings would be similar for thrombosis of the superior sagittal sinus, which is less common.

The condition is classed as a variety of **idiopathic intracranial hypertension.**[1902] It was first described by Quincke,[4559] but this term was introduced (and later withdrawn) by Sir Charles **Symonds.**

otoconia   Crystals of calcium carbonate within the utricles, floating in the endolymph and thus sensitive to gravitational forces. When they settle in the cupula of the posterior semicircular canal, they may be responsible for causing position-related sensations of imbalance by stimulating the hair cells also within the fluid.

otofaciocervical syndrome   A congenital dysmorphic syndrome, characterized also by skeletal deformi-

ties, conductive deafness, winged scapulae, and mental and developmental delay.[4360]

otolithic catastrophe   Acute episodes of vertigo with abrupt atonia and falling, without loss of consciousness, considered to reflect an undetermined inner ear disorder.[5665]

otoliths   Small calciferous granules in the semicircular canals of the inner ear. Their gravitational effect upon the hair cells leads to afferent responses signalling acceleration in the various dimensions of space.

otopalatodigital syndrome   A recessively inherited dysmorphic syndrome characterized by dwarfism, broad nasal root, hypertelorism, frontal and occipital bossing, small mandible, cleft palate, digital anomalies, abnormal bony ossification, conductive deafness, and mental and motor delay.[1540] See **Taybi syndrome.**

otosclerosis   A dominantly inherited syndrome with variable penetrance, characterized by the onset of slowly progressive conductive symmetrical hearing loss of variable severity in the second or third decade, with tinnitus but normal vestibular responses.[3124]

outliers   Motor unit action potentials that have values for amplitude, duration, or number of phases far outside the mean; their analysis provides information of diagnostic value in both neuropathic and myopathic muscle diseases.[5312]

out-of-phase signals   Two waves of opposite phases.

oval pupils   A transient sign of damage to the oculomotor nerve or nucleus in the setting of acute, severe intracranial vascular disease. As a result of this there is nonuniform paresis of the sphincter pupillae.[1851]

overbreathing   See **hyperventilation.**

overflow myoclonus   See **ballistic movement overflow myoclonus.**

overlap myasthenic syndrome   The coexistence of **myasthenia gravis** and **Lambert-Eaton myasthenic syndrome.**[4213]

overlap neuropathy   The coalescence of the areas of motor or sensory deficit resulting from multiple mononeuropathies, which may give the appearance of a peripheral polyneuropathy at first sight. See **vasculitic neuropathy.**

overlap syndrome   1. (polymyositis or dermatomyositis associated with connective tissue disorder) The concurrence of signs of polymyositis or dermatomyositis with evidence of one of the connective tissue disorders, such as systemic lupus erythematosus, mixed connective tissue disease, rheumatoid arthritis, **Sjögren syndrome**, rheumatic fever, or progressive systemic sclerosis. The only clinical difference from typical polymyositis is the frequent concurrence of sclerodactyly and Raynaud phenomenon.[3687] 2. A vasculitis in which the features combine those of **polyarteritis nodosa, allergic angiitis,** and **granulomatosis** and **hypersensitivity vasculitis.**[1750]

overuse syndromes (repetitive overuse syndrome, repetition strain syndrome) Injuries presumed to be caused by the cumulative effects on tissues of repetitive physical stress that exceeds physiological limits. These usually affect the muscle-tendon unit in the arms, and are common in, for example, musicians, but spinal and other joint disease, pulmonary disease, nerve entrapment syndromes, and dystonias are other examples.[3312,3450]

Oxford stroke classification   Four clinically identifiable subgroups of cerebral infarction: large anterior circulation infarcts with both cortical and subcortical involvement with a large or medium-sized cortical infarct or a large subcortical infarct in middle cerebral arterial (MCA) territory (total anterior circulation infarcts, TACI); restricted and predominantly cortical infarcts or a large subcortical infarct in anterior cerebral arterial (ACA) or MCA territories (partial anterior circulation infarcts, PACI); infarcts clearly associated with the vertebrobasilar arterial territory (posterior circulation infarcts, POCI); and small infarcts confined to the territory of the deep perforating arteries (lacunar infarcts, LACI).[324,5843]

5-oxoprolinemia (glutathionine synthetase deficiency) A diffuse encephalopathy due to a deficiency of glutathione synthetase and characterized by metabolic acidosis with mental retardation and increased urinary excretion of 5-oxoproline.[5912]

oxycephaly (Gr, sharp + head) 1. A congenital deformity of the skull, which is high and conical from too early closure of the posterior part of the sagittal, the metopic, or the sagittal and both coronal sutures, such that it resembles a wedge with the long axis lying above the sagittal suture. The term was first used by Aristophanes. The *tête en poire* of King Louis XVI was presumably caused in this way. Increased intracranial pressure, optic atrophy, and exophthalmos are commonly found. 2. A late-appearing synostosis affecting the coronal sutures and leading to recession of the supraorbital rim backward, including the forehead, and to elevation of the top of the head.

In *harmonious oxycephaly*, the suture is fused but the shape of the head remains normal.

oxytocin   A hormone secreted by the magnocellular cells in the supraoptic and paraventricular nuclei of the posterior pituitary.

P

P 300 evoked potential A high-amplitude, positive waveform (an event-related potential) of limbic origin, recorded over the parietal regions following detection of a sensory event in any channel for which the individual has been primed. The waveform increases in latency and diminishes in amplitude with age and in dementing states.[2193]

Pacchioni, Antonio (1665–1726) Italian professor of anatomy at Rome, who in 1705 described the granulations named for him, and who described the anatomy of the meninges in 1724. He erred in considering the granulations to have lymphatic functions[5204] and was corrected by Fantoni in 1738.

Pacchionian granulation seizures A syndrome of uncertain validity, reported as occurring in early life and characterized by focal convulsions beginning in the leg or shoulder which occur chronically over many years without associated neurological signs. Anomalous pacchionian granulations extending into the precentral gyrus or primary motor areas are considered to be the cause.

The original description recounted the performance of an operation to divide the anomalous granulations; an attendant reduction in seizure frequency was claimed.[4939]

Pacchionian granulations The larger arachnoid villi projecting into the superior sagittal sinus, constituting a lock on the "canal" of CSF circulation and filtering the CSF from the subarachnoid space to the venous circulation. Hypertrophy of the granulations is described secondary to raised CSF pressure, sometimes producing local lytic lesions of the overlying skull. The radiological differences from sagittal sinus thrombosis have been listed; the occurrence of hypertrophic granulations in the lateral transverse sinuses, normal dural sinus blood flow, and local bony lysis are the most obvious distinguishing features.[2125]

Pace sign Resisted abduction of the thigh while the patient is seated or lying with the painful side up, and the painful leg semiflexed. The patient then abducts the thigh against slight resistance. Weakness, faltering, and reproduction of pain during resisted abduction and external rotation of the hip may be observed in the **piriformis syndrome.** (HJM)[409,4287]

Paced Auditory Serial Addition task A test of the efficiency of information processing in which the subject hears 60 single numbers presented at various speeds and is required to sum the last two numbers heard, over four trials. There is thus both a need to recall the previous number, adding it to the new one without distraction from the mental operation of successive addition.[2288] The test has been used particularly in patients with **postconcussional syndrome** and **multiple sclerosis.**

pachycephaly (Gr, thick + head) A rare craniofacial dysplasia in which there is hypoplasia and flattening of the occiput due to premature fusion of the lambdoid sutures, with or without the involvement of other sutures. When occurring alone, it is seldom of consequence.[4]

pachyencephalia Abnormal thickness of the vault of the skull.

pachygyria A developmental disorder due to abnormalities of neuronal migration, characterized by abnormally few, thickened and wide cerebral gyri, and the presence of histological abnormalities in the claustrum, medulla, and cerebellum. The condition is also associated with both **agyria** and **microgyria.**[2409]

pachymeninges (Gr, thick + membrane) The dura mater, the thicker meningeal covering of the brain which separates it from the skull and the spinal cord from the spine.

pachymeningitis A term (now seldom used) to refer to inflammation of the thicker outer coverings of the brain. *Pachymeningitis externa* is such inflammation resulting from local infection in the cranial bones; *pachymeningitis interna* is due to infections spreading outwards from the arachnoid; *pachymeningitis serosa* is the term for a subdural serous effusion. *Pachymeningitis hemorrhagica interna* (Virchow) represents a subdural hematoma and *pachymeningitis externa spinalis* or *peripachymeningitis* constitutes an inflammatory process (usually syphilitic) occurring outside and around the spinal dura mater, sometimes causing hyperplasia and secondary compression of the nerve roots or the spinal cord.

Syphilis, sarcoidosis, and tuberculosis are the most common identified causes, and headaches, cranial nerve palsies, and ataxia are the leading clinical features, along with inflammatory changes in the CSF. In *idiopathic intracranial pachymeningitis*, no cause is found.[3684]

A local form also occurs in the **superior orbital fissure syndrome** (Tolosa-Hunt syndrome). Inflammation of the other meninges may be referred to as **arachnoiditis** or as **leptomeningitis,** but meningeal inflammation usually affects all three layers, at least to some extent.

pachymeningitis cervicalis hypertrophica Thickening of all the meninges in the cervical region as a result of **meningovascular syphilis.**

pachymeningitis externa See **spinal epidural abscess.**

pachymeningitis hemorrhagica interna See **chronic subdural hematoma.**

Pacini, Filippo (1812–1883) Italian anatomist who re-described the sensory organs described by Vater, but now bearing his name.

Pacinian corpuscles   The sensory endings of some cutaneous and other nerves, which had been mentioned by Vater a century before their description by Pacini, although the data had been lost.[5204] They are widely distributed in the skin, especially of the hands and feet, but are also found in the periosteum, the joints, and many other areas. Steady mechanical pressure leads to a rapidly adapting response, although they were at first thought (by **Adrian**) to be organs for signalling static pressure.

pack palsy   See **rucksack palsy.**

PADL   See **Performance of Activities of Daily Living test.**

Page syndrome   Blotchy red areas on the face, neck, and upper trunk, seen usually in young women who are embarrassed. Other sympathetic evidence of anxiety, including transient elevations of blood pressure, may accompany the rash.[4292]

The condition has been elevated beyond its dignity by the term *hypertensive diencephalic syndrome*; the latter term is also used for **Penfield syndrome,** which is an accepted entity with a few similar features.

Paget disease   (osteitis deformans) A dominantly inherited disease with variable penetrance, characterized by variable degeneration and regeneration of the membrane bones of the skull and of the bones of the limbs. The condition is manifested in later life and leads to bony softening, overgrowth, and deformity due to absorption and rarefaction, and sometimes to sarcomatous change.

Compression of nervous tissue at cranial or spinal levels results in a proportion of cases, leading to deafness, hemifacial spasm, trigeminal neuralgia, pyramidal signs resulting from basilar invagination, or myelopathy.[1045] Basilar impression may also cause other cranial nerve palsies, compression of the cerebellum and medulla, and hydrocephalus with dementia, while shallow orbits may be responsible for proptosis. Paget described the disease in 1876.[3124]

Paget, Sir James   (1814–1899) English surgeon.

pagophagia   Ice eating, a form of pica which may indicate an iron deficiency state. (HJM)

pain   1. An unpleasant subjective sensory and emotional experience associated with or described in terms of actual or potential tissue damage. Varieties can be classified as *neuropathic, nocioceptive,* or *psychogenic.*[4493] 2. A localized form of sorrow (Spinoza).

Pain   The Journal of the International Association for the Study of Pain, published by Elsevier. Web site: http://www.halcyon.com/iasp/journal.html.

pain asymbolia   (insensitivity to pain) The term of Schilder for loss of the psychic reaction to pain despite retention of the sensation of painful stimuli.[2858,4963]

pain asymbolia with auditory imperception   See **congenital pain asymbolia.**

pain density   A measure of the severity of chronic pain, in which numerical values are assigned to severity and frequency and are then multiplied to yield a score.[176]

pain disorder   A persistent syndrome in which pain is appreciated despite the absence of continuing demonstrable pathology considered adequate to cause it, and accompanied by behavioral chnages relevant to the perception.

DSM-IV diagnostic criteria are as follows:
A. Pain in one or more anatomical sites is the predominant focus of the clinical presentation and is of sufficient severity to warrant clinical attention.
B. The pain causes clinically significant distress or impairment in social, occupational, or other important areas of functioning.
C. Psychological factors are judged to have an important role in the onset, severity, exacerbation, or maintenance of the pain.
D. The symptom or deficit is not intentionally produced or feigned (as in factitious disorder or malingering).
E. The pain is not better accounted for by a mood, anxiety, or psychotic disorder and does not meet criteria for dyspareunia.

Code as follows:
307.80 **Pain disorder associated with psychological factors:** psychological factors are judged to have the major role in the onset, severity, exacerbation, or maintenance of the pain.
307.89 **Pain disorder associated with both psychological factors and a general medical condition:** both psychological factors and a general medical condition are judged to have important roles in the onset, severity, exacerbation, or maintenance of the pain.

Reprinted by kind permission from American Psychiatric Association, *Diagnostic and Statistical Manual of Mental Disorders,* 4th ed. (DSM-IV TR).[150] Washington, DC: © American Psychiatric Association, 2000. See DSM-IV TR for full criteria.

pain reflex   Dilation of the pupil in response to painful stimuli. See **ciliospinal reflex.**

pain spots   Areas in the skin where pain can be appreciated, surrounded by areas in which it cannot. The existence of such places was proposed by **von Frey,** but the idea was discredited by those who did not try hard enough to find them.

Paine syndrome   (hypoplasia of the cerebellum and pons) An X-linked syndrome of recessive microcephaly, seizures, psychomotor retardation, various skeletal deformities, and spasticity occurring in the presence of brainstem and cerebellar hypoplasia and accompanied by generalized aminoaciduria.[2439,4297]

Paine-Efron syndrome   A spinocerebellar degeneration characterized by the onset of mild but slowly progressive cerebellar signs in childhood or adult life. Diffuse telangiectasia or pigmented nevi also appear but the other features of **Louis-Bar syndrome** are not found.[4298]

painful arms and moving fingers A syndrome of pain in the arm with discontinuous, involuntary, irregular, repetitive contractions of the small hand muscles, producing a writhing, pseudoathetotic appearance, described in the setting of brachial plexus neuritis following radiotherapy[5750] or following relatively slight arm trauma.

painful feet See **burning feet syndrome.**

painful jumping amputation stumps See **stump spasm.**

painful legs and moving toes A chronic syndrome characterized by deep, pulling, gnawing, or aching pains of variable severity in the feet or legs, accompanied by spontaneous, purposeless, wriggling movements of the toes. The pain is worsened by movement but is sometimes relieved temporarily by sympathetic block.[5281]

The underlying pathology is not understood, but the phenomenon has been recorded after root or nerve lesions, following minor trauma to the legs, and with lateral plantar nerve lesions. The nature of the central or peripheral cause is at present unknown.

Along with **painful arms and moving fingers,** this condition should probably be subsumed under the heading of *painful limbs and moving digits.* See also **cramp-fasciculation syndrome.**

painful lumbar plexopathy A syndrome of painful deficits in lumbar or sacral regions associated with an elevated erythrocyte sedimentation rate (ESR) and cuffing of epineurial blood vessels by mixed inflammatory cells on sural nerve biopsy specimens, in the absence of other evidence of an autoimmune disorder and of vasculitis or cancer.[699] See also **idiopathic lumbosacral plexopathy.**

painful ophthalmoplegia syndrome See **superior orbital fissure syndrome.**

painful penile erections Awakenings from rapid eye movement sleep periods occasioned by painful sensations resulting from normal rapid eye movement sleep–related penile erections.[2930,3705] (See also Chart S–6 and ASDA Diagnostic Classification,[234] **sleep disorders.**)

painful sensory neuropathy with antisulfatide antibodies See **immune mediated neuropathies.**

painless legs and moving toes The occurrence of painless semicontinuous involuntary movements of the toes of the foot similar to those seen in **painful legs and moving toes**. EMG and nerve conduction studies show only a predominant co-contraction of the foot flexors and extensors at 0.6–1.2 Hz in a pattern sometimes seen in painful legs and moving toes. The etiology is undetermined.[5835a]

painless whitlows (panaris analgésique de Morvan) Infection of the terminal parts of the digits in limbs that lost their thin-fiber sensory innervation, as in **hereditary sensory and autonomic neuropathy** or **syringomyelia.**

paintbrush sign The myelographic appearance in the case of extradural compression at the level of the cauda equina. The column of contrast becomes less and less homogeneous as it is followed from above downward to the level of the compression; the dye is drawn out into vertical lines similar to those left by a paintbrush, its paint progressively yielded up to the surface along which it is drawn.

painter's palsy Radial nerve palsy. See **lead palsy.**

paint-sniffer's encephalopathy (glue-sniffer's neuropathy) An irreversible syndrome resulting from long-term toluene inhalation and characterized by cerebellar ataxia, tremor, and cognitive defects, and by disturbances in very long–chain fatty acid metabolism.[2652]

Paired Associated Learning test A traditional test of new learning, in which subjects are required to associate the two words of a pair presented, so that, when one is given after an interval, the other will be recalled and reproduced. The test is sensitive to early changes in short-term memory function.[5888,5889]

paired discharge Two action potentials occurring consistently in the same relationship with each other. Compare with **double discharge.**[146]

paired stimuli Two consecutive stimuli delivered in a time-locked fashion. The time interval between the two stimuli and the intensity of each stimulus can be varied but should be specified. The first stimulus is called the *conditioning stimulus* and the second stimulus is the *test stimulus*. The conditioning stimulus may modify tissue excitability, which is then evaluated by the response to the test stimulus. (From the 2001 Report of the Nomenclature Committee of the American Association of Electromyography and Electrodiagnosis.[10] Used by permission, copyright © 2001, AAEM.)

Pal, Jakob Budapest physician and neuropathologist who with Weigert introduced a staining reaction for myelinated fibers.

palatal fricative A consonant made by partially blocking the air flow between the palate and tongue, causing air turbulence and resulting in a sound; for example, /sh/ as in shoe.[3505]

palatal myoclonus (bulbar myoclonus, myoclonique de la calotte, palatal myokymia, palatal tremor, oculopalatal myoclonus) An uncommon irreversible, involuntary movement disorder characterized by continuous, rapid, regular, and rhythmic quivering of the soft palate, larynx, and other structures derived from the embryonic branchial arches (face, neck, and diaphragm) occurring at about 10 Hz and probably due to denervation hypersensitivity of the inferior olive. The movements persist in sleep. Audible clicks may be the presenting symptom.[2318,3703] **Ocular bobbing** may accompany the palatal movements,[6065] in which case the condition is known as **oculopalatal myoclonus.**

Despite the name, this is not true myoclonus at all, but is a form of **myokymia.** The pathology is usually infarction involving the **Guillain-Mollaret triangle,** particularly the contralateral inferior olivary nuclei, which may be hypertrophic.

Variants include the following:

Palatal myoclonus and ataxia A dominantly inherited syndrome with adult onset characterized by dysarthria, branchial (palatal) myoclonus, nystagmus, ataxia, and spastic paraparesis.[1429]

Complicated palatal myoclonus A progressive, dominaantly inherited disorder with onset in the third decade, characterized clinically by palatal myoclonus, ataxia, bulbar weakness, and spastic quadriparesis and pathologically by the presence of **Rosenthal fibers** and myelin loss. Differentiation from the last entry is speculative.[2668]

palatal myokymia   See **palatal myoclonus.**

palatal tremor   See **palatal myoclonus.**

palatopalpebral reflex   Blinking in response to palatal stimulation, described by Imperartori in 1930. See **palpebral reflex.**

palencephalography   (Gr, to shake + the brain) A technique for recording cephalic vibrations at 1–20 Hz in an attempt to localize intracranial lesions.[345] It is now superseded by more precise methods.

paleo-   (Gr, ancient).

paleocerebellar syndrome   Ataxic gait, limb ataxia, and disturbance of postural reflexes with muscle hypotonia, due to a lesion of the anterior lobe of the cerebellum.[292]

paleocerebellum   The anterior lobe of the cerebellum, consisting of the vermis and the paravermian cortex.

paleocerebrum   The second oldest part of the cerebellum (the archicerebellum is phylogenetically more ancient), differentiated from the **neocerebrum** by **Edinger** in 1885.

paleostriatal syndrome   See **dyssynergia cerebellaris myoclonica.**

paleostriatum   The globus pallidus, caudate, and putamen situated lateral to the internal capsule.

paligraphia   (Gr, again + to write) Perseveratory writing of a word or phrase that has already been written once.[1178]

palilalia   (from Gr, again + language) 1. The phenomenon whereby the patient repeats the last word or two of a verbal statement, the words trailing off in a diminuendo fashion and with increasing rapidity.[1172]

2. Repetition by the patient of a phrase spoken by the examiner, with or without a change in pronoun; a morbid, obsessive, involuntary reiteration of spoken words, both spontaneously and in reply to questions. It is not heard when the patient recites or reads aloud, nor in singing.

The condition which **Brissaud** called *autoecholalia* is probably the same as palilalia, the name supplied in 1908 by **Souques** in a lecture to the Société de Neurologie in Paris.[5265] It is observed especially in demented patients, and in the settings of postencephalitic parkinsonism, paramedian thalamic infarcts, and diffuse cerebrovascular disease.

palilaliopraxia   See **signing tics.**

palilogia   An oratorical device whereby emphasis is attained by repetition.

palindromic   (from Gr, a running back) Relapsing.

palinesthesia   The persistence or recurrence of tactile sensations after the exciting stimulus has been withdrawn.

palinopsia   (paliopsia) (Gr, again + vision) The persistence or brief recurrence of a visual image for minutes or hours after the exciting stimulus has been extinguished. This may occur in either seeing or blind fields.

The phenomenon has been considered to be a form of release hallucination and suggests the presence of a structural lesion in the parieto-occipital cortex, but many other causes have been implicated.[4487] See also **visual perseveration, polyopia, allesthesia.**

paliopsia   See **palinopsia, visual perseveration.**

palipraxia   Complex hyperkinesias including psychomotor forms, in which small, patterned fragments of movement are performed stereotypically (patting the hands, touching or stroking objects, and so on), and others in which the movement appears to be a deliberate volitional action that is perseverated long after the initial stimulus has passed.

palipsychism   (from Gr, again + soul) The superimposition of mental activities that are normally processed sequentlially, such that a subject may offer biographical information while working on a calculation test.[2090]

pallanesthesia   Loss of the appreciation of vibration.

pallbearer's palsy   An upper brachial plexus lesion. See **rucksack palsy.**

pallesthesia   The appreciation of vibration. See **vibratory sensation.**

pallid breath-holding spells   See **breath-holding spells.**

pallidal atrophies   A group of hereditary or sporadic diseases characterized clinically by various movement disorders, including parkinsonism, chorea, and dystonia. They include **pure pallidal atrophy, pallidonigral degenerations,** and combinations of pallidal atrophy with other system degenerations.

pallidal degeneration   It is doubtful whether this condition exists as an entity separate from **pallidal atrophies** or from the next entries.[2094]

pallidal polyglucosan bodies in cerebral palsy   One of the group of **pallidonigral degenerations** in which cerebral palsy due to perinatal hypoxia presents in childhood with chorea and dystonia, accompanied by the finding of polyglucosan bodies in the neuronal cytoplasm of cells in the pallidum.[6059]

pallidoluysian atrophy   (pure pallidoluysian atrophy) A system degeneration presenting in adult life and characterized by generalized dystonia, dysarthria, loss of postural reflexes, gait disorder, supranuclear vertical gaze palsy, and bradykinesia without either tremor or rigidity.

Pathologically, atrophy of the lateral segment of the globus pallidus and that of the subthalamic nucleus are the only notable features.[6036]

pallidonigral degeneration with spinal muscular atrophy   One of the group of pallidonigral degenerations in which these two findings coincide.[5075]

pallidonigral degenerations   (idiopathic subcortical degenerations) A group of rare conditions united by this singular abnormality and their production of complicated akinetic-rigid syndromes. They include **dentatorubropallidoluysian degeneration, Hallervorden-Spatz disease, hereditary (holotopistic) striatal degeneration, idiopathic calcification of the basal ganglia, infantile neuroaxonal dystrophy, pallidal polyglucosan bodies in cerebral palsy,** and **pallidonigroluysian atrophy.**[2094]

Other *variants* are **pallidonigral degeneration with spinal muscular atrophy** and *amyotrophic lateral sclerosis with* **pallidonigroluysian atrophy.**[2094] See **motor neuronal diseases.**

pallidonigroluysian atrophy   One of the group of **pallidonigral degenerations** in which akinesia, rigidity, dystonia, tremor, and dementia appear sporadically in adults.

In some cases the picture resembles **progressive supranuclear palsy;** in others, **amyotrophic lateral sclerosis** has been associated.[2094] See **pallidonigral degenerations** (*variants*).

pallidopyramidal disease   See **juvenile parkinsonism syndrome.**

pallidostriatonigral degeneration   See **system degenerations, pallidonigroluysian atrophy.**

Pallister syndrome   An X-linked recessive, congenital dysmorphic syndrome manifesting also skeletal anomalies, seizures, pyramidal signs, and mental and developmental delay.[4307]

Pallister-Hall syndrome   See **Hall syndrome.**

Pallister-Hawes-Landon syndrome   A disorder due to vitamin B deficiency, probably identical to **Strachan syndrome.**

pallium   (Lat, cloak) The cerebral cortex, covering the rest of the brain like a cloak.[5204]

palmar grasp   See **palmar reflex, developmental reflexes.**

palmar reflex   (palmar grasp) Flexion of the fingers in response to gentle stroking of the palm of the hand. The sign is present at birth and normally disappears by 2 months of age. When enhanced, it forms the basis of the **grasp reflex.**

palmaris brevis sign   Wrinkling of the ulnar side of the palm due to retained contraction of the palmaris brevis, which is spared in the case of lesions of the ulnar nerve at the pisohamate ligament (Guyon's canal), but not with those at more proximal sites.[4462] A **palmaris brevis spasm syndrome** may accompany this.

palmaris brevis spasm syndrome   Isolated, spontaneous, brisk, tonic involuntary contractions of this muscle leading to dimpling of the ulnar side of the hand and usually seen in older males with proximal ulnar nerve or root lesions. The syndrome is benign and slowly progressive over years.[5072]

palmar-plantar erythrodysesthesia   A syndrome of dysesthesias and tenderness of the hands and feet with swelling and redness of the skin, described as a complication of 5-fluouracil therapy and usually responsive to pyridoxine.[326]

palmomental reflex   (Marinesco-Radovici reflex) Contraction of the mentalis muscle causing wrinkling of the chin with elevation and protrusion of the lower lip when the skin over the thenar eminence is scratched.[4642]

This is a nonspecific sign of diffuse cerebral dysfunction (although often detectable in infancy and in the normal elderly), first described by Marinesco and Radovici in 1930.

palmus   See **Bamberger disease.**

palpebra   Latin for "eyelids."

palpebral reflex   (menace reflex) Blinking in response to a variety of stimuli, such as loud noises, menace, bright lights, or sensory stimulation of the face or buccal mucosa. See **orbicularis oculi reflex.**

palpebromandibular synkinesis   (spontaneous corneomandibular reflex) A centrally initiated synkinesis characterized by the association of bilateral eyelid closure with anterolateral deviation of the mandible to the opposite side, in response to spontaneous eye-blinks, in patients with bilateral cerebral or brainstem disease.[4544,4545]

palpebro-oculogyric reflex   See **Bell phenomenon.**

palsy   (derived from Middle English, *parlesie*, and from French, *paralysie*[5204]) Lack of power, paralysis.

Palthe reflex   Arrest of respiratory and swallowing movements in response to cold stimulation of structures supplied by the second division of the fifth cranial nerve, such as a sudden cold stimulus to the face. It is presumed to have a protective function that serves to discourage the ingestion of harmful substances into the pharynx.[4314]

pamplegia   (from Gr, all + a stroke) (panplegia) Generalized weakness following a stroke.

Pan-African Association of Neurological Sciences An organization seeking to further neurological sciences and the exchange of ideas for neurologists in Africa and worldwide. Address: P.O. Box 20413, Nairobi, Kenya. Web site: http://www.bioline.org.br/ns.

panaris   French for "whitlow."

panaris analgésique de Morvan   See **painless whitlows.**

panautonomic failure   See **pandysautonomia.**

Panayiotopoulos syndrome   A fairly common and benign form of childhood epilepsy characterized by the occurrence of clusters of seizures with ictal vomiting, deviation of the eyes, impaired consciousness, and progression sometimes to tonic clonic convulsions. The peak age of onset is 5 years; remission occurs usually within 2 years. Many of the attacks are nocturnal. The EEG shows **occipital spikes.**[4318] See also **childhood epilepsy with occipital paroxysms.**[485]

Pancoast, Henry Khunrath   (1875–1939) American radiologist and radiotherapist, occupant of the first American chair in radiology, at the University of Pennsylvania and the leader of that branch of the profession in his lifetime.

Pancoast syndrome   (Pancoast-Tobias-Ciuffini syndrome, Hare syndrome) A painful lower brachial plexopathy with an added **Horner syndrome** occurring as a result of infiltration of these nerve trunks by an apical carcinoma of the bronchus or other malignancy.[4320]

Pancoast-Tobias-Ciuffini syndrome   See **Pancoast syndrome.**

PANDAS   See **pediatric autoimmune neuropsychiatric disorders associated with streptococcal infection.**

pandiculation   (from Lat, to stretch oneself) A compound automatic movement consisting of extension of the legs, elevation and stretching of the arms, and extension of the head and trunk with yawning. It is generally physiological and related to drowsiness and waking, but may occur preceding a paroxysm of malaria.[4512]

Pandy test   A test for the concentration of globulin in the CSF; it is not of current value.

pandysautonomia   (panautonomic failure) 1. A syndrome of acquired failure of both sympathetic and parasympathetic functions; it is most often due to **multiple system atrophy, primary autonomic failure,** or **hereditary motor and sensory neuropathy, type 3** when slow in onset; the syndrome also occurs acutely in **acute inflammatory demyelinating polyneuropathy** and as a **paraneoplastic syndrome.** The pathogenesis is unknown. It occurs most commonly in adults and is characterized clinically by widespread autonomic failure involving the pupils, skin, and blood pressure, with added trigeminal and bulbar weakness, dysarthria, sensorimotor peripheral neuropathy, and spontaneous pain. See also **postural tachycardia syndrome, neurocardiogenic syncope, multiple system atrophy, familial amyloid neuropathy, diabetic neuropathy, Shy-Drager syndrome.** 2. Also described as pseudo-obstruction syndrome, heat intolerance. 3. A relationship to **chronic fatigue syndrome** is also suggested.

panoramic looking   Overall gaze that precedes seeing.[1398] Its pathway involves posterior parietal area 7, an area dominantly important in visual attention.

panoramic nystagmus   See **optokinetic nystagmus.**

panplegia   See **pamplegia.**

Pansini, Sergio   (1860–1918) Italian neurologist who trained at Naples and practiced there, eventually as professor of clinical semeiology. His publications covered numerous areas including myotonia, acromegaly, the innervation of the diaphragm, and infectious diseases.

Pansini syndrome   A cerebellar syndrome with marked dysarthria, reported as a complication of malaria.[4321]

pantanencephalia   (Gr, complete + absence + the brain) A synonym of **anencephaly.**

pantomime   Movements made for semiotic or referential purposes within the context of communicating information.[1169] Movements carried out in silence with strict deliberation in order to express an idea or feeling.[1172]

Disturbances in the comprehension of such activity are another result of damage to the dominant hemisphere.

pantomime agnosia   The ability to imitate pantomimes that are not comprehended, reported as accompanying amnesia and alexia and associated with a lesion of the inferior visual association cortex.[4816]

Panum's fusional area   That part of space encompassing the **horopter,** where binocular vision is preserved (although always containing points that have some retinal disparity).

Paper test   A test of verbal comprehension introduced by Pierre **Marie,** stated as follows: "Here are three papers, a big one, a medium-sized one and a small one. Take the biggest and rumple it up and throw it on the ground. Take the medium one and give it to me. Put the smallest one in your pocket."

Papez, James Wenceslaus (1883–1958) American neurophysiopsychologist at Cornell University, whose insights led to the realization of the functions of the limbic system in 1937.[4325] The "Papez circuit" (hippocampus–fornix–mammillary body–anterior nucleus of the thalamus–bundle of Vicq d'Azir–cingulate gyrus) is essentially synonymous with the limbic system.

papill- (Gr, projection) Prefix denoting projection.

papillary meningioma See **meningioma.**

papilledema (Lat, teat + Gr, swelling) Swelling of the optic nerve head due both to axonal swelling and the presence of extraaxonal fluid, and occurring as a result of increased intracranial pressure.[431] **Jackson** defined four stages (Chart P–1).

Chart P–1. The Four Stages of Papilledema

The *early* stage is characterized by blurring of the nerve fiber layer with indistinctness of the superior and inferior disk margins, retinal venous distension, loss of spontaneous venous pulsations, splinter hemorrhages in the nerve fiber layer at or close to the disk margin, and retention of the optic cup.

The *fully developed* stage consists of opacification of the nerve fiber layer, which prevents visualization of vessels crossing the rim of the disk; elevation and expansion of the disk, with an increase in the size of the blindspot; flame hemorrhages; infarcts of the nerve fiber layer; retinal edema (**macular star**); marked venous distention; and hyperemia of the disk.

In the *chronic* stage, the optic cup is obliterated and the disk takes on the shape of a button mushroom, surrounded often by hard exudates.

Eventually the disk becomes gliotic, *atrophic* (secondary optic atrophy), pallid, and flattened, with associated field defects due to damage to the retinal nerve fiber layer.[5]

papillitis Inflammation of the head of the optic nerve, thus visible with the ophthalmoscope. The swelling may be mistaken for **papilledema,** but in papillitis the visual acuity is significantly reduced and a central scotoma is present, rather than enlargement of the blind spot, with or without constriction of the outer fields.

papillomacular bundle The tract of myelinated fibers running from the macula to the optic nerve head, visibly pallid when demyelinated, as in some patients with multiple sclerosis. Because the tract enters the optic disk on the temporal side, that side appears paler than the nasal side in such cases, leading to the appearance of temporal pallor, but this is also the case in normal subjects and the determination of abnormal pallor is sometimes an artistic judgment.

papillophlebitis (optic disk vasculitis) A benign and self-limited condition characterized by mild, protracted, monocular visual impairment, swelling of the optic disk, retinal venous engorgement, and perivenous retinal hemorrhages in young people, without evidence of optic neuropathy. The other eye is normal and the cause is unknown.[1637] See also **retinal vasculitis, big blind-spot syndrome.**

pa-ping An endemic form of periodic paralysis with hypokalemia and vacuolar myopathy described in China, where it was due to barium poisoning.[3301]

papulosis atrophicans maligna A severe, progressive atrophic and necrotic skin disease, rarely associated with features of necrotizing cerebral and spinal vasculitis.[1038]

para- (Gr, beside)

para-abducens center The brainstem center for lateral gaze, situated ventral to the median longitudinal fasciculus and lateral to the abducens nucleus.

paraballism 1. Bilateral hemiballism, caused in some cases not by lesions of the subthalamus but of the caudate nucleus and putamen; a rare and possibly lethal condition, most often occurring as a lacunar syndrome.[2887,3452] See **ballism.** 2. A form of chorea in childhood induced by oral contraceptive ingestion.

Paracelsus (Gr, beside Celsus) Aureolus Threophrastus Bombastus von Hohenheim (1493–1541), an eccentric Swiss physician from Zurich who trained first in Vienna and then in medicine at Ferrara. He adopted the name of Aulus Celsus, a Roman historian, in a (successful) attempt at self-glorification. The name Bombastus was a similar addition, but he did not actually use the name "Paracelsus" himself.

He attacked the teachings of Galen, advocating the replacement of these mythologies with a new, scientific and empirical system, and encouraged scientific experiment. On the basis both of experiment and cogitation he introduced the use of mercurials for the treatment of syphilis and he was the inventor of laudanum, an extract of morphia. Paracelsus also described congenital syphilis and the manifestations of hysteria; linked endemic goiter and cretinism; produced anesthetic ether; and described chorea. His collected writings, published in 1658, spurred the investigative approach of such English physicians as Boyle, **Willis,** and **Sydenham.**[2686]

paracentral scotoma A scotoma, the edge of which passes through the fixation point, bisecting the line of central vision.

parachiasmal mass lesions Tumors of the sphenoid or petrous temporal bones or of the overlying meninges, an aneurysm of the internal carotid artery, granulomas, or other masses in the region of the cavernous sinus that may compress the chiasm on its medial aspect.[1231]

parachute reflex (parachute response) Extension of the arms of an infant suspended prone and dropped, still in the examiner's hands, toward a table below, the movement made as if to grab onto something to break the fall. This appears at 5–9 months and normally persists, but is absent in the setting of neuromuscular disease, spastic diseases, and mental retardation. Asymmetry of the response suggests the presence of a local upper or lower motor neuron lesion. See also **developmental reflexes.**

parachute response   See **parachute reflex.**

paraclinical evidence   (of a multiple sclerosis lesion) Demonstration by means of various tests and procedures of the existence of a lesion of the CNS which has not produced *signs* of neurological dysfunction but which may or may not have caused *symptoms* in the past. Such tests and procedures include the **hot bath test,** evoked response studies, oligoclonal banding in the CSF, tissue imaging procedures (MRI), and expert urological assessment.[4504,4505]

paracrusis   (Gr, playing a discord) Mild delirium.

paracusis   (Gr, next to + hearing) 1. Distortion of the loudness of sounds heard. 2. Paradoxical improvement in hearing in the presence of background noise, as recorded by Thomas **Willis.**

paracusis of Willis   (paracusis Willisiana) The state of only being able to hear in the presence of loud background noise, as in the case of the deaf woman who could only hear while a drum was beating, described by Thomas **Willis** in his *De Anima Brutorum.* The phenomenon is a feature of otosclerosis.

paracusis Willisiana   See **paracusis of Willis.**

paradigm of Sternberg   A memory test in which the subject is required to determine whether a word presented by the examiner was or was not included in word lists presented immediately before.[5346]

paradoxical ankle reflex   (of Bing) Tapping the extensor aspect of the ankle between the malleoli produces plantar flexion of the foot in patients with pyramidal lesions.

paradoxical dystonia   See **dystonia.**

paradoxical flexor reflex   See **Gordon reflex.**

paradoxical foot phenomenon of Westphal   Involuntary and persistent contraction of the tibialis anterior, extensor digitorum longus, and peronei when the ankle is passively dorsiflexed; a dystonic feature seen in some patients with parkinsonism.[574]

paradoxical myotonia   Myotonia that increases with repeated muscle contractions, unlike the more common finding of a reduction in improvement in the myotonia in that situation.

This phenomenon represents a major feature of **paramyotonia congenita.**

paradoxical pain   Pain generated as a result of neural dysfunction, not following classical pain pathways and without any stimulation of peripheral nociceptors. Chronic nociceptive pain of this nature does not respond to morphine.[3991]

paradoxical patellar reflex   Contraction of the thigh adductors in response to a tap on the quadriceps tendon, as a result of disinhibition of the spinal cord at levels adjacent to L2, 3 in the presence of pyramidal tract lesions above those sites, or in response to transmitted vibration to the adductor muscle.

paradoxical pupil phenomenon   See **Westphal-Piltz phenomenon.**

paradoxical pupillary dilatation   (of Byrne) The pupil with sympathetic denervation, especially of the third neuron, exhibits **denervation hypersensitivity** to circulating catecholamines and thus may dilate under stress (when the levels of such substances are increased). Thus the pupil is usually smaller than in **Horner syndrome,** but may be larger in stressful conditions. The phenomenon represents a **pain reflex** mediated by sympathetic pathways. See also **Westphal-Piltz phenomenon.**

paradoxical reflexes   Occasional *variant* forms of the usual muscle stretch reflexes, modified in certain conditions by the underlying disorder and the method of elicitation,[5858] as with the **paradoxical triceps reflex.**

paradoxical sleep   Rapid eye movement sleep, so called because the EEG resembles that of wakefulness but the subject is asleep. See **rapid eye movement sleep.**

paradoxical triceps reflex   (olecranon reflex) Contraction of the elbow flexors when the triceps tendon is tapped, as a result of a lesion at C7 (8), which causes depression of the triceps response. The tap leads to a slight stretch of the biceps, which is followed by contraction of that muscle.[5858]

parafoveal region   The region of the macula immediately about the fovea contralis.

paraganglioma   1. A neuronal tumor, usually arising in the cauda equina and characterized by the presence of neurons within the uniform mass of polygonal cells.[6] 2. (chemodactoma) See **glomus jugulare tumor.**

paraganglioma-ganglioneuroma   A neuronal tumor.

parageusia   See **dysgeusia.**

paragonimiasis   A trematodal infestation characterized clinically by meningoencephalitis, seizures, focal neurological deficits, visual disturbances with optic atrophy, and dementia. Intracerebral calcifications are common.[2567]

paragraphia   A syndrome characterized by writing errors that occur when one-half of a word is neglected; thus *bus-stop* may be written as *stop.* It may occur in patients with right hemispheric neglect syndromes. See also **paralexia, neglect syndromes.**

parainfectious inflammatory encephalomyelitis   A form of encephalitis clinically indistinguishable from direct viral encephalitis, but in which the organism (such as Epstein-Barr virus, *Mycoplasma*, or influenza virus) cannot be cultured from the brain but is detected as a result of a rise in antibody titers. The CSF contains an increased number of white cells.[4763] See also **acute disseminated encephalomyelitis, opsoclonus-myoclonus syndrome.**

parainfectious noninflammatory encephalomyelitis (acute toxic encephalopathy, acute nonsuppurative encephalitis, acute brain swelling) A form of encephalopathy characterized by acute brain swelling without inflammation or glial reaction, occurring usually in children who present with acute confusion, coma, and seizures, and who manifest a marked increase in intracranial pressure due to cerebral edema, without cells in the CSF.[4763]

The condition was first described by Dr. James **Putnam.** See also **Reye syndrome, acute disseminated encephalomyelitis.**

paralalia   The substitution of other distinct sounds for those which cannot be pronounced as a result of **mogilalia.** The pronunciation of "Th" for "S" (lisping) and "W" for "R" are examples.

paralanguage   Nonverbal methods of communication, including gesture and music.[1172]

paraleresis   Mild delirium.

paralexia   1. The occurrence of substitutions in reading aloud. 2. Inability to attend to the words on one side of a page, as may be seen in **neglect syndromes.** The reading errors occur because one-half of a word is neglected; thus *tenant* may be read as *ant*. This may occur in patients with right hemispheric neglect syndromes.[3650] See also **paragraphia.**

paralgesia   Diminished sensibility of painful stimuli.

paralimbic areas   Mesocortical areas better differentiated than **allocortex** but still lacking the six-layered structure of the **neocortex.** These areas include the insula, orbitofrontal cortex, temporal pole, the parahippocampal and cingulate gyri, and the paraolfactory areas.

paralinguistic communication   The use of gestures and facial expressions to enhance verbal understanding.

paralysie des amants   Radial nerve paralysis following prolonged compression of the nerve by the head or body of an actual or intended sexual partner. The lesion usually involves that portion of the radial nerve in the mid-forearm, so that triceps function is spared and the other individual can be pushed away.

paralysis   (from Gr, weakness, disabling) Loss of motor function.

paralysis agitans   Dr. James **Parkinson**'s name for the disease now bearing his.[4339] See **Parkinson disease.**

paralysis agitans mercurialis   Basal ganglion disease due to chronic mercury poisoning. See **hatters' shakes.**

paralysis vacillans   (from Lat, paralysis + to stagger) Chorea.

paralytic pontine exotropia   An internuclear ophthalmoplegia with paralytic monocular exotropia of the eye on the other side; the combination of a unilateral horizontal gaze palsy and internuclear ophthalmoplegia, caused by a single paramedian lesion of the pons. In the acute phase, one eye deviates laterally while the other is immobile in the primary position of gaze.[5100] See also **one-and-a-half syndrome.**

paralytic postural syncope   Syncope due to impairment of autonomic reflexes, including the vasovagal reflex, which leads to impairment in the redistribution of blood flow with alterations in posture, such that venous return to the heart (and so cardiac output) is reduced.

paralytic pupil   A dilated and unreactive pupil, occurring as a result of damage to the preganglionic parasympathetic nerves running with the third cranial nerve and supplying the pupillary sphincter. Ptosis and either complete or partial third nerve extraocular palsy are usually present as well. See also **pupillary sparing.**

paralytic rabies   See **dumb rabies.**

paralytic shellfish poisoning   A severe illness resulting from inhibition of the voltage-dependent sodium channel due to **saxitoxin** poisoning. The condition occurs mainly (in North America) on the northern and Alaskan coasts. After an incubation period of $^1/_2$–3 hours, patients experience paresthesias of the mouth, face, and limbs, usually with nausea, vomiting, and diarrhea and a "floating" sensation. Severe intoxication leads to dysphonia, ataxia, and systemic weakness progressing to ventilatory failure within 2–12 hours. Most deaths occur within the first 12 hours; those surviving 24 hours will recover. Symptoms persist overall for about 3 days. The case fatality rate varies from 1% to 12%.[3015]

paralytic strabismus   Those forms of strabismus which result from a lesion of cranial nerves III, IV, or VI.

Paralyzed Veterans of America   A charitable organization also concerned with advocacy for its members. Address: 801 18th Street, NW, Washington, DC 20006. Tel: 202-872-1300, 800-424-8200. Web site: http://www.pva.org/.

Paralyzed Veterans of America Spinal Cord Research Foundation   A charitable organization providing support and information on this condition. 801 18th Street, NW Washington, DC 20006. Tel: 202-416-7659.

paramagnetic   Possessed of an uneven number of particles (nucleons). When placed in a magnetic field that is sufficiently intense, some of the paramagnetic nuclei in a substance align themselves with that field and are susceptible to further alterations of their axes when a radiofrequency signal is applied to them, returning to their former position at various rates when it ceases. This represents the basis of MRI scanning.

paramagnetic agents Chemical substances which, when injected into the patient, enhance the quality of the images produced by **magnetic resonance imaging.**

paramedian diencephalic syndrome (syndrome of the thalamoperforating artery of Foix and Hillemand, syndrome of the basilar communicating artery of Percheron, syndrome of the mesencephalic artery, thalamosubthalamic infarction syndrome). The combination of fluctuating hypersomnolent apathy, an amnesic syndrome, impaired vertical (mainly downward) gaze, and often aphasia and palilalia, resulting from bilateral diencephalic infarctions.[3815] See also **top of the basilar syndrome.**

paramedian infarction Bilateral thalamic infarctions resulting from occlusion of the thalamosubthalamic arteries, producing a syndrome of acute transient coma, followed by drowsiness, asterixis, hypersomnia, vertical gaze paresis, and, in some cases, persistent amnesia.[2303] See also **paramedian diencephalic syndrome.**

paramedian pontine infarction One of three types of pontine infarction described by Foix in 1926 (the others being short circumferential and tegmental) producing hemiplegia worse in the arm with mild dysarthria and due either to a large lacune or numerous small lacunes, sometimes bilateral.[1867]

parameningeal infections (meningite de voisinage, Dupré syndrome) Infectious processes situated within the dura mater (sinus thrombophlebitis) or outside the meninges completely (epidural abscess, otitis, sinusitis) but which cause a meningeal reaction by virtue of their proximity.[1556] Some authorities would also include intracerebral abscesses within this category.

paramnesia (Gr, beside + memory) A psychiatric condition characterized by the misinterpretation of events or locations. See also **reduplicative paramnesia.**

paramyoclonus multiplex (Kny disease, convulsive tremor) (from Gr, beside + a muscle + a tumult) A dominaantly inherited myoclonic disorder characterized by involuntary contractions of single muscles or groups of synergic muscles, resulting in sudden, paroxysmal, symmetrical, clonic spasms at 10–50 per minute, occurring mainly in males and at any age. Voluntary movements and alcohol intake may suppress them, but they persist in sleep and are increased by activities requiring fine coordination such as writing, and by conscious attempts to inhibit them.[1960] See also **Friedreich disease, hereditary essential myoclonus.**

The movements involve the arms, legs, trunk, and neck, but particularly the arms and neck, and are most frequent and intense proximally; the diaphragm may be involved. They are always rapid and brief and are sometimes asynchronous. The accompanying EMG electrical activity lasts less than 500 msec. This was the original term applied by **Friedreich** in 1881[1959] and by Kny 7 years later[3104] to a condition characterized by bursts of irregular myoclonus in the trunk and limbs lasting several minutes.

It has been suggested[3570] that the onset of paramyoclonus (bilaterally symmetrical jerks often inhibited by movement) before the age of 20, with dominant inheritance and a benign course, without generalized seizures, dementia, or ataxia and with a normal EEG constitute diagnostic criteria.

paramyotonia Intermittent myotonia induced by repetitive use of muscles and increased by exposure to cold or (rarely) to heat. It is most obvious in the face, neck, and distal extremities. Attacks usually last for hours.

Compare with **myotonia,** in which the abnormal muscle contraction tends to lessen with exercise or with warmth, and with **paradoxical myotonia.**

paramyotonia congenita (Eulenberg disease, myotonic periodic paralysis, congenital myotonia) A rare, dominantly inherited syndrome of intermittent, nonprogressive tonic contraction (myotonia) of the facial, bulbar, and distal muscles precipitated by exposure to cold for short periods, with episodic flaccid weakness of the limbs and areflexia occurring after longer exposure. The onset is in infancy. The responsible gene maps to chromosome 17q13.1–q13.5. The physiological basis is disruption of inactivation of the fast sodium channel (the SCN4A subunit), though some mutations also disrupt the slow Na^+ channel. Numerous point mutations of the *SCN4A* gene have been held responsible.

There are no dystrophic features, but a tendency toward muscle hypertrophy is notable clinically, as is a variation in muscle fiber size histologically. No other laboratory abnormalities coexist, but EMG reveals that repetitive muscular contractions lead to a decreasing recruitment pattern, and after cooling the hand in ice water, the myotonia disappears and the hand enters a state of electrically silent contracture.[1362,4132] **Paradoxical myotonia** may also occur.[5573]

The disease was described in 1886 by Eulenberg who was aware of its occurrence in six generations of the family that he studied.[1710] Becker suggested the term *paralysis periodica paramyotonica*[418] to refer to those patients in whom the weakness is associated with hyperkalemia, and in whom prolonged, repeated movements stimulate the myotonia and fatigability is noted.

Variant conditions include the following:

Myotonia fluctuans

Myotonia permanens

Acetazolamide-responsive myotonia

Paramyotonia congenita without cold paralysis A dominantly inherited myotonic syndrome in which the symptoms begin in childhood. The myotonia is easily provoked by exercise and elicited by percussion, but not by cold.[1362]

Potassium-aggravated myotonia A form in which the attacks are precipitated by a potassium load, and in which there is no weakness. Weakness precipitated by hypokalemia resembles paramyotonia congenita but without the cold paralysis.

Paramyotonic periodic paralysis A dominantly inherited syndrome of percussion and paroxysmal myotonia induced by exercise, warmth, and cold, and associated with weakness and easy fatigability.[197] This may or may not be the same condition as paramyotonia congenita. See **familial periodic paralysis.**

Temperature-sensitive sodium channelopathy with heat-induced myotonia and cold-induced paralysis A rare dominantly inherited syndrome with these findings due to a mutation in the skeletal muscle sodium channel.[5408]

paraneoplastic acute ascending polyneuropathy An illness indistinguishable from **acute inflammatory demyelinating polyneuropathy,** occurring in some patients with **Hodgkin disease.**

paraneoplastic acute necrotizing myopathy A rare complication of remote carcinoma, characterized by rapidly or subacutely progressive symmetrical proximal muscle weakness and atrophy due to both neuropathy and muscle inflammation.[5438]

paraneoplastic amyotrophic lateral sclerosis A disorder almost indistinguishable from **amyotrophic lateral sclerosis** except for a potential for improvement following the elimination of the malignancy. See **amyotrophic lateral sclerosis** (*variants*).

paraneoplastic antibodies See **anti-Yo, anti Hu, anti-Ri.**

paraneoplastic autonomic neuropathy Sympathetic and parasymptathetic failure as a reslt of remote malignancy. Varieties include the following:[5394]

Acute pandysautonomia
Paraneoplastic intestinal pseudo-obstruction
Dysautonomia complicating **paraneoplastic encephalomyelitis**
Impaired sweating and postural hypotensiion with **paraneoplastic sensorimotor peripheral neuropathy**
Local autonomic dysfunction with root infiltration
Autonomic effects as a result of therapy (e.g., vincristine) or in the **Lambert-Eaton syndrome**

paraneoplastic dementia An acute or slowly developing dementing syndrome usually accompanying other paraneoplastic disorders. See also **paraneoplastic limbic encephalitis.**

paraneoplastic dermatomyositis (paraneoplastic polymyositis) The appearance of clinical signs of polymyositis or dermatomyositis in the presence of overt or latent malignancy, especially small-cell carcinoma of the lung or alimentary carcinomas in men and carcinomas of the ovary or breast in women.[3687]

paraneoplastic encephalomyelitis Diverse subacute syndromes complicating remote malignancy (usually bronchogenic carcinoma), and listed under **paraneoplastic syndromes** (carcinomatous encephalomyeloneuropathy). Lymphocytic infiltrates in the meninges and parenchyma, glial nodules, and perivascular lymphocytic cuffing are characteristic pathological findings[1498] and both motor and sensory neuronopathies may be associated. Anti-Hu antibodies may be detected.

paraneoplastic encephalomyelitis with bulbar involvement A syndrome of meningoencephalitis with subacute cerebellar degeneration, myelitis, ganglioradiculitis, ophthalmoplegia, nystagmus, and peripheral neuropathy, occurring mainly in males with an underlying malignancy (usually oat-cell carcinoma of the bronchus),[1498] but also in women with breast or uterine carcinomas.

paraneoplastic limbic encephalitis A subacute amnestic dementing syndrome in which there are varying degrees of anxiety, confusion, and memory impairment, complicating small-cell carcinoma of the lung or other malignancies. Pathologically, amygdaloid and hippocampal degenerative changes and widespread inflammation in other parts of the CNS are usually detected;[1136] antineuronal antibodies are also detectable.

paraneoplastic motor neuronopathy A syndrome of slowly developing lower motor neuron–type weakness without sensory changes in patients treated with irradiation for **Hodgkin disease** or other lymphomas. A potential for recovery after successful treatment of the malignancy has been described. See **subacute motor neuronopathy, amyotrophic lateral sclerosis** (*variants*).

paraneoplastic myopathy Muscle disease occurring as a remote effect of malignancy. Varieties include[5399] **dermatomyositis, acute (necrotic) myopathy, carcinoid myopathy, steroid nyopathy, and cachectic myopathy.**

paraneoplastic myeloradiculoneuropathy A mixed syndrome with elements of both **paraneoplastic subacute necrotic myelopathy** and **paraneoplastic sensorimotor peripheral neuropathy.** Clinically, radicular pain, sensory loss, lower motor neuron disease, and areflexia are typical findings and the CSF is almost always abnormal.

paraneoplastic myopathies Muscle disorders occurring in association with a remote carcinoma. These include **paraneoplastic dermatomyositis/polymyositis, Lambert-Eaton myasthenic syndrome, paraneoplastic acute necrotizing myopathy,** and **cachectic myopathy.**

paraneoplastic neuropathies Disorders of the peripheral nervous system occurring as remote effects of distant carcinoma. These include the following:[5394]

1. Motoneuron disorders
   a. **Amyotrophic lateral sclerosis**–like syndrome
   b. **Paraneoplastic motor neuronopathy**

c. Anterior horn cell disease with **paraneoplastic encephalomyelitis**
2. Radiculopathies
   a. **Paraneoplastic myeloradiculoneuropathy**
   b. Neuritis, e.g., herpes zoster
3. Plexopathies
   a. Neoplastic **plexopathies**
   b. **Radiation-induced plexopathies**
4. Other neuropathies
   a. **Paraneoplastic sensory neuronopathy**
   b. **Paraneoplastic sensorimotor peripheral neuropathy**
   c. Autonomic neuropathies
   d. Mononeuropathies, especially of the median and common peroneal nerves
   e. Radiation-induced schwannomas
   f. Neuropathies resulting from chemotherapy (vincristine, platinum, cytosine arabinoside, procarbazine etc.)

See also **dysproteinemic neuropathy, antineuronal antibodies.**

paraneoplastic optic neuritis A rare complication of remote carcinoma, presenting with progressive visual loss and swelling of the optic nerve head.

paraneoplastic polymyositis See **paraneoplastic dermatomyositis.**

paraneoplastic retinopathy (cancer-associated retinopathy) A syndrome of retinal photoreceptor degeneration leading to rapid visual deterioration, accompanied by narrowing of the retinal arterioles, visual field defects, nyctalopia, and absence of the electroretinographic response, and occurring in association with lung, breast, uterine, or renal carcinomas.[3083]

paraneoplastic sensorimotor peripheral neuropathy A mixed acute, subacute, or chronic axonal peripheral neuropathy, often with secondary demyelination, complicating carcinomas of the lung, breast, and gastrointestinal tract and associated with raised CSF protein levels and with the presence of antimyelin antibodies in the serum.[2544] This is perhaps the most common of the neuropathies due to distant malignancy.[1186,1187,5394] Raised CSF protein levels are usual.[2545] The appearance of symptoms may preceed evidence of the malignancy by years or may follow it. See also **gammopathic neuropathy.**

Variants are *acute inflammatory demyelinating polyneuropathy* seen with Hodgkin disease or lung cancer; a form of **chronic acute inflammatory demyelinating polyneuropathy;** and a vasculitic form of polyneuritis. Cachectic neuropathy may also occur. See also **paraproteinemia.**

paraneoplastic (carcinomatous) sensory neuronopathy (or ganglionopathy, or ganglionitis) A severe, immunologically mediated, acute or subacute, painful, pure sensory neuronopathy, most commonly seen in female patients with small-cell lung cancer and presenting with distal paresthesias, dysesthesias and numbness, pain and hyporeflexia, later suffering generalized sensory loss, pseudoathetosis, and sensory ataxia. Even though anti-Hu antibodies staining neuronal nuclei may be detected, the usual small-cell lung or other cancer may not appear until up to 3 years after the time of presentation of the neuropathy. Other paraneoplastic syndromes such as limbic encephalitis may coexist.[5394]

The spinal ganglion cells are destroyed as a result of a presumed autoimmune attack.[1391,2664] The CSF protein levels are raised and other cerebellar, autonomic, or cerebral paraneoplastic syndromes are also present in about half the cases.[957] The sensory nerve action potentials are small or absent and sensory evoked potentials are delayed or absent.

In a *variant* form, the same condition occurs with added **polymyositis.**

paraneoplastic stroke Stroke (affecting any vessel) occurring in association with mucin-induced coagulopathy in patients with carcinomas that are not necessarily mucin secreting.[153]

paraneoplastic subacute cerebellar degeneration with bulbar involvement A rare complication associated with ovarian, small-cell lung, or breast carcinomas, or with **Hodgkin disease,** and presenting with ptosis, ophthalmoplegia, **opsoclonus,** and facial weakness.[711] Deafness due to degeneration of the cochlear nerve may also occur as a component of the syndrome.

Anti-Purkinje cell antibodies are detectable in the serum. See also **subacute cortical cerebellar degeneration.**

paraneoplastic subacute necrotic myelopathy A rapidly progressive syndrome of myelopathic motor and sensory loss ascending to thoracic levels in some patients with carcinoma of the bronchus.[2411]

paraneoplastic syndromes (nonmetastatic syndromes) Rare, distant, nonmetastatic complications of underlying malignant disease, such as small-cell carcinomas of the lung or ovarian carcinomas, which may appear before the tumor is detected. They may be due in part to the immunological response of the host to the tumor protein, the immunoglobulins cross-reacting with antigens on certain subsets of neurons. See the preceding 23 entries, **paraneoplastic vasculitis,** and **hyperviscosity syndromes.**

The clinical syndromes described are listed in Chart P–2.

Chart P–2. The Paraneoplastic Syndromes

1. Carcinomatous encephalomyeloneuropathy
   Subacute cortical cerebellar degeneration
   Paraneoplastic subacute cerebellar degeneration with bulbar involvement
   Lower brainstem (bulbar) encephalitis
   Paraneoplastic limbic encephalitis or encephalomyelitis
   Acute intrinsic myelopathy
   Paraneoplastic subacute necrotic myelopathy (necrotizing myelitis with predilection for anterior horn cells)
   Psychological disorders
   Opsoclonus-myoclonus syndrome

Paraneoplastic dementia
Neuromyotonia, stiff-man syndrome
2. Myopathic-myasthenic syndromes
   Lambert-Eaton myasthenic syndrome
   A syndrome resembling **myasthenia gravis**
   Paraneoplastic polymyositis/dermatomyositis
   Acute necrotizing myopathy
   Myotonia
3. **Progressive multifocal leukoencephalopathy**
4. Opthalmological disorders
   Cancer-associated retinopathy (paraneoplastic retinopathy, CAR syndrome)
   Nutritional amblyopia
   Uveomeningitic syndrome
   Paraneoplastic optic neuritis
5. Neuropathies (reviewed by Grisold and Drlicek, 1999)[2285]
   Paraneoplastic sensory neuronopathy and subacute sensory neuropathy
   Paraneoplastic sensorimotor neuropathy
   Subacute pure **motor neuronopathy**
   Paraneoplastic vasculitis with multiple mononeuropathy
   Monoclonal **gammopathic neuropathy**
   Neuropathy with insulinoma
   Paraneoplastic acute ascending polyneuropathy
   Paraneoplastic amyotrophic lateral sclerosis
   Pandysautonomia

paraneoplastic vasculitis   A multiple mononeuropathy in which wallerian degeneration is associated with microvasculitis, usually complicating a small-cell carcinoma of the lung.[2867] Clinically, the disorder presents as a mixed sensorimotor neuropathy with autonomic signs.

paraneurons   Endocrine brothers of neurons which produce substances that are either the same as or related to neurotransmitters or neurohormones; they possess neurosecretory-like and/or synaptic vesicles or granules and have receptosensory functions.[1979]

paranoia   (from Gr, beside + mind; hence out of one's mind) From ancient Greek times to the Middle Ages it was the term for all forms of madness, being restricted to the endogenous psychoses in the nineteenth century and then incorporated as a type of dementia praecox by Kraepelin early in this century. The term is now used for the delusional belief that one is the target of unwarranted hostility.

paraparesis   1. Weakness of the legs, usually as a result of bilateral pyramidal tract lesions. 2. Incomplete paraplegia.

paraphasia   (Gr, beside + speechlessness) 1. The tendency to utter words that are distorted although similar to the correct words sought; the incorrect use of words, within the context of a dysphasic condition.

The phenomenon is a manifestation of patients with aphasias whose utterances are distortions of normal words. *Literal* and *phonemic* forms are distinguished. In *verbal paraphasias*, whole words or phrases are substitutes for those intended.

2. The evocation of an inappropriate sound in place of a desired word or phrase; the replacement of a desired word with an articulate sound devoid of conventional meaning.

paraphonemia   An inability to distinguish between phonemes that are somewhat similar in their acoustic properties.[1172]

paraphrasia   Incoherent or disordered speech.

paraphrenesis   Dementia or delirium (eighteenth century).

paraphrenia   A paranoid state occurring in the elderly.

paraphysial cyst   Colloid cysts arising from the ependyma of the paraphysis, a vestigial third ventricular structure.

paraplegia   (from Gr, beside + a stroke) (paraplexia) "A palsy which seizeth all parts of the Body below the Head" (Blancard's *Dictionary*, 1693; quoted by Skinner[5204]). Now taken to mean complete paralysis of the legs, as from a spinal cord lesion or severe neuropathy.

paraplegia dolorosa   Paraplegia with pain, usually due to spinal cord compression from spinal tumors **Cruveilhier.**

paraplegia-in-extension   A posture of the legs consequent upon a pyramidal lesion, in which resting tone is greater in the extensor muscles than in the flexors; usually an entity in which the severity of the lesion is less than that which occurs in cases of **paraplegia-in-flexion.**[3648]

paraplegia-in-flexion   The result of unantagonized flexor reflex action giving rise to a rigid posture of the legs, which is intermittent and thus gives rise to involuntary movements; it is consequent upon a pyramidal lesion. In this state, resting tone is greater in the flexor muscles than in the extensors. Absent or reduced knee and ankle jerks and an extensor response accompany these findings.

Its presence usually indicates that the severity of the lesion is greater than that occurring in cases of **paraplegia-in-extension.**[3648,5829] The term was introduced by **Babiński.**

paraplegin   A mitochondrial metalloproteinase, a mutation of which is responsible for a recessive form of **hereditary spastic paraparesis.**

paraplexia   See **paraplegia.**

paraplexy   A state of paralysis due to apoplexy or perhaps to other causes. The word was used by early Greek physicians and is probably synonymous with the term **paraplegia** as we use it.[1046]

paraproteinemia   The presence of elevated amounts of abnormal immunoglobulins in the plasma, due either to plasma cell malignancies or to nonmalignant conditions. Polyneuropathies complicate the syndrome in up to a third of cases.[3301] See **gammopathic neuropathy.**

pararhinal sclerosis   See **mesial temporal sclerosis.**

parasagittal   In a plane parallel to the anteroposterior midline axis.

parasagittal cerebral injury   A syndrome of usually bilateral and symmetrical cortical and subcortical ischemic injury in the **watershed zones** of the brain as a result of a reduction in cerebral perfusion pressure. In the newborn, the clinical characteristics include hypotonia and weakness in the arms and legs, later developing into spastic quadriparesis.[1146]

parasellar lesions   Those lesions which are located alongside the pituitary fossa, such as those within the cavernous sinus, and including meningiomas, aneurysms, etc.[1231] See **parachiasmal mass lesions.**

parasite potential   See **satellite potential.**

parasomnias   Recurrent physiological or abnormal motor, behavioral, or experiential phenomena representing disorders of arousal, partial arousal, and sleep transition, which intrude into the sleep process and reflect activation of the CNS.

In Chart P–3 the conditions are listed as classified by the **American Sleep Disorders Association.**[234]

Chart P–3. The Primary Parasomnias

A. Arousal disorders
 1. **Confusional arousals**
 2. **Sleepwalking**
 3. **Sleep terrors** (pavor nocturnus)
B. Sleep–wake transition disorders
 1. **Rhythmic movement disorder**
 2. **Sleep starts**
 3. **Sleeptalking**
 4. **Nocturnal leg cramps**
C. Parasomnias usually associated with rapid eye movement sleep
 1. **Nightmares** (dream anxiety attacks)
 2. **Sleep paralysis**
 3. **Impaired sleep-related penile erections**
 4. **Sleep-related painful erections**
 5. **Rapid eye movement sleep–related sinus arrest**
 6. **Rapid eye movement sleep behavior disorder**
D. Other parasomnias
 1. Sleep **bruxism**
 2. Sleep **enuresis**
 3. **Sleep-related abnormal swallowing syndrome**
 4. **Nocturnal paroxysmal dystonia**
 5. **Sudden unexplained nocturnal death syndrome**
 6. Primary **snoring**
 7. Infant **sleep apnea**
 8. **Congenital central hypoventilation syndrome**
 9. **Sudden infant death syndrome**
 10. **Benign neonatal sleep myoclonus**
 11. Sudden onset of sleep in Parkinson disease
 12. **Catathrenia**
 13. Other parasomnias not otherwise specified

Adapted from The International Classification of Sleep Disorders Diagnostic and Coding Manual. Rochester, *MN: American Sleep Disorders Association,* © *1990. Reproduced by kind permission of the American Academy of Sleep Medicine.*

Restless limb syndrome, periodic limb movements in sleep, and **hypnagogic and hypnapompic hallucinations** could equally well be included in this list.

Secondary parasomnias include nocturnal epilepsy syndromes, various headache disorders, nocturnal muscle cramps, nocturnal panic attacks, and certain respiratory and gastrointestinal conditions.[5370]

paraspinal mapping   An electromyographic technique in which the EMG needle probes in many directions from each of five specified paraspinal sites, in order to sample activity from multifidus muscles at different levels in the precise diagnosis of radiculopathy.[2371]

parasympathetic system   The procreative, vegetative division of the autonomic nervous system, comprising the unmyelinated fibers of the vagus nerve and the sacral outflow at S2, 3, 4. See **autonomic function tests.**

parathymia   Brain exhaustion (nineteenth century).

paratonia   (paratonic or arteriosclerotic rigidity, pure motor negativism, gegenhalten) An increase in muscle tone proportional to the amount of force used to achieve passive movement of a limb (usually the leg), and often worsened by exhortations made to the patient to relax; such resistance to movement may be a consequence of a dyspraxia.[5673] See **Foerster syndrome.**

It occurs as a result of diffuse bifrontal disease (when the legs are involved) and in association with dyspraxias (when it occurs in the arms).[3081]

paratonic rigidity   An inability to relax a group of muscles, occurring together with brisk reflexes and extensor plantar responses (Dupré). See also **paratonia.**

paratrigeminal oculosympathetic syndrome   See **Raeder paratrigeminal syndrome.**

paredrine test   See **hydroxyamphetamine test.**

parencephalis   Antique term for the cerebellum.

parencephalocele   A congenital malformation in which there is herniation of a cyst of the posterior fossa through a defect in the occipital bone.

parenchymatous cortical cerebellar atrophy   (late cortical cerebellar atrophy, Thomas atrophy)[179] See **olivopontocerebellar atrophy, autosomal dominant cerebellar ataxias, Marie-Foix-Alajouanine syndrome.**

parenchymatous syphilis   That form of tertiary syphilis which affects the substance of the nervous system directly, as opposed to **meningovascular syphilis. General paresis, tabes dorsalis,** and syphilitic optic atrophy are the three varieties of this form.

paresis   (Gr, a slackening) Partial paralysis or weakening of muscle power.[5204] The word is used almost interchangeably with **paralysis,** but is generally used to indicate a less severe degree of weakness than the latter.

paresthesias   (Gr, beside + sense perceptions) 1. Abnormal sensations as of tingling or burning in regions to which the nerve supply is impaired but not lost, and due to the generation of ectopic nerve impulses in dysfunctional axons.

The contraction of *paraesthesia* to *paresthesia* is usual in North America, but the dipthong is retained in the United Kingdom. To retain a certain quasi-authenticity, the plural may be written *paresthesiae*, but the -*s* ending is used here for simplicity, the author having little Latin and less Greek.

2. An illusion of sensation, affecting any sense channel (nineteenth century).

paretic   Of or belonging to a **paresis.**

paretic nystagmus   Nystagmus that occurs when a subject attempts to deviate the eyes voluntarily in the direction of action of a weak extraocular muscle. The same phenomenon may occur in subjects with conjugate gaze paresis.

parietal   (from Lat, concerning a wall) The wall of a cavity, or, in neurology, the covering of the ventricles; thus the parietal lobe or (relating to the wall or side of a cavity) the parietal bone. The syndromes of the parietal lobe have been reviewed by Critchley.[1171]

parietal apraxia   See **apraxia.**

parietal ataxia   (parietal kinetic ataxia, pseudocerebellar ataxia) Ataxia resembling that due to cerebellar disease, occurring in the absence of clinical weakness or any sensory deficit and due to a lesion of the contralateral parietal lobe.[199,1171]

The original report of **Claude** and **Lhermitte** in 1918 documented gait ataxia resulting from bilateral parietal lobe lesions, but pathological studies were not performed.

parietal foramina-cleidocranial dysplasia   A congenital dysmorphic syndrome manifesting also absent auditory canals, hypertelorism, absent clavicles, dolichocephaly, and macrocephaly with parietal foramina. The foramina can also occur in isolation.

parietal kinetic ataxia   See **parietal ataxia.**

parietal lobe epilepsies   Location-related epileptic syndromes usually characterized by simple partial and secondarily generalized seizures. Most seizures arising in the parietal lobe remain as simple partial seizures, but complex partial seizures may arise out of simple partial seizures and occur with spread beyond the parietal lobe. Seizures arising from the parietal lobe have the following features: the symptoms are predominantly sensory; and positive phenomena consist of tingling and a feeling of electricity, which may be confined or may spread in a Jacksonian manner. There may be a desire to move a body part or a sensation as if a part were being moved. Muscle tone may be lost. The parts most frequently involved are those with the largest cortical representation (e.g., the hand, arm and face). There may be tongue sensations of crawling, stiffness

or coldness, and facial sensory phenomena may occur bilaterally. Occasionally, an intraabdominal sensation of sinking, choking, or nausea may occur, particularly in cases of inferior and lateral parietal lobe involvement. Rarely, there may be pain, which may take the form of a superficial burning dysesthesia, or a vague, very severe, painful sensation.

Parietal lobe visual phenomena may occur as hallucinations of a formed variety. Metamorphopsia with distortions, foreshortenings, and elongations may occur, and are more frequently observed in cases of nondominant hemisphere discharges. Negative phenomena include numbness, a feeling that a body part is absent, and a loss of awareness of a part or a half of the body, known as *asomatognosia.* This is particularly the case with nondominant hemisphere involvement. Severe vertigo or disorientation in space may be indicative of inferior parietal lobe seizures. Seizures in the dominant parietal lobe result in a variety of receptive or conductive languages disturbances. Some well-lateralized genital sensations may occur with paracentral involvement. Some rotatory or postural motor phenomena may occur. Seizures of the paracentral lobule have a tendency to become secondarily generalized. (From the revised ILAE Classification,[1114] reproduced by kind permission from Blackwell Science.) The more common of these experiences are somatosensory (occasionally painful) sensations, disturbances of body image, visual illusions, vertiginous sensations, aphasic aura, feeling of inability to move one extremity, complex visual or auditory hallucinations, elementary visual hallucinations, conscious confusion, and cephalic or epigastric sensations.[4884]

In addition, complex partial seizures with loss of contact and automatisms, or asymmetric tonic seizures may occur.[5985] Ictal SPECT studies are a preferred way of localizing the originating discharges.[2593]

parietal lobe syndrome   See **Déjèrine syndromes.**

parietal stroke   Infarcts of a parietal lobe, often producing one of three sensory syndromes: the **pseudothalamic sensory syndrome,** the **cortical sensory syndrome,** or an **atypical sensory syndrome** in addition to or in place of the **Déjèrine syndromes.**[383]

Parinaud, Henri   (1844–1905) French neuroophthalmologist whose doctoral thesis (University of Paris) was on the subject of papilledema in meningitis. He described the syndrome named for him (in a paper describing all forms of gaze pareses) in 1883,[4331] localizing the lesion to the pons and midbrain without autopsy verification. This article concerned convergence and divergence impairment as well as horizontal and vertical gaze abnormalities, and he was not certain about the localization of the lesion (whether in the ocular motor nuclei or the corpora quadrigemina). He later suggested that the center for vertical gaze is in the frontal lobes, but also that the lesion causing failure of upward gaze was of the quadrigeminal plates. His professional appointment at the **Salpêtrière** gave him access to the patients of **Charcot** and so provided him with huge experience in disorders of eye movement, strabismus, and binocular vision; he wrote on all of these subjects extensively. He is properly regarded as the father of neuro-ophthalmology.

Parinaud syndrome 1. See **dorsal midbrain syndrome.** 2. The oculoglandular syndrome in cat-scratch disease.

Parkes-Weber syndrome See **Klippel-Trenaunay-Weber syndrome.**

Parkes-Weber-Dimitri disease See **Sturge-Weber syndrome.**

parkin One of half a dozen gene loci identified in monogenic forms of **Parkinson disease,** described as responsible for autosomal recessive juvenile parkinsonism in Japanese families. In forms associated with this mutation, Lewy bodies are seldom found.[3924]

Parkinson disease The name applied by **Charcot** to the prototypical form of parkinsonism; a chronic progressive degenerative disease initially described by James **Parkinson** under the rubric "shaking palsy," and manifesting the triad of tremor, bradykinesia, and rigidity, with a shuffling, festinating, or propulsive gait; stooped posture; and (in its advanced stages) loss of postural reflexes, **hypophonia,** dysphagia, cachexia, and dementia.

Additional manifestations include torsion spasms, thermal paresthesias, chronic constipation, impotence, orthostatic hypotension, and seborrhea. Neuronal degeneration in the perikaryon or surviving neurons and in the parenchyma is the main histological feature. The Lewy bodies may also occur in neurons in the peripheral autonomic ganglia, Auerbach's and Meissner's plexuses, the intermediolateral cell column of the thoracic spinal cord, the hypothalamus, the amygdala, the hippocampus, and, in some cases, the cerebral cortex diffusely. In patients with diffuse cortical Lewy bodies (and in those without, at a late stage), dementia may be the predominant clinical manifestation. A screening questionnaire for community use has been developed.[962] An excellent review is found at www.aafp.org/afp/990415ap/2155.html.

The etiology is unknown; most cases are apparently sporadic but familial occurrence has been reported, and both exogenous environmental and genetic factors are suspected. [RCD]

Numerous other disorders also give rise to one or more of these manifestations as well as other features, including **oculogyric crises,** depression, ophthalmoplegia, motor neuropathy and ataxic syndromes; these conditions are subsumed under the general heading of **parkinsonism-plus.** Inclusion and exclusion criteria have been suggested by Koller,[3118] and are given in Chart P–4.

Chart P–4. Inclusion and Exclusion Criteria for the Diagnosis of Parkinson Disease

Inclusion Criteria

1. The presence for a year or more of two of the following three cardinal signs: resting or postural tremor, bradykinesia, rigidity
2. Responsiveness to L-dopa therapy (at least 1 g/day for a month) given the degree of improvement is moderate or marked and the duration of improvement is 1 year or more

Exclusion Criteria

1. Abrupt onset of symptoms
2. Remitting course
3. Stepwise progression
4. Neuroleptic therapy within the last year
5. Exposure to any substance known to cause parkinsonism
6. History of encephalitis
7. Oculogyric crises
8. Supranuclear downward or lateral gaze palsy.
9. Cerebellar, lower motor neuron or unexplained pyramidal signs
10. Severe autonomic failure
11. Dementia from the onset of the disease
12. Postural instability/falling early in the course of the disease
13. Evidence of cerebrovascular disease
14. Unilateral dystonia associated with apraxia or cortical sensory loss

From Koller WC. How accurately can Parkinson's disease be diagnosed? Neurology 1992;42(Suppl):6–16. Reproduced by kind permission.

A simpler set of diagnostic categories has been proposed by Calne et al.[875]

Clinically possible The presence of any one of the salient features: postural or resting tremor of recent onset, bradykinesia, or rigidity.

Clinically probable A combination of any two of the cardinal features: resting tremor, bradykinesia, rigidity, or impaired postural reflexes. Alternatively, asymmetrical resting tremor, asymmetrical rigidity, or asymmetrical bradykinesia are sufficient.

Clinically definite Any combination of three of the following features: resting tremor, bradykinesia, rigidity, or impaired postural reflexes. Alternatively sufficient are two of these features, with one of the first three above displaying asymmetry.

Variant forms of Parkinson disease include the following:

A *dominantly inherited* form with numerous Lewy bodies.[5869] This form is due to a mutation in the α-synuclein gene.

A *familial autosomal dominant* form in which signs of **amyotrophic lateral sclerosis** are also found. See **motor neuronal diseases.**

Dominantly inherited early-onset parkinsonism A form with onset in the third decade, characterized by the typical clinical features of Parkinson disease with the frequent addition of dystonias and without Lewy bodies or neurofibrillary tangles in the brain and mapped to 4q21-23.[1566,2158]

Autosomal recessive juvenile parkinsonism A form due to degeneration of the substantia nigra, not accompanied by Lewy body formation. The condition has its onset between the ages of 6 and 35 years. The phenotype resembles that of typical Parkinson disease and results from a mutation of the "parkin" gene at 11p.[3924]

Autosomal recessive juvenile parkinsonism with diurnal fluctuation linked to 6q25.2–27

Benign early-onset Parkinson disease

Segawa disease

Despite this clean classification, it should be appreciated there are at least six autosomal dominant and three autosomal recessive genes responsible for dopa-responsive parknsonism.[4020]

For other *variants*, see **parkinsonism-plus.** See also **American Parkinson Disease Association, Michael J. Fox Foundation for Parkinson's Research, National Parkinson Foundation, Parkinson Alliance, Parkinson's Action Network, Parkinson's Institute,** and **Parkinson's Resource Organization.**

Parkinson Alliance A charitable organization in this field. Address: 211 College Rd. East, 3rd Floor, Princeton, NJ 08540. Tel: 609-688-0870; 800-579-8440. E-mail: admin@parkinsonalliance.net. Web site: http://www.parkinsonalliance.net/.

Parkinson Disease Disability scales Rating scales designed to record changes in patients with Parkinson disease. The **Hoehn and Yahr** scale,[2598] UCLA disability scale, New York University Parkinson disease disability scale, Columbia scale,[1726] **Parkinson disease impairment index,** and Northwestern University disability scale are commonly used; unfortunately, the correlations between them are imperfect.[1430]

Parkinson Disease Impairment Index An instrument designed to quantitate the impairment suffered by patients with Parkinson disease, including arbitrary scores as to the presence of depression and dementia.[3745]

Parkinson Education program A charitable educational trust. Address: 1800 Park #302, Newport Beach, CA 92660.

Parkinson, James (1755–1824). English physician, social activist, ethicist, and amateur paleontologist, practicing in Hoxton in the East End of London. He was apprenticed to his father and at the age of 29, his name appearing on a list of surgeons approved by the Corporation of that city. Parkinson's career was overshadowed by his involvement in a variety of social and philanthropical, even revolutionary, causes, and he wrote many pamphlets, most appearing under the pseudonym "Old Hubert," in his radical capacity. Perhaps because he was a member of the London Corresponding Society, a genteel club devoted both to gastronomy and to revolution, he was haled before the Privy Council as an agitator on more than one occasion, but it appears he was not punished. In keeping with his strong religious beliefs, he spent considerable time in attempting to ease the burden of the poor, regulate the conduct of mental asylums, provide more Sunday schools, and reform the method of parliamentary representation.[4378,6060]

His medical works included books on family medicine for lay audiences (one of which went to six editions), a handbook of chemistry, a textbook of geology, and memoirs of his days as a hospital pupil, as well as works on trusses, fevers, appendicitis (written with his son), and the gout. His *Essay on the Shaking Palsy* (**Parkinson disease**) was published in 1817;[4339] he referred to the preceding descriptions of the condition by Galen, Boetius, and others in the first chapter. In this work, he paid little attention to rigidity and claimed that the senses and intellects were uninjured (both errors corrected by Trousseau), wrote that the tremor was severe in sleep, and considered that the likely lesion was in the cervical cord, but otherwise his observations have stood the test of time. It is of some interest that the first of the cases he described, and that one in the greatest detail, would now be classified as a case of **multiple system atrophy.** Half of the patients he reported on had been seen only on the street and never examined, but his description of the progression of the disease over years is so convincingly accurate that he must have had further experience of it either within his practice or in that of his father. Parkinson also noted that paralysis from stroke inhibited the tremor, antedating later attempts at surgical relief.[5047,6060]

Parkinson-ALS-dementia complex of Guam See **Lytico-Bodig.**

Parkinson Society Canada A charitable organization in this field. Address: 4211 Yonge St., Suite 316, Toronto, Ontario M2P 2A9. Tel: 416-227-9700; 1-800-565-3000. E-mail: General.info@parkinson.ca. Web site: http://www.parkinson.ca/home.html.

parkinsonian ataxia See **frontal gait disorder.**

parkinsonian gait Walking that is delayed and slowed, with a tendency to accelerate and to fall forward, the subject often taking many little steps (*marche à petits pas*) on tiptoe and showing a posture of flexion affecting the upper and lower limbs as well as the trunk. The arms swing less than normally or not at all. **Freezing** is common, especially at a doorway or when an obstacle has to be negotiated. **Propulsion** and **retropulsion** are occasionally seen.

parkinsonian hand The resting posture of the hand in some patients with parkinsonism, characterized by wrist dorsiflexion, flexion at the metacarpophalangeal joints, extension of the fingers with adduction, and ulnar deviation of the wrist.

parkinsonism A clinical syndrome of tremor, bradykinesia, rigidity, stooped posture, and impaired postural reflexes due to degeneration or dysfunction of the nigrostriatal neuronal system, or to pharmacological blockade or loss of striatal dopamine receptors; thus, a syndrome of striatal dopamine deficiency. Most commonly it is due to **Parkinson disease,** but the syndrome may also occur as part of the clinical expression of many other disorders such as **progressive supranuclear palsy, multiple-system atrophy,** various types of cerebral vascular disease, **Lytico-Bodig, Wilson** and **Huntington diseases,** and as a sequel to encephalitis (**postencephalitic parkinsonism**). It may also be produced by various pharmacological agents, notably the neuroleptic drugs, and by the dopaminergic neurotoxin **MPTP.** [RCD] Yet other causes have been listed.[3118]

Parkinsonism & Related Disorders   The official journal of the World Federation of Neurology Research Committee on Parkinsonism and Related Disorders, published by Elsevier. Web site: http://www.elsevier.com/homepage/sah/wfn-rced/doc/main_frm.html/.

parkinsonism-dementia   The combination of some features of these two syndromes, as occurs in **Alzheimer disease, progressive supranuclear palsy, Hallervorden-Spatz disease, corticobasal degeneration, vascular dementia, communicating hydrocephalus, progressive subcortical glial dystrophy,** variants of **Pick disease, Lytico-Bodig,** and **sporadic amyotrophic lateral sclerosis.**[2095]

A *variant form* is *dominantly inherited dementia and parkinsonism with non-Alzheimer amyloid plaques,* a dominantly inherited syndrome of adult onset characterized by severe dementia and parkinsonism with extracellular hyaline eosinophilic and congophilic amyloid plaques in the cerebral cortex, basal ganglia, thalamus, and substantia nigra.[4792]

parkinsonism-plus   A group of disorders in which the signs of parkinsonism are accompanied by others, including myoclonus, pyramidal signs, dementia, autonomic failure, and cerebellar signs. The conditions are listed in Chart P-5.

Chart P-5. Disorders Comprising Parkinsonism-Plus

Familial extrapyramidal disease with peripheral neuropathy A dominantly inherited sensorimotor peripheral neuropathy with distal weakness, muscle atrophy and areflexia, and stocking hypoesthesia occurring in association with Parkinson disease. Axonal degeneration is more common than demyelination as the underlying pathology.[860]

A syndrome of **amyotrophic lateral sclerosis** accompanying the parkinsonism, without dementia, inherited as an autosomal dominant characteristic. See also **Creutzfeldt-Jakob disease.**[713]

Tic, Parkinson disease, motor neuron disease, and acanthocytosis A syndrome with childhood onset, characterized by acanthocytosis with self-mutilation, rigidity, motor neuropathy and a burst-suppression pattern on the EEG. See **neuroacanthocytosis.**

Parkinsonism with anosmia A rare dominantly inherited syndrome of young adult onset characterized by anosmia

in association with rigidity and tremor. See **Kallmann syndrome.**

Familial parkinsonism–dementia (Lewy body) syndrome See **diffuse Lewy body disease.**

Fatal parkinsonism, alveolar hypoventilation, and depression A rare syndrome of adults manifesting respiratory difficulties, depression, bulbar pareses, tremor, seizures, and early death.[4546]

Parkinsonism with cerebellar ataxia A rare association of unknown significance.

Parkinsonism with cerebellar ataxia and peripheral neuropathy See **hereditary motor and sensory neuropathy, type 2.**

Juvenile parkinsonism A rare syndrome in which pyramidal signs, rigidity, dystonia, and tremor occur before the age of 20 years.[2099] See also **young-onset Parkinson disease.** The autosomal recessive juvenile form is mapped to 11p.

Parkinsonism, depression, and taurine deficiency A rare dominantly inherited syndrome of adult onset characterized by these features.[4415]

Parkinsonism-dystonia See **juvenile parkinsonism syndromes.**

Rapidly progressing autosomal dominant parkinsonism and dementia with pallidopontonigral degeneration A progressive syndrome of parkinsonism with dystonia, frontal release signs, pyramidal features, urinary incontinence, and perseverating vocalizations.[6050] Linkage to 4q21–23 has been established in at least one kinship.

Rapid-onset dystonia-parkinsonism A dominantly inherited disorder characterized by the rapid onset of parkinsonian signs and dystonia, involvement more of the bulbar and arm muscles than of the legs, lack of response to levadopa, and normal cranial imaging.[4457]

X-linked dystonia parkinsonism (Lubag) A complicated form mapped to Xq12-13.1

Such associations are also found in Parkinson disease with ALS, **corticobasal ganglionic degeneration; Lytico-Bodig; Hallervorden-Spatz disease; Huntington disease; neuroacanthocytosis; neuronal ceroid lipofuscinosis; normal-pressure hydrocephalus; olivopontocerebellar degeneration; progressive pallidal atrophy; progressive supranuclear palsy; Shy-Drager syndrome; striatal necrosis; strionigral degeneration;** and **Wilson disease.**

Parkinson's Action Network   A charitable organization in this field. Address: 300 North Lee St., Suite 500, Alexandria, VA 22314. Tel: 800-850-4726; 703-518-8877. California: 707-544-1994. E-mail: info@parkinsonsaction.org. Web site: http://www.parkinsonsaction.org/.

Parkinson's Disease Foundation, Inc.   A charitable organization. Address: 710 West 168th Street, New York, NY 10032. Tel: 1-800-457-6676. Web site: http://www.parkinson.org/onlinpub.htm.

Parkinson's Disease Society   A charitable organization. Address: 215 Vauxhall Bridge Road, London SW1V 1EJ, UK. Tel: 020 7931 8080. Web site: http://www.parkinsons.org.uk/.

Parkinson's Institute   A charitable organization in this field. Address: 1170 Morse Ave., Sunnyvale, CA

94089-1605. Tel: 408-734-2800; 800-786-2958. E-mail: outreach@parkinsonsinstitute.org. Web site: http://www.parkinsonsinstitute.org/.

Parkinson's Resource Organization   A charitable organization in this field. Address: 74-090 El Paseo, Suite 102, Palm Desert, CA 2260-4135. Tel: 760-773-5628;   310-476-7030;   877-775-4111.   E-mail: info@parkinsonsresource.org. Web site: http://www.parkinsonsresource.org/.

paroniria   The disturbance of sleep by disagreeable dreams.

parosmia   Distortion of the sense of smell, almost invariably interpreted as unpleasant.

paroxysm   (from Gr, to excite, hence a severe attack of disease) A periodic fit or attack of a disease, or of certain symptoms that occur periodically; the increase of symptoms to a maximum, with succeeding decline, their severity being less emphasized than their tendency to abrupt recurrence.

paroxysmal aphasia   Intermittent language disorders classified as *dysphasic seizures* (paroxysmal posterior aphasia) and *phonatory seizures* (paroxysmal anterior aphasia), almost always due to a discharging lesion in the left hemisphere.[49]

paroxysmal ataxia and vertigo   A dominantly inherited cerebellar ataxia; a *variant* of **May-White syndrome.**[3715]

paroxysmal choreoathetosis   (extrapyramidal seizures) A syndrome of abnormal involuntary movements resembling chorea, athetosis, or dystonia, variously considered to be due to dystonia or, in the past, to subcortical seizures. They were first described by Mount and Reback[4019] but were also known to **Gowers** as "reflex epilepsy."

The *variants* were classified by Lance[3234] as follows:
Familial paroxysmal dystonic choreoathetosis A dominantly inherited syndrome with onset in childhood in which the movements occur in prolonged attacks lasting between 2 minutes and 4 hours and may be complicated by spasticity. They are only seldom triggered by voluntary activity.[4019] The condition has been mapped to chromosome 1p.
Intermediate form A dominantly inherited syndrome in which the attacks of abnormal movements last between 5 and 30 minutes after precipitation by heavy exertion.
Paroxysmal choreoathetosis after craniocerebral trauma[1514]
Paroxysmal kinesigenic choreoathetosis

paroxysmal choreoathetosis and spasticity   A dominantly inherited variant of **paroxysmal dystonic choreoathetosis** in which the attacks are precipitated by exercise. Spastic paraplegia, perioral psaresthesias, diplopia, headache, and myoclonus are associated features.[256]

paroxysmal depolarization shift   An alteration in the charge of a neuronal cell body causing a sudden, high-amplitude burst of high-frequency action potentials and producing locally synchronous sustained depolarization and prolonged after-hyperpolarization. If this occurs synchronously in a number of adjacent neurons, an isolated spike may be recorded on the EEG and this may be the basic neurophysiological abnormality underlying the production of focal spikes in epilepsy. The term was introduced by Ajmone-Marsan in 1964.

paroxysmal dyskinesias   A heterogeneous group of acute, transient movement disorders, seven of which have been differentiated. They include **paroxysmal dystonic choreoathetosis, familial paroxysmal dystonic choreoathetosis, paroxysmal exertion-induced dyskinesia, nocturnal hypogenic paroxysmal dyskinesia, paroxysmal choreoathetosis and spasticity,** *infantile convulsions and paroxysmal choreoathetosis,* and *rolandic epilepsy, paroxysmal exercise-induced dystonia, and writer's cramp.*[5760]

paroxysmal dystonia   See **familial paroxysmal dystonic choreoathetosis, nocturnal paroxysmal dystonia.**

paroxysmal dystonic choreoathetosis   (paroxysmal nonkinesigenic dyskinesia) A channelopathy presenting as attacks of abnormal involuntary movements such as ballism, chorea, and dystonic postures, sometimes triggered by voluntary activity, occurring first in childhood.[543,1514] The attacks are of long duration (up to 6 hours) and are induced by a variety of factors including coffee, tea, alcohol, and fatigue but not by sudden movement. The gene for familial PDC has been linked in two families to chromosome 2q34 but sporadic cases also occur. See **familial paroxysmal dystonic choreoathetosis, paroxysmal kinesigenic choreoathetosis.**

In a *variant* dominantly inherited form, there is added spasticity.[541]

paroxysmal exertion-induced dystonia   A similar dominantly inherited condition in which the movements are induced by prolonged or sustained exercise The attacks lasted from a few minutes to up to 2 hours, and patient ages at onset range from 2 to 30 years. Hemidystonic attacks, bilateral leg involvement, and single leg involvement have all been described.[543]

paroxysmal hemicranias   Frequent short-lasting attacks of unilateral pain usually in the orbital, supraorbital, or temporal region that typically last minutes. The attack frequency usually ranges from 5 to 40 attacks per day. The pain is severe and associated with autonomic symptoms such as conjunctival injection, lacrimation, nasal congestion, rhinorrhoea, ptosis, or eyelid edema. Almost all reported cases respond to treatment with indomethacin.

Forms with marked autonomic activation include **chronic** and **episodic paroxysmal hemicrania, short-lasting unilateral neuralgiform headache with conjunctival injection and tearing** (SUNCT syndrome), and **cluster headache.** Those without autonomic activation are **hypnic headache,** and persistent headache with milder autonomic features such as **hemicrania continua.**

paroxysmal hypnogenic dyskinesia   See **paroxysmal hypogenic dystonia.**

paroxysmal hypogenic dystonia (paroxysmal hypnogenic dyskinesia) The occurrence of multiple, brief tonic flexor or extensor spasms in several extremities, waking the patient from non–rapid eye movement sleep and not diminishing consciousness. The ictal and interictal EEG record is normal but some patients also have seizures. The condition may be either familial or sporadic.[3314] See **dyskinesias.**

paroxysmal kinesigenic choreoathetosis (Mount-Reback syndrome, familial paroxysmal choreoathetosis, paroxysmal dystonic choreoathetosis, periodic dystonia, reflex epilepsy, seizures induced by movement, conditionally responsive extrapyramidal syndrome, hereditary kinesthetic reflex epilepsy) A sporadic or dominantly inherited syndrome of uni- or bilateral dystonic posturing of the trunk, eyes, and limbs without alteration of consciousness, occurring in the waking state and usually lasting 5 minutes but possibly up to 2 hours (the "reflex epilepsy" of **Gowers**). These choreoathetotic or ballistic movements are provoked by startle or by sudden movement. The movements may be suppressed by anticonvulsant drugs.[541,3017,3234] The condition has been mapped to 2q33–35. In a *variant* of this condition, a focal brain lesion can be identified.

Despite some of the names attached, this is not an epileptic syndrome at all; it could be an ion-channel disorder. It was first described by **Gowers** in the second edition of his book *Epilepsy and Other Chronic Convulsive Diseases* (London, 1801), but was then forgotten for 40 years until re-described in 1940.[4019]

See also **paroxysmal choreoathetosis, paroxysmal dystonic choreoathetosis.**

paroxysmal kinesigenic and nonkinesigenic dystonias   See **dystonia.**

paroxysmal kinesigenic dyskinesia   See **dyskinesias.**

paroxysmal lacrimation syndrome   See **crocodile tears.**

paroxysmal movement disorders   See **paroxysmal dyskinesias.**

paroxysmal myoclonic dystonia with vocalizations A movement disorder characterized by paroxysmal bursts of involuntary, regular, repetitive, rhythmic, bilateral, stereotypical, and severe myoclonus with vocalizations, often associated with tonic movements and interfering with voluntary activity. Mild **attention-deficit hypcractivity disorder,** learning disabilities, and resistance to treatment with haloperidol are other features of the condition.[1765]

paroxysmal nocturnal dystonia A syndrome characterized by sleeptalking, stereotypical movements in sleep with autonomic excitation, and transient arousals leading to the complaint of excessive daytime sleepiness.[3540] In some cases dominant inheritance is suggested with a mutation of the neuronal acetylcholine receptor gene (*CHRNA4*) on chromosome 20q and this may be the same condition as **autosomal dominant nocturnal frontal lobe epilepsy.** See also **dystonia.**

paroxysmal nocturnal hemaglobinuria (Marchiafava-Micheli syndrome) A rare, sporadic hematological disorder characterized by a deficiency in blood cell membrane glycoproteins, causing intravascular hemolysis, pancytopenia, and frequently intravascular (cerebral arterial or venous) thrombosis.[101]

paroxysmal nocturnal hemidystonia   See **dystonia.**

paroxysmal nonkinesigenic dyskinesia   See **dyskinesias.**

paroxysmal polyspike activity with arousal   See **pure tonic seizures with arousal.**

paroxysmal positional nystagmus   See **benign positional vertigo.**

paroxysmal positional vertigo A common and benign symptom of peripheral vestibular dysfunction occurring spontaneously or following head trauma, and probably due to **cupulolithiasis.**

paroxysmal tonic upgaze A benign neuro-ophthalmological syndrome of infancy characterized by prolonged episodes of sustained tonic upward deviation of the eyes, often with incomplete downward saccades (resembling nystagmus) on downgaze and sometimes accompanied by ataxia, speech, and learning disability and developmental delay. The condition is worsened by fatigue and remits during sleep. It usually follows infection or vaccination but is likely heterogeneous.[2491]

paroxysmal torticollis in infancy   See **benign paroxysmal vertigo of childhood.**

paroxysmal vertical ocular dyskinesia Paroxysmal, spontaneous, rapid, involuntary, vertical, and pendular eye movements lasting some 5 minutes, suppressed by horizontal movement, depressed by eye opening, made more regular with eye closure, and maximal in the mid-position of gaze. They are thought to be due to a supranuclear defect in vertical gaze control, the lesion resembling that of the **sylvian aqueduct syndrome.**[3557]

Parrot, Joseph-Marie-Jules (1829–1883) French physician and anthropologist who trained in Paris, where he later became professor of medical history and then of pediatrics. He described syphilitic pseudoparalysis (characterized by a disinclination to move because of osteitic pain, occurring in infants[4343]) as well as achondroplasia and the following two signs.

Parrot nodes Frontal and parietal bossing of the skull in congenital syphilis, leading to a "natiform" skull shape rather resembling that of a hot cross bun.[4344]

Parrot sign   1. See **hot cross bun skull.** 2. Dilation of the pupil when the skin of the neck is pinched, a normal response, though once thought diagnostic of meningitis.[4345] See **ciliospinal reflex.**

Parry, Caleb Hillier   (1755–1822) English physician who practiced in Bath. He was the first to describe facial hemiatrophy (**Parry-Romberg syndrome),** his notes being published posthumously in 1825, while **Romberg**'s account appeared in 1846. These notes also contained excellent descriptions of Hirschsprung disease, exophthalmic goiter, and angina.[1829]

Parry syndrome   A congenital dysmorphic syndrome of sparse, prematurely gray hair, sensorineural deafness, pigmentary abnormalities of the iris, cataract, abnormal teeth and nails, hypogonadotropic hypogonadism, arthritis, hyperkeratosis, depigmented skin, and psychomotor retardation.[337]

Parry-Romberg syndrome   (Romberg disease, [progressive] hemifacial atrophy, localized linear scleroderma, Wartenberg syndrome) A rare syndrome of unknown cause, in which atrophy of the skin and subcutaneous tissues of one side of the face occurs during the second (seldom the first) decade of life. The tongue, gums and soft palate, and the cartilage of the nose, ear, larynx, and eyelid are all affected. The condition may represent localized scleroderma.[239]

Associated abnormalities have included heterochromia iridis, alopecia, vitiligo, pigmented facial nevi, facial pain, optic atrophy, enophthalmos, strabismus, ptosis, miosis, uveitis, ataxia, and focal motor epilepsy.[4755] Cerebral lesions (cystic encephalomalacia) demonstrable by CT scan, ophthalmoparesis, involvement of other cranial nerves, and numerous other neurological signs appear less commonly.[4346] Some patients have café-au-lait spots, although this condition has nothing to do with **neurofibromatosis.**

Parry described it in 1825; Romberg, in 1846; and Wartenberg, in 1945.[5857]

Parsonage-Turner syndrome   See **neuralgic amyotrophy.**

Parsons, Sir John   (1868–1957) English physician who introduced the word **papilledema** to refer to the appearance of the swollen optic disk in patients with raised intracranial pressure—properly displacing the term *optic neuritis*, previously applied by von **Graefe.**

partial complex seizures   See **complex partial seizures.**

partial continuous epilepsy   (epilepsia partialis continua) An epileptic syndrome characterized by the association of variable, repetitive, clonic, focal, asymmetrical muscular twitching or jerks localized to a limited area on one side of the body without alteration of consciousness, lasting hours, days, or months and often associated with Jacksonian seizures. They are almost al-

ways the result of a vascular or mitotic lesion involving the rolandic cortex.[3146]

The EEG may show spike activity or other nonspecific abnormalities. The seizure episodes sometimes occur as a result of encephalitis of acute or chronic types, and in mitochondrial encephalopathies.[325] See also **Kozhevnikoff syndrome.**

partial convulsive status epilepticus   See **status epilepticus.**

partial epilepsy   See **epilepsy, localization-related epilepsies, and syndromes.**

partial epilepsy with auditory features   An unusual localization-related epilepsy syndrome, probably a variant of lateral temporal lobe epilepsy, characterized by auditory hallucinations and other sensory symptoms and linked to a mutation at 10q22–24.[6002]

partial epilepsy with pericentral spikes   A benign familial epilepsy syndrome linked to chromosome 4p15, and characterized by many variable seizure types (hemiclonic, hemitonic, generalized tonic-clonic, and complex partial) with onset in or after the first decade and manifesting spikes or sharp waves in the pericentral regions on the EEG.[3056a]

partial epilepsy with variable foci   (OMIM 600512) A dominantly inherited, localization-related epileptic disorder of childhood manifesting various seizure types and deafness, with normal cognition, mapped to 10q22–q24.[4516]

partial nonconvulsive status epilepticus   See **status epilepticus.**

partial optic aplasia   See **optic nerve hypoplasia.**

partial seizures   A seizure should be classified as partial when there is evidence of a clinical partial onset, regardless of whether the seizure is secondarily generalized. The aura (the first clinical signs of a seizure) has high localizing value and results from the anatomical or functional neuronal activation of part of one hemisphere.

When alertness and ability to interact appropriately with the environment are maintained, the seizure is classified as a *simple partial seizure.*

When impairment of consciousness, amnesia, or confusion during or after a seizure is reported, the seizure is classified as a *complex partial seizure.*

When a seizure becomes secondarily generalized, the seizure is classified as *partial seizure, secondarily generalized (simple or complex).*

When the distinction between simple and complex partial seizure cannot be made from information provided by history and medical records, the seizure is classified as *partial epileptic seizure of unknown type.*

When a patient has several types of partial seizure, each should be separately categorized.[1115]

Classifications provided by the Commission of Epidemiology and Prognosis I. Guidelines for epidemiological studies in epilepsy. *Epilepsia* 1993;34:592-6, by kind permission of Blackwell Science.

The selection of the word *partial* in this context suggests that the committee selecting it operated under a communal linguistic challenge. The word would have been equally incorrect appearing in the definitions of other such absolute entities as, for example, pregnancy or death. *Focally* or *locally originating seizures* would have been more appropriate.

partial syndrome   Incomplete, minor manifestations of typical dominantly inherited **myotonic dystrophy** carrying the same prognosis for transmission of the disorder. Isolated cataracts, few colored lens specks or minor EMG abnormalities are typical of these isolated manifestations.[4539]

Partington syndrome   (Russell-Silver–like syndrome) A congenital dysmorphic syndrome, possibly inherited as an X-linked dominant trait and manifesting low birth weight, short stature, patchy skin pigmentation, facial weakness, and delayed closure of the fontanelles.[337]

parturition palsy   Compressive neuropathy of the femoral nerve due to prolonged hyperflexion of the hips during childbirth.

parvo-   (Gr, small) Prefix denoting small.

PAS stain   (periodic acid-Schiff stain) A stain used to demonstrate the glycogen in, for example, muscle biopsy specimens. When the sample is stained using PAS stain with and without diastase, the glycogen content is both displayed and quantified. However, mucoproteins, mucolipids, glycoproteins, and glycolipids are also stained purple in histological preparations using this method.

Pascual-Castroviejo   syndrome   (cerebrofaciothoracic dysplasia) A congenital dysmorphic syndrome manifesting also short neck, hypertelorism, brachycephaly, flat occiput, kyphoscoliosis, vertebral anomalies, a high or Sprengel shoulder, strabismus, intracranial calcifications, callosal abnormalities, and mental and developmental delay.[337]

passibility   (from Lat, to suffer + able) Unpleasant sensations; a term used in the nineteenth century for **hyperesthesia.**

Passow syndrome   The association of **Horner syndrome** with **heterochromia iridis,** kyphoscoliosis, cervical rib, and spina bifida. Optic atrophy, facial hemiatrophy, trigeminal sensory loss, and generalized muscle weakness may also be found.

Dr. Arnold von Passow (1888–1966) was a German ophthalmologist.

Passwell syndrome   The association of congenital ichthyosis, erythroderma, mental retardation, dwarfism, and generalized aminoaciduria. Spastic paraparesis may also occur.[4355]

past pointing   1. (kinetic deviation) The subjects (with eyes closed) extend their arm to touch the examiner's finger with their own, and repeatedly lower and raise their arm again; progressive deviation to one side may be seen in patients with labyrinthine disease.

2. In the **finger–nose–finger test,** the subject's finger repeatedly veers off to one side of the target, and thus fails to come to a stop when the target is reached. This sign is usually sought in patients with disease of a cerebellar hemisphere.

Pasteur, Louis   (1822–1895) French bacteriologist and physiologist who determined that **rabies** was an infectious disease, although he never saw it. He also introduced preventive vaccination at a time when such prevention only existed for smallpox, his vaccine experiments having shown that the virulence of the virus was reduced with successive passage through a tribe of monkeys, or through rabbits. He later used a drying technique to reduce the virulence of the organism.

His therapy was at first controversial, partly on account of the immune reactions caused by the injection of foreign neural tissue; but the huge reduction in mortality resulting from use of the vaccine eventually quieted doubts, if not anxieties.

Patau syndrome   See **trisomy 13 syndrome.**

patellar clonus   Repetitive contraction of the quadriceps muscle after elicitation of its muscle stretch reflex in states of reflex hyperexcitability.

The absurd name is derived from the fact that the movements of the patella are the most obvious, at least to the untrained eye.

patellar relex   See **knee jerk.**

Paterson-Brown-Kelly syndrome   See **sideropenic dysphagia.**

pathoclisis   (Gr, disease + a tendency) An unusual vulnerability of certain neuronal systems to specific pathogenic agents.

pathological affect   See **emotionalism.**

pathological emotionality   The expression of strong emotion without the appropriate experience of joy or sadness; usually evidence of diffuse lesions affecting the brainstem and occasionally the cortex. See **emotionalism.**[116]

pathological fall   An unintended change in position occurring when unhealthy homeostatic mechanisms fail to preserve normal postural integrity. This typically occurs in **Parkinson disease.**

pathological laughter   Involuntary and inappropriate laughter, occurring as a result of cerebral disease. Three varieties are defined: *forced laughter* (or crying) may occur in patients with pseudobulbar or bulbar palsies, with or without awareness of the affect portrayed; **gelastic** *laughter* is an epileptic manifestation; and *inappropriate laughter* may occur in psychotic patients, one hopes in accord with their inner thoughts.[595]

Patin syndrome   See **myositis ossificans.**

Paton-Gowers-Kennedy syndrome See **Foster Kennedy syndrome.**

Patrick, H.T.   (1860–1938) American neurologist and psychiatrist, and professor at Northwestern University, Chicago. He was a founder and editor of the *Archives of Neurology and Psychiatry.*[1829]

Patrick sign   (FABERE test) Pain felt in the hip when the painful leg is flexed at the hip and knee, the heel placed on the opposite knee and pressed downward and laterally causing the abduction and external rotation. This maneuver does not cause pain in patients with root irritation, but is intensely painful in those with hip joint disease. The acronym FABERE is derived from **F**lexion, **AB**duction, **E**xternal **R**otation, and **E**xtension.

Patrick trigger areas   Trigger points in the distribution of the fifth cranial nerve which, when touched, induce paroxysms of pain in patients with trigeminal neuralgia.

pattern   A form recognizable by contrast with a background. A model or standard from which other models may be made or recognized by exact reproduction. Within neurology, it may be regarded as the space–time relationships of theoretically deducible and operationally detectible changes in the nervous system.[2187]

pattern theory   The theory that there are no specific fibers or receptors for sensation; what leaves the skin as a result of cutaneous stimulation is a complex spatially and temporally dispersed pattern of impulses, and this, or something like it, is what arrives in the brain.[5180]

pattern-sensitive seizure   An epileptic syndrome characterized by the occurrence of absence, myoclonic, or other seizures upon viewing a contrasting pattern. Most subjects also show clinical and electrical sensitivity to flicker.[56]

Patterson pseudoleprechaun syndrome   A congenital dysmorphic syndrome also manifesting low birth weight, dwarfism, hirsutism, cutis laxa, bronzed skin, a Cushingoid appearance, kyphoscoliosis, genu valgum, osteoporosis, delayed skeletal maturation, wide metaphyses, and seizures.[4364] See also **leprechaunism.**

pause (omnipause) neurons   Neurons which, with burst neurons, are found in the paramedian pontine reticular formation and whose tonic high-frequency activity, which normally inhibits the burst neurons, is interrupted before saccades occur in either a specific or any direction.

Pavlov, Ivan Petrovich   (1849–1936) Russian physiologist who trained in medicine at St. Petersburg, where he later became professor at the Army Medical Academy and director of the Institute of Experimental Medicine.

He is best remembered by neurologists for his studies of reflex action, particularly conditioned reflexes. He also enunciated the law of dynamic localization, which introduced the concept of graded or variable localization of function in the cortex, allowing different areas the potential for more than one function (pluripotentiality). He was awarded the Nobel prize in 1904, largely for his studies of the autonomic nervous system.

Pavlov reflexes   Conditioned reflexes (learned behavior patterns displayed in response to a stimulus repeatedly presented in association), first fully described by Pavlov in his *Lectures on Conditioned Reflexes* (New York, 1928).

pavor nocturnus   One or two-minute episodes of **night terror** occurring in children more often than in adults, which occur within the first half-hour of nocturnal sleep (in non–rapid eye movement stages 3 or 4). The child awakens screaming or moaning with the usual autonomic accompaniments of extreme fear.

PCB neuropathy   A toxic sensory polyneuropathy accompanied by headache and dysequilibrium and resulting from exposure to polychlorinated biphenyls.[1006]

Peabody picture vocabulary test   A test of comprehension, in which the subject is supplied with a word and is required to identify the corresponding picture from among four choices at different levels of complexity.[1551] As a test of receptive vocabulary it is used in children over the age of 2 years and in adults.

peacock trunk   A form of focal or axial dystonia affecting the truncal muscles and leading to a gait pattern resembling that of the peacock.

peak latency   the interval between the onset of a stimulus and a specified peak of the evoked waveform.

peak-dose chorea   A hyperkinetic form of fluctuation in parkinsonian patients on long-term L-dopa therapy, in whom choreic movements occur as the L-dopa levels rise.

peak-dose dyskinesia   See **peak-dose dystonia.**

peak-dose dystonia   (peak-dose dyskinesia) A dystonic form of fluctuation in parkinsonian patients on long-term L-dopa therapy in which dystonic movements appear as the L-dopa levels rise.

pectoral reflex   Contraction of the pectoral muscle when its tendon is tapped in the anterior axillary line, or when the tap is on the seventh rib. The reflex is normally present but is palpable rather than visible. It is enhanced in the setting of pyramidal lesions located above the C5 cord level.

pectoralis minor syndrome   Weakness and discomfort precipitated by manual labor, due to compression of the axillary veins below the pectoralis minor, which causes a syndrome (*venous claudication*) resembling intermittent claudication in the legs.[4063]

pedal   Relating to the foot.

pedialgia   Pain in the foot. See **Morton metatarsalgia.**

pediatric autoimmune neuropsychiatric disorders associated with streptococcal infections (PANDAS) A spectrum of childhood behaviors arising as a result of postinfectious autoimmune mechanisms through molecular mimicry. Clinical manifestations include fragments of Tourette syndrome, including obsessive-compulsive features, myoclonus, and attention-deficit hyperactivity disorder.[3195]

Pediatric MIDAS scale A questionnaire designed to assess the disability suffered by children with migraine.[2556] See also **MIDAS** scale.

Pediatric Neurology A subspecialty journal published by Elsevier. Web site: http://www.elsevier.nl/inca/publications/store/5/2/4/9/0/4/.

peduncle (from Lat, a foot stalk) A stalk-like process by which an anatomical part is joined to the main organ. Such an appearance led to the terms *cerebral* and *cerebellar peduncles.*

peduncular hallucinosis (red nucleus hallucinatory syndrome) The occurrence of vivid, colored, variable, non-threatening visual **pseudohallucinations** of patterns, places, or moving images, in association with lesions of the mesencephalon, pons, thalamus, or cerebral peduncles. They are accompanied in most cases by paresis of upward gaze, skew deviation, horizontal gaze paresis, nystagmus, choreoathetosis, cerebellar signs sleep disturbance, or other signs of posterior fossa dysfunction.[3399]

It was first described by J-J. **Lhermitte** in 1922 in a 75-year-old woman with a mesencephalic infarct who saw animals and people in the room with her, especially at nightfall (*vesperal hallucinations*); they appeared absurd to her, but aroused neither psychic nor motor reactions. Lhermitte regarded these as manifestations of diurnal dreaming (rapid eye movement dream material in wakefulness),[3398] an interpretation which is not much different from their current explanation as a release phenomenon related to damage to the ascending reticular activating system. The name was supplied by van Bogaert in 1924.[1862]

peek sign Myasthenic fatigue leads to weakening of the orbicularis oculi muscle during sustained tight eye closure, so that the subject's eyes open a little and the subject "peeks."[4266]

PEHO syndrome An X-linked syndrome of mental retardation, with marfanoid habitus, methyl-microcephaly, epilepsy, hypsarrhythmia, and coarse facial features. The basis of the disorder appears to be an increase in the endogenous production of nitric oxide.[5731]

Peiper optic reflex The occurrence of **opisthotonos** in response to stimulation with bright light; a normal response in the newborn.

Pel crises (tabetic ciliary neuralgia) Paroxysmal crises of orbital pain with lacrimation and photophobia, eventually leading to glaucoma and occurring in **tabes dorsalis.**

Pel, Pieter Klazes (1852–1919) Dutch physician and professor of pathology and medicine at Amsterdam University, who in 1898 described the crises now named for him.[4979]

pelagic paralysis See **paralytic shellfish poisoning, scombroid, ciguatera.**

Pelizaeus, Friedrich (1847–1929) German neurologist who in 1885 first described the features of the syndrome named for him.

Pelizaeus-Merzbacher disease (OMIM 312080) A rare, X-linked recessive, degenerative myelinopathy (a sudanophilic **leukodystrophy**) in which there is preservation of some myelin islands among widespread demyelination, with sparing of the cortical U fibers, due to mutations of the proteolipid protein (*PLP*) gene.

Clinically, the condition appears in infants or young children who manifest slowly progressive mental deterioration, arrhythmic nystagmus, bradylalia, choreoathetosis, seizures, spastic paraparesis, and both parkinsonian and cerebellar signs.[4393] A syndrome of spinal muscular atrophy (see **hereditary motor neuropathy**) is also described. The original gene location was to chromosome Xq21.2–q22. See also **Merzbacher E.**

Six varieties have been differentiated[5053] (see Chart P–6).

Chart P–6. Varieties of Pelizaeus-Merzbacher Disease

Pelizeus-Merzbacher disease type 1 (classic form) A congenital syndrome, usually inherited as an X-linked recessive trait and manifesting short stature, optic atrophy, nystagmus, dysarthria, microcephaly, pyramidal and cerebellar signs, choreoathetosis, and psychomotor delay. White matter hypodensities are seen on CT scans. Death occurs by the age of 25 years.[5866]

Pelizaeus-Merzbacher type 2 (Seitelberger disease, connatal disease) A congenital recessive or X-linked syndrome in which there is severe CNS dysmyelination to the extent that there may be no stainable myelin, although the axons are spared. Clinically, the condition is characterized by cataract, absent phalanges, hypotonia, microcephaly, nystagmus, spasticity, extrapyramidal signs, and severe psychomotor delay or arrest. White matter hypodensities are seen on CT scans.[5053]

Pelizaeus-Merzbacher type 3 (transitional form) A sporadic syndrome in which the findings are transitional, resembling both of the above two types.

Pelizaeus-Merzbacher type 4 (adult form, Lowenberg-Hill disease) A dominantly inherited syndrome characterized by tremor, ataxia, pyramidal signs, and dementia with onset in mature adult life.[3491]

Pelizaeus-Merzbacher type 5 A *variant* form in which there is only patchy demyelination.

Pelizaeus-Merzbacher type 6 A form characterized by microcephaly, dwarfism, mental retardation, ataxia, retinal pigmentation, cataract, facial thickening, joint contractures, and peripheral neuropathy. See **Cockayne syndrome.** "Jimpy" mice probably suffer from this condition.

pellagra   (Ital, skin + rough) (mal de rose, maidism, mal de sole, malattia della miseria) A syndrome of vitamin B (nicotinic acid) deficiency, characterized by a red, scaly, photosensitive dermatitis; dementia; depression; diarrhea; glossitis; insomnia; irritability; fatigue; depression; and anorexia. The rash is first seen in a necklace distribution—the *"Casal collar."*

The condition was first described by Gaspar Casal (1691–1759) and is still seen in alcoholics, patients with **Hartnup disease,** and in people who subsist on a diet of maize, from which the nicotinic acid may not be easily extractable. The myelopathy and skin rash respond to treatment with nicotinic acid; when present, an accompanying sensory neuropathy responds to thiamine.

pellagra encephalopathy   A syndrome of confusion, paratonia, and myoclonus, seen in patients with chronic alcoholism and multiple vitamin B deficiencies, in this case, particularly of niacin.[5759] See also **Wernicke-Korsakoff encephalopathy, Marchiafava-Bignami disease, acquired hepatocerebral encephalopathy.**

pellagrinoid   Suffering from **pellagra.**

Pellizzi disseminated cortical dysplasia   See **tuberous sclerosis.**

Pellizzi-Bourneville disease   See **tuberous sclerosis.**

pelvic floor syndromes   Myofascial pain syndromes affecting the muscles of the pelvic floor and causing pain in the buttocks, coccyx, hip, and posterior thigh regions. Per rectal massage has been recommended as treatment.

pelvic thrusting   Repetitive forward pelvic jerks resembling those characteristic of sexual activity but clinically manifested as evidence of underlying frontal or temporal lobe or of pseudo- (nonepileptic) seizures.[2086]

Pena-Shokeir 1 syndrome   See **Pena-Shokeir phenotype.**

Pena-Shokeir phenotype   (Pena-Shokeir 1 syndrome) A lethal recessively inherited, congenital syndrome, characterized by camptodactyly, severe fetal hydrops, multiple ankyloses, facial anomalies, pulmonary hypoplasia, hypokinesia in utero, and resulting arthrogryposis.[4399] See also **fetal akinesia malformation sequence,**[3929] **cerebro-oculofacioskeletal syndrome.**

The *multiple contracture syndrome, Finnish type,* is probably the same condition, except that it is fatal in the neonatal period.

Pendred syndrome   (deafness and goiter) The association of congenital bilateral sensorineural deafness, mutism, and goiter, inherited recessively.[4400]

pendular knee jerk   See **hypotonia.**

pendular macro-oscillations   See **square-wave pulses.**

pendular nystagmus   (undulatory nystagmus, talantropia; [from Gr, to oscillate]) That form of nystag-mus in which there are two equal-velocity slow phases of the abnormal deviations of the eyes, with no jerk component.

In the more common *congenital* form, the movements are usually horizontal and complaints of **oscillopsia** are rare; the lesion is considered to involve the dentate-rubro-olivary pathway. In the less common *acquired* form, the movements are rapid at 2–6 Hz and omnidirectional, and oscillopsia is usual. Numerous disorders of the brain and brainstem or cerebellum (especially demyelinating diseases) are considered to be the most common causes.[3330]

pendular pseudonystagmus   Spontaneous pendular oscillations of the eyes, made worse by reading, concentration, or trivial head movement and leading to complaints of blurred and shimmering vision or of oscillopsia. The vestibulo-ocular reflex is absent.

The condition is considered to reflect an imbalance in ocular compensation for an **essential tremor** affecting the head.[770]

Penfield syndrome   (autonomic diencephalic epilepsy) An unusual variety of seizure in which major autonomic (sympathetic) manifestations occur due to hypothalamic lesions.

Penfield's original case was of a woman who died with an encapsulated tumor that compressed the thalamus. Intermittent episodes of vasodilation, lacrimation, sweating, salivation, hypertension, piloerection, tachycardia, hypothermia, exophthalmos, hiccuping, shivering, and Cheyne-Stokes respirations were the clinical features of the attacks recorded. Most other cases have occurred in young males, among whom headache, abdominal pain, and evidence of autonomic arousal are the features most frequently recorded.[4401] See also **diencephalic autonomic seizures.**

Penfield, Wilder   (1891–1973) American-Canadian neurosurgeon who was an undergraduate at Princeton and was awarded a Rhodes scholarship, after which he graduated in medicine from Johns Hopkins in 1918 and later trained in surgery at Harvard, New York, Edinburgh, and London Universities. He practiced in New York for some years before moving to Montreal in 1928, when he was appointed professor of neurology and neurosurgery at McGill University. An internationally respected figure, he was honored by governments and universities in many countries.

The advances in neurosurgical technique which he made over the few years after his arrival in Montreal led the Rockefeller Foundation to provide funds to establish the Montreal Neurological Institute, with Penfield as its first director. Over his professional life, his research particularly concerned cerebral cortical localization, epilepsy, and the surgical approaches to its treatment. As well as numerous papers, he published books on the cytology of the CNS and on military surgery, *Epilepsy and Cerebral Localization* (1941), *The*

Cerebral Cortex of Man (1950), and *Epilepsy and the Functional Anatomy of the Human Brain* (1954), authored alone or in conjunction with colleagues at the Institute. He also wrote works of fiction.

Penfield-Ward syndrome   Calcifying cerebral hemangiomas.[4404]

PEP syndrome   See **POEMS.**

Pepper syndrome   See **Hutchinson tumor.**

peptides   (Gr, digest) Single-chain, low-molecular-weight amino acid compounds distributed widely throughout the CNS in selective neuronal pathways. Over 30 such compounds are known to act as neurotransmitters; *vasoactive intestinal peptide* exerts influence on the cerebral circulation, *substance P* and *opioid peptides*, on pain pathways; *cholecystokinin*, on appetite control; and *vasopressin* and *adrenocorticotrophic hormone*, on memory functions.

Perceived Deficits Questionnaire   A subjective measure of cognitive function designed for assessment of mental activity in patients with **multiple sclerosis.**[5410]

perception   The qualitative experience of a conscious person, evoked by a series of events including the unconscious reception, selection, differentiation, and integration of afferent stimuli. It depends upon alterations in the strength and rate of impulses derived from a peripheral organ and transmitted centrally.[2187] Perception thus denotes the identification of the source, significance, and emotional connotation of sensory stimuli. A percept stripped of meaning is merely a sensation.

perceptual cortex   The name given by **Penfield** to the upper lateral portion of the temporal lobe, stimulation of which led to **perceptual illusions** in the subjects he studied.

perceptual speed test   A digit cancellation task dependent upon psychomotor speed and sensitive to brain damage.[3967]

percussion myotonia   Contraction of muscle fibers with delayed relaxation, not under voluntary control, induced by tapping the muscle. This is a constant feature in myotonic syndromes.

percutaneous rhizotomy   Blind surgical section of posterior nerve roots, usually performed in an attempt to relieve spasticity or pain.

percutaneous transluminal angioplasty   A surgical technique for clearing an artery of a stenotic obstruction, employing a double lumen balloon catheter which is inflated within the vessel at the site of the obstruction.

peregrinating problem patients   See **Munchausen syndrome.**

Perez reflex   Pressure upward along the spine of the normal neonate lying prone leads to flexion of the limbs, extension of the neck, and crying.

Performance of Activities of Daily Living test (PADL) An objective instrument used especially in the elderly at home for determining physical functional abilities such as self-care, mobility, and transfers, with regard to their future management and need for care, and assessing some aspects of cognitive capacity.[3166]

performance scales   A self-report tool used in multiple sclerosis research, inquiring into the patient's perception of their capacities in mobility, hand function, fatigue, cognitive functions, bladder–bowel control, and sensory and spasticity symptoms.[5019]

perfusion pressure   The difference between the mean systemic arterial pressure and the cerebral venous pressure.

peri-   (Gr, around) Equivalent to the Latin *circum.*

periarteritis   See **polyarteritis nodosa.**

periaxin   A constituent protein of neural plasma membranes, its various mutations causing a wide range of genetically determined neuropathies.

pericranium   The membranous covering of the skull, or periosteum, first described by Galen.

perifascicular atrophy   The presence of myofibrils with an abnormally reduced diameter in the peripheral rather than the central parts of a muscle fascicle. Such an appearance is a characteristic of **dermatomyositis.**

perikaryon   The cell body.

perimetry   The mapping of visual fields, introduced in 1856 by von **Graefe** and subsequently refined by **Holmes** and **Traquair.** The subjects fixate on a central point and respond when they are made aware of a stimulus emanating from some point outside the area of fixation. See also **static perimetry, kinetic perimetry.**

perinatal telencephalic leukoencephalopathy   A condition due to damage to the white matter in neonates, possibly inflicted by endotoxins, and marked by the presence of hypertrophic astrocytes or acutely damaged glial cells in the neonatal telencephalon.[3380]

perineurial cyst   See **Tarlov cyst.**

perineurioma   1. A solitary intramuscular tumor composed of perineurial cells, but containing neither nerve fibers nor onion bulb lesions and unattached to a nerve trunk. 2. Perineurial cell accumulations within the nerves in **localized hypertrophic neuropathy.**[3915]

perineuritis   Inflammation of the perineurium with thickening of that membrane and degeneration of its cells with an associated lymphocytic inflammatory reaction; a well-recognized finding in patients with dysimmune sensory or sensorimotor multiple neuropathy of various etiologies.[5260] See also **sensory perineuritis.**

periodic alternating gaze   (ping-pong gaze) A disorder of ocular movement usually noted in patients in coma due to structural cerebral damage or drug toxicity. It consists of slow, rhythmic, and pendular conjugate horizontal deviations of the eyes that alternate from one extreme of gaze to the other every 3 to 7 seconds.[5066] Compensatory head turning to the opposite side for 1–2 minutes also occurs, followed by a midline changeover period lasting 15 seconds or so.

The phenomenon is seen in some comatose patents with severe bilateral hemispheric[5066] or hindbrain disease.

periodic alternating nystagmus (and aperiodic alternating nystagmus) Most commonly an acquired horizontal or oblique jerk nystagmus, present in the primary position and occurring in cycles lasting between 1 and 2 minutes, in which the direction of the fast component changes after a few seconds pause, persisting in this alternation.[6109]

Posterior fossa lesions of all kinds (usually located in the dorsal medulla or cerebellum) and drug toxicity have been incriminated as causes. The phenomenon reflects disordered activity within a γ-amino butyric acid inhibitory pathway, as confirmed by its inhibition by baclofen. An elegant elucidation of the mechanisms has been presented by Leigh et al.[3328]

In a *variant* form, the phases are irregular and occur in association with bilateral severe visual loss, which is usually congenital.

periodic alternating skew deviation A variant form of **skew deviation** in which the direction of the ocular deviations reverses spontaneously. It is sometimes associated with **periodic alternating nystagmus**.[3386]

periodic ataxia A dominantly inherited syndrome characterized by episodes of ataxia, vertigo, nystagmus and dysarthria responsive to acetazolamide. The same problem can occur as a complication of multiple sclerosis, in which case they are frequent and brief but do not cease with acetazolamide treatment.[1490,2016]

periodic downbeat nystagmus An unusual complication of hypomagnesemia, reported as $1^1/_2$ minutes of downbeating nystagmus separated by a period of 2 minutes.[1553]

periodic dystonia See **paroxysmal kinesigenic choreoathetosis.**

periodic hypersomnia (recurrent hypersomnia) A disorder characterized by recurrent episodes of hypersomnia that typically occur weeks or months apart. Diagnostic criteria have been suggested[234] and are given in Chart P–7.

Chart P–7. Diagnostic Criteria for Periodic Hypersomnia

A. A complaint of excessive sleepiness
B. The episodes of somnolence last for at least 19 hours a day.
C. The excessive sleepiness recurs at least once or twice a year, lasting a minimum of 3 days and up to 3 weeks.

D. The disorder occurs predominantly in males, with an age of onset typically in adolescence.
E. Associated features during the episodes include at least one of the following:
   1. Voracious eating,
   2. Hypersexuality, or
   3. Disinhibited behaviors such as irritability, aggression, disorientation, confusion, and hallucinations.
F. Polysomnographic monitoring during an episode demonstrates:
   1. A high sleep efficiency,
   2. Reduced NREM stages 3 and 4 sleep,
   3. Reduced sleep latency and rapid eye movement latency, and
   4. A multiple sleep latency test that demonstrates a mean sleep latency of less than 10 minutes.
G. The symptom is not associated with other medical or psychiatric disorders, such as epilepsy or depression.
H. The symptom is not associated with other sleep disorders, such as narcolepsy, sleep apnea syndromes, or periodic limb moment disorder.

From ASDA Diagnostic Classification Steering Committee. The International Classification of Sleep Disorders Diagnostic and Coding Manual. Rochester, MN: American Sleep Disorders Association, 1990.

See also **Klein-Levin syndrome.**

periodic hypersomnia associated with menstruation Intervals of severe, excessive daytime sleepiness and elevated total sleep time lasting for about a week after the onset of menstruation, sometimes also associated with depression.[2321]

periodic lateralized epileptiform discharges (PLEDs) Recurrent uniform spike– or sharp-wave discharges localized to part of one hemisphere on the EEG, occurring regularly at 0.5–2 Hz or irregularly. In adults they involve a large area of one hemisphere and are associated most commonly with acute destructive lesions of the brain caused by tumors or cerebral infarct; in children, chronic diffuse lesions of the CNS are most often responsible. They are often accompanied by disturbed consciousness and seizures.[990]

periodic leg movements See **periodic limb movement disorder.**

periodic limb movement disorder (periodic leg movements, nocturnal myoclonus, periodic limb movements in sleep, leg jerks, sleep myoclonus, periodic sustained anterior tibial contractions with arousal, night starts, sudden bodily jerks on falling asleep) A disorder characterized by periodic episodes of repetitive and stereotyped, semipurposeful limb movements that occur during stages 1 and 2 of non–rapid eye movement sleep or in the period of relaxed wakefulness immediately prior to sleep,[1100,1101,5456] consisting of single, body-wide jerks of unknown cause, unassociated with known neurological disease, immediately restoring the subject to wakefulness. Extension of the hallux, dorsiflexion of the ankle, and flexion of the knee and hip are the usual movements recorded (a pattern reminiscent of the **Babinski reflex**).

The bursts of electrical activity underlying them last 2–15 seconds (unlike other forms of positive **myoclonus**) and recur with marked periodicity.[1101] A disorder of the CNS dopaminergic systems producing increased excitability of segmental spinal flexor reflexes is considered to be the underlying pathophysiology.

Despite the alternative names, these movements are seldom as fast as true myoclonus. They are associated with both **narcolepsy** and the **restless legs syndrome.** Daytime somnolence and nocturnal insomnia may also result. See also **sleep myoclonus.**

Diagnostic criteria have been suggested[234] and are given in Chart P–8.

Chart P–8. Diagnostic Criteria for Periodic Limb Movement Disorder

A. A complaint of insomnia or excessive sleepiness. Occasionally the patient will be asymptomatic and the movements are noticed by an observer.
B. Repetitive highly stereotyped limb muscle movements occur, which in the leg are characterized by extension of the big toe in combination with partial flexion of the ankle, knee, and sometimes hip.
C. Polysomnographic monitoring demonstrates:
   1. Repetitive episodes of muscle contraction (0.5–5 seconds in duration) separated by an interval typically of 20–40 seconds
   2. Arousal or awakenings may be associated with the movements.
D. There is no evidence of a medical or psychiatric disorder that can account for the movements.
E. Other sleep disorders may be present but do not account for the movements, e.g., obstructive sleep apnea syndrome.

From ASDA Diagnostic Classification Steering Committee. The International Classification of Sleep Disorders Diagnostic and Coding Manual. Rochester, MN. American Sleep Disorders Association, © 1990, by kind permission of the American Academy of Sleep Medicine.

periodic migrainous neuralgia of Wilfred Harris Yet another term for **cluster headache,** but this one more comfortably euphonious, if rather lengthy. At least it recognizes the uncertainty that yet remains as to whether the pathogenesis of this condition is neural, vascular, or both.

periodic miosis (intermittent oculosympathetic paresis) Periodic pupillary constriction with conjunctival injection, lasting from minutes to months.[5425]

periodic movements in sleep See **periodic limb movements of sleep.**

periodic paralysis A dominantly inherited syndrome characterized by episodic bouts of acute, progressive, symmetrical, flaccid weakness, mainly in the limbs and lasting hours to days, with areflexia, due to genetically determined abnormalities in potassium metabolism. See **familial periodic paralysis.**

The attacks follow a carbohydrate load or exertion, and insulin or adrenalin administration. Depolarization of the muscle fibers and impaired Na^+-K^+ activity in muscle may predispose. In the setting of hyper-

thyroidism, the condition is mainly recorded in male Japanese.

periodic somnolence with morbid hunger See **Kleine-Levin syndrome.**

periodic sustained anterior tibial contractions with arousal See **periodic limb movement disorder.**

periodic syndromes 1. A childhood syndrome of typical adult migraine or a combination of one or more of the following symptoms: cyclic vomiting or repeated bilious attacks; recurrent vague abdominal pain; recurrent headaches; dizzy spells; periodic attacks of fever; and periodic attacks of limb and joint pains or stiffness ("growing pains"). The prevalence of this condition alone may be 4.5%. The syndrome most likely includes many cases of juvenile **migraine,** particularly when headache is present.[359]

2. Recurrent episodes of neurological deficit in children, which may be precursors to or associated with migraine (migraine equivalents). There are two varieties, and the following diagnostic criteria are suggested by the Headache Classification Committee of the International Headache Society[1051] (Chart P–9).

Chart P–9. Diagnostic Criteria for the Periodic Syndrome

Benign paroxysmal vertigo of childhood A probably heterogeneous disorder characterized by brief attacks of vertigo in otherwise healthy children.
A. Multiple, brief, sporadic episodes of dysequilibrium, anxiety, and often nystagmus or vomiting
B. Normal neurological examination findings
C. Normal electroencephalogram
Alternating hemiplegia of childhood Attacks of hemiplegia occurring in infants, involving each side alternately, and often associated with other paroxysmal phenomena and mental impairment.
A. Onset before 18 months of age
B. Repeated attacks of hemiplegia involving both sides of the body
C. Other paroxysmal phenomena, such as tonic spells, dystonic posturing, choreoathetoid movements, nystagmus, or other ocular motor abnormalities, autonomic disturbances associated with the bouts of hemiplegia or occurring independently.
D. Evidence of mental or neurological deficits

From Headache Classification Committee of the International Headache Society. Classification of headache disorders, cranial neuralgias and facial pains; and diagnostic criteria for primary headache disorders. Cephalalgia 1988;8(suppl):1–96 by kind permission of Blackwell Science.

periodic vestibulocerebellar ataxias Dominantly inherited conditions of adult onset manifested by diplopia and intermittent attacks of vestibular dysfunction and ataxia. See **cerebellar ataxias.**

periodic-acid Schiff stain See **PAS stain.**

periodic/aperiodic nystagmus See **periodic alternating nystagmus.**

perioptic neuritis   (optic perineuritis) An inflammatory disorder of the optic nerve sheaths; when explained, it is usually due to syphilis, sarcoidosis, or other inflammatory conditions.[3609]

perioral reflexes   Contraction of various facial and cervical muscles in response to a tap on the lips or the perioral regions, or as a result of other stimuli to the face. Both proprioceptive and nociceptive stimulation produces such responses, which are present in most normal subjects but which may be exaggerated in the presence of diffuse cortical dysfunction.[1628,5858] See also **corneomandibular reflex, orbicularis oris reflex.**

periosteal reflexes   A misnomer, the periosteum having no receptor stimulation that leads to reflex muscle contraction. The numerous "reflexes" described with this suffix are muscle stretch reflexes, and are only entered as such in this book. See **muscle stretch reflex.**

peripheral neurofibromatosis and peroneal muscular atrophy   See **hereditary motor and sensory neuropathy** (*variants*).

peripheral neuropathy   A disorder of the motor and/or sensory nerves, as opposed to the fiber tracts within the CNS. Involvement of cranial nerves below the optic nerve and of the autonomic nervous system is subsumed.

Primary disease of the cells of the motor nuclei of cranial and spinal nerves might be supposed to indicate the presence of a CNS disorder, but the effects are the same as those of other, more distal, neural pathologies and are generally classified under the heading of *peripheral neuropathy*.

peripheral neuropathy affecting the arms   A dominantly inherited syndrome of distal neurogenic arm weakness and wasting with early adult onset.[3249]

Peripheral Neuropathy Association   See **Neuropathy Association.**

Peripheral Neuropathy Symptom Questionnaire   A validated tool for the detection of neuropathy in neuroepidemiological studies.[1945] The following questions are asked:
> How often have you had any of the following conditions in the past 4 weeks?
> Cramps in the muscles of the arms or legs
> Twitching in the muscles of the arms or legs
> Need for help getting out of a chair
> Difficulty in opening screw top lids on jars
> Tingling or pins and needles sensations in the hands, arms, feet, or legs
> Numbness
> A burning sensation in the arms or legs
> Pain in the arms after work, when resting
> A need to strain in order to start urine flowing
> A need to push on the abdomen to start or keep the urine flowing

peripheral neuropathy with hepatic disease   A demyelinating peripheral neuropathy complicating cirrhosis, portosystemic shunt, or hepatic necrosis, considered most likely to be due to a toxic metabolite or to disordered insulin metabolism as a result of the hepatic damage.[1318]

peripheral nystagmus   A form of conjugate, direction-fixed nystagmus often with both horizontal and rotatory components, caused by a lesion of the vestibular system outside the CNS.

When it is induced by head movements (**Bárány test**), there is a delay of some seconds before it occurs, and it fatigues with time and with repetition. Unlike **central nystagmus,** its amplitude is lessened by visual fixation. See also **direction-fixed nystagmus.**

peripheral vertigo   That form of vertigo due to a lesion of the end-organ of the vestibular system or of the vestibular nerve, giving rise to **peripheral nystagmus.**

peripheral vestibular paroxysmia   (disabling peripheral vertigo) A tentative syndrome considered likely due to neurovascular crossovers between the eighth nerve and a brainstem artery such as the AICa. Clinically, it presents as as a series of short attacks or a series of rotational or to-and-fro-vertigo, sometimes related to changes in head position and often with hypacusis and tinnitus.[5391]

peripheral vestibulopathy   A syndrome of single or recurrent episodes of vertigo lasting for hours to days, unassociated with hearing loss or other neurological dysfunction.

The clinical syndrome encompasses various nonspecific disorders, the most notable being **vestibular neuronitis.**[1511]

periphlebitis retinae   See **Eales disease.**

perisylvian syndrome   A congenital syndrome characterized by bilateral perisylvian micropolygyria with multiple seizure types, cognitive deficits, and pseudobulbar (faciopharyngomasticatory) palsy.[3204]

perithelial small cell sarcoma   See **primary CNS lymphoma.**

perivascular plaques   (Scholz plaques) Amyloid deposits in the walls of cerebral arterioles.

perivascular sarcoma   See **primary CNS lymphoma.**

periventricular leukomalacia   (periventricular lucencies) Damage to the white matter, particularly in the occipital radiation and close to the foramen of Monro, involving the centrum semiovale at the junction of the corpus callosum and the internal and external capsules.

They are typically caused by **watershed infarcts** of the (as yet unmyelinated) white matter. When occurring in infants as a result of hypoxic-ischemic injury, some form of **cerebral palsy** with motor deficits, cognitive and visual impairment, and seizures is the usual clinical result. The condition is common in the brains of neonates of low birth weight who survive severe clinical insults in the perinatal period for only a few days.[5146] **Leukoaraiosis** has a similar distribution in adults.

periventricular lucencies See **periventricular leukomalacia.**

Perlia nucleus A small group of cells medial to the third cranial nerve nuclear complex, described in 1889. They probably represent a center for the control of ocular convergence, but the existence, let alone the function, of this "nucleus" has been called into question.

Perlia, Richard German ophthalmologist.

permanent global amnesia A rare, severe, selective, and stable memory disorder of adult life affecting both new learning and recall, and associated with selective hippocampal atrophy, probably on an ischemic basis.[3164] See also **transient global amnesia.**

permanent persistent postconcussive syndrome The prolonged experience of symptoms common in the immediate phase after mild traumatic brain injury (concussion) including dizziness, headache, unusual sensitivity to most or all sensations, impairment of memory, attention, and executive functions, and emotional symptoms such as irritability, depression, and resentment.[96]

permanent unconsciousness See **persistent vegetative state.**

peroneal compartment syndrome Ischemic necrosis of the muscles with resultant compression of the nerves in the peroneal compartment, either as a result of primary vascular occlusion or following overexertion, which may lead to muscle swelling beneath the strong fascial membrane delimiting the compartment, thus inducing secondary occlusion of the blood vessels within it.

Clinically, pain, swelling, weakness, and sensory loss in the territory of the common peroneal nerve are the major findings.[4666] See **anterior tibial syndrome.**

peroneal muscle reflex Contraction of the anterior compartment muscles when the examiner's finger, placed on the dorsum of the foot, is tapped with a reflex hammer. The contraction is increased in the presence of pyramidal lesions and decreased with lesions of the L5 or S1 reflex arcs.[510]

peroneal muscular atrophy See **hereditary motor and sensory neuropathy, types 1** and **2.**

peroneal sign See **Lust phenomenon.**

peroneus (from Gr, a leg bone; the same as the Latin word *fibula*, the bone over which the peroneal nerve and muscles overlie) The relationship of the tibia to the fibula was considered similar to that of a brooch and its pin.

peroxidase deficiency A dominantly inherited form of **neuronal ceroid lipofuscinosis;** a corencephalopathy.[619]

peroxisomal disorders Inborn errors of metabolism affecting multiple organ systems and caused by disorders of these intracellular organelles in which the enzymatic utilization of oxygen and the production of hydrogen peroxide occur.[3307,3951,4611] Disorders involving these entities are due to absence of a specific peroxisomal enzyme or to a failure to form peroxisomes, resulting in a generalized deficiency of these enzymes (peroxisomal biosynthesis disorders). Peroxisomes are responsible for the catabolism of very long–chain fatty acids, dicarboxylic acids, and pipecolic and phytanic acids, and for the biosynthesis of bile acids.[3]

Clinically, severe mental retardation and both visual and auditory defects are constant symptoms in those peroxisomal diseases with congenital presentations, as in Group 1 in Chart P–10, which lists those of neurological interest identified to date.

Clinical features suggesting the possible presence of a disorder of this type are presented in the table below.

Prevalence	Clinical Features
Invariable	Psychomotor retardation
Over 75% of cases	Low, broad nasal ridge
	Encephalopathy
	Impaired hearing
	Hepatomegaly
	Neonatal hypotonia
	Seizures
	Abnormal electroretinogram
50%–70% of cases	Large fontanelles
	Epicanthus
	Congenital cataracts
	Peripheral neuropathy in early childhood
	Failure to thrive after 6 months of age
	Shallow orbital ridges
	Pigmentary retinopathy

Precise listings of symptoms related to age are presented by Baumgartner et al.[397] and by Theil et al. (cited by Moser[4011]). The genetic correlations of the various disorders have been nicely reviewed by Barth et al.[379] and more recently by Raymond.[4614]

Chart P–10. The Peroxisomal Disorders

1. Single-enzyme defects with normal peroxisomal structure and abnormalities of a single peroxisomal function. Examples are:

   X-Linked adrenoleukodystrophy and the *Naidu variant*
   X-linked adrenomyeloneuropathy
   Acyl CoA oxidase deficiency (pseudoneonatal adrenoleukodystrophy)
   Pseudo-**Zellweger disease**
   Adult Refsum disease (**hereditary motor and sensory neuropathy, type 4**)
   Other adult-onset polyneuropathies
   Rhizomelic chondrodysplasia and variant phenotypes
   Hyperoxaluria type 1
   Acatalasemia
   Mevalonic aciduria; hyper-IgD syndrome[379]
   Glutaric aciduria type 3

2. *Disorders of peroxisomal dysgenesis* Disorders in which peroxisomes are present but two peroxisomal functions are disturbed, and there are multiple enzyme disorders. These devastating diseases are characterized by failure to

thrive, mental retardation, seizures, blindness, deafness, and liver failure due to deficiency in multiple peroxisomal enzymes.[3541] Examples are:

Leber optic atrophy
Zellweger syndrome
Pseudo-Zellweger disease
Rhizomelic chondrodysplasia punctata
Neonatal **adrenoleukodystrophy**
Infantile Refsum disease

A benign *variant* is *ataxia and peripheral neuropathy*, which is a childhood syndrome of ataxia, hyporeflexia, and hypotonia with panperoxisomal dysfunction in the plasma, fibroblasts, and liver.[3541,4011]

peroxisomal polydystrophy syndromes The syndromes of **infantile Refsum disease,** neonatal **adrenoleukodystrophy,** and **hyperpipecolic acidemia.**[2999]

peroxisomes Subcellular single-membrane bound organelles within nucleated cells that generate H_2O_2 in the course of oxidizing a large number of substrates including immunoacids, hydroxyacids, and fatty acids. They also contain catalase, an enzyme that breaks down H_2O_2. These ubiquitous organelles house the proteinaceous *impedimenta* of numerous metabolic pathways, most involving brain more than peripheral nervous system functioning.

Chemical abnormalities associated with peroxisomal defects include elevated concentrations of very-long–chain fatty acids, excessive pipecolate in blood and urine, and reduced tissue concentrations of plasmalogenes.[2167]

per-rotational response Nystagmus induced by the onset of a velocity-step stimulus.[3330]

perseverance (persistence) The laudable ability of an individual to stick to a task in hand.

perseveration The involuntary continuance or recurrence of a purposeful response that is more appropriate to a preceding stimulus than to the succeeding one just given, which is essential to provoke it.[116] More simply, it is the continuation or recurrence of an experience or activity without the appropriate stimulus.

It is not spontaneous; two or more stimuli are required to demonstrate it. It is seen in normal subjects at the extremes of age, but is also a sign of any kind of diffuse or focal organic brain disease.

Three varieties have been defined:[4908]
1. Recurrence of a previous response with a subsequent stimulus within the context of an established set (*recurrent perseveration*). This is most closely associated with left hemisphere lesions.
2. Inappropriate maintenance of a category or framework of activity (*stuck-in-set perseveration*), associated with frontal-subcortical and mesolimbic lesions.
3. Abnormal prolongation or the continuation without cessation of current behavior (*continuous perseveration*), for which right hemisphere lesions are most commonly responsible.

The term was introduced by Neisser in 1895. Wilson described perseveration as follows: "The persistence of certain impressions may become a fertile source of error in the execution of complex movements; a patient may recognise an object and use it correctly, but be unable to prevent himself from repeating this act when a different object is shown to him."[6000]

Perseveration is a reliable sign of organic mental dysfunction at any time after infancy.[1946]

persistence See **perseverance.**

persistent conditioned insomnia See **persistent DIMS.**

persistent DIMS (disorders of initiation or maintenance of sleep, persistent conditioned insomnia, internal arousal insomnia, psychophysiological arousal) A disorder of sleep initiation and maintenance (i.e., falling asleep and staying asleep) as a result of chronic somatized tension combined with conditioned reinforcers of sleeplessness (see also ASDA Diagnostic Classification[249]).

persistent DOES (**D**isorders **O**f **E**xcessive **S**leep) Chronic sleepiness following a prolonged period of emotional stress. See also **general adaptation syndrome** and the ASDA Diagnostic Classification.[249]

persistent idiopathic hyperCKemia When muscle biopsy samples of the vastus lateralis are obtained for histologic analysis and contracture testing with halothane and caffeine show that half are positive, unexplained persistently increased CK levels in an otherwise healthy patient should alert the anesthesiologist to the possibility of malignant hyperthermia syndrome and/or myopathy.[5892]

persistent infantile sleep apnea Congenital failure of the automatic control of respiration, leading to alveolar hypoventilation in the presence of normal function of the lungs and heart and normal metabolism; one likely cause of the **sudden infant death syndrome.**

persistent pain of cranial nerve origin Diagnostic criteria have been suggested by the Headache Classification Committee of the International Headache Society[1051] and are reproduced in Chart P–11. See also the review of Portenoy et al.[4494]

Chart P–11. Diagnostic Criteria for Persistent Pain of Cranial Nerve Origin

A. Pain in the distribution of one or more cranial nerves and/or cervical roots 2 and 3, with or without projection to neighboring areas
B. There is demonstration of a relevant lesion.
C. Onset of pain is temporally related to the onset of a cranial nerve lesion.
D. If the lesion can be effectively treated or remits spontaneously, pain abates or disappears.
Compression or distortion of cranial nerves and second or third cervical roots Headache or facial pain caused by a lesion directly compromising one or more of the afferent nerves supplying pain sensation to the head and neck (namely,

the trigeminal, nervus intermedius, glossopharyngeal, vagus, and cervical roots 2 and 3).

Optic neuritis (retrobulbar neuritis)

A. Pain is felt.

B. Central vision becomes impaired because of a central or paracentral scotoma.

C. No extrinsic lesion can be demonstrated.

Infarction of cranial nerves

Diabetic neuritis Pain around the eye and forehead associated with an oculomotor (third cranial nerve) palsy of diabetic origin.

A. Pain is felt around the eye on the affected side.

B. Pain is of acute onset, developing over a few hours.

C. There is a partial or complete oculomotor nerve palsy.

D. The patient suffers from diabetes mellitus.

E. No extrinsic lesion can be demonstrated.

Inflammation of cranial nerves

Chronic postherpetic neuralgia Facial pain developing during the acute phase of herpes zoster infection and persisting more than 6 months thereafter.

A. Pain is restricted to the distribution of the affected cranial nerves or divisions thereof.

B. Pain persists more than 6 months after the onset of herpetic eruption.

From Headache Classification Committee of the International Headache Society. Classification of headache disorders, cranial neuralgias and facial pains and diagnostic criteria for primary headache disorders. Cephalalgia 1988;8(suppl):1–96 by kind permission of Blackwell Science.

persistent vegetative state (wakefulness without awareness, akinetic mutism, apallic state, alpha coma, chronic coma, coma vigil[e], irreversible coma, neocortical death, permanent unconsciousness) A form of eyes-open permanent unconsciousness in which the patient has periods of wakefulness and physiological sleep–wake cycles within 1 to 2 weeks following the initial coma, but the subject is at no time aware of the self or the environment, although blinking may occur in response to threat or loud noises. Cognition, recognition, and meaningful interaction with the environment are absent and thought, reason, memory, speech, affect (and any of the other qualities conventionally characteristic of human nature or personhood) are lost. As far as can be determined, neither pain nor suffering is experienced. Wandering, conjugate eye movements return but sustained visual pursuit does not occur. Brainstem functions such as breathing, chewing, swallowing, and cranial/spinal reflexes are preserved and occasional nonpurposive movements may be performed. Sphincter control is lost.

The condition results from diseases that lead to the total loss of cerebral cortical functions, while those of the brainstem are retained. Most commonly, it follows severe anoxic or traumatic brain disease, but it can also occur as an end stage in chronic dementing or other neurological disorders.

Its characteristics have been defined by committees of the American Academy of Neurology[142] and the American Neurological Association,[148] the latter being reproduced in Chart P–12 in a slightly adapted form. A further major review has been published.[5529]

Chart P–12. Diagnostic Criteria for Persistent Vegetative State

To allow the diagnosis, the following slightly adapted criteria must be met:

A. The patient displays no evidence of awareness of self or surroundings, although reflex or spontaneous eye opening may occur.

B. No meaningful and consistent auditory or written communication between the examiner and the patient can be established. (Target stimuli are not usually followed visually, but visual tracking can occasionally occur.) The patient shows no emotional response to verbal input.

C. There is no comprehensible speech nor mouthing of words.

D. Smiling, frowning, and crying can occur, but are inconsistently related to any apparent stimulus.

E. Sleep-wake cycles are present.

F. Brainstem and spinal reflex activity is variable. Sucking, rooting, chewing, and swallowing reflexes may be preserved. Pupillary reactivity to light, oculocephalic reflexes, grasp reflexes, and muscle stretch reflexes may be present.

G. The presence of voluntary movements or behavior, no matter how rudimentary, is a sign of cognition and is incompatible with the diagnosis of persistent vegetative state. There is no motor activity suggesting learned behavior and no mimicry. Rudimentary movements (such as withdrawal or posturing) may be seen with noxious or disagreeable stimuli.

H. Blood pressure control and cardiorespiratory functions are usually intact. Incontinence of bladder and bowel is present.

Adapted from the American Neurological Association Committee on Ethical Affairs. Persistent vegetative state. Ann Neurol 1993;33:386–390 by kind permission.

Despite such confident assertions, a problem is that one can only say that the condition is actually persistent in retrospect, because we do not yet have the power of accurate prognosis for this condition. How long it takes for this syndrome to be labeled "persistent" with justification is a question removed from the practice of medicine and best left to the family, the lawyers, the ethicists, and the administrators of the hospital where the metabolizing patient lies dead to the world. Some suggest 1 year; this author's living will specifies a week. The simpler term "vegetative state" avoids the issue but at least makes fewer assumptions.

persistent wakefulness A disorder of sleep (dyssomnia) characterized by an inability to sleep, and due to a pre-trigeminal midpontine lesion or to psychophysiological mechanisms.[2478]

perte de la parole (Fr, loss of words) The earliest term for what we now know as **aphasia,** used by Bouillaud in 1825.[678]

pertussis neurotoxic syndrome A supposed neurological complication following the administration of whole-cell pertussis vaccine. It is characterized clinically by screaming, ataxia, irritability, convulsions, or coma, occurring several hours after injection of the vaccine into an infant.[4521]

pervasive developmental disorders   A heterogeneous collection of disorders affecting young children's social interaction and ability to communicate, commonly combined with stereotyped behavioral patterns. See **Prader-Willi syndrome; inv dup (15) syndrome.**

perverse pupillary reaction   Pupillary dilation on attempted near-gaze. It is thought to be a psychosensory response to the examiner's enthusiastic encouragement.[5824]

perverted nystagmus   Vertical nystagmus resulting from unilateral caloric stimulation.[3330] See **vestibular nystagmus.**

pes cavus   A common congenital or acquired deformity of the foot, in which the anteroposterior measurement is decreased, the arch high, and the toes flexed at the distal, and extended at the proximal, interphalangeal joints.

In a third of the cases the abnormality is not associated with any neurological deficits, but it is a frequent finding in patients with **spinocerebellar degenerations** and with the **hereditary motor and sensory neuropathies** and other genetically determined neuropathies.[741]

pes planus   Flat foot, either mobile or fixed in that position.

Pescia epileptogenic encephalopathy   A congenital syndrome manifesting seizures, microcephaly, cerebral atrophy, callosal agenesis, and mental and developmental delay.[337]

PET scan   A test of regional cerebral metabolic function. See **positron emission tomography.**

petalias   Indentations on the inner table of the skull due to asymmetrical compression by the asymmetrical brain during development.

Petges syndrome   See **dermatomyositis.**

petit mal   See **three-Hz spike-and-slow waves, atypical repetitive spike-and-slow waves.**

petit mal epilepsy   See **absence epilepsy** (minor seizures).

petit mal seizures with focal components   Attacks differing from other forms of typical absence attack by virtue of a later age of onset, the frequent presence of cerebral lesions (usually frontal), and a poor response to treatment.[1247]

petit mal status   See **status epilepticus, absence status.**

petit mal triad   The combination of akinetic and absence seizures with myoclonus.

petit mal variant   See **atypical repetitive spike-and-slow waves.**

Petren gait   A disorder of motility in which the patient becomes unable to continue walking after the first few steps have been taken. The condition is usually considered to indicate the presence of frontal lobe pathology.

The phenomenon is a version of **astasia trepidante.** See also **isolated gait ignition failure.**

petrosal ganglion   A ganglion associated with the ninth cranial nerve, which contains the cell bodies of fibers which pass to the nucleus solitarius.

petrosphenoidal space syndrome   See **Jacod syndrome (triad).**

petrous apical syndrome   See **Gradenigo syndrome.**

petrous neuralgia   (Gardner neuralgia) Intermittent bouts of severe pain in the cheek and lateral parts of the eyebrow, with lacrimation and rhinorrhea.

The condition resembles, and is probably a variant of, **cluster headache,** but also contains elements of **trigeminal neuralgia.**

Pfaundler-Hurler syndrome   See **mucopolysaccharidoses.**

Pfeiffer scale   A short, portable mental status questionnaire for the assessment of organic brain deficit in elderly patients.[4429]

Pfeiffer syndrome   (acrocephalosyndactyly type 4, congenital ataxia with choroidal coloboma) A congenital dysmorphic syndrome characterized by craniosynostosis affecting the coronal suture, with turri-brachycephaly and kleeblattschädel (cloverleaf malformation of the skull), ocular hypertelorism, broad thumbs, syndactyly, proptosis, strabismus, deafness, elbow joint synostosis, and developmental delay.[3661] See **acrocephalopolysyndactyly.**

PGO waves   See **pontogeniculo-occipital waves.**

phakomatoses   (from Gr, mark on the skin) (neurocutaneous syndromes, neuroectomesodermoses, genoneurodermatoses, ectomesodermal blastomatoses, congenital neuroectodermal dysplasias) A heterogeneous collection of inherited ectodermal disorders which have in common the involvement of the skin and of the nervous system.

The name was bestowed by van der Hoeve (1923). See **neurocutaneous syndromes.**

Phalen sign   Compression of the median nerve by the exertion of finger pressure over the carpal tunnel leads to the complaint of paresthesias in the median nerve distribution in many patients with **carpal tunnel syndrome.** The incidence of positive results with this sign varies rather widely between different series.[4430]

Dr. George Phalen was an orthopedic surgeon who practiced at the Cleveland Clinic.

phantom   (from Gr, to make invisible). A mental illusion.

phantom limb   The subjective perception of the presence of a body part when it is in fact absent, because of either amputation or congenital absence. The size of the limb perceived may slowly diminish over the years following amputation, or it may remain unaltered, sometimes enlarging during intercurrent illnesses. In *variant* forms, a patient with sensory or motor loss may feel the paretic limb moving when it is not doing so, or may experience a phantom as part of a sensory seizure.

Such a perception might well have been regarded as evidence of possession in medieval times, but it was recognized as a medical problem by Ambrose Paré (1551), Réne Descartes, and Sir Charles **Bell.** Admiral Lord Nelson believed that his awareness of the phantom fingers of his amputated arm provided direct proof of the existence of the soul. More modern descriptions are those of **Weir Mitchell,**[3909,4685] drawing from his experiences in the American Civil War, and of Herman Melville ("a dismasted man never loses the feeling of his old spar but it will still be pricking him at times").

phantom (limb) pain   Persistent but variable cramping, burning, or aching pain, made worse by any emotional or physical stimuli and by attempted "movement" and felt in a phantom part, especially the arm, and especially by patients who experienced severe pain in their limb prior to its removal. Such pain is experienced by less than 5% of all amputees. It is sometimes relieved by sympathetic block, suggesting a peripheral origin.[2534]

phantom optic nerve   An artifact on CT scanning, whereby an optic nerve which has been removed nevertheless appears to be present in horizontal sections of orbital scans.[5123]

phantom petit mal   See **phantom spike and wave.**

phantom spike and wave   (Phantom petit mal, wave-and-spike phantom) Generalized, bilateral, brief bursts of low-voltage spike-and-wave discharges on the EEG which run at about 6 Hz, mainly in frontocentral regions (but occasionally seen posteriorly) and which are activated by diphenhydramine.[5834] The appearance is rare, although it is more common in adult women and has been linked, with incomplete confidence, to various other EEG abnormalities and to the occurrence of clinical seizures, headaches, and some psychiatric disorders. The discharge is, however, probably physiological and no more than an electrophysiological curiosity.[3604] See **six-Hz spike-and-slow waves.**

phantom tics   The extracorporeal projection of the premonitory sensations preceding motor tics in Tourette syndrome as a result of mental projection of sensory impression to other people, inanimate objects, or even nonexistent objects, partially relieved by touching those that do exist.[2935]

phantom vision   The transient belief that visual sensations are present and seen by an eye which is in fact absent.[1092]

pharmacological pupillary testing   The use of drugs in low concentrations to assess the innervation of the pupils. Thus, 4% *cocaine* dilates the pupil so long as postganglionic sympathetic activity is intact; 0.1% *adrenaline* has no effect on a normal pupil but causes dilatation when there is postganglionic failure, due to denervation supersensitivity; 1% *hydroxyamphetamine* dilates a normal pupil by releasing norepinephrine, while its failure to do so signifies a lesion of the second or third neuron; and both 2.5% *methacholine* and 0.125% *pilocarpine* have no effect on a normal pupil but constrict one with pre- or postganglionic parasympathetic denervation, again due to supersensitivity. See **autonomic function tests.**

pharyngeal dystonia   A rare, idiopathic dystonic syndrome presenting in adult life with dysphagia.[3639]

pharyngeal nystagmus   See **ocular myoclonus.**

pharyngeal-cervical-brachial variant of acute inflammatory polyradiculoneuropathy   See **acute inflammatory demyelinating polyneuropathy.**

pharyngismus   Spasm of the pharyngeal constrictor muscles. While this is usually a psychogenic problem (**globus hystericus**), it is also seen in **rabies** and as a result of local irritation. See also **cricopharyngeal spasm.**

phase   1. (In electromyography) That portion of a waveform that occurs between the departure from and the return to, the baseline. 2. The time or angular relationships between a point on a wave and the onset of the cycle of the same wave. This is usually expressed in degrees or radians. (From 1974 report of the Committee on Terminology, IFCN. In: Chatrian GE, Bergamini L, Dondey M, et al. A glossary of terms most commonly used by clinical electroencephalographers. *EEG Clin Neurophysiol* 1974;**37**:538–548[989]) with permission from Elsevier Science.

phase advance   The movement of a subject's period of sleeping or waking to a position earlier in the 24-hour cycle.

phase delay   The movement of a subject's period of sleeping or waking to a position later in the 24-hour cycle. See **delayed sleep phase syndrome.**

phase lag   See **delayed sleep phase syndrome.**

phase reversal   The opposite polarity of the spike discharge on each side of an electrically discharging lesion in the CNS. This site, where no spike at all is seen, is regarded as **equipotential.** See **true phase reversal, instrumental phase reversal.**

phase transition   The two junctures of the major sleep and wake phases in the 24-hour cycle.

phasic reflexes   Those reflexes which chiefly employ the limb flexor muscles and which give rise to phasic (or clonic) reflex movements. Their origin is at the spinal level (Sir Charles **Sherrington**).[5120] The hind-limb flexion response reflex is an example.

phase-shift disorders   Conditions arising as a result of mismatch between the real time and the personal body-clock time, as after a journey across numerous time zones and in certain experimental situations.

phenobarbitone   The first drug for the treatment of epilepsy possessing an acceptable therapeutic ratio, introduced by Alfred Hauptmann (1881–1948) in 1912.

phenylketonuria   (Fölling syndrome, phenylpyruvic oligophrenia; OMIM 261600) A recessively inherited dysmetabolic syndrome due to lack of phenylalanine hydroxylase. As a result of this, the subject cannot oxidize phenylalanine to tyrosine. The gene responsible is mapped to chromosome 12q–24.1.

Clinically, the condition typically manifests neonatal feeding problems, mild microcephaly, fair hair, hyperkinesia and irritability; seizures, spasticity, aminoaciduria, and mental and developmental delay are evident by the end of the first year of life. The condition was described by **Fölling** in 1934. A recent complete review was by Pietz in 1998.[4442]

Variants of the syndrome include the following:
Dihydropteridine deficiency (PKU II) A rare condition characterized by high phenylalanine levels in which feeding disturbances from infancy lead rapidly to death.[5225] Seizures and both physical and mental retardation are notable. The gene responsible for the lack of dihydropteridine reductase maps to chromosome 4q16.1–p15.1.
Biopterin deficiency A progressive degenerative disorder of infants characterized by rigid hypertonia and later hypotonia, parkinsonism, myoclonus, seizures, and upper and lower motor neuron signs.[1982,2966]
Spinal muscular atrophy with phenylketonuria
Progressive spastic paraparesis with dementia A rare adult phenotype.[2948]

phenylpyruvic oligophrenia   See **phenylketonuria.**

pheochromocytoma   A benign tumor of the adrenal medulla secreting norepinephrine. It usually occurs in isolation but may also be a feature of **neurofibromatosis** and of the pluriglandular syndrome (**multiple endocrine neoplasia**).

Philippson reflex   See **crossed extensor reflex.**

Phillips thoracic dysplasia with retinal aplasia   A congenital dysmorphic syndrome manifesting also optic atrophy; retinal aplasia with pigmentation and macular colobomas, leading to blindness; nystagmus; pectus carinatum; cleft palate; digital abnormalities; and mental and developmental delay.[4432]

phobic postural vertigo   A form of psychogenic vertigo with the following characteristics, as defined by Brandt.[725]

1. Dizziness and subjective disturbance of balance while standing or walking despite normal clinical balance tests such as Romberg, tandem walking, balancing on one foot, and routine posturography

2. Fluctuating unsteadiness in episodes lasting seconds to minutes or momentary perceptions of illusory body perturbations

3. Although the attacks can occur spontaneously, there is usually a perceptual stimulus (bridge, staircase, empty room, street) or social situation (department store, restaurant, concert, crowd) from which the patients have difficulty withdrawing and they recognize as a provoking factor. There is a tendency for rapid conditioning, generalization, and avoidance behavior to develop.

4. Anxiety (57%) and distressing vegetative symptoms occur during or after vertigo. Most patients have attacks both with and without anxiety.

5. Obsessive-compulsive type personality, labile affect, mild depression

6. Onset of the condition frequently follows a period of particular emotional stress, after a serious illness, or following an organic vestibular disorder.

phonation   (from Gr, the sound of the voice) The expression of sounds by the larynx.

phone   The actual sound produced in speech.

phoneme   The minimum distinctive sound feature into which any given flow of speech can be separated;[1172] a distinct sound unit recognized by speakers of a language, and the most elementary unit of speech, existing only as constituents of words. A phoneme is a category of sounds which embraces all **phones,** (since different people pronounce each different phoneme differently).

There are 46 phonemes in the English language: 9 vowels and 37 consonants.[3505]

phonemic dyslexia   See **deep dyslexia.**

phonemic errors   Disturbances of speech consisting of substitutions of words and/or syllables, known as literal or verbal **paraphasias,** respectively.

phonetic errors   Disturbances of speech affecting the formation and articulation of the words themselves; errors are thus **dysarthrias.**

phonetic palsy   Aphonia due to disease affecting the tenth cranial nerve.

phonetics   The science of spoken speech.

phonographie   See **hypergraphia.**

phonological agraphia   The condition resulting from damage to the **phonological system** in which patients cannot spell nonwords such as CHOSP but can spell those with which they are already familiar. The lesion is thought to be in the left precentral gyrus.[5088]

phonological dyslexia   See **deep dyslexia.**

phonological memory   One of two postulated passive auditory–verbal short-term memory storage systems concerned with the memorization and repetition of lists, as opposed to the other (lexical) system, which is concerned with the comprehension of language.[3730]

phonological system   One of two functional systems used by human beings for spelling. It employs sound–

letter (phoneme) conversion rules, and is used when spelling unfamiliar words or pronounceable nonwords.

The other is the **lexical** system, which compares what is read or heard to a bank of previously acquired visual word-images of learned word spellings in order to achieve comprehension. Either can be damaged in isolation. Damage to the phonological system leads to an inability to spell nonwords, although the ability to spell known real words remains (**deep dyslexia**).

phonological–syntactical syndrome A mixed expressive-receptive disorder resembling Broca aphasia in which the speech is nonfluent, the articulation faulty, and the syntax simplistic.

phonology The speech sounds of a language and the rules followed by speakers when combining and pronouncing speech sounds.[3505]

phoria The normal tendency for a slight misalignment of the visual axes of the two eyes during monocular viewing. This is normally overcome by fusion mechanisms when the eyes are both viewing; thus, a phoria is a latent, not usually overt, deviation of the visual axes of the eyes. See **heterophorias**.

phosphatide A combination of phosphoglyceric acid with fatty acids and a base such as choline or ethanolamine.

phosphenes Positive visual sensations (light spots or patterns) perceived in the absence of visual (luminous) stimuli. They may occur in the presence of disease of the striate cortex or optic nerve and may be triggered by alerting stimuli.[4269,4293] See also **movement phosphenes**.

phosphoethanolaminuria See **hypophosphatasia**.

phosphofructokinase deficiency (Tarui disease) A recessively inherited form of glycogen storage disease due to complete or partial deficiency of this enzyme, leading to complaints of fatigability, exertional muscle weakness, cramps, and pain and in some cases to hyperuricemia and hemolytic anemia.[3303] See **glycogen storage diseases**.

phosphoglucomutase deficiency See **glycogen storage disease**.

phosphoglycerate kinase deficiency An X-linked recessive disorder due to the presence of a phosphoglycerate kinase variants (*PGK New Jersey, PGK North Carolina*[5657]) that impair the second stage of the glycolytic process within muscle. This leads to the clinical complaints of weakness and exercise-induced muscle pain with myoglobinuria, as occur in McArdle disease, but with the added features of mental retardation and hemolytic anemia.[1450] See **glycogen storage diseases** (type 9).

phosphoglycerate mutase deficiency A recessive syndrome with onset in youth, in which lack of the enzyme impairs the glycolytic process within muscle and

leads to the clinical complaints of weakness and exercise-induced muscle pain with myoglobinuria as occur in **McArdle disease**.[1457] However, lactate production is maintained during aerobic exercise. See **glycogen storage diseases** (type 10).

phosphohexoisomerase deficiency See **glycogen storage diseases**.

phosphorylase An enzyme with numerous isoenzymes, existing in both active and inactive forms. For its normal function in active form, adenyl cyclase, cyclic AMP, protein kinase, and phosphorylase kinase are necessary enzymes.

Myophosphorylase cleaves glucose from glycogen within muscles, thus allowing the use of glycogen as a source of energy. Its absence may be due to a condition inherited as either a dominant or recessive characteristic. See **glycogen storage diseases**.

phosphorylase *b* kinase deficiency A rare deficiency of an enzyme initiating glycogenolysis, leading to the clinical syndrome of weakness, exercise-induced muscle pain, and myoglobinuria in adults, and to weakness and hepatomegaly in children.[1057] See **glycogen storage diseases**.

photic driving (photoentrainment) A physiological response recorded on the EEG, consisting of rhythmic activity elicited over the posterior regions of the head by repetitive photic stimulation at frequencies of about 5–30 Hz.

The term should be limited to refer to activity time-locked to the stimulus and at a frequency identical to, or harmonically related to, the stimulus frequency. Photic driving should be held in contradistinction to the visual evoked potentials elicited by isolated flashes repeated at very low frequencies. (From the Report of the Committee on Terminology, IFCN. In: Chatrian GE, Bergamini L, Dondey M, et al. A glossary of terms most commonly used by clinical electroencephalographers. *EEG Clin Neurophysiol* 1974;37:538–548[989] by kind permission of Elsevier Science.)

photic reflex myoclonus A form of stimulus-sensitive myoclonus of cortical origin, manifest as myoclonic jerks elicited at a fixed latency by photic stimulation.[2918] See **myoclonus**.

photic sneeze reflex (**A**utosomal Dominant **Co**mpelling **H**elio-**O**phthalmic **O**utburst syndrome [ACHOO], photosternutatory reflex) Sneezing when a bright light is shone into the eyes; a normal reflex in infants, but seen in adults as well. It is likely to be dominantly inherited. Parasympathetic overactivity has been suggested as a mechanism,[1720] but the cause is not known.[5951]

The acronym is slightly forced, but remains, in the author's opinion, the best of the last decade.

photic stimulation Delivery of intermittent flashes of light to the eyes of a subject as an EEG activation procedure.

photisms Transient "positive" anomalies of vision consisting of simple but brightly colored spectral phenomena, often of a geometrical character, and occurring in the context of epilepsy and migraine.

photoconvulsive response A generalized paroxysmal EEG discharge, usually at 3 Hz, evoked by intermittent photic stimulation. See **photoparoxysmal response.**

photoelectric oculography Techniques for measuring the displacement of the ocular globe, using a light source directed upon the cornea and equipment responsive to the light reflected from it.

Horizontal rather than vertical ocular deviations are measured because of eyelid interference in recordings of the latter. See also **electrooculogram.** An infrared method is also available.[5]

photoentrainment See **photic driving.**

photogenic epilepsy A tendency toward recurring seizures triggered only by exposure to a flickering light source.[335] See also **photosensitive epilepsies, photoparoxysmal response.**

photomotograph A photoelectric device for recording the speed of muscle contraction and relaxation, usually applied to the ankle jerk.[5117] It was most often employed in the assessment of hypothyroidism, in which slowness of relaxation (the "hung-up" reflex) is common, but it is not now in general clinical use.

photomyoclonic response (photomyoclonus) An anteriorly located EEG discharge accompanied by facial, periocular, and occasionally arm myoclonic jerks and time-locked to flashes of light during intermittent photic stimulation.[557] See **photomyogenic response.**

photomyoclonus See **photomyoclonic response.**

photomyoclonus, diabetes mellitus, nephropathy, and deafness A dominantly inherited syndrome characterized by these features and by dementia. This condition may be a lipidosis.[335]

photomyogenic response (photomyoclonic response, photomyologic response)[3075] A response to intermittent photic stimulation, characterized by brief, repetitive spikes derived from muscle over the anterior regions of the head. These often increase gradually in amplitude as stimuli are continued and cease promptly when the stimulus is withdrawn.

This response is frequently associated with flutter of the eyelids and vertical oscillations of the eyeballs and sometimes with discrete jerking mostly involving the musculature of the face and head. (From the 1974 Report of the Committee on Terminology, IFCN. In: Chatrian GE, Bergamini L, Dondey M, et al. A glossary of terms most commonly used by clinical electroencephalographers. *EEG Clin Neurophysiol* 1974;**37**:538–548[989], with permission from Elsevier Science.)

photomyologic response See **photomyogenic response.**

photoparoxysmal response (photoconvulsive response) A response to intermittent photic stimulation characterized by spike-and-wave and multiple spike-and-slow-wave complexes. These are bilaterally synchronous, symmetrical, and generalized, and may outlast the stimulus by a few seconds.

This response may be associated with impairment of consciousness and brisk jerks involving the musculature of the whole body, most prominently that of the upper extremities and head. (Adapted from the 1974 Report of the Committee on Terminology, IFCN. In: Chatrian GE, Bergamini L, Dondey M, et al. A glossary of terms most commonly used by clinical electroencephalographers. *EEG Clin Neurophysiol* 1974;**37**:538–548[989], with permission from Elsevier Science.)

photophobia (Gr, light + dread) Pathological discomfort experienced as eye pain and excessive glare in light conditions which, by definition, are comfortable for others. Photophobia is evidence of inflammation or irritation of ocular structures including the optic nerve, but is also extremely common with migraine and related headaches.

photophthalmia (snow blindness, desert blindness, ultraviolet keratitis) The occurrence of photophobia, burning ocular pain, itching, lacrimation, blepharospasm, and blurred vision following exposure to intense ultraviolet radiation.

photoplethysmography A method of detecting the volume of pulsation in the frontal and supraorbital arteries using an infrared photosensor placed over the area of skin they supply. Compression maneuvers of the facial, temporal, and carotid arteries can be used to increase the sensitivity of the test, which is otherwise not as accurate as more sophisticated methods; it is now rarely used.[4141]

photopsias Visual disturbances that accompany migraine attacks.

photosensitive epilepsies Seizure disorders in which the convulsion is associated in time with visual stimulation. Four types are recognized (see Chart P–13).[56]

Chart P–13. The Photosensitive Epilepsies

Pure photosensitive epilepsy The occurrence of seizures (usually of the generalized tonic-clonic variety) exclusively as a result of environmental flicker stimulation. *Television epilepsy* and *space-invaders epilepsy* are forms of this, in which the attacks are precipitated when the subject sits close to a television screen.[2821]

Photosensitive epilepsy with spontaneous seizures A variant of the above, in which seizures also occur without such provocation.[2821]

Eyelid myoclonia with absences A syndrome characterized by upward jerking of the eyes and eyelids on eye closure in well-lit surroundings. Spike (or polyspike)-and-wave patterns are seen on the EEG with eye closure in the dark.[2820]

Self-induced photosensitive epilepsy A syndrome of absence seizures or myoclonic epileptic attacks as a consequence of self-induced flicker stimulation, as accomplished by oscillating the hands with the fingers outstretched in the line of sight to a bright light source.

photosensitive epilepsy with spontaneous seizures See **photosensitive epilepsies.**

photosensitive myoclonic epilepsy A syndrome in which myoclonic absences, myoclonic jerks, and generalized clonic convulsions all occur.[1515]

photosensitivity Genetically determined precipitation of neurological phenomena (such as generalized seizures) by flashing light stimuli.[6019]

photosternutatory reflex See **photic sneeze reflex.**

photostress test See **light stress test.**

phrenesis An ancient term for any affection capable of inducing delirium.

phrenic (Gr, the seat of the mind; the diaphragm). The techniques for electrophysiological study of the phrenic nerves supplying the two sides of the diaphragm have been described.[996]

phrenitis (Gr, the seat of the mind + Lat, inflammation) The term of Celsus and Galen for what we know colloquially as madness. The term *phrenopathia* is synonymous. Both are defunct.

phrenology (cranioscopy) A system introduced by Franz **Gall,** an anatomist in the latter part of the eighteenth century, who postulated that the brain was the organ of mind, with its mental and moral faculties localized to various parts of the cortex. A deficiency or a surfeit of each faculty could be determined by palpating the bumps on the cranium, and maps were published showing the positions of the relevant area for each. As Clarke and Dewhurst[1048] remark, it is curious that the faculties are all represented by bumps, because deficiency in one of them should presumably have led to a depression. Neither the system of faculties nor the localizations of those which are acceptable to us today have stood the test of time.

The organs (faculties) that Gall identified as common to humans and animals are listed in Chart P–14.

Chart P–14. Gall's Organs (Faculties)

1. Instinct for reproduction
2. Love of offspring
3. Friendship
4. Self-defense and courage
5. Carnivorous instinct, tendency to murder
6. Cunning, cleverness
7. Ownership, covetousness, tendency to steal
8. Pride, love of authority
9. Vanity, ambition, love of glory
10. Caution, forethought
11. Memory of things and facts
12. Sense of places and space
13. Memory and sense of people
14. Memory of words
15. Sense of language and speech
16. Sense of color
17. Sense of sound, music
18. Sense of numbers, mathematics
19. Sense of mechanics, architecture

Those Occurring Only in Humans

20. Wisdom
21. Sense of metaphysics
22. Satire, witticism
23. Poetical talent
24. Kindness, compassion, morality
25. Mimicry
26. Religion
27. Firmness of purpose, obstinacy, or constancy

phthinodes (from Gr, to waste away + form) Tissue wasting.

physaliphorous cells (Gr, bubble + cary) (bubbly cells) Tumor cells found in **chordomas** which contain "bubbles" of non-staining material.

physical ADL See **activities of daily living.**

Physical and Mental Impairment of Function Evaluation A 77-item scale providing a comprehensive behavioral assessment of institutionalized geriatric patients and allowing scores on 10 factors, including self-care, dependency, confusion, anxiety, behavioral deterioration, withdrawal, paranoia, etc.[2337]

Physical Self-Maintenance scale An instrument on which an observer rates toileting, feeding, dressing, grooming, physical ambulation, and bathing on a 5-point scale. A 3-point scale is used when these functions are self-rated by the patient.[3298]

physiological hypnic myoclonus Small-amplitude, irregular, and asynchronous twitches, mainly affecting the orofacial and the distal muscles during stage 1 non–rapid eye movement and during rapid eye movement sleep and relaxed wakefulness. Electrically, they may be composed of isolated simple potentials or of brief tonic discharges.[1365]

physiological myoclonus See **myoclonus.**

physiological nystagmus (end-point nystagmus, fatigue nystagmus) That form of nystagmus induced in normal subjects by rotation, by caloric irrigation, or by optokinetic stimuli, and representing an automatic resetting of the position of the eyes to compensate for the normal reflex tendency of the eyes to move in a direction contrary to, and during, bodily movement with the purpose of maintaining clear vision.

This form of horizontal jerk nystagmus is commonly elicited by sustained lateral deviation of the eyes and lasts for 15–25 seconds. Some subtypes are the following:

1. *Fatigue nystagmus* A form of jerk nystagmus seen in both eyes symmetrically in normal subjects who maintain far-lateral deviations of the eyes. This tends to be of greater amplitude in the adducting eye.
2. Micro-oscillations of the eyes occurring during precise high-resolution eye movement recordings. See **ocular flutter.**
3. *End-point nystagmus* A few lateral jerks of the eyes normally occurring on far-lateral gaze.
4. *Sustained end-point nystagmus* Persistent lateral jerks of the eyes normally occurring on far-lateral gaze.[5]

Other varieties of physiological nystagmus listed under **vestibular nystagmus** are *positional alcohol, positioning, postrotational,* and *pseudo-caloric* forms.

physiological tremor A normal and usually asymptomatic small-amplitude oscillation of all body parts. When a limb is supported, cardioballistic thrust is the most important mechanism, combined with the mechanical resonance of that body part. During maintenance of a posture, the tremor depends on the initial firing rate of motor units, which is usually around 8 Hz.

Such oscillations are made worse by fatigue, recent physical exercise, or increased adrenergic tone, as occurs with emotion or in hyperthyroidism. **Essential tremor** is an exaggerated form.

physiological vertigo Those forms of vertigo induced by external stimulation of the normal vestibular, visual, or somatosensory systems. **Motion sickness, space sickness,** and **height, visual, somatosensory, auditory, head-extension,** and **bending-over vertigo** are examples.

physostigmine An inhibitor of cholinesterase which crosses the blood–brain barrier, having no quaternary amine group.

phytanic acid (3,7,11,15 tetramethylhexadecanoic acid) A fatty acid found in dairy products, meat, and fish oils that accumulates in Refsum disease (**hereditary motor and sensory neuropathy, type 4**), **infantile Refsum disease, Zellweger disease,** neonatal **adrenoleukodystrophy,** and **rhizomelic chondrodysplasia punctata.**

phytanic acid storage disease See **hereditary motor and sensory neuropathy, type 4.**

pia mater (Lat, soft + mother; *mater* because of the ancient Arabian belief that the meninges gave rise to all the body's membranes[5204]) The innermost and thinnest of the three membranes (meninges) covering the brain.

pianist's cramp An **overuse syndrome** or focal occupational **dystonia,** in which the performer's digits cease to obey his or her will and take up an extended position for a few seconds.

piblokto (arctic hysteria) Screaming, removal of clothing, and wild running with succeeding amnesia, considered to be a dissociative state. The similarity to **amok** in the Malays is notable.[746]

pica (Lat, a magpie) Depraved appetite; abnormal eating behavior in which the subject ingests objects that are not acceptable food substances.

Pick, Arnold (1851–1924) Austrian-Czechoslovakian neuropathologist and psychiatrist. He was born in Moravia and studied in Iglau, Vienna, Berlin, and Prague, where he was eventually elected professor of psychiatry in 1886, retaining that position until his retirement in 1921. He published over 350 contributions to the medical literature, but is best known for his studies on early-life dementia.

Pick was both the first to put **Wernicke**'s ideas of aphasia on a sound anatomicopathological basis and to demonstrate the origin of the fibers of the spinocerebellar tract in the axis-cylinder processes of the cells of Clarke's column. He also described various spinal cord abnormalities, established with Kohler the clinical picture of combined systemic disease, associated hemichorea and hemiathetosis occurring with thalamic and lenticular lesions, and conducted important studies on apraxia and agrammatism.[5047]

Pick bodies Spherical neurofilamentous argyrophilic and eosinophilic intracytoplasmic inclusions, found in hippocampal neurons (**Pick cells**) in some cases of **Pick disease.**

Pick cells Swollen eosinophilic neuronal cell bodies with a peripherally displaced nucleus and argyrophilic inclusions, found in the neocortex, hippocampus, basal ganglia, and brainstem in **Pick disease.**

Pick complex disorder See **frontotemporal dementia.**

Pick disease (Pick lobar atrophy, Pick complex disorder, lobar sclerosis, circumscribed cortical atrophy, dementia with lobar atrophy and neuronal cytoplasmic inclusions) See **frontotemporal dementia.** Pick disease Internet Web sites of value are www.picksdisease.org/pick and www.bhoffcomp.com/coping/picks.html.

Pick disease without Pick bodies See **frontal lobe dementia.**

Pick, Ludwig (1868–1944) German physician who graduated from Königsberg University and later trained further in pathology in Berlin where he was eventually elected professor of pathological anatomy. His paper, distinguishing what we know as **Niemann-Pick disease** from **Gaucher disease,** was published in 1927. He died in a concentration camp for Jews in 1943.

Pick lobar atrophy See **Pick disease.**

Pick sign Lid nystagmus induced by convergence movements of the eyes; an uncommon feature in some posterior fossa lesions.[1291]

Pick syndrome See **aphasia-agnosia-apraxia syndrome.**

Pickwickian syndrome Somnolence, periodic respiration, polycythemia, pulmonary hypertension, cor pulmonale, diminished respiratory drive in response to increases in pCO_2, and excessive appetite with obesity as complications of the obstructive sleep apnea syndrome. The somnolence can be traced to alveolar hypoventilation. The syndrome takes its name (applied by Osler) from Charles Dickens' character Joe, the fat boy in *The Pickwick Papers*.[851]

pico- (Gr, small) Prefix denoting small.

pictorial test of intelligence A cognitive test appropriate for children with severe motor and speech impairment.

picture arrangement A subtest on the **Wechsler Adult Intelligence Scale** sensitive to disturbances of function of the right parietal lobe.

picture completion A subtest on the **Wechsler Adult Intelligence Scale** (revision) sensitive to parietal lobe disorders.

pied en griffe (Fr, claw foot) Weakness with atrophy of the intrinsic muscles of the foot leads to unopposed action of the long toe extensors, which causes dorsiflexion of the proximal phalanges while the long flexors shorten the foot and produce plantar flexion at the distal interphalangeal joints.

Piepkorn short rib–polydactyly syndrome A congenital dysmorphic syndrome manifesting also skeletal and visceral anomalies, brachydactyly and polydactyly, brachycephaly, craniosynostosis, delayed closure of fontanelles, and ossification defects of the skull.[337]

Pierre Robin syndrome A congenital syndrome of mental retardation, cleft palate, facial dysmorphism (notably a small receding chin causing glossoptosis), flattening of the nasal bridge, low-set ears, microphthalmos, congenital glaucoma, cataract, myopia, and a tendency toward congenital heart disease.[4724]

Pierre Robin (1867–1950) was professor of dental surgery in Paris.

pierres de la peau See **Profichet syndrome.**

Pietrantoni syndrome The occurrence of **infraorbital neuralgia** and facial hypoesthesia as a complication of infiltrating nasopharyngeal tumors.[4441]

Pietrowski, A. (b. 1878) German neurologist.

Pietrowski sign See **anterior tibial sign.**

pigment variety of amaurotic idiocy A pigmented variety of **neuronal ceroid lipofuscinosis,** characterized by the onset in childhood of progressive mental and neurological deterioration with ubiquitous lipid infiltration of neurons and extracellular pigmentation of the globus pallidus and substantia nigra.[5055]

pigmentary retinal degeneration See **pigmentary retinopathy.**

pigmentary retinopathy (pigmentary retinal degeneration) A hereditary, noninflammatory, degenerative

retinal dystrophy marked by gliosis and the deposition of melanin derived from the retinal pigmented epithelium within the walls of blood vessels in the neurosensory retina. Clinically, the condition is characterized by marked constriction of the visual fields with retention of some central vision, arteriolar narrowing, disk pallor, and frequently (but not invariably) pigmentary deposition in the retina.

Central and *sectorial* types are described, as is another *variant* in which the same changes occur without any pigment deposition (*retinitis pigmentosa sine pigmento*). In a further *variant* form, only certain sectors of the retina are affected.

See also **cone dystrophy, retinitis pigmentosa.**

pili torti Kinky hair. When combined with deafness this is known as *Björnstadt syndrome*.[592] See **Menkes disease.**

pill-rolling tremor See **resting tremor.** This is a classic error in terminology, since early pharmacists did not make pills by rolling the ingredients between their fingers and thumbs but between two flat wooden boards. The term was not used by **Parkinson** nor by **Gowers** but appeared in the early part of this century.[1940]

pilocarpine test Instillation of a drop of 0.1% pilocarpine into the conjunctival sac of the normal eye has no effect; constriction of the pupil within 15 minutes, lasting for up to 2 hours, suggests the presence of denervation hypersensitivity resulting from a lesion of the parasympathetic supply to the iris, as with the **Adie pupil.** See also **methacholine test, pharmacological pupillary testing.**

pilocytic astrocytoma See **astrocytoma.**

pilomotor seizure A rare manifestation of partial seizures in which paroxysmal piloerection ("gooseflesh") occurs following an **epigastric aura,** without alteration in consciousness.[767] A right hemisphere lesion has been responsible in the few cases reported.[2264]

Pilotto syndrome A congenital dysmorphic syndrome manifesting also short stature, scoliosis, fusion of vertebrae, hemivertebrae, patent ductus arteriosus, brachycephaly, microcephaly, and pyramidal signs.[337]

Piltz, Jan (1870–1931) Polish neurologist who studied in Switzerland and Russia and, after graduation, studied psychiatry and neurology at the **Salpêtrière** and in Zurich. He concluded his career as professor of neurology and psychiatry at Krakow University.

Piltz reflex 1. The consensual light reflex. 2. Constriction of the pupil when a person's attention is drawn to an object, not necessarily requiring ocular convergence.[4447]

pincer grasp Use of the thumb and forefinger to grasp a small object. This facility is normally present by 7 to 10 months of age, and persists.

pinch sign   When patients are asked to make a hollow square by putting the tip of the index finger onto the tip of the thumb, they cannot do so because of weakness of the long flexors of the finger and of the thumb, and make a triangle instead. The sign is typically positive in the **anterior interosseous nerve syndrome.** See also **Froment sign.**

pinch-press test   A test of the sense of passive movement of the skin in which the examiner variously pinches or presses upon the skin and the patient reports which sensation is felt.[1349a]

pincushion effect   A distortion of vision caused by the wearing of **Fresnel's glasses.**

pineal   (from Lat, a pine-cone) Resembling a pine-cone.

pineal apoplexy   An acute hemorrhagic upper brainstem lesion in the pretectal region.[203]

pineal cyst   A cyst containing fluid with the density of CSF, located within the pineal gland, regarded as a normal variant when detected on MRI scanning.[1436]

pineal gland   A dorsal midline outgrowth of the diencephalon. In lower vertebrates it was light sensitive; its function in humans is still not understood, although it may have a role in modifying skin pigmentation through the production of melanotropin. Descartes proposed it as the seat of the soul, in which the imagination resided.

The tendency of the gland to calcify relatively early in life was useful as a sign of midline shift before the advent of echoencephalography, a test which itself is redundant since the development of CT and MRI scanning.

pineal shift   A radiological sign, indicating shift of the hemispheres across the midline, thus pushing the (calcified) pineal gland with them. It was first described by Arthur Schuller.

pinealoblastoma   A malignant, invasive **primitive neuroectodermal tumor** resembling the **medulloblastoma** histologically as well as in its aggressive local and metastatic spread.

pinealocytoma   A rare tumor arising in the pineal gland in young adult life and composed of small cells arranged in ribbons or lobules, often with argyrophilic and eosinophilic polar cytoplasmic processes.[6]

pinealoma   Any tumor of the pineal gland.

Pinel, Philippe   (1755–1826) French psychiatrist at the Bicêtre and later at the **Salpêtrière,** who established new standards for the humane care of the mentally ill and who made the first systematic attempt to classify mental illness.

He wrote repeatedly that he owed most of his experiences and insights into the dynamics of insanity to the French Revolution, which showed him the tremendous wealth of reactions that the human may show under the stress of exceptional situations. Initially, however, he had taken to psychiatry after a friend lost his reason and ran into the woods, where he was eaten by wolves.[1829,4453]

ping-pong ball depression   A small, depressed skull fracture resulting from compression by forceps or with molding during delivery.

ping-pong gaze   (short-cycle periodic alternating gaze deviation) A disorder of ocular movement consisting of rhythmic and pendular conjugate horizontal deviations of the eyes which alternate from one extreme of gaze to the other every 3 to 8 seconds. This is usually noted in patients in coma due to structural cerebral damage, drug toxicity, or other causes of metabolic encephalopathy.[5066] See **periodic alternating gaze.**

pinhole test   A simple method of correcting for, and thus diagnosing, the presence of refractive errors. The subject reads from a test card, first without and then with a cover pierced by a small hole placed in front of the eye; an improvement in acuity suggests the presence of a refractive error, since the focal length of a lens system is increased as its aperture is diminished, and the elimination of light coming in from an angle with retention of that coming straight (and thus subject to little or no refraction anyway) allows more precise focusing on the macula. Subjects with macular disease will see nothing at all through the pinhole.

The test was devised by Christoph Scheiner (1575–1650), a German physicist, in 1619.[4979]

pink disease   (acrodynia, Feer disease, mercuric encephalopathy) A syndrome of scaly erythema of the skin with coldness and redness of the cheeks and extremities, perspiration, alopecia, insomnia, irritability, convulsions, peripheral sensorimotor neuropathy, tachycardia, stomatitis, pruritus, tremor, hypotonia, a flexed posture, and photophobia, resulting from mercury encephaloneuropathy in infants.

The cause was chronic mercury poisoning, coming from the calomel in teething powder that loving parents placed on the gums of their physiologically unwell babies.[4360] The condition was described by Dr. E. Feer (1864–1911), a Swiss pediatrician, but he did not recognize its etiology.[1829]

pinky finger sign   Reflex movements of the fifth finger that are elicited when the patient extends and abducts the fingers of one hand, after which the second, third, and fourth fingers are flexed at the metacarpophalangeal (MCP) joints against the examiner's resistance. Normal subjects and patients with a pyramidal lesion affecting the limb hyperextend the fifth finger at the MCP joint while patients with pseudodementia (depression) psychogenic hemiparesis and whiplash-induced upper limb monoparesis flex the fifth finger at the MCP joint during resisted finger flexion.[4208]

Pinocchio syndrome A rare form of reflex epilepsy in which partial seizures are triggered by the enunciation of terminological inexactitudes.

pinpoint pupils The term for pupils that are each about 1 mm in diameter but still react to light. Such extreme pupillary constriction occurs with morphine poisoning and with complete loss of sympathetic innervation of the pupil, as with pontine lesions.

pinwheel photopsias Visual hallucinations resembling fireworks, occurring in patients with irritative temporal lobe lesions.[1073]

Piotrowski sign (antagonistic anterior tibial reflex) Percussion of the tibialis anterior muscle leads to plantar flexion of the toes in the presence of pyramidal lesions, presumably as a result of vibration transmitted to the gastrocnemius muscle. This response was described by Piotrowski in 1912. See also **anterior tibial sign.**

A variant stimulus is percussion of the external malleolus, described by Balduzzi in 1925. The (slight) utility of both signs has been reviewed.[4876]

pipecolic acidemia See **hyperpipecolic acidemia.**

pipestem capillaries Thickening of the capillaries in muscles affected by necrotizing myopathy complicating underlying carcinoma or arteritis.[1651]

piriformis syndrome (Lat, a pear + shape). 1. A sciatica-like syndrome considered due to periarthritis involving the anterior sacroiliac ligament, the piriformis muscle, and the adjacent sciatic nerve.[1949,4727,6077] The similarity of symptoms to those of lumbar radiculopathy, including positive Lasègue signs, can lead to misdiagnosis and ineffective lumbar surgery. Correct anatomic localization is indicated by the consistent occurrence of sciatic notch tenderness. The Freiberg and **Pace** signs may also be present. (HJM)[3173,4349]

Nerve conduction studies and needle EMG are usually normal; in the occasional case with true denervation the findings are those of a mild axonal sciatic mononeuropathy at the level of the sciatic notch, with or without an inferior gluteal mononeuropathy.[1872] In such cases there may be a fibrous band or aberrant artery compressing the sciatic nerve in the region of the piriformis muscle.

The validity of the syndrome is considered to be controversial by those who have not experienced it themselves (H.J. Moore, personal communication, 2002). See also **wallet neuritis** and **hip pocket neuropathy.**[6096]

2. A myofascial pain syndrome manifested by external rotation of the leg and some response to local anesthetic injection into the piriformis muscle. The buttock pain may be referred to the thigh and there is exquisite point tenderness over the sciatic notch elicited externally and on rectal or pelvic examination, with or without back pain.[3173] The pain is maximal during prolonged sitting (such as while driving or cycling),

bending at the waist, or activity that requires hip adduction and internal rotation such as cross-country skiing. The Trendelenberg test is positive. Weakness, reflex changes, and definitive sensory loss are absent. Rotation or abduction of the hip joint causes pain (but this is not specific for this condition). Lumbar MRI does not show disc disease.

Although the first syndrome is thought to reflect neuropathy and the second "myofascial pain," the distinction between the two is at best blurred.

Pisa syndrome Tonic flexion to one side with rotation of the trunk, unaccompanied by other dystonic signs. The condition is a dystonia, noted after the ingestion of drugs.

The name reflects the leaning position of the subject.[6071]

pitcher's arm An electrodiagnostic anomaly probably representing the result of repetitive strain to the brachial plexus of professional baseball pitchers, characterized by a reduction in the amplitude of sensory nerve action potentials in the throwing arm. There appears to be no deficit in performance as a result, however.[3467]

pithiatism (from Gr, suggestion + curable) The term coined by **Babiński** for diseases that are curable by persuasion; it was used by **Charcot** to replace the word **hysteria,** but it failed to do so.

Pitres, Albert (1848–1928) French neurologist and histologist, professor of medicine at Bordeaux University, who trained with **Charcot** and Ranvier and whose major works concerned cortical localization and aphasia. His book on neuroanatomy and physiology with Testut, *Les Nerfs en Schemas* (Paris, 1925), was quickly regarded as a classic.

Pitres' law (1895) The language that the patient used most before onset of aphasia will be recovered best. The rule has not been validated.

Pitres sign Loss of deep pain sensation, assessed by the response to squeezing of the testicles. The sign was described in patients with **tabes dorsalis,** some of whom are reputed to have benefited financially as a result of winning bets on their capacity to tolerate such insults.

Pitt syndrome A recessively inherited congenital dysmorphic syndrome manifesting also short stature, respiratory difficulties, clubbing of the fingers, abnormal skin creases, pes cavus, seizures, microcephaly, and mental and developmental delay.[4455]

pituitary (from Lat, phlegm [mucous secretion], one of the humors) The pituitary gland was first described in 1524 by Berengarius, and was thought by Vesalius to secrete mucus into the nose, an opinion held until the seventeenth century.[5204]

pituitary adenomas Circumscribed benign tumors arising from cells within the pituitary gland and in many cases extending upward or eroding laterally, and thus causing clinical effects by compression. Secreting and nonsecreting forms are defined. The former usually secrete prolactin; less commonly they secrete growth hormone, follicle-stimulating hormone, and luteinizing hormone.

pituitary apoplexy   A rare, life-threatening syndrome resulting from acute infarction of the pituitary gland, usually in the presence of an adenoma or as a component of **Sheehan syndrome.** The clinical manifestations include a history suggesting dyspituitarism; severe retro-orbital headache with meningism; ocular palsies; rapidly advancing visual impairment, especially bitemporal field loss; altered consciousness; and involvement of the first division of the fifth cranial nerve. Vasospasm or compression of the internal carotid may lead on to seizures or focal deficits. However, the condition may also occur silently after asymptomatic hemorrhage into a pituitary adenoma.

Surviving patients show evidence of pituitary failure with loss of lactation, amenorrhea, lethargy, and sometimes diabetes insipidus. The syndrome and its many predisposing causes have been reviewed.[4637]

pituitary gigantism   (Launois syndrome, Maurois syndrome, Marie syndrome) Increased growth due to excessive production of growth hormone by a pituitary adenoma prior to closure of the epiphyses, first described by Launois in 1904, but described in greater detail by the authors whose names are variously attached to the syndrome.

pituitary tumor without acromegly but with genital arrest   See **Frölich syndrome.**

placing reaction   When the normal infant is lifted up and the dorsum of the foot brought into contact with the underside of, for example, a table top, the infant's leg flexes at the hip and knee so that the foot is lifted and placed on the upper surface of the table.[3552]

The sign is present after the 34th week of gestation and disappears at 2 months of age.

plagiocephaly   (from Gr, sideways + the head) (wry head) 1. A craniofacial malformation resulting from asymmetrical premature fusion of a coronal or lambdoid suture on one side, causing the skull to have its longest axis on the diagonal.[4] There is thus abnormal flattening of one side of the head (and compensatory bulging of the other side) with flattening of the forehead on the affected side and elevation of the orbit and distortion of the root of the nose. Radiologically, the orbits are obviously asymmetrical, the affected orbit being triangular in its upper and outer part, producing a "devil's eye" or "harlequin" appearance.

2. Also given this name is the persistent deviation of the head to one side in infancy, due to the posture assumed by a child lying supine for most of the day.

planotopokinesia   The term suggested in 1922 by Pierre **Marie** for **visuospatial agnosia.**

plantar grasp reflex   (Lat, sole of the foot) Stroking of the palmar surface of the foot causes flexion of the toes.[6064] The sign is present from birth until 2 months of age. See also **grasp reflex of the foot, developmental reflexes.**

plantar muscle reflex   (Rossolimo reflex) Extension of the hallux when the sole is tapped with a reflex hammer, a toe is flicked upward, or the plantar surfaces of a number of toes are percussed with the ankle dorsiflexed.

This is a muscle stretch reflex, the counterpart of the **finger flexion reflex** in the arm and not a true variant of the **Babiński response.** Tapping on the heel may also elicit toe flexion as the result of vibration transmitted to the plantar muscles.

plantar neuroma   See **Morton metatarsalgia.**

plantar push   An alternative way of eliciting the **Babiński response.** A ballpoint pen (retracted) or an orange stick is pressed onto the sole of the foot and rotated. This questionable method (enthusiastically promulgated but never published by this author) has a low yield of positive results (upgoing toes) compared with the **Stransky** response.

plantar reflex   (plantar response) See **Babiński signs.**

plantar response   See **Babiński signs.**

planum temporale   The isthmus of the temporal lobe—the region on the superior surface of the temporal lobe between Wernicke's language area and Heschl's gyrus.

plaques   1. (in **multiple sclerosis**) Zones of demyelination within the white matter of the CNS, most common in the periventricular and periaqueductal regions, the optic nerve, and the spinal cord. Histologically, acutely formed plaques are characterized by the presence of intact axons, myelin breakdown products within foamy macrophages, a proliferation of hypertrophic reactive astrocytes, local and circumferential round-cell infiltration, and perivascular cuffing, as well as by a paucity of oligodendrocytes. Chronic "burntout" plaques are circumscribed regions within the white matter which lack myelin but show intense gliosis without inflammatory cells.

2. (in **Alzheimer disease**) Various forms are defined:
Classic plaques (senile, amyloid or discrete plaques) Areas close to the capillaries in the neuropil and consisting of a densely stained core of amyloid surrounded by argentophilic rods and granules derived from dystrophic neuronal processes.
Primitive plaques (amorphous or neuritic plaques) Small clusters of distended neurites without a discrete central core. See **neuritic plaques.**
Burnt-out plaques (compact plaques) Amyloid deposits in the neuropil without other distinguishing features.
Diffuse plaques A network of fibrillar or granular material without amyloid content.[66]

3. See **perivascular plaques.**

plasma exchange See **plasmapheresis.**

plasmapheresis (Gr, form + removal) (plasma exchange) The mechanical separation of certain protein fractions of plasma from whole blood by centrifugation, followed by the replacement of the blood without such elements but with the addition of volume expanders.

The procedure is established as beneficial in **myasthenia gravis,** presumably because of the removal of antiacetylcholine receptor antibodies; in **acute inflammatory demyelinating polyneuropathy;** and in some **gammopathic neuropathies.** Its value in the treatment of **Lambert-Eaton myasthenic syndrome, amyotrophic lateral sclerosis, multiple sclerosis, polymyositis, Fabry disease,** and other conditions remains under study.[1297]

plateau waves See **intracranial pressure waves.**

platelet-activating factor An endogenous phospholipid with a role in the mediation of many physiological reactions, including vasoconstriction and hemostasis. In the brain, where it is released after injury, it may act directly or through other mediators to cause vasospasm, disruption of the blood–brain barrier, and cerebral edema.[3419]

platy- (Gr, flat) Prefix denoting flatness.

platybasia An increase in the breadth (obtuseness) of the basal angle of the skull (the angle made by the intersection of the plane of the sphenoid with the plane of the clivus) to >150°.

The term is attributed to **Virchow,** and has been used by anthropologists interested in craniometry for over 100 years. It is not the same thing as **basilar impression.**[5282]

platycephaly (Gr, flat + the head) An abnormal skull shape in which the vertical height of the skull is reduced.

platysma phenomenon (Signe de Peaucier) Failure of the platysma muscle on the side of a hemiparesis to contract when a subject opens his or her mouth widely against resistance.

PLEDs See **periodic lateralized epileptiform discharges.**

pleoconial myopathy A familial muscular disorder presenting with slowly progressive weakness, attacks of flaccid paralysis, and a craving for salt from infancy. The characteristic pathological feature is an excess of mitochondria and morphological inclusions within such organelles.[5151]

pleocytosis A pathological overabundance of cells.

pleomorphic xanthoastrocytoma See **astrocytoma.**

pleonosteosis A dominantly inherited diffuse encephalopathy characterized by abnormal, unusually early ossification of the epiphyses, with dwarfism, broad digits, flexion contractures, a mongoloid facial appearance, and mental retardation. See **Leri syndrome.**

pleurodynia (Gr, side + pain) (Devil's grippe, epidemic myalgia, Bornholm disease) A syndrome of chest wall and often other myalgic pain (the former made much worse by deep breathing) and fever, without the clinical or radiological features of pleurisy. Infection with the Coxsackie B virus is the usual cause.

pleurothotonos Muscular spasm leading to lateral flexion of the trunk.

plexiform neuroma Peripheral neural tumors that resemble schwannomas and that appear in childhood and adolescence, increasing in size and number during pregnancy and with aging.

plexiform sarcoma See **cylindroma.**

plexitis Inflammation of the brachial or lumbosacral plexuses.

plexopathy Any disease of the brachial or, less commonly, the lumbosacral plexus. *Neoplastic plexopathies* affect mainly the lower brachial plexus, causing pain in the shoulder girdle and medial aspect of the forearm and hand and often a **Horner syndrome.** Arm lymphedema is uncommon. See also **Pancoast syndrome.**

Lumbosacral plexopathies are most often due to direct extension of a tumor of the colon or cervix, and present mainly with pain and sensory and motor findings according to the level of the plexus infiltrated. Sphincter disturbance is uncommon. See also **radiation plexopathy.**

plexus (from Lat, a braid or weaving; to intertwine) The complex rearrangements of the nerve roots into peripheral nerves. The term is also applied to networks of blood vessels.

Plicz sign Tight eye closure leads to constriction followed by dilation of the pupils. Presumably this is determined by infrared photography.

PLO-SL See **polycystic lipomembranous osteodysplasia with sclerosing leukoencephalopathy.**

Plott laryngeal abductor paralysis–retardation syndrome A congenital syndrome of optic atrophy, facial weakness, stridor, tracheolaryngeal anomalies, and mental and developmental delay.[337]

plumbism (Lat, lead) Lead poisoning. See **Remak paralysis.**

Plummer-Vinson syndrome See **sideropenic dysphagia.**

plurideficiency malnutrition syndrome See **kwashiorkor.**

plus-minus lid syndrome Unilateral ptosis with contralateral retraction of the eyelid, due to a small lesion in the paramedian mesencephalon causing damage to the third cranial nerve nucleus involving the ipsilateral levator palpebrae fascicles as they emerge from the central caudal nucleus. Overactivation of the contralateral levator palpebrae muscle accompanies this because of a failure of inhibition.[2064]

PNET   See **primitive neuroectodermal tumors.**

pneumatic nystagmus   See **vestibular nystagmus.**

pneumatic tourniquet paralysis   See **tourniquet paralysis.**

pneumocele   The presence of air within the cranium, usually as the result of trauma.

pneumocephalus   (cranial aerocele) Gas (usually air) within the head, resulting from skull fractures, infection, tumor, or surgical trauma.[1239]

pneumoencephalocele   A gas-containing cyst within the brain.

pneumoencephalography   The introduction of air into the lumbar subarachnoid space in order to visualize radiographically the basal cisterns and ventricular system outlined by the air after it has ascended through the CSF. The test was introduced in 1919 and was valuable in its day. That day has passed.[1271]

pneumogastric nerve   The **vagus nerve.**

pneumotaxic and apneustic centers   Cell collections within the pons responsible for synchronization and modulation of respiratory effort.

pocket sign   The ability of patients with pseudo-kyphosis (due to severe weakness of the thoracic muscles) to attain spinal extension by bracing their extended arms against their upper thighs.[6022] Why this term was chosen remains a mystery to this author.

POEMS   (**P**olyneuropathy, **O**rganomegaly, **E**ndocrinopathy, **M**onoclonal gammopathy, and **S**kin changes; PEP syndrome, Crow-Fukase syndrome, Tatasuki syndrome, osteosclerotic myeloma) A rare, dominantly inherited plasma cell dyscrasia of adult life manifesting recurrent episodes of flaccid weakness and areflexia due to partial depolarization of the muscle fiber membrane in the context of symmetric demyelinating sensorimotor polyneuropathy, sparing the cranial nerves but progressing centrally from its initial distal location. Hepatosplenomegaly, lymphadenopathy, hypogonadism, hypoadrenalism, hypothyroidism, and diabetes are the main endocrine features, and hypercalcemia is present in those cases in which the condition complicates osteosclerotic myeloma. The skin is thickened and hyperpigmented, with hirsutism and angiomas. The associated neoplasm is more often an osteosclerotic than an osteolytic myeloma, and it can sometimes cause myelopathy.

Intracranial hypertension with papilledema, infiltrative orbitopathy, peripheral edema, pleuritis, and bone lesions may also accompany the findings indicated by the acronym.[348] The condition has been reported mainly from the Orient.

poikiloderma congenitale   (Rothmund-Thompson syndrome) A recessively inherited diffuse encephalopathy manifesting mental retardation, juvenile cataract, small genitalia, short stature, macrocephaly, abnormal hands and feet, atrophy and pigmentation of the skin with photosensitivity, and later hyperkeratosis.[5570]

point apophysiaire   A tender spot overlying the spinous process of a vertebra corresponding (roughly) to the level of irritation of a nerve root, described by **Trousseau.** See also **cellulalgia.**

pointe-onde   (Fr, spike and wave)

pointing test   See **Barany test.**

Poisoned Food Problem task   (of Arenberg). A test measuring problem-solving skills.

Poland anomaly   See **Poland syndrome.**

Poland syndrome   (Poland anomaly) Congenital unilateral absence of part of the sternomastoid or of one or both pectoral muscles, usually with scoliosis, syndactyly, and hypoplasia of the ipsilateral arm and hand, occurring sporadically but perhaps dominantly inherited in some cases.

The condition was described in 1841 by Alfred Poland of Guy's Hospital.[4476] Other associated signs include short fingers, absence of some digits, herniation of the lung, and absence or hypoplasia of the breast.[1309] See also **muscle aplasia, Souques syndrome.**

In a *variant* form, the features of **Möbius syndrome** are also found.[2651]

polar spongioblastoma   A **primitive neuroectodermal tumor** that resembles an astrocytoma, but differentiates along the lines of neuroglia. It tends to occur in early life, arising close to the ventricles and spreading through CSF pathways.

polarization   In clinical neurophysiology, the presence of an electrical potential difference across an excitable cell membrane. The potential across the membrane of a cell when it is not excited by an input or spontaneously active is termed the *resting potential*; it is at a stationary nonequilibrium state with regard to the electrical potential difference across the membrane. *Depolarization* describes a reduction in the magnitude of the polarization toward the zero potential. *Hyperpolarization* refers to an increase in the magnitude of the polarization relative to the resting potential. *Repolarization* describes an increase in polarization from the depolarized state toward, but not above, the normal resting potential. (Adapted from the 1987 Report of the Nomenclature Committee of the American Association of Electrodiagnostic Medicine. AAEE glossary of terms in clinical electromyography. *Muscle Nerve* 1987;**10S:** G5–G23. Copyright 1987 by John Wiley and Sons, Inc. Reprinted by permission of John Wiley and Sons, Inc.)

policeman's tip   See **porter's tip position.**

polio-   (Gr, gray - hence gray matter).

Polio Connection of America   A charitable organization in this field. Address: P.O. Box 182, Howard Beach, NY 11414. Tel: 718-835-5536. E-mail: w1066polio@hotmail.com. Web site: http://www.geocities.com/w1066w/.

Polio Survivors Association   A charitable organization providing support and information on this condition. Address: 12720 La Reina Avenue Downey, CA 90242. Tel: 562-862-4508. Web site: http://www.polio-association.org/.

polioencephalitis   (from Gr, gray + brain + inflammation) Inflammation of the gray matter of the brain.

polioencephalitis hemorrhagica superior   See **Wernicke-Korsakoff encephalopathy.**

polioencephalomyelopathy   See **Creutzfeldt-Jakob disease.**

poliomyelitis   (from Gr, gray + marrow + inflammation) (Heine-Medin disease, acute anterior poliomyelitis, infantile paralysis, morning paralysis) An acute systemic viral illness caused by the picornavirus poliovirus types 1, 2, or 3, which is usually spread by the fecal-oral route. The gene responsible for susceptibility to poliomyelitis maps to chromosome 19q12–13.2.

Clinically, it only sometimes affects (but then often devastates) the nervous system. The greatest effects of the disease are on the anterior horn cells or cranial nerve motor nuclei in the gray matter of the spinal cord or brainstem, respectively. Most commonly a febrile *minor illness* occurs without progression to neurological involvement; but in some 2% of the cases, this is followed by a *major illness*, characterized by features of **aseptic meningitis,** which in some cases progresses further to a paralytic stage, typically affecting the limbs proximally and asymmetrically with myalgia, tenderness, weakness, fasciculations, loss of muscle stretch reflexes, and eventual muscle atrophy. Bulbar involvement occurs in some 10% of the cases of paralytic disease.[393] Signs of autonomic involvement and encephalitis, meningitis, or cerebellar ataxia are also described, but rarely.

The first modern description was that of Jacob Heine in 1840,[2522] but Dr. Michael Underwood (1737–1820) gave a very adequate account in his *Treatise on the Diseases of Children* in 1789 and the effects of the disease were carved in Egyptian relics in 1500–1400 B.C. The name of Karl Medin, a Swedish physician (1847–1927), also used to be associated with this disease, following his observation that the disease ran in epidemics. The virus has a particular predilection for the anterior horn cells of the cord and for the cranial nerve motor nuclei, as was first demonstrated by **Charcot.** Major epidemics occurred in the United States in 1890, 1907, and in the following two decades, but ceased after an effective vaccine was introduced by Salk in 1955.[4369]

In *variant* forms, a polio-like syndrome occurs in association with infection by enteroviruses 70 and 71.

In *acute hemorrhagic conjunctivitis*, a severe painful peripheral neuropathy with acute paralysis of the legs, areflexia, and sensory loss are the usual neurological findings. The enterovirus-70 responsible appears to attack the lumbar anterior horn cells or these and the anterior and posterior roots preferentially.[5796]

Enterovirus 71 infection may also cause an aseptic meningitis, *hand, foot, and mouth disease*, or a poliomyelitis-like illness with encephalitic signs.[6030]

poliosis   Premature graying of the hair.

POLIP syndrome   A progressive and potentially fatal neurological disorder characterized by sensorimotor **P**eripheral neuropathy, external **O**phthalmoplegia, **L**eukoencephalopathy, deafness, and chronic **I**ntestinal **P**seudo-obstruction due to visceral neuropathy.[5170]

Pollitt syndrome   A recessively inherited congenital dysmorphic syndrome manifesting also low birth weight; dwarfism; sparse, fine, brittle hair; cataract; premature aging; hypogonadotropic hypogonadism; microcephaly; seizures; cerebellar signs; spasticity; osteosclerosis or osteopetrosis, ichthyosis; and mental and developmental delay.[1144]

poly-   (Gr, many) Prefix denoting many.

polyarteritis nodosa   (periarteritis, systemic necrotizing vasculitis) An inflammatory disease of the large and medium-sized arteries described by Adolf Kussmaul (1822–1902) and Rodilg Maier (both German physicians) in 1866.[4979] Three conditions are regarded as variants: the classic form, the **Churg-Strauss syndrome,** and an **overlap syndrome.**[2414]

The classic form is complicated by painful multiple mononeuropathies, cutaneous neuropathies, or sensorimotor polyneuropathies, and less often by radiculopathies or brachial plexopathies. Focal or multifocal cerebral or spinal cord lesions and diffuse encephalopathies are also common.[2414]

polyclonia   See **Friedreich disease.**

polycystic lipomembranous osteodysplasia with sclerosing leukoencephalopathy   (PLO-SL; OMIM 221770) A recessively transmitted disorder characterized by the onset of bone pain in the twenties, dementia and successively agnosic-aphasia-apraxic syndromes and seizures, and then death within the following two decades.

CT scans reveal atrophy with calcification of the basal ganglia and X-ray studies show cysts in the small hand bones.[585]

polydactyly   The presence of six or more digits on a limb. In *preaxial polydactyly*, the extra digit is on the radial side of the hand, the thumb or index finger being duplicated, and in *postaxial polydactyly* it is on the ulnar side of the hand or the fibular side of the foot. The malformation is usually dominantly inherited.

polyglucosan bodies   Small, non–membrane-bound cytoplasmic structures, composed of unusual polymers of glucose. Lafora bodies, Bielschowsky bodies, and corpora amylacea are all composed of such polymers[6059] found within neuronal and astrocytic processes in various pathological conditions such as **Lafora body disease,** adult **polyglucosan body disease,** and many others, as well as in normal aged brains.[3461]

polyglucosan body disease   An inherited storage disease with onset in adult life, manifesting cerebral atrophy with dementia, pyramidal signs, sensorimotor peripheral neuropathy with loss of pain, vibration and proprioception, axonal neuropathy (nerve conduction studies also show myelinated fiber loss), neurogenic bladder, myopathy, and hypodensities in the white matter on CT scanning.[3475] See **adult polyglucosan body disease.**

polygraphic recording   The simultaneous monitoring of multiple physiological functions such as the EEG, the EKG and EMG, respirations, eye movements, galvanic skin resistance, and blood pressure.

polygyria   A developmental abnormality of the cerebrum, characterized by the presence of many small but true gyri.

polymicrogyria   A congenital developmental abnormal or neuronal migration within the cerebrum or cerebellum, in which the number of gyri is increased but their size is reduced. Cytomegalovirus infection has been incriminated as a cause. **Schizencephaly** is likely to be associated.

Clinically, the anomaly is associated with disordered intellectual maturation. Bilateral opercular or perisylvian polymicrogyria constitutes a part of the **Foix-Chavany-Marie syndrome;** bilateral parasaggital (parieto-occipital) polymicrogyria is a localized and sporadic condition. Bilateral frontal polymicrogyria is symmetrical and associated clinically with developmental delay, mild spastic quadriparesis, language impairment, and occasionally seizures.[2308] A classification has been suggested.[358] and is reproduced here, amended from Guerrini R, Barkovich AJ, Sztriha L, et al. Bilateral frontal polymicrogyria. *Neurology* 2000;**54:**909–13, by kind permission.

Classification of the Polymicrogyrias and Schizencephalies
A. Polymicrogyria and schizencephaly
 1. Bilateral polymicrogyria syndromes
  a. Bilateral diffuse polymicrogyria
  b. Bilateral frontal polymicrogyria
  c. Bilateral perisylvian polymicrogyria (autosomal dominant [22qll.2 and others], recessive, or X-linked)
  d. Bilateral parieto-occipital polymicrogyria
  e. Bilateral mesial occipital polymicrogyria

 2. Schizencephaly (polymicrogyria with clefts)
  a. Isolated schizencephaly
  b. Septo-optic dysplasia–schizencephaly syndrome
  c. Other rare schizencephaly syndromes
 3. Polymicrogyria with other brain malformations or abnormalities
  a. Polymicrogyria with abnormal white matter
 4. Polymicrogyria or schizencephaly as part of multiple congenital anomaly/mental retardation syndromes
  a. Adams-Oliver syndrome
  b. **Aicardi syndrome**
  c. Arima syndrome
  d. Delleman syndrome (oculocerebrocutaneous syndrome)
  e. Galloway-Mowat syndrome
  f. Micro-syndrome

polymodal nociceptor   A sensory nerve ending that signals the presence of any of the various potentially damaging stimuli to tissue, such as extreme temperature, physical insults, or chemical damage, along C fibers.

polymyalgia rheumatica   A systemic disease marked by inflammation of the intramuscular septa and restricted to people over the age of 50 years, who complain of stiffness of the girdle muscles (which is much worse in the mornings), fatigue, malaise, anorexia, weight loss, and low-grade fever. The erythrocyte sedimentation rate (ESR) is almost always greatly raised. The syndrome is at one end of a spectrum, at the other end of which is **giant cell arteritis,** but it responds to a lower dose of steroids and is eventually self-limiting.[341]

The following diagnostic criteria have been suggested:[4149]
 1. Bilateral muscle pain lasting for more than 2 weeks in more than two of the following areas: neck, shoulders, or shoulder girdle, upper arms, hips or pelvic girdle, and thighs
 2. Normal serum muscle enzyme levels
 3. ESR >40 mm/hr
 4. No swelling of the joints of the hands
The presence of all four of these is practically diagnostic of the condition.

polymyoclonia   See **opsoclonus.**

polymyositis   A group of acquired, subacutely progressive, idiopathic, inflammatory, noninfectious, nongranulomatous proximal myopathies of adults. When a skin rash is associated, the term **dermatomyositis** is used.

The condition was first described by Wagner in 1863. The definition of the term is currently in evolution; while once all generalized inflammatory myopathies of presumed autoimmune, paraneoplastic, or collagen-vascular etiology were subsumed under the heading, two major categories of **infective myopathies** and **idiopathic inflammatory myopathies** are now recognized, the latter including both *generalized* and *localized* varieties. Polymyositis is included in the *generalized* category.

Classification of the varieties of polymyositis or dermatomyositis has been achieved[637,638] and amended.[3687,3688] They are listed in Chart P–15.

Chart P–15. Varieties of Polymyositis and Dermatomyositis

1. **Primary idiopathic (isolated) polymyositis**
2. **Primary idiopathic (isolated) dermatomyositis**
3. **Paraneoplastic dermatomyositis or polymyositis**
4. **Childhood (juvenile) dermatomyositis** or polymyositis associated with vasculitis
5. Polymyositis or dermatomyositis associated with connective tissue disorder (**overlap syndrome**)
6. **Drug-induced polymyositis or dermatomyositis**[922]
7. Infantile polymyositis
8. **Inclusion body myositis**
9. Idiopathic giant cell polymyositis[4071]
10. *Secondary polymyositis* The occurrence of inflammatory changes in muscles showing also evidence of denervation or of noninflammatory myopathy.[2839]

Criteria for diagnosis of polymyositis and dermatomyositis have been formulated and are given in Chart P–16.

Chart P–16. Criteria for the Diagnosis of Polymyositis and Dermatomyositis

1. Clinical
   A. Proximal muscle weakness, myalgia, and muscle tenderness, usually symmetrical, progressing during weeks or months, with or without muscle pain. The bulbar and neck muscles are typically involved.
   B. Arthralgia, fever, and the Raynaud phenomenon are commonly present and in cases of dermatomyositis, dermatological manifestations will be present.
2. Pathological
   Muscle fiber necrosis and regeneration and mononuclear cell infiltration are present. Perifascicular atrophy is sometimes present.
3. Biochemical
   Raised ESR and serum CK (MM isoenzyme), aldolase, or myoglobin levels; frequently polyclonal hypergammaglobulinemia is found.
4. EMG
   There are multifocal EMG features of myopathy; spontaneous activity is often present at rest.

Adapted from Hudgson P, Peter JB. Classification (of polymyositis) Clin Rheum Dis 1984;10:3–8.

Variant forms include the following:

Acute myoglobinuric polymyositis with virus-like crystals An acute, degenerative, necrotic muscle disease presenting with fever and muscle hypotonia and accompanied by myoglobinuria, probably due to influenza B6 virus infection.[1022,1987]

Chronic focal polymyositis A chronic, sporadic, inflammatory myopathy of adult life with insidious onset, affecting the quadriceps, the forearm flexors, and the brachioradialis muscles, associated with raised serum CK levels and with typical muscle biopsy specimen appearances.[540]

Inflammatory myopathy with COX-negative muscle fibers A slowly progressive proximal myopathy affecting mainly the quadriceps.[3379]

See also **scapuloileoperoneal atrophy with cardiomyopathy and inflammatory myopathy, congenital inflammatory myopathy, acne fulminans with inflammatory myopathy.**

polyneuritis cranialis   1. A demyelinating disorder affecting the lower cranial nerves (V, VII, IX, X, and XII) and considered to represent a localized form of **acute inflammatory demyelinating polyneuropathy.** In some cases, ophthalmoplegias, ataxia, or weakness of the limbs and trunk is also present. The CSF protein level is raised.[4486] 2. See **superior orbital fissure syndrome.**

polyneuropathy, organomegaly, endocrinopathy, monoclonal gammopathy, and skin changes.   See **POEMS.**

polyneuropathy with acromicria   A recessively inherited demyelinating peripheral neuropathy accompanied by retardation of intellectual function, premature menopause, unusual smallness of the extremities, and shortness of stature.[3518]

polyneuropathy–skin pigmentation–hepatosplenomegaly syndrome   A syndrome with onset in early adult life, characterized by papilledema, gynecomastia, hepatosplenomegaly with ascites, lymphadenopathy, demyelinating sensorimotor neuropathy, edema, skin hyperpigmentation, and cavernous hemangiomas.[337]

polyopia   The perception of multiple images with a single visual stimulus. This occurs occasionally in patients with right-sided occipital lobe disease who see multiple images of moving targets in the defective field of vision. In such cases, the polyopia closely resembles, and may actually represent, **visual perseveration.** See also **cerebral diplopia.**

polyosotic fibrous dysplasia   See **McCune-Albright syndrome.**

polyphagia   Excessive ingestion of food without hunger; often a compulsion, to be distinguished from morbid hunger.

polypharmacy   The practice of prescribing more than one drug for the same condition, notably the use of multiple anticonvulsant agents in the treatment of intractable forms of epilepsy.

polyphasic action potential   An action potential with four or more baseline crossings, producing five or more phases. See **phase.** cf. **serrated action potential.** (From the 2001 Report of the Nomenclature Committee of the American Association of Electromyography and Electrodiagnosis.[10] Used by permission, copyright © 2001, ΛΛEM.) See also **diphasic wave, triphasic wave.**

polyporencephaly   See **multicystic encephalopathy.**

polyradiculitis   (polyradiculopathy, polyradiculoneuropathy) Disorders affecting the spinal nerve roots at many levels. Most are inflammatory, often as a result of autoimmune attack, as in the case of **acute inflammatory demyelinating polyneuropathy.**

polyradiculitis with cellular infiltrates   See **neurolymphomatosis.**

polyradiculoneuritis   See **acute inflammatory demyelinating polyneuropathy.**

polyradiculoneuropathy   See **polyradiculopathy.**

polyradiculopathy   1. Any disease involving numerous spinal roots. 2. An EMG diagnosis made in patients with clinical evidence of disease affecting multiple roots and with normal or near-normal motor and sensory nerve conduction study findings but EMG evidence of **denervation** in a multiple-root distribution, either bilaterally or in three or more levels on one side.

polysclerosis   See **multiple sclerosis.**

polysomnogram   (polysomnography) The concurrent recording during sleep of such physiological variables as EEG, EOG, EKG, ear oximetry, respiratory rate and excursion, nasal air flow, and surface EMG of the anterior tibial and submental muscles.

polysomnography   See **polysomnogram.**

polyspike complex   See **multiple spike complex.**

polyspikes   See **generalized multiple spikes.**

polysynaptic reflex arc   A spinal reflex arc in which interneurons are involved between the afferent and efferent neurons. Most nociceptive reflexes and some postural reflexes are of this type.

Pompe disease   (glycogenosis type 2) See **glycogen storage diseases.**

Pompe disease of children   See **glycogen storage diseases.**

Pompe disease of infants   See **glycogen storage diseases.**

Pompe, J. C.   (1901–1945) Dutch pathologist who described the disease named for him in his Amsterdam University graduation thesis. He was shot by the German occupying forces for his resistance activities.

pons   (or pons varioli) (Lat, a bridge) The section of the brainstem between the medulla and the midbrain. The first published description was that of **Variolus** in 1573.

pontine disconnection syndrome   See **locked-in syndrome.**

pontine locked-in syndrome   See **locked-in syndrome.**

pontobulbar palsy with deafness   (Brown-Vialetto–Van Laere syndrome) A rare recessive syndrome of bilateral nerve deafness and nonfunctioning labyrinths with progressive weakness of all the muscles supplied by the cranial nerves below the fifth cranial

nerve, occurring in early childhood. Spinal motor neurons and the pyramidal tract may also be affected.[2010]

pontocerebellar hypoplasia   (pontoneocerebellar hypoplasia) A rare congenital disorder characterized by hypoplasia, mainly of the lateral lobes of the cerebellum, manifested clinically in neonatal life with feeding problems and respiratory distress, microcephaly, ataxia, spasticity, and mental and developmental delay. Callosal agenesis is commonly found as well. This condition is similar to **olivopontocerebellar atrophies** in that spastic paraparesis may also be found; it is incompatible with life after a few years.[4159] See **cerebellar ataxias** (*variants*), **Paine syndrome.**

Variants are *spinal muscular atrophy with* **pontocerebellar hypoplasia;** *pontocerebellar hypoplasia type 1,* a recessively inherited form associated with infantile spinal muscular atrophy and gross developmental delay without extrapyramidal features; and *pontocerebellar hypoplasia type 2,* a recessively inherited form associated with microcephaly and extrapyramidal dyskinesia.[378]

pontogeniculo-occipital waves   (PGO waves) Cortical signals recorded in animals during rapid eye movement sleep, accompanied by muscular twitching, autonomic changes, and irregular respirations.

These electrical discharges arise from the gigantocellular field in the pons and pass to many brain areas, as a result of disinhibition during rapid eye movement sleep. They have been considered to underlie the desynchronization of the EEG, the eye movements, and the instability of the autonomic nervous system during rapid eye movement sleep.[249] They are also occasionally recorded in the human EEG immediately before the onset of rapid eye movement sleep.[2005]

pontoneocerebellar hypoplasia   See **pontocerebellar hypoplasia.**

pontopseudocoma   See **locked-in syndrome.**

pontosubicular necrosis   Neuronal injury limited to the pontine nuclei and hippocampus occurring in premature infants born between 26 and 36 weeks gestation who suffer hypoxia and acidosis and who are subsequently exposed to high oxygen concentrations.[360]

Pool, James Lawrence   (b. 1906) New York neurologist who described myeloscopy (in 1942) and the following sign.

Pool-Schlesinger sign   (leg phenomenon) A sign of latent **tetany;** the induction of painful spasms in the knee extensors and ankle plantar flexors when the hip is maintained in flexion with the knee extended. The same phenomenon occurs in the forearm and hand when the shoulder is held in a position of elevation and forced abduction.

Popeye effect   The appearance of the wasted proximal part of the arm compared with the less-affected forearm in certain forms of muscular dystrophy, notably **facioscapulohumeral** dystrophy. The phenomenon is named for the cartoon character drawn thus.

Popeye syndrome   A form of brachial plexus palsy in which there is proximal (upper arm) muscle atrophy with retention of muscular bulk more distally, as may occur with C5–6 lesions.

A similar finding is occasionally seen in patients with **limb-girdle muscular dystrophy.**

popliteal angle   Part of the Dubowitz battery of tests for assessing **gestational age.**[1528] With the infant supine and the pelvis flat on the examining couch, the thigh is held in the knee-chest position by the examiner's left index finger and thumb supporting the knee. The leg is then extended by gentle pressure from the examiner's right index finger behind the ankle, and the popliteal angle (between the femur and the lower leg) is measured—the smaller the angle, the greater the degree of hypertonia.

Popplelreuter task   A test of right hemispheric visual perceptual processing, in which the subject is required to identify each of two superimposed line drawings of common objects.[4489]

Porch index of communication ability   A standardized and reliable (but complex) instrument for the assessment of a sample of language functions, praxis, and other communication skills, requiring substantial training on the part of the interviewer, in which patients are made to see, hear, or feel common objects, and their spoken and written naming responses are recorded.[4491]

porencephaly   The replacement of cerebral tissue by fluid, usually as the result of a localized ischemic lesion in the pre- or perinatal periods (type 1) or as a familial developmental disorder (type 2). The condition was recognized by **Cruveilhier,** but was named this by **Heschl** in 1859. Clinically, hemiparesis, seizures and intellectual impairment are the usual features. Radiological criteria have been defined.[1638]

poriomania   Wandering, as a manifestation of a clouded or confused state in complex partial seizures. The term was introduced by Emil Kraepelin.[3719]

porphyria   A group of dominantly inherited disorders in the biosynthesis of heme, leading to the excessive production and excretion of porphyrins. Hepatic and erythropoietic forms are differentiated, neurological complications occurring only in the former. See **acute intermittent porphyria, variegate porphyria,** and **hereditary coproporphyria.**[363,1164]

In a classic exercise in medical detection, Macalpine and Hunter[3538] concluded that porphyria has affected members of the royal houses of the United Kingdom (and their European relatives), back at least to Mary, Queen of Scots, but most prominently, King George III.

porter's tip position   That position of the arm assumed by patients with Erb palsy (C5–6 or upper trunk brachial plexopathy). The arm hangs adducted and pronated, with the fingers in slight flexion because of weakness of the shoulder abductors, the elbow flexors and supinators, and the long extensors of the wrist.

In previous eras, porters were available to carry luggage. Today, regrettably, the alternative name of *policeman's tip* is perhaps more appropriate.

Porteus maze test   A test of planning behavior, assessing largely the function of the frontal lobes, in which the subject is required to trace with a pencil the paths through progressively more complicated printed mazes.[4496]

portmanteau word   The fusion of part or whole of two or more words to form a hybrid neologism.[1172]

portosystemic shunt encephalopathy   See **acquired hepatocerebral encephalopathy.**

Portuguese neuropathy   See **Andrade neuropathy.**

Poser criteria   Criteria for the diagnosis of multiple sclerosis, the first to introduce the concept of laboratory evidence as support for the clinical diagnosis (see Chart P–17).[4504] Dr. Charles M. Poser is a contemporary American neurologist.

Chart P–17. The Poser Criteria for the Diagnosis of Multiple Sclerosis

Category	No. of Attacks	No. of Lesions Clinical		Paraclinical	CSF
A. Clinically Definite					
CDMS A1	2*	2*,†		NA**	NA
CDMS A2	2*	1	and	1**	NA
B. Laboratory-Supported Definite					
LSDMS B1	2*	1	or	1	+
LSDMS B2	1	2*		NA	+
LSDMS B3	1	1	and	1*	+
C. Clinically Probable					
CPMS C1	2*	1		–	–
CPMS C2	1	2*		–	–
CPMS C3	1	1	and	1*	–
D. Laboratory Supported Probable					
LSPMS D1	2*	–		–	+

*All attacks are separated in time and in location of the lesion.

†One of the clinical attacks can be historical only if the information is reliable.

**Separate location of the lesion.

Diagnostic Criteria for Multiple Sclerosis

The proposed classification of multiple sclerosis (MS) for use in research protocols consists of two major groups, definite and probable, each with two subgroups, clinical and laboratory supported. The traditional possible MS group is not included because patients so labeled would not be acceptable for research studies.

A. *Clinically definite MS (CDMS)*
 1. Two attacks and clinical evidence of two separate lesions
 2. Two attacks; clinical evidence of one lesion and paraclinical evidence of another, separate lesion

The two attacks must involve different parts of the CNS, must be separated by a period of at least 1 month, and must each last a minimum of 24 hours.

Certain historical information may be substituted for clinical evidence of one of the two lesions (in category 1), if it fulfills the following conditions: the information is reliable, it is adequate to localize a lesion typical of MS, and it has no other explanation. Examples include a **Lhermitte sign** in any person under the age of 50 years who does not have radiologically demonstrable evidence of cervical spine disease; a useless hand due to severe impairment of position sense causing severe stereoanesthesia; a typical optic neuritis occurring before the age of 50 with loss of vision and with pain on motion of the eye or, if no substantial loss of vision has occurred, with description of visual field defect or alteration of color vision; transient paraparesis with paresthesias; **oscillopsia;** typical diplopia (in the absence of thyroid disease or a prior history of orbital trauma) that is abolished by closing either eye; and trigeminal neuralgia with onset before the age of 40. Extreme caution must be exercised in making such a substitution. If possible, confirmation by a relative or friend should be obtained if the attack was not observed and recorded by a physician.

Paraclinical evidence of CNS lesions may be elicited by a variety of means, including induced hyperthermia, evoked potential studies, CT and MRI scans, or special urological studies. Findings on neuropsychological evaluation conducted by an expert examiner indicate definite cognitive impairment in a patient under the age of 50 may be suggestive and helpful, but not yet specific enough to be fully diagnostic. No other explanation for these lesions must be evident. Use of the procedures and evaluation of results must follow the guidelines.

B. *Laboratory-supported definite MS (LSDMS)*

The laboratory support consists of demonstration in CSF of IgG oligoclonal bands (OBs) or of increased CNS synthesis of IgG. The OBs must not be present in the patient's serum, in whch the IgG level must be normal. This assumes that other conditions causing CSF changes, such as syphilis, subacute sclerosing panencephalitis, sarcoidosis, collagen vascular disease, and similar disorders, have been ruled out.
 1. Two attacks; either clinical or paraclinical evidence of one lesion; and CSF OB/IgG. The two attacks must involve different parts of the CNS and be separated by a minimum of 1 month, each having lasted at least 24 hours. One of the episodes must involve a part of the CNS distinct from that demonstrated by the clinical or paraclinical evidence.
 2. One attack; clinical evidence of two separate lesions; and CSF OBs/IgG
 3. One attack; clinical evidence of one lesion and paraclinical evidence of another, separate lesion; and CSF OBs/IgG

Historical information cannot be substituted for the clinical evidence. Regardless of whether the evidence is clinical or paraclinical, both lesions must not have been present at the time of the first examination and must be separated by at least 1 month. This separation in time is designed to reduce the possibility of including a case of acute disseminated encephalomyelitis. In a patient with the so-called progressive form of MS, (i.e., without remissions and exacerbations), evidence of clinical or paraclinical optic nerve involvement, for example, should not have been present at the time the paraparesis first appeared. Under those circumstances, and only if steady progression has taken place for at least 6 months, may such a case be accepted as MS.

C. *Clinically probable MS (CPMS)*
 1. Two attacks and clinal evidence of one lesion. The two attacks must involve separate parts of the CNS. Historical information cannot be considered as a substitute for the clinical evidence.
 2. One attack and clinical evidence of two separate lesions
 3. One attack; clinical evidence of one lesion and paraclinical evidence of another, separate lesion

D. *Laboratory-supported probable MS (LSPMS)*
 1. Two attacks and CSF OBs/IgG. The two attacks must involve different parts of the CNS, must be separated by a minimum of 1 month, and must each have lasted at least 24 hours.

*From Poser CM, Paty DW, Scheinburg L, et al. New diagnostic criteria for multiple sclerosis: guidelines for research protocols. Ann Neurol 1983;**13**:227–231. Reproduced by kind permission.*

positional alcohol nystagmus The occurrence of nystagmus and vertigo in the presence of levels of blood alcohol above 0.4 g/L. This occurs because of the diffusion of alcohol into the cupula within the ampulla of the semicircular canals, where it alters the relative densities of the cupula and the endolymph, transforming the semicircular canals into gravity-sensitive receptors.[727] See also **vestibular nystagmus.**

positional nystagmus Nystagmus induced by changes in the position of the head, usually tested by getting the patient to move quickly from an upright to a head-down position. It may have either *central* (brainstem) or *peripheral* (eighth cranial nerve and vestibular apparatus) causes. The phenomenon was regarded by Nylen as the surest and simplest sign of disturbance of the vestibular system.

Most cases have a peripheral cause (**benign paroxysmal positional vertigo**); there is a latency of 5–30 seconds before the nystagmus appears with assumption of the provocative position, the nystagmus fatigues after some seconds, habituation occurs on re-testing, the direction of the nystagmus is always to one side only (although a torsional component may be present), and the accompanying vertigo may be severe. None of these features is present when the lesion is central.

In a variant form, *persistent direction-changing positional nystagmus,*[315] fatigue does not occur but the nystagmus persists as long as the position is held but changes direction with different head positions.

positional vertigo See **benign positional vertigo.**

positioning nystagmus A common form of nystagmus occurring as a result of rapid head movement, seen in many patients with lesions of the vestibular system of any type and at any site. See **vestibular nystagmus.**[5]

positive myoclonus   See **myoclonus.**

positive occipital sharp transients of sleep   (lambdoids) Sharp, transient, single, or repetitive EEG waves with maximal amplitude over the occipital regions, positive relative to other areas, and occurring apparently spontaneously during sleep. Their amplitude varies but is generally below 50 Uv. (Adapted from the 1974 Report of the Committee on Terminology, IFCN[989] and reproduced by kind permission).

positive sharp wave   A biphasic, positive then negative action potential of a single muscle fiber. It is initiated by needle electrode movement (insertional or unsustained positive sharp wave) or occurs spontaneously. Typically the discharge is in a uniform, regular pattern at a rate of 1 to 50 Hz; the discharge frequency may decrease slightly just before cessation of discharge. The initial positive deflection is rapid <1 msec), its duration is usually less than 5 msec, and the amplitude is up to 1 mV. The negative phase is of low amplitude, and its duration is 10 to 100 msec. A sequence of positive sharp waves is commonly referred to as a *train of positive sharp waves*. These are assumed to be recorded from a damaged area of a muscle fiber. This configuration may result from the position of the needle electrode, which is believed to be adjacent to the depolarized segment of a muscle fiber injured by the electrode. Note that the positive sharp waveform is not specific for muscle fiber damage. Positive sharp waveforms may occur in association with fibrillation potentials and are thought by some to be equivalent discharges. Motor unit action potentials and potentials in myotonic discharges may have the configuration of positive sharp waves. (From the 2001 Report of the Nomenclature Committee of the American Association of Electromyography and Electrodiagnosis.[10] Used by permission, copyright © 2001, AAEM.)

positive supporting reaction   A postural reflex consisting of extension of the leg in response to pressure applied upward on the sole of the foot, said to be increased in primates after resection of the anterior lobe of the cerebellum but normally present at birth and persisting for about 6 months thereafter.

positive symptoms   Those symptoms caused by abnormal electrical activity within the nervous system as opposed to those due to the cessation of normal electrical activity. Hughlings-**Jackson** pointed out that destructive lesions never cause positive effects, but may induce a negative condition that permits positive symptoms to appear.[3857]

Those positive symptoms arising from motor axons include fasciculations, cramps, and spasms; those from sensory axons, pricking or tingling (paresthesias) and sensations of tightness, crawling, heat and cold, and pain.[1568]

positive wave   See **positive sharp wave.**

positron emission tomography   (PET) An investigational technique for the creation of images using radioactive isotopes that decay with the emission of positively charged electrons (positrons) to map the physiological, biochemical, hemodynamic, and pharmacological processes of the body.

Radioisotopes emitting positrons, produced in a cyclotron, such as the isotopes of oxygen, carbon, nitrogen, and fluorine, are incorporated into molecules with known biological behavior, and tomographically produced cross-sectional images of the distribution of these agents within the body are created, making use of the same principles as in CT scanning. Such images indicate underlying biochemical or pharmacological processes in defined anatomical loci. Over 500 compounds have been labeled with these isotopes for use as PET tracers.

Brain metabolic variables that can be mapped regionally by PET include blood flow and volume, pH, the oxygen extraction fraction, and the rates of consumption of glucose and oxygen. Tracers are also available for measuring the transport and metabolism of amino acids, free fatty acids, and glucose metabolites, and for the assessment of protein synthesis and molecular diffusion. Specific receptor ligands labeled with positron emitters have been used to map dopamine, serotonin, benzodiazepine, cholinergic, opioid, and adrenergic binding sites. Positron emitting–labeled medications including antiepileptics, neuroleptics, and agents suitable for mapping enzyme distribution can also be produced.[4526]

Cerebral glucose metabolism has been the most studied using, for example, fluorine[18]-labeled fluoro-2-deoxyglucose, but oxygen[15]-labeled water or gases such as carbon[15]-labeled carbon dioxide also allow assessments of cerebral blood flow, oxygen utilization, etc. Neurotransmitters may also be labeled to allow mapping of their distribution and activity. The technique has been employed in the preoperative evaluation of patients with refractory seizures, and in subjects with dementia, movement disorders, and brain tumors.[145,780]

possible multiple sclerosis   A diagnostic category in the 1954 definitions of Allison and Millar,[117] now largely replaced by the **Schumacher,** the **Poser,** or the **McDonald criteria.**

post-   (Lat, after)

Post, Wright   (1766–1822) American surgeon who was the first to ligate the carotid artery, in a patient with aneurysm (1814).

postactivation   The period following voluntary activation of a nerve or muscle. Contrast with **post-tetanic potentiation.** (From the 2001 Report of the Nomenclature Committee of the American Association of Electromyography and Electrodiagnosis.[10]

postactivation depression   A reduction in the amplitude and area of the M wave(s) in response to a single stimulus or train of stimuli that occurs within a few minutes following a 10- to 60-second strong voluntary contraction. (From the 2001 Report of the Nomenclature Committee of the American Association of Electromyography and Electrodiagnosis.[10] Used by permission, copyright © 2001, AAEM.)

postactivation exhaustion   The cellular mechanisms responsible for the observed phenomenon of **postactivation depression.**

The term is also used to describe the reduction of the M wave following a tetanus, which should logically be termed *post-tetanic depression.* (From the 2001 Report of the Nomenclature Committee of the American Association of Electromyography and Electrodiagnosis.[10] Used by permission, copyright © 2001, AAEM.)

postactivation facilitation   See **facilitation.**

postactivation potentiation   An increase in the force of contraction (mechanical response) after a strong voluntary contraction. See also **facilitation.**

postanesthetic apnea   Prolonged depolarization of muscles following succinylcholine usage during anesthesia, leading to flaccidity and weakness, most prominently manifest as apnea. The responsible gene maps to chromosome 3q21–q26. See **succinylcholine sensitivity.**

postanoxic myoclonus (chronic posthypoxic myoclonus)   Multifocal cortical **action myoclonus** with cerebellar ataxia and frequently a reduction in cognitive capacity, due to subcortical ischemic anoxia. Typically this follows a period of cardiorespiratory arrest.[3240]

The condition presents with the major feature of multifocal cortical action myoclonus that is often stimulus-sensitive. The cognitive deficits are usually mild. An exaggerated startle response and brainstem reticular reflex myoclonus are also described. See **Lance-Adams syndrome.**

postchalastic fits   See **sleep paralysis.**

Postconcussion Syndrome checklist   An instrument recording the experience of cognitive, emotional, and physical symptoms of subjects following concussion.[2087]

postconcussional syndrome   A persistent syndrome commonly following head trauma (not always sufficiently severe to result in loss of consciousness) and including such disparate somatic symptoms as headache; fatigue; diplopia; convergence insufficiency; dizziness (seldom true vertigo); tinnitus; hearing loss or hyperacusis; insomnia; reduced tolerance to stress, emotional excitement and alcohol; anergy, blurred vision, and photophobia; cognitive disturbance such as difficulty in concentrating and performing mental tasks (especially those involving information processing); impairment of memory, slowed thinking and reaction times; and

emotional disturbances including irritability, lack of spontaneity, reduced initiative, and both anxiety and depression, all occurring in the absence of physical signs.[1845,4338]

At least three of the features described should be present for a definite diagnosis. Careful evaluation with laboratory techniques (EEG, brainstem evoked potentials, brain imaging, oculonystagmography) may yield objective evidence to substantiate the symptoms but results are often negative.

The complaints are not typically motivated by thoughts of compensation.

See also **Paced Auditory Serial Addition Task, Glasgow Coma scale,** and **chronic fatigue syndrome,** the symptoms of the latter being similar in nature.

postcontusion seizure syndrome   See **traumatic spreading depression syndrome.**

postconvulsive palsy   See **Todd paralysis.**

postdural puncture headache   See **postlumbar puncture headache.**

postencephalitic parkinsonism   A parkinsonian syndrome occurring years after the illness **encephalitis lethargica,** and characterized by especially severe rigidity and facial impassivity, the occurrence of **oculogyric crises,** psychiatric features such as dementia, personality change, psychosis, and akinetic states, and the remarkable feature of the return to active mobility for short periods under extreme emotional stimulation.[4571]

postencephalitic parkinsonism with amyotrophy   The occurrence of progressive atrophy of the spinal muscles many years after the onset of parkinsonism of the postencephalitic type. There is degeneration in the pons, oculomotor nuclei, and anterior horn cells of the cervical and dorsal levels of the spinal cord, without tract degeneration.[2271]

postencephalitic syndrome   A syndrome of residual behavioral change following recovery from either viral or bacterial encephalitis. Symptoms are nonspecific and vary from individual to individual, from one infectious agent to another, and, most consistently, with the age of the individual at the time of infection. The principal difference between this disorder and the organic personality disorders is that it is often reversible.[150]

The old DSM-III APA guidelines suggested that the manifestations may include general malaise, apathy or irritability, some lowering of cognitive functioning (learning difficulties), altered sleep and eating patterns, and changes in sexuality and in social judgement. There may be a variety of residual neurological dysfunctions, such as paralysis, deafness, aphasia, constructional apraxia, and acalculia.

postepileptic headache   A migraine-like headache following generalized tonic-clonic seizures experienced by many epileptic patients.[4990]

postepileptic paralysis   See **Todd paralysis.**

posterior agraphia   See **agraphia.**

posterior aprosodia   A receptive form of **aprosodia,** in which subjects are unable to discern the emotive content of the spoken speech that they hear. The lesion is situated in the posterior right temporoparietal area or in the thalamic and adjacent regions.[4801]

posterior canal benign positional vertigo   The most common form of **benign positional vertigo.**

posterior cerebral artery syndrome   Clinical syndromes resulting from occlusion of the posterior cerebral artery by embolism or thrombus. The clinical features, visual and nonvisual, resulting from occlusions at proximal and distal sites have been summarized by Fisher[1857] and are given in Chart P–18.

Chart P–18. Clinical Features of the Posterior Cerebral Artery Syndromes

Proximal occlusions may lead to visual signs, including third cranial nerve palsy, **Parinaud syndrome,** vertical gaze paresis, paralysis of downward gaze, bilateral ptosis, oval pupils, blepharospasm, **retraction nystagmus,** tucking of eyelids, anterior **internuclear ophthalmoplegia,** pseudo-paralysis of the sixth cranial nerve, decreased or absent spontaneous blinking with retained reflex blink to light and sound, absence of slow roving eye movements, absence of horizontal saccades, delayed eye closure on falling asleep, and ocular tremor, and to other signs including **abulia,** drowsiness, brief wake–sleep cycles, coma, dementia, **tachyphemia,** hemiparesis, **decerebrate posture, Horner syndrome,** cerebellar ataxia, **rubral tremor, Weber, Claude,** or **Benedikt syndromes, hemiballismus, asterixis,** and **Cheyne-Stokes respirations.**

Distal occlusions may lead to visual signs, including hemianopia, unilateral and bilateral; **Anton syndrome; alexia without agraphia;** color anomia; **dyschromatopsia;** simple, complex, formed and unformed hallucinations; **central photophobia; visual perseveration; polyopia;** tilted vision; visual spread; migrainous features (scintillations, blindness, and blurring); **prosopagnosia; topographic agnosia; visual agnosia; peduncular hallucinosis;** checkerboard fields and **metamorphopsia,** and to other signs, including sensory deficits; the **Déjèrine-Roussy syndrome** of thalamic pain; choreoathetosis; confusion; agitation; impairment of memory; anomia for proper names; isolated **dysgraphia;** unsteadiness or lightheadedness; and hemorrhagic infarction secondary to brain herniation. From Fisher CM. The Posterior Cerebral Artery Syndrome. *Can. J. Neurol. Sci.* 1986;**13**:232–9,[1857] reproduced by kind permission.

posterior cervical sympathetic syndrome   A constellation of subjective complaints including occipital head pain, vertigo resulting from head turning, tinnitus, hazy vision without objective abnormality, and fatigability. The condition was considered by Barré[373] to result from cervical joint disease. See **cervical migraine, Barré syndrome.**

posterior column ataxia   see **Biemond syndrome.**

posterior column sensations   **Déjèrine** wrote that with posterior column lesions, "Even if tactile sensibility is almost normal, the sense of localization, the notion of weight, the sense of tactile discrimination (two-point) are greatly altered; and finally astereognosis is frequent." Wartenberg noted that the posterior columns mediate spatial functions as the recognition by feeling of forms (e.g., numerals) traced on the skin.

There is now evidence that the posterior column and the anterolateral tracts together subserve at least touch and pressure sensibility, and that the disturbance of position sense leads to many of the other impairments of discrimination.[4077] Other authorities consider **directional cutaneous kinesthesia** to be the only sensation properly named.[451]

posterior columns   (Wall)[5814] See **dorsal columns.**

posterior compartment syndrome of the thigh   Sciatic neuropathy following prolonged sitting.[4490]

posterior cortical atrophy   (posterior cortical dementia, De Renzi–Benson syndrome) A syndrome of slowly progressive dementia with initial alexia, anomia, asomatognosia, and object agnosia, followed by a **Balint** or a **Gerstmann syndrome, constructional apraxia,** visuospatial disorientation, and transcortical sensory aphasia, considered to be due to bilateral, asymmetrical parieto-occipital atrophy.[465,1408]

The syndrome may be seen in patients with **Alzheimer disease** but also in those with **Pick disease, progressive subcortical gliosis,** or **Creutzfeldt-Jakob disease.** It was described first by Rosenfeld in 1909 but more completely by Benson and by De Renzi in the last decade. See also **progressive biparietal atrophy.**

posterior cortical dementia   See **posterior cortical atrophy.**

posterior diencephalic autonomic epilepsy syndrome   See **de Morsier syndrome.**

posterior femoral cutaneous neuralgia   A syndrome of pain in the scrotal and perineal area, radiating to the adjacent thigh, associated with damage to the posterior femoral cutaneous nerve.[1035]

posterior fossa compression syndrome   The occurrence of apnea and coma with continuous cardiac function due to a primary failure of the respiratory center, as a result of compression as a result of posterior fossa disease.[4742]

posterior fossa stare   See **Collier sign.**

posterior inferior cerebellar artery syndrome   See **lateral medullary syndrome.**

posterior internuclear ophthalmoplegia   Conjugate gaze palsy recovering to leave paresis of the lateral rectus on that side, while the contralateral medial rectus regains its function. One cause is an infarct of the brainstem just above the abducens nucleus.[4818]

posterior interosseous syndrome (supinator channel syndrome, radial tunnel syndrome, deep radial nerve paralysis, dorsal interosseous syndrome) Deficits of this major terminal branch of the radial nerve, which supplies the extensor muscles of the forearm.

Compression of the nerve in the arcade of Frohse or by, for example, lesions at the level of the radioulnar joint lead to complaints of proximal forearm pain, worsened by forced supination and resembling that of tennis elbow or tenosynovitis; weakness of wrist, finger, and thumb extension with a radial drift; and occasionally wasting of the forearm extensor muscles, with minimal sensory deficit in the forearm, wrist, or hand.[5921] Most cases are idiopathic, but trauma or local mass lesions may be responsible.

The **supinator syndrome** is considered to be a special form of this syndrome.[903,1157,1745]

posterior lacerocondylar syndrome Involvement of the twelfth cranial nerve, usually with involvement of nerves IX, X, and XI as well, due to a lesion such as a primary or secondary tumor at the base of the skull. See **Collet-Sicard syndrome.**

posterior leukoencephalopathy A reversible syndrome likely due to capillary leakage and characterized by headache, altered mental functioning, seizures, and loss of vision associated with findings indicating predominantly posterior leukoencephalopathy on imaging studies. Patients may be receiving immunosuppressive therapy, or have eclampsia or acute hypertensive encephalopathy. Clinical findings include headaches, vomiting, confusion, seizures, cortical blindness, and other visual abnormalities and motor signs. CT and MRI studies show extensive bilateral white matter abnormalities suggestive of edema in the posterior regions of the cerebral hemispheres, the characteristic of subcortical edema without infarction; changes may also involve other cerebral areas, the brainstem, or the cerebellum. Reversible, predominantly posterior leukoencephalopathy may develop in patients who have renal insufficiency or hypertension or who are immunosuppressed.[2577]

posterior peroneofemoral reflex See **external hamstring reflex.**

posterior retroparotid syndrome See **Villaret syndrome.**

posterior retropharyngeal syndrome See **Villaret syndrome.**

posterior scarf sign See **scarf sign.**

posterior temporal lobe epilepsy A seizure syndrome arising from a focus usually in the basal region of the temporal lobe, seen most often in children and characterized clinically by initial behavioral arrest followed by tonic contraversive movements and then motor signs. Automatisms are late appearing and a minor feature only.[1539]

posterior thalamic syndrome See **thalamic syndrome.**

posterior tibial neuropathy A syndrome of weakness and wasting of the gastrocnemius-soleus and of the intrinsic muscles of the foot as a result of damage to the posterior tibial nerve fibers, either while still a part of the sciatic nerve in the pelvis or more distally in isolation. Lesions of the main trunk of the nerve in the thigh are usually a result of compression, trauma, or ischemic disease and cause sural sensory and lower motor neuron lesions in the gastrocnemius, soleus, and plantar muscles. Distally, the problem could be located at any point along its course, but, becauase of the protection afforded by overlying structures at higher levels, it is usually at a point below the medial malleolus, in which case only the foot muscles and sensation in the sole of the foot are affected. See **tarsal tunnel syndrome.**

posterior tibiofemoral reflex See **internal hamstring reflex.**

posterior vermal split syndrome Impairment of tandem gait with relative retention of other cerebellar functions, following surgical transection of the posterior inferior cerebellar vermis.[386]

posterolateral sclerosis See **subacute combined degeneration of the cord.**

postfixation An anatomical variant of the optic chiasm such that it lies posteriorly in relation to the sella turcica, and above the dorsum sella.

postfixational blindness Loss of vision distal to a point of close fixation in patients with bitemporal hemianopia, due to approximation of the blind half-fields that occurs as the eyes converge. The subject thus retains a cone of vision immediately anterior to the face, but can see nothing behind this.

postganglionic cholinergic dysautonomia The rare occurrence of pure postganglionic cholinergic dysfunction which presents as internal ophthalmoplegia, impaired secretion of tears and saliva, anhidrosis, and hypertension without the sympathetic involvement present in **autonomic neuropathy** (definition 1). The condition may have an autoimmune or postinfectious etiology.[2452]

postganglionic fibers Those neurons of the parasympathetic and sympathetic systems arising from the peripheral ganglia and passing to their respective end-organs.

The name was bestowed by J.N. **Langley.**

posthemiplegic chorea (postparalytic chorea) Chorea following stroke, first described by Silas Weir **Mitchell** in 1874.

posthemiplegic dystonia The occurrence of dystonic movements (or athetosis) years after a stroke. The responsible lesions are of the contralateral caudate nucleus, the thalamus, or both.

postherpetic neuralgia A chronic painful condition in which burning and jabbing pain persists for longer than a month in the distribution of the skin eruptions of prior herpes zoster, such as a thoracic dermatome or a division of the trigeminal nerve (usually the first). The pain, which can be either a burning hyperesthesia or lancinating stabs, occurs both spontaneously and following any stimulus to the affected skin; it may be intractable. It is more common in females and increases both in severity and frequency with advancing age. Scarring of the skin and sensory loss are also common in the affected regions. The therapies in current use have been reviewed.[3141]

posthyperventilation apnea A period of apnea not normally exceeding 12 seconds, occurring after a period of voluntary hyperventilation, such as five deep breaths. When it lasts longer, bilateral hemispheric disease is suggested.[4465]

A mechanism linked to vigilance and to the respiratory control centers acts to prevent this apneic pause in normal, awake humans, but is disturbed itself in states of diminished consciousness, leading to a period of apnea that is prolonged.

postictal hemiplegia Weakness of one side of the body lasting for periods of up to days, usually following prolonged somatomotor seizures but also occurring after partial seizures without motor manifestations. See also **Todd paralysis.**

postictal hemisyndrome See **Todd paralysis.**

postictal nose rubbing A behavioral pattern strongly suggesting an ipsilateral temporal lobe location of seizure origin.[5916]

postictal psychosis Paranoid or schizophrenia-like psychoses developing after a flurry of complex partial or generalized seizures, and also seen sometimes following right temporal lobectomy performed for the control of intractable partial seizures.[3586] The EEG does not show seizure activity during such psychotic episodes.[3460]

postinfection fatigue syndrome (myalgic encephalomyelitis, benign encephalomyelitis, chronic Epstein-Barr virus infection, Icelandic disease, epidemic neuromyasthenia, **Royal Free disease**) A syndrome of persistent, profound fatigue precipitated by minimal physical exertion, occurring after a viral or other infection, almost invariably associated with some emotional disturbance. There is little or no objective abnormality revealed by EMG, isometric strength testing, or muscle biopsy.[3446]

The syndrome may be episodic or sporadic. What combination of organic and functional factors interact to cause it remains the subject for intermittent dispute,

except among its sufferers, who reject angrily any hint of a psychological etiology. Despite this, their symptoms much resemble the somatic complaints of patients with depressive illnesses.

Criteria for diagnosis have been suggested[3446] and are given in Chart P–19.

Chart P–19. Criteria for the Diagnosis of Postinfection Fatigue Syndrome

To fulfill the criteria, the patient must have chronic persisting or relapsing fatigue of a generalized nature, causing disruption of usual daily activities, present for greater than 6 months, *and* two major criteria *or* one major and three minor criteria, as follows:

1. Symptoms: persistent for at least 6 months continuously, or relapsing on three or more occasions with a similar pattern, over 6 months or more:

Major	*Minor*
Concentration or memory impairment	Myalgia
Arthralgia	
Headaches	
Depression	
Tinnitus	
Paresthesias	

2. Signs: present on at least one occasion subsequent to the initial illness:

Major	*Minor*
Lymphadenopathy	Pharyngitis
Localized muscle tenderness	

3. Immunological assessment:

Major	*Minor*
T4 or T8 lymphopenia (absolute count)	
Cutaneous anergy *or*	Hypoergy

*From Lloyd AR, Hales JP, Gandevia SC. Muscle strength, endurance and recovery in the post-infection fatigue syndrome. J Neurol Neurosurg Psychiatry 1988;**51**:1316–22,[3446] reproduced by kind permission.*

postinfectious autoimmune neuropsychiatric disorders associated with streptococcal infection (PANDAS) The occurrence of tic and/or obsessive-compulsive disorder (OCD) following group A β-hemolytic streptococcal (GABHS) infections in children or adolescents. The likely pathophysiology is the development of antistreptococcal antibodies that cross-react with the basal ganglia of genetically susceptible hosts. See also **Sydenham chorea.** The following diagnostic criteria have been proposed:

1. Pediatric onset: symptoms of the disorder first become evident in the majority of patients between 3 years of age and the beginning of puberty.
2. Presence of tics and/or OCD: symptoms must meet lifetime diagnostic criteria for OCD and/or a tic disorder.
3. An episodic clinical course: onset of a specific symptom exacerbation can often be assigned to a particular day or week, at which time symptoms seemed to "explode" in severity. Symptoms may resolve completely between episodes, or continue at lesser severity.
4. Symptom exacerbations must be associated with a GABHS infection. Since streptococcal infections and tics

are common in childhood, confirmation of an association between them can only be made by following the children over time, observing at least two exacerbations occurring shortly after GAS infections.

5. During symptom exacerbations, patients may have adventitious movements (motor hyperactivity and/or choreiform movements).

The tics may be severe, involving head, limb, or whole-body jerks, with no prior history of the more typical eye-blinking or facial movements. Most children with PANDAS have normal premorbid personalities.[2038,3195]

postinfectious cerebellar ataxia   (acute benign cerebellar ataxia) an uncommon self-limiting syndrome of limb and gait ataxia, nystagmus, or opsoclonus following viral infections such as measles and varicella in children.[3084]

postinfectious encephalomyelitis   A multifocal immunological, inflammatory, and demyelinating polioencephalopathy considered to result from allergy to an infectious agent.

The syndrome evidences widespread acutely or subacutely evolving cerebral and spinal cord disease following a viral or other infection, such as measles, mumps, varicella, or rubella, and presents with fever, headache, seizures and focal neurological signs, alteration in consciousness, slow activity on the EEG, and modestly increased CSF protein levels and mononuclear cell counts, while signs of meningeal irritation are less common.[3003,4763] The patients usually recover. See also **postvaccinial encephalomyelitis.**

postinfectious encephalopathy   See **toxic hydrocephalus.**

postinfectious polyneuropathy   See **acute inflammatory demyelinating polyneuropathy.**

postinfective   See **postinfectious.**

postinfluenzal myositis   (benign acute childhood myositis) A mild necrotizing, inflammatory myopathy occurring in epidemic or sporadic forms, and manifesting pain, tenderness, and swelling of calf and thigh muscles in the week following an attack of influenza or parainfluenza A or B, with spontaneous resolution.

postirradiation myelopathy   See **radiation myelopathy.**

post–lumbar puncture headache   (low-pressure headache, post–dural puncture headache, postmyelogram headache, drainage headache) A postural headache felt mainly in the neck and occipital regions with forward radiation, relieved quickly by recumbency and occurring within 48 hours of lumbar puncture. The headache is considered to be due to traction on pain-sensitive intracranial structures as a result of an alteration in fluid dynamics from the continuing escape of CSF through the dural puncture site.[5277]

The condition was first described in 1898 by Augustus Bier, the "father of spinal analgesia," who developed one himself while studying the effects of subarachnoid cocaine.

The following diagnostic criteria are suggested by the Headache Classification Committee of the International Headache Society[1051] (Classification of headache disorders, cranial neuralgias and facial pains; and diagnostic criteria for primary headache disorders. *Cephalalgia* 1988;**8**[suppl]:1–96).

Bilateral headache develops less than 7 days after lumbar puncture.

Headache occurs or worsens less than 15 minutes after assuming the upright position, and disappears or abates less than 30 minutes after resuming the recumbent position.

Headache disappears within 14 days after lumbar puncture (if duration exceeds 14 days, consider **low–CSF pressure headache**).

postmyelogram headache   See **post–lumbar puncture headache.**

postoptokinetic nystagmus   See **optokinetic afterinduced nystagmus.**

postparalytic chorea   See **post hemiplegic chorea.**

postpartum cerebral angiopathy   A true inflammatory vasculitis or transient vasoconstriction related to the hormonal events of pregnancy and the postpartum period and a cause of hemorrhagic stroke in young women. Cerebral angiography demonstrates diffuse irregularity of branches of the middle cerebral arteries consistent with a diffuse vasospastic process or classic vasculitis. Neurological deficits resolve after high-dose corticosteroids.[5693]

postpertussis encephalopathy   A potentially fatal polioencephalopathy characterized by fever, alterations in consciousness, seizures, and focal neurological signs, occurring rarely during the paroxysmal stage of pertussis, usually in young children. Whether the cause is hypoxic or immunological is uncertain.[6030]

postpolio syndrome   See **postpoliomyelitis muscular atrophy.**

postpoliomyelitis muscular atrophy   (postpolio syndrome) A condition characterized by slowly progressive, asymmetrical impairment of muscle function after a documented attack of poliomyelitis with succeeding functional stability or recovery that has lasted at least 15 years. Residual atrophy, fasciculations, weakness and areflexia in at least one limb, normal sensation, a combination of acute and chronic denervation changes on EMG testing, and the presence of new muscle weakness and neuromuscular symptoms unrelated to other intercurrent disorders are other suggested criteria. The muscle pain and cramping are noted where none were present previously.

Clinically, the new weakness occurs 30–40 years after the original illness and in most cases is asymmetrical and predominantly focal. Fatigue, myalgias, and atrophy are common. Fasciculations are occasional accompaniments, but are increased by exercise. The course is slow, stepwise, and unpredictable, but the weakness and decreasing levels of function are progressive, although there are long periods of subjective stability. Upper motor neuron signs are not present.[1243] See also **postpoliomyelitis syndromes.**

postpoliomyelitis syndromes   Conditions regarded as either the direct effects of progressive muscle weakness or the indirect effects of the late results of poliomyelitis; the appearance of new, slowly progressive symptoms, including muscle pain and increasing weakness and fasciculations in muscles formerly weak as a result of poliomyelitis, and sometimes in those spared. The conditions are considered to result from the accelerated aging and death of individual nerve terminals, but an intrathecal immune response to the poliovirus is frequently present.[5096]

The major symptoms include complaints of fatigue; cramps and fasciculations;[1805] progressive musculoskeletal deformity; pain; **postpoliomyelitis muscular atrophy;** and sleep apnea. The usual latency following prior poliomyelitis is a quarter of a century or more. The condition probably represents the exhaustion of overstressed motor neurons as they try to maintain innervation of the unusually large number of myofibrils in the few remaining motor units.[1245]

post-pump chorea   The development of choreic and athetoid movements in up to 18% of small children within 2 weeks of cardiopulmonary bypass operations when deep hypothermia is used. The clinical accompaniments range from mild learning disability to profound hypotonia and lethal obtundation.[3802]

postrotational nystagmus   See **vestibular nystagmus.**

postrotational response   Nystagmus induced by sudden cessation of a velocity-step rotation.[3330]

postsaccadic drift   See **glissade.**

post-sinocibal syndrome   See **Chinese restaurant syndrome.**

post-stroke depression   The occurrence of long-lasting depression as diagnosed using the DSM-IV criteria and present in about a third of subjects following a stroke. The site of the lesion seems to have little effect in determining the occurrence of the depression.[912]

post-sympathectomy neuralgia   A pain syndrome appearing within 2 weeks of sympathectomy, characterized by deep, boring pain in the proximal part of the affected limb, with local tenderness and lasting a few weeks.[371]

post-tetanic   The period following tetanus.

post-tetanic depression   See **postactivation depression.**

post-tetanic facilitation   See **facilitation, potentiation.**

post-tetanic potentiation   1. The incrementing mechanical response of muscle during and after repetitive nerve stimulation. 2. In CNS physiology, enhancement of excitability or reflex outflow of neuronal systems following a long period of high-frequency stimulation. See also **facilitation, potentiation.** (From the 2001 Report of the Nomenclature Committee of the American Association of Electromyography and Electrodiagnosis.[10] Used by permission, copyright © 2001, AAEM.)

post-traumatic amnesia   A period of time following a concussion during which subjects are unable to make a permanent record of their experiences. The period ends when their capacity to retain information continuously is regained. Its duration is regarded as a crude but reliable indicator of the severity of the cerebral trauma sustained.

post-traumatic angiospasm   See **reflex sympathetic dystrophy.**

post-traumatic apoplexy   The occurrence of an intracerebral hematoma days after cerebral trauma.

post-traumatic dysesthesia   A neurogenic dysesthetic pain syndrome occurring some months after paraplegia caused by trauma at any level of the cord, including cordotomy.[5944]

post-traumatic edema   See **reflex sympathetic dystrophy.**

post-traumatic encephalopathy   A prolonged period of impaired intellectual functioning with variable somatic complaints occurring after craniocerebral trauma.[2831]

post-traumatic epilepsy   The occurrence of seizures related to a previous episode of head injury sustained more than a week before.

Factors identified as increasing the risk of subsequent seizures include dural penetration or loss of consciousness at the time of the original trauma; the occurrence of neurological deficit; wounds in the centroparietal area; intracerebral, extradural, or subdural hemorrhage; and seizures occurring during the first week after the injury.[1761]

Two forms are defined: *early*, the more common form, in which partial motor or generalized tonic-clonic seizures occur within a week of head trauma and usually in the first 24 hours; and *late*, in which generalized tonic-clonic, complex partial, or partial motor seizures occur after that time. Either penetrating or nonpenetrating injuries may be responsible in either case.[2842,2843]

post-traumatic headache   There are two types of post-traumatic headache, acute and chronic, and within each type two forms are defined. The criteria for the acute type are given in Chart P–20, and those for the chronic type are given in Chart P–21.

Chart P–20. Diagnostic Criteria for Acute Post-traumatic Headache

With significant head trauma and/or confirmatory signs:
A. Significance of head trauma documented by at least one of the following:
   1. Loss of consciousness
   2. Post-traumatic amnesia lasting more than 10 minutes
   3. At least two of the following reveal relevant abnormality: clinical neurological examination, X-ray of skull, neuroimaging, evoked potentials, CSF examination, vestibular function test, neuropsychological testing
B. Headache occurs less than 14 days after regaining consciousness (or after trauma if there has been no loss of consciousness)
C. Headache disappears within 8 weeks after regaining consciousness (or after trauma if there has been no loss of consciousness)

With minor head trauma and no confirmatory signs:
A. Head trauma that does not satisfy criteria for **acute post-traumatic headache**
B. Headache occurs less than 14 days after injury
C. Headache disappears within 8 weeks after injury

From Headache Classification Committee of the International Headache Society. Classification of headache disorders, cranial neuralgias and facial pains; and diagnostic criteria for primary headache disorders. Cephalalgia 1988;8(suppl):1–96,[1051] *by kind permission of Blackwell Science.*

Chart P–21. Diagnostic Criteria for Chronic Post-traumatic Headache

With significant head trauma and/or confirmatory signs:
A. Significance of head trauma documented by at least one of the following:
   1. Loss of consciousness
   2. Post-traumatic amnesia lasting more than 10 minutes
   3. At least two of the following exhibit relevant abnormality: clinical neurological examination, X-ray of skull, neuroimaging, evoked potentials, spinal fluid examination, vestibular function test, neuropsychological testing
B. Headache occurs less than 14 days after regaining consciousness (for after trauma, if there has been no loss of consciousness)
C. Headache continues more than 8 weeks after regaining consciousness (or after trauma, if there has been no loss of consciousness)

With minor head trauma and no confirmatory signs:
A. Head trauma that does not satisfy criteria for **chronic post-traumatic headache**
B. Headache occurs less than 14 days after injury
C. Headache continues more than 8 weeks after injury

From Headache Classification Committee of the International Headache Society. Classification of headache disorders, cranial neuralgias and facial pains; and diagnostic criteria for primary headache disorders. Cephalalgia 1988;8(suppl):1–96,[1051] *by kind permission of Blackwell Science.*

post-traumatic hypersomnia Excessive sleepiness that occurs as a result of a traumatic event involving the CNS, characterized clinically by complaints of excessive sleepiness, frequent daily sleep episodes, the onset temporally associated with head trauma, and with normal timing, quality, and duration of sleep. The **minimal sleep latency test** shows a mean latency of less than 10 minutes, and less than two sleep-onset rapid eye movement periods as recorded by polysomnography.[234]

post-traumatic movement disorders Tremors, parkinsonism and generalized or segmental axial dystonias of central or peripheral origin, occurring either as a direct result of the trauma on the nervous system or by acceleration of a preexisting condition.[2806]

post-traumatic neuralgia (cold pain) Intense, deep, throbbing pain in the hand or foot, referred proximally and resembling the normal person's sensation of intense cold, brought on by cold or by deep pressure in the area bordering the zone of complete anesthesia following a peripheral nerve injury. This is a variant of Head's **hyperesthesia,** but differs from **causalgia** in its restriction to the innervation territory of the affected nerve and in the response to cooling.[1396]

post-traumatic neurosis See **disability neurosis.**

post-traumatic osteoporosis See **reflex sympathetic dystrophy.**

post-traumatic pain syndrome See **reflex sympathetic dystrophy.**

post-traumatic Parkinson disease Criteria for the diagnosis have been suggested:[1200]
A. Trauma is sufficiently violent to cause concussion.
B. The time between the trauma and the onset of parkinsonism must be short.
C. An uninterrupted course of Parkinson disease should follow.

post-traumatic paroxysmal choreoathetosis A syndrome characterized by the occurrence of attacks of typical paroxysmal choreoathetosis within a month or two after recovery of consciousness from a head injury without abnormal EEG activity or imaging evidence of lesions of the basal ganglia.

A reported response to anticonvulsants suggests that the condition may have an epileptic basis.[1514]

post-traumatic stress disorder (shellshock, nostalgia) A multisymptom complex occurring in some subjects following severe and distressing physical or emotional trauma outside the range of normal human experience.

Diagnostic criteria have been suggested by the American Psychiatric Association[150] (Chart P–22)

Chart P–22. Post-traumatic Stress Disorder

1. The patient has experienced an event that is outside the range of usual human experience and that woud be markedly distressing to almost anyone.
2. The traumatic event is persistently re-experienced in at least one of the following ways:
   Recurrent and intrusive distressing recollections of the event
   Recurrent distressing dreams of the event
   Sudden acting or feeling as if the traumatic event were recurring
   Intense psychological distress at exposure to events that

symbolize or resemble an aspect of the traumatic event, including anniversaries of the trauma

3. Persistent avoidance of stimuli associated with the trauma or numbing or general responsivensss (not present before the trauma), as indicated by at least three of the following:

Efforts to avoid thoughts or feelings associated with the trauma

Efforts to avoid activities or situations that arouse recollections of the trauma

Inability to recall an important aspect of the trauma

Markedly diminished interest in significant activities

Feeling of detachment or estrangement from others

Restricted range of affect

Sense of a foreshortened future

4. Persistent symptoms of increased arousal (not present before the trauma) as indicated by at least two of the following:

Difficulty falling or staying asleep

Irritability or outbursts of anger

Difficulty concentrating

Hypervigilance

Exaggerated startle response

Physiologic reactivity upon exposure to events that symbolize or resemble an aspect of the traumatic event

5. Duration of above symptoms for at least 1 month

Reprinted with permission from the Diagnostic and Statistical Manual of Mental Disorders, *Fourth edition, text revision copyright 2000 American Psychiatric Association.*

post-traumatic syndrome   A condition of asthenia, irritability, diminished concentration, depression, and frequently headache following head trauma that was severe enough to have caused at least a brief period of unconsciousness. See also **de Morsier syndrome.**

post-traumatic syringomyelia   The occurrence of a syrinx, usually at thoracic or cervical levels, months or years after spinal cord injury.[1629,5013]

post-traumatic tremor   Postural and kinetic tremor of the hands and head occurring 1–4 weeks after mild head injury, often accompanied by myoclonic-like jerking. The tremor resembles that of **essential tremor.**[547]

post-tussive syndrome   See **cough syncope.**

postural deviation   Tilting or movement of the whole body in the direction of the flow of endolymph, provoked by caloric testing or by intrinsic disease of the vestibular system. This is noted when the subject walks heel-to-toe or along a straight line on the floor.

postural orthostatic tachycardia syndrome   (POTS) A mild and treatable form of autonomic dysfunction presenting with modest falls in blood pressure that are insufficient to cause full syncope, but produce near-syncope with vertigo, dizziness, disabling fatigue, exercise intolerance, and lightheadedness accompanying postural tachycardia. Diagnosis is facilitated by head-upright tilt table testing, which should demonstrate a heart rate increase of ≥30 beats/minute (or a maximum heart rate of 120 beats/minute) within the first 10 minutes upright

(unassociated with profound hypotension), with reproduction of symptoms. Central serotonergic mechanisms appear to participate in the pathogenesis of recurrent neurally mediated syncope.[2293,5531]

postural reflexes   Involuntary patterns of muscle contraction designed to compensate for shifts in gravity with alterations in body position. Such neural equilibratory mechanisms are of two kinds: *anticipatory postural responses* are truncal adjustments made immediately preceding a limb movement to preserve balance; *reactive postural responses* are sequential postural reactions to a shift of the center of gravity of the body when standing.[4180]

Postural control declines with age, as assessed by counting the number of steps a (forewarned) patient takes backward in response to a modest thrust on the sternum; 2–4 steps is considered evidence of moderate impairment.[5896] See also **rescue reactions, protective reactions.**

postural syncope   (areflexic syndrome) Reduction in consciousness as a result of reduced cerebral perfusion after attaining the upright posture. The mechanisms of this may be either vasovagal or an impairment of autonomic reflex function.

postural tremor   Tremor present when the subject voluntarily maintains a position against gravity. When it appears, usually during the performance of visually guided tasks, it may be called *position-specific postural tremor.* See **cerebellar tremors, tremor.**

posturography   A standardized quantitative laboratory method of studying vestibulo-ocular function, in which patients with dysequilibrium stand on a platform and the amount of body sway is analyzed when standing level or with anteroposterior or lateral tilt of the platform and with the eyes open and closed.[14,1813]

postvaccinial encephalomyelitis   A multifocal immunological, inflammatory, and demyelinating polioencephalopathy occurring as a complication of vaccination, but otherwise identical with **postinfectious encephalomyelitis.**

postventilatory paretic syndrome   An acquired syndrome of unknown cause occurring in adults or in children, characterized by neurogenic or myopathic weakness due to axonal neuropathy, and developing after a period of assisted ventilation for asthma or other severe pulmonary or meningitic illness. See **Hopkins syndrome, acute myopathy,** and **critical illness polyneuropathy,** the conditions variously considered to be responsible.[2582,3218]

postviral asthenia   See **chronic fatigue syndrome.**

potassium depletion myopathy   An acute myopathy associated with endogenous or drug-induced potassium loss, and presenting with flaccid muscle weakness without sensory loss, myalgia, polyuria, and polydipsia. Serum creatine kinase levels are markedly raised. Atrophy of type 2 fibers is observed on muscle biopsy specimens. The condition reverses with potassium repletion.[1112]

potassium exercise test   A standardized exercise test designed to show that increases in serum potassium levels as a result of exercise (80–100 watts on a bicycle ergometer) are less than normal in subjects with the hypokalemic variety of **familial periodic paralysis.**[2920]

potassium-sensitive myotonia   See **myotonia fluctuans.**

potential   1. A difference in charges, measurable in volts, that exists between two points. Most biologically produced potentials arise from the difference in charge between two sides of a cell membrane. 2. A term for a physiologically recorded waveform. (From the 2001 Report of the Nomenclature Committee of the American Association of Electromyography and Electrodiagnosis.[10] Used by permission, copyright © 2001, AAEM.)

potential field   The amplitude distribution of an EEG wave at the surface of the head or of the cerebral cortex or in the depth of the brain, measured at a given instant in time, and usually represented in diagrams by equipotential lines. (From Chatrian GE, Bergamini L, Dondey M, et al. A glossary of terms most commonly used by clinical electroencephalographers. *EEG Clin Neurophysiol* 1974;**37:**538–48, with permission from Elsevier Science.)

potentiation   Physiologically, the enhancement of a response. The convention is to use the term to describe the incrementing mechanical response of muscle elicited by repetitive nerve stimulation, e.g., post-tetanic potentiation, whereas the term *facilitation* is used to describe the incrementing electrical response elicited by repetitive nerve stimulation, e.g., postactivation facilitation. (From the 2001 Report of the Nomenclature Committee of the American Association of Electromyography and Electrodiagnosis.[10] Used by permission, copyright © 2001, AAEM.)[5588] See also **incrementing response.**

potomania   An abnormal desire to drink. (HJM)

Pott paraplegia   Paraplegia due to compressive myelopathy, the latter resulting from tuberculous spondylitis (caries of the vertebral column), local accumulations of tuberculous pus or granulation tissue, or vertebral collapse or dislocation.[4509] See also **chronic spinal meningitis.**

Pott, Sir Percival   (1714–1788) English surgeon at St. Bartholomew's Hospital. Pott's fracture was that of the fibula, originally described in himself following a fall from a horse. He also described cancer of the scrotum in chimney-sweep children, and wrote on hernias and head injury as well as the preceding condition, in 1779.

Potter syndrome   (oligohydramnios syndrome) A recessively inherited congenital dysmorphic syndrome, characterized by oligohydramnios prior to birth, and thereafter by growth retardation, lung hypoplasia, bilateral renal agenesis, dry skin, micrognathia, limb deformities, defects of neuronal migration with cerebellar heterotopias, and, in some cases, hydrocephalus.[2297]

Potzl, Otto   (1877–1962) Austrian psychiatrist who graduated from Vienna University, where he spent most of his professional life, latterly as professor of neurology and psychiatry.

Potzl syndrome   Word blindness with hemianopia and disturbance of the recognition of colors.[4510]

Pourfour du Petit, Francois   (1664–1741) French ophthalmologist, anatomist, and army surgeon who described contralateral innervation as a result of the decussation of the pyramids in his *Lettres d'un médecin des hopitaux* (Naumur, 1710) as well as the anatomy of the sympathetic chain and the ocular signs resulting from damage to it, as in the following syndrome, which he observed in soldiers wounded by sabres in the Napoleonic wars.

Francois Pourfour du Petit

Pourfour du Petit syndrome   (cervical sympathetic irritation syndrome) Mydriasis, exophthalmos, widening of the palpebral fissure, and increased intraocular pressure as a result of irritation of the sympathetic chain in the neck. The inverse of **Horner syndrome.**[1554]

Powassan encephalitis   A tick-borne direct infection of the brain by a flavivirus member of the togavirus group of arboviruses, and representing another member of the **Russian spring-summer encephalitis** complex but characteristically causing only sporadic (but severe) encephalitis with convulsions, respiratory failure, coma, and frequently death.

The condition is described rarely, mainly affecting children, in all parts of the Northern United States and Southern Canada.[5997]

Practical Neurology   A neurology digest journal covering current research, practice and thinking in neurology, published by Blackwell Science. Web site: http://www.blackwell-science.com/~cgilib/jnlpage.bin?Journal=pnr&File=pnr&Page=aims.

Prader syndrome   (pseudodeficiency rickets) A congenital dysmorphic syndrome manifesting also short stature, dental and skeletal anomalies, aminoaciduria and renal tubular acidosis, hypocalcemia, multiple fractures, hypotonia, seizures, and delayed closure of the fontanelles.[337]

Prader-Willi syndrome   (hypotonia, hypomentia, hypogonadism, obesity syndrome, HHHO syndrome) A complex multisystem chromosomal disorder. The diagnostic features (present in over 90% of cases) include congenital mental retardation; cerebellar ataxia; infantile hypotonia; short stature; obesity after infancy; cryptorchidism; hypogonadism; diabetes, strabismus, and various musculoskeletal and dysmorphic deformities, including ocular hypertelorism; low-set ears with overlapping helix; high-arched palate; micrognathia; microdontia; defective dental enamel; and partial syndactyly of the toes. Most affected subjects have a chromosome 15 deletion at 15q11.[937,1090]

prae- (pre-)   (Lat, in front of, before) Prefix denoting before.

pragmatic decoding   The utilization of nonlanguage cues to assist in decoding verbal meaning.

prandic epilepsy   See **eating epilepsy.**

praxis   The function of performance, as of a manual task; the execution of a learned movement in response to an appropriate stimulus, in the presence of normal afferent and efferent functions and without lack of attentiveness or cooperation.

This may be assessed formally by, for example, the block design test, using patterned cubes, by constructional tasks, and by having the patient perform complex movements on command or in imitation.

preacher's hand   (main de prédicateur) Extension of the metacarpophalangeal joints, flexion of the interphalangeal joints, and flattening of the thumb, as a result of combined median and ulnar nerve pareses, which put the hand into the position traditionally assumed by priests during the act of blessing.

preangular alexia   (anterior alexia) See **alexia.**

precentral area   See **motor cortex.**

prechiasmal syndrome   (Lat, before + Gr, decussation) Compression of an optic nerve and of the olfac-

tory, as by a presellar meningioma, which later grows back to involve the optic chiasm. Initially there is involvement of one optic nerve, including the fibers within **von Willebrand's knee;** at a later stage, a **Foster Kennedy syndrome** may be also present.

precocious Alzheimer disease   See **congophilic angiopathy.**

precommunal posterior cerebral artery   That segment of the artery proximal to the posterior communicating artery.

precordial catch syndrome   See **Texidor twinge.**

predormital myoclonus   See **sleep starts.**

prefixation   An anatomical variant in which the optic chiasm is situated unusually anterior with reference to the sella turcica, such that it lies above the tuber cinereum.

prefixation blindness   The inability to see objects introduced into the space between the subject and the point of fixation, as the result of overlap of the two blind hemifields when the eyes of a patient with binasal hemianopia converge.[4445]

prefrontal leukotomy   See **prefrontal lobotomy.**

prefrontal lobotomy   (prefrontal leukotomy) An operation introduced by Egas Moniz, designed to free schizophrenic patients from the torment of their disordered thinking. Latter it was found of some use in the management of obsessive-compulsive states and of depressive illnesses, but its wide use, frequently in cases where the blunting of affect and the dilution of personality characteristics were more troublesome than the original disorder of mentation, led to its vilification and eventual disuse.[1612,1947]

preganglionic neurons   Those neurons of the parasympathetic and sympathetic systems arising from the CNS and passing to the peripheral ganglia. The name was attached by J.N. **Langley.**

preherpetic neuralgia   Severe, burning radicular pain felt in the dermatomal regions destined to bear the acute lesions of herpes zoster between a week and 3 months later.[2115]

preictal pseudosleep   A state behaviorally resembling normal sleep in that the subject is motionless with the eyes closed, although the EEG shows a persisting alpha rhythm. It is recorded as preceding the appearance of **pseudoseizures** (nonepileptic seizures).[446]

premature aging with telangiectasias   See **Breathnach syndrome.**

premature senility syndrome   (Hutchinson-Gilford syndrome) See **progeria.**

premaxillary agenesis   A congenital, sporadic, dominantly or recessively inherited dysmorphic syndrome reflecting disordered embryonal differentiation and characterized by midline cleft lip, microcephaly, flattened nose, hypotelorism, mental and developmental delay, seizures, spastic quadriparesis, and impaired vision with colobomas. Hypopituitarism is commonly associated.

The chromosomal abnormalities include trisomy 13 or 18, deletions at 18p- and 13q-, etc.[1089]

premotor area   An arbitrary term for that area of brain lying immediately anterior to the **motor cortex;** its posterior border is ill-defined and its functions and those of the motor cortex overlap or may even be the same, except that damage to this region leads to motor apraxia rather than to hemiplegia. Damage to the areas immediately anterior to it give rise to slowness of movements and perseveration.

premotor syndrome   According to **Fulton,** a syndrome bearing witness to the effects of lesions of the premotor cortex. This syndrome has four main components: inability to perform skilled movements, particularly with the digits, without gross impairment of motor power; spasticity and an increase in the muscle stretch reflexes; forced grasping; and vasomotor disturbances, often with Jacksonian seizures in addition. **Walshe,**[5830] however, criticized this formulation and considered that apraxia of movement was the only important consequence of such lesions.

presbyophrenia   Dementia occurring with advancing age.

presbyopia   (from Gr, old man + eye) Impairment of the power of accommodation with aging.

presenile dementia   A term with no useful meaning, there being no notable difference in the characteristics of a disease attacking humankind after as opposed to before the age of 65 years, nor in the people themselves. The term is best reserved as a pejorative for political opponents rather than as one bundling together such entities as early-onset **Alzheimer disease,** the **frontotemporal dementias, dementia with Lewy bodies,** and prion disorders such as **Creutzfeldt-Jakob disease**.

presenile dementia–motor neuron disease   (ALS-parkinson-dementia syndromes) A dementing syndrome of adult onset manifesting behavioral and speech disturbances, bulbar palsies, pyramidal signs and cerebral atrophy with gliosis, and spongy changes in the cerebral cortex. See **amyotrophic lateral sclerosis.**

Present State Examination   A semistructured psychiatric interview used mainly in the diagnosis of dementia.[6004]

presque vu   (Fr, almost seen) An internal feeling of patients with visual field defects that they are going to see something within the blind field, a feeling not borne out by subsequent experience.

pressor nerves   Those sympathetic nerves which, when stimulated, lead to arteriolar vasoconstriction, and thus to an increase in blood pressure.

pressure palsy   Weakness as a result of conduction block occurring in a peripheral nerve compressed as a result of internal derangements caused by external forces; the loss of function of a peripheral nerve due to incidental compression. The compression has presumably led to ischemia with local conduction block; it is usually reversible within months unless the severity of compression has led to **axonotmesis.**

A *variant* familial form occurs, with onset at any age, in which weakness and sensory loss with autonomic dysfunction occur randomly in peripheral nerves in the presence of relatively minor compressive lesions.

pressure sensation   The awareness of deep, non-painful compressive distortion of a body part. This function is mediated by the same pathways that subserve discriminative touch sensation, and uses the larger myelinated fibers in the peripheral and the posterior columns of the CNS. The term *touch-pressure sensation* underscores the similarity of the two modalities, which indeed may form a continuum.

pressure-volume index   That volume of CSF required to produce a 10-fold increase in CSF pressure; a calculation of value physiologically in assessing CSF formation and absorption rates and clinically in prognosticating the outcome after severe head injuries.[3673]

pretectal pseudobobbing   Involuntary, repetitive, rapid, arrhythmic, downward, and inward eye movements with a faster downstroke than upstroke, occurring at slow rates and associated with pretectal rather than with pontine lesions, such as acute obstructive hydrocephalus. A blink precedes most of the movements, which may represent a form of spontaneous convergence nystagmus.[2979]

pretectal syndrome   A collection of ocular changes associated with lesions of the dorsal brainstem at the level of the superior colliculus, characterized by limitation of downward gaze; retraction of the upper lid; convergence–retraction eye movements; paralysis of convergence; dysjunctive eye positions including esotropia and skew deviation; and nystagmus. The pupillary abnormalities include diminished light response, light-near dissociation, and anisocoria.[2983] See **dorsal midbrain syndrome.**

pretraumatic amnesia   See **retrograde amnesia.**

pretrigeminal neuralgia   A mild "toothache" or "sinus-like" pain felt in the distribution of the fifth cranial nerve, triggered by jaw movement or drinking hot or cold liquids and preceding by days or years acute episodes of trigeminal neuralgia in the same facial region.[1971]

Preus syndrome   A congenital dysmorphic syndrome characterized also by low birth weight, small mouth, cleft palate, dwarfism, coarse hair, hernias, skeletal anomalies, sensorineural deafness, cryptorchidism, hypotonia, myoclonic seizures, and mental and developmental delay.[337]

Prevent Blindness America A charitable organization. Address: 500 E. Remington Road, Schaumberg, IL 60173. Tel: 1-800-331-2020. Web site: http://www.preventblindness.org/.

Prévost sign (Vulpian sign) Conjugate deviation of the head and eyes toward the side of an acute cerebral lesion and away from the paralyzed side.[4522] See also **conjugate eye deviation, Vulpian sign.**

priapism (from Lat, Priapus, the god of procreation) Sustained penile erections, as may occur in men with incomplete spinal cord lesions or on walking, when it may be a sign of spinal canal stenosis.

primary adhalinopathy See **myopathy** (*severe childhood muscular dystrophy*).

primary alcoholic dementia A non-entity.[5759] See instead **Wernicke-Korsakoff encephalopathy, pellagra encephalopathy, Marchiafava-Bignami disease,** and **acquired hepatocerebral encephalopathy.**

primary aldosteronism See **Conn syndrome.**

primary alveolar hypoventilation syndrome See **congenital central hypoventilation syndrome.**

primary amnesia A monosymptomatic cognitive disorder in which there is slowly developing amnesia in the absence of other signs of cortical functional impairment, such as that of language, praxis, perception, or calculation.[3503]

primary angiitis of the CNS See **isolated angiitis of the nervous system.**[1158]

primary antiphospholipid syndrome The occurrence of clinical thrombotic disease and/or fetal loss in association with thrombocytopenia and the presence of antiphospholipid antibodies in the blood. Young adults are predominantly affected; noninflammatory thrombotic occlusion of large or small arteries or veins causes, variously, spontaneous abortion, migraine, seizures, multi-infarct dementia, chorea, **amaurosis fugax** or retinal artery occlusion, cardiac murmurs, mitral valve lesions, and livedo reticularis.[2562]

primary autonomic failure See **progressive autonomic failure.**

primary basilar impression A bony deformity characterized by indentation of the floor of the posterior fossa by the atlas, diminishing its volume, and not due to bone disease such as osteomalacia or Paget disease.

The condition may be asymptomatic or else associated with features suggesting the **Chiari** malformation.

primary cerebrovascular amyloidosis See **congophilic angiopathy.**

primary chronic cluster headache See **chronic cluster headache.**

primary chronic insomnia An idiopathic syndrome of lifelong fragmentation of sleep with daytime fatigue, tension, and depression, sometimes associated with signs of minimal brain damage.

primary CNS lymphoma (reticulum cell sarcoma, perivascular sarcoma, microglioma, perithelial small-cell sarcoma, primary [malignant] cerebral lymphoma, immunoblastic sarcoma) A fatal primary neurological malignancy characterized by the presence of multiple deep intracerebral (periventricular) or submeningeal lymphomatous masses, their histological appearance similar to that of systemic non-Hodgkin lymphoma, and consisting of large lymphoid cells, perivascular histiocytes, microglia, plasma cells, and various (mainly B) forms of lymphocytes with multiplication of the basement membranes of those blood vessels involved by the lymphomatous process. The B-cell and T-cell types can be differentiated by immunocytochemistry.[4242]

Clinically, the tumor produces the clinical syndromes of confusion, dementia, increased intracranial pressure, or focal CNS signs and seizures; uveocyclitis is unusually common. Both progressive and relapsing-remitting courses are described. Such features are increasingly seen in this decade as a complication of immunosuppression, as in **AIDS**,[3728] as well as of congenital immunodeficiency syndromes, drug therapy, and collagen vascular diseases, but in the past the tumor was found to affect mainly males during later adult life. Enhancement of a mass in the gray matter or the corpus callosum without surrounding edema and contrast-enhancing lesions in contact with the subarachnoid space and without necrosis are characteristic findings on CT or MRI scans. They sometimes appear well before the clinical manifestations of the disease (*sentinel lesions*).[6032] The tumor is exquisitely sensitive to steroid treatment, which induces cell lysis.

primary degeneration of the granular layer of the cerebellum A congenital developmental abnormality leading to cerebellar ataxia. See **Lhermitte-Duclos disease.**

primary degenerative dementia Those forms of dementia caused by disease processes that primarily affect the CNS but which are neither infectious nor due to vasculopathy.[6041]

Other organs may also be affected. The disease causes progressive dysfunction and degeneration of neurons and other cells. Three subgroups are defined (see Chart P–23).[2341]

Chart P–23. Subgroups of Degenerative Dementia

Frontotemporal Cortical Predominance

Pick disease
Frontal lobe dementia
Amyotrophic lateral sclerosis with dementia
Atypical Alzheimer disease
Rare familial forms

Temporoparietal Cortical Predominance

Alzheimer disease with early onset
Alzheimer disease with late onset
Down syndrome with dementia of Alzheimer type
Subcortical dementias

Other Forms

Parkinson disease with dementia
Diffuse Lewy body disease

After Gustafson L. Clinical classification of dementia conditions. Acta Neurol Scand *Suppl 1992;139:16–20.*

primary dementias   Those dementing conditions due to degenerative disease of the brain affecting primarily the nerve cells.

primary deviation   A phenomenon observed during the performance of the **Alternate Cover test** in a patient with a lesion of one of the oculomotor nerves causing muscle paresis.

When patients direct their gaze in the direction of action of the affected muscle, deviation of the covered paretic eye away from the target is known as *primary deviation*. When patients direct their gaze so that the paretic eye fixes on the target, the deviation of the covered normal eye is known as *secondary deviation*. The latter is of greater amplitude. See **Cover test.**

primary diffuse leptomeningeal gliomatosis   A rare, fatal syndrome characterized by extensive basal and chronic infiltration of the meninges by tumor cells arising from heterotopic cell nests, without parenchymal involvement. The clinical presentation is typically with headache, raised intracranial pressure, and encephalopathy. Elevated CSF levels of protein and low glucose with moderate mononuclear pleocytosis are usual, and in the absence of direct evidence of neoplasia, commonly lead to a diagnosis of chronic meningitis. Meningeal biopsy may assist in making the diagnosis.[410]

primary generalized epilepsies   Seizure disorders without macroscopic pathological features, inherited either as polygenic or as autosomal dominant characteristics with age-dependent penetrance and characterized by **generalized tonic-clonic, myoclonic,** or **generalized absence** seizure types, either alone or in combination.

primary generalized epilepsy of adolescence   See **typical absence epilepsy of adolescence.**

primary generalized epileptic myoclonus   A fragment of primary generalized epilepsy usually manifesting as small focal muscle jerks (**minipolymyoclonus**) or as generalized and precisely synchronized bodily jerks.

The origin of the electrical discharge is considered to be an area of hyperexcitable cortex driven to synchrony by ascending impulses from subcortical regions.[2384]

primary hyperaldosteronism   (Conn syndrome) Excessive secretion of aldosterone by the adrenal cortex, leading to hypertension, sodium retention, hypokalemic alkalosis, muscle weakness, tetany, and, in some cases, to features of **familial periodic paralysis** (hypokalemic form).

primary hyperoxaluria   Two rare recessive disorders of glyoxalate metabolism characterized clinically by recurrent calcium oxalate nephrolithiasis leading to chronic renal failure with death from uremia. The pathological mechanism responsible is the deposition of calcium oxalate crystals within the kidney and within the walls of arterioles and venules in other organs.

An associated neuropathy with both axonal degeneration and segmental demyelination has been reported rarely.[2377]

primary idiopathic dermatomyositis   A form of **idiopathic inflammatory myopathy** in adults, considered to be due to a disorder of the immune system.

The condition is much less common than **primary idiopathic polymyositis,** which it otherwise resembles, but shows in addition various skin changes, including erythema affecting the butterfly area of the face and extensor limb surfaces and trunk, violet discoloration of the eyelids with periorbital edema, periungual hyperemia, telangiectasia, sclerodactyly, keratosis, and skin edema.

primary idiopathic polymyositis   (isolated polymyositis)   An acute inflammatory myopathy due to a disorder of the immune mechanisms. Clinically, the condition is characterized by acute, subacute, or chronically progressive proximal weakness and Raynaud phenomenon, with maximal incidence in childhood and again in mid-adult life. Arthralgia, bulbar and respiratory muscle involvement, and muscle pain are unusual and the skin is not involved.

Muscle biopsy specimens show little vascular change but there is marked invasion of myofibrils by cytotoxic lymphocytes and macrophages and scattered muscle fiber necrosis is notable.[2936] The presence of skin changes should dictate the diagnosis of **dermatomyositis.**

The following diagnostic criteria have been suggested:[2684] From Hudgson P, Peter JB. Classification (of Polymyositis). *Clin Rheum Dis* 1984;**10:**3–8, by kind permission.

A. Predominantly or exclusively proximal, usually symmetrical muscle weakness, progressive over weeks or months, with or without myalgia and with or without compatible dermatological features

B. Biopsy evidence of muscle fiber necrosis, regeneration, and mononuclear cellular infiltrate (perifascicular and intrafascicular), with or without perifascicular atrophy

C. Elevated serum creatine kinase (MM isoenzyme), aldolase, or myoglobin levels

D. Multifocal EMG changes typical of myopathy (small, short-duration polyphasic motor potentials), with or without increased insertional activity and spontaneous potentials

Definite polymyositis is diagnosed when all four criteria are satisfied; three criteria allow a diagnosis of *probable polymyositis.*

primary intraventricular hemorrhage   The uncommon occurrence of hemorrhage without spread into periventricular regions, usually as a result of bleeding from an arteriovenous malformation in a lateral ventricle, or as a result of **moyamoya disease.**[1282]

primary lateral sclerosis   A syndrome of progressive generalized spasticity, typically asymmetric in onset and progression, starting most commonly in the legs, but sometimes in the arms or with speech as progressive spastic dysarthria, and resulting from circumscribed atrophy of the precentral gyrus with complete loss of Betz cells, decreased numbers of pyramidal neurons, and laminar gliosis in the external and internal pyramidal cell cortical layers. There are no lower motor neuron lesions.

All patients eventually develop a severe spastic dysarthria and may progress to anarthria. Other features include saccadic breakdown of smooth pursuit eye movements (in most) and urinary incontinence (in about half). Patients become wheelchair bound after several years, but the rate of progression is variable. Cognitive impairment is absent but emotional lability is common. MRI scans may show atrophy of the precentral gyrus.

Frontal lobe patterns of dementia, including both **Pick disease** and frontal lobe dementia, have been associated on rare occasion with **amyotrophic lateral sclerosis,** but that condition is not associated with primary lateral sclerosis. In 1875 **Erb** considered this to be a rare variant of amyotrophic lateral sclerosis, characterized by the isolated appearance of slowly progressive upper motor neuron lesion signs affecting all four limbs in the absence of any lower motor neuron signs and of disorder of cognition, but that view is not now held. Excellent reviews are those of Pringle et al. and of Miller Fisher.[1849,4529]

Pathological confirmation of the diagnosis has seldom been achieved in life, and confusion with cervical spondylotic myelopathy, stroke, **multiple sclerosis,** or **hereditary spastic paraparesis** is likely in many of the reported cases.[404] See also **amyotrophic lateral sclerosis.**

primary malignant (cerebral) lymphoma   See **primary CNS lymphoma.**

primary memory   See **short-term memory.**

primary orthostatic tremor   (supermarket tremor, cocktail party tremor, **orthostatic tremor**) A high-frequency, synchronized tremor in the legs and axial muscles occurring within seconds after standing up and increasing in amplitude over time until relieved by walking, sitting, or lying down again. The patients usually complain of unsteadiness or imbalance. The frequency of the tremor runs between 14 and 18 Hz.[2516] It is sometimes possible to see and to hear with a stethoscope (or detect with EMG) a 16-Hz tremor in the quadriceps muscle after the patient has been standing for a few seconds. It may occur in isolation or with cerebellar disease.

primary pallidal atrophy   A basal ganglion syndrome characterized by involvement of the subthalamic nucleus, globus pallidus, and cerebellum.[2703] See **pure pallidal atrophy.**

primary parasomnias   Sleep disorders occurring without associated pathology. Sleep and wakefulness are not mutually exclusive—for example, sleep drunkenness, microsleeps, and automatic behavior. Rapid eye movement sleep has both tonic and phasic components, and these may persist into wakefulness; such disorders are subsumed under this heading.

primary partial epilepsies   Focally originating, age-dependent seizure disorders of congenital or childhood origin without macroscopic pathology. The group includes **benign rolandic epilepsy, benign partial epilepsy with occipital sharp waves, benign sensorimotor epilepsy with parietal spikes,** and **atypical benign parietal epilepsy of childhood.** See also **primary generalized epilepsies.**

primary position   The position of the eyes at rest, looking directly forward in parallel. See also **secondary position.**

primary position upbeat nystagmus   A downward drift of the eyes when the patient attempts to maintain the primary position of gaze, interrupted by saccadic movements that correct the position of the eye back toward the primary position. It is due to intraaxial lesions, usually of the pons or of the superior cerebellar vermis.[1836]

primary progressive aphasia   A focal cerebral cortical degenerative syndrome characterized by a slow but relentless deterioration of language abilities with sparing of cognitive and behavioral functions, due to focal spongiform degeneration in the left perisylvian region, confirmed by imaging techniques.[3849] Although usually sporadic, an autosomal dominant form has been described.[967]

The language deficit most often resembles **Broca aphasia** in its agrammaticism and nonfluency, but other dysphasic types are also described. The difference between this condition and **slowly progressive aphasia,** in which dementia eventually supervenes, appears to be largely a function of time. The relationship with **Alzheimer disease** is unclear, but, on the basis of current neuropathological data, seems unlikely to be close,[3061] and the pathology may resemble that of Pick disease;[3021] thus it is best regarded as an **asymmetric cortical dengeneration syndrome.**

The following diagnostic criteria have been proposed:[3853] (From Mesulam M-M. Primary Progressive Aphasia. *Ann Neurol* 2001;**49:**425–32, by kind permission.)

1. Insidious onset and gradual progression of word-finding, object-naming, or word-comprehension impairments

as manifested during spontaneous conversation or as assessed through formal neuropsychological tests of language

2. All limitation of daily living activities attributable to the language impairment, for at least 2 years after onset

3. Intact premorbid language function (except for developmental dyslexia)

4. Absence of significant apathy, disinhibition, forgetfulness for recent events, visuospatial impairment, visual recognition deficits, or sensory-motor dysfunction within the initial 2 years of the illness (This criterion can be fulfilled by history, survey of daily living activities, or formal neuropsychological testing.)

5. Acalculia and ideomotor apraxia may be present even in the first 2 years. (Mild constructional deficits and perseveration [as assessed in the go–no go task] are also acceptable as long as neither visuospatial deficits nor disinhibition influences daily living activities.)

6. Other domains are possibly affected after the first 2 years, but language remains the most impaired function throughout the course of the illness and deteriorates faster than other affected domains

7. Absence of "specific" causes such as stroke or tumor as ascertained by neuroimaging

See also **Pick disease, corticobasal ganglionic degeneration.**

primary progressive multiple sclerosis   That form of multiple sclerosis in which the disease manifests a progressive course from its onset. It usually presents in later life with paraparesis, although visual distubances, hemiparesis, or brainstem syndromes may also occur in this form. It may manifest a reduced number of MRI lesions and be associated with a specific heterozygous *Taq*-1 HLA-DQ β restriction fragment, unlike **secondary progressive multiple sclerosis.**[5560] The following diagnostic criteria for primary progressive multiple sclerosis have been suggested:[5561] (From Thompson AJ, Montalban X, Barkhof F, et al. Diagnostic Criteria for Primary Progressive Multiple Sclerosis: A Position Paper. *Ann Neurol* 2000;**47**:831–5, by kind permission.)

Definite Primary Progressive Multiple Sclerosis

1. Clinical progression for at least 1 year *and*
2. Positive CSF evidence *and*
3. Positive MRI evidence *or* equivocal MRI evidence *and* a delayed visual evoked potential

Probable Primary Progressive Multiple Sclerosis
Either

1. Clinical progression for at least 1 year *and*
2. Positive CSF evidence *and*
3. Equivocal MRI evidence *or* delayed visual evoked potential

or

1. Clinical progression for at least 1 year *and*
2. Positive MRI evidence *or* equivocal MRI evidence *and* a delayed visual evoked potential (but CSF evidence either unavailable or negative)

Possible Primary Progressive Multiple Sclerosis

1. Clinical progression for at least 1 year *and*
2. Equivocal MRI evidence *or* delayed visual evoked potential

primary reading epilepsy   A dominantly inherited form of **reflex epilepsy** with symptoms beginning in the second decade, in which seizures are triggered by reading or by the eye or jaw movements commonly associated with that activity. An EEG pattern of left frontotemporal wave discharges is a common concomitant. See **reading epilepsy.**

primary rhinencephalic epilepsy   Seizure disorders with initial involvement of the hippocampal and amygdaloid structures. Their clinical features include olfactory hallucinations, visceral motor symptoms, elementary automatisms, apnea, cardiovascular changes, tonic somatomotor manifestations, and disturbances of memory.[56]

primary sensory area   The principal somatosensory area of the cerebral cortex comprising Brodmann's areas 3, 2, and 1.

primary sensory neuropathy   See **subacute sensory neuronopathy.**

primary systemic amyloidosis   See **amyloidosis.**

primary subcortical gliosis   A dementing syndrome of adult life with progressive and insidious course, differing from **Pick disease** only in the general atrophy of the cortex and in the absence of Pick cells. The usual histological features of **Alzheimer disease** are also absent, but there is widespread gliosis of the brainstem, basal ganglia, and subcortical white matter.[4104] See also **frontal lobe dementias.**

primary suppurative myositis   See **pyomyositis.**

primary thrombocythemia   See **thrombocythemia.**

primary writing tremor   A task-specific tremor; a variant of essential tremor in which the unwanted movement appears only with attempts to write or assumes the writing position.[2898,4187,4819] Dystonia may be associated.

prime movers   (agonists, protagonists) Those muscles whose action is to perform precisely a movement in question. See also **antagonists, synergists, muscles of fixation.**

primitive neuroectodermal tumors   (PNETs) Rare, highly malignant embryonal neuroectodermal tumors found in children and young adults and characterized histologically by small cells with a high nuclear/cytoplasmic ratio; fine fibrillary processes; small, oval hyperchromatic nuclei; frequent mitotic figures; and evidence of glial, neuronal, or ependymal differentiation. They usually occur above the tentorium and seed widely through the neuraxis.[2465] **Medulloblastoma, medulloepithelioma, cerebral** and **abdominal neuroblastoma, esthioneuroblastoma, retinoblastoma, medulloblastoma, pinealoblastoma, ependymoblastoma,** and **polar spongioblastoma** have been regarded as examples of PNETs.[6]

primitive reflexes (frontal release signs, release symptoms) "A mechanism by which a particular type of response is brought about by either the activity of a single nervous arc or several nervous arcs, such reflexes as have been observed in embryonic and later life in lower forms of animals and in human beings. . . . The reflexes appearing earliest in the order of functional development are apt to be the last to disappear in the process of functional disintegration. In a similar manner, the last to be acquired are likely to disappear early in the course of the dementia" (Buckley, 1927, quoted by Landau[3246]).

Swallowing, sucking, grasp, palmomental, corneomandibular, glabellar, nuchocephalic, and flexor reflexes are considered to be examples,[2783] but these are not usually present in patients who had frontal lobotomies, and to attribute such reflexes to lack of inhibition resulting from a single lesion is inappropriate. See also **developmental reflexes.**

primrose syndrome A congenital dysmorphic syndrome manifesting also calcification of the ear cartilages, cataract, joint contractures, hydrocephalus, proximal and distal myopathy with atrophy, and mental and developmental delay.[337]

principle of compensation A theory of Hughlings-Jackson: when any loss of function ensues from a lesion of the nervous system, recovery takes place, not because other units have taken on functions they never had before but because those units, having functions closely similar to those of the units destroyed, can perform nearly as well for the functions of both. On this basis, compensation can never be absolute, as is clinically obvious.

Pringle, J.J. (1855–1932) English dermatologist on the staff of the Middlesex Hospital, London.

Pringle-Bourneville disease See **tuberous sclerosis.**

prion diseases (transmissible spongiform encephalopathies, slow virus diseases) Dementing illnesses involving the transmission of an aberrant isoform of prion protein, which also makes up the content of amyloid plaques.

Such human transmissible, noninflammatory, neurodegenerative conditions include **kuru; iatrogenic, familial,** and **sporadic Creutzfeldt-Jakob disease; Gerstmann-Straussler-Scheinker syndrome; fatal familial insomnia;** and some other atypical dementing diseases (*prion dementia without characteristic pathology; dementia with spastic paraparesis*), while in animals, **scrapie,** chronic wasting disease of elk, transmissible mink encephalopathy, and **bovine spongiform encephalopathy** are typical conditions. Two recent major review were those of Prusiner.[4533,4534]

prions Small, proteinaceous, infectious particles that contain little or no nucleic acid and in which a host protein is a major and necessary component. The molecular properties of these unconventional agents distinguish them from viruses.

pro- (Gr, and Lat, before, for, or on behalf of) Prefix denoting before or for.

probable multiple sclerosis That form of multiple sclerosis characterized by relapsing-remitting symptoms with only neurological signs commonly associated with multiple sclerosis, or a documented single episode with signs of multifocal white matter disease and with signs of partial recovery; with no better explanation.[5011]

This diagnostic category is now largely replaced by the **Poser or McDonald criteria.**

Probst bundle An anomalous bundle of fibers that would normally have crossed in the corpus callosum but that pass rostrocaudally, parallel to the cingulate bundle, in cases of agenesis of the corpus callosum.

procedural learning The learning of manual skills rather than of words and facts. These skills are lost early in patients with lesions of the caudate nuclei. The differentiation is made because patients with dementing conditions such as **Alzheimer disease** and those given scopolamine may retain these abilities even though **declarative learning** is severely limited.

Procerus sign An astonished, reptile-like, or worried facial expression shown by subjects with progressive supranuclear palsy, likely resulting from focal dystonia of the procerus muscle, reduced blinking, spasticity, lid retraction, and gaze palsy.

The muscle originates on the nasal bone and inserts into the skin of the central forehead.

Prochaska, Georg (1749–1820) Professor of anatomy and of ophthalmology variously at Prague and Vienna Universities. He was the first to ascribe different (motor and sensory) functions to the anterior and posterior nerve roots, in 1812. He also made one of the earliest suggestions that reflexes occur in considering that the cerebrum acts as the *sensorium commune* in receiving afferent impulses, which it reflects into the periphery again to the motor nerves (1780–1784).

proctalgia fugax (Gr, anus + pain and Lat, fleeting) Severe pain arising as a result of cramp of the levator ani, often during sleep, and lasting 5–30 minutes with spontaneous resolution. The condition was described by MacLennon in 1917.

prodrome Clinical events that herald worse clinical events, with which they share a common cause.

Profichet syndrome (calcinosis universalis, pierres de la peau) The slow development of widespread subcutaneous calcifications in adults. Muscle atrophy and sensory changes are the usual neurological features.[1563]

Profile of Mood States A self-report questionnaire evaluating mood states in psychiatric patients and assessing changes in affective status.[3785]

Profile of Nonverbal Sensitivity Test   A test of the ability to comprehend nonverbal, emotional aspects of human communication, in which the subject describes the message portrayed in a set of standard videotapes.[4798]

Patients with right hemisphere lesions are likely to do poorly on this test.

profile perimetry   See **static perimetry.**

progeria   (Lat, before + Gr, old age) (Hutchinson-Gilford syndrome, Variot-Pironneau senile dwarfism; in adults, **Werner syndrome**) Recessively inherited dwarfism with accelerated aging supervening after a normal early childhood. Apart from the changes in physical appearance which suggest advanced age (such as gray hair, baldness, thinness, arthritis, loss of eyebrows and teeth, cataract, a seemingly small face, atrophic skin, loss of subcutaneous fat, and narrow chest), premature atherosclerotic changes lead to angina and strokes.[2717] Myopathy,[1685] spastic paraparesis, and polyneuropathy are yet other complications.

A *neonatal* form exists as a congenital dysmorphic syndrome, manifesting also low birth weight, muscular build, sparse hair, premature aging, delayed closure of fontanelles, and deficient/absent adipose tissue.[337] **Cockayne syndrome** (trisomy 10, Neil-Dingwall syndrome) is similar.[1064]

progressive adult-onset bulbar paresis   See **Fazio-Londe syndrome.**

progressive alcoholic dementia   See **Marchiafava-Bignami disease.**

progressive amusia and aprosody   A focal cortical degeneration syndrome.[1116]

progressive anarthria   A focal cortical degeneration syndrome.[787]

progressive aphasia without dementia   See **primary progressive aphasia.**

progressive apraxia   A focal cortical syndrome characterized by isolated apraxia or visual agnosia, which may progress to dementia but which has been distinguished from **Alzheimer disease.**[277,1408]

progressive ascending spinal paralysis   (Mills disease) See **amyotrophic lateral sclerosis.**

progressive ataxia, retinal degeneration, peripheral neuropathy, myopathy, and mental subnormality   See **cerebellar ataxias** (5. of unknown etiology).

progressive autonomic failure   (idiopathic orthostatic hypotension, primary or pure autonomic failure) A part of the syndrome of **multiple system atrophy,** characterized by idiopathic degeneration of the central, peripheral, and autonomic nervous systems in elderly people. However, a more distal site of pathology has also been suggested in some cases.

Clinically, orthostatic hypotension with drop attacks, dizziness, weakness, anhidrosis, sphincter disturbances, and impotence are most obvious, but forms with associated parkinsonism (PAF-P) or multiple system atrophy (PAF-MSA, Shy-Drager syndrome[5148]) also occur. There is evidence that this represents a postganglionic failure, both of sudomotor and of other adrenergic fibers.[3776,5540,5541]

A *variant* is *familial orthostatic hypotension,* characterized by autonomic failure, upper and lower motor neuron signs, ataxia, and parkinsonism.[3387,5541]

progressive axial muscle rigidity of infancy   A syndrome characterized by rigidity of the axial and proximal limb muscles, occurring in infancy and leading to ventilatory failure. EMG studies reveal continuous muscle firing in apparently normal motor units, unaffected by neuromuscular blockade and without evidence of CNS abnormality.[3600]

progressive biparietal atrophy   A focal cortical dementing syndrome considered to precede the more typical manifestations of **Alzheimer disease** and likely to represent the dorsal form of **posterior cortical atrophy.** Clinical manifestations are early visuospatial problems, peripheral or apraxic agraphia, and difficulties with bimanual tasks, but with only minor impairments of memory or language in the early stages, although these do supervene later and a full Alzheimer-type dementia picture may develop eventually. MRI and SPECT studies reveal local biparietal involvement.

progressive bulbar palsy   (Duchenne paralysis) A form of **amyotrophic lateral sclerosis** described by **Duchenne** in 1858 as "labioglossolaryngeal paralysis," of which the earliest features are lower motor lesions of the bulbar muscles and in which the prognosis tends to be worse than that in the forms with predominant upper motor neuron lesions.[1536] In rare instances, ophthalmoplegia or deafness has been associated. See also **motor neuronal diseases.**

Variants include the following:
Fazio-Londe disease (progressive bulbar palsy of children)
Vialetto–van Laere syndrome (progressive bulbar paralysis and nerve deafness) A recessively inherited syndrome characterized by the onset of progressive deafness in childhood followed by visual loss and amyotrophy of cranial and upper limb muscles; signs of corticospinal tract involvement appear later.[74]
Progressive pure bulbar paralysis A dominantly inherited syndrome characterized by the occurrence of progressive bulbar paralysis in advanced adult life without other evidence of neurological dysfunction.[3483]

progressive bulbar paralysis of childhood   See **Fazio-Londe syndrome.**

progressive cerebral poliodystrophy   See **Alpers disease.**

progressive CNS deterioration   A slowly progressive deterioration of CNS function seen in some premature infants treated with ventilatory assistance and continuous positive airway pressure for over 28 days, and characterized by loss of developmental milestones, increasing hypotonia, EEG changes, and death; or by progressive apnea, bradycardia, and sudden death.[1643]

Pulmonary hypertension, hypoxemia, hypercapnia, and acidosis are considered to be the relevant etiological factors.

progressive cramp Increasing difficulty in performing new tasks because of the presence of hand cramps.[1082]

progressive dementia with photosensitivity See **neuronal ceroid lipofuscinosis.**

progressive diaphyseal dysplasia (Engelmann disease) A recessively inherited syndrome characterized by increased density of the bones of the skull and thickening of the diaphyseal cortex of the limb bones, the former leading to optic atrophy and deafness in youth or young adult life.[3769] Proximal myopathy with a waddling gait is another common feature. See **Camurati-Engelmann syndrome.**

progressive diffuse encephalopathy A neurological complication of **HIV** infection, characterized pathologically by diffuse demyelination, astrocytic proliferation, and multinucleated giant cells.

progressive dystonia with diurnal fluctuation A dystonic syndrome of childhood or early adult life, characterized by emotional lability, pyramidal signs, rigidity, dystonias, chorea, and resting tremor, all of which are worse during the daytime.[5052] See **Segawa dystonia.**

progressive encephalomyelitis with rigidity (PEWR, subacute myoclonic spinal neuronitis) A rare progressive, incapacitating, and ultimately fatal syndrome of tonic muscular rigidity producing abnormal postures, accompanied by myoclonus and painful stimulus-sensitive muscle spasms (thus resembling the **stiff-man syndrome**), but associated also with changes in the brainstem and cervical cord, suggesting encephalomyelitis with destruction of spinal internuncial neurons.[5947]

progressive external ophthalmoplegia (chronic progressive external ophthalmoplegia, von Graefe syndrome, PEO) A heterogeneous syndrome appearing in adult life, comprising progressive symmetrical ptosis and limitation of ocular motility, as shown by a reduction in the velocity of the saccadic movements (if any are possible at all).

The syndrome may occur in isolation or in association with other neurodegenerative disorders, including ataxia, pigmentary retinopathy, mitochondrial myopathy, optic atrophy, cardiac conduction defects, spasticity, deafness, organic mental changes, small stature, and elevated CSF protein levels.[5785] Ragged red fibers are found in muscle biopsy specimens. See also **Kearns-Sayre syndrome, oculopharyngeal muscular dystro-phy, centronuclear myopathy, myotonic dystrophy, mitochondrial diseases.**

Variants include the following:

Progressive external ophthalmoplegia with immunological abnormality A syndrome of adult life comprising ophthalmoplegias and myopathic muscle atrophy, with ragged red fibers present in muscle biopsy specimens.

Autosomal dominant progressive external ophthalmoplegia with multiple deletions of mtDNA This form has been mapped variously to 10q23.3–24.3 and to 3p14.1–21.2. Clinically, muscle weakness, depression, and personality disorders accompany the usual features of the condition.[5420]

Autosomal recessive progressive external ophthalmoplegia.

Progressive external ophthalmoplegia with floppy mitral valve A progressive cardioneurological syndrome characterized by the concurrence of mitral valve prolapse and ophthalmoplegia.[1292]

progressive facial hemiatrophy See **Parry-Romberg syndrome.**

progressive familial encephalopathy A syndrome with congenital or infantile onset, comprising bilateral spasticity and dystonia, microcephaly, a rapid course to death, basal ganglion calcification, and persistent CSF lymphocytosis.[61]

progressive familial myoclonic epilepsy See **Unverricht-Lundborg-Lafora syndrome.**

progressive hemifacial atrophy See **Parry-Romberg syndrome.**

progressive hereditary diaphyseal dysplasia See **Camurati-Engelman syndrome.**

progressive hypertrophic interstitial neuropathy (Déjèrine-Sottas syndrome) See **hereditary motor and sensory neuropathy, type 3.**

progressive infantile poliodystrophy See **Alpers disease.**

progressive juvenile bulbar palsy A rare syndrome manifesting ocular, facial, and bulbar weakness in childhood, leading to weakness and atrophy of the trunk and limb muscles with selective degeneration of the bulbar and spinal motor nuclei.[2180] See **Fazio-Londe disease.**

progressive lenticular degeneration See **Wilson disease.**

progressive multifocal leukoencephalopathy An acquired, fatal demyelinating disease of adult life, caused by a papovavirus and characterized by widely disseminated small perivascular foci of myelin sheath destruction, these foci becoming confluent. Astrocytic hypertrophy and basophilic staining of the nuclei of oligodendrocytes are other pathological features. The condition appears to be a complication of disturbed cellular immune systems.

Clinically, the presentations include progressive cognitive and personality changes and focal neurological signs such as hemiparesis, facial paresis, incoordination, language, visual deficits, and occasionally seizures. The condition has been reported as a **paraneoplastic syndrome** in association with systemic Hodgkin disease and leukemia, and as a complication of sarcoidosis, tuberculosis,[250] and now HIV,[5662] in which case progression to death is usually rapid.

In those patients with HIV infection, diagnostic criteria include rapid onset (<2 weeks) of multifocal neurological signs and symptoms, advanced immunosuppression and asymmetric uni- or multifocal white matter lesions without mass effect, contrast enhancement, or cortical atrophy on MRI. Mean survival is a few months. Human polyoma virus JC (JCV) polymerase chain reaction (PCR) in the CSF demonstrates a considerable rate of possible cerebral co-infection with HIV-1 and JCV as well as subclinical infection with JCV. Routine stereotactic brain biopsy is not necessary to confirm the diagnosis.[5782]

progressive muscle spasms, alopecia, and diarrhea
See **Satoyoshi syndrome.**

progressive muscular atrophy See **amyotrophic lateral sclerosis.**

progressive muscular rigidity See **stiff-man syndrome.**[3930]

progressive myelopathy See **chronic myelopathy, progressive necrotic myelopathy.**

progressive myoclonic ataxia A mitochondrial encephalopathy syndrome presenting with myoclonus and progressive "cerebellar" ataxia. Epileptic seizures are infrequent and cognitive decline is not notable.[3647] The condition overlaps **progressive myoclonic epilepsy.**

progressive myoclonic ataxic syndrome with celiac disease. A progressive neurological syndrome dominated by action and stimulus-sensitive myoclonus of cortical origin with mild ataxia and infrequent seizures, following the gastrointestinal and other manifestations of celiac disease while on a gluten-free diet, in the absence of overt features of malabsorption or nutritional deficiency.

progressive myoclonic epilepsy (OMIM 254800) A rare group of recessively inherited neurodegenerative conditions presenting with myoclonus and generalized seizures, in which there is progressive neurological decline that usually takes the form of ataxia, visual loss, and dementia.[3647,4740] Abnormalities of somatosensory evoked potentials are commonly demonstrable.[5130] The responsible gene maps to chromosome 21q22.3. The most common form is EPM1, a recessively inherited disorder

Such stimulus-sensitive cortical reflex myoclonic diseases include some that are recessively inherited and some that are acquired, and are either degenerative or

metabolic in pathogenesis. **Unverricht-Lundborg disease** (Baltic myoclonus), **Lafora body disease, sialidosis,** dominant **cerebellar ataxia** (SCA 2), **neuronal ceroid lipofuscinosis,** the **encephalomyelopathies** (Fukuhara syndrome), **dentatorubro-pallidoluysian atrophy,** and **May-White syndrome** are examples.

A *variant* is *progressive myoclonic epilepsy, seizures, scoliosis, pes cavus, retinopathy, cardiac involvement, ophthalmoplegia, and dementia,*[3458] which in almost every way resembles **mitochondrial cytopathy** except for the absence of ragged red fibers.

progressive myoclonic epilepsy, degenerative type
See **Baltic myoclonus.**

progressive myoclonic epilepsy, with Lafora bodies
See **Lafora body disease.**

progressive necrotic myelopathy A disease of unknown cause affecting adults who present with paresthesias and burning in the limbs or ill-defined pains in the trunk, worsening subacutely over months and culminating in para- or tetraplegia. The CSF protein levels are increased, with or without pleocytosis, but oligoclonal bands are not detected. The condition does not respond to immulomodulation.

The following clinical diagnostic criteria have been suggested:[2952]

Regional loss of reflexes, flaccidity, and muscle atrophy
Shrunken or cavitated cord shown on MRI scan, without evidence of arteriovenous malformation
Denervation over several cord segments shown by EMG, while sensory nerve action potentials may be retained
Absence of evidence of systemic disease, including malignancy

See also **Devic disease.**

progressive neuronal degeneration of childhood
See **Alpers disease.**

progressive neuronal degeneration of childhood with liver disease See **Alpers disease.**

progressive, nonfamilial hypertrophic neuritis See **Roussy-Cornil syndrome.**

progressive nuclear ophthalmoplegia syndrome (Levic syndrome, nigrospinodentatal degeneration with nuclear ophthalmoplegia) A genetically determined, extensive degenerative process, characterized by bilateral facial weakness, congenital external near-complete ophthalmoplegia with ptosis (but sparing the pupil), scrotal tongue, progressive chorioretinal sclerosis, and intellectual deficit.[3367,6033]

Motor neuron involvement, ataxia, spastic paraplegia, dystonia, retinitis pigmentosa, and peripheral neuropathy have also been described in a few cases; the condition is unlikely to consist of a single entity.

progressive ophthalmoplegia, glycogen storage, and abnormal mitochondria A mitochondrial disease presenting with facial and proximal limb weakness in childhood and with progressive ophthalmoplegia. See also **glycogen storage diseases.**

progressive ophthalmoplegia in Kugelberg-Welander disease See **hereditary motor neuropathy** (*variants*).

progressive pallidal atrophy A basal ganglion syndrome presenting with Parkinsonian features, of which at least four variants are recorded: **pure pallidal atrophy;** *pallidal atrophy with atrophy of the subthalamic nucleus,* consisting of extended pallidal atrophy with striatal and nigral involvement; *pallidal atrophy in association with degeneration of other neuronal systems;*[2829] and *progressive pallidal degeneration with pigmentary retinopathy.*[6005]

See also **hereditary dentatorubropallidoluysian atrophy.**

progressive pallidal degeneration See **Hallervorden-Spatz disease.**

progressive pontobulbar palsy with deafness See **Vialetto-van Laere syndrome, progressive bulbar palsy.**

progressive possible multiple sclerosis See **McDonald-Halliday Criteria.**[3744]

progressive probable multiple sclerosis See **McDonald-Halliday Criteria.**[3744]

progressive proximal spinal and bulbar muscular atrophy See **bulbospinal neuronopathy.**

progressive proximal spinal and bulbar muscular atrophy of late onset (Kennedy-Alter-Sung syndrome) An X-linked recessive anterior horn cell disease manifesting after the age of 30 years and characterized by cramps, low backache, proximal muscle weakness and wasting, fasciculations, and bulbar muscle weakness, with hyporeflexia but without pyramidal tract or sensory involvement. The course is only slowly progressive, and life span is not diminished.[3006]

progressive pseudorheumatoid arthropathy of childhood A syndrome of childhood manifesting irregular end-plates to vertebrae, platyspondyly, arthropathy, proximal and distal myopathic weakness, and stippled or fragmented epiphyses.[337]

progressive pure anomia A form of progressive fluent aphasia in the presence of selective atrophy of the left temporal cortex, presenting as a profound progressive anomia while semantic knowledge is unaffected.[2254]

progressive pyramidopallidal degeneration A slowly progressive degenerative condition manifesting a pseudobulbar palsy, mild pyramidal signs in the limbs, and postural rigidity with akinesia and chorea, and with cell loss and gliosis in the putamen, globus pallidus, and pyramidal tracts.[3400]

The condition appears to resemble **Hallervorden-Spatz disease.** See also **Lhermitte-Cornil-Quesnel syndrome.**

progressive rigidity with apraxia See **corticobasal degeneration with neuronal achromasia.**

progressive rubella panencephalitis A severe progressive encephalitis, clinically resembling **subacute sclerosing panencephalitis,** apart from the presence of clinical cerebellar involvement, histological evidence of vasculitis, and an absence of detectable viral antigen.[1153]

progressive senile scoliosis Increasing scoliosis documented in elderly women in the absence of osteoporotic vertebral body crush fractures. The common underlying mechanism appears to be asymmetric loading of the spine which can be caused by a previously established scoliosis, spondylolysis/ spondylolisthesis, lumbosacral anomalies, or leg length discrepancy. Subsequent factors causing increasing curvature include degenerative disc disease with lateral disc space narrowing, soft tissue failure, and osteoporosis.[2116]

progressive sensory neuropathy See **subacute sensory neuropathy.**

progressive sensory radiculopathy A benign and reversible syndrome due primarily to lesions of the preganglionic sensory roots, characterized by slowly progressive pansensory loss spreading proximally to involve the whole body, with mild weakness, incoordination, and areflexia. The CSF protein levels are raised, electrodiagnostic studies suggest the presence of an axonal motor neuropathy, and sural nerve biopsy findings are normal.[1040]

The condition appears to be responsive to steroid therapy and may be presumed to have a similar etiology to that of **chronic inflammatory demyelinating polyneuropathy** and **chronic idiopathic ataxic neuropathy.**

progressive spatial disorientation A focal cortical syndrome resulting from right hemisphere degeneration and leading to loss of memory for people.[4592]

progressive (spinal) muscular atrophy 1. (Aran-Duchenne disease) A form of **amyotrophic lateral sclerosis** in which the earliest features are lower motor neuron lesions of the spinal musculature.[204]

Variants are *progressive muscular atrophy with malignant course,* a form that is fatal within 1 year, but that is not clearly different from autosomal dominant **amyotrophic lateral sclerosis;** and *progressive muscular atrophy with amyotrophic lateral sclerosis;* this entity is not clearly different from peroneal muscular atrophy with pyramidal features. See **amyotrophic lateral sclerosis.**

2. See **hereditary motor neuropathy, type 1**

progressive spinal muscular atrophy with chorea and deafness See **hereditary motor neuropathy** (*variants*).

progressive subcortical arteriosclerotic encephalopathy See **Binswanger disease.**

progressive subcortical glial dystrophy (progressive subcortical gliosis) A rare sporadic or dominantly inherited dementing illness with onset between 35 and 50 years, mapped to chromosome 17.[4423] Personality change and impaired social abilities with disinhibition and depression delusions appear first, with disturbances of visual perception, reduced speech output, echolalia, auditory hallucinations, and features of the **Kluver-Bucy syndrome** following.[3272,4104] The pathological hallmark is astrogliosis at the junction of cortex and white matter. The condition may be indistinguishable in life from **progressive supranuclear palsy** and may represent a variety of **frontotemporal dementia.**

progressive subcortical gliosis See **progressive subcortical glial dystrophy, frontotemporal dementia.**

progressive supranuclear palsy (PSP; Steele-Richardson-Olszewski syndrome) A slowly progressive dementing syndrome of later adult life exhibiting ocular and neurological signs, the cause of which is unknown. The cardinal clinical features include those of **subcortical dementia,**[82] with early postural instability and falls, supranuclear vertical gaze palsy, akinetic-rigid parkinsonism, axial dystonia in extension, pseudobulbar palsy, vertical (later horizontal) gaze pareses, and a poor response to L-dopa therapy. Moderate to severe postural instability and falls during the first year after onset of symptoms are typical features. Defects in fixation, saccades, pursuit, convergence, and vestibulo-ocular reflexes are also notable.[1565,5328] Apathy is a common manifestation but irritability, agitation, and anxiety are not. Segmental dystonia and myoclonus, but not aphasia nor alien limb syndrome, are described. The eponymous title recalls the syndrome's more recent descriptors, although a similar condition was described by W.C. Posey in 1904.

The unstable gait, absence of tremor-dominant disease, and absence of a response to levodopa differentiate PSP from **Parkinson disease;** however there is notable pathological evidence to differentiate the two conditions. Clinically, the supranuclear vertical gaze palsy, gait instability, and the absence of delusions distinguish it from **diffuse Lewy body disease;** the supranuclear vertical gaze palsy and increased age at symptom onset distinguish it from **multiple system atrophy;** the gait abnormality, severe upward gaze palsy, bilateral bradykinesia, and absence of **alien limb** syndrome separate it from **corticobasal degeneration;** and the postural instability separates it from **Pick disease.**[3439]

A valuable website is at www.psp.org/.

Criteria for the neuropathologic[2480] and clinical diagnosis of PSP have been defined (see Chart P–24).

Chart P–24. NINDS-SPSP Suggested Criteria for the Diagnosis of Progressive Supranuclear Palsy (PSP)

Definite Progressive Supranuclear Palsy

Clinically probable or possible PSP and histologically typical PSP

Probable Progressive Supranuclear Palsy

Mandatory inclusion criteria:
Gradually progressive disorder
Onset at age 40 or later
Vertical supranuclear (either upward or downward gaze abnormalities) ophthalmoparesis and prominent postural instability with tendency to falls in the first year of symptom onset

Possible Progressive Supranuclear Palsy

Mandatory inclusion criteria:
Gradually progressive disorder
Onset at age 40 or later and either
  a. Vertical supranuclear (either upward or downward gaze abnormalities) ophthalmoparesis *or*
  b. Slowing of vertical saccades and prominent postural instability with falls within 1 year of symptom onset

Mandatory Exclusion Criteria (for Both Probable and Possible Progressive Supranuclear Palsy)

History compatible with **encephalitis lethargica**
Alien hand syndrome, cortical sensory deficits, focal frontal or temporoparietal atrophy
Hallucinations or delusions unrelated to dopammergic therapy
Cortical dementia of Alzheimer's type (severe amnesia and aphasia or agnosia, NINCDS-ADRDA criteria)
Prominent cerebellar symptomatology or unexplained **dysautonomia** (early, prominent incontinence, impotence, or symptomatic postural hypotension)
Severe asymmetry of **parkinsonian** signs (bradykinesia)
Neuroradiologic evidence of relevant structural abnormality (basal ganglia or brainstem infarcts, lobar atrophy)
Whipple disease, confirmed by polymerase chain reaction, if indicated

Supportive Features (Not Required for Diagnosis)

Symmetric akinesia or rigidity, proximal more than distal
Retrocollis
Poor, absent, or transient response of parkinsonism to levodopa therapy
Early dysarthria and dysphagia
Early cognitive impairment, including at least two of the following: apathy, impaired abstract thought, decreased verbal fluency, "imitation" behavior, or frontal release signs.

From Litvan I, Agid Y, Calne DB, et al. Clinical research criteria for the diagnosis of progressive supranuclear palsy (Steele-Richardson-Olszewski syndrome). Neurology 1996;47:1–9, by kind permission.

A diagnostic algorithm has been suggested[1108] in which prerequisites for the diagnosis are onset age over 40 years; no family history; insidious onset and progressive course; no relevant structural lesions on neuroimaging, the presence of supranuclear downgaze paralysis and three of the following signs; prominent early postural instability with frequent falls and five of the following signs; or both of these and two of the following signs, all in the absence of exclusionary criteria (below).

The added required signs are the following:
Bradykinesia
Staring, non-blinking facies
Retrocollis or dystonic arm
Babiński signs
Pseudobulbar signs (two of dysarthria, dysphagia, pathological emotionality)

Rigidity in the neck more than arms
Wide-based, shuffling gait
Sitting en bloc
Dementia or personality change
   Verification is obtained with a history of 2 years of minimal or unsustained response to levadopa.
   Exclusionary criteria are the following:
Prominent and early dysautonomia, especially orthostatic hypotension
Prominent polyneuropathy
Pronounced rest tremor
Cortical sensory loss
Alien limb sign
Unilateral presentation or pronounced asymmetry.

From Collins SJ, Ahlskog JE, Parisi J, et al. Progressive supranuclear palsy: neuropathologically based diagnostic clinical criteria. J. Neurol. Neurosurg. Psychiatry 1995;58:167–73, by kind permission.

Variants of the syndrome are listed in Chart P–25.

Chart P–25. Variants of Progressive Supranuclear Palsy

Progressive supranuclear palsy with action myoclonus and seizures A progressive neurological disease characterized by dysarthria, facial action myoclonus with correlated EEG spikes, generalized convulsions, pseudobulbar signs, and late eye movement disorder. The condition differs from progressive supranuclear palsy in the conspicuous presence of action myoclonus and seizures, the late appearance of the eye movement disorder, and the absence of rigidity and conspicuous dementia. The pathological characteristics include neuronal loss, gliosis, loss of neurofibrils, and secondary demyelination with occasional perivascular cuffing with lymphocytes mainly affecting the cerebral cortex but not the globus pallidus, subthalamic nuclei, substantia nigra, or red nuclei.[3193]

Recessive progressive supranuclear palsy-like syndrome A condition resembling the classic disease, except for the presence of neurofibrillary tangles, predominantly in the limbic system.[4220]

Autosomal dominant progressive supranuclear palsy-like syndrome A form in which the clinical and pathological lesions are those of the sporadic variety, but in which dominant inheritance is postulated.[792]

Progressive Supranuclear Palsy Association A charitable organization in this field. Address: The Old Rectory, Wappenham, Nr. Towcester, Northamptonshire, UK. NN12 85Q. Tel: + 44 1327 861007. E-mail: psp.eur@virgin.net. Web site: http://www.pspeur.org/. See also **Society for Progressive Supranuclear Palsy.**

progressive systemic sclerosis See **scleroderma.**

progressive unilateral hypertrophic myopathy A condition characterized by the occurrence of complex repetitive discharges within a group of muscles, the histological appearances of which suggest the presence of myopathy.
   Clinically, stiffness and cramps occur within the hypertrophied muscles.[4444]

progressive vascular myelopathy A syndrome of progressive amyotrophy due to ischemia of the anterior horns of the spinal cord.[2830]

projected patterns Abnormal EEG activities believed to result from a disturbance at a site remote from the recording electrodes. (From Chatrian GE, Bergamini L, Dondey M, et al. A glossary of terms most commonly used by clinical electroencephalographers. *EEG Clin Neurophysiol* 1974;37:538–48, with permission from Elsevier Science.)[989]

projected rhythms An EEG pattern showing intermittent bursts of bilaterally synchronous rhythmic slow waves, seen in the frontal or occipital regions in patients with metabolic disease, diffuse cerebral diseases or deep midline cerebral lesions.[3075] See **frontal intermittent rhythmic delta activity, occipital intermittent rhythmic delta activity.**

projection (tactile projection) The sensation of a touch in a place distant from that place which was actually touched by the examiner. See also **alloesthesia.**

prolactinoma (Lat, before + milk + tumor) A prolactin-secreting benign pituitary basophil adenoma.

proliferating systematized angioendotheliomatosis See **malignant angioendotheliosis.**

proliferative myositis A syndrome with a benign course characterized by the appearance of a rapidly growing, localized, painless muscle swelling at any site, lasting up to 2 months without ossification. Histologically, bundles of degenerating muscle fibers with an excessive fibrous reaction are found. The cause is unknown.[3009]
   The myositis seldom recurs after excision.[1683] See also **focal nodular myositis, pseudomalignant myositis ossificans.**

prolonged exercise test 1. A standardized exercise test involving 2 hours of exercise on a bicycle ergometer set at half the subject's maximal tolerated work load. Measurements of serum lactate, creatine kinase, and fatty acid levels allow the differentiation of metabolic and mitochondrial myopathies from psychogenic states.[774] 2. A mode of demonstrating paresis in **paramyotonia congenita** or familial hyperkalemic periodic paralysis. The patient spreads his or her fingers maximally for 20 seconds at a time, then relaxing them for 2–3 seconds after each contraction repetitively over about 4 minutes. In normal control subjects there may be a small decline or a small increase (pseudofacilitation) in the compound muscle action potential following the exercise, but the potentials return to their normal shape within several minutes. In those with periodic paralysis, a progressive decline of the compound muscle action potential occurs for 20 to 40 minutes after the exercise.[3780]

prolonged Q-T syndrome A cardiac condition associated with ventricular tachyarrhythmias and sudden death. It may also present as epilepsy.[4289] See **syncope.**

pronation sign See **Neri signs.**

pronation–supination test   The patient is asked to make rapid repetitive rotatory movements of the forearm; such movements cannot be performed fluently in a subject with a cerebellar lesion affecting the arm because of slowness of movement, lack of rhythm, irregularity of range, loss of postural tone, and imperfect timing of the arrest of movement.

pronator   (from Lat, turned or inclined forward) Each of the two forearm muscles (pronator teres and quadratus) that function to rotate the arm internally on the elbow.

pronator catch   A temporary resistance to passive pronation, evidencing hypertonia of the muscles in an arm affected by a pyramidal lesion.

pronator drift   Slow movement of the outstretched arm downward and laterally with pronation of the forearm and slight flexion of the elbow, wrist, and fingers; a sign of mild pyramidal weakness of the arm, but also recorded in the setting of chorea and with cerebellar lesions.[1349a]

pronator reflex   Pronation of the forearm in response to a tap on the volar aspect of the radius, the arm lying in the neutral position. The contraction is enhanced in the presence of pyramidal lesions and states of increased emotional tension, and is reduced by lesions at C6.

pronator sign   The tendency of the arms to rotate into a pronated position when extended above the head or while in recumbency. In the former case, this is a nonspecific sign of basal ganglion disease; in the latter, it suggests pyramidal disease. See also **pronator drift.**

pronator teres syndrome   (high median neuropathy) Compression of the median nerve at the level of the pronator teres muscle at the elbow (between the two heads of which it passes), leading to weakness of the forearm muscles supplied by the anterior interosseous nerve and of the median-supplied hand muscles, and to paresthesias in the hand.

The clinical diagnosis is confirmed by EMG studies and decompression may relieve the symptoms.[3994]

See also **anterior interosseous nerve syndrome.**

propagation velocity of a muscle fiber   The speed of transmission of a muscle fiber action potential.

propaxic postural tremor   See **cerebellar tremors.**

propositional language   Aspects of verbal communication, including lexicon, grammar, and articulation; a left hemisphere function.

propositional speech   Speech containing a judgement; a term and concept important within Aristotelian logic. Though a sentence is a significant portion of speech, not every sentence is a proposition; propositions are those which have in them either truth or falsity. Such speech may be internal and unenunciated or external and enunciated, but the two forms are different only in degree.

Propositions and thought have been considered identical, leading to the classification of aphasia as a thought disorder by Hughlings-**Jackson.**[4691]

propping reaction   Extension of the arm toward the side to which the sitting normal infant of 5–6 months is pushed.

proprioception   (from Lat, one's own + to receive) The term of **Sherrington** (1900) for the ability to recognize the position of joints in space. It depends on a reduplicated system (one pathway reaching consciousness, the other not) informing the brain as to the angulation of joints and therefore the position of body parts in space, and contributing to the individuals' image of their own body—the body schema. Alternative terms are *enteroception* and *eomesthesis*, the latter especially pointing out the subjects' awareness of their own body. Both static and kinetic types of proprioception exist—the former giving information on the momentary position of limbs, the latter informing about the movement at joints.

proprioceptive ataxia   See **sensory ataxia.**

proprioceptive, exteroceptive   (Lat, self + receive: Lat, outside + receive) The terms of **Sherrington** denoting the sense organs whose adequate stimuli come from inside and outside the body, respectively. See also **proprioception.** *Interoceptive* sensations are those mediated by sense organs, in this case within the alimentary canal with relationships to local musculature. *Exteroceptive* sensations are subdivided between those stimulated by objects in contact with the body and those stimulated by distance receptors such as the eyes and ears.

proprioceptive tricks   Maneuvers which, as patients suffering from dystonia have learned, may inhibit the abnormal posture. Thus, a touch on the face or head may restore the cranial posture to normal in a patient with spasmodic torticollis. See also **geste antagonistique.**

proprionic acidemia   A lethal, recessively inherited syndrome characterized by episodic vomiting, lethargy, coma, seizures, chorea, hypertonia, and respiratory insufficiency with ketotic hyperglycinemia, occurring in neonates and infants as a result of deficiency of proprionyl coenzyme A carboxylase. The responsible gene for the B form maps to chromosome 3q13J.3q22, that for the A form to chromosome 13. Hypoglycemia, platelet abnormalities, hyperammonemia, organic aciduria, and low densities in the white matter on CT scans are also found.[719] See **ketotic hyperglycinemia.**

propriospinal myoclonus   That form of focal and segmental spinal myoclonus in which the abnormal movements in axial muscles originate from discharges in slowly conducting spinal tracts, such as the long propriospinal pathways.

Clinically, the movements are limited to the thoracoabdominal muscles, predominantly on one side and especially at times transitional between wakefulness and sleep. See also **segmental myoclonus** (that form of spinal myoclonus in which the discharges originate in a few adjacent spinal segments).[1019]

proptosis   (Lat, forward + Gr, falling) Protrusion of the eye, most commonly due to dysthyroid ophthalmopathy in adults.

propulsion   Forward inclination of the body in **Parkinson disease,** leading to a tottering, almost running gait, as though the patient were trying to chase his or her own center of gravity.

propulsive petit mal   See **myoclonic astatic seizures.**

proscencephalon   Those parts of the brain formed from the foreparts of the anterior cerebral vesicle, thus including the cerebral hemispheres, corpora striata, and olfactory lobes.

prosody   (Gr, modulation) 1. (chanson de parler) The timing, stress, intonation, accent, and overall individual melodic quality of spoken speech, conveying both linguistic and affective information. Impairment of this function is known as *dysprosodia*, while absence of such melody in speech (as in parkinsonism) is *aprosodia*. Excessive use of speech inflections, etc., is *hyperprosody*; it is heard in some patients with Broca aphasia and in most Shakespearean actors.

The right hemisphere plays a dominant role in the modulation of the affective components of language. Affective language is tested by examining spontaneous speech and the patient's enunciation of speech in different affective styles, and by his or her comprehension and identification of affectively charged speech and pantomime.

2. The fluctuations in rhythm and timbre of articulated speech.

prosopagnosia   An unusual impairment of perception, characterized by the inability to recognize known faces or individual members of a group, always in association with some visual field deficit. Thus, a farmer may lose the ability to identify his cows, or any person her own belongings or even her own face. Lord Salisbury, an English prime minister, is reported once to have failed to recognize the face of his own son. The cause is the presence of bilateral lesions of the central visual system, often in mesial occipitotemporal regions and more marked on the right side, but right or left hemisphere lesions have also been held responsible. Dressing apraxia, topographic agnosia, unilateral spatial agnosia, achromatopsia, **Balint syndrome,** visual neglect, and impairment of nonverbal learning are often present as well.[1262,1263]

The word was coined by Bodamer in 1947, although the phenomenon had been recognized by **Jackson** and **Charcot** at the end of the nineteenth century.[1094]

Prosopagnosia is not specific for faces, relating to all visual items and to topography; but the patient may be able to read unless there is a lesion of the deep left occipitotemporal and occipital white matter. The most common cause is a vascular (embolic) lesion; tumors and **herpes simplex encephalitis** are others. See also **agnosia.**

prosopalgia   (Gr, the face + pain) (prosopodynia) Facial pain.

prosopodiplegia   (Gr, face + double + blow) Bilateral facial paralysis.

prosopodynia   See **prosopalgia.**

prosopoplegia   Unilateral facial paralysis.

protagonists   See **prime movers.**

protective reactions   Automatic limb responses brought into play to prevent injury when falling is occurring as a result of the failure of other mechanisms to maintain equilibrium.[4180]

protein C deficiency   A dominantly inherited anomaly mapped to 2q13–q14 and associated with an increased tendency to stroke.

protein S deficiency   A dominantly inherited anomaly mapped to 3p11.1–q11.2 and associated with an increased tendency to stroke.

protein-calorie malnutrition   Marked growth retardation as a result of prolonged starvation. See **kwashiorkor.**

proteus syndrome   (hemihypertrophy-nevi-hamartoma) A dominantly inherited combination of plantar hyperplasia ("moccasin feet"), macrocephaly, exostoses, asymmetrical limbs and lipomas, hemangiomas, epidermal nevi, and varicosities, leading in some cases to a fearful appearance. Tall stature, thick calvarium, macrocephaly, strabismus, ptosis, asymmetrical hypertrophy of arms and legs, hypocalcemia, osteoporosis, seizures, and muscle atrophy are other features described.

Tibbles and Cohen[5580] have suggested that this was the condition from which Joseph Merrick (the "Elephant Man," befriended by Sir Frederick Treves) suffered. The syndrome is named for the Greek god who appeared in polymorphous guises.

proto-   (Gr, the first) Prefix denoting first.

proton magnetic resonance spectroscopy   An MRS technique providing signals for phospholipids, creatine, n-acetyl aspartate, etc. and allowing estimation of the relative amounts of demyelination and axonal injury in brain regions.

protopathic pain   More vivid but less acute sensation of superficial skin pain coupled with more extreme heat and cold sensation, as may be experienced after incomplete nerve injury.[2500]

protopathic sensory loss   A disorder of superficial sensation in the area between that in which there is total thermoanesthesia and the surrounding area in which sensation is normal, following peripheral nerve injury. In this area, cotton wool touch is not perceived, discrimination of small changes in temperature and in two-point sensation is diminished, and pinprick leads to a most unpleasant ill-localized and persistent sensation.

Henry **Head** originally proposed that this group of sensory modalities was subserved by a distinct system of sensory nerve fibers, but in fact the problem is a qualitative reduction in sensitivity, not a separate system.

protopathic system   The sensory system envisaged by Henry **Head** as being capable of responding to painful cutaneous stimuli and to extremes of heat and cold; it is characterized by high threshold, long latencies, poor localization, an inability to adapt, and an intense response to stimulation.

protoplasmic astrocytoma   See **astrocytoma.**

Proust-Lichtheim maneuver   A method whereby the patient, who is unable to evoke an appropriate word, can nevertheless indicate how many syllables are entailed—for example, by squeezing the examiner's hand or by tapping the table the appropriate number of times.

proved multiple sclerosis   That form of the disease in which the diagnosis is established at autopsy.

provoked nystagmus   See **induced nystagmus.**

provoked seizures   (acute symptomatic seizures) Seizures occurring in close temporal association with an acute systemic, metabolic, or toxic insult or in association with an acute CNS insult (infection, stroke, cranial trauma, intracerebral haemorrhage, or acute alcohol intoxication or withdrawal). They are often isolated epileptic events associated with acute conditions, but may also be recurrent seizures or even status epilepticus when the acute conditions recur—for example, in alcohol withdrawal seizures. See also **situation-related seizures.**

proximal chronic inflammatory polyneuropathy with multifocal conduction block   See **multifocal inflammatory demyelinating neuropathy.**

proximal intentional neglect   A failure to move toward or in proximal space, associated with a right parietal lesion.[2159]

proximal lower motor neuron syndrome   An acquired proximal motor axonal neuropathy with adult onset, initially affecting the arms, and frequently associated with the presence of antibodies to asialo-GM$_1$ and to galactose β-1-3Ga1NAc-disaccharide.

proximal myotonic myopathy   (PROMM; OMIM 600109) A dominantly inherited multisystem disorder resulting from an abnormality on chromosome 3q.21 at a locus similar to that of **myotonic dystrophy** (DM2) but without the CTG repeat found in that condition.

Clinically, the onset is in adult life with asymmetric muscle enlargement and weakness (facial and distal strength are normal), which can vary over hours and is worse with warming; stiffness (myotonia); and pain. Muscle atrophy and cognitive failure are not features. Cataracts and cardiac arrhythmias have been described. MRI may show white matter hyperintensities on T2-weighted images. Serum CK levels are modestly raised and muscle biopsy findings are nonspecific.

Electrically, the myotonia shows no decrement. Repetitive stimulation may provoke "myopathic" motor unit potentials.[4679] The exercise test reveals that there is no decrement in compound motor action potential amplitude or area immediately following exercise, unlike the situation in classical myotonic dystrophy.[4896]

Further *variants* are *proximal myotonic myopathy,* with both myotonic and myopathic features;[3840] *proximal myotonic dystrophy,* characterized by the same and added dystrophic features;[5680] and *myotonic dystrophy type 2* (OMIM 602688), another multisystem myotonic disorder clinically closely resembling classic myotonic dystrophy, but again without the CAG repeat.

proximal symmetrical motor neuropathy   See **diabetic neuropathies.**

prune belly syndrome   (triad syndrome) A rare condition characterized by the absence of normal abdominal musculature, megaureter, and undescended testicles. Associated anomalies include polydactyly and syndactyly; malformations of the jaw, intestines, heart, eyes, ears, and nose; spina bifida or meningomyelocele; congenital dislocation of the hip; and congenital myopathy.[51]

pruritis   See **itch.**

psammoma bodies   (Gr, sand + tumor) (corpora arenacea, acervuli) Small spheres composed of concentric layers of calcification within collagen, seen within some **meningiomas** and in the normal pineal gland. The resemblance of these calcific deposits to sand was noted by **Virchow.**

Pseudopsammoma bodies are intra- or extracellular periodic acid-Schiff–positive protein droplets secreted by meningothelial cells.

psammomatous meningioma   See **meningioma.**

pseudo-   (Gr, false)

pseudoabducens palsy   1. Impairment of lateral deviation of a sound eye in the presence of a lesion of the third cranial nerve nucleus.[3667] 2. Impairment of lateral deviation of the eye due to **convergence spasm,** in which case the accompanying miosis suggests the diagnosis.[5643] 3. Paresis of voluntary ocular abduction while abduction is possible with, e.g., ice-water caloric stimulation and thus not due to a lesion of the sixth cranial nerve. A rostral mesencephalic lesion is the usual cause.

pseudoaneurysm   (fibrous globes, fibrin globes) Arteriolar outpouchings in the deep white matter and basal ganglia, consisting of a platelet plug at the end of an occluded arteriole and limited by a condensation of fibrin and white cells.

pseudo-anterior interosseous syndrome The production of the usual features of compression of the anterior interosseous nerve by a partial lesion of the main trunk of the median nerve at a point above its branching.[5928]

pseudo–Argyll Robertson pupil see **Holmes-Adie syndrome.**

pseudoathetosis Random involuntary movements of a limb deficient in proprioceptive sensory function, but without any primary involvement of motor control systems. The afferent lesion may be at any site in the sensory pathway from peripheral nerve to cortex.[5097]

pseudo–Babiński sign Permanent dorsiflexion of the hallux, seen in some basal ganglion disorders such as the later stages of parkinsonism and of pallidal degenerations. See also **dystonic foot response.**

pseudoblastoma See **orbital pseudotumor syndrome.**

pseudobobbing See **pretectal pseudobobbing.**

pseudobulbar affect See **emotionalism.**

pseudobulbar palsy 1. Bilateral upper motor neuron lesions affecting the bulbar musculature, and thus located at or above the level of the pons. 2. A form of **amyotrophic lateral sclerosis** in which the earliest features are those of upper motor neuron lesions affecting the bulbar musculature.[980]

The term is regrettable, for, as **Wartenberg** pointed out, there is nothing "pseudo" about the paralysis. *Spastic bulbar palsy* would be a far better term.

pseudobulbar palsy and mental retardation See **bilateral central macrogyria.**

pseudocaloric nystagmus Horizontal jerk nystagmus of mild intensity, beating in the appropriate direction (away from the irrigated ear) in response to caloric irrigation of an ear in which vestibular function has, however, been lost. The fast phase beats away from the diseased ear, regardless of whether warm or cold stimuli are used. The cause is unknown, but it may represent unmasking of **latent nystagmus** by the alerting effect of the stimulation.[416]

pseudo–carpal tunnel syndrome (sublimis syndrome) A neuropathy of the median nerve proximal to the carpal tunnel, caused by compression of the nerve by the lateral border of the belly of the sublimis muscle, clinically mimicking the true syndrome.[2021]

pseudocataplexy Transient loss of muscle tone immediately following laughter, but not other emotional perturbations, occurring as a seizure manifestation (*gelastic-atonic seizures*) in subjects without any other features of the **narcolepsy** tetrad.[2792]

pseudocele See **cava septi pellucidi et vergae.**

pseudocerebellar ataxia See **parietal ataxia.**

pseudocervical cord syndrome A central cord pattern of weakness resembling paraparesis, reported in the context of **hepatic encephalopathy.**[3742]

pseudocholinesterase deficiency See **myasthenia gravis.**

pseudoclaudication syndrome See **lumbar spinal stenosis.**

pseudocoma See **locked-in syndrome.**

pseudocyst (nerve sheath myxoma) A benign intracranial tumor characterized by its mucinous content. It usually occurs on the common peroneal or ulnar nerves, suggesting a traumatic etiology. See also **ganglion.**

pseudodecrement An artifact produced by movement of the stimulating or recording electrodes during repetitive nerve stimulation. The amplitude and area of the M wave can vary in a way that resembles a decrementing response, however, the responses are generally irregular and not reproducible. (From the 2001 Report of the Nomenclature Committee of the American Association of Electromyography and Electrodiagnosis.[10] Used by permission, copyright © 2001, AAEM.)

pseudodeficiency rickets See **Prader syndrome.**

pseudodementia Cognitive disorders resulting from functional disorders; a group of conditions in which features suggesting dementia are not associated with any organic illness.[4866] The following characteristics are usually described:

1. The impairment of memory, learning, and related cognitive functions is caused by a psychiatric illness.
2. The impairment is nonprogressive and is likely to be reversible if the primary illness is treated.
3. Any neuropathological process present is considered to be minor and insufficient to explain the severity of the cognitive defects.

Depression, mania, and malingering are the usual antecedents. See also **Ganser syndrome.**

pseudodrusen Multiple refractile bodies, representing degenerated axons, situated close to the optic nerve head and sometimes seen in patients with chronic papilledema.[2590] See also **drusen.**

pseudoepileptic seizures See **pseudoseizures.**

pseudoepileptiform patterns EEG patterns containing spikes which occur in bursts or trains, and which are not associated with clinical seizures. Such abnormalities are more likely to occur in non–rapid eye movement sleep stages 1 or 2.

pseudofacilitation See **incrementing response.**

pseudo–Foster Kennedy syndrome Unilateral optic atrophy with contralateral optic nerve swelling as a result of conditions other than tumors compressing that eye with the atrophic optic nerve.[2069] See also **pseudo-pseudo–Foster Kennedy syndrome.**

pseudoglaucoma   A dominantly inherited syndrome with onset in young adult life, characterized by a deep optic cup and slowly progressive visual loss with constriction of the visual fields in a pattern resembling that seen in glaucoma, but with normal intraocular pressure.[4909]

pseudo–Graefe phenomenon   (Fuchs sign) Elevation of the upper eyelid on downward movement of the eyes; a synkinesis in which the action of the levator palpebrae is linked with that of the inferior rectus as a result of aberrant regeneration of the third cranial nerve after injury. Miosis on down-gaze may be associated.[5789,5825]

See also **Gowers signs.**

pseudohallucinations   Vivid, usually visual, hallucinations, which the patient realizes are unreal. Those hallucinations resulting from organic brain disease and without any alteration in consciousness are commonly of this type.

pseudo–Horner syndrome   Unilateral miosis with lid drooping, not due to sympathetic damage, as pharmacological testing yields normal results. The condition may have no underlying pathology or may be due to any of numerous causes of miosis and ptosis, as reviewed by Thompson et al.[5562]

pseudo–Huntington disease   A rare variant of **dentatorubropallidoluysian atrophy** characterized by dementia and chorea.[335]

pseudo–Hurler disease   See **GM$_1$ gangliosidosis.**

pseudo–Hurler polydystrophy   See **sialidosis.**

pseudohydrophobia   An infectious bulbar paralysis described in Hungary and in Brazil, where it is known as the "scratching pest."[262]

pseudohypertrophic muscular dystrophy   See **Duchenne muscular dystrophy.**

pseudohypertrophy   Increase in the size of an organ despite a loss in the size or number of its constituent cells, which is usually due to the replacement of normal components by exogenous infiltrates, fat, or other connective tissue.

pseudohypoparathyroidism   (Martin-Albright syndrome) A rare metabolic disorder due to end-organ unresponsiveness to parathyroid hormone. Neurological features include seizures, headache, photophobia, blurred vision, weakness, lethargy, muscle cramps, paresthesias, and numbness; the **Trousseau** and **Chvostek** signs are positive. Classically, the patients have round faces and short, wide digits with an absence of knuckles.[87]

A normocalcemic form (pseudo-pseudohypoparathyroidism) was also described by Albright, but the two conditions are now considered to be but *variants* of each other.

pseudohypoparathyroidism with parkinsonism   A rare autosomal or X-linked dominant syndrome resulting from end-organ resistance to parathyroid hormone and characterized by the above features, without calcifications of the basal ganglia.[1713]

pseudoinsomnia   See **subjective DIMS complaint without objective findings.**

pseudoisochromatic plates   (Isihara plates) Colored surfaces printed with dots reflecting a mixture of wavelengths that appear different in color to a normal ("trichromatic") observer, who can thus read numbers, etc., on the surfaces, but which appear identical to a dichromatic person suffering a defect in the retinal cones' pigment, so that no numbers, etc., can be discerned. This is the standard portable test for **color blindness.**[4381]

pseudokyphosis   Trunkal flexion resulting from severe weakness of the thoracic musculature.

pseudolarval electrographic seizure of the elderly   See **subclinical rhythmic discharges of adults.**

pseudolymphoma   Generalized lymphadenopathy, joint swelling, hepatosplenomegaly, and skin rash due to an idiosyncratic reaction to long-term treatment with diphenylhydantoin. Lymph node biopsy specimens show replacement of the normal architecture by large reticuloendothelial cells and the presence of germinal centers. The condition usually abates when the offending drug is withdrawn.[5001]

pseudomalignant myositis ossificans   Rapidly growing, localized painless swelling in a muscle, due to inflammation and thus resembling **proliferative myositis,** except that in this condition the process leads to ossification.[4588] See **proliferative myositis.**

pseudo–Marfan syndrome   See **Dinno syndrome.**

pseudomeningitis   See **idiopathic intracranial hypertension.**

pseudomigraine with temporary neurological symptoms and lymphocytic pleocytosis   A migraine variant most commonly seen in young males, some with a history of migraine and some after a viral-like illness up to 3 weeks prior to the onset of the syndrome. The clinical picture consists of episodes of changing variable neurological deficits accompanied by moderate-to-severe headache and sometimes fever. The headaches are typically throbbing and bilateral, lasting less than a day, while the transient neurological deficits last a mean of 5 hours. Sensory symptoms are most common, followed by aphasia and motor symptoms. Visual symptoms appear rarely. Patients are asymptomatic between episodes. Lymphocytic pleocytosis has ranged from 10 to 760 lymphocytic cells/mm^3 CSF (mean, 199), and protein is increased in almost all cases, brain CT and MRI are normal, but EEG frequently shows focal slowing.[2183]

pseudomyasthenic syndrome See **Lambert-Eaton myasthenic syndrome.**

pseudomyelia paresthetica Sensations perceived as though coming from phantom extremities.[5897]

pseudomyoclonic seizures Tonic or atonic seizures in which the patient suddenly falls to the ground as a result of lack of tone or generalized abnormal contraction of those muscles normally responsible for the maintenance of posture.

pseudomyopathic spinal muscular atrophy See **hereditary motor neuropathy, type 3.**

pseudomyotonia (myotonia acquisita, Hoffman syndrome) 1. The association of muscle hypertrophy with painful stiffness, worse in the cold; electrically silent **myoedema;** presence of the Woltman sign (hung-up reflexes); and affection of speech and gait more than of the face.

The slow, weak, painful sustained contractions and slow relaxation of muscles reflect a reduction in myosin ATPase activity and impaired calcium uptake by the sarcoplasmic reticulum. On muscle biopsy specimens, type 1 fiber atrophy, decreased oxidative enzyme activity, and increased glycogen content are the usual findings. The condition is not the same as **paramyotonia.** The complex rhythmic discharges are pseudomyotonic and thus are not worse with rest nor better with exercise, and there is no percussion myotonia but rather silent myoedema. Hyperparathyroidism may also contribute to the proximal weakness and fatigability, which abate with restoration of normal parathyroid hormone levels and vitamin D replacement. See also **acid maltase deficiency, neuromyotonia.** 2. See **pseudomyotonic discharge.**

pseudomyotonia and pseudotetany See **idiopathic neuromyotonia.**

pseudomyotonic discharge See **complex repetitive discharge.**

pseudoneurogenic thoracic outlet syndrome The occurrence of the typical clinical features of the **thoracic outlet syndrome** including focal atrophy and weakness, resulting, however, from disease of the contralateral cerebral hemisphere.[5176]

pseudonystagmus 1. A rare form of psychogenic eye movement disorder characterized by rapid, fine, pendular horizontal movements, accompanied by blepharospasm, convergence spasm, and miosis in almost all cases. 2. Abnormal pendular eye movements described in patients with vestibular failure and head tremor.[633]

pseudo-ophthalmoplegia See **Roth-Bielschowsky syndrome.**

pseudopalisading The radial arrangement of the adjacent nuclei of tumor cells around areas of necrosis; a characteristic appearance in **glioblastoma multiforme.**[6]

pseudopapilledema (pseudoswelling of the disk) A benign congenital anomaly characterized by elevation and enlargement of the optic nerve head on each side, not due to increased intracranial pressure but rather to excessive myelination at the margins of the optic disk, so that the nerve fibers appear to be elevated and the disk edge blurred. The finding may be dominantly inherited and may occur without accompanying features or in the presence of hyperopia or skull deformities. Clinical manifestations (if they occur at all) may include transient visual obscurations, retinal hemorrhages, or arcuate field defects. The blind spot is commonly increased in area. Venous pulsations are present. Hyaline bodies in the disk are a common cause. See **drusen.**

Criteria for differentiating true and pseudopapilledema have been defined by Glaser,[5] and are presented in Chart P–26 in adapted form.

Chart P–26. Diagnostic Features of Pseudopapilledema

In pseudopapilledema

A. The central cup is absent and the disk diameter tends to be small;
B. Hyperemia is not present;
C. Vessels arise from the central apex of the disk;
D. Anomalous branching of vessels, an increased number of major disk vessels, and venous pulsations are present;
E. The disk may be transilluminated, with a glow appearing from hyaline bodies (if they are present);
F. The disk margins are irregular, with derangement of the peripapillary retinal epithelium;
G. The nerve fiber layer is not opaque;
H. Superficial capillary telangiectasias, hemorrhages, exudates, and **cotton-wool spots** are absent; and
I. Retinal folds are uncommon and choroidal folds absent.

Adapted from Glaser JS. Neuro-ophthalmology, 2nd ed. Philadelphia, J.B. Lippincott, 1990.

pseudoparalysis Apparent weakness of ocular muscles, the appearance being produced not by nerve lesions but by mechanical problems with certain muscles, such as fibrosis of the inferior rectus in **dysthyroid orbitopathy,** of the lateral rectus in **Duane syndrome,** and of any of the ocular muscles after years of strabismus. Convergence spasm is another possible cause.

pseudoparalytic syndrome See **myasthenia gravis.**

pseudophakia The presence within the eye of an artificial lens in place of the natural one.

pseudoplegia A term denoting dissociation of voluntary and emotional movements, such as those of the face, jaws, throat, and larynx in the **anterior operculum syndrome.**[3601] See **diplegia with dissociation, oral-buccal apraxia.**

pseudopolymyelia The delusion of reduplication of parts of the body, usually occurring in those with left hemiparesis. The condition is regarded as a syndrome of parietal lobe origin involving disruption of the body schema.[5897]

pseudopolyneuropathy   Sensory disturbances in a pattern resembling that of peripheral neuropathy but found in patients with cervical spondylotic myelopathy at C5–C7, and in **multiple sclerosis.** Nerve conduction studies and F-wave latencies are normal. The anatomical substrates for this type of sensory impairment could be caused by combination of the dorsal horn/anterior commissure lesions for the upper limbs, and the anterolateral funiculi lesions for the lower limbs.[6083]

pseudopolyphasic action potential   See **serrated action potential.**

pseudoprogeria   A congenital dysmorphic syndrome manifesting also short stature, atrophy of the skin, glaucoma, ptosis, skeletal anomalies, osteoporosis, seizures, microcephaly, pyramidal signs, and mental and developmental delay.[337]

pseudopsammoma bodies   See **psammoma bodies.**

pseudo-pseudo–Foster Kennedy syndrome   The clinical picture of progressive visual loss suggesting pseudo–Foster Kennedy syndrome due to nonarteritic anterior ischemic optic neuropathy, but here due to a compressive lesion situated posteriorly.[2069]

pseudo-pseudohypoparathyroidism   See **Albright syndrome.**

pseudo-pseudoulnar claw hand   The appearance of **pseudoulnar claw hand** but in this case due to cervical radiculopathy at C8 or other proximal lesions.[884]

pseudoptosis   1. The appearance of unilateral ptosis in an eye that is in fact healthy, because of the presence of proptosis (with consequential eyelid retraction) of the other. 2. See **apraxia of eyelid opening.**

pseudoradicular syndrome   Numbness and paresthesias felt in an apparent radicular distribution such as C8, in association with a lesion of the contralateral sensory cortex or thalamus.

pseudorelapse   A temporary deterioration in the clinical status of a patient with **multiple sclerosis** as the consequence of a concurrent (usually febrile) illness.

pseudorosettes   Clear rings around blood vessels due to the centripetal extension of fine fibrillary processes from the ependymal tumor cells surrounding them.

pseudo-Schnabel cavernous degeneration of the optic nerve   Degeneration of the optic nerve occurring in glaucoma; the "pseudo" form is that in which a similar appearance is found in association with local silicone injections.[5132]

pseudosclerosis   The term of **Westphal** for a disease (actually **Wilson disease**) in which the signs resemble those of **multiple sclerosis** but the pathology does not.

pseudoseizures   See **nonepileptic seizures, factitious epilepsy.**

pseudosixth   Failure of ocular abduction not due to a lesion of the sixth cranial nerve but rather to a mesencephalic lesion. The sign is frequently bilateral and is accompanied by **hyperconvergence.** See **pseudoabducens palsy, Duane syndrome, ocular myasthenia. Graves orbitopathy,** old squint, medial rectus entrapment, and convergence spasm also enter the differential diagnosis.

pseudospasticity   An increase in muscular resistance to passive stretch and in muscle activity, leading to the adoption of abnormal postures, as a consequence of peripherally generated continuous motor unit discharges. The pathogenesis may involve a reduction of ionized calcium levels in the presence of an axonal motor neuropathy.[4520]

pseudo–status epilepticus   Simulated status epilepticus, differentiated from the true condition by the frequent occurrence of retained consciousness; pelvic thrusting; flailing, asynchronous or rolling limb movements; gaze aversion; resistance to passive movements; frequency of induction by suggestion; gradual onset; and avoidance of a hand falling onto the face. Cyanosis, tongue and other injuries, and abnormal ictal or postictal EEG records are uncommon.[2671]

pseudoswelling of the disk   See **pseudopapilledema.**

pseudotabes   (peripherica) A syndrome in which the clinical features (sensory ataxia, pupillary changes, **Charcot joints,** etc.) resemble those of tabes dorsalis, but their cause is not syphilis. Diabetes mellitus is the classic example, but alcoholic and diphtheritic neuropathies may do the same. See **Oppenheim disease.**

pseudotabetic pupillotonia   The preferred term of **Wartenberg** for **Adie syndrome,** which did not find favor, perhaps in part because of the decline in the incidence of **tabes dorsalis.**

pseudotabetic syndrome   The occurrence of **Argyll Robertson pupils** with areflexia and proprioceptive disturbance, occurring either as a complication of diabetes or in the **Holmes-Adie syndrome.**

pseudo–tetanus of d'Espine   Tonic spasm of all limbs or opisthotonos in children with markedly increased intracranial pressure, who cry or are stimulated externally, and perhaps due to spasmodic decorticate posturing.

pseudothalamic syndrome   Unpleasant radiating sensations resembling thalamic pain, but in this case due to lesions of the opercular part of the postcentral gyrus.[1400]

Touch, pain, temperature, and vibration sensations in the contralateral face, arm, and leg are lost when the lesion (which is usually a stroke) involves the anterior-inferior part of the parietal lobe. See also **parietal stroke.**

pseudothalidomide syndrome   A recessively inherited syndrome of symmetrical reductive limb defects, flexion contractures, scanty blond hair, hypoplastic ears and nose, and sometimes seizures and mental retardation.[2552] See **Roberts syndrome.**

pseudotonic pupillotonia   See **Adie pupil.**

pseudotumor cerebri   See **idiopathic intracranial hypertension.**

Pseudotumor Cerebri Society   A charitable organization in this field. Address: 750 East Adams St., c/o Dr. D. Friedman, Syracuse, NY 13210. Tel: 315-464-3937.

Pseudotumor Cerebri Support Network   A charitable organization in this field. Address: 8247 Riverside Dr., Powell, OH 43065. Tel: 614-794-0442. E-mail: sondra@sprynet.com. Web site: http://www.pseudotumorcerebri.com/.

pseudotumor orbiti   An autoimmune disorder in which inflammation of the orbital contents with striking edema and round cell infiltration is associated with proptosis, painful ocular palsies, and visual deterioration. See **orbital pseudotumor syndrome.**

pseudoulnar claw hand   Hyperextension at the fourth and fifth metacarpophalyngeal joints with distal flexion, due to a partial lesion of the radial or posterior interosseous nerves.[3618]

pseudoxanthoma elasticum   (Gr, false + yellow + tumor + driven) A rare, recessively inherited disorder characterized by loosening of the skin, abnormalities of blood vessels such as early calcification, and the formation of aneurysms and **angioid streaks** of the retina with hemorrhages. Neurologically, intracranial hemorrhages, infarcts, dementia, calcification of the falx, and seizures have all been reported.[2749]

pseudo-Zellweger syndrome   A **peroxisomal disorder** that clinically and biochemically is identical to **Zellweger syndrome** but in which there are abundant liver peroxisomes and the β-ketothiolase is defective. Clinically, it is characterized by dysmorphisms, expressionless face, facial weakness, a cat-like cry, ventricular septal defect, large liver and kidneys, multiple renal cysts, adrenal hypoplasia, recurrent infections, and seizures.[2167]

psittacosis   (Gr, parrot) (ornithosis) Infection with *Chlamydia psittaci*, a unique form of intracellular parasite, following the inhalation of dust from dried bird excreta. The disease mainly affects the lungs, but in some cases, fever, chills, diffuse headaches, myalgia, and eventually encephalomyelitis with coma are described.[920]

psoas insufficiency syndrome   A syndrome of tightness and weakness of the psoas muscles, found almost exclusively in gymnasts and dancers, and resulting from the use of the muscles mainly to pull the lumbar spine into a position of flexion and lordosis.[4860]

psoriatic myopathy   A chronic proximal myopathy; an unusual complication of the skin disease.[3946]

psychiatric dizziness   (space and motion discomfort) Both the occurrence of anxiety symptoms as a result of imperfect processing of environmental clues and the precipitation of the sensation of imbalance as a result of anxiety, each witnessing the close functional association of the vestibular and limbic systems. Furman and Jacob[1995] have reviewed the subject.

psychic paralysis of visual fixation   See **Balint syndrome.**

psychic pillow   The appearance of some patients with schizophrenia or Parkinson disease who lie supine in bed with the neck flexed off the mattress, as though there were a pillow supporting the head.

psychic variant   See **affective-psychic seizures.**

psychical hallucinations   Those formed hallucinations produced by stimulation of the temporal or parietal cortex anterior to area 19, and considered by Penfield and Jasper to be re-evocations of prior perceptions elicited from the experiential cortex.

psychogalvanic reflex   (electrodermal response, sympathetic skin response, Tarchanov phenomenon) A test of sudomotor function, measuring the change in skin resistance to the passage of a constant current with psychic (or with sensory) stimuli and which can normally be evoked by electrical stimulation of a peripheral nerve in subjects less than 60 years old. The presence of the reflex indicates that pre- and postganglionic sympathetic functional innervation of sweat glands is intact.[3223] See **galvanic skin response.** Charles Féré[1785] noted in 1888 that the electrical resistance in the body, measured with a galvanometer, was variable with emotional fluctuations, as did Ivan Romanovich Tarchanov (1848–1909), a Russian physiologist, in 1890, but the first mention was by **Waller,** who thought that it was an artefact.

psychogenic disease   See **hysteria.**

psychogenic dystonia   Atypical dystonia without response to the usual medications and with a protracted course. Differences between this entity and structurally based torsion dystonia have been summarized and are presented in the table below[3262] listing the features that help to distinguish psychogenic dystonia from idiopathic torsion dystonia.

Pyschogenic Dystonia	Idiopathic Torsion Dystonia
Onset with resting dystonia	Onset with action dystonia
Adult-onset leg involvement common	Leg involvement rare with adult onset
Often fixed spasm	Mobile spasms
Rapid progression and spread to maximum disability early in the course of disease	Slow progression
Dystonic movements inconsistent over time	Consistent over time (*caution: in rare cases patients with cervical dystonia may change the direction of dystonia after a remission*)

No geste antagoniste	Geste frequent
Selective disabilities or abilities inconsistent with fixed spasms	Surprising abilities despite severe movements and postures (*caution: action dystonia may result in selective disabilities; some patients with "paradoxical dystonia" improve with action*)
Painful (often with pronounced tenderness to touch and exaggeration with passive movement)	Usually painless (*caution: patients with cervical dystonia do have pain*)
No improvement after sleep	Symptoms often improve briefly after sleep
Attempted voluntary movement to command in the opposite direction of the dystonic posturing may activate antagonists with little apparent action in agonist muscles (limb or digit may do the opposite of what is requested by the examiner)	Voluntary movement and attempts to overcome the dystonia often result in further cocontraction of agonists and antagonists with variable changes in the dystonic posturing
Paroxysmal dystonia (isolated or mixed with persistent dystonia) and/or other paroxysmal movements	Paroxysms not a feature (*caution: exclude other causes of paroxysmal dystonia/ dyskinesias*)
Other psychogenic movement disorders Other nonorganic neurological features	Other movements possible (e.g., tremor, myoclonus) (*caution: important to consider a psychogenic movement disorder or other psychogenic features superimposed on an organic movement disorder*)
Precipitant common	Precipitant uncommon
Remissions: spontaneous or with nonphysiological treatments	(*caution: spontaneous remissions occasionally occur, especially in cervical dystonia*)
No family history	Family history not uncommon.

From Lang AE. Psychogenic Dystonia: a review of 18 Cases. Can J Neurol Sci 1995;22:136–43, by kind permission.

psychogenic flutter (psychological nystagmus, hysterical flutter, hysterical nystagmus, voluntary flutter, ocular fibrillation, ocular shudderings) A form of saccadic intrusion or oscillation characterized by back-to-back saccades occurring at high frequency, usually induced voluntarily during attempted convergence.[3830] See also **voluntary nystagmus.**

poychogenic headache See **episodic tension-type headache.**

psychogenic myoclonus Segmental, generalized, or focal myoclonus for which no structural or biochemical cause can be elucidated.

Clinically, incongruous clinical presentations of the myoclonus or of associated motor or sensory features, evidence of underlying psychopathology, and improvement with distraction or placebo have been suggested as useful points in diagnosis.[3950]

psychogenic pseudoneuropathy A syndrome comprising positive and negative motor and sensory complaints and vascular symptoms and considered to result from psychological dysfunction. The incorrect diagnosis of **reflex sympathetic dystrophy** is commonly made.[4193]

psychogenic seizures Attacks in which geotropic (earthward) eye and head movements occur even when the body is turned 180°. Other features suggesting the presence of this entity include asynchronous movements of the legs and arms, pelvic thrusting or rocking, holding on to a bed-rail, puffed-out cheeks with breath-holding, and the preferred occurrence in hospital at times of nursing shift change.

psychogenic tremor Tremors starting abruptly with maximal deficit at onset, present at rest, maintaining a posture and with action, with a static or fluctuating course and unassociated with demonstrable CNS lesions. One limb is initially affected in most cases but diffusion occurs. Spontaneous resolution and recurrence, distractibility, response to suggestion, and lack of response to conventional therapies are other common features.[3042]

psychogenic unresponsiveness A nonorganic coma-like state. Physical signs helpful in making the diagnosis include the following: opposition to eye opening; the presence of Bell's phenomenon; retention of corneal reflexes; inhibition of eye movement with oculocephalic maneuvers as a result of visual fixation (in true coma, the eyes "roll" with oculocephalic maneuvers, unless there is a brainstem lesion); when the subject's hand is dropped so as to hit the face, it is steered away; the patient placed in uncomfortable postures spontaneously assumes a more natural and comfortable resting posture; breath-holding when spirits of ammonia are kept under the nostril; nystagmus, not just tonic deviation of the eyes, in the cold caloric test; retention of optokinetic nystagmus; an avoidance reaction when a vibrating tuning fork is touched to the nostrils or air is blown up the nostril with a syringe; and a normal alpha pattern with the eyes closed that attenuates when the eyelids are elevated.

psychogenic vertigo A common diagnosis but an uncommon syndrome, most patients with a psychogenic basis to their symptoms having basic organic (structural) lesions as well, either demonstrable at the time or subsequently. The subject has been reviewed.[1995]

psychological fatigue Failure of motivation to perform a muscular task with the full power available.[777]

psychological nystagmus See **psychogenic flutter.**

psychomotor retardation Slowing of the thought processes and of the initiation and execution of voluntary movements, either in the context of a depressive reaction or of generalized depression of cortical function stemming from any cause.

psychomotor seizures A term introduced by **Gibbs** in 1937 for those seizures originating within a temporal lobe, with alteration in consciousness and affective upsurges as components. See **pseudoseizures, affective-psychic seizures, complex partial seizures.**

psychomotor variant Rhythmic mid-temporal bursts of theta activity which are benign and not associated with an epileptic process. See **rhythmic temporal theta burst of drowsiness.**

psychomyogenic headache See **episodic tension-type headache.**

psychopathy See **hysterical personality.**

psychophysiological arousal See **persistent DIMS.**

psychophysiological insomnia A disturbance of initiating or maintaining sleep which is not due to an underlying structural or to a major psychiatric cause, in which tension and anxiety insufficient to allow a diagnosis of anxiety state lead to a learned pattern of sleep disorder through the association of poor sleep with the habitual sleeping environment. Although most commonly transient (*adjustment sleep disorder*), a persistent variety also occurs.[2478]

Diagnostic criteria have been defined[234] and are listed in Chart P–27.

Chart P–27. Diagnostic Criteria for Psychophysiological Insomnia

A. A complaint of insomnia combined with a complaint of decreased functioning during wakefulness

B. Indications of learned sleep-preventing associations are found:
  1. Trying too hard to sleep, suggested by an inability to fall asleep when desired, but ease of falling asleep during other relatively monotonous pursuits, such as watching television or reading
  2. Conditioned arousal to bedroom or sleep-related activities, indicated by sleeping poorly at home, but sleeping better away from home or when not carrying out bedtime routines

C. Evidence for increased somatized tension, e.g., agitation, muscle tension, increased vasoconstriction

D. Polysomnographic monitoring demonstrates:
  1. An increased sleep latency
  2. Reduced sleep efficiency
  3. An increased number and duration of awakenings

E. No evidence of other medical or psychiatric disorder that would account for the sleep disturbance

F. Other sleep disorders can coexist with the insomnia, e.g., inadequate sleep hygiene, obstructive **sleep apnea** syndrome, etc.

From ASDA Diagnostic Classification Steering Committee. The International Classification of Sleep Disorders Diagnostic and Coding Manual. Rochester, MN: American Sleep Disorders Association, 1990. Reproduced by kind permission of the American Academy of Sleep Medicine.

psychosis A class of mental illness in which there is gross impairment of reality testing, usually evidenced by such features as delusions, hallucinations, or seriously disorganized behavior. The individual with gross impairment revealed by reality testing incorrectly evaluates the accuracy of his or her perceptions and thoughts, and makes incorrect inferences about external reality, even in the face of contrary evidence.

Two forms are usually differentiated: the *organic psychoses*, in which physical disease (primarily or secondarily of the brain) is present; and the *functional psychoses*, which include schizophrenia and manic-depressive psychosis.[5839]

The term is, however, loosely used and, in the absence of complete understanding of causes, the term could well be dropped from the vocabulary.

PTAH stain See **Mallory stain.**

ptarmus See **sneezing.**

pterygocorneal reflex See **Wartenberg winking jaw phenomenon.**

pterygoid reflex (Gr, wing-like) Contraction of the medial pterygoid muscle in response to a downward tap on the chin. The reflex can only be assessed electrically with an EMG needle in the muscle. It is said to inform about the status of neuronal pools in the pontomesencephalic region,[2645] but the clinical utility of the technic requires further study.

pterygopalatine fossa syndrome 1. Pain in the second and later the third divisions of the fifth cranial nerve, numbness in the territory of the infraorbital nerve, paresis of the soft palate and of the pterygoid muscles, deafness resulting from compression of the eustachian tube, blindness resulting from optic nerve compression, and lateral rectus, pterygoid, and palatal palsies, all occurring as a result of malignant infiltration of the fossa, usually by a nasopharyngeal tumor.[240] See also **Trotter syndrome.** 2. See **cluster headache.**

pterygopalatine ganglion The ganglion in association with the ninth cranial nerve, within the fossa of the same name, through which pass fibers conducting taste impulses from the palate.

ptosis (from Gr, a falling) (blepharoptosis) Drooping of the upper eyelid, as with myasthenia gravis, myopathy, or third nerve palsy. In **Horner syndrome,** the lower lid rises a little as well and the ptosis is not severe; while in the other conditions, the upper lid may descend completely, occluding the eye.

Cerebral (supranuclear) ptosis is uni- or bilateral and is thought to be due to damage to pyramidal fibers rather than to the third cranial nerve or due to damage to the sympathetic fibers supplying the eye.[895]

pubic reflex The **abdominal reflex,** obtained in this case by tapping the symphysis pubis. The induced vibration also leads to contraction of the hip adductors in some cases.

pudendal (from Lat, shameful) The parts that should be covered; the genitalia.[5204]

pudendoanal reflex   Contraction of the external anal sphincter in response to stimulation of the dorsal nerve of the penis or the clitoris, with a normal latency of around 40 msec. This latency is increased in subjects with neurogenic lesions affecting the external anal sphincter.[5743] The bulbocavernosus muscle is similarly stimulated to contract by this maneuver.

Pudenz valve   A plastic valve placed subcutaneously under the scalp and attached to a slit valve, allowing the bubble to be pumped in order to check intracranial pressure and clear partial obstructions.

puerperal hemiplegia   The sudden onset of headache, convulsions, coma, and hemiplegia in a woman days to weeks after delivery, as a result of cerebral venous sinus thrombosis.

puffer fish toxin   See **tetrodotoxin.**

pugilistic encephalopathy   See **punch-drunk syndrome.**

Pulfrich phenomenon   When subjects view a pendulum swinging in a plane perpendicular to the line of vision (i.e., side to side) with one of their eyes covered by a filter or smoked glass, the pendulum appears to trace an elliptical path, coming toward them as it goes one way and away from them as it goes the other, the direction varying according to which eye is covered. The illusion is due to delayed perception in the covered eye, as with **optic neuritis.**[1610]

pulsatile tinnitus   An intracranial murmur synchronous with the heartbeat and due to disorders of the arterial or venous systems in the cranium or to idiopathic intracranial hypertension.[5807]

pulse   A burst of neuronal activity with precise onset and offset.

pulse dysmetria   An abnormality of saccadic control in which the rapid initial (pulse) part of the saccade is too great or too small. See also **glissade.**

pulse sequence   A set of radiofrequency (and/or gradient) magnetic field pulses and time spacings between these pulses used in conjunction with gradient magnetic fields and MRI signal reception to produce magnetic resonance images.

pulse-delay oculoplethysmography   A technique for measuring the arrival of pulses in the vessels of the eye and the earlobe. Severe internal carotid artery stenosis is suggested by a delay in arrival of the pulse wave between the eye and ipsilateral ear, or in the different times of arrival of the pulse wave in the two eyes. External carotid artery stenosis is documented by a delay in arrival of the ear pulse compared with the ocular pulse.[4141]

pulseless disease   See **aortic arch disease.**

pulseless saccade   See **hypometric saccade.**

PULSES profile   A global assessment of disability in which *physical condition, upper and lower limb functions, sensation, and bladder and bowel functions* are rated on 4-point scales. The instrument's limitation in scope is offset by reliability in usage.[925]

pulse-step control   A motor neuronal control signal comprising initially a phasic, high-frequency burst of activity in the motor nerve leading to the activation of agonist and the inhibition of antagonist muscles (the pulse), followed by a steady-state or tonic neuronal firing rate (the step), as seen in the extraocular muscles, in which the duration of the pulse is normally half that of the whole saccade.[290] These represent two components of the **controller signal** managing eye movements.[291]

pulvinar   (from Lat, a cushion) The elevated posterior projection of the thalamus. This is the largest and most posterior of the thalamic nuclei, having a role in motor functions and also in the processing of certain sensory signals.

pulvinar sign   The presence of T2-weighted MRI hyperintensities in the posterior thalamus, recorded in patients with new variant Creutzfeldt-Jakob disease.[1964]

punch-drunk syndrome   (dementia puglistica, pugilistic encephalopathy) A chronic encephalopathy presenting as a dementing illness, usually with added parkinsonian features and evidence of cerebellar and pyramidal disease, resulting eventually from the cumulative effect of repeated head injuries as incurred in professional **boxing.**[2882] It is characterized pathologically by perforation of the septum cavum, lesions of the substantia nigra, and the presence of scattered neurofibrillary tangles in the cortex and brainstem, and by diffuse cerebral atrophy on CT scans.

punding   Stereotyped motor behavior in which there is a protracted occupation with repetitive purposeless activity such as disassembling mechanical objects, jotting down figures, sorting or arranging, tidying up, or grooming or picking at one's self. Punding is observed among stimulant abusers and may be a result of excess dopamine stimulation. (HJM)[1792,4862]

pupil   (from Lat, pupilla, an orphan girl) The aperture of the eye, surrounded by the iris. It has been said that the aperture is called this because a tiny image of the beholder is therein reflected.

pupil cycle time   The time taken between constriction and dilation of the pupil stimulated with a light beam shone through a slit-lamp. The light causes the pupil to constrict, reducing the retinal stimulus so the pupil redilates; this leads to the repeated light stimulation of the retina and to pupillary constriction, and so on. The duration in seconds of 100 such cycles is recorded and the mean determined; the average cycle time is 840 msec.

Abnormal slowing indicates a lesion of the parasympathetic efferent pathway in the absence of an afferent pathway defect.[3664] The test is of value in cases of bilateral compressive optic neuropathy in which the optic nerves are symmetrically affected, so that a relative afferent pupillary defect is not easily demonstrated.[3889] See also **hippus.**

pupillary dilatation lag　See **dilatation lag.**

pupillary escape　The re-dilation of the pupil on the side of an afferent defect (a lesion of the optic nerve or retina) elicited by the swinging flashlight test. The mechanism, as explained by Levatin, is diminished stimulation of the pupilloconstrictor center when the light swings across from the normal to the abnormal eye, and thus diminished constriction occurs.

The phenomenon also occurs with continued light stimulation of an eye in the presence of an afferent defect. The clinical utility of the test is not established.[1151]

pupillary reflex　Constriction of the pupils in response to light stimulation.

pupillary sparing　The retention of normal pupillary reactions to light in the presence of a third cranial nerve palsy causing paresis of the extraocular muscles. Small-vessel disease is determined as the cause in three-quarters of such patients, but aneurysms and tumors are also, though rarely, responsible.[4055]

pupillography　A technique whereby infrared light is used to record the size of the pupils in such conditions as sleep.

pupillotonia　The tonic pupillary reaction as seen in the **Adie pupil.**

pupillotonic pseudotabes　See **Adie pupil.**

puppenkopfphänomenon　See **oculocephalic reflex.**

puppet-like gait　A stiff, uncoordinated, and jerky gait adopted by some patients with leg spasticity in association with the myelopathy of hepatic disease.

pure affective deafness　(pure prosodic deafness) A rare syndrome comprising motor aprosodia, loss of emotional gesturing, impaired repetition, and comprehension of affective prosody but normal comprehension of emotional gesturing, due to an anterior right hemisphere lesion.[4801]

pure agraphia　See **agraphia.**

pure akinesia syndrome　A rare syndrome characterized by freezing of gait, speech, and handwriting without accompanying limb rigidity, tremor, dementia, or ophthalmoplegia, unresponsive to L-dopa therapy but strikingly responsive to treatment with L-threo-3,4 dihydroxyphenylserine (L-DOPS).[4073] The condition may represent an atypical presentation of **progressive supranuclear palsy.**

pure alexia　A modality-specific disconnection syndrome. See **alexia without agraphia, pure word blindness.**

pure autonomic failure　See **progressive autonomic failure.**

pure autonomic variant of acute inflammatory polyradiculoneuropathy　See **autonomic neuropathy,** definition 1.

pure axonal neuropathy　A syndrome with the onset in youth of axonal motor and both thick-fiber and thin-fiber sensory neuropathy, accompanied later by dementia and pyramidal and cerebellar signs, and with spongy/cavity/cystic changes in the CNS. This condition may be a *variant* of **hereditary motor and sensory neuropathy, type 2.**

pure cholinergic dysautonomia　See **autonomic neuropathy.**

pure dysarthria　Dysarthria (usually with obvious lower-quadrant facial weakness) occurring as a **lacunar syndrome.**[1853,1867]

pure motor demyelinating neuropathy　See **chronic inflammatory demyelinating polyneuropathy.**

pure motor hemiparesis　(pure motor stroke) A **lacunar syndrome** manifesting complete or incomplete paralysis of the face, arm, and leg on one side, unaccompanied by sensory disturbances, visual deficits, aphasia, or apractagnosia. In the case of brainstem lesions, the patient will be free of vertigo, tinnitus, deafness, diplopia, cerebellar ataxia, and gross nystagmus.[1867] In 15% of cases, however, another stroke cause is detected.

The disorder is due to a small infarct of the basis pontis, in the middle part of the cerebral peduncle or in the posterior limb of the internal capsule. *Variant forms* follow.

> *Pure motor hemiparesis sparing the face* See **lacunar syndromes.**[1853,1867]
> *Pure motor hemiparesis with confusion* See **lacunar syndromes.**[1853,1867]
> *Pure motor hemiparesis with crossed third nerve palsy* (Weber syndrome) See **lacunar syndromes.**[1853,1867]
> *Pure motor hemiparesis with crossed sixth nerve palsy* (Foville syndrome) See **lacunar syndromes.**[1853,1867]
> *Pure motor hemiparesis with horizontal gaze palsy* See **lacunar syndromes.**[1853,1867]

pure motor monoparesis　Isolated corticospinal deficits in one limb only, of sudden onset and usually due to a mass lesion in the contralateral cerebral hemisphere.[242]

pure motor negativism　See **paratonia.**

pure motor stroke　A **lacunar syndrome** usually due to a lesion in the basis pontis or in the internal capsule. See **pure motor hemiparesis.**[1853]

pure motor variant of acute inflammatory polyradiculoneuropathy　See **acute inflammatory demyelinating polyneuropathy.**

pure pallidal atrophy　(Hunt–van Bogaert syndrome) A progressive familial degenerative system disease of young adult life, manifesting parkinsonian features, the tremor later disappearing and the rigidity and hypokinesia remaining. Pathologically, there is degeneration of the motor neurons of the pallidal system.[2703] See also **progressive pallidal atrophy.**

pure pandysautonomia Virtually complete but reversible paralysis of both sympathetic and parasympathetic functions in the absence of other features of neurological disease.[6094] See **acute autonomic neuropathy.**

pure photosensitive epilepsies Epileptic syndromes in which the seizures are induced exclusively by exposure to light, no attacks occurring spontaneously.[56] See **photosensitive epilepsies.**

pure progressive aphemia Severe anarthria or apraxia of speech, reported as a manifestation of primary progressive aphasia or vascular lesions affecting the inferior left premotor cortex.[1083]

pure prosodic deafness See **pure affective deafness.**

pure sensory stroke (hemisensory syndrome) A common **lacunar syndrome** characterized by complaints of intermittent or persistent numbness occurring unilaterally in the face, arm, and leg without other complaints.

The lesion was originally described as being in the ventroposterolateral thalamic nucleus,[1844] but posterior cerebral artery infarctions and lacunes in the thalamocortical pathways may also produce the syndrome.

pure sensory variant of acute inflammatory demyelinating polyneuropathy See **acute inflammatory demyelinating polyneuropathy.**

pure tone audiometry A quantitative test of auditory function employing electrically generated pure tones delivered by air or bone conduction. The threshold of acuity is determined at different frequencies and compared to an arbitrary standard.

pure tonic seizures with arousal (paroxysmal polyspike activity with arousal) Nocturnal seizures presenting solely with arousal from sleep, but with **excessive daytime sleepiness** as a related complaint. Daytime seizures seldom occur in such patients.[4392]

pure typical absence epilepsy of childhood (pyknolepsy) A syndrome characterized by the daily occurrence of frequent simple and complex absence attacks, with onset between the ages of 3 and 9 years. Typical spike-and-wave complexes are recorded on the EEG during the attacks.[807]

pure visual associative agnosia Failure to recognize or demonstrate the functions of objects seen but without any impairment of verbal facility.

pure word blindness (agnosic alexia, pure alexia, subcortical visual aphasia) A condition in which there is an inabilty to read but writing and oral language are preserved. Essentially, language activities are normal except for the recognition of written symbols, so that reading is somewhat impaired, although letters can be comprehended.[69] See also **alexia, pure alexias.**

pure word deafness (subcortical auditory aphasia, isolated speech deafness, auditory verbal agnosia) A rare aphasic disconnection syndrome in which the pathway from the auditory area to Wernicke's area is interrupted, leading to lack of auditory comprehension, and of being able to write from dictation and repeat spoken language, but with normal fluent spontaneous speech, reading, and comprehension ability, both of written language and of all nonverbal sounds.[462] In some cases, auditory agnosia is also present. Cortical deafness may precede the development of the problem.

The condition is due to disconnection (isolation) of Wernicke area (the posterior part of area 22 in the posterior part of the dominant superior temporal gyrus) from the left auditory radiation and from the callosal fibers from the opposite auditory region, within the temporal lobe, thus preventing it from receiving auditory stimulation. This may occur with bilateral lesions in the auditory association areas or with unilateral left-sided lesion interrupting transcallosal input. The syndrome was first described by Liepman in 1898.[2080]

pure word dumbness See **aphemia.**

Purine Research Society A charitable organization in this field providing information and support. Address: 5424 Beech Ave., Bethesda, MD 20814-1730. Tel: 301-530-0354. E-mail: purine@erols.com. Web site: http://www2.dgsys.com/~purine/. See also **Lesch Nyhan syndrome.**

Purkinje cells Constituents of the middle layers of the cerebellar cortex, described by Purkinje in 1837.[5204] Pure atrophy of the cells was described by André-Thomas.[179]

Purkinje, Johannes Evangelista von (Purkyne, Jan) (1787–1869) Bohemian priest and professor of physiology at Breslau and Prague. He was known as the "gypsy physiologist" perhaps both because of his race and because his areas of research were eclectic—the effects of poisoning by various agents; digestive and visual physiology; fingerprints; the use of the microtome, Canada balsam and glass slides; staining methods with potassium bichromate and carmine; vertigo; deafness; ciliary movement; and both cardiac and CNS histology being areas in which he made important contributions, for example, the identification in 1837 of the cerebellar cortical neurons named for him.

His enthusiasm for the experimental method led him to induce seizures in himself by the administration of camphor in 1835.[1104] After years of ostracism on account of his fervid nationalism and his individualistic approach to medicine, he was appointed professor of physiology at Prague University and thereafter to the Czech parliament, while still holding an appointment as newspaper editor, thus combining service both to the third and fourth estates.

Purkinje images The shadows of one's own retinal vasculature, visible to a subject in a dark environment when a bright light is shone onto the conjunctiva.

Purkinje phenomenon Fields of equal brightness but with different colors, appearing unequally bright when the intensity of the illumination is decreased.[2995]

purple glove syndrome A rare, generally benign and self-limited syndrome of distal limb edema with discoloration and local pain, recorded following the administration of dilantin intravenously, less often orally. Skin necrosis and limb ischemia resulting from the compression of vascular structures have also been documented in this condition.[4191]

pursuit Ocular deviations performed in order to maintain fixation upon a moving target.

pursuit defect nystagmus A form of horizontal jerk nystagmus seen in patients with a hemispheric lesion, in which there is a constant drift of the eyes toward the intact hemisphere and a failure of pursuit movements toward the damaged one. The nystagmus occurs with the fixation of moving and static objects. It is thought to be due to an imbalance in drives from the smooth pursuit system.[5099]

pursuit eye movements Smooth, reflexly controlled eye movements with speeds of up to 60° to 70° per second which maintain the image of a moving target upon the fovea after it has been placed there by a refixation saccade.

Disturbances in this function in all directions (*omnidirectional pursuit paresis*) suggest the presence of diffuse cerebral disease; disturbances in one direction only suggest the existence of a lesion of the cortical, subcortical, or cerebellar structures on the same side. See also **smooth pursuit system.**

pursuit gain See **gain of pursuit eye movements.**

pursuit imbalance nystagmus Conjugate drifting of the eyes toward the side of the intact hemisphere, seen in patients with parietal lobe disease during the performance of **pursuit movements.**

pursuit rotor test An instrument for the quantification of motor skills, in which the subject is required to follow a moving target with a hand-held stylus.[1132]

Purves-Stewart sign Spontaneous flexion of the toes of one foot while walking—an early sign of **Parkinson disease.**[4547]

pusher syndrome See **contraversive pushing.**

pushing palsy Self-induced bilateral peroneal palsies incurred during natural childbirth (without instrumentation or analgesia) as a result of compression of the nerves caused by the patient's pulling the hips and knees into maximal flexion.[45]

putamen (Lat, a paring—hence rind or tree bark.) The outermost portion of the lenticular nucleus.

Putnam acroparesthesia See **carpal tunnel syndrome.**

Putnam, James Jackson (1846–1918) An American neurologist who trained at Harvard and studied thereafter in Germany and in England with Hughlings-Jackson. He was the first neurologist appointed to the Massachusetts General Hospital (1872), and one of the first professors of neurology at Harvard. He was a founder of the American Neurological Association and one of its early presidents.

He described subacute combined degeneration of the cord,[4549] athetosis, and hypothyroidism following hyperthyroidism, and published with G.A. Waterman *Studies in Neurological Diagnosis* (Boston, 1902) and a book on ethics in 1915.

Putnam sign Apparent lengthening of the involved limb occurring with hysterical weakness.

Putnam syndrome Delirium following spinal injury; usually a fatal sign.[4550]

Putnam-Dara syndrome See **subacute combined degeneration of the cord.**

Puusepp little toe reflex Slow abduction of the little toe when the outer border of the foot is lightly stroked; a phenomenon said to occur in disorders of the extrapyramidal system, especially of the striatum. Puusepp's original patients had tumors or epidemic encephalitis.[5047]

Puusepp, Ludwig Martinovich (1879–1942) Russian-Estonian neurologist who trained in St. Petersburg and, after military service, with Bekhterev. He became professor of clinical neurology but moved to Estonia after the Russian Revolution and to Germany at the start of World War II. His publications covered topics in both neurology and neurosurgery.

pyknodysostosis (Maroteaux-Lamy syndrome) A recessively inherited congenital dysmorphic syndrome of macrocephaly with frontal and occipital bossing of the skull, delayed closure of the fontanelles, osteoporosis, multiple fractures, micrognathia and underdevelopment of the facial bones, deformed teeth, dwarfism due to defective and shortened long bones, and sometimes kyphoscoliosis. About a quarter of the affected subjects show a degree of mental retardation as well.[3635]

pyknolepsy (Gr, frequent + seize) A term not currently employed but originally used to refer to the frequent brief spells of unawareness observed in childhood petit mal epilepsy (simple absence seizures). It was introduced by Max Friedmann, a German neurologist in 1906.[1957] See **pure typical absence epilepsy of childhood, absence seizures, childhood absence epilepsy.**

Pyle disease A dominantly inherited cochleovestibular atrophy in which progressive neural or conductive deafness occurs in infancy, accompanied by metaphyseal dysplasias and sometimes optic atrophy and facial palsy.[4553] See **craniometaphyseal dysplasia.**

pyomyositis   (Gr, discharge + muscle + inflammation) (primary suppurative myositis, tropical pyomyositis) Acute or subacute infection of muscles by pyogenic bacteria giving rise to the usual systemic and focal signs of inflammation; a rare condition in temperate climates.[3301] See **acute suppurative myositis.**

pyramidal   (Gr, conical; a pyramid: "a solid resting on a plane base with three or more sides, each of which is triangular and rises to an apex"[5204]) The pyramidal tract was described by Paul Emil Fleschig in 1876, and its functions were most critically discussed by **Walshe.**[5831]

pyramidal decussation syndrome   (crossed hemiplegia syndrome, cruciate hemiplegia) Paresis of one arm and the other leg with sparing of the face, due to a lesion within the pyramid at a point below the decussation of the fibers destined for the arm and above that of the fibers destined for the leg.[992]

pyramidal lesion   See **upper motor neuron lesion.**

pyramidal myoclonus   See **focal reflex myoclonus.**

pyramidal pathways   All those corticospinal fibers that arise from the pyramidal cells in the fifth layer of the precentral cortex and, traversing the medullary pyramid, decussate or remain uncrossed and make up the crossed or uncrossed pyramidal tracts, respectively, of the spinal cord. Functionally, this is the pathway whereby the sensory system initiates and continuously directs willed movements.[5831]

pyramidal tract   (corticospinal tract) A fiber pathway comprising a bundle of about a million descending fibers that arise from the Betz cells of the motor cortex and traverse the medullary pyramids *en route* to the anterior horn cell pools in the spinal cord. Despite this, the term *pyramidal* is conventionally applied to all descending motor pathways, even those which play on the cranial motor nerve nuclei and which obviously do not pass though the pyramids. Moreover, the term is used synonymously with *corticospinal*, although some of the fibers traversing the pyramids do not arise from the motor cortex.

In monkeys at least, lesions of the pyramids in the medulla cause flaccid paralysis of the appropriate limbs and an upgoing plantar response; the remainder of what is generally called the *pyramidal syndrome* must, in humans, be due to associated lesions of other other descending pathways.

The tract was discovered by Ludwig Turck in 1851, its decussation by Duverney.

pyramid-hypoglossal syndrome   See **Déjèrine syndromes.**

pyridoxine deficiency   A potential cause of seizures (Hunt epilepsy) and of peripheral neuropathy.[2700]

pyridoxine dependency seizures   (OMIM 266100) A recessively inherited syndrome linked to 2q31 and characterized by increased fetal movements and intractable neonatal seizures due to glutamate acid decarboxylase deficiency, and responsive to high-dose pyridoxine therapy, required for life.[1049]

pyridoxine overdose neuropathy   A severe sensory neuropathy resulting from a massive overdose of vitamin B_6; a milder form is characterized by paresthesias, hyperesthesias, bone pains, muscle weakness, numbness, and fasciculations, all of which are most marked in the extremities and usually bilateral.

It is also seen in women who take lower doses (up to 200 mg/day). The symptoms remit when the ingestion ceases.[1255]

pyruvate decarboxylase deficiency   A rare recessive disorder usually manifesting in the first year of life and characterized by episodic anorexia, nausea, and vomiting with failure to thrive, ataxia, respiratory difficulties, hypoglycemia, hypotonia, microcephaly, seizures, CNS demyelination, aminoacidemia, disturbances of lactate and pyruvate metabolism with severe lactic acidosis, lipid myopathy, and mental and developmental delay.[254,3735] The responsible gene maps to chromosome 11q. Neuropathy, including optic neuropathy, choreoathetosis, and abnormal eye movements, are other features reported.[2439] See also **cerebellar ataxias.**

pyruvate dehydrogenase deficiency   An inherited intermittent ataxic syndrome due to a failure of the PDH complex of enzymes responsible for the conversion of pyruvate to acetyl coenzyme A, and involved in the synthesis of acetylcholine and lipids. Depending on the severity of the enzyme deficiency, different phenotypes include fulminant neonatal acidosis; **Leigh disease;** chronic ataxic encephalopathy, hypotonia, and weakness; and mental and motor delay.

Clinically, the deficiency presents congenitally or during infancy with combinations of optic atrophy, feeding problems, lethargy, hypotonia, apneic spells, seizures, microcephaly, ophthalmoplegia, ataxia, spasticity, chorea, and athetosis during fevers, accompanied by organic acidosis with high pyruvate and lactate levels. Dysmorphic features are usually evident. Many of the children also develop a peripheral neuropathy[2439] and cerebral atrophy; callosal agenesis and heterotopias may also be present.[600]

A *variant* is *familial intermittent ataxia*, an X-linked ataxic syndrome with onset in infancy, also characterized by dysarthria, neurodegenerative regression, and abnormal lactate and pyruvate metabolism.[337]

pyruvic acidemia   Abnormal levels of serum pyruvate, found in some cerebellar ataxic syndromes and in **Leigh disease.**

Pythagoras   Greek mathematician who was the first to record his opinion that the brain was charged with the power of reasoning.

Q

Q fever An acute, self-limited febrile illness due to infection with *Coxiella burnetii*. The primary infection is occasionally complicated by the **Miller Fisher syndrome,** encephalitis, meningitis, or myelopathy. Chronic endocarditis, hepatitis, and osteomyelitis are other reported associations.[2720] The "Q" derives from Queensland, the Australian state where the disease was first characterized.

qNP See **quantified neurophysiology.**

Q-SART See **quantitative sudomotor axon reflex test.**

quadrantanopia (Lat, quarter + Gr, loss of vision) Loss of vision in one-quarter of the visual field. This occurs with parietal (inferior quarter-field loss) or temporal (superior quarter-field loss) lobe lesions, because of the differing courses of the various fibers from the retina that pass through these two lobes, respectively.

Restricted occipital lobe lesions may also produce quadrantanopia. See **Meyer loop.**

quadrantic hemianopia See **hemianopia.**

quadraplegia See **quadriparesis.**

quadriceps myopathy a dominantly or recessively inherited, slowly progressive syndrome of myopathic weakness and wasting solely of the quadriceps muscles, with adult onset.

Late spread to other regions in some cases suggests that this condition is a variant of **limb-girdle muscular dystrophy**[5441] or, when there is abnormal staining for **dystrophin,** a forme fruste of **Becker muscular dystrophy.**

Variants are a neurogenic form with juvenile onset, and sporadic *chronic neurogenic atrophy of the quadriceps.*

quadriceps reflex See **knee jerk.**

quadrilateral space An anatomical artefact described as bounded by the teres major muscle below, the long head of the triceps medially, the neck of the humerus laterally, and the subscapularis muscle above, while the teres minor lies behind. The axillary nerve passes through this space.

quadrilateral space syndrome Compression of the axillary nerve in this space, sometimes associated with compression of the posterior circumflex artery and presenting clinically with deltoid weakness and wasting and hypoesthesia in C5 distribution.[4303]

quadriparesis Weakness of all four limbs. By common usage, this term is used when the degree of that weakness is incomplete.

quadriparesis, deafness, and mental retardation A rare syndrome, probably of autosomal recessive inheritance but possibly X-linked, characterized by facial weakness, mental retardation, spastic quadriparesis, impaired hearing, and diffuse, coarse pigmentary retinopathy.[2204]

quadripedal reflex see **Brain reflex.**

quadriplegia (quadraplegia) More or less complete paralysis of all four limbs, due either to an upper or to a lower motor neuron lesion.

quadriplegic myopathy (acute necrotizing myopathy of intensive care, floppy-person syndrome, thick filament myopathy, acute quadriplegic myopathy) An acute, generalized myopthy occurring in patients admitted to intensive care units with nonneuromuscular problems and treated with steroids and nondepolarizing muscle blockers.[2611,6134] The pathological characteristics are muscle fiber atrophy (often type 2), vacuolar muscle necrosis, and loss of myosin thick filaments. See **acute quadriplegic myopathy.** See also **postventilatory paretic syndromes.**

quadruple sectoranopia A visual deficit in which a thin strip of visual activity is spared around the horizontal meridian of a blind field. This is noted in some patients with infarction in the territory of the anterior choroidal artery and is considered to be diagnostic of infarction of the lateral geniculate body.[1963]

quail myopathy An acute myoglobinuric syndrome associated with the eating of quail, perhaps as a result of the prior ingestion of hemlock (the plant that killed Socrates) by the birds, for which it appears to be nutritious.

It has also been suggested that the plague affecting the Jews during their exodus from Egypt was of this nature.[4280]

quality extinction test A method of determining hemisphere malfunction which evaluates the verbal answers of a blindfolded subject to the simultaneous brushing of the palm of each hand with two different common materials which the subject has examined previously.[5018]

quality of life (quality of life index, quality of well-being scale) An attempt to express in a single statement a composite of all of those factors which determine the extent to which a person is able to participate in activities capable of providing pleasure or fulfilment. These might include relationships with family and friends, the health of the person and of those important to him or her, finances, housing, independence, leisure activities, religion, and social life.

Disease- and treatment-related symptoms; self-care, mobility, and physical activity levels; cognitive and emotional factors (including a sense of physical and psychological well-being); and social activity are the four areas considered central to this assessment.

Ten of the instruments currently most favored for this purpose are reviewed by de Haan et al.[1333] There follows a selection of scales with a similar purpose.

Frenchay Activities Index A measure of disability and functional handicap in stroke patients, assessing

1. (In the last 3 months) Abilities related to preparing main meals; washing-up; washing clothes; light and heavy housework; local shopping; social outings; walking outside for longer than 15 minutes; actively pursuing a hobby or interest, and driving.
2. (In the last 6 months) Ability to go on outings; gardening; household or car maintenance; reading books; and gainful work.[2612]

Nottingham Ten-point Activities of Daily Living Index A simple rating scale of items of daily living, used originally in stroke patients, to assess such activities as eating and drinking from a cup; transferring; washing; dressing; and preparing simple foods.[1599]

Nottingham Extended Activities of Daily Living Index A rating scale of items of daily living, used originally in stroke patients, to assess activities under the headings of mobility, kitchen work, domestic tasks, and leisure.[4174]

Karnofsky Performance Scale A simple if arbitrary score, given in percentages, reflecting the overall ability of a subject to cope with working and domestic or self-care activities.[2934] However, at all levels below 50% the subject is so greatly in need of assistance that the sensitivity of the scale, and thus its value, is lessened.

Sickness Impact Profile A reliable and valid inventory assessing best the effects of illness on day-to-day functions. Its physical dimension contains three subscales measuring ambulation, mobility, and body care and movement, which have been used especially in the detrermination of disability in subjects with multiple sclerosis.[5278]

quality of life index   See **quality of life.**

quality of well-being scale   See **quality of life.**

quantal squander   See **neuromyotonia.**

quantified neurophysiology   (qNP) Topographic EEG mapping; a computerized technique using the waveforms recorded over different areas of the scalp to produce a composite picture of the electrical activity of different brain regions.

The degree to which this represents a technical advance and how much an expensive (but professional) toy, is disputed.

quantitative cisternography   A technique for the indirect measurement of CSF flow using intrathecally injected radio-iodinated albumin and repetitive scintigraphic scanning.

quantitative electromyography   (QEMG) A systematc method for measuring the recordings made by an intramuscular needle electrode. Measurements include motor unit action potential characteristics such as amplitude, duration, and phases, or interference pattern characteristics. See **turns analysis.** (From the 2001 Report of the Nomenclature Committee of the American Association of Electromyography and Electrodiagnosis.[10] Used by permission, copyright © 2001, AAEM.)

quantitative muscle testing   Techniques for evaluating the strength of muscle contractions, in which a mechanical myometric system is employed to allow objective measurement of the muscular force generated.[5035] See **quantitative neurological examination.**

Quantitative Neurological Examination   A structured clinical examination emphasizing the findings in the motor system[1306] (see Chart Q–1).

Chart Q–1. The Quantitative Neurological Examination

Lateral Gaze

Pursuit. Hold index finger or pointer about 18 inches from the patients eye and ask the patient to follow it as it is slowly moved laterally.

  A. Range
    0 = Normal
    1 = Incomplete
    2 = No pursuit
  B. Smoothness of movement
    0 = One continuous movement
    1 = "Catch" or jerky; may stop mid-movement and look the other way
    2 = No pursuit

Vertical Gaze

Pursuit. As the patient moves his or her eyes up and down, it is useful for the examiner to hold the eyelids up for a better view of smoothness.

  A. Extent
    0 = Normal
    1 = Incomplete
    2 = No pursuit
  B. Smoothness of movement
    0 = One continuous movement
    1 = "Catch" or jerky
    2 = No pursuit

Saccades

Examiner holds up both index fingers about 18 inches (45 cm) from the patient at the extremes of lateral gaze and asks the patient to look from one finger to the other as quickly as possible.

  A. Speed
    0 = Normal
    1 = Slow
    2 = Cannot execute command
  B. Blink suppression: If the patient blinks while performing saccades, ask the patient to stop.
    0 = Does not blink or can stop.
    1 = Cannot stop
    2 = Cannot execute command
  C. Smoothness of movement
    0 = One smooth lateral movement
    1 = Attains goal by series of short movements
    2 = Cannot execute command
  D. Head moves laterally (ask not to move head)
    0 = None
    1 = Head moves with eyes
    2 = Cannot do saccades

Gaze Holding

Ask the patient to keep his or her eyes on a target at the lateral extreme of gaze, several meters away.

0 = Keeps eyes firmly on the target
1 = Eyes keep wandering off the target.
2 = Cannot execute command

Forceful Eye Closure

Ask patient to close his or her eyes tight, burying the eyelids. Score normal if patient does so even momentarily.

0 = Buries lids
1 = Cannot bury lids
2 = Cannot execute command

Facial Mimicking

Ask the patient to mimic the examiner's performance of the following movements.

a. Blow out both cheeks at once, keeping mouth closed.
b. Put tongue in cheek with enough force to make the cheek "pouch out."
c. Frown (knit brows).
d. Wink (non-winking eye may move but not close).
e. Rapid tongue movements.
  0 = Can perform
  1 = Cannot perform

(Ask the patient to touch the tip of the tongue to each corner of his lips alternately. There should be at least 4 touches/second performed smoothly to score 0.)

Motor Impersistence

(This item rates the patient's ability to sustain voluntary movement.)

A. Eye closure. Ask the patient to close his or her eyes and to keep them closed.
  0 = Maintains eyes closed for 20 seconds
  1 = Opens eyes before 20 seconds
  2 = Cannot execute command
B. Tongue. Ask the patient to protrude the tongue. The patient may not hold it out by using the teeth.
  0 = Maintains tongue out for 20 seconds
  1 = Retracts tongue before 20 seconds
  2 = Cannot execute command

Speech: Repeated Syllables

Ask the patient to repeat the following syllables after the examiner.

Rhythm (rh):	0 = regular	1 = irregular
Rate (ra):	0 = >4 syllables/ second	1 = 4 syllables/ second
Clarity (cl):	0 = each syllable clear	1 = syllables run together

Add 1 to each category if the patient is mute (total = 12).

a. La-la-la . . .
b. Go-go-go . . .
c. Kitty-kitty-kitty . . .
d. Attenuation (ask the patient to count to 20—or may be scored if noted in conversation).
  0 = No
  1 = Yes
  2 = If mute

Conversational Speech

This should be rated as the interview and examination progress.

A. Rhythm
  0 = Smooth with expected pauses and transitions
  1 = Unexpected pauses; speech comes in bursts
  2 = Mute
B. Rate
  0 = Normal
  1 = Speech is either too fast or too slow
  2 = Mute
Note: This seems subjective but is easily noted when present.
C. Clarity
  0 = Speech is normally understandable
  1 = The examiner must listen carefully but does not need to ask the patient to repeat him- or herself if speech is "jerky."
  2 = The patient must often try more than once, but can be understood
  3 = Speech is almost or entirely incomprehensible
  4 = Mute

Tone

(Examine tone in wrists and elbow and neck. Code arms and neck separately.)

0 = Normal
1 = Decreased
2 = Increased

Strength

Test biceps and strength of grasp, unless more extensive examination is indicated by clinical symptoms.

0 = Normal
1 = Decreased
2 = Cannot test because of advanced disease

Muscle Stretch Reflexes

Assess the composite score of the biceps, knee, and ankle jerks.

0 = Normal
1 = Absent
2 = Very brisk but no clonus
3 = Brisk with clonus at the ankle (or throughout)

(If asymmetrical, draw a diagram on the coding sheet showing the findings.)

Plantar Response

(Score the left and right responses separately.)

0 = Flexor
1 = Extensor

Asymmetry: Tone, Strength, Reflexes

0 = Symmetrical
1 = Asymmetry present

Finger–Nose

(Ask the patient to make a pointer with his or her finger and to touch the examiner's finger and then his or her own nose.

The examiner's finger should be held far enough away so that the patient must completely extend the arm.)

    0 = Quick, smooth, accurate (finger–nose–finger in 1 second)
    1 = Slow but accurate
    2 = Dysmetria
    3 = Cannot execute command

Finger–Thumb Tap

(Ask the patient to tap his or her index or third finger with the thumb quickly. Score each hand separately.)

    0 = >4 taps/second, smooth
    1 = 3 taps/second or faster but arrhythmic
    2 = <2 taps/second
    3 = Cannot perform

Diadochokinesis

(Ask the patient to pronate and supinate his or her hand alternately, patting the other palm on the ipsilateral knee. Score each hand separately.)

    0 = >3 pats/second smoothly executed
    1 = 2 pats/second or faster but arrhythmic
    2 = <2 pats/second
    3 = Cannot perform

Also ask the patient to stand with the feet together, eyes closed, arms out 90°, palms down, and fingers apart. Note balance as well as any tremor or chorea of the finger tips. Score tremor or chorea.

Tremor

(If the patient cannot stand, ask the patient to hold the arms at 90° while sitting. Tremor will not be scorable in patients with severe chorea.)

    0 = None
    1 = Mild
    2 = Marked
    3 = Cannot test because of chorea or poor concentration

Chorea

(Notice all body parts and make a summary rating. Chorea is a fairly quick, jerky movement which is not as stereotyped as a tic. It may be of any amplitude. It is not as quick as ballismus, which is also not usually symmetrical.)

    0 = Absent
    1 = Mild, occasional
    2 = Frequent but low amplitude
    3 = Frequent or continuous with moderate amplitude
    4 = Continuous, severe, but patient can carry out some voluntary movements
    5 = So severe as to be totally incapacitating

Note: All patients should have chorea scored at rest and with stress. Score as above in the following situations:

    a. With arms out at 90°
    b. Ask patient to hold as still as possible while sitting, hands in lap, or lying in bed
    c. During conversation
    d. During voluntary movement (e.g., walking)
    e. During stress (e.g., calculating)

Posture

(Rate standing or seated if unable to stand.)

    0 = Normal
    1 = Somewhat stooped
    2 = Very stooped with downward gaze or rigid and extended

Standing

(Observe for 10–15 seconds.)

    0 = Normally still or slight weaving
    1 = Widened base to stay in one place
    2 = Cannot stand still for 10 seconds or cannot stand

Walking

    0 = Normal gait, narrow base (heels should approximate a straight line)
    1 = Wide base
    2 = Wide base with deviation from a straight line
    3 = Walks with assistance (person, walker, leans on wall)
    4 = Unable to walk

Stopping

    0 = Stops on command
    1 = Stops but body lurches forward or takes a step
    2 = Takes 2 or more steps before stopping
    3 = Unable to walk

Turning

    0 = Pivots on a narrow base
    1 = Hesitates, widens base, or moves feet
    2 = Turns slowly and awkwardly
    3 = Cannot walk

Tandem Walk

Four practice steps, then 10 paces, heel touching toes at each stop.

    0 = No deviations or weaving after practice
    1 = 1–3 deviations or excessive truncal weaving
    2 = More than 3 deviations, but completes 10 paces
    3 = Cannot complete the task although tries
    4 = Cannot attempt task

Snout

Tap middle of closed lips with reflex hammer. Do not score random choreic movement.

    0 = Absent
    1 = Present

Grasp

Stroke patient's palm, with patient's palm down. Ask the patient not to grasp the examiner's hand.

    0 = Absent
    1 = Patient grasps the examiner's hand

Bradykinesia

0 = Voluntary movements at normal speed
1 = Mild slowness of gait, speech, task completion
2 = Marked slowness
3 = In bed without movement

Motor Impairment Scale

Eye closure (0–2)
Clarity or repeated syllables (0–4)
Finger–nose (0–3)
Diadochokinesis
right (0–3)
left (0–3)
Plantar response (0–2)
Gait (0–4)
Tandem walk (0–4)
Bradykinesia (0–3)
Maximum score = 28.

From David AS, Jeste DV, Folstein MF, et al. Voluntary movement dysfunction in Huntington's disease and tardive dyskinesia. Acta Neurol Scand 1987;75:130–139. ©1987 Munksgaard International Publishers, Ltd. Reproduced by kind permission of Blackwell Science.

Quantitative Neuromuscular examination A protocol that examines total muscle strength in terms of the MRC (Medical Research Council) Scale score based on a clinical assessment of 32 groups of muscles using the 6-point MRC grading: the force of 8 selected muscle groups measured on a myometer; a motor ability score based on 20 consecutive motor activities; walking times over 28 and 150 feet; and a recording of muscle contractures. See also **muscle testing in ALS**[177] and **Hammersmith scale**.

quantitative oculopneumoplethysmography A method of measuring absolute ophthalmic systolic blood pressure and the amplitude of the pulsations, capable of identifying stenoses reducing the diameter of the arterial lumen by more than 60%.

The technique employs scleral cups to raise the intraocular pressure and to interrupt the circulation; when the vacuum is removed, returning pulsations are detected by a sensor in the cup. Severe stenosis is suggested when the ophthalmic and brachial systolic blood pressures, the intraocular systolic blood pressures of the eyes, or the relative amplitudes of the ocular pulsations are abnormal.

This is the most widely used of the oculoplethysmographic tests and is the most accurate, but it does suffer from deficiencies in distinguishing occlusion from severe stenosis, and bilateral severe disease may also be difficult to identify with this method.[4141]

quantitative phonoangiography A technique whereby the frequency content of bruits is analyzed and related to the residual lumen diameter of the internal carotid artery.

It does this accurately in patients who have bruits, but suffers from the fact that about half of all patients

with severe disease do not have one, and it provides no information about the features of the vessel wall itself.

quantitative sensory testing The instrumented techniques used to measure the intensity of stimuli needed to produce specific sensory perceptions; methods of testing absolute sensory thresholds, designed for the assessment of the deficits in patients with peripheral neuropathy.

Vibratory detection thresholds, thermal perception, light touch, pain thresholds, and autonomic functions can all be quantitated using standardized methods,[8,1568,1575] but standardization has not yet been achieved.[4412]

Quantitative Somatosensory Thermotest A mechanical method of assessing the function of the A delta and C fibers responsible for transmitting impulses concerned with the appreciation of temperature sensation, using a technique for determining warming and cooling thresholds.[5749]

quantitative sudomotor axon reflex test (QSART) A method of measuring sweat production in a specific skin area in response to acetylcholine iontophoresis, in order to assess postganglionic sympathetic cholinergic function.[3486] The drug should induce sweating in preganglionic but not in postganglionic sympathetic disorders and is thus useful in the estimation of C-fiber function.

Antidromic transmission of the impulse from the nerve terminals reaches a branch point, then travels orthodromically to release acetylcholine from the nerve terminals, inducing a sweating response. In small fiber polyneuropathy, the response may be reduced or absent. In painful neuropathies, and in reflex sympathetic dystrophy, the response may be excessive and persistent or reduced. (Adapted from the 2001 Report of the Nomenclature Committee of the American Association of Electromyography and Electrodiagnosis.[10] Used by permission, copyright © 2001, AAEM.)

Queckenstedt, Hans Heinrich Georg (1876–1918) German physician who graduated from Leipzig and practiced in Heidelberg and Rostock. He became head of the German army medical services in Hamburg during World War I. His life was ended suddenly when he was thrown off his horse and under a munitions truck, 2 days before the end of the war and 1 year after his two publications—one on changes in CSF pressure with coughing, straining, and jugular vein compression, and the other on high protein levels in acellular CSF in cases of **acute inflammatory demyelinating polyneuropathy** and sciatica.[4557,4558]

Queckenstedt test Compression of the jugular veins causes elevation of the intraspinal fluid pressure as measured by a manometer, the pressure falling again when compression ceases. These pressure changes are dampened or absent in the presence of spinal block.[4557]

The sign was doubtless valuable in its day; the rationale for performing it now that safer and far more precise diagnostic tests are available is doubtful at best.

In the *reversed Queckenstedt test*, saline is injected into the lumbar theca and the consequent pressure changes are monitored through a needle placed in the cisternal space. Failure of the pressure to increase indicates an obstruction to the flow of CSF between the lumbar and cervical regions.

quiet sleep   See **non–rapid eye movement sleep.**

Quincke, Heinrich Irenaeus   (1842–1922) German physician who trained at Berlin, Wurzurg, and Heidelberg Universities and who quickly became professor of medicine, first at Bern and later at Kiel and Frankfurt. He made contributions in all fields of internal medicine and was the first to describe angioneurotic edema, but he is remembered in neurology for having successfully performed lumbar puncture in 1891, describing both the pressure changes and the constituents of CSF.[4559] He was not the first to do so, however, as Walter **Wynter** had published an account of lumbar puncture in the *Lancet* in the same year, while Corning in New York had described the operation in 1889.[5863]

Unlike **Wynter**'s patients who all had meningitis and who all died, many of Corning's patients lived (one at least probably having meningism rather than meningitis and others having hydrocephalus; however, it is not certain that Corning actually entered the subarachnoid space). Quincke also published on the topics of cerebral palsy, the physiology of the choroid plexus, and puncture of the anterior fontanelle in infants.

Quincke meningitis   See **idiopathic intracranial hypertension.**

quinolinic acid   A neurotoxic endogenous tryptophan metabolite that acts through the *N*-methyl-D-aspartate set of glutamate receptors to produce axon-sparing lesions similar to those in **Huntington disease.**

Quinquaud, Charles-Eugène   (1841–1894) French hematologist and dermatologist who studied in Limoges and Paris where he became chief of service at the Hôpital St-Louis. A "modest, honest, indulgent, sympathetic and great savant" (Maridort), he was elected a member of the French Academy of Medicine in 1891, by which time he had become well known as a brilliant dermatologist and for his publications on many topics in dermatology, pathology, and hematology, in the latter applying the principles of physics and chemistry to medicine. He died prematurely, "a victim of overwork."[5047]

Quinquaud sign   Tremor felt by the examiner when the patient's abducted fingers are firmly placed vertically on the examiner's palm. The sign was first described in alcoholics, and a description of it published by Quinquaud's pupil, Dr. P. Maridort, 6 years after Quinquaud's death. He recounted that "the Master forcibly applied the palm of his right hand to the tip of the extended fingers of his pupils. He looked at two of them (a point there is no need to labor) with a slight irony and made a negative sign to the others. Early in the ensuing month the beloved professor died and no one after him could determine what pressure on the tip of the extended fingers could reveal. . . . He carried his secret to the grave." [Translated by Awtin Seckerson.][5047]

Maridort, however, determined that "little shocks, as if the bones of each finger were being pushed back suddenly and were striking your palm" indicated that the patient suffered from alcoholism.[3612]

quisqualic acid   An excitotoxin.

quitarian epilepsy   Seizures in which the subject weeps. Quiritian was a Roman citizen, but the word *quitarian* probably derives from the Latin, to shout out loud. See **dacrystic epilepsy.**

quiver eye movement   (postsaccadic glissade) A backward drift of the eyes, interrupting the completion of a saccade as a result of fatigue of the myofibrils in the extraocular muscle.[3330]

quix test   The patient stands with both arms extended horizontally, and the fingers pointing at the examiner's shoulders. Drift of both hands consistently in any direction when the patient's eyes are closed is abnormal and suggests disease of the vestibular apparatus.[1511]

R

R1, R2 waves See **blink responses.**

rabbit syndrome See **rabbit tremor.**

rabbit tremor (rabbit syndrome) Fast, chittering movements of the lips and jaw with the mouth held slightly open; a feature in some cases of **tardive dyskinesia,** but also occurring at rest in some patients with parkinsonism.

rabies (from Lat, rage) (hydrophobia, lyssa, la rage; also St. Hubert disease) An acute viral encephalomyelitis resulting from infection by a member of the rhabdovirus family transmitted by foxes, wolves, raccoons, and dogs in North America and Europe; by wolves, jackals, and small carnivores in Asia and Africa; and by vampire bats in the Caribbean and South America. Transmission is almost always the result of the bite of an infected animal, the virus being found in its saliva, but airborne transmission has also occurred.

The incubation varies from a week to several years, but is usually less than 3 months after an animal bite, and the occurrence of the disease in *spelunkers* (facultative cave dwellers) suggests that the virus may infect after inhalation through the olfactory mucosa; this is followed by prodromal symptoms of a flu-like illness, pain, and paresthesias at the site of the bite; later by anxiety, agitation, and insomnia, and then by either the *furious* or the *dumb* form of rabies. Three cases of rabies have been reported in which the patient lived. The remainder of the 15,000 or more cases occurring annually in the word die as a result of the disease.[6030] **Negri bodies** are found in the brain in most cases. The condition was recognized in the third century B.C., but the usual term used to refer to it up to the seventeenth century was *hydrophobia.*

In the *furious* form, there is an encephalopathy with at least some mental disturbance, but this is overshadowed by the intermittent inspiratory and pharyngeal spasms and attacks of terror which are precipitated by attempts to drink (or even the thought of doing so), and which may lead to seizures and respiratory arrest. Cranial nerve palsies, pyramidal signs, involuntary movements and meningism, and autonomic disturbances are also typical. Laryngeal spasm may lead to respiratory arrest and death. Hyperexcitability with hallucinations and delirium occurs, interspersed with periods of normal cognitive functioning. Meningism and bulbar palsies precede coma and eventual death.

The unusual *dumb (paralytic)* form closely resembles **acute inflammatory demyelinating polyneuropathy** and is characterized by progressive pareses beginning in the limb that was bitten, but ascending to produce respiratory and bulbar weakness.[3876] Muscle spasms and hydrophobia develop terminally in these patients prior to death.

Vaccination is possible using a human diploid fibroblast culture vaccine, which is safe and effective, having been successful even when used after exposure.

Rabot epilepsy A form of benign familial myoclonic epilepsy due to a hereditary error of metabolism.

raccoon eyes Periorbital bruising, occurring bilaterally in most cases after fractures of the anterior cranial vault.

racemose aneurysm See **arteriovenous malformation.**

racemose angioma See **arteriovenous malformation.**

rachialgia (Gr, the spine + pain) "Spinal irritation . . . local pain and tenderness referred to the spinal column itself" (Sir William **Gowers**).[2240]

rachischisis (Gr, the spine + splitting) (dysraphism) Disorders of fusion of the dorsal midline structures of the primitive neural tube. **Spina bifida, meningocele, meningomyelocele, tethered cord,** and **diastematomyelia** are examples.

rad The basic unit of absorbed radiation in tissue.

radial aplasia See **Baller-Gerold syndrome.**

radial bending reflex See **bending reflex.**

radial deviation Inclination of the hand toward the radial side when the subject with a posterior interosseous nerve lesion attempts to make a fist.

Sparing of the extensor carpi radialis longus (innervated by the radial rather than by the posterior interosseous nerve) is responsible for this.[2586]

radial neglect A visual vertical neglect syndrome in which the subjects fail to bisect accurately radial lines extending from a midpoint.[3058] See also **line bisection test.**

radial reflex See **brachioradialis reflex.**

radial tunnel syndrome Entrapment of the posterior interosseous nerve by an abnormal fibrous band or by the edge of the extensor carpi radialis brevis tendon or its origin, causing pain in the lateral part of the elbow and forearm.[4746] See **posterior interosseous syndrome.**

radialis sign Inability to make a fist without marked extension of the wrist. The sign was described by **Strümpell** and is present with pyramidal lesions and in tetany.

radian An arc or segment of a circle with a length equal to the radius of the circle. The term is included because it has been suggested that cerebral concussion, in the absence of impact, approximated 330 radians/

second over at least 20 msec and about half of that with concussive injuries.[2587]

radiary nystagmus   See **circular nystagmus.**

radiation damage to the nervous system   Transient or permanent neurotoxicity resulting from direct or incidental irradiation of the nervous system. The neurological complications of such radiotherapy have been reviewed and classified by Keime-Guibert et al. (1998).[2989]

Acute (minutes to 1 week)	Early-delayed (4–16 weeks)	Late-delayed (4 months to years)
Acute encephalopathy	Somnolence syndrome Increased focal signs, worsening MRI findings **Rhombencephalopathy**	Radiation necrosis Late cognitive dysfunction, dementia Endocrinopathy Radiation arteriopathy Radiation-induced tumor
Paraesthesias	Transient cognitive dysfunction **Anosmia Lhermitte** sign **Ageusia** Hearing loss	Transverse myelopathy (see **radiation encephalomyelopathy** Hemorrhagic myelopathy Motor neuron syndrome Visual loss Hearing loss, hair cell damage Lower cranial nerve paralysis
Brachial or lumbosacral	Brachial or lumbosacral reversible **plexopathy**	Brachial or lumbosacral late plexopathy Radiation-induced tumors

From Keime-Guibert F, Napolitano M, Delattre J-Y. Neurological complications of radiotherapy and chemotherapy. J Neurol 1998;245:695–708, reprinted by permission.

radiation encephalomyelopathy   (postirradiation myelopathy) Insidiously progressive evidence of damage to the spinal cord occurring 3 months to 5 years after its irradiation.

Slowly progressive paraparesis with spinothalamic sensory loss and a **Brown-Séquard syndrome** are the usual syndromes developing after cervical irradiation. A painless motor neuropathy may occur when the cauda equina is included in the field but almost any syndrome of myelopathy can be produced. In the most common form, with cervical disease, pain in the neck and shoulders, and sensory disturbances such as numbness, paresthesias, **Lhermitte** symptom, and thermoanalgesia in the legs are the usual presenting complaints.[4616]

These features may be *early and transient* (in the first 6 months after irradiation) or may go on to the *chronic (late-delayed) progressive* form in which after 6 months there appear typical motor and sensory signs of partial cord transection with sphincter involvement; these are irreversible.

Variant syndromes such as *arrested radiation myelopathy, disseminated demyelination in the CNS causing encephalopathy,* and *acute paraplegic* and *lower motor neuron* types have also been recorded.[3187,4310]

radiation of pain   The experience of pain at a distance from the site from which it is perceived to emanate, but within the distribution of the sensory nerve or root supplying the painful part. See also **referred pain.**

radiation plexopathy   (radiation-induced peripheral neuropathy) A syndrome of paresthesia in the fingers, hypoesthesia, and weakness, the last affecting mainly muscles innervated by C5 through C7, occurring months or years after irradiation with 6000 cGy or more to a field including the brachial plexus, usually for the treatment of breast cancer. A **Horner syndrome** is seldom seen.[5365] Lymphedematous swelling of the arm is a common associated sign and, electrically, myokymia is often found in the affected muscles.

Lumbosacral plexopathy is a less common result of radiation therapy. Other causes of plexopathy have been reviewed.[5394]

radiation radiculopathy   A subacute or slowly progressive syndrome of muscle atrophy and weakness with paresthesias occurring between 3 months and 3 years after irradiation of the spinal column, particularly at lumbosacral levels.[700]

radiation-induced peripheral neuropathy   See **radiation plexopathy.**

radicular compression   The result of degenerative changes of the spinal column, whereby spinal nerve roots are distorted or compressed. The clinical criteria establishing the diagnosis comprise a local muscle spasm causing stiffness of the neck or a decrease in straight-leg raising, postural and gait disturbances, and motor or sensory neurological deficits appropriate to the roots compressed.

radicular deficit   See **radiculopathy.**

radicular myelopathy associated with spinal neuronitis   See **chronic spinal meningitis.**

radicular reflex myoclonus   A myoclonic disease in which the jerks appear to originate from the brainstem reticular substance.

radiculitis   (spinal neuritis) Inflammation of the roots of the spinal nerves. This occurs with viral infections such as herpes zoster, and may also be due to toxic agents.

The word is sometimes used to describe the state of the nerve roots irritated by local mechanical disease, such as occurs with a prolapsed intervertebral disk.

radiculomeningitis   Inflammation of the spinal arachnoid meninges with consequent compression and inflammation of the nerve roots traversing these, usually due to collagen vascular diseases such as **ankylosing spondylitis** or rheumatoid arthritis.

Clinically, lumbar pain, atrophy, and weakness or a full **cauda equina syndrome** is the more common presentation.

radiculomyelopathy The association of long-tract signs due to cervical cord disease with evidence of root lesions at higher cervical levels, in conjunction with anomalies of the spinal column such as **atlantoaxial dislocation;** a disorder reported from India.[5795]

radiculoneuritis See **acute inflammatory demyelinating polyneuropathy.**

radiculopathy (radicular deficit, root lesion) A clinical syndrome resulting from lesions of the anterior or posterior spinal nerve roots. Motor features include complaints of weakness, with wasting and hyporeflexia in the territory of the roots affected; sensory symptoms include pain and sensory dysfunction such as hypoesthesias, dysesthesias, and paresthesias, again restricted typically to the appropriate territory. The pathophysiology, clinical manifestations, and diagnostic methodologies have been reviewed.[5965]

From the viewpoint of electrodiagnosis, this is an axonal and/or demyelinating disorder affecting the nerve fibers exclusive to one spinal nerve root or spinal nerve. It may affect the anterior (motor) or posterior (sensory) spinal nerve roots, or both, at one spinal cord segment level. The resulting clinical syndrome may include pain, sensory loss, parethesia, weakness, fasciculations, and muscle atrophy. If more than one spinal root is involved, the term *polyradiculopathy* may be used as a descriptor. (From the 2001 Report of the Nomenclature Committee of the American Association of Electromyography and Electrodiagnosis.[10] Used by permission, copyright © 2001, AAEM.)

The classification in Chart R–1 is closely based on that of the World Federation of Neurology. See also **neuromuscular diseases.**

Chart R–1. Classification of Radiculopathies

Disorders of Motor Nerve Roots

A. *Congenital*
   1. Associated with **meningomyelocele** and other anomalies
   2. **Arthrogryposis multiplex congenita** (radicular type)
B. *Acquired disorders*
B1. *Physical causes*
   1. Laceration, contusion, distraction, or avulsion of roots
   2. Compression of roots by vertebral osteoarthritis, prolapsed intervertebral disk, **Paget disease,** tumor in the spinal canal or intervertebral foramina, or vertebral collapse
B2. *Ischemia*
B3. *Radiation*
B4. *Toxic agents* (injected local anaesthetics, phenol, etc.)
B5. *Infective* (e.g., radiculopathy in meningitis, syphilis, AIDS,[1135] granulomatous arachnoiditis from other causes (including spinal tuberculosis and sarcoidosis), bilharziasis

B6. *Postinfective, allergic, or immunologically mediated*
   1. **Acute inflammatory demyelinating polyneuropathy** (polyradiculoneuropathy)
   2. Polyradiculoneuropathy after inoculation
   3. **Serum neuropathy**
   4. **Neuralgic amyotrophy**
   5. Radiculopathy of **Lyme disease**
   6. Radiculopathy in **HIV** infection[1135]
B7. *Neoplastic* (e.g., neurofibroma, meningioma, metastases, reticulosis)
B8. *Vascular malformation*

Adapted from the World Federation of Neurology Classification Subcommittee Classification of neuromuscular diseases. J Neurol Sci 1988;86: 333–360. The classification used here is adapted by kind permission of the World Federation of Neurology, and uses the same enumeration.

radioperiosteal reflex A misnomer. See **brachioradialis reflex.**

radiosurgery A therapeutic method in which intense beams of gamma radiation are collimated and focused on deep-seated inoperable brain lesions such as arteriovenous malformations in a single session.

radius (Lat, a ray, hence the spokes of a wheel[5204]) The name for the smaller of the two bones of the forearm, applied by Celsus.

Radovici sign The **palmomental reflex,** first described by J. Radovici (b. 1868), a Romanian neurologist and a pupil of **Marinesco.**[1829]

Raeder paratrigeminal syndrome (middle cranial fossa syndrome, paratrigeminal syndrome) The occurrence of oculosympathetic paresis with evidence of trigeminal sensory loss or motor weakness, the trigeminal involvement usually presenting with facial or temporal pain in the distribution of the first (but occasionally the second) division of the fifth cranial nerve.[4569] This is not merely a painful **Horner syndrome.**

The presence of head or face pain was not regarded originally as part of the syndrome, although sometimes it is considered so today. If pain were to be included as a criterion, it should be neuralgic rather than, for example, vascular in type. The sign localizes a lesion to the middle cranial fossa; in Raeder's (1918) cases, diplopia and systemic features such as vomiting and anorexia also occurred; tumor and trauma were the only definite etiologies identified.[3939] Dr. G. Raeder was a Norwegian ophthalmologist.

In *variants* of the syndrome, optic nerve involvement, oculomotor pareses or dysgeusia occur with the signs just described.

ragged red fibers An appearance on muscle biopsy specimens stained with Gomorri trichrome, in which subsarcolemmal clumps of red-staining mitochondria impart an uneven, granular appearance to the edge of the type 1 myofibrils.

The biochemical defect in the muscle is also expressed in the brain. The condition is a marker for the presence of mitochondrial oxidation defects, especially in those diseases associated with a clinical myopathy such as **cytochrome-*c* oxidase deficiency,**[1448] but is not invariably present and is not a criterion for the diagnosis of **mitochondrial diseases**.

ragged-red fiber mitochondrial disease   See **mitochondrial encephalopathy.**

railway nystagmus   See **optokinetic nystagmus.**

railway spine   (delayed posttraumatic myelitis of Gowers) Symptoms supposed to result from concussion of the brain and spinal cord as a result of traveling in railway carriages in the nineteenth century. Such a problem was accepted as genuinely organic in the early days of railway travel, and received much support in England and the United States from the writings of **Erichsen.**

The absence of such symptoms stemming from travel in stagecoaches appears not to have been remarked.

Raimistes signs   1. Flexion at the wrist in an arm affected by pyramidal tract lesion, when extended. 2. When the hemiparetic patient lies prone with the legs separated and tries to adduct or abduct the sound leg against resistance, the paretic leg adducts or abducts also.[4723]

Rainbow Foundation for Brain Tumor Research, Inc.   A charitable association in this field. Address: Box 327 Highland Mills, New York 10930. Tel: 914-928-8683. Web site: http://www.thorstenbaye.com/cause05.htm.

Ramachandran sign   (mirror agnosia) When subjects with a right parietal lesion are asked to look into a mirror held to their right side and to reach out to grasp a pen held up on their left side, they reach repeatedly into the mirror, thus mistaking the mirror for the object even though they are aware of the nature and properties of the mirror itself.[4574]

Ramon y Cajal, Santiago   (1852–1934) Spanish anatomist and neurohistologist who trained at Saragossa. He was appointed professor of anatomy at Valencia at the age of 29, but transferred to Bologna and then returned to Spain as professor of histology and morbid anatomy in Madrid. His major work, *Histologie du systeme nerveuse de l'homme et des vertebres* (Paris, 1909–1911), established him as the father of neurohistology, although some of the credit belongs to Camillo **Golgi,** a modification of whose silver stain Cajal used, and with whom he shared the Nobel prize in 1906.

He also introduced a silver nitrate stain to show the content of neuronal cytoplasm; this stain was used by **Alzheimer** to demonstrate neurofibrillary tangles. Among his students or collaborators were **Lorento de No, Lafora,** and Wilder **Penfield.**

Cajal used the brains of small immature animals such as embryonic mice, bats, and rats for study, because in them the relative lack of myelin allowed better staining of the cellular elements. With these techniques he revolutionized the understanding of the form and nature of the cell populations of the nervous system. He was the first to show that the processes of cells are not linked indiscriminately within a reticulum, but have specific sites of termination on the dendrites or bodies of other cells. He enunciated his neuronal theory in three parts. First, nerve cells are independent elements that do not anastomose (as in a synctium) but make contact with others only at specific points. Second, nervous impulses are always transmitted from the cell body out to the axon. And third, the axon conducts away from the cell body.

His collected opinions appeared in his *Manual de anatomia patologica general* (Madrid, 1909) and in the translated *Studies on Degeneration and Regeneration in the Nervous System* (London, 1928). His autobiography has recently been published.[4579]

Ramsay Hunt, James   (1872–1937) American neurologist who trained in Philadelphia and then in Paris and Berlin, returning to Cornell University and later becoming professor of nervous diseases at Columbia.

He was the first to describe in detail the effects of internal carotid artery occlusion and of damage to the deep palmar branch of the ulnar nerve, as well as to report the following conditions.

James Ramsay Hunt

Ramsay Hunt paralysis   See **juvenile Parkinson disease.**

Ramsay Hunt syndromes   1. **dyssynergia cerebellaris myoclonica,** a recessively inherited cause of **progressive myoclonic epilepsy** producing the clinical triad of severe action and stimulus-sensitive myoclonus, progressive ataxia, and grand mal seizures, with onset in childhood or youth.[2704] Other clinical features include dysarthria and pes cavus.

Variants include the following:

A *dominantly inherited* form with seizures, chorea, dementia, and mental and physical delay

Ramsay Hunt syndrome with peripheral neuropathy A rare variant of the preceding one, with the onset in youth of speech defects, dementia, seizures and myoclonus, cerebellar signs, and peripheral neuropathy. Spongy changes, demyelination, and gliosis in the brain are the pathological hallmarks.[337]

Other forms complicated by central neurogenic hypoventilation, mental retardation, and morphological mitochondrial changes in skeletal muscle. See **MERRF.**

This syndrome is not a single entity; **Unverricht-Lundborg progressive myoclonic epilepsy, neuronal ceroid lipofuscinosis, sialidosis, biotin-responsive encephalopathy,** malabsorption secondary to celiac disease, **action myoclonus–renal failure syndrome, mitochondrial encephalopathies** and many of the **multisystem degenerations** are all causes.

2. *Geniculate herpes.* Herpes zoster of the external ear and the oral mucosa with homolateral facial paralysis, due to infection of the facial nerve (actually distal to the geniculate ganglion), causing severe lancinating pains felt deep in the external auditory meatus.[2701] The peripheral ganglia of cranial nerves VIII, IX, and X may also be infected, with resulting paresis. Tinnitus, hearing loss, nausea, and vomiting may be associated. The prognosis for recovery in this form of facial palsy is worse than in the case of the more common **Bell palsy.** In a small number of cases, the rash does not appear.[5447] See also **geniculate neuralgia.**

3. **Dentatorubral atrophy.**[2703]

ramus communicans   (Lat, a branch + communicating) The sympathetic fibers running between the spinal roots and the sympathetic chain in the thoracolumbar outflow. White rami are lightly myelinated efferent fibers; gray rami are scantily myelinated and afferent.

Rancho Los Amigos levels of cognitive functioning
A universal scale of cognitive functioning applicable to head-injured patients.

1. No response to stimuli
2. Generalized response to stimuli
3. Localized response to stimuli
4. Confused, agitated
5. Confused, inappropriate—not agitated
6. Confused, appropriate
7. Automatic, appropriate
8. Purposeful, appropriate

random epilepsy   Generalized seizures occurring independently of the sleep–wake cycle.

Rankin scale   A popular scale for the assessment of the burden of stroke[4588] in which the first and last points are objective, the remainder subjective. It appears in Chart R–2 in a modified form.

Chart R–2. The Rankin Scale[323]

Grade	Description
0	No symptoms
1	Minor symptoms that do not interfere with activities of daily living
2	Minor handicap, symptoms that lead to some restriction in lifestyle but do not interfere with the patient's capacity to continue self-care
3	Moderate handicap, symptoms that significantly restrict lifestyle and prevent independent existence, although the patient can walk without assistance
4	Moderately severe handicap, symptoms that clearly prevent independent existence (the patient cannot walk unaided and needs assistance with personal bodily needs), though not requiring constant attention
5	Severe handicap, totally dependent (bedridden, incontinent). The patient requires constant attention night and day.
6	Death

From Bamford JM. Interobserver agreement for the assessment of handicap in stroke. Stroke *1989;20:828, reproduced by permission.*

Ranvier, Louis-Antoine   (1835–1922) French histologist, who trained in medicine in Paris and was selected by Claude **Bernard** to lead the histological service at the Collége de France. Ranvier was soon appointed professor of general anatomy there and published on many areas of histology. In 1878, he described the **nodes** named for him.[5204]

RAPD   See **relative afferent pupillary defect.**

raphe   (Gr, a seam) A place where it appears as though adjacent structures had been sewn together.

Rapid Disability Rating Scale   An instrument for assessing the activities of daily living, disabilities, and special problems in elderly subjects.[3422]

rapid eye movement sleep   See **REM sleep.**

rapid time zone change syndrome   (jet lag, acute phase shift of sleep) A transient desynchronization of an individual's sleep–wake cycle as a result of rapid travel across multiple time zones. Clinically, excessive sleepiness and irritability with impaired memory occur during waking periods, and insomnia occurs during the normal sleep period of the new environment. The normal circadian patterns for cortisol levels and temperature are also affected.[3750]

Readjustment occurs at the rate of 88 minutes/day going west and 55 minutes/day going east (see also ASDA Diagnostic Classification[234]).

rapidly progressive aphasic dementia and motor neuron disease   A rare syndrome characterized by the occurrence of speech and language impairment, including severe nonfluent dysphasia, as the initial features of rapidly progressing **amyotrophic lateral sclerosis.**[936]

rapidly progressive parkinsonism and dementia with pallidopontonigral degeneration   An autosomal dominant neurodegenerative disease characterized by progressive parkinsonism with dystonia unrelated to medications, as well as dementia, abnormal ocular motility, pyramidal tract dysfunction, frontal lobe release signs, perseverative vocalizations, and urinary incontinence.

The course is exceptionally aggressive, with symptom onset and death consistently occurring in the fifth decade.

rapid-onset dystonia-parkinsonism   A dominantly inherited movement disorder characterized by the onset over hours to days of parkinsonism and **dystonia** together, with a subsequently stable course and with minimal response to dopamine agonists or other therapies. Dysarthria and bradykinesia are prominent features and the condition affects the bulbar and arm muscles more than those of the legs. Focal or segmental dystonia precedes the onset of the disorder in some cases.[1483,5441] The following diagnostic criteria have been suggested:[728]

Typical Rapid-onset Dystonia-Parkinsonism
  Autosomal dominant inheritance
  Sudden onset of combined dystonia and parkinsonism with
      stabilization in less than 4 weeks
  Bulbar symptoms including dysarthria and dysphagia
  Bulbar and arm involvement greater than legs
  Moderate to no response to levodopa/carbidopa or dopamine
      agonists
  Normal brain CT or MRI
  Low CSF HVA levels (not required for diagnosis)
Other Rapid-onset Dystonia-Parkinsonism Phenotypes
  Family history of classical rapid-onset dystonia-parkinsonism
  Gradual or sudden onset of dystonia (± subtle parkinsonism)
  Moderate or no response to levodopa/carbidopa or dopamine
      agonists
  Normal brain CT or MRI
  Low CSF HVA levels (not required for diagnosis)

From Brashear A, DeLeon D, Bressman SB, et al. Rapid-onset dystonia-parkinsonism in a second family. Neurology 1997;**48**:1066–9, reproduced by permission.

Rappaport disability rating scale   A rating scale designed for the continuing assessment of patients with severe head injury throughout the course of recovery.

Three items in the scale reproduce the **Glasgow Coma scale,** while others deal with *toileting, grooming, feeding, overall level of functioning,* and *employability.*[4596]

RAS   See **reticular activating system.**

Rasdolsky syndrome   Contracture and paresis of the masseter and facial muscles as a result of a neoplasm of the homolateral pontine tegmentum.[4598]

Rasmussen encephalitis (chronic unilateral encephalitis of Rasmussen; OMIM 30-59915) A chronic, progressive, smoldering focal encephalitis of unknown etiology but perhaps autoimmune, presenting (usually in children) with intractable epileptic seizures (**epilepsia partialis continua**), dementia, and varied neurological and psychiatric disturbances.[4607] The early occurrence of uveitis suggests a role for a viral pathogen, and about half the patients have a history of some infectious or inflammatory illness prior to the onset of their seizures; cytomegalovirus has been particularly incriminated.[3772] Rasmussen described the condition in 1958.[4607] It's etiology is probably autoimmune, but even that remains as uncertain today as when Wilder **Penfield,** doubting a primary inflammatory cause in 1956, offered a new hat to anyone who could prove him wrong.

Simple or complex partial seizures, epilepsia partialis continua, and secondarily generalized tonic-clonic seizures are described and status epilepticus can be the presenting manifestation. EEG and MRI findings indicate patchy, multifocal involvement primarily of one hemisphere, especially in perisylvian regions.

Stages of development of the condition have been defined. Stage 1 involves the evolution of a hemiparesis on the afflicted side. Seizures usually are simple partial or complex partial with occasional episodes of epilepsia partialis continua. The usual duration of this stage is about 3 years. During stage 2, there continues a steady deterioration of neurologic function. Seizures may tend to generalize more frequently. This stage has an average duration of 4 years. Stage 3 consists of an end stage of function. Typically, there is a hemiparesis or hemiplegia with a visual field hemianopia. Seizures tend to be less severe but still intractable and with overt loss of intellectual function.

The CSF is either normal or contains a few lymphocytes/monocytes with or without elevation of protein. The EEG reveals focal slowing over the affected hemisphere with multifocal epileptiform discharges and/or periodic lateralized epileptiform discharges (PLEDs) interictally. CT and MRI eventually show perisylvian atrophy. There are abnormal T2-weighted signal abnormalities in the white matter early in the course of the illness. Single photon emission tomography and positron emission tomography demonstrate decreased blood flow and metabolism in the affected area. Pathologically, frontotemporal cortical areas show chronic inflammatory changes with microglial nodules, neuronal loss, gliosis, and cortical dysplasias in the affected areas and with perivascular collections of round cells without inclusions.[4607]

See also **American Autoimmune Related Diseases Association.**

Rasmussen, Theodor   Contemporary Canadian neurosurgeon.

raster   A method of displaying a free-running sweep on the cathode ray oscilloscope by off-setting each successive sweep below the last.

Rathke cleft cyst Cysts within the sella turcica derived from Rathke's pouch, pathological in humans but common in certain other species. They are usually asymptomatic but may rarely cause chiasmal compression or hypophysial dysfunction.[4701]

Rathke, Martin H. (1793–1860) German anatomist and physiologist, professor at Dornat and then at Königsberg, who described the anatomy of the pituitary region and the "pouch" in 1838.

Rathke's pouch A diverticulum from the embryonic buccopharyngeal area which gives rise to the anterior part of the pituitary gland.[5204]

Raven Progressive Matrices A standard nonverbal test of visual perception and analogue reasoning, in which the subject is required to determine which of a set of alternative patterns completes the sequence of patterns printed on a card.[4608]

A variant is the simpler **colored progressive matrices.**[4609] A more difficult set has been designed for those of high native intelligence.

raw EMG Unprocessed EMG signals recorded with surface or intramuscular electrodes.

Fulgence Raymond

Raymond, Fulgence (1844–1910) French neurologist with a strong interest in neuropathology, practicing in Paris at the **Salpêtrière,** where he succeeded **Charcot** as professor for a few years before handing over his position to **Marie.**

He continued the Tuesday demonstrations, filling those of the first 6 months following the death of **Charcot** with a biography of the Master. Apart from describing the syndromes in the following, entries, he wrote extensively on the topic of spinal diseases and collaborated with Pierre Janet in studies of the neuroses.

Raymond syndrome See **Raymond-Cestan syndrome.**

Raymond-Cestan syndrome 1. (dissociation of lateral gaze, superior Foville syndrome, alternating abducent hemiplegia) A syndrome seen with lesions of the rostral-tegmental pons, characterized by homolateral sixth nerve palsy with contralateral hemiparesis. It has also been also described as the combination of paralysis of conjugate gaze horizontally or vertically with internuclear ophthalmoplegia, contralateral hemiparesis, hemianesthesia, and athetosis.

These signs were considered by the original authors to indicate the presence of lesions of the paramedian regions of the pons and upper medulla,[4613] as they originally reported the case of a young woman with syphilis whose illness began with dysphasia and right hemiparesis affecting the lower face and limbs, but who later showed prosopagnosia and both partial left third and sixth cranial nerve palsies; they localized the disease to the lower pons and considered that a sixth nerve palsy and alternating hemiplegia were the hallmarks of the condition, in this case due to a gumma. The syndrome now known by this eponym is thus somewhat suspect, although MRI scanning has confirmed that a lesion at the mesial pontomedullary junction can indeed produce homolateral sixth nerve palsy with contralateral hemiparesis.

2. Lateral rectus palsy with crossed hemiparesis, resulting from a lesion of the caudal-ventral pons.[5162]

Raymond-Foville syndrome See **Foville syndrome.**

Raynaud, Maurice (1834–1881) French physician who in his Paris graduation thesis described the phenomenon named for him as "local syncope," and correctly ascribed it to autonomic dysfunction.

He did not have a particularly notable professional career thereafter, although he was regarded as a fine clinician and was elected to the French Academy of Medicine.

Raynaud phenomenon The successive appearance of pallor, cyanosis, and redness of the extremities (in that order), lasting minutes or hours, the final phase being extremely painful. It is a result of excessive sympathetic vasoconstrictor activity.

The syndrome is especially common in women who are otherwise generally healthy. Its occurrence is stimulated by exposure to cold and tobacco use, and by the use of vibrating instruments, but it may also be symptomatic of small vessel disease such as the collagen vascular diseases or cryoglobulinemia.[2267,4615]

Reaction Level scale (RLS 85) An 8-point scale rating patients on factors included in the **Glasgow Coma scale** and adding an overall assessment of drowsiness and orientation.[5322]

1 Alert; no delay in response

2 Drowsy or confused; responsive to light stimulation

3 Very drowsy or confused; responsive to strong stimulation

4 Unconscious; localizes but does not ward off pain

5 Unconscious; withdrawal movements on pain stimulation

6 Unconscious; stereotyped flexion movements on pain stimulation

7 Unconscious; stereotyped extension movements on pain stimulation

8 Unconscious; no response to pain stimulation

See also **coma scales.**

reaction time   The interval between a stimulus (such as a click) and a learned manual response to it. Such an interval is increased in both hands with cerebral lesions, especially those of the nondominant hemisphere.

reactive myotonia   Local myotonia produced by muscle percussion.

reactivity   The susceptibility of individual rhythms or the EEG as a whole to change following sensory stimulation or other physiologic actions. (Adapted from the 1974 report of the Committee on Terminology, IFCN. In: Chatrian GE, Bergamini L, Dondey M, et al. A glossary of terms most commonly used by clinical electroencephalographers. *EEG Clin Neurophysiol* 1974;**37**: 538–548.[989])

reading epilepsy   (primary reading epilepsy) An induced seizure disorder in which subjects complain that their jaw snaps or opens when they read, especially aloud. Abnormal focal or generalized EEG discharges accompany the myoclonus-like movements of the mouth and throat, which progress to a generalized seizure if the subjects persist in reading thereafter.[556,558]

The mechanism may lie in afferent stimulation derived from the neural mechanisms controlling eye movements. Sporadic and likely dominantly inherited cases have been described.[1257]

Rebeitz-Kolodny-Richardson syndrome   See **corticobasal degeneration.**

rebound   A phenomenon noted by Sir Gordon **Holmes;** when the extended arm is depressed by the examiner against the patient's resistance and the pressure is suddenly removed, the subject's arm travels upward for a short distance and then recoils downward again. This last correction is the rebound or **check reflex.**

Although the upward excursion is greater in patients with cerebellar disease, the real rebound is actually the final downward corrective movement and is normally present, being reduced or lost in the presence of cerebellar disease and increased in spastic limbs.[5357]

rebound headache   (**medication-induced headache** analgesic, narcotic abstinence headache, refractory headache, rebound headache, ergotamine headache, drug-induced headache) A common, persistent, daily-occurring headache afflicting chronic migraine or tension-type headache sufferers who have, over the long term, taken to consuming acetylsalicylic acid, acetaminophen, nonsteroidal anti-inflammatory agents, benzodiazepines, ergot compounds, caffeine, narcotics, barbiturates, or combinations of these agents in increasing doses and on a regular basis, usually daily or near-daily.[4595]

The headaches have the clinical characteristics of both **migraine** and **tension-type headaches,** and are frequently increased in the mornings on waking. They are partially relieved by ingestion of the subject's usual medication. Their mechanism is unknown, but the morning accentuation of the symptom would support the existence of chemical dependence, such that headaches are triggered by falling levels of the offending drug. This perpetuates and worsens instead of alleviating the headaches, and is assumed to be the result of some alteration in the setting of serotonin 1_D receptors occasioned by frequent use of the serotonergic drugs listed.

rebound nystagmus   1. A form of horizontal jerk gaze–paretic nystagmus usually associated with cerebellar disorders. The nystagmus is seen on sustained lateral gaze; it fatigues and reverses the direction of its fast component after some seconds; on return to the center, jerk nystagmus appears with its fast component in the direction opposite the previous direction of gaze and lasts several seconds.[2636]

2. A form of gaze-evoked horizontal jerk nystagmus which is not present in the primary position but which beats transiently in the opposite direction after relaxation of sustained lateral gaze to one side. The first of these types may be followed by the second. A lesion in the cerebellum and phenytoin intoxication are the most common causes.[2636]

rebound phenomenon   See **rebound headache.**

receptive amusia   Defects in the perception and recognition of tones and melodies, due to disease of one or other temporal lobe.[821]

receptive field   That region of the skin, position of a joint, or location of an initial stimulus which, when stimulated appropriately, give rises to activity within a particular neuron.

recessive absence of tibia and deafness   A recessively inherited syndrome characterized by congenital absence of one or both tibias and severe deafness.[918] See also **Berant syndrome.**

recessive atopic dermatitis and neural deafness   A nonprogressive, recessively inherited syndrome manifesting moderate neural deafness associated with atopic dermatitis involving only the trunk and arms. Vestibular function is normal.[3124]

recessive congenital moderate deafness A recessively inherited syndrome characterized by congenital symmetrical, nonprogressive, moderate neural hearing loss, but normal vestibular function.[3124]

recessive congenital severe deafness A recessively inherited syndrome characterized by congenital severe neural hearing loss and normal vestibular function.[3124]

recessive deafness, mental deficiency, ataxia, and hypogonadism See **Richards-Rundle syndrome.**

recessive distal muscular dystrophy A recessively inherited myopathic disorder with onset in young adult life, characterized by conspicuous distal muscle weakness and atrophy affecting especially the calf muscles but spreading proximally. The arms are affected late but the small hand muscles are spared. Serum creatine kinase levels are raised and the muscle biopsy specimen changes (fiber necrosis and active regeneration) are similar to those of **Duchenne dystrophy.**[3921]

recessive early-onset neural deafness A recessively inherited syndrome characterized by early-onset severe neural hearing loss, in which essentially no hearing remains after 6 years of age, but the vestibular responses are normal.[3833]

recessive generalized myotonia See **myotonia congenita.**

recessive goiter and deafness A recessively transmitted disease manifesting severe sensorineural deafness and goiter due to a failure of iodination of tyrosine.[3124] See **Pendred syndrome.**

recessive malformed low-set ears and conductive deafness A recessively inherited disease characterized by uni- or bilateral malformed pinnae, mild to severe conductive hearing loss, and low-set ears in about half of those affected.[3124]

recessive myopia and deafness A recessively inherited syndrome of congenital severe myopia, nonprogressive neural deafness, and mild intellectual impairment.[4223]

recessive optic atrophy, hearing loss, and juvenile diabetes A recessively transmitted syndrome manifesting progressive optic atrophy, neural deafness, and diabetes mellitus from the time of childhood.[350]

recessive osteodysplasty See **Danks syndrome.**

recessive pili torti and deafness A recessively inherited syndrome characterized by congenital pili torti and neural deafness.[4628]

recessive retinal changes, deafness, muscular wasting, and mental retardation A recessively transmitted syndrome manifesting congenital deafness, retinal detachment, marked mental retardation, severe muscle wasting and weakness, and the retinal changes characteristic of **Coates disease.**[5213]

recessive retinal degeneration See **Alstrom-Hallgren syndrome.**

recessive retinitis pigmentosa with congenital deafness See **Usher syndrome.**

recessive split-hand and foot syndrome A recessively inherited syndrome characterized by the congenital absence of phalanges or syndactyly, severe deafness, and impaired vestibular function.[5969]

reciprocal contralateral leg sign See **Brudzinski signs.**

reciprocal inhibition Inhibition of a motor neuron pool secondary to the activation of the motor neuron pool of its antagonist. It is one of several important spinal mechanisms of motor control that help to make movements smoother and utilize less energy. There are multiple mechanisms for reciprocal inhibition, including one mediated by the Ia inhibitory interneuron that activates Ia afferents and disynaptically inhibits the muscle that is antagonist to the source of the Ia afferents. (From the 2001 Report of the Nomenclature Committee of the American Association of Electromyography and Electrodiagnosis.[10] Used by permission, copyright © 2001, AAEM.)

Recklinghausen disease See **neurofibromatosis.**

Friedrich Daniel von Recklinghausen

Recklinghausen, Friedrich Daniel von (1833–1910) German pathologist who trained in Berlin and was then assistant to **Virchow,** later becoming professor of pathological anatomy, in order, at Königsberg, Würzburg, and Strasbourg. He described the disease bearing his name in 1882, although a Scottish physician, Robert Smith, had published an excellent illustrated account of the same condition in 1849.[4979]

Von Recklinghausen also described osteitis fibrosa cystica, hemochromatosis, the periostitis of congenital syphilis, and fibroids, and he contributed numerous other papers to medical journals.

recognition memory test   An instrument for assessing visuoverbal and nonverbal memory, in which subjects are asked to recall which of a set of printed letters or photographs of people had been shown to them on a previous run.[5850]

recording electrode   Device used to record electric potential difference. All electric recordings require two electrodes. The electrode close to the source of the activity to be recorded is called the *active* or *exploring electrode*, and the other recording electrode is called *the reference electrode*. Active electrode is synonymous with input terminal 1, or E-1 (or older terms whose use is discouraged, grid 1and G1). Reference electrode is synonymous with input terminal 2, or E-2 (or older terms whose use is discouraged, grid 2 and G2). In some recordings it is not certain which electrode is closer to the source of the biologic activity, e.g., recording with a bifilar needle recording electrode, or when attempting to define far-field potentials. In this situation, it is convenient to refer to one electrode as input electrode 1, or E-1, and the other as input electrode 2, or E-2. By present convention, a potential difference that is negative at the active electrode (input terminal 1, E-1) relative to the reference electrode (input terminal 2, E-2) causes an upward deflection on the display screen. The term *monopolar recording* is not recommended, because all recordings require two electrodes; however, it is commonly used to describe the use of one type of intramuscular needle electrode. A similar combination of needle electrodes has been used to record nerve activity and also has been referred to as *monopolar recording.* (From the 2001 Report of the Nomenclature Committee of the American Association of Electromyography and Electrodiagnosis.[10] Used by permission, copyright © 2001, AAEM.)

recovery nystagmus   A form of spontaneous nystagmus seen to change direction as the initial stimulus producing the nystagmus (e.g., otolithic stimulation) diminishes with time.

recruitment   The successive activation of the same and additional motor units with increasing strength of voluntary muscle contraction. (From the 2001 Report of the Nomenclature Committee of the American Association of Electromyography and Electrodiagnosis.[10] Used by permission, copyright © 2001, AAEM.)

recruitment frequency   Firing rate of a motor unit action potential (MUAP) when a different MUAP first appears during gradually increasing voluntary muscle contraction. This parameter is essential to assessment of recruitment pattern. (From the 2001 Report of the Nomenclature Committee of the American Association of Electromyography and Electrodiagnosis.[10] Used by permission, copyright © 2001, AAEM.)

recruitment interval   The interdischarge interval between two consecutive discharges of a motor unit action potential (MUAP) when a different MUAP first appears during gradually increasing voluntary muscle contraction. The reciprocal of the recruitment interval is the recruitment frequency. See also **interdischarge interval.** (From the 2001 Report of the Nomenclature Committee of the American Association of Electromyography and Electrodiagnosis.[10] Used by permission, copyright © 2001, AAEM.)

recruitment pattern   A qualitative and/or quantitative description of the sequence of appearance of motor unit action potentials during increasing voluntary muscle contraction. The recruitment frequency and recruitment interval are two quantitative measures commonly used. See **interference pattern, early recruitment, reduced recruitment pattern** for qualitative terms commonly used. (From the 2001 Report of the Nomenclature Committee of the American Association of Electromyography and Electrodiagnosis.[10] Used by permission, copyright © 2001, AAEM.)

recruitment spasm   The spread of tonic spasm from one muscle to adjacent muscle groups, as in **tetanus.**

rectal crises   Paroxysmal rectal pain in tabetic patients.

rectocolic reflex   Distention of the rectum prior to evacuation precipitates the colonic contractions designed to refill it.

rectosphincteric reflex   Contraction of the external sphincter in response to rectal distension.

rectus abdominis syndrome   1. Abdominal wall pain made worse by head elevation in the supine position, and thought to be due to compression of the intercostal nerves by the rectus abdominis muscle.[3122]

2. Acute rhabdomyolysis of the rectus muscles following excessive use, as with the performance of repetitive sit-ups. Local pain, rigidity, and tenderness with an increase in serum creatine kinase values are the main findings.[4981]

recurrent   Turned back so as to lie or run in a direction opposite to the former one.

recurrent brachial neuritis and cleft palate   A dominantly inherited syndrome characterized by sudden attacks of pain in the shoulder, arms, and hands, with persisting paresthesias and weakness, winging of the scapulas, and some sensory loss in association with facial asymmetry and hypotelorism.[1697]

recurrent hypersomnia   See **periodic hypersomnia.**

recurrent inhibition   Decreased probability of firing of a motor neuron pool mediated by Renshaw cells. Renshaw cells are activated by recurrent collaterals from the axons of α-motoneurons. Such inhibition influences the same cells that originate the excitatory impulses and their neighbors. (From the 2001 Report of the Nomenclature Committee of the American Association of Electromyography and Electrodiagnosis.[10] Used by permission, copyright © 2001, AAEM.)

recurrent laryngeal nerve   That branch of the tenth cranial nerve which innervates almost all of the intrinsic laryngeal muscles. The name acknowledges the long course of the nerve, which on the left side runs below the aorta before ascending again to the larynx.

recurrent optic neuromyelitis and endocrinopathies   A demyelinating syndrome of uni- or bilateral optic neuropathy and acute or subacute myelopathy in the cervical and thoracic segments causing dissociated sensory loss, the whole culminating in blindness and paraplegia. Amenorrhea, galactorrhea, diabetes insipidus, hypothyroidism, or hyperphagia are associated problems. See also **Devic disease**.[5754]

recurring utterances   See **stereotypy.**

red boy   See **kwashiorkor.**

red ear syndrome   A disorder described by James Lance[3238] characterized by attacks of migraine-like headache with or without aura accompanied by redness and burning of the ear. Upper cervical disorders, temporomandibular joint dysfunction, atypical trigeminal and glossopharyngeal neuralgia, and local axon reflexes have been implicated in this syndrome, whose pathophysiological explanation is still not completely elucidated but it may be caused by vasodilatator peptides released during activation of the trigeminovascular system.

red glass test   Assessment of vision with a red screen placed before one of the patient's eyes. In the presence of diplopia, both a red and a white image of the light are seen by the subject, allowing in turn determination of the muscles, which are paretic according to the **rules for diplopia.**

red migraine   See **cluster headache.**

red muscles   The dark-colored striated muscles, best seen in animals or birds, composed mainly of type 1 myofibrils. They contain substantial amounts of myoglobin and oxidative enzymes, and have a slow-twitch capacity and tonic contraction functions. Compare with **white muscles.**

The back muscles in humans are representative of this type.

red nucleus hallucinatory syndrome   See **peduncular hallucinosis.**

red nucleus syndrome   See **Foix syndrome.**

red nucleus tremor   See **rubral tremor.**

red orbit syndrome   The association of redness of the eye and of the periorbital tissues with proptosis, accompanied by diplopia and/or visual loss.[5070]

red reflex   The red color normally visible through the pupil when the eye is examined with the ophthalmoscope from a distance. The presence of a cataract or of another lesion obstructing light obliterates the reflex, which is thus used for quick determination of the transparency of the ocular media.

red-and-black tremor   See **midbrain tremor.** The term derives from the supposition that the tremor is caused by damage to both the red nucleus and the substantia nigra.

red-green test   See **Lancaster red-green test.**

red-eyed shunt syndrome   Vascular dilatation of the scleral and conjunctival vessels in the presence of a **caroticocavernous fistula.**[4431]

Redlich, E.   (1866–1930) Austrian neurologist practicing in Vienna. He described **narcolepsy** independently of **Gélineau,** and his name has also been attached to that disorder.

Redlich encephalitis (Redlich-Flatau syndrome, Munch-Petersen encephalomyelitis) A poorly defined entity, either a mild but protracted form of epidemic disseminated encephalomyelitis[5047] or a presentation of **encephalitis lethargica.** Redlich and Flatau described it in the populations of Poland and Austria during 1927–1928. The nature of the infectious agent is speculative.[1884]

Redlich-Fischer plaques   "Senile" plaques found in the brain in patients with **Alzheimer disease** and **Down syndrome.**

Redlich-Flatau syndrome   See **Redlich encephalitis.**

RED-M syndrome   The combination of **R**etinopathy, **E**ncephalopathy, and **D**eafness with **M**icroangiopathy; a condition of unknown cause.[3674]

redressement du tronc   Extension of the hips and elevation of the trunk when pressure is placed on the soles of a baby seated with his or her back to the examiner.

reduced recruitment pattern   A descriptive term for the interference pattern when the number of motor units available to generate a muscle contraction are reduced. One cause for a reduced interference pattern. See **interference pattern, recruitment pattern.** (From the 2001 Report of the Nomenclature Committee of the American Association of Electromyography and Electrodiagnosis.[10] Used by permission, copyright © 2001, AAEM.)

reducing body myopathy   A progressive and fatal congenital myopathy characterized by the presence of sarcoplasmic inclusion bodies possessed of sulfhydryl groups, RNA, and glycogen, which stain positively with menadione-nitroblue-tetrazolium.

The clinical characteristics of the disorder include motor delay; hypotonia; severe, progressive proximal and distal muscle weakness; muscle contractures; and cardiorespiratory failure.[778]

In *variant* forms the myopathy is nonprogressive and benign,[4219] or occurs at a later age, in association with mitral valve prolapse and scoliosis.[4151] See also **congenital myopathies.**

redundant carotid artery syndrome   The condition in which transient ischemic attacks occur, leading to the performance of arteriography which in turn demonstrates tortuosity of the carotid artery, without ulceration or stenosis. This deviation from the assumed normal has thus been regarded as pathological.[4711] Whether it is or not is quite unproved.

reduplicative paramnesia   A specific memory disturbance (a "delusional misidentification syndrome") characterized by the subject's certainty that a familiar place, person, object, or body part has been duplicated; hence, the confabulation of the existence of two or more places with almost similar attributes, although only one exists in reality. The syndrome was first described by Arnold **Pick** in 1903.[4438]

Reduplication of time is also described and may accompany any other form, all reduplicative phenomena having as their basis diffuse dysfunction of the cerebrum.[5897] The causative lesions were considered to involve the right hemisphere (altering spatial coding of the environment) or bifrontally (preventing awareness of this deficit), but specific lesions of the anterior part of the right fusiform gyrus have now been shown capable of causing the syndrome.[2687]

The same mechanism is likely to exist when an individual believes that he or she has a double (a *Doppelgänger*); see **Frégoli syndrome, Capgras syndrome.**

reference electrode   (grid 2, G2) The recording electrode farthest from the source of the biological activity to be recorded; in general, any electrode against which the potential variations of another electrode are measured. Specifically, a suitable reference electrode is any electrode customarily connected to the input terminal 2 of an EEG amplifier and so placed as to minimize the likelihood of its picking up the same EEG activity as that recorded by an exploring electrode usually connected to the input terminal 1 of the same amplifier, or its picking up other activities.

Whatever the location of the reference electrode, the possibility that it might be affected by appreciable EEG potentials should always be considered. A reference electrode connected to the input terminal 2 of all or several EEG amplifiers is called a **common reference electrode.** See also **recording electrode, input terminal 2.** (Adapted from the Committee on Terminology, IFCN[989] ©1974, with kind permission from Elsevier Science.)

referential derivation   A recording made from a pair of electrodes consisting of an exploring electrode generally connected to the input terminal 1 and a reference electrode usually connected to the input terminal 2 of an EEG amplifier. See also **exploring electrode, reference electrode, referential montage, common reference montage.** (Adapted from the Committee on Terminology, IFCN[989] ©1974, with kind permission from Elsevier Science.)

referential montage   An EEG montage consisting of referential derivations. A referential montage in which the reference electrode is common to multiple derivations is called a **common reference montage.** (Adapted from the Committee on Terminology, IFCN[989] ©1974, with kind permission from Elsevier Science.)

referred headache   Headache or facial pain associated with disorders of the cranium, neck, eyes, ears, nose, sinuses, teeth, mouth, or other facial or cranial structures. The diagnostic criteria in Chart R–3 are suggested by the Headache Classification Committee of the International Headache Society.[1051]

Chart R–3. Diagnostic Criteria for Referred Headache

A. Clinical and/or laboratory evidence of disorder in the cranium, neck, etc. (specify)
B. Headache located in the affected facial or cranial structure and radiating to surroundings. Pain may or may not be referred to more distant areas of the head.
C. Headache disappears within 1 month after successful treatment or spontaneous remission of the underlying disorder.

Cranial Bone

Osteomyelitis, Paget disease, and multiple myeloma are possible causes of such headaches.

Neck

Cervical spine
A. Pain localized to neck and occipital region. May project to forehead, orbital region, temples, vertex, or ears.
B. Pain is precipitated or aggravated by special neck movements or sustained neck posture.
C. At least one of the following is present:
 1. Resistance to or limitation of passive neck movements
 2. Changes in neck muscle contour, texture, tone, or response to active and passive stretching and contraction
 3. Abnormal tenderness of neck muscles
D. Radiological examination reveals at least one of the following:
 1. Movement abnormalities in flexion/extension
 2. Abnormal posture
 3. Fractures, congenital abnormalities, bone tumors, rheumatoid arthritis, or other distinct pathology (not spondylosis or osteochondrosis)

Eyes

Acute glaucoma
A. Acute glaucoma diagnosed by appropriate investigations
B. Pain in the eye and behind or above it

Refractive errors
A. Uncorrected refractive errors, e.g., hypermetropia, astigmatism, presbyopia, wearing of incorrect glasses
B. Mild headaches in the frontal region and in the eyes themselves
C. Pain absent on awakening, and aggravated by prolonged visual tasks at the distance or angle where vision is impaired

Heterophoria or *heterotropia* (latent or manifest squint)
A. Heterophoria or heterotropia is demonstrated.
B. Mild to moderate constant headache in the frontal region
C. At least one of the following is present:
   1. Headache occurs or worsens during a visual task, especially when tiring
   2. Intermittent blurred vision or diplopia
   3. Difficulty adjusting focus from near to distant objects or vice versa
D. Relief or reduction in symptoms by closing one eye

Ears

Headache referred from middle ear disease.

Nose and Sinuses

Temporomandibular joint disease
A. At least two of the following are present:
   1. Pain in the jaw precipitated by movement and/or clenching
   2. Decreased range of movement
   3. Noise during joint movements
   4. Tenderness of the joint capsule
B. Positive X-ray and/or isotope scintigraphic findings
C. Pain is mild to moderate and located in the temporomandibular joint and/or radiating from there.

From *Headache Classification Committee of the International Headache Society. Classification of headache disorders, cranial neuralgias and facial pains; and diagnostic criteria for primary headache disorders. Cephalalgia 1988;8(suppl):1–96, reproduced by kind permission of Blackwell Science.*

referred itch   (Fr, synalgies; Ger, *Mitempfindungen:* [associated feelings]) 1. The phenomenon in which scratching an irritation may produce an itch elsewhere, almost always on the same side. The first modern description was that of Kovalesky, professor of physiology in Kazan, in 1885,[1717] but the original phenomenon was first described in 1733 by the English cleric and experimental physiologist, Rev. Stephen Hales.

The sensations of the stimulus and the response differ, but are always ipsilateral. The response is pinpoint, immediate, transient, and reproducible, and is usually experienced at a higher segmental level than the stimulus. The mechanism is unknown. One might speculate that this may have something to do with acupuncture points.

2. The peculiar sensation of referred itching in which a sensory stimulus in one part of the body is followed by awareness of an ipsilateral sensation akin to a sudden itch elsewhere, possibly as a result of impulses traveling through the variable spinocervical tract.[4993]

referred pain   Pain felt at a distance from the site of nociceptive stimulation, in an area innervated at the same segmental levels.

Such pain is felt deeply rather than superficially, and is often accompanied by hyperalgesia of the skin at the referred site and sometimes by muscle spasm and tenderness.[2596]

referred trigeminal syndrome   A syndrome of constantly lateralized pain lying entirely within the sensory cutaneous territory of the trigeminal nerve, in association with evidence of pathology at the level of the craniovertebral junction (Dr. C.J.F. Davis, personal communication).

reflex   (Lat, to turn back) Stereotyped, unlearned, involuntary motor responses to stimuli. Erb described "tendon reflexes" in 1875. **Westphal** published his account of the phenomenon in the same issue of the same journal (of which he was the editor), but he rejected **Erb**'s contention that the responses were reflexes.

reflex acoustic nystagmus   Jerk nystagmus induced by sudden loud noise.

reflex action   The mechanism whereby a sensory stimulus elicits a motor response without conscious participation or influence.

Reflexes were known to Descartes, Stephen Hales, and Robert **Whytt**,[5595] but the concept of reflex action was further realized by Prochaska in 1784, who stated (in his essay on the functions of the nervous system) that ["the impressions of the sensitive nerves are reflected into the motor nerves"]. **Marshall Hall**[2381] further developed the concept for clinical use. The word was used first by Johann August Unzer (1727–1799) of Halle.

reflex anoxic seizure   A paroxysmal event triggered by a painful or frightening stimulus which, by vagal stimulation, causes pronounced bradycardia or even cardiac arrest, and consequently relative cerebral ischemia, thereby inducing an anoxic seizure.

See also **breath-holding spells, febrile reflex anoxic seizures.**

reflex atrophy   The rapid and severe wasting of muscles around an inflamed or tender joint, associated with hyporeflexia.

reflex dystrophy   See **causalgia.**

reflex epilepsies   See **evoked seizures, paroxysmal choreoathetosis, paroxysmal kinesiogenic choreoathetosis, stimulus-sensitive epilepsies.**

reflex hammer   The trademark of the neurologist, much as the mirror is to the ear-nose-throat surgeon and the couch to the psychiatrist. The hammer was introduced by J. Madison Taylor and S. **Weir Mitchell** in the 1880s and a similar version (the rubber "tomahawk") is still made. **Babiński** coated a metal disk on a short handle with rubber in 1912. The hammer used by Sir Gordon **Holmes** was a disk of ivory circled by a rubber pessary, mounted upon a hollow ebony stem, allowing its alternative use as a stethoscope. The Queen Square hammer was devised in 1925 by a nursing sister at the **National Hospital** and is the standard one used in English neurology, while the German Troemner hammer is that favored on the European continent and the Taylor tomahawk finds favor in the United States. A history of the reflex hammer has been published.[3271]

reflex incontinence   The passage of urine due to contraction of the bladder wall in response to stretch, occurring in patients with severe or complete upper or lower motor neuron lesions. This forms the basis of automatic micturition. See **automatic bladder.**

reflex muscle atrophy   Unusually rapid atrophy of muscles adjacent to an inflamed or painful joint, often with loss of their stretch reflexes and due to an unidentified mechanism operating in the spinal cord.

reflex myoclonus   See **stimulus-sensitive myoclonus, cortical myoclonus.**

reflex neurogenic bladder   See **autonomous bladder.**

reflex neurovascular dystrophy   See **reflex sympathetic dystrophy.**

reflex of spinal automatism   See **flexor reflex.**

reflex sensory nystagmus   Jerk nystagmus induced by painful cranial stimulation.

reflex sympathetic dystrophy   See **complex regional pain syndrome.**

Reflex Sympathetic Dystrophy Syndrome Association   An organization founded to promote awareness of the condition, distribute information, finance research, and collect data, and organize support groups in the United States. The organization also provides referral services and publishes a quarterly newsletter. Address: P.O. Box 502, Milford, CT 06460. Tel: 203-877-3790. E-mail: jwbroatch@aol.com. Web site: http://www.rsds.org/.

reflex syncope   Brief fainting due to a vagal reflex inducing dilation of intramuscular capacitance vessels and thus reducing venous return to the heart, cardiac output, and cerebral blood flow. This is the most common form of syncope, and is usually precipitated by pain, standing for a long period, hot surroundings, or coughing. Graying of vision, collapse, pallor, sweating and cold skin, and muscular flaccidity with occasional brief myoclonic jerks are the usual features and recov-

ery is quick without confusion. See also **vasovagal syncope.**

Breath-holding attacks   in children are considered to be a form of reflex syncope.

reflexe des raccourcisseurs   See **flexor reflex.**

reflexive memory   Probably the same as **procedural memory**—a noncognitive learned motor response, similar to learned habits.

reflexology   A system of alternative medicine, the practitioners of which believe that, by digital compression of certain regions of the soles of the feet, beneficial changes can be induced in distant organs.

refractory period   General term for the time following an action potential when an excitable membrane cannot be stimulated to produce another action potential. The *absolute refractory period* is the time following an action potential during which no stimulus, however strong, evokes a further response. The *relative refractory period* is the time following an action potential during which a stimulus must be abnormally large to evoke a second response. The *functional refractory period* is the time following an action potential during which a second action potential cannot yet excite the given region. (From the 2001 Report of the Nomenclature Committee of the American Association of Electromyography and Electrodiagnosis.[10] Used by permission, copyright © 2001, AAEM.)

refractory period of transmission   Interval following an action potential during which a nerve cannot conduct a second one. Distinguish from refractory period, as commonly used, which deals with the ability of a stimulus to produce an action potential. (From the 2001 Report of the Nomenclature Committee of the American Association of Electromyography and Electrodiagnosis.[10] Used by permission, copyright © 2001, AAEM.)

refrigeration palsy   So called because of a supposed association between exposure to cold or drafts and the onset of the seventh cranial nerve paresis. See **Bell palsy.**

Refsum disease   A recessively inherited syndrome of polyneuropathy, pigmentary retinopathy, and cerebellar ataxia. See **hereditary motor and sensory neuropathy, type 4.**

Infantile Refsum disease is a neonatal variant of this condition and is a **peroxisomal disorder** with features resembling a mild form of **Zellweger syndrome**, such as facial dysmorphism, failure to thrive, hypotonia, pigmentary retinopathy, nerve deafness, seizures, hepatomegaly, and developmental delay. The possibility that adult Refsum disease may also be a peroxisomal disease thus arises. **Hyperpipecolic acidemia** is probably the same condition.[2060]

Refsum, Sigvald   (1907–1991) Norwegian neurologist who studied medicine at Oslo, where he went on to train in neurology and psychiatry. He was professor of neurology successively at Bergen and Oslo Universities, and was president of the World Federation of Neurology for 8 years. His major academic contribution was the description and elucidation of much of the abnormal biochemistry of the hereditary neuropathy named for him, but he also published widely on other aspects of neurology, especially hereditary diseases and migraine, and on electroencephalography.

regeneration The restoration of anatomical and physiological integrity through the regrowth of nerve elements following injury. It occurs to a minimal degree in the CNS; that it occurs at all in the peripheral nervous system was first recognized in 1776 by William Cruickshank (1745–1800), who worked as a dissector for John Hunter and who sectioned the vagus nerves serially in dogs; when the dogs did not die following the second (delayed) section, he deduced that nerve regeneration had occurred, and went on to demonstrate the nerve swelling and repair at the site of the first section.[4195]

regional curare test A diagnostic maneuver for **myasthenia gravis,** in which a small dose of curare is injected into the veins of the wrist and allowed to diffuse regionally, the local circulation being occluded. Standard electrical end-plate testing is then performed; in the presence of myasthenia, unusual sensitivity to the curare produces abnormal test results (**decrementing response**) where they were normal before.[1899]

Reichert syndrome See **glossopharyngeal neuralgia.**

Reil, Johann Christian (1759–1813) Danish physiologist, anatomist, and psychiatrist who was professor of medicine at Halle and later at Berlin University. He first described the insula or island of Reil, the triangular area forming the floor of the space within the insula in 1796.

He is also remembered for his descriptions of the lobes of the cerebellum and for applying the term *vegetative nervous system* to the **autonomic nervous system.**

reinforcement The augmentation of muscle stretch reflex responses as a result of slight contraction within the muscle before the stimulus is applied.

This can be achieved by getting the subject to tighten other muscles (**Jendrassik maneuver**), cough, do mental arithmetic, grasp the examiner's arm, or concentrate on anything; or it can be elicited by applying any sensory stimuli to the patient immediately before the necessary stimulus.

reinforcement sign (of **Babiński**) Extension of the paretic leg when the subject sits with the legs hanging free and pulls the hands against each other; a sign of a pyramidal tract lesion affecting that side.

rejection behavior Strong withdrawal or refusal to be touched on the face or head even if this would not produce pain; a behavioral pattern resulting occasion-

ally from lesions involving temporoparietal regions bilaterally.[3987]

rejection encephalopathy A syndrome of headache, confusion, seizures, and evidence of increased intracranial pressure occurring in renal transplant recipients during rejection episodes. The severity of the encephalopathy parallels the severity of the rejection, as estimated by serum creatinine levels.[2291]

relapse In the context of **multiple sclerosis,** the new occurrence of symptoms or signs or the recurrence or worsening of those previously existing, lasting more than 24 hours and then stabilizing or resolving, and not resulting from intercurrent fever.

relapsing corticosteroid-dependent polyneuritis See **chronic inflammatory demyelinating polyneuropathy.**

relapsing eosinophilic perimyositis A syndrome of relapsing muscle pain with biopsy and EMG findings of myositis, the biopsy specimens latter demonstrating a perimysial infiltrate, sometimes with peripheral blood eosinophilia.

The condition differs from **eosinophilic fasciitis** in the absence of pseudosclerodermic skin changes, its prompt response to anti-inflammatory agents, and the occurrence of relapses.[5073]

relapsing fever See **neuroborreliosis.**

relapsing hypertrophic neuritis See **chronic inflammatory demyelinating polyneuropathy.**

relapsing inflammatory polyradiculoneuropathy A form of **acute inflammatory demyelinating polyneuropathy** in which recurrences occur.[220]

relapsing ischemic encephaloenteropathy and cryoglobulinemia A rare complication of cryoglobulinemia characterized by recurrent encephalopathy and symptoms of gastrointestinal ischemia. The cryoglobulinemia is seldom ascertained in life. Autopsy examination shows diffuse cerebral, enteral, and systemic small vessel lesions immunoreactive for immunoglobulins and typical of mixed essential cryoglobulinemia.[2734]

relative afferent pupillary defect (RAPD) An impaired light response in one pupil relative to the other, although the consensual response is normal. This latter finding rules out an efferent lesion as the cause, and so allows a diagnosis of optic nerve disease on the side of the defective pupil response. See **Gunn pupil.**

Relative Assessment of Global Symptomatology A rating instrument for use by a close relative or a friend of a patient, assessing the latter's behavior in the community. In this assessment, the caregiver determines to what extent the subject needs help in certain activities of daily living, participates in activities or shows evidence of abnormal psychopathology or cognitive disturbance. In all, 21 items are rated.[4600]

relative refractory period   See **refractory period.**

relaxation times   (MRI) After excitation, the spins tend to return to their equilibrium distribution, in which there is no transverse magnetization and the longitudinal magnetization is at its maximum value oriented in the direction of the static magnetic field. In the absence of an applied radiofrequency, the transverse magnetization decays toward zero with a characteristic time constant (T2), and the longitudinal magnetization returns to the equilibrium value with a characteristic time constant (T1).

release hallucinations   Visual hallucinations occurring in areas of visual loss stemming from any cause.[822]

release symptoms   See **primitive reflexes.**

REM atonia   The lack of muscle (other than eye muscle) activity, characteristic of rapid eye movement sleep.

REM density   A measurement of the frequency of eye movements during rapid eye movement sleep.[249]

REM intrusion   The isolated and inappropriate intrusions of components of rapid eye movement sleep (such as eye movements or inhibition of EMG activity) into non–rapid eye movement (NREM) sleep or wakefulness, accounting for many of the symptoms of **narcolepsy,** such as **cataplexy** and **sleep paralysis.** NREM sleep intrusions (e.g., automatic behavior in patients with narcolepsy) may also occur.[249]

REM nightmare   See **nightmare.**

REM percent   The proportion of the total sleep time that is constituted by rapid eye movement sleep.

REM rebound   (REM sleep recovery) A lengthening and increase in the frequency and density of rapid eye movement sleep (REM) sleep periods following a period of REM sleep deprivation.

REM recovery   See **REMS rebound.**

REM sleep   (active sleep, desynchronized sleep, paradoxical sleep, D-state) A sleep period occurring 3 to 6 times nightly, during which the brain's metabolism is increased as physiological activity is enhanced; rapid eye movements (REMs) are recordable discontinuously, but EMG activity in most other muscle groups is inhibited, and there is total relaxation of postural muscles with dropping of the head.[235]

The EEG activity in this sleep stage is characterized by low-voltage, fast (not alpha) activity and saw-toothed waves. REM sleep occupies some 20%–25% of the total sleep time. *Tonic* stages (paralysis with muscle atonia, increased cerebral blood flow, high arousal threshold, penile erections, cortical EEG desynchronization, and hippocampal theta activity) and *phasic* stages (muscle twitching, bursts of eye movements, hypopnea, variable pulse and blood pressure, and pontogeniculooccipital spike activity) are differentiated. **Dreaming** and **nightmares** also occur during REM sleep.

REM sleep behavior disorder   A **parasomnia** characterized by abnormal activity during rapid eye movement (REM) sleep in which muscle tone is restored even though the patient is in the REM phase of sleep; this facilitates the release of stereotypic behavior during dreaming.

Such behavior occurs during the middle third of nocturnal sleep at any age, but mainly in elderly men with brainstem disease. The bizarre behavior, which may lead to physical injury of others, may represent the acting-out of dreams. The responsible lesion is considered to be in the pontomesencephalic tegmentum. In a few patients, **narcolepsy** is associated.[3575,4954]

Minimal diagnostic criteria have been suggested and are given in Chart R–4.

Chart R–4. Diagnostic Criteria for REM Sleep Behavior Disorder[3575]

A. *Polysomnographic abnormality*   At least one of the following must be noted during REM sleep:
   1. Excessive augmentation of chin EMG tone
   2. Excessive chin and/or limb phasic EMG twitching, irrespective of chin EMG tone
B. *Documentation of abnormal REM sleep behaviors*   At least one of the following must be observed:
   1. Excessive limb and/or body jerking
   2. Complex behaviors
   3. Vigorous or violent behaviors, *or*
History of problematic sleep behaviors   At least one of the following must apply:
   1. Harmful or potentially harmful behaviors
   2. Behaviors disruptive of sleep continuity
C. *Lack of evidence for seizure activity on EEG*

From Mahowald MW, Schenck, CH. REM sleep behavior disorder. In: Kryger MH, Roth T, Dement WC, eds. Principles and Practice of Sleep Medicine. Philadelphia: W.B. Saunders, 1989, with kind permission from Elsevier Science.

REM sleep intrusions   The isolated and inappropriate occurrence of components of REM sleep during wakefulness.[3576] They include components of the narcolepsy tetrad and REM dreaming during the transition between wakefulness and sleep.

REM sleep phasic events   Rapid eye movements, middle ear muscle activity, and somatic muscle twitching.[3576]

REM sleep recovery   See **REM rebound.**

REM sleep tonic events   Desynchronization of the EEG, muscle atonia, and penile tumescence.[3576]

REM sleep-related sinus arrest   A cardiac rhythm disorder that is characterized by sinus arrest during rapid eye movement sleep in people without cardiac, medical, or other sleep disorders. No sleep complaints occur, but the person may have vague chest discomfort during the day and infrequently syncope at night, should they get up.[4018]

Remak cell   Cells with functions similar to those of **Schwann cells,** the cytoplasm of which, however, surrounds numbers of unmyelinated axons. Named for Robert **Remak.**

Remak, Ernest Julius (1848–1911) German neurologist, son of Robert **Remak**. He graduated from Berlin and practiced there for most of his life, finally as professor of neurology. He remarked (but did not appreciate) the plantar response before **Babiński**.

Remak fibers Nonmedullated fibers described by Robert **Remak** in 1838.

Remak paralysis (plumbism, saturnine palsy) A peripheral motor neuropathy named after E.J. **Remak**, affecting the nerves/muscles most used, thus usually the radial forearm extensors producing wrist-drop; potentially any muscle group could be involved, however. Tremor, delirium, and somnolence witness the presence of an associated encephalopathy due to the chronic lead poisoning.[4657] See **lead palsy**.

Remak reflex Extension of the knee and plantar flexion of the toes on the side on which the thigh is stroked. This is a sign of pyramidal disease and is named after E.J. **Remak**.

Remak, Robert (1815–1865) German physiologist and professor of neurology in Posen. In his graduating thesis (University of Berlin, 1838), he described non-medullated fibers, the axis cylinder, and the origin of axons from the nerve cell, thus introducing the modern concept of the autonomic nervous system. He was also the first to define the endoderm, mesoderm, and ectoderm (in 1851), and was a pioneer of electrotherapy. He also described the **Horner syndrome** in animals, although the first description in humans was that of Claude **Bernard** in 1852.

Robert Remak

Remak sign A double sensation experienced with a single peripheral painful stimulus in the setting of **tabes dorsalis**. Named after E.J. **Remak**.

reminiscence The process of remembering events and activities, usually discursively.

remission (of multiple sclerosis) A definite abatement of signs, symptoms, or both that has been present for at least 24 hours. A remission must last for at least 1 month to be considered significant.[4504]

Remote Memory Questionnaire A multiple-choice recognition test containing questions about news items dating between 1930 and 1970, grouped by decade. The test is sensitive to dementia and its severity.[5305]

remote memory tests See **retrograde memory tests**.

renal tubular acidosis with periodic paralysis, optic atrophy, or calcification of the basal ganglia A syndrome characterized by these features and due to carbonic anhydrase deficiency II, with the responsible gene mapping to chromosome 8q32.

Renaut bodies Loosely textured, whorled structures containing few cells, found in the subperineurial space of normal peripheral nerves, especially at sites of compression.[227]

Rendu tremor A coarse tremor of the limbs, increased by attempted movement and thus resembling that of cerebellar disease, but in this case hysterical in origin. It was described in 1888 by Henri-Jules-Louis Rendu (1844–1902), a French physician at the Hôpital Necker in Paris.

Rendu-Osler-Weber hemangiomatosis A dominantly inherited syndrome of facial hemangiomas and telangiectasias in the skin, lung, and brain with cerebral arteriovenous malformations. See **hereditary hemorrhagic telangiectasia**.

Renier syndrome (adrenal hypoplasia with mental retardation and muscular dystrophy) The occurrence of short stature, adrenal hypoplasia, mental and developmental delay, and proximal and distal myopathic weakness in the presence of muscle hypertrophy.[337]

Renshaw cells Small neurons in proximity to the anterior horn cells, recurrent collaterals of which activate them to inhibit the parent motor neuron pool and the Ia inhibitory interneurons that are responsible for the reciprocal inhibition of the antagonist muscles. The cells thus dampen agonistic contraction, both directly and indirectly. They were described by Birdsey Renshaw (1911–1948), an American neurophysiologist.

reo- (Gr, behind, backward) Prefix denoting behind.

repeated dream arousals **See** repeated REM sleep interruptions.

repeated REM sleep interruptions (repeated dream arousals) A pattern of insomnia in which the subject awakens for 2–3 minutes or more during at least 75% of all nocturnal rapid eye movement sleep periods and with less than 20% of occurrences during non–rapid eye movement sleep periods[2266] (see also ASDA Diagnostic Classification[234]).

reperfusion nerve injury   An acute inflammatory response occurring when ischemic tissues are re-perfused, as a result of the enhanced production of inflammatory mediators, increased adherence, and emigration of leukocytes in postcapillary venules and leakage of proteins from the vessels. Local nerve demyelination results.[4179]

repetition   A faculty allowing the rehearsal of speech that has been heard, dependent upon normal functioning in an "arch," suggested by **Wernicke** and comprising the primary auditory reception area, Wernicke's area, Broca's area, and the primary motor area. Repetition is faulty in all forms of aphasia apart from the anomic and transcortical forms.

repetitive discharge   General term for the recurrence of an action potential with the same or nearly identical form. It may refer to recurring potentials recorded in muscle at rest, during voluntary contraction, or in response to a single nerve stimulus. See **double discharge, triple discharge, multiple discharge, myokymic discharge, complex repetitive discharge, neuromyotonic discharge, cramp discharge.** (From the 2001 Report of the Nomenclature Committee of the American Association of Electromyography and Electrodiagnosis.[10] Used by permission, copyright © 2001, AAEM.)

repetitive nerve stimulation   (repetitive stimulation test) The technique of repeated supramaximal stimulation of a peripheral motor nerve at 2–50 Hz with continuous recording of the **evoked muscle action potentials** resulting, commonly used to assess the integrity of neuromuscular transmission in the presence of disease of the motor end-plate. The abnormal response may be either a decrement or an increment in the amplitudes of these potentials.

The number of stimuli and the frequency of stimulation should be specified, as should the activation procedures performed prior to the test, such as sustained voluntary contraction or contraction induced by nerve stimulation. If the test is performed after an activation procedure, the time elapsed after the activation procedure was completed should also be specified.

For a description of specific patterns of responses, see **incrementing response, decrementing response, facilitation,** and **postactivation depression.** (Adapted from the 1987 Report of the Nomenclature Committee of the American Association of Electrodiagnostic Medicine. AAEE glossary of terms in clinical electromyography. *Muscle Nerve* 1987;**10S**:G5–G23. Copyright 1987 by John Wiley and Sons, Inc. Reprinted by permission of John Wiley and Sons, Inc.)

repetitive overuse syndrome   See **overuse syndrome.**

repetitive stimulation test   See **repetitive nerve stimulation.**

repetitive strain injury   A clinical disorder unsupported by demonstrable pathology, thought to be characterized by musculotendinous injuries caused by overload of a particular muscle group as a result of repeated use or by the maintenance of contraction.

The chief clinical features are pain (which is usually aching, burning, or boring, and which leads to easy fatigue and a decline in work performance), subjective swelling, cramping, tightness, stiffness, numbness and tingling, and impairment of dexterity and finger control, accompanied by marked tenderness to palpation and increased discomfort with limb manipulation or voluntary use.[805] See also **chronic fatigue syndrome.**

replay phenomenon   The spontaneous intrusion into consciousness of the recollection of part of a melody recently heard, silently but with exact precision; similarly, some seconds of recent scenes witnessed may be re-enacted within the inner imagination just before the onset of sleep at night.[1860]

repolarization   A return in membrane potential from a depolarized state toward the normal resting level. See also **polarization.**

Reporters test   A sensitive test to detect expressive language disturbances in aphasic patients.[1409,1410]

representation   1. The assignment of responsibility for directing motor or sensory functions of an anatomical part to a region of the brain. Thus, the function of speech is represented in the left speech area, and of discriminatory sensations in the left arm in the right parietal sensory cortex. 2. An aspect of knowledge, corresponding to the way in which this information is recorded, stored, or expressed; a coded form of information. Thus, the printing of this sentence *represents* the meaning that is to be conveyed. The next stage is to *process* the information in order to use it in cognitive tasks. 3. The mental and physiological trace of a psychological or physiological event. See **engram.**

reptilian stare   An imaginative name applied to the unblinking gaze of the patient with **Parkinson disease.**

rescue reactions   Automatic limb responses brought into play when **anticipatory** or **reactive postural reflexes** fail to maintain equilibrium.[4180]

Research Group on Motor Neuron Diseases   The World Federation of Neurology Research Group on motor neuron diseases. Membership is open to physicians with an interest in clinical or scientific aspects of motor neuron diseases, including amyotrophic lateral sclerosis. Membership provides the Research Group's official journal *Amyotrophic Lateral Sclerosis and Other Motor Neuron Disorders.* Web site: http://www.wfnals.org/.

residual latency The calculated time difference between the measured distal latency of a motor nerve and the expected latency, calculated by dividing the distance between the stimulating cathode and the active recording electrode by the maximum conduction velocity measured in a more proximal segment of the nerve. It is due in part to neuromuscular transmission time and to slowing of conduction velocity in terminal axons due to decreasing diameter and the presence of unmyelinated segments. (From the 2001 Report of the Nomenclature Committee of the American Association of Electromyography and Electrodiagnosis.[10] Used by permission, copyright © 2001, AAEM.)

resistance-capacitance coupled amplifier An amplifier in which successive stages are connected (coupled) by networks consisting of capacitors and resistors.

resistant tennis elbow Pain in the region of the lateral epicondyle that does not respond to rest, anti-inflammatory drug therapy, or local injections of anesthetics since it is due (in most cases) to entrapment of the posterior interosseous nerve at a point just below the epicondyle.

respirator brain (brain death with autolysis) The changes characteristic of cerebral autolysis in subjects whose vital support systems are artificially maintained following the death of brain cells, due to anoxia/ischemia. Swelling or congestion of the cerebral cortex, softening of the brain, and cerebellar and pituitary destruction are typical features.

Arrest of the cerebral circulation due to extremely high intracranial pressure is the supposed basis for the initial cell death.[4010]

respiratory alternans A ventilatory pattern occurring when there is a reduction in central respiratory drive and characterized by alternation of rib cage and abdominal movements.

respiratory apraxia Selective abnormalities of voluntary breathing due to increased respiratory center responsiveness to CO_2, suggesting that medullary centers are disinhibited, as may occur in patients with bilateral cerebrovascular disease.[4119]

respiratory chain An intracellular metabolic pathway comprising four functional units (complexes), disorders of which are common forms of inborn errors of metabolism, leading to heterogeneous symptom complexes ranging from isolated myopathy to severe multisystem disease with death in the neonatal period. Four complexes are presently defined:

Complex I (NADH-coenzyme Q reductase) Defects of this pathway lead to myopathy with exercise intolerance and weakness with onset in youth, or to encephalomyopathy or liver disease. Syndromes include **MELAS, Leber optic neuropathy, Leigh disease, Alpers disease, Huntington disease, Parkinson disease, dystonia, Kearns-Sayre syndrome,** cardiomyopathy, cataracts, hepatopathy, and tubulopathy.[3057]

Complex II (succinate-coenzyme Q reductase)
Complex III (reduced coenzyme Q–cytochrome-*c* reductase) Deficiency of this combination leads to myopathy or encephalomyopathy. Multiple phenotypes exist, including confusional states, **progressive external ophthalmoplegia,** pyramidal signs, and exercise intolerance.
Complex IV (cytochrome-*c* oxidase) Defects of this pathway are those most commonly detected. They are found in **benign** and in **fatal infantile mitochondrial myopathies; Menkes disease; Leigh** and **Alpers diseases;** and in the **Kearns-Sayre syndrome.**[1448]

respiratory patterns Characteristic patterns of ventilatory activity, such as **Cheyne-Stokes, Biot,** and **Kussmaul** breathing, and **central neurogenic hyperventilation.**

respiratory syncope See **cough syncope.**

response An activity elicited by a stimulus.

response-to-next-patient stimulation Perseveratory verbal or gestural activity in response to the stimulation of other patients in the immediate environment, the patient replying to questions or obeying commands when the physician has actually addressed these to, for example, a patient in an adjacent bed. The syndrome suggests severe right hemisphere damage in dextrals.[630]

In this context, one may wonder at the practice of hospitals crowding together the sickest and most vulnerable people into a single room, while charging perhaps 10 times the going rate for a hotel where such exposure would be socially unacceptable.

restiform body (Lat, a rope + a shape) The inferior cerebellar peduncle, named by Humphrey Ridley, an English anatomist, in 1665.

resting membrane potential Voltage across the membrane of an excitable cell in the absence of a stimulus. See **polarization.**

rest(ing) tremor Tremor occurring in a distal part of the body despite complete relaxation and physical support; a characteristic feature in parkinsonism.[1819] See **tremor.**

restless eyes (ocular agitation) Rapid, violent, and abrupt oscillations of the eyes at up to 100 Hz as a result of released brainstem activity following bilateral hemispheric lesions.[1847]

restless legs DIMS syndrome See **restless legs syndrome** (see also ASDA Diagnostic Classification[234]).

restless legs DOES syndrome The equivalent (near-identical) syndrome as **restless legs DIMS syndrome,** except for the patient's leading complaint, which here is of excessive daytime sleepiness rather than of insomnia. See ASDA Diagnostic Classification.[234]

restless (limbs) legs syndrome (Ekbom syndrome, fidgety feet, irritable legs, dyslysis, anxietas tibiarum, restless legs DIMS syndrome, Wittmaack-Ekbom syndrome, Allison leg jitters) An exasperating intermittent compulsion to move the legs, usually occurring sporadically, but sometimes in association with iron deficiency or peripheral neuropathy. The unpleasant nocturnal paresthesias or creeping sensations of the legs absolutely require the subject to move them. Weakness or clumsiness while walking and a sensation of cold in the legs are other occasional symptoms, all occurring in the absence of physical signs.[1623,1624,2460]

Urges such as these crop up variously; when suppressed they are known (at least by psychiatrists) as *obsessions*, but when acted out, as *compulsions*. Neurologists naturally subclassify them; compulsions to move the legs are called the *restless legs syndrome of Ekbom*; compulsions to utter and to make facial or limb movements signify that the patient has **Tourette syndrome.**

The fully developed syndrome comprises irresistible restlessness; paresthesias, prickling, tension, or aching of the legs, from which relief is gained only by moving the limbs; accentuation of the symptoms at night with resulting sleep disturbance; **periodic limb movements of sleep;** and dyskinetic or myoclonic movements while awake. The family history is often positive.[3956] A disorder of central dopaminergic systems appears to be responsible, since relief is often obtained by treatment with dopamine agonists.

Two forms are recognized: *asthenia crurum paresthetica*, which is painless; and *asthenia crurum dolorosa*, which is not. Although many diseases have been associated, no causal connection has been proved.

The following diagnostic criteria have been suggested:[5836]

A desire to move the limbs, usually associated with para- or dysesthesias

Motor restlessness

Symptoms are worse or exclusively present at rest; partial or temporary relief occurs with activity.

Symptoms are worse in the evenings or at night.

Additional features include sleep disturbance, periodic limb movements in sleep, normal CNS examination findings, a positive family history, and chronicity of symptoms with exacerbations and remissions.

Although Ekbom[1624] is to be credited with the fullest modern description in 1945, the condition was also well reported by Thomas **Willis** in 1685, thus; "Wherefore to some, when being abed, they betake themselves to sleep, presently in the Arms and Leggs, Leapings and Contractions of the Tendons and so great a Restlessness and Tossings of their members ensue that the diseased are no more able to sleep than if they were in a Place of the greatest Torture."[5988]

Variants include *familial restless legs syndrome*, a dominantly inherited form in which the typical symptoms begin in childhood; and a form in association with lipomas, ataxia, and MERRF.[872]

Restless Legs Syndrome Foundation   A charitable organization providing support and information on this condition. Address: PO Box 7050, Rochester, MN 55902–2985. Web site: www.rls.org.

restless red legs syndrome   The association of the **restless legs syndrome** with arborizing telangiectasia of the limbs, of unknown cause.[3854] See also **National Sleep Foundation.**

restrictive ophthalmopathy   The prevention of full and free ocular excursions within the orbit as a result of disease of the extraocular muscles, which either prevents their relaxation or reduces their elasticity. See also **Brown syndrome, forced duction.**

ret   A measure of the biologic effect of ionizing radiation, derived from the total dose of radiation in rads, the number of fractions in which it was given, and the time over which this irradiation took place.

Retardation–hyperkeratosis–spastic paraplegia syndrome   See **Fitzsimmons syndrome.**

rete mirabile   (Lat, a net + wonderful) 1. Galen's term for the network of blood vessels at the base of the brain in ungulates, which was also known as the *marvellous net* by Herophilus. It was considered by Galen to receive pneuma from the lungs and heart by way of the internal carotid artery, which it refined to animal spirits, the life force, for storage in the ventricles, while the unrefined material (*pituita*) was excreted into the nose and pharynx. From the ventricles the animal spirits were thought to be transported inside hollow nerves throughout the body.

The rete is not normally present in rodents nor in primates such as humans, but, since Galen's dissections were mainly performed on sheep, he was not to know that. **Vesalius'** pictures showed it in 1538, but he accepted the earlier opinion of Berengarius in denying its existence in humans 5 years later.

2. A fine network of new blood vessels emanating from the inner retinal surface.

reticular activating system   (RAS) Those parts of the lower brainstem which in the myelin-stained preparation are characterized by an interlacing network of fiber bundles, thus including all the gray masses of the tegmentum of the medulla, pons, and midbrain which do not belong to either the normal nerve nuclei or the relay nuclei of the lemniscal systems.[4003]

The system is neither an anatomical unit nor a physiological entity, although it has complex and varied relationships with consciousness. Functionally, its direct stimulation desynchronizes the EEG in a manner simulating wakening from sleep or alerting to attention. Collaterals from all afferent paths to the cortex turn into this subcortical system and EEG arousal induced by afferent stimulation can be shown to be mediated through it.

reticular reflex myoclonus   (subcortical reflex myoclonus) A fragmentary type of generalized epilepsy, in which myoclonic jerks typically affect the whole body or a segment of it, spontaneously or with movement or somatic stimulation. Muscles which are proximal or flexor are affected more than those which are distal or extensor. The origin of the abnormal movement may lie in hyperexcitability of the caudal brainstem reticular formation.

When provoked by stimulation, the condition is regarded as one form of **stimulus-sensitive myoclonus** (the other being **cortical reflex myoclonus**). It is seen most commonly in **postanoxic states** and in **progressive myoclonic epilepsy**.[2384,5127]

reticular theory   The contention of Golgi, Gerlach, and Weigert that the cells of the cerebral gray matter were in continuity, forming a reticulum or nerve net. **Cajal**'s use of Golgi's own silver stain allowed the disproof of the theory.

reticulosis of the nervous system   See **neurolymphomatosis**.

reticulum cell sarcoma   See **primary CNS lymphoma**.

retinal abiotrophy   See **Leber congenital amaurosis**.

retinal angiomatosis   See **Von Hippel–Lindau disease**.

retinal blur   Imprecise images occurring as a result of the inexact focusing of light on the retina.

retinal dysplasia   See **Krause syndrome**.

retinal dysplasia with hydrocephalus   See **Walker-Warburg syndrome**.

retinal infarction   Acute, painless, and persistent (more than 24 hours) monocular loss of visual acuity or of the visual field, with the ophthalmoscopic findings consisting of pallor of all or a section of the posterior pole of the retina.

Additional findings may include the presence of an afferent pupillary defect, embolic material in the retinal arteries or arterioles, and a cherry-red spot over the fovea in cases of central retinal artery occlusion.[2416]

retinal migraine   Repeated attacks of monocular scotoma or blindness lasting less than an hour and associated with headache. An ocular or structural vascular disorder must be ruled out. The Headache Classification Committee of the International Headache Society suggests the following diagnostic criteria (from Classification of headache disorders, cranial neuralgias and facial pains; and diagnostic criteria for primary headache disorders. *Cephalalgia* 1988;**8**[suppl]:1–96[1051]), by kind permission of Blackwell Science.

  A. At least two attacks fulfilling B and C
  B. Fully reversible monocular scotoma or blindness lasting less than 60 minutes and confirmed by examination during attack or (after proper instruction) by the patient's drawing of the monocular field defect during an attack

  C. Headache follows visual symptoms with a free interval of less than 60 minutes, but may precede them.
  D. Normal ophthalmological examination findings outside of attack. Embolism is ruled out by appropriate investigations.

retinal slip   The difference between the speed of eye movement and the speed of movement of an object viewed; this represents the input signal that controls the velociy of pursuit eye movements.

retinal slits   Defects in the retinal nerve fiber layer, best visualized close to the optic nerve head through the ophthalmoscope using red-free light. They arise as a result of atrophy of several small adjacent nerve fiber bundles, as occurs in optic atrophy stemming from various causes.

Sector defects are wedge-shaped areas in which the atrophy of the nerve fiber layer is yet more extensive, as in glaucoma, nutritional amblyopia, and retinal infarcts.[4116]

retinal vasculitis   1. A benign syndrome characterized by monocular visual blurring, swelling of the optic disk with enlargement of the blind spot, dilated retinal veins, and multiple small hemorrhages into the retinal nerve fiber layer, lasting a year or two and then regressing. The condition may be a *variant* form of **central retinal vein occlusion** but is not obviously an inflammatory disorder.[4895] See **big blind spot syndrome**. 2. The presence of focal or extensive retinal vascular sheathing or occlusion, retinal infiltrates or hemorrhages, cellular debris in the vitreous humor, and vascular leakage demonstrated on fluorescein angiography, in association with multiple sclerosis or autoimmune, granulomatous, or systemic inflammatory disease.[4903] See **papillophlebitis**.

retinal vein pulsations   Pulsations of the retinal veins at the disk head, seen through the ophthalmoscope and present in about 90% of normal subjects. Their presence is a reliable indicator that the intracranial pressure is <180 mm CSF, while the absence of such pulsations may be found in the presence of normal intracranial pressure but usually indicates increased pressure, as with obstructed venous drainage.[3369]

retinitis pigmentosa   (retinal dystrophy, rod-cone dystrophy, pigmentary retinopathy or degeneration) A heterogeneous group of noninflammatory ocular disorders, usually genetically determined and characterized by a progressive loss of photoreceptor and pigment epithelium function. All forms of genetic transmission have been described.[5129]

Clinically, the early symptoms are night blindness and clumsiness due to constriction of the visual fields. Central visual acuity is preserved in relation to peripheral acuity but there is early impairment in color discrimination. Myopia, lens and vitreous opacities, disk pallor, and retinal arteriolar narrowing are usual, but the characteristic abnormality is the deposition throughout the equatorial region of the ocular fundus of patches of black pigment with the shape of bone spicules, although this may not appear in the early stages. Electroretinography shows defective rod responses from the earliest stages.

The following diagnostic criteria have been formulated:[4295]

1. Bilateral involvement
2. Loss of peripheral vision
3. Rod dysfunction, evidenced by rod final threshold on dark adaptation and/or rod responses on electroretinography that are reduced in amplitude and prolonged in implicit time, or are not detectable
4. Progressive loss of photoreceptor function

Retinitis pigmentosa is a feature of a large number of syndromes, including those characterized by sensorineural deafness (see **Usher syndrome**), ataxia, or mental retardation; storage diseases; mitochondrial diseases; peroxisomal disorders; mucopolysaccharidoses; and skeletal dysplasias. The topic has been reviewed by Pagon.[4295]

Different forms occur according to the inheritance pattern:

Dominant A mild and slowly progressive form with onset in youth, mapped to 3q. A peripherin-related form is mapped to 6p21.1.

Recessive The most common form; it is more severe and rapidly progressive with onset in youth, and often associated with cataract and macular degeneration. Much less common is a milder, slowly progressive recessive form that has its onset in early adult life.

X-linked A rare type, intermediate in severity between the previous two.

In all, visual fields are constricted and night blindness is an early complaint. Visual fields are affected in proportion to the extent of macular involvement.

retinitis pigmentosa, ataxia, and neuropathy A sporadic autosomal or X-linked recessively transmitted condition characterized by clinical features resembling Refsum syndrome (**hereditary motor and sensory neuropathy, type 4**) but with normal serum phytanic acid levels. Sensorineural deafness and evidence of cerebellar atrophy have also been detected in such patients.[5660] See also **cerebellar ataxias** (*variants*), **NARP syndrome.**

retinitis proliferans Neovascularization extending from the retina into the vitreous. See **Eales disease.**

retinoblastoma See **primitive neuroectodermal tumor.**

retinocephalic angiomatosis See **Wyburn-Mason syndrome.**

retinocerebellar degenerations A phenotypically diverse, dominantly inherited syndrome manifesting any combination of signs consistent with retinal rod, cone, and ganglion cell atrophy; neuronal loss in the brainstem and spinal cord; pyramidal lesions; and olivo-cerebellar and dentatorubral pathway disease of early or late onset.[3653]

retinocochleocerebral arteriolopathy A syndrome of deafness, encephalopathy, and blindness due to retinal arteriolar occlusions. The cause is unknown.[626]

retinoic acid embryopathy A malformation syndrome characterized by hydrocephaly, dysplastic calvaria, ocular hypertelorism, micrognathia, and congenital cardiac defects.[4]

retino-orbicular reflex See **Descartes reflex.**

retinopathy, Raynaud syndrome, and migraine A dominantly inherited syndrome characterized by these features but without apparent linkage to the *CACNA1* gene.[5527]

retinotopy The functional topographical anatomy of the retina as represented in the visual cortex.

retraction bulbs Eosinophilic or argyrophilic axonal swellings seen in the subcortical white matter and the corpus callosum in brains affected by **diffuse axonal injury.**

retraction nystagmus (retraction–convergence nystagmus, nystagmus retractorius) A form of nystagmus in which all the extraocular muscles contract synchronously and intermittently, so that the eyes retract into the orbits with each beat.[4891]

The cause is usually a lesion such as a pinealoma in the region of the sylvian aqueduct, compressing the mesencephalon. Vertical and convergence nystagmus, pupillary abnormalities, and convergence spasm may be associated (Koerber-Salus-Elschnig syndrome).[2764]

retraction–convergence nystagmus See **retraction nystagmus.**

retro- (Lat, behind or backwards) Prefix denoting behind or backwards.

retrobulbar neuritis Inflammation of the optic nerve behind the globe of the eye, and thus invisible on ophthalmoscopy.

retrocollis A focal dystonia characterized by sustained involuntary contractions of the neck muscles, which result in abnormal extension of the head on the neck. See **cervical dystonia.**

retrograde amnesia 1. Loss of memory for remote events. 2. (pretraumatic amnesia) Loss of memory for events during a period that preceded a neurological event, such as head injury.

retrograde memory tests (remote memory tests) Psychological tests that assess a subject's memory for events acquired normally at times prior to the onset of the subject's illness—traumatic or other. See also **retrograde amnesia.**

retrolisthesis Backward displacement of a vertebra upon the one below as a result of degeneration of the facet joints.

retroparotid space syndrome   See **Villaret syndrome.**

retropharyngeal tendinitis   Constant pain in the back of the neck and head that becomes maximal within 3 weeks. The pain is aggravated by retroflexion of the neck. Swelling of the prevertebral soft tissues seen on X-ray studies and full recovery after treatment with nonsteroidal anti-inflammatory drugs are features in every case. The Headache Classification Committee of the International Headache Society suggests this definition and the following diagnostic criteria (from Classification of headache disorders, cranial neuralgias and facial pains; and diagnostic criteria for primary headache disorders. *Cephalalgia* 1988;**8**[suppl]:1–96[1051]), by kind permission of Blackwell Science.

   A. Pain in the back of the neck radiates to the back of the head or to the whole head.
   B. Pain is nonpulsating, uni- or bilateral, and aggravated severely by bending the head backwards.
   C. Prevertebral soft tissues in adults measure >7 mm at the level between C1 and C4 (special X-ray techniques may be required).
   D. Pain is alleviated within 2 weeks of treatment with nonsteroidal anti-inflammatory drugs in recommended doses.

retropulsion   The tendency for patients with Parkinson disease to move backward, as if unable to straighten up and thus to halt. The sign is iatrogenic, seldom occurring except when the physician pushes back on a patient who then takes small, fast steps (as is the case with the opposite but forward movement, **propulsion**), as if chasing his or her center of gravity.

retropulsive absences   See **tonic absences.**

Rett syndrome   A condition characterized by a progressive loss of cognitive and motor skills, autism, and the development of stereotypic hand movements, occurring after an apparently normal initial 6 to 18 months of development. It was described by Dr. Andreas Rett of Vienna in 1966 and is inherited as an X-linked dominant trait, lethal in males. An *MECP2* mutation is present in all or almost all subjects with the disorder.[158,5698]

   Repetitive movements resembling hand washing are a prominent feature, though not specific to it. The condition is not all that uncommon, but was only identified comparatively recently. Diagnostic criteria have been established[4667,5633] and are given in Chart R–5. See also **International Rett Syndrome Association.**

Chart R–5. Diagnostic Criteria for Rett Syndrome

A. Necessary criteria.*
   1. Apparently normal prenatal and perinatal period
   2. Apparently normal psychomotor development through the first 6 months†
   3. Normal head circumference at birth
   4. Deceleration of head growth between the ages of 5 months and 4 years
   5. Loss of acquired purposeful hand skills between the ages of 6 and 30 months, temporally associated with communication dysfunction and social withdrawal
   6. Development of severely impaired expressive and receptive language and presence of apparent severe psychomotor retardation
   7. Stereotypical hand movements such as hand wringing/squeezing, clapping/tapping, mouthing, and "washing"/rubbing automatisms appearing after purposeful hand skills are lost
   8. Appearance of gait apraxia and truncal apraxia/ataxia between the ages of 1 and 4 years
   9. Diagnosis tentative until 2 to 5 years of age
B. Supportive criteria
   1. Breathing dysfunction
   2. Periodic apnea during wakefulness
   3. Intermittent hyperventilation
   4. Breath-holding spells
   5. Forced expulsion of air or saliva
C. EEG abnormalities
   1. Slow waking background and intermittent rhythmical slowing (3–5 Hz)
   2. Epileptiform discharges, with or without clinical seizures
   3. Seizures
   4. Spasticity, often with associated development of muscle wasting and dystonia
   5. Peripheral vasomotor disturbances
   6. Scoliosis
   7. Growth retardation
   8. Hypotrophic small feet
D. Exclusion criteria*
   1. Evidence of intrauterine growth retardation
   2. Organomegaly or other signs of storage disease
   3. Retinopathy or optic atrophy
   4. Microcephaly at birth
   5. Evidence of perinatally acquired brain damage
   6. Existence of identifiable metabolic or other progressive neurological disorder
   7. Acquired neurological disorders resulting from severe infections or head trauma

*Modified from Hagberg et al.[2367]

†Development may appear to be normal for up to 18 months.

From Trevathan E, et al. Diagnostic criteria for Rett Syndrome. Ann Neurol 1988;**23**:425–8. ©1988. Reprinted by permission of John Wiley and Sons. Inc.

Described *variants* include[5181] *a forme fruste* with delay in the appearance of symptoms until late childhood; a late childhood regression variant, in which there is early psychomotor delay but the major features appear only at school age; a *congenital variant*, without the initial period of normality; a *familial variant*; a *preserved speech variant*; and a *male variant*.

Rett Syndrome Research Foundation   A charitable organization in this field. Address: 4600 Devitt Dr., Cincinnati, OH 45246. Tel: 513-874-3020. E-mail: mail@rsrf.org. Web site: http://www.rsrf.org/.

Retzius, Gustav Magnus   (1842–1919)   Swedish anatomist whose anatomical studies of the cerebrospinal fluid pathways and physiology laid the foundations of current knowledge.

reversal sign   A decrease in the CT scan density of gray matter and relatively increased density of white matter in the brain following hypoxic brain damage.[715]

reverse Chaddock sign   A variant of the **Babinski response** in which the stimulus consists of stroking the dorsum of the foot from the medial to the lateral side, especially with stimulation of the sural nerve territory, while the normal and abnormal responses are the same as those elicited in the classic maneuver.[5494]

reverse Marcus Gunn phenomenon   See **Wartenberg winking-jaw phenomenon.**

reverse ocular bobbing   (atypical ocular bobbing, inverted ocular bobbing) Abnormal spontaneous eye movements complicating metabolic encephalopathy or pontine hemorrhage, in which the fast phase is in an upward direction and the slow return in a downward direction. See also **ocular bobbing, ocular dipping.**

reverse ocular dipping   See **ocular dipping.**

reverse optokinetic nystagmus   That form of **optokinetic nystagmus** in which the fast phases of eye movements beat in the same direction as the movement of the stimulus, explained as the patient's own gaze-modulated spontaneous (congenital) nystagmus which is shifted to the primary position of gaze by optokinetic stimulation.[2392]

reverse postoptokinetic nystagmus   See **optokinetic after-induced nystagmus.**

reverse pursuit   A phenomenon seen in some patients with congenital nystagmus, in whom the ocular movements stimulated by the moving visual stimulus are in the direction opposite to that normally expected.

reverse straight-leg raising   See **femoral stretch test.**

reversible ischemic neurological deficit   (RIND) A minor stroke of which there remains no clinical signs after the (arbitrary) period of 3 weeks. Such stroke syndromes have a degree of severity uncomfortably situated between **transient ischemic attacks** and **ischemic infarction,** the "reversible" part of the term indicating that clinical examination demonstrates improvement in the clinical condition; an improvement that (though clinically real) may be belied by the appearances on CT or MRI scanning, which sometimes show infarction that is not appreciable to even the most talented observer.

Revilliod, Jean-Leoprard-Adolf   (1835–1918) Swiss physician who trained in Geneva and Paris and became professor of clinical medicine in Geneva in 1876.

Revilliod sign   (Herey-Simoneau sign) Inability to close only that eye on the affected side in the presence of upper motor neuron facial weakness.[4669]

revised behavior problem checklist   An inventory scale for the assessment of child behavioral disturbances.[4556]

Revue Neurologique   (*Rev. Neurol.*) A French neurological journal. Web site: http://www.info-presse.fr/fiches/revue-neurologique_1791_pro.htm/.

Rey Auditory Verbal Learning test   A complex test of learning, of the effects of interference, and of the adequacy of recognition, in which subjects are required to recall as many of a list of 15 words read out to them as they can, then to do so again with a second list, and then to recall words from the first list again. Finally, they are asked to identify whether words that the examiner reads out were or were not on the first list.[4671]

The amount of proactive and retroactive interference can be assessed as the subject supplies words variously from the wrong list.

Reye, Ralph Douglas Kenneth   (1912–1977) Australian physician who graduated from the University of Sydney and became director of pathology at the Royal Alexandra Hospital for Children. He recognized the syndrome named for him in 1951 and published an account of 20 cases of it in 1963.[1829]

Reye syndrome   (encephalopathy and fatty degeneration of the viscera, white-liver disease) A noninflammatory encephalopathy with cerebral edema and fatty degeneration of the liver and kidneys following a viral infection in small children, also facilitated by their exposure to aspirin.

Clinically, the condition is characterized by irritability, lethargy, and persistent vomiting following upper respiratory infections with influenza B, varicella, or other viral illnesses. Coma ensues, with hypoglycemia, acidosis, hyperammonemia, and ketonuria. Increased intracranial pressure due to brain edema, hyperpyrexia, hypotension, gastrointestinal hemorrhage, pancreatitis, and seizures are other potential complications and in some cases there is clinical evidence of myopathy.[4672] The condition is frequently fatal.

Intermyofibrillar edema, mitochondrial disruption, and swelling of the vascular endothelium are demonstrated in muscle biopsy specimens.[2427] Pan-lobar fatty metamorphosis of the liver with severe ultrastructural changes in the mitochondria also occurs.

Suggested diagnostic criteria (in the appropriate context) are as follows:

1. A clinical history of a preceding viral-like prodrome and a biphasic illness
2. Less than 10 cells/mm^3 in the CSF
3. Serum transaminase levels exceeding 200% of normal, and blood ammonia levels exceeding 150% of normal
4. Exclusion of other causes of encephalitis with hepatocellular dysfunction

Logically, fulfillment of the last criterion should be sufficient by itself. See also **ornithine transcarbamylase deficiency, systemic carnitine deficiency,** and **medium and long chain AcylCoA dehydrogenase deficiency,** and **National Reye's Syndrome Foundation.**

Reynolds, Russell J. (1828–1896) English physician who became professor of medicine at University College, London and later president of the Royal College of Physicians and a Fellow of the Royal Society. He first came to prominence when only 30 years old, upon his publishing a clear account of the then-current knowledge of the nervous system.

Rey-Osterreith test (Complex Figures test) A method of examining visual memory, perceptual organization, and constructional abilities, in which the subject is required to reproduce on paper a complex and meaningless pattern, after having studied it for a short time.[4670,4671]

rhabdo- (Gr, rod)

rhabdoid tumor A rare, highly malignant neoplasm occurring in early childhood, usually arising from the kidney but occasionally in the CNS.[4039]

rhabdomyolysis The process of breakdown of the muscle fiber membrane, resulting in a clinical syndrome characterized by pain, weakness, and swelling of skeletal muscles with myoglobinuria. The syndrome has numerous inciting causes, such as excessive exertion, toxins, ischemia, certain primary muscle disorders, and metabolic defects.

In some cases (**idiopathic rhabdomyolysis, paroxysmal myoglobinuria**) no cause can be detected, although there are forms in which the rhabdomyolysis recurs in adolescent males who have recently engaged in very strenuous exercise, and another in which it follows a benign febrile illness in childhood but is not recurrent. It involves damage to the membranes of the myofibrils, leading to spillage of the fluid contents of the myofibrils, myoglobin and creatine kinase being the ones most easily measured.

rhabdomyoma A rare tumor of muscle composed of or containing striated muscle fibers.

rhabdomyosarcoma A rare, primary, highly malignant tumor of voluntary muscle, often metastasizing to the orbit. *Adult pleomorphic, embryonal botroid* and *embryonal alveolar* types are differentiated; however, the tumor is usually seen in children.

Rhazes (869–962) Arabian physician who recognized and described nocturnal and febrile seizures as well as **night terrors.**

rhencospasm See **snoring.**

rheobase See **strength–duration curve.**

rheoencephalography (Gr, flow + brain + write) The use of electrical impedance plethysmography to determine changes in cerebral circulation, and indirectly to monitor changes in intracranial pressure.[3758] The procedure is now obsolete.

rheumatic chorea See **Sydenham chorea.**

rheumatic palsy See **Bell palsy.**

rheumatoid neuropathy A group of peripheral neuropathies associated with this vasculitic disease, including mononeuropathies of the upper or lower limbs, digital neuropathy, distal sensory neuropathy, and distal sensorimotor polyneuropathy.[4306]

Both pressure and intrinsic arthritis of the vasa nervorum are considered to be causal.[5282]

rhinencephalic seizures See **amygdalohippocampal seizures.**

rhinencephalon (Gr, nose + brain) That most anciently derived part of the cortex, functionally related to olfaction, memory, and emotion—thus the **limbic system.**

rhino- (Gr, nose) Prefix indicating nasal.

rhinolalia Nasal speech, as is heard in patients with weakness of the soft palate.

rhinorrhea Discharge of fluid from the nose. When serous, this is trivial and is usually due to sinusitis; but, when clear and with a measurable glucose content, it suggests CSF leakage and is thus an ominous finding.

rhizalgia Pain occurring due to irritation of spinal nerve roots.

rhizo- (Gr, a root). A root.

rhizomelia A congenital deformity consisting of disproportionate shortness of the proximal limb bones.

rhizomelic chondrodysplasia punctata (Spranger syndrome) A rare **peroxisomal disorder,** resulting from deficiency of DHAP-acyltransferase. The condition is recessively inherited, and is characterized by dysmorphisms, dwarfism, microcephaly, cataract, ichthyosis, vertebral coronal clefts occupied by cartilage, tracheal or laryngeal calcification, rhizomelia of the arms and legs, joint contractures, microcephaly, spasticity, and mental and developmental delay. Affected infants usually die within a year of birth.[2563]

rhombencephalitis Brainstem encephalitis, caused in some cases by *Listeria.*[1544] See also **Bickerstaff brainstem encephalitis.**

rhythm EEG activity consisting of waves of an approximately constant period.

rhythmias Coordinated, repetitive, seemingly purposeful and partly voluntary abnormal movements usually seen in young children or subjects with mental retardation; they include head rolling, shaking, or nodding, as well as swaying and rocking movements of the body which are regularly repeated. The anatomical basis for the movements is not known.

rhythmic movement disorder Sleep–wake transition parasomnias in which stereotyped movements occur such as head banging, head rolling, body rocking, and similar sleep-related stereotypical repetitive movements of the head, neck, or large muscle groups, often associated with rhythmic vocalization.[234]

Such features occur mainly in children during any stage of sleep. The cause and the remedy are each unknown.[3574]

rhythmic nystagmus   See **jerk nystagmus.**

rhythmic temporal theta burst of drowsiness   (psychomotor variant pattern) Extended runs of 4- to 7-Hz EEG activity frequently notched by faster waves, occurring over the temporal regions of the head during drowsiness.

The clinical significance of this pattern would be controversial, were it important enough to be so.

rhythmie du sommeil   See **jactitatio capitis nocturna.**

riboflavin-responsive lipid myopathy with carnitine deficiency   See **lipid myopathies.**

Ribot law   (law of regression) The events that occurred closest to the onset of amnesia (as in **Wernicke-Korsakoff syndrome**) are recalled least well.[85]

Ribot's rule   (1883) The language best recovered by the polyglot should be the mother tongue.

Richards-Rundle syndrome   (ataxia-hypogonadism-deafness; recessive deafness, mental deficiency, ataxia, and hypogonadism) A recessively inherited syndrome of childhood characterized by progressive hearing loss, mental deterioration, weakness, ataxia, distal muscle wasting, hyporeflexia, hypogonadism with failed development of the secondary sex characteristics, keto-aciduria, and decreased excretion of steroids.[4675]

Richardson, J. Clifford   (1909–1986) Canadian neurologist and professor of neurology in Toronto, remembered internationally for his description[5328] of **progressive supranuclear ophthalmoplegia** (Steele-Richardson-Olszewsky syndrome) and nationally for his leadership of Canadian neurology during his lifetime.

Riche-Cannieu anastomosis   An anastomosis between the median nerve in the palm and the deep branch of the ulnar nerve. As a result, the thenar muscles retain their innervation in the presence of a palmar lesion of the median nerve.[4858]

Richieri-Costa syndrome   A congenital dysmorphic syndrome comprising short stature, hypotelorism, prominent teeth, brachydactyly, camptodactyly, clinodactyly or skin syndactyly, microcephaly, and mental and developmental delay.[337]

A *variant* is *Richieri-Costa Schwartz–Jampel like syndrome* that has the added features of platyspondyly and myotonia.[337]

Richner-Hanhart syndrome   (tyrosinemia II) An autosomal recessive syndrome mapping to chromosome 16 q22.1–q22.3, in which a deficiency of hepatic tyrosine aminotransferase causes the subject to suffer palmoplantar keratoderma, keratitis, mental retardation, and any of a wide variety of neurological deficits.[4296]

Riddoch, George   (1888–1947) Scottish physician who trained at Aberdeen and, during the World War I, worked with Henry **Head** at a wartime neurological unit, where he studied traumatic brain disease and its effects on visual perception and the reflex functions of the damaged spinal cord.[4683] His administrative abilities being recognized, his research declined and the latter years of his career were spent in wartime clinical and governmental activities.

George Riddoch

Riddoch mass reflex   See **mass reflex.**

Riddoch reflex   See **nociceptive reflex.**

Riddoch syndrome   The ability to discriminate visual stimuli presented in the blind field following a lesion affecting the primary visual cortex.[4684] See **visual disorientation.**

Rieder paralysis   (Knapsack paralysis) Paralysis of the muscles supplied by the upper fibers of the brachial plexus due to prolonged compression, as from the straps of a knapsack or a hod.[4687] See **upper brachial plexus palsy.**

Riegel, Wilhelm   (fl. 1900) German neurologist and ophthalmologist, practicing in Nuremberg.

Riegel symptom   (sprung pupil) Alternating constriction and dilation of one pupil with retained light and accommodative reactions between the episodes of dilatation.[4688]

Rieger syndrome A dominantly inherited congenital dysmorphic syndrome manifesting also myotonic dystrophy, iris dysplasia, glaucoma, corneal opacities, optic atrophy, and dental anomalies.[4689]

rifle-sling palsy A compression neuropathy of the radial nerve at the level of the axilla.

right eye closure Excessive closure of the right eye ipsilateral to the side of a middle cerebral artery infarct, with slight closure of the left as well. The pathogenesis is not known.

righting reflexes Coordinated synergistic patterns of muscle contraction triggered by visual, vestibular, tactile, and proprioceptive stimuli, and designed to bring the head and the body into an upright position in order to facilitate stance and locomotion.[2435]

Such postural reflexes, normally appearing in defined order during the first year of life, are lost or suppressed in spastic states. They include:

1. *Neck righting reflex* Turning of the head to one side is followed by body movements. This is present at birth and maximal by 3 months of age.
2. *Labyrinthine righting reflex* Extension of the neck of the infant suspended prone, or flexion of the neck in the supine infant. This is present at 2 months and is maximal at 10 months of age.
3. *Body righting reflex* A modification of the neck righting reflex, appearing at 7–12 months of age.[2732]

rigid spine syndrome A relatively benign, nonprogressive myopathy affecting children who show marked limitation of flexion (and later extension) of the cervical and dorsolumbar spine due to myopathic shortening of the spinal extensor muscles. Less important signs include mild and nonprogressive proximal muscle weakness, flexion contractures, waddling gait, scoliosis, and a reduction in subcutaneous fat.[5736] Nocturnal hypoventilation is a dangerous complication recorded in some cases. EMG shows myopathic changes and serum creatine kinase are moderately raised.

A type 1 fiber myopathy is usually the basis of the syndrome but that it represents a single pathological entity is unlikely. It was described first by Dubowitz in 1965.[1530] The same phenotype occurs in **nemaline myopathy, Emery-Dreifuss syndrome, acid maltase deficiency** and **Bethlem myopathy,** and in a late-onset myopathy with spinal extensor contractures, seen in adults. See also **congenital muscular dystrophy.**

Variants include the following:

An *autosomal recessive neurogenic* form with facioscapuloperoneal atrophy[4312]

A *recessively inherited* form This form is characterized by the onset of symptoms in childhood, as in the usual form, and by the presence of autophagic vacuoles, muscle spindle swelling, and type 1 fiber predominance on muscle biopsy specimens.[3477]

A form that is not benign, characterized by pronounced weakness of the vertebral column and limb girdles, severe respiratory muscle weakness, including weakness of the diaphragm, paraspinal wasting, and diffuse proximal weakness, which are accompanied by a myopathic appearance on EMG. Muscle biopsy specimens show inclusions similar to those seen in mitochondrial myopathy, with marked variability in appearance and fiber size.[6007]

A *lethal, dominantly inherited* variety, otherwise clinically similar to the preceding form.[4474]

Familial mixed congenital myopathy with rigid spine phenotype An autosomal dominant form characterized by the early onset of a slowly progressive myopathy and rigid spine syndrome and pathologically by cytoplasmic bodies, tubulofilamentous inclusions, increased desmin storage, and microscopic features of reducing body myopathy.[4635]

rigidity (from Lat, stiff) Increased involuntary resistance to passive stretching of muscles throughout the range of movement. Three major types are described: *plasticity*, in which the degree of resistance is constant and does not change throughout the range of movement tested; *cogwheel rigidity*, in which a ratchet-like sensation is transmitted to the examiner's hand; and *paratonia* (**gegenhalten**), in which the resistance increases in proportion to the stretching force applied.

From the viewpoint of electrodiagnosis, rigidity is defined as a velocity independent increase in muscle tone and stiffness with full range of joint motion as interpreted by the examiner. It is often associated with simultaneous low-grade contraction of agonist and antagonist muscles. Like muscle spasticity, the involuntary motor unit action potential activity increases with activity or passive stretch but it does not seem to change with the velocity of stretch and, on passive stretch, the increased tone has a "lead pipe" or constant quality. It is a cardinal feature of central nervous system disorders affecting the basal ganglia. (Adapted from the 2001 Report of the Nomenclature Committee of the American Association of Electromyography and Electrodiagnosis.[10] Used by permission, copyright © 2001, AAEM.)

rigor (Lat, stiffness. Gr, shuddering) Both meanings of the term are in use today, the Latin for continuous stiffness (**rigor mortis**) and the Greek for intermittent contractions, as with a rigors as part of a febrile illness.

Riley-Day syndrome (familial dysautonomia) A recessively inherited syndrome of sensory neuropathy with autonomic dysfunction, seen mainly in Jewish children and mapped to 9q31–33. The main clinical features are lack of tearing, blotchy red skin marks, postural hypotension, febrile episodes, hyperhidrosis, indifference to pain as a result of the somatic sensory neuropathy, ageusia, lack of tongue papillae, and speech disorder. Few patients survive beyond adolescence.[4695]

Nerve biopsy specimens show marked reduction in the number of unmyelinated fibers and of large myelinated fibers above 12 μm.[53] See **hereditary sensory and autonomic neuropathy, type 3.**

Riley-Schwachman syndrome A syndrome of abnormal gait, pyramidal signs in the legs, easy fatigue, anorexia with emaciation, and symmetrical areas of increased density and dilatation of the bony shafts of the long bones with lucencies seen on X-ray films.[4696]

Riley-Smith syndrome   A dominantly inherited syndrome of congenital macrocephaly, pseudopapilledema with normal vision, and multiple subcutaneous angiomata.[4698]

rimmed vacuoles   Nonstorage autophagic cytoplasmic vacuoles exhibiting lipid and granular staining in their periphery and surrounded by filaments. Though characteristic of the **familial periodic paralyses,** they are also found in the settings of inclusion body myositis, oculopharyngeal dystrophy, distal myopathy, and neurogenic muscle atrophies.[1283]

RIND   See **reversible ischemic neurologic deficit.**

ring chromosome 20 syndrome   A syndrome presenting with a confusional state (nonconvulsive status epilepticus) or refractory seizures lasting minutes to hours with abnormal EEG findings (bilateral slow waves with occasional spikes), mapped variously to 20p.13q3; p13q.13p; and p13q13.33.[4516]

ring scotoma   A scotoma that encircles the central part of the visual field. This is most commonly seen in glaucoma and in pigmentary retinal degenerations, but may also be produced by the wearing of strong positive lenses.

ring scotoma with nasal step   A ring scotoma formed by the fusion of arcuate defects that do not join perfectly at the equator, giving rise to the "step" on the nasal side of the disk.

ringebinden   See **ringed fibers.**

ringed fibers   (ringebinden, rinngbande) Striated myofibrils surrounded by an aberrant spiral of cross-striated myofibrils ("spiral annulets"), which in cross section appear as a circle. They are found most commonly in muscles containing sarcoplasmic masses (e.g., **myotonic dystrophy**), but also in normal muscles.[534]

Rinne test   A bedside hearing test comparing air and bone conduction. A vibrating tuning fork (512 Hz) is held first with its foot on the mastoid process and, when the subject can no longer hear the hum, beside the ear. Normally, the subject hears the ringing more loudly when the fork is in the second of these positions (air better than bone conduction). In patients with middle ear (conductive) deafness, the sound is heard more loudly when the fork is applied to the mastoid process (so that bone is better than air conduction).

The test was described by H.A. Rinne (1819–1868), a German otolaryngologist.[4708a] See also **Weber** and **Schwabach tests.**

rinngbande   See **ringed fibers.**

Rio-Hortega, Pio del   Spanish histologist, remembered for his stains for microglia, oligodendroglia, and nerves.

Rio-Hortega stain   A glial metallic implant method using ammoniacal silver nitrate and formalin, of particular value in demonstrating astrocytes, oligodendroglia, and microglia.

Rip van Winkle syndrome   The process of adaptation to major environmental change that has occurred during the subject's prolonged absence from familiar surroundings. Refuge from the environment obtained by sleeping is a prominent feature.

In the story of Washington Irving, van Winkle slept for 20 years; many patients discharged from long-term care institutions into a "caring" environment have been away longer than that, but difficulty in adaptation to home and work with subsequent depression is also described in young patients discharged after only a few months in hospital.[4518]

A similar syndrome of hypersomnia may be familial, and is also a feature in some patients after stroke.

rippling muscle disease   (OMIM 600332) A rare dominantly inherited or sporadic disorder of muscle due in some cases to a mutation at chromosome 1q41, presenting with painful muscle stiffness and cramps, mainly in the legs and worse with exercise, slowly moving self-propagating ("rippling") contractions of these muscles in response to stretch, and painful mounding of muscles after percussion, resembling myotonia except for the absence of accompanying electrical discharges.[849,4682] Serum CK levels are raised. The phenomenon may evidence stretch-activated channels in human skeletal muscle.

A variant is *sporadic rippling muscle syndrome*, which is the same syndrome associated with thymoma and myasthenia gravis. A caveolin-3 mutation has been detected in one case.

RISA cisternography   The injection of radio-iodinated serum albumin (RISA) into the lumbar subarachnoid space, with serial scintillation scanning of the spine and cranium to determine the rate and pattern of CSF flow.[1432]

RISA ventriculography   The injection of radio-iodinated serum albumin into the lateral ventricles, with serial scintillation scanning of the cranium to determine the rate and pattern of CSF flow.[1432]

The many false-positive and false-negative results have led to uncertainty about the value of the test in the diagnosis of **normal-pressure hydrocephalus.**

rise time   The interval from the onset of a change in polarity of a potential to its peak.

risus sardonicus   Spasm of the facial muscles as in tetanus, drawing the mouth open, narrowing the palpebral fissures, and elevating the eyebrows, and thus giving the appearance of a forced smile. "A sneering grin was thought of old to resemble the effect of Sardinian ranunculus, which on being chewed, contorted the face of the eater".[6000]

Ritchie Russell, W. (1903–1980) English neurologist, professor of clinical neurology at the University of Oxford. His most respected research was that on craniocerebral trauma, performed at the military Head Injury Center situated in Oxford during and after the World War II, and on the management of poliomyelitis. He was also a teacher who built up the Oxford neurological school to a position of eminence, and served as editor of the *Journal of Neurology, Neurosurgery and Psychiatry.*

ritualistic movements Patterned movement sequences, commonly slow, squirming hand movements frequently accompanied by a blank stare and withdrawal of the child from any interaction with the environment. The ritual can, however, be interrupted by stimulation and the condition is not epileptic in origin. It is seldom seen outside the age range of 2–4 years.

river blindness See **onchocerciasis.**

Rivermead Activities of Daily Living scale An instrument for the assessment of residual functions in patients after stroke. Sixteen items to do with self-care (e.g., shaving, washing, and combing hair) and 15 household activities (e.g., making a hot drink or a snack, making a bed, vacuuming) are scored.[3415]

Rivermead Behavioral Memory test An instrument for assessing nonverbal memory.[5993]

Rivermead Mobility index A scale assessing overall mobility within the context of any neurological disorder such as stroke or **multiple sclerosis.** The patient is asked the questions, listed in Chart R–6, and the response scored.[1102]

Chart R–6. The Rivermead Mobility Index

1. Turning over in bed: Do you turn over from your back to your side without help?
2. Lying to sitting: From lying in bed, do you get up to sit on the edge of the bed on your own?
3. Sitting balance: Do you sit on the edge of the bed without holding on for 10 seconds?
4. Sitting to standing: Do you stand up (from any chair) in less than 15 seconds and stand there for 15 seconds (using hands, and with an aid if necessary)?
5. Standing supported: Observe the patient standing for 10 seconds without any aid.
6. Transfer: Do you manage to move from the bed to the chair and back without any help?
7. Walking inside, with an aid if needed: Do you walk 10 meters, with an aid if necessary, but with no standby help?
8. Stairs: Do you manage a flight of stairs without help?
9. Walking outside (even ground): Do you walk around outside on the sidewalk without help?
10. Walking inside, with no aid: Do you walk 10 meters inside, with no walker, splint, or aid and without standby help?
11. Picking off floor: If you drop something on the floor, do you manage to walk 5 meters, pick it up, and then walk back?
12. Walking outside (uneven ground): Do you walk over uneven ground (grass, gravel, snow, ice, etc.) without help?
13. Bathing: Do you get in and out of the bath or shower unsupervised, and can you wash yourself?
14. Up and down four steps: Do you manage to go up and down four steps with no rail, using an aid if necessary?
15. Running: Can you run 10 meters without limping in 4 seconds? (a fast walk is acceptable).

A score of 1 is given for each "yes" answer.

From Lincoln N, Leadbitter D. Assessment of motor function in stroke patients. Physiotherapy 1979;**65**(2):48–51, by permission.

Rivermead Motor assessment An instrument for assessing motor function in patients who have suffered stroke. Gross motor function, leg and trunk movements, and arm functions are rated after clinical enquiry and physical examination.[3413]

Rivers, William Halse (1864–1922) English physician who experimentally sectioned a peripheral nerve of Henry **Head** (at Sir Henry's request).[4713]

Roaf sign Tilting of the neck, a posture adopted by patients with a spinal cord injury complicated by root avulsion.[4716]

Roberts syndrome (pseudothalidomide syndrome) A congenital dysmorphic syndrome characterized by short stature, sparse depigmented hair, dysplastic ears, hypertelorism, proptosis, cloudy corneas, cataract, blue sclerae, facial hemangiomas, cleft lip and palate, congenital heart disease, multiple renal cysts, digital deformities, syndactyly, hypoplastic thumbs, microcephaly, encephalocele, cranial meningocele, hydrocephalus, and mental and developmental delay.[337] See **cleft lip–palate and tetraphocomelia.**

Robertson, D.M.C.L.A. See **Argyll Robertson.**

Robin, Charles (1821–1885) French histologist who described the perivascular lymphatic spaces in 1868. **Virchow** demonstrated that, in the brain, these contained CSF. They are now known as **Virchow-Robin spaces.**

Robin, Pierre See **Pierre Robin.**

Robinson ectodermal dysplasia A dominantly inherited congenital dysmorphic syndrome manifesting also dental anomalies, hypoplastic nails, and sensorineural deafness.[4730]

robotic speech A disorder of enunciation in which the syllables are separated, slowing the flow. It resembles the "scanning" speech described in patients with cerebellar disease.[2109]

Rochon-Duvigneau syndrome Dysfunction of cranial nerves III, IV, VI, and of the first division of cranial nerve V, with blindness, exophthalmos, and some vegetative disturbances, as a result of a tumor in the superior orbital fissure.

Nevertheless, Rochon-Duvigneau described this syndrome in patients with syphilis.[4734] See **superior orbital fissure syndrome.**

Rocky Mountain spotted fever   A rickettsial infection with a tick vector, most commonly found in northern California and the eastern part of the United States. The clinical disease is seasonal, with maximum incidence in the spring and summer, and is the result of widespread vasculitis.

Clinically, fever, chills, headaches, myalgia, conjunctival injection, photophobia, skin rash, and features of encephalitis with delirium, convulsions, focal neurological deficits and coma may occur, and in many cases these persist after recovery. The Weil-Felix reaction shows agglutination of strains OX 19 and OX 2, but the specific diagnosis can be made using complement fixation tests.[3882]

rod bodies   Tetragonal filaments in structural continuity with thin filaments, detected within muscle fiber sarcoplasm, which originate from the Z-disk and in which the periodic lines are perpendicular and parallel to the long axis.[1656]

They are seen in nemaline myopathy, polymyositis, and certain forms of limb-girdle dystrophy.

rod body myopathy   See **nemaline myopathy.**

rod monochromatism   See **cone dystrophy.**

rod-cone dystrophy   See **retinitis pigmentosa.**

Rodiet-Cans sign   Corneal anesthesia occurring in chronic alcoholic patients.[4736]

Roger sign   Numbness of the chin. See **numb chin syndrome.**[3681]

rolandic seizures   See **benign childhood epilepsy with centrotemporal spikes** and *variants.*

rolandic spikes   See **central-midtemporal spikes.**

rolandic vein occlusion   (Merwarth syndrome) A progressive pyramidal syndrome primarily affecting the leg, due to occlusion of this cortical vein.[3847]

Rolando, Luigi   (1773–1831) Italian professor of anatomy in Sardinia and later at Turin, who first described the substantia gelatinosa, the central sulcus or fissure in 1825 (named for him by Leurat in 1839), and the motor area lying anterior to it. However, the ascription of his name to the latter structures was in error, Leurat being unaware of their earlier description by **Vicq d'Azir.** Following animal experiments, Rolando also demonstrated the homolateral motor functions of the cerebellum in humans, in 1809.

benign focal epilepsy with centrotemporal spikes, popularly known as *rolandic epilepsy,* is named for the anatomy, not the anatomist.[5733]

Rolex sign   The effect of hypokinesia upon self-winding watches, leading to the complaint that the watch does not keep proper time. This is of occasional value in the diagnosis of early Parkinson disease.

roller coaster headache   Head pain due to the generation of a chronic subdural hematoma by the gravitational stresses imposed when riding giant roller coasters.[1791]

Dissection of the internal carotid or vertebral arteries represents another complication of this search for liberation from gravity.

rollers   See **dancing mania.**

Rollet syndrome   (orbital apex syndrome, Tolosa-Hunt syndrome) See **superior orbital fissure syndrome.**[4747]

rolling arm test   See **forearm rolling test**

Romano-Ward syndrome   See **familial Q-T prolongation syndrome.**

Romberg disease   See **Parry-Romberg syndrome.**

Romberg, Moritz Heinrich   (1795–1873) German physician, professor at the University of Berlin. He was the author of the first textbook emphasizing neurological symptoms and signs (*Lehrbuch der Nervenkrankheiten des Menschen,* 1840–1846), but although he named **tabes dorsalis** and gave a good description of achondroplasia, the **Argyll Robertson pupil, facial hemiatrophy,** and numerous other disease states well recognized today, he is best remembered for his test of conscious proprioception (see **Romberg test**).

The correct spelling of his surname (without an "h") is a neurological shibboleth.

Romberg sign (test)   A test of conscious proprioception, in which the patient stands and the amount of body sway is compared when his or her eyes are open to that which occurs when they are closed. Increased sway or unsteadiness actually amounting to a tendency to fall when the eyes are closed indicates proprioceptive failure. Gross swaying *without* falling frequently has a psychogenic basis.

Romberg published his accounts of the sign in his *Lehrbuch der Nerven-Krankheiten des Menschen* between 1840 and 1846, considering it diagnostic of tabes dorsalis.[4754] The origination of the sign has been reviewed.[3273]

Romberg spasm   A form of masticatory spasm of unknown cause, probably dystonic.

Romberg syndrome   A syndrome that is usually sporadic, comprising facial hemiatrophy with onset in childhood, contralateral focal sensory or motor seizures, trigeminal neuralgia, and changes in the eyes and hair.[4753] See **Parry-Romberg syndrome.**

Rommen syndrome   A congenital dysmorphic syndrome also characterized by short stature, Fallot tetralogy, thyroglossal cyst, skeletal deformities, seizures, brachycephaly, microcephaly, plagiocephaly, and mental and developmental delay.[337]

room tilt illusion   The transient perception of a 90° shift in the environment following vestibular stimulation in subjects with skew deviations due to brain stem lesions.[5586]

Roos test   The patient is asked to raise the arms into the "stick-up" position, causing abduction and external rotation at the shoulder, and to open and close the hands repeatedly. Pallor and lack of pulsations in the limb suggests the presence of a vascular thoracic outlet syndrome. Pain and numbness in C8 distribution may accompany the vascular signs.[3418]

root lesions   Lesions that impinge upon the spinal nerve roots, leading to either sensory or motor features. Prolapsed intervertebral disks and tumors are the more common examples. See **radiculopathy.**

rooting reflex   (search reflex) Exploration of the mother's skin by the normal full-term baby's mouth in an effort to locate the nipple, stimulated by the touch of her skin on the baby's cheek or lips; a developmental reflex.[4370] Similarly, touching the cheek of the infant with the tip of the index finger induces opening of the mouth and turning of it toward the stimulus.[6064]

The reflex appears at 30 weeks' gestation and normally disappears at 1 year of age. See also **developmental reflexes.**

Roque sign   Left pupillary dilatation and mild proptosis in association with aneurysmal dilation of the aorta. This, the opposite of **Horner syndrome,** may have been what **Pourfour Du Petit** described; it is presumably due to irritation of the sympathetic chain.

Rosai-Dorfman disease   (sinus histiocytosis with massive lymphadenopathy) A histiocytic proliferative disorder usually presenting with massive cervical lymphadenopathy but capable of invading, skin, sinuses, and many other sites including the intracranial compartment.[4428]

Rose disease   (Rose-Villar syndrome, Janin tetanus, Klemm tetanus) Tetanus confined to the muscles of the head following a head wound, manifesting spasmodic dysphagia and facial paresis. It carries a prognosis even more deadly than other forms of tetanus.[4775] See **cephalic tetanus.**

Rose tetanus   See **cephalic tetanus.**

Rosen neuralgia   Tic-like neuralgic pain in the territory of the chorda tympani; a variant of **glossopharyngeal neuralgia.**[4777]

Rosen scale   A modification of the **Hachinski scale,** shortened without apparent loss of reliability, which scores only the following: abrupt onset, stepwise deterioration, history of stroke, focal neurological signs, emotional incontinence, and somatic complaints.[4780]

Rosenbach, Ottomar   (1851–1907) Silesian physician who trained at the University of Berlin. After graduation he worked with Nothnagel and then practiced in Breslau, eventually as professor, until induced to go to Berlin. He analyzed the abdominal reflexes in 1876.

Rosenbach sign   1. Fine tremor of the gently closed eyelids in the presence of dysthyroid ophthalmopathy. 2. Absence of the abdominal reflexes on the side of a hemiparesis[4781] and also in the presence of acute abdominal disease.

Rosenberg-Bertstrom disease   A dominantly inherited condition manifesting ataxia, deafness, renal insufficiency, and hyperuricemia.[4783]

Rosenberg-Chutorian syndrome   A recessively inherited condition with onset in infancy or childhood, manifesting optic atrophy, **hereditary motor and sensory neuropathy,** and progressive nerve deafness.[4791]

Rosenthal, Curt   (fl. 1930) German neuropsychiatrist at the University of Breslau. He described sleep paralysis in 1927, but noted that earlier reports of the same condition were known since 1903; his paper called attention to the overwhelming fear that may attend this experience.

Rosenthal fibers   Cylindrical, hyaline astrocytic processes staining with acid dyes, found in areas of fibrillary gliosis, diffusely in the brain in **Alexander disease,** and in the more indolent gliomas and ependymomas such as pilocytic astrocytomas or ependymomas.[6] See also **palatal myoclonus.**

Rosenthal syndrome   (Munzer-Rosenthal syndrome, cataleptic hallucinatory fear syndrome) See **sleep paralysis.**

Rosenthal-Melkersson syndrome   See **Melkersson-Rosenthal syndrome.**

Rose-Villar syndrome   See **cephalic tetanus.**

Ross syndrome   The combination of the tonic (**Adie**) pupil, areflexia, and segmental hypohidrosis, leading to fever, tachycardia, tachypnea, and even exhaustion (heat stroke) when the patient gets very hot.[4800] The autonomic dysfunction may, however, be more widespread than this description suggests.

A *variant* is *Ross syndrome plus*, in which there is also a **Horner syndrome.**[5135]

Rossolimo, Grigoryi Ivanovitch   (1860–1928) Russian physician, who described "myotonia atrophica" in 1902,[4807] 7 years before Steinert, whose name is often given to the disease.

Rossolimo reflex   1. (Rossolimo-Goldflam reflex) See **plantar muscle reflex.** 2. The **anal reflex** 3. (Rossolimo reflex of the hand) Percussion of the volar aspect of the flexed fingers leads to further flexion of the fingers and supination of the forearm in patients with pyramidal lesions affecting the arm.[1349a]

Rossolimo-Goldflam reflex   See **plantar muscle reflex.**

rostral basilar artery syndrome   Rostral brainstem, diencephalic, and posterior hemisphere dysfunction as a result of vascular occlusive disease of the rostral basilar artery.

Clinically, numerous named and unnamed syndromes may result, although an acute confusional state initially seems invariable. **Déjèrine-Roussy, Benedikt, and Weber syndromes;** thalamic amnesia; visual field defects; limb anesthesia or dysesthesia; and a variety of motor signs affecting the face and arm more than the leg are all examples. In many such cases the clinical features are reversible.

Subcortical aphasia, hemiballism, acute amnestic syndromes; Balint syndrome; hemispatial neglect; hemispatial agnosia; internuclear ophthalmoplegia; visual associative agnosia; color agnosia, anosognosia; dysorthographia, topographic agnosia, peduncular hallucinosis; vertical gaze paresis; delirium; and **preangular alexia** are also described.[3807]

rostral dominance   Of two touches simultaneously applied to the face and the hand, it is the former that is normally more likely to be perceived.

rota-   (Lat, wheel)

rotary nystagmus   See **torsional nystagmus.**

rotary pursuit   A motor learning task in which the subject's ability to hold a stylus continually to a rotating target is measured in the two hands successively.[1132] See **pursuit rotor test.**

rotation test   A method for assessing the side of a diseased labyrinth; the patient, who is seated on a revolving chair, is rotated 10 times in 20 seconds with the head bent forward at 30°; the nystagmus that results is assessed after such rotations in each direction. It is greater in severity and duration when the rotation occurs in the direction of the affected side.

rotational nystagmus   (perrotational response, postrotational response) A physiological form of horizontal jerk nystagmus of the peripheral vestibular type induced by endolymphatic movement as a result of rotatory acceleration of the subject, which causes asymmetrical stimulation of the labyrinths.

During the rotation, the fast phase of the nystagmus is in the direction of rotation; after rotation ceases, the fast phase is in the opposite direction.[5] See also **vestibular nystagmus.**

rotatory nystagmus   That form of nystagmus with a torsional component about the anteroposterior axis of the eye. It is usually due to brainstem lesions but may be congenital. See **torsional nystagmus.**

rotatory seizures   (circular, volvular, or gyratory seizures) Generalized or partial seizures during which the subject turns around one or more times. The direction of turning has no localizing value.[4881]

Roth spots   Pale areas representing organized leukocytes and fibrin following hemorrhage in the retina, as in bacterial endocarditis, described by M. Roth (1839–1914), a Swiss pathologist in Basel. See **white-centered retinal hemorrhages.**

Roth, Vladimir K.   (Rot, V.K.) (1848–1916) Russian neurologist, a pupil of **Korsakoff.**

Roth-Bernhardt disease   See **meralgia paresthetica.**

Roth-Bielschowsky syndrome   (pseudo-ophthalmoplegia) Paralysis of conjugate gaze in one direction, but with retention of the slow phase of conjugate deviation on caloric testing. This is evidence of a supratentorial lesion affecting the pathways for conjugate gaze in the tectum.[1076]

Rothmund-Thompson syndrome   See **poikiloderma congenitale.**

Roussy, Gustave   (1874–1948) Swiss-French neuropathologist who trained in Geneva and Paris, and became professor of pathological anatomy at the University of Paris and later dean of the faculty and rector there.

He published on the thalamic syndrome bearing his name and that of **Déjèrine** (to whom he was assistant) while he was still an intern, and wrote also on the topics of hypothalamic lesions, syringomyelia, and other spinal lesions, as well as neurophysiology. The other two syndromes to which his name is attached are defined in the next two entries.

Gustave Roussy

Roussy-Cornil syndrome   (progressive, nonfamilial hypertrophic neuritis) A demyelinating sensorimotor peripheral neuropathy with onset usually after the third decade, affecting the upper limbs more than the lower. Sensory ataxia, lancinating pains, generalized areflexia, and intention tremor may also be evident.[4822]

This condition resembles **hereditary motor and sensory neuropathy,** for example of type 3, but has its onset in adult life and is sporadic.

Roussy-Levy syndrome (hereditary areflexic dystasia; OMIM #180800) A dominantly inherited condition associated with partial duplication at chromosome 17p11.2. related to the spinocerebellar degenerations and manifesting pes cavus, sensory and gait ataxia, areflexia, awkward movements, and a mild cerebellar intention tremor, but no nystagmus, present from the time of infancy. Kyphoscoliosis, sensory changes, extensor plantar response, and typical cerebellar signs are absent.

The presence of pyramidal signs was hinted at, but Roussy and Levy did not describe the pathology in their original paper in 1926.[4823] The syndrome is now thought to represent a combination of **hereditary motor and sensory neuropathy** (HMSN) with **benign essential tremor.** Confusion with **Friedreich ataxia** is less likely when it is recalled that the latter is inherited in an autosomal recessive manner, so that most patients have no affected relative (but a few HMSN type 1 kinships also show recessive inheritance). See **hereditary motor and sensory neuropathy, type 1.**[259]

Rowland-Payne syndrome The association of recurrent laryngeal and sympathetic nerve palsies due to their compression by lymph nodes in the neck at the level of C6.

Royal Free disease See **chronic fatigue syndrome, postinfection fatigue syndrome.**

R-R interval variation A measure of vagal influences upon the heart, derived from continuous electrocardiographic recordings obtained during deep breathing or with the Valsalva maneuver. With deep breathing, the variation between the maximal and minimal heart rate is normally 15 beats per minute or more; 10 beats per minute or less is definitely abnormal. With the Valsalva maneuver, the normal ratio is 1.21 or more and less than 1.20 is abnormal.[1722] See **autonomic function tests.**

RSD See **reflex sympathetic dystrophy.**

rub epilepsy A form of reflex epilepsy induced by prolonged or repetitive stimulation of the skin or (as with toothbrushing) of mucosal surfaces. The site of excitation is usually on the left side and leads to a sensory Jacksonian march of symptoms starting at the site stimulated, but a motor march may occur with toothbrushing. The phenomenon is considered to reflect the effect of propagation of epileptic discharges from the post-central to the supplementary motor area.[2914]

rubbing nose sign The tendency of subjects with frontal lobe tumors to rub the nose repeatedly. The same phenomenon may occur in those with temporal lobe neoplasms, and in those with caudate lesions.

rubeosis iridis Proliferation of new blood vessels on the anterior surface of the iris, leading frequently to glaucoma.

rubi- (Gr, red) Prefix denoting red.

Rubinstein-Taybi syndrome A dysmorphic syndrome of broad, short thumbs and halluces, dwarfism, microcephaly, psychomotor retardation, high-arched palate, refractive error, ptosis, strabismus, antimongolian slant to the eyes, nevus flammeus in half the cases, and unusual susceptibility to chest infections.[4839,5504]

Seizures, callosal agenesis, and pyramidal signs have also been described. See also **microcephaly.**

rubral tremor (red nucleus tremor Holmes tremor, midbrain or thalamic tremor, myorhythmia) A large-amplitude, rotatory tremor of the limbs or head, present at rest and increased when maintaining a posture and with voluntary movements, with which it interferes. Random movements of the hands and abnormal head postures may be associated. It is thought to occur as a result of damage to the red nucleus. See **cerebellar tremors, midbrain tremor, Benedikt syndrome.**

rubrospinal tract (von Monakow bundle) A diffuse network of fibers that descend from the red nucleus, crossing in the anterior tegmental decussation to reach the lower brainstem and upper cervical spinal cord; identified in the dog by von Monakow in 1883, but small to the point of near-disappearance in humans below the cervical level.[4076]

rucksack palsy (trekkers shoulder, Erb palsy, pallbearers palsy, pack palsy) The syndrome of upper brachial plexus (Erb) palsy brought about by compression from the shoulder straps of a heavy rucksack (or other compressive objects).

Clinically, weakness, atrophy, depressed reflexes, and sensory loss are found in the territories, variously, of the suprascapular, axillary, radial, and musculocutaneous nerves. The median nerve is minimally affected and the ulnar nerve is spared.[1298] See **upper brachial plexus palsy.**

Rud syndrome A sporadic **neurocutaneous syndrome** characterized by congenital ichthyosis, hypogonadotropic hypogonadism, dwarfism, mental retardation, deafness, seizures, and polyneuropathy.[4845]

Macrocytic anemia, pigmentary retinopathy, arachnodactyly, and muscular atrophy are associated features.[2764,3665]

rudimentary athetosis Athetosis that can only be detected by its appearance during voluntary movements.

Ruffini, Angelo (1874–1929) Italian anatomist who trained and practiced in the Bologna-Siena-Florence region, settling down as professor of histology in Bologna.

Ruffini corpuscles Deep sensory cutaneous nerve endings, described by Ruffini in 1898.

Ruggeris' sign Tachycardia on attempted adduction of the eyes, in the setting of hyperthyroidism.

Rulandus, Martinus (1582–1602) Bavarian physician and court physician at the ducal palace; the original descriptor of **benign focal epilepsy with centro-**

temporal spikes (confusingly known as **rolandic seizures**) in 1597.[5733]

rule of the Bs   A mnemonic defining the factors requiring the closest attention in patients following a head injury—namely breathing, bleeding, brain, bladder, bowel, and bone.

rules for diplopia   1. The peripheral image is the false image. 2. The separation of images is greatest in the direction of action of the affected muscle(s). 3. The false image is less distinct that the true image.

rum thumb   A mnemonic indicating that three nerves (the radial, ulnar, and median) innervate, in order, the abductor pollicis longus, the adductor pollicis, and the abductor pollicis brevis muscles of the thumb.

run   See **montage.**

runners' headache   A form of **benign exertional headache** related to this form of exercise.[2735]

running fits   See **epilepsia cursiva.**

runs of rapid spikes   See **generalized paroxysmal fast activity.**

rushes   A **migraine** *variant* described in children, characterized by subjective distortions of time such that sounds or other perceptions of the environment appear to rush by abnormally fast. This suggests cortical dysfunction occurring as a feature of the aura.[1495] See also **Alice in Wonderland syndrome.**

Russell, A.   Contemporary English pediatrician.

Russell, Dorothy   (1895–1983) Australian pathologist who was trained at Cambridge and the London Hospital where she was neuropathologist until her retirement, apart from the war years, which she spent in Oxford. Her most lasting work was in neuro-oncology. She characterized the pinealoma as a teratoma, recognized primary CNS lymphoma (to which she gave the name **microgliomatosis**), and published, with Lucien Rubinstein, the landmark *Pathology of Tumours of the Nervous System* (1959),[4852a] as well as authoring important papers on hydrocephalus, methodologies in neuropathology, etc.

Russell, James Samuel Risien   (1863–1939) English physician who with **Batten** and **Collier** described and named **subacute combined degeneration of the cord**[4856] although **Dana** had already described that condition.

Russell syndrome   1. See **diencephalic syndrome**. 2. (Russell-Batten-Collier syndrome, neuroanemic syndrome) See **subacute combined degeneration of the cord.**

Russell-Batten-Collier syndrome   See **subacute combined degeneration of the cord.**

Russell-Silver syndrome   A dominantly inherited syndrome of dwarfism, hemihypertrophy, smallness of the facial bones (pseudohydrocephalus), short stature, and craniofacial dysostosis.[2613]

Blue sclerae, facial dysmorphism, asymmetrical arms and legs, clinodactyly, finger clubbing, hypoglycemia, delayed closure of the fontanelles, and delayed skeletal maturation are other features of the condition.

Russell-Silver–like syndrome   See **Partington syndrome.**

Russian spring-summer encephalitis   A direct infection of the brain by a flavivirus member of the togavirus group of arboviruses. The condition occurs epidemically and presents with severe headaches, fever, meningism, and extreme damage to the anterior horns and cranial nerve motor nucleus cells in the cervical cord and bulbar regions.[6030]

Rust phenomenon   The use of the hands to support the head, seen in patients with high cervical spinal cord injuries (and with tuberculosis and rheumatoid arthritis). It was described by J.N. Rust (1775–1840), a German surgeon with a wide experience in war injuries.[1829]

Rutledge cerebellar-renal-ocular-limb syndrome   A congenital dysmorphic syndrome also characterized by short stature; ocular, cardiac, pulmonary, tracheal, and other visceral abnormalities; rhizomelia of the arms; polydactyly; pes cavus; craniosynostosis; hydrocephalus; and cerebellar atrophy.[337]

Ruvalcaba-Myhre-Smith syndrome   (macrocephaly–intestinal polyps–genital pigmentation) A congenital dysmorphic syndrome characterized by high birth weight, macrocephaly, myopathic weakness, myotonia, acanthosis nigricans, ocular abnormalities including the presence of visible nerve fibers in the cornea, lobulated tongue, pectus excavatum, gastrointestinal tumors, and genital pigmentation.[4859]

Ruzika syndrome   (ichthyosis-deafness-brachydactyly) A congenital dysmorphic syndrome characterized by ichthyosis, sensorineural deafness, myopia, oligodontia, extra ribs, brachydactyly, clinodactyly, thyroid tumors, and mental and developmental delay.[337]

Ryukyuan muscular atrophy   A rare, recessively inherited form of **hereditary motor neuropathy** with onset in early infancy, and characterized by proximal symmetrical muscle atrophy, more severe in the pelvic girdle. Fasciculations, kyphoscoliosis, contractures, and pes cavus are associated. The prognosis for prolonged survival is good.

The condition has been detected only in the residents of the Ryukyuan islands of northern Japan. It has been ascribed to a single mutation occurring before the fourteenth century.[3123]

S

S aneurysm See **megadolichobasilar anomaly.**

S state Slow-wave sleep. See **non–rapid eye movement sleep.**

S-100 protein A soluble cytoplasmic protein present almost exclusively in neuroectodermal cells. Stains for this protein are useful in the diagnosis of **schwannomas** and metastatic melanocarcinomas.

Sabinas syndrome (trichoonycho-oligophrenia—Gr, hair + nail + few + mind) A congenital dysmorphic syndrome manifesting also brittle hair, dysplastic nails and skin, pigmentary retinal degeneration, and mild mental delay.[205] The condition is named after the Mexican community in which the first cases were recognized.

Sabin-Feldman syndrome An acquired infection of early childhood, leading to extensive cerebral damage with disseminated calcification, microphthalmia, optic atrophy, and chorioretinitis. The condition resembles toxoplasmosis in every way, except that the serological findings are negative.[3771]

saccade velocity test A method for the rapid, quantitative measurement of saccade amplitude, duration, and velocity using DC electro-oculography. The technique is of particular value in the determination and assessment of subclinical disturbances of eye movement.[321]

saccades (from Fr, a twitch or jerk) Rapid voluntary eye movements lasting less than 100 msec, including voluntary refixations, the fast components of optokinetic nystagmus and vestibular nystagmus. They represent the mechanism for turning the eyes rapidly and voluntarily upon a target in any direction. This demands an initial *pulse*, which overcomes the inertia of the eyes and moves them in the required direction, followed by a *step*, which maintains the eyes in the appropriate position now achieved. *Volitional, reflexive,* and *spontaneous* types are described.[3330]

With a *normometric* saccade, a single-step refixation occurs because the pulse and the step signals are appropriate for the desired change in fixation. *Hypometric* single-step saccades occur when the pulse portion of the controller signal is too small for the eye to reach the target and it slides to its required new position (**glissade**) as a result of the step signal; thus the eye does not deviate as far as it should in search of the target. *Slow* saccades are hypometric saccades with a very low velocity due to absence of the pulse signal.

Hypermetric saccades are those which overshoot the target as a result of incorrect dynamic or glissadic steps as the eye deviates in the direction of the target. The occurrence of two or more dynamic saccadic components underlies *multiple-step dysmetric* saccades.[291]

The word was formerly applied to involuntary jerking movements occurring as part of the act of swallowing. See also **microsaccades, catch-up saccades, corrective catch-up saccades, express saccades,** and the following entries.

saccadic contrapulsion A disorder of ocular movement occurring in patients with cerebellar disease, and characterized by saccades that overshoot the target on the opposite side and undershoot it on the same side as the cerebellar lesion.[3330] See also **saccadic lateropulsion.**

saccadic delay Prolongation of the latency of saccadic eye movements; a feature of congenital ocular apraxia and of lesions of the visual afferent and central oculomotor systems, the cerebrum, or the basal ganglia at various sites.

saccadic double pulses Intrusions of fixation composed of two back-to-back saccades without any intervening latent period, occurring in normal subjects.

saccadic dysmetria (saccadic overshoot/undershoot) Inaccurate saccades as a result of excessive or inadequate pulses initiating them, respectively. They may be caused by lesions of the cerebellar pathways, the median longitudinal fasciculus, the end-plate, or the sixth cranial nerve.[6112]

saccadic intrusions Abnormal, extraneous, saccadic eye movements that occur during, and disrupt, normal saccades and thus impair the fixation of an object by the macula. See **square-wave jerks, square-wave pulses, ocular flutter, opsoclonus, macrosaccadic oscillations, saccadic double pulses, saccadic lateropulsion, superior oblique myokymia.**

saccadic ipsipulsion See **saccadic lateropulsion.**

saccadic lateropulsion (ipsipulsion, saccadic ipsipulsion) A dramatic form of saccadic intrusion or oscillation characterized by overshoot of voluntary saccadic movements (hypermetria) toward the side of a medullary lesion, with undershoot (hypometria) in the other direction.[1163]

saccadic nystagmus A sustained conjugate horizontal ocular dyskinesia of moderate amplitude at a frequency of 2–3 Hz, dependent on visual fixation.

This is one of many ocular dyskinesias that occur in the presence of brainstem or cerebellar disease.[124] See also **square-wave pulses.**

saccadic oscillations Bursts of high-frequency, to-and-fro movements of the eyes, as with **voluntary nystagmus.** See **square-wave pulses, oscillations, square-wave jerks.**

saccadic overshoot/undershoot See **saccadic dysmetria.**

saccadic paralysis   (selective saccadic palsy) Inability to trigger saccadic eye movements in a direction away from the side of an acute cerebral lesion, or toward the side of a lesion of the pontine tegmentum, due in the latter case to damage to the paramedian pontine reticular formation.

saccadic pulses   (abduction nystagmus, ataxic nystagmus, saccadic intrusions, saccadic oscillations, stepless saccades) Intrusions of fixation resulting from burst cell discharges without the usual step. Saccades are off-target and are corrected by a glissade back to the desired point of fixation.[1368]

saccadomania   See **opsoclonus**.

saccharopinuria   A defect in the catabolic pathway of lysine, resulting in a clinical syndrome consisting of short stature, mild intellectual impairment, and progressive pyramidal signs. Plasma lysine levels and urinary lysine and saccharopine levels are greatly raised.[928]

saccular miliary aneurysm   See **microaneurysm**.

saccule   A statokinetic receptor in the inner ear, responsible for detecting linear displacement of the body.

Sachs, Bernard Parney   (1858–1944) German-American pediatric neurologist. After obtaining a B.A. degree from Harvard, he went to Europe and studied medicine in Strasbourg. Thereafter he did the usual rounds of European centers (Berlin, Vienna, Paris, London), and then returned to America, eventually becoming professor of medicine and of neurological diseases at the New York Polyclinic and a consultant at other New York hospitals. He was at one time the owner of the *Journal of Mental and Nervous Diseases.*

He is best remembered for his descriptions, first in 1887, and independently of Warren Tay, of the gangliosidosis which has for a century or so been named for them,[4867] which he recognized when in general practice and for which he suggested the name *amaurotic familial idiocy*. The term *cherry-red spot* was first used by Herman Knapp, a New York ophthalmologist who saw Sachs' patient. Among Sachs' most important publications were *A Treatise of Nervous Diseases of Children* (1895), the first textbook of child neurology in English, and a monograph on normal childhood development.

Sack syndrome   The occurrence of cerebrovascular accidents in patients with **Ehlers-Danlos syndrome,** such as result from caroticocavernous fistulas or from vertebral or carotid branch aneurysms.[3064]

sacral agenesis   A syndrome characterized by aplasia of the bony structures of the lower spine and sacrum, usually associated with severe motor deficits in the pelvic and leg muscles, mild sensory losses, and visceral anomalies. Apart from agenesis of the sacrum, typical features are absence of the coccyx and aplasia of the lumbar facets and of vertebrae at higher levels.[4920] See **caudal regression syndrome.**

sacral lipomatosis   (Schmidt-Voigt syndrome) An entity of doubtful provenance, allegedly characterized by the presence of dense, palpable lumps in the lumbar and sacral regions of women of early middle age who complain of local pains that are worse with movement. See **myofascial pain syndromes.**[1563]

sacral sparing   The absence of sensory loss in the S2–4 dermatomes in the presence of uni- or bilateral hypoesthesia in, for example, L4–5, S1 territory (but no lower). The causal lesion is usually a disk or tumor that compresses the outermost fibers of the cauda equina but spares those from lower cord levels, which are situated more centrally. See also **saddle anesthesia.**

sacralization   Fusion of the L5 with the S1 vertebra, thus enlarging the sacrum. This condition may cause subacute low back pain or may be symptomless.[1974]

sacralization-scoliosis-sciatica syndrome   See **Bertolotti syndrome.**

saddle anesthesia   Reduced sensation in the territory of the conus medullaris, which includes the natal cleft and buttocks and the posterior upper thighs. This is classically a sign of damage to the S2–4 segments of the cord or, less often, to those roots after they have left the cord. In clinical terms, the phenomenon represents the reverse of **sacral sparing.**

SADS   See **Schedule for Affective Disorders in Schizophrenia.**

Saenger sign   Return of the lost pupillary light reflex when the patient is placed in a darkened room; described as a sign in cerebral syphilis but not present in **tabes dorsalis.**

Dr. Alfred Saenger (1860–1921) was a German neurologist in Hamburg.[4872,5047]

Saenger syndrome   See **Adie pupil.**

Saethre-Chotzen syndrome   A dominantly inherited congenital dysmorphic syndrome manifesting also ptosis, asymmetrical craniosynostosis with plagiocephaly or brachycephaly, syndactyly, and sometimes mental delay.[4874] It is mapped to chromosome 7p. See **acrocephalosyndactyly** *type III*; **craniosynostosis.**

safety factor   The physiological excess in the amplitude of an electrical stimulus, in the concentration of transmitter in a chemical transmission system or in the extent of the available receptor pool. Thus, in the case of myelinated nerve fibers, the safety factor is the ratio of the current available to stimulate a given node to the minimum current required for that purpose.

sagittal   (from Lat, an arrow) The anteroposterior suture of the skull, crossing the coronal suture as an arrow sits upon a bow.

It would be churlish to complain that, in this case, the arrow is not only on the wrong side of the bow but is pointing in quite the wrong direction.

St. Anthony's dance   Synonym for St. Vitus' dance (**chorea**).

St. Avertin's disease   An antique name for epilepsy.

St. Avisius' disease   An antique name for deafness.

St. Guy's dance   Synonym for St. Vitus' dance (**chorea**).

St. Hubert disease   See **rabies**.

St. Job's disease   Syphilis.

St. John's dance   See **dancing mania**.

St. John's evil   An antique name for epilepsy.

St. Lazarus' disease   Leprosy.

St. Louis encephalitis   Direct infection of the brain by a flavivirus member of the togavirus group of arboviruses. The condition is mosquito-borne and occurs in all parts of South America, the United States and southcentral Canada in particular.

Clinically, the condition is most common in subjects over 50 years of age. The condition is usually asymptomatic, but fever and headaches as well as meningitis and encephalitic syndromes are recorded, the latter presenting with altered consciousness, tremors, dysarthria, and seizures.[717]

St. Mathurin's disease   An antique name for epilepsy, and also for insanity.

St. Modestus' dance   Synonym for St. Vitus' dance (**chorea**).

St. Paul   (Saul of Tarsus) (c. 10 B.C.–48 A.D.) Initially in the employ of the Jewish anti-Christian establishment, he was converted to Christianity during a journey to Damascus where (as described in Acts 9 and 22) he was suddenly blinded by a bright light, fell to the ground, and received the remonstrances of God. This episode has been interpreted as evidence of a complex partial seizure,[3259] especially as Paul wrote of a persistent "thorn in the flesh," and thus perhaps of a tendency to some such recurrent problems, but the conflicting evidence in the similar experiences of others in his party, the more usual occurrence of postictal blindness after generalized rather than after partial seizures, and the retention of insight into his sightlessness have led to some scepticism regarding the epileptic basis of this extraordinary event.

St. Sement's disease   Syphilis.

St. Valentine's disease   An antique name for epilepsy.

St. Vitus' dance   St. Vitus was a young Sicilian martyr, dying under the Roman Emperor Diocletian. He prayed that all who commemorated the day of his death should be protected against the **dancing mania,** a disease (probably a form of mass hysteria) which is no longer fashionable. In 1418, sufferers from this condition prayed successfully to the Saint for relief at his chapels in Zabern, near Strasbourg.

Although **Sydenham** described chorea in 1675, the association between dancing mania and chorea (St. Vitus' dance) has been maintained to some degree, quite incorrectly since the two are completely different conditions. See **Sydenham chorea**.

Sahs, Adolph L.   (1906–1986) American neurologist, born in Iowa, where he received his medical training and where he practiced for most of his life, becoming chairman of the Department of Neurology at the University of Iowa in 1948.

He was president of both the American Neurological Association and the American Academy of Neurology (of which latter he was a founding member) and as editor further developed *Grinker's Textbook of Neurology*. The most influential research on which he published was on the subject of intracranial hemorrhage.

Sakati-Nyhan-Tisdale syndrome   (acrocephalopolysyndacyly type 2) A sporadic dysmorphic syndrome characterized by craniosynostosis affecting all of the sutures and leading to turri-brachycephaly. Acrocephalopolysyndactyly, short limbs, congenital heart disease, anomalous ears, alopecia, and atrophic skin are other features described.[4] See **craniosynostosis**.

salaam attacks   The term applied by Sir Charles Clarke to the movements in **West syndrome.** In the words of Dr. West, the forward bobbings of his affected infant son's head "become so frequent and powerful as to cause a complete heaving of the head forwards toward his knees, and then immediately relaxing into the upright position... These bowings and relaxings would be repeated alternately at intervals of a few seconds and repeated from ten to twenty or more times, for two or three minutes; he sometimes has two, three or more attacks in the day . . . Just before they come on he is all alive and in motion, making a strange noise, and then all of a sudden down goes his head and upwards his knees; he then appears frightened and screams out."[5929] See also **flexor spasms**.

Saldino-Mainzer syndrome   A recessively inherited syndrome characterized by pigmentary retinopathy, ataxia, cone-shaped epiphyses of the digits, and short limbs.[4886]

Salih syndrome   A congenital dysmorphic syndrome manifesting also pellagrinoid skin lesions, cataract, cerebellar signs, microcephaly, and mental and developmental delay.[337]

Salinas syndrome   A congenital dysmorphic syndrome manifesting also clefting of the mandible, face, and palate; acrocephaly; and microcephaly.[337]

Salivo-Sudipar syndrome   See **gustatory sweating**.

Salla disease   See **sialidosis** (*type 3*).

salmon patch   See **nevus flammeus**.

Salpêtrière   (from Fr, *salpêtre*, gunpowder) A large hospital in southeast Paris, formerly an ammunition storehouse, and now a general hospital attached to the Hôpital Pitié. During the nineteenth century its function as a house of asylum for the insane was changed so that it became a neurological as well as psychiatric hospital, in large measure due to the influence of J.-M. **Charcot,** who was appointed to its staff in 1862.

salt and pepper on the face   Painful dysesthesias, or stinging or burning sensations due to damage to the quintothalamic tract at its decussation, usually as a result of ischemia.[902]

salt wasting syndrome   Hyponatremia and polyuria with substantial loss of cations, especially sodium, leading to hypovolemia and occurring as a complication of subarachnoid hemorrhage. The condition may result from excessive production of atrial natriuretic peptide, but is not the result of inappropriate ADH secretion.[4036]

saltatory spasm   (Lat, a dancer + Gr, spasm) (static reflex spasm) "Applied to a rare form of clonic spasm in the legs which comes on when the patient attempts to stand, and causes springing or jumping movements, whence the name" (Sir William **Gowers**).[2240]

A manifestation of flagrant hysteria, it was first described by Bamberger in 1859[322] but now seems to have died out. See **Bamberger disease.**

San Francisco syndrome   A craniofacial malformation characterized by synostosis affecting the coronal suture, ptosis, midface hypoplasia, bulbous nose, and small ears.[4]

Sanchez-Corona syndrome   A congenital dysmorphic syndrome manifesting also abnormalities of the hair, speech defects, scoliosis, cerebellar signs, and mental and developmental delay.[337]

Sanderson syndrome   A congenital dysmorphic syndrome manifesting also abnormalities of the genitalia and hair, microcephaly, and cerebral atrophy.[337]

Sandhoff-Jatkiewicz disease   See **GM₂ gangliosidosis.**

Sandifer, Paul   (1908–1964) English neurologist who trained at the Middlesex Hospital and then at the **National Hospital,** Queen Square. He practiced at the National and Royal National Orthopedic Hospitals and at the Hospital for Sick Children as pediatric neurologist; his publications dealt mainly with the *floppy infant* syndrome, **cerebral palsy,** and cerebral degenerative diseases, and he first characterized the **opsoclonus syndrome** (dancing eyes–dancing feet) as well as the syndrome described in the next entry.

Sandifer syndrome   A pseudodystonic syndrome presenting with torticollis and neck extension in different directions, occurring in infants and small children as a response to the sensations arising from a hiatal hernia and the accompanying esophagitis. The condition was first recognized by Sandifer but was further described by Kinsbourne and others.[541,3053]

Sandoz Clinical Assessment Geriatrics scale   (SCAG) A highly reliable clinician-rated instrument designed to differentiate between early senile deterioration and depression in elderly people, and to evaluate the effects of drug treatment on dementia.

The scale examines a broad spectrum of cognitive, affective, and behavioral manifestations; the items deal with confusion, impaired mental alertness, impaired recent memory, disorientation, anxiety, depression of mood, emotional lability, irritability, impaired self-care, anxiety, lost motivation, bothersomeness, hostility, fatigue, appetite, responsiveness to the surroundings, sociability, cooperativeness, fatigue, and dizziness, and allow an overall impression to be gained by the rater.[5086]

Sanfilippo disease A, B, C   See **mucopolysaccharidoses.**

Sanger Brown   (1852–1928) American psychiatrist and neurologist who, after his initial training, studied the functions of the occipital lobe with Schafer. Returning to Chicago he eventually became professor of clinical neurology at the College of Physicians and Surgeons there but later went into private practice.[1829]

Sanger Brown ataxia   (Brown ataxia) A dominantly inherited hyperreflexic spinocerebellar degeneration with juvenile or adult onset, and with added chorea, dementia, optic atrophy, and ophthalmoplegia. The condition thus resembles some of the olivopontocerebellar ataxias, but it is pathologically heterogeneous. The condition was reported by Sanger Brown in 1892 but is now classified as an **autosomal dominant cerebellar ataxia** of late onset.[2438,2439]

Santavuori disease   See **neuronal ceroid lipofuscinosis** (infantile type),[4912] **muscle, eye, brain disease.**

Sao Paulo south coast epidemic encephalitis   Encephalitis caused by *Rocio flavivirus*, a new group B arbovirus capable of attacking the gray matter throughout the neuraxis and producing acute encephalopathy with behavioral disturbances, cerebellar signs, intracranial hypertension, and sometimes coma.[4776]

saphenous neuropathy   An uncommon entrapment neuropathy, usually presenting with pain in the distribution of the nerve on the medial aspect of the lower leg, and causing tenderness at the site where the nerve exits from the femoral canal.[5624]

Sarbo sign   Anesthesia in the distribution of the peroneal nerve, once thought specific for **tabes dorsalis.**

sarco-   (Gr, flesh) Prefix denoting flesh, hence *sarcoma*, a fleshy tumor. The term is now restricted to describe tumors of connective tissue.

sarcoglycanopathies   A class of slowly progressive muscle disease affecting especially the gluteus maximus and thigh adductors, pelvic and shoulder girdle muscles with calf contractures causing toe walking, a rigid spine syndrome, elevated serum CK levels, and myopathic muscle biopsy findings. See also **severe childhood autosomal recessive muscular dystrophy** and http://www.neuro.wustl.edu/neuromuscular/maltbrain.html.

sarcoid myelopathy A rare subacute myelopathy with intense focal enhancement of the C6–7 cord, resembling the appearances of an intramedullary tumor.[6098]

sarcoid myopathy A chronic proximal myopathy resulting from the presence of noncaseating granulomas within the muscle in the context of systemic sarcoidosis. However, in many cases, the presence of such granulomas does not produce any symptoms.[2025]

sarcoid neuropathy Multiple fluctuating and remitting cranial nerve pareses, involving especially cranial nerve VII and less often cranial nerves I, II, V, and XI, or peripheral multiple mononeuropathy.[3706]

A subacute or chronic axonal sensorimotor neuropathy without cranial neuropathy, beginning months to years after established systemic sarcoidosis, is also described, as are diaphragmatic weakness and atypical neuropathies such as acute Guillain-Barré syndrome, unilateral lumbosacral plexopathy, and a subacute symmetric sensory polyneuropathy, all able to appear before systemic sarcoidosis becomes evident.[6139]

sarcoidosis (Besnier-Boeck-Schaumann disease) A multisystem granulomatous disorder of unknown etiology, most commonly affecting young adults and presenting most frequently with bilateral hilar lymphadenopathy, pulmonary infiltration, and skin or eye lesions. Less than 10% of cases have neurological involvement.

The diagnosis is supported by histological evidence of widespread noncaseating epithelioid cell granulomas in more than one organ, and by a positive Kveim-Siltzbach skin test result.[2800] See also **neurosarcoidosis.**[4177]

sarcolemma (Gr, flesh + rind, peelings) (myolemma) The most intimate limiting membrane of the myofibril.

sarcoma A malignant tumor arising from muscle or nerve. In the latter case, the context is most often the syndrome of **neurofibromatosis.** Neural sarcomas cause pain, swelling, and motor and sensory deficits in the appropriate territory; in muscle, local pain, swelling, and weakness are the usual complaints.

The human herpesvirus 8 is found in *Kaposi's sarcoma*, a definitive marker for AIDS. *Ewing's sarcoma* is a peripheral primitvie neuroectodermal tumor that can arise from the intracranial leptomeninges. Primary CNS, meningeal, osteosarcomas, chondro- leiomyolipo- and angoiosarcomas are also recognized.

sarcosinemia An aminoaciduria characterized by mental retardation in some cases, with increased levels of sarcosine and ethanolamine in the blood and urine as a result of a deficiency of sarcosine dehydrogenase.[2849]

sarcotubular myopathy A rare, benign, recessively inherited, nonprogressive myopathic syndrome characterized by onset in early childhood, myopathic facial and proximal weakness and atrophy, and the presence of multiple empty membrane-bound vacuoles in type 2 myofibrils in muscle biopsy specimens, representing dilatation of the sarcotubular system.[6,2851]

sartorius (from Lat, a tailor) The tailor's muscle; it flexes the knee and laterally rotates the thigh, thus allowing the traditional cross-legged position to be adopted.

satellite potential A small action potential separated from the main motor unit action potential by an isoelectric interval which fires in a time-locked relationship to the main action potential. It usually follows, but may precede, the main action potential. Less preferred terms include *late component, parasite potential, linked potential,* and *coupled discharge.* (From the 2001 Report of the Nomenclature Committee of the American Association of Electromyography and Electrodiagnosis.[10] Used by permission, copyright © 2001, AAEM.)

satellitosis An increase in the numbers of oligodendrocytes clustering around the larger neurons of the basal ganglia and the fourth, fifth, and sixth layers of the cerebral cortex. The pathological significance of this is not known.

Satoyoshi syndrome (progressive muscle spasms, alopecia, and diarrhea, myospasm gravis) A sporadic syndrome with onset in childhood or youth characterized by frequent painful, progressive, intermittent episodes of rigid muscle cramps beginning in the legs (*myospasm gravis*) and then several years after onset, the neck, trunk, and masticatory muscles become affected.

Associated features include alopecia, diarrhea, short stature, multiple bony abnormalities, intestinal malabsorption, a flat oral glucose tolerance curve, amenorrhea, and sometimes retardation of growth. The cramps result from synchronized motor unit discharges at 40–50 Hz and at 4–10 mV amplitude.[4924,4927] Intestinal polyposis was present in the two patients originally studied; the condition is considered to be a specific variety of malabsorption.

In a *variant form,* **myasthenia gravis** is associated. See **glycogen storage diseases, oculopharygodistal muscular dystrophy.**

Saturday night palsy 1. Radial nerve compression palsy in the spiral groove of the humerus, usually therefore sparing the branches to the triceps muscle. The term is applied because the disorder is occasionally seen in young men whose chivalry has extended to supporting the head of their girlfriend for a period of an hour (or even a night), with resultant ischemic compression of the nerve. Since this is usually a neurapraxia, recovery is often both early and complete. 2. Sciatic nerve compression palsy as a result of prolonged compression of the buttocks and thighs wedged into a toilet seat while the street-drugged subject is unconscious.[5675]

Saturday night retinopathy   Unilateral visual loss related to ocular pressure caused by the person remaining in the recumbent position while deeply intoxicated, or by wearing an anesthetic mask.[2819]

saturnine encephalopathy   (Lat, pertaining to lead) Any kind of cerebral syndrome caused by lead poisoning. Coma, delirium, toxic psychoses, aphasias, seizures, and pareses are mentioned by Kinnier **Wilson.**[6000]

saturnine palsy   See **lead palsy, Remak paralysis.**

saturnism   Weakness due to lead poisoning.

satyriasis   (Gr, satyr + lewd person) 1. Exceedingly great sexual desire in the male. 2. An old term for **leprosy,** on account of the malformations produced by it, leading the patient to resemble the mythical satyrs who were represented as being extremely ugly.

Saul syndrome   1. A congenital dysmorphic syndrome manifesting also tall stature, dislocation of the lens, ectopic pupils, arachnodactyly, seizures, and mental and developmental delay.[337] 2. A congenital dysmorphic syndrome manifesting also pigmentary skin disorders, microcephaly, seizures, extrapyramidal lesions, and mental and developmental delay.[337]

Saunders, William   (1743–1817) British physician who was born in Scotland and who trained at the University of Edinburgh, but practiced in London as physician to Guy's Hospital. He was very involved in the activities of the Royal College of Physicians. His unpublished descriptions of **delirium tremens** were recognized by Thomas **Sutton,** who named the condition thus in his tract of 1813,[5429] in which he also gave a definitive description. Saunders did publish, however, on the topics of hepatitis, other diseases of the liver, the treatment of ague, and the dissolution of renal stones.

Saunders-Sutton syndrome   See **delirium tremens.**

Sauvineau, Charles   (b. 1862) French ophthalmologist in Paris who first described **internuclear ophthalmoplegia.**[4931]

Sauvineau syndrome   See **internuclear ophthalmoplegia.**

savant syndrome   A precocious ability to function superbly in certain tasks, set against a background of intellectual mediocrity at best. The syndrome is classified by the nature of the skill exhibited; exceptional memory, language, mathematical skills, the visual arts, and musical talents are described.

saxitoxin neuropathy   Paralytic shellfish poisoning, first recognized by Captain Vancouver in 1801. The toxin is a sodium channel blocker and is contained in certain protozoa ingested by the molluscs. The local discoloration of the water that is produced has led to the term *red tide.*

Clinical symptoms include burning in the mouth, paresthesia, and numbness with ataxia and sometimes brainstem involvement. See also **ciguatera poisoning.**[119]

saxophone headache   Severe episodic headache associated with an increase in intrathoracic or intraabdominal pressure, reported in patients with **Chiari malformation** (type 1) but with the same character as the head discomfort commonly occurring as a result of performing a sustained Valsalva maneuver.[1757,2413]

Say syndrome   A congenital dysmorphic syndrome in which skeletal abnormalities and microcephaly are the other main features.[4936]

SCAG   See **Sandoz Clinical Assessment Geriatrics scale.**

scalenus anticus syndrome   See **thoracic outlet syndrome.**

scallop pupils   Irregularities in the edge of the pupil, usually associated with amyloidosis or other disease of the short ciliary nerves leading to sector atrophy of the iris.[3363]

scalp   (Dutch, a shell) The shell or covering of the head.

scalp electrode   A recording electrode held against, attached to, or inserted into the scalp.

scalp electroencephalogram   A record of electrical activity of the brain made by means of electrodes placed on the surface of the head. This term and its abbreviation should be used only to distinguish between scalp and other EEGs such as depth EEGs. In all other instances, a scalp EEG should be referred to simply as an *EEG.* (Adapted from the 1974 report of the Committee on Terminology, IFCN. In: Chatrian GE, Bergamini L, Dondey M, *et al.* A glossary of terms most commonly used by clinical electroencephalographers. *EEG Clin Neurophysiol* 1974;**37:**538–548[989] by kind permission of Elsevier Science.)

Scandinavian Neurological Stroke Scale   A reliable instrument for the stratification of stroke patients and for the evaluation of long-term outcome. The scale rates nine factors (consciousness, eye movements, arm motor power, hand motor power, leg motor power, orientation, speech, facial palsy, and gait) and derives from these both prognostic and long-term scores. Neglect and visual field deficits are not scored, increasing the reliability of the scale.[3417]

scanning EMG   A technique by which a needle electrode is advanced in defined steps through muscle while a separate single-fiber-EMG electrode is used to trigger both the display sweep and the advancement device. The scanning EMG provides temporal and spatial information about the motor unit. Distinct maxima in the recorded activity are considered to be generated by muscle fibers innervated by a common branch of an axon. These groups of fibers form a motor unit fraction. (From the 2001 Report of the Nomenclature Committee of the American Association of Electromyography and Electrodiagnosis.[10] Used by permission, copyright © 2001, AAEM.)

scanning speech Separation of the syllables of words so that speech sounds disjointed, somewhat resembling that of partially literate schoolchildren made to recite poetry, thus damaging the reputations of both author and interpreter.

It is due to an inability to change the positions of the vocal muscles rapidly, as occurs with disorders of the cerebellum. With nystagmus and ataxia, it formed the **Charcot triad** of signs of **multiple sclerosis** (all of which are, however, merely signs of cerebellar disease).

scanpaths The pathways along which vision is directed during stereotypical visual scanning of the critical stimulus features of a studied image.[4714]

scaphocephaly (Gr, hull + head) A developmental defect in skull shape with a long and narrow configuration as a consequence of premature fusion of the sagittal suture, such that it resembles an upturned boat, the keel lying along the suture. This, the most common form of **craniosynostosis,** also produces lowering and narrowing of the parietal level with a compensatory projection of the frontal and occipital areas; the face is little affected and hypertelorism is absent.[4]

A similar deformity occurs in premature neonates as a result of skull moulding during birth.

scapular reflex Stroking of the skin overlying the scapula leads to contraction of the underlying muscles. This is usually present but invisible, although it may be felt. Augmentation of the response occurs in the presence of a pyramidal lesion above C5. See **interscapular reflex.**

scapular winging Backward protrusion, often with rotation, of the scapula as a result of lesions of the long thoracic nerve, the C7 root, or the eleventh nerve branch to trapezius, but also occasionally due to a proximal myopathy.[3583]

scapulocostal syndrome A painful condition ascribed to myofascitis of the shoulder muscles and thought to be caused by altered posture, prolonged immobilization of the shoulder region, or fixed scapular/spinal deformities.[4260,6106]

scapulohumeral reflex Contraction of various muscles of the shoulder girdle, particularly those supplied by C5–6, in response to a tap on the medial border of the scapula. Unilateral absence of the reflex indicates a lesion at the level of C5.

scapuloilioperoneal atrophy with cardiopathy and inflammatory myopathy A dominantly inherited syndrome of slowly progressive muscle weakness with a scapuloileoperoneal distribution and cardiopathy, with onset in young adult life. Muscle biopsy specimens show neurogenic and myopathic changes with inflammatory cell reactions and perivascular cuffing.[2839]

scapuloperoneal atrophy (Kaeser syndrome, Stark-Kaeser syndrome) A dominantly inherited syndrome representing a *variant* form of **hereditary motor neuropathy.** See also **scapuloperoneal syndrome.**

scapuloperoneal atrophy, cardiopathy, and inflammatory myopathy See **hereditary motor neuropathy** (*variants*).

scapuloperoneal syndrome (Davidenkow syndrome) A heterogeneous syndrome of muscle weakness and wasting affecting the scapular and peroneal muscles first and most, although arm, neck, ocular, other cranial and trunk muscles may be affected later. The onset is at any time after childhood. It is usually dominantly inherited, but all forms of inheritance patterns and also sporadic cases have been described.[5026,5544]

The syndrome represents a combination of the features of the **hereditary motor neuropathies** (spinal muscular atrophies) and of the girdle dystrophies.[2900] The pathological findings and results of electrical studies constitute the usual features of either neurogenic or myopathic disease, or of both. The course is generally benign unless cardiac complications ensue, as in the **Emery-Dreifuss syndrome.**[5544] It was described first by Brossard in 1886, but more fully by Davidenkow in 1939,[1310] who commented that the signs in the legs resemble those of Charcot-Marie-Tooth neuropathy while the atrophy of the shoulder girdle muscles is like that of Erb muscular dystrophy.

The typical form (*scapuloperoneal muscular atrophy with sensory disturbance*, adult-onset scapuloperoneal myopathy, Davidenkow syndrome) is a dominantly or recessively inherited scapuloperoneal syndrome with juvenile or young adult onset, and is characterized by facial, bulbar, proximal, and distal myopathic weakness, often with pseudohypertrophy, ophthalmoplegias, sensory disturbances, and pes cavus.[1310,6076]

Variant subtypes are listed in Chart S–1.

Chart S–1. Subtypes of Scapuloperoneal Syndrome

Scapuloperoneal muscular atrophy without sensory disturbance (Stark-Kaeser syndrome, scapuloperoneal atrophy) A dominantly inherited syndrome of early or mid-adult life manifesting ophthalmoplegias, facial and bulbar weakness, and neurogenic girdle muscle atrophy.[5320] X-linked recessive inheritance of this condition has also been reported.[335]

Scapuloperoneal muscular atrophy without sensory disturbance, recessive form A congenital or childhood scapuloperoneal syndrome manifesting only neurogenic muscle atrophy and weakness.

Scapuloperoneal muscular dystrophy, X-linked A severe congenital scapuloperoneal syndrome manifesting both myopathic and neurogenic muscle atrophy, contractures, weakness, and cardiomyopathy, with unusual sparing of the extensor digitorum brevis muscles.[5550] See **Emery-Dreifuss syndrome.**

Scapuloperoneal muscular dystrophy, X-linked, without contractures A severe congenital scapuloperoneal syndrome manifesting both myopathic and neurogenic muscle atrophy, weakness, and severe cardiomyopathy.[496] See **Emery-Dreifuss syndrome.**

Scapuloperoneal muscular dystrophy, cardiomyopathy, and mental retardation A myopathic syndrome manifesting in childhood with cardiomyopathy, syncope, and neurodegenerative regression.[2839]

Benign muscular dystrophy with contractures[295]

Other neuromuscular syndromes that may present with this distribution include **myotonic dystrophy,** acid maltase, or phosphofructokinase deficiency, and various **congenital myopathies.**

scarf sign Abnormal mobility of the arms of the supine infant, as shown when the examiner is able to pull the infant's hand across the chest, around the neck, and possibly back around the opposite shoulder.

Using the scoring system of Dubowitz et al.[1530] for assessing **gestational age,** score 0 if the elbow reaches the opposite axillary line; 1 if the elbow can be moved to a point between the midline and the opposite axillary line; 2 if the elbow reaches to the midline; and 3 if the elbow does not reach the midline. In the *posterior scarf sign,* the hand is drawn toward the opposite acromion but behind the neck. In hypotonic states, the hand can be led unusually far, constituting a positive response.[2732]

Scarff syndrome A syndrome characterized by early-onset focal seizures affecting the legs first, with minimal neurological deficit. The condition was thought by the original author to be due to the large pacchionian granulations that were detected at operation and that had extended into the primary motor areas.[4939]

Scarpa, Antonius (1747–1832) Italian professor of surgery in Modena and afterwards of anatomy in Pavia. He was widely travelled, and was a fellow of the Royal Colleges of England, Edinburgh, and Ireland, as well as a Fellow of the Royal Society. A superb artist, he illustrated his own work on the inner ear, ocular disease, and other subjects. He described (Scarpa's) canal in the inner ear, and the nerve, canal, fascia, and triangle to which his name is also given. He was also the first to identify disease of the medial wall of arteries as the basis of aneurysms.[3893]

Scarpa's ganglion A ganglion on the vestibular nerve in the internal auditory meatus.

scelotyrbe festinans (from Gr, leg + perturbation, and Lat, hurrying; hence *festinating gait*) The classic gait disturbance of parkinsonism, in which, in the words of Trousseau, "[the patients] center of gravity is thus displaced, he is obliged to run after himself, as it were, so that he keeps trotting and hopping on."[5648]

SCHAD deficiency See **short-chain acyl–coenzyme A dehydrogenase deficiency.**

Schaefer reflex An alternative method of seeking the **Babinski response,** in this case by pinching the Achilles tendon or the skin overlying it.[4942] **Babinski** himself had mentioned this method in a paper published the year before Schaefer's report.

Schedule for Affective Disorders in Schizophrenia (SADS) A complex interviewer- and observer-rated scale designed to establish research and other diagnostic criteria for specific depressive disorders.[1653]

Scheibe defect (membranous cochleosaccular dysplasia) An inherited dysplasia of the inner ear with atrophy of both the cochlear and vestibular divisions of the eigth cranial nerve.

Scheie disease See **mucopolysaccharidoses.**

schema (Gr, form) 1. A preconscious phenomenon, not amounting to a mental image (which is consciously appreciated). 2. The term of Sir Henry **Head** for a pattern of response in the realms of both speech and sensation, based on previous responses of the organism but occurring outside awareness.[1173]

Scheuermann disease A benign epiphyseal disease of the spine, causing complaints of mild pain on exercise in adolescents over the course of a few (usually 2–4) years.

Schilder disease (encephalitis periaxialis diffusa) A term for disorders with different etiologies, characterized by diffuse sclerosis of the cerebral white matter. The patients reported by Schilder[4962] suffered from different conditions; he himself pointed out that "diffuse sclerosis" was not a single entity.

Some such cases are due to **multiple sclerosis** (*demyelinating form*) and the remainder to a disturbance of abnormally constituted myelin (*dysmyelinating form*).[4499] The condition now regarded as that most likely affecting the patients described by him is **adrenoleukodystrophy;**[4501] the term *Schilder disease* is best taken to refer to diffuse sclerosis occurring as a subacute condition in children, while transitional sclerosis is most likely to be a form of multiple sclerosis. See also **diffuse sclerosis.**

Schilder myelinoclastic diffuse sclerosis See **neuromyelitis optica.**

Schilder, Paul Ferdinand (1886–1940) Austrian neurologist and psychiatrist who trained in Vienna, where he soon obtained a staff position in the university hospital. He continued there (except for a period of War service) until he emigrated to the United States in 1929. He worked at Bellvue hospital in New York and later became associate professor of psychiatry at the New York Medical College.

His description of the syndrome named for him was published in 1912; his remaining 300 or so publications concerned psychiatric and philosophical topics, but in neurology, his papers on involuntary movements, aphasia, other disorders of language, consciousness and the syndromes described in the following entries were especially notable.

Paul Ferdinand Schilder

Schilder variant of multiple sclerosis A form of multiple sclerosis characterized clinically by the presence of dementia and pathologically by the presence of cerebral atrophy, ventricular dilatation, and shrinkage of the white matter associated with the presence of multiple chronic **plaques.** See **neuromyelitis optica.**

Schilder-Flatau disease See **Schilder-Foix disease.**

Schilder-Foix disease (Marie-Foix syndrome, Schilder-Flatau disease, intracerebral symmetrical lobar sclerosis) A nonprogressive condition due to perinatal anoxic encephalopathy, in which gliotic lesions are distributed throughout the cerebral white matter. Marie, Foix,[3617] and Flatau further analyzed some of the cases of Schilder and separated this condition from diffuse sclerosis.

Schimke syndrome An X-linked recessive congenital syndrome characterized by short stature, deafness, extraocular palsies, microcephaly, chorea, pyramidal signs, myopathy, and mental and developmental delay.[4968]

Schinzel syndrome (trisomy chromosome 13) A congenital dysmorphic syndrome manifesting also postaxial polydactyly with duplication of the halluces, macrocephaly, callosal agenesis, and severe mental and developmental delay.[4971] See **acrocallosal syndrome.**

Schiotz tonometry A method of assessing intraocular pressure by measuring the compressibility of the cornea. The normal pressure is up to 15 mmHg.

Schirmer, O.W.A. (1864–1917) German ophthalmologist.

Schirmer syndrome A variant of **Sturge-Weber syndrome** in which glaucoma occurs unusually early.

Schirmer test A test of tear formation, in which a 5-mm-wide strip of absorbent filter paper is hooked around the lower lid so that one end lies in the inferior conjunctival sac. The length of the paper wetted by normal tear formation during 5 minutes is measured, and the two sides are compared with each other and with the normal result (which is 15 mm or more). In Sjögren syndrome, the length of the paper wetted is less than this.

Schirmer-Sturge-Weber syndrome See **Sturge-Weber syndrome.**

schistosomiasis A common protozoal infection with *Schistosoma japonicum, haematobium,* or *mansoni,* occurring in Africa, South America, and the Orient. Neurological complications are seldom the presenting problem, but seizures and myelopathy may result from the granulomas that form in reaction to the presence of the ova in the brain or spinal cord.

schizencephaly (Gr, split + brain) A congenital primary neuronal migration defect of the brain in which the cerebral mantle is not formed in the regions of the major (especially the sylvian) fissures.

The condition appears in infancy or up to early adult life, and is characterized by microcephaly, hemiplegia, infantile spasms, and mental and developmental delay in association with deep symmetrical cerebral clefts with infolding of cortical gray matter along them, and abnormalities of the ventricular system, including hydrocephalus.[3879]

Schizophrenia Society of Canada A charitable organization. Address: 75 Donway West #814, Don Mills, Ontario M3C 2E9, Canada.

schizophrenia-like psychosis of epilepsy A chronic paranoid psychosis occurring in some patients with a long-standing history (mean: 14 years) of complex partial seizures originating in the temporal lobe. No important differences exist between the psychological symptoms of this condition and those of schizophrenia without an accompanying seizure disorder.[5208] The prevalence of schizophrenia in epileptic people is substantially higher than that in a control population.

schlaftrunkenheit See **confusional arousals.**

Schlemm, Friedrich (1795–1858) German anatomist. The canal of Schlemm is a small opening at the junction of the cornea and the sclera.

Schlesinger sign Strong passive inversion of the hip leads to extreme extension of the leg and inversion of the foot in **tetany.**[374]

Schmidt, Adolf (1865–1918) German neurologist.

Schmidt, Henry D. (1832–1888) American pathologist practicing in New Orleans. His description of the clefts in the nerve sheaths (1874) preceded that of Lantermann by 3 years.

Schmidt, Johann Baptist (1823?–1884) German obstetrician who trained at Würzburg and whose paper on aphasia (1871) was drawn upon by **Wernicke** in his classic description of the syndrome 3 years later.[643]

Schmidt syndrome (vagoaccessory syndrome) Unilateral paresis of the muscles supplied by the tenth and eleventh cranial nerves (vocal cord, soft palate, trapezius, and sternomastoid) with contralateral hemiplegia, due to a medullary lesion that is usually vascular.[5431] It is thus a variant of the **Jackson-Mackenzie syndrome,** but without the tongue paralysis.[4976] The syndrome is named after A. **Schmidt.**

Schmidt-Lantermann clefts Conical interruptions in the myelin sheath (intersegmental clefts) seen by light microscopy; named after H.D. Schmidt.

Schmidt-Rimpler test Subjects complaining of loss of vision are asked to look at their own hand.[1349a] Those with true blindness will turn their eyes in the appropriate direction; those with simulated blindness will look randomly in any direction, unless they have the wit to realize that this is a test of conscious proprioception at least as much as of vision. The test is named after A. **Schmidt.**

Schmidt-Voigt syndrome See **sacral lipomatosis.**

Schnabel optic atrophy Mucoid degeneration of the optic nerves occurring in patients with glaucoma, and described by Dr. Isidor Schnabel (1842–1908). See also **pseudo–Schnabel cavernous degeneration of the optic nerve.**

Schneider disease A virus infection occurring in the spring and fall, causing high fever, chills, nasopharyngitis, arthralgia, malaise, headache, and vomiting for about 4 days, followed by a latent period, and then either by serous meningitis and complete recovery or by a more severe meningoencephalitis with hyperkinesia, sensory disorders, tics, and seizures, but with full recovery. Rarely, the meningoencephalitis produces signs resembling those of poliomyelitis.

The nature of the disorder is uncertain and these syndromes may be nonspecific complications of different viral infections.[4983]

Scholz plaques See **perivascular plaques.**

Scholz syndrome See **metachromatic leukodystrophy.**

Scholz, Willibald (b. 1889) German psychiatrist, neurologist, and neuropathologist at Tübingen, Leipzig, and Munich, who developed the concept of glial insufficiency in metachromatic leukodystrophy (sulfatide lipidosis) in 1925; his name has been attached to the disease as a result.

Schrijver-Bernhard reflex Plantar flexion of the toes in response to a tap on the tibia or the overlying mus-

cles; a sign of pyramidal tract or basal ganglion disease. See **distant toe flexor reflex.**

Schroeder tetrad A child from a rural area in good general health with marked intracranial hypertension and with ill-defined focal neurological signs. The presence of these four features strongly suggests the diagnosis of cerebral hydatid disease.[5003]

Schüller, Artur (1874–1957) Viennese radiologist who published the first X-ray atlas of the skull and described the signs of increased intracranial pressure on the sella turcica. He also contributed data leading to the definition of **Hand-Schüller-Christian disease.**

Schulman syndrome See **eosinophilic fasciitis.**

Schultze acroparesthesia (Schultze-Nothnagel syndrome, Putnam-Schultze syndrome) The concurrence of acroparesthesia, anesthesia, and pain in the arms without vasomotor symptoms. The condition probably represents a severe form of **carpal tunnel syndrome.**

Dr. Frederick Schultze (1848–1934) was a German physician.

Schultze syndrome Meningeal neurofibroblastomatosis.

Schultze test Percussion of the skin of the face overlying the facial nerve between the angle of the jaw and the zygoma. Twitching of the middle part of the face in response is a positive result, indicating the presence of latent **tetany.**[374]

A *variant* test is to tap the protruded tongue. In tetany and **myotonic dystrophy,** dimpling or rising-up of the part tapped may occur. See also **Chvostek test,** of which this is but a modification, although perhaps increasing the sensitivity.

Schumacher, G.A. Contemporary American neurologist.

Schumacher Panel criteria Criteria for the diagnosis of definite **multiple sclerosis,** published in 1965 and, in the opinion of some physicians, still the least disputatious.[5011] The criteria are as given in Chart S–2.

Chart S–2. Schumacher Panel Criteria for the Diagnosis of Multiple Sclerosis

1. Neurological examination must reveal objective abnormalities that can be attributed to dysfunction of the CNS.
2. Examination of the case history must supply evidence that two or more parts of the CNS are involved.
3. Evidence of CNS disease must reflect predominant involvement of white matter—that is, long-tract damage.
4. Involvement of the neuraxis must have followed one of two time patterns:
   a. Two or more episodes of worsening, each lasting at least 24 hours and each at least a month apart
   b. Slow or stepwise progression of signs and symptoms over at least 6 months
5. At onset, the patient must be between 10 and 50 years old.*

6. A physician competent in clinical neurology should decide that the patient's condition could not be better attributed to another disease.

It is now generally held that this criterion is not obligatory. (From Schumacher GA, Beebe G, Kibler RF, et al. problems of experimental trials of therapy in multiple sclerosis: report by the panel on the evaluation of experimental trials of therapy in multiple sclerosis. Ann NY Acad Sci 1965;122:522–568.)

schusterkrampf   (Ger, shoemaker cramps) Tetany.

Schwab, Robert S.   (1903–1972) American neurologist, educated at Harvard and Cambridge Universities, who trained in neurology at the Boston City and Massachussetts General Hospitals, where he established a reputation as a clinician-researcher, becoming well known as an expert in Parkinson disease, the EEG, epilepsy, and myasthenia gravis.

Schwabach test   The direct comparison of a patient's ability to hear a vibrating tuning fork placed on the mastoid process with the ability of the examiner to do so. The test has elements of both the **Rinne** and of the **Weber** tests; when the examiner hears the sound for longer than the patient, the latter is suspected to have sensorineural deafness.

Schwalbe, Gustav   (1844–1916) Professor of anatomy at Strasbourg. He gave his name to a number of anatomical features, the most memorable being the medial vestibular nucleus.

Schwalbe's nucleus   The principal (medial) vestibular nucleus.

Schwann cell   A macrophage, the supporting cell providing myelin insulation for the axons of peripheral nerves.

Schwann, Theodor   (1810–1882) Prussian physician, professor of anatomy, physiology, or comparative anatomy at various northern European universities, notably Liège and Louvain. He was an early proponent of the neuronal theory of the nervous system and of the cellular doctrine of tissues in general, and was the discoverer of pepsin as well as of the cell named for him (1838).

schwannoma   (neurilemmoma, neurinoma, acoustic neuroma, neurofibroma, lemmoma, perineurial fibroblastoma, endothelioma, gliofibrosarcoma) A benign, solitary, sporadic, lobulated, encapsulated tumor of the nerve sheath, arising usually from the vestibular portion of the eighth cranial nerve or from the sensory roots of other cranial or spinal nerves, usually in adult life. Histologically these tumors are characterized by the presence of a rich reticulin network, **Antonini type A** and **B** areas, **Verocay bodies,** and positive staining for S-100 protein.

Most clinical symptoms arise as a result of compression of local structures; neural hearing loss, vertigo, facial numbness and weakness, dysphagia, ataxia, and hydrocephalus are the more common problems encountered when the tumor arises from the eighth nerve; pain and segmental sensorimotor deficits, when it arises from a spinal nerve root. Malignant transformation can occur. In rare instances, the tumor is part of the **neurofibromatosis 2 syndrome,** a dominantly inherited disorder mapping to chromosome 22.

The tumor was first described by Sandifort in 1777.

schwannomatosis   The occurrence of multiple schwannomas in people whose disorder does not meet criteria for **neurofibromatosis type 2.** The condition is manifest later and is seldom familial, the prognosis is better, and the tendency for other tumors to develop is much less than in that condition.[3542]

Schwartz disease   See **syndrome of inappropriate ADH secretion.**

Schwartz, Henry Gerard   (b. 1909) American surgeon practicing in St. Louis. He was the first to describe the operation of medullary tractotomy for the relief of intractable pain.[5022]

Schwartz, W.B.   Contemporary American physician.

Schwartz-Jampel syndrome   (myotonic chondrodystrophy, chrondrodystrophic myotonia, oculochondromuscular dystrophy) A rare, recessively inherited dysmorphic condition of early childhood, mapped to chromosome 1p34–p36, manifesting dwarfism; metaphyseal and epiphyseal dysplasias; ocular, genital, and skeletal abnormalities; blepharophimosis; and muscle weakness, stiffness, and contractures with small muscle mass despite the unique feature of the presence of myotonia and continual high-frequency muscle fiber activity, as recorded on the EMG at rest.[1924]

In a *variant* form, the condition is dominantly inherited.[4351]

Both Drs. Oscar Schwartz and R. Jampel are contemporary American ophthalmologists.

Type 1A has onset in childhood of myotonia, bone dysplasia, micrognathia, platyspondyly, cleft vertebrae, small stature, contractures, myopia, hirsutism, and small testes. There is an icreased risk of malignant hyperthermia.

Type 1B has onset at birth and resembles type 1A except that there is more severe bone dysplasia.

Type 2 is recessively inherited. This is probably the same entity as Stuve-Wiedemann syndrome (SWS) with congenital onset of hypotonia, respiratory and feeding difficulties, and recurrent episodes of hyperthermia. The EMG shows complex repetitive discharges.

Schwarz-Lelek syndrome   A syndrome of massive internal bowing of the femurs (genu valgum) with radiolucent splaying of the metaphyseal area and hyperostosis and sclerosis of the skull,[5020] described by Dr. L. Schwarz in 1960. See **craniometaphyseal dysplasia.**

Schweiz Gesellschaft für Muskelkrankheiten   (SGMK) A member society of the European Alliance of Muscular Dystrophy Societies based at: Lenggstrasse 67, Ch-8008 Zurich, Switzerland.

Schweizerische Gesellschaft für Neurologie   A professional organization. Address: c/o Dr. A. Steck, CHUV, 8011, Lausanne, Switzerland.

sciatic   (from Gr, the hip joint, later Lat, pains in that region) The condition of **sciatica** indicates irritation of the sciatic nerve with pain felt in the distribution of the nerve. The first description was that of **Cotugno** in 1764.

sciatic list   The distance between a plumb line dropped from the cervicodorsal spine and the gluteal cleft. With radiculopathy, this deformity remains during forward bending, while psychogenic lists usually disappear with spinal flexion.[1150]

sciatic neuralgia   See **sciatica.**

sciatic neuropathy   Pain, weakness, wasting, and sensory disturbances in the territory of the nerve as a result of damage to it in the pelvis; but, for reasons unknown, clinically more likely to damage the peroneal rather than the posterior tibial portion.

Lesions above the piriformis muscle affect also the glutei, tensor fascia lata, and possibly the paraspinal muscles; below it but within the pelvis, the hamstrings; and below the sciatic notch, the structures innervated by the two major branches of the nerve according to the relative damage done to each branch.

Presenting features include numbness and paresthesias, distal dysesthesias, subjective and objective weakness, reduced or absent ankle jerks, and elctrodiagnostic evidence of denervation in the EDB, tibialis anterior, or abductor hallucis and reduced or absent sural or superficial peroneal sensory nerve action potentials.[6096]

See also **piriformis syndrome, posterior tibial neuropathy, common peroneal neuropathy, hunkering.**

sciatica   (Cotugno disease, sciatic neuralgia) The popular name for pain radiating in sciatic nerve distribution as a result of root irritation.[1142] Drs. William J. Mixter and Joseph S. Barr showed in 1934 that this was frequently due to nerve root irritation by a prolapsed intervertebral disk.

The pain is sharp, continuous, or lancinating, felt in the region innervated by the damaged nerve fibers and worsened by spinal movements. It is usually accompanied by paresthesias and by motor and sensory deficits when the cause is radicular compression. However, deep, aching pain may be referred in the same distribution without paresthesias as a result of distortion or inflammation of structures close to the spinal column. See also **Cotugno, D.**[6096]

sciatique spasmodique   Sciatic nerve irritation with spasm of the contralateral erector spinae muscles, leading to scoliosis. The sign was described by **Brissaud;** it is found in patients with severe sciatica and also in those with **facet syndromes.**

scintillating scotomas   (Lat, spark + Gr, darkening) Areas of visual loss with superimposed positive visual phenomena such as showers of sparks and twinkling lights, occurring as a result of retinal or occipital lobe ischemia, as in migraine. These were first described thus by Dianon in his 1875 Paris graduation thesis, but had been recorded earlier by Fothergill, Wilks, Parry, Living, and many other migraineurs.

scintillations   Hallucinated persistent or transitory shimmering or flickering lights, seen by patients with lesions of the calcarine cortex and suggesting the presence of ischemia in the territory of the posterior cerebral artery.[1847]

scleral show   Sclera visible below the iris of the eye, suggesting weakness of the orbicularis oculi muscle, a sign occurring in facial nerve palsies and in those muscular dystrophies which affect the facial muscles. See **Dalrymple sign.**

sclero-   (Gr, hard) Prefix denoting hard.

scleroderma   (progressive systemic sclerosis) A multisystem collagen-vascular disease characterized by inflammation and fibrosis of small blood vessels and of the dermal layers, and by fibrosis and atrophy of smooth muscle and connective tissue.

The major neurological complication is neuropathy, most evidently of the trigeminal nerve but occasionally of the peripheral nerves,[3032] while CNS complications are usually due to hypertension or to any associated vasculitis. Proximal, symmetrical myopathy, inflammatory polymyositis, and neuropathic weakness are also described.[2566]

scleromalacia perforans   Thinning and sometimes perforation of the sclera, as may occur in rheumatoid arthritis.

sclérose en plaques   See **multiple sclerosis.**

sclerosis   Accumulation of glial scar tissue in the brain and spinal cord, there being no fibroblasts present to allow fibrosis to occur.

sclerosis disseminata dolorosa   Neuralgic or other pains occurring in the course of **multiple sclerosis.**

sclerostosis   A recessively inherited craniotubular hyperostotic syndrome, characterized by osteopetrosis, syndactyly, severe facial dysmorphism, increased intracranial pressure, optic atrophy, and cranial nerve palsies affecting the seventh and eighth cranial nerves in particular.[5651]

sclerotome   The deep somatic structures which share innervation by a single spinal segment and to which pain may be referred when some part of the sclerotome is damaged.

The area of referred pain is somewhat variable between subjects, and the concept of fixed sclerotomes, akin to **dermatomes,** has been criticized.

scoliosis   (Gr, curvature or twisting) The word used by Hippocrates for a spinal curvature; today it signifies more specifically a lateral curvature of the spine, with rotation in cases of fixed or structural spinal disease.

scombroid   A relatively common icthyotoxicosis resulting from the ingestion of fish (or cheese) in which there has been bacterial decarboxylation of histidine to histamine. Within minutes up to an hour after ingestion, the patient complains of abdominal cramps, nausea, burning in the mouth and throat, headache, and dizziness. Flushing is usual, bronchospasm and respiratory distress are occasional. Untreated, the condition lasts but a few hours and is seldom fatal.

scotoepilepsy   A form of seizure disorder in which visual fixation can suppress the paroxysms. The clinical features resemble those of **benign occipital epilepsy.**[3512]

scotoma   (Gr, darkening, an eclipse) An island of blindness in a sea of vision. An *absolute scotoma* is an area in which not even light can be perceived. A *relative scotoma* is that form in which the subject can see form or movement but not color. *Negative scotomas* are imperceptible to the patient, while *positive scotomas* are appreciated as areas of darkness, as in the case of lesions situated anterior to the retina. See also **central, paracentral, ring,** and **centrocecal scotoma.**

scoto-sensitive epilepsy   Seizures precipitated by a decrease in ambient illumination.

Scott palsy   (Scott-Strachan disease) See **Strachan syndrome.**

Scott syndrome   A congenital X-linked dysmorphic syndrome characterized also by obesity, short stature, acanthosis nigricans, deafness, genital and skeletal abnormalities, microcephaly, and mental and developmental delay.[5032]

Scott-Strachan disease   See **Strachan syndrome.**

scrapie   A chronic, naturally occurring transmissible demyelinating disease of sheep due to a subvirus particle (virion) which induces a spongiform encephalopathy.

The name derives from the tendency of the sheep to scrape alongside fences and other field furniture as a result of their progressive ataxia.

Scratch 'n Sniff test   A commercial smell identification test in which a series of familiar odors is presented in the form of impregnated cards that release each odor when abraded.

scratching pest   See **pseudohydrophobia.**

Scripps neurological rating scale   A scale designed for the assessment of subjects with **multiple sclerosis.**[5191]

scrivener's palsy   A focal (occupational) dystonia. See **dystonia, writer's cramp.**

scrotal tongue   A ridged appearance to the tongue, reminding some of the dermal anatomy in baser regions.

scrotal reflex   Vermicular contraction of the dartos muscle, not causing elevation of the testicle, normally seen in response to gentle stimulation of the perineum.

scrub typhus   (tsutsumagushi fever) An infection caused by *Rickettsiae tsutsumagushi,* prevalent in eastern and southern Asia and transmitted by mites.

Clinically after a 1- to 3-week incubation period, an eschar develops at the site of the bite, and this is followed in order by the appearance of regional lymphadenopathy, fever, conjunctival injection, severe headache, myalgia, and frequently a rash. Neurological complications comprise features of encephalitis, including restlessness, delirium, tremors, seizures, and papilledema. Deafness and bulbar signs have also been described. The Weil-Felix reaction shows agglutination of O-K but the immunofluorescent test is more precise in diagnosis.[6030]

SDEEG   See **stereotactic (stereotaxic) depth electroencephalogram.**

sea shell sound   (sea shell roar or noise) The fanciful (though acceptably appropriate) name given to the continuous background activity sometimes recorded during electromyography, and representing **end-plate activity.**

sea-blue histiocytosis   The presence of large macrophages in which the cytoplasm is packed with granules staining blue-green or blue on Wright-Giemsa staining, particularly in the spleen, liver, and bone marrow. The granules may contain, for example, ceroid, lipofuscin, sphingomyelin, or other phospholipids. See **sphingomyelin storage disorders.**

The condition has been associated with a number of neurological, hematological, and other diseases; in the former category, albinism, **Hallervorden-Spatz disease, neuroaxonal dystrophies, Niemann-Pick disease,** peripheral neuropathy, posterior column dysfunction, and a multisystem CNS and anterior horn cell disease are examples.[243]

seamstresses' cramp   A focal (occupational) dystonia. See **dystonia.**

search reflex   See **rooting reflex.**

Seashore measure of musical talents   A test of pitch, loudness, rhythm, time, timbre, discrimination, and tonal memory. The evocative name, however, is merely that of the inventor.[5044]

seat-belt syncope   Syncope, mainly in the elderly, due to pressure of a seat-belt worn too high and pressing upon the carotid sinus.

Sebire syndrome   A pediatric encephalopathy characterized by the subacute appearance of movement disorders such as orofacial dyskinesias and chorea or limb dystonias, loss of motor skills, global aphasia, CSF pleocytosis, and sometimes seizures, with spontaneous recovery.[5045]

Seckel bird-headed dwarfism   (Virchow-Seckel syndrome, nanocephalic dwarfism, bird-like face syndrome) A recessively transmitted disease of children in which the head is small, the eyes apparently large, the nose beaked, and the mandible underdeveloped, all in association with severe mental retardation.

High-arched or cleft palate, prominent low-set or lobeless ears, antimongolian slant, epicanthic folds, kyphoscoliosis, sternal defects, absent patellae, congenital dislocation of the hip, and disorders of bone maturation are other features described.[5046] Apart from the dysmorphism, and sometimes feeding problems due to temporomandibular ankylosis, the condition may be complicated by hypersomnia, periodic obstructive apneic periods during sleep, and alveolar hypoventilation.

The first description of the condition was actually that of **Virchow** in 1882.

Seckel, H.P.G.   (b. 1900) Swiss pediatrician.

second impact syndrome   An unusual syndrome of uncertain provenance in which diffuse brain swelling occurs with delayed deterioration in cerebral function after repeated concussions, the second event occurring before the effects of the first one have subsided. It has usually been described in the context of sports played by young people. Both a failure in cerebral vascular autoregulation and true cerebral edema have been speculated as underlying the condition. The following diagnostic criteria have been formulated:[3738]

1. Medical review after a witnessed first impact
2. Documentation of ongoing symptoms following the first impact up to the time of the second impact
3. Witnessed second head impact with a subsequent rapid cerebral deterioration
4. Neuropathologic or neuroimaging evidence of cerebral swelling without significant intracranial hematoma or other cause for edema

See also **pugilistic encephalopathy, ding.**

second messenger   A substance mediating the transduction of a usually external cellular stimulus or signal and a given cellular response, such as muscle contraction, and neurotransmitter release, etc.

second sensory area   An area of cortex lying along the upper bank of the sylvian fissure with crude somatotopic representation, not including the face.[3504]

second sensory seizures   Epileptic seizures arising from a focus within the second sensory region, characterized by pain in the trunk and limbs.[6087]

second visual system   A system involving the pathway between the colliculus, the pulvinar, and the parietal lobe, which is concerned with directed visual attention (the detection of events, their location in space, and the control of orienting responses to them for subsequent identification by the first system). The control of orienting responses involves the geniculostriate pathway and is concerned with identification rather than detection.[6128]

second wind   Adaptation to exercise following an initial transient period of progressive fatigue and weakness of the affected muscles, first described in myophosphorylase deficiency but to some degree a normal phenomenon.

The mechanisms of re-invigoration include an increase in cardiac output and thus in muscle blood flow, increased EMG activity, and an alteration in the metabolic pathways, such that hexose phosphates, free fatty acids, and blood-borne glucose can be utilized to supply energy.[697]

secondary bilateral synchrony   The occurrence of sequential focal spikes of sharp waves on the EEG that lead on to bilaterally synchronous epileptiform paroxysms within 500 msec.[612]

secondary carnitine deficiency   Low levels of carnitine in the muscles of patients suffering from generalized systemic disease, other myopathies, or renal disease. The role of the reduced carnitine levels in the genesis of weakness in such situations is unproved.

secondary chronic cluster headache   See **chronic cluster headache.**

secondary dementias   Those dementing conditions due to pathological conditions affecting the brain or other organs other than primary degenerations.

secondary (ocular) deviation   See **primary deviation, cover test.**

secondary hypersomnolence   See **hypersomnolence.**

secondary optic atrophy   Optic atrophy following previous papilledema. Unlike the stark white disk of primary optic atrophy, the appearance in this condition is of a ragged, yellowish disk, sometimes with pigmentary deposits evidencing previous hemorrhage. See **consecutive optic atrophy.**

secondary phase nystagmus   See **vestibular nystagmus.**

secondary position   The position of the eyes when in adduction or abduction, elevation, or depression—that is, directed anywhere away from the straight-ahead primary position.

secondary syringomyelia   The formation of cavities within the spinal cord as a result of hemorrhage, tumor, or trauma.

secondary wave   A visible wave of contraction slowly progressing through a healthy muscle after it has been tapped or firmly stroked. The phenomenon was first described in 1857 by Schiff in Berne.[4053]

sector defects   See **retinal slits.**

sector scotoma   Holmes' term for homonymous loss of vision in the ipsilateral field due to lesions of the calcarine cortex, in which the loss lies along the vertical axes through the fixation points, either above or below the meridian and generally becoming wider toward the upper or lower limits of the fields.

sectoral hemianopia   See **hemianopia.**

sectoranopia   (sector defects) Loss of a section of the visual field, as a result of retinal lesions or of infarcts of the lateral geniculate body. See **retinal slits.**

Sedgwick-Boder syndrome   See **Louis-Bar syndrome.**

seducible nystagmus   See **gaze-evoked nystagmus.**

Seeligmüller neuralgia   Bilateral auriculotemporal neuralgia, in which the pain is felt from ear to ear over the vertex of the skull, especially pain elicited by pressure on the head, described in syphilis.[5050]

Seeligmüller, Otto Ludwig Gustav Adolf   (1837–1912) German neuropathologist who graduated from the University of Halle, studied neurology in Vienna and Paris, and was an associate professor in Halle. He is best remembered for his studies on childhood spastic states,[5049] but also for the observations in adjacent entries.

Otto Ludwig Gustav Adolf Seeligmüller

Seeligmüller sign   Mydriasis on the side affected in trigeminal neuralgia. The mechanism is uncertain.

Seemenova syndrome   A recessively inherited congenital dysmorphic syndrome, characterized also by short stature, T-cell and immunoglobulin deficiency, and microcephaly.[5051]

seesaw anisocoria   See **springing pupil.**

seesaw nystagmus   A rare ocular oscillation induced by an unstable visuovestibular interaction control system (likely due to disruption of chiasmal crossing fibers) in which there is rapid, rhythmic, opposed alternation of the vertical positions of the eyes. The movements are pendular and torsional with a vertical component, but are asymmetrical; the intorting eye rises while the other, extorting, eye falls. The condition is not actually a true nystagmus.[1368] The most common cause is a caudal diencephalic lesion, such as a parasellar tumor expanding into the third ventricle, in which case a bitemporal field defect is also commonly found. Trauma, multiple sclerosis, and brainstem vascular diseases are other causes.[4065]

A *congenital form* is similar, but it lacks the torsional component. See also **ocular tilt reaction, hemi-seesaw nystagmus.**

seesaw winking with orofaciodigital signs   A congenital dysmorphic syndrome, characterized also by dental and skeletal abnormalities, strabismus, and mental and developmental delay.[337]

Segawa dystonia   (hereditary progressive diurnal dystonia, progressive dystonia with diurnal fluctuation) A dominantly inherited dystonic syndrome mapped to 14q21–22.2, with onset in childhood and also characterized by the diurnal occurrence of the abnormal movements, usually accompanied by parkinsonian features. The condition responds well to L-dopa therapy.[1403,5052] See also **dopa-responsive dystonia.**

Segelman syndrome   A congenital dysmorphic syndrome characterized by skeletal abnormalities, multiple cavernous hemangiomas, recurrent infections, and mental and developmental delay.[337]

segmental demyelination   Selective, discontinuous damage to Schwann cells, rendering them unable to maintain that segment of myelin for which they are responsible and leading to the disruption and removal of myelin in the segments between two nodes of Ranvier; loss of portions of the myelin sheath surrounding peripheral axons.

Depending on both the number of adjacent Schwann cells so affected and their position in relation to the node of Ranvier, **conduction block** may or may not occur.

segmental dystonia   Dystonia that affects more than one body area, such areas being contiguous.

segmental hyperhidrosis   Increased sweating in the skin supplied by one or more spinal segments uni- or bilaterally and usually indicating irritation or infiltration of preganglionic sympathetic fibers or of the sympathetic chain. See also **Ross syndrome.**[5010]

The same problem can also occur in trigeminal nerve territory.

segmental instability   A spinal disorder, possibly a cause of recurrent low back pain and scoliosis, characterized by narrowing of the disk space, the presence of numerous **traction spurs,** and shifts in spinal alignment seen on radiographs taken in flexion and extension.[1975,4054] However, the very existence of the syndrome is controversial.[1974]

segmental myoclonus Myoclonus of cranial or spinal origin, which thus affects a group of muscles innervated by one cranial nerve (as with hemifacial spasm) or affects one or more than one adjacent spinal segment. The movements may be irregular or periodic, and may be stimulus-sensitive. See **spinal myoclonus.**

segmental neuralgia See **intercostal neuralgia.**

segmental neurofibromatosis See **neurofibromatosis.**

segmental spinal muscular atrophy A sporadic or dominantly inherited syndrome of weakness and atrophy which affects especially the distal upper extremities.[4390] This condition may be the same as **de Grouchy syndrome.**

Séguin, Edouard Onesimus (1812–1880) French psychiatrist who trained under Esquirol and was later an instructor at the Bicêtre. Encouraged by the example of **Itard** with the "Wild Boy of Aveyron", he espoused the cause of the mentally retarded, employing the principle that the senses could be made to compensate for each other when any one was impaired. From his unit at the Bicêtre he published his *Traitement moral, hygiene et éducation des idiots et des autres enfants arrières* in 1846, an account of his pioneering experiences in the training of mentally retarded people.

His political activities made it advisable for him to emigrate from France on the ascent of Louis Napoleon, and he chose the United States, where successively in Cleveland, Pennsylvania, and New York he introduced new methods in the management of the mentally ill and the mentally defective, using his refinements of the methods of Esquirol. The spirit of these endeavors was adopted by Mme. Montessori in her schools.

Séguin, Edward Constant (1843–1898) British physician who described the autopsy findings in **multiple sclerosis** and **papilledema.**

Séguin sign Contraction of a local group of muscles immediately before a generalized tonic-clonic convulsion,[4723] and thus evidence of a focal origin of the seizure.

Seitelberger disease 1. See **infantile neuroaxonal dystrophy, glioneuronal dystrophies.** 2. See **Pelizaeus-Merzbacher disease.**

seizure arrest The process whereby the further development of a partial seizure is aborted by a specific activity of the patient.

Gowers pointed out that ligatures placed about the upper arm of a patient of his who suffered Jacksonian seizures in that arm successfully stopped his seizures at that point, with greater effect as the exercise was repeated. In other cases, strong odors have been found effective in arresting complex partial seizures.

seizure pattern, EEG The occurrence of repetitive EEG discharges with a relatively abrupt onset and termination and with a characteristic pattern of evolution, lasting at least several seconds. The component waves or complexes vary in form, frequency, and topography. They are generally rhythmic, and frequently display increasing amplitude and decreasing frequency during the same episode. When focal in onset, they tend to spread subsequently to other areas.

EEG seizure patterns unaccompanied by a clinical epileptic manifestation detected by the recordist and/or reported by the patient should be referred to as *subclinical.* See also **epileptiform pattern.** (Adapted from the 1974 report of the Committee on Terminology, IFCN. In: Chatrian GE, Bergamini L, Dondey M, et al. A glossary of terms most commonly used by clinical electroencephalographers. *EEG Clin Neurophysiol* 1974; **37:**538–548, by kind permission of Elsevier Science.)

seizure rating scales Attempts to quantify the impact and severity of seizures, most assessing seizure frequency, type and duration, postictal events and their duration, automatisms, seizure clusters, known patterns, warnings, tongue biting, incontinence, resulting injuries, and functional impairment. Those in current use, reviewed by Cramer and French (2001),[1155] include the **Veterans Administration (VA), Chalfont-National Hospital, Liverpool, Hague,** and occupational hazard scales.

seizures Combinations of motor, sensory, and psychical events occurring as the result of occasional, sudden, rapid, local, and excessive discharges of gray matter (after J. Hughlings-**Jackson**).

seizures induced by movement See **paroxysmal kinesigenic choreoathetosis.**

seizures with multiple independent spike foci An epileptic syndrome seen in younger children, characterized by the frequent occurrence of polymorphic bilateral seizures, including generalized atonic-clonic seizures, myoclonic jerks, atypical absences, and tonic or clonic bilateral motor seizures or partial motor seizures, associated with neurological signs, including mental retardation. Three or more spike foci are recorded in both hemispheres on the EEG.[610]

selective amnesia Restricted failure of memory resulting from unilateral damage to the limbic system. The defect resulting is material-specific (verbal or nonverbal), according to the side of the lesion.

selective attention evoked potential A negative potential shift recorded from scalp electrodes positioned at the vertex, lasting less than a second and occurring during directed attention to auditory, visual, or somatosensory stimuli presented from one side as opposed to the other.[3851]

selective neuronal necrosis   Cellular damage following ischemia of selectively susceptible cells, usually due to cardiac arrest. The affected cells (for instance, of the hippocampus, striatum, or neocortex) show pyknosis, nuclear swelling, and cytoplasmic eosinophilic change.

selective neuronal vulnerability   The variable response of certain neurons and discrete areas of the brain to a generalized metabolic insult, such as hypoxia; to which, for example, the third, fifth, and sixth cortical cell layers, Sommers' sector of the hippocampus, the Purkinje and basket cells of the cerebellum, and parts of the amygdala are especially sensitive, while the spinal cord is relatively immune.

selective saccadic palsy   See **saccadic paralysis.**

selective signature dysgraphia   A selective inability to sign one's name, in the absence of other cognitive disorders, first described by one of the original authors following his left parietal lesion.[4633]

selective sleep stage deprivation   The process whereby the functions of rapid eye movement or non–rapid eye movement sleep are studied by repetitively waking the patient when such a stage is entered.

self-grasping   The grasping of one forearm with the other hand, a sign indicating the presence of a contralateral frontal or parietal lobe lesion.[4765]

self-induced photosensitive epilepsy   See **photosensitive epilepsies.**

sella turcica   (Lat, a Turkish saddle) The fossa in the skull base in which the pituitary gland lies.

Selye, Hans   (1907–1952) Austrian physician, philosopher, and physiologist who trained in Vienna, Paris, Rome, and Prague. He emigrated to Canada and became director of the Institute of Experimental Medicine at the Université de Montréal.

His philosophy was overt rather than institutional, and led (among other things) to his concept of the **general adaptation syndrome.**[5061]

Selye syndrome   See **general adaptation syndrome.**

semantic anomia   See **anomia.**

semantic aphasia   The term of Sir Henry **Head** for that form of speech disorder characterized by a disturbance in the capacity to comprehend and retain the general significance of a word or phrase as part of a complete act of language. The single word may be understood but its ultimate meaning within the context of the sentence is lost. It stems from a lesion of the supramarginal gyrus. The term is now seldom employed.[2496]

semantic dementia   A fluent variety of primary progressive aphasia (**frontotemporal dementia**) in which patients lose semantic memory and the comprehension of the meaning of words but retain normal articulation and syntax.

semantic jargon   Speech in which the correct words are replaced by those which are acceptable but semantically faulty in that context. This occurs in **transcortical** and in **Wernicke aphasias.**

semantic memory   A type of long-term memory comprising the store of all the information required in order to use language, including the words, their meanings, and what they represent, as well as grammatical, mathematical, and factual rules and related data.

semantic paralexia   The substitution of synonyms for the written words read aloud.

semantic pragmatic syndrome   A disorder of higher language processing leading to impairments in answering questions of the why? when? or how? type and in prosody and fluency, despite retention of phonological and syntactical skills, and the ability to answer questions of the yes/no variety. It was described first in hydrocephalic children.[5451]

semantic retrieval-organization syndrome   A disorder of higher language processing leading to impairments in fluency due to difficulties in word finding and syntax, especially in elicited as opposed to spontaneous speech.

semantics   1. The meanings in words and phrases. For example, in English it would be unacceptable to say "bachelor's wife," since the phrase contains a contradiction in meaning. Further, the sentence "The baseball bat bit the girl " is unacceptable, since a baseball bat is an inanimate object.[3505,5852] 2. The rules governing meaningful verbal dialogue; that branch of linguistics which deals with meaning.[1178]

semi-   (Lat, half; the Greek form is *demi*). Prefix denoting half.

semicircular canals   The three curved, endolymph-containing channels situated at right angles to one another, which open into the utricle and saccule within, and constitute, the inner ear. They were described by Fallopius in 1561.

semilunar ganglion   (Gr, half + moon) The main sensory ganglion (**gasserian ganglion**) of the trigeminal nerve, lying on the medial end of the petrous portion of the temporal bone.

semiotics   (semantics) A system of symbols manipulated according to certain conventions, such as numbers, letters, morse code, and chessmen.

semimembranosus reflex   See **internal hamstring reflex.**

Seminars in Neurology   (*Semin. Neurol.*) A neurological review journal. Address: Thieme Medical Publishers, 381 Park Ave. South, New York, NY 10016. Web site: http://www.thieme.com/SID1993373986839/journals/pubid2017629976.html.

seminoma-like tumor   See **germinoma.**

semipurposeful automatisms   See **sleepwalking.**

semitendinosus reflex   Contraction of this muscle in response to a tap on its tendon on the medial side of the popliteal fossa. The reflex has little clinical importance, although the biceps femoris reflex is of value since it informs uniquely about the state of the L5 reflex arc. The tendon of this latter muscle is on the lateral side of the popliteal fossa.

Semliki forest encephalitis   Direct infection of the brain by an alphavirus member of the togavirus class of arboviruses, occurring in southern and eastern Africa.

Semon, Sir Felix   (1849–1921) German-English laryngologist who trained in Heidelberg and Berlin but went to England in 1875 and practiced in London, where he worked at the **National Hospital** and other hospitals and collaborated with **Horsley.**

He showed that adductor paralysis of the larynx could be due to psychosomatic states, myasthenia, or other muscle diseases, and that nerve lesions affecting the larynx affected the abductors first.

Semon's law   The abductor fibers of the recurrent laryngeal nerve are affected by disease sooner than the adductor fibers. Thus, with partial lesions of the vagus (recurrent laryngeal) nerve, the paretic cord tends to lie in a position of adduction.[5063]

Semont liberatory maneuver   (manoeuvre libératoire) A technique for relieving the symptoms of **benign positional vertigo**[5064] (see Chart S–3).

Chart S–3. The Semont Liberatory Maneuver

1.A. Starting with the patient sitting straight up on the examining table, swing the patient down quickly, with the offending ear down and the head slightly declined. If the nystagmus appears (it should be torsional with the fast phase beating toward the down ear), keep the patient there until the nystagmus disappears, and then wait another 2–3 minutes.

1.B. If the nystagmus doesn't appear in A, turn the patient's head so that the face is up 45° from the horizontal. The nystagmus should then appear. Again, keep the patient in this position for 2–3 minutes after the nystagmus stops.

2. Hold the patient's head and neck with both hands and swing the patient quickly to the opposite side. The speed of the head must be 0 at the moment it touches the examining table.

3.A. If you are dealing with a classic case of benign positional paroxysmal vertigo (BPPV), a rotatory nystagmus will develop with the fast phase still beating toward the offending ear (the top ear). If it is beating toward the down ear, all bets are off and you are not dealing with BPPV. The typical BPPV nystagmus generally has a greater amplitude but lower frequency than the nystagmus with the bad ear down.

3.B. If no nystagmus develops after the turn to the oppo-site ear, move the head slowly to 90° facing up, and then turn the head in the opposite direction 135° so that it is 45° facing down below the horizontal (with the sick ear up). The nystagmus should then occur.

3.C. Hold the patient in the nystagmus-inducing position for at least 5 minutes, and then bring the patient back to a sitting position very, very slowly.

4. Have the patient keep the head absolutely vertical during the next 48 hours, day and night. See the instructions to patients, below.

5. After the 48-hour interval, patients are prohibited from sleeping on their vertigo-generating side for a week. If the maneuver is not successful, it is performed again a week later.

There is an 84% positive success rate with one maneuver and 90% positive success rate after a second maneuver 1 week later. The recurrence rate is 4.2%.

Instructions to patients after the liberatory maneuver: Whatever the position of your body, you must keep your head vertical for the next 48 hours. Imagine your head being hung by an invisible string to the ceiling. You must not bend your head forward nor backward. You must not go to the barber, hairdresser, or dentist. No exercise. When men shave under their chins, they should bend the body forward in order to tense the skin and keep the head vertical. Do not instill eyedrops. Only shampoo when under the shower. At night, lie on your back with plenty of pillows to keep your head vertical while your trunk is 30°–45° elevated off the bed. Put something at the bottom of the bed in order not to slip down during the night.

From Semont A, Freyss G, Vitte E. Curing the BPPV with a liberatory maneuver. Adv Otorhinolaryngol 1988;42:290–293. Reprinted with the kind permission of Karger (Basel).

Senator disease   See **polymyositis.**

Senator, Hermann   (1834–1911) American neurologist.

Senger syndrome   A congenital dysmorphic syndrome inherited as an X-linked recessive trait and characterized by obesity, short stature, hypogenitalism, hydrocephalus, and mental and developmental delay.[337]

senile   A pejorative term of no clinical worth, there being no known physical alteration affecting people at the time of their 65th birthday. Even the euphemistic "of later life" is preferable to this author.

senile chorea   A rare condition of later life characterized by the appearance of generalized and progressive chorea that is unaccompanied by mental changes or any family history of **Huntington disease,**[88] although the pathological changes in the caudate nucleus are similar.

senile dementia   See **Alzheimer disease.**

senile dementia of the Alzheimer type   See **Alzheimer disease.**

senile dementia of the Binswanger type   See **Binswanger disease.**

senile gait   See **cautious gait.**

senile macular degeneration   Bilateral retinal degenerative changes, including the formation of subretinal fibrovascular plaques, hemorrhages, pigmentation, and proliferative retinopathy, occurring as an age-related change in the macular region as a result of microvascular disease.

senile plaques   See **neuritic plaques.** They were regarded by Rio Hortega as resembling rooks' nests in winter elms.

senile psychosis   A term that is irritating because of use of the word *senile* and imprecise because of use of the word *psychosis*, but that is used variously to refer to the dementias of later life and for presbyophrenia (a paranoid state probably arising from a depressive illness in elderly people).

senile thenar atrophy   A focal muscle atrophy described by Marie and Foix well before the delineation of the **carpal tunnel syndrome,** which is the usual cause.

Senior-Loken syndrome   (familial retinal-renal dystrophy) A rare, recessively inherited syndrome characterized by pigmentary retinal degeneration with visual failure, psychomotor retardation, anemia, and renal impairment leading eventually to renal failure.[5012]

Both congenital and adult forms are described, the latter of lesser severity and longer course.

sensation, cortical   Modes of awareness, depending on the presence of the analytic powers of the cortex. These include **graphesthesia, stereognosis, tactile discrimination,** and **tactile localization.**

sense of obstacles   See **facial vision of the blind.**

Sensenbrenner syndrome   See **craniosynostosis.**

sensitivity   The ratio of the input voltage to the output pen deflection in an EEG channel. Sensitivity is measured in microvolts per millimeter (uV/mm). Thus:

$$\text{Sensitivity} = \frac{\text{Input Voltage}}{\text{Output Pen Deflection}} = \frac{50 \text{ uV}}{10 \text{ mm}} = 5 \text{ uV/mm}$$

sensorimotor perineuritis   A rare sensorimotor peripheral neuropathy with prominent motor deficits, accompanied by marked slowing of nerve conduction velocities, histological evidence of inflammatory perineurial thickening, and deposits of immunoglobulin G and M on perineurial cells.[684] See also **sensory perineuritis, gammopathic neuropathy.**

sensorimotor psychological syndrome   Hemianesthesia with psychological and motor disturbances accompanied by visual, auditory, and vestibular symptoms including hallucinations, and involuntary movements, all affecting the same side of the body and considered by de Morsier to be due to some disturbance of the hypothalamic system.[1381]

sensorimotor stroke   (thalamocapsular stroke) A **lacunar syndrome** characterized by the association of hemiparesis with hypoesthesia or dysesthesia involving one side of the mouth and the arm on that side, or the whole of that side of the body. The site of the lesion is variable—it may be either deep in the basal ganglia or in the corona radiata.[5899]

sensorineural deafness   Deafness resulting from genetic, neoplastic, inflammatory, vascular, traumatic, or other lesions of the cochlear branches of the eighth cranial nerves. Such deafness may also complicate systemic autoimmune diseases, and autoimmunity has been proposed as the basis of some cases of **Ménière disease** and acute vertigo.

sensorium commune   The entire central nervous system—the common seat of the mechanism of sensation. See also **sensus communis.**

sensory and autonomic neuropathy   A rare syndrome characterized by features otherwise typical of progressing **hereditary sensory and autonomic neuropathy,** but with onset during adult life and without the appearance of the disease in other family members.[4229]

sensory aprosodia   An inability to perceive the emotive content of language heard, despite retention of normal spontaneous affective prosodic variation and gesture. It is a sign of a right parietotemporal lesion[4801] (inferior divisional infarction of the right middle cerebral artery). See **aprosodia.**

sensory ataxia   (proprioceptive ataxia) Awkwardness of voluntary movements as a result of impaired conscious proprioception. The syndrome is characterized by poor directional control of movement, made worse by eye closure, **fantaisiste ataxia,** and disorganization of movement rather than true incoordination.

sensory ataxia–optic atrophy syndrome   A nutritional disorder resulting from vitamin B complex (B_1, B_2, B_3, B_5, and B_6) deficiency.[5794] The leading clinical features are sensory ataxia due to peripheral neuropathy and visual failure with optic atrophy.

sensory ataxic ganglionopathies   See **sensory ganglionitis.**

sensory chronic inflammatory demyelinating neuropathy   A variant of **chronic inflammatory demyelinating neuropathy** presenting with distal painful pansensory loss, which is minimal if there is any distal weakness and electrical evidence of demyelination. See http://www.wustl.edu/neuromuscular.

sensory competition   A sign of parietal lobe dysfunction. The inability to appreciate one of two stimuli presented simultaneously. The test is most often performed with bilateral stimulation, but double stimuli on the one side may also show an abnormality in which only one is perceived, although each is appreciated when presented in isolation. See **extinction.**

sensory dermatomes   The area of skin supplied by a single sensory root. Overlap on the trunk makes the determination of the dermatomes difficult, but the areas supplied in the limbs are relatively constant and overlap between segments is much less.

sensory end-organ   An apparatus by which a sensory nerve fiber is rendered distinctly amenable to some particular physical agent, and at the same time rendered less amenable to, that is, is shielded from, other excitants (Sir Charles **Sherrington**). The definition thus accepts both the concepts of receptor specificity and of the adequate stimulus.

sensory fusion   The ability to fuse two retinal images together using cerebral cortical mechanisms.

sensory ganglionitis   (autoimmune ataxic neuropathies; sensory ataxic ganglionopathies) Immune-mediated disorders in which inflammatory changes affect the dorsal root ganglia and lead to the clinical picture of sensory axonal neuropathy. It may occur as a **paraneoplastic syndrome,** in the **sicca syndrome,** and in **idiopathic sensory neuronopathy.** Toxic, deficiency, and hereditary causes are also described. Clinically, losses of thick fiber function lead to prominent sensory ataxia with loss of motor control.[4231]

See also **Miller-Fisher syndrome, acute demyelinating neuropathy, chronic idiopathic ataxic neuropathy, chronic inflammatory dysimmune polyneuropathy, hereditary sensory and autonomic neuropathy, olivopontocerebellar atrophy.**

sensory inattention   See **inattention.**

sensory Jacksonian seizures   Attacks of paresthesia occurring spasmodically in a certain part of the body and spreading in a certain order, not always in keeping with the accepted geography of the sensory homunculus on the postcentral gyrus.

According to Arnold **Pick,** the term was first employed by Krafft-Ebing, who described sensory paralytic attacks in his book on **general paresis.**

sensory latency   The interval between the onset of a stimulus and the onset of the negative deflection of the compound sensory nerve action potential. This term has been used loosely to refer to the sensory peak latency. It may be qualified as proximal sensory latency or distal sensory latency, depending on the relative position of the stimulus. (From the 2001 Report of the Nomenclature Committee of the American Association of Electromyography and Electrodiagnosis.[10] Used by permission, copyright © 2001, AAEM.)

sensory loss   See **alternating, cortical, hysterical, suspended,** and **thalamic sensory loss.**

sensory modalities   Different sensory perceptions, mediated by patterns of neuronal input which vary in time and space but which are not exclusively associated with a particular afferent pathway. Thus ascription of pain and temperature function to the spinothalamic tract is but a convenient approximation.

sensory nerve   A nerve containing only sensory fibers, composed mainly of axons innervating cutaneous receptors.

sensory nerve action potential   (SNAP) See compound sensory nerve action potential.

sensory nerve conduction velocity   The speed of propagation of action potentials along a sensory nerve.

sensory neuronopathy   See **subacute sensory neuropathy.**

sensory neuropathy with hereditary ataxia   See **hereditary sensory and autonomic neuropathy** (*variants*).

sensory paralytic bladder   Afferent denervation of the bladder, with anesthesia, dilatation, retention, and overflow incontinence but without loss of the ability to initiate micturition consciously. Lesions of the pelvic nerves or of the posterior columns may be responsible.

sensory peak latency   Interval between the onset of a stimulus and the peak of the negative phase of the compound sensory nerve action potential.

sensory perineuritis   A sensory peripheral neuropathy or multiple mononeuropathy with the pathological finding of chronic inflammatory and fibrotic changes limited to the perineurium of the affected nerves.

Clinically, patients complain of pain and sensory loss in a glove-and-stocking distribution. No systemic disease is detected and the cause is not known,[230] but the condition may respond to steroid therapy. See also **migrant sensory neuritis, sensorimotor perineuritis.**

sensory starts   Sudden paroxysmal awareness of stimulation of one sensory channel on falling asleep; the sensory equivalent to **hypnic jerks.**

sensory system   All of the afferent pathways informing the organism about the disposition of the internal and external environments.

sensory tics   Uncomfortable, involuntary, transient, and recurrent somatic sensations felt in the skin and relieved only by vocalization or other movements in **Tourette syndrome.** They are variously described as feelings of pressure, tickle, warmth, cold, or other sensations, and are usually localized to the upper half of the body.[993,5092]

sensory trick   See **geste antagonistique.**

sensus communis   (sensorium commune) A primary faculty of perception; the gathering of all specific sense impressions to allow the appreciation of magnitude, motion, and time, according to Aristotle. This overall appreciative sense was termed **coenesthesis** by Reil in 1794, who noted its obscure, immediate, compound nature, and who considered it to be the basis for self-awareness and personal identity, localized somewhere, he knew not where, in the cerebrum. And nor do we.

sentinel headache   (warning headache) An acute head pain, usually felt posteriorly and resembling the pain of **subarachnoid hemorrhage,** though less severe and commonly lasting for less time. The pathogenesis is, however, the leaking of blood into the CSF, usually from an aneurysm, and the headache demands the same attention and management as that for the full-blown condition, since catastrophic rupture of an aneurysm may follow at any time.

SEPs   See **somatosensory evoked potentials.**

septic aneurysm   See **mycotic aneurysm.**

septic embolism   An infected embolus occluding an artery. The consequences of this include infarction or septic infarction of the territory supplied by that vessel; a focal arteritis which may spread into surrounding tissues to cause (in the brain) a local cerebral abscess or focal meningitis; and weakening of the vessel wall, which may lead on to the formation of a **mycotic aneurysm.**

septic encephalopathy   A heterogeneous syndrome of altered consciousness with paratonia and impairments in attention, orientation, concentration, and writing, occurring early in the course of sepsis, trauma, or burns, with multiple organ dysfunction ("critical illness") developing later. Frank delirium occurs later still. Focal or multifocal seizures, multifocal myoclonus, cranial nerve palsies, and asterixis are *not* typical clinical features of the condition.

The underlying mechanisms include **central pontine myelinolysis,** microabscesses, microhemorrhages, multiple cerebral infarctions, and direct toxic or metabolic causes.[2770]

septic myopathies   Disorders of muscle complicating severe septic illnesses and possibly burns and severe trauma. These include cachexia, commonly; myositis and myoglobinuria due to panfascicular muscle fiber necrosis, and **acute suppurative myositis,** a condition of multiple purulent abscesses within muscles, occur rarely.[649]

septo-optic dysplasia   A congenital syndrome, sometimes recessively inherited, characterized by hypoplasia of the optic nerve, hypoglycemia, hypopituitarism, seizures, small sella turcica, avum septi pellucidi, and both physical growth retardation and psychomotor delay.[604]

Callosal abnormalities, schizencephaly, hydrocephalus, encephalocele, and cerebral atrophy have also been reported in this rare syndrome.[335] See **de Morsier syndrome.**

septum pellucidum   (septum lucidum) A thin membrane between the fornix and the corpus callosum, first described by Galen.

sequential ultrasonic arteriography   A technique whereby either pulsed or continuous-wave Doppler sonography is used to construct an image of blood vessels, disease being detected by the finding of defects in the image itself and by spectral analysis (as in duplex ultrasonography). The method accurately identifies severe disease, but is insensitive to minor lesions.[4141]

serial recitation tests   Tests of attention, in which the subject is required to count in 3's, to subtract numbers serially (serial sevens), or to recite the days or months in forward or reverse order.

serial seizures   A series of epileptic attacks in which consciousness is regained between each.[56]

serotonin   5-Hydroxytryptamine (5-HT), a vasoactive (variously constrictor or dilator) substance that is also involved in mood, appetite, sleep, and pain pathways.

serotonin receptors   Receptors present both in cerebral blood vessels and central pain pathways. 5-HT1a, 1b, 1c, 1d, and 5-HT2 sites are identified with certainty, and more are likely to be detected.

serotonin syndrome   A syndrome resulting from central serotonergic hyperstimulation, typically as a result of combining serotonergic drugs with monoamineoxidase inhibitors (MAOIs). It may also occur when combinations of L-tryptophan, clomipramine, bromocriptine, L-dopa, demerol, or dextromorphan are given at the same time as MAOIs, carbamazepine, pentacozine, or selective serotonin reuptake inhibitors (SSRIs), because of enhancement of serotonin activity through blockade of its reuptake, thus increasing presynaptic release.

Clinically, it is characterized by mental status and behavioral changes (agitation, excitement, confusion, hypomania, obtundation), motor system involvement (myoclonus, hemiballismus, tremor, hyperreflexia, motor weakness, dysarthria, akathisia, incoordination) and autonomic symptoms (fever, chills, diarrhea, sweating, shivering). The syndrome has been reported exclusively in patients on medications for psychiatric illness and parkinsonism, and in those taking one or more serotonomimetic agents for migraine prophylaxis (sertraline, paroxetine, lithium, imipramine, amitriptyline) or acute therapy (a triptan or dihydroergotamine). Typical combinations of drugs reported to produce the syndrome include L-tryptophan and SSRIs or MAOIs; SSRIs and carbamazepine, pentacozine, or MAOIs (or alone); venlafaxine and MAOIs; clomipramine and MAOIs (or alone); bromocriptine and L-dopa; and demerol or dextromorphan and MAOIs. Lithium worsens all features of the syndrome.

Symptoms are usually transient with full recovery on withdrawal of the responsible agents; but high fever, nystagmus, oculogyric crises, dysarthria, pyramidal syndrome, myoglobinuria, renal failure, disseminated intravascular coagulation, cardiac arrhythmias and death have been reported, rarely.[618,3695]

The following diagnostic criteria have been determined:[5344, 5345]

1. The symptoms must coincide with the introduction or dosage increment of a known serotomimetic agent.
2. At least three of the following signs and symptoms must be present.
   Mental status changes such as confusion or hypomania
   Myoclonus
   Diaphoresis
   Tremor
   Poor coordination
   Agitation
   Hyperreflexia
   Shivering
   Diarrhea
   Fever
3. Other etiologies must be ruled out, such as infection, metabolic disturbance, and substance abuse or withdrawal.
4. **Neuroleptic malignant syndrome** should be excluded from the differential diagnosis (a neuroleptic agent should not have been initiated or increased in dose prior to the onset of signs and symptoms).

serous meningitis (minor pseudomeningitis) See **idiopathic intracranial hypertension.** The term is now largely discarded, though once it was used to denote meningeal irritation without evidence of such in the CSF and so usually indicated the presence of a parameningeal focus of inflammation or a nonpurulent (lymphocytic) meningitis.

serrated action potential A waveform with several changes in direction (turns) which do not cross the baseline. The term is most often used to describe a motor unit action potential. It is preferred to *complex motor unit action potential* and *pseudopolyphasic action potential.* See also **turn** and **polyphasic action potential.**[10]

serum sickness A form of hypersensitivity vasculitis. Neurological complications may include encephalopathy with coma and seizures, brachial plexopathy, and (rarely) symmetrical peripheral neuropathy.[1506]

set test A test of verbal fluency in which subjects are asked to name as many examples as they can recall in each of four categories—animals, colors, fruits, and towns—to a maximum of 10 each; scores of under 15 are considered to indicate a loss of verbal fluency.[2751]

setting sun sign Tonic downward deviation of the eyes in association with retraction of the upper lid (**posterior fossa stare**); a sign of compression of the dorsal midbrain, as in infants with hydrocephalus.

setting-in nystagmus See **gaze-evoked nystagmus.**

Seven Minute screen A sensitive screening tool to help identify patients who merit evaluation for Alzheimer disease, using a series of questions to assess different types of intellectual functionality and claimed to be able to distinguish between cognitive changes due to the normal aging process and those due to dementia.

Four tests are included: *orientation* (awareness of the current year, month, date, day of the week, and time);

memory (recall of 16 pictures, presented four at a time on individual flash cards. A cue is offered when the patient is asked to recall each set of pictures; while healthy individuals benefit from this hint, persons with Alzheimer disease do not.); *clock drawing*, in which subjects are asked to draw the face of a clock, with the hands set to 3:40 P.M.); and *verbal fluency*, in which the subject is asked to name as many items as possible in a specific category (such as "vegetables") within 1 minute. The test is available at: http://www.7minutescreen.com/html/works.html.

severe childhood autosomal recessive muscular dystrophy (SCARMD; OMIM 253700) A polygenic, recessively inherited form of congenital muscular dystrophy (an **adhalinopathy/dystrophinopathy**) resembling **Duchenne dystrophy** except for its autosomal recessive inheritance pattern. All components of the sarcoglycan complex are absent in the muscles.[4285] The condition is mapped variously to 13q and 17q.

For a confident diagnosis, the parents of the subject should be healthy and consanguineous and their male and female children should exhibit calf pseudohypertrophy and other Duchenne muscular dystrophy–like symptoms. See also **autosomal recessive muscular dystrophy, limb-girdle muscular dystrophy.**

severe congenital encephalopathy A fatal familial disease due to a primary disorder of axonal development, leading to a reduction in interneuronal synaptic contacts.

Clinically, a profound disorder of mental and motor development, hypotonia, secondary microcephaly, and agenesis of the corpus callosum are characteristic features; necrotizing myopathy, cardiomyopathy, cataracts, and failure to thrive are others.[3532]

Severe Impairment battery A scheme for assessing the retained capabilities of patients with advanced dementia using simple verbal commands with gestural reinforcement.[4935]

severe infantile neuraminic acid storage disease, French type See **sialuria.**

severe infantile sialidosis See **nephrosialidosis.**

severe muscular dystrophy in girls A rare, recessively inherited condition in which there is severe muscular dystrophy presenting in infancy or early childhood with delayed motor milestones, predominant early toe-walking, and more weakness of the deltoid muscles and a slower and milder course than in the case of **Duchenne dystrophy.** There is no cardiac involvement. The distribution and nature of the other symptoms are similar to those of Duchenne dystrophy, but the serum creatine kinase levels are raised only to between 7 and 70 times the normal levels.[2024]

severe myoclonic epilepsy of infancy A recently defined syndrome, the characteristics of which include a family history of intractable epilepsy or febrile convulsions, normal development before onset, seizures beginning during the first year of life in the form of generalized or unilateral febrile clonic convulsions, secondary appearance of myoclonic jerks, and often partial seizures.

The EEG shows generalized spike–waves and polyspike–waves, early photosensitivity, and focal abnormalities. Psychomotor development is retarded from the second year of life on, and ataxia, pyramidal signs, and interictal myoclonus appear. This type of epilepsy is very resistant to all forms of treatment. (From the revised ILAE Classification,[1114] reproduced by kind permission from Blackwell Science.) See also **myoclonus.**

severe postural cerebellar tremor   See **cerebellar tremors.**

sex-linked diseases   See **X-linked** diseases.

Seyffrath syndrome   See **pronator teres syndrome.**

SFEMG   See **single fiber electromyography.**

shadow plaque   Incomplete staining of newly formed myelin in a plaque of **multiple sclerosis** in the brain.

shagreen patch   A flattened plaque of skin with an orange peel or pigskin texture, overlying a region of subepidermal fibrosis, usually in lumbosacral regions; a diagnostic finding in **tuberous sclerosis.**

shaken infant syndrome   An encephalopathy resulting from shaking injuries that caused cortical and subcortical contusions, hemorrhages, hypoxic/ischemic and axonal damage, and/or severe edema. These findings, however, usually resolve within 6 months but may result in multicystic encephalomalacia, porencephaly, generalized white matter attenuation, diffuse cortical atrophy, microgyria, ulegyria, hydrocephalus ex vacuo, progressive cortical dysplasia with cytoarchitectural disorganization, laminar obliteration, morphologic and functional (synaptic reorganization) neurofilament immunoreactivity.[3625]

shaking palsy   The term applied by Dr. James Parkinson to what is now known as **Parkinson disease.**

shaky legs syndrome   See **orthostatic tremor.**

sham mirth   Release of the controlling mechanisms for activity of the laughter center (wherever that is) in the absence of the appropriate stimulus, usually either as a manifestation of epilepsy or in cases of bilateral pyramidal tract disease, sometimes actually before the establishment of a stroke or subarachnoid hemorrhage (*Le fou rire prodromique* of Féré, 1903).

The anatomy of the lesions is unclear, but the hypothalamus appears to be involved in most cases.[3655] See **spasmodic laughter.**

sham rage   A state in which an animal deprived of its cerebral hemispheres (or of the amygdaloid nuclei bilaterally) reacts to all stimuli with the behavioral and autonomic manifestations of extreme anger.

Shapiro syndrome   See **corpus callosum agenesis with recurrent hypothermia.**

shark mouth   The appearance of the upper lip of some children with **myotonic dystrophy,** the lip being tented upward like a circumflex accent.

sharp wave   A transient wave on the EEG clearly distinguished from background activity, with a pointed peak at conventional paper speeds and with a duration of 70–200 msec. Its main component is generally negative relative to other areas and its amplitude is variable. The term applies neither to distinctive physiologic events such as **vertex sharp transients, lambda waves,** and **positive occipital sharp transients of sleep,** nor to sharp transients poorly distinguished from background activity, nor to sharp-appearing individual waves of EEG rhythms.

Sharp waves should be differentiated from spikes— that is, transients having similar characteristics but shorter duration, but this distinction is largely arbitrary and serves primarily descriptive purposes. Practically, in ink-written EEG records obtained at 3 cm/second, sharp waves occupy more than 2 mm of paper width and spikes 2 mm or less. See also **spike.** (From Chatrian GE, Bergamini L, Dondey M, et al. A glossary of terms most commonly used by clinical electroencephalographers. *EEG Clin Neurophysiol* 1974;37:538–48,[989] with permission from Elsevier Science.)

sharp-and-slow-wave complex   The sequence of a sharp wave and a slow wave recorded on the EEG, especially as a characteristic of **absence seizures.**

The hyphenation facilitates the use of the term in the plural form: sharp-and-slow-wave complexes or sharp-and-slow-waves.

shearing injury   See **diffuse axonal injury.**

sheathing   The appearance of the retinal veins in some cases of sarcoid or multiple sclerosis, in which the veins are outlined by a white streak on either side as a result of preceding periphlebitis.

Sheehan syndrome   Postpartum pituitary necrosis leading to the cessation of lactation, amenorrhea, and hypopituitarism, described by H.L.D Sheehan (b. 1900), professor of pathology at Liverpool.[5109]

shellshock   See **Brissaud syndrome.**

Sherlock epiloia   See **tuberous sclerosis.**

Sherrington, Sir Charles   (1857–1952) English physiologist, linguist, philosopher, and poet, "the most profound student of the nervous system that the world has yet known" (Fulton), educated at Cambridge and St. Thomas' Hospital, and later in Spain, Italy, and Germany. His physiological studies began while he was an undergraduate working with Langley, and were continued while on the staff at St. Thomas' Hospital in London, then at the University of Liverpool (where **Cushing** learned from him) and, from the age of 56, as

Sir Charles Scott Sherrington

Waynflete Professor of Physiology at Oxford. He was elected a Fellow of the Royal Society in 1893 on the basis of his work on nerve roots and reflexes, and was its president from 1920 to 1925. He was knighted in 1922 and with E.D. (Lord) Adrian, was awarded the Nobel prize for medicine in 1932 for his studies of the physiology of the nervous system.

The central problem which motivated him was, in the words of **Denny-Brown:** "how the relationship between a network of myriads of nerve cells and fibers, each functioning in terms of transmitting nerve impulses, could develop the properties of self-awareness, mind and memory. . . . The conclusion was that a dualism between nerve function and mind is a natural mystery, insoluble by prevailing scientific knowledge." Starting with anatomical studies of dermatomes and myotomes, he quickly branched into neurophysiology, discovering or illuminating (and often naming) reciprocal innervation, decerebrate rigidity, inhibitory reflex effects, the final common pathway, cortical reactivity, synaptic activity (he coined the term *synapse* in 1897), excitation, and inhibition.

He was the first to investigate the proprioceptive system in depth; in his studies of sensory functions, he introduced the terms *exteroception, enteroception,* and *nocioception.* His analysis of **decerebrate rigidity** paralleled that of **Magnus,** while his stimulation and ablation experiments on the cortex were at least as precise as those of clinical scientists such as **Ferrier** and **Horsley.**

He regarded the brain as a manager of muscle, a thoroughfare for nerve action passing on its way to the motor animal, and an input-output signaling system.[5121] His view that the function of the brain was to coordinate the activities of the rest of the organism and his studies on decerebrate rigidity,[5118] reciprocal innervation, and cortical reactivity were all summarized in his book *The Integrative Action of the Nervous System* (published in 1906), still a classic neurophysiology text,[5119] as is his *Selected Writings,* edited by **Denny-Brown** (London, 1939).[5122]

At the end of his academic life and in retirement, he published books of verse and literary criticism as well as biographies of Goethe and Jean Fernel.[1600]

Sherrington's law   The posterior spinal nerves supply their own skin territories but overlap with adjacent territories.

shift-work sleep disorder   A syndrome of either insomnia or excessive sleepiness that occurs as a transient phenomenon in relation to altering work schedules.[234]

Shiga toxin   A substance produced by some *Escherichia coli* strains capable of causing hemorrhagic colitis, hemolytic-uremic syndrome, and acute encephalopathy with severe autonomic dysfunction.

shingles   (from Lat, cingulum, a belt) An English corruption, denoting the dermatomal spread of the painful rash of herpes zoster.

Shipley Institute of Living Scale   A compound measure of global psychological functioning. The abstraction subtest examines verbal analogic reasoning, the subject being required to complete unfinished verbal series.[5137]

Shirres, David Alexander   A Scottish physician, the first neurologist appointed as such in Canada (at the Montreal General Hospital in 1902) and the first physician anywhere to attempt spinal cord transplantation (performed in a human suffering from traumatic division of the cord; without success).[4717]

shock optic neuropathy   Bilateral blindness resulting from optic atrophy is an unusual complication following shock and cardiorespiratory arrest. One report describes a patient with acute respiratory failure due to pneumococcal pneumonia treated with very high levels of positive end expiratory pressure who developed bilateral blindness following cardiac arrest or hemodialysis-associated hypotension. This unfortunate complication most likely resulted from increased intraocular pressure and low systemic perfusion pressure synergistically causing ischemia of the optic nerves.[994]

Shokeir syndrome   See **Pena-Shokeir phenotype.**

Shoni No Noshinkei   (*Nervous System in Children*) A Japanese journal of pediatric neurology, founded in 1976.

Short Care scale   An instrument for the brief assessment of cognitive impairment and depression performed by interview.[3166]

short ciliary nerves   Small myelinated postganglionic parasympathetic nerves running from the ciliary ganglion to the iris sphincter muscle.

Short Exercise test   A method of demonstrating transient weakness following physical rest in patients with myotonic syndrome. The hand is immobilized and the ulnar nerve stimulated every minute, the compound muscle action potential (CMAP) being recorded from the hypothenar muscles.

Maximum voluntary isometric exercise is performed for 10 seconds, the patient spreading the fingers maximally. The ulnar nerve is stimulated again after the exercise and again every 10 seconds for 1 minute. Both the size of the evoked CMAP and twitch tension decrease as a result of this exercise, the detriment being caused by transient inexcitability of the muscle fiber membrane in the absence of any abnormality at the motor end-plate itself.[5378, 5379]

Short Portable Mental Status questionnaire   A formalized, short, bedside screening test for overall cognitive impairment, containing 10 items, with emphasis being placed on orientation and personal and remote memories. It is most suitable for the detection of the more disabled subjects but like similar tests has a substantial false-negative rate.[4429]

short rib–polydactyly   (Majewski syndrome) A lethal congenital dysmorphic syndrome manifesting these anomalies, in which numerous other skeletal, genital, and ocular abnormalities occur, accompanied by macrocephaly.[3582]

Other short rib–polydactyly syndromes also occur, without notable neurological features.

short sleeper   The condition in which a normal subject feels adequately refreshed by shorter periods of (normal pattern) sleep than are regarded as normal for age[2470] (see also ASDA Diagnostic Classification, **sleep disorders**[234]).

Short Wisconsin Card Sort   A modified card sorting test sensitive to frontal lobe dysfunction.[4091] See **Wisconsin Card Sorting test.**

short-chain acyl–coenzyme A dehydrogenase deficiency   (SCHAD deficiency) A rare, genetically determined enzyme disorder of infancy, the genetic defect resulting in failure to thrive, developmental delay, episodic juvenile-onset recurrent myoglobinuria, hypoketotic hypoglycemic encephalopathy, myopathy, and hypertrophic cardiomyopathy triggered by fasting.[5516]

short-chain specific 3-ketothiolase defect   See **beta-ketothiolase deficiency.**

short-cycle peiodic alternating gaze deviation   See **ping-pong gaze.**

shortening reaction   1. The paradoxical contraction of a muscle when it is passively shortened, described first by Westphal in 1877. The phenomenon is only commonly detected in patients with parkinsonism, athetosis, dystonia, or cerebellar disease, but it is in fact present in normal subjects as well.[181] 2. A tonic contraction supervening on the initial contraction of, for example, the quadriceps when its tendon is tapped, which normally checks the momentum of the falling leg. The absence of such a reaction leads to unchecked swinging of the leg—the **pendular reflex.**

Short-Increment Sensitivity index   (SISI) An auditory test in which the subject responds to small (1 decibel) increments of an intermittent tone superimposed upon a background continuous tone at the same frequency. In normal subjects and those with retrocochlear lesions such increments cannot be identified, but they can in those with cochlear lesions.

short-lasting unilateral neuralgiform headache attacks with conjunctival injection and tearing   See **SUNCT syndrome.**

short-latency reflex   A reflex with one (monosynaptic) or few (oligosynaptic) synapses. Used in contrast to long-latency reflex.

short-latency somatosensory evoked potential   (SSEP) That portion of the waveforms of a somatosensory evoked potential normally occurring within 25 msec after stimulation of the median nerve in the upper extremity at the wrist, and 40 msec. after stimulation of the posterior tibial n. at the fibular head. (From the 2001 Report of the Nomenclature Committee of the American Association of Electromyography and Electrodiagnosis.[10] Used by permission, copyright © 2001, AAEM.) The characteristics of SSEPs in various nerves are summarized in Chart S–4.

Chart S–4. Short-Latency Somatosensory Evoked Potentials

1. *Median nerve SSEPs:* Normal short-latency response components to median nerve stimulation are designated P9, P11, P13, P14, N20, and P23 in records taken between scalp and noncephalic reference electrodes, and N9, N11, N13, and N14 in a cervical spine-scalp derivation. Potentials having opposite polarity but similar latency in spine-scalp and scalp-noncephalic reference derivations do not necessarily have identical generator sources.

2. *Common peroneal nerve SSEPs:* Normal short-latency response components to common peroneal stimulation are designated P27 and N35 in records taken between scalp and noncephalic reference electrodes, and L3 and T12 from a cervical spine-scalp derivation.

3. *Posterior tibial nerve SSEPs:* Normal short-latency response components to posterior tibial nerve stimulation are designated as the PF potential in the popliteal fossa, P37 and N45 waves in records taken between scalp and noncephalic reference electrode, and L3 and T12 potentials from a cervical spine-scalp derivation.

SSEP, Short-latency somatosensory evoked potential. (From the 1987 Report of the Nomenclature Committee of the American Association of Electrodiagnostic Medicine. AAEE glossary of terms in clinical electromyography. Muscle Nerve 1987;10S:G5–G23. Copyright 1987 by John Wiley and Sons, Inc. Reprinted by permission of John Wiley and Sons, Inc.)

short-period alternating nystagmus   A benign and self-limited form of **periodic alternating nystagmus** with an unusually short (4–9 second) cycle, occurring in association with ataxia and dysarthria in patients with brainstem encephalitis.[4643]

short-term memory   (primary memory, immediate memory, working memory) The present content of thought; the mental tasks that a person is currently working on or thinking about. In this form of memory, seven to nine words or objects are stored for immediate access, in order to allow other mental operations to proceed. If rehearsal is not allowed, significant decay occurs. Variable amounts of the material contained may be transferred to long-term memory stores, depending on their significance and on the amount of reinforcement given.

This term is not a synonym for *recent memory*, a non-specific phrase used clinically.

shoulder girdle disk   Weakness and wasting of shoulder girdle muscles, associated with cervical spondylosis producing cord compression at C3–4 or with root compression below this level.[4434]

shoulder girdle neuritis   See **neuralgic amyotrophy.**

shoulder girdle syndrome   See **neuralgic amyotrophy.**

shoulder-hand syndrome   See **complex regional pain syndrome.**

Shprintzen-Goldberg syndrome   A congenital craniofacial malformation syndrome, characterized also by skeletal and cardiac abnormalities, optic atrophy, strabismus, craniosynostosis with dolichocephaly, mitral valve prolapse, and mental and developmental delay.[4]

shuddering attacks in infants   An uncommon movement disorder characterized by frequent, paroxysmal tremors of the head, elbows, trunk, and knees, with adduction of the arms and legs, but without alteration of consciousness or EEG abnormality, occurring in infants and young children who then develop normally. They occur perhaps 100 times daily.[829,2629] The cause is unknown, but ingestion of monosodium glutamate has been incriminated.

Shulman syndrome   See **eosinophilic fasciitis.**

Shy, George Milton   (1919–1967) American neurologist who trained at the University of Oregon and, after the war, at the **National Hospital,** Queen Square, and McGill University, Montreal. After a short period on the faculty at Oregon, he became the first clinical director of the National Institute of Neurological and Communicative Disorders and Stroke (NINCDS), where he was later associate director. He was professor and chairman at the University of Pennsylvania and moved, just before his untimely death, to the College of Physicians and Surgeons of Columbia University.

He is best remembered for his discoveries or descriptions of a number of congenital myopathies, of **idiopathic orthostatic hypotension,** and of the Kearns-

Shy syndrome; he edited and prepared for publication the first of the important books published in the last two decades relating clinical and basic science neurology, but died suddenly, before its appearance.

George Milton Shy

Shy-Drager syndrome   A constituent disorder within the group of diseases comprising **multiple system atrophy,** representing a progressive multisystem degeneration. Clinically, it presents as a combination of **parkinsonism** and autonomic failure (orthostatic hypotension, anhidrosis, pupillary failure, loss of bladder and bowel sphincter function, and iris atrophy) in the presence of certain signs, such as unresponsiveness to L-dopa and the existence of pyramidal or cerebellar signs, which are atypical for idiopathic **Parkinson** disease. Other signs noted include extraocular pareses, rigidity, and tremor, as well as evidence of damage to lower motor neurons.[5148]

Pathologically, the condition is marked by neuronal loss in the intermediolateral cell columns, the substantia nigra, the striatum, and the cerebellum. The syndrome is not identical to **idiopathic orthostatic hypotension,** either alone or in combination with idiopathic Parkinson disease and autonomic signs.[4560,5148] See also **progressive autonomic failure, Lewy body disease.**

The condition is named for the late Dr. G.M. Shy and for Dr. Glenn Drager, who is also an American neurologist. A review of their original paper suggests inconsistencies, leading to the suggestion that rectal incontinence, iris atrophy, gaze palsies, fasciculations, distal wasting, and evidence of a lower motor neuron lesions shoud not be regarded as typical of the syndrome which should encompass only autonomic failure, pyramidal and cerebellar signs, and parkinsonism.[4561]

Shy-Drager/Multiple System Atrophy Support Group, Inc. A charitable organization providing information and support in this field. Address: 2004 Howard Lane, Austin, TX 78728. Tel: 866–737–4999: 800–288–5582. E-mail: Don.Summers@shy-drager.com. Web site: http://www.shy-drager.com/.

Shy-Gonatas syndrome A form of complicated progressive external ophthalmoplegia with added ataxia, myopathy, and neuropathy, resembling **Kearns-Sayre syndrome.**[5150] See **mitochondrial myopathies.**

Shy-Magee syndrome See **central core disease.**

SIADH See **syndrome of inappropriate ADH scretion.**

sialidoses (Gr, saliva) (mucolipidoses; OMIM 256550) A group of recessively inherited sphingolipid and mucopolysaccharide lysosomal storage disorders associated with α-N-acetyl-neuraminidase deficiency, in which excessive amounts of sialo-oligosaccharides are excreted in the urine and lipid-like and polysaccharide-like material is deposited in the tissues.[3488] They are mapped to 6p21.2

Clinical presentations, usually between the ages of 8 and 15 years, include visual failure with a cherry-red macular spot and myoclonus; intelligence is normal and there are neither somatic nor bony abnormalities. A classification of the sialidoses is given in Chart S–5.

Chart S–5. Classification of Sialidoses

1. Sialidoses with isolated sialidase deficiency
   Congenital sialidosis
   Severe infantile sialidosis
   Nephrosialidosis
   Cherry red spot-myoclonus syndrome (*sialidosis type 1*) See below.
2. Sialidosis with additional β-galactosidase deficiency
   Goldberg syndrome (mucolipidosis 1, infantile sialidosis)
3. Other forms
   Fucosidosis
   Mannosidosis
   Aspartyl-glycosaminuria
   Mucolipidosis type 1 (see below)
   Mucolipidosis, other types

Sialidosis type 1 (cherry red spot-myoclonus syndrome, normosomatic type) A lysosomal storage disease in which sialo-oligosaccharides accumulate. The clinical syndrome is characterized by the onset (after the age of 10 years) of **progressive myoclonic epilepsy** with severe, progressive, stimulus-sensitive action and intention myoclonus and tonic-clonic seizures.[4593] Cerebellar signs and mental deterioration are also described. Lens and corneal opacities, pyramidal signs, and a mild peripheral neuropathy are less constant signs.[1758] The retinal spot appears later. Beta-galactosidase levels are normal. The EEG shows photosensitive responses, paroxysmal discharges, and fast polyspike discharges over central regions during rapid eye movement sleep.[1672]

The association of such abnormalities also occurs in **Tay-Sachs disease, Nieman-Pick disease, GM₁** gangliosidosis, **metachromatic leukodystrophy,** and the **glycogenoses.**

A *variant* is *mild infantile sialidosis* (lipomucopolysaccharidosis), an inherited lysosomal storage disease characterized by a deficiency of neuraminidase and the accumulation of sialo-oligosaccharides. The clinical features include short stature and the onset in infancy of mental retardation, ataxia, deafness, seizures, and myoclonus, with coarse facies, corneal clouding, cherry-red spot, visceromegaly, and dysostosis.

Sialidosis type 2 (mucolipidosis type 1; Goldberg syndrome; gangliosialidosis, dysmorphic type) Forms in which action myoclonus, tonic-clonic seizures, cherry-red spots, gargoyle-like coarsening of the facial features, dementia, hearing loss, mental impairment, pyramidal and cerebellar signs, multiple dysostoses, hepatosplenomegaly, and deafness occur between the ages of 10 and 30 years, mainly in subjects of Japanese ancestry. In this group, deficiency of β-galactosidase may be present in cases with juvenile onset, leading to the designation *galactosidosis.*[505] When onset is in infancy, the galactosidase levels are normal.

I-cell disease

Sialidosis type 3 (Salla disease, Finnish-type lysosomal storage disorder) A recessively inherited lysosomal storage disease due to a deficiency of oligosaccharide-specific neuraminidase, leading to lysosomal storage of sialic acid and oligosaccharides.

Clinically, the onset is in early childhood; severe and progressive mental retardation with early onset, coarse facies, speech failure, short stature, strabismus, myoclonus and other seizures, and pyramidal, cerebellar, and basal ganglion signs are the most notable features. An increased urinary excretion of free sialic acid is a diagnostic pointer. The condition has been reported mainly from Finland.[263]

Sialidosis type 3a. Pseudo-Hurler polydystrophy An inherited lysosomal storage disease, characterized by deficiency of β-galactosidase, α-L-fucosidase, and neuraminidase, and by the accumulation of mucopolysaccharides, gangliosides, and oligosaccharides. This is a congenital dysmorphic syndrome marked by the accumulation of mucolipids and sphingolipids as a result of an inherited enzyme failure. Clinically, the syndrome presents at the age of 2 to 5 years with stiffness of joints and muscle contractures, carpal tunnel syndrome, bony changes, corneal clouding, mild mental retardation, coarsening of facial features, short stature, platyspondyly, arthropathy, epiphyseal dysplasia, acne, ataxia, mental and developmental delay, deafness, visceromegaly, and aortic or mitral valve disease.[5510]

Sialidosis type 4 See **sialuria.**

Berman type A recessively inherited lysosomal storage disease of Ashkenazi Jews, characterized by deficiency of ganglioside neuraminidase and the accumulation of mucopolysaccharides, phospholipids, and gangliosides. The clinical features include the onset in infancy of mild mental retardation and corneal clouding, optic atrophy, pigmentary retinopathy, hypotonia, pyramidal signs, athetosis, and dystonia in Ashkenazi Jewish children.[514]

In a *variant* form, there is an added congenital myopathy with proximal and distal weakness and hypotonia, with joint contractures, spasticity, athetosis, and mental and developmental delay.

sialuria (mucolipidosis or sialidosis type 4; severe infantile neuraminic acid storage disease, French type;

Tondeur syndrome) A recessively inherited, congenital, generalized lysosomal storage disease, characterized by corneal clouding, optic atrophy, and retinopathy leading to impaired vision, mucopoly/oligosaccariduria, pyramidal and extrapyramidal signs, and psychomotor retardation. Levels of free sialic acid in urine and cultured fibroblasts are increased[5605] but conjunctival or skin biopsy showing cytoplasmic inclusions is the easier diagnostic method.[1948]

Siber syndrome   A congenital dysmorphic syndrome characterized by ocular and genital abnormalities and microcephaly, seizures, cerebellar and pyramidal signs, aqueduct stenosis with obstructive hydrocephalus, callosal agenesis, and mental and developmental delay.[337]

Sicard, Jean-Athenase   (1872–1929) French neurologist, born in Marseille, who trained in medicine in Paris where he was influenced by **Brissaud** to enter neurology. He became chef-de-clinique under Brissaud and spent most of the rest of his professional career at the Hôpital Necker in Paris, where he was elected professor of pathology in 1923 and from which he made numerous basic contributions to neurology in the short time remaining before his early death.

With Jacques Forestier in 1922, he introduced radio-opaque iodized oil (lipiodol) for the investigation of intraspinal disease, and he contributed significantly to the techniques of angiography and pneumoencephalography. He also wrote on syphilis, encephalitis, and toxic neuropathies, and collaborated with others in the description of brainstem stroke syndromes, one of which is named for Collet and himself.

Sicard sign   Aggravation of the back pain induced during straight-leg raising as a result of passive dorsiflexion of the hallux.[374] See also **Bragard sign.**

Sicard spasm   See **hemifacial spasm.**

Sicard-Brissaud syndrome   See **Brissaud syndrome.**

Sicard-Collet syndrome   See **Collet-Sicard syndrome.**

Sicard-Hagueman syndrome   See **Meige syndrome.**

Sicca syndrome   See **Sjögren syndrome.**

sick sinus syndrome   A clinical state characterized by a primary disorder of the atrial pacemaker, presenting first as sinus bradycardia and later progressing to sinus arrest or sinoatrial block. Some patients alternate between attacks of bradycardia and tachycardia. Clinically, syncope, dizziness, convulsions, and possibly sudden death in childhood are recognized neurological complications.[5034]

sickle-cell disease   A sickling hemoglobinopathy of black people, which may manifest in a homo- or heterozygous form. Painful crises, jaundice, anemia, leg ulcers, and hepatomegaly are common symptoms; stroke syndromes, myelopathy, cognitive impairment,

headaches, retinopathy, stupor or coma, and seizures are the main neurological complications[4518a,6029] and are due to the occlusion of small blood vessels by sickle cells.

Sickness Impact profile   A self-report, general health status measure of the dysfunction experienced as a result of disease. *Psychosocial factors* such as social interaction, alertness, emotional behavior, and communication; *physical factors* such as mobility, ambulation, and body care; and *other* areas of concern (communication, bodily functions, activities of daily living) are assessed through the subjects' responses to about 140 questions.[499, 4480] See **quality of life.**

sideropenic dysphagia   (Gr, iron + shortage + difficulty in eating) (Plummer-Vinson syndrome, Paterson-Brown-Kelly syndrome) An acquired syndrome of dysphagia with the usual clinical accompaniments of chronic hypochromic anemia, occurring in adult life, usually in women.[2670]

siderophilia   A tendency to accumulate iron or calcium and other metals, seen in both neurons and astrocytes in the settings of **Hallervorden-Spatz** disease and **Fahr** disease, and occurring in areas adjacent to leaked blood.

siderosis   See **superficial siderosis of the central nervous system.**

SIDS   See **sudden infant death syndrome.**

Siegrist streaks   Pigmented lines on the fundus, seen in some patients with chronic uremia.

Siemens syndrome   A recessively inherited syndrome seen mainly in males, and characterized by anhidrosis, skin pallor, hypotrichosis, cataract, corneal dystrophy, and mental retardation.[5155]

Siemens-Bloch pigmented dermatosis   See **incontinentia pigmenti.**

Siemerling-Creutzfeldt disease   See **adrenoleukodystrophy.**

Sierpinski-Bart syndrome   A congenital dysmorphic syndrome characterized by skeletal and genital abnormalities, retinitis pigmentosa, myopia, strabismus, kyphoscoliosis, optic atrophy, microcephaly, and mental and developmental delay.[337]

Sieveking, Sir Edward H.   (1816–1904) English physician at the **National Hospital,** who reported the impression of **Locock** that bromides were effective in the treatment of hysterical seizures, and so advocated their use in organic ones in his book *On Epilepsy and Epileptiform Seizures* (London, 1858).

SIF cells   See **small intensely fluorescent cells.**

sigma nystagmus   See **optokinetic nystagmus.**

sigma rhythm   See **sleep spindles.**

signe de journal   See **Froment sign.**

signe de la pensée douloureuse   The precipitation of headaches by intensive mental concentration, considered by Josue to be a sign of cerebral vascular insufficiency,[574] although today such disorders would probably be classified as **tension-type headaches.**

signe de l'éventail   See **Babinski signs.**

signe de Peaucier   See **platysma phenomenon.**

signing tics   The use of gestures to replace the usual speech accompaniments (phonic tics) of tic disorders such as **Tourette syndrome.** Such complex learned movements parallel the performance of verbal symptoms such as coprolalia, echolalia, and palilalia; the terms *coprolaliopraxia, echolaliopraxia,* and *palilaliopraxia* have naturally been coined for them.[3263]

signpost phenomenon   If a subject with **Parkinson disease** rests his elbows on the table with the forearms vertical, and lets the arms and wrists relax, the wrists nevertheless remains in partial extension and do not fall as in the normal, so that the hand assumes a position near the horizontal.

silent period   A pause in the electrical activity of a muscle, such as that seen after its rapid unloading.[146] Such reflex inhibition of muscle electrical activity typically follows a twitch contraction for about 100 msec and is due to direct inhibition of the reflex arc by Renshaw cells, with withdrawal of afferent muscle spindle facilitation. It is normal in the **stiff-man syndrome** but is shortened or absent in **tetanus.**[3301]

silent pituitary apoplexy   Nonsymptomatic hemorrhage within pituitary adenomas.

silent stroke   The CT or MRI appearances of stroke that are unaccompanied by historical or clinical evidence of transient ischemic attack or of stroke deficit. **Leukoaraiosis** or bilateral periventricular lucencies alone are insufficient for the diagnosis.

Silver disease   See **hereditary spastic paraplegia.**

simian crease   A single palmar crease.

simian hand   (Lat, monkey-like) See **ape hand.**

simian stance   A posture characterized by slight flexion of the knees, hips, and lumbar spine, and by loss of the normal lumbar lordosis. This is seen in **lumbar spinal stenosis** and in **Parkinson disease,** but in the latter case there is also flexion of the neck and upper limbs.

similarities test   A subtest of the **Wechsler Adult Intelligence Scale** in which the subject is asked in what way two items (eating–sleeping, pen–pencil) are alike (i.e., share common properties).

Simmerlin dystrophy   See **limb-girdle muscular dystrophy.**

Simmonds syndrome   Panhypopituitarism, occasionally complicating pituitary tumors or following **pituitary apoplexy.** See **Sheehan syndrome.**

Simon sign   Incoordination of the intercostal and diaphragmatic movements, said to be a sign of early meningitis.[4723]

Simon-Binet tests   See **Binet, intelligence tests.**

simple aphasia   See **aphemia.**

simple central anisocoria   Asymmetry in the size of the pupils, measuring a constant 0.5-mm difference or less in both bright and dim illumination. See also **Horner syndrome.**

simple cramp   Difficulty in performing a single specific task due to the presence of focal hand cramps.[5110]

simple partial seizures   Partial seizures, often without accompanying EEG changes, in which there are elementary symptoms, consciousness is not impaired, and later recollection is undistorted. They are further subdivided according to the nature of the symptoms; thus, motor, sensory, autonomic, cognitive, affective, and mixed components occur variously. Rapid generalization to generalized tonic-clonic seizures may occur.

simple tremor   See **cerebellar tremors.**

Simpson's test   A sign in myasthenia gravis, which is positive when the patient staring up at the ceiling develops worsening ptosis within 1 minute. An extended form requires 3 minutes of up-gaze.

simultagnosia   The inability to perceive more than one object in a particular sensory channel at one time, most commonly seen in patients with bilateral or right parietal lobe disease.

The term was suggested by Wolpert in 1924,[3857] but the defect is better considered a form of visual disorientation. See **visual disorientation.**

sin-cib-syn   (sinocibal syndrome) See **Chinese restaurant syndrome.**

sincipital   At the junction of the frontal and ethmoidal bones of the skull.

sinciput   The anterior protuberance of the cranium, as opposed to the occiput.

singing paraplegia   Intermittent leg weakness occurring as the result of increased venous pressure transmitted to a spinal dural arteriovenous fistula, with resultant cord compression and ischemia.[3031a]

single fiber electromyography   (SFEMG) A general term referring to the technique and conditions that permit the recording of action potentials from single muscle fibers.[146] A review of the technique and its value has been published.[4901]

single fiber electromyographic jitter   See **jitter.**

single fiber needle electrode   A needle electrode with two small recording surfaces (usually 25 μm in diameter) which permits the recording of single muscle fiber action potentials between the active recording surface in the bevel at the tip of the cannula and that face laterally through a side port situated more proximally.[146]

single (isolated) seizure One or more epileptic seizures occurring in a 24-hour period.[1115]

single-photon emission computed tomography (SPECT) A technique for imaging cross sections of the body and for measuring focal intracerebral blood flow, in which isotopes emitting single photons are detected using the same principles of image reconstruction as those used in CT, but employing a rotating gamma camera. Single photon-emitting isotopes of carbon, hydrogen, oxygen, or nitrogen do not exist; hence, SPECT is not directly useful for metabolic imaging based on these biologically important atoms.

At present, SPECT is used principally for brain perfusion imaging. Commonly employed tracers are ^{123}I-iodoamphetamine, ^{99m}Tc-hexamethyl-propylene-amine oxime (HMPAO), and ^{99m}Tc-bicisate. These diffuse into the brain tissue at a rate proportional to regional perfusion rates and thus to the rate of local cerebral metabolism.

SPECT tracers are highly lipophilic and therefore cross the blood–brain barrier easily. Once in the brain, some tracers such as HMPAO are metabolized to less lipophilic compounds and leave the brain slowly. Their distribution preserves a record of the regional cerebral blood flow (rCBF) at the time of injection, which can be imaged at any time within the next several hours. However, tracers that are not metabolized (e.g., xenon 133) demonstrate rCBF by the kinetics of their entry into or departure from the brain, and must be imaged at the time that occurs.[4471,4526]

singultus See **hiccoughs.**

sinistrality (Lat, left-handedness) Although the word, meaning **left-handedness,** is occasionally regarded as a pejorative (sinister), the Book of Judges in the Old Testament refers to an army of 700 left-handed slingers, who never missed.

sinistrosis See **Brissaud syndrome.**

sinking pitch sign A reduction in the pitch of the voice occasioned by fatigue of the laryngeal adductor muscles in myasthenia gravis.[5809]

sinus arrhythmia A physiological alteration of heart rate which depends on cardiac parasympathetic activity such that the decreased vagal activity occurring with inspiration leads to an increase in the heart rate. When a subject breathes at 6 respirations per minute, the electrocardiogram should show differences of 15 bpm; less than 10 bpm change is abnormal.[3368]

Quantitation of the normal response has been achieved. The **expiratory/inspiratory ratio** (the mean of the longest R-R interval during expiration divided by the mean of the shortest R-R interval during inspiration) should exceed 1.2 in patients aged less than 40 years.[1722]

sinus headache See **acute sinus headache.**

sinus of Morgagni syndrome See **Trotter syndrome.**

sinus pericranii A persistent venous connection between the superior sagittal sinus and the scalp veins in the parieto-occipital region, seen in some infants. The fluctuant mass swells with crying, but this is only dangerous in the event that it should bleed.

sinus thrombosis Partial or complete occlusion of an intracranial venous sinus, often leading to venous infarction of the subjacent brain. Septic and aseptic causes are recognized.

The condition was recognized by **Gowers**[2240] in association with pregnancy and wasting diseases, but it also occurs in conjunction with hematological conditions, cardiac failure, oral contraceptive therapy, and dehydration; with local infections such as mastoiditis; and without a known cause.

The clinical features of superior sagittal sinus thrombosis include headache with signs of raised intracranial pressure, seizures, nausea, and vomiting, aphasia, focal deficits affecting mainly the legs, and reduced level of consciousness.[685,686]

sinus thrombosis causing intracranial hypertension See **otitic hydrocephalus.**

Sipple syndrome See **multiple endocrine neoplasia.**

Siriraj score A bedside instrument for assessing the likelihood of intracerebral hemorrhage in stroke patients while awaiting computed tomography, assessing consciousness, vomiting, headache within 2 hours, diastolic blood pressure, and atheroma markers such as diabetes, angina, and intermittent claudication.[945] See also **Allen score.**

Calculation of Siriraj Score

Variable	Clinical Feature	Score
Consciousness (×2.5)	Alert	0
Drowsy, stupor		1
Semicoma, coma		2
Vomiting (×2)	No	0
	Yes	1
Headache within 2 hours (×2)	No	0
	Yes	1
Diastolic blood pressure (×0.11)		
Atheroma markers (×3)	None	0
(diabetes, angina, intermittent	One or more	1
claudication)		
Constant		−12

A score >1 indicates cerebral hemorrhage, while a score <−1 indicates cerebral infarct; the score between −1 and +1 is equivocal and a CT scan is needed.

(From Celani MG, Righetti E, Migliacci R, et al. Comparability and validity of two clinical scores in the early differential diagnosis of acute stroke. Brit Med J. 1994;308:1674–6, reproduced by kind permission.)

Siris-Coffin-Wegienka syndrome   See **Coffin-Lowry syndrome.**

SISI   See **short increment sensitivity index.**

Sisto sign   Constant crying in children with congenital syphilis. Dr. G. Sisto was an Argentinean pediatrician.

site-of-injury headache   A form of post-traumatic headache in which the pain is localized to the site of the original injury, probably because of local soft-tissue trauma and entrapment of sensory nerves in scar tissue.[5764]

sitki   See **oroya fever.**

situational syncope   The provocation of syncope by certain activities or by normal activities performed in particular situations. **Cough, swallow, micturition,** and **defecation syncope** are examples.

situation-related seizures   (provoked seizures) Seizures that occur within a week of acute metabolic disorders, heavy alcohol consumption or withdrawal, or stroke or head trauma, or with cerebral tumor or infection.[3462]

six-element test   A test of planning ability in which the subject is asked to carry out six open-ended tasks in a fixed time. The tasks include dictating details of a journey, performing arithmetic, and writing down the names of pictures presented.[5089]

six hertz spike-and-slow-waves   (phantom spike-and-wave, fast spike–wave) Spike-and-slow-wave complexes at 4–7 Hz (but mostly at 6 Hz), occurring generally in brief bursts bilaterally, synchronously, symmetrically, or asymmetrically and either confined to or of larger amplitude over the posterior or anterior regions of the head. Their amplitude is variable but is generally smaller than that of spike-and-slow-wave complexes repeating at slower rates. The clinical significance of this pattern is controversial. (From Chatrian GE, Bergamini L, Dondey M, et al. A glossary of terms most commonly used by clinical electroencephalographers. *EEG Clin Neurophysiol* 1974;**37**:538–48,[989] with permission from Elsevier Science.)

This EEG pattern is seen mainly in young adults and is not usually associated with seizures; it is more likely to be benign when it occurs in **F**emales, predominantly **O**ccipitally, with **L**ow amplitude, and during **D**rowsiness (FOLD), but this may not be so when the pattern occurs during **W**aking, with **H**igh Amplitude, predominantly **A**nteriorly, and in **M**ales (WHAM). Such discharges have an uncertain relationship with any clinical epileptic syndrome.[5539]

sixth nerve pseudopalsy   See **pseudo–sixth nerve palsy.**

sixth sense   See **facial vision of the blind.**

Sjäastad syndrome   See **chronic paroxysmal hemicrania.**

Sjögren, Henrik Samuel Conrad   (b. 1899) Swedish ophthalmologist, practicing in Stockholm.

Sjögren syndrome   (keratoconjunctivitis sicca, sicca syndrome, Mikulicz-Gougerot-Sjörgren syndrome) A collagen-vascular disease characterized by dryness of the mouth and eyes, ichthyosis, keratitis, corneal ulceration, recurrent salivary gland enlargement, rheumatoid arthritis, and sometimes relapsing and remitting neurological signs.[5201] Anemia, leukopenia, and a raised ESR are common. The condition occurs mainly in postmenopausal women, either alone or in association with other autoimmune disorders.

The neurological features include seizures; focal or multifocal CNS signs including cerebellar or spinal cord syndromes, ophthalmoplegia, dementia, meningoencephalitis, migraine, myalgias and fatigue, and psychoses or "organic brain syndromes." Sensory (ganglionopathy), sensorimotor, and pure motor neuropathies are other complications but are rarely of clinical significance. A few patients develop trigeminal sensory neuropathy or involvement of the third and eighth cranial nerves. Intracerebral or subarachnoid hemorrhage is probably the most specific indicator of vasculitis, but ischemic lesions can also occur. Subacute or chronic aseptic meningitis or meningoencephalitis manifesting as dementia or encephalopathy may also rarely be seen.

Serum anti Ro/SS-A, anti-La/SS-B, and anti-Hu antibodies, polyclonal hyperglobulinemia, and positive tests for cryoglobulins may be detected.[2667] A minority has antibodies to Ro (SSA).

Diagnostic criteria have been reviewed:[4232]

A. Positive **Schirmer test** results

B. Positive result from the Rose Bengal dye test for keratoconjunctivitis, or

C. Abnormal minor salivary gland biopsy findings

Alternative criteria require the same but with the demonstration of antinuclear factor or rheumatoid factor and objective evidence of diminished salivary flow in place of the salivary gland biopsy.

Although the clinical and MRI findings may suggest a resemblance to **multiple sclerosis,** screening of all patients who are suspected of having multiple sclerosis for Sjögren syndrome is unwarranted, since the latter syndrome is so uncommon.

In *variant forms,* **polymyositis, dermatomyositis,**[4703] or a syndrome indistinguishable from **idiopathic sensory neuronopathy** (found almost exclusively in women) occur in conjunction.

Sjögren-Larsson syndrome   (ichthyosis-Little disease; OMIM 270200) A recessively inherited leukodystrophy characterized by congenital ichthyosiform erythroderma (scaly hyperkeratosis), pigmentary retinopathy, dental enamel dysplasia, deficient scalp hair, spastic paraparesis, seizures, speech defect, and mental retardation.[5202] Impaired oxidation of long-chain fatty alcohols due to deficiency of the enzyme FALDH (fatty aldehyde dehydrogenase) carried on chromosome 17p11.2 may be the underlying mechanism.

Ichthyosis and neurological signs also occur together in **Rud** and **Refsum syndromes.**

skeletal dysplasia–unusual facies–mental retardation   See **CAT syndrome.**

skeletal myoclonus   See **myorhythmia.**

skew deviation   (Hertwig-Magendie syndrome) An acquired nonparetic ocular divergence in the vertical plane due to an imbalance of prenuclear inputs—a supranuclear lesion involving the brainstem tegmentum at any level between the medulla and the diencephalon. It is characterized by downward and inward rotation of one eye, accompanied by upward and outward rotation of the other, and by nystagmus.[4511]

The following criteria for the diagnosis have been suggested:[5233]

A. Sudden onset of vertical diplopia, usually in adults
B. Significant vertical deviation, comitant or noncomitant
C. No preceding strabismus
D. A laterally comitant deviation (no deviation in left gaze, for example, but vertical deviation in right gaze, essentially equal both up and right and down and right, and essentially the same in amount with either eye fixing in these positions)
E. Associated signs and symptoms
F. Clinical evidence of a brachium pontis lesion
G. Exclusion of third and fourth cranial nerve disease, orbital fractures, etc.
H. Noncomitant **skew deviation** mimicking inferior or superior rectus or inferior oblique palsies or primary overaction of an oblique most commonly, but without other evidence of third or of fourth cranial nerve disease.

It is regarded as a sign of disease of the utricle (upward deviation of both eyes with different amplitudes); of the dorsal medulla (hypertropia of one eye); of the midbrain tegmentum (simultaneous hypertropia of one eye and hypotropia of the other, and inferred when pupillary or third cranial nerve abnormalities are also present); or of intrinsic brainstem or cerebellar disease (on the side of the lower eye).

A *variant* is *slowly alternating skew deviation,* in which one eye descends as the other ascends over 30–60 seconds, and which is a sign of a pretectal lesion.[1128]

The condition was first recognized in laboratory animals by **Magendie** in 1824 and by Henry Hertwig 2 years later, but it was only reported in humans following the carnage of the World War I.

skin roll test   Gentle pinching or rolling of the skin of the neck or head leads to a complaint of unusual pain in patients with migraine; in fibromyalgia the pain is increased in areas overlying the tender muscle trigger points. The problems with the method are the variability of the stimulus and the subjectivity of the estimate of pain felt.

skin wrinkling   The ridged appearance of skin immersed for a period in warm water. This depends on the capacity of keratin to bind water, which in turn requires the presence of salt. As this is derived from sweat, the phenomenon occurs only in the presence of an intact sympathetic system; its absence is suggested as a simple test of sympathetic function.[703]

skinache syndrome   A syndrome of uncertain validity characterized by chronic pain of unknown etiology with numerous cutaneous trigger points and responsive to injection of local anesthetic.[384]

Skre syndrome   See **hereditary spastic paraplegia.**

SKT test battery   A scale designed to measure recent memory and attention in patients with cognitive impairment, containing nine manually administered subtests, available in five alternate forms, and completed within 10 to 15 minutes. The test has been used frequently in treatment trials that include patients with **Alzheimer disease.**[1701]

skull   (Old Engl, skulle) The protective bony covering of the brain and organs of special sense, consisting of the cranium and the face.

skull noise   Murmurs heard over the skull, as in patients with cervical or cranial vascular disease or intracranial arteriovenous communications, and in many normal children and others with anemia or with increased cerebral blood flow stemming from other causes. See also **cephalic bellows sound.**

sleep   A heterogeneous and complicated physiological condition in which consciousness and activity are altered, occurring cyclically due to reductions in the activity of systems promoting wakefulness such as the ascending reticular activating system, and the activation of other systems responsible for non–rapid eye movement sleep (median forebrain area, serotonergic median raphe nuclei) or for rapid eye movement sleep (gigantocellular tegmental field in the pons).

SLEEP   The official publication of the *American Academy of Sleep Medicine* (Web site: http://www.aasmnet.org/) and the *Sleep Research Society* (Web site: http://www.sleepresearchsociety.org/srs/index.php).

sleep apnea   A condition in which repetitive nocturnal apneas result in recurrent hypoxemia and sleep disruption. The occurrence of at least 15 apneic or hypoapneic episodes per hour of sleep in association with symptoms, including restless nocturnal sleep with repeated awakenings, excessive daytime sleepiness, attacks of choking during the night, morning headaches, nocturia, and irritability, suggests the diagnosis of sleep apnea syndrome.[5954]

The cessation of ventilatory movements during sleep is due to a prolonged pause in the central brainstem upper airway motor neuron output at the end of expiration. Clinically, the condition presents most often with snoring, abnormal sleep behavior, excessive daytime sleepiness, intellectual deterioration, personality change, morning headache, and sleep disturbances. It occurs in association with a wide range of primary neurological diseases, most of which affect the brainstem or the brain in a diffuse manner.

Four types of sleep apnea have been defined (see Chart S–6), although all have the same neurological basis. The **Pickwickian syndrome** and **idiopathic hypoventilation** may also be classified as sleep apnea syndromes.

Chart S–6.   The Four Types of Sleep Apnea

1. *Central sleep apnea syndrome* Respiratory movements cease so that there is no oronasal air flow. The disorder is characterized by a cessation or decrease of ventilatory effort during sleep, usually with associated oxygen desaturation. The following diagnostic criteria have been suggested:[234]
   A. The patient has a complaint of either insomnia or excessive sleepiness. Occasionally the patient may be unaware of clinical features observed by others.
   B. Frequent episodes of shallow or absent breathing during sleep
   C. Associated features include at least one of the following:
      1. Gasps, grunts, or choking during sleep
      2. Frequent body movements
      3. Cyanosis during sleep
   D. Polysomnographic monitoring demonstrates:
      1. Central apneic pauses greater than 10 seconds (20 seconds in infancy) in duration, and one or more of the following:
      2. Frequent arousals from sleep associated with the apneas
      3. Bradytachycardia
      4. Oxygen desaturation in association with the apneic episodes, with or without:
      5. A mean sleep latency test that demonstrates a mean sleep latency of less than 10 minutes
   E. Other sleep disorders can be present, e.g., periodic limb movement disorder, obstructive sleep apnea syndrome, or central alveolar hypoventilation syndrome.
2. *Obstructive sleep apnea syndrome* A disorder characterized by repetitive episodes of upper airway obstruction that occur during sleep and are usually associated with a reduction in blood oxygen saturation. In this form, the diaphragm and chest wall move with variations in intrathoracic pressure, but there is no air flow at the nose or mouth. The problem is due to facial/palatal malformations, upper airway disease, or collapse of the muscular wall of the pharynx.[3044] The following diagnostic criteria have been suggested:[234]
   A. The patient has a complaint of excessive sleepiness or insomnia. Occasionally the patient may be unaware of clinical features that are observed by others.
   B. Frequent episodes of obstructed breathing during sleep
   C. Associated features include the following:
      1. Loud snoring
      2. Morning headaches
      3. A dry mouth upon awakening
      4. Chest retraction during sleep in young children
   D. Polysomnographic monitoring demonstrates:
      1. More than five obstructive apneic episodes, greater than 10 seconds in duration, per hour of sleep and one or more of the following:

2. Frequent arousals from sleep associated with the apneas
3. Bradytachycardia
4. Arterial oxygen desaturation in association with the apneic episodes, with or without:
5. An mean sleep latency test that demonstrates a mean sleep latency of less than 10 minutes
   E. Can be associated with other medical disorders, e.g., tonsillar enlargement
   F. Other sleep disorders can be present, e.g., periodic limb movement disorder or narcolepsy.
3. *Mixed* Respiratory movements and air flow are absent early in the episode but are followed by unsuccessful attempts at breathing.
4. *Subobstructive* There is reduced air flow with increased respiratory effort.

Another *variant* is *infantile sleep apnea*, which is defined as the occurrence of central or obstructive apneas during sleep in infants.[219] The following diagnostic criteria have been suggested:[234]
A. Clinical presentation includes one or more of the following:
   1. An episode of cessation of breathing during sleep
   2. An episode characterized by:
      a. Color change (pallor or cyanosis)
      b. Tone change (limpness, rarely stiffness)
   3. Noisy breathing during sleep
B. Central or obstructive apneas occurring during sleep
C. Age of infant at presentation either:
   1. Less than 37 weeks postconceptional age
   2. Greater than 37 weeks postconceptional age
D. Polysomnographic monitoring demonstrates one or more of the following:
   1. Prolonged central apnea >20 seconds
   2. Obstructive apnea >10 seconds
   3. An apnea accompanied by cyanosis
   4. An apnea accompanied by transient bradycardia (defined as a drop in heart rate to levels below 50 bpm, a heart rate below 60 bpm lasting more than 10 seconds or a drop below 60 bpm with a duration exceeding 30 seconds below baseline heart rate)
   5. Arterial oxygen saturation <85% during sleep
   6. Sustained hypoventilation (end tidal carbon dioxide partial pressure [PETCO$_2$] >45 mmHg) during sleep
E. An identifiable cause for the apnea was either:
   1. Found following a thorough diagnostic evaluation, and is believed to be the cause of the apnea, or
   2. Not found following a thorough diagnostic evaluation.

From ASDA Diagnostic Classification Steering Committee. The International Classification of Sleep Disorders Diagnostic and Coding Manual. *Rochester, MN. American Sleep Disorders Association,* © *1990, by kind permission of the American Academy of Sleep Medicine.*

Narcolepsy, cervical cordotomy, **Chiari malformation,** kyphoscoliosis, bulbar polio, and brainstem infarct or tumor are other causes of sleep-related apnea, and may be accompanied by disturbed sleep with abnormal movements, hypnagogic hallucinations, enuresis, and somnambulism.[2321]

sleep apnea DIMS (disorders of initiating or maintaining sleep) syndrome   Cessation of ventilation during sleep due to central causes (sometimes with obstructive causes as well), leading to complaints of insomnia as a result of multiple awakenings.[1383] This was the terminology of the original American Sleep Disorders Association (ASDA) diagnostic classification of **sleep disorders.**[249]

sleep apnea DOES (disorder of excessive sleep) syndrome (sleep apnea, obstructive sleep apnea syndrome) A syndrome characterized by multiple obstructive or mixed apneas during sleep, loud snoring, and excessive daytime somnolence. Additional symptoms include **sleep drunkenness** and dulling of the sensorium; cardiac arrhythmias may occur and may cause death.[2322] This was the terminology of the original American Sleep Disorders Association (ASDA) diagnostic classification of **sleep disorders.**[249]

sleep apnea headache   See **sypoxic headache.**

sleep architecture   The disposition of rapid eye movement and non–rapid eye movement sleep periods relative to one another.

sleep attacks   Overpowering attacks of sleepiness, occurring typically as part of the **narcolepsy** syndrome.

sleep deprivation   Unusual prevention of sleep, leading to decreased vigilance and creative efficiency, increase in microsleeps, improved affect, and a reduction in seizure thresholds. If sleep deprivation is prolonged, delirium may occur. Afterward, delta and later rapid eye movement sleep times increase.

sleep disorders   A subspecialty within neurology, the problems subsumed including those in Chart S–7 as listed by Hauri[2477] and in the 1990 International Classification of Sleep Disorders.[234]

Chart S–7. Sleep Disorders

1. **Dyssomnias** (disorders associated with difficulty in initiating or maintaining sleep, or with excessive sleepiness)
   A. **Intrinsic sleep disorders**
   B. **Extrinsic sleep disorders**
   C. **Circadian rhythm sleep disorders**
2. **Parasomnias**
   A. Arousal disorders
   B. **Sleep–wake transition disorders**
   C. Parasomnias usually associated with rapid eye movement sleep
   D. Other parasomnias
3. **Sleep disorders associated with medical/psychiatric disorders**
4. **Proposed sleep disorders**
   A. **Short sleeper**
   B. **Long sleeper**
   C. Subwakefulness syndrome
   D. **Fragmentary myoclonus**
   E. Sleep hyperhidrosis
   F. Menstrual-associated sleep disorder
   G. Pregnancy-associated sleep disorder
   H. Terrifying hypnagogic hallucinations
   I. Sleep-related neurogenic tachypnea
   J. Sleep-related laryngospasm
   K. Sleep choking syndrome

From ASDA Diagnostic Classification Steering Committee. The International Classification of Sleep Disorders Diagnostic and Coding Manual. Rochester, MN. American Sleep Disorders Association, © 1990, by kind permission of the American Academy of Sleep Medicine.

sleep disorders associated with medical/psychiatric disorders   The classification in Chart S–8 is suggested by the American Sleep Disorders Association (ASDA).[234]

Chart S–8. Sleep Disorders Associated with Medical/Psychiatric Disorders

A. Associated with mental disorders:
   1. Psychoses
   2. Mood disorders
   3. Anxiety disorders
   4. Panic disorder
   5. Alcoholism
B. Associated with neurological disorders:
   1. Cerebral degenerative disorders
   2. Dementia
   3. Parkinsonism
   4. **Fatal familial insomnia**
   5. **Sleep-related epilepsy**
   6. **Electrical status epilepticus of sleep**
   7. **Sleep-related headaches**
C. Associated with other medical disorders:
   1. Sleeping sickness
   2. Nocturnal cardiac ischemia
   3. Chronic obstructive pulmonary disease
   4. Sleep-related asthma
   5. Sleep-related gastroesophageal reflux
   6. Peptic ulcer disease
   7. Fibrositis syndrome

From ASDA Diagnostic Classification Steering Committee. The International Classification of Sleep Disorders Diagnostic and Coding Manual. Rochester, MN. American Sleep Disorders Association, © 1990, by kind permission of the American Academy of Sleep Medicine.

sleep drunkenness   (somnolentia) A **parasomnia** of adult life characterized by clouding of the sensorium with confusion and inappropriate impulsive behavior occurring during an abnormally prolonged period of transition between the states of being asleep (commonly in a deep non–rapid eye movement sleep stage) and of being awake. Tiredness, impaired concentration, ataxia, headache, and drowsiness are other symptoms described.[4812] See also ASDA Diagnostic Classification,[234] **sleep disorders, confusional arousals.**

sleep efficiency   The ratio of the total sleep time to the time designed for sleep by an individual.

sleep epilepsy   Generalized or complex partial seizures occurring during any phase of sleep.

sleep fragmentation   Repetitive interruption of sleep by arousals and awakenings.[249]

sleep hiccough   The unusual occurrence of hiccups during sleep, recorded in a patient following severe head injury.[247]

sleep hypochondriasis   See **subjective DIMS complaint without objective findings.**

sleep inertia   The apparent paradoxical decrement in psychometric performance following a brief sleep, associated with the feeling of grogginess and non-restoration on awakening. During this state, the EEG features of light non–rapid eye movement sleep are mingled with those of wakefulness.[785]

sleep latency   The time between subjects' composing themselves for sleep and attaining it.

sleep maintenance insomnia   The occurrence of frequent nocturnal arousals after initially falling asleep. This is usually due to incidental parasomnias or to anxiety.[249]

Sleep Medicine   A subspecialty journal published by Elsevier Science. Web site: http://www.elsevier.com/inca/publications/store/6/2/0/2/8/2/.

sleep mentation   The imagery, thinking, and emotion experienced during sleep, most vividly in dreams and during the first entry into and last exit from non–rapid eye movement sleep.[249]

sleep myoclonus   (periodic movements in sleep) Periodic, repetitive, brief, rhythmic myoclonic movements due to contraction of the tibialis anterior and more proximal muscles, occurring during any stage of non–rapid eye movement sleep in adults and afterward accompanied by features of the **restless legs syndrome**.[1101]

The condition was first reported by Symonds in 1953. See **periodic limb movement disorder.**

sleep onset   The transition from the waking state to sleep, usually non–rapid eye movement stage 1, but, in infancy and in narcolepsy, into rapid eye movement sleep (see ASDA diagnostic classification,[249] **sleep disorders**).

sleep paralysis   (catalepsy of awakening, daymares, waking cataplexy, postchalastic fits, nocturnal hemiplegia, Rosenthal syndrome) A dissociated rapid eye movement sleep inhibitory process, characterized by periods of flaccid paralysis of all but the respiratory and extraocular muscles with areflexia, occurring for minutes during the waking stage immediately preceding or succeeding sleep and terminated by sleep or by sensory stimulation. The experience is frequently frightening.

This may represent the tonelessness of normal rapid eye movement sleep occurring in the conscious state. **Cataplexy** is the equivalent in the waking state. The syndrome may occur in isolation or as a component of the **narcolepsy** syndrome. The following diagnostic criteria have been suggested:[234]

A. A complaint of inability to move the trunk or limbs at sleep onset or upon awakening
B. Presence of a brief episode of partial or complete skeletal muscle paralysis
C. Episodes can be associated with hypnagogic hallucinations or dreamlike mentation

D. Polysomnographic monitoring demonstrates at least one of the following:
   1. Suppression of skeletal muscle tone
   2. A sleep-onset rapid eye movement period
   3. Dissociated rapid eye movement sleep
E. Not associated with other medical or psychiatric disorders, e.g., hysteria or hypokalemic paralysis

From ASDA Diagnostic Classification Steering Committee. *The International Classification of Sleep Disorders Diagnostic and Coding Manual.* Rochester, MN: American Sleep Disorders Association, 1990. Reproduced by kind permission of the American Academy of Sleep Medicine.

The condition was described by the American Dr. R. McNish in 1837, but Weir **Mitchell** in 1876 gave a more professional account.[3911] *Variants* include familial and sporadic or "isolated" cases in which an attack occurs in otherwise normal subjects, and those linked with the **Pickwickian syndrome.** The first description may have been that told in the childrens' story of the *Sleeping Beauty*, who awoke from her slumber at the touch of the Prince's kiss. More mundane stimuli, however, are equally effective. See also **narcolepsy.**

sleep rebound   The increase in the proportion of rapid eye movement sleep which occurs following a period of selective deprivation of that stage.

Sleep Research Society   An American professional society composed of members with research interests in the realm of sleep. Address: One Westbrook Corporate Center, Suite 920, Westchester, IL 60154. Tel: 708 492-0930. E-mail: Jyore@aasmnet.org. Web site: http://www.sleepresearchsociety.org/contact/index.php/.

sleep reversal   Wakefulness during darkness and sleep during the day; a phenomenon occurring in some demented patients and in the context of South African trypanosomiasis (**sleeping sickness**).

sleep spindles   (sigma rhythm) Recurring bursts of increasing- and then decreasing-amplitude EEG activity at 11–16 Hz (but mostly at 12–14 Hz), lasting 0.5–2 seconds, signaling the onset of stage 2 non–rapid eye movement sleep. They are generally diffuse but of higher voltage over the central regions of the head. Their amplitude is variable but is mostly below 50 uV in the adult. (From ASDA Diagnostic Classification Steering Committee. *The International Classification of Sleep Disorders Diagnostic and Coding Manual.* Rochester, MN. American Sleep Disorders Association, © 1990, by kind permission of the American Academy of Sleep Medicine.)

sleep stages   Periods of sleep with individual distinguishing characteristics, as recorded with the measures used in **polysomnography,** in which stereotyped patterns of EEG, electrooculographic, and EMG activity allow distinction between non–rapid eye movement (**NREM**) and **rapid eye movement** (REM) stages. Precise guidelines for scoring and naming these stages are available.[4620] Non-rapid eye movement stages are defined as shown in Chart S–9.

Chart S–9. Non–Rapid Eye Movement Sleep Stages

Stage 1. A stage of sleep following directly upon wakefulness and characterized by the EEG appearance of low-voltage activity with alpha activity constituting less than 50%, with beta activity and vertex spikes, and with slow rolling eye movements. This usually comprises some 5% of total sleep time.

Stage 2. A stage of sleep characterized by the appearance of sleep spindles and K complexes on a low-voltage mixed-frequency background and with delta activity constituting up to 20% of the stage. This stage usually comprises some 50% of the total sleep time.

Stage 3. A stage of sleep characterized by the appearance of high-amplitude delta waves (>75uV, <2 Hz) for between 20% and 50% of the time, which occurs in the first third of the sleep period.

Stage 4. A stage of sleep characterized by the appearance of high-amplitude delta waves (>75uV, <2 Hz) for more than 50% of the time and comprising, with NREM stage 3, slow-wave or delta sleep.

Adapted from Rechtschaffen A, Kales A. A Manual of Standardized Terminology, Techniques and Scoring for Sleep Stages of Normal Subjects. Washington, DC: Department of Heath, Education and Welfare, 1968.

The first indication of the existence of different types of sleep was given by **von Economo,** who noted that drowsy postencephalitic patients had lesions in the posterior hypothalamus and mesencephalic tegmentum while those who were insomniac had lesions in the forebrain. See also **rapid eye movement sleep.**

sleep starts   (hypnagogic jerks, hypnic jerks, predormital myoclonus, somnolescent starts) A sleep–wake transition parasomnia in the form of a partial arousal response, manifest as generalized, single, asymmetrical bodily jerks on falling asleep, unassociated with clinical or EEG abnormalities and of no pathological significance. They are occasionally accompanied by a perception of falling or a flash of dream prior to intense arousal, with return of alpha rhythms on the EEG.[4274]

These brief, spontaneous, generalized, or localized nonperiodic myoclonic movements of the trunk and limbs occur mainly at the onset of the first periods of stages 3 and 4 of non–rapid eye movement sleep. They last less than a quarter of a second, mainly affect the legs, resemble the startle reaction of wakefulness,[234] and occur in many normal people, usually during sleep onset. A positive family history is frequently found.

Diagnostic criteria have been suggested[234] and are reproduced in Chart S–10.

Chart S–10. Diagnostic Criteria for Sleep Starts

A. A complaint of either difficulty initiating sleep or of an intense body movement at sleep onset

B. Sudden brief jerks at sleep onset, mainly affecting the legs or arms

C. Associated with at least one of the following:
  1. A subjective feeling of falling
  2. A sensory flash
  3. A hypnagogic dream

D. Polysomnographic monitoring during an episode demonstrates one or more of the following:
  1. Brief, high-amplitude muscle potentials during the transition from wakefulness to sleep
  2. Arousals from light sleep
  3. Tachycardia following an intense episode

E. Absence of any medical or psychiatric disorder that could produce the disorder, e.g., **hyperekplexia**

F. Can occur in the presence of other sleep disorders producing insomnia

From ASDA Diagnostic Classification Steering Committee. The International Classification of Sleep Disorders Diagnostic and Coding Manual. Rochester, MN. American Sleep Disorders Association, © 1990, by kind permission of the American Academy of Sleep Medicine.

In a *variant* form, the jerks are excessive and repeatedly interrupt sleep, without evidence of **hyperekplexia.**[784]

See also **physiological hypnic myoclonus.**

sleep state misperception   A disorder in which there is a complaint of insomnia or excessive sleepiness without objective evidence of disturbance of sleep. Polysomnography reveals a normal sleep latency and the multiple sleep latency test demonstrates a mean sleep latency of greater than 10 minutes.[234]

sleep terrors   See **night terrors.**

sleep test   A diagnostic procedure for **myasthenia gravis,** in which a temporary remission in ptosis and ocular muscle paresis is seen after resting for some 30 minutes in a quiet, dark room, the differences being ascertained by photography.[6008]

sleeping sickness   1. (African trypanosomiasis) Infection by the *Trypanosoma brucei gambiense* or *brucei rhodesiense* as a result of a bite of the tsetse fly.

Neurological complications of the *West African* form include a chronic meningitis with focal gliosis. Clinically, this leads to neurological complications after a year of systemic symptoms, with evidence of progressive chronic encephalitis characterized particularly by tremor, ataxia, involuntary movements, and dementia. In the *East African* form, a more acute illness occurs as a result of infection by *T. brucei rhodesiense.* Involvement of the nervous system occurs early with fever and evidence of diffuse encephalopathy, usually with associated cardiac involvement. The condition is usually fatal.[6030]

2. See **encephalitis lethargica.**

sleep-onset association disorder   A condition of impaired sleep onset as a result of the absence of a certain object or set of circumstances. This is mainly a disorder of childhood and is eventually self-limiting.

sleep-onset insomnia   (prolonged sleep latency) The occurrence of a delay in going to sleep of 30 minutes or more. This is usually due to psychological or environmental factors. See **delayed sleep phase syndrome.**

sleep-onset REM sleep period   (SOREMP) The occurrence of rapid eye movement sleep without a preceding period of non–rapid eye movement sleep, as in infancy and with depressive illness and **narcolepsy.**[4337]

sleep-related abnormal swallowing syndrome   A disorder in which inadequate swallowing of saliva results in aspiration, with coughing, choking, and brief arousals or awakenings from sleep. The following diagnostic criteria have been suggested:[234]

A. A complaint of sudden awakenings associated with choking, or of insomnia

B. Choking during sleep associated with gurgling sounds from the upper airway

C. Polysomnography demonstrates frequent arousals from sleep associated with gurgling sounds.

D. Absence of any medical or psychiatric disorder that could account for the symptoms, e.g., panic attacks

E. Does not meet the diagnostic criteria for any other sleep disorder that could account for the symptoms, e.g., obstructive sleep apnea syndrome or sleep-related gastroesophageal reflux

(From ASDA Diagnostic Classification Steering Committee. The International Classification of Sleep Disorders Diagnostic and Coding Manual. Rochester, MN. American Sleep Disorders Association, © 1990, by kind permission of the American Academy of Sleep Medicine.)

sleep-related bruxism   See **bruxism.**

sleep-related enuresis   (idiopathic enuresis) A disorder of partial arousal in which involuntary micturition occurs during the first period of nocturnal non–rapid eye movement stage 3 or 4 sleep in children more than 3 years old. See also ASDA Diagnostic Classification,[234] **sleep disorders.**

sleep-related epilepsy   The occurrence of seizures with particular frequency at night as opposed to by day. Any form of seizure can occur nocturnally, but benign focal epilepsy of childhood, seizures of "partial" origin, and **juvenile myoclonic epilepsy** are most likely to occur at night.[5338]

sleep-related head banging   See **jactatio capitis nocturna.**

sleep-related myoclonus DIMS syndrome   (nocturnal myoclonus) The occurrence of repetitive stereotyped attacks of leg myoclonus, starting during sleep but leading to multiple awakenings and complaints of insomnia, usually in adults. The movements occur every 20–120 seconds, last between 0.5 and 10 seconds, and occur in groups of 30 or more jerks.[3514] See also **hypnic jerks, myoclonus,** and the ASDA Diagnostic Classification,[234] **sleep disorders, periodic limb movement disorder.**

sleep-related myoclonus DOES syndrome   (nocturnal myoclonus) The occurrence of repetitive stereotyped attacks of leg myoclonus, starting during sleep but leading to multiple awakenings and complaints of excessive daytime sleepiness, usually in adults. The movements occur every 20–120 seconds, last between 0.5 and 10 seconds, and occur in groups of 30 or more jerks. The sleepiness is the sole feature differentiating

this from the equivalent DIMS syndrome.[3514] See also **hypnic jerks, myoclonus,** the ASDA diagnostic classification,[234] **sleep disorders, periodic limb movement of sleep.**

sleep-related painful erections   The occurrence of prolonged, painful erections, subsiding over minutes and often recurring during the same night usually during rapid eye movement sleep periods, leading to arousal; without associated deficits in sexual functioning. Erections during wakefulness are painless.[2930]

sleeptalking   (somniloquy) The utterance of speech or sounds during sleep without simultaneous subjective detailed awareness of the event. Such talking during rapid eye movement sleep may represent the vocal expression of dream experiences, but it also occurs during transient arousals from non–rapid eye movement sleep.

The following diagnostic criteria have been suggested:[234]

A. Speech or utterances during sleep

B. Episodes are not associated with subjective awareness of talking.

C. Polysomnography demonstrates episodes of sleeptalking that can occur during any stage of sleep.

D. Can be associated with psychiatric or medical disorders, e.g., anxiety disorders or febrile illness

E. Can be associated with other sleep disorders, e.g., sleepwalking, obstructive sleep apnea syndrome, or rapid eye movement sleep behavior disorder

(From ASDA Diagnostic Classification Steering Committee. The International Classification of Sleep Disorders Diagnostic and Coding Manual. Rochester, MN: American Sleep Disorders Association, 1990. Reproduced by kind permission of the Assocaition and Dr. Michael Thorpy.)

Sleep–Wake Disorders (Canada)   A charitable organization providing support and information on this condition. Address: 5385 Yonge St., P. O. Box 45034, North York, ON M2N 5R7. Tel: 416–787–4848, 416–787–5374. Web site: http://swdca.org/.

sleep–wake transition disorders   Sleep disturbances which occur in the transition from wakefulness to sleep, in the transition from sleep to wakefulness, or occasionally in transitions from between different sleep stages. These include **rhythmic movement disorder, sleep starts, sleeptalking,** and **nocturnal leg cramps.**

sleepwalking   (somnambulism, semipurposeful automatisms) A sequence of complex behaviors during clouded consciousness which occur during the first nocturnal periods of non–rapid eye movement sleep stages 3 or 4, which are not thereafter recalled by the subject, and which may end with confused awakening or with a return to normal sleep.[2907] Sitting up in bed, perseverated simple movements, and complex automatic activities such as walking, descending stairs, and opening doors may occur; attempts to restrain the subject usually lead to avoidance behavior.[4620] Such abnormal behavior is seen less in adults than in children, among whom it may be associated with **enuresis** and **night terrors.**[249]

The following diagnostic criteria in Chart S–11 have been suggested:[234]

Chart S–11. Diagnostic Criteria for Sleepwalking

A. Ambulation that occurs in sleep
B. The onset typically occurs in prepubertal children.
C. Associated features include:
   1. Difficulty in arousing the patient during an episode
   2. Amnesia following an episode
D. Episodes typically occur in the first third of the sleep episode.
E. Polysomnographic monitoring demonstrates the onset of an episode during stage 3 or 4 sleep.
F. Other medical and psychiatric disorders can be present but do not account for the symptom.
G. The ambulation is not due to other sleep disorders, such as rapid eye movement sleep behavior disorder or sleep terror

---

From ASDA Diagnostic Classification Steering Committee. The International Classification of Sleep Disorders Diagnostic and Coding Manual. Rochester, MN. American Sleep Disorders Association, © 1990, by kind permission of the American Academy of Sleep Medicine.

slimmers' paralysis   A neuropathy affecting the peroneal nerves in subjects on a weight-reducing diet.

While the most likely reason would seem to be an unusual susceptibility of the nerve to the effects of compression when the knees are crossed,[3658] a local cause has been considered unlikely by other authors.[5261]

slipping clutch gait   See **isolated gait ignition failure.**

slit ventricle syndrome   The occurrence of scattered pyramidal signs following the collapse of formerly enlarged ventricles, as a result of surgical shunting.[2295]

slit ventricles   Abnormally narrow ventricles occurring in children with raised intracranial pressure, whose shunts are blocked. The ventricles are not expanded probably because of the presence of subependymal gliosis that has resulted from repeated distension of their walls in the past, stiffening them.[1673]

slow activity   All EEG activity at a frequency lower than that of alpha rhythms (8–13 Hz).

slow alpha variant rhythms   EEG rhythms at 3.5–6 Hz (mostly at 4–5 Hz) recorded most prominently over the posterior regions of the head. They generally alternate or are intermixed with alpha rhythms, to which they are often harmonically related. Their amplitude is variable but is frequently close to 50 uV and they are blocked or attenuated by attention, especially visual and mental effort.

Slow alpha variant rhythms should be held in contradistinction to posterior slow waves, which are characteristic of children and adolescents and are occasionally seen in young adults. (Adapted from the 1974 report of the Committee on Terminology, IFCN. In: Chatrian GE, Bergamini L, Dondey M, et al. A glossary of terms most commonly used by clinical electroencephalographers. *EEG Clin Neurophysiol* 1974;**37**:538–548.[989]

slow channel syndrome   (slow ion channel defect) A congenital, dominantly inherited, myasthenic syndrome of selective weakness and fatigability in the face, neck, and arms, not responding to edrophonium or pyridostigmine, but with a decrementing response to repetitive nerve stimulation (which also causes a repetitive response to a single shock). It is also seen in infancy and childhood.

The characteristic laboratory features are prolonged decay phases of end-plate potentials and of minature end-plate potentials, repetitive compound motor action potentials, and degenerative changes of the postsynaptic membrane.

The pathophysiology is considered to be a prolongation of the "open time" of the acetylcholine-induced ion channel, with a reduction in the safety factor being due to decreased amplitudes of the normal miniature end-plate potentials.[1658,1670] See also **myasthenia gravis.**

slow downward ocular bobbing   See **dipping.**

slow eye movements   See **pursuit eye movements, optokinetic nystagmus.**

slow fusional adaptive mechanism   See **fusion.**

slow ion channel defect   See **slow channel syndrome.**

slow motor neuron disease   Those forms of **amyotrophic lateral sclerosis** in which patients survive for longer than 5 years.

slow saccades   Reduction in the velocity of the saccadic movements of the eyes, due to focal or diffuse lesions in the pontine tegmentum. See **hypometric saccades.**

slow spike-and-wave activity   See **generalized sharp-and-slow-wave discharges.**

slow stroke syndrome   An ischemic stroke syndrome that is atypical because of its extended and gradual progression toward completion over weeks without the more usual stepwise deteriorations characteristic of multiple emboli.

slow syndrome   The term of Plum[4464] for the somnolent, hypokinetic, apathetic state characterizing **thalamic dementia.**

slow upward ocular bobbing   A variety of ocular bobbing seen in patients with pontine infarcts, in which the eye moves upwards slowly, returning fast to the mid-position. See **ocular bobbing.**

slow wave   An EEG waveform with a duration longer than that of alpha waves.

slowly alternating skew deviation   A form of dysconjugate eye movement in which the findings resemble those of **skew deviation** but in which the cycles take 30–90 seconds. Mesodiencephalic lesions are responsible.[1128]

slowly progressive aphasia   A syndrome in which the first symptom is typically an anomic, dysfluent dysphasia with phonemic paraphasic errors and relatively retained comprehension, resulting from initial involvement of the left perisylvian region. Eventually, other cognitive losses appear, indicating the presence of a dementing illness (Pick, Alzheimer, spongiform or other types).[3832,3849]

slow-virus syndrome   See **prion disease.**

slow-wave sleep   The alternate of rapid eye movement sleep, in which a gradual reduction in the frequency and amplitude of the EEG rhythms occurs. Sleep spindles, vertex sharp waves, and kappa complexes also appear on this theta and delta background.

Sluder, Greenfield   (1865–1928) American laryngologist, who practiced in St. Louis. He believed that disease of the sphenopalatine ganglion was responsible for various facial and cranial pains.

Sluder syndrome   (sphenopalatine neuralgia, lower-half headache) Persistent pain felt intermittently in the face at the root of the nose and in the frontal region, temples, eye, occiput, mastoid, teeth or hard palate, associated with homolateral reduction in the sense of taste, facial flushing, lachrymation and salivation, and often following sphenoid or ethmoid sinusitis.

Sluder reported that this pain could be relieved by cocainization of the sphenopalatine ganglion. Its etiology is obscure; it may be a form of **cluster headache** but the (incomplete) descriptions given suggest that it is quite unlike any of the usual types of that disease,[5209] although later authors, in reviewing the condition, have incorporated features which Sluder did not describe.

Sly disease   See **mucopolysaccharidoses.**

Small disease   A recessively inherited syndrome of deafness, mental retardation, muscle atrophy with weakness and clumsiness, and vascular retinopathy.[5213] See also **Coats syndrome.**

small fiber sensory neuropathies   Those neuropathies that selectively affect the small-diameter myelinated and unmyelinated fibers, leading to spontaneous neuropathic pains and reduced thermal and pain sensitivity while proprioception and power are unaffected. Causes include **hereditary sensory neuropathy, Fabry disease, amyloidosis, HIV** infection, and certain toxins. See also **QSART.**

small intensely fluorescent cells   (SIF cells) Ganglion cells capable of releasing dopamine and epinephrine.

small sharp spikes   (big/large sharp spikes, SSS, benign sporadic sleep spikes, **benign epileptiform transients of sleep**) Stereotyped unilateral, low-amplitude, brief, diphasic, single but repeated, transient needle-sharp spikes, recorded sporadically, mainly over temporal regions during non–rapid eye movement sleep stages 1 and 2 in normal adults and shifting between the two sides of the brain. These waveforms have no significance with regard to epilepsy.[3075,5943]

Smell Identification test   A multiple-choice "scratch and sniff" test using over three dozen odors. Although it also requires that the patient's language and memory be intact, it correlates well with other tests of olfactory thresholds.[1501]

smile-wink phenomenon   The tendency for one eyelid to descend in patients with contralateral infarcts when they smile, if they smile.[3040]

Smith cramp   A focal (occupational) dystonia. See **focal dystonia.**

Smith syndrome   1. (macular colobomas and dwarfism) A congenital dysmorphic syndrome characterized by short stature, macular pigmentation, colobomas of the retina, skeletal deformities, and pendular nystagmus.[5222] 2. (dwarfism, mental retardation and dysmorphism) A congenital dysmorphic syndrome characterized by low birth weight, short stature, proportionate but prominent ears, strabismus, ptosis, seizures, dolichocephaly, and mental and developmental delay.[5222]

Smith-Lemli-Opitz syndrome   A relatively common congenital, recessively inherited syndrome of dwarfism, microcephaly, holoproscencephaly, micrognathia, psychomotor retardation, ptosis, genital abnormalities, spasticity or hypotonia, seizures, and variable other musculoskeletal anomalies such as dwarfism[5223] due to a defect in cholesterol biosynthesis. In the brain, polymicrogyria, small brainstem and cerebellum, and absence of the corpus callosum are described.

The authors are American pediatricians and geneticists.

SMON   See **subacute myelo-opticoneuropathy.**

smooth endoplasmic reticulum   A structural component of the axon, continuous distally from the perikaryon and responsible for the rapid transfer of large-molecular-weight proteins.

smooth pursuit system   A reflex mechanism, not therefore under voluntary control, whereby the eyes track a mobile target so as to keep the image of that target on the fovea. The pathways responsible are not precisely known but must involve the frontal eye fields and the occipital cortex as well as subcortical connections. See also **fixation, saccades, optokinetic nystagmus, pursuit eye movements.**

Sneddon syndrome   A thrombotic vasculopathy leading to the rare association of idiopathic livedo reticularis and cerebrovascular accidents, the latter being due to a noninflammatory arteriopathy affecting small and medium-sized vessels. Seizures and dementia are also described as part of the syndrome.

The condition appears in youth or adult life and is probably dominantly inherited. Complicated obstetrical histories, cardiac lesions, venous thromboses, thrombocytopenia, and disturbed sexual function in men are other features described.[4618,5242]

In a *variant* form, a vascular dementing syndrome without livedo reticularis occurs in the presence of **antiphospholipid antibodies.** See also **Worster-Drought syndrome.**

sneeze center   A cell cluster in the rostral dorsolateral pontomedullary area, damage to which may result in abortion of the normal sneezing phenomena.[1826]

sneeze reflex   See **nasal reflex.**

sneeze syncope   Fainting produced by sneezing (or other methods of performing the Valsalva maneuver), and noted rarely as a complication of the **Chiari malformation.**[1127]

sneezing   (ptarmus, sternutatio convulsiva) A compound reflex with various adequate afferent stimuli that induce involuntary spasmodic inspiration, followed by explosive expiration with initial brief nasopharyngeal closure and closure of the eyes. It is mediated by the fifth and seventh cranial nerves and brainstem respiratory centers.

The Talmud describes sneezing as a pleasure sent from God, while Pope Gregory (540–604) regarded it as a sign of impending plague and, following his lead, the benediction "God bless you" is commonly offered to a person who sneezes. Intractable sneezing is usually psychogenic but may have an epileptic or local basis.[1060] See also **ACHOO.**

Snellen, Hermann   (1834–1908) Dutch ophthalmologist who in 1862 devised the first standard test types for assessing visual acuity. He also described the aural hyperemia that occurs with stimulation of the auriculotemporal nerve.

Sniffin' Sticks   A proprietary test of olfactory functions assessing odor threshold, discrimination, and identification.

snoring   (rhencospasm) (from Gr, snore + spasm) The occurrence of loud upper airway breathing sounds during sleep without episodes of apnea or hypoventilation, occurring mainly in males with large tonsils. Retrognathia, depression of the CNS, nasal congestion, and obesity also predispose to snoring. Although snoring is also a feature of forms of **sleep apnea,** the primary form is not associated with these conditions.[234]

snout response   Puckering or protrusion of the lower lip and depression of the corner of the mouth, elicited by a light tap below the nose or brief pressure above the upper lip. This is a developmental reflex (an aug-

mentation of the **oral** reflex) which is present in cases of anterior cerebral artery occlusion, hepatic coma, toxic and traumatic states, and dementias[4370] and in subjects with diffuse cortical disease or bilateral corticobulbar tract lesions. See **buccal reflex.**

snouting   See **buccal reflex.**

snow blindness   See **photophthalmia.**

snowbanking   Accumulation of the products of inflammation in the lower half of the anterior chamber of the eye as a result of gravity.

S-O syndrome   See **sphenoidal fissure–optic canal syndrome.**

soap-bubble tumor   A name suggested by the CT appearance of lymphoplasmacytoid lymphoma (cerebral immunocytoma).[5489]

sobbing spasms   See **breath-holding spells,** of which these attacks represent a *variant*, characterized by prolonged sobbing up to the point that the infant is performing a Valsalva maneuver.[2055]

Social Ties checklist   A 10-item scale that assesses the quantity and quality of social supports. Scores range from 0 to 10, higher scores indicating better social supports.

Sociedad Espanola de Neurologia   A professional organization. Address: c/o Dr. I Picornell, Darder Paseo de la Castellana 244 28046 Madrid, Spain. Web site: http://www.medynet.com/index.html.

Society for Neuro-Oncology   A professional organization. Web site: http://www.soc-neuro-onc.org/.

Society for Progressive Supranuclear Palsy, Inc.   An advocacy and mutual support group. Address: Woodholme Medical Bldg., Suite 515, Baltimore, MD 21208. Tel: 410–486–3330, 1–800–457–4777. Web site: http://www.psp.org/.

Society for Research into Hydrocephalus and Spina Bifida   A charitable organization. Web site: http://www.demon.co.uk/charities/srhsb/.

Society of British Neurological Surgeons   A professional organization. Address: Dept. of Neurosurgery, Walgrave Hospital, Coventry, England CV2 2DX.

Society of Neurological Surgeons   A professional organization. Address: Southwest Medical Schools, 5323 Harry Hynes Blvd., University of Texas, Dallas, TX 75235. Web site: http://www.societyns.org/.

Society of Neurosurgical Anesthesia and Critical Care   A professional organization. Address: P.O. Box 11086, Richmond, VA 23230–1086. Tel: 804–673–9037. Web site: http://www.snascc.org.

Socioeconomic Scale   An instrument designed to identify the socioeconomic needs of patients with **multiple sclerosis,** in which working ability; financial/economic status; residence; dependence; transportation; therapy services; psychosocial status; problem-solving capacity; and memory are each rated on a 6-point scale.[3820] See also **environmental status scale.**

SOD1   Copper/zinc superoxide dismutase, the gene for which appears remarkably likely to undergo mutations causing various phenotypic varieties of **amyotrophic lateral sclerosis,** etc.

sodium amytal test   (Wada test) The intracarotid injection of sodium amylobarbitone for the purpose of producing reversible inhibition of the functions of the ipsilateral hemisphere.

The test was introduced by Dr. Jun Wada while at the Montreal Neurological Institute, in an attempt to determine the side where speech function is localized—important information in candidates for temporal lobectomy.

Soederbergh pressure reflex   Flexion of the second, third, and fourth fingers when the ulna is firmly stroked in a downward direction. When this is done over the radius, the thumb flexes. The phenomenon is seen in some cases of pyramidal and perhaps basal ganglion disease. Similar muscle contractions in response to pressure upon other bony prominences are also described.

Soemmerring, Samuel Thomas von   (1755–1830) Prussian anatomist, professor of anatomy and surgery at a number of German universities, who in 1778 reclassified **Willis'** scheme of the cranial nerves into one recognizing 12 pairs, which is the system accepted today, albeit with some reluctance. He gave priority to Vicq d'Azir for discovering the substantia nigra but was an early describer of the difference between the gray and white matter of the cerebrum, described the macula lutea, and the substantia gelatinosa, and reported a case of achondroplasia.

soft exudates   Organized edema fluid in the retina, the whitish clumps having ill-defined margins.

soft neurological signs   Clinical departures from the normal which, because of their imprecision, inconstancy, or isolation, are not adequate to convince the examiner of the presence of disease.

soma-   (Gr, the body). Prefix denoting body.

Somagyi sign   Dilation of the pupils with full inspiration and constriction with full expiration. The feature is physiological but small in extent.

somatization disorder   (conversion disorder, hysterical neurosis, dissociative/conversion disorder, Briquet syndrome) The expression of psychological conflicts as physical complaints, *or* "a tendency to experience and communicate somatic distress and symptoms unaccounted for by physical findings, to attribute them to physical illness and to seek medical help."[4757] The di-

agnostic criteria proposed in the *DSM-IV* are given in Chart S–12.

Chart S–12. Diagnostic Criteria for Somatization Disorder

A. There is a history of many physical complaints, beginning before age 30 years, that occur over a period of several years and result in treatment being sought or significant impairment in social, occupational, or other important areas of functioning.

B. Each of the following criteria must have been met, with individual symptoms occurring at any time during the course of the disturbance:

1. *Four pain symptoms*: a history of pain related to at least four different sites or functions (e.g., head, abdomen, back, joints, extremities, chest, rectum, during menstruation, during sexual intercourse, or during urination)

2. *Two gastrointestinal symptoms*: a history of at least two gastrointestinal symptoms other than pain (e.g., nausea, bloating, vomiting other than during pregnancy, diarrhea, or intolerance of several different foods)

3. *One sexual symptom*: a history of at least one sexual or reproductive symptom other than pain (e.g., sexual indifference, erectile or ejaculatory dysfunction, irregular menses, excessive menstrual bleeding, vomiting throughout pregnancy)

4. *One pseudo-neurological symptom*: a history of at least one symptom or deficit suggesting a neurological condition not limited to pain (conversion symptoms such as impaired coordination or balance, paralysis or localized weakness, difficulty swallowing or lump in throat, aphonia, urinary retention, hallucinations, loss of touch or pain sensation, double vision, blindness, deafness, seizures; dissociative symptoms such as amnesia; or loss of consciousness other than fainting)

C. Either

1. After appropriate investigation, each of the symptoms in criterion B cannot be fully explained by a known general medical condition or the direct effects of a substance (e.g., a drug of abuse or a medication), *or*

2. When there is a related general medical condition, the physical complaints or resulting social or occupational impairment are in excess of what would be expected from the history, physical examination, or laboratory findings.

D. The symptoms are not intentionally feigned or produced (as in factitious disorder or malingering).

somatoform disorder   See **conversion disorder, hysteria.**

somatofugal axonal atrophy   The process whereby altered synthesis of neurofilaments in the cell body of an axon leads to the delivery of axoplasm containing a low concentration of neurofilament protein to the distal part of the axon, which causes the axon to shrink.

somatognosia   The conscious awareness of the presence, disposition, and orientation of the parts of the body, forming a scheme or image of the body in the mind. This distinct body function is localized in the right hemisphere. This distinct psychological function is concerned with bodily orientation corresponding to body image or to the "body schema" of **Head** and **Holmes** and represents "A spatial quality in the awareness of various sensory impressions of the body" (Bonnier, 1905).[4472]

somatomotor seizures A form of simple partial seizure characterized by localized unilateral clonic movements affecting particularly the distal and the bulbar muscles.

In a *variant* form, the attacks begin with a brief period of tonic contraction and then become clonic.

somatosensory blink response A blink response elicited by electrical stimulation of a peripheral nerve such as the median, recording from the inferior orbicularis oculi muscles. It represents a release phenomenon transmitted through the brainstem reticular activating system. Miwa et al.[3919] suggest the following criteria:

The latency to the onset of the EMG response of the orbicularis oculi muscle ranges from 35 to 60 msec.

The EMG response is a bilateral response (at times, its appearance can be slightly more pronounced on the side ipsilateral to the stimulation).

The EMG response is a phasic response with a duration of less than 100 msec.

If three consecutive electrical stimulations at intervals of at least 10 seconds fail to elicit any obvious EMG discharges, the somatosensory blank response is considered negative.

The amplitude of the obtained EMG response is at least threefold greater than the baseline activities of the orbicularis oculi muscles by inspection.

somatosensory evoked potentials (SEPs) Electrical waveforms of biological origin elicited by electrical stimulation or physiological activation of peripheral sensory fibers, for example, of the median, common peroneal, or posterior tibial nerves.

The normal SEP is a complex waveform, with several components that are specified by polarity and the average peak latency. The polarity and latency of individual components depend on the following:

1. Subject variables, such as age and sex
2. Stimulus characteristics, such as intensity and rate of stimulation
3. Recording parameters, such as amplifier time constants, electrode placement, and electrode combinations

Adapted from the 1987 Report of the Nomenclature Committee of the American Association of Electrodiagnostic Medicine. AAEE glossary of terms in clinical electromyography. *Muscle Nerve* 1987;**10S**:G5–G23. Copyright 1987 by John Wiley and Sons, Inc. Reprinted by permission of John Wiley and Sons, Inc.

See also **spinal evoked potential.**

somatosensory nystagmus See **arthrokinetic induced nystagmus.**

somatosensory seizures Simple partial seizures in which paresthesias or abnormal somatognosis occurs, usually spreading through a geographical area of the body on one side.[3712]

somatosensory vertigo 1. A physiological illusion of bodily rotation which occurs when limbs are passively rotated about a vertical axis at the hips or shoulder joints. The phenomenon may be accompanied by **arthrokinetic-induced nystagmus.** 2. Vague sensorimotor symptoms occurring in patients with peripheral sensory neuropathy, especially when there is an abnormality in another afferent channel.[727] See **multisensory syndrome.**

somatostatin (growth hormone inhibitory factor) A neuropeptide transmitter substance found in the striatum and hypothalamopituitary axis. It inhibits the secretion of growth hormone but also depresses the secretion of insulin and glucagon. It is also found in the spinal cord, where it may act as a modulator of the pain pathway.

somatotopic localization The representation of particular regions of the body within specific areas of the CNS.

somesthesis The sensation of the static position or of movement of a part of the body.

somesthetic temporal discrimination The ability to perceive as separate two successive somesthetic stimuli applied to the same or different places on the skin. The somatosensory pathways and parietal cortex, the supplementary motor area, and subcortical regions are all normally involved in such discrimination.[3220]

Sommer sector Ammon's horn, a part of the hippocampus, in which the pyramidal cells are unusually sensitive to oxygen deprivation. It was described by Wilhelm Sommer (1852–1900), a German physician.

Sommer syndrome A congenital dysmorphic syndrome of modern description, characterized by dysplasia of the iris, renal agenesis, hydrocephalus, wide cranial sutures, and mental and developmental delay.[337]

somnambulism See **sleepwalking.**

somniloquy See **sleeptalking.**

somnolence See **excessive daytime sleepiness, hypersomnia.**

somnolence syndrome A reversible syndrome of lethargy, nausea, and headache with slowing of the EEG patterns, occurring in children treated as with methotrexate and irradiation for leukemia. See also **necrotizing leukoencephalopathy.**[1943]

somnolentia See **sleep drunkenness.**

somnolescent starts See **sleep starts.**

sonogenic reflex epilepsy See **musicogenic epilepsy.**

sopor- (Lat, deep sleep) Prefix denoting sleep.

soporific (from Lat, deep sleep + making) Inducing sleep.

sorbinil An aldose reductase inhibitor, currently under scrutiny as a treatment for diabetic peripheral neuropathy.

sorbitol An alcohol sugar, the level of which is increased in the peripheral nerves of those with diabetes.

Sotos syndrome See **cerebral gigantism.**

Sotos Syndrome Support Association A charitable organization in this field. Address: Danada Sq. East, PMB #235, Wheaton, IL 60187. Tel: 888–246–7772. E-mail: sssa@well.com. Web site: http://www.well.com/user/sssa/.

Sottas, J. (1866–1953) French neurologist. See **hereditary motor and sensory neuropathy, type 3.**

soul-deaf Totally destitute of hearing and of all reminiscence of sounds previously heard.

Souques, Achille-Alexandre (1860–1944) French neuropsychiatrist who switched from the study of law to that of medicine at the Université de Paris. He worked under **Charcot,** eventually becoming *chef de clinique* under **Brissaud** and **Raymond** after Charcot's death. After some years spent elsewhere, he returned to the **Salpêtrière,** where he remained until his retirement in 1925.

He described **palilalia,** the **inversion** of reflexes, and hypophyseal infantilism, but published principally on the topics of parkinsonism, multiple sclerosis, epilepsy, **camptocormia,** and medical history.

Achille-Alexandre Souques

Souques disease (functional bent back) See **camptocormia.**

Souques signs 1. Elevation and extension of a paretic arm causes extension and spreading of all the fingers.[3953,5264] See also **digiti quinti sign.** 2. (Leg sign) When a parkinsonian patient seated on a chair is suddenly tipped backwards on the chair, the subject's legs do not extend because of the lack of the normal associated movements.[1829] 3. See **Gordon sign.** See also **pinky finger sign.**

Souques syndrome 1. See **palilalia.** 2. Congenital absence of the pectoral muscles, usually unilaterally.[5263] Hypotrophy of the corresponding arm may be associated.

South American trypanosomiasis (Chaga disease) A zoonosis caused by *Trypanosoma cruzi,* a protozoan organism with an animal reservoir in the southern United States and South America.

In the chronic phase of the infection, parasympathetic degeneration occurs as a result of massive degeneration of autonomic ganglia, leading to digestive disturbances, motor neuropathy, and cardiac signs including sudden death. Clinically, an acute, mild febrile illness leads to asymptomatic infection or to cardiomyopathy, with or without systemic myositis.[6030] See also **sleeping sickness** (West African trypanosomiasis).

South Indian paraplegia See **Madras neuropathy.**

space sickness Motion sickness generated by active head movements under conditions of weightlessness, due to inequality of the weight of the otoliths or to an intravestibular mismatch between the otoliths and the semicircular canals.[727]

space-occupying lesions See **mass lesions.**

Spanish toxic oil syndrome A clinical syndrome of myalgia, joint limitation, weight loss, cramps, progressive weakness and wasting, sensory disturbances, and changes in the skin due to a progressive mixed axonal neuropathy affecting both proximal and distal muscles. The condition was due to the ingestion of cooking oil adulterated with triorthocresyl phosphate and was described in Spain in 1981.[1208]

sparganosis Infection with the larvae of tapeworms belonging to the genus *Spirometra,* presenting usually as a solitary cyst in muscle containing the worm *Spirometra mansoni* or *Diphyllobothrium latum.* Ptosis and orbital cellulitis are other complications described.[103]

sparing of fixation (macular sparing) Retention of the central 5° of the visual field in the presence of occipital lobe infarction. This is considered to be due to the supplementary supply of blood through the middle cerebral artery to the occipital pole (which is the projection area for the macula), rather than to the bilateral representation of macular function.

spasm   (Gr, muscular contraction) Involuntary reflex muscle contractions with accompanying electrical activity that is either normal or resembles that occurring in **tetany.** The cramps may be tonic or clonic, and are usually painful. Prolonged muscle contraction and ischemia are the more common causes.

spasm faciale mediane   See **cranial dystonias.**

spasm of conjugate gaze   Conjugate deviation of the eyes when the patient attempts to close them against resistance. This is a sign of parietal lobe disease, the eyes deviating away from the side of the lesion. The sign would be of greater localizing value were it not often present also with some lesions of the brainstem.[1073]

spasm of the near reflex   Intermittent and painful attacks of convergence, accommodation, and miosis with failure of lateral movement of the globes. The condition resembles bilateral sixth cranial nerve palsies except that there is miosis of the putative abducting eye on attempted lateral gaze.[1072] See **convergence spasm.**

spasmodic crying   See **emotionalism.**

spasmodic dysphonia   (spastic dysphonia, inspiratory speech) A laryngeal dystonia leading to a form of speech that is constrained, harsh, and monotonous; enunciated *staccato* with variable but uncontrolled volume and accompanied by spillover movements of the face and bulbar muscles. Other descriptions note quiet, tremulous, hoarse, strangulated, or whispered speech, interrupted by irregular stoppages or catches. Whispering may, however, be relatively normal. The features of **Meige syndrome** or of other **dystonias** may coexist. The condition was first described by Traube in 1871.

Although all of the speech is uttered during expiration, the sound effect is unnatural and suggests the picturesque but incorrect title given it. A good example will be given if the reader enunciates this entry during inspiration rather than expiration. No single pathology is suggested by such speech, which has parallels in certain other languages.[1168]

spasmodic laughter   (Homeric laughter, sham mirth) Emotional expression in the absence of emotional experience, as occurs in some patients with brainstem or frontal lobe disease, intracranial hemorrhage, or **Lytico-Bodig.**

Uncontrollable weeping without appropriate affect is a similar phenomenon.[3655]

spasmodic torticollis   A common form of focal or segmental dystonia, characterized by involuntary tonic or intermittent spasms of the neck muscles, which typically lead to a deviation of the head from its normal position and which may be painful.

The condition was first described in detail by Jean **Cruchet** in 1907. Other dystonias and tremor are found

in a proportion of patients and the condition may be a *forme fruste* of idiopathic torsion **dystonia.** It has also been detected in fossil dinosaurs.[3640,4758]

Although there assuredly exists organic disease of the basal ganglia in this condition, which may also complicate cervical spinal lesions, the precise nature of this is not known. See also **cervical dystonia, antecollis, retrocollis.**

spasmophilia   1. (latent **tetany**) An increased tendency to suffer tetanic attacks, as in patients with hypocalcemia. 2. (**hyperventilation syndrome**) A state characterized by hyperventilation and anxiety.

spasmus nictitans   (nictitatio, blepharoclonus) Clonic spasms of the eyelids, seen in dystonias and in **hemifacial spasm.**

spasmus nutans   (head nodding) The rare association of ocular oscillations at 2.4 Hz, head-nodding, tilt, and torticollis occurring in the first 2 years of life. It seldom lasts longer than 3 years, except in the unusual case in which it is due to a tumor in the region of the third ventricle. An accompanying pendular horizontal nystagmus is frequently bilateral but asymmetrical.[5268]

spastic ataxia of Charlevoix-Saguenay   See **Charlevoix-Saguenay spastic ataxic syndrome.**

spastic diplegia   See **Little disease.**

spastic dysphonia   See **spasmodic dysphonia.**

spastic eyelids   Uninhibited tonic lid elevation leading to the maintenance of eye opening in the unconscious state without blinking, associated with increased levator tone and thought to indicate the presence of a pontine lesion.[2975]

spastic paraplegia   The syndrome of pyramidal signs with a defined upper level corresponding to a spinal level, usually taken as below C8. The causes include **hereditary spastic paraparesis,** spinal tumors, transverse myelopathy, **multiple sclerosis,** and spinal trauma, as well as a range of less common conditions, but it may also occur after multiple cerebrovascular episodes, indicating that not all cases are of spinal origin.[5687]

Spastic Paraplegia Foundation   A charitable organization in this field. Address: P.O. Box 1208, Forston, GA 31808. Tel: 888–572–7934. Web site: http://www. sp-foundation.org/.

spastic paraplegia, ataxia, mental retardation (SPAR)   See **hereditary spastic paraparesis.**

spastic paretic facial contracture   A chronic, persistent, unilateral facial contracture resulting from persistent **myokymia,** associated with facial weakness and due to intrinsic pontine disease.[5252] See also **Rasdolsky syndrome.**

spastic pelvic floor syndrome   A disorder due to persistent contraction of normal pelvic floor muscles, causing a functional outlet obstruction during straining and resulting in severe constipation.[3184]

spastic pseudosclerosis   See **Wilson disease.** The term has also been used for **Creutzfeldt-Jakob disease.**

spastic spinal paralysis   (Erb spastic paraparesis) See **Erb-Charcot syndrome.**

spasticity   "A motor disorder characterized by a velocity-dependent increase in tonic stretch reflexes (muscle tone) with exaggerated tendon jerks, resulting from hyperexcitability of the stretch reflex, as one component of the upper motor neuron syndrome".[3235,3236]

Loss of supraspinal control leads to excessive activity of motoneurons and lack of normal reciprocal innervation, and thus to the firing off of agonists and antagonists at the same time, either spontaneously or as a response to stimulation. Hyperreflexia, clonus, and extensor spasms are associated.

This definition is but one among many; some others (in which the term denotes proprioceptive reflex release, generalized reflex release, the upper motor neuron syndrome, dystonic-rigid states, etc.) are reviewed by Landau.[3244]

spasticity of conjugate gaze   The term of Cogan for ocular deviation contralateral to the side of a hemispheric (especially parietotemporal) lesion with attempted eye closure.[5409]

spät apoplexy   (Ger, late + Gr, stroke) Delayed intracerebral hemorrhage following cranial trauma, which may be minor.[2351] The mechanisms suggested for it include an acute rise in blood pressure, suddenly increased intracerebral blood flow after the relief of a focal obstruction, and reperfusion of ischemic regions.

spatial agnosia   See **spatial neglect.**

spatial agraphia   See **agraphia.**

spatial neglect   (agnosia for the opposite half of space, spatial agnosia) Inattention to half of visual space—almost always the left half and occurring in patients with a right hemisphere lesion in the region of the parieto-occipitotemporal junction which interferes with spatial analysis and visual perception of the left side. See also **extinction, neglect.**

spatial summation   A phenomenon of synaptic transmission, whereby two inadequate impulses converging upon a synapse may together form an adequate stimulus for excitation or suppression at that site.

Spatz, H.   (1888–1969) German neurologist, experimental neuropathologist, and neuroanatomist, who worked in Kraepelin's clinic in Munich, where **Hallervorden** studied the brain of a girl who had died with the syndrome until now known by their names.

Captured by the American forces after World War II, both were pressed into serving the Allied forces' medical services, and were later installed in a laboratory in Vienna for the remainder of their professional careers.

special sensory ataxia   Sensory ataxia caused by loss of muscle spindle (proprioceptive) afferent input to the cerebellum.

specificity theory of sensation   The original concept of **von Frey** that four somatesthetic senses were mediated by four receptor types in the skin. This is now considered to be untenable, but the **pattern theory,** which in contradistinction stated that there were neither specific fibers nor receptors, has also been found wanting. A synthesis has been achieved by Melzack and Wall.[3825]

SPECT   Acronym for **S**ingle **P**hoton **E**mission **C**omputed **T**omography, a technique for measuring cerebral perfusion rate by using ^{99}Tc HMPAO or Iofetamine ^{123}I as the tracer agents, with computerized reconstruction of the isotopic emissions recorded by a rotating gamma camera.

spectaclar shrinking deficit   The dramatic improvement in the clinical appearance of a patient with cardiogenic brain embolism, occurring over the course of minutes to hours and considered to be due to rapid dissolution of the embolus within a large artery in the carotid system, with consequent re-establishment of adequate cerebral perfusion.[3935]

speech   1. The enunciation of "words referring to one another in a particular manner" (Hughlings-**Jackson**) according to grammar, which allows a meaning to be derived over and above the sum of the meanings of the individual words uttered. 2. The expression and reception of ideas and feelings by way of verbal symbols such as words or other verbal tools. See also **propositional language** and **speech.**

speech apraxia   Selective impairment in ability to produce speech sounds.[3138]

speech audiometry   The assessment of auditory perception using phonemically balanced word lists. Typically, patients with neural lesions exhibit a particular difficulty in hearing speech sounds, as opposed to pure tones.[662]

speech dyspraxia   See **dysprosody.**

speech questionnaire   A rating scale of communication impairment, completed during an interview of the relative(s) of a subject with aphasia, such as that occurring after a stroke. The scale consists of 19 questions relating to expressive speech and comprehension, but ignores repetition and naming abilities.[3414]

spelling agraphia   An agraphic syndrome characterized by a disturbance of letter choice, although the actual form of the written letters remains intact.[399]

spelling alexia   Inability to read words and phrases with relative sparing of the ability to read individual letters.[5090]

Spens, Thomas (1769–1842) Edinburgh physician whose account of bradycardia with syncope antedated that of Stokes by over half a century.[5274]

spermatic neuralgia   Severe unilateral paroxysms of pain radiating between the testis and the inguinal canal, with no known cause.[574]

sphenocavernous syndrome   An inclusive term for the orbital apex, cavernous, and **superior orbital fissure syndromes.** The clinical features include involvement of the third, fourth, sixth, and first two divisions of the fifth cranial nerves, and sometimes of the optic and oculosympathetic nerves as well, with or without proptosis and pain.[2431]

sphenocephaly   A malformation due to persisting patency of the anterior fontanelle and the metopic suture, characterized by prominence of the bregma and by frontal bossing.[4]

sphenoid   (Gr, like a wedge) Wedge-shaped. The sphenoid bone is so-named because it is placed as though "wedged" between its neighbors.

sphenoid sinus   A rectangular midline structure within the sphenoid bone, bounded by the pituitary fossa above, the ethmoid sinus and nasal cavity in front, the nasopharynx and eustachian tube below, the clivus and brainstem behind, and the superior orbital fissure, cavernous sinuses, and petrous temporal bone at the sides.

sphenoid sinus carcinoma   Rare primary carcinomas, usually presenting in adult males who complain of severe, deep-seated, boring headaches and visual loss, and who show features of the **sphenocavernous syndrome,** diplopia due to isolated sixth cranial nerve paresis, or visual obscurations due to optic nerve or chiasmal infiltration.[2431]

sphenoidal electrodes   Long EEG recording wires that can be introduced through the mandibular notch to lie beneath the floor of the middle cranial fossa. They are used the better to record discharges emanating from the inferomedial aspect of the temporal lobe. The technique was originated by H.H. **Jasper.**

sphenoidal fissure syndrome   (Tolosa-Hunt syndrome, orbital apex syndrome, Rollet syndrome, Rochon-Duvigneau syndrome, painful ophthalmoplegia) A syndrome of retroorbital pain, oculomotor palsies, and sometimes visual impairment, often with acute onset following trauma or a viral infection, but also commonly with a slower onset and then usually due to a neoplasm or to granulomatous inflammation.[4747] See **superior orbital fissure syndrome.**

sphenoidal fissure–optic canal syndrome   (S-O syndrome, orbital apex syndrome) Involvement of cranial nerves II, III, IV, and VI and of the ophthalmic division of the fifth nerve; sympathetic fibers; and the ophthalmic artery and vein by an infiltrating malig-

nancy in this region, such as a nasopharyngeal carcinoma. The **superior orbital fissure syndrome** is probably the same thing.

sphenopalatine neuralgia   One of the 17 terms for **cluster headache** listed by Kudrow,[3177] suggesting, as does the term *periodic migrainous neuralgia*, that a neurogenic basis may be found for the condition. It may but it has not yet been.

sphenopetrosal fissure syndrome   See **superior orbital fissure syndrome.**

spheroid body myopathy   A rare, dominantly inherited, benign myopathy (a desminopathy) characterized by the onset in youth of proximal weakness, pain, and atrophy in the legs and by the presence of filamentous spheroid bodies in type 1 fibers on muscle biopsy specimens. Serum CK levels are normal.[2148] See also **myofibrillar (desmin-storage) myopathy,** and for further data see http://www.neuro.wustl.edu/neuromuscular/maltbrain.html.

sphingolipidoses   A group of lysosomal storage diseases characterized by the accumulation, variously, of gangliosides, sulfatides, cerebrosides, or sphingomyelin as a result of genetically determined enzymatic failure. They include **Fabry disease, Farber disease, Gaucher disease, GM$_1$** and **GM$_2$ gangliosidoses, Krabbe disease,** the **mucosulfatidoses, sphingomyelin storage disorders** such as Niemann-Pick disease, and the **sulfatidoses.**

sphingomyelin   A diaminophosphatide derived from sphingosine.

sphingomyelin lipidosis   See **sphingomyelin storage disorders.**

sphingomyelin storage disorders   (sphingomyelin lipidoses) A group of uncommon, recessively transmitted lysosomal storage diseases affecting sphingomyelin metabolism and causing the deposition of sphingomyelin and cholesterol in the endothelial, mesenchymal, and parenchymal cells of all body organs. Six varieties are described. Types A, B, and F have detectable deficiency of sphingomyelinase and storage of sphingomyelin. In types C, D, and E, the sphingomyelinase activity is normal or only mildly reduced. The features of the different types of the disease are summarized in Chart S–13. All are characterized by the presence of Niemann-Pick cells in the bone marrow and a greater or lesser deficiency of sphingomyelinase.

Chart S–13. Summary of the Sphingomyelin
Storage Disorders

I. *Type A. Classical infantile Niemann-Pick disease, acute neuropathic form* A familial condition marked by sphingomyelin storage in the viscera and nervous system, and clinically manifesting mental and motor deterioration beginning in the first year of life, with seizures, hypotonia, and later hypertonia, gait disturbance, Mongoloid facies, emaciation, hepatosplenomegaly, and sometimes a cherry-red macular spot with visual failure.[4134] This form is the most common. It occurs mainly in Jewish infants and is marked by the accumulation of foamy cells throughout the reticuloendothelial system, heart, spleen, and liver, and the deposition of sphingomyelin, gangliosides, and cholesterol in the CNS, leading to demyelination, gliosis, and atrophy.

II. *Type B. Juvenile, non-neuropathic* or chronic *visceral format* A form in which there is visceral involvement only; neurological abnormalities have only been described in adults.[1525]

III. *Type C. Juvenile chronic neuropathic form* (downgaze paralysis–ataxia–foam cell syndrome; juvenile dystonic lipidosis; supranuclear vertical gaze palsy with sea-blue histiocytosis; neurovisceral storage disease with vertical supranuclear ophthalmoplegia) The phenotype originally described, this chronic form is recessively inherited and occurs in late infancy with neurological involvement (vertical supranuclear ophthalmoplegia and disorders of other saccadic movements; and variable mental and motor retardation, seizures, rigidity, ataxia, and dementia). The presence of foamy storage cells (sea-blue histiocytes) in the bone marrow, the occurrence of sphingomyelin storage in the spleen, and the presence of sphingomyelinase are also notable. Three phenotypes are described:

1. An early-onset, rapidly progressive form with severe hepatic dysfunction and psychomotor delay in infancy, and with the later development of vertical gaze pareses, peripheral neuropathy, ataxia, spasticity, and dementia.[3257]

2. A delayed-onset form with a slower course, characterized by mild intellectual impairment in childhood, vertical gaze pareses, ataxia and variable dementia, seizures, and extrapyramidal defects. See **dystonic juvenile lipidosis.**

3. A late (adult-onset) slowly progressive form otherwise resembling the last.[1824] It may present as a schizophrenia-like psychosis, but dementia, ataxia, dysarthria, and gaze palsies later appear.[5008] This form is also known as type F.

IV. *Type D. Nova Scotia variant* A late-onset, slowly progressive form affecting only families of Acadian extraction from the southwest part of that Canadian province. Clinical features are macular degeneration, hypotonia, gait disturbance, early jaundice, and sphingomyelin storage in the spleen. The hepatic involvement is more severe[1185] but otherwise the differences from type C are minimal.

V. *Type E. Chronic Niemann-Pick disease with neurological involvement* In this form, dementia and peripheral sensorimotor neuropathy are the leading features. It resembles the infantile form in its onset and features but the juvenile form in its course, when it affects the nervous system at all.

VI. *Type F.* The adult form of type C.

L. Pick (1868–1935) was a German pathologist working in Berlin who re-described Niemann's patients in fuller detail, and referred to the disease with both of their names attached.[4439]

sphingomyelinase An enzyme responsible for breaking down sphingomyelin, absent in some **sphingomyelin storage disorders** such as **Niemann-Pick disease.**

sphingosine The base of the sphingolipids, so named by Johann Ludwig **Thudichum** (1829–1901) who left his native Germany when he was 25 years old and who eventually became director of chemistry at St. Thomas' Hospital, London.

Because the substance remained insoluble in ether, and in commemoration of the many enigmas that it presented, he chose a name derived from that of the sphinx, another enigma (although that word comes from the Greek term for *squeeze* or *strangle*).[1940]

spiegelschrigft See **mirror writing.**

Spielmeyer, Walther (1879–1935) German neuropsychiatrist who graduated from Halle and trained in psychiatry and pathology. In 1905 he reported the variant of **neuronal ceroid lipofuscinosis** to which his name is attached, and he produced a book on cerebral histology during this period of his training. In 1912 he succeeded **Alzheimer** as professor at Munich at the invitation of **Kraepelin** and continued his work, which now included studies of the peripheral nervous system. He concluded his professional career as director of the Kaiser Wilhelm Institute, though in some danger of displacement on account of his antipathy to the Nazi régime.[1829]

Spielmeyer-Sjögren disease See **neuronal ceroid lipofuscinosis.**

Spielmeyer-Stock disease See **neuronal ceroid lipofuscinosis.**

Spielmeyer-Vogt disease See **neuronal ceroid lipofuscinosis.**

Spielmeyer-Vogt-Sjögren syndrome See **neuronal ceroid lipofuscinosis.**

spike 1. In cellular neurophysiology, a short-lived (usually 1–3 msec), all-or-none change in membrane potential that arises when a graded response passes a threshold.

2. The electrical record of a nerve impulse or similar event in muscle or elsewhere.

3. In clinical EEG recordings, a wave with a duration of less than 80 msec (usually 15–80 msec).[146] Its main component is generally negative relative to other areas and its amplitude is variable. EEG spikes should be differentiated from **sharp waves,** i.e., transients having similar characteristics but longer durations, but this distinction is largely arbitrary and serves primarily descriptive purposes. In practical terms, spikes occupy 2 mm or less of paper width and sharp waves more than 2 mm in ink-written EEG records taken at 3 cm/sec.

Such spikes are associated with clinical seizures states. They should be held in clear contradistinction to the brief unit spikes recorded from single cells with microelectrode techniques. (From Chatrian GE, Bergamini L, Dondey M, et al. A glossary of terms most commonly used by clinical electroencephalographers. *EEG Clin Neurophysiol* 1974;**37**:538–48, with permission from Elsevier Science.)

spike-and-slow-wave complex   An EEG pattern consisting of a spike regularly followed by a slow wave.

spike–wave stupor   See **status epilepticus, twilight state, absence status.**

Spillane syndrome   See **neuralgic amyotrophy.**

Spiller syndrome   (epidural ascending spinal paralysis) A syndrome resembling transverse myelitis, but resulting from thrombophlebitis of the meningeal veins in the presence of pachymeningitis, and leading to cord compression, pain in the back and chest, and the motor and sensory deficits of acute (ischemic) myelopathy.[5285] See **hypertrophic spinal meningitis.**

Spiller, William Gibson   (1863–1940) American neurologist, pathologist, and psychiatrist who trained at the University of Pennsylvania and then in Europe with **Déjèrine, Gowers,** and **Edinger.** After his return to the United States he became professor of neuropathology and later head of the Department of Neurology at the University of Pennsylvania and held senior academic appointments in that city until his retirement in 1932. He edited the *Journal of Nervous and Mental Diseases* from 1902 to 1913. His publications were mainly on the topics of brainstem vascular diseases, extraocular movements, facial pain and weakness, and on **Spiller syndrome,** which he described in 1911.

spina   (Lat, a thorn).

spina bifida   Nonfusion of the laminas of the spinal arches. When the fusion defect is yet more severe, **meningocele** or **meningomyelocele** results.

Spina bifida occulta is the term for nonfusion of the arches without any clinical manifestations unless a dermoid cyst or lipoma is also present, or if there is **diastematomyelia.** *Spina bifida manifesta* indicates the presence of some neurological or local evidence of disease.

The disorder was described and named by the Dutch physician Dr. Nicholas **Tulp** in his *Medical Observations* (1641), although he is better remembered as being the inspiration for Rembrandt's picture "The Anatomy Lesson of Dr. Tulp."

Spina Bifida Association of America   A charitable association in this field. Address: 4590 MacArthur Blvd., NW. Ste. 250, Washington, DC 20007. Tel: 202–944–3285 or 1–800–621–3141. Web site: http://www.sbaa.org.

Spina Bifida/Hydrocephalus Association of Canada   A charitable organization providing support and information on this condition. Address: #977–167 Lombard Ave., Winnipeg, Manitoba R3B OV3, Canada. Tel: 204–925–3650, 1–800–565–9488. Web site: http://www.sbhac.ca/.

spinal adductor reflex   See **spinaoadductor reflex.**

spinal adhesive arachnoiditis   See **spinal arachnoiditis.**

spinal and bulbar muscle atrophy   See **bulbospinal neuronopathy.**

spinal angioma   An arteriovenous malformation involving the spinal cord, where it causes a slowly progressive myelopathy due to local ischemia, the angioma acting as a shunt. See **subacute necrotizing myelitis.**

spinal arachnoid cyst   See **arachnoid diverticula.**

spinal arachnoiditis   (chronic spinal meningitis, adhesive spinal arachnoiditis, meningitis serosa circumscripta spinalis, spinal adhesive arachnoiditis) A rare condition of localized or generalized scarring of the leptomeninges. The condition usually follows meningeal infection, lumbar disk disease, spinal surgery, or repeated lumbar punctures performed for the administration of intrathecal drugs or for diagnostic purposes.

Bilateral sciatic pain, clinical evidence of multilevel radiculopathy, and paraparesis are the more common presentations.[5104]

spinal arachnoiditis ossificans   A rare form of arachnoiditis in which bone is deposited within the inflamed arachnoid membrane. Clinically, the condition may remain asymptomatic or may cause spinal cord or optic nerve compression.[6010]

spinal block   Obstruction to the flow of CSF beside the spinal cord as a result of occlusion of the subarachnoid space by a lesion within the cord (*intramedullary* or *intrinsic*), outside the cord but within the dura mater (*intradural*), or outside the dura mater (*extradural*). See **Froin syndrome.**

spinal cholesterolosis   A myelopathic syndrome resulting from heavy deposits of cholesterol within the spinal canal.[5705] See **Thiébaut syndrome.**

Spinal Cord.   The official Journal of the *International Spinal Cord Society* published by Nature Publishing Group. Web site: http://www.naturesj.com/sc/index.html.

spinal cord gliomas   Primary malignancies of the spinal cord, including pilocytic and diffuse fibrillary astrocytomas and ependymomas.[2539]

Spinal Cord Society   A charitable organization providing support and information on this subject. Address: 19051 County Highway 1, Fergus Falls, MN 56537. Tel: 218–739–5252. Web site: http://www.users.aol.com/scsweb.

Spinal Cord/Spinal Injuries Society of Canada   A charitable organization providing support and information on this condition. Address: 37 Wenonah Drive Mississauga, Ontario L5G 3W4 Canada. (905) 271-0589. See also **National Spinal Cord Injury Hotline.**

spinal dural arteriovenous fistula   The most common vascular anomaly affecting the spinal cord, causing slowly progressive myelopathy as a result of impaired venous drainage. See also **Foix-Alajouanine syndrome.**

spinal dysraphism   Congenital defects in closure of the neural tube.

spinal epidermoid tumor   A benign tumor resulting from the implantation of superficial tissue into the spinal canal during prior lumbar puncture. Local and radicular pain and radiculopathic signs are the usual clinical features.[2105]

spinal epidural abscess   (pachymeningitis externa) Pyogenic infection in the epidural space as a result of hematogenous spread or direct local extension from an adjacent infection, such as vertebral osteomyelitis.[4623] Clinically, the usual picture consists of the progression of back and radicular pain to weakness and paraparesis. The most common infecting organism is *Staphylococcus*.

spinal epidural hematoma   Extravasation of venous blood into the epidural space, usually in low cervical or thoracolumbar areas and most often associated with local arteriovenous malformations or malignancy, or with coagulopathies in adults or birth injury in neonates.

The clinical effect is usually acute myelopathy, which must be handled as an emergency if cord function is not to be lost permanently. MRI is the diagnostic procedure of choice.

Subacute or chronic presentations with evidence of cord compression may also occur.[3293]

spinal epidural lipomatosis   An increase in the amount of epidural fat in lumbar or thoracic regions, occurring in Cushing's disease, in patients treated with steroids for a prolonged period, and occasionally without a known cause as a form of **lipoma.** Clinically, gradually progressive paraparesis, back pain and radiculopathy are the usual syndromes resulting.[2923]

spinal evoked potential   Electrical waveforms of biological origin recorded over the sacral, lumbar, thoracic, or cervical spine in response to electric stimulation or physiological activation of peripheral sensory fibers.[146] See **somatosensory evoked potential.**

spinal monomelic amyotrophy   See **monomelic amyotrophy.**

spinal muscular atrophy   (SMA) A group of heterogeneous conditions with the common factor of damage to the anterior horn cells of the spinal cord and/or the bulbar nuclei, leading to denervation of muscles in variable distributions.

Those SMAs with a genetic basis are classified under the **hereditary motor neuropathies.** Acquired forms may have an acute onset (acute anterior **poliomyelitis,** *Coxsackie,* other enterovirus infections) or may be chronic (**amyotrophic lateral sclerosis,** anterior horn cell disease in the spinocerebellar degenerations, **Creutzfeldt-Jakob disease, Huntington disease, parkinsonism,** Shy-Drager syndrome [**multiple system atrophy**], Joseph disease, and with remote neoplasms as a **paraneoplastic syndrome).**

spinal muscular atrophy, optic atrophy with deafness   See **hereditary motor neuropathy** (*variants*).

spinal muscular atrophy, Ryukyuan type   See **hereditary motor neuropathy** (*variants*).

spinal muscular atrophy with calf hypertrophy   See **hereditary motor neuropathy** (*variants*).

spinal muscular atrophy with deafness   See **hereditary motor neuropathy** (*variants*).

spinal muscular atrophy with mental retardation   See **hereditary motor neuropathy** (*variants*).

spinal muscular atrophy with microcephaly and mental retardation   See **hereditary motor neuropathy.**

spinal muscular atrophy with myoclonus   See **hereditary motor neuropathy** (*variants*).

spinal muscular atrophy with oculopharyngeal muscular atrophy   See **hereditary motor neuropathy** (*variants*).

spinal muscular atrophy with ophthalmoplegia   See **hereditary motor neuropathy** (*variants*).

spinal muscular atrophy with pallidonigral degeneration   See **hereditary motor neuropathy** (*variants*).

spinal muscular atrophy with retinitis pigmentosa   See **hereditary motor neuropathy** (*variants*).

spinal muscular atrophy, with retinitis pigmentosa and hereditary spastic paraplegia   See **hereditary motor neuropathy** (*variants*).

spinal myoclonus   (focal myoclonus) Sudden, involuntary, near-rhythmic focal muscle jerks of the arms or legs, usually at about 1 Hz, occurring during rest in the awake state and during sleep and anesthesia, without an accompanying EEG abnormality and not precipitated by sensory or motor stimuli. Their electrical origin is in the spinal cord at sites of ischemic damage, myelitis, degenerative or traumatic cord lesions, or tumors.[2648] See **segmental myoclonus.**

spinal nerve   That portion of the nerve fiber pathway issuing from the spinal cord which lies outside the intradural space.

spinal nerve root   That portion of the nerve fiber pathway which issues from the spinal cord and which is still within the extramedullary, intradural space.

spinal neuritis   See **radiculitis.**

spinal schistosomiasis   A myelopathy or radiculopathy resulting from granulomatous involvement of the spine and underlying dura mater, usually with *Schistosoma mansoni* or *haematobium*.[582]

spinal shock   A condition lasting days or weeks during which the severely traumatized spinal cord conducts no impulses, consequent upon the sudden withdrawal of the normal tonic excitation playing down upon it from higher levels.

The phenomenon was first noted by Robert **Whytt,** but was so named by Marshall **Hall.**

spinal stenosis   A syndrome of compression of the spinal nerve roots, usually at lumbar levels and as a result of soft tissue intrusion or disc prolapse into a congenitally narrow spinal canal with reduction in its caliber. Degenerative osteophyte formation, spondylosis, or spondylolisthesis, and developmental abnormalities such as achondroplasia are other causes.

Low back pain, poorly localized referred pain on exercise (**neurogenic claudication**), paresthesias, a flexed posture, weakness (footdrop or waddling gait), and areflexia in lumbar and sacral segments on exercise, relieved by rest, are the leading clinical features.

The *central* type often presents as drop attacks, back pain, and pain in the shins with prolonged standing or walking. At night, the patient may experience cold or rubbery legs, and neurological deficits may appear with exercise.

In *lateral spinal stenosis*, the patient complains of radicular pain provoked by exercise, but the usual signs of root irritation are absent.

spinal subdural hematoma   Extravasation of blood into the subdural space of the spine, usually as a result of birth injury in the newborn or of other trauma in older subjects. Clinically, radicular pain and local tenderness, often with evidence of myelopathy, are the major features.

spinal xanthomatosis   A variant of cerebrotendinous xanthomatosis manifesting a slowly progressive, chronic myelopathy. MRI demonstrates white matter abnormalities in the lateral and dorsal columns of the spinal cord.[5756]

spindle   A group of rhythmic waves on the EEG, characterized by a progressively increasing then gradually decreasing amplitude. See also **sleep spindles.**

spindle coma   The occurrence of physiological patterns of non–rapid eye movement sleep such as sleep spindles, vertex sharp waves, K complexes, and background theta and delta activity on the EEG following CNS trauma, or metabolic, infectious, or hypoxic problems.[2817] Spindle coma may represent a combination of true sleep and coma, the latter accounting for the failure of arousal attributed to impairment of the activating ascending reticular formation. The causative lesion is in the hypothalamic or upper mesencephalic regions. In post-traumatic cases, the prognosis for recovery may be good, but in nontraumatic cases, it is significantly worse.[2428] The presence of spindles, vertex waves, and K complexes indicates relative integrity of the cerebral hemispheres.[1375]

spindle vertigo   That state of fearfulness and "dizziness" reflecting a distortion of muscle sense and seen particularly in the aged in association with a loss of 1A afferent fiber (proprioceptive) activity or with of age-related changes in the intramuscular nerve terminals.

spindles   Groups of encapsulated special muscle fibers within somatic muscles with the function of assessing the rate and force of stretch as a result of the contraction of surrounding muscle, and thus modulating the strength of further muscle contraction. Two forms are described, according to their shape, as resembling either a *bag* or a *chain.*

spin-lattice relaxation time   (T1, longitudinal relaxation time) The characteristic time constant for spins to achieve an equilibrium alignment within an applied magnetic field.[779,6028]

spinoadductor reflex   (Tschlenow reflex, spinal adductor reflex) Bilateral contraction of the adductors of the leg in response to the vibration set up by a tap over the spine. It is said to be present in normal subjects but increased in the setting of pyramidal disease.

This reflex is the corollary of the **scapulohumeral reflex** in the upper limb and has the same slight importance.

spinobulbar muscular atrophy   See **bulbospinal neuronopathy** (Kennedy disease).

spinocerebellar ataxia and pupillary paralysis   See **cerebellar ataxias** (*variants*).

spinocerebellar ataxia with dementia and plaque-like deposits   See **Gerstmann-Straussler-Scheinker syndrome.**

spinocerebellar ataxias   See **cerebellar ataxias**   A heterogeneous group of neurodegenerative disorders characterized by features of degeneration in the brainstem, cerebellum, and spinal cord.

spinocerebellar degeneration with motor system involvement.   See **cerebellar ataxias** (*variants*).

spinocerebellar degenerations   A group of progressive diseases characterized clinically by disturbances in the coordination of movement, or ataxia, and pathologically by degeneration of those afferent and efferent neuronal systems upon which the smooth and efficient regulation of movement depends.[2270] See **cerebellar ataxias** (*variants*).

spino-olivocerebellar degeneration and ophthalmoplegia   See **cerebellar ataxias** (*variants*).

spinopontine atrophy   A dominantly inherited, progressive ataxic syndrome characterized by the onset in youth or young adult life of optic atrophy; dementia; cerebellar, pyramidal, and posterior column signs; and myoclonus.

It may be classified with the progressive late-onset **cerebellar ataxias** of unknown cause until the underlying biochemical defect is ascertained.[647] See also **Joseph disease.**

spinoscopy   A method of assessing spinal movements using a high-resolution television camera that records the varying relative positions of markers placed on a subject's back during forward and lateral flexion, allowing the estimation of movement at the facet joints and at the intervertebral disk spaces. Despite the pretentious name, the operator does not look at (and even less so into) the spine by this method.

spinothalamic system   (anterolateral system) One of two somatosensory systems (the other is the posterior or **lemniscal**), comprising the ascending fiber pathway, which arises from the dorsal root cells concerned with the conduction of impulses subserving the sensations of pain, heat, and cold as well as sexual sensation, although the system also contains a number of lemniscal fibers. Its fibers terminate in the reticular activating system, in the intralaminar and centromedian thalamic nuclei, and in the ventrobasal thalamic complex.

The system is characterized by wide receptive fields, lack of modality specificity, and slow adaptation. It was first described by **Edinger** but more fully by **Brown-Séquard.**

spin-spin relaxation time   (T2, transverse relaxation time) The characteristic time constant for loss of phase coherence among spins oriented at an angle to the static magnetic field, due to interactions between the spins, with resulting decay of the transverse magnetization and MRI signal. Starting from a finite value, the transverse magnetization will decay so that it loses 63% of its initial value in time (T2).[779,6028]

spiral nerve bands of Fontana   Zig-zag or spiraling lines most easily visible on the surface of nerves, using oblique lighting; the optical expression of the arrangement of nerve fibers in the nerve.[1047]

splenium   The posterior third of the corpus callosum.

split brain   The condition resulting from the severance of the neocortical commissures, leading to the inability to exchange information between the hemispheres and to the existence of two independent cognitive systems within the same brain. The right hemisphere thus appears to have some function in the processing of language.

The retention of abilities related to calculation, spatial orientation, and lexical decision making support the view that the brainstem is implicated in the transfer of some cognitive processing.[5069]

split hand syndrome   Preferential denervation of the thenar muscles and the first dorsal interosseus as opposed to the hypothenar muscles, recorded in some cases of **amyotrophic lateral sclerosis** and with distal ulnar lesions. The name was applied because of the involvement mainly of the muscles on the lateral side of the hand,[5967] such as the thenar muscles and the FDI.

split notochord syndrome   See **diastematomyelia.**

spondyl-   (Gr, a vertebra) Prefix denoting vertebral.

spondylalgia   Pain in the spine.

spondylitis   (Gr, a vertebra + inflammation) Inflammatory disease of the vertebrae.

spondylolisthesis   (Gr, a vertebra + a slippage) The name given by Killian in 1852 to the forward slippage of one vertebra upon the one below (usually L4 on L5, but in his case, L5 on S1), either due to a defect in the isthmus of the pars interarticularis (*true spondylolisthesis*) or to degeneration of the disk and facet joints (*degenerative spondylolisthesis*).

Lumbar spinal stenosis is a possible result, but in many cases, its occurrence causes no symptoms.[1974]

spondylolysis   A defect in the pars interarticularis of the vertebra, and thus a cause of **spondylolisthesis.**

spondylopathy   Any disease of the vertebra.

spondylosis   A degenerative hypertrophy of the ligamentous, bony, and articular structures of the spinal column which occurs with aging. The unwanted effects of this may include compression of the emerging nerve roots and possibly of the spinal cord itself.

spongiform encephalopathies   A group of slowly progressive, transmissible cerebral diseases affecting humans and animals, with the shared characteristic of cortical spongy change, neuronal loss, an accumulation of **prion** protein, and gliosis. They include **Creutzfeldt-Jakob disease, scrapie, kuru, fatal familial insomnia,** and **Gerstmann-Straussler-Scheinker syndrome.**[5977]

spongiform encephalopathy with white matter changes   See **Creutzfeld-Jakob disease,** of which this is a *variant.*

spongioblast   (Gr, a sponge + a germ) A cell of ectodermal origin which is the precursor of glial cells.

spongioblastoma polare   (polar spongioblastoma) A malignant but relatively slowly growing cerebral tumor composed of primitive spongioblasts, occurring mainly in the cerebellum, brainstem, and optic chiasm.[3011] See also **primitive neuroectodermal tumors.**

spongy degeneration   The histological appearance of brain tissue that contains round, empty spaces separated by bands of more or less intact neural tissue. The agonal production of CO_2 from glycogen reservoirs just after the cessation of blood flow has been suggested as the cause.[1763]

Such an appearance is also seen in many other metabolic, degenerative, and infectious conditions. See **Canavan leukodystrophy.**

spongy degeneration of infancy   See **Canavan leukodystrophy.**

spongy glioneuronal dystrophy   A familial degenerative disorder of the nervous system of unknown cause, marked by spongy change in the thalamus, dentate nucleus, and cortex with sparing of white matter. The disease closely resembles **Alpers disease.**

Clinical characteristics are the onset between the ages of 1 and 5 years of intellectual failure, seizures, myoclonus, involuntary movements, cerebellar signs, blindness, deafness, and eventual decerebration and death.[2650,2832] See **glioneuronal dystrophies.**

spontaneous activity   Electrical activity recorded from muscle or nerve at rest after insertion activity has subsided and when there is no voluntary contraction or external stimulus. Compare with **involuntary** (**EMG**) **activity.**

spontaneous corneomandibular reflex   See **palpebromandibular synkinesia.**

spontaneous intracranial hypotension   (primary or **idiopathic intracranial hypotension,** aliquorrhoea) A syndrome of postural frontal and cervical headache relieved by recumbency; low CSF pressure; and often other features such as nausea, vomiting, vertigo, tinnitus, altered auditory acuity, photophobia, neck stiffness, diplopia due to sixth cranial nerve palsy, and bradycardia.

The syndrome results from a persistent leak of CSF (usually from the spinal axis) through a meningeal defect, as after lumbar puncture. The problem may rarely be complicated by subdural fluid collections.[1033,4585] Diagnosis is best made by MRI, which typically shows dural enhancement, or by isotope cisternography.

spontaneous nystagmus   Those forms of nystagmus that occur without provocation, as, for example, those elicited by **optokinetic** stimuli.

spontaneous periodic hypothermia   A rare disturbance of thermoregulation leading to severe sweating and persistently low body temperatures, usually arising in patients with other evidence of hypothalamic damage. The condition has been considered to represent a form of diencephalic epilepsy.[1926]

spoon test   Variable resistance is normally felt when a soup spoon is drawn across the skin, but the resistance is smooth and unopposed when the spoon crosses (anhidrotic) areas of sympathetic denervation.[5655]

sporadic degenerative visceral neuropathy   Alteration in bowel function due to damage to the myenteric plexus of the colon in association with inflammatory conditions and paraneoplastic disorders.[6006]

sporadic juvenile amyotrophic lateral sclerosis   See **amyotrophic lateral sclerosis** (*variants*).

sporadic myoclonic encephalopathy   See **opsoclonus-myoclonus syndrome, Ohtahara syndrome.**

sporadic olivopontocerebellar degeneration   See **cerebellar ataxias** (autosomal dominant, late-onset forms).[1346]

sporadic progressive thalamic atrophy   The rare occurrence of isolated atrophy of any of the thalamic nu-

clei without other neurological disorders, such as **Wernicke-Korsakoff syndrome, cerebellar ataxias,** or distant carcinoma. Abulia and dementia are the clinical accompaniments reported, but the very existence of the syndrome as an entity is unproved. See also **multisystem atrophies.**

sporadic spongiform encephalopathies with myoclonus   See **Creutzfeldt-Jakob disease.**

Spranger syndrome   See **rhizomelic chondrodysplasia punctata.**

spread of comitance   The reduction in the degree of primary and secondary deviation of the eyes in a patient with strabismus, as a function of time.

spreading depression of Leao   Marked, enduring reduction in the electrical activity of the cortex (of rabbits) following an excitation wave produced by weak faradic or mechanical stimulation of the exposed cerebrum, associated with markedly increased blood flow in the surface arterioles and veins, and followed by increased fast activity on the EEG.[3308]

Sprengel deformity   A sporadic or dominantly inherited syndrome resulting from maldevelopment occurring during embryogenesis, in which the scapulas fail to migrate to their usual position. Scapular elevation, rotation, and winging result.

The condition was first described by Dr. O.G.K. Sprengel (1852–1915), a German surgeon.

springende pupille   See **springing pupil.**

springing pupil   (seesaw anisocoria, mydriasis à bascule, springende pupille) A term variously employed, but generally taken to indicate the presence of periodic alternating dilation of the pupils of unknown cause (*type 1*), but often in a pupil affected by long-standing **Horner syndrome.** In *type 2*, unilateral iris paresis (as in **Adie syndrome**) leads to the appearance of unilateral pupillary dilation during accommodation and in bright light conditions. *Type 3* is synonymous with **cyclic oculomotor spasm.**[2388]

springlike phenomenon   See **rebound.**

sprouting   The growth of new nerve fibers (neurites) in large numbers from the proximal end of a cut nerve in the process of repair.

sprung back   The condition of rupture or stretching of the supra- and interspinous ligaments, usually at low lumbar levels, associated with both aging and prolapse of intervertebral disks. Whether the problem is a cause or an effect has yet to be determined.[4117]

sprung pupil   See **Riegel symptom.**

spurious diabetes   See **diabetes insipidus.**

spurious hydrocephalus   See **Hall syndrome.**

Spurling sign   1. Accentuation of the pain felt during **straight-leg raising** elicited by dorsiflexion of the ankle or the hallux, thus causing slight further traction on the sciatic nerve. This sign represents a combination of the signs of **Sicard** and of **Bragard.** 2. Pain in the shoulder or arm occurring with lateral flexion of the neck to that side; a sign of acute (or of severe chronic) cervical disk herniation.

Spurway syndrome   See **Apert syndrome.**

Spurzheim, Johann Caspar (1776–1832) French physician and iconoblast. He forsook the study of theology for that of medicine in order to become a student (and a highly partial proponent of the theories) of F.J. **Gall,** with whom he presented a major treatise on the anatomy of the brain to the *Institut de France* in 1808, and produced between 1810 and 1819 a superb four-volume text on the anatomy and physiology of the nervous system and of the brain, containing accounts of many new and definitive dissections. He lectured on **phrenology** on both sides of the Atlantic, but his enthusiastic and uncritical claims for that discipline (quite unlike the reserved and scholarly productions of **Gall** himself) could not be substantiated, and he thus accelerated the rejection of Gall's theories. Spurzheim withdrew from participation in the writing of Gall's major work after 4 years of labor because of disagreements between them.[5280]

sputtering positive potentials   Small, irregular, positive potentials resembling nerve potentials, recorded on EMG in normal distal muscles. They are artifactual and have no clinical significance.[4440]

square window   The angle between the hypothenar eminence and the plane of the forearm, made when the infant's wrist is passively flexed to the maximal extent, normally up against the forearm. Less acute angles suggest prematurity.

The same maneuver can be applied at the ankle, and scored according to the key provided in Dubowitz's test procedure.[1527]

square-wave jerks   (square-wave oscillations, gegenrucke, hopping nystagmus, lightning eye movements, ocular myoclonus, saccadic intrusions, saccadic oscillations, zickzakbewegungen) Involuntary, 0.5° to 3° conjugate horizontal saccades occurring at 1–4 Hz, moving the eyes away from a point of fixation for 200 msec and followed after about 200 msec by a corrective saccadic return to the original fixation position, these cycles occurring at about 2 Hz.[1287]

The term is applied because of the rectangular waveform of the tracing of eye movements. They occur sometimes in normal subjects with the eyes closed, but more usually and obviously in patients with **progressive supranuclear palsy** or with cerebellar disease whose eyes are open. See also **macro–square-wave jerks.**[23]

square-wave oscillations   See **square-wave jerks.**

square-wave pulses   (kippdeviationen, kippnystagmus, pendular macro-oscillations, saccadic nystagmus, saccadic oscillations, saccadic intrusions) See **macro–square-wave jerks.**

squat-jump myoglobinuria   The occurrence of myoglobinuria following this provocative exercise as a result of excessive or unaccustomed use of the leg muscles.

squint   (Old Engl, to escape or avoid) Lack of parallelism of the ocular axes so that the eyes look in different directions. See **strabismus.**

squint syndrome of Braun   See **Swan syndrome.**

SREDA   See **Subclinical Rhythmic Excitatory Discharges of Adults;** an orphan EEG phenomenon.

SSEP   See **short-latency somatosensory evoked potential.**

S-shaped lid   The appearance of the upper lid in patients with a neurofibroma in its outer part which droops as a result, while the inner half remains in its usual position.

SSS   See **small sharp spikes.**

stable stroke   A form of stroke in which there is little change in the deficit over a specified period of time.[4141]

Staehli pigment line   A crescent of brown pigment in the lower central quadrant of the cornea found in some elderly patients, in the region where the arcus senilis usually begins.

staircase phenomenon   The progressive increase in the force of a muscle contraction in response to continued low rates of direct or indirect muscle stimulation.[146]

This phenomenon may be produced by the increasingly efficient mobilization of acetylcholine quanta from the nerve terminals during muscular activity over a finite period.

stammering   Abnormal speech in which the flow of words is interrupted by hesitations, during which the muscles of articulation function in the absence of laryngeal speech sounds. See also **stuttering.**

stamping gait   The gait of a subject with **sensory ataxia,** which is markedly worse in dark places and on rough ground. The hips and knees are flexed to an unusual extent, and the regularity and precision with which they are brought down again to the ground are both impaired.

standard electrode placement   The EEG electrode location(s) on the scalp determined by the **ten-twenty system.**

Stanford Sleepiness scale   A long and complicated instrument for assessing and rating sleepiness.[2597]

Stanford-Binet tests   A test battery modifying and expanding upon the original intelligence scales developed in France by Alfred **Binet.**

Stanley syndrome   (proctalgia fugax) (Gr, anus + pain + fleeting) A benign but uncomfortable condition of severe intermittent attacks of rectal pain, said to be common in elderly, myopic lexicophiles and caused by remaining in the sedentary position for long periods (J. Stanley, cited by Jablonski[2764]).

stapedius myokymia   Repetitive contractions of the stapedius muscle for reasons unknown, causing tinnitus.

stapedius reflex   Bilateral reflex contraction of the stapedius muscles with sound stimulation of one ear, this contraction measurably altering the acoustical impedance of the middle ear.

stapedius reflexometry   Measurement of the contractions of the stapedius muscle by means of an electroacoustic impedance bridge, the threshold and decay of the reflex allowing estimation of the degree or weakness and fatigability of the muscle, as in **myasthenia gravis.**

star walking   Subjects with mild left vestibular disease who walk sets of three paces forward and three back with the eyes closed will angle their course anticlockwise, and those with right-sided disease will veer clockwise (provided, of course, that they do not fall down in the meantime).[730] See also **stepping test.**

stare nystagmus   See **look nystagmus.**

Stargardt, K.B.   (1875–1927) German ophthalmologist who graduated from Kiel and trained further both there and at Strasbourg and Bonn. He succeeded **Bielschowsky** as professor and director of the eye clinic at Marburg.

Stargardt syndrome   (familial juvenile macular degeneration) A recessively inherited syndrome of insidious deterioration of vision first detectable in infancy, leading eventually to total blindness. Bilateral macular pigmentation is the earliest sign, followed by the appearance of coalescing yellow retinal spots and pigmentary retinal degeneration of the outer layers of the retina.[5319]

Stark-Kaiser syndrome   See **scapuloperoneal syndromes.**

startle   A basic alerting reaction seen in all mammals, consisting in humans of a stereotyped facial grimace, flexion of the head, trunk, elbows, and knees; and elevation of the shoulders in response to sudden stimuli, but diminishing somewhat with the repetition of such stimuli. The reflex is enhanced by tension, fatigue, and the expectation of the causal stimulus.[167,661]

Though a normal motor pattern, it may become excessive, in which case the disease is known as **hyper-**

ekplexia, or **jumping** or **startle epilepsy,** and it may be a precipitant of myoclonus or other seizures.[165]

The disorders named **latah** in Malaysia, **myriatchit,** *ikota,* or *amurakh* in Siberia, and *ainu imu* elsewhere in Asia, *jauns* in Burmah, *bah-tsche* in Thailand, *mali mali* or *silok* in the Philippines, *panic* in Lapland, and the Bantu or southwest African disorder are also considered by some to represent the same condition.

startle disease   See **startle epilepsy.**

startle disorder   See **hyperekplexia.**

startle epilepsy   (startle disease) An unusual form of reflex epilepsy in which the seizures are precipitated by sudden, unexpected stimuli, and comprise an abrupt startle response followed by a phase of tonic posturing involving the paretic side, or by a generalized seizure.[3589] They are poorly responsive to antiepileptic drugs.

The condition may also complicate the **Lennox-Gastaut syndrome,** perinatal anoxic encephalopathy, porencephaly, Down syndrome, or other known cerebral disorders. It was first described by Gowers in 1881.[2239,4873]

In a dominantly inherited *familial* form (**hyperekplexia,** congenital stiff-man syndrome, hereditary stiff-baby syndrome), the responsible gene is located on chromosome 5q.

startle reflex   Flexion of the arms in response to a sudden loud noise, normally present in babies up to 3 months of age.[798]

startle-induced seizures   A syndrome seen in some children with brain damage of any kind, comprising brief motor seizures characterized by sudden flexion of the neck, trunk, and limbs, elicited by visual, auditory, or proprioceptive stimuli, and followed by tonic flexion of the arm and extension of the leg on the hemiparetic side. Consciousness is minimally affected.

The EEG shows a muscle artifact corresponding to the seizure, followed by temporary suppression of activity. The attacks lessen with increasing age.[56]

startle-induced tics   The occurrence of tics with this precipitant as part of Tourette syndrome of late onset.[5585]

start-stop-start phenomenon   A pattern of electrographic activity in which the abnormal activity representing an electrographic seizure appears for a few seconds, disappears, and then recurs, usually from the same site.[613]

stasi-basophobia   Immobility in the standing position due to a pathological fear of walking,[5286] usually in association with severe bilateral frontal cortical disease.

static embryopathy   A pathological state occurring during fetal life, caused by viral infections in utero, and leading to developmental abnormalities of the brain which do not progress after birth. Cytomegalovirus, varicella, and rubella viruses are the best-known causative agents.

static encephalopathy (nonprogressive encephalopathy) A chronic, nonprogressive, genetic or developmental brain disorder resulting from lesions of the brain sustained before, during, or after birth. The clinical features are essentially those of **cerebral palsy,** with intellectual functions and motor development most affected. Basal ganglion calcification and dystonia are also common findings.

static perimetry (profile perimetry) That form of perimetry in which the contrast of a stimulus at given points in the visual field is gradually increased up to the threshold of perception. The technique is of particular value in the quantitative assessment of retinal sensitivity.[1636] See also **kinetic perimetry.**

The test is most accurately performed with the aid of a computerized program that monitors fixation and provides false-negative and false-positive scores, in which the target is of fixed size and is illuminated at different points programmed by the computer with variable and increasing intensity.

static positional nystagmus A form of nystagmus that persists during the maintenance of a particular position of the head, of no localizing value, though seen most often in the context of peripheral vestibular disease. Positional alcohol nystagmus is an example.

static reflex spasms See **saltatory spasm.**

static reflexes Those reflexes which employ the extensor muscles of the limbs in the maintenance of posture, their origin being in the mesencephalon. They are best expressed in decerebrate preparations and are lost in spinal animals (Sir Charles **Sherrington**).

static seizures See **myoclonic astatic seizures.**

static tremor See **cerebellar tremors.**

stationary night-blindness A familial syndrome, variably inherited, and characterized by an inability to see at night as a result of absent secondary rod or cone adaptation. The fundi are normal.

Vision is unaffected in the dominantly inherited form, but it is abnormal in the recessively inherited and X-linked varieties (in part due to myopia).[917]

statognosia The appreciation of the position of a limb in space.

statokinetic dissociation A difference in visual sensitivity for moving targets compared with that for stationary targets. In the presence of optic atrophy, dissociation is increasingly marked, the subject having a higher sensitivity for moving targets.[5891]

status dissociatus A severe form of **REM sleep behavior disorder** in which elements of REM and NREM sleep are mixed together, the sleep interrupted by dreaming, twitching, and vocalizations. Alcohol withdrawal, narcolepsy, and brainstem diseases have been associated.[4955]

status dysmyelinatus A congenital disorder of the lenticular nuclei characterized by loss of neurons and myelinated fibers, leading to athetosis in childhood and additional severe rigidity later. This may be the underlying mechanism of **juvenile paralysis agitans.**

The condition was described by the **Vogts** in 1919–1920, but the pathogenesis is still uncertain. See **double athetosis.**

status epilepticus 1. Any seizure state lasting longer than half an hour; *or* a single epileptic seizure >30 minutes in duration or a series of epileptic seizures during which function is not regained between ictal events in a >30-minute period.[1115]

2. Recurrent seizures that occur without an intervening period of conscious awareness.

3. An epileptic seizure that is sufficiently prolonged, or repeated at sufficiently brief intervals, so as to produce an unvarying and enduring epileptic condition.

Operationally, the simplest definition is "any seizure state which is not self-limiting." Generalized status may be convulsive (tonic/clonic/myoclonic) or nonconvulsive (absence). Partial status may comprise simple (somatomotor, aphasic) or complex partial seizures.[56] The various forms of status have been classified by Gastaut[2052] and these are summarized in Chart S–14.

See also **serial seizures.**

Chart S–14. Classification of Status Epilepticus

Convulsive tonic-clonic and clonic status are the more common forms, in which the seizure type is as indicated by the name. *Tonic status* is less common but very prolonged; it is usually seen in children with **Lennox-Gastaut syndrome.**

Myoclonic status is rare, and consists of the unremitting repetition of massive myoclonic jerks with retained consciousness, unless it is accompanied by generalized tonic-clonic or absence attacks.

Partial convulsive status is the persistence of convulsive activity within a restricted area on one side of the body.

Generalized nonconvulsive status epilepticus (absence status, petit mal status, minor epileptic status, spike–wave stupor, epilepsia minoris continua, epileptic twilight state) is characterized by some degree of clouding of mental processes, accompanied by bilateral spike–wave discharges on the EEG.

Partial nonconvulsive status epilepticus may present as recurrent typical complex partial seizures without normalization of mental activity between seizures; or as prolonged continuous episodes of mental confusion and behavioral disturbance, with or without automatisms.[56]

*Adapted from Gastaut H. Classification of status epilepticus. Adv Neurol 1983;**34:**75.*

status hemiparalyticus See **hemiparetic seizures.**

status marmoratus (Lat, state + marble) A pathological appearance of the basal ganglia in patients with hypoxic-ischemic cerebral injury (asphyxia neonatorum), characterized by irregular and excessive myelination of these structures, producing a marbled appearance. Clinically, this is associated with the later development of dystonia, chorea, spastic quadriparesis, and mental retardation. See **double athetosis, état marbré.**

status migrainosus   Attack of migraine in which the headache phase lasts more than 72 hours, despite treatment. Headache-free intervals of less than 4 hours (sleep not included) may occur. This definition and the following diagnostic criteria are suggested by the International Headache Society[1051] (Classification of headache disorders, cranial neuralgias and facial pains; and diagnostic criteria for primary headache disorders. *Cephalalgia* 1988;**8**[suppl]:1–96, by kind permission of Blackwell Science.)

A. The patient fulfills criteria for migraine with or without aura.

B. The present attack fulfills criteria for one form of migraine except that headache lasts more than 72 hours whether treated or not.

C. Headache is continuous throughout the attack, or interrupted by headache-free intervals lasting less than 4 hours. Interruption during sleep is disregarded.

For practical purposes, this is a disabling headache of the migraine type, lasting for over 72 hours, refractory to the usual analgesics and requiring hospitalization or repeated visits to the emergency room.

Steele-Richardson-Olszewski syndrome   (heterogeneous system degeneration) A dementing illness with the added features of impairment of vertical gaze, especially downwards; parkinsonism; dystonic axial rigidity; and variable corticospinal and cerebellar signs. See **progressive supranuclear palsy.** The condition was described by these Canadian physicians in 1964.[5328]

steely hair disease   See **Menkes syndrome.**

Steinbrocker disease   (shoulder-hand syndrome) See **reflex sympathetic dystrophy.**

Steinert disease   (Steinert-Batten-Curschmann disease) See **myotonic dystrophy.**

Steinert, Hans   German physician who practiced in Leipzig and whose description of **myotonic dystrophy** was published in 1909.

Steinert-Batten-Curschmann disease   See **myotonic dystrophy.**

Steinfeld syndrome   (holoprosencephaly and limb defects) A congenital dysmorphic syndrome characterized also by optic atrophy, seizures, microcephaly, and holoprosencephaly or arhinencephaly with skeletal and visceral maldevelopments.[337]

Stellwag, Karl   (1823–1904) Austrian ophthalmologist.

Stellwag sign   Infrequent and incomplete blinking, with retraction of the upper eyelid and resultant widening of the palpebral fissure seen in **dysthyroid ophthalmopathy,** but also noted in **Parkinson disease.**

Stengel syndrome   The association of constructional apraxia, loss of spatial orientation, and all four features of **Gerstmann syndrome.**[5332]

stenosis   (from Gr, to make narrow) The pathological narrowing of a hollow viscus or bony conduit.

Stephens syndrome   A familial syndrome characterized by the combination of **chronic progressive external ophthalmoplegia,** cerebellar ataxia, and peripheral neuropathy resembling **hereditary motor and sensory neuropathy, type 2.**[5334]

stepless saccades   See **saccadic pulses.**

steppage gait   The gait of subjects with drop foot on one or both sides, who are aware that in order to prevent their feet catching on obstacles or irregularities on the ground, each must be lifted higher than is normal before being brought down again in front of them.

stepping response   (walking reflex) When the held infant is lowered so that the feet touch the table, the infant makes stepping movements.[6064] The response normally appears after at least 34 weeks gestation and disappears by 6 months of age.

stepping test   The subject is asked to take 60 steps in place with the eyes closed and the arms held parallel to the ground. In the presence of unilateral vestibular disease, the subject tends to rotate more than 45° toward the affected side. With bilateral lesions, the tendency is to move forward or backward. See also **star walking.**

stereoanesthesia   Lack of recognition of the shape or form of objects handled, due to lesions of the contralateral parietal lobe or of the ascending sensory pathways in the spinal cord.

stereognosis   Three-dimensional tactile feeling; the ability to perceive objects in three dimensions or in a spatial relationship within a depth of field. In the visual form, this requires sight in each eye; in the tactile forms, this requires normal parietal lobe function. In each case the peripheral pathway is assumed to be functioning normally.

stereomorphometry   Measurement of the distance between neuronal cell bodies in three dimensions.

stereopsis   The ability to discriminate depth (i.e., three-dimensional perception) as a result of binocular vision, a function dependent upon normal activity in both cerebral hemispheres.

stereotactic (stereotaxic) depth electroencephalogram   (SDEEG) A recording of the electrical activity of the brain by means of electrodes implanted within the brain substance according to stereotactic measurements. (From Chatrian GE, Bergamini L, Dondey M, et al. A glossary of terms most commonly used by clinical electroencephalographers. *EEG Clin Neurophysiol* 1974;**37**:538–48,[989] with permission from Elsevier Science.)

stereotypy   An involuntary, patterned, repetitive, continuous, coordinated, purposeless or ritualistic movement, posture, or utterance (recurring utterances, verbal automatism, monophasia, formula speech).

Stereotypy may be simple, as exemplified by repetitive tongue protrusions or body-rocking movements, or complex, such as self-caressing, crossing and uncrossing of the legs, marching in place, and pacing.[5308]

Sterling reflex   The **Rossolimo reflex** applied to the fingers.[5336]

Sterling sign   Adduction of the normal shoulder against resistance, accompanied by involuntary adduction of the opposite shoulder, indicating the presence of a pyramidal tract lesion affecting the latter side.

Sterling-Flatau progressive torsion spasm   An alternate name for primary torsion **dystonia.**

Sternberg-Cushing-Oppenheim syndrome   See **Oppenheim disease.**

Sternberg-Oppenheim syndrome   See **Oppenheim disease.**

Stern-Garcin syndrome   A rapidly progressive dementing illness without focal cortical symptoms, first described by Dr. K. Stern in a 41-year-old patient admitted to the **National Hospital** under Dr. F.M.R. Walshe (and by Raymond Garcin in 1962) as "severe dementia associated with bilateral symmetrical degeneration of the thalamus," although the temporal and parietal cortices were gliotic and showed neuronal loss. Garcin hinted that this may be the same condition as **Creutzfeld-Jakob disease,** but Stern rejected that possibility.[3783,5341] See **familial myoclonic dementia.**

sternomastoid reflex   Contraction of this muscle in response to a tap on its tendon at its insertion into the clavicle. The reflex is diminished in the presence of lesions of C3, 4 and augmented with pyramidal tract lesions above that level.

sternospinal reference   A noncephalic reference achieved by interconnecting two electrodes, one placed over the right sternoclavicular junction and the other over the spine of the seventh cervical vertebra, the voltage between them being balanced by means of a potentiometer in order to reduce ECG artifact. (Adapted from the 1974 report of the Committee on Terminology, IFCN. In: Chatrian GE, Bergamini L, Dondey M, et al. A glossary of terms most commonly used by clinical electroencephalographers. *EEG Clin Neurophysiol* 1974;**37**:538–548.[989])

sternotomy-related brachial plexopathy   A lower trunk brachial plexopathy in which the ulnar sensory and motor amplitudes are the most affected responses.

The predominant damage is in C8 distribution, suggesting that the focus of the lesion is localized at the level of the anterior primary rami of the cervical roots rather than in the lower trunk of the brachial plexus.[3372]

sternutation convulsiva   See **sneezing.**

sternutatory reflex   See **nasal reflex.**

steroid myopathy   A syndrome of proximal muscle weakness and wasting preferentially affecting the legs. Type 2 fiber atrophy is the characteristic pattern on muscle biopsy. Plasma creatine kinase activity is at the lower end of the normal range. A myopathic electromyogram and a raised 24-hour urinary 3-methylhistidine/creatinine ratio on a creatine-free diet are also typical findings.[3029]

steroid-responsive myositis   See **dropped head syndrome.**

steroid-responsive recurrent polyneuropathy   See **chronic inflammatory demyelinating polyneuropathy.**

stethoscope loudness imbalance test   A bedside test of stapedial muscle function. A strongly activated tuning fork placed close to the bell of a stethoscope worn by the subject with seventh cranial nerve palsy affecting the nerve to stapedius leads to a louder sound on the side of stapedius paresis. Quieter vibrations are not so lateralized.[3523]

stethoscope neuropathy   Compression of the greater auricular nerves by the metal arms of a stethoscope held in a resting position on the neck.

Clinically, this presents with a sensation of increased warmth, numbness, burning, and paresthesias bilaterally along the posterior service of the auricle and lobule of the ears and over the retroauricular mastoid areas in the distribution of the nerves.[4622]

Stewart, J.P.   (1869–1949) English neurologist.

Stewart-Holmes syndrome   See **Jackson cerebellar fits.**[5357]

Stewart-Morel-Morgagni syndrome   A benign condition of increased thickness of the skull in the frontal regions, with which no neurological features are clearly associated. See **hyperostosis frontalis interna.**

Stickler syndrome   (hereditary arthro-ophthalmopathy) A dominantly inherited congenital syndrome characterized by conductive and sensorineural deafness, cataract, detached retina, skeletal deformities including platyspondyly, and mental and developmental delay.[5359]

stick-man dystrophy   A slowly progressive nonspecific myopathy with onset in early childhood, characterized by marked wasting of the limb muscles with retention of a surprising degree of power, and by contractures. See also **Emery-Dreifuss syndrome, congenital muscular dystrophy.**

stick-man syndrome   See **congenital muscular dystrophy.**

stiff-baby syndrome   (hereditary startle syndrome) A rare, dominantly inherited, congenital disease characterized by muscle stiffness, maximal at birth and tapering slowly during childhood.[3420] See **startle epilepsy.**

stiff-leg syndrome   A syndrome of adults manifest as symmetric stiffness and spasms of the legs induced by voluntary movements and reflex stimuli. The remainder of the nervous system is normal.[799]

stiff-man syndrome   (Moersch-Woltman syndrome, stiff-person syndrome, progressive muscular rigidity) A rare syndrome with onset in adult life of persistent, progressive, painful rigidity with powerful muscular spasms of spinal origin, mainly affecting the axial and pelvic girdle muscles and inducing hyperlordosis. The spasms are triggered by stretching, emotion, and sensory stimuli. The cause is considered to be diminution of activity in a spinal descending inhibitory pathway as a result of an (autoimmune?) attack on glutamic acid decarboxylase, a precursor of GABA.

The spasms, which may be strong enough to break underlying bones, may be evoked by many exteroceptive stimuli and are at first intermittent but later become more or less continuous. They are worsened by any attempt at active or passive movement or by noise, but diminish in sleep. The EMG shows a pattern resembling normal maximal contractions. The spasms may be reduced by high doses of diazepam, curare, baclofen, or sodium valproate.[3930] Associated disorders described include seizures, diabetes mellitus, type 1, breast or lung cancer, thymoma, and other immune disorders such as thyroiditis, pernicious anemia, myasthenia gravis, and ovarian or adrenal failure. Sudden death may occur due to cardiac arrhythmias or restrictive respiratory arrest. For further analysis, see http://www.wustl.edu/neuromuscular.

EMG findings are of continuous action potentials indistinguishable from voluntary activity with superimposed brief bursts of 5–6 Hz rhythmic synchronous activity.

Separation into three categories has been suggested. In the first two the course is slow and the manifestations either distal (stiff-limb syndrome) or axial stiff trunk (man) syndrome. In the last, the course is rapidly progressive to death within months (progressive encephalomyelitis with rigidity).[351]

Variants include the *jerking stiff-man syndrome,* in which it is myoclonic jerks that are triggered by such stimulation; *congenital stiff-man syndrome;*[4897] *stiff-man syndrome with tremor;*[1463] and an association with thymoma and myasthenia gravis. See also **stiff-baby syndrome, startle epilepsy.**

Focal lesions of the spinal cord may imitate this constellation of clinical features.[797]

stiff-person syndrome   See **stiff-man syndrome.**

stiff-skin–lipoma syndrome   A familial congenital syndrome characterized by generalized hirsutism, lipomas, conjunctivitis, scleroderma-like stiffness of the skin, digital flexion contractures, dental abnormalities, stomach ulcers, renal stones, arthropathy, strabismus, deafness, bulbar weakness, and loss of pain sensation.[1707]

stigmatic electrode   The term of **Sherrington** for the **active,** or exploring, electrode.

Stiller disease   (asthenia universalis congenita) An ill-defined entity comprising constitutional visceroptosis, neurasthenia, and vasomotor instability.

Stilling, Benedict   (1810–1879) German anatomist and surgeon who described the solitary bundle and tract in the medulla in 1843 and who demonstrated the innervation of the walls of blood vessels. He published detailed accounts of the anatomy of the spinal cord, medulla, and pons, data which he acquired from his use of serial sections in three dimensions, using the microtome which he had introduced in 1824.

Employing this technique, he described and differentiated almost all the cranial nerve nuclei recognized today. On the clinical side, he described various surgical procedures, but also wrote on psychosomatic symptoms, which he considered to be due to spinal cord irritation.

Stilling, Jakob   (1842–1915) German ophthalmologist who graduated from Marburg and trained further in Paris, Berlin, and Vienna, returning to practice ophthalmology in Strasbourg for most of his career.

Stilling syndrome   (ocular retraction syndrome) See **Duane syndrome.**

Stilling-Turk-Duane syndrome   A syndrome of complete or partial failure of abduction; partial or complete adduction with retraction of the affected eye into the socket when it is adducted; an oblique movement of the eye up and in or down and in when it is adducted; and deficiency of convergence. See **Duane syndrome.**

The account by Duane[1522] is complete, but was published 18 years after Stilling's original definition of the condition, which he acknowledged.

Stimmler syndrome   (alaninuria-microcephaly-dwarfism-diabetes) A congenital dysmorphic syndrome characterized also by short stature, dental abnormalities, diabetes, aminoaciduria, ataxia, microcephaly, and mental and developmental delay.[337]

stimulant-dependent sleep disorder   A disorder characterized by a reduction of sleepiness or suppression of sleep caused by central stimulants and resultant alterations in wakefulness following drug abstinence.[234]

stimulating electrode   Device used to deliver electric current. All electric stimulation requires two electrodes; the negative terminal is termed the *cathode,* and the positive terminal is the *anode.* By convention, the stimulating electrodes are called *bipolar* if they are encased or attached together and are called *monopolar* if they are not. Electric stimulation for nerve conduction studies generally requires application of the cathode in the vicinity of the neural tissue to produce depolarization. (From the 2001 Report of the Nomenclature Committee of the American Association of Electromyography and Electrodiagnosis.[10] Used by permission, copyright © 2001, AAEM.)

stimulation   single fiber electromyography (stimulation SFEMG) Use of electrical stimulation instead of voluntary activation of motor units for the analysis of single fiber electromyography. The method is used in patients who are unable to produce a steady voluntary muscle contraction. The stimulation can be delivered to intramuscular axons, nerve trunks, or muscle fibers. (From the 2001 Report of the Nomenclature Committee of the American Association of Electromyography and Electrodiagnosis.[1] Used by permission, copyright © 2001, AAEM.)

stimulation-produced analgesia   Lack of pain discrimination produced by stimulation of the ventrolateral periaqueductal gray matter of the midbrain.

stimulus   (Lat, goad) Any external agent, state, or change that is capable of influencing the activity of a cell, tissue, or organism. In clinical nerve conduction studies, an electric stimulus is applied to a nerve. It may be described in absolute terms or with respect to the evoked potential of the nerve or muscle. In absolute terms, it is defined by a duration (msec), a waveform (square, exponential, linear, etc.), and a strength or intensity measured in voltage (V) or current (mA). With respect to the evoked potential, the stimulus may be graded as subthreshold, threshold, submaximal, maximal, or supramaximal. A threshold stimulus is one just sufficient to produce a detectable response. Stimuli less than the threshold stimulus are termed *subthreshold*. The maximal stimulus is the stimulus intensity after which a further increase in intensity causes no increase in the amplitude of the evoked potential. Stimuli of intensity below this level but above threshold are submaximal. Stimuli of intensity greater than the maximal stimulus are termed *supramaximal*. Ordinarily, supramaximal stimuli are used for nerve conduction studies. By convention, an electric stimulus of approximately 20% greater voltage/current than required for the maximal stimulus is used for supramaximal stimulation. The frequency, number, and duration of a series of stimuli should be specified. (From the 2001 Report of the Nomenclature Committee of the American Association of Electromyography and Electrodiagnosis.[10] Used by permission, copyright © 2001, AAEM.)

stimulus-sensitive epilepsies   (reflex epilepsies) Seizures that are regularly and reproducibly evoked or facilitated by specific motor, sensory, or psychic stimuli. Visual stimuli are the most common of these. See also **photoconvulsive response.**

More complex stimuli occasionally provoking seizures include music, hot water, eating, and thinking. Thus, *language-induced epilepsy* is that form in which seizures are induced by reading, writing, or speaking.[56]

stimulus-sensitive myoclonus   (reflex myoclonus) Myoclonus, often of the action or intention variety, which appears abruptly when a voluntary movement is initiated or during its performance. Such movements are often those requiring precision for their proper accomplishment.

stinger   The term of football players for the direct trauma causing upper trunk brachial plexopathy.

Stingle syndrome   The association of loss of spatial orientation with the major features of **Gerstmann syndrome.**[5360a]

Stocker sign   The patient in typhoidal delirium fumbles with and tends to turn down or push away the bedclothes. In the presence of tuberculous meningitis, the patient is said to try to replace them.[4723]

Stock-Speilmeyer-Vogt disease   See **neuronal ceroid lipofuscinosis.**

Stokes, William   (1804–1878) Irish physician who practiced in Dublin. His description of syncopal attacks in association with a permanently slow pulse[5363] led to the attachment of his name to the syndrome, although **Spens** in Edinburgh had described the same thing 50 years before. See **Adams-Stokes-Morgagni syndrome.**

Stokes-Adams syndrome   See **Adams-Stokes-Morgagni syndrome.**

stop   See **voiceless bilabial.**

Storandt battery   A screening instrument comprising a group of tests for intellectual impairment including some taken from other scales. The battery consists of two trailmaking tests, the Wechsler logical memory test, and a test of mental control, but is under revision.

Stormorken syndrome   A dominantly inherited syndrome characterized by dyslexia, ichthyosis, short stature, migraine-like headache, photophobia, extreme miosis, impaired upward gaze, muscle fatigue, distal myopathic weakness, slow relaxation of muscle, absence of the spleen, thrombocytopathia, and red cell abnormalities.[5372]

strabismic amblyopia   Visual failure in one eye due to an abnormality in neuronal maturation as a consequence of lack of use of the eye for fixation in early development. The usual reason for the neglect of the eye is muscular imbalance—a **strabismus.**

strabismus   (from Gr, a squinting) Lack of parallelism of the ocular axes caused by the incoordinate action or developmental malposition of the extraocular muscles.

The name was given by the Alexandrians to the geographer Strabo, who was so afflicted. See also **diplopia, ductions, phoria, tropia, vergence, versions.**

Strachan syndrome (Strachan-Scott disease, Jamaican neuritis) A nutritional neuropathy resembling **pellagra,** manifest as the combination of amblyopia due to optic neuritis, painful areflexic sensorimotor neuropathy with sensory ataxia, hearing loss, and orogenital dermatitis.

The syndrome was originally described in the residents of Jamaica[5376] in 1897 but occurs in malnourished people with low levels of riboflavin regardless of where they live. The epidemic neuropathy found in Cuba today may reflect the result of malnourishment occasioned by the economic embargo placed on that country.

See also **Cuban optic neuropathy.**

Strachan, William Henry Williams (1857–1921) English physician, attached to the British West Indian garrison in Jamaica in the late nineteenth century.

Strachan-Scott disease See **Strachan syndrome.**

straight-leg raising A maneuver described by **Lasègue** in which the extended leg is passively flexed at the hip, thereby pulling on the sciatic nerve. Normally this is painless, but with meningeal irritation or root compression, pain is felt in the low back and in the back of the leg when the flexion reaches 60°, and spasm of the hip extensors occurs to prevent further flexion.[3306]

straight-thumb sign Inability to flex the terminal joint of the thumb when making a grasping movement. This is seen in the presence of anterior interosseous palsy, and is due to weakness of the flexor pollicis longus.[1000] See also **Froment sign.**

Stransky nystagmus See **arthrokinetic-induced nystagmus.**

Stransky sign An alternative method of eliciting the **Babinski response,** whereby the little toe is pulled laterally and suddenly released. Its value is in its diminished tendency to cause withdrawal of the foot. See also **Allen reflex.**

Stransky syndrome A congenital dysmorphic syndrome characterized by short stature, aminoaciduria, renal tubular acidosis, osteoporosis, distal myopathy, and mental and developmental delay.[337]

strategic-infarct dementia Persistent cognitive impairment occurring as a result of a single left-sided cerebral infarct. This has been described following an acute syndrome of confusion, abulia, fluctuating alertness, inattention, memory disturbance, and psychomotor retardation, due to a small infarct in the lowest part of the genu of the internal capsule, causing thalamocortical disconnection.[5497]

strategy application disorder The inability to plan and execute complex tasks, requiring articulation of goals, specification of plans, self-monitoring, and the evaluation of outcomes. This disorder may reflect uni- or bilateral frontal lobe lesions.[5089]

strength testing See **functional muscle tests.**

strength–duration curve Graphic presentation of the relationship between the intensity (Y axis) and various durations (X axis) of the threshold electric stimulus of a nerve or muscle. The rheobase is the intensity of an electric current of infinite duration necessary to produce a minimal action potential. The chronaxie is the time required for an electric current twice the rheobase to elicit the first visible action potential. Measurement of the strength–duration curve is not a common practice in modem electrodiagnostic medicine. (From the 2001 Report of the Nomenclature Committee of the American Association of Electromyography and Electrodiagnosis.[10] Used by permission, copyright © 2001, AAEM.)

strephosymbolia (Gr, turn + symbol) The occurrence of reversals of single letters such as "P" and "Q"; or of words (e.g., *ten* and *net*), as seen in patients with **dyslexia.**

stress 1. Any condition which poses a potential threat to the comfort or integrity of an organism or its constituents. 2. Accentuation of a spoken syllable.

stress convulsions Epileptic attacks in subjects without previous unprovoked seizures who have been exposed to stresses in the period immediately preceding the attack. Such stresses include lack of sleep, physical exhaustion, and emotional stress. The EEG is unhelpful in diagnosis or prognosis, and the incidence of epilepsy at follow-up is little higher than the rate in normal subjects.[1961]

stress headache See **episodic tension-type headache.**

stretch reflex The reflex contraction of a muscle following sudden stretch, as by a tap on its tendon. The first physiological explanation was supplied by Sir Charles **Sherrington** in 1927.

The reflex is produced by passive lengthening of a muscle. The principal sensory stimuli come from group la and group II muscle spindle afferents. It consists of several phases. The earliest component is monosynaptic and is also called the **myotatic reflex,** or **tendon reflex.** There are also long-latency stretch reflexes. See also **muscle stretch reflex, T wave.** (From the 2001 Report of the Nomenclature Committee of the American Association of Electromyography and Electrodiagnosis.[10] Used by permission, copyright © 2001, AAEM.)

stria (Lat, a furrow) A stripe or line, both elevated (ridges) and depressed lines (furrows) being so named.

stria terminalis A fiber pathway carrying impulses from the amygdala to the medial hypothalamic nuclei.

striatal foot   See **dystonic foot response.**

striatal hemiplegia   An uncommon syndrome of athetosis proceeding to a fixed dystonic hemiplegia and resulting from lesions of the putamen and caudate nucleus.[1394]

striatal necrosis   A syndrome with congenital or early childhood onset, characterized by cerebral atrophy with pyramidal and extrapyramidal signs, seizures, apathy, depression, and mental and developmental delay. See also **Hallervorden-Spatz disease, infantile bilateral striatal necrosis, Wilson disease, Leigh disease, cerebral palsy.** A similar syndrome may complicate wasp-stings.

striate cortex   That area of cortex at the occipital pole, forming the banks of the calcarine fissure in which the striae Gennarii are visible, and which receives input from the entire retina, relayed through the lateral geniculate bodies.

striate pseudobulbar palsy   The state in which multiple lacunar infarcts lead to severe weakness of the bulbar muscles—in the opinion of **Wartenberg** it is sufficient to cause virtual anarthria.[574]

striatocapsular infarction   A stroke syndrome in the territory of the lateral striate arteries, infarcting the head of the caudate and the anterior limb of the internal capsule and due to complete or partial occlusion of the proximal part of the middle cerebral artery.

The usual clinical presentation is with arm weakness accompanied by such cortical signs as dysphasia, neglect, or dyspraxia.[1491]

striatonigral degeneration   (striopallidonigral degeneration) A rare, sporadic, degenerative, akinetic-rigid syndrome of adult life, involving primarily the putamen and substantia nigra and leading to the clinical syndrome of parkinsonism, with marked and progressive bradykinesia, rigidity, apathy or depression, and urinary incontinence. Pyramidal and cerebellar signs are often detectable.[37,5716]

The clinical features suggested as most indicative of the diagnosis include the occurrence of unexplained falls, autonomic dysfunction, absence of rest tremor, and poor response to L-dopa treatment.[1754] See also **multisystem atrophies.**

In a *variant* form, the condition is dominantly inherited.[4794,4795]

striatopallidal calcification   (Fahr syndrome, idiopathic familial intracerebral arterial calcification, symmetrical cerebral calcification, dominant basal ganglion calcification, brain ferrocalcinosis) A rare heterogeneous group of conditions in which, bilaterally, the capillaries of the basal ganglia, dentate nucleus, and deeper cortical layers are affected by nonarteriosclerotic calcification of the vessels. The condition was first described in 1850; the later contribution of Fahr has been belittled and the eponym is no longer used.

Clinically, the condition may be asymptomatic, or it may be associated with any combination of dementia, seizures, evidence of raised intracranial pressure, and pyramidal, cerebellar and extrapyramidal syndromes, including parkinsonism, dystonia, or solitary tremor in young or middle adult life,[1734] coupled with evidence of parathyroid disturbance in the endocrine cases. Both dominantly and recessively inherited familial varieties, often with added ataxia and pigmentary retinal degeneration,[5380] are also delineated and have been reviewed by Baraitser.[335]

Idiopathic, pseudo-, and pseudo-pseudohypoparathyroidism are present in most sporadic cases, but the mineral deposition (not always calcium) may also be seen in various other neurological or metabolic diseases such as **Cockayne syndrome, Down syndrome, AIDS, Hallervorden-Spatz disease, mitochondrial myopathy, Aicardi syndrome, Kearns-Sayre syndrome,** and **osteopetrosis.**[1639,3494,4015]

Variant forms are given in Chart S–15.

Chart S–15.   Variants of Striopallidal Calcification

Basal ganglion calcification, mental retardation, and steatorrhea A recessively inherited syndrome characterized by these features.[1065]

Basal ganglion calcification with hypoparathyroidism A recessively inherited syndrome characterized by these features.[4000]

Familial basal ganglion calcification with neurological features A dominantly inherited syndrome of dense symmetrical calcification in the basal ganglia, with ataxia, spasticity, and mental deterioration and without evidence of pseudo- or pseudo-pseudohypoparathyroidism or evidence of infectious, toxic, or metabolic disease; and with normal serum calcium and phosphate levels and a renal tubular response to parathyroid hormone.[1901,4015]

Familial basal ganglion calcification with pseudo-hypoparathyroidism A dominantly inherited syndrome in which the endocrine features are accompanied by calcium deposition in the lenticular nuclei.[4127]

Familial calcifications of the brain, iron storage, and porphyria A condition in which calcifications are accompanied by deficient serum iron transport, hemochromatosis, and porphyria.[405]

Familial encephalopathy and basal ganglion calcification A recessively inherited congenital syndrome of microcephaly, seizures, spasticity, dystonia, abnormal eye movements, and lymphocytosis in the CSF.[61]

Idiopathic familial calcification of the basal ganglia A recessively inherited syndrome of dense basal ganglion, occipital lobe, and dentate nucleus calcification with (variously) parkinsonism in middle life, dementia, spasticity, contractures, and athetosis, ataxia, or dystonia.[335]

Striatopallidal calcification with ataxia A rare variant, also manifesting pigmentary retinopathy, described by Strobos et al.[5380]

striatum   The caudate, putamen, and globus pallidus. This group of structures is called this because of their striped appearance in fresh sections, as a result of the layers of fibers crossing the internal capsule to connect the caudate and putamen.

string sign   An extended region of almost, but not quite, total occlusion of a major artery, seen on angiograms in patients with dissection of the carotid artery in the neck.

striatocapsular infarcts   Small infarcts of the caudate, anterior of limb of internal capsule, or the putamen resulting from middle cerebral artery occlusion embolus, atheroma, arteritis, dissection, etc. and causing hemiparesis with neuropsychological dysfunction and arm weakness greater than that in the face or leg. Cortical signs may be minimal or absent. CT/MRI shows comma-shaped signals in the striatum.

striopallidodentate calcification   The appearance of diffuse metallic signals from the basal ganglia. The causes include hypoparathyroidism and pseudohypoparathyroidism, familial striopallidodentate calcification,[5380] and infantile or familial cases associated with microcephaly, pigmentary macular degeneration, and progeria. The appearances of iron deposition resemble those of calcium on CT scans. In another *variant* syndrome, leukodystrophy and parenchymal brain cysts are associated.[3214]

Clinical features include seizures, EEG abnormalities, mental deterioration, signs of Parkinson disease, pyramidal signs, and endocrinological symptoms.[3494]

See also **mitochondrial myopathies, Urbach-Weithe disease, lipomembranous polycystic osteodysplasia.**

striothalamic hand   See **thalamic hand.**

Strohl, André   (b. 1887) French physician who studied in Paris, where he was later elected professor of physical medicine. Most of his work was on the circulatory system, electrophysiology, and respiratory functions. He was, with Guillain and Barré, an author of the classic description of **acute inflammatory demyelinating polyneuropathy.**

Stroke   A professional journal of the American Heart Association, publishing reports on clinical and basic investigation of any aspect of the cerebral circulation and its diseases. Address: American Heart Association, 7272 Greenville Avenue, Dallas TX 75231–4596. The journal does not follow the Vancouver style for references. Web site: http://stroke.ahajournals.org/.

stroke   (cerebrovascular disease)   A neurological deficit secondary to cerebral arterial or venous disease. This is a generic term for all neurovascular syndromes, whether due to infarction, hemorrhage, or subarachnoid hemorrhage.[4141]

Classifications of stroke have been suggested;[2355,4080] The scheme of Prof. Hachinski is reproduced in Chart S–16.

Chart S–16. Classification of Stroke

A. Presumed stroke
   Presumed TIA
   Other
B. Anatomical classification
   By axial location:
      Supratentorial
         Lobar (specify)
         Centrencephalic (specify)
      Infratentorial
         Cerebellar (specify)
         Brainstem (specify)
   By vascular territory:
      Carotid (specify)
      Vertebrobasilar (specify)
C. Etiological classification
   By result
   Cerebral infarct:
      Arterial
      Arteriolar (lacunar)
      Venous
   Cerebral hemorrhage:
      Intraparenchymal
      Subarachnoid
      By cause
   Ischemia:
      Extracranial vascular disease
      Embolism
      Other
   Hemorrhage:
      Hypertension
      Amyloid angiopathy
      Vascular malformation
      Other
D. Management classification
   TIA and minor stroke
   Major stroke
   Deteriorating stroke
   Stroke in the young
   Stroke in the elderly

TIA, transient ischemic attack. (From Hachinski VC. Classification of stroke for clinical trials. Stroke 1990;21 suppl. II:II-27–II-29, by permission.)

Stroke Association   http://www.stroke.org.uk/ A charitable organization in the UK.

Stroke Center   A web resource for information about stroke care and research at www.strokecenter.org/. Another excellent web resource is at www.neuro.wustl.edu/stroke/.

stroke databank   A study initiated in 1978 by the National Institute of Neurological and Communicative Disorders and Stroke to amass information from a large number of patients as a data source for clinical research in stroke.[3190]

stroke delirium   An acute confusional state following infarction of the lower division of the middle cerebral artery in the nondominant hemisphere.

stroke scales   Semiquantitative rating scales of the deficits resulting from stroke. Some of those most commonly employed are described more fully in this book (see **Canadian Neurological scale, Mathew scale, Rankin scale, Frenchay Activities Index, Barthel Index of Activities of Daily Living, NIH Stroke Scale**). Van Gijn[5728] has reviewed 41 such scales in an assessment of outcome measures and de Haan has dissected five of them.[1334] See also **disability scales.**

stroke-in-evolution   See **evolving stroke.**

stroke-like episodes and leukoencephalopathy   A dominantly inherited syndrome characterized by the occurrence in mature adulthood of completed subcortical strokes or transient ischemic attacks, migraine-like headaches, and evidence from CT or MRI scanning of widespread white matter disease.[5617] See also **MELAS.**

Stroke-TIA.org   A Web site providing data on cerebrovascular diseases to health professionals, at http://www.stroke-tia.org/stroke-tia/professional.html.

strongyloidiasis   Infection with *Angiostrongylus cantonensis*, a nematode usually acquired from tropical snails, with a tendency to invade all body tissues, including the brain and spinal cord. Clinical neurological signs of infection include headache, meningism, sixth and seventh cranial nerve palsies, and occasionally coma as a result of a chronic granulomatous encephalomyelitis, the response of the nervous system to the presence of the dead nematodes. The CSF shows an eosinophilic pleocytosis.

Stroop Word Color test   A test of perseverance and concentration, based on the fact that normal subjects read a word faster than they name an object or color associated with that word. In the test, subjects first read color words, then name the colors of dots, and finally name the color in which each of 100 words is printed—but these colors do not match the word. Thus the word RED may be printed in green ink, and the correct response is "green").[5384] The test has been used extensively in the identification of simulated (malingering) syndromes. A computerized form is available.

Strümpell disease   1. Acute polioencephalomyelitis; the cerebral form of poliomyelitis, with convulsions and hemiplegia added to the peripheral motor effects of the poliovirus.[5387] 2. See **Erb-Charcot syndrome.** 3. See **cerebral infantile paralysis.**

Strümpell, Ernst Adolf Gustav Gottfried von (1853–1925) Russian physician who studied philosophy, psychology, and the violin before turning to medicine, graduating from Leipzig in 1879 and later succeeding **Erb** as Director of the Medical Clinic at Heidelberg. He was finally elected professor of medicine at Leipzig University in 1910.

Strümpell published extensively on the topics of tabes dorsalis, neuritis, muscular atrophy, **multiple sclerosis,** and traumatic disease, and gave the first description of pure **hereditary spastic paraplegia** in 1880,[5386] completing this in 1886.[5388] He also published a classic study of polioencephalomyelitis and described spastic pseudosclerosis and (ankylosing) spondylitis deformans. The first of the 30 editions of his textbook of medicine was published in 1883, when he was 31.

Ernst Adolf Gustav Gottfried von Strümpell

Strümpell hereditary spastic paraplegia (Strümpell-Lorrain syndrome) See **hereditary spastic paraplegia.**

Strümpell signs   1. Contraction of the tibialis anterior as an associated movement during hip flexion.[5390] See **tibialis phenomenon.** 2. Strong passive flexion of the forearm normally leads to pronation as well but this is increased in the presence of an upper motor neuron lesion. 3. Dorsiflexion of the hallux with leg paresis. (The preceeding three signs were noted in patients with pyramidal disease.) 4. (**radialis sign**) Inability to close the hand without dorsiflexion of the wrist, as seen in both spasticity and tetany. 5. An alternative method of producing the **Babinski response,** whereby the examiner firmly runs his or her finger and thumb down the spine of the tibia.

Strümpell-Liechtenstern disease   See **acute disseminated encephalomyelitis, acute hemorrhagic leukoencephalitis.**

Strümpell-Lorrain disease See **hereditary spastic paraplegia.**

Struthers ligament A band of aponeurotic tissue arising from the humerus and inserted into the medial epicondyle, occasionally compressing the median nerve and producing impairments resembling the **pronator teres syndrome** except for the absence of involvement of that muscle, innervation of which is achieved at a higher level.

Sir John Struthers was an English physician-anatomist.

Stuart syndrome (Stuart-Bergstrom syndrome) A congenital dysmorphic syndrome characterized also by nerve deafness, papilledema, vascular abnormalities of the retina, callosal agenesis, and cutaneous pustules.[5392]

Stuart-Bergstrom syndrome See **Stuart syndrome.**

stuck-in-set perseveration Persistent and inappropriate repetition of a motor task; a sign of frontal lobe or mesolimbic disease.

stump dyskinesia The occurrence of motor sequelae such as chorea, dystonia, repetitive jerking spasms, and tremor in the stump after amputation, frequently associated with pain.[3626]

stump pain A sharp, jabbing pain felt locally in the site of amputation of a limb and worsened by local pressure. A neuroma of the cut nerve endings is held to be responsible.

stump pressure The intraarterial pressure distal to the site of arterial occlusion.

stump spasm (convulsive movements of the stump, painful jumping amputation stumps, trepidation du moignon) Myoclonic or choreic movements of the remaining stump of an amputated limb, not always actually painful. The pathophysiology is unknown.[3186]

stunned brain Brain tissue within the **ischemic penumbra** surrounding a region of infarction, which is not now functioning but which may be expected to do so in time.

stupidity 1. The term of **Willis** for amentia or **dementia;** Failure of the imagination, memory, and judgement [in which] the eye of the intellect is . . . dulled. 2. Inability to share the insights of the observer.

stupor (Lat, insensibility) A state of reduced consciousness in which the subject retains the ability to make limb motor and vocal but not verbal responses to vigorous stimulation; the range of awareness is markedly diminished but not lost, and there is little or no spontaneous activity. On the **Glasgow Coma Scale,** the scores will be 3–5–3.

Sturge, William Allen (1850–1919) English physician, who trained at University College Hospital, Lon-

don, and worked at the **National Hospital,** Queen Square, and in Paris with **Charcot,** returning to a staff position at the Royal Free Hospital. For the sake of his wife's health, he removed to Nice in France, practicing there for nearly 30 years, and only returning to England after his wife's death and his remarriage. His published output was small, papers on **amyotrophic lateral sclerosis** and on the disease bearing his name being those of lasting record.

In 1879, he presented a patient with a port-wine stain and focal motor seizures to a London medical society meeting, suggesting that the seizures were a result of an underlying lesion upon the brain, but he was not believed. Further details of the **Sturge-Weber syndrome** were provided by Parkes Weber in 1925.

Sturge-Kallischer-Weber disease See **Sturge-Weber syndrome.**

Sturge-Weber Foundation An organization which acts as a clearinghouse of information on the disorder for patients and professionals, and which maintains a registry of patients. It is based at; PO Box 418, Mt. Freedom, NJ 07970. Tel: 973–895–4445 or 1–800–627–5482. Web site: http://www.sturge-weber.com./.

Sturge-Weber syndrome (Sturge-Weber-Dimitri syndrome, Crouzon-Crostophy-Gaucher syndrome, neurocutaneous angiomatosis, Cushing-Bailey-Cobb syndrome, cutaneocerebral angioma, encephalofacial or encephalotrigeminal angiomatosis, Parkes-Weber-Dimitri disease, Sturge-Kallischer-Weber disease, Schirmer-Sturge-Weber syndrome, Brushfield, Hebold, Krabbe, Lawford, Luschka, Milles, Jahnki, or Wyatt syndrome; Weber himself called it *Sturge-Kallischer disease*) Venous angiomas of the meninges with overlying dermal angiomas (port-wine stain) in the trigeminal nerve distribution, frequently associated with atrophy of the underlying cortex, hemiparesis, and seizures, described by Sturge in 1879[5396] and by Weber in 1922. Choroidal angiomas may lead to glaucoma and visual loss.

Skull radiographs may show **tramline calcification** in the affected cortical layers; this calcium is also well seen on CT scans. The clinical features of note are the presence of a vascular nevus (port-wine stain) in the territory of the trigeminal nerve, and of capillary and cavernous hemangiomas within the brain, the tendency to suffer recalcitrant seizures, glaucoma, macrocephaly, and mental or developmental delay.

Jablonski[2764] lists 36 separate names for this condition, indicating that either many physicians have rushed into print without adequate familiarity with the literature or the desire to coin Latin neologisms is an addiction of neurologists.

The *variants* of the syndrome have been classified by Francois[1930] and are shown in Chart S–17.

Chart S–17. Classification of Sturge-Weber Syndrome

Complete, Three Signs

Sturge-Weber (with glaucoma)
Jahnki (without glaucoma but with choroidal angioma)

Incomplete

A. *With ocular and cutaneous signs only*
Schirmer (with early glaucoma and buphthalmos)
Lawford (with late glaucoma, not buphthalmos)
Milles (with choroidal angioma)

B. *With two signs, one neurological*
Krabbe (with encephalotrigeminal angioma and bulbospinal symptoms)
Crouzon-Crostophy-Gaucher (with minor CNS signs only)
Cushing-Bailey-Cobb (with cutaneomedullary angiomatosis)
Arieti-Gray (with arterial aneurysms, multiple angiomatosis, mental deficiency, intracranial calcification, and seizures)
van Bogaert–Divry (with corticomeningeal telangiectatic angiomatosis) (infantile meningeal angiomatosis) Λ syndrome comprising seizures, spastic paraplegia or quadriplegia, and associated with an increased incidence of meningioma or sarcoma in the brain.

Other *variant forms* in which there is an association with **von Hippel–Lindau disease, neurofibromatosis,** or **tuberous sclerosis** are noted by Baraitser.[335]

Sturge-Weber-Dimitri syndrome   See **Sturge-Weber syndrome.**

Sturge-Weber Foundation   A charitable organization providing support and information on this condition. Address: P.O. Box 418, Mount Freedom, NJ 70970. Tel: 973–895–4445, 1–800–627–5482 (USA).

stuttering   Involuntary repetition, prolongation, or arrest of sounds in conversational speech. The precise etiology is unknown, but acquired forms may commence in association with traumatic or degenerative brain disease or aphasia and may be transient or persistent. They show no adaptation effect: any syllable of any type of word may be affected; and there is no concurrent abnormal motor activity, but certain visuospatial and alternating motor tasks may be poorly performed by subjects suffering from acquired stuttering.

Aphasic stuttering may be etiologically linked; *stuttering with aphasia* is an emotional reaction to the lesion; and *dysarthric stuttering* occurs during recovery from expressive forms of dysphasia.[2525]

Stuttering Foundation of America   A charitable organization providing support and information on this condition. Address: 3100 Walnut Grove Road, Suite 603, P.O. Box 11749, Memphis, TN 38111-0749. Tel: 901–452–7343, 1–800–992–9392. Web site: http://www.stuttersfa.org/.

stylohyoid process syndrome   See **Eagle syndrome.**

styloradial reflex   See **brachioradialis reflex.**

Suarez-Kelly syndrome   See **dropped head syndrome.**

sub-   (Lat, under, beneath) Prefix denoting beneath.

subacute AIDS encephalitis   See **HIV-associated dementia complex.**

subacute angioendotheliopathy   See **subacute diencephalic angioencephalopathy.**

subacute arteriosclerotic encephalopathy   See **Binswanger disease.**

subacute cerebellar degeneration   See **subacute cortical cerebellar degeneration.**

subacute cerebral degeneration   See **Creutzfeldt-Jakob disease.**

subacute combined degeneration of the cord   (Dana syndrome, posterolateral sclerosis, Putnam-Dana syndrome) Demyelination of the lateral columns and the posterior columns of the spinal cord as a result of deficiency of vitamin B_{12}. In the case of the posterior columns, the demyelination reflects primary damage to the large dorsal root ganglion cells, whose centripetal processes originate there.[4856]

A pyramidal syndrome obscured by hyporeflexia, and diminution or loss of proprioception, discriminative touch, and vibration are the classic findings; they are often accompanied by optic atrophy.[1268]

The condition was described by Lichtheim in 1887. The first clue as to the etiology was found by Minot, who observed improvement in a patient who ate liverwurst on a daily basis.

subacute cortical cerebellar degeneration   (Lichtheim syndrome, subacute cerebellar degeneration) A rare **paraneoplastic syndrome** characterized by the acute or (more usually) subacute development of pancerebellar and brainstem dysfunction, sometimes with evidence of paraneoplastic **subacute motor neuronopathy** and dementia,[711] but usually without other motor or sensory signs. The syndrome is associated with small cell carcinomas of the lung, with ovarian carcinoma, and with Hodgkin disease more commonly than with other malignancies. Progressive incoordination of gait and limb movements bilaterally, dysarthria, nystagmus, and oscillopsia are the major clinical features.

Pathological examination reveals severe loss of the cerebellar Purkinje cells and perhaps lymphocytic infiltration of the meninges. A misdirected immune attack is considered the most likely etiology;[4508] high titers of anti-Hu and/or anti-Yo antibodies are typically detected.

subacute degeneration of the thalamus   See **fatal familial insomnia.**

subacute degenerative polioencephalopathy of the presenium   See **Creutzfeldt-Jakob disease.**

subacute demyelinating polyneuropathy   See **chronic inflammatory demyelinating polyneuropathy.**

subacute diencephalic angioencephalopathy   (subacute angioencephalopathy) A syndrome of progressive impairment of intellect and memory, behavioral disturbances, abnormality in consciousness, apathy or depression, and myoclonus, associated with bilateral destructive lesions of the thalamus due to proliferative inflammatory lesions of the small blood vessels.[1328]

subacute encephalitis   See also   **HIV-associated cognitive/motor complex.**

subacute (brainstem) encephalomyelitis   A slowly progressive syndrome of distal more than proximal stiffness at its onset progressing to lower brainstem involvement manifest as nystagmus and ophthalmoplegia, deafness, blindness, and long tract signs. The CSF contains inflammatory cells. The brainstem and cord pathology is that of inflammation and gliosis.

subacute encephalomyelitis   Acquired inflammatory disease of the brain due to direct viral invasion or to postinfectious autoallergic responses, leading to a slowly progressive deterioration in functions. **Rabies, shingles, polymyoclonia, Reye syndrome,** and **acute cerebellar ataxia** are examples of such disorders.

subacute encephalomyelopathy   See **Leigh disease.**

subacute familial thalamic atrophy   A slowly progressive dementing disease, also characterized by sleep disturbances, and associated with atrophy of the dorsomedial and anterior thalamic nuclei.[2891] See also **Stern-Garcin syndrome.**

subacute idiopathic demyelinating poly(radiculo)-neuropathy   A neuropathic syndrome which clinically and pathologically resembles mild **chronic inflammatory demyelinating polyneuropathy,** but which has a slowly progressive phase lasting 1–3 months,[2697] although "lumpers" would not allow this as an adequate differentiating feature.

subacute inclusion body encephalitis   A form of encephalitis characterized by the presence of type A intranuclear inclusion bodies in the CNS. See **subacute sclerosing panencephalitis.**

subacute motor neuronopathy   A **paraneoplastic syndrome** occurring as a remote effect of Hodgkin disease or of other lymphomas, and manifested as a subacute, painless, progressive lower motor neuron syndrome affecting the legs more than the arms, often asymmetrically. The symptoms may remit if the underlying cause is treated successfully.[4987,5394]

subacute myelo-opticoneuropathy   (SMON, acrodermatitis enteropathica) A central-distal axonopathy induced by the ingestion of clioquinol, in which axonal degeneration is found in the optic nerves, the distal corticospinal tracts, and the gracile columns at the cervicomedullary junction (the distal part of the central extension of the dorsal root ganglion cells).[5397,5650]

Clinical features of note when the disease was extant included painful distal hypoesthesia and paresthesias, hyperreflexia, visual loss, ataxia, signs of autonomic neuropathy, seizures, and abdominal complaints. Also notable was the finding that the tongue and feces were stained green.[5620]

subacute myoclonic spinal neuronitis   See **progressive encephalomyelitis with rigidity.**

subacute necrotizing encephalomyelopathy   See **Leigh disease.**

subacute necrotizing myelitis   A slowly progressive ischemic myelopathy, usually in the thoracic regions, due to an arteriovenous malformation or to obliterative sclerosis of the small vessels of the cord in the affected areas causing cord necrosis, and leading to the usual motor, sensory, and autonomic signs of transverse myelitis extending upward from the legs. The initial spasticity is later replaced by flaccid paraparesis and the dissociated sensory alteration by complete loss of all modes.

The CSF protein level is increased but the cell counts remain low. Thrombophlebitis of the spinal thoracic and lumbosacral veins appears to be the most likely pathology.[1896] See **Foix-Alajouanine syndrome.**

subacute necrotizing myopathy   A syndrome of muscular weakness with histological changes of muscle necrosis without inflammation. Whether this is a **paraneoplastic syndrome** or a *variant* of acute **polymyositis** is not determined.[5692]

subacute necrotizing polioencephalopathy   A fatal progressive disease of the cortex and brainstem of unknown cause, marked by disseminated areas of focal necrosis without inflammatory change.[4875]

subacute presenile polioencephalopathy   See **Creutzfeldt-Jakob disease.**

subacute presenile spongy atrophy   See **Creutzfeldt-Jakob disease.**

subacute reversible motor neuron disease   See **amyotrophic lateral sclerosis.**

subacute sclerosing leukoencephalitis   A slowly progressive form of encephalitis in which there is conspicuous gliosis of the white matter of the CNS.[5703] See **subacute sclerosing panencephalitis.**

subacute sclerosing panencephalitis   (van Bogaert encephalitis, Dawson encephalitis, subacute inclusion body encephalitis, subacute sclerosing leukoencephalitis) A fatal progressive encephalitis of children following exposure to the measles virus at an early age, the agent now acting as a slow virus.

The clinical picture is initially that of a slight behavior disorder, but it is followed by mental deterioration and impairment of speech, leading to generalized and partial seizures, myoclonus, ataxia, dementia, decerebration, and death.

Pathologically, there is both neuronal and white matter damage; eosinophilic inclusions are seen in neurons and oligodendroglia; and viral antigen is detectable in neurons in all parts of the brain except the cerebellum. The white matter lesions (perivascular edema, inflammation, and demyelination) are identical to those seen in progressive rubella encephalitis, subacute AIDS encephalomyelitis, tropical spinal paraparesis due to HTLV-1, and visna of Icelandic sheep, and deposits of immune complexes can be demonstrated in the walls of small cerebral blood vessels. The EEG appearance of paroxysmal slow-wave dysrhythmias (**burst–suppression**) is characteristic. A high titer of anti-measles antibodies is found in the CSF.[4503,5703]

subacute sensory neuropathy (primary sensory neuropathy, malignant sensory neuropathy, ganglioradiculitis, progressive sensory neuropathy, sensory neuronopathy) A **paraneoplastic syndrome** typically associated with small cell carcinoma of the lung most commonly among adult white female smokers, but also occurring in **Sjögren syndrome,** as a result of toxicity[2963] and with Epstein-Barr virus infections.

Clinically, it is characterized by the subacute but progressive asymmetrical centripetal loss of all sensory modes, mainly in the limbs, with pain and dysesthesias but good motor power and with raised CSF protein levels. Sensory ataxia, pseudoathetosis, and frequently other signs of neurological dysfunction such as limbic encephalitis, seizures, cerebellar, myelopathic, or autonomic signs, a myasthenic syndrome, and inappropriate ADH secretion are also described. The pathological hallmark is inflammation and widespread degeneration of the dorsal root ganglia.[2664] The presence of anti-Hu antibodies staining neuronal nuclei is a marker for the small cell carcinoma.

The condition was first recognized by **Denny-Brown** in 1948.

subacute spongiform encephalopathy See **Creutzfeldt-Jakob disease.**

subarachnoid bolts Devices inserted through the skull to monitor intracranial pressure.

subarachnoid hemorrhage (meningeal apoplexy) The extravasation of blood into the subarachnoid space as a result of rupture of a berry aneurysm on an artery close to the circle of Willis, or as a result of bleeding from an arteriovenous malformation; less commonly other causes are responsible.

The first recorded incident was probably that described in 2 Kings 4:18, in which a boy became moribund after a sudden violent headache, and was revived by the prophet Elisha, who apparently used mouth-to-mouth respiration. It was, however, Sir Charles **Symonds** who gave the most complete account of the findings in 1924–1925.

Suggested criteria for the clinical diagnosis[4300] include the following:

1. The demonstration by CT scan of blood in the sylvian fissure, the basal cisterns, the interhemispheric sulcus, or a ventricle, *or*
2. Any combination of
   Blood in the CSF (after a nontraumatic tap) or xanthochromia, *and* the presence of
   Severe headache at onset or on awakening after the ictus, *or*
   Depressed level of consciousness, *or*
   Clinical signs of meningeal irritation, *or*
   Retinal hemorrhages, *or*
   Focal neurological signs.

subarachnoid hemorrhage grading scale A scale designed to describe change in an individual patient at different times, estimate prognosis, and standardize assessment and management in different groups of patients. It emphasizes level of consciousness (assessed with the **Glasgow Coma scale**) and the presence or absence of hemiparesis or aphasia[1513] (see Chart S–18).

Chart S–18. The Subarachnoid Hemorrhage Grading Scale

Grade	Glasgow Score	Motor Deficit
1	15	Nil
2	14–13	Nil
3	14–13	+
4	12–7	+/-
5	6–3	+/-

*From Drake CG. Report of a World Federation of Neurosurgeons committee on a universal subarachnoid hemorrhage scale. J Neurosurg 1988;**68**:1985–1986, by kind permission.*

subclavian steal syndrome (brachial-basilar insufficiency) Symptoms of brainstem ischemia (vertebrobasilar insufficiency) occurring because of reversal of the flow of blood that has ascended in one vertebral artery and down the other one, rather than continuing up the basilar artery. This occurs as a result of stenosis of the first part of the subclavian artery proximal to the take-off of the vertebral, so that blood cannot ascend in that vessel. When that arm is exercised, its demand for blood increases, but the demand cannot be met across the proximal stenosis, so flow is diverted down the vertebral artery on that side to supply the arm, thus stealing from the basilar.[4656] The syndrome may only cause symptoms when flow in the carotid system is also reduced.

Symptoms include vertigo, limb paresis, binocular visual changes, paresthesias, ataxia, diplopia, syncope, and monocular visual changes, in that order of frequency.[1811]

subclinical rhythmic excitatory discharges of adults (SREDA; pseudolarval electrographic seizure of the elderly) A rare EEG pattern resembling an epileptic discharge but without any known clinical association.[3075]

subclinical seizure   A paroxysmal event without clinical behavioral or cognitive changes produced by an "epileptic" discharge on the EEG.

subcortical aphasia   Forms of aphasia consequent upon circumscribed infarctions in the neostriatum and thalamus (territory supplied by the lenticulostriate branches of the middle cerebral artery) on the dominant side.

The characteristics of the resulting aphasic syndromes vary between cases, but, at least in those cases with thalamic infarctions, may resemble those of the **transcortical aphasias**.[1262] See also **subcortical motor aphasia**.

subcortical arteriosclerotic encephalopathy   See **Binswanger disease**.[282]

subcortical auditory aphasia   See **pure word deafness.**

subcortical band heterotopia   See **diffuse cortical dysplasia.**

subcortical dementia   Dementia occurring in association with degenerative disorders involving the subcortical structures. The major clinical features include forgetfulness; marked slowing of thought processes; alterations of personality with inertia, apathy, and depression; occasional irritability or euphoria; inappropriate emotional display; and impaired ability to manipulate abstract knowledge (e.g., poor abstraction ability and calculation). Dysarthria and motor signs are also common.

These changes are thought to stem from a primary problem of excessive delay in the performance of intellectual tasks. **Parkinson disease, progressive supranuclear palsy, Huntington disease, progressive subcortical gliosis, Hallervorden-Spatz disease, multisystem atrophy,** paramedian thalamic infarctions,[2951] and **normal-pressure hydrocephalus**[82] are representative disorders.

Clinically, the condition may be suspected when the dementia is accompanied by prominent motor disturbances, while typically "cortical" signs such as aphasias, apraxias, agnosias, and visual field deficits are less evident[2680] and memory loss is relatively slight. Verbal and perceptual–motor abilities are also relatively well preserved if the subject is not pressed for time.[82]

Criticisms of this clinical differentiation have been reviewed, with the conclusion that its validity is as yet unproved.[5945]

subcortical dysequilibrium   (tottering, astasia-abasia, thalamic astasia) A gait disorder characterized by prominent dysequilibrium with absent or ineffective postural responses. Sometimes the postural responses are inappropriate; for example, the patient may hyperextend the trunk and neck and fall backward. Other pa-

tients appear inattentive to their posture and unable to generate postural responses, although EMG recordings show that there are postural responses, though ineffective. Locomotion is primarily impaired because of the dysequilibrium. There is thus an inability to stand in the absence of muscle weakness or marked sensory loss, due usually to a unilateral vascular lesion.

The pattern is associated with lesions of the midbrain, thalamus, or basal ganglia, and associated signs include ocular palsies (vertical gaze palsies and pupillary abnormalities), dysarthria, and extrapyramidal signs. (Adapted from Nutt JG, Marsden CD, Thompson PD. Human walking and high-level gait disorders, particularly in the elderly. *Neurology* 1993;43:268–279, and from Masdeu and Gorelick.[3668])

subcortical functions   Those endowments which preferentially serve fundamental functions, such as arousal, motivation, and mood. Dysfunction is considered to lead to slowing of information processing, with disturbance of memory, cognition, mood, and behavior. The memory disturbance, however, is mainly a difficulty in spontaneous recall rather than in encoding or storing new material, so memory assisted by clues and cues is better than free recall.

subcortical junctional infarcts   Infarcts in the periventricular regions, resulting from distal middle cerebral artery occlusions (usually due to extracranial carotid artery disease) and causing hemipareses with hemisphere-specific neuropsychological dysfunction.

subcortical laminar heterotopia   An X-linked or dominantly inherited neuronal migration disorder giving a "double cortex" appearance on MRI scans.[4448] See also **lissencephaly, pachygyria.**

subcortical motor aphasia   An aphasic syndrome characterized by the acute onset of mutism, progressing to hypophonia with dysarthria and paraphasia, while comprehension, naming, and reading are variably affected or spared and repetition may be good, with progressive reduction in paraphasic errors. The likelihood of ultimate recovery is high.

Hemiparetic and hemisensory deficits are usually present in the early stages at least. See **aphemia, subcortical aphasia.**

subcortical neglect   Neglect produced by subcortical lesions. Compare with **neglect.**

subcortical reflex myoclonus   See **reticular reflex myoclonus.**

subcortical sensory aphasia   See **Lichtheim aphasia.**

subcortical visual aphasia   See **pure word blindness.**

subdural abscess   See **subdural empyema.**

subdural effusion   A collection of fluid beneath the cranial dura mater. The term is used to describe acute, subacute, or chronic subdural hemorrhage, subdural hygroma, and subdural empyema. The fluid contained is usually xanthochromic and may be hemorrhagic, but is usually sterile.

The effusion is commonly the result of birth or other head injuries, meningitis, or cranial surgery, usually stemming from the organization of a subdural hematoma. Its clinical features include seizures, vomiting, irritability, and failure to thrive in infants who are found to have a bulging fontanelle, hyperactive reflexes, and enlargement of the head, sometimes with evidence of the fluid-containing cyst shown by transillumination.

In adults, the clinical features are those of subdural hematoma.[3699]

subdural empyema   (subdural abscess, cortical abscess, circumscript meningitis, internal purulent pachymeningitis) Pyogenic infection of the meninges in which the pus lies between the arachnoid and dural membranes.

The condition was first recorded in 1886. It is usually a complication of chronic otitic or sinus infection with adjacent osteomyelitis, and presents clinically with rapidly progressive local symptoms, headache, fever and meningism, alteration of consciousness, and focal seizures and neurological signs, depending on the site of the empyema.[3175]

subdural grid electrodes   A line of electrodes placed on the cortex at open operation in an attempt to determine the precise origin of abnormal electrical discharges in epileptic patients. **Magnetometry** may in the future accomplish the same thing better and noninvasively.

subdural hematoma   (subdural hemorrhage) A collection of blood or blood products beneath the dura of the skull or in the spinal cord, stemming from rupture of the bridging veins, usually due to trauma. Both *acute* and *chronic* forms exist. Clinically, these are signs of increased intracranial pressure, focal signs, and occasionally seizures due to compression of the underlying cortex.

The presence of hemiparetic signs on the side opposite the skull lesion was first noted in the Edwin Smith Papyrus, and appears again in Hippocratic writings, with a description of post-traumatic seizures. Ambrose Paré described the underlying pathology and most of the physical signs resulting, although LeDran was the first to comment on the **lucid interval** (which, however, is more common with **epidural hematoma**). Pupillary dilatation as a result of compression of the third cranial nerve was drawn by Hans Wachtlin of Basel in 1527, but the sign was not recognized further until noted by Richard **Bright** in 1827, again in a case of epidural hematoma. Jonathan **Hutchinson** gave a full account of the stages of pupillary dilation in 1867.[1879]

subdural hemorrhage   See **subdural hematoma.**

subdural hygroma   A collection of fluid in the subdural space, usually remotely following trauma and presenting with symptoms similar to those of chronic subdural hematoma.[4059]

subependymal cell plate   See **germinal zone.**

subependymal giant cell astrocytoma   See **astrocytoma.**

subependymal zone   See **germinal zone.**

subependymoma   An uncommon, slowly growing, malignant primary neuroectodermal cerebral tumor, likely a variant of **ependymoma,** occurring mainly in males. It is usually located in the fourth ventricle, less often in periventricular regions of the brain, and rarely in the spinal cord. It carries a fair prognosis if completely removed, and in some cases remains asymptomatic.

Pathologically, the lobulated tumor is characterized by the presence of nests of fibrillary astrocytes with round nuclei containing chromatin, separated by areas filled with glial processes and by the presence of calcium and hyalinized, partly obliterated vessels within it.[4951] The underlying glial layer also proliferates.

subjective DIMS complaint without objective findings   (pseudoinsomnia, sleep hypochondriasis) Complaints of insomnia (and of its usual associated symptoms) that cannot be verified by polysomnography (see ASDA diagnostic classification,[249] **sleep disorders**).

subjective tinnitus   See **tinnitus.**

sublimis syndrome   See **pseudo–carpal tunnel syndrome.**

submandibular, rectal, and ocular pain and flushing   A dominantly inherited syndrome of infancy characterized by severe, brief attacks of pain in the eyes, rectum, and submandibular regions, with local skin flushing and bowel movement. The cause is not known.[2487]

submedullary syndrome   See **Opalski syndrome.**

subnormal period   A time interval that immediately follows the supernormal period of nerve which is characterized by reduced excitability compared to the resting state. Its duration is variable and is related to the refractory period. (From the 2001 Report of the Nomenclature Committee of the American Association of Electromyography and Electrodiagnosis.[10] Used by permission, copyright © 2001, AAEM.)

subpial cerebral siderosis   The deposition of iron-containing pigment within the subpial layers of the CNS following previous bleeding into the subarachnoid space stemming from any cause.[3753]

substance P   A vasoactive oligopeptide hormone found in the hypothalamus and elsewhere in the CNS, in the dorsal horn of the spinal cord, and in the gastrointestinal tract. It functions as a primary sensory neurotransmitter in the pain pathways and is capable of activating pain receptors. Its release is inhibited by morphine and by the endorphins.

substantia gelatinosa   A curved band capping the posterior part of the dorsal horn of gray matter in the spinal cord, distinguished from the surrounding structures by its transparency and consistency. It receives the bulk of the C-fiber afferent projections in the cord as well as many small myelinated afferent fibers.

Described first by the Italian anatomist **Rolando** in 1824, this is the only structure in the spinal cord extending continuously from the brainstem to the filum terminale. While its relevance to pain in the transmission of impulses is a keystone of the **gate theory,** other authors have concluded that its function is still unknown and have cast doubt upon its role as a functional entity.[949]

substantia nigra   (Lat, substance + black) A pigmented area in the mesencephalon dorsal to the crura cerebri, but ventral to the red nuclei.

subtentorial lesions   Lesions within the posterior fossa, beneath the tentorium, and above the foramen magnum. Their clinical effects are manifest through their effects on the brainstem, the cerebellum, and the passage of CSF.

subthalamic nuclear degeneration   See **dentatorubropallidoluysian atrophy.**

subthalamic syndrome   The clinical features following occlusion of the thalamoperforating arteries, comprising extension at the interphalangeal joints, most marked at the fifth finger and progressively less toward the thumb; slight flexion at the metacarpophalangeal joints; and choreoathetotic movements of the hand, and including tremor, ataxia, and choreoathetosis but minimal sensory disturbances.[574]

subtle seizures   (fragmentary seizures) See **automatism, minimal seizures.**

subwakefulness syndrome   A rare form of hypersomnolence of unknown cause, characterized by excessive daytime sleepiness with repetitive non–rapid eye movement stage 1 or 2 sleep episodes but normal nocturnal sleep patterns.[249,4021] See **idiopathic CNS hypersomnolence.**

succinylcholine sensitivity   A recessive condition with a locus on chromosome 3, in which exposure to succinylcholine as a muscle relaxant in anesthesia leads to prolonged muscle paralysis with apnea. Screening tests for the disorder use quantitative assays of plasma pseudocholinesterase, which are low.

succinylpurinemic autism   An inherited syndrome due to deficiency of adenylsuccinase for which the responsible gene maps to chromosome 22.

succubus   A female devil, thought in the Middle Ages to be seeking sexual intercourse with men during their sleep. See also **incubus.**

sucking reflex   Stimulation of the lips by a finger introduced between them (or stimulation of the cheek) elicits sucking movements involving the lips, tongue, and jaw, and turning of the head toward the stimulus. The reflex is normally present from 30 weeks' gestation, is lost by 4 months, and reappears only in the presence of diffuse bilateral cortical disease or bilateral corticobulbar lesions.[6064]

sudanophilic (orthochromatic) leukodystrophies   A group of congenital dysmyelinating syndromes characterized by optic atrophy, seizures, nystagmus, spasticity, low densities in the periventricular white matter on T2-weighted MRI scans, and the accumulation of sudanophilic lipids in microglia and astrocytes.[4516] See **adrenoleukodystrophy.**

sudden bodily jerks on falling asleep   See **periodic limb mvement disorder.**

sudden infant death syndrome   (SIDS) A syndrome of uncertain cause, one candidate being failure of the automatic control of respiration, leading to periodic apnea, alveolar hypoventilation, and death. Structural changes in the brainstem affecting the neural controlling mechanisms are present in a number of infants dying from this cause. **Ondine's curse** is a similar condition in adults. See also the ASDA classification[234] and **sleep disorders.**

sudden unexpected death in epilepsy   Deaths occurring either directly as a result of seizures or without that explanation. Some of the latter may, however, be due to unwitnessed seizures, leading to cardiac arrhythmias, pulmonary edema, or respiratory arrest. Occurrence of tonic-clonic seizures, treatment with more than two anticonvulsants, and a full-scale IQ of less than 70 are identified risk factors.[5804]

sudden unexplained nocturnal death syndrome   The occurrence of sudden death during sleep in young adults previously considered healthy. This is most commonly seen in subjects of Southeast Asian decent, and appears to be based on episodic ventricular fibrillation.

Diagnostic criteria have been suggested[234] and are given in Chart S–19.

Chart S–19.   Diagnostic Criteria for Sudden Unexplained Nocturnal Death Syndrome

A. Sudden cardiorespiratory arrest during sleep
B. Occurs in persons of Southeast Asian descent
C. Associated features include one or more of the following:
   1. Male sex
   2. Choking, gurgling, gasping, or labored breathing during the episode
   3. The episode occurs during the habitual sleep period.
   4. A history of prior sleep terror episodes

D. Polysomnograhic monitoring of survivors has not been reported.

E. Cardiac studies of survivors have demonstrated spontaneous ventricular fibrillation after initial resuscitation.

F. No evidence of any medical or psychiatric disorder that could account for the features, e.g., ischemic heart disease

G. May be associated with sleep terrors. Does not meet the criteria for other sleep disorders producing a risk of cardiopulmonary arrest, e.g., obstructive sleep apnea syndrome or rapid eye movement sleep–related sinus arrest.

From ASDA Diagnostic Classification Steering Committee. The International Classification of Sleep Disorders Diagnostic and Coding Manual. Rochester, MN: American Sleep Disorders Association © 1990, by kind permission of the American Academy of Sleep Medicine.

Sudeck atrophy See **reflex sympathetic dystrophy, causalgia.**

Sudeck, Paul Hermann Martin (1866–1938) German surgeon, professor at Hamburg.

Sugiura sign Depigmentation within the corneal limbus, seen in patients with **uveomeningoencephalitic syndrome.**

sulfatide lipidosis See **metachromatic leukodystrophy.**

sulfatidoses Forms of sphingolipidosis characterized by the accumulation of sulfatides and, in some cases, steroid, heparan, or dermatan sulfate; they include the various forms of **metachromatic leukodystrophy** and **mucosulfatidosis.**

sulfite oxidase deficiency (sulfituria) A syndrome of severe neurological dysfunction with mental retardation, microcephaly, seizures, blindness, and extrapyramidal and pyramidal signs, also characterized by dislocation of the lenses and the excretion of inorganic sulfite, thiosulfite, and *S*-sulfocysteine.[791]

sulfituria See **sulfite oxidase deficiency.**

Suliman syndrome A congenital dysmorphic syndrome characterized by short stature, ptosis, skeletal and genital abnormalities, and mental and developmental delay. See also **Marden-Walker syndrome,** which is similar.

Sulzberger-Bloch disease See **incontinentia pigmenti.**

summation hyperpathia The awareness of excessive pain during stimulation of the same area in two modes. The lesion may be in either the thalamus or the cerebral cortex.[3864]

Summerskill sign Widening of the palpebral fissure in patients with hepatic insufficiency.[5413]

Summitt syndrome A recessively inherited congenital syndrome characterized by craniosynostosis, syndactyly, obesity, strabismus, and high-arched palate.[5414] See **craniosynostosis, acrocephalopolysyndactyly.**

sunbath polyneuritis A subacute sensory polyneuropathy with photosensitivity usually resulting from treatment with phenothiazines or their derivatives with a good prognosis. Seventh cranial nerve palsy may be associated.[4738]

SUNCT syndrome (**S**hort-lasting **U**nilateral **N**euralgiform headache attacks with **C**onjunctival injection and **T**earing) A distinctive, rare, trigeminal-autonomic cephalalgia characterized by intermittent head pains (unilateral neuralgia-like paroxysms lasting 5–250 [mean, 50] seconds) up to about 20 times daily accompanied by marked autonomic activation such as conjunctival injection, tearing, rhinorrhea, subclinical sweating, raised intraocular pressure, and bradycardia, the attacks being precipitated by stimulation of regions innervated by the fifth cranial nerve.[5199] They seldom occur at night.[2142]

sundown syndrome The onset or exacerbation of delirium during the evening or night, with reduction or disappearance of the delirium during the day. Reduced ability to maintain attention to external stimuli, disorganized thinking and speech, restlessness and agitation, perceptual disturbances such as illusions, and hallucinations and emotional disturbances are common features. The problem is common in the setting of dementing illnesses.[5771]

sunflower cataract The appearance of the cataract in **Wilson disease.**

sunflower syndrome Heliotropism (Gr, the sun + movement; thus an attraction toward strong light) followed by the performance of movements of the arm on the side to which the gaze is directed, perhaps to induce flickering of the solar image and leading to heterogeneous (photosensitive) epileptic attacks, which presumably either induce pleasurable sensations or blot out unpleasant ones—the subjects are amnesic for the events during the seizures.[152]

sunrise (sunset) sign Depression of the eyeball with failure of upward gaze and retraction of the upper lid, such that only the upper rim of the cornea shows above the lower lid margin; seen in children with pressure on the mesencephalic tegmentum due to hydrocephalus.

super- (Lat, above) Prefix denoting above.

superficial anal reflex A superficial reflex manifested by contraction of the anal sphincter in response to stroking or scratching the perianal skin. The reflex arc employed is at S4–5.

superficial radial nerve palsy Damage to the nerve, causing pain, numbness, and paresthesias in the space between the thumb and the index finger, most commonly as a result of **handcuff** or watch-strap pressure[5368] or within the syndrome of **multiple mononeuropathy.** See **cheiralgia paresthetica.**

superficial reflexes Reflex muscle contraction elicited by stimulating cutaneous receptors. Such reflexes are relatively long in latency and duration, are graded in proportion to the strength of the stimulus, and show both summation and exhaustion; in all of these characteristics they differ from the **muscle stretch reflexes.** See also **cutaneous reflexes.**

superficial siderosis of the central nervous system A disorder characterized by deposition of hemosiderin in the leptomeninges and the subpial tissue following repeated episodes of bleeding into the subarachnoid space from any cause, after treatment of cerebellar tumors or without known cause.

Clinically, the disease causes any combination of myelopathy, sensorineural deafness, cerebellar ataxia, and dementia.[2694] The diagnosis may be suggested by the MRI findings of hypointensities overlying the brainstem, cerebellar vermis, eighth cranial nerve, spinal cord, and sometimes the cerebral cortex, and in the basal cisterns, as a result of the deposition of iron-containing compounds such as hemosiderin.[3112] Anterior horn cell disease has also been reported.

superior canal dehiscence syndrome A variant of the typical perilymph fistula presenting as recurrent attacks of vertigo and oscillopsia as a result of stimuli changing the intracranial or inner ear pressures, and due to dehiscence of bone overlying the superior semicircular canal, creating a window additional to the oval and round windows.[3902]

superior cerebellar peduncle syndrome See **cerebellar tremors.**

superior cerebellar peduncle tremor See **cerebellar tremors.**

superior Foville syndrome See **Raymond-Cestan syndrome.**

superior gluteal nerve entrapment syndrome A syndrome of aching gluteal pain and weakness of the gluteus medius muscle causing weakness of leg abduction and limping, and considered to be due to compression of the nerve by the piriformis muscle.[4599] See also **piriformis syndrome.**

superior laryngeal nerve syndrome See **Avellis syndrome.**

superior laryngeal neuralgia (Arnold syndrome, auriculotemporal neuralgia) A rare syndrome of severe lancinating paroxysmal pain in the side of the neck, extending up to the face as high as the zygoma, down to the upper portion of the thorax and medially perhaps as far as the mid-larynx, almost invariably unilateral and triggered by swallowing, yawning, coughing, or stretching the neck. The attack lasts from seconds to a minute or more.[5235] The syndrome was first described fully by Avellis[269] in 1891. The following diagnostic criteria are suggested by the Headache Classification Committee of the International Headache Society.[1051] (From Classification of headache disorders, cranial neuralgias and facial pains; and diagnostic criteria

for primary headache disorders. *Cephalalgia* 1988; 8[suppl]:1–96). With kind permission from Blackwell Science.

A. Pain paroxysms felt in the throat, submandibular region, or under the ear, lasting for minutes or hours
B. Paroxysms are triggered by swallowing, straining the voice, or head turning.
C. Susceptibility continues for days or weeks.
D. A trigger point is present on the lateral aspect of the throat overlying the hypothyroid membrane.
E. Exclusion of a structural lesion

superior oblique myokymia A variant form of **saccadic intrusion,** characterized by a rapid, intermittent, small-amplitude, torsional, vertical jerk nystagmus in one eye, as a result of repetitive contraction of the superior oblique muscle. This leads to complaints of oscillopsia and often of oblique diplopia.

The condition was first described by Duane in 1906. It is not really myokymia at all, but a chronic microtremor[4787] caused by any form of partial damage to the fourth cranial nerve.

superior oblique tendon syndrome (Brown syndrome) A restrictive ophthalmopathy in which fibrosis and shortening with tethering of the superior oblique tendon within its sheath causes failure of elevation of the adducted eye due to prevention of the normal upward and inward movement of the globe of the eye. It is caused by contraction of the inferior oblique muscle and gives the impression of paresis of that muscle.

The condition is usually congenital, but has also been described as an acquired and intermittent problem.[2168,2764]

superior orbital fissure syndrome (intermittent painful ophthalmoplegia, superior orbital fissuritis, anterior cavernous sinus syndrome, Colio syndrome, Rollet syndrome, orbital apex syndrome, Tolosa-Hunt syndrome, sphenoidal fissure syndrome, cavernous sinus–lateral wall syndrome, cavernous sinus syndrome of Raeder, syndrome of Bonnet and Bonnet, sphenopetrosal fissure syndrome) A syndrome of episodic acute or subacute orbital pain associated with paralysis of one or more of the muscles supplied by the third, fourth, or sixth cranial nerves, which resolves spontaneously but may relapse and remit. It is considered to result from a nonspecific inflammatory process affecting the structures traversing the superior orbital fissure, including the three oculomotor nerves, the first division of the fifth cranial nerve, and the sympathetic and parasympathetic fibers destined for the eye. Involvement of the optic nerve has also been recorded.[4747] Trauma, neoplasm, and aneurysm affecting the superior orbital fissure may produce identical findings.[3082]

The symptoms include painful unilateral ophthalmoplegia, headache, ocular pain, and sensory loss on the upper face and scalp. The condition resembles **orbital pseudotumor syndrome** in its responsiveness to steroids and may represent the same pathology located more posteriorly.

No conclusive diagnostic test exists,[2389,5600] but the following diagnostic criteria are suggested by the Headache Classification Committee of the International Headache Society[1051] (from Classification of headache disorders, cranial neuralgias and facial pains; and diagnostic criteria for primary headache disorders. *Cephalalgia* 1988;**8**[suppl]:1–96).

A. Episode or episodes of unilateral orbital pain for an average of 8 weeks if untreated
B. Association with paralysis of one or more of the third, fourth, or sixth nerves, which may coincide with the onset of the pain or follow it by a period of up to 2 weeks
C. Pain is relieved within 72 hours after initiation of corticosteroid therapy.
D. Exclusion of other causative lesions by neuroimaging and (not compulsory) carotid angiography

Hunt (an American neurosurgeon in Columbus, Ohio) proposed that the diagnostic criteria should include the presence of a **Horner syndrome,** involvement of the first division of the fifth cranial nerve, spontaneous remission and recurrence, and the absence of features suggesting the presence of lesions outside the cavernous sinus; and he contributed six new cases. Collier gave an account of such features in 1921. Steroid responsiveness was suggested as another criterion in 1966. Other features reported include chemosis, proptosis, papilledema, and irregular constriction of the carotid syphon on angiography (**arterial stationary wave**). The causes vary; both vasculitis and nonspecific granulomas of the retro-orbital region have been described.[2141,2420,5600]

An identical condition is unusually common in Asia, where it is known as *polyneuritis cranialis*.[5502,5794]

superior orbital fissuritis   See **superior orbital fissure syndrome.**

superior thoracic aperture syndrome   See **thoracic outlet syndrome.**

supermarket neuropathy   Proper digital neuropathies causing numbness and tingling of the fingers, occasioned by the constricting effects of the handles of filled plastic shopping bags.[4263]

supernormal period   A time interval that immediately follows the refractory period which corresponds to a very brief period of partial depolarization. It is characterized by increased nerve excitability and is followed by the subnormal period. (From the 2001 Report of the Nomenclature Committee of the American Association of Electromyography and Electrodiagnosis.[10] Used by permission, copyright © 2001, AAEM.)

supernumerary first rib   A harmless condition until detected during the search for a cause of the complaints of dragging pain, discomfort, paresthesias, and minor vascular changes in an arm or hand, usually a feminine disorder. But when found, it is cast in the role of male-

factor, for which nothing but radical extirpation will suffice. When symptoms persist thereafter, treatment of a **carpal tunnel syndrome** often provides relief.

superoxide dismutase   A cell enzyme inactivating superoxide.

supination   (from Lat, bent back, lying on the back) The posture of the body lying with the face up and the arms externally rotated and thus also facing up.

supinator channel syndrome   See **posterior interosseous syndrome.**

supinator reflex   See **brachioradialis reflex.**

supplementary motor area aphasia   See **transcortical aphasia.**

supplementary motor cortex   An area situated on the mesial surface of the frontal lobe of the human brain, above the cingulate gyrus and anterior to the primary motor areas of the foot and leg (part of Brodmann's area 6).[4406] It is considered to play an important role in the intentional process, whereby internal thought content sparks the elaboration of action.

Goldberg suggests that the area is crucial in the programming and fluent execution of extended action sequences. It was defined by Penfield and Welch[4406] on the basis of the motor responses obtained with electrical stimulation which differed from those produced by stimulating the primary motor cortex.[2160,4405]

supplementary motor epilepsy   An epileptic syndrome in which the seizure patterns are postural, focal and tonic, with vocalization, speech arrest, and fencing postures. (From the revised ILAE Classification,[1114] reproduced by kind permission from Blackwell Science.)

The seizures begin abruptly and occur frequently, without warning. They consist of tonic posturing of one or more limbs and twisting truncal movements, with vocalization and speech arrest, ending with rhythmic or clonic movements of the extremities, such as the elevation of one arm (fencing posture). Awareness is preserved even though all four limbs may be affected. The seizures are highly resistant to current medical treatment.[3994]

This form of seizure was first described by **Penfield** and colleagues. An increase in seizure frequency during rapid eye movement sleep is also described. The interictal EEG record is usually normal.

supplementary sensation   Retention of pressure sensation in an area insensitive to pinprick after nerve injury.[2500]

supporting reactions   The involuntary contraction of the antigravity muscles which allows the body to maintain the upright position.[4180]

supporting response   If an infant is held vertically above a table and the feet allowed to come into contact with its surface, there will be simultaneous contraction of the leg flexors and extensors as if to provide standing support for the body. This is a normal reflex, persisting from birth. See also **stepping response.**

supra- (Lat, above) Prefix denoting above.

supramarginal gyrus Area 40 of Brodmann, located at the junction of the frontal, parietal, and temporal lobes. Lesions in this region are associated with **Wernicke aphasia** and with the **Gerstmann syndrome.**

suprameatal triangle See **MacEwen triangle.**

supramodal 1. Attending to more than one single sensory channel. Thus the parietal lobe considers both visual and auditory **representations** in the analysis of information about spatial relationships. 2. Processes that are above the perceptual modalities, such as vision, hearing, and touch.

supranuclear gaze palsy See **progressive supranuclear palsy, sphingolipidoses.**

supranuclear upgaze paresis A form of dysconjugate eye movement in which there is limitation of elevation of one eye in all positions of horizontal gaze, due to a contralateral pretectal lesion.

supraorbital neuralgia See **cluster headache.**

supraorbital reflex See **orbicularis oculi reflex, glabellar tap.**

suprapatellar reflex Contraction of the quadriceps with extension of the knee in response to a tap on the top of the patella, with the knee flexed.

This is just another way of obtaining the knee jerk, and is best seen in patients with hyperactive muscle stretch reflexes due to a pyramidal lesion.

suprarubral syndrome A syndrome of intention tremor, ophthalmoparesis, and disturbed conjugate eye movements occurring as a result of **multiple sclerosis** or of a vascular lesion in the basilar artery territory, in subthalamic regions.[1013]

suprascapular neuropathy Wasting and weakness of the supra- and infraspinatus muscles as a result of entrapment of the nerve. This usually occurs at the upper trunk of the brachial plexus or at the suprascapular notch; less commonly it is more distal, at the spinoglenoid notch,[3128] in which case only the infraspinatus muscle is affected.

suprasellar cysts Benign tumor masses having the same site and origin as **craniopharyngiomas,** but lined with keratinizing squamous epithelium and thus also resembling epidermoid cysts elsewhere.[6]

supratentorial cavernous hemangioma See **cavernoma.**

sural neuropathy A syndrome of numbness on the lateral aspect of the foot as a result of damage to the sural nerve, due to compression or stretch at the popliteal fossa or in the calf, or due to direct local trauma.[3045]

surface electrode A conducting device for stimulating or recording when placed on the surface of the skin.

Surgical Neurology A neurosurgical journal published by Elsevier. Web site: http://www.elsevier.com/locate/surneu.

sursumduction See **ductions.**

Susac syndrome (arterial occlusive retinopathy and encephalopathy; retinocochleocerebral arteriolopathy) A rare microangiopathy of the brain and retina occurring in young women with features resembling multiple sclerosis and with added hearing loss, usually remitting within 2 years. The etiology is unknown.[5422] See also **RED-M syndrome.**

sustension Sustained forward extension of the upper limbs against gravity, used to demonstrate drifts or abnormal movements or tremors. The term may also be applied to other sustained motor activities, such as vocal sustension. (HJM)

suspended sensory loss See **hanging sensory loss.**

Sutton, Thomas (1767–1835) English physician practicing in Kent, who wrote *Tracts on Delirium Tremens* (1813),[5429] in which he gave the first definitive description of the condition and named it, although he noted the prior contributions of Thomas **Saunders.**

His peculiar familiarity with the disease was, as he recognized, due to its frequency among those who, living on the Kentish coast, were able to procure alcohol smuggled in from France at knock-down prices.

swallow syncope A rare occurrence of syncope during or immediately after swallowing, and due to reflexly enhanced vagal tone and thus sinus bradycardia, in patients with esophageal or cardiac abnormalities when they eat.[2302] See **deglutition syncope.**

Swan syndrome 1. (squint syndrome of Braun) A physiological method for the abolition of diplopia by turning the head 12°–18°. This allows light from the object viewed to fall on the physiological blind spot of the deviating eye, thus eliminating the false image.[5434] 2. The association of insufficiency of the inferior oblique muscle with proptosis, entropion, epicanthus, and hypotelorism.[5435]

sweat testing See **quantitative sudomotor axon reflex test, thermoregulatory sweat test.**

Swedenborg, Emanuel (1688–1772) Swedish scientist, visionary, and philosopher (but some have said psychotic) whose accomplishments in neurology included the identification of the cortical motor areas and the localization of representation in them. He also ascribed motor functions to the basal ganglia and differentiated upper from lower motor neuron lesions.

Swediaur disease See **achillodynia.**

swim-goggle headache A headache described as feeling like a tight band constricting the head, probably because it is due to a tight band constricting the head, in this case the elastic strap of the goggles. See **external compression headache.**

swimmer's migraine   Acute, benign, pulsating headache related to swimming; a form of **effort headache.**[2735]

swimming reflex   When a baby is supported in water in the prone position, rhythmic movements of all extremities and the trunk are made.[6064]

swinging flashlight test   A most sensitive clinical test for afferent lesions of the anterior visual pathway. A bright flashlight is directed into one eye and then swung rapidly across to the other one. When the normal eye is stimulated, both direct and consensual pupillary constriction occurs. When the light passes across from a normal eye to an eye with an afferent defect, the stimulus to constrict is less effective, and so both pupils dilate; but the examiner is looking at the illuminated one, which is said to dilate "paradoxically."[1196]

The phenomenon of dilatation of the pupil being examined in this circumstance is wrongly named for **Marcus Gunn,** the test having been described by Levatin.

Swiss syndrome   See **familial Cushing syndrome, Carney complex.**

switching-on, switching-off   Fluctuations in the clinical state of parkinsonian patients on long-term L-dopa therapy in which the facilitation or inhibition of movements occurs at times of rising or falling L-dopa levels, respectively.

Sybert syndrome   A congenital dysmorphic syndrome characterized by skeletal and cutaneous abnormalities, short stature, optic atrophy, pigmentary retinopathy, microcephaly, and mental and developmental delay.[337]

Sydenham chorea   (chorea minor, rheumatic chorea, infectious chorea, **St. Vitus' dance,** danse de St. Guy) Acute, benign, and self-limited chorea, incoordination of voluntary movement, and muscle weakness occurring in the limbs, face, and trunk of children; carditis (which is much less benign) may also be found.[5452]

The condition may complicate group A β-hemolytic *Streptococcus* infection and is due to the formation of autoantibodies against the caudate nucleus and endothelium. Girls are more commonly affected. **Wilson**[6000] quoted the saying that a choreic child is punished thrice before her condition is recognized—once for general fidgetiness, once for breaking crockery, and once for making faces at her grandmother.

Sydenham cough   Spasm of the respiratory muscles, as an hysterical manifestation. It was described by Thomas **Sydenham** in his *Epistolary Dissertation to Dr. Cole* in 1682 as follows: "When it falls on the lungs, the patient coughs continually, but without spitting; and although this cough may not shake the chest so much

as the true convulsive sort, the fits are much more frequent, and the patient is less able to master them. Women with an excess of phlegm are most liable to this cough; which, otherwise, is very rare."

Sydenham, Thomas   (1624–1689) Prominent English physician, born in Dorset. He attended the University of Oxford for a short spell, leaving to enter military service on the side of Parliament (as opposed to the Royalist cause), but returned, graduated, and succeeded in being elected to a Fellowship of All Souls College upon the expulsion of a Royalist member.

Before the restoration of legal government, he had moved to France and then to London, where he remained in practice for the rest of his life. He was known as the English Hippocrates, his reputation resting upon his first-hand accounts of diseases such as hysteria, gout, dysentery, scarlatina, smallpox, malaria, tuberculosis, and rheumatism, but he is best remembered today for his account of chorea minor (1686), now named for him.[7]

syllogomania   The compulsion to hoard rubbish; usually a sign of a failing brain.

Sylvester disease   A dominantly inherited syndrome of progressive deafness with optic atrophy, cerebellar ataxia, and muscle wasting, mainly of the shoulder girdle and hands, with onset in childhood.[5453]

sylvian aqueduct   The pathway for CSF drainage from the third ventricle to the fourth.

sylvian aqueduct syndrome   (Kestenbaum syndrome, Koerber-Salus-Elschnig syndrome) Light-near dissociation, anisocoria, impaired conjugate upward gaze, convergence and retraction nystagmus, vertical nystagmus on up- or down-gaze, and extraocular palsies, occurring due to lesions of the rostral periaqueductal gray matter, usually tumors.[1647,3113]

Salus' first case had a *Cysticercus* cyst in the aqueduct and rostral fourth ventricle.[4891] See **Parinaud syndrome.** The aqueduct itself was first described by Jacobus Sylvius (1478–1555), a French anatomist. See **dorsal midbrain syndrome.**

sylvian epilepsy   See **benign childhood epilepsy with centrotemporal spikes.**

sylvian fissure   (lateral fissure) The first fissure to be described, it separates the frontal lobe before and above from the temporal and parietal lobes behind and below. It was named after Sylvius (who did not write about it until 1663) by Caspar Bartholin, a Danish anatomist, in 1641.

sylvian spikes   See **central-midtemporal spikes.**

Sylvius   (François de la Böe, 1614–1672) A physician of French origin but born in Germany, training in medicine in Sedan, Leiden, and Basel. As professor of medicine in Leiden his most significant publications were on cerebral anatomy, even though most of the structures now named after him had been identified previously.[1478] He did, however, break new ground in proposing that the cerebral cortex, rather than the ventricles, was responsible for brain function.

Symbol-Digit Modalities test A simple oral test assessing the speed of information processing, and not requiring the patient to make any nonverbal motor responses.[5214] See also **Wechsler Adult Intelligence Scale.**

symmetrical calcification of the basal ganglia with familial ataxia and pigmentary macular degeneration A syndrome of symmetrical basal gangulion calcifications, usually recessively inherited. It is associated with progressive ataxia, impairment of central vision due to macular degeneration, and onset in the fourth decade.[5380] See **striatopallidal calcification.**

symmetrical cerebral calcification See **striatopallidal calcification.**

symmetrical degeneration of the neostriatum See **infantile bilateral striatal necrosis.**

symmetrical proximal lower extremity motor neuropathy See **diabetic amyotrophy.** Such convoluted appellations emphasize the relevance of eponyms.

symmetry 1. The approximately equal amplitude, frequency, and form of EEG activities over homologous areas on opposite sides of the head. 2. The approximately equal distribution of potentials of unlike polarity on either side of a zero isopotential axis (see also **true phase reversal**). 3. The approximately equal distribution of EEG waves about the baseline. (From Chatrian GE, Bergamini L, Dondey M, et al. A glossary of terms most commonly used by clinical electroencephalographers. *EEG Clin Neurophysiol* 1974;**37**:538–48,[989] with permission from Elsevier Science.)

Symonds, Sir Charles Putnam (1890–1978) English neurologist who trained as a postgraduate at the **National Hospital,** Queen Square, and was subsequently appointed the first physician for diseases of the nervous system at Guy's Hospital and later at the National Hospital as well. His clinical analyses of disease were outstanding, as typified by his correct diagnosis of a ruptured berry aneurysm in a patient of **Cushing,** made while Symonds was on a traveling fellowship to the United States; this was the first occasion on which such a diagnosis had been made in a living patient.

Many of his classic publications on head injury, cluster headache, multiple sclerosis, neuropathies, myelopathies, **idiopathic intracranial hypertension,**[5455] and other topics have been preserved in his *Studies in Neurology.*[5461] During World War II, he rose to the rank of Air Vice Marshal (in WWI he had been wounded as a dispatch rider) and was later knighted. He retired in 1970.

Symonds syndrome See **idiopathic intracranial hypertension.**

sympathalgia See **reflex sympathetic dystrophy.**

sympathetic delirium See **delirium.**

sympathetic dyspraxia The appearance of dyspractic responses on the left side in a patient with a right hemiparesis. See **apraxia.**

sympathetic skin response Electrical potential resulting from electrodermal activity in sweat glands in response to both direct and reflex peripheral or sympathetic trunk stimulation of autonomic activity. See **psychogalvanic response.**

sympathetic system The division of the autonomic nervous system originating in the hypothalamus, its second-order neurons departing from the spinal cord through white rami exclusively at thoracic and upper lumbar levels and then running to relay in ganglia of the sympathetic chain.

Galen had recognized the existence of the structure that **Willis** called the *intercostal nerves.* The current name was first applied by Winslow in 1732, when he described the nerves to the heart and gastrointestinal tract as sympathetic because they regulated the "sympathies" of the body using nervous energy.[2764] Their anatomy was well delineated by Dr. Benjamin Kent in his 1831 thesis presented to Edinburgh University. In 1885 Gaskell noted that the three outflows (bulbar, thoracolumbar, and sacral) are organized into two antagonistic systems, and named them the *involuntary nervous system.* The term **autonomic nervous system** was the invention of Langley in 1889.

sympathotonic orthostatic hypotension A syndrome in which receptor insensitivity leads to orthostatic hypotension accompanied by tachycardia, without other evidence of central or peripheral nervous system disease.[4477]

symphysis pubis reflex Contraction of the lower abdominal muscles in response to a tap over the symphysis pubis. If the stimulus is applied more laterally, the hip adductors may also contract (*puboadductor reflex*).[1349a]

symphysis sign See **Brudzinski signs.**

symptomatic diabetic neuropathy A stage of diabetic neuropathy in which any of the features listed in Chart S–20 appear, but not to the extent that they produce **disabling diabetic neuropathy.**

Chart S–20. Features of Symptomatic Diabetic Neuropathy

Motor

  1. Symptoms of muscle weakness in acts of daily living

Sensory

  1. Absence of feeling: reported deficiency of tactile, thermal, or nociceptive sensation encountered in acts of daily living

2. Sensory ataxia: reported unsteadiness in walking
3. Numbness or paresthesia ("dead asleep," "prickly asleep," "like hand gone asleep," "tightly bound feeling," etc.), judged by its distribution, persistence, and duration to be due to neuropathy and not due to physiological compression, as occurs in acts of daily living or entrapment syndromes
4. Neuropathic pain: burning, aching, excessive discomfort of feet or hands with use, and lancinating pain

Autonomic

Any of the following symptoms due to diabetes mellitus and not to medications, psychologic disturbance, intercurrent illness, disease of the organ, or previous injury or surgery: gastric atony; urinary retention; urinary incontinence; rectal incontinence; diarrhea; impotence in males <65 years of age, postural hypotension, light-headedness, or fainting (with postural decrease of systolic BP >30 mmHg)[1568]

Adapted from Dyck PJ. Detection, characterization and staging of polyneuropathy: asseses in diabetics. Muscle Nerve 1988;11:21–32. © 1988. Reprinted by permission of John Wiley and Sons, Inc.

symptomatic generalized epilepsies and syndromes Epilepsies most often occurring in infancy and childhood, and characterized by generalized seizures with clinical and EEG features different from those of idiopathic generalized epilepsies. There may be only one type, but more often there are several, including myoclonic jerks, tonic seizures, atonic seizures, and atypical absences. The EEG expression is bilateral but less rhythmic than that seen in idiopathic generalized epilepsies, and it is more or less asymmetrical.

The interictal EEG abnormalities differ from those of idiopathic generalized epilepsies, appearing as suppression bursts, hypsarrhythmia, slow spike–waves, or generalized fast rhythms. Focal abnormalities may be associated with any of the above. There are clinical, neuropsychological and neuroradiologic signs of a usually diffuse, specific, or nonspecific encephalopathy. (From the revised ILAE Classification,[1114] reproduced by kind permission from Blackwell Science.)

"*Symptomatic seizures or epilepsies*"[1115] are seizures arising as a consequence of known or suspected cerebral dysfunction.

symptomatic internal carotid artery The internal carotid artery supplying the territory of that eye or that side of the brain manifesting dysfunction due to ischemia.[2416]

The actual internal carotid artery might not, however, actually be the site of the causal pathology; for example, the middle cerebral artery is the site of the lesion in some cases.

symptomatic migraine Headaches that fulfill the Internationa Headache Society diagnostic criteria but that are considered to arise as a result of the presence of such disorders as meningioma or hydrocephalus.

symptomatic myoclonus See **myoclonus.**

synalgies See **referred itch.**

synapse The term of Foster and Sherrington (1897) for their functional conception of the structure that forms the junction of two or more neurons. This represented the final seal of approval of the neuron theory, contradicting the idea that neurons are in substantial continuity.

Sherrington had considered *syndesm*, but abandoned that name in favour of synapse (from Gr, a clasp), as advised by Verrall, a Greek scholar with whom he was acquainted.

synaptic dysgenesis The abnormal formation of synapses as a result of environmental insults or defective genetic control of neuronal proliferation and differentiation.[417]

synaptosomes Specialized sites in the membranes of cells adapted for the reception of nerve transmission.

synchysis scintillans Showers of glistening particles composed of cholesterol, falling within the eye with ocular movement.

synchronized fibrillation See **complex repetitive discharge.**

synchronized sleep Non–rapid eye movement sleep, in which the EEG shows waveforms are more regular or sinusoidal in all areas.

synchrony The simultaneous occurrence of EEG waves over regions on the same or opposite sides of the head.

synclonus (Gr, together + great shaking) Continuous repetitive contractions of muscle groups.

syncopal migraine See **basilar migraine.**

syncope (Gr, a cutting short) A transient reduction in consciousness due to global diminution in cerebral perfusion and accompanied by visual and postural impairments. The most common causes are excessive vagal tone leading to bradycardia (vasovagal, vasodepressor or **reflex syncope**) and, in the elderly, orthostatic hypotension or cardiac dysrhythmias. Various specific types have been named according to their antecedent causes, such as **swallow, micturition, defecation, cardiac, respiratory,** and **cough syncope** as well as the **carotid sinus syndrome.** See also **neurocardiogenic syncope, oculocardiac reflex.**

Differentiation from seizures may be difficult since multifocal and generalized myoclonus, incontinence, head injury, tonic body extension, automatisms, vocalizations, eye deviations, and visual and auditory hallucinations can occur in both conditions. With syncope, however, the predominant movement pattern consists of multifocal arrhythmic jerks in proximal and distal muscles, generalized myoclonus being frequently superimposed. Head turns, oral automatisms, and righting movements are also common. The eyes usually remain open and initial upward deviation is usual. Such motor elements have led to the use of the term *convul-*

sive syncope; it occurs in about 10% of syncopal episodes, especially those that are vasovagal in origin.[3341,3342]

syndactylic craniovertebral anomalies   A group of syndromes linked by the common characteristics of syndactyly and premature fusion of the cranial sutures. See **craniosynostosis.**

syndrome   (Gr, to run with, or together) "A group of symptoms constantly associated in a particular disease and together presenting a characteristic picture of that disease or condition".[5204]

In philosophical terms, a syndrome is a chain of physiological processes which, when interrupted, produces the same impairment of bodily functions, as opposed to it occurring as a result of specific disease factors. Thus a further definition might be: a recurrent association of clinical signs for which a single pathogenesis or localization may be postulated.

Some syndromes are eponymic, some descriptive. The first use of the word was in Copland's translation of Galen.[1563]

syndrome de spasmes en flexion   See **flexor spasms.**

syndrome of approximate answers   See **Ganser syndrome.**

syndrome of Bonnet and Bonnet   See **superior orbital fissure syndrome.**

syndrome of caudal regression   See **caudal regression syndrome.**

syndrome of Charles Bonnet   (ophthalmopathic hallucinations) See **Bonnet syndrome.**

syndrome of inappropriate ADH secretion   (SIADH, Schwartz syndrome) Excessive, nonphysiological secretion of antidiuretic hormone by the posterior pituitary, in the absence of the usual stimuli of hyperosmolality or hypervolemia, leading to dilutional hyponatremia as a result of impaired water excretion at a time that sodium excretion is normal.

Essential diagnostic features include hyponatremia, hypo-osmolality of the serum, inappropriately high urinary osmolality, normovolemia, and urinary sodium levels >20 mEq/L in the presence of normal acid base and potassium balance and normal renal, adrenal, and thyroid function.

Clinically, it presents with fatigue, anorexia, headache, nausea, and vomiting, progressing, if untreated, to a confusional state, agitated delirium, convulsions, coma, and death.[4774] The condition may complicate many neurological diseases affecting both the central and peripheral nervous systems, or it may occur as a paraneoplastic syndrome or as a reaction to certain drugs.

syndrome of Jacobson's nerve and plexus   See **tympanic neuropathy.**

syndrome of Mount and Reback   See **familial paroxysmal dystonic choreoathetosis.**

syndrome of Rochon–du Vigneau   See **orbital pseudotumor syndrome.**

syndrome of the basilar communicating artery of Percheron   See **paramedian diencephalic syndrome.**

syndrome of the cerebral peduncle   See **Weber syndrome.**

syndrome of the corpus striatum   See **Vogt syndrome.**

syndrome of the decussation   See **hemiplegia cruciata.**

syndrome of the interpeduncular space   Bilateral third cranial nerve palsies with quadriparesis, due to large central mesencephalic lesions, or to others affecting the cerebral peduncles bilaterally.

syndrome of the mesencephalic artery   See **top of the basilar syndrome.**

syndrome of the mesencephalic gray matter   (aqueduct syndrome, Lyle syndrome) A periaqueductal lesion causing bilateral third cranial nerve palsy, bilateral mydriasis, somnolence, and vertical nystagmus or gaze palsy. Irritative phenomena may include miosis and convergence spasms. See **mesoencephalothalamic syndrome.**

syndrome of the neural crest   See **neural crest, hereditary sensory and autonomic neuropathy.**

syndrome of the paramedian thalamic arteries   Sudden alteration of consciousness followed by fluctuating hypersomnia and bilateral ophthalmoplegia due to asymmetric, paramedian thalamic, and midbrain lesions as a result of emboli to the rostral basilar artery originating from a fibrillating heart.[568]

syndrome of the posterior commissure   External ophthalmoplegia due to a central mesencephalic lesion; the association of a reduction in conjugate upward gaze movements with lid retraction (**Collier** sign), gaze disturbances including spasm and retraction nystagmus and frequently impaired saccades on downward gaze, downbeat nystagmus, light-near dissociation of the pupillary reactions, and skew deviation of the eyes. The horizontal movements remain intact. See **Parinaud syndrome.**

syndrome of the posterior-inferior cerebellar artery   See **lateral medullary syndrome.**

syndrome of the sea-blue histiocyte   See **sea-blue histiocytosis.**

syndrome of the thalamoperforating pedicle of Foix and Hillemand   See **paramedian diencephalic syndrome.**

syndrome paralytique unilateral global des nerfs craniens   See **Garcin syndrome.**

synechiae   Intraocular adhesion(s) classified as anterior (iridicorneal) and posterior (iridolenticular).

synergist   A muscle which by its contraction assists the action of an **agonist** muscle, either by stabilizing the joint or by exerting a weaker action in the same direction as that of the agonist.

synergy   (Gr, with + work) The term of **Babinski** for the ability to accomplish simultaneously all of those movements which together are required to execute a purposeful movement. Failure to do so results in **decomposition of movement.**

synesthesia   (Gr, together + perception) A permanent, involuntary spillover of sensory impressions such that stimulation of one sensory channel leads to a perception in another one or more than one. From *synesthetes*, the clause "I see what you're saying" could be taken literally. The condition is reported to have affected the composers Scriabin, Sibelius, and Rimsky-Korsakov, for some of whom certain keys evoked particular colors.[5849]

The condition was reported in 1690 in a studious blind man who perceived sound-induced colored visions, understanding scarlet to be the sound of a trumpet, and again by by Thomas Woolhouse (an English ophthalmologist).[1237] Erasmus Darwin and Isaac Newton next experimented with its production, resulting in the *clavacin oculaire*, an instrument that produces sound and light simultaneously. Modern electronic versions are available.

Clinical examples of synesthesias include geometrically shaped taste and colored smells, but the evocation of colors following the presentation of sounds is the most common form and is known as *chromesthesia*.[1237] In the idiopathic form, non–right-handers predominate; the condition is extant in childhood and may be an autosomal dominant trait with incomplete penetrance. It is more common in women and can probably be localized in the left hemisphere, since many synesthetes display elements of **Gerstmann syndrome** without other neurological abnormalities other than phenomenal memories while mathematical and spatial navigational skills suffer.

The phenomena are distinguished from imagery by five criteria:
1. The sensations are involuntary and insuppressible.
2. They are perceived as external and real.
3. They are discrete and few in number.
4. They are highly memorable.
5. They are accompanied by strong emotion.

Synesthesia can also occur during epileptic seizures involving the hippocampus, with hallucinogenic intoxication, with brainstem lesions, and sometimes following concussion, in which case sudden noises or bright lights may actually cause pain.[1238]

syngnathia with fusion of the gums and jaws   A congenital developmental anomaly in which fusion of the maxilla and mandible is accompanied by facial weakness, microcephaly, nystagmus, hemivertebrae, an atrial septal defect, and mental and developmental delay.[337]

synkinesis   (Gr, together + movement) Involuntary movements made by muscles distant from those being activated voluntarily due to aberrant reinnervation and/or ephaptic transmission, as during recovery after facial neuropathy in some cases.

synkinetic blepharoclonus   A benign, sporadic, or familial condition manifesting blepharoclonus with eye closure, vertical gaze, speech, or postural changes, sometimes with other movement disorders such as tremor, myoclonus, or restless legs.[2789]

synophrys   The condition of hair growth linking the eyebrows across the **glabella;** it is of no known pathological significance, although to the timid it appears mildly threatening.

synoptophore   A device for testing the normal fusion of visual images when these are presented separately to the eyes

syntactic alexia   A failure to recognize relational words in the presence of preserved recognition of substantive words (written in this case), as occurs in **anterior alexia;** the inability to comprehend graphically presented sentences when their meaning depends on the syntax.

Although the condition often occurs with **Broca aphasia,** the usual cause is considered to be a lesion in the dominant supramarginal gyrus.[4815]

syntactic aphasia   The term of Sir Henry **Head** for that form of speech disturbance in which the internal balance of a word as an orderly rhythmic expression is disturbed, and jargon results. Articulation, speech rhythm, and grammaticism are severely affected.[2496] See **Wernicke aphasia.**

syntactic structure   Descriptions of the structural relationships between words in a sentence—the representations of the grammatical pattern of sentence; for example, "The man is going to the store" consists of a noun phrase + auxilliary + verb -*ing* + preposition + noun phrase.[3505]

syntactic transformations   Rules that serve to define the structures of different sentence types in a language and describe the relationships between words, the overall form of sentences, and how simple sentences are changed from one type to another, such as questions, commands, passives, and embedded sentences.

For example, transformations of the sentence "You are holding the boy up" might include: "Are you holding the boy up?" (question); "Hold the boy up" (command); "The boy is being held up by you" (passive); and "I can see that you are holding the boy up" (embedded sentence).[3505]

syntax   The ordering of words, their alteration, and the insertion among them of qualifying words in accordance with a set of grammatical rules peculiar for each language.

synucleopathies   A diverse group of neurodegenerative disorders that share the characteristic of aggregates of the protein α-synuclein in certain vulnerable populations of neurons and glia. The filaments produced are toxic and lead to degeneration in certain brain regions in such conditions as familial **Parkinson disease, dementia of Lewy body type,** and **multisystem atrophy.**[2013]

Synuclein is a member of the nonamyloid component of proteins within the plaques of **Alzheimer disease.** While important in the learning processes of singing birds, its presence within **Lewy bodies** is toxic to neurons in humans. See also **tauopathies.**

syphilis   (Gr, a hog + to love) 1. A wayward shepherd, a character in *Morbus Gallicorum,* a book of poetry published by Girolamo Fracastoro in 1530. The book was described as a call to righteousness and piety as well as a medical text, since in it he described the transmission and manifestations of the disease at some length. The author dedicated the book to the College of Cardinals in Rome. 2. Infection by the spirochete **treponema pallidum,** classified by Kinnier **Wilson,**[6000] as shown in Chart S–21.

Chart S–21. Classification of the Forms of Syphilis

1. **Syphilitic meningitis**
2. *Spinal syphilis*
   Meningomyelitis, leading to any syndrome of myelopathy **Erb-Charcot syndrome** (spinal syphilitic paralysis, a slowly progressive spastic paraparesis)[1693]
   Systematized spinal sclerosis, a pure pyramidal syndrome
   Systemic amyotrophy resembling **amyotrophic lateral sclerosis**
3. *Cerebral syphilis*
   General, a mild dementing or delirious syndrome
   Local (basal, convexity, intracerebral, midbrain), leading to cranial nerve palsies and hydrocephalus, focal signs, or a parkinsonian syndrome
4. *Cerebrospinal syphilis* (disseminated syphilitic sclerosis)
   Any form of cerebral and spinal syphilis in combination such as **tabes dorsalis, general paresis,** or **syphilitic optic atrophy**
5. Syphilitic neuroses
6. **Syphilitic optic atrophy**
7. **Syphilitic neuritis,** syphilitic osteitis

From Wilson, SAK. Neurology. London: Edwin Arnold, 1940.

See also **congenital syphilis, gumma, Erb-Charcot syndrome.**

syphilis serology   (serological tests for syphilis) A set of tests used to confirm syphilitic infection and to measure the activity of the disease.

Nontreponemal tests such as the **Veneral Disease Research Laboratory test** detect nonspecific antibodies (reagins) that react with the lipoidal antigens of *Treponema pallidum* or others produced by interaction with the host.

Treponemal tests detect antibodies that are specific for the organism and include the **FTA-Abs, TPI** and the **TPHA,** or **MHA-TPA.** More recently, specific assays of treponemal immunoglobulin antibodies have become available.

syphilitic amyotrophy   (syphilitic neuritis) A widespread lower motor neuron degeneration with onset in the small hand muscles and radial extensors, occurring in patients with the meningovascular form of tertiary syphilis.

The classic description indicated an absence of myelopathic signs, but the existence of such a syndrome is disputed today, as a lower motor neuron syndrome associated with syphilitic myelopathy (**Erb-Charcot syndrome**) does occur, which must be the same condition.

syphilitic meningitis   Latent, acute, chronic patchy, or generalized inflammation of the spinal or cerebral membranes. See **meningovascular syphilis, syphilitic amyotrophy.**

syphilitic myelitis   See **Erb-Charcot syndrome.**

syphilitic neuritis   See **syphilitic amyotrophy.**

syphilitic optic atrophy   A form of primary optic atrophy characteristically seen alone or in the setting of **tabes dorsalis** or **general paresis** as a manifestation of tertiary **syphilis.** It does not differ from other forms of primary optic atrophy except in its association with **Argyll Robertson pupils.**

syphilitic "osteitis"   A manifestation of congenital **syphilis,** characterized by severe pain in the limb bones with disinclination of the child to move the limb as a result of syphilitic osteochondritis. The condition was described by **Parrot** in 1871.

syphilitic wristdrop   Weakness of the radial extensors of the forearm occurring in the setting of **syphilitic amyotrophy.**[2502]

syringal hemorrhage   Slow bleeding into hydrosyringomyelia, perhaps due to tearing of an intraspinal vein, described first by Gowers in 1904. A condition of extreme rarity.[4413]

syringobulbia   A condition in which brainstem signs are detectable in patients with syringomyelia resulting from distortion of the hindbrain due to pressure differences acting downward upon it. Clefts may extend from the fourth ventricle into the substance of the medulla oblongata, or may occur as a result of upward impulsive fluid movements from the cavity in the cervical cord. Hydrocephalus is commonly associated.

In descending order of frequency, the most common clinical signs are headache, vertigo, dysphonia or dysarthria, facial paresthesias, dysphagia, diplopia, and palatal and lingual palsies.[3976]

syringomeningocele (Gr, a pipe + a membrane + a rupture) Protrusion of a cystic mass composed of the membrane and posterior wall of the dilated central canal of the spinal cord through a spinal defect (spina bifida).

syringomesencephalia A cystic cavity in the CNS extending through the brainstem into the mesencephalon, and possibly representing a diverticulum from the aqueduct. The condition is far less common than syringomyelia or syringobulbia.[4893]

syringomyelia (Gr, a pipe + the marrow) The formation of an elongated fluid-containing cavity running from the center of the spinal cord posterolaterally beside a posterior horn, expanding the cord. The abnormality occurs most often in the cervical or thoracic regions.

The term was first applied by **Chiari** in 1888. Clinically, signs of compromise of the spinothalamic and pyramidal tracts, and of the cord and the anterior horn cells at the levels of the cavity, are the usual features; the triad of dissociated sensory loss, distal arm weakness, and pyramidal signs in the legs is classic. **Gull** gave the first account of the clinical manifestations in 1862.[2329] See also **secondary syringomyelia, hydromyelia.**

A *variant* familial form is also reported.[4040]

syrinx (Gr, a pipe) The fluid-filled abnormal cavity in the spinal cord in the setting of **syringomyelia.** The name was applied by Ollivier d'Angers in 1824, but the condition had been recognized by Estienne in 1546.

system A whole compounded of several parts; a compounding of things assembled to create a complex functioning scheme.

system degenerations 1. Selective atrophy or demyelination of distinct anatomical fiber pathways in the CNS. These may be genetic (e.g., **Friedreich ataxia**) or acquired (e.g., **subacute combined degeneration of the cord, tabes dorsalis**). A more restricted definition is that of Oppenheimer,[4255] who lists autonomic nervous system failure (**idiopathic orthostatic hypotension**), olivopontocerebellar atrophy (**late-onset cerebellar ataxias**), **striatonigral degeneration,** and **dentatorubropallidoluysian atrophy,** to which Baraitser[335] suggests the addition of **pure pallidal atrophy, pallidoluysian atrophy,** and **pallidostriatonigral degeneration.**

2. A heterogeneous group of neurological diseases characterized by cell loss and variable gliosis occurring in one or more neuronal groups (or "systems"). These disorders are characterized by the spontaneous dysfunction and death of certain systems within the nervous system. Almost all are inherited.

The syndromes resulting appear to be the functional result of various combinations of localizable lesions within the neuraxis, including retinal degeneration, optic atrophy, mid-brain lesions with pupillary dysreflexia, or progressive external ophthalmoplegia; atrophy of the cerebellar nuclei, pons, or olives; degeneration of the cochleas, the posterior columns, the spinocerebellar or the pyramidal tracts, the anterior horn cells or roots, or the dorsal ganglion cells.[1062] See also **multisystem atrophies.**

systemic achromic nevus See **hypomelanosis of Ito.**

systemic angiomatosis See **Ullmann syndrome.**

systemic carnitine deficiency A fatal disorder of lipid metabolism in which the effects of carnitine deficiency include recurrent attacks of metabolic encephalopathy (resembling that of **Reye syndrome**), hypoketotic hypoglycemia, cardiomyopathy, and a proximal lipid-storage myopathy with muscle weakness and failure to thrive. Carnitine levels in red cells, muscle, and liver are low, and those in the serum are variable.[2938,4619] See **carnitine deficiency.**

systemic histiocytosis See **histiocytosis.**

systemic late infantile lipidosis See **GM$_1$ gangliosidosis.**

systemic lupus erythematosus A relapsing and remitting multisystem inflammatory disease of unknown cause, characterized by dermal, vascular, serosal, and neural manifestations.

The American Rheumatological Association has suggested the following criteria, any four of which must be present for the diagnosis to be made:[5479] malar skin rash; discoid photosensitivity; oral or nasal ulceration; non-erosive peripheral polyarthritis; pleurisy or pericarditis; renal disorder (with proteinuria or cellular casts); neuropsychiatric disorder; hematological disorder (hemolytic anemia, leukopenia, lymphopenia, thrombocytopenia); immunological disorder (LE cells, anti-DNA antibodies, anti-sM antibodies, false-positive test for syphilis); and antinuclear antibody.

The neurological features more commonly reported reflect the effects of widespread vasculitis or of scattered demyelination and include cognitive dysfunction; seizures; focal stroke-like syndromes; psychoses and affective disorders; diffuse encephalopathy; cranial neuropathy; retinal vasculitis; papilledema; brainstem disorders; chorea, parkinsonism, or ataxia; headache; aseptic meningitis; transverse myelopathy; syndromes resembling almost any form of multiple sclerosis; and multiple mononeuropathy or polyneuropathy.[62,3895]

systemic mastocytosis A generalized disorder with headaches and autonomic features such as hypotension, flushing, and lacrimation as potential neurological complications.[3131] See **mastocytosis.**

systemic sclerosis   See **progressive systemic sclerois.**

systemic necrotizing vasculitis   See **polyarteritis nodosa.**

systemic vasculitic neuropathy   A multiple mononeuropathy resulting from multifocal vasculitis causing occlusion of epineurial arterioles.[1570]

Szabo sign   Diminished sensation in only one small cutaneous nerve territory at a time in patients with sciatic nerve lesions. The sign was described by a Hungarian physician whose other contributions are less well recorded.

T

T wave   A compound muscle action potential evoked from a muscle by rapid stretch of its tendon, as part of the muscle stretch reflex.[146]

T1 spin-lattice   (longitudinal relaxation time). A term in MRI for the characteristic time constant for spins to achieve an equilibrium alignment, returning to their original position within the external magnetic field. In the case of water, this may be as long as 500 msec.

T1 weighting   (inversion-recovery) An MRI image generated by a pulse sequence that does not allow the magnetization of the tissues of interest to attain their equilibrium values. Contrast in the image is determined by the differential T1 values of the tissues, with short T1 tissues, such as fat, appearing bright. The grayscale brightness is inversely proportional to T1. This sequence provides the greatest T1 weighting with a short T1 value. Using this technique, H$^+$ protons (as in water) show as lucencies.[779]

T2 spin-spin   (transverse relaxation time) The characteristic time constant for the loss of phase coherence among proton spins, due to lack of homogeneity of the magnetic field. It is from to interactions between the spins, with resulting decay of the transverse magnetization and the MRI signal. This is much shorter than the T1 time constant, and is usually less than 100 msec.

T2-weighted image   (spin-echo) An MRI image generated by a pulse sequence with a long repetition time and long echo time, so that only those tissues with a sufficiently long T2 value will still have any remaining transverse magnetization to contribute to the signal. Using this technique, H$^+$ protons (as in water) are bright.

When the TE value is extended beyond 100 msec, the image obtained is referred to as a *heavily T2-weighted image*. This gives improved demonstration of brain lesions, tumor, and edema because of the longer T2 values relative to normal brain.[779]

tabes dorsalis   (Lat, wasting + back) Wasting (of the dorsal columns), the most noticeable pathological abnormality in the most common form of tertiary neurosyphilis, much more commonly seen in men. It is characterized clinically by a triad of symptoms (lightning pains, ataxia, and urinary incontinence with dysuria) and a second triad of signs (Argyll Robertson pupils, areflexia, and loss of joint position sense), but also by other acute (lightning) pains (**crises**),[979] paresthesias, patchy sensory loss, deafness, impotence, and rectal incontinence and by optic atrophy, Charcot joints, painless perforating ulcers of the feet, ptosis, and oculomotor palsies. The CSF is usually abnormal.[5172]

Although **Romberg** had described the condition well in 1846, the term was first applied by **Remak**.[4657] That tabes is a form of syphilis was the initially controversial opinion (1876) of Jean Alfred Fournier (1832–1914), a French physician.

The major damage is incurred by the large dorsal root ganglion cells, the central processes of which run in the posterior columns; their atrophy led to the name given. **Duchenne** (1858) called it *locomotor ataxia;* his description[1535] was so complete that the condition was known as *Duchenne disease* for many years.

Many signs once regarded as specific for tabes (**Frankel, Gowers, Pitres, Remak, Sarbo, Westphal**) are no longer considered to be so. The lightning pains and arthropathies were first recorded by **Charcot** and Bouchard in 1866[979] and Delamarre described gastric crises in the same year. The arthropathy was described independently in 1869 by the English physician Thomas Clifford Allbutt (1836–1925).

tabetic ciliary neuralgia   See **Pel crises.**

tache cérébrale   Excessive dermal hyperemia along the track scratched by a finger, described by **Trousseau** in the setting of meningitis, but in fact not specific to that condition.

tachistoscope   A device for the instantaneous presentation of visual images.

tachyphemia   See **cluttered speech.**

tachyphylaxis   (Gr, fast + guard) Increasing tolerance to the pharmacological effect of a drug.

tactile   (Lat, touching) Of or to do with the sense of touch.

tactile agnosia   (agraphesthesia) Loss of the power of appreciating size, shape and form in three dimensions, as well as consistence and texture,[2498] due to a lesion in the contralateral hemisphere which is usually postrolandic.

tactile aphasia   The inability to name objects felt by one hand or foot, although they can be named when heard or seen, in the presence of normal spontaneous speech. This represents a disconnection syndrome in which somatesthetic impulses fail to cross to the opposite hemisphere because of a lesion in the anterior part of the corpus callosum.[2080]

tactile apraxia   Impairment of hand movements for the use of and interaction with an object, in the presence of preserved intransitive movements.[3138] See **apraxia.**

tactile discrimination   The ability to recognize unseen objects by touch. It is usually tested on the hands or fingers with a two-point discriminator or a pair of compasses, but figure-writing on the palms tests the same function. Loss of tactile discrimination in the absence of peripheral or spinal lesions suggests damage to the contralateral parietal lobe. See also **direction of scratch test.**

tactile form recognition test   A test of visual perceptual function in which the subject touches an unseen cutout of a shape and must then select the matching figure from a group of visually presented drawings.[474]

tactile hallucinations   (haptic hallucinations) Hallucinations of touch; an uncommon phenomenon in the settings of partial epilepsy or delirious states. See **haptic hallucinations.**

tactile perception of direction   (direction of scratch) A specific sensory function of the dorsal columns, which appears to be alone in providing a centripetal pathway that transmits impulses concerning the direction of a moving cutaneous stimulus. Clinical findings suggest that the length of the scratch should be 2 cm.[2415] although 2 mm can usually be discerned on the palms. See **direction of scratch test.**

tactile perseveration   Continued perception of a tactile stimulus after its removal; a sign of right parietal lobe lesions.

tactile projection   See **projection.**

tacts   Comments made about external stimuli.[1178] See also **mands.**

tadpole pupil   Intermittent spasm of one segment of the pupillodilator muscle, causing the pupil to assume a comma-shaped appearance. The pupil is often of the **springing** type. The condition is benign.[5566]

Takayasu disease   See **aortic arch disease.**

talantropia   See **pendular nystagmus.**

talipes equinovarus   (Lat, to walk on the ankles) Clubfoot.

Talma disease   (myotonia acquisita) Myotonia occurring for the first time in adult life, without a positive family history.[5476]

Talma, Sape   (1847–1918) Dutch surgeon and physician who graduated from Utrecht and practiced in that city as professor of pathological anatomy or medicine.

Tamari-Goodman upper limb–cardiovascular syndrome   A congenital dysmorphic syndrome characterized also by short stature, strabismus, kyphosis, atrial septal defect, pulmonary stenosis, winged scapulae, radioulnar synostosis, microcephaly, and mental and developmental delay.[337]

Tamminga marfanoid syndrome with leukodystrophy   A congenital dysmorphic syndrome characterized also by tall stature; ocular, cardiac, and skeletal

anomalies; hypotonia; cerebral atrophy; hydrocephalus; and mental and developmental delay.[337]

tandem Romberg test   The subject stands with one foot directly in front of the other with the arms folded and the eyes closed. A normal subject can maintain this position for at least 5 seconds. Failure to do so indicates impairment of conscious proprioception.

tangent screen   A piece of black material, upon which a grid is faintly marked and with a central point for gaze fixation. Hand-held stimuli are brought in from the periphery toward the center by the examiner, allowing charting of the central 25° of the visual field.

Tangier disease   (analphalipoproteinemia, high-density lipoprotein deficiency) An inherited clinically heterogeneous multisystem disease with two main forms:

1. A slowly progressive peripheral neuropathy, clinically resembling syringomyelia with dissociated sensory loss and facibrachial weakness
2. Prominent but relapsing-remitting multiple mononeuropathies[1676]

Both varieties are characterized by hepatosplenomegaly, diarrhea, tonsillar enlargement, and low serum cholesterol and α-lipoprotein levels, but raised triglycerides.

The name comes from the small island in Chesapeake Bay (United States) where the disorder was first recognized by Fredrickson in 1961.[1939,4485]

tapetoretinal degeneration   A form of retinal pigmentary degeneration, usually dominantly inherited but expressed more commonly in boys, who complain of impaired twilight vision (**nyctalopia**) which progresses in some cases to blindness.

Tapia, Antonio Garcia   (1875–1950) Spanish otolaryngologist in Madrid, who in 1904 described the syndrome named for him, his patient being a matador who had suffered an occupational injury.

Tapia syndrome   (ambiguohypoglossal paralysis) Unilateral damage to the ninth, tenth and eleventh cranial nerves in the brainstem, usually as a result of vascular disease, or due to lesions at the base of the skull or in the retroparotid space, such as infiltration by tumors.[5490] Paralysis of the pharynx, larynx and tongue results but the trapezius and sternomastoid are spared. However, some instances of Tapia syndrome (possibly including Tapia's original case) may be the result of dissection of the external carotid artery, thus signifying imminent endangerment of the internal carotid artery as well.[2870a]

Differentiation between the syndromes of **Avellis, Collet, Jackson, Schmidt, Tapia,** and **Vernet** is an exercise in grand roundsmanship but is clinically irrelevant.[4986]

tapping test   1. A test of repetitive motor abilities using agonist and antagonistic muscles. The subject is required to tap the wrist, elbow, and shoulder and then with the ankle, knee, and hip on each side with his or her finger, the number of taps completed at each site on each side in 30 seconds being counted. 2. The subject is asked to tap out rhythms, such as groups of double or triple taps, changing between them on command. Difficulty in executing the taps rhythmically suggests a lesion of (usually the left) prefrontal area.

tarantism See **dancing mania.**

Tarchanov phenomenon See **psychogalvanic reflex.**

tardive akathisia (Lat, late + Gr, not sitting) A form of chronic **akathisia** that occurs at a late stage of neuroleptic therapy, coinciding with a reduction in the dose of the drug.[843]

tardive dyskinesia (cervicolinguomasticatory syndrome, Tarnow-Kulenkampff syndrome) An involuntary movement disorder (dystonic, choreic, or athetotic) complicating the prolonged ingestion of dopamine antagonists such as the butyrophenones, reserpine, or the phenothiazines.[2026]

Research diagnostic criteria have been formulated[4992] and are given in Chart T–1.

Chart T–1. Diagnostic Criteria for Tardive Dyskinesia

Prerequisites

1. A history of at least 3 months total cumulative neuroleptic exposure, continuous or discontinuous (Patients who have failed to meet this criterion should receive the appropriate diagnosis with the qualification "less than 3 months' neuroleptic exposure".)
2. The presence of at least moderate abnormal involuntary movements in one or more body areas or at least mild movements in two or more body areas (face, lips, jaw, tongue, upper extremities, lower extremities) because of the variability of the movements associated with tardive dyskinesia (TD). If the examination reveals movements that are only minimal or mild in only one body area, the examination should be repeated in 1 week to confirm their presence. Determination of the presence of these movements should be made using a standarized examination procedure and a rating scale such as the **Abnormal Involuntary Movement scale** or the **Tardive Dyskinesia Rating scale.**
3. Absence of other conditions that might produce abnormal involuntary movements

Diagnosis of Clinical Types

1. *Probable tardive dyskinesia* The patient needs three of the above prerequisites.
2. *Masked tardive dyskinesia* The patient meets the criteria for probable TD but within 2 weeks following an increase in dosage in the case of concurrent neuroleptics or reinstitution of neuroleptic treatment in the case of a neu-

roleptic-free patient (movements no longer meet the second prerequisite).
3. *Transient tardive dyskinesia* The patient meets the criteria for probable TD, but, on subsequent examination within 3 months, movements meeting the second prerequisite are no longer observed and neuroleptic treatment has not been reinstituted nor the dose increased.
4. *Withdrawal tardive dyskinesia* The patient does not meet the second prerequisite while receiving neuroleptics, but does so within 2 weeks following their discontinuation. If within 3 months of drug withdrawal the movements meeting the second prerequisite are no longer observed, the diagnosis stands.
5. *Persistent tardive dyskinesia* The patient meets the criteria for probable TD and continues to do so over a 3-month period. The diagnosis may be qualified as "concurrent neuroleptic" if the patient has been receiving the neuroleptics continuously during the 3-month period; as "neuroleptic-free" if the patient has received no neuroleptics during the 3-month period or has met the criteria for withdrawal TD, but the movements meeting the second prerequisite have persisted for at least 3-months with no neuroleptic administration; or as "unspecified" if the patient has received neuroleptics for part but not all of the 3-month period.
6. *Masked persistent tardive dyskinesia* The patient meets the criteria for persistent TD, but, within 3 weeks following an increase in dosage or reinstitution of neuroleptic treatment for movements, no longer meets the second prerequisite.

From Schooler NR, Kane JM. Research diagnoses for tardive dyskinesia. Arch Gen Psychiatry 1982;39:486–487. Copyright, American Medical Association.

Tardive Dyskinesia Rating scale A 43-item scale scoring abnormal movements in five general body areas (face, neck and trunk, upper extremities, lower extremities, and entire body) with an attached list of definitions of the abnormal movements that can occur.[5179]

An abbreviated form of the scale has also been validated; its 16 items examine the periocular areas (blinking, eyelid tremor); lip movements; chewing; the **bonbon sign;** tongue protrusion and tongue tremor; **rabbit syndrome;** axial hyperkinesia; rocking movement; torsion movements; head and neck movements; movements of fingers and wrists, and of ankles and toes; stamping movements; repetitive thumb movements; and **akathisia.**

Tardive Dyskinesa/Tardive Dystonia National Association A charitable organization providing support and information on this condition. Address: 4244 University Way, NE, P.O. Box 45732, Seattle, WA 98145-0732. Tel: 206–522–3166.

tardive dystonia 1. Persistent late-onset dystonia occurring as a result of the ingestion of antipsychotic drugs at least within the previous 2 months, in the absence of a positive family history of dystonia and of evidence of any other known cause. Opisthotonos, retrocollis, torticollis, scoliosis, and isolated limb dystonias have been the movements described.[841,5478] 2. The same, occurring after head injury.

tardive myoclonus   Sudden brief, shock-like movements, occurring singly or repetitively, after a period of treatment with dopamine receptor blocking drugs.

tardive stereotypy   A common form of **tardive dyskinesia** characterized by involuntary, patterned, repetitive, continuous, coordinated, purposeless, or ritualistic movements, postures, or utterances, occurring after prolonged treatment with dopamine receptor blocking agents.[5308] See also **stereotypy.**

tardive tremor   An involuntary oscillatory movement disorder, the tremor having a frequency range of 3–5 Hz, appearing at all times but especially during maintenance of a posture and induced by long-term neuroleptic treatment. Other tardive movement disorders (see previous entries) are also frequently present.[5309]

tardy ulnar palsy   Ulnar nerve paresis developing slowly after trauma to that nerve at the elbow. See **cubital tunnel syndrome.**

target fibers   Myofibrils, usually of type 1, found in ATPase preparations, in which a densely stained ring of tissue is interposed between an inner core, which does not take up the stain, and a normally stained outer ring of tissue. The appearance is due to streaming of the Z-disk material and to alterations in the distribution of muscle enzymes.

The fibers represent a variant of the muscle **cores** seen in slowly progressive denervating diseases, in which there appear three concentric zones composed of a central mass, a light halo, and a surrounding region of normal myofibrils. They are most commonly seen in slowly progressive denervating diseases and after tenotomy.[1674]

Tarlov cyst   A perineurial cyst compressing the sacral roots and capable of causing sciatic pain.[5491]

Tarnow-Kulenkampff syndrome   (cervicolinguomasticatory syndrome) See **tardive dyskinesia.**

tarsal tunnel syndrome   Compression of the posterior tibial nerve in the fibro-osseous compartment beneath the flexor retinaculum at the medial malleolus, leading to complaints of pain, weakness, and sensory loss in the distribution of one or all of the three branches (medial, lateral plantar, calcaneal) of that nerve.[1609] In the *anterior* form of the syndrome, there is pain and sensory loss in the distal parts of the dorsum of the foot. The *posterior* type presents with pain in the sole of the foot. Entrapment of the medial calcaneal branch leads to chronic pain in the heel.

The electrodiagnostic features have been described.[1364]

tarsophalangeal response   See **dorsal foot response.**

Tarui disease   (phosphofructokinase deficiency) See **glycogen storage diseases.**

task-specific tremor   Tremor of the limbs occurring during the performance of specific activities, such as writing (**primary writing tremor**). Other task-specific tremors include the **yips** observed in golfers, while tremors occurring in musicians may be associated with the later appearance of signs of essential tremor or of **Parkinson disease.**[2898] See also **tremor.**

taste disorders   See **ageusia, dysgeusia.**

Tatasuki syndrome   See **POEMS.**

tau (τ) protein   A microtubule-associated protein capable of aggregating and accumulating within the microtubules, causing metabolic dysfunction, which is expressed pathologically as neurofibrillary tangles. Various dementia syndromes are associated with the many mutations of the gene that have been described. See **tauopathies.**

tauopathies   Conditions associated with the presence of mutated tau protein; they include *dementia lacking distinctive histopathology* and *progressive subcortical gliosis* (**frontotemporal dementia** linked to chromosome 17 with the dementia-predominant or the parkinsonism-predominant phenotype); **Alzheimer** and **Pick** diseases, variant **Creutzfeldt-Jakob disease, corticobasal degeneration,** and **progressive supranuclear palsy.** See also **synucleopathies.** Other conditions with defined tau pathology are reviewed by Delacourte and Buée (2000)[1352] and by Arvanitakis and Wszolek (2001).[225]

Hallervorden-Spatz disease, postencephalitic parkinsonism, dementia pugilistica, Down syndrome, subacute sclerosing panencephalitis, parkinsonism-dementia complex of Guam, Niemann-Pick disease type C, some forms of **muscular dystrophy,** and **inclusion body myositis** are other conditions in which tau pathology is found.

Tay sign   The cherry-red foveal spot seen in certain **gangliosidoses.**[5503] The term *cherry-red spot*, however, originated with Herman Knapp, a New York ophthalmologist.

Tay syndrome   (ichthyosiform erythroderma) A recessively inherited dysmorphic syndrome, characterized also by congenital ichthyosis, dermal atrophy, brittle hair, physical and mental retardation, hypogonadism, and frequently skin photosensitivity. Neurological complications are variable, but may include microcephaly, intracerebral calcifications, seizures, and pyramidal and cerebellar signs.

The condition was originally reported from Singapore,[5501] but is not confined to the Orient.

Tay, Warren (1843–1927) English ophthalmologist who trained at the London Hospital, where he was later appointed to the staff. He was also surgeon at Moorfields Eye Hospital and thus a colleague of Jonathan **Hutchinson.**

In 1880 he described the ocular findings in the disease named in part for him, in the first volume of the *Transactions of the London Ophthalmological Society*, of which he was a founding member.

Warren Tay

Taybi syndrome A form of generalized skeletal dysplasia, manifesting also mental retardation, small stature, conductive deafness, thin frontal skull, hypotelorism, cleft palate, and limited extension of the elbows.[5504] See **oropalatodigital syndrome.**

Taybi-Rubinstein syndrome See **Rubinstein-Taybi syndrome.**

Tay-Sachs disease See **GM$_2$ gangliosidosis.**

tea party epilepsy Seizures occurring as a result of hyponatremia induced by excessive water intake, as in primary polydipsia.[4467] The same syndrome has been observed in the residents of Labrador and Scandinavia as a result of the excessive consumption of low sodium–containing beer. See **hyponatremic encephalopathy.**

teakettle calves The appearance of the calves in pseudohypertrophic muscular dystrophy (Sir William **Gowers**).

tectocerebellar dysraphia with encephalocele A congenital dysmorphic syndrome, manifesting also ventricular septal defect, encephalocele, hydrocephalus, cerebellar lesions and neuronal heterotopias.[337]

tectorial (Lat, covering or roofing over) Covering like a roof.

tectorial membrane Part of the cochlea in which the cilia of the hair cells are embedded.

tectospinal tract (Lowenthal's tract [or bundle], predorsal bundle) An extrapyramidal motor pathway first identified by Wilhelm Lowenthal (1850–1894), a German physician.[4001]

tectum (Lat, a roof) A lid or roof.

tegmen (Lat, a covering) A covering or coating.

tegmental mesencephalic paralysis See **Benedikt syndrome.**

tegmental syndrome See **Benedikt syndrome.**

teichopsia (Gr, *teichos*, a wall + seeing) The experience of visual hallucinations as part of the migraine aura, in which blurred vision leads to bilateral homonymous paracentral scotomata which expand with a jagged edge, likened to the plan of some northern European medieval castles. The term was introduced by Dr. Hubert Airy in 1870.

Tel-Hashomer camptodactyly A recessively inherited, congenital dysmorphic syndrome characterized also by dwarfism, frontal bossing, telecanthus, high-arched palate, winged scapulae, abnormal palmar creases, camptodactyly, syndactyly, clubfoot, joint laxity, brachycephaly, absent muscles, and myopathic muscle atrophy.[2197]

The condition was described in Jewish children of Bedouin descent; the name is that of the hospital in Israel where it was identified.[2764]

tela choroidea (Lat, a web + Gr, membrane) The layer of pia mater inside the ventricles forming the choroid plexus.

telangiectasia (Gr, the end + a vessel + an extension) A congenital dilatation of capillaries and other small vessels.

telecanthus (Gr, far + corner of the eye) A congenital malformation consisting of an increase in the distance between the medial canthi, as commonly seen with **Waardenburg syndrome, meningoencephalocele** or **blepharophimosis.**[4]

telegrammatism See **telegraphic speech.**

telegraphic speech (telegrammatism) That type of aphasic speech or writing in which propositions, articles, and conjunctions tend to be omitted, while nouns, verbs, and adjectives (which are usually more concrete in their nature) tend to be spared; thus, the type of speech which results after the sacrifice of the shorter terms, which are less heavily charged with reference, function, or meaning.[1172]

Such agrammatical, nonfluent speech resembles the typical style used in telegrams, only the words with the highest substantive content being included and the filler words that form the grammatical mesh being omitted. The same form of speech is beloved of Hollywood dialogue experts when writing parts for native people ("Me write more book"). See **agrammatism.**

telegraphist's cramp   A focal (occupational) dystonia. See **occupational cramp.**

telencephalon   (Gr, end + brain) The cerebrum.

telencephalosynapsis   See **holoprosencephaly.**

teleopsia   A visual distortion, in which objects appear to have receded into the distance. When unilateral, local retinal disease or chiasmal diseases are usually found, but when bilateral, temporal lobe lesions are the most common pathology.

teleorbitism   See **hypertelorism.**

television epilepsy   One of the more common types of **photosensitive epilepsy.** *Video game epilepsy* is a small-screen variant.

Telfer syndrome   A dominantly inherited cochleo-vestibular atrophy characterized by variable depigmentation of the skin, white forelocks, mild deafness, mental retardation, and ataxia.[5519]

temperature sensation   A misnomer, since, between the limits of a physiological range (21°–38°C), the body registers not absolute temperature but the rate of loss or gain of heat.

temple   (from Lat, temple) The anterior portion of the lateral side of the head. Hair in this region is the first to go gray and, as the Greeks considered time to be an isolated portion of eternity, and the temple a place where a blow might well be fatal, the structures in this area are called *temporal.* The word has been in use in English for some 700 years.

temporal arteritis   See **giant cell arteritis.**[933] The alternative term is preferred in recognition of the fact that involvement of the temporal arteries in this condition is the least serious complication of a disorder that can involve any or all branches of the carotid system.

temporal crescent   The extreme temporal peripheral field, with only monocular representation, in the occipital lobe. It extends some 45° further laterally than the binocular field, which subtends about 120° horizontally. Nasal retinal and postgeniculate lesions lead to impairment of vision in this region, best identified with Goldman perimetry.

temporal dispersion   Relative desynchronization of components of a compound muscle action potential due to different rates of conduction of each synchronously evoked component from the stimulation point to the recording electrode. It may be due to normal variability in individual axon conduction velocities, especially when assessed over a long nerve segment, or to disorders that affect myelination of nerve fibers. (From the 2001 Report of the Nomenclature Committee of the American Association of Electromyography and Electrodiagnosis.[10] Used by permission, copyright © 2001, AAEM.)

temporal lobe epilepsy   See **temporal lobe syndromes.**

Temporal Lobe Rating scale   A system for assessing localized atrophy on MRI scans.[2012]

temporal lobe syndromes   (temporal lobe epilepsy) A seizure syndrome characterized by simple partial seizures, complex partial seizure, and secondarily generalized seizures, or any combination of these. Their onset is frequently in childhood or young adult life. The seizures occur in clusters at intervals or randomly; frequently there is a history of febrile seizures.

On metabolic imaging (e.g., positron emission tomography), hypometabolism is frequently observed. Uni- or bilateral temporal lobe spikes are common on EEGs. Memory deficits may occur.

Features which, when present, are strongly suggestive of the diagnosis include:

1. Simple partial seizures which are typically characterized by autonomic and/or psychic symptoms and certain sensory phenomena such as olfactory and auditory hallucinations or illusions. Most common are the often rising epigastric sensation (the **epigastric aura**) and déjà vu phenomena.
2. Complex partial seizures which often (but not always) begin with motor arrest, typically followed by oroalimentary automatisms; other automatisms frequently follow. They typically last longer than 1 minute. Recovery is gradual, often with postictal confusion and amnesia for the ictal events. *Amygdalohippocampal* and *lateral temporal* varieties are defined on the basis of EEG and surgical studies.[1114]

In interictal periods, the subject may have no psychiatric morbidity, but, in a few cases, a schizophrenia-like psychosis occurs[5208] and psychosis may also arise after temporal lobectomy.[3586] Facial asymmetries are described,[4658] but there are seldom other neurological signs peculiar to the more common temporal lobe lesions causing seizures.

Electroencephalographic characteristics are also used to make the diagnosis. The interictal scalp EEG may show:

1. No abnormality
2. Slight or marked asymmetry of the background activity
3. Temporal spikes, sharp waves, and/or slow waves, which are unilateral or bilateral, and usually synchronous but also asynchronous. These findings are not always confined to the temporal region.
4. In addition to scalp EEG findings, intracranial record-

ings may allow better definition of the intracranial distribution of the interictal abnormalities.

Various EEG patterns may accompany the initial clinical ictal symptomatology, including a unilateral or bilateral interruption of background activity and temporal or multilobar low-amplitude fast activity, rhythmic spikes, or rhythmic slow waves.

The onset of the EEG disturbance may not correlate with the clinical onset, depending on the methodology used. Intracranial recordings may provide additional information regarding the chronological and spatial evolution of the discharges. (Adapted from Commission for Classification and Terminology, ILAE. Proposal for revised classifications of epilepsies and epileptic syndromes. *Epilepsia* 1989;**30**:389–399.[1114]) See also **amygdalo-hippocampal seizures.**

A *variant* is *mesial temporal lobe epilepsy*, the characteristics of which have been defined by Engel.[1672a]

A. History
There is an increased incidence of complicated febrile convulsions or a family history of epilepsy.
  The onset is in the latter half of the first decade of life. Auras are common and occur in isolation.
  Secondarily generalized seizures occur infrequently. Seizures often remit for several years until adolescence or early adulthood, but in time often become medically intractable. Interictal behavioral disturbances can occur (most commonly depression).

B. Clinical seizure
  1. An aura is usually present; most common is epigastric rising, often with other autonomic or psychic symptoms including emotion (e.g., fear). Olfactory or gustatory sensations lasting several seconds are also described.
  2. The complex partial seizures often begin with arrest and stare; oroalimentary automatisms and complex automatisms are also common. Posturing of one upper extremity may occur on the side opposite the ictal discharge and last 1 to 2 minutes.
  3. The postictal phase usually includes disorientation, recent memory deficit, amnesia for the event, and dysphasia if the seizure began in the language-dominant hemisphere, and lasts several minutes.

C. The neurologic examination is generally normal, although recent memory deficit may be detected.

D. EEG
  1. Unilateral or bilateral independent anterior temporal spikes are recorded with their maximum amplitude in the basal electrodes.
  2. There may be intermittent or continuous rhythmic slowing in one mesial temporal area.
  3. Extracranial ictal activity appears only with complex partial symptoms, and usually consists of initial or delayed focal-onset pattern of 5–7/second rhythmic activity with its maximum amplitude in one basal temporal derivation.
  4. Depth electrode studies show that the onset of the ictus is usually with high-amplitude rhythmic spikes or sharp waves. Low-voltage waves or suppression are less common.
  5. Propagation to the contralateral side is slow (>5 seconds, and may be minutes) or may not occur at all.

E. Usual focal functional deficits
  1. Temporal lobe hypometabolism is seen on interictal FDG-PET, often involving the ipsilateral thalamus and basal ganglia as well.
  2. Temporal lobe hypoperfusion is documented on interictal SPECT and there is a characteristic pattern of hypo- and hyperperfusion on ictal SPECT.
  3. Material-specific memory disturbances are shown by neuropsychological testing, and contralateral intracarotid sodium amylobarbitone injection produces amnesia.
  4. Mesial temporal lobe slowing and attenuation of normal rhythms can be seen with scalp/sphenoidal electrodes, but are shown better with depth electrodes. This is exacerbated by IV thiopental administration.

F. Structural imaging
  MRI scans may show a reduction in size of the hippocampus and temporal lobe with enlargement of the temporal horn on one side.

G. Pathophysiology
  1. Hippocampal sclerosis (>30% cell loss with specific patterns)
  2. Sprouting of dentate granule cell mossy fibers
  3. Selective loss of certain hilar neurons (somatostatin and NPY-containing cells)
  4. Hamartomas and heterotopias may occur as dual pathology
  5. Microdysgenesis is common.
  6. Seizures may originate in sclerotic hippocampi but a much larger area appears to be included in the epileptogenic region.

H. Features that cast doubt on the diagnosis
  1. A history of severe head trauma, encephalitis, or other specific causal events
  2. The occurrence of focal motor or specific sensory symptoms at seizure onset or postictally
  3. Interictal focal neurologic deficits
  4. Marked cognitive impairment on neuropsychological testing
  5. Bilaterally synchronous, generalized, or extemporal focal EEG spikes
  6. Diffuse or extratemporal focal EEG slowing
  7. The presence of any cerebral lesion other than hippocampal sclerosis on MRI scans

From Engel J Jr. Update on surgical treatment of the epilepsies. Summary of the Second International Palm Desert Conference on the Surgical Treatment of the Epilepsies (1992). Neurology. 1993;43(8):1612–7, by permission.

temporal lobectomy Resection of the anterior 5–6 cm of a temporal lobe in the treatment of medically intractable complex partial seizures. Other stereotactic or surgical approaches are also available.

temporolimbic epilepsy See **temporal lobe syndromes.**

temporomandibular dysfunction (Costen syndrome [?], Schwartz syndrome, craniomandibular disorder) A painful syndrome arising from dysfunction of the temporomandibular (TM) joint, characterized by facial or jaw pains, tenderness of the masticatory muscles, clicking arising from the TM joints, and restriction of jaw opening. The syndrome has been critically reviewed.[4089]

temporomandibular joint pain A persistent, dull, aching, but sometimes severe pain in the masticatory muscles, worse with mouth opening and chewing, often spreading to involve that side of the face or head.

Temtamy syndrome A dominantly inherited congenital syndrome characterized by brachydactyly, affecting mainly the second and fifth digits of the hand and the lateral four toes.[2764] Obesity, hirsutism, blindness, scoliosis, platyspondyly, sclerosis of the skull, optic atrophy, pendular nystagmus, metaphyseal dysplasia, and skin atrophy have also been described in association.

tenalgia Pain arising from tendons of muscles overtaxed by protracted contraction. See **repetitive strain injury, overuse syndromes.**

tenascin An extracellular matrix glycoprotein expressed predominantly on glioma tissue in the CNS. Its assay may be useful in the evaluation and monitoring of the progress of brain tumors.[6082]

tendinous xanthomatosis See **cerebrotendinous xanthomatosis.**

tendon reflex (deep tendon reflex) See **muscle stretch reflexes.**

That the percussion of a tendon should lead to reflex contraction of that muscle was not appreciated until 1875, when the German physicians **Erb** and **Westphal** each described the phenomenon. Despite the fact that Erb introduced this term, it remains a misnomer, as tendons have no part to play in the generation of the reflex, except for providing a convenient place to hit the patient. See also **deep tendon reflex,** an even worse misnomer.

TENDS See **transient episodes of neurological dysfunction.**

tennis elbow See **lateral epicondylitis.**

tensilon See **edrophonium.**

Tensilon test The observation of a patient with suspected **myasthenia gravis,** who shows fatigability after exercise and who is then given an intravenous injection of edrophonium chloride (Tensilon®; an inhibitor of cholinesterase) in an attempt to reverse the fatigability temporarily.

A 2-mg dose is usually injected first, and, if there are no untoward effects within 2 minutes, more is given, either as one 8-mg dose or as two doses (3 mg followed by 5 mg). Salivation, sweating, and fasciculations are common; hypotension and bradycardia are less common side effects. Cardiac arrhythmias and asthma are contraindications. Atropine should be available in the event of marked bradycardia. Cynics give a placebo dose of saline first.

Improvement in ocular signs is the easiest to assess clinically, though better accuracy is obtained with the **Lancaster red-green test.** Unfortunately, ptosis and oculomotor weakness do not respond to the Tensilon in all cases of **myasthenia gravis.**[1288,5082]

tensilon tonography A test for **myasthenia gravis** in which increased ocular pressure occurs after the intravenous injection of Tensilon (edrophonium chloride) in myasthenic patients as a result of contraction of the extraocular muscles in response to the drug; no such increase is seen in normal subjects.[6046]

tension (-type) headache See **episodic tension-type headache.** A class of headaches subdivided as follows in the International Headache Society Classification:
2.1 **Episodic tension-type headache**
  2.1.1 Episodic tension-type headache associated with disorder of pericranial muscles
  2.1.2 Episodic tension-type headache unassociated with disorder of pericranial muscles
2.2 **Chronic tension-type headache**
  2.2.1 Chronic tension-type headache associated with disorder of pericranial muscles
  2.2.2 Chronic tension-type headache unassociated with disorder of pericranial muscles
2.3 Headache of tension-type not fulfilling above criteria

From Classification of headache disorders, cranial neuralgias and facial pains; and diagnostic criteria for primary headache disorders. *Cephalalgia* 1988;8(suppl): 1–96),[1051] by kind permission of Blackwell Science.

tensor (from Lat, to stretch) A muscle that tightens or stretches a body part.

tensor fascia lata reflex Contraction of this muscle in response to a tap applied at its origin from the anterior superior iliac spine. The reflex informs about the state of the reflex arcs between L4 and S1.

tentorium (Lat, a tent, from Lat, to stretch) The tentorium cerebelli is indeed shaped similarly and forms a roof for the posterior fossa.

ten-twenty system A standardized system of scalp electrode placement recommended by the International Federation of Societies for Electroencephalography and Clinical Neurophysiology. According to this system, electrode placements are determined by measuring the head from external landmarks and taking 10% or 20% of each such measurement. (From Chatrian GE, Bergamini L, Dondey M, et al. A glossary of terms most commonly used by clinical electroencephalographers. *EEG Clin Neurophysiol* 1974;37:538–48,[989] with permission from Elsevier Science.)

tephromalacia The term of **Marie** for softening of the anterior part of the spinal cord in patients thought to have syphilitic arteritis.

teratoid tumor of head or neck See **dermoid cyst.**

teratoma A rare, slowly growing tumor containing a range of tissue components as a result of differentiation along various embryonic lines. They occur mainly in the region of the pineal, in the posterior fossa, or within mixed germ cell tumors.[6]

The term *malignant teratoma* (teratocarcinoma) is used both for embryonal carcinomas and for regions of malignancy within an otherwise well-differentiated teratoma.

terminal innervation ratio (TIR) The ratio of the number of terminals at the distal ends of **neurites** to the number of motor end-plates innervated. The ratio is normally 1:1, but, in the process of regeneration following axonal section, there are temporarily excessive numbers of neurites; in chronic atrophic diseases, the few surviving axons each innervate an unusually large number of motor end-plates. Thus, only a small minority of healthy axons innervate more than one muscle fiber. The innervation ratio increases in the presence of motor neuropathies and in **myotonic dystrophy.**[1067]

The ratio is a histological measurement of axonal branching within muscles; the *absolute TIR* is the number of subterminal motor arborizations arising from a given number of motor axons, and the *functional TIR* is the number of muscle fibers innervated by these axons.

terminal latency The interval between the stimulation of a nerve distally and the muscle's response.

terminal latency index An electrographic measure of demyelination in peripheral nerves, calculated as follows:[135]

$$TLI = \frac{distal\ distance}{(proximal\ conduction\ velocity \times distal\ latency)}$$

terminal transverse with orofacial manifestation Inherited syndromes characterized by the presence of cranial nerve palsies associated with a variety of craniofacial and limb malformations. These include **Möbius syndrome, Duane syndrome,** and single sixth and seventh cranial nerve palsies.[3885]

Terson syndrome Intraocular hemorrhage (retinal, subhyaloid, or vitreous) following a sudden increase in intracranial pressure, as occurs with **subarachnoid hemorrhage** or trauma.[5526]

tertiary position The position of the eyes when they have deviated from the primary position to any position other than that obtaining with pure adduction, abduction, elevation, or depression.

Tesla The preferred unit of measurement of a magnetic field. One Tesla is equal to 10,000 gauss, where the Earth's magnetic field has a strength of about 1 gauss.

Tesla, Nikola Yugoslavian physicist, who worked for much of his life in the United States, mainly in the area of magnetic fields. The units of magnetic field strength are named for him. As a result of his scientific achievements, he was offered the Nobel prize, but refused it.

Test for Severe Impairment A validated measure that is sensitive to cognitive changes in severely demented patients with **Alzheimer disease.**[79]

test types Samples of print of different sizes, standardized such that the smallest print which can be read by a subject allows the assignment of a score that reflects the subject's acuity relative to the normal acuity of the population.

tetanic contraction The contraction produced in a muscle through repetitive maximal direct or indirect stimulation at a sufficiently high frequency to produce a smooth summation of successive maximum twitches. The term may also be applied to maximum voluntary contractions in which the firing frequencies of most or all of the component motor units are sufficiently high that successive twitches of individual motor units fuse smoothly. Their combined tensions produce a steady, smooth, maximum contraction of the whole muscle. (From the 2001 Report of the Nomenclature Committee of the American Association of Electromyography and Electrodiagnosis.[10] Used by permission, copyright © 2001, AAEM.)

tetanic neuromyopathy syndrome Strong tetanic muscle contractions with encephalopathy and myoclonus occurring as part of the syndrome of uremic encephalopathy.[1721]

tetanoid chorea The term of Gowers for **athetosis.**

tetanus 1. Maximal and unphysiological tonic contraction of muscle fibers, as a result of repetitive stimulation of the muscle itself or of its nerve. This was first achieved by Volta in 1792, using electrical stimulation. 2. A disease caused by the exotoxin of *Clostridium tetani* which selectively blocks inhibitory interneuronal transmission in the brainstem and spinal cord. The condition was known in Egypt 3000 years ago and was well described by both Hippocrates and Aretaeus; the nature of the underlying disorder was elucidated by Rosenbeck in 1887.

Clinically, after an incubation period of up to 3 weeks following a breach of the skin or mucosa, the patient manifests muscle rigidity, hyperreflexia, and later strong, painful intermittent spasms in a localized or generalized distribution, involving the agonist and antagonist muscles and precipitated by any form of sensory stimulation initially, though later spontaneous. The spinal extensors and face are particularly affected, the former leading to stiffness of the neck and opisthotonos, and the latter to the *risus sardonicus*. (It should be noted that facial involvement is not a feature of the **stiff-man syndrome.**) Rigidity of the chest and abdominal muscles and laryngeal spasm are other features of note. The muscle spasm and secondary myofibrillar damage may lead to myoglobinuria and renal failure.[1721] The condition itself[1747] and the electrophysiological manifestations of diseases associated with excessive motor unit activity have been reviewed.[261]

Variants include the following:

Chronic tetanus A protracted form of tetanus occurring in partially immune subjects and presenting with risus sardonicus, trismus, and stimulus-sensitive spasms of somatic muscles, and causing denervation with reinnervation of the affected muscles.[4712]

Neonatal tetanus Infants are infected through the umbilical cord, and present within 2 weeks of birth with failure to suck, restlessness, muscle stiffness, opisthotonos, fever, and seizures.

See also **trismus, local tetanus, cephalic tetanus.** A *hemiplegic* form is also described.

tetanus-like seizures See **diencephalic autonomic seizures.**

tetany Involuntary tonic muscle contraction as a result of excessive spontaneous repetitive activity in the motor nerve, as occurs with hypocalcemia or alkalosis, causing a reduction in ionized calcium levels. Clinically, this is seen preferentially in distal muscles (*carpopedal spasm*), including those of the face (**Chvostek sign, Schultze sign**). Muscle twitching, cramps, and carpal and pedal spasm are manifestations of peripheral and central nervous system nerve irritability stemming from several causes. Tetany is the only neuromuscular complication of hypoparathyroidism, but hypocalcemia, the usual cause, may be asymptomatic until the nerve is made ischemic (see **Trousseau sign**) or until the patient hyperventilates (*latent tetany*).[2753]

In these conditions, repetitive discharges (double discharge, triple discharge, multiple discharge) occur frequently with voluntary activation of motor unit action potentials or appear as spontaneous activity, enhanced by systemic alkalosis or local ischemia. Tetany was first described by **Erb** in 1873 and by **Trousseau** in 1861,[5648] although Walter Harris (1647–1732) was the first to use calcium (in the treatment of infantile tetany) in 1689. George Kellie (1777–1846), a Scottish physician, first described the laryngospasm in this condition.[4979] Twelve eponymous signs are listed by Robertson and Robertson,[4723] all manifesting the excessive irritability of peripheral nerves to mechanical or electrical stimulation, but only the **Chvostek** and **Trousseau** signs are regarded as important today.

tethered cord syndrome (tethering, filum terminale syndrome) A midline embryological defect in which there is anchoring of the conus medullaris within the confines of the sacrum, usually by a lipomatous growth. The condition is considered to be a form of spinal **dysraphism.**

Clinically, progressive neurological defects in the legs, scoliosis, enuresis, foot ulcers and deformities appear, usually when the child attains the erect posture or during the rapid pubertal growth phase,[6070] but presentation may be delayed until adult life. In some cases, muscle hypertrophy is noted in the affected regions.[528] See also **diastematomyelia.**

tethering See **tethered cord syndrome.**

tetra-amelia with multiple malformations (Gr, four + no + limb) See **Zimmer syndrome.**

tetrahydrobiopterin Defects in the metabolism of this substance lead to raised levels of phenylalanine in infants, in whom myoclonic seizures, rigidity, and dystonia develop. See **phenylketonuria.**

tetraphasic action potential Action potential with three baseline crossings, producing four phases.

tetrodotoxin (puffer fish toxin) A potent inhibitor of the initiation and propagation of the action potentials of excitable cells, through its absolute inhibition of the passage of sodium ions across cell membranes.[3116] It occurs after the ingestion of improperly prepared puffer fish or salamanders. The clinical syndrome comprises facial paresthesias, numbness, peculiar sensory experiences, nausea, sweating, pallor, salivation, and hypotension, leading to areflexia and ventilatory failure, and is potentially lethal.

Texidor twinge (precordial catch syndrome) A recurrent, acute, brief, and self-limited pain localized to the anterior left chest wall, associated with the slouched position and relieved by standing erect or by taking a deep breath. The etiology is unknown, but unless the subjects agree to full cardiological investigation, the condition is harmless.[3877]

thalamencephalon (Gr, an inner chamber + the brain) Those parts of the brain around the third ventricle which are derived from the first primary vesicle.

thalamic amnesia An acute, persistent, amnesic syndrome caused by bilateral paramedian thalamic infarction due to occlusion of a thalamosubthalamic artery supplying both medial thalami. Clinically, after a period of transient coma, the patient enters an apathetic and hypersomnolent state, accompanied by severe anterograde verbal and visual amnesia and bilateral vertical gaze palsies, evolving to a condition of **subcortical dementia.**[2303]

thalamic aphasia A fluent dysnomic aphasia, complicated by fluctuations of attention and of performance, resulting from thalamic hemorrhagic or ischemic strokes. This is not necessarily a causative association, however, as all patients studied more recently have had evidence of diminished cortical perfusion or the cortical effects have been interpreted in terms of the interruption of neural connections.

thalamic astasia See **subcortical dysequilibrium.**

thalamic ataxia Unilateral ataxia, coarse action tremor, hemisensory loss, and mild hemiparesis as a result of contralateral midthalamic or posterior thalamic infarction.[3602,5254]

thalamic Creutzfeld-Jakob syndrome See **thalamic dementia.**

thalamic degeneration with multiple system atrophy See **thalamic dementia.**

thalamic dementia   Global psychological defects in adult patients with paramedian diencephalic lesions.

The syndrome is characterized clinically by optic atrophy, ophthalmoplegias, myoclonic seizures, dystonias, spasticity, and autonomic disturbances. Mental signs include impairment of attention and mental control with apathy, poor motivation, slowness in response, amnesia, and emotional lability.[633]

Three types have been defined:

Selective thalamic degeneration includes familial or sporadic types, characterized by severe thalamic atrophy without pathology elsewhere. This may be the same condition as **fatal familial insomnia.**[4422]

Thalamic degeneration with multiple-system atrophy include sporadic or familial cases in combination with with cerebellar ataxia or **hereditary motor neuropathy.**

Thalamic **Creutzfeld-Jakob syndrome** comprises those sporadic cases in which there is substantial gliosis or spongy change in the cerebral cortex as well as the thalamic pathology.[4422]

The condition may also occur as a **lacunar syndrome.**[1853,1867]

See also **Stern-Garcin syndrome, subcortical dementia.**

thalamic esotropia   Sustained convergence of the eyes as a result of acute thalamic disease.[2179]

thalamic hand   1. Permanent sensory loss of part of the arm, down into the hand, in association with a small thalamic infarction (pseudoradicular infarction). 2. (striothalamic hand) The flexed, pronated, and adducted posture of the hand and fingers in some patients with basal ganglion disorders.

thalamic infarcts   Small infarcts resulting from in situ disease of small vessels or at the mouth of the parent artery; or from cardioembolism and producing a variety of syndromes with mild to moderate contralateral motor and sensory signs, memory impairment, dysphasia (if the left thalamus is involved), and neglect (if the right is involved). Other clinical features include confusion, behavioral changes, eye movement disorders, and contralateral ataxia. Posterior choroidal artery infarcts may produce an isolated homonymous horizontal sectoranopia.

thalamic neglect   A neglect syndrome resulting from a lesion of the medial thalamic nuclei which, like the mesencephalic reticular activating system, are involved with tonic arousal.[5874]

thalamic overreaction   The occurrence of spontaneous pains and of **hyperpathia** following thalamic lesions.[574]

thalamic pain   Unilateral facial pain and dysesthesia attributed to a lesion of the quintothalamic pathway or the thalamus, usually on the right side. The symptoms also involve the trunk and limbs on the same side. This definition and the following diagnostic criteria are suggested by the Headache Classification Committee of the International Headache Society[1051] and are reproduced by kind permission.

A. Pain and dysesthesia of one half of the face, associated with impaired sensation to pinprick, not explicable by a lesion of the trigeminal nerve

B. One or more of the following:

1. A history of sudden onset suggesting a vascular lesion
2. A remitting and relapsing history of symptoms in the face or elsewhere suggesting multiple sclerosis
3. The demonstration of a lesion in an appropriate site by CT or MRI

From: Classification of headache disorders, cranial neuralgias and facial pains; and diagnostic criteria for primary headache disorders. *Cephalalgia* 1988;**8**(suppl): 1–96, by kind permission of Blackwell Science.

allodynia, hypoesthesia and **hypalgesia, dysesthesia,** and motor and sensory signs are also commonly found, and symptoms more commonly affect half the body than the face alone. Déjèrine and Roussy described the pains as follows: "lively pains on the hemiparetic side which are persistent, paroxysmal, often intolerable and refractory to any analgesic therapy". See also **central pain.**

thalamic sensory loss   More or less complete loss of all forms of sensation of the contralateral side of the face and body as a result of a lesion of the posterior thalamic nuclei.

thalamic syndrome   (Déjèrine-Roussy syndrome, capsulothalamic syndrome) **Thalamic pain** following lesions of the ventroposterior thalamic nuclei (occlusion of thalamogeniculate branches of the posterior cerebral artery) or of the deep white matter of the parietal lobe. This usually succeeds a period of mild contralateral hemiparesis, hemiataxia and choreoathetosis, complete astereognosis, and persistent hemianesthesia, although superficial sensation may be more or less spared.

The severe, persistent, paroxysmal and often intolerable pain is variously described with a wealth of verbal detail. Any outside stimulus appears capable of aggravating it. Therapy is seldom effective.[1344] The various thalamic infarct syndromes have been reviewed.[633]

Isolated anterior thalamic infarctions lead to acute, severe perseverative behavior in thinking, speech, and memory tasks with increased sensitivity to interference and **palipsychism,** anterograde memory impairments with impairment of delayed recall, and difficulty in programming motor sequences.[2090]

See also **paramedian thalamic artery syndrome.**

thalamic tremor   Unilateral resting and postural 3 Hz tremor of the upper limb, occurring as a delayed manifestation of thalamic stroke.[3918]

thalamocapsular stroke   See **sensorimotor stroke.**

thalamosubthalamic infarction syndrome   See **paramedian diencephalic syndrome.**

thalamus   (Gr, room or inner chamber) (optic thalamus) The name applied by Galen to the final major relay station in the ascending sensory pathways and reaffirmed as such by **Willis** in 1664.

thalassemic myopathy   (Gr, sea + blood + muscle + disease) A myopathic syndrome occurring uncommonly in patients with (homozygous) thalassemia major and presenting with proximal weakness (mainly in the legs) and a myopathic EMG pattern.[3459]

thallium poisoning   A syndrome of peripheral neuropathy, ataxia, somnolence, seizures, and sometimes cranial nerve palsies, including optic neuritis, resulting from the ingestion of thallium-containing substances (usually pesticides). Ataxia and some degree of dementia may be permanent sequelae.[941]

thanatophoric dwarfism   (Gr, death + bringing) (nanism) A rare, congenital, asphyxiating syndrome of skeletal deformities resulting from complicated achondroplasia. The clinical features of note include dwarfism and platyspondyly, anal atresia, kleeblattschädel (cloverleaf malformation of the skull), widened cranial sutures and fontanelles, and heterotopias with CNS dysplasias.[3147]

thanatophoric dysplasia   A dominantly inherited lethal congenital syndrome of craniosynostosis and short-limbed dwarfism, mapped to chromosome 4p.

thanos syndrome   A congenital dysmorphic syndrome characterized by myopia, macrocephaly, craniosynostosis, thickened calvarium, sclerosis of the skull bones, epidermoid nevi, and mental and developmental delay.

Thaysen syndrome   See **proctalgia fugax, familial rectal pain.**

The Neurologist   A review journal focusing on clinically relevant issues, published by Lippincott, Williams and Wilkins. Web site: http://www.theneurologist.org/.

Theile syndrome   A congenital dysmorphic syndrome characterized also by scoliosis, cryptorchidism, microcephaly, and mental and developmental delay.

thenar   The flat part or hollow of the hand. The name was used by Homer, Hippocrates and Galen for the small hand muscles, but the separation into thenar muscles (at the base of the thumb) and hypothenar muscles (on the ulnar side) was the choice of Riodan in 1649.[5204]

thenar hypoplasia   A sporadic developmental anomaly characterized by the occurrence of hypoplastic thenar muscles on one or both sides. The differential diagnosis of this condition from **carpal tunnel syndrome** is not easy, especially because it may not lead to referral for medical care until adult life; but there are no sensory changes in this anomalous form.[943]

therapeutic embolization   The intraarterial injection of foreign substances with the aim of obliterating a vascular lesion such as an arteriovenous malformation or an aneurysm fed by the appropriate artery.

The precise indications for the procedure are still in the process of determination.[1925]

thermanesthesia   Loss of temperature sensation.

thermesthesia   Temperature sensation.

thermhypesthesia   Partial loss of temperature sensation.

thermography   A technique for the measurement of skin temperature using either a liquid-crystal device applied to the skin or infrared detection equipment. Its reliability in the diagnosis of radiculopathies and of neuropathies is disputed. An American Academy of Neurology subcommittee concluded that it is of limited value in characterizing neurological dysfunctions.[141,894] Those who possess a machine, however, find its use profitable.

thermoregulatory sweat test   A technique for assessing the integrity of the central and peripheral efferent sympathetic pathways. It consists of measuring the sweat distribution using an indicator powder while applying a controlled heat stimulus to raise body temperature sufficient to induce sweating.

In performing the test, the naked patient is heated by 1°C, and coated with starch powder and iodine; in the presence of moisture (sweat) the starch-iodine reaction causes a dark blue-gray color change. See **autonomic function tests.**

Thermotest   A commercial device (Somedic, Sweden) useful in the assessment of small fibre neuropathies.

theta rhythm   An EEG rhythm with a frequency of 4 to <8 Hz.

theta wave   A waveform recorded on the EEG, with a duration of less than 0.25 second and more than 0.125 second.

Thévenard disease   (l'acropathie ulcéro-mutilante familiale) Neurogenic plantar ulceration, as may occur in **hereditary sensory and autonomic** and **alcoholic neuropathies, syringomyelia, tabes dorsalis,** the **cerebellar ataxias,** and low spinal cord lesions.[5534]

thiamine-dependent lactic acidemia   A rare congenital or childhood syndrome characterized by mental retardation, episodic ataxia, choreoathetosis, hypotonia with areflexia, and chronic lactic acidosis. The condition is considered a manifestation of **pyruvate decarboxylase deficiency.**[1557] See also **Leigh disease.**

thiamine-dependent maple syrup urine disease   (thiamine-responsive branched-chain ketoaciduria) A milder variant of **maple syrup urine disease** in which there is an error in the degradation of the branched-chain amino acids leucine, isoleucine, and valine and presenting with ketoacidosis and seizures in the neonatal period. The clinical disease resolves in those infants treated permanently with thiamine.[1557]

thiamine-dependent megaloblastic anemia, sensorineural deafness, and diabetes mellitus A rare syndrome of unknown cause characterized by the combination of these features.[2484]

thiamine-responsive branched-chain ketoaciduria See **thiamine-dependent maple syrup urine disease.**

thick-filament myopathy See **acute quadriplegic myopathy.**

Thiebaut syndrome (spinal cholesterolosis) A syndrome of spastic paraparesis with hypercholesterolemia and large tendinous masses. It is probably a form of **cerebrotendinous xanthomatosis** but has so far been reported only without pathological verification.[5535]

Thiebaut-Refsum disease See **hereditary motor and sensory neuropathy** (type 4, Refsum disease).

thigmesthesia General tactile sensibility, the receptors for which are around the hair follicles and in Merkel's disks.

third alexia See **alexia.**

third and fourth pharyngeal pouch syndrome See **DiGeorge syndrome.**

third circulation The CSF system, this term being suggested by **Cushing** in 1926.

third occipital headache A constant, aching occipital or suboccipital head pain worsened by neck movement and resulting from irritation of the third occipital nerve (a branch of the C3 root) by pressure from osteophytes around the C2–3 zygapophyseal joints[621] and following whiplash injury.[3472]

thirty:fifteen ratio The ratio of the pulse rates at 30 compared to 15 beats after standing; a measure of parasympathetic autonomic function.[2736] Normally the ratio is 1.04 or more; 1.00 or less is definitely abnormal. See also **expiration-inspiration ratio, autonomic function tests.**

Thomas, André See **André-Thomas.**

Thomas atrophy See **olivopontocerebellar atrophies.**

Thomas disease (André-Thomas disease, pure cerebellar cortical atrophy) An ataxic syndrome best classified as an **olivopontocerebellar atrophy** even though described separately[5536] from that on which André-Thomas and **Déjèrine** had published an account 5 years before.[1346]

Thomas reflex A rather different method of eliciting the **Babinski** plantar response, in which the examiner smartly rubs the sole of the patient's foot with the back of the knuckles two or three times. The particular indications for this technique are not defined.

Thomsen disease Dominantly inherited myotonia with secondary hypertrophy of muscles and without loss of power, unlike **paramyotonia.** See **myotonia congenita.**

Thomsen, Julius (1815–1896) Danish physician and lyric poet, who suffered from **myotonia congenita** (Strümpell, 1881) the disorder subsequently named after him by **Westphal** (1883). His family history was strongly positive over five generations (not surprisingly in a condition with frequent autosomal dominant inheritance) but he refrained from publishing his observations on "'Ataxia Muscularis'" or "'Tonic Cramp'" until 1876, when his son, who was also affected, was accused of feigning symptoms in order to avoid military service.[2863,5569]

The production of muscle spasms by emotion led Thomsen to consider the condition a disease of the central rather than of the peripheral nervous system. Unknown to him, Ernst **Leyden** had published a good account of the same disorder 2 years before, and Wilhelm **Erb** wrote an exhaustively complete account of it 10 years later.

Thompson syndrome A congenital form of optic atrophy.

Thompson test The patient kneeling with the foot hanging over the edge of a couch, the calf is pinched just below its widest point. Passive plantar flexion of the foot is the normal response, but this is absent in the presence of rupture of the Achilles' tendon.[1812]

thoracic inlet syndrome See **thoracic outlet syndrome.**

thoracic outlet An anatomical artefact, variously described as including the interscalene triangle, the costoclavicular passage, and the axillary passage, through which passes the neurovascular bundle composed of the brachial plexus and the subclavian artery and vein as it leaves the chest to enter the arm.

thoracic outlet syndrome (Falconer-Weddell syndrome, scalenus anticus syndrome, costo-clavicular syndrome, hyperabduction syndrome, Naffziger syndrome, neurogenic or vascular thoracic outlet compression syndromes, thoracic inlet syndrome, superior thoracic aperture syndrome) A collection of disorders, linked by the common (but thin) thread of supposed compression of the brachial plexus and subclavian vessels along the costoclavicular passages by, e.g., a cervical rib at C7, a fibrous band passing from the scalenus medius to the first rib, or the scalenus anterior muscle itself. *Neurogenic* and *vascular* (both arterial and venous) forms are described.[1210] The description by Falconer and Weddell[1737] of the "costo-clavicular compression syndrome" is among the most complete.

Clinically, combinations of aching pain in the forearm or shoulder, reproduced by traction on the arms; paresthesias in the medial part of the forearm, weakness and occasionally wasting of the hand, and coldness and color changes are the more common symptoms. Supraclavicular bruits and sensory or motor findings appropriate to compression of the lower fibers of the brachial plexus may be found, but the diagnosis is suggested by the symptoms rather than by the signs, of which there may be none.

The *neurogenic* form is characterized by pain and sensory disturbance in the ulnar side of the forearm and hand, made worse by use of the arm, combined with weakness and wasting of the intrinsic hand muscles (especially the abductor, flexor and opponens of the thumb). The presence of a cervical rib assists in the diagnosis but a long C7 transverse process and a fibrous band (visible only to surgeons) have also been incriminated as causal.[3321] Its electrophysiological signs are inconstant and disputed, although abnormal medial antebrachial cutaneous sensory studies are reported as being abnormal in all such cases.[3142] A recent dispassionate review was by le Forestier et al. (1998)[332]

The *vascular* form presents with evidence of arterial insufficiency in the hand, presumed to be as a result of subclavian artery or vein compression.

A host of names has been ascribed to the syndrome of arm pain and subjective sensory disturbance and these will not be recounted here. The syndrome represents a major source of controversy because the pathology can exist without any symptoms, the clinical features are not specific, the operation is attended by potential important complications, and there exists no definitive confirmatory test. Thus the condition perplexes neurologists, vexes electromyographers and activates surgeons. Recent disputations have been published.[4761,5964] In 30 years of EMG practice, this author has encountered two patients in whom both the clinical evidence was complete and the surgical intervention beneficial. See also **droopy shoulder syndrome.**

thoracic radiculopathy   See **diabetic truncal neuropathy.**

thoracic-pelvic-phalangeal dystrophy   See **Jeune syndrome, Langer-Gierdon syndrome.**

thoracoabdominal neuropathy   See **diabetic truncal neuropathy.**

Thorburn phenomenon   Involuntary muscle contractions associated with mechanical or other insults to adjacent regions of the spinal cord; adoption of a position of abduction of the shoulders and flexion of the elbows as a result of bilateral C7 lesions. See **Bradborn sign.**

As an example, the tragic shooting of President Kennedy caused an immediate initial elevation of his shoulders and flexion of his arms (C5, 6 activation) when the bullet pierced the cord at C6.

thought   Conscious mental content, whether in linguistic form or not.

three paper test   A test of reading comprehension using verbal instruction, introduced by Pierre **Marie.** The patient is given a piece of paper on which is written: "When you have finished reading this, tear the paper into three. Give one piece to me. Throw a second piece on the floor. Put the third piece in your pocket."

three words, three shapes test   A test of verbal and nonverbal memory in which the subject copies three simple shapes, each labeled with an unrelated word, and then attempts to reproduce these without further stimulation after various intervals.[3851]

three-Hertz spike-and-slow waves   A paroxysm of EEG activity consisting of a regular sequence of spike-and-slow-wave complexes which repeat at 3–3.5 Hz (measured during the first few seconds of the paroxysm). They are bilateral in their onset and termination, generalized, and usually of maximal amplitude over the frontal areas, and are approximately synchronous and symmetrical on the two sides of the head throughout the paroxysm. Their amplitude is variable but can reach values of 1000 uV. See also **atypical repetitive spike-and-slow waves.** (From Chatrian GE, Bergamini L, Dondey M, et al. A glossary of terms most commonly used by clinical electroencephalographers. *EEG Clin Neurophysiol* 1974;**37**:538–48,[989] with permission from Elsevier Science.)

threshold   In any context, the level at which a clear and abrupt transition occurs from one state to another. The term is generally used to refer to the voltage level at which an action potential is initiated in a single axon or muscle fiber or a group of axons or muscle fibers. (From the 2001 Report of the Nomenclature Committee of the American Association of Electromyography and Electrodiagnosis.[10] Used by permission, copyright © 2001, AAEM.)

Throckmorton sign   Extension of the hallux when the metatarsophalangeal region is repeatedly struck just medial to the tendon of the extensor hallucis longus. This is a variant of the **Babinski reflex,** but of rather less utility. It was described by T.B. Throckmorton (b. 1885), an American neurologist.

thrombocythemia   (primary thrombocythemia) A condition characterized by platelet counts greater than >400 × 10⁹/L and an increase in the number of clustered mature megakaryocytes in bone marrow biopsy specimens, in the absence of any cause for reactive thrombocytosis.

Neurological complications include transient ischemic attacks and other evidence of microvascular disease such as erythromelalgia, presenting with burning paresthesias and pains in the extremities, and painful acrocyanosis, but the peripheral pulses are normal.[3866]

thrombophlebitis, cerebral   See **cerebral venous thrombosis.**

thrombosis   Occlusion of a blood vessel as a result of coagulation of the blood contained in it, triggered either by hematological disease or by disease of the vessel wall. See **cavernous sinus thrombosis, cerebral thrombosis, cerebral venous thrombosis.**

thrombotic microangiopathy   See **Moschcowitz disease.**

thrombotic thrombocytopenic purpura   See **Moschcowitz disease.**

Thudichum, Johann Ludwig Wilhelm   (1828–1901) German physician and neurochemist who emigrated to England and was appointed to the staff of St. Thomas' Hospital in London in 1853. He studied the normal chemical composition of the brain, isolating and naming the phosphatides, sphingomyelin, sulfatides, cerebrosides, and cholesterol, in many cases giving an account of their chemical composition. His overview of his research results[5574] laid the foundations of modern neurochemistry but his observations were not well received in his time.

He also invented a nasal speculum and published on gastronomy.

thumb adductor response   Adduction and flexion of the thumb in response to gentle stroking of the ulnar side of the palm; seen in patients with pyramidal tract lesions. The reflex was described by **Marie** and **Foix.**

thumb reflex   Tapping the tendon of the flexor pollicis longus above the pronator quadratus leads to flexion of the distal phalanx. This reflex is usually appreciated only in patients with pyramidal tract disease.

thumb sign   Protusion of the thumbs over the ulnar aspect of the palm when the fist is clenched; a sign in **Marfan syndrome** resulting both from elongation of the phalanges and metacarpals and hypermotility of the joints. See also **arachnodactyly.**

thumb-chin reflex   Contraction of the mentalis muscle when the underside of the patient's thumbnail is flicked up by the index finger nail of the examiner; a variation of the **palmomental reflex,** with the same significance.

thunderclap headaches   Paroxysmal, excruciatingly severe, generalized headaches presenting with extreme abruptness. The pathophysiology is unknown but the condition appears to be benign. Headaches of this nature suggest subarachnoid hemorrhage, but here there is no evidence of intracranial bleeding.

Diagnostic criteria suggested by Dodick[2002] include the instantaneous or hyperacute onset of very severe pain lasting for up to 30 seconds. Appropriate investigations will exclude the presence of an underlying cause such as subarachnoid hemorrhage, cerebral venous sinus thrombosis, pituitary apoplexy, arterial dissection, spontaneous intracranial hypotension, and acute hypertensive crisis.

Dodick also pointed out that the attacks may be spontaneous or precipitated by the Valsalva maneuver, sexual activity, or strenuous exercise, and that they may recur infrequently over 1–2 weeks. Their occurrence is also described in **migraine** (*crash migraine*). In all cases, full investigation is urgently required.

See also **Call-Fleming syndrome, sentinel headache,** and **coital cephalgia** (headache associated with sexual activity, benign sex headache) each of which, like cervical spinal disorders, may present with pain of a similar nature.[1317]

thunderstruck disease   An antique colloquialism for apoplexy.

thymectomy   Removal of the thymus gland, first performed by Alfred Blalock (b. 1899), an American surgeon, for the treatment of **myasthenia gravis.**

thymoma   (Gr, thymus + cutting out) A tumor of the thymus gland, usually benign, and frequently without any associated symptoms. The tumor is usually in the lateral lobes of the thymus, and is characterized by mixed epithelial or lymphothelial cell nests with many lymphocytes, rosettes, and some gland-like formations. A relationship with **myasthenia gravis** is established.

thyrocerebrorenal syndrome   A recessively inherited congenital dysmorphic syndrome, characterized by sensorineural deafness, goiter with hypothyroidism, platelet abnormalities, seizures, and cerebellar signs.[1235]

thyroid ophthalmopathy   See **dysthyroid orbitopathy.**

thyroid storm   See **thyrotoxic crises.**

thyrotoxic crises   (thyroid storm, acute thyrotoxic encephalomyelopathy) An agitated delirious state with tremor and hyperkinesia, and later lethargy, obtundation, or coma. Pyramidal signs, aphasia, chorea, bulbar palsy, and respiratory insufficiency are also recorded.

Other features include insomnia, fever, tachycardia, diarrhea and vomiting, atrial fibrillation and cardiac failure. The disorder is precipitated by infection, trauma, and hot summer weather, and may occur in hypothyroid subjects given too much thyroxine.

The best early description was that of Waldenström in 1945; he also pointed out the difficulty in deciding whether the bulbar weakness was due to myopathy or to encephalopathy.

thyrotoxic myopathy   A syndrome of symmetrical proximal muscle weakness and wasting, found almost universally in patients with hyperthyroidism.

thyrotoxic periodic paralysis   (Kitamura syndrome) Recurrent attacks of flaccid paralysis of the limbs more than the trunk, lasting for between 2 and 72 hours, in association with hypokalemia. The condition is described mainly in young Japanese, Chinese, and Thai males with hyperthyroidism.[2014,4166]

thyrotropin releasing hormone   A hypothalamic hypophysiotropic peptide hormone, one of the first to be identified. Like other brain peptides, it is localized within nerve terminals, is released as a result of depolarization, and acts as a supplementary neurotransmitter—in this case to cause the release of thyrotropin.

TIAS   See **transient ischemic attacks.**

tibial neuropathy   Lesions of the main trunk of the nerve, usually in the thigh, as a result of compression, trauma, or ischemic disease and causing sural sensory and lower motor neuron lesions in the gastrocnemius, soleus and plantar muscles. See **posterior tibial neuropathy.**

tibialis anterior hypertrophy   A syndrome of localized painful hypertrophy of this muscle in association with persistent complex repetitive discharges within it, arising neurogenically.[4145]

tibialis anterior reflex   The contraction of the tibialis anterior in response to sudden stretch resulting from a tap on the dorsal aspect of the hallux. The reflex is not usually visible in the healthy subject, but can be recorded electromyographically.[5314] At the bedside, therefore, the clinician has to rely on the lateral hamstrings to provide a site for the assessment of the L5 reflex arc.[5314]

tibialis phenomenon   (Strümpell sign) Marked dorsiflexion at the ankle when the patient attempts to flex the thigh on the hip; a pathological associated movement seen in patients with pyramidal lesions.

tibialis posterior reflex   The contraction of the tibialis posterior in response to sudden stretch resulting from a tap on its tendon above and behind the medial malleolus. The contraction is not usually visible in the healthy subject, but can be recorded electromyographically. The reflex informs about the state of the reflex arcs at L5 and S1.

tic   A sudden, brief, stereotyped, more or less complex, repetitive, normally coordinated but inappropriate movement which can be suppressed for a period by an effort of will, but only at the expense of rising psychic tension (which in turn is only relieved by expression of the tic).[2163] In brief, these are irresistible, inapposite involuntary movements.

Motor (including vocal) and sensory tics are described; these may be either simple or complex, and represent either *transient* or *chronic tic disorders.* See also **coprolalia, palilalia, echolalia**).[2807]

The international classification[6038] distinguishes between elementary, complex, and generalized tics. Examples of the *elementary* forms are mimicking, blinking, sniffing, tooth-grinding or swallowing, stuttering, neck, shrugging, trunk and leg, and vocal tics, the last including barking, shouting, grunting, and swearing. Any of these in, combination are regarded as *complex tics,* while the *generalized tic* category includes those tics affecting a number of separate body areas, with or without vocal expression. All of these forms are met with in

Tourette syndrome.[2163] A rating scale for the disorder has been devised.[2155]

tic convulsif   See **trigeminal neuralgia.**

tic disorder   Diseases of unknown origin (but with a genetic predisposition) in which tics are manifested as a major feature. Criteria for this diagnosis[3194] are listed in Chart T–2, but see also **Tourette syndrome.**

Chart T–2. Research Diagnostic Criteria for Tic Disorders

A–1. Definite **Tourette syndrome**
1. Both multiple motor and one or more phonic tics have been present at some time during the illness, although not necessarily concurrently.
2. The tics occur many times a day (usually in bouts), nearly every day, or intermittently throughout a period of more than a year.
3. The anatomical location, number, frequency, complexity, type, and severity of the tics change over time.
4. Onset is before age 21 years.
5. Involuntary movements and noises cannot be explained by other medical conditions.
6. Motor and/or phonic tics must be witnessed by a reliable examiner directly at some point in the illness, or be recorded by videotape or cinematography.

A–2. **Tourette syndrome** *by history*
1. Both multiple motor and one or more phonic tics have been present at some time during the illness, although not necessarily concurrently.
2. The tics occur many times a day (usually in bouts), nearly every day, or intermittently throughout a period of more than a year.
3. The anatomical location, number, frequency, complexity, type, and severity of the tics change over time.
4. Onset is before age 21 years.
5. Involuntary movements and noises cannot be explained by other medical conditions.
6. Tics have not been witnessed by a reliable examiner, but tics were witnessed by a reliable family member or close friend, and the description of the tics as demonstrated is accepted by a reliable examiner.

B–1. Definite chronic multiple motor or phonic tic disorder
1. Either multiple motor or phonic tics, but not both, have been present at some time during the illness.
2. The tics occur many times a day (usually in bouts), nearly every day, or intermittently throughout a period of more than a year.
3. The anatomical location, number, frequency, complexity, type, and severity of the tics change over time.
4. Onset is before age 21 years.
5. Involuntary movements or noises cannot be explained by other medical conditions.
6. Motor and/or phonic tics must be witnessed by a reliable examiner directly at some point in the illness, or be recorded by videotape or cinematography.

B–2. Chronic multiple motor or phonic tic disorder by history
1. Either multiple motor or phonic tics, but not both, have been present at some time during the illness.
2. The tics occur many times a day (usually in bouts), nearly every day, or intermittently throughout a period of more than a year.

3. The anatomical location, number, frequency, complexity, type, and severity of the tics change over time.

4. Onset is before age 21.

5. Involuntary movements or noises cannot be explained by other medical conditions.

6. Tics have not been witnessed by a reliable examiner, but were witnessed by a reliable family member or close friend, and the description of the tics as demonstrated is accepted by a reliable examiner.

C. Chronic single motor or phonic tic disorder (by history)

1. Same as B-1 (and B-2), but with single motor or phonic tic

D–1. Definite transient tic disorder

1. Single or multiple motor and/or phonic tics

2. The tics occur many times a day (usually in bouts), nearly every day for at least 2 weeks, but for no longer than 12 consecutive months.

3. The anatomical location, number, frequency, complexity, type, and severity of the tics change over time.

4. There is no history of Tourette syndrome or chronic motor or phonic tic disorder.

5. Onset is before age 21 years.

6. Motor and/or phonic tics must be witnessed by a reliable examiner directly at some point in the illness or be recorded by videotape or cinematography.

D–2. Transient tic disorder by history

1. Single or multiple motor and/or phonic tics

2. The tics occur many times a day (usually in bouts), nearly every day for at least 2 weeks, but for no longer than 12 consecutive months.

3. There is no history of Tourette syndrome or chronic motor or phonic tic disorder.

4. Onset is before age 21 years.

5. Tics have not been witnessed by a reliable examiner, but tics were witnessed by a reliable family member or close friend, and the description of the tics as demonstrated is accepted by a reliable examiner.

E–1. Definite nonspecific tic disorder

1. Tics that do not meet the criteria for a specific tic disorder. An example is a tic disorder with onset in adulthood.

2. Motor and/or phonic tics must be witnessed by a reliable examiner directly at some point in the illness or be recorded by videotape or cinematography.

E–2. Nonspecific tic disorder by history

1. Tics that do not meet the criteria for a specific tic disorder. An example is a tic disorder with onset in adulthood.

2. Tics have not been witnessed by a reliable examiner, but tics were witnessed by a reliable family member or close friend, and the description of the tics as demonstrated is accepted by a reliable examiner.

F. Definite tic disorder, diagnosis deferred

1. The disorder meets all criteria for a tic disorder, but duration of illness has not yet extended to 1 year, so that a distinction between a chronic and transient tic disorder cannot be made.

*G. Probable **Tourette syndrome***

Type 1. Fulfills all criteria for definite Tourette syndrome (A–1) completely, except for criteria 3 and/or 4.

Type 2. Fulfills all criteria for definite Tourette syndrome (A–1) except for criterion 1. This type can be either a single motor tic with phonic tics or multiple motor tics with possible phonic tic(s).

Subjects can be assigned to more than one diagnostic category. For example, an individual with definite chronic motor tics, but possible phonic tics, may be classified as having a definite chronic motor tic disorder, probably Tourette syndrome.

From Kurlan R. Tourette's syndrome: current concepts. Neurology *1989;**39**:1625–1630. Reprinted by permission.*

In a *variant* form, a familial tic disorder is accompanied by signs of Parkinson disease, motor neuron disease, and acanthocytosis.[5296] See also **neuroacanthocytosis.**

tic douloureux   See **trigeminal neuralgia.**

tick paralysis   A syndrome of neuromuscular blockade, capable of inducing a subacute generalized flaccid paralysis starting in the legs, with areflexia, respiratory and bulbar paralyses, and death, usually in children, due to envenomation by the ticks *Ixodes holocyclus* or *Dermacentor andersoni* or *variabilis*, which are most commonly hidden in the hair. Sensory functions are normal. The clinical features have been ascribed to both impairment of nerve conduction and of neurotransmission.[999]

ticq   A seventeenth-century French term denoting unsightly muscular activity.

Tietz syndrome   See **dominant albinism and congenital deafness.**

Tietze syndrome   A syndrome of acute chest wall pain, probably due, for example, to coxsackie virus infection.

tigroid demyelination   A mottled appearance of the white matter caused by the sparing of perivascular myelin in the context of dysmyelinating disease such as **Pelizaeus-Merzbacher disease.**

tilt test   (tilt-table test) The measurement of sequential 30-second periods of heart rate and blood pressure, recorded both with the subject supine and with upright tilt to 65° after an initial 15 minutes lying supine. The normal response is for both heart rate and diastolic blood pressure to increase, while systolic pressure declines. The test examines aspects of sympathetic autonomic function. See also **neurocardiogenic syncope.**

tilted disks   An ocular anomaly occurring when the optic nerve leaves the globe at an unusually oblique angle. Focal ectasia or hypoplasia of the inferonasal retina is the underlying defect. The syndrome is characterized by high myopia and angulation of the optic disks which now point nasally and/or inferiorly, and which may lead to incomplete field defects, usually bitemporally.[6095]

tilting reaction   Large labyrinthine postural reactions affecting the whole body and excited by bodily instability, especially angular displacement of the supporting base relative to the horizontal plane. They are designed to maintain the center of gravity of the individual within the vertical projection of its base.

Such reactions are impaired or lost in the settings of parkinsonism and other diseases of the basal ganglia.[3656]

time agnosia   The illusionary appreciation of the passage of time without impairment of orientation in other spheres and in an otherwise unclouded sensorium, occurring as a feature of a chronic organic psychosyndrome without precise localization.[1311]

time constant, EEG channel   (TC) The product of the values of the resistance (in megohms) and the capacitance (in microfarads) which make up the time constant control of an EEG channel. This product represents the time required for the pen to fall to 37% of the deflection initially produced when a D.C. voltage difference is applied to the input terminals of the amplifier and is expressed in seconds (sec).

For a simple R-C coupling network, the time constant is related to the percentage reduction in sensitivity of the channel at a given stated low frequency by the equation TC = 1/2 f, where f is the frequency at which a 30% (3 Db) attenuation occurs at 0.5 Hz. Thus, either the time constant or the percentage attenuation at a given stated low frequency can be used to designate the same position of the low-frequency filter of the EEG channel. See also **low frequency filter.** (From Chatrian GE, Bergamini L, Dondey M, et al. A glossary of terms most commonly used by clinical electroencephalographers. EEG Clin Neurophysiol 1974;**37:**538–48,[989] with permission from Elsevier Science.)

time dotting test   A test of repetitive motor activity, in which the subject is required to place dots in small squares with the right and left hands separately, in each case for 30 seconds.

time zone change syndrome   (jet lag) A condition characterized by difficulty in initiating or maintaining sleep, excessive sleepiness, decrements in subjective daytime alertness and performance, and somatic symptoms following rapid travel across multiple time zones.[234]

timed functional testing   Tests of the capacity of patients (with neuromuscular disease) to perform complex movements that reflect activities of everyday living and that compose part of the battery of **functional tests.**

The trials employed vary slightly for various diseases; thus, in **Duchenne dystrophy,** the ability to stand, climb 4 steps, and walk 30 feet (9 meters) are examined; in **amyotrophic lateral sclerosis,** the ability to stand, climb 4 steps, and walk 15–20 feet (4.5–6 meters), speech rate, and pegboard test results are assessed; in **hereditary motor neuropathy,** the tests comprise the time taken to drink 4 ounces (120 ml) of water, to stand, climb 4 steps, and walk 30 feet, and pegboard tests; while in **myotonic dystrophy,** standing, climbing four steps, walking 30 feet, and cutting out a 3-inch (7.5 cm) square are the activities examined.[4022]

timed manual performance test   An instrument for assessing the performance of structured fine and gross manual motor tasks, based on observations of activities performed under timed conditions.[5983]

Tinel, Jules   (1879–1952) French neurologist who trained in Rouen and Paris, becoming a student of **Landouzy** and of **Déjèrine** during his further training. He became chef de clinique at the **Salpêtrière** but left to perform military service.

His description of the sign of regenerating nerve fibers appeared in his book on gunshot injuries to nerves, and arose from his experiences in the World War I. Before World War II he reduced active practice because of cardiac disease but, along with all his family, played an active role in the Resistance, for which his son paid with his life.

Tinel sign   Paresthesias felt in the distal distribution of a sensory nerve when it is percussed, indicating the presence of regenerating nerve fibers at the site percussed.[5590] A motor variant has been described[3955] in which tapping a motor nerve leads to twitching of distal muscles supplied by that nerve.

Hoffmann also described the sign in 1915, a few months before Tinel did, but from the opposing side and at a time when it was not literature that was being exchanged.

tinnitus   (Lat, ringing in the ears) (tinnitus aurium, subjective tinnitus) Hallucinatory sounds caused by disturbance of the cochlea or eighth cranial nerve (in 80% of cases) or occurring with disease in the CNS (in 20% of cases).[3311] In either case, it is the perception of sounds originating from inside the head. Such sounds may be constant or intermittent, steady or pulsatile, and may be described as humming, buzzing, whistling, or ringing.[3525] The causes are legion, but the pathophysiology is poorly defined, with both neural and cochlear mechanisms being suggested. In most cases, some hearing loss is associated.

Objective tinnitus signifies the presence of such sounds appropriately heard by a patient with, for example, carotid artery stenosis, an arteriovenous communication such as a **glomus jugulare tumor** or **palatal myoclonus.**

tinnitus aurium   See **tinnitus.**

tip-of-the-tongue phenomenon   A form of anomia or word-finding difficulty in which the subject is keenly aware that the word sought is partially recalled and close to discovery, but still cannot be brought forth without facilitatory phonetic or semantic cues.

The phenomenon occurs in normal subjects and in those with parkinsonism.[3698] See also **word production anomia.**

tired arm syndrome   See **Wartenberg cheiralgia paresthetica.**

Tissot, Simon-André (1728–1797) Swiss physician who trained in Geneva and Montpelier before entering practice in Lausanne, where his early fame rested on his success in combating an outbreak of the smallpox, using Jennerian vaccination. In 1750 he published *Traité de l'onanisme*, a work strongly condemning masturbation; this was widely successful on account of its popular appeal and brought him a pension, membership of the Royal Society of London, and an international reputation, which would not quite have been justified by his other publications on psychiatric topics—although many of his ideas seem to have antedated those of Freud and he did give the first recorded descriptions of simple absence and of myoclonic seizures.

titubation (from Lat, to stagger) 1. A rhythmic anteroposterior (to-and-fro) or side-to-side head or body tremor at about 2–5 Hz resulting from cerebellar lesions. 2. Restlessness, a staggering gait, and incoordination due to cerebellar disease (nineteenth century).

tobacco-alcohol amblyopia (nutritional optic neuropathy) Optic atrophy resulting from deficiency of B complex vitamins, initially confined to the papillomacular bundle, described first by Dr. Wordsworth, an English physician, in 1863. See **nutritional amblyopia.**

Tobey, George Loring (1881–1947) American otolaryngologist.

Tobey-Ayer test Failure of the CSF pressure (measured at lumbar puncture) to rise during compression of one jugular vein, while pressure on the other one does cause a pressure increase. It suggests the presence of lateral sinus thrombosis on that side where compression does not change the CSF pressure. See also **Crowe test.** The MRI is a much better guide, however.

Todd paralysis (postepileptic paralysis, postconvulsive palsy, postictal hemisyndrome) A neurological deficit in a body part following a focal epileptic seizure, associated with focal or generalized slowing or absence of EEG activity and lasting for up to 36 hours. The paralysis (or aphasia, or sensory deficit) is in many cases an aid to the localization of the underlying lesion and a confirmation of the focal rather than the generalized nature of the seizure.[5597] Todd described both hemiparesis and hemianesthesia as postepileptic manifestations in his patients, but the phenomenon had already been described by J.C. Prichard in 1822. It would be reasonable to regard the confusion and generalized weakness that follow generalized tonic-clonic (grand mal) seizures as having exactly the same mechanism, namely either active inhibition due to postictal hyperpolarization or else functional exhaustion of the overstimulated area due to local (or generalized) cortical anoxia.[3861]

Todd, Robert Bentley (1809–1860) Irish physician who trained in medicine in Dublin with **Graves** and at Oxford and was afterwards appointed professor of physiology and morbid anatomy, and later dean of King's College, London, while continuing the practice of medicine.

He is remembered by neurologists for his (1854) description of postepileptic paralysis in a volume of clinical lectures in neurology, which was followed by two others on general medical topics. His full descriptions of the neurological symptoms, signs, and syndromes led to his depiction as "the greatest neurologist that Britain had produced until the time of Hughlings-**Jackson**" (Collier, cited by Spillane[5280]).

toe reflex Forcible flexion of the hallux leads to tightening of all the leg muscles below the knee in normal people, but more so in patients with pyramidal tract lesions.

1. The *great toe phenomenon of Edelmann* consists of dorsiflexion of the hallux in response to passive flexion of the hip when the knee is extended. It is a minor sign of meningeal irritation.[1349a]

2. The *little toe reflex of Puusepp* consists of slow adduction of the little toe when the outer border of the foot is stroked.[1349a] Although a sign of extrapyramidal disease, it has no precise localizing value.

toe walking Tightness of the heel cords (Achilles' tendon), either as an isolated problem or as a manifestation of muscle contracture in severe dystrophies.[773]

toilet seat neuritis See **Saturday night palsy.**

Token test A test for latent receptive dysphasia in patients with hemispheric lesions, the results yielded correlating strongly with the results of tests of auditory verbal comprehension.[1412]

In the test, subjects are instructed verbally to touch or otherwise manipulate large and small, round and square counters of five different colors in response to commands of increasing complexity.[644,1412]

Tollner syndrome A congenital dysmorphic syndrome characterized by atrioventricular septal defect, horseshoe kidneys, polydactyly, macrocephaly, and hydrocephalus.[5598]

Tolosa, Eduardo Spanish neurosurgeon in Barcelona who described the **superior orbital fissure syndrome** in 1954.[5600]

Tolosa-Hunt syndrome See **superior orbital fissure syndrome.**

toluene encephaloneuropathy See **glue sniffers' neuropathy.**

tomaculae String-of-sausage-shaped swellings in peripheral nerves, representing segmental expansion of the damaged myelin sheath.

tomaculous neuropathy (from Lat, a sausage) A pathological feature in some neuropathies, consisting of sausage-shaped thickenings of the myelin sheaths of between 80 and 250 μm, affecting fibers of all sizes and usually accompanied by segmental demyelination with remyelination and early onion bulb formation.

The clinical accompaniments include recurrent brachial plexus neuropathy, pressure-sensitive neuropathy or sensorimotor polyneuropathy;[4395] in most cases there is a genetic basis.[4898] See **hereditary pressure-sensitive neuropathy.**

Tondeur syndrome   See **sialuria.**

tone   (tonus) 1. The resistance of muscles to passive stretch. 2. A defined frequency of vibration. 3. A manner of behavior.

tone decay   A hearing test using pure tone audiometry in which continuous tones are repeatedly presented at threshold intensity. Patients with cochlear nerve lesions, but not those with lesions of the cochlea itself, perceive such tones as decreasing in loudness and eventually disappearing.

tongue-blade sounds   See **linguals.**

tongue-point sounds   See **linguals.**

tonic   (from Gr, pitch or tension) 1. See **tone** (definition 1). 2. Continuously occurring.

tonic absences   (retropulsive absences) Atypical absences accompanied by mild tonic contractions, especially in the neck muscles.

tonic arousal   A state of alert arousal for which the mesencephalic venticular activating system (RAS) is responsible. Unilateral lesions of that structure produce contralateral neglect, while bilateral lesions cause coma.[5874]

tonic cerebellar fits   1. Acute attacks of vertigo, with clouding of consciousness seen in patients with cerebellar tumors, described by Sir Gordon **Holmes** in 1904. 2. Attacks of retraction of the head, arching of the back, flexion and supination of the elbows, and plantar flexion of the toes, occurring in association with tumors of the cerebellar vermis and likely to be a form of decorticate response.

tonic convergence reaction of pupils   See **Holmes-Adie syndrome.**

tonic foot response   Persistent plantar flexion of the ankle as a result of diffuse cerebral disease. It interferes with walking, as the foot may remain "stuck" to the ground—the *magnetic foot.*

tonic innervation   The term of **Wilson** and **Walshe**[6001] for a delay in the relaxation of a voluntary contraction, resulting in an inability to relax the grasp in the paretic arm of a patient affected by hemiparesis due to frontal lobe lesions affecting the premotor area (area 6 of Brodmann).

Differentiation from **gegenhalten** and **perseveration** is difficult, but tonic innervation is often associated with motor apraxia and always with pyramidal

signs. **Grasping** and **groping** reactions are often associated.

tonic inverse masticatory activity   Contraction of a muscle that normally closes the mouth only when the subject is trying to open it. This may be a form of **dystonia** and is seen with lesions in the cerebello-pontine angle.

tonic labyrinthine reflexes   Extension of the neck of babies lying in the supine position, and flexion of the neck when lying in the prone position; also, extension of the arms of the prone child aged more than 4 months when the chin is passively raised.

Children of this age with cerebral palsy may respond to chin elevation with flexion of the arms or tonic extension of the arms and flexion of the legs.[2732]

tonic neck reflex   1. *Asymmetrical response:* extension of the arm on turning of the head to one side while the normal baby is lying quietly in the supine position. The arm may extend fully with further rotation of the neck. This reflex is normally lost by the third month but persists in children with spasticity. 2. *Symmetrical response:* extension of the arms with flexion or extension of the neck.[6064] Such postural changes induced by afferent stimuli from the neck muscles were first demonstrated by Magnus and de Kleijn in animals after total labyrinthine extirpation. See also **developmental reflexes.**

tonic palmar reflex   Slow flexion and adduction of the thumb, flexion of the other fingers, and increased palmar concavity in response to linear tactile stimulation of the palm going from proximal to distal.[671]

tonic perseveration   The term of Liepmann for the inability to relax any muscle group or groups owing to the presence of a central lesion. Wilson and Walshe[6001] substituted the term **tonic innervation.**

tonic plantar response   Slow and persistent flexion and adduction of the toes and of the ankle in response to gentle stroking of the sole of the foot. This is a sign of extrapyramidal disease, but is otherwise not localizing.

tonic pupil   See **Holmes-Adie syndrome.**

tonic seizures   Epileptic seizures lasting 10–20 seconds and predominantly occurring during the night, almost exclusively during NREM sleep in children, and consisting of tonic contractions of various muscle groups without progression to any clonic phase but sometimes causing the child to fall to the ground as a result of leg flexion. Respiratory arrhythmias, tachycardia, mydriasis, flushing, salivation, and loss of consciousness, accompanied by slow-spike and slow-wave complexes on the EEG are other features. During the tonic seizure, the EMG shows muscle activity similar to that occurring during voluntary contraction.

This seizure pattern is seen most commonly in the

Lennox-Gastaut syndrome among individuals who are intellectually impaired and who may manifest multiple other seizure types.[2058]

tonic status epilepticus   See **status epilepticus.**

tonic tics   See **tics.**

tonic torsion neurosis   See **dystonia.**

tonic vibration reflex   Tonic muscle contraction normally evoked by the effect of vibration on primary spindle endings. It is diminished on the side of a hemiparesis and lost below a spinal cord lesion.[839]

tonotopy   Functional localization in the auditory cortex, in which there is spatial representation of different tones.

tonsillar herniation   Downward extrusion of the cerebellar tonsils into the foramen magnum, leading to compression of the caudal medulla. This typically results from expansion of a mass lesion in the posterior fossa.

Reduction in conscious level, neck rigidity, skew deviation of the eyes, and vomiting are the associated clinical signs, preceding the appearance of irregular respirations, apnea, bradycardia, and death.

tonus   See **muscle tone.**

Tooth, Howard Henry   (1856–1926) English neurologist who trained at Cambridge and St. Bartholomew's Hospital, where he was later appointed physician. He was also on the staff at the **National Hospital,** and was active in army medicine during the Boer and First World wars.

He described **hereditary motor and sensory neuropathy** as *the peroneal type of progressive muscular atrophy* (London, 1886) and wrote on the pathology of spinal cord degeneration and on cerebral tumors.

toothed trochlea phenomenon   See **Negro sign.**

top of the basilar syndrome   A stroke syndrome characterized by visual, oculomotor, and behavioral abnormalities, often without significant motor dysfunction, in which the lesions are confined to the territory of the distal branches of the posterior cerebral artery (or arteries). Rostral brainstem infarction produces oculomotor and pupillary signs identical to those in thalamic hemorrhage, sometimes with somnolence, vivid hallucinations, and dreamlike behavior. Temporal and occipital infarctions are often accompanied by hemianopia with distinctive characteristics such as fragments of the **Balint syndrome,** amnestic dysfunction and agitated behavior. The cause is usually embolic.[896]

Two major forms are defined:

1. *Rostral brainstem infarction* (the syndrome of the mesencephalic artery) is characterized by disorders of vertical gaze, **convergence spasm** on attempted lateral gaze, **convergence retraction nystagmus, pseudo-sixth, Collier sign,** lightning-like oscillations of the eyes, **skew deviation** of the eyes, and **corectopia** with loss of the pupillary responses.

2. *Posterior cerebral artery* territory hemispheric infarction commonly leads to partial hemianopia with awareness of the deficit and complaints of surrounding scintillations, visual perseveration, and anomic aphasia, **alexia without agraphia,** or visual agnosia when the infarct is unilateral. With bilateral infarcts, **asimultagnosia,** apraxia of gaze, **metamorphopsia,** memory deficits, sensory loss, and agitated delirium are typical findings.[896]

topesthesia   (Gr, a place + sensation) Local sensibility to touch.

topognosis   (locognosis) Localization of a point of contact on the body; a function identified by A.W. Volkmann in 1844.

topographic amnesia   (topographical disorientation) A disorder of finding one's way about familiar environments and of learning to navigate new ones. The problem may represent the effect of a disorder of spatial memory coupled with a failure to recognize places and has been described in a patients with right temporal lobe disease.[3729]

topographic disorientation   See **topographic amnesia.**

topographical agnosia   (body image agnosia) 1. Failure of localization of a point of contact on the body. 2. Failure to identify the proper placing of cities, etc., on a map, inability to find defined places within a town, or to locate a specific room in a house.

The disturbance in visuospatial memory is a form of visual agnosia, and is associated with bilateral or right-sided posterior (occipitoparietal) lesions.

topography   The distribution of the amplitudes of EEG activity at the surface of the head, in the cerebral cortex or in the depths of the brain.

TOPOSCOUT   A user-friendly computer-based system designed to analyze the presenting clinical features in a case of cerebrovascular disease in order to identify the most likely stroke territory.[5297] See also **microstroke.**

torcular Herophili   (Lat, wine-press, from the verb *to twist*) The confluence of the dural venous sinuses posteriorly.

Toriello-Carey syndrome   A rare syndrome comprising agenesis of the corpus callosum, telecanthus, small palpebral fissures, Pierre Robin sequence, abnormal ears, nuchal laxity, and cardiac defects.[52a]

Torkildsen shunt   The operation of ventriculocisternostomy, performed as a palliative procedure for aqueductal stenosis. It was introduced by A. Torkildsen, a Norwegian neurosurgeon, in 1939.[5612]

tornado epilepsy   (epilepsia rotatoria) A form of seizure disorder characterized by recurrent vertigo and falling; it is only differentiated from **benign paroxysmal vertigo of childhood** by the greater age of the patient and by the abnormality in the EEG, which usually suggests the presence of a lesion in a temporal lobe.

The condition was first described (as *epilepsia rotatoria*) by Arnold Pick in 1903.[4131]

Tornwaldt disease   The presence of a cyst formed by occlusion of the orifice of a nasopharyngeal bursa, leading to local abscess formation and nasopharyngeal stenosis and presenting clinically with occipital headache or glossopharyngeal neuralgia.[5342] Dr. Gustav Tornwaldt (1843–1910) was a German physician.

Toronto Stenosis index   A method of determining the degree of narrowing of the internal carotid artery (ICA) from angiograms in which the diameter of the stenotic region is compared with the expected diameter of the ICA as assessed by its usual relationship (120%) to that of the common carotid artery.[598]

torosity   (from Lat, muscular sheath) Muscular strength.

torpescence   See **torpor.**

torpid   (Lat, to be sluggish) Dull, stupid, or inactive.

torpor   (torpescence) The state in which a part of the body or the whole organism becomes numbed, unreactive to external stimuli, and disinclined to move.

torsion dystonia   See **dystonia.**

torsion dystonia with basal ganglion lucencies   See **dystonia.**

torsion dystonia, X-linked   A *variant* X-linked dystonic syndrome of childhood or early adult onset, manifesting also sensorineural deafness and mental and developmental delay. See **dystonia.**

torsion spasm   Slow, forceful, twisting dystonic movements at the neck, shoulder, hip, and trunk, representing proximal dystonic movements.[6038]

torsional nystagmus   (rotary nystagmus) That form of central vestibular nystagmus in which the movement of the globe is about the anteroposterior axis, increases after active rotation of the head, and is suppressed by convergence.

The upper pole of the iris usually beats away from the damaged side. The disorder may be congenital in origin, but is also seen with thalamic, pontine or lateral medullary lesions disrupting central vestibular connections.[3999,4168] See also **rotatory nystagmus.**

torticollis   (from Lat, twist + a neck) (wry-neck) A focal dystonia causing intermittent or persistent rotation of the neck, and frequently part of a generalized dystonic state. Cruchet gave the first modern description.[1203] In infancy, torticollis may occur in association with hematomas of the sternomastoid.[3406] Guillaume **Dupuytren** (1823) in France and W.W. Keen (1891) in America advised respectively section of the sternocleidomastoid muscle and of the spinal accessory nerve for its relief.[4976]

In a *variant* form, the torticollis is associated with sternomastoid myopathy and neuropathy of the spinal accessory nerve.[4919] See **spasmodic torticollis.**

torulosis   *Cryptococcus neoformans* meningitis, often combined with granulomatous pulmonary, dermal, and mucosal lesions. See **cryptococcal meningitis.**

The condition was described first in humans by James L. Stoddard (b. 1899) and Elliott C. Cutler, both American pathologists.

total lipodystrophy   An uncommon condition characterized by the complete loss of body fat and sometimes associated with diabetes mellitus, hepatomegaly, hyperpigmentation, hyperlipidemia, and renal disease.

Peripheral neuropathy is an occasional complication.[5661]

Total Neuropathy score   A composite measure of peripheral nerve function, scoring sensory and motor and autonomic symptoms, pinprick and vibration sensibility, motor power, muscle stretch reflexes, quantitative vibratory sensory testing, and the amplitude of sural and peroneal sensory nerve action potentials.[1134]

total sleep period   The period of time from the onset of sleep to final awakening, and including the time spent in brief arousals.

total sleep time   The total amount of time spent asleep during a sleep period, *not* including the time spent in arousals.

tottering gait   See **subcortical dysequilibrium.**

touch epilepsy   A form of stimulus-sensitive seizure disorder, tactile stimuli being capable of inducing an attack.[539]

touch sensation   The faculty of awareness of the contact of an object with the skin. Though not obviously subdivisible, nevertheless the sensation is bipartite, consisting both of a crude awareness of a contact and a discriminative perception of the nature of the object. Impulses subserving the former are considered to be carried centrally in the spinothalamic tracts, and possibly even perceived at the thalamic level; those for the latter ascend in the posterior columns and relay in the thalamus, since they require the discriminatory functions of the parietal cortex.

Toulouse reflex   See **buccal reflex.**

Tourette, George-Edmond-Albert-Brutus Gilles de la   (1857–1904) A colorful and versatile French neuropsychiatrist who was born in Vienne and died in Lausanne. Described as a clever but unruly boy, he studied medicine in Poitiers and afterwards went to Paris, becoming a favorite pupil of **Charcot** at the **Salpêtrière,** but (like **Babiński**) he was never appointed to its faculty. He was prolific in his literary output in medicine (concentrating upon syphilis, hysteria, and neurasthenia), and also published on social and political reform, literature, forensic medicine, and aspects of medical history. In 1884, the year he joined Charcot, he described jumping, latah and myriatchit, considering all to be the same condition, and, in the following year, gave a complete description of the syndrome that bears his euphonious name, stimulated by his reading of George **Beard**'s account of jumping disease (**hyperekplexia**). The disease, however, had already been described by **Itard** in 1825.

In 1893, two tragedies occurred from which Tourette never fully recovered—his son died and he himself was shot by a paranoid female patient in his consulting room, but he returned to active practice and to historical and other writing until his death.[5047]

Tourette syndrome (maladie des tics compulsifs/impulsifs, compulsive tics, multiple tic syndrome, imubacco) A dominantly inherited syndrome with incomplete penetrance, characterized by recurrent, involuntary, repetitive, rapid, purposeless motor movements of variable intensity affecting several muscle groups; similar involuntary utterances occur at some time during the duration of the disorder, which lasts for over a year. The tics can be suppressed voluntarily for a short time. They often occur daily, with variable location, severity, and complexity, and last a lifetime. The responsible gene maps to 18q22.1.

The first recorded sufferer was the French Prince of Condé, who had to stuff cloths into his mouth to stop himself from barking at King Louis XIX. In 1825, Dr. J-M-G Itard reported the case of the Marquise de Dampierre, who had begun to tic at the age of 7 and later uttered bizarre cries and meaningless phrases; her symptoms abated with milk-bath treatments in Switzerland, but worsened after her marriage, and from then on included severe coprolalia, forcing her to become a recluse for the rest of her life. She died, still cursing, at the age of 85. **Trousseau** mentioned her case briefly in his *Clinique médicale* of 1867.

Tourette gave a long, broad, but incomplete description of the syndrome in 1885,[5615] while a 28-year-old student of **Charcot,** and the eponym was granted when C.L. **Dana** attributed it in the following year, even though Tourette had incorporated Itard's case into his paper. In the same year, Georges Guinon described five further cases, commenting on the abnormal mental state but not emphasizing the compulsive behavior. Ten years later, **Brissaud** described "chorea variabilis," which is now considered to be Tourette syndrome. In 1899, Tourette wrote a summary paper, accepting that mental symptoms were also characteristic of the disease. Despite Tourette's original title, **latah, myriachit** and **jumping** (the jumping Frenchmen of Maine) are different diseases.

American Psychiatric Association Diagnostic Criteria for Tourette Syndrome

Both multiple motor and one or more vocal tics have been present at some time during the illness, although not nec-essarily concurrently. (A tic is a sudden, rapid, recurrent, nonrhythmic, stereotyped motor movement or vocalization.)

The tics occur many times a day (usually in bouts) nearly every day or intermittently throughout a period of more than 1 year, and during this period there was never a tic-free period of more than 3 consecutive months.

The disturbance causes marked distress or significant impairment in social, occupational, or other important areas of functioning.

The onset is before age 18 years.

The disturbance is not due to the direct physiological effects of a substance (e.g., stimulants) or a general medical condition (e.g., Huntington's disease or postviral encephalitis).

Dysarthria or involuntary movements, depressed mood and guilt, or obsession may also be present.

Reprinted with permission from the *Diagnostic and Statistical Manual of Mental Disorders,* Fourth edition, Text Revision Copyright 2000 American Psychiatric Association.

echolalia (Gr, echo + speech) (the repetition of words or phrases) is also common, but **coprolalia** (the uttering of obscenities) occurs in only a third of patients, though it captures the imagination of everybody. Associated obsessive-compulsive behavior, attention-deficit disorder, and sleep disturbances are other characteristics.[150] Tic disorders other than Tourette syndrome are distinguishable only by the absence of coprophenomena and of vocalizations. Whether they are regarded merely as partial expressions of a dominant condition depends on the attitude of the observer rather than on evidence. See also **tic disorder.**

Tourette Syndrome Association A national, non-profit organization dedicated to finding the cause and cure of Tourette syndrome. Address: 42–40 Bell Blvd., Bayside, NY 11361. Tel: 718–224–2999. Web site: http://www.tsa-usa.org/.

Tourette Syndrome Diagnostic Confidence index A weighted diagnostic schedule rating coprolalia, echo phenomena, complex tics, temporal features, subjective experiences, tic severity, and duration and confirmatory features.[4721]

Tourette Syndrome Foundation of Canada A charitable organization providing support and information on this condition. Address: 194 Jarvis Street, #206, Toronto, ON M5B 2B7 Canada. Tel: 416–861–8398, 1–800–361–3120.

Tourette Syndrome Global scale A scale attempting to give semiquantitative ratings of the various phenomena of Tourette syndrome such as simple and complex motor tics or rituals, simple or complex phonic tics, and aspects of social functioning such as behavior in the company of other people, motor restlessness, and difficulties in school or at work.[2432]

Tourette Syndrome "Plus" A Web site providing information and support in this disease area, is at http://www.tourettesyndrome.net/.

Tournay sign (Gianelli sign) Dilation of the pupil of the abducting eye after about 5 seconds of extreme lateral deviation, seen in normal people and in those with **Horner syndrome.**[4723] The sign has no known diagnostic value.

Dr. A. Tournay (b. 1878) was a French ophthalmologist who described the sign in 1917, 10 years after Gianelli did.

tourniquet paralysis (pneumatic tourniquet paralysis) Persisting conduction block at the upper and lower edges of an area of compression of peripheral nerves due to compressive ischemia, as occurs with the use of a tourniquet, which disrupts the myelin sheath of the nerves and causes conduction block.[648,3940]

tourniquet test A test of pain tolerance and perception in which the subject is required to perform precisely graded manual exercise during occlusion of the circulation to the arm.[5224]

tower skull (turricephaly) Vertical enlargement of the skull as a result of premature fusion of the coronal and lambdoid sutures. See **Crouzon syndromes.**

toxic encephalopathy See **Dupré syndrome.**

toxic hydrocephalus (postinfectious encephalopathy, serous meningitis) Raised intracranial pressure following nasopharyngeal or otitic infections, occurring in children and adolescents. See **idiopathic intracranial hypertension, otitic hydrocephalus.**

toxic leukoencephalopathy White matter damage resulting from exposure to drugs, irradiation, chemicals, or environmental toxins and clinically causing variable degrees of cognitive deficit, impairment of consciousness, and reduction in movement. Pathological features progress from white matter edema through demyelination to axonal loss, particularly affecting white matter tracts devoted to higher cognitive functions.[1817]

toxic oil syndrome (Spanish toxic oil syndrome) A syndrome of fever, pneumonitis, headache, myalgia, hepatitis, and eosinophilia, causing appreciable mortality in the acute stage and leading on to chronic sensorimotor peripheral neuropathy.

Adulteration of the olive oil used for cooking by aniline-treated rapeseed oil led to an epidemic of the disease in Spain in 1980.[5464] In other outbreaks in which cooking oil has been poisoned (for instance, in Jamaica and in Algeria), acrylamide or TOCP was the offending toxin.

toxic pseudomeningitis See **idiopathic intracranial hypertension.**

toxic psychosis An encephalopathy produced by metabolic disease or intoxication, presenting as a paranoid, delusional, or hallucinatory state in which the psychotic disturbance rather than inattention is the most salient feature. See **confusional state.**[3851]

toxic shock syndrome An acute illness induced by staphylococcal exotoxins, characterized by mucosal and skin lesions, upper respiratory symptoms, hypotension, nausea, vomiting and diarrhea, myalgia, and delirium, proceeding in some cases to coma and death. Laboratory abnormalities include evidence of hepatic and renal damage, thrombocytopenia, and raised serum CK and myoglobin levels (in cases with muscle destruction).[1002]

toxic-nutritional amblyopia A form of optic neuropathy leading to subacute loss of the central fields, in some cases due to cyanide poisoning as a result of excessive tobacco exposure; in others it is due to the ingestion of alcohol or of other toxins.

toxin-induced sleep disorder A disorder characterized by either insomnia or excessive sleepiness produced by poisoning with heavy metals or organic toxins.[234]

toxocariasis (visceral larva migrans) A systemic infection due to ingestion of the eggs of *Toxocara canis*, the developing larvae of which migrate extensively within the body. Encephalitis, myelitis, optic neuritis, and/or seizures are the usual clinical manifestations of neurological involvement, which is, however, uncommon. Some cases of **acute inflammatory demyelinating polyneuropathy** have been ascribed to this organism.[4435,5258]

toxoplasmosis Infection with the protozoon *Toxoplasma gondii*. Acquired CNS toxoplasmosis was highly uncommon (except in immunosuppressed patients) before the AIDS epidemic, but syndromes of diffuse encephalopathy with or without seizures, of meningoencephalitis, or of progressively enlarging intracerebral mass lesions are now well-recognized neurological presentations.[1588,4828,5619] The usual systemic illness comprises an acute febrile illness with which lymphadenopathy and uveitis may be associated.

An association with **polymyositis** or **dermatomyositis** has been suggested but not proved. Congenital toxoplasmosis is an important cause of mental retardation with microcephaly and chorioretinopathy.[100]

TPHA, MHA-TP (*Treponema pallidum* hemagglutination test, microhemagglutination *Treponema pallidum* test) Treponemal tests for syphilis which are more sensitive and more specific than the **VDRL,** and which, unlike that test, are persistently reactive following infection.[5172]

TPI (*Treponema pallidum* immobilization test) A specific diagnostic test for syphilis in which the motility of treponemes exposed to the patient's serum is recorded. Though sensitive, it is hard to perform and is not widely available.[5172]

trace alternant An EEG pattern of sleeping newborns, characterized by bursts of slow waves at times intermixed with sharp waves and intervening periods of relative quiescence. (From Chatrian GE, Bergamini

L, Dondey M, et al. A glossary of terms most commonly used by clinical electroencephalographers. *EEG Clin Neurophysiol* 1974;**37**:538–48,[989] with permission from Elsevier Science.)

tract (Lat, a pathway) An anatomically defined bundle of nerve fibres.

traction headache The headache of raised intracranial pressure.

traction response That flexion of the neck occurring when the infant lying supine is pulled gently and slowly up to the sitting position.

Such flexion is usually seen by the end of the first month of life; by 3 to 5 months, the infant can pull against the examiner, flexing the arms at the elbow and holding the neck and trunk in a straight line without any head lag.[3,6064]

traction spurs Osteophytes projecting away from the disk space, as seen in the **segmental instability** syndrome.

tractotomy Surgical section of a specific fiber pathway in the spinal cord or medulla, usually for the relief of pain. High spinothalamic tractotomy was introduced by Achille Mario Dogliotti (1897–1966), an Italian neurosurgeon, for this purpose in 1938, the same year as Carl Sjoqvist (b. 1901) reported medullary trigeminal tractotomy.[3999]

Trailmaking test A test of concentration, conceptual shifting, perceptual motor speed, and resistance to interference, in which the subject first connects successive printed numbers with a pencil, and then connects 13 numbers/letters (e.g., 1-A-2-B-3-C and so on), thus continually alternating response strategies. As a result, it provides a sensitive indicator of the presence of **perseveration.**

The Trailmaking test is a part of the Halstead-Reitan Battery, and is sensitive to brain damage in either hemisphere. It is used mainly in the assessment of aging and dementia.[4653,5842]

train nystagmus See **optokinetic nystagmus.**

train of stimuli A group of successive stimuli.

tramer reflex (contralateral abdominal proprioceptive reflex) Contraction of the abdominal muscles on the side opposite that on which a tap was made on the upper abdominal wall, described as a sign of basal ganglion disorders such as **Huntington disease.**[5621]

transcortical aphasias Those aphasias that are caused by large lesions of the cortex in the watershed areas, as occur after severe global reduction in cerebral perfusion, and which are characterized by preserved repetition with variably impaired comprehension and spontaneous output. They represent **disconnection syndromes,** the language areas now being out of touch with concepts and memories stored elsewhere in the brain. Three types are described, and are summarized in Chart T–3.

Chart T–3. The Transcortical Aphasias

Motor form Spontaneous speech is nonfluent, effortful, and sparse with poor naming and a reduction in the drive to speak, but articulation, repetition, and comprehension are unaffected. The anomia is for category naming; object naming may be unimpaired. The causative lesion, anterior and superior to Broca's area, disconnects the frontal perisylvian speech zone from the supplementary motor area.[1941]

Sensory form Speech is fluent and paraphasic, but comprehension and naming are impaired, as in Wernicke aphasia; repetition is retained. The lesion is usually at the border between the parietal and temporal lobes.[2517]

Mixed form (isolation of the speech area) The findings resemble those of global aphasia, in that spontaneous speech is nonfluent or nonexistent, and comprehension, naming, reading and writing are severely impaired and semantic paraphasias are evident. Repetition is retained, however, to the extent that the totality of the patient's speech echoes that of the examiner. The lesion is at the watershed areas between the middle and the anterior and the posterior cerebral arteries,[3025] and may be due to internal carotid occlusion with both pial and watershed infarcts.

Supplementary motor area aphasia is probably an identical condition.

transcortical aprosodia See **aprosodia.**

transcortical syndromes See **disconnection syndromes.**

transcranial Doppler sonography (TCD) The extension of the principles used in **continuous-wave Doppler sonography** of the carotid bifurcation to the basal cerebral arteries.

A low-frequency pulsed Doppler sound wave is sent through the temporal bone, the orbit, and the foramen magnum, allowing determination of the direction and character of blood flow in the circle of Willis. Two- and three-dimensional representations of the velocity of blood flow in various vessels can be obtained by the newer machines, noninvasively.

TCD is used chiefly to detect cerebral vasospasm and evaluate of the intracranial collateral pathways, but also to assess the degree of any intracranial vasoconstriction, detect arteriovenous malformations, and demonstrate absent blood flow in the case of suspected brain death.[1427,4141]

transcranial electrical stimulation (TES) Stimulation of the cortex of the brain through the intact skull and scalp by means of a brief, very high-voltage, electrical stimulus. Activation is more likely under the anode rather than the cathode. Because it is painful, this technique has largely been replaced by transcranial magnetic stimulation. (From the 2001 Report of the Nomenclature Committee of the American Association of Electromyography and Electrodiagnosis.[10] Used by permission, copyright © 2001, AAEM.)

transcranial magnetic stimulation Stimulation of the cerebral cortex by the creation of a brief intense magnetic field in the order of 1 to 2 Tesla generated by a bank of capacitors beside the cranium, which induces an electrical field in the subjacent tissues, capable of depolarizing neurons and dendrites presynaptically. The procedure is thus able to provide measurements of **central conduction time** from the cortex to the spinal cord and to the muscles from which standard recordings of the compound muscle action potentials are made. (From the 2001 Report of the Nomenclature Committee of the American Association of Electromyography and Electrodiagnosis.[10] Used by permission, copyright © 2001, AAEM.)

The procedure is easily tolerated (each stimulus feels like a brisk blow to the head of a person wearing an army helmet) and apart from a possible risk of causing deafness, appears safe. Normative data for typical recording modes have been published.[1619]

transformed migraine A headache syndrome that represents an alteration in the pattern of previous migraine headaches, usually as a result of the too-frequent ingestion of agents that can cause medication-induced headache. Proposed criteria for the diagnosis are as follows:[5157]

A. Daily or almost-daily (>15 days/month) head pain for >1 month
B. Average headache duration of >4 hours/day (if untreated)
C. At least one of the following:
   1. History of episodic migraine meeting any International Headache Society (HIS) criteria 1.1 to 1.6.
   2. History of increasing headache frequency with decreasing severity of migrainous features over at least 3 months
   3. Current headache meets IHS criteria for migraine 1.1 to 1.6 other than duration
D. At least one of the following:
   1. There is no suggestion of one of the disorders listed in the HIS diagnostic groups 5–11.
   2. Such disorder is suggested, but it is ruled out by appropriate investigations.
   3. Such disorder is present, but first migraine attacks do not occur in close temporal relation to the disorder.

From Classification of headache disorders, cranial neuralgias, and facial pains; and diagnostic criteria for primary headache disorders. *Cephalalgia* 1988;8 [suppl]: 1–96), reproduced by kind permission.

transformational migraine See **migraine with interparoxysmal headaches.**

transient and situational DIMS A period of sleep disturbance related to a psychologically disturbing situation and lasting less than 3 weeks after this has ended, as defined in the ASDA Diagnostic Classification.[249] See also ASDA Diagnostic Classification,[234] **sleep disorders.**

transient and situational DOES The condition in which the normal sleep–wake pattern is disrupted as a result of a psychological disturbance related to life stress; the subject has trouble staying awake or is aware of an abnormal need to sleep, although the sleep architecture remains normal. The ASDA Diagnostic Classification[249] defined this state as occurring only for a maximum of 3 weeks after the initiating events. See also ASDA Diagnostic Classification,[234] **sleep disorders.**

transient CNS deficits A common, benign syndrome in young adults. The neurological deficits last less than 24 hours. Loss of vision, power, balance, or coordination are those most commonly noted. Although the same definition may be used for **transient ischemic attacks,** in this context the term refers to episodes of neurological dysfunction unaccompanied by evidence of vasculopathy in young people who, over a median 5-year follow-up, exhibit no other evidence of neurological disease.[3381]

transient epileptic amnesia A syndrome of youth or young adult life, characterized by multiple brief (<1 hour) episodes of pure amnesia, often preceded by an aura and occurring usually after a period of sleep. Affected subjects frequently have a personal or past medical history of seizures, and a history of past or current lesions of the brain in or near the temporal lobes.

Despite the lack of responsiveness, inappropriate speech and behavior, involuntary stereotyped movements, and reduction in ability to retain new information presented during the period of the event, some recollection of the episode may be possible afterwards. Bilateral mesial temporal lobe dysfunction is considered to be responsible and sleep EEGs may show bilateral temporal lobe discharges.[2928] See also **transient global amnesia.**

transient episodes of neurological dysfunction (TENDs) The author's inclusive term for a symptom complex characterized by the occurrence of neurological deficits with a definable onset and termination and with periods of normality intervening.

The term is proposed to recall the differential diagnosis of typical **transient ischemic attacks.** Events due to **migraine,** labyrinthine disorders, **papilledema,** cerebral tumor, seizure manifestations, **narcolepsy,** glaucoma, and **multiple sclerosis** are thus included.

transient global amnesia An acquired syndrome characterized by the sudden onset of inability to form memories (and thus inability to recall newly presented information), and of uncertainty with regard to the current situation, leading to futile repetitive questioning of companions. It occurs in elderly people and lasts for minutes up to about 4 hours, with a variable period of retrograde amnesia ensuing. There is no loss of consciousness, personal identity, nor insight, and the patient remains alert and may be able to perform complex activities. There are no physical signs.

Although once considered a manifestation of epilepsy, transient ischemia of the mesial temporal lobe structures is now considered the likely pathophysiology, perhaps as a manifestation of migraine. The first description was that of Bender,[448] but two years later Fisher and Adams[1865] proposed the term now used. The following diagnostic criteria are modified from those of Caplan.[898] From Caplan LR. TGA criteria: what's in a name? *Neurology* 1986;**36**:1625 reprinted by permission.

A. Attacks must be witnessed and reported by a capable observer present during the attack.

B. Anterograde amnesia occurs during the attack.

C. Consciousness is not clouded and there is no loss of personal identity; the cognitive impairment is limited to amnesia.

D. No focal neurological symptoms are present during the attack, nor significant neurological signs afterward.

E. No epileptic features occur.

F. The attack resolves within 24 hours.

G. The patient does not have an active seizure disorder, and has not suffered a recent head injury.

A *variant* familial form has been reported.[1161,4309]

transient headache with neurologic deficits and CSF lymphocytosis (HaNDL) A syndrome of unknown cause characterized by recurrent episodes of severe headache with temporary neurological deficits in various parts of the brain and increased CSF lymphocytes (and sometimes pressure). The patients are typically normal between attacks.[489]

transient idiopathic dystonia of infancy A form of segmental dystonia affecting infants in the first year of life, who present with an abnormal posture of one arm or on one side of the body while at rest. The problem disappears usually by the age of 18 months. The etiology is unknown.[5979]

transient ischemic attacks (from Lat, temporary + Gr, shortage + blood) (TIA) Acute episodes of focal cerebral or ocular dysfunction lasting less than 24 hours (actually usually 2–15 minutes) and caused by ischemia of the appropriate part of the cerebrum or retina. Such ischemia may be due either to thromboembolism or spasm of the arterial wall. Denny-Brown[1393] reviewed the phenomenology of such transient cerebrovascular episodes.

The attacks can usually be localized to that portion of the brain supplied by one vascular system (left or right carotid or vertebrobasilar system).[4141]

The following diagnostic criteria (Chart T–4) have been suggested:[1389]

Chart T–4. Diagnostic Criteria for Transient Ischemic Attacks

Time course The symptoms should have developed within a few seconds, affecting several different parts of the body (e.g., face, arm, leg) at the same time with no "march"; symptoms must resolve completely within 24 hours.

Symptoms of carotid TIA Hemiparesis, aphasia or transient loss of vision in one eye only.

Symptoms of vertebrobasilar TIA Bilateral or alternating weakness or sensory symptoms. Vertigo, diplopia, dysphagia, ataxia, and drop attacks are accepted only if two or more symptoms occur together. Sudden bilateral blindness occurs in patients over 40 years of age.

Symptoms of uncertain arterial territory Hemianopia alone or dysarthria alone.

Symptoms explicitly not acceptable as TIA Syncope, loss of consciousness or confusion, convulsion, incontinence of urine or of feces, dizziness, focal symptoms associated with migrainous headache, scintillating scotomata.

From Dennis M, Bamford JM, Sandercock JM, Warlow CP. A comparison of risk factors and prognosis for transient ischemic attacks and minor ischemic strokes. Stroke 1989;20:1494–1499, reprinted by permission.

transient lone bilateral blindness The occurrence in youth or young adult life of transient bilateral blindness with abrupt onset over seconds, unaccompanied by any other features, lasting minutes and with a benign outcome. The cause is unknown but is precipitated usually by exercise or postural change.[693]

transient monocular blindness (amaurosis fugax) Sudden temporary failure of sight; a term introduced by Posey in 1902, and now preferred to the alternative one named here.[1861] The usual cause is the presence of emboli from the carotid artery that have migrated to the retinal circulation, but glaucoma, migraine, and raised intracranial pressure are among the other causes.

transient movement disorders See **epilepsy, myoclonus, palatal essential tremor, jitteriness, shuddering attacks, transient idiopathic dystonia of infancy, spasmus nutans, benign paroxysmal torticollis of infancy, benign paroxysmal tonic upgaze, benign myoclonus of the newborn, benign myoclonus of infancy,** and **transient tic disorder.**[1795]

transient neonatal myasthenia See **neonatal myasthenia.**

transient tic disorder A condition with the same diagnostic criteria as **Tourette syndrome,** except that the tics have occurred for less than a year at the time of examination. It is a common event in schoolaged children, and probably represents partial expression of the same condition, which is itself not uncommon.[3196]

transient topographical amnesia A benign cognitive disorder of later adult life without sequelae or known cause, manifest as a temporary difficulty in finding one's way in a familiar place.[5375] See **topographic amnesia; transient global amnesia.**

transient tumor attacks The occurrence of episodes of nonepileptic, reversible cerebral dysfunction as a result of the presence of an intracranial tumor. The episodes include loss of vision, motor power, sensation, speech, or posture and last between minutes and 2 or 3 days. They allow no conclusion as the to nature or localization of the tumor, and their pathophysiology is also uncertain.[4803]

transient visual obscurations   Painless and fleeting reductions in vision of one or both eyes, classically in association with raised intracranial pressure but also occasionally due to other causes of elevated pressure in the optic nerve head.[4871]

transient wave   Any isolated EEG wave or complex which can be distinguished from background activity.

transillumination test   Applicable to the paranasal sinuses as well as to the head, the test compares the amount of light passing through the part examined to that transmitted in a normal subject. This subjective determination does not invalidate the test, so long as it has been performed and verified on numerous prior occasions. Increased transillumination of the skull suggests hydrocephalus. Decreased transillumination of the sinuses suggests local tumor or infection.

transitional diffuse sclerosis   A leukoencephalopathy. The term is probably best regarded as a synonym for **adrenoleukodystrophy.**

transitional meningioma   See **meningioma.**

transitional progressive multiple sclerosis   An unusual presentation and course of multiple sclerosis.[1815] See **multiple sclerosis.**

transmantle pressure   The difference between the ambient pressure in the subarachnoid space over the convexity, and the intraventricular pressure. The difference is greatest with obstructive, and least with communicating, hydrocephalus.

transmissible dementias   Prion diseases that involve an aberrant isoform of prion protein, present within the amyloid plaques of patients with such conditions, and causing encephalopathy in animals and humans. These include **scrapie** (in sheep and goats), **transmissible mink encephalopathy, chronic wasting disease** (in deer and elk), sporadic and familial **Creutzfeldt-Jakob disease, Gerstmann-Straussler syndrome, kuru,** and **bovine spongiform encephalopathy.**

transmissible mink encephalopathy   A slow virus disease characterized by spongy changes and gliosis of the gray matter, occurring in mink and possibly analogous to **Creutzfeldt-Jakob disease** and **kuru** in humans.

transmissible spongiform encephalopathies   See **prion diseases.**

transneuronal degeneration   See **transsynaptic degeneration.**

transsynaptic degeneration   (transneuronal degeneration) Secondary atrophy of neurons, whose cell bodies receive major excitatory influences from other neurons in the CNS, which themselves have atrophied as a result of disease. It is thus the result of a loss of afferent impulses.

An example is the degeneration of some lower motor neurons in the spinal cord that occurs after a stroke in the contralateral hemisphere, and thus involves damage to the descending pyramidal tracts. The precise mechanism of the change is not known. See also **diaschisis.**

transtentorial herniation   (clivus edge syndrome) See **uncal syndrome, Kernohan notch syndrome.**

transthyretin   (prealbumin) An abnormal form of this substance polymerizes into amyloid fibrillary protein, deposited in the tissues of patients with **familial amyloid neuropathy.**

transverse bipolar montage   See **coronal bipolar montage.**

transverse myelitis   Segmental inflammation of the spinal cord, usually viral or postviral in nature, or as a manifestation of **multiple sclerosis.** Clinical diagnostic criteria might include the following:

A. Acute onset of motor and sensory pareses with sphincter involvement
B. A spinal segmental sensory level can be detected.
C. The subsequent course is stable.
D. There is no evidence of compression of the spinal cord.
E. Pain is felt at the level of involvement.

transverse myelopathy   An acute intrinsic ("intramedullary") dysfunction of the spinal cord occurring bilaterally, affecting numerous segments and appearing without prior evidence of cord disease.

Ropper and Poskanzer[4771] have summarized the causes as infectious, peri- or postinfectious, or vaccinial, vascular, demyelinating, paraneoplastic, post-irradiative, and secondary to vascular malformations.

transverse relaxation time   See **T2 spin-spin.**

transverse temporal gyri   See **Heschl gyri.**

trapezius   (from Gr, a four-sided figure with no two sides parallel) A large superficial muscle of the upper back and neck.

trapezius hump   A mound of the muscle which can be seen like the sunrise over the middle third of the clavicle in patients with girdle atrophy, both at rest and with arm elevation, when the trapezius contracts in an effort to fix the scapula.

trapshooter's cramp   An occupational dystonia of the trigger finger occurring in competitive marksmen, the finger not obeying the willed command to squeeze the trigger at the appropriate time.[64] See **dystonias, yips, bowlers' cramp.**

Traquair, Harry Moss   (b. 1876) Scottish ophthalmologist.

Traquair scotoma   (junctional scotoma) A central scotoma superimposed upon a bitemporal hemianopia because of compression of the optic chiasm.[5625]

Traub-Hering waves   See **C waves.**

traumatic brain (injury) disease Brain injury following head trauma, usually as a result of abrupt deceleration. It may be diagnosed in the presence of the following:

A. Loss of consciousness of any duration following head injury

B. Evidence of a neurological deficit following the trauma

C. Evidence of focal brain damage revealed by clinical or laboratory methods

The severity of brain injuries has been classified[1908] (see Chart T–5).

Chart T–5. Classification of Traumatic Brain Disease

Mild brain injury Following a transient loss of consciousness there is no focal neurological deficit and consciousness is regained rapidly. PTA is less than 1 hour.

Moderate brain injury There is still impaired consciousness or disorientation 1 hour after injury but the patient can obey commands; or is alert but shows evidence of a focal deficit. PTA is from 1 to 24 hours.

Severe brain injury The patient cannot follow commands after the injury and, if able to speak, words are used inappropriately. The best motor response is the ability to localize stimuli. PTA of 1–7 days is usual.

Very severe brain injury The patient's eyes are closed soon after the injury, despite intense stimulation; words cannot be uttered nor commands followed, and the best motor response is posturing. The threat to life is severe; if death does not occur, a **persistent vegetative state** may ensue. PTA is longer than 7 days, if it can be assessed.

PTA, post-traumatic amnesia.

In *severe traumatic brain injury* the combination of focal and diffuse brain lesions leads to a complex syndrome characterized by disorders of memory, attention, and executive function, slowed information processing and changes in personality and behavior, correlating poorly with the results of brain imaging studies.[1908]

traumatic neuralgia See **causalgia.**

traumatic neuroma (amputation neuroma) A bulbous mass at the end of an injured peripheral nerve, largely composed of neurites and fibrous tissue.

traumatic spreading depression syndrome (postcontusion seizure syndrome, juvenile head trauma syndrome) Early convulsions following mild or trivial head injuries in infants and young children, or other transient neurological signs (headache, nausea, somnolence, vomiting, confusion, alteration in consciousness, aphasia, hemiparesis) occurring in the same context but following a lucid (asymptomatic) interval in children and adolescents, with complete recovery.

The condition is considered by Ohtahara *et al.*[4226] to represent the clinical effects of the **spreading depression of Leao.**

Treacher Collins syndrome See **mandibulofacial dysostosis.**

Tredgold, Alfred Frank (1870–1952) English physician who trained at the London Hospital and devoted his life to the subject of mental retardation. His book *Mental Deficiency* (1908) was a landmark, consolidating knowledge to that time. In it, Tredgold gave the first account of *idiots savants.*

trefoil canal The fancied cloverleaf shape of the spinal canal in a congenital variant of the normal, or as a result of degenerative hypertrophy of the lumbar facets.

In either case, the cross-sectional area of the canal is diminished, and symptoms of **spinal stenosis** may appear.[222]

Treft syndrome A dominantly inherited syndrome of childhood characterized by optic atrophy, visual failure, ophthalmoplegia with ptosis, and deafness.[4831]

Trekker's shoulder See **upper brachial plexus palsy, rucksack palsy.**

tremblement affirmatif A vertical or nodding movement of the head, in which the amplitude of the oscillations increases rather than decreases with voluntary movement. It is seen in **essential tremor,** but also in some elderly people who have no other evidence of that condition.

tremblement negatif A horizontal shaking movement of the head, in which the amplitude of the oscillations increases rather than decreases with voluntary movement. It is seen in **essential tremor,** but also in some elderly people who have no other evidence of that condition.

tremor (Lat, to shake) Involuntary rhythmic and regular oscillations of a body part in any plane, due to the alternate or synchronous action of groups of muscles and their antagonists.

Tremors may be regular or irregular in rate and amplitude. They are classified according to the state of motor activity of the body part when they occur—**rest tremor, postural tremor,** or tremor during goal-directed activity (**intention** or action tremor) or at the completion of a complex and skilled activity. Using etiology as the basis for a classification, **cerebellar, dystonic, essential, flapping, functional, neuropathic, parkinsonian, physiological, postural,** and **wing-beating** (hepatic) forms are defined.[6038]

A classification suggested by Jankovicz is adapted in Chart T–6 with some definitions after Bain.[299] See also Movement Disorder Society Consensus Statement.[1422]

Chart T–6. A Classification of Tremors

A. *Rest tremor* (tremor occurring when the limb is supported against the effects of gravity and in which muscle contraction is voluntarily inhibited)

1. Parkinsonian tremor (**Parkinson disease**, other parkinsonian disorders; **parkinsonism-plus**)

2. **Spasmus nutans**

3. **Hereditary chin quivering (tremor)**

4. Other: **midbrain (rubral) tremor, severe essential tremor,** and tremors in **Roussy-Lévy syndrome, Wil-**

son disease, acquired hepatocerebral degeneration, myorhythmia, tardive tremor

B. *Action tremor* (tremor that occurs during any voluntary muscle activation)
  1. *Postural* (tremor that occurs when a posture is maintained voluntarily)
      A. **Physiologic tremor**
        1. Normal physiologic tremor
        2. **Accentuated physiologic tremor** (stress-induced, endocrine, drugs, toxins)
      B. **Essential tremor**
        1. Autosomal dominant
        2. Sporadic
        3. With **hereditary motor and sensory neuropathy** (see **Roussy-Lévy syndrome**)
        4. With other movement disorders (e.g., dystonia, parkinsonism, myoclonus)
        5. With metabolic disorder (e.g., vitamin E deficiency)
      C. Re-emergent action tremor of parkinsonism[2811]
      D. **Neuropathic tremor**
      E. Cerebellar (hypotonic) postural tremor (**titubation**)
      F. **Rubral tremor** (of midbrain origin)
      G. **Dystonic tremor**
  2. *Kinetic (intention)* (tremor occurring during the performance of a voluntary movement; *terminal tremor* is that form of kinetic tremor in which the amplitude of the tremor is increased at the end of the goal-directed movement.)
      A. **Cerebellar tremors**
      B. Cerebellar outflow tremor with midbrain lesions (**rubral tremor**)
  3. *Other tremors*
      A. Psychogenic tremor. Abnormal repetitive movements that do not fit the patterns described here, occurring in patients with suspected disorders of personality or emotional control. Many with adequate follow-up turn out to have organic neurological disease.
      B. **Task-specific tremor,** in which the tremor occurs only during one or more particular highly skilled activities, such as playing a musical instrument or writing (primary handwriting tremor) and in certain sports (see **bowlers cramp,** yips).
      C. **Isometric tremor,** occurring when muscle activity is exerted at maximal force against an unyielding object, or against the antagonists of the muscle in question
      D. **Orthostatic tremor** Isometric tremor, present when muscles contract against an unyielding force.

After Dr. Joseph Jankowic' personal communication (2002), with many thanks.

tremor saturninus   A fine, irregular, distal tremor of the fingers and lips, seen in the setting of lead and other heavy metal poisoning.

tremorgenic encephalopathy   A syndrome of kinesigenic tremor and reversible dementia, thought to occur as a result of the inhalation of neurotoxins derived from the fungi within moldy silage.[2206] Such toxins may be produced by *Aspergillus flavus, fumigatus,* and *clava-*

tus, and *Penicillium cyclopium* and *claviceps;* in animals, they are recognized as able to produce a syndrome of transient tremor and weakness. See also **woodtrimmers disease.**

trench foot   (immersion foot) A syndrome of ulceration, maceration, and trophic changes in the skin of the legs and feet consequent upon prolonged immersion in cold water, as occurred in soldiers fighting from the trenches during World War I. The cold injury also damages both the arterial supply and the nerves in the legs, resulting in ischemia and distal sensorimotor neuropathy.

Trendelenburg, Friedrich   (1844–1924) German surgeon.

Trendelenburg gait   A waddling gait, due to weakness in the pelvic girdle muscles.[5630]

Trendelenburg test   When the patient stands on one foot, the buttock of the unsupported foot usually rises, but falls in patients with weak gluteal muscles, as in radiculopathy, high sciatic neuropathy, and the **piriformis syndrome.**

Trends in Neurosciences   (*Trends Neurosci*) A basic science neurological journa. Web site: http://www.elsevier.nl/locate/tins.

trepanning   See **trephining.**

trephining   (trepanning) The surgical opening of the skull. The original word was *trepan* (Gr, a gimlet); *trephine* was introduced by Woodall in 1628 as the name for an instrument he had devised for this purpose.

  Osler stated that this operation is the oldest known surgical procedure, but it is likely to have been preceded by circumcision.

trepidant abasia   (from Lat, fearful + Gr, not + going) See **isolated gait ignition failure.**

trépidation du Moignon   See **stump spasm.**

triad syndrome   See **prune belly syndrome.**

triangular bipolar montage   A montage consisting of derivations from pairs of electrodes in a group of three electrodes arranged in a triangular pattern. (From Chatrian Ge, Bergamini L, Dondey M, et al. A glossary of terms most commonly used by clinical electroencephalographers. *EEG Clin Neurophysiol* 1974;**37:**538–48, with permission from Elsevier Science.)

triceps   (from Lat, three + heads) 1. The major extensor muscle of the elbow (triceps brachii). 2. The gastrocnemius and soleus muscles (triceps surae).

triceps surae reflex   The correct name for the Achilles reflex or **ankle jerk,** use of the term being a custom honored entirely in the breach rather than the observance, perhaps in part because there is no alternative to the name of **triceps reflex** in the arm.

The reflex is obtained by tapping the tendon of the muscle itself or, with the ankle in slight passive dorsiflexion, the sole of the foot or the belly of the tibialis anterior muscle (**Gowers' frontal tap**).

trichinosis Muscle infection by the larvae of the nematode *Trichinella spiralis*, the pork tapeworm, most often as a result of eating measly meat.

The condition is usually subclinical, but the larvae may encyst in muscles after oral ingestion, causing diffuse myalgia, eosinophilia, and systemic signs such as periorbital edema, ocular pain, chemosis, a generalized maculopapular rash, and eosinophilia. Encephalitis is a rare complication.[1314]

tricho-onycho-oligophrenia   See **Sabinas syndrome.**

trichopoliodystrophy   (Gr, hair + gray + wrong + growth) See **Menkes disease.**

trichopsia   Central blindness with scintillating scotomata, as in **migraine.**

trichotillomania   (Gr,   hair + pluck + madness) Compulsive pulling-out of the hair, leading to patchy baldness. The patients may also eat the hair pulled out. **Bulimia** is associated in some cases.[5446]

trickle angiography   A technique for visualizing blood clots in the carotid bulb and internal carotid artery, introduced by Hugh in 1970.[2689]

trident tongue   See **triple-furrowed tongue.**

trientine   A chelating agent of value in the treatment of **Wilson disease.**

trifacial neuralgia   See **trigeminal neuralgia.**

trigeminal nerve   (Lat, three + twins; thus triplets, appropriate since the nerve has three branches) The fifth cranial nerve, described by Fallopius.

trigeminal neuralgia   (tic douloureux, trifacial neuralgia, facial chorea, Fothergill syndrome, tic convulsif) A syndrome of brief facial pains, one of the most severe afflicting humans. It occurs in patients older than 55 years, is unilateral, and is felt in the second or third divisions of the fifth cranial nerve; when any of these conditions is not met, symptomatic trigeminal neuralgia is diagnosed and a structural lesion along the path of the nerve is sought.

The condition was known to Galen and Avicenna, and was described by **Fothergill,** first in 1776 and again (more fully) in his book 30 years later.[1915] However, Johannes Fehr and Elias Schmidt were probably describing the same condition in their 1671 eulogy of Dr. Johannes Bausch who had died suffering from this condition.[4979]

Two forms (*idiopathic* and *symptomatic*) are described by the Headache Classification Committee of the International Headache Society[1051] and their definitions and diagnostic criteria are reproduced in Chart T–7.

Chart T–7. Definition and Diagnostic Criteria for Trigeminal Neuralgia

Idiopathic trigeminal neuralgia A painful unilateral affliction of the face, characterized by brief electric shock-like (lancinating) pains limited to the distribution of one or more divisions of the trigeminal nerve. Pain is commonly evoked by trivial stimuli including washing, shaving, smoking, talking, and brushing the teeth, but may also occur spontaneously. The pain is abrupt in onset and termination, and may remit for varying periods. The diagnostic criteria are as follows:

A. Paroxysmal attacks of facial or frontal pain which last a few seconds to less than 2 minutes
B. Pain has at least four of the following characteristics:
1. Distribution along one or more divisions of the trigeminal nerve
2. Sudden, intense, sharp, superficial, stabbing, or burning in quality
3. Pain intensity severe
4. Precipitation from trigger areas, or by certain daily activities such as eating, talking, washing the face, or cleaning the teeth
5. Between paroxysms, the patient is entirely asymptomatic.
C. No neurological deficit
D. Attacks are stereotyped in the individual patient.
E. Exclusion of other causes of facial pain by history, physical examination, and special investigations when necessary.
Symptomatic trigeminal neuralgia (compression of the trigeminal root or ganglion) The diagnostic criteria are as follows:
A. Pain as described above for trigeminal neuralgia with or without persistence of aching between paroxysms and signs of sensory impairment in the distribution of the appropriate trigeminal division
B. The demonstration of a causative lesion by special investigations or posterior fossa exploration[1051]

(From Classification of headache disorders, cranial neuralgias and facial pains; and diagnostic criteria for primary headache disorders. Cephalalgia 1988;8(suppl):1–96), by kind permission of Blackwell Science.

Central lesions can cause a similar pain. See also **Hellsing syndrome.**

Trigeminal Neuralgia Association   A nonprofit, voluntary organization founded in 1990, providing information and support to patients with trigeminal neuralgia and their families through informational mailings, a support network, and support groups. The association also endeavors to increase public and professional awareness of this disorder. Address: 2801 SW Archer Road, Suite C, Gainesville, FL 32608. Tel: 352–376–9955. Web site: http://www.tna-support.org/.

trigeminal sensory neuropathy   A benign syndrome of slowly progressive sensory loss affecting one or more branches of the fifth cranial nerve, sometimes preceded by paresthesias and mild pain and accompanied by impairment of taste sensation but with the corneal reflex preserved.[5284]

The clinical syndrome is the same in isolation as it is when accompanying various connective tissue diseases, particularly progressive systemic sclerosis and mixed connective tissue disease.

In a *variant* form with degeneration and amyloid deposition in the trigeminospinal system, nasal ulceration and myelopathy accompany the facial numbness.[5283]

trigeminobrachial reflex   Flexion and supination of the forearm in response to stimulation of the contralateral side of the face, as seen in patients with bilateral corticobulbar tract disease.

trigeminocervical reflex   1. Rotation of the neck in the direction away from the side on which the face is stimulated; a sign of bilateral corticobulbar tract disease. 2. A short latency reflex that can normally be recorded from the sternocleidomastoid muscle after electrical stimulation of the infraorbital nerve. It may be absent with medullary lesions.[1445]

trigemino-encephalo-angiomatosis   See **Sturge-Weber syndrome.**

trigeminofacial reflex   The **blink reflex,** elicited by electrical stimulation of the supra- or infraorbital nerves. The reflex is employed clinically in the study of brainstem reflex circuits. See **orbicularis oculi reflex.**

trigemino-ocular synkinesis   See **Gunn phenomenon.**

trigemino-orbicularis reflex   See **palpebral reflex.**

trigeminopalpebral reflex   See **palpebral reflex.**

trigeminosympathetic neuralgia   See **trigeminal neuralgia, Bonnet syndrome.**

trigeminovascular system   A network of intracranial and extracranial blood vessels innervated by the fifth cranial nerve. Stimulation leads to the release of vasoactive peptides in the arterial walls, considered responsible for the pain of migraine headaches.[4014]

trigger zone   An area which, when excited by any stimulus, precipitates acute severe pain, usually in the same area.

trigonocephaly   (Gr, triangle + head) An unusual cranial malformation characterized by synostosis of the midline frontal (metopic) suture, giving the forehead a triangular, pointed shape. Radiologically, the orbits are closer than normal with parallel inner walls.

The malformation is sometimes associated with arhinencephaly and hypotelorism.[4] See also **Opitz-Frias syndrome.**

trihexose ceramide lipidosis   See **Anderson-Fabry disease.**

trilaminar muscle fiber disease   A rare congenital myopathy presenting with weakness at birth, manifested as poor sucking and swallowing as well as limb weakness, but abating with time.[6] Trichrome stains of muscle fibers reveal three concentric rings, the center zone (which contains no contractile elements) staining red, the (normal) middle zone staining green, and the outside (containing variously glycogen, mitochondria, and lipid) staining purple.[4706]

trilateral retinoblastoma   The concurrence of **pinealoblastoma** and **retinoblastoma.**

trinucleotide repeat disorders   Conditions due to unstable mutations, in most of which there is an expansion of the CAG repeat in the coding sequence of a gene. See **cerebellar ataxias, (X-linked spinal-bulbar muscular atrophy, fragile X syndrome, FRAXE mental retardation, myotonic dystrophy, Huntington disease, dentatorubropallidoluysian atrophy.** See also **triplet repeat diseases.**

triorthocresylphosphate   An organophosphate with a strong anticholinesterase effect and with a delayed neurotoxic effect causing a motor neuropathy. See **toxic oil syndrome.**

triose phosphate isomerase deficiency   An inborn error of metabolism (a corencephalopathy) in which the enzyme is deficient in muscle, skin fibroblasts, and blood cells. Clinically, denervation atrophy of muscles, pyramidal signs, tremor, and dystonia with hemolytic anemia develop in young children.[4478]

triphasic action potential   Action potential with two baseline crossings, producing three phases.

triphasic wave   An EEG manifestation consisting of a waveform with an initial negative (upward), then a major downward deflection followed by a second upward deflection before return to baseline. Such waves are common in all metabolic encephalopathies, such as those due to hepatic or renal failure, in which they are said to have an earlier onset in frontal regions, and in **Alzheimer disease,** hyperthyroidism, and **Mollaret meningitis** as well as after strokes.[1904]

triple discharge   (triplet) Three motor unit action potentials of the same form and nearly the same amplitude occurring consistently in the same relationship to one another and generated by the same axon. The interval between the second and third action potentials often exceeds that between the first two, and both are usually in the range of 2 to 20 msec. See also **double discharge, multiple discharge.** (After the 2001 Report of the Nomenclature Committee of the American Association of Electromyography and Electrodiagnosis.[10] Used by permission, copyright © 2001, AAEM.)

triple E syndrome   Bilateral posterior fracture-dislocations of the shoulders, as a result of sudden extreme extensor and internal rotator contractions of the shoulder girdle musculature. The more common causes of this are **E**pilepsy, **E**xtreme trauma, and **E**lectrocution.[698]

triple response   The formation of a weal, surrounded by a tache and flare at the site of a linear scratch on the skin, due to local axon reflex activity, described by Lewis.

The existence of such a response indicates that the smallest cutaneous nerve fibers are intact.

triple symptom complex   See **Behçet syndrome.**

triple-furrowed tongue   (trident tongue) The presence of three longitudinal fissures in the tongue, said to be characteristic in **myasthenia gravis.**

triplet   See **triple discharge.**

triplet repeat disease   Any of several familial diseases resulting from expansion in length of a segment of repeated nucleotide triples within an affected gene (see tables below). Many (but not all) of the triplet repeat diseases arise from expansion of a repeated cytosine-adenine-guanine $(CAG)_n$ triple in an exon of the gene, which causes a corresponding increase in length of a polyglutamine $(Gln)_n$ segment of the affected protein. This expanded $(Gln)_n$ tract can produce a toxic gain of function, and the mutant protein often has a propensity to coalesce as intracellular inclusion bodies. The triplet repeat of the gene may be prone to increase in length during replication so that each affected generation possesses a successively longer expansion. This results in genetic anticipation, in which each generation expresses the phenotype of the disease at a successively younger age. Note however that triplet repeat expansions can also occur within an intron, or within an altogether untranslated segment of the gene, and in these cases the resulting disease arises by some other mechanism. Expansions of runs involving other triplet combinations including thymine (T) also occur. (HJM)

The following tables are by courtesy of Dr. Homer J. Moore.

Triplet Repeat Diseases*

Disease	Gene Locus	Affected Protein	Number of Triplet Repeats		Mechanism/Inheritance*
			Normal	Diseased	
I. Diseases Caused by $(CAG)_n$ Expansions					
Haw River syndrome (dentatorubropallidoluysian atrophy, [DRPLA])	12p13.31	Atrophin-1	6–35	49–88	$(Gln)_n$/AD Ant
Huntington disease	4p16.3	Huntingtin	6–35	36–121	$(Gln)_n$/AD Ant
Kennedy disease (spinobulbar muscular atrophy, [SBMA])	Xq13–21	Androgen receptor	9–36	38–62	$(Gln)_n{}^a$/SLR
Spinocerebellar ataxia type 1[†]	6p23	Ataxin-1	6–44	39–82	$(Gln)_n{}^b$/AD Ant
Spinocerebellar ataxia type 2[†]	12q24.1	Ataxin-2	15–31	36–63	$(Gln)_n$/AD Ant
Machado-Joseph disease (spinocerebellar ataxia type 3[†])	14q32.1	Ataxin-3	12–40	55–84	$(Gln)_n$/AD Ant
Spinocerebellar ataxia type 6[2†]	19p13	α_{1A}-voltage-dependent Ca^{2+} channel subunit	4–18	21–33	$(Gln)_n$/AD Ant ?
Spinocerebellar ataxia type 7[†]	13p12–13	Ataxin-7	4–35	37–306	$(Gln)_n$/AD
Spinocerebellar ataxia type 12[6†]	5q31–33	PP2A-PR55β	7–28	66–78	5′ UTR/AD
Spinocerebellar ataxia type 17	6q27	TATA-binding protein	24–42	47–55	
II. Diseases Caused by Other Trinucleotide Expansions					
Fragile X syndrome (FRAXA)/CGG	Xq27.3	FMR-1	6–53	>230	5′ UTR/SLR
Fragile XE syndrome (FRAXE)/GCC	Xq28	FMR-2	6–35	>200	5′ UTR/SLR
Friedreich ataxia/GAA	9q13–21.1	Frataxin	7–34	>100	intron 1/AR
Myotonic dystrophy/CTG	19q13.3	Dystrophia myotonica protein kinase (DMPK)	5–37	>50	3′ UTR/AD Ant
Oculopharyngeal muscular dystrophy/GCC	14q11	PABP2	6	8–13	$(Ala)_n$/AD
Spinocerebellar ataxia type 8/CTG (SCA 8)	13q21	KLHL1	16–37	>110	3′ UTR/AD

*Modified from Tables 1 and 2 in Cummings et al. (2000).[1212a]

[†]See **cerebellar ataxia.**

Mechanism/Inheritance

(Gln)$_n$ This (AG)$_n$ repeat occurs in an exon of the affected gene and encodes a (Gln)$_n$ tract in the protein product, resulting in toxic gain in function. Carrier females may be protected by random X-chromosome inactivation and by lower levels of circulating androgen. Longer CAG repeats in normal alleles are interrupted by CAT triplets, whereas disease alleles contain only CAG.

(Ala)$_n$ This (GCG)$_n$ repeat occurs in an exon of the affected gene and encodes an polyalanine tract in the protein product, resulting in toxic gain of function; the (GCG)7 allele is intermediate and worsens disease expression in heterozygotes with the disease allele, but acts as an autosomal recessive mutation for late-onset disease in homozygotes.

intron 1 the (GAA)$_n$ repeat occurs in intron 1 of the gene and inhibits gene expression.

3′ UTR The triplet repeat expansion occurs in the 3′ untranslated region of the gene, causing disease by a complex mechanism which may include mRNA toxic gain of function.

5′ UTR the triplet repeat expansion occurs in the 5′ untranslated region of the gene and affects expression of the gene.

AD, autosomal dominant; Ant, genetic anticipation; AR, autosomal recessive; SLR, sex-linked recessive

trismus   (Gr, grinding) Involuntary, painful spasm of the masseter muscles leading to an inability to open the mouth.

Classically, it is a sign of **tetanus,** but it also occurs with dystonic reactions to drugs, with local disease of the muscles or joints and in psychogenic disease.

trismus nascentium   Neonatal **tetanus.**

trisomy 8 syndrome   An uncommon congenital chromosomal disorder with marked phenotypic variation. Dysmorphic facies, skeletal deformities, clino- and camptodactyly, mental and motor delay, agenesis of the corpus callosum, and the presence of deep furrows on the palms and soles are characteristic and representative findings.[3] See **Warkany syndrome.**

trisomy 9p   A relatively common syndrome of mental retardation, seizures, microcephaly, short stature, kyphosis, other dysmorphic features, and extra chromosomal material on the short arm of chromosome 9.[5340]

trisomy 12p syndrome   A congenital dysmorphic syndrome manifesting hypotonia, enlarged fontanelle, turricephaly, hypertelorism, severe mental retardation, and a seizure disorder resembling **progressive myoclonic epilepsy** accompanied by 4-Hz slow waves and polyspikes on the EEG.[2309]

trisomy 13 syndrome   (Patau syndrome, chromosome 13 trisomy syndrome) An uncommon congenital chromosomal dysmorphic syndrome in which the extra chromosome is responsible for causing microcephaly, physical and mental retardation, feeding difficulties, breath-holding spells, atypical minor motor seizures with **hypsarrhythmia,** agenesis of the olfactory apparatus, optic atrophy, deafness, **holoprocencephaly,** microphthalmia, congenital cardiac and genital malformations, polydactyly, and multiple other skeletal anomalies.

Numerous other associated anomalies, such as cleft lip or palate, capillary hemangiomas of the scalp, and genital anomalies, have been described in a minority of cases.[5221] A report of Bartholin (a Danish physician) in 1657 probably concerned the same condition.[4356]

trisomy 18 syndrome   (Edwards syndrome) An uncommon congenital chromosomal dysmorphic syndrome, characterized by low birth weight, cardiac and skeletal anomalies (e.g., micrognathia, long narrow head, flexed fingers, and pelvic and foot deformities), and hypoplasia of the cerebellum, anterior commissure, and corpus callosum. Mental retardation, seizures, and spasticity are common. Most affected infants die before they are 3 months old.[1608]

trisomy 21 syndrome   See **Down syndrome.**

TRISS   An acronym derived from **TR**auma score and **I**njury **S**everity **S**core, noting also the age of the patient and whether the injury is blunt or penetrating, in order to provide a measure of the probability of survival.

The *injury scale* is derived from the Abbreviated Injury Scale Booklet (AIS, 1990) obtainable from the Northwestern Injury Research Centre, University of Manchester, Hope Hospital, Salford, England, M6 8HD.

The *trauma score* combines coded measurements of respiration, systolic blood pressure, and the **Glasgow Coma scale** to provide a general assessment of physiological derangement.[6073]

tritanopia   Dominantly inherited yellow-blue color blindness.

In a *variant* rare, dominantly inherited syndrome, the tritanopia is associated with optic atrophy.[3162,6049]

triton tumor   A rare, high-grade malignant tumor of the peripheral nerve sheath showing rhabdomyosarcomatous degeneration, commonly in the context of **neurofibromatosis.**[781]

trochanter reflex   The **adductor reflex** elicited by the vibration set up by a tap over the greater trochanter.

trochlear nerve   (from Lat, a pulley) The fourth cranial nerve, described by Alessandro Achillini (1463–1512), an Italian anatomist.

TROG   Acronym for the **T**est for the **R**eception **O**f **G**rammar, an instrument for assessing language comprehension in which the child is asked to select which of four pictures best fits the verbal cue given by the examiner.

Trolard, Paulin   (1842–1910) Professor of anatomy in Algiers.

Trolard's vein   The great annectent vein of the cerebral cortex, described by Trolard in his graduation thesis (University of Paris) in 1868.

trombone tongue   Repetitive protrusion and replacement of the tongue, seen characteristically in **Huntington disease** and other choreic states, but also in tertiary syphilis.

Trömner reflex   Flexion of the fingers in response to a tap on the volar surface of the tip of the patient's second or third finger; a sign with the same significance as the **finger flexion reflex,** of which it is a *variant.*

Trömner-Hoffman reflex   See **Hoffmann reflex.**

trophic   1. Causing movement. 2. Stimulating growth.

trophic influences   Factors causing growth or differentiation of the targeted structures.

tropias   Manifest deviation of the eyes (with misalignment of the visual axes), present when both eyes are viewing a target. See **heterotropia, phoria.**

tropical ataxic neuropathy   See **Nigerian neuropathy.**

tropical neuropathy   See **brucellosis, leprosy, Nigerian neuropathy, HIV, HTLV, cassava, ciguatoxin, scombroid.** Poisoning by coyotillo and gloriosa suberba may also cause acute neuropathies.[5543]

tropical nutritional ataxia   See **Nigerian neuropathy.**

tropical pyomyositis   See **pyomyositis.**

tropical spastic paraparesis   (HTLV-1-associated myelopathy [HAM]) An insidiously progressive paraparesis occurring in the third to fifth decades as a result of cytotoxic T cell–mediated demyelination following infection with HTLV-1. Clinically, the major features include "burning feet" and later spastic gait, spastic bladder, and impotence in men. Additional features include lumbar girdle pains, leg spasticity and hyperreflexia, myoclonic jerks, and slowly progressing loss of vibration and common sensation in the feet with paresthesia in both the hands and the feet. The ankle reflexes are diminished at a later stage.[4750,4751]

The disease is more prevalent in tropical, rainforested countries such as India, the Seychelles, Jamaica, and Colombia and in Africa, but has extended with the spread of the virus elsewhere in the world. The clinical features resemble those of pure spinal multiple sclerosis.[1206]

tropical sprue   A malabsorption syndrome of unknown cause, seen particularly in India and Africa. Clinical features include steatorrhea with xylose malabsorption, and (later) progressive muscle weakness, sensory neuropathy, and features of both **tetany** and **subacute combined degeneration of the cord.**[5488]

tropomyosin   A protein constituent of muscle with contractile properties, manifest when contacted by troponin.

Trotter syndrome   (Sinus of Morgagni syndrome) Malignant infiltration of the lower cranial nerves uni-laterally by a malignant tumor in the lateral pharyngeal recess, producing facial pain and numbness, palatal paresis, and weakness of the masticatory and facial muscles with conductive deafness due to infiltration of the eustachian tube.[5645] See also **pterygopalatine fossa syndrome.**

Trotter, Wilfred Batten Lewis   (1872–1939) English physician.

trouble du sens de l'éspace   See **visuomotor ataxia.**

Trousseau, Armand   (1801–1867) French physician who was trained in medicine and practiced in Paris. He introduced the procedure of tracheotomy; wrote two successful textbooks on medicine and therapeutics; and described what is now known as Hodgkin disease independently in 1864, hemochromatosis in 1859, his sign in tetany in 1861, and the occurrence of thrombophlebitis in association with a visceral carcinoma (in himself) shortly before his death.[1829]

Trousseau sign   1. A test for latent **tetany;** the appearance within 3 minutes of paresthesias, muscle tightening, and **carpopedal spasm** distal to a blood pressure cuff inflated to 20 mmHg above the systolic blood pressure in the arm. 2. The **tâche cérébrale.**

Troyer syndrome   (hereditary spastic paraparesis with wasting and growth retardation) A recessively inherited syndrome of **hereditary spastic paraparesis** with onset in early childhood, complicated by **pseudobulbar palsy,** distal muscle wasting, choreoathetosis, and short stature, and detected in the Amish people of Ohio.[1196]

true Broca aphasia   See **Broca aphasia.**

true myoclonic epilepsy   See **centrencephalic myoclonic-astatic epilepsy.**

true phase reversal   The occurrence of simultaneous pen deflections in opposite directions in two referential derivations using a suitable common reference electrode and displaying the same wave. This phenomenon is rarely observed in scalp EEGs, but when demonstrated beyond doubt in appropriate recording conditions, it indicates a 180° change in phase of an EEG wave between adjacent areas of the brain on either side of a zero isopotential axis. See also **instrumental phase reversal.** (From Chatrian GE, Bergamini L, Dondey M, et al. A glossary of terms most commonly used by clinical electroencephalographers. *EEG Clin Neurophysiol* 1974;**37**:538–48, with permission from Elsevier Science.)

trunk control test   See **motricity index.**

trunk extension test   The subject extends the spine while standing. Pain felt in the back, radiating to the leg, indicates the presence of root compression at lower lumbar levels.

trunkal dystonia   Rare, isolated, focal dystonias affecting the trunk alone, and causing trunk flexion, extension, scoliosis, or torsion, often increased by walking.[3641]

trunkal incurvation   See **developmental reflexes, Galant reflex.**

trunkal mononeuropathy   See **diabetic truncal neuropathy.**

trunk-thigh sign   Flexion of the thigh with elevation of a paretic leg from the bed when the subject attempts to sit up from the supine position without using the arms for support. The normal response is for the legs to remain in contact with the bed during this movement.

trypanosomiasis (African)   See **sleeping sickness.**

trypanosomiasis (American)   See **Chagas disease.**

tryptophan-eosinophilia-myalgia syndrome   A form of **eosinophilic fasciitis** presenting as a scleroderma-like syndrome, and caused by the oral ingestion of tryptophan products. Whether the cause of the syndrome is the tryptophan or something in the excipient is not determined.

tryptophanuria   A rare syndrome resulting from a block in the pathway of tryptophan metabolism. The clinical features resemble those of **Hartnup disease** and include cerebellar ataxia, dermal photosensitivity, small stature, and mental retardation.[1248]

tsara'ath   See **leprosy.**

tschlenow reflex   See **spinoadductor reflex.**

tsiminakis syndrome   Chorea.

tsutsugamshi fever   An infectious disease manifesting rash, fever, meningoencephalitis, and a positive Weil-Felix reaction.

The disease is frequently complicated by peripheral neuropathy, seizures, and residual nerve deafness.[4147] See **scrub typhus.**

tuberculoid leprosy   (maculoanesthetic leprosy) That form of the disease in which the body's immune response to the bacillus is relatively successful. Clinical manifestations include raised anesthetic maculopapules involving the face, buttocks, and limb extensor surfaces and a nodular hypertrophic multiple mononeuropathy.[4863] See **leprosy.**

tuberculoma   (tuberculous granuloma) Encapsulated nodules of granulation tissue which range in size from millimeters to centimeters in diameter. They are composed of acid-fast bacilli; necrotic caseous material; lymphoid, epitheliomatous, and plasma cells; histiocytes; and giant cells, and are surrounded by a zone of vascularity in the periphery.[5486]

Tuberculomas result from the hematogenous spread of *Mycobacterium tuberculosis* to any part in the body.

tuberculoma dolorosa   The **glomus tumor.**

tuberculous alcoholic polyneuritis   See **Lemierre-Boltanski-Justin-Besançon syndrome.**

tuberculous encephalopathy   A rare syndrome of diffuse brain damage, apparently restricted to children and characterized by edema of the white matter with perivascular demyelination and sometimes hemorrhagic leukoencephalopathy. The condition is considered due to an allergic reaction to proteins released by the mycobacteria.[1296]

tuberculous granuloma   See **tuberculoma.**

tuberculous meningitis   A chronic basal meningitis characterized by the usual features of meningeal irritation, increased intracranial pressure, and involvement of the cranial nerves, usually with a protracted but accelerating course culminating in death if untreated. The infection of the meninges proceeds from the spillage of acid-fast bacilli from a small tuberculoma anywhere within the nervous system.

The first description was that of Robert **Whytt** (1714–1766), a Scottish physician, published posthumously in 1768.

tuberous sclerosis   (tuberose sclerosis, Bourneville disease, Bourneville-Brissaud disease, Bourneville-Pringle disease, Brushfield-Wyatt disease, Bourneville-Pellizzi disease, Sherlock epiloia, Pellizzi disseminated cortical dysplasia; OMIM 191090, 1911092)[5047] A complex syndrome inherited as an irregular autosomal dominant trait, and manifesting mental deficiency, multifocal seizures including infantile spasms, and **adenoma sebaceum.** Bourneville's early description made all the important clinical points.[682] The responsible genes map variously to 9q34.1–9q34.2, 11q14–q23, or 16p13.3.

Complications of the numerous calcifying subependymal tubers and of those scattered elsewhere in the brain include focal neurological signs and obstructive hydrocephalus. Simian hands, short in-curved little fingers, accessory thumbs, deformities of the ears, rhabdomyoma of the heart, hypernephroma, spina bifida, dental enamel abnormalities, cardiac tumours, honeycomb lung, renal cysts, renal tumors, osteosclerosis, skeletal cysts, and thickened calvarium may also be found.[683,1165,2179]

Bourneville noted the first case of the disease at the **Salpêtrière** in 1867, and published his observations in 1880, the same year as the condition was described by Hartgeden from Germany. Pringle described the skin signs in 1890.

In a *variant form*, tuberous sclerosis is associated with the **Klippel-Trenaunay-Weber syndrome** in childhood. The clinical features include pseudogliomas of the retina, seizures, bony abnormalities, and mental and developmental delay.

Diagnostic criteria have been proposed[4715] and are summarized in Chart T–8.

Chart T–8. Diagnostic Features of Tuberous Sclerosis

Major Features	Minor Features
Facial angiofibromas or forehead plaque	Multiple, randomly distributed pits in dental enamel
Nontraumatic ungual or periungual fibroma	Hamartomatous rectal polyps
Hypomelanotic patches (three or more)	
Shagreen patch (connective tissue nevus)	Bone cysts
Multiple retinal nodular hamartomas	Cerebral white matter radial migration lines
Cortical tuber	Gingival fibromas
Subependymal nodule	Nonrenal hamartoma
Subependymal giant cell astrocytoma	Retinal achromatic patch
Cardiac rhabdomyoma, single or multiple	"Confetti" skin lesions
Lymphangiomyomatosis	Multiple renal cysts
Renal angiomyolipoma	

Definite tuberous sclerosis complex: Two major or one major and two minor features

Probable: One major and one minor feature

Possible: Either one major or two or more minor features

From Roach ES, Gomez MR, Northrup MH. Tuberous sclerosis complex consensus conference: Revised clinical diagnostic criteria J Child Neurol 1998;13:624–8, by permission of BC Decker.

tubular aggregate myopathies (myopathy with tubular aggregates) Rare, slowly progressive, dominantly or recessively inherited myopathies presenting in adult life.

Clinical complaints include cramps, muscle stiffness, and myalgias that are brought on by exertion and relieved by prolonged rest, as well as proximal muscle weakness[2112] and fatigability without atrophy. Compact collections of tubules are seen on electron microscopy preparations in the subsarcolemmal regions of some of the muscle fibers of each type (especially type 2), associated with some type 2 fiber atrophy.[3984,3985,4743] This pathological change may also be a feature of the **familial periodic paralyses**.[773]

tubular aggregates Densely packed, subsarcolemmal, basophilic tubules with doubled walls, found in type 2b myofibrils, which stain red on trichrome staining.[3985] They derive from proliferations of the sarcoplasmic reticulum and are detectable in a variety of diseases, including a myasthenic syndrome, dominantly and recessively inherited myopathies (**tubular aggregate myopathies),** a syndrome of myalgias and cramps without other pathological change,[4788] familial and nonfamilial myopathies and hyperornithinemia, and after poisoning with diazepam or alcohol.[4743]

tubular constriction See **gun-barrel constriction of the visual fields.**

tubulomembranous inclusion disease A progressive myopathy of youth resembling limb-girdle dystrophy, with facial involvement, marked fatigability, and elevated serum creatine kinase, in which these inclusions are seen on electron microscopy preparations of muscle.[1984]

tucked-lid sign Retraction of the upper eyelid, with scleral show; a finding in **Parinaud syndrome.** See **Collier sign.**

Tuck-McLeod syndrome A sporadic disorder characterized by onset in childhood or middle adult life of a predominantly sensory peripheral polyneuropathy, cerebellar ataxia, and sensorineural hearing loss without distinguishing biochemical abnormalities.[5660]

Tufts Quantitative Neuromuscular Examination A 28-item protocol assessing the neuromuscular deficit at various levels of the neuraxis in **amyotrophic lateral sclerosis.** The items include the results of pulmonary function tests, tests of bulbar function, timed functional tests of hand activities and measurements of isometric strength. To date, it has been used mainly in research studies (see Chart T–9).[177]

Chart T–9. The Tufts Quantitative Neuromuscular Examination

Pulmonary Function

1. Forced vital capacity; best of two trials
2. Maximum voluntary ventilation

Oropharyngeal

1. Time (seconds) to say "pa" 20 times
2. Time (seconds) to say "pata," 15 times

Timed Motor Activities

1. Dialing 764–7172 on a spring-loaded dial phone
2. Number of pegs placed on the Purdue peg board in 30 seconds
3. Time (seconds) taken to walk 15 feet (4.5 meters) with any aid or assistance as needed

From Andres PL, Hedlund W, Finison L, et al. Quantitative assessment in amyotrophic lateral sclerosis. Newrology 1986;36:937–941, reproduced by permission.

Isometric arm and leg strength scores are also awarded on the basis of assessments of maximum voluntary isometric contractions, which reliably quantitate motor unit losses.

tullidora See **buckthorn neuropathy.**

Tullio phenomenon Vertigo, nystagmus, and postural instability induced by high-intensity sound stimulation in patients who are congenitally deaf or who have labyrinthine fistulas. The effect is due to physical activation of the vestibular system by the sound vibrations.[727,5875]

Tulp, Nicholaas (Claes Pieteszoon, 1593–1674) Physician of Amsterdam who trained in Leyden. He gave the first full description of **spina bifida** in his *Observationes medicae* (1641),[7] but is better remembered because his anatomy lesson at the Amsterdam surgeon's guild was painted by Rembrandt in 1631.

Tumarkin otolithic crisis   See **otolithic catastrophe.**

tumor   (Lat, swelling) See **brain tumor** and specific entries.

tumor circoidius   See **arteriovenous malformation.**

Tunbridge-Paley syndrome   A recessively inherited syndrome of progressive deafness with pigmentary retinopathy, optic atrophy, and diabetes mellitus, commencing in the first decade of life.[5666]

tunnel vision   Symmetrical constriction of the visual fields as though the subject were looking down a hollow cylinder. The diameter of the field is identical whether the target object is close or far away, unlike the physiological "funnel vision" in which the field's diameter increases with distance.

turban tumors   See **cylindromatosis.**

Turck, Ludwig   (1810–1868) Austrian anatomist and chief of a neurology service in Vienna, who showed in 1851 that degeneration in a nerve fiber corresponds to the direction in which it conducts impulses physiologically, ascending tracts being above the lesion and descending tracts, below.[4001]

The bundle of Turck comprises the motor fibers that run from the parietotemporal cortex through the posterior limb of the internal capsule to the cerebral peduncle, and then to the pons. Turck also described the anterior corticospinal tract in 1849.

Turcot syndrome   (intestinal polyposis and glioma) A rare, genetically transmitted (dominant or recessive) syndrome, characterized by the occurrence of multiple colorectal tumors with cerebral glioblastoma or medulloblastoma.[2406]

turn   The point of change in polarity of a waveform and the magnitude of the voltage change following the turning point. It is not necessary that the voltage change pass through the baseline. The minimal excursion required to constitute a change should be specified. (From the 2001 Report of the Nomenclature Committee of the American Association of Electromyography and Electrodiagnosis.[10] Used by permission, copyright © 2001, AAEM.)

Turner, William   (1832–1916) Professor of anatomy at the University of Edinburgh, noted for his description of the gyri, fissures, and lobes of the cerebral cortex in today's accepted form.

turns analysis   An automated method of analyzing EMG activity during isometric voluntary contraction whereby the number of positive and negative potential changes exceeding 100 uV is counted over a specific period. The method provides some data distinguishing primary myopathic from neurogenic muscle disease.[2019]

turns-amplitude analysis   A computerized method of assessing the muscle recruitment patterns recorded by EMG. The parameters studied are the maximal number of turns to mean amplitude (peak ratio or PR); the mean amplitude; and the number of time intervals between turns at different degrees of voluntary contraction. The technique assists in the EMG diagnosis of myopathy.[5313]

turricephaly   (Lat, tower + Gr, head) See **tower skull.**

turtle headache   A condition described only in colder climates, characterized by the occurrence of dull, generalized matutinal headaches, presumed to be due to the hypercapnia resulting from sleeping completely under the bedclothes.

tussive syncope   (Lat, cough + Gr, faint) (laryngeal vertigo) See **cough syncope.**

twilight state   (absence status, état confusionnel simple, spike–wave stupor, fugue state) A syndrome characterized by prolonged confusion, diminished responsiveness, speech arrest, automatic behavior, and subsequent amnesia as a result of petit mal or subconvulsive complex partial seizure (psychomotor) status.

In the former, diffuse, irregular 1.5- to 4-Hz multispike-wave complexes are recorded, there is no complete loss of responsiveness, and the episode represents one single prolonged attack. In the latter, the episode is due to repetitive, discontinuous attacks; total unresponsiveness may ensue; and the EEG patterns are variable and include both fast- and slow-wave discharges, rhythmic diffuse bilateral spikes and anterior temporal sharp waves.[436] Twilight states may also occur as postictal manifestations.[1703]

twitch-convulsive syndrome   A symptom of uremic encephalopathy in the setting of other metabolic disorders such as delirium tremens, diabetes, and lupus erythematosus. Clouding of consciousness, seizures, and multifocal myoclonus occur, the latter in any area of the body in both the waking and sleeping states.

two-point discrimination   The discrimination of two points of simultaneous contact on the skin or mucosa.

TWUD index   (Time Wasted in Unnecessary Discussion) The relationship between the frequency with which a condition is considered and the frequency with which it is actually present. Informal, introspective analysis suggests a TWUD index of 4800 for **normal-pressure hydrocephalus,** 320 for **Creutzfeldt-Jakob disease,** and 15 for **Bell palsy.** The occurrence of bedsores in demented patients has a negative score.

tylosis-optic atrophy   A rare syndrome of adult life consisting of thickening of the palms and soles and the later development of optic atrophy.[1460]

tympanic neuropathy   (syndrome of Jacobson's nerve and plexus) Loss of secretion by the parotid gland as a result of damage to the nerve, usually as a result of cranial trauma.[3374]

tympanic plexus neuralgia   See **glossopharyngeal neuralgia.**

type grouping   The presence of unusually large numbers of fibers (50 or more) of the same histochemical type, arranged contiguously in groups within a microscopic preparation of muscle. The appearance is considered to indicate the collateral sprouting of motor axons in cases of chronic motor neuropathy.[2941] See **fiber type grouping.**

type 1 acrocephalosyndactyly   See **Apert syndrome.**

type 1 fiber atrophy   Selective atrophy of type 1 muscle fibers, found in numerous conditions such as nemaline myopathy, congenital fiber-type disproportion,[772] and myotonic dystrophy and also as a lone familial occurrence when it presents with congenital nonprogressive muscle wasting and weakness.[4925]

type 1 fiber hypotrophy with central nuclei   An X-linked recessive disorder characterized by this microscopic appearance, which is associated clinically with congenital severe diffuse weakness and hypotonia and enlargement of the tongue, the disease resembling **hereditary motor neuropathy, type 1.**[1679] Biopsy specimens show fiber hypertrophy or hypotrophy with central nuclei and the presence of cytoplasmic bodies.[337]

type 1 fiber predominance   The appearance on muscle biopsy specimens when the number of histochemically type 1 fibers shown exceeds the normal for the muscle biopsied. For the vastus lateralis, >55% would be abnormal.

The finding is present in cases of **congenital** and **Duchenne muscular dystrophies,** various **congenital myopathies, hypothyroid myopathy,** and **benign congenital hypotonia,** and also in some children with hypotonia without other evidence of neuromuscular disease.[3211]

type 1 myofibrils   Slow-twitch muscle fibers containing substantial amounts of myoglobin and staining well for dehydrogenases. ATPase stains at pH 9.4 stain these fibers poorly, but they stain dark at pH 4.35.

type 2 myofibrils   Fast-twitch muscle fibers staining well for phosphorylase, glycogen, and α-glycerophosphate dehydrogenase. ATPase stains at pH 9.4 stain these fibers dark. At pH 4.35 they are unstained and at pH 4.63, two fiber subtypes (colorless 2a and intermediate 2b) can be differentiated.

type-specific atrophy   Selective atrophy of type 1 or type 2 myofibrils. Type 2b atrophy is seen in the settings of cachectic wasting, or systemic malignancy or prolonged immobilization.

type/token ratio   A measure of verbal diversification in which the number of times a particular word appears in a block of language is expressed as its ratio to the total number of words in the block. All the words in the block are counted (*tokens*), but the count of the number of different words is the *type*. In the shortest and simplest sentences, in old age and in dementia, the ratio is low (e.g., <0.5).[1180]

typhus   A louse-borne *rickettsial* infection causing generalized vasculitis. Clinical features consist of fever, headache, vomiting, respiratory symptoms, conjunctival injection and diarrhea, followed by the appearance of a purpuric rash.

The neurological complications are those of a meningoencephalitis causing delirium and stupor, and any of many possible focal deficits, occurring either during or following the acute illness.[2548]

typical absence attacks   See **typical absence epilepsy.**

typical absence epilepsy   (typical absence attacks) A term applied to a number of epileptic syndromes including frequent absence attacks occurring in isolation between the ages of 4 and 10 years (**pyknolepsy**); typical absence epilepsy of adolescents, sometimes with associated tonic-clonic seizures, etc; petit mal epilepsy; myoclonic absences (clonic absences); and typical absence epilepsies with unusual EEG features. The latter include adversive absence, absences occurring with focal clinical features, absence with evidence of a brain lesion, and absences induced by visual stimuli.[56]

Simple typical absences are characterized by sudden stress or a marked decrease in mental functioning of brief duration, usually 5 to 15 seconds, with abolition or diminution of awareness, responsiveness, and memory for the event when the subject returns from this period of unawareness and unresponsiveness. Hyperventilation and stimulation are strong precipitants.

In *complex typical absences*, the impairment of consciousness is associated with motor manifestations, including gaze deviation, head rotation, clonic jerks, or decreased muscle tone.

typical absence epilepsy of adolescence   (primary generalized epilepsy of adolescence) A syndrome of repetitive absences clustering within the hour following awakening, in which the attacks are shorter and less frequent than the similar syndrome in younger children, and sometimes without complete loss of contact with the surroundings. Generalized tonic-clonic seizures also occur in some cases.[6018] See also **juvenile myoclonic epilepsy of Janz.**

tyramine infusion test   A test of postganglionic sympathetic fiber integrity, in which tyramine is infused intravenously at rates of 60 to 500 μg/min until there is an elevation of systolic blood pressure of 15 mm Hg or more.

An exaggerated response (e.g., with 300 μg/min) suggests the presence of denervation hypersensitivity, and an impaired response, severe postganglionic damage.[330]

The test is based on the fact that normally the tyramine is taken up by sympathetic vesicles and leads to the secretion of norepinephrine, and hence an increase in blood pressure.[330]

tyrosine hydroxylase   The rate-limiting enzyme in catecholamine synthesis.

tyrosinemia I   (OMIM 276700) A rare recessively inherited disorder of amino acid metabolism due to a deficiency of the gene for fumarylacetoacetate hydrolase, leading to hepatic disease, neuropathy, and other neurological features resembling those of porphyria.[2287]

tyrosinemia II   A diffuse encephalopathy presenting with cataracts, skin lesions, and mental delay.[3907] The responsible gene maps to 16q22.1–q22.3. See **Richner-Hanhart syndrome.**

tyrosinosis   A recessively inherited dysmetabolic state seen in neonates, and due to impairment of hepatic tyrosine transaminase function. The condition is characterized by hepatic and renal impairment, vitamin D–resistant rickets, blepharospasm, and mental and motor delay in the survivors.[6102]

U

U fibers The longitudinal (*arcuate*, from Lat, bow-shaped) myelinated fibers of the cerebral cortex which course beneath the sulci. They are spared in **Binswanger disease,** in some leukodystrophies, and in **cerebral amyloid angiopathy.**

ubiquitin An abnormal protein component of neuronal inclusions in **Alzheimer, Parkinson,** and **Pick diseases.**

UBOs See **unidentified bright objects.**

Udorn encephalopathy A syndrome described in the population of Thailand which closely resembles **Reye syndrome,** but which is due to aflatoxin poisoning.[4234]

Uhthoff symptom (hot-bath sign) Deterioration of neural function in association with a rise in local body temperature.[5683] It is seen in patients with demyelinating disease as a result of the increased conduction block occurring at higher temperatures, and is usable as a sign of demyelination when nystagmus, motor power, or visual acuity are measured before and after heating a patient by as little as 1°C. While present in many patients with multiple sclerosis, the sign is not diagnostic of that condition. Dr. Wilhelm Uhthoff (1853–1927) was a German physician who described the phenomenomn in 1889.

An *inverse Uhtoff sign* has been reported, in which vision improves with warming.[131]

ulcerative mutilating acropathy with abnormal CSF aminoacids A rare *variant* of **hereditary sensory and autonomic neuropathy.**

ulceromutilating acropathy (mutilating acropathy) The trophic changes, including impaired circulation and loss of hair, nonhealing ulceration of the skin, and infection of soft tissues and bone, occurring usually in the distal parts of limbs as a result of peripheral sensory neuropathies impairing pain sensation and autonomic functions. See **hereditary sensory and autonomic neuropathy, familial amyloid neuropathy.**

Lesions of the conus medullaris and central cord may do the same. Compare with **Charcot joint** (in which the damage is more proximal).

ulegyria (mantle sclerosis, nodular cortical sclerosis) A localized destruction of the deepest parts of the cortical wall in the sulci with relative sparing of the cortex at the surface. The abnormality may be generalized or localized, but in either case is usually a result of perinatal hypoxia.

Ullmann syndrome (systemic angiomatosis) A heterogeneous syndrome characterized by the presence of cavernous and telangiectatic angiomas in the brain with associated dural abnormalities. The condition is probably a form of **Osler-Rendu-Weber disease.**

Ullrich muscular dystrophy See **congenital muscular dystrophy** (*atonic-sclerotic type*).

Ullrich, Otto (1894–1957) German pediatrician who practiced in Essen, Berlin, and Rostock, and who described what is now known as *Turner syndrome* and *hypophosphatemic renal rickets* as well as the syndromes described in the following entries.

Ullrich syndrome 1. See **congenital muscular dystrophy** (*atonic-sclerotic type*). 2. A benign form of muscular dystrophy associated with hyperexcitability in the CNS. See **minimal change myopathy.**

Ullrich-Noonan syndrome See **Noonan syndrome.**

ulnar flexion maneuver Flexion of the elbow and flexion and ulnar deviation of the wrist increase paresthesias in the fourth and fifth digits in cases of ulnar nerve entrapment beneath the flexor carpi ulnaris.[1821]

ulnar nerve palsies Sensory deficits with weakness and wasting of the muscles supplied by the ulnar nerve, usually as a result of its compression in the cubital tunnel or distally, in **Guyon's canal.** The former is far more common (**cubital tunnel syndrome**); the interossei, adductor pollicis, and hypothenar muscles are affected, and there is reduced common sensation in the ulnar palm and the ulnar 1 1/2 digits. The **Tinel sign** is frequently positive at the cubital tunnel. Damage to the *deep palmar branch* of the nerve in **Guyon's canal** occurs in carpenters, cobblers, cyclists, and others who repeatedly compress the nerve there in the course of work or play. Weakness and wasting of the interossei and adductor pollicis without hypothenar muscle involvement and without sensory changes are the characteristic findings. The most useful electrodiagnostic test compares the latencies of the median and ulnar mixed nerve action potentials between the wrist and the elbow.[3844]

Isolated damage to the *dorsal sensory branch* of the nerve on the dorsum of the hand is a rarity, and almost always due to local trauma. See also **all ulnar hand.**

ultimum moriens The superior portion of the trapezius muscle, which **Gowers** considered to be remarkable in that it did not atrophy in certain myopathic states, when other muscles did.

ultraterminal sprouting The growth of neuronal shoots at the motor nerve terminal to innervate orphaned end-plates, seen when the release of acetylcholine from the terminal is blocked, as in **botulism.**

ultraviolet keratitis See **photophthalmia.**

umami The savory taste associated with cured meats, Parmesan cheese, and monosidium glutamate, additional to the usually regonized sweet, salt, sour, and bitter quartet.

uncal herniation (Lat, hook + rupture) (lateral transtentorial herniation) Downward displacement of the uncus and parahippocampal gyrus through the tentorial opening due to increased intracranial pressure, as may result from an expanding mass in the temporal lobe.

uncal syndrome The clinical effect of herniation of the uncus downward through the tentorium cerebelli as a result of increased intracranial pressure, usually resulting from a temporal lobe mass on the same side. Lateral displacement of the brainstem may be as important as the downward shift, however.[4769]

The herniating tissue compresses the brainstem at the level of the peduncles and distorts the third cranial nerve, leading to third nerve palsy, diminution in conscious level, Cheyne-Stokes respirations, and direct compression of the same and secondary compression of the opposite cerebral peduncle, leading to ipsi- and contralateral hemiparesis with a grave prognosis.[4466]

Compression of the posterior cerebral artery may lead to occipital infarction, the resultant homonymous hemianopia then representing a false localizing sign.

uncinate (Lat, hooked) To do with the uncus.

uncinate fits Complex partial seizures in which olfactory hallucinations occur as part of the consciously appreciated manifestations of the seizure, and assumed to be due to electrical excitation of the uncus and olfactory cortex.[1256]

The name was applied by Hughlings-**Jackson** in 1899: "There is at the onset of the paroxysm a crude sensation of smell or of taste or in which there are movements of chewing, smacking of the lips, and sometimes spitting, etc." Jackson was aware of the research of **Ferrier** showing that the functions of smell and taste in animals are localized in the uncinate gyrus.

uncrossed diplopia That form of diplopia which results from **esotropia,** and in which the false image is displaced toward the side of the paretic eye. See also **crossed diplopia.**

Underwood, Michael (1737–1820) English physician, pediatrician, and obstetrician, who gave the first modern account of **poliomyelitis** in 1789.[4369]

undifferentiated jargon See **jargon.**

undulatory nystagmus See **pendular nystagmus.**

unformed hallucinations Visual hallucinations, the images not being recognizable as people or objects, or, in the case of auditory hallucinations, those in which the sound heard does not resemble that from any recognized source.

unidentified bright objects (UBOs) Areas of brightness on T2-weighted (long spin-echo) MRI scans indicating the presence in those areas of high concentrations of H^+ protons (i.e., water or glial cells); such areas

may be multiple sclerosis plaques, infarcts, or other pathologies.

Unified Form for Neurological Stroke scales A combination scale constituting reconciliations of the Neurological Scale for Middle Cerebral Artery Infarction (MCANS) and the Scandinavian Stroke Scale (SNSS). It also allows the generation of scores on the **Canadian Stroke scale.**[4258] (see Chart U–1).

Chart U–1. Unified Form for Neurological Stroke Scale

Item	SNSS	MCANS
Consciousness		
Normal/fully conscious	6	15
Somnolent/drowsiness	4	10
Reacts to verbal command	2	10
Stupor (reacts to pain only)	0	5
Coma	0	0
Speech/Verbal Communication		
Normal/No aphasia	10	10
Limited vocabulary or incoherent speech/difficult	6	5
More than yes-no but not longer sentences/difficult	3	5
Only yes-no or less/extremely difficult or impossible	0	0
Eye Movements/Eyes and Head Shift		
No gaze/palsy/none	4	10
Gaze palsy/gaze failure	2	5
Conjugate eye deviation/forced	0	0
Facial Palsy		
None/dubious/slight paresis.	2	5
Present/paralysis or marked paresis	0	0
Arm: Motor Power/Raising		
Raises with normal strength/normal	6	10
Raised with reduced strength/possible	5	10
Raises with flexion in elbow/incomplete	4	5
Can move but not against gravity/impossible	2	0
Paralysis	0	0
Hand: Motor Power/Movements		
Normal strength/normal	6	15
Reduced strength/skilled	4	10
Fingertips do not reach palm/useful	2	5
Paralysis/useless	0	0
Leg: Motor Power/Raising		
Normal strength	6	15
Raises with reduced strength/against resistance	5	10

Raises with flexion of knee/ against gravity	4	5
Can move, but not against gravity/ impossible	2	0
Paralysis	0	0

Foot Dorsiflexion

Against resistance/normal	—	10
Against gravity	—	5
Foot drop	—	0

Upper Limb Tone

Normal (even if brisk reflexes)	—	5
Overtly spastic or flaccid	—	0

Lower Limb Tone

Normal (even if brisk reflexes)	—	5
Overtly spastic or flaccid	—	0

Orientation

Correct for time, place, and person	6	—
Two of these	4	—
One of these	2	—
Completely disoriented	0	—

Gait

Walks at least 5 m without aids	12	—
Walks with aids	9	—
Walks with help of another person	+6	—
Sits without support	3	—
Bedridden/wheelchair	0	—
Total		

From Orgogozo JM. A unified form for neurological scoring of hemispheric stroke with motor impairment. Stroke 1992;23:1678–1679, by permission.

unipolar needle electrode   See **monopolar needle recording electrode.**

Unified Rating Scale for Parkinsonism   (Version 3.0) A popular and comprehensive scale for the determination of disability in Parkinson disease.[5343] The scale is reproduced in Chart U–2.

Chart U–2. Unified Rating Scale for Parkinsonism

1. Mentation, Behavior, and Mood

1. Intellectual impairment
   0. None
   1. Mild. Consistent forgetfulness with partial recollection of events and no other difficulties.
   2. Moderate memory loss, with disorientation and moderate difficulty handling complex problems. Mild but definite impairment of function at home with need of occasional prompting.
   3. Severe memory loss with disorientation for time and often to place. Severe impairment in handling problems.
   4. Severe memory loss with orientation preserved to person only. Unable to make judgments or solve problems. Requires much help with personal care. Cannot be left alone at all.

2. Thought disorder (due to dementia or drug intoxication)
   0. None
   1. Vivid dreaming
   2. "Benign" hallucinations with insight retained
   3. Occasional to frequent hallucinations or delusions, without insight. Could interfere with daily activities.
   4. Persistent hallucinations, delusions, or florid psychoses. Not able to care for self.

3. Depression
   0. Not present
   1. Periods of sadness or guilt greater than normal, never sustained for days or weeks
   2. Sustained depression (1 week or more)
   3. Sustained depression with vegetative symptoms (insomnia, anorexia, weight loss, loss of interest)
   4. Sustained depression with vegetative symptoms and suicidal thoughts or intent

4. Motivation/initiative
   0. Normal
   1. Less assertive than usual; more passive
   2. Loss of initiative or disinterest in elective (non-routine) activities
   3. Loss of initiative or disinterest in day-to-day routine activities
   4. Withdrawn, complete loss of motivation

2. Activities of Daily Living (determine for "on–off")

5. Speech
   0. Normal
   1. Mildly affected; no difficulty being understood
   2. Moderately affected; sometimes asked to repeat statements
   3. Severely affected; often asked to repeat statements
   4. Unintelligible most of the time

6. Salivation
   0. Normal
   1. Slight but definite excess of saliva in mouth; may have night-time drooling
   2. Moderately excessive saliva; may have minimal drooling
   3. Marked excess of saliva with some drooling
   4. Marked drooling; requires constant tissue or handkerchief

7. Swallowing
   0. Normal
   1. Rare choking
   2. Occasional choking
   3. Requires soft food
   4. Requires nasogastric tube or gastrostomy feeding

8. Handwriting
   0. Normal
   1. Slightly slow or small
   2. Moderately slow or small; all words are legible
   3. Severely affected; not all words are legible
   4. The majority of words are not legible

9. Cutting food or handling utensils
   0. Normal
   1. Somewhat slow and clumsy, but no help needed
   2. Can cut most foods, although clumsy and slow—some help needed
   3. Food must be cut by someone, but can still feed slowly
   4. Needs to be fed

10. Dressing
   0. Normal
   1. Somewhat slow, but no help needed
   2. Occasional assistance with buttoning, or with getting arms in sleeves
   3. Considerable help required, but can do some things alone
   4. Helpless
11. Hygiene
   0. Normal
   1. Somewhat slow, but no help needed
   2. Needs help to shower or bathe; or very slow in hygienic care
   3. Requires assistance for washing, brushing teeth. combing hair, going to the bathroom
   4. Foley catheter or other mechanical aids
12. Turning in bed and adjusting bed clothes
   0. Normal
   1. Somewhat slow and clumsy, but no help needed
   2. Can turn alone or adjust sheets, but with great difficulty
   3. Can initiate, but not turn or adjust sheets alone
   4. Helpless
13. Falling (unrelated to freezing)
   0. None
   1. Rare falling
   2. Occasionally falls, less than once per day
   3. Falls on average of once daily
   4. Falls more than once daily
14. Freezing when walking
   0. None
   1. Rare freezing when walking; may have start-hesitation
   2. Occasional freezing when walking
   3. Frequent freezing; occasionally falls from freezing
   4. Frequent falls from freezing
15. Walking
   0. Normal
   1. Mild difficulty. May not swing arms or may tend to drag leg
   2. Moderate difficulty, but requires little or no assistance
   3. Severe disturbance of walking, requiring assistance
   4. Cannot walk at all, even with assistance
16. Tremor
   0. Absent
   1. Slight and infrequently present
   2. Moderate; bothersome to patient
   3. Severe; interferes with many activities
   4. Marked; interferes with most activities
17. Sensory complaints related to parkinsonism
   0. None
   1. Occasionally has numbness, tingling, or mild aching
   2. Frequently has numbness, tingling, or aching; not distressing
   3. Frequent painful sensations
   4. Excruciating pain

3. Motor Examination

18. Speech
   0. Normal
   1. Slight loss of expression, diction, or volume
   2. Monotone, slurred but understandable
   3. Marked impairment, difficult to understand
   4. Unintelligible

19. Facial expression
   0. Normal
   1. Minimal hypomimia, could be normal "poker face"
   2. Slight but definitely abnormal diminution of facial expression
   3. Moderate hypomimia; lips parted some of the time
   4. Masked or fixed facies with severe or complete loss of facial expression; lips parted 1/4 inch or more
20. Tremor at rest
   0. Absent
   1. Slight and infrequently present
   2. Mild in amplitude and persistent; or moderate in amplitude but only intermittently present
   3. Moderate in amplitude and present most of the time
   4. Marked in amplitude and present most of the time
21. Action or postural tremor of hands
   0. Absent
   1. Slight; present with action
   2. Moderate in amplitude, present with action
   3. Moderate in amplitude with posture holding as well as action
   4. Marked in amplitude; interferes with feeding
22. Rigidity (judged on passive movement of major joints with patient relaxed in sitting position; cogwheeling to be ignored)
   0. Absent
   1. Slight or detectable only when activated by mirror or other movements
   2. Mild to moderate
   3. Marked, but full range of motion easily achieved
   4. Severe, range of motion achieved with difficulty
23. Finger taps (patient taps thumb with index finger in rapid succession with widest amplitude possible, each hand separately)
   0. Normal
   1. Mild slowing or reduction in amplitude
   2. Moderately impaired. Definite and early fatiguing; may have occasional arrests in movement.
   3. Severely impaired. Frequent hesitation in initiating movement or arrests in ongoing movement.
   4. Can barely perform the task
24. Hand movement (patient opens and closes hands in rapid succession with widest amplitude possible, each hand separately)
   0. Normal
   1. Mild slowing and/or reduction in amplitude
   2. Moderately impaired. Definite and early fatiguing. May have occasional arrests in movement.
   3. Severely impaired. Frequent hesitation in initiating movement or arrests in ongoing movement.
   4. Can barely perform the task
25. Rapid alternating movements of hands (pronation-supination movements of hands, vertically or horizontally, with as large an amplitude as possible, both hands simultaneously)
   0. Normal
   1. Mild slowing or reduction in amplitude
   2. Moderately impaired. Definite and early fatiguing. May have occasional arrests in movement.
   3. Severely impaired. Frequent hesitation in initiating movements or arrests in ongoing movements.
   4. Can barely perform the task

26. Leg agility
    0. Normal
    1. Mild slowing and/or reduction in amplitude
    2. Moderately impaired; definite and early fatiguing. May have occasional arrests in movement.
    3. Severely impaired. Frequent hesitation in initiating movements or arrests in ongoing movement.
    4. Can barely perform the task
27. Arising from chair (patient attempts to arise from a straight-backed wood or metal chair with arms folded across chest)
    0. Normal.
    1. Slow; or may need more than one attempt
    2. Pushes self up from arms or seat
    3. Tends to fall back and may have to try more than one time but can get up without help
    4. Unable to arise without help
28. Posture
    0. Normal erect
    1. Not quite erect, slightly stooped posture; could be normal for older person
    2. Moderately stooped posture, definitely abnormal; can be slightly leaning to one side
    3. Severely stooped posture with kyphosis; can be moderately leaning to one side
    4. Marked flexion with extreme abnormality of posture
29. Gait
    0. Normal
    1. Walks slowly, may shuffle with short steps, but no festination, short steps, or propulsion
    2. Walks with difficulty but requires little or no assistance; may have some festination, short steps, or propulsion
    3. Severe disturbance of gait, requiring assistance
    4. Cannot walk at all, even with assistance
30. Postural stability (response to sudden posterior displacement produced by pull on shoulders when patient is erect with eyes open and feet slightly apart; patient is prepared)
    0. Normal
    1. Retropulsion, but recovers unaided
    2. Absence of postural responses; would fall if not
    3. Very unstable, tends to lose balance spontaneously
    4. Unable to stand without assistance
31. Body bradykinesia and hypokinesia (combining slowness hesitancy, decreased arm-swing, small amplitude, and poverty of movement in general)
    0. None
    1. Minimal slowness, giving movement a deliberate character; could be normal for some persons. Possibly reduced amplitude.
    2. Mild degree of slowness and poverty of movement that is definitely abnormal. Alternatively, some reduced amplitude.
    3. Moderate slowness, poverty, or small amplitude
    4. Marked slowness, power, or small amplitude of movement

4. Complications of Therapy (in the past week)

   A. Dyskinesias

32. Duration: What proportion of the waking day are dyskinesias present? (historical information)
    0. None

1. 1%–5% of day
2. 26%–0%
3. 51%–75%
4. 76%–100%
33. Disability: How disabling are the dyskinesias? (historical information)
    0. Not disabling
    1. Mildly disabling
    2. Moderately disabling
    3. Severely disabling
    4. Completely disabled
34. Painful dyskinesias: How painful are the dyskinesias?
    0. No painful dyskinesias
    1. Slight
    2. Moderate
    3. Severe
    4. Marked
35. Presence of early morning dystonia
    0. No
    1. Yes

   B. Clinical fluctuations

36. Are any off periods predictable as to timing after a dose of medication?
    0. No
    1. Yes
37. Are any off periods unpredictable as to timing after a dose of medication?
    0. None
    1. Yes
38. Do any of the "off" periods come on suddenly (e.g., over a few seconds)
    0. No
    1. Yes
39. What proportion of the waking day is the patient "off" on average?
    0. None.
    1. 1%–25%
    2. 26%–50%
    3. 51%–75%
    4. 76%–100%

   C. Other complications

40. Does the patient have anorexia, nausea, or vomiting?
    0. No
    1. Yes
41. Does the patient have any sleep disturbances (e.g., insomnia, hypersomnolence)?
    0. No
    1. Yes
42. Does the patient have symptomatic orthostasis?
    0. No
    1. Yes

Record the patient's blood pressure, pulse, and weight on the scoring form.

From Stern MB. The clinical characteristics of Parkinson's disease and parkinsonian syndromes: diagnosis and management. In: Stern MB, Hurtig HM, eds. The Comprehensive Management of Parkinson's Disease, pp. 33–41. New York: PMA Publishing, 1988, by permission.)

   See also **Hoehn and Yahr scale,**[2598] **Columbia rating scale,**[1726] **Parkinson Disease Impairment index.**

uniform fiber-type myopathy   A form of muscle disorder in which histochemical staining demonstrates that more than 99% of the muscle fibers belong to one histochemical type.[4212]

unihemispheric sleep The biological changes of sleep occurring in but one of the cerebral hemispheres; an attribute of dolphins.

For a human to be "half-asleep," however, suggests the presence of stage 1 non–rapid eye movement sleep on both sides.

unilateral atonic seizures See **hemiparetic seizures.**

unilateral jaw and masticatory spasm A focal dystonic syndrome with onset in youth or early adult life, characterized by spasm and secondary hypertrophy of the masseters. See **oromandibular dystonia.**

unilateral juvenile muscular atrophy of upper limbs See **monomelic amyotrophy.**

unilateral lobar atrophy A form of unilateral frontotemporal atrophy causing slowly progressive aphasia without dementia, and associated with neuronal loss, gliosis, and spongiform change in the affected cortical region.[3061]

unilateral pursuit paresis The association of saccadic (rather than smooth) pursuit when the eyes follow toward the side of a hemispheric lesion, and contralateral homonymous hemianopia.[5575]

unilateral spatial agnosia Massive neglect of the left half of visual space, leading to loss of topographical orientation and caused by a lesion of the right parietal region.

unimacular nystagmus See **latent nystagmus.**

unimodal apraxia Any form of apraxia that is specific to actions demonstrated in a single modality, e.g. visual but not auditory.[3138] See **apraxia.**

uniocular nystagmus Vertical oscillations of one eye in association with long-standing visual loss. The amplitude of the oscillations ranges between 3° and 50° and the frequency between 0.1 and 5 cycles/second, inversely correlated with the amplitudes.[4530]

unipolar See **referential derivation.**

United Cerebral Palsy Association A charitable organization. Address: 1660 L Street, NW, Suite 700, Washington, DC 20036. Tel: 202-776-0406, 800-872-5827. Web site: http://www.ucpa.org/.

United Leukodystrophy Foundation A charitable association in this field. Address: 2304 Highland Dr., Sycamore, IL 60178. Tel: 815-895-3211, 800-728-5483. Web site: http://www.ulf.org/.

United Mitochondrial Disease Foundation An American charitable association promoting research and supporting families of people with mitochondriopathies. Address: 8085 Saltsburg Road, Suite 201, Pittsburgh, PA 15239. Tel: 412-793-6477. Web site: www.umdf.org/.

United Parkinson Foundation An organization dedicated to funding research on Parkinson disease, publishing educational materials for patients and health-care professionals, and providing support for patients with the disease. Address: 833 West Washington Blvd., Chicago, IL 60607. Tel: 312-733-1893.

unloading reflex A biphasic response characterized by an initial reduction or absence of electrical potentials recorded on the EMG, followed by an abrupt increase in electrical activity, when a muscle is contracted against an external load and the load is then suddenly removed.[126]

unprovoked seizures of unknown etiology Cases of unprovoked seizures for which no clear antecedent etiology can be detected. One form comprises the *idiopathic epilepsies*, which are defined by the ILAE[1115] as certain partial or generalized epileptic syndromes with particular clinical characteristics and with specific EEG findings; the term should not be used to refer to epilepsy or seizures without obvious cause.

Unverricht, Heinrich (1853–1912) German physician, practicing in Jena, Austria. His graduating thesis, in which he asserted that all seizures required the presence of cortex, aroused great interest, and within 6 years he had been appointed professor of medicine at Dorpat. He published his account of familial myoclonic epilepsy in 1891.

Unverricht-Lundborg-Lafora syndrome (Lafora body epilepsy, Baltic or Nordic myoclonus, myoclonic encephalopathy with progressive cranial nerve palsies, progressive familial myoclonic epilepsy)[505,5689] A recessively inherited **mitochondrial encephalomyelopathy** presenting between the ages of 8 and 13 years with tonic-clonic seizures; spontaneous, stimulus-sensitive, and action myoclonus (**cortical myoclonus**); drop attacks; ataxia; rigidity; cerebellar signs; and, later, progressive mental deterioration. Repetitive morning myoclonus is a common complaint and is the most common cause of progressive myoclonic epilepsy. The biochemical cause is not known but the responsible gene maps to chromosome 21q22.3.

The Marseilles consensus group defined the condition as follows: "Myoclonus with epileptic seizures and progressive neurological decline, particularly ataxia and dementia." The syndrome was first reported by Unverricht in 1891 and appears to occur mainly in the populations of eastern Sweden and Finland, determining the name *Baltic*, but it has also been reported from distant shores. It is probably the same condition as many (but not all) cases of the **dyssynergia cerebellaris myoclonica** of **Ramsay Hunt.**[5496] Lundborg contributed to understanding of the syndrome, by adding new cases, demonstrating autosomal recessive inheritance and confirming that the disease is indeed progressive, by demonstrating the presence of intracytoplasmic inclusions (**Lafora bodies**) within the nervous system.

Myoclonic encephalopathy with progressive cranial nerve palsies is a *variant* form,

See also **progressive myoclonic ataxias, dentatorubropallidoluysian atrophy.**

Unverricht-Wagner syndrome   See **dermatomyositis.**

upbeat nystagmus   A form of central vestibular jerk nystagmus in which the fast component is upward and which is present in the primary position but increases on upward gaze. Defective upward pursuit but intact vestibulo-ocular movements are characteristic accompaniments.

Bilateral lesions of the ventral tegmental pathways at the pontomesencephalic junction or in the caudal brainstem close to the perihypoglossal nuclei and lesions of the anterior vermis are most commonly incriminated.[2984,4583]

up-gaze palsy   Failure of conjugate upward deviation of the eyes as a result of a pretectal lesion in which the posterior commissure is damaged. Other features of the **Parinaud syndrome** are usually present as well.

upper airway resistance syndrome   Anatomical constriction of the airways at levels above the larynx, considered relevant in the genesis of some cases of **idiopathic hypersomnia.**[91]

upper brachial plexus palsy   (Erb palsy, Duchenne-Erb palsy, **rucksack palsy,** knapsack palsy, **pallbearers' palsy**) Weakness and atrophy of the muscles supplied by C5–6 through the upper trunk of the brachial plexus, leading to the posture of the arm described as the "porter's tip" position. It is commonly caused by violent falls on the shoulder, excessive traction on the head during delivery, or direct injury to the upper fibers of the brachial plexus.[1687]

Erb's name is popularly attached to this condition, although he attributed its delineation to **Duchenne,** whose adequate account had been provided 19 years before.[5069] Another, by William Smellie, a Scottish obstetrician, had been published in 1768.

upper motor neuron lesion   (pyramidal lesion, corticospinal tract lesion) A lesion of the descending motor pathways between the cortex and the brainstem or spinal cord, producing a relatively constant syndrome of postural disturbance, increased tone (spasticity), decreased power especially in the arm extensors and the leg flexors, hyperreflexia of the muscle stretch reflexes and loss of superficial reflexes, and an upgoing plantar (positive Babinski) response. Both the corticospinal and the corticoreticulospinal pathways are considered to be involved.

The alternative term *pyramidal lesion* is used synonymously, but could be considered inappropriate in those cases in which the lesion affects the corticopontine fibers, because obviously these do not go as far as the pyramids. Lesions of the extrapyramidal pathways are also upper motor neuron lesions, but the syndrome resulting is different and by convention such disturbances are not included under this heading.

On electromyographic examination of weak muscles, there is slow motor unit action potential firing at maximal effort.

upper syndrome of the brainstem tegmentum   Infarction of the nucleus of the fourth cranial nerve, and perhaps of the third; with superior cerebellar peduncle and medial lemniscus involvement.

upside-down ptosis   The elevation of the lower lid accompanying drooping of the upper lid in **Horner syndrome.**

upward transtentorial herniation   Upward herniation of the cerebellum through the tentorial incisura, usually due to a cerebellar tumor, abscess, or hemorrhage, but lesions of the cerebellopontine angle, pons, or medulla may occasionally be responsible. Forward compression of the brainstem and downward herniation of the cerebellar tonsils precede the upward movement.

Clinically, the patients are in a coma with unreactive miotic pupils, loss of vertical doll's head movements, asymmetrical or absent caloric responses, and decerebrate posturing.[1219]

Urbach-Wiethe disease   (hyalinosis cutis et mucosae) A rare, recessively inherited lipid storage disorder, characterized by hoarse voice, waxy infiltration of the skin and mucous membranes, skin nodules over the upper body, photosensitivity, alopecia, short stature, ocular and dental abnormalities, intracranial calcifications, seizures, rage attacks, and memory disturbances (sometimes without other evidence of dementia).[4122] See **lipoid proteinosis.**

ureal diabetes   See **diabetes insipidus.**

uremic myopathy   A syndrome of proximal weakness and wasting with myopathic EMG findings, occurring in patients with chronic renal failure.[1890]

uremic polyneuropathy   A progressive peripheral sensorimotor axonal neuropathy complicating chronic renal failure.[232]

urethral crisis   Acute paroxysms of pain felt along the course of the urethra in patients with **tabes dorsalis.**

urethral reflex   The fancied gripping of a catheter or sound passed into the penile lumen. The mechanism and purpose of this reflex are equally obscure.

urogenital triangle   The anatomical space whose floor is the deep transverse perineal muscles and the external sphincter, forming the urogenital diaphragm. On each side are the bulbocavernosus (perineal nerve) and ischiocavernosus muscles, while the base is formed by the superior transverse perineal muscles.

useless hand   Lack of control of the hand or arm as a result of sensory deafferentation, despite the retention of normal power and seen most usually as a result of a multiple sclerosis in the posterior column at cervical cord level. The condition was first described by Oppenheim in 1910.[1099]

Usher syndrome (Hallgren syndrome, recessive retinitis pigmentosa with congenital deafness) The recessively inherited combination of progressive visual loss resulting from retinitis pigmentosa (tapetoretinal degeneration), moderate to severe congenital sensorineural deafness, vestibular impairment, cerebellar atrophy, and mental retardation or other mental disorders.[3115,5694]

Both *severe (type 1)* and *mild (type 2)* forms of the condition are described. Although vision is preserved until later life and there are no vestibular symptoms in the type 2 form, it is uncertain whether this is a single condition or more than one.[3756]

utilization behavior A disturbance in the response to external stimuli, which indicates an exaggerated and disinhibited dependency on the environment for behavioral clues, and which indicates the presence of damage to one or both frontal lobes, with loss of frontal inhibition of posterior perceptual and perceptuomotor processing.[3393] Paramedian thalamic infarcts have also been described as leading to this behavior.

Such activity can be considered an extension of bimanual grasping behavior (**magnetic apraxia**), in which the patient appears compelled to grasp and use any object presented visually or through touch; it is associated with uni- or bilateral lesions of the frontal lobe. See also **forced hyperphasia.**

utilization time See **latency of activation.**

utricle A part of the labyrinthine structures, with the saccule and semicircular canals. It contains specialized sensory epithelium from which the hair cell processes project into mucilaginous material within it, where they are stimulated by the movement of otoliths.

uveal tract The iris, ciliary body, and choroid in the eye.

uveitis Inflammation of the uvea, classified as *anterior* (inflammation of the iris and/or the ciliary body, i.e., iritis, cyclitis, iridocyclitis) and *posterior* (inflammation of the choroid, i.e., choroiditis).

uveomeningitic syndrome See **uveomeningoencephalitic syndrome**.

uveomeningoencephalitic syndrome (Vogt-Koyanagi-Harada syndrome) A multisystem disorder comprising uveitis or sympathetic ophthalmia, dysacousis, alopecia, leukoderma, whitening of the eyelashes and eyebrows, and acute encephalitic and fluctuating meningitic signs.[5775]

The initial acute meningitic phase may be complicated by delirium, cranial nerve palsies and other pareses, and loss of sphincter control, and is accompanied by pleocytosis in the CSF. Acute bilateral uveitis with widely dilated pupils then supervenes and retinal detachment and acute glaucoma may ensue. Deceased visual acuity, macular edema, papillitis, and visual field defects are common findings. The remaining systemic features of the disease, listed above, appear during the convalescent phase. Abortive forms also occur.[5] Sarcoidosis is an important cause of the uveomeningitic syndrome (without the encephalitis); **Behçet disease** and viral infections are others. Other uveomeningeal syndromes occur in acute or chronic infections and in **multiple sclerosis** or as a **paraneoplastic syndrome** associated with breast carcinoma.

Vogt gave the first modern report in 1906, but the condition was described in part at least by Ali-ibn-Isa (940–1010), an Arabian physician.[4367]

The clinical features and stages have been delineated[2742] and are given in Chart U–3.

Chart U–3. Stages of Uveomeningoencephalitic Syndrome

1. *Early acute stage* (uveoauditomeningitis)
   1. Bilateral uveitis
      Loss of visual acuity
      Cells in the anterior chamber
      Exudative retinal detachment
      Multifocal dye leakage from retinal pigment epithelium on angiography
   2. Auditory disturbance
      Tinnitus, vertigo
      Nerve deafness
   3. Meningitis
      Headache, nausea
      CSF pleocytosis
2. *Recovery stage* (oculodermal depigmentation)
   1. Ocular depigmentation
      Depigmentation of the iris
      Depigmentation of the ciliary body
      Sunset glow fundus
      Dalen-Fuchs nodules
      Multiple window defects of retinal pigment epithelium with angiography
      Perilimbal vitiligo (**Sugiura sign)**
   2. Dermal depigmentation
      Poliosis in eyebrow and eyelash
      Alopecia
      Vitiligo of face, chest, hands and back

From Inomata H, Kato M. Vogt-Koyanagi-Harada disease. In Bruyn GW, Vinken PJ, eds. Handbook of Clinical Neurology, *pp. 611–626. Amsterdam: Elsevier, 1989, by permission.*

uveoparotid fever A variety of sarcoidosis. See **Heerfordt syndrome.**

V pattern deviation   A nonparalytic form of horizontal strabismus or **tropia** in which the visual axes are directed to closer objects (**esotropia**) as the subject looks down, or separate (**exotropia**) as the subject looks up. The phenomenon is described in patients with mesencephalic lesions. See also **A pattern deviation.**

V wave   See **vertex sharp transient.**

vacor   An organophosphate rodenticide capable of inducing neuropathy and neuromuscular junction disease.

vacuolar myelopathy   See **HIV-associated myelopathy.**

vacuolar myopathies   Disorders of muscle in which the occurrence of widespread irregular vacuoles with a well-defined wall is the major or the only histological abnormality.

Such myopathies include those due to **glycogen storage diseases, familial periodic paralysis,** steroid myopathy, and myopathies complicating collagen vascular diseases. A recessive X-linked form is also described, with juvenile onset and slow progression of proximal myopathic weakness. Pathologically there is vacuolation of muscle fibers without necrosis but with excessive autophagy. In a second form, cardiomyopathy and mental retardation are associated.[264]

vacuoliting megalencephalitic leukoencephalopathy (OMIM 604004)   A rare, recessively inherited leukodystrophy with infantile onset, characterized by diffuse swelling of the white matter, large subcortical cysts, and megalencephaly. The condition has been mapped to chromosome 22qtel.[5607]

vagal neuralgia   A form of neuralgia resembling **glossopharyngeal neuralgia,** but in which the pain is felt rather in the throat and laryngeal regions.

vagal stimulation   A technique whereby chronic stimulation of one vagus nerve by an implanted electrode is used to reduce the frequency of generalized and partial epileptic seizures. The precise mode of action of this intervention remains undetermined but it appears to be effective for the treatment of uncontrolled partial seizures, Lennox-Gastaut syndrome, and depression.

vagal syncope   See **carotid sinus syncope.**

vaginismus   Retentive spasm of the vagina, described by a certain Y. Davis. Davis was supposed at the time to be a real person but in fact the name was but the pseudonym of Sir William **Osler** in a mellow mood. The condition, fortunately, does not exist either.

vagoaccessory syndrome   See **Schmidt syndrome.**

vagus nerve   (pneumogastric nerve) A mixed nerve, supplying the entire cranial parasympathetic outflow as well as having somatic motor and sensory functions. It was described by Marinus in about 100 A.D. as the sixth cranial nerve and was known to Galen, but was named by Domenico di Marchetti of Padua (1626–1688). The nerve's long course and wide distribution led to the derivation of the name from the Latin word *vagari* (a wanderer).

Vail neuralgia   See **vidian neuralgia, cluster headache.**

Vail vidian neuralgia   See **cluster headache.**

valgus   Having the calf of the leg bent outward. "Applied originally to a bow-legged man, the meaning [became] reversed and the term *genu valgum* is now used for a knock-kneed person."[5204]

Valleix, François-Louis-Isidore   (1807–1855) French physician who trained in Toulouse and Paris, but whose advancement in the Paris hospitals was disappointing, although he published over a hundred papers before his early death from diphtheria contracted from a patient. He described the points on nerves, now named for him, in his book *Traité des névralgies ou affections douloureuses des nerfs* (Paris, 1841).

Valleix points   1. Local areas of tenderness along the course of peripheral nerves both proximal and distal to a site of compression, which persist between paroxysms of neuralgia.[5697] 2. Regions where nerves are accessible to palpation. As is known to exponents of Oriental martial arts, such points are extremely sensitive to pressure, but, in cases of nerve irritation or neuralgia, even light pressure may be agonizing, which suggests the presence of such nerve pathology.

Valleix sign   Tenderness of the sciatic nerve in the buttock or posterior thigh. The sign is said to be positive with root irritation, but muscle tenderness is easily confused with nerve pain.

Valsalva, Antonio Mario   (1666–1723) Italian anatomist who trained in Bologna, where he was later professor of anatomy. In 1704 he described the increase in intrathoracic pressure as a means to express pus from the middle ear in otitis. Valsalva also observed that hemiparesis occurs on the side opposite a hemispheric stroke.

Valsalva maneuver   Forcible expiration against a closed glottis, as by exhaling hard against resistance, leading to an increase in intrathoracic pressure to about 30–40 mmHg, usually maintained for 10 seconds in the test situation. In the normal subject this results in a substantial rise in intrathoracic pressure and a transient increase in blood pressure (*phase 1*); a reduction in venous return to the heart and in blood pressure with an increase in the pulse rate (*phase 2*); further increase in pulse rate and decrease in blood pressure occurring immediately after the pressure is released (*phase 3*); and a restitution of blood pressure after an initial overshoot, with a fall in pulse rate, following this (*phase 4*). Absence of any of these changes suggests disturbance in the parasympathetic system. See **autonomic function tests.**

Valsalva ratio   A test of baroceptor afferent and both sympathetic and parasympathetic efferent functions. The maximum heart rate generated by the Valsalva maneuver is divided by the minimum heart rate occurring within 30 seconds of the maximum, measured by a continuously running ECG. The ratio of the longest R-R interval to the shortest should be 1.45 or more in healthy young people. The measurement is more accurate using invasive techniques.[3777] See also **thirty:fifteen ratio, autonomic function tests.**

Van Allen, Maurice   (1918–1986) American neurologist, born in Iowa where he received his early training in medicine, who before and again after wartime service trained in neurosurgery and neurology, although his practice was in the latter discipline. He became professor at the University of Iowa in 1965 and later chairman of the Department of Neurology.

His greatest impact was as editor of the *Archives of Neurology* from 1976, but his introductory text on the neurological examination was also hugely successful. See also **familial amyloid neuropathy** (type 3).

van Bogaert encephalitis   See **subacute sclerosing panencephalitis.**

Ludo van Bogaert

van Bogaert, Ludo   (1897–1989) Belgian neurologist who trained in Brussels and who later studied in Paris under Pierre **Marie** and Marcel Labbé. His graduation thesis was on the mental changes that occur in **amyotrophic lateral sclerosis.** He practiced as a neurologist and neuropathologist in Belgium, developing a spe-

cial interest in neurometabolic disorders, multiple sclerosis, and hypothalamic tumors, as well as the subjects suggested by the following entries.

van Bogaert syndrome   (Divry–van Bogaert syndrome, corticomeningeal diffuse angiomatosis, Hozay–van Bogaert syndrome) A recessively inherited or sporadic syndrome of mental retardation, seizures, spastic paraparesis, extrapyramidal disorders, hemianopia, marbled skin, and telangiectasia[5706] associated with diffuse, noncalcifying angiomatosis of the cortex and meninges and demyelination of the centrum semi-ovale,[2035] resembling the changes in **Binswanger disease.** Death usually occurs within 20 years of presentation.

van Bogaert–Bertrand disease   The same condition as **Canavan disease.** See **glial degenerations, glioneuronal degenerations.**

van Bogaert–Divry syndrome   See **Sturge-Weber syndrome, Van Bogaert syndrome.**

van Bogaert–Nissen-Pfeiffer syndrome   See **metachromatic leukodystrophy.**

van Bogaert–Scherer-Epstein syndrome   See **cerebrotendinous xanthomatosis.**

van Buchem syndrome   See **hyperostosis corticalis generalisata familiaris.**

van Deen, Isaac   (1805–1869) Danish physician who graduated from the University of Leyden in Holland. An ingenious experimenter, he demonstrated that in frogs the posterior columns of the cord carry sensory impulses and the anterior columns, motor impulses, conclusions which assisted **Brown-Séquard** in the elucidation of the basis of cord lesions. He was eventually appointed professor of physiology at Groningen.[3111]

van der Hoeve phakomatosis   1. (Ekbom-Lobstein syndrome) A dominantly inherited cochleovestibular atrophy with onset between 10 and 30 years of age, and manifesting progressive conductive deafness, blue sclerae, and the other features of osteogenesis imperfecta.[5717] 2. Pediculate tumors on the optic nerve head associated variously with **Sturge-Weber disease, tuberous sclerosis, von Hippel–Lindau disease,** and **neurofibromatosis.**

van der Hoeve syndrome   See **Apert syndrome.**

van der Hoeve–Halbertsma-Waardenburg-Klein syndrome   See **Waardenburg syndrome.**

van der Kolk's law   The sensory fibers of a mixed nerve are distributed to parts that are moved by muscles supplied with motor fibers from the same nerve.

van Dyke–Hanson syndrome   A rare syndrome of contractures with continuous muscle discharges, titubation, and episodic ataxia. See **hereditary myokymia with periodic (episodic) ataxia.**

vanillylmandelic acid   The product of the metabolism of norepinephrine, used as a marker of norepinephrine production since it is a stable substance and is freely excreted in the urine.

vanishing white matter (VWM) disease See **fatal infantile leukodystrophy**

vapours A term commonplace in Victorian England for a state of reluctance to engage in any exertion on account of a sense of extreme fatigue; and also used for presyncope, usually with an emotional cause. In those days, such affections were considered evidence of exalted sensibility. Today, see **chronic fatigue syndrome.**

variant hereditary motor and sensory neuropathy The association of retinitis pigmentosa, ataxia, and peripheral neuropathy without any increase in the serum phytanic acid level. Sensorineural deafness and radiological evidence of cerebellar atrophy are occasional features. Sensory conduction is more affected than motor conduction. Biopsy specimens show a reduction of myelinated fibers without onion bulb formations.

The cases reported resemble Refsum disease (**hereditary motor and sensory neuropathy,** type 4) but have neither detectable biochemical abnormality nor peripheral nerve hypertrophy.[5660]

varicella-zoster myelitis A self-limiting motor paraparetic syndrome, sometimes with a relapsing–remitting course, with variable sensory and sphincter involvement, occurring after acute varicella or zoster infection and considered to be a postinfectious myelitis. More severe and acute syndromes are also described.[2114]

variegate porphyria A dominantly inherited form of **porphyria** in which protoporphyrin is not converted into heme and coproporphyrin is continuously excreted in the stools. The disorder is most common in South Africans (Afrikaaners).[1164,4756]

Neurological features complicate some acute attacks, and include the acute or subacute occurrence of proximal motor neuropathy affecting the arms more than the legs (often asymmetrically) and also the face and autonomic system, in the setting of other features of the disease, including skin photosensitivity, abdominal pain, vomiting, tachycardia, hypertension, and often seizures and delirium.

Variot-Pironneau senile dwarfism See **progeria.**

Varoli, Costanzo (1543–1575) Italian anatomist, who described the pons (in a book published posthumously in 1591) and named the hippocampus.

varus Bent or grown inward, knock-kneed (Lat), but the meaning is now reversed and the term is used to describe bowleggedness.[5204]

vascular dementia (multi-infarct dementia) Progressive cognitive disturbance due to thromboembolic cerebrovascular disease. This was an early definition; other forms of cerebrovascular disease such as hypoperfusion, subdural hematoma, vasculitis, and subarachnoid hemorrhage are equally capable of leading to

cognitive impairment and the same may be true for states of chronically impaired cardiac output.

Erkinjuntti et al.[1698] regard vascular dementia as that form in which there is a history of focal or acute signs and symptoms referable to disturbed cerebral circulation, and they suggest the following subcategories. *Vascular dementia of hemodynamic type* is that form of dementia evolving in connection with cardiac arrhythmias and systemic hypotension. *Probable vascular dementia* is that form clinically considered to be related to disturbances of the cerebral circulation without any clear temporal connection with the evolution of the dementia, and without evidence of multiple vascular lesions on the CT scan. This group includes patients with combined degenerative and vascular dementias. *Multi-infarct dementia* is that form which evolves in connection with acute neurological symptoms and signs and/or CT scan findings indicating multiple cortical or deep vascular lesions of the brain.

For dementia to result from vascular disease, it is estimated that at least 100 ml of brain tissue has to have been destroyed. A high **Hachinski ischemic score** may be helpful in predicting the presence of cerebral infarcts, but does not predict the pathology causing the dementia in any given case.[4950] There are no clinical clues to the presence of vascular as opposed to other pathologies to be gleaned from the features of the dementia itself.

Two of at least five sets of criteria extant for the diagnosis (CERAD,[3903] APA-DSM,[150] Hachinski,[2356] Chui et al.,[1031] and the NINCDS-AIREN Workshop[4752]) are presented in Charts V–1 and V–2; the critique of Drachman[1510] should be imbibed prior to their ingestion. A suggested data collection form has been published.[4735] See also **multi-infarct dementia.**

Chart V–1. Criteria for the Diagnosis of Vascular Dementia

Vascular dementia is a complex disorder characterized by cognitive impairment resulting from ischemic or hemorrhagic stroke or from ischemic-hypoxic brain lesions.

The clinical criteria for the diagnosis of probable, possible, and definite VaD are summarized below.

I. Criteria for the clinical diagnosis of *probable VaD* include all of the following:

  1. Dementia defined by cognitive decline from a previously higher level of functioning and manifested by impairment of memory and of two or more cognitive domains (orientation, attention, language, visuospatial functions, executive functions, motor control, and praxis), preferably established by clinical examination and documented by neuropsychological testing. Deficits should be severe enough to interfere with activities of daily living, and not be due to physical effects of stroke alone.

Exclusion criteria include cases with disturbance of consciousness, delirium, psychosis, severe aphasia, or major sensorimotor impairment precluding neuropsychological testing. Also excluded are systemic disorders or other brain diseases such as AD that in and of themselves could account for deficits in memory and cognition.

2. Cerebrovascular disease, defined by the presence of focal signs on neurological examination consistent with stroke, with or without a history of stroke, and evidence of relevant CVD by brain imaging (CT or MRI), including multiple large-vessel infarcts or a single strategically placed infarct (angular gyrus, thalamus, forebrain, or posterior or anterior cerebral artery territories) as well as multiple basal ganglia and white matter lacunes or extensive periventricular white matter lesions or combinations thereof.

3. A relationship between the above two disturbances manifested by one or more of the following: (*a*) onset of dementia within 3 months following a recognized stroke; (*b*) abrupt deterioration in cognitive functions; or fluctuating, stepwise progression of cognitive deficits.

II. Clinical features consistent with the diagnosis of *probable VaD* include the following:

1. Early presence of a gait disturbance (small-step gait or marche à petits pas, or magnetic, apraxic-ataxic or parkinsonian gait);

2. History of unsteadiness and frequent, unprovoked falls;

3. Early urinary frequency, urgency, and other urinary symptoms not explained by urologic disease;

4. Pseudobulbar palsy; and

5. Personality and mood changes, abulia, depression, emotional incontinence, or other subcortical deficits including psychomotor retardation and abnormal executive function.

III. Features that make the diagnosis of VaD uncertain or unlikely include:

1. Early onset of memory deficit and progressive worsening of memory and other cognitive functions, such as language (transcortical sensory aphasia), motor skills (apraxia), and perception (agnosia), in the absence of corresponding focal lesions on brain imaging;

2. Absence of other focal neurological signs other than cognitive disturbance; and

3. Absence of cerebrovascular lesions on brain CT or MRI scans.

IV. Clinical diagnosis of *possible VaD* may be made in the presence of dementia (section I-1) with focal neurological signs in patients in whom brain imaging studies to confirm definite CVD are missing; or in the absence of clear temporal relationships between dementia and stroke; or in patients with subtle onset and variable course (plateau or improvement) of cognitive deficits and evidence of relevant CVD.

V. Criteria for the diagnosis of *definite VaD* are as follows:

1. Clinical criteria for probable vascular dementia;

2. Histopathological evidence of CVD obtained from biopsy or autopsy;

3. Absence of neurofibrillary tangles and neuritic plaques exceeding those expected for age; and

4. Absence of other clinical or pathological disorder capable of producing dementia.

VI. Classification of vascular dementia for research purposes may be made on the basis of clinical, radiological, and neuropathologic features for subcategories or defined conditions such as cortical vascular dementia, subcortical vascular dementia, Binswanger dementia, and thalamic dementia.

The term *AD with CVD* should be reserved to classify patients fulfilling the clinical criteria for possible AD and who also present clinical or brain imaging evidence of relevant CVD. Traditionally these patients have been included with VaD in epidemiological studies. The term *mixed dementia*, used previously, should be avoided.

*AD, Alzheimer disease; CVD, cerebrovascular disease; VaD, vascular dementia.(From Román GC, Tatemichi TK, Erkinjuntti T, et al. Vascular dementia: diagnostic criteria for research studies. Neurology 1993;**43**:250– 260, reprinted by permission.*

Chart V–2. Diagnostic Criteria for Ischemic Vascular Dementia (IVD)

Probable Ischemic Vascular Dementia

A. The criteria for the clinical diagnosis of probable IVD include all of the following:

1. Dementia

2. Evidence of two or more ischemic strokes by history, neurological signs, and/or neuroimaging studies (CT or T_1-weighted MRI); or occurrence of a single stroke with a clearly documented temporal relationship to the onset of dementia; and

3. Evidence of at least one infarct outside the cerebellum by CT or T_1-weighted MRI.

B. The diagnosis of probable IVD is supported by:

1. Evidence of multiple infarcts in brain regions known to affect cognition;

2. A history of multiple transient ischemic attacks;

3. History of vascular risk factors (e.g., hypertension, heart disease, diabetes mellitus); and

4. Elevated **Hachinski Ischemia** scale score (original or modified version).

C. Clinical features that are thought to be associated with IVD, but await further research, include:

1. Relatively early appearance of gait disturbance and urinary incontinence;

2. Periventricular and deep white matter changes on T_2-weighted MRI that are excessive for age; and

3. Focal changes in electrophysiological studies (e.g., EEG, evoked potentials) or physiological neuroimaging studies (e.g., SPECT, PET, NMR spectroscopy).

D. Other clinical features that do not constitute strong evidence either for or against a diagnosis of probable IVD include:

1. Periods of slowly progressive symptoms;

2. Illusions, psychosis, hallucinations, delusions; and

3. Seizures.

E. Clinical features that cast doubt on a diagnosis of probable IVD include:

1. Transcortical sensory aphasia in the absence of corresponding focal lesions on neuroimaging studies;

2. Absence of central neurological symptoms/signs, other than cognitive disturbance.

Possible Ischemic Vascular Dementia

A clinical diagnosis of possible IVD may be made when the following are present:

1. Dementia, and one or more of the following:

2a. A history or evidence of a single stroke (but not multiple strokes) without a clearly documented temporal relationship to the onset of dementia, or

2b. Binswanger's syndrome (without multiple strokes) that includes all of the following:

i. Early-onset urinary incontinence not explained by urological disease, or gait disturbance (e.g., parkinsonian, magnetic, apraxia, or senile gait) not explained by peripheral cause;

ii. Vascular risk factors; and

iii. Extensive white matter changes on neuroimaging.

Definite Ischemic Vascular Dementia

A diagnosis of definite IVD requires histopathological examination of the brain, as well as:

1. Clinical evidence of dementia; and

2. Pathological confirmation of multiple infarcts, some outside of the cerebellum.

If there is evidence of Alzheimer's disease or some other pathological condition that is thought to have contributed to the dementia, a diagnosis of **mixed dementia** should be made.

IVD, ischemic vascular dementia. (From Chui HC, Victoroff JI, Margolin D, et al. Criteria for the diagnosis of ischemic vascular dementia proposed by the State of California Alzheimer's disease diagnostic and treatment centers. Neurology 1992;42:473–480.) Reprinted by permission.

vascular malformations   Collections of abnormal blood vessels of various sizes, most often found in the cerebral lobar white matter, and ranging in size from small capillary telangiectasias through **venous** and **cavernous angiomas** to **arteriovenous malformations.**

They represent occasional causes of intraparenchymal or intraventricular hemorrhage in the CNS, especially in younger patients, but are often asymptomatic.

vascular thoracic outlet compression syndrome   See **thoracic outlet syndrome.**

vasculitic neuropathy   Mononeuropathies, multiple mononeuropathies, or polyneuropathies associated with systemic vasculitic diseases. These have been classified by Scott.[5033]

Diagnostic criteria for clinically probable vasculitic neuropathy in patients lacking biopsy-proven necrotizing vasculitis have been suggested and are presented below.[1107]

Diagnosis requires at least three of the first five criteria for nonsystemic vasculitic neuropathy; criterion 6 is also mandatory for systemic vasculitis.

1. Clinical presentation typical for a vasculitic neuropathy
   Asymmetric or multifocal, painful, sensorimotor neuropathy
   Acute/subacute relapsing, progressive, or relapsing progressive course
   No spontaneous remission

2. Elevated sedimentation rate or other laboratory evidence of a systemic inflammatory state

3. Electrodiagnostic evidence of an active, asymmetric, axonal, sensorimotor neuropathy

4. Suggestive neuromuscular pathology
   Vascular thickening or sclerosis, narrowing or oblit-

eration of the vascular lumen, thrombosis, periadventitial capillary proliferation, hemosiderin deposits, nonrandom nerve fiber loss, or wallerian-like degeneration

5. Clinical response to immunosuppressive therapy

6. Clinicopathologic evidence of a systemic/secondary etiology
   Concurrent condition known or suspected to predispose to vasculitis (connective tissue diseases, certain infections, certain drugs, malignancies/paraproteinemias, cryoglobulinemia)
   Simultaneous multiorgan, nonperipheral nerve involvement
   Biopsy-proven vasculitis in other tissues

vasculitis   Inflammation and necrosis of the walls of blood vessels, as part of a multisystem disease that is drug-related, or isolated within the CNS.

The various syndromes have been classified; the one in Chart V–3 is freely modified from Moore and Cupps.[3962]

Chart V–3. Classification of the Vasculitides

1. *Systemic necrotizing vasculitis*
   Classic **polyarteritis nodosa**
   Allergic angiitis and granulomatosis (**Churg-Strauss disease**)
   Wegener granulomatosis
   Overlap syndromes
   Cerebral vasculitis with ulcerative colitis

2. *Hypersensitivity vasculitis*
   Henoch-Schönlein purpura
   Serum sickness
   Vasculitis associated with infections, connective tissue disease, or malignancy
   Drug-induced vasculitis (amphetamines, heroin, cocaine)

3. *Giant cell arteritides*
   Cranial arteritis
   Takayasu **aortic arch arteritis**

4. *Localized vasculitis*
   Isolated peripheral nervous system vasculitis (nonsystemic neuropathy)
   Isolated angiitis of the nervous system
   Cutaneous polyarteritis
   Essential mixed cryoglobulinemia
   Lymphomatoid granulomatosis
   Behçet disease.

After Moore PM, Cupps TR. Neurological complications of vasculitis. Ann Neurol 1983;14:155. © 1983, John Wiley and Sons, Inc. Reprinted by permission of John Wiley and Sons, Inc.

vasoactive intestinal peptide   (VIP) A peptide hormone found in the gut and CNS of humans, with its highest concentrations in the cerebral cortex, where it acts as a modulator of vasodilation, as well as having a release function for growth hormone and prolactin and a neurotrophic action on neuronal survival.

vasoconstriction syncope   See **Gowers syndromes.**

vasogenic cerebral edema   An increase in the volume of the brain's extracellular space due to the accumulation of water, electrolytes, and protein within it, as a result of damage to the **blood–brain barrier.** This occurs most typically in the tissue surrounding cerebral tumors, infarcts, abscesses, and contusions.

vasopressin (antidiuretic hormone) A peptide with highest concentration in the supraoptic and paraventricular nuclei of the hypothalamus and in their nerve terminals in the posterior pituitary gland, with effects on learning as well as on renal water excretion.

vasoregulation The process whereby blood vessels adapt to the metabolic needs of the tissues they supply. Carbon dioxide and oxygen tensions and pH are the most effective stimuli leading to alterations in the caliber of the cerebral arterioles.

vasovagal syncope Cerebral ischemia resulting from vagal inhibition of cardiac action, leading in turn to bradycardia and hypotension, and thus decreased cerebral perfusion. Other manifestations include malaise, anxiety, visual darkening, pallor, and brief convulsive movements during the period of unconsciousness.

The mechanism was described in 1932 by Thomas Lewis (1881–1945), an English cardiologist.[4979] See also **encephalosyncope, reflex syncope.**

Vater, Abraham (1684–1751) German anatomist, the first to describe the encapsulated nerve endings now named for **Pacini.**

VDRL See **Venereal Disease Research Laboratory test.**

Vegas neuropathy An ulnar neuropathy at the elbow, resulting from leaning the elbow on the edges of gaming tables for prolonged periods.[2816]

vegetative nervous system See **autonomic nervous system.**

vegetative state A state of altered consciousness occurring as a residuum from severe brain injury in which wakefulness appears to be present because the eyes are opened and a sleep–wake cycle is retained, but in which there is no evidence of conscious awareness, the patients neither speaking nor obeying commands given in any modality nor showing evidence of emotional awareness. There is thus arousal without awareness. The **Glasgow Coma scale** scores will be 4–4–2 or worse.

The condition is seen usually after severe head injury or hypoxic-ischemic injury. See also **persistent vegetative state.**[4466]

vein of Galen A large, deep cerebral vein draining into the straight sinus. It is subject to massive dilation as a congenital anomaly (**aneurysm of the vein of Galen**) which may lead to compression of the midbrain, bleeding, seizures, macrocephaly with hydrocephalus, and, by virtue of the volume of blood shunted, heart failure in infants.[3958]

vein of Labbé See **Labbé's vein.**

vein of Trolard See **Trolard's vein.**

Venereal Disease Research Laboratory Test (VDRL) A nontreponemal test for syphilis, detecting flocculation in reaction to nonspecific antibodies of, or in response to, *Treponema pallidum* infection of the host.

Though widely used as a screening test, the result is negative in up to a quarter of the cases of tertiary syphilis and may be positive in collagen-vascular disease, after other infections or recent immune challenges, in leprosy and in old age.[5172] See also **TPI.**

Venezuelan equine encephalitis Direct brain infection by an arthropod-borne alphavirus of the togavirus group, causing cycles of encephalitic disease throughout Central and South America and the southern United States.

Clinically, adults exhibit an influenzal disease with marked myalgia, fevers, nausea and vomiting, headaches, conjunctivitis, and pharyngitis. A few children suffer severe neurological complications such as seizures, paralysis, and coma.[1615]

venoarteriolar reflex Arteriolar constriction in the skin and muscles of the legs reducing blood flow during limb dependency (when venous pressure is raised by 25 mmHg) as a result of a local sympathetic C-fiber reflex.[4023]

venous angiomas Rare tumor-like masses comprising dilated veins with slight or no arterial contribution. See **venous malformation.**

venous infarction Ischemic damage to tissues resulting from impairment of their venous drainage. This occurs most often in the retina and in the spinal cord, and as a result of thrombosis of the dural venous sinuses. See **central retinal vein thrombosis, Foix-Alajouanine syndrome, sinus thrombosis, cerebral venous thrombosis.**

venous lakes Benign demineralized areas of the skull seen on either side of the midline on plain X-ray and CT studies, and of no pathological import, unless they prompt invasive investigations.

venous malformation A congenital **vascular malformation** consisting of a mass of dilated venous channels, within or on the surface of the cerebrum.

Bleeding may be clinically inapparent and lesions may be detected fortuitously, especially if they calcify. See **venous angiomas, arteriovenous malformation.**

venous sinus thrombosis Occlusion of the superior sagittal or the transverse sinus, usually as a result of infection or dehydration. See **sinus thrombosis.**

venous stasis retinopathy A syndrome of unilateral, slowly progressive visual loss with a funduscopic picture of venous engorgement and dot-and-blot hemorrhages, with low central retinal artery pressure, resulting from central retinal vein occlusion and usually associated with severe carotid artery disease. Anterior segment ischemia may also be present.[2985]

ventral brainstem syndrome   See **locked-in syndrome.**

ventral cerebellum   See **inverse cerebellum.**

ventral pontine syndrome   See **locked-in syndrome.**

ventral suspension   A test of motor abilities used in determining **gestational age,** in which the infant is suspended in the prone position with the examiner's hand under the infant's chest (one hand in a small infant, two in a large infant).

Normally, there will be obvious extension of the neck and lower spine with some flexion of the arms and legs.[1528]

ventricle of Arantius   See **cava septi pellucidi et vergae.**

ventricles   (Lat, a small belly) A hollow part of an organ. The paired lateral and the third and the fourth ventricles were considered to be "cells" by the ancient Greeks, in which mental functions resided. The ventricular contents were considered to be animal spirits that were pumped out through small tubes to the rest of the body. Hierophilus of Alexandria in 300 B.C. located the seat of the soul in the fourth ventricle. These concepts remained essentially unaltered until the sixteenth century.

ventricular germinal zone   See **germinal zone.**

ventriculitis   Inflammation of the cerebral ventricles, usually as a complication of **leptomeningitis.**

ventriculography   A procedure for outlining the internal proportions of the cerebral ventricles with X-radiography after the introduction of air or contrast medium at operation. The procedure was introduced by **Dandy** in 1913,[1270,4979] after Dr. W.H. Luckett had published an account of intraventricular air following a compound skull fracture.

ventriculostium   A communication between the cerebral ventricles and the subarachnoid space, occurring spontaneously.[2915]

VEP   See **visual evoked potential.**

verb phrase   The part of a sentence which contains the verb (the predicate) as well as all words, clauses, and sentences modifying the verb.[3505]

verbal adynamia   See **dynamic aphasia.**

verbal alexia   Inability to interpret the written word, although isolated letters can be identified. The phenomenon is seen in patients with dominant angular gyrus lesions.[1178]

verbal aphasia   (motor aphasia) The term of Sir Henry **Head** for that form of speech disturbance (a defect in word formation) in which words are evoked with

difficulty and tend to be abnormal in structure and the vocabulary restricted. See **Broca aphasia.**

verbal asomatognosia   Distorted awareness of a body part, manifested as verbal denial of ownership of a limb, accompanied by hemispatial neglect. The lesion is considered to lie in the right supramarginal gyrus.[1764]

verbal auditory agnosia   See **word deafness.**

verbal automatism   See **stereotypy.**

verbal dysdecorum   A syndrome resulting from focal damage to the medial, sagittal, and/or dorsal convolutions of the right frontal lobe, in which patients voice bizarre and caustic descriptions of themselves, of everyday occurrences, and of those about them, and fail to monitor the undesirable effects of this output and to inhibit it.[462]

verbal paraphasia   The substitution of incorrect words within sentences; a characteristic of dysphasic syndromes.

verbal perseveration   Repetition of the same word or phrase. See **verbigeration.**

verbal standstill   The interruption of flowing speech because the correct word fails to come to mind. When it is offered by another, it is immediately recognized as correct and speech continues. Paraphasic errors and substitutions do not occur.

This occurs commonly in elderly people and in those of any age who are under stress or fatigued.[1180]

verbal sterotypy   See **stereotypy.**

Verbiest syndrome   See **lumbar spinal stenosis.**

verbigeration   The meaningless repetition by the patient of the same words or phrases over and over again, with appropriate gestural accompaniment; an example of verbal stereotypy.

vergence   (Lat, turn downward) (disjunctive eye movements) Simultaneous movements of the eyes, but in different directions. This is usually seen as an in-turning of the eyes (which thus lose the parallelism of their axes), in order to allow focused close vision. Refixation movements and visual tracking movements are of this type, and other forms are described.[2133]

Four components of vergence are described:

1. *Tonic vergence* determines the baseline alignment of the visual axis in darkness.
2. *Accommodator vergence* is an involuntary in-turning of the eyes induced by blurring of vision.
3. *Fusional vergence* is induced by retinal disparity.
4. *Proximal vergence* (nearness) is induced by a sense of distance of the target and is based on a number of sensory cues.[5958]

See also **versions.**

Verger, Theodore-Paul-Henri   (1873–1930) French neurologist who trained in Bordeaux, **Pitres** being one of his teachers. He was appointed in succession to the chairs of forensic and then internal medicine. He wrote on proprioceptive sensation and the functions of the parietal lobe, experimental thalamic syndromes, neuralgias, encephalitis, syringomyelia, the traumatic neuroses, and medical ethics.

Verger-Déjèrine syndrome (Déjèrine syndrome, Déjèrine-Mouzon syndrome, Claude topoanesthesia) A syndrome of the parietal lobe in which discriminative tactile sensations and proprioception are lost, while sensations of pain, temperature, vibration, and crude light touch remain intact.[1343]

vermis (Lat, worm-like) The appearances of the folia of the cerebellar vermis bear a fanciful resemblance to the segmented body of a worm.

Vernant syndrome (recurrent optic neuromyelitis with endocrinopathies) A syndrome described in young black women in the West Indies, comprising recurrent optic neuritis, cervical myelopathy with a syringomyelia-like syndrome, and amenorrhea with galactorrhea. The cause is not known,[5754] but tuberculous neuropathy and hemorrhagic fevers may be associated.[4748]

vermis syndrome (Bailey syndrome) Disturbance of equilibrium with nystagmus and some degree of limb ataxia as a result of a lesion of the vermis of the cerebellum. Depending on the cause, there may also be evidence of increased intracranial pressure.

Vernet, Maurice (b. 1887) French neurologist, who described the following syndrome in his graduation thesis (University of Lyon) in 1916.

Vernet syndrome (Vernet-Sargon syndrome, Collet-Sicard syndrome) Unilateral paralysis of cranial nerves IX, X, and XI, due to a lesion at the level of the jugular foramen in front of the anterior occipital condyles. The clinical consequences of this include loss of taste in the posterior third of the tongue; paresis of the vocal cords and palate with resulting dysarthria, dysphagia, and dysphonia; anesthesia of the soft palate and throat; and weakness of the trapezius and sternomastoid muscles.[5431,5755]

The pathology is usually a malignancy, aneurysm, or fracture. See also **jugular foramen syndrome.**

Vernet-Sargon syndrome See **Vernet syndrome.**

vernicomyelia The presence of the contents of the amniotic fluid sac in the spinal subarachnoid space, accompanied by a foreign-body giant cell reaction in the leptomeninges.

The condition may complicate a lumbar meningomyelocele in infants.[2780]

Verocay nodule A mass of nuclei of fusion formed by polar cells seen within neurinomas, tightly opposed in palisades and forming a nodule within the tumor; the arrays of palisaded cells within **schwannomas.**[6]

Verocet neurilemmoma See **schwannoma.**

versions Normal, conjugate deviations of the eyes in any direction, in parallel. *Fast versive eye movements* of this type include **saccades,** microsaccades, saccadic pursuit, the fast phase of jerk nystagmus, **saccadic intrusions, saccadic oscillations,** and the rapid eye movements of (paradoxical) **REM sleep.**[2133] *Slow versive eye movements* include **pursuit eye movements, microdrift, glissades,** the slow phase of jerk nystagmus, and the movements of **pendular nystagmus.** Other forms are also recorded.[2133] See also **vergence.**

verruga peruana See **Oroya fever.**

versive movements See **versive seizures.**

versive seizures (versive movements) A variety of simple partial seizures involving conjugate deviation of the head and eyes, usually but not invariably away from the side of the hemispheric discharge.[56] They are evidence of a frontal lobe lesion in most cases, but disease of other cortical regions may occasionally be responsible.

Nonversive movements are smaller-amplitude, ill-sustained, and wandering eye movements in any direction, and although likely to be electrically driven, have no localizing significance.[6055]

Compare with **Vulpian sign.**

vertebra prominens The (longest) spinous process, of C7, and thus that which is most easily palpated or seen in the low neck.

The longest (middle) finger is also innervated by C7.

vertebral dysplasia–spinal dysraphism (Curry syndrome) A congenital dysmorphic syndrome characterized by dwarfism, short webbed neck, kyphosis, platyspondyly, spina bifida occulta, skeletal deformities of the thorax and sacrum, inguinal hernia, absent testes, and cutis gyrata of the scalp.[337]

vertebrobasilar Ds A mnemonic to assist the recall of common symptoms of hind-brain ischemia: dysphagia, dysarthria, diplopia, drop attacks, dysmetria, and dysesthesia.

vertebrobasilar insufficiency (Millikan-Siekert syndrome) Transient ischemic attacks in the territory of the posterior circulation, first recognized in 1955.[3892]

The symptoms may be precipitated by extrinsic compression of the vertebral artery, by spasm or dissection of its wall, by emboli within the lumen, or by diversion of blood (as in the **subclavian steal syndrome**). The clinical localization of the vascular lesion is frequently incorrect.

The diagnosis is suggested by the finding of any two of the following motor or sensory symptoms or both occurring bilaterally in one attack: ataxia of gait or clumsiness of both extremities; diplopia; dysphagia; and bilateral homonymous hemianopia.[265,5937]

vertebrobasilar insufficiency nystagmus See **cervical nystagmus.**

vertebrobasilar migraine   See **basilar migraine.**

vertex sharp transient   (vertex sharp wave, V wave) A sharp potential, maximal at the vertex, usually negative in relation to other areas and occurring apparently spontaneously during sleep or in response to a sensory stimulus during sleep or wakefulness. It may be single or repetitive and its amplitude varies but rarely exceeds 250 uV. See also **K complex.**

vertex sharp wave   See **vertex sharp transient.**

vertical gaze paresis   Inability to deviate the eyes voluntarily in the vertical plane as a result of a mesencephalic lesion involving the posterior commissure, or bilaterally. See **dorsal midbrain syndrome.**

vertical nystagmus   A form of central vestibular nystagmus resulting from an imbalance in central vestibulo-ocular reflex pathways, in which the deviations of the eyes are in the vertical plane. See **upbeat nystagmus, downbeat nystagmus.**

If purely vertical, nystagmus is never of peripheral origin.

vertical one-and-a-half syndrome   1. The combination of paralysis of up-gaze in both eyes and of down-gaze in one of them.[1360] 2. A supranuclear down-gaze paralysis with monocular paralysis of elevation.

In each case, the precise nature of the responsible brainstem lesion is unknown.

vertical retraction syndrome   A rare syndrome characterized by limitation of elevation or depression of the globe of the eye, with retraction and narrowing of the palpebral fissure.

The condition is likely to be a synkinesis due to aberrant reinnervation following injury to the third cranial nerve.[5]

vertical vestibulo-ocular reflex   Ocular deviation resulting from vertical head movement or bilateral caloric stimulation. Bilateral cold stimulation induces downward deviation of the eyes and warm stimulation, upward deviation, the corrective fast component (taken as the direction of the nystagmus) naturally being in the opposite direction in each case.

vertige épileptique   See **affective-psychic seizure.**

vertige larynge of Charcot   See **cough syncope.**

vertige paralysant   (Kubisagari) The acute onset of vertigo and pareses of the elevators of the eyes and weakness of the neck and limbs, occurring in those who work in and around stables in Geneva and Japan. The cause of the condition is not known. See **Gerlier disease.**

vertiginous epilepsy   Brief seizures which include a sensation of rotational or linear vertigo accompanied by versive movements of the head, eyes, and body. They are usually due to a focus in the temporal or parietal lobe.[333]

vertigo   (Lat, dizziness) A hallucination of movement; the distortion of static gravitational orientation, or the erroneous perception of movement of the self or of the environment, frequently accompanied by nystagmus, ataxia, and nausea. Episodic or paroxysmal; sustained; and positional forms are differentiated.[5391]

It represents a mismatch between the sense of motion provided by the vestibular apparatus and that provided by visual or proprioceptive inputs. Its presence may be **physiological** or pathological, the latter indicating dysfunction in the vestibular, visual, or somatosensory systems or (rarely) in the cortex of the superior temporal gyrus. *Central* (brainstem) and *peripheral* (vestibular apparatus) forms exist, the difference at a clinical level being the absence of nausea in many cases of central vertigo, and the form of the accompanying nystagmus.

See **benign positional vertigo, central nystagmus, peripheral nystagmus, motion sickness, space sickness, auditory vertigo, bending-over vertigo, head-extension vertigo, height vertigo, somatosensory vertigo,** and **visual vertigo.**

Vesalius, Antonio   (1514–1564) Belgian anatomist After study at the Universities of Louvain, Montpelier, and Paris, he worked in Venice and Madrid and was successively professor of anatomy at Padua, Bologna, and Pisa, and at one time was surgeon to the Emperor Charles V.

He introduced eponyms into anatomy, but is thus remembered himself only for a small bone and a foramen, although his monumental book *De humani corporis diffusa libri septum* (Basel, 1543) assured him a permanent monument as one of the greatest anatomists of all time. In the fourth and seventh books, he corrected Galen's error that the human has a rete mirabile and that the vapor rather than the fluid was the important part of the third (CSF) circulation, though he agreed with the flow pattern suggested.

He began to reject what is now called the *medieval cell doctrine* on the basis of his human dissections, which latter led him to be the first to describe internal hydrocephalus.

vesical crises   (Lat, bladder + Gr, sudden change) Acute paroxysmal neuralgic pain in the bladder region experienced by patients with **tabes dorsalis.** The same may occur in the larynx and the abdomen. See also **gastric crises, rectal crises.**

vesical reflex   Stimulation of the bladder mucosa through bladder distension leads to contraction of the detrusor muscle, relaxation of the internal sphincter, and voiding of the bladder contents. The reflex is mediated through reflex arcs at S2–4.

vesperal hallucinations   (Lat, evening + wandering in mind) Hallucinations occurring at nightfall, as is typically the case with **peduncular hallucinations.**

vespers curse   Pain in the low back and legs with features of the **restless limb syndrome,** waking the subject from sleep in the early morning. The mechanism is considered to be the combination of congestive cardiac failure and lumbar spinal stenosis, the increased right atrial filling pressure being transmitted to the epidural venous plexus and causing increased pressure in the constricted spinal canal.[3213]

Vestibular Disorders Association   A charitable organization. Address: PO Box 4467, Portland, OR 97208–4467. Tel: 503–229–7705. Web site: http://www.verstibular.org/.

vestibular epilepsy   (vestibulogenic epilepsy) 1. A variety of sensory-evoked epilepsy precipitated by excessive provoked or spontaneous stimulation of the vestibular apparatus.[333] 2. Recurrent, transient postepileptic vertigo, possibly a variant of that form of epilepsy in which the seizures are provoked by excessive spontaneously arising discharges of the vestibular apparatus.[430]

vestibular migraine   The occurrence of rotational or to-and-fro vertigo lasting minutes to hours in adults, often without currently accompanying headache.[1443]

vestibular neuronitis   A form of recurrent unilateral labyrinthine dysfunction presenting as acute severe rotatory vertigo with postural imbalance, nausea, and vomiting lasting for about a week, without cochlear or other neurological symptoms.[1474,5391] A viral etiology is suspected in some cases, but the unique identity of the syndrome is not universally agreed on. See **acute peripheral vestibulopathy.**

vestibular nystagmus   (electrical nystagmus) A class of acquired horizontal, horizontal-rotatory, or vertical jerk nystagmus resulting from dysfunction of the central or peripheral vestibular system and commonly associated with the clinical complaint of vertigo.

Its amplitude is increased with gaze in the same direction as the fast phase, and, when due to peripheral end-organ disorder, the fast phase is away from the side of the lesion. When due to *peripheral lesions,* the nystagmus is unidirectional, the fast phase is away from the side of the lesion, a rotatory component is common, visual fixation tends to inhibit it, the nystagmus is not always reproducible with testing, and the vertigo is usually marked.

By contrast, in the presence of *central lesions,* the nystagmus is uni- or bidirectional, it is usually purely vertical or rotatory, fixation has no effect on the amplitude, and any accompanying vertigo is mild.[5]

Forms described include **apogeotropic,** alternating current, **Bechterew, caloric, after-caloric, compensatory,** compression, faradic, galvanic, **geotropic, head-shaking,** induced, L-, **labyrinthine,** perverted, pneumatic, **positional,** positioning, **postrotational,** pseudocaloric, **rotational, upbeat, downbeat,** and secondary phase nystagmus.

vestibular schwannoma   See **schwannoma.**

vestibular vertigo   Vertigo due to disorders affecting the semicircular canals or the otoliths in the utricle and saccule.

The first of these causes a spontaneous rotational vertigo of the self or the surroundings, associated with spontaneous nystagmus with the fast phase beating away from the side of the lesion; and with severe nausea, postural imbalance, and homolateral horizontal canal paresis on irrigation.

The second produces more of a sensation of tilt or levitation, with postural imbalance, vibration oscillopsia, and moderate nausea, but without nystagmus, although there is diminution of ocular counter-rolling on head tilt.[727]

vestibule   (Lat, a room within an entrance) A cavity leading into another of larger size.

vestibulitis   An acute acquired, presumably viral, infection of the vestibular apparatus, leading to acute vertigo, nystagmus, nausea and vomiting, and imbalance. See also **vestibular nystagmus, vestibular vertigo, vestibular neuronitis.**

vestibulocephalic response   See **vestibulocerebral response.**

vestibulocerebral response   (oculocephalic response, vestibulocephalic response, doll's head response) Ocular deviation, with or without nystagmus, occurring as a result of head movements causing labyrinthine stimulation.

vestibulocollic reflex   Short-latency contractions in the anterior neck muscles in response to auditory click-stimuli.[1096] A cochlear component would appear likely as well.

vestibulogenic epilepsy   A variety of sensory-evoked seizure, the stimulus here being of the peripheral labyrinth. See **vestibular epilepsy.**

vestibulo-ocular reflex   (VOR) A short-latency reflex ensuring stability of the position of the eyes (and thus stable retinal imaging) during rapid changes in head position, through the execution of smooth, conjugate, restitutive, slow eye movements.

The pathway runs from the semicircular canals to the superior vestibular nuclei in the brainstem and then to the oculomotor nerve nuclei. The reflex and its mechanisms and disturbances are fully reviewed by Leigh and Zee.[3330] See **oculovestibular reflex.**

vestibulo-oculogyric reflex   (labyrinthine reflex) Lateral deviation of the eyes, with or without nystagmus, away from the side of stimulation of one labyrinth, as in **caloric testing** using cold water. See **oculovestibular response.**

vestibulopathy   Any affection of the vestibular apparatus.

A dominantly inherited *familial vestibulopathy* is described in which episodic vertigo is succeeded by gait imbalance and oscillopsia in the presence of normal hearing.[319]

vestibulopupillary response   Dilation of the pupil in response to labyrinthine stimulation.

Veterans Administration (VA) Seizure Frequency and Severity scale   A scale recording the frequency and severity of partial seizures based on the reports of the patient and of observers.[1551]

Vialetto–van Laere syndrome   (bulbar spinal muscular atrophy with deafness, bulbar palsy with deafness) A recessively inherited form of bulbar palsy seen in children and occurring in two forms:

1. Eighth nerve deafness and bulbar palsy accompanied by extraocular palsies and facial weakness; the condition is fatal within 18 months of onset.[5934]
2. A form that has similar clinical features, but its onset is in the second decade and the deafness and facial, bulbar, and truncal neurogenic weakness may progress slowly enough to allow life until the fourth decade.

   Madras neuropathy   may be identical. See also **progressive bulbar palsy.**

vibrameter   A device that emits continuous sinusoidal vibrations at frequencies and intensities under the control of the operator. The subject is exposed to such varying stimuli in the bedside quantitation of large-diameter afferent fiber conduction or the assessment of posterior column function.

vibration oscillopsia   Reduced visual acuity during walking due to damage to the otoliths in the utricle and saccule.[727]

vibratory sensation   (pallesthesia) (from Gr, shake + sensation) A sensory mode considered at the end of the nineteenth century to be a discrete modality, with receptors in the periosteum conveying the "shocks of locomotion." (The ability of the penis, cheek, breast, and skin of the abdominal wall to feel vibration was not considered.) The modality was first examined in the clinical context by Rumpf in 1889; it had not been noticed by Gowers in his textbook the previous year.

   von Frey   believed that vibration was mediated by pressure receptors, and pacinian corpuscles are now regarded as the relevant end-organs. The central transmission pathway includes a route through the posterior columns and almost certainly others, perhaps even in the lateral columns and spinocerebellar tracts, which would support the suggestion that from the skin, the pathway is the same as that for touch, but, from deeper structures, the pathway is the same as that for postural sensibility.

   The sensation of vibration itself represents the temporal modulation of tactile sense, analogous to the relationship between flicker and vision. Loss of vibratory sense is due to the desynchronization of the afferent pattern of impulses in demyelinated peripheral nerves or in the central processes of the large dorsal root ganglion cells.[874] The tuning fork was invented by John Shore, an English musician, in 1711.

vibration white finger   See **hand-arm vibration syndrome.**

vibration-induced nystagmus   Nystagmus induced by a vibrating tuning fork placed on the mastoid process, with the fast component away from the side of the vestibular lesion.

Vicq d'Azir, Felix   (1748–1794) French physician and comparative anatomist, physician to the French Queen Marie Antoinette and secretary of the French Academy of Medicine. He gave a rudimentary account of the lobes of the cerebrum, his anterior, middle, and posterior lobes corresponding to the frontal, parietal, and occipital, but the temporal lobe was only differentiated by **Arnold** in 1838. He also described the insula well before Reil, the substantia nigra ("locus niger crurum cerebri") in 1786, and the mammillothalamic tract (bundle of Vicq d'Azir), although this observation was not published until 1805.

Victor, Maurice   (1920–2001) Canadian neurologist who trained initially in Winnipeg and later in Utah and Boston. He accompanied Dr. Raymond Adams to the Massachussetts General Hospital in 1951 and moved to Cleveland in 1962. An outstanding teacher and clinician, he wrote on many neurological topics, especially on those related to alcohol abuse, but is most widely remembered for his joint authorship of a textbook, *Principles of Neurology* (with Dr. Raymond Adams), to which he brought huge knowledge, perspicacity, and common sense in its descriptions of the basic and clinical aspects of the discipline.

vidian neuralgia   (Vail neuralgia, **cluster headache**) A syndrome of facial pain resembling **Sluder syndrome,** the pain radiating as far back as the ear, mastoid, neck, and shoulder (as it may also in the latter condition; the distinction between the two is too fine for this author to perceive).[5695]

   The condition may represent another form of **cluster headache.** Vidus Vidius (1500–1569) was an Italian physician to King Francis I of France and later professor of medicine at Pisa.

Viets test   Manual compression of the jugular veins until the subject feels a fullness in the head. Increased pain radiating from the back into the legs represents a positive result, suggesting irritation of the lumbosacral nerve roots.

   The **Naffziger test** is similar except that it employs a blood pressure cuff around the neck, inflated to 40 mmHg for 10 minutes, whereby the patient is made to suffer extreme discomfort in order to add a degree of spurious precision to an observation of minor diagnostic importance.

Vieusseux, Gaspard Swiss physician who himself suffered a lateral medullary syndrome (**Vieusseux-Wallenberg syndrome**), his case being discussed and reported in 1810. He gave the first description of bacterial meningitis in 1806, in Geneva.

Vieusseux, Raymond (1641–1716) French physician, professor of anatomy at Montpelier. He described the inferior olives, the pyramids, the centrum ovale, and the semilunar ganglion.

Vieusseux-Wallenberg syndrome See **lateral medullary syndrome.**

vigilance The ability to sustain sensory attention. A state of the nervous system manifested at all levels and capable of either local or general depression; the high-grade physiological efficiency in those neural structures responsible for certain activities and allowing diverse and varying modes of response. Conscious processes would thus be the expressions of physiological vigilance.[2496]

Villar-Rose syndrome See **cephalic tetanus.**

Villaret, Maurice (1877–1946) French physician and physiologist with major interests outside medicine, who wrote on cirrhosis and the portal circulation and was an expert in the therapeutic value of spas.[1829]

Maurice Villaret

Villaret syndrome (retroparotid space syndrome, posterior retropharyngeal syndrome, posterior retroparotid syndrome) Unilateral paralysis of the muscles supplied by cranial nerves IX, X, XI, and XII, and sometimes cranial nerve VII, with **Horner syndrome,** as a result of compression of these nerves in the posterior retroparotid space, usually by a malignancy.[5766]

The difference between this and the **Collet-Sicard syndrome** is minimal. The cranial nerves affected in other syndromes resulting from disease of this area include **Jackson syndrome** (complete unilateral X, XI, XII); **Mackenzie syndrome** (IX, X, XI, XII); **Collet-Sicard syndrome** (IX, X, XI, XII); **Avellis syndrome** (X); **Schmidt syndrome** (X, XI); **Tapia syndrome** (XI, XII); **Lannois and Jouty syndrome** (IX, X, XI, XII); and **Vernet syndrome** (VII,IX, X, XI, XII with or without involvement of the cervical sympathetic pathway and hemiparesis).[5431]

Vincent sign The **Argyll Robertson pupil.**

Vineland Adaptive Behavior scale A set of scales measuring self-help skills such as communication, daily living skills, socialization, motor skills, and maladaptive behavior, based on a questionnaire and a structured interview. The instrument is appropriate for cognitively impaired people at all ages from infancy to adult.[5269]

violaceous hue The light purple color of the skin of the eyelids in some patients with **dermatomyositis** or with the skin lesions of morphoea. The French word *mauve* would be equally appropriate, if less memorable.

violinists' cramps Focal (occupational) dystonias occurring in either the hand fingering the strings or that holding the bow. See also **musician overuse syndrome.**

viral myoglobinuria The occurrence of rhabdomyolysis with spilling of myoglobin into the urine, as a result of viral (e.g., influenzal, Coxsackie) infections.

Virchow disease Acute congenital encephalitis. The nature of this condition is now uncertain.[5770]

Virchow, Rudolf Ludwig Karl (1821–1902) German pathologist who graduated from Berlin University. After he reported that the cause of a typhus epidemic into which he had been sent to inquire was largely social and directly the fault of the government, he was dismissed from his posts in Berlin, but was appointed at once as professor of pathological anatomy at Würzburg and eventually was able to return to Berlin as professor in 1856.

The father of modern pathology, particularly cellular pathology, he founded *Virchow's Archives*, the prestigious journal of pathology, in 1847, and was a pre-eminent medical scientist, historian, and politician during his active career. He first identified the neuroglia in 1846, and also described thrombosis, infarction, vascular emboli, subdural hematomas, spina bifida occulta, and leontiasis ossea. The terms *agenesis, heterotopia, ochronosis,* and *leukocytosis* were initially his, and Virchow's name is also given to the following two items.

Virchow spaces (Virchow-Robin spaces) Gaps around blood vessels in the brain, described by Virchow 4 years after they had been identified by Charles-Philippe Robin (1821–1885), a French physician.

Virchow-Seckel syndrome See **Seckel syndrome.**

virile reflex See **bulbocavernosus reflex.**

visceral epilepsy Epigastric auras consisting of indescribable feelings, pain (**Moores syndrome**), and cardiac, respiratory, or gastrointestinal symptoms as manifestations of partial epilepsies.[4034]

visceral larva migrans See **toxocariasis.**

visceral neuropathy See **familial visceral neuropathy.**

visceromotor symptoms Lip-smacking, swallowing, or chewing movements, most commonly recognized as part of a seizure originating in the temporal lobe. See **temporal lobe syndromes.**

viscosity 1. Stickiness of thought processes, leading to a tendency to talk repetitively and circumstantially on a narrow range of topics. 2. Enhanced intrapersonal adhesiveness; a tendency to cling to certain other people. In each case, the trait is associated with temporal lobe epilepsy, especially with left-sided or bilateral foci.[4591]

vision (from Lat, the sense of seeing) The faculty of sight.

visual adaptation The disappearance of a stationary visual target after the subject has gazed at it for a few seconds. The phenomenon is occasionally found with some cases of lesions of the optic radiations.[401]

visual agnosia A disorder of recognition confined to the realm of vision in which alert, intelligent, and nondysphasic patients with normal visual perception fail to comprehend the nature or meaning of nonverbal visual stimuli which formerly had been understood.

Two forms are recognized: In *visual apperceptive agnosia*, the subject cannot name, copy, or match an object, although the visual fields are full and acuity is unaffected. The lesion, usually ischemic, affects the calcarine cortex bilaterally, or its pathways.[672] In *visual associative agnosia*, discrimination is retained but identification fails. Thus, the subject can recognize or draw an object named and presented among others, but cannot recognize objects visually without such cues.[4446]

visual agnosia or apraxia without dementia A progressive syndrome in which there is an impairment of visuoperceptive abilities in the absence of dementia or oral language disorders, starting in adult life and with slow progression. The relationship to other primary progressive dementias is not yet clarified.[1408] See also **agnosia.**

visual allesthesiae The transfer of visual images from one half-field to the other, thus a form of **palinopsia.**[2782]

Visual Analog Mood scale A method of assessing mood levels whereby subjects select a point along a visually presented scale corresponding to their assessment of their level of, for example, happiness–sadness.[1906]

Visual Analog test A method for scoring the amount of pain felt, whereby subjects are required to mark on a line the place corresponding to the intensity of their pain, from *no pain* to *the worst pain I ever felt.*[650]

visual apperceptive agnosia See **visual agnosia.**

visual associative agnosia See **visual agnosia.**

visual axis A line between the fovea and the point of fixation.

visual confusion A visual error consisting of the perception that two different objects are occupying the same position in space. See also **diplopia.**

visual disorientation (Holmes syndrome, Riddoch syndrome) Defective visuospatial orientation as a result of lesions in the region of the supramarginal and angular gyri; there is, thus, an inability to localize objects in the three planes of space, and especially to estimate absolute and relative distances. When occurring in a single homonymous half-field, it is due to a contralateral parietal lobe lesion.[4684] See **simultagnosia.**

visual dysesthesia The tendency for stimuli in one half-field to to have an unpleasant quality, tending to elicit an exaggerated startle reaction; an uncommon manifestation in disease of the visual cortex.

visual evoked potential (visual evoked response) Electric waveforms of biologic origin recorded over the cerebrum and elicited in response to visual stimuli. They are classified by stimulus rate as transient or steady state, and they can be further divided by stimulus presentation mode. The normal transient VEP to checkerboard pattern reversal or shift has a major positive occipital peak at about 100 msec (PI 00), often preceded by a negative peak (N75). The precise range of normal values for the latency and amplitude of P100 depends on several factors: (*1*) subject variables, such as age, gender, and visual acuity; (*2*) stimulus characteristics, such as type of stimulator, full-field or half-field stimulation, check size, contrast, and luminescence; and (*3*) recording parameters, such as placement and combination of recording electrodes. (From the 2001 Report of the Nomenclature Committee of the American Association of Electromyography and Electrodiagnosis.[10] Used by permission, copyright © 2001, AAEM.)

visual evoked response See **visual evoked potential.**

visual field That portion of space in which objects are visible at the same moment during steady fixation of the gaze in one direction.[5626] See also **field of vision.**

visual grasp reflex The return of gaze to a target despite commands to look elsewhere. Reflex saccadic movements are made toward a transiently presented visual stimulus, while gaze is meant to be directed upon a different, fixed target.[1886]

visual hallucinations Perception of visual images in the absence of objective stimuli. See **ophthalmopathic hallucinations, hemianopic hallucinations, peduncular hallucinosis, hypnagogic hallucinations.**

The subject has been reviewed in depth by Miller Fisher.[1862]

visual illusions of movement   The appearance of movement or displacement of the visual field with respect to an observer when no such movement has occurred.

Three forms are differentiated:

1. *Autokinetic illusions* are the apparent wanderings of a small light source in a dark environment.
2. *Oculogyral illusions* arise when the observer experiences the stimulus of angular acceleration, again best seen when the observer fixes a small light source in a dark place.
3. *Oculogravic illusions*, linked with the stimulus of linear acceleration, can be seen in any condition of illumination, and consist of illusions of tilt and movement.

All three forms have been ascribed to small, involuntary, and physiological eye movements resulting from labyrinthine activity.[5948]

visual inversion   Transient complete 180° inversion of the visual image. It occurs as a result of ischemic, traumatic, or inflammatory pathology in the occipital lobes.[3808]

visual neglect   A defective ability to attend to one or more components of the total visual environment as a result of lesions of one or other cerebral hemisphere, especially the right.

Accompanying visual field defects are not always demonstrable. The area of neglect is more frequently central or bilateral than contralateral to the site of the cerebral lesion. It occurs with either left or right hemisphere damage but is more severe after right. It is also more common in the center of the page or bilaterally than unilaterally and so is probably a bilateral phenomenon and it may occur without a visual field defect.[80]

Visual Neglect Recovery index   A battery of tests modified from the **Behavioral Inattention test** and used to evaluate visual and other forms of neglect following acute stroke, and to predict recovery.[5366]

visual object agnosia   A failure of generic class recognition—even worse than the usual visual agnosia. See also **agnosia.**

visual orbicularis reflex   (of Descartes) (palpebral reflex) See **orbicularis oculi reflex.**

visual paraesthesia   A disagreeable quality of sensations coming from the affected side in patients with partial hemianopias.

visual perseveration   (paliopsia) 1. Recurrence of visual perceptions after the stimulus-object has been removed. A variety of this affection (*illusory visual spread*) comprises an illusory extension of the visual perception over an area greater than that which the stimulus-object would be expected to excite; thus, a metamorphopsia in which objects appear elongated in one di-

mension only. The causative lesion is in the posterior part of the hemisphere, on either side.[1170] 2. A phenomenon characterized by the prolonged persistence of a visual image without late recurrences, in the presence of evidence of ictal activity but without any associated hemianopia.[1216] See also **palinopsia.**

visual reproduction test   A test of visuospatial praxis in which the subject has to reproduce increasingly complex geometric figures after a 10-second study period, and then to copy the stimulus figures (to assess visuoperceptual dysfunction).[4854]

visual static agnosia   Impaired recognition of statically presented stimuli, with relatively retained recognition of those that are moving.[673]

visual vertigo   1. (optokinetic motion sickness) The physiological effect of a mismatch between the visual sensation of movement and the concomitant vestibular and somatosensory inputs which signal that movement is not occurring—as occurs when viewing chase scenes on a wide-angle cinema screen. 2. Vertigo induced by distorted visual input, as with incorrect refraction, strong plus-lenses after cataract surgery, or oculomotor paresis (ocular vertigo).[769]

visual-constructive derangement   See **visuospatial agnosia.**

visual-palpebral reflex   See **palpebral reflex.**

visual-verbal test   A test of abstraction ability in which the subject is required to determine the common attributes of three of the four patterns printed on cards, there being two sets, each card with three patterns sharing such attributes.[1776]

visuomotor ataxia   (disturbance in visual orientation, *trouble du sens de l'éspace*) A disorder of the visual control of motor activity despite intact motor, cerebellar, and somatosensory functions, and with normal praxis and visual perception. One or both half-fields and the contralateral or the homolateral hand may be affected; bilateral involvement indicates the presence of a callosal lesion; unilateral involvement, a lesion of the occipitofrontal pathways subserving the visual control of movement.[4759] See **optic ataxia.**

visuospatial ability   The capacity to recognize the presence, position, and spatial relationships of objects seen, and to manipulate them appropriately in space.

visuospatial acalculia   See **acalculia.**

visuospatial agnosia   (planotopokinesia, apractagnosia for spatial orientation, visual-constructive derangement) A defect in the analysis of spatial relationships and in the execution of constructional tasks under visual control, particularly those demanding a fine appreciation of spatial structure such as drawing, copying, and the manipulation of patterns, caused by a lesion of the "minor" hemisphere parietal lobe,[4641] due in part to unilateral visual inattention.

visuospatial agraphia   See **agraphia.**

visuospatial neglect   A relative imperception of objects in one half of the visual field, most commonly occurring with right hemisphere lesions in the early stages after, for example, stroke, but later found with equal incidence after lesions of either hemisphere.

visuovestibulo-ocular response   A combination of the **vestibulo-ocular response** and **optokinetic nystagmus,** providing the mechanism for the stability of the retinal image when not only the head but also the object of fixation is moving.

vitamin E deficiency   A consequence of chronic malabsorption syndromes in which dysarthria, an ataxic syndrome with or without musculoskeletal changes (especially in children), an areflexic sensorimotor peripheral neuropathy, and extensor plantar responses have been described.[2444] Other manifestations may include cranial neuropathy with ophthalmoplegia and dysarthria, psychomotor impairment, posterior column dysfunction, myopathy, and pigmentary retinopathy. This deficiency has been held responsible for the neurological syndromes of children with severe chronic liver disease and of **hypo-** and **a-betalipoproteinemia.** The syndrome resembles **Friedreich ataxia,** but in that condition plasma α-tocopherol levels are normal and there is no response to vitamin E supplementation.

Isolated vitamin E deficiency is inherited as an autosomal recessive disease mapped to chromosome 8q13 and presents with cerebellar and peripheral neuropathic signs.[2771]

vitamin E deficiency myopathy   A syndrome complicating chronic cholestasis, in which low serum vitamin E levels, absent reflexes, mild weakness, ataxia, and sensory loss in the arms and legs occur in association with the presence of multiple autofluorescent inclusions within skeletal muscle fibers, showing strong acid phosphatase reactivity.[4108]

vocal agnosia   Difficulty in recognizing a known human voice due to bilateral temporal lobe damage.

vocal cord abductor paralysis   A potential life-threatening complication of multisystem atrophy through its ability to cause nocturnal airway obstruction.[2757]

vocal spasmodic dystonia   A primary focal dystonia affecting phonation, the speech having a "strangled" or tight quality.

Vogt, A.   (1879–1943) Swiss ophthalmologist working in Zurich.

Vogt, Cécile   (1875–1931) French neuroanatomist, who trained in Paris and worked for a year with **Marie** at the **Salpêtrière,** where she met Oskar **Vogt,** whom she later married. Her earlier interests were in myelination, but she and her husband later concentrated on **cytoarctitectonic** and stimulation studies in primates, which led to the differentiation of 100 separate cortical areas—minutiae no longer accepted as meaningful. She also studied the basal ganglia and was the first to ascribe a specific disease state (double athetosis) to disease of the striatum and to apply the term **état marbré.**

Vogt, Heinrich   (1875–1937) German psychiatrist who graduated from Heidelberg University and became professor of psychiatry in Göttingen. He described the features of the juvenile form of **neuronal ceroid lipofuscinosis** (Spielmeyer-Vogt disease) before, but published after, Spielmeyer.[7]

Vogt, Oskar   (1870–1959) Danish-German neuroanatomist and neuropathologist. He was born in Schleswig-Holstein and trained with **Binswanger** and **Forel, Marie,** and the **Déjèrines** in biological sciences and neurology. His goal was to found an institute where scientists of various disciplines could work together on problems of the nervous system, and he did so with the founding of the Neurologische Zentralstation in Berlin (1898), later incorporated into the University of Berlin and in 1931 becoming the Kaiser Wilhelm-Institut with over a hundred staff members and himself as director, funded in large part by the Rockefeller Foundation.

Political factors led to his removal in 1937 to a smaller institute in Neustadt, from which he was called up for military service as a private soldier at the age of 69. However, he proved intractable and was discharged to resume his cytological studies on the huge collection of brains collected in the Institut by Bielschowsky, Brodmann, Foerster, Liepmann, Oppenheim, and others, and preserved over the years.

Both Oskar and Cecile Vogt had as their goal the correlation of normal and abnormal behavior with brain morphology, and to this end they published their works on cytoarchitectonics from 1903, assisted by **Brodmann,** and on myeloarchitectonics in numerous animals as well as in humans.

The Vogts also studied the variable susceptibility to disease manifested by different brain areas, noting that the vulnerability of each neuron system is determined by the distinctive physicochemical composition of its cells (pathoclisis).[2490,5047]

Vogt syndrome   1. (Wilson-Vogt syndrome, congenital chorea, syndrome of the corpus striatum) A form of cerebral palsy with athetosis, chorea, and eventually dystonias, and usually with mental retardation, characterized by the abnormal presence of myelinated fibers in the corpus striatum (**état marbré**).[5776]

The clinical syndrome results from destruction of the cells of the caudate nucleus and putamen, leading to spastic diplegia without pyramidal tract involvement, dysarthria, athetosis, rhythmic oscillations, and pseudobulbar palsy as a consequence of damage to all cell types in the neostriatum.[5776] See also **double athetosis.**

2. A form of **acrocephalosyndactyly** once regarded as type 2, but so similar to type 1 (**Apert syndrome**) that the difference is illusory.

Vogt-Koyanagi syndrome   See **uveomeningoencephalitic syndrome.**

Vogt-Koyanagi-Harada syndrome   See **uveomeningoencephalitic syndrome.**

Vohwinkel syndrome   See **deafness, keratopachydermia, and digital constrictions.**

voice-induced epilepsy   A form of **reflex epilepsy** in which the seizures are triggered by a certain quality of the voice heard.[1912]

voiceless bilabial   (stop) A consonant made by occluding air flow completely at the lips, letting pressure build up, then releasing it in a sudden burst. The only voiceless bilabial stop in English is "P".[3505]

volitional activity   Activity performed as a result of conscious decision.

volitional facial palsy   Weakness of the lower quadrant of one side of the face for the performance of willed movements, as a result of damage to some of the corticobulbar fibers supplying the seventh cranial nerve nucleus.

Compare with **mimetic facial palsy.**

Volkmann ischemic contracture   Muscle fibrosis and sensorimotor neuropathy with distal muscle atrophy resulting from prolonged compressive ischemia, as in the **compartment syndromes** and thus most commonly seen in forearm and pretibial muscles after vascular injury due, for example, to supracondylar fractures. Features of **Sudeck atrophy** are also commonly present.[5778]

Volkmann, Richard von   (1830–1889) German surgeon who graduated in Berlin and later became professor of surgery in Halle.

Vollmer reflex   Lordosis of the spine, flexion of the limbs, and a loud cry occurring when the spine of the infant held in ventral suspension is firmly stroked. This reflex is normally present for the first 3 months of life.[6064]

voltage   The potential difference between two sites, expressed in volts (V) or millivolts (mV).

volume conduction   The propagation of electrical currents from external sources within the body, but through extraneural tissues.[1547]

voluntary   (from Lat, of free will) Under conscious control.

voluntary activity   In electromyography, the electric activity recorded from a muscle with consciously controlled contraction. The effort made to contract the muscle may be specified relative to that of a corresponding normal muscle, e.g. minimal, moderate, or maximal. If the recording remains isoelectric during the attempted contraction and equipment malfunction has been excluded, it can be concluded that there is no voluntary activity. (From the 2001 Report of the Nomenclature Committee of the American Association of Electromyography and Electrodiagnosis.[10] Used by permission, copyright © 2001, AAEM.)

voluntary flutter   See **psychogenic flutter.**

voluntary nystagmus   A series of repetitive, conjugate eye movements (back-to-back saccades) which are consciously induced. They can seldom be sustained for more that 15 seconds at a time and usually occur horizontally at high frequency, often accompanied by facial grimacing.

Rarely, the same can be seen in one eye only. The condition has also been reported to occur as a dominant characteristic, but in such cases the movements do not represent true nystagmus.[233,3316] See also **psychogenic flutter.**

volvular epilepsy   A form of complex partial seizure in which the patient walks around in small circles; a generalized tonic-clonic attack may or may not follow. The seizure focus is in the temporal or frontal region.[1489]

vomiting reflex   Reverse peristalsis of the esophagus with vomiting in response to stimulation of the posterior pharyngeal wall, or anywhere in the upper part of the gastrointestinal tract. This is a normal response unless markedly disinhibited.

von Ammon syndrome   See **Apert syndrome.**

von Angyal syndrome   A variant of **Gerstmann syndrome,** characterized by right–left confusion, dysgraphia, and thumb-mouth agnosia.[5779]

von Békésy, Georg   (1899–1972) Hungarian otologist and physicist whose work (mainly at Harvard) clarified the functions of the cochlea, for which he was awarded the Nobel Prize for Physiology in 1961. He invented the patient-controlled audiometer that bears his name.

von Bekhterev reflex   See **carpometacarpal reflex.**

von Bonsdorff technique   A method of increasing the yield in the **Trousseau** test, whereby a blood pressure cuff on the arm is inflated to just below the diastolic pressure for 10 minutes, after which the patient hyperventilates for a minute. Tetany in the arm tested represents a positive result.

von Burdach, Karl Friedrich   See **Burdach.**

von Economo encephalitis   See **encephalitis lethargica.**

von Economo, Konstantin   (1876–1931) Austrian neurologist and neuropathologist. Born in Romania of wealthy Greek parents, he grew up in Trieste and studied engineering in Vienna before commencing medical studies. After graduation he trained with Pierre **Marie** in Paris, but later returned to Vienna and eventually became professor of psychiatry and neurology in 1921. Having numerous other interests, however, he refused further promotion. He was passionately interested in aeronautics (and was the first Austrian to hold an international pilot's licence) and in ballooning.

He published on the topics of pontine tumors, the trigeminal nerve, sleep, **Wilson disease,** and cortical cytoarchitecture, his 1925 treatise clarifying much of the prevailing confusion about the extent of the different areas and their characteristics. As a result of a paper on accelerated dementia, von Economo narrowly escaped having his name attached to what is now known as **Creutzfeldt-Jakob disease.** His published account of **encephalitis lethargica** (May 10, 1917)[5780] immediately followed that of **Cruchet** of Bordeaux (April 27, 1917) and the latter began a squabble, loudly claiming that precedence which was then considered important; as delicately adjudicated by **van Bogaert,** he failed in his claim, since von Economo had defined the condition as a single disease entity, which Cruchet and his colleagues had not.[5709]

Konstantin von Economo

von Frey hairs   Bristles of varying thicknesses, mounted upon suitable holders, for the semiquantitative examination of the sense of touch.

von Frey, M.   Originator (1895) of the specificity theory of sensation, he considered that heat, cold, touch, and pain were the four specific modalities, each subserved by specific receptors and fibers. He believed that skin receptors are differentiated with respect to the lowest threshold to particular energy categories: Meissner corpuscles and hair cells for touch, Ruffini end-organs for warm, Krause end-bulbs for cold, and free nerve endings for pain—opinions which are no longer held.

von Gierke disease   (glycogenosis type 1) A recessively inherited deficiency of glucose-6-phosphatase, leading to the deposition of glycogen in the liver and kidneys. Clinically, obesity, hepatomegaly, renal impairment, lactic acidosis, and failure to thrive are the most obvious features; seizures represent the only neurological problem.[5781] See **glycogen storage diseases.**

von Graefe cramp   See **blepharospasm.**

von Graefe, Friedrich Wilhelm Ernst Albrecht   See **Graefe.**

von Graefe sign   Lid lag—the failure of the upper lid to maintain its normal position relative to the globe during down-gaze, although the lid descends normally with eye closure. The sign is an inconstant feature of hyperthyroidism, and is also seen in facial nerve palsy (in which, however, there is ptosis of the brow) and in **myasthenia gravis.**[5784a] See also **pseudo–von Graefe sign.**

von Graefe syndrome   See **chronic progressive external ophthalmoplegia, progressive external ophthalmoplegia.**

von Graefe–Sjögren syndrome   (Hallgren syndrome) A recessively inherited condition characterized by pigmentary retinal degeneration, deafness, and spinocerebellar ataxia, often with mental retardation.[5784]

von Gudden, Bernhard Aloys   (1824–1886) See **Gudden.** He demonstrated the presence of both crossed and uncrossed fibers in the optic nerve and showed secondary thalamic atrophy to occur after a lesion of the occipital cortex.

von Hippel, Eugen   (1867–1939) German ophthalmologist who trained in Heidelberg, where he became assistant to **Leber,** working mainly on angiomatosis retinae. He later became professor at Halle and then at Göttingen Universities.

Von Hippel did not report the autosomal dominant inheritance of the condition named for him, nor its intracranial complications, nor occurrence of pancreatic cysts, pheochromocytomas, and renal and pancreatic tumors, which may also be features of the disorder; these insights were the work of Arvid Lindau (1926).

von Hippel–Lindau disease (cerebroretinal an-giomatosis; OMIM 193300) A rare, dominantly inher-ited, multisystem tumor syndrome with variable ex-pression, in which diffuse hemangiomatoses are found (in descending order of frequency) in the retinas, ad-renal glands, cerebellum, spinal cord, and kidney.[2578] The gene is carried on the short arm of chromosome 3 at 3p25–p24.

Renal carcinoma, solid or cystic hemangioblastoma anywhere in the neuraxis, and pheochromocytoma are important and specific complications; cerebral tumors are detected by enhanced MRI in 70% of cases. En-dolymphatic sac tumors, which can cause tinnitus or deafness, are also described.

The diagnosis is likely if a patient with a family his-tory of von Hippel–Landau disease (VHL):

A. Has more than one retinal or cerebellar hemangioblas-toma; or

B. Has an isolated lesion in association with a visceral man-ifestation of the disease such as renal cell carcinoma or pheochromocytoma, and, possibly, multiple pancreatic cysts; or

C. When there is only one manifestation in the presence of a positive family history.

In the absence of a family history of VHL, the presence of two or more retinal or cerebellar hemangioblas-tomas, or one hemangioblastoma with one visceral tu-mor, is required for diagnosis.

The condition was first described in England by Collins in 1894, but it was von Hippel who 10 years later recognized that the lesions were hemangioblas-tomas,[2714] while Lindau reported the cerebellar fea-tures.

von Mickulicz disease Sarcoidosis affecting the parotid glands.

von Monakow see **Monakow.**

von Monakow bundle See **rubrospinal tract.**

von Monakow reflex See **lateral foot reflex.**

von Monakow syndrome See **anterior choroidal ar-tery syndrome.**

von Recklinghausen disease See **neurofibromatosis.**

von Recklinghausen, Friedrich Daniel See **Reck-linghausen.**

von Soemmerring, Samuel Thomas See **Soemmer-ring.**

von Stein tests 1. Performance of the **Romberg test** while the patient stands on one leg or with one foot in front of the other. This adds sensitivity but subtracts specificity. 2. Tilt-table tests.

von Stockert phenomenon The prompt induction of sleep by certain visual stimuli in subjects who have re-covered from an acute attack of **encephalitis lethar-gica.**

von Strümpell, E.A.G.G. See **Strümpell,** E.A.G.G.

von Willebrand's knee A looping-forward of cross-ing fibers in the optic chiasm, such that a lesion of the posterior part of the homolateral optic nerve also af-fects these fibers, causing a field defect in the opposite eye.

vorbeireden (Ger, talking past [or beside] the point). Although this word is used to describe the characteris-tic feature of Ganser syndrome, Ganser never used it himself, preferring *vorbeigehen*, translated as "to pass by," which actually gives a better feeling for the abnor-mal verbal output.

Vulpian, Edmé-Felix-Alfred (1826–1887) French physician, a pupil of Flourens who assisted him to en-ter medical school in Paris. Vulpian later worked with **Charcot** at the **Salpêtrière,** where he later succeeded **Cruveilhier** as professor of pathological anatomy.

A retiring man, he was somewhat overshadowed by Charcot, although considered an outstanding teacher. His research output included studies of peripheral nerve regeneration, the **scapuloperoneal syndrome,** the chromaffin system, the motor end-plate, and the pathological anatomy of the spinal cord.[1829]

Vulpian sign (Prévost sign) The tendency of the eyes to turn toward the side of a cortical lesion and thus away from the paralyzed side, as after a hemispheric stroke. The integrity of the frontal eye fields appears necessary for normal deviations to occur in either di-rection, but the sign does occur with some more pos-terior lesions in the right hemisphere and, according to the original publications, with deep lesions as well.[2200]

Vurpas reflex See **buccal reflex.**

Waaler anomaly (hydrocephalus, costovertebral dysplasia with Sprengel deformity) A dominantly inherited congenital dysmorphic syndrome characterized by white forelock, deafness, and numerous musculoskeletal abnormalities affecting the face, ribs, spine, and limbs.

Waardenburg, Petrus Johannes (1886–1979) A Dutch ophthalmic geneticist working in Utrecht.

Waardenberg syndrome 1. (van der Hoeve–Halbertsma-Waardenburg-Klein syndrome) A relatively common dominantly inherited syndrome characterized by nerve deafness, heterochromia iridis, confluence of the eyebrows (**synophrys**), a white forelock, lateral displacement of the lacrimal canthi, abnormal skin pigmentation, and impaired vestibular responses.[5789,5790]

In a *variant* form, *Mende syndrome*, the features of **Down syndrome** are also present.

2. A singularly rare form of **acrocephalosyndactyly** (variously *type III* or *V*), characterized by hypertelorism, facial dysmorphism, syndactyly of the hands, and abnormal genitalia.[5522] See also **Apert syndrome.**

Wada test The intracarotid injection of sodium amylobarbitone, given in order to ascertain the lateralization of the speech centers in patients under consideration for excision of a temporal lobe for the management of intractable seizures.[2846]

By causing temporary (10 minute) inactivity of the injected hemisphere, the functions of the other one can be assessed. The technique was described in 1949 by Dr. Jun Wada of Vancouver, Canada. Questions to do with its interpretation have been discussed,[3794] but it is likely that the use of functional MRI will make it obsolete in the foreseeable future.

Waddell signs Physical findings that suggest that the back pain complained of by a patient has its root in some behavioral disturbance. The signs are grouped into five classes:

1. Tenderness which is superficial (dermal) or nonanatomical. See also **cellulalgia, skin roll test.**
2. Simulation tests, which give the patient the impression that a test is being performed, when actually it is not. Back pain felt with downward compression on the head or rotation of the patient's shoulders and pelvis in the same plane are examples.
3. Distraction tests, such as the examination of straight-leg raising with the patient in the lying and then in the sitting position
4. Regional disturbances. "Giving way" of many muscle groups that cannot be explained on a localized neurological basis and sensory disturbances following a glove-and-stocking rather than a dermatomal distribution are examples.
5. Behavioral and verbal overreaction to the manipulations of the examiner

After Waddell G, McCulloch JA, Kummell E, et al. Nonorganic physical signs in low back pain. Spine 1980;5:117–25. Reproduced by permission of the Journal of Neurosurgery; Spine.

Such signs were shown to correlate with each other, but not with the presence of organic causes for back pain.[5791]

Wadia-Swamy spinocerebellar degeneration A dominantly inherited cerebellar ataxic syndrome, characterized also by unusually slow saccades and pursuit movements of the eyes.[5797]

Wagener retinopathy See **Keith-Wagener scale.**

Waggoner syndrome A recessively inherited syndrome characterized by mental retardation and agenesis of the cerebral white matter.[5800]

Wagner, Ernst Leberecht (1829–1888) German physician who described acute generalized polymyositis in 1863.[5801]

Wagner syndrome (Wagner-Unverricht syndrome, Wagner-Hepp disease, Potain dermatomyositis, Bergouignan edematous polymyositis) See **dermatomyositis.**

Wagner von Jauregg, Julius (1857–1940) German physician, awarded the Nobel prize in 1927 for his introduction of malarial treatment for **general paresis.**

Wagner-Hepp disease See **Wagner syndrome.**

Wagner-Unverricht syndrome See **Wagner syndrome.**

WAGR syndrome A rare syndrome characterized by the association of **W**ilms tumor, **A**niridia, **G**enital abnormality, and mental **R**etardation. The responsible gene maps to 11–p13.

Waida dystrophy See **benign X-linked muscular dystrophy.**

WAIS, WAIS-R Acronyms for the **Wechsler Adult Intelligence Scale** (Revised), the most used of all the comprehensive intelligence tests available.

wakefulness without awareness See **persistent vegetative state.**

wake-up stroke The first awareness of a neurological deficit when a patient wakes, usually due to an ischemic infarct that had occurred during sleep.

wake-up test A procedure used most commonly in spinal surgery. During critical portions of an operation in which the spinal cord is at risk for injury, the level of general anesthesia is allowed to decrease to the point where the patient can respond to commands. The patient is then asked to move hands and feet, and a movement in response to commands indicates the spinal cord is intact. This procedure is used routinely in some centers. Somatosensory evoked potential monitoring has supplanted its use in most centers, except sometimes in the situation where they indicate the possibility of spinal cord injury. (From the 2001 Report of the Nomenclature Committee of the American Association of Electromyography and Electrodiagnosis.[10] Used by permission, copyright © 2001, AAEM.)

waking cataplexy   See **sleep paralysis.**

waking epilepsy   Generalized seizures occurring only during the waking hours.

Waldenström macroglobulinemia   (hyperviscosity syndrome) A syndrome characterized by excessive IgM production and circulation following the uncontrolled proliferation of lymphocytes and plasma cells. It occurs either in isolation among elderly men (primary macroglobulinemia) or as a **paraneoplastic syndrome** associated with multiple myeloma and leukemia.

Clinical characteristics include easy bruising and bleeding, anemia with systemic malaise and fatigue, chorioretinopathy with retinal hemorrhages, optic disk edema, focal cerebral deficits, sensorimotor peripheral neuropathy, hepatosplenomegaly, lymphadenopathy, and Raynaud syndrome.

Laboratory findings include anemia, raised ESR, abnormal protein immunoelectrophoresis, and hyperviscosity of the serum.[5806]

Waldenström syndrome   See **acute thyrotoxic encephalomyelopathy.**

Waldeyer, Heinrich   German physician who formulated the concept that the unit structure of the nervous system is the "neuron," which he so named in 1881.

Walker effect   Induced fatigabilty of remote muscles (e.g., ptosis) after the forearm muscles have been exercised repeatedly with an inflated blood pressure cuff occluding the arm circulation, and then removed. Temporarily high lactic acid levels have been suggested as the cause.

Walker, Mary Broadfoot   (1888–1974) English physician who discovered the beneficial effect of physostigmine in **myasthenia gravis** in 1934. For some months she had been trying the effect of a number of different agents on a close friend with the disease[5810] but experimented with this one on a hospital patient after discussing the similarity of myasthenic symptoms to those of curare poisoning with Dr. D. **Denny-Brown,** who was then consultant to the hospital in which she was a junior staff member.[2988]

She was also first to describe hypokalemia in periodic paralysis.

Walker syndrome   See **Marden-Walker syndrome.**

Walker-Warburg syndrome   (lissencephaly, encephalo-optic dysplasia; oculocerebral malformative syndrome; muscle-eye-brain disease; cerebro-ocular dysgenesis; cerebro-oculomuscular syndrome; retinal dysplasia with hydrocephalus; hydrocephalus, agyria, retinal dys-plasia, and encephalocele/HARD + E syndrome, Fukuyama-type muscular dystrophy) A lethal, recessive, congenital neurodysplastic syndrome, characterized by cortical agyria with a lack of cortical laminations (type 2 **lissencephaly**), congenital muscle dystrophy, cerebellar aplasia, callosal agenesis, hydrocephalus, ocular abnormalities such as buphthalmos, micro-ophthalmia, corneal opacities, and retinal dysplasia and detachment in the absence of such known causes as toxoplasmosis or cytomegalovirus or other viral disease.[663,5949] The condition has been mapped to 9q31–33, as have some of the other conditions listed above.[5595] Diagnostic criteria have been suggested.[1479]

The **Dandy-Walker malformation, encephalocele,** aqueductal stenosis and hydrocephalus, and mental and developmental delay are also commonly found. HARD ± E is the acronym for **H**ydrocephalus, **A**gyria and absent cortical laminar structure, **R**etinal **D**ysplasia ± **E**ncephalocele.[5814]

walking reflex   (stepping response) When a baby is supported upright over a table and the feet allowed to come into contact with the surface of the table, reciprocal flexion and extension of the legs is induced, simulating walking. The reflex normally disappears after the age of 6 weeks.

Wallenberg, Adolf   (1862–1949) German neurologist who graduated from Heidelberg University and worked in Danzig, where he was elected titular professor of neurology. Forbidden to publish by the Nazi régime, he left Germany for Oxford, moving to the United States in 1943. The syndrome named for him is his major legacy, but he also published important work on poliomyelitis, cerebellar vascular disease, and neuroanatomy.

Wallenberg syndrome   (Vieusseux-Wallenberg syndrome) See **lateral medullary syndrome.**[5816]

Waller, Augustus Volney   (1816–1870) English physician and physiologist who lived in France for much of his childhood, graduating from medical school in Paris. He practiced in London for a few years and continued his physiological research, studying nerve regeneration in the frog (1860) and pointing out that a divided nerve fiber will only survive when it retains its continuity with its cell body, and that degeneration thus will only occur distal to the site of injury. He left England in 1851 to work with Budge in Berlin on pupillary innervation before going in turn to Paris, Birmingham, and finally Geneva, where he died.

Waller's law   "If a spinal nerve be divided, the peripheral parts degenerate completely. If the anterior root be divided, the peripheral fibres degenerate. If the posterior root be divided, the central fibres degenerate. If the ganglion on the posterior root be divided, both central and peripheral nerve fibres degenerate. Hence it is assumed that the trophic center for the fibres in the anterior root lie in the multipolar cells of the anterior grey cornu of the cord, and the trophic center for the fibres of the posterior root in the cells of the ganglion in this root."

No more succinct description has yet been provided.

wallerian degeneration   (axonal degeneration) Those changes occurring distal to the site of transection of a nerve fiber, and thus in that part of an axon separated from its perikaryon. They are characterized by fragmentation, dissolution, and removal of the myelin sheath and the subsequent departure of Schwann cells, and by the dissolution of the axis cylinder distally, as a result of failure of the energy processes required to maintain the exclusion of calcium ions from the interior of the cell. Similar changes also occur for a very short distance in a proximal direction, and the neuronal cell body swells and shows a degree of **chromatolysis.**

These events were first observed in 1850 by Waller[5818] in the glossopharyngeal nerve of the frog.

wall-eyed bilateral internuclear ophthalmoplegia syndrome   (WEBINO syndrome) Lateral deviation of both eyes (exotropia) and loss of the power of convergence, with bilateral internuclear ophthalmoplegia, as a result of bilateral midbrain lesions affecting the nuclei of both medial recti and both median longitudinal fasciculi.[5381]

Walsh, Frank Burton   (1895–1978) Canadian neuro-ophthalmologist, born and trained in Manitoba, who was invalided out of the army after active service in World War I. He later trained in ophthalmology, from which he developed the specialty of neuro-ophthalmology at the Willmer Eye Institute, Baltimore, where he was in his later years professor emeritus. Described as an "optimath" (one who never ceases to learn), he provided the world with superb teaching in his subspecialty, epitomized by his classic book *Clinical Neuro-Ophthalmology,* which reached its third edition before his death; by his co-authored *Neuropathology of Vision;* and by over a hundred original clinical papers.

Walshe, Sir Francis   (1886–1973) English neurologist, philosopher, writer, and critic, the outstanding intellectual of British neurology in his time. He trained in medicine at University College Hospital, where he was at one time house surgeon to Sir Victor **Horsley,** and with **Sherrington** at Oxford. He was later appointed to the staff of University College Hospital and of the **National Hospital,** Queen Square. He was at various times in his career the editor of *Brain,* president of the Royal Society of Medicine and of the Association of British Neurologists, which he had helped to found, and he was elected to fellowship of the Royal Society.

He was a devout admirer of Hughlings-**Jackson** and, like him, was a supremely capable clinical observer who deduced physiology where he did not experiment in the laboratory to demonstrate it. His books, in particular his textbook of neurology and *Critical Studies in Neu-*

rology, reflect his precise critical analyses of neurological mechanisms and phenomena.

A highly principled man, he accepted no government salary for his hospital work because he remained unreconciled with the concept of the British National Health Service. He was a towering figure in neurology; yet, it must be accounted as a regrettable loss to the advancement of learning that he was also a polemicist of mean repute whose emotional defense of his opinions did nothing to encourage the uncertain, while his barbed comments, commonly appearing in academic journals, provided brief entertainment for the reader but must have inhibited constructive discourse. Nevertheless, seven of his publications are referenced in this book.[5827,5828,5829,5830,5831,5832,5833]

waning discharge   A repetitive discharge gradually decreasing in frequency or amplitude before it stops. cf. **myotonic discharge.**

Warburg syndrome   See **Walker-Warburg syndrome, HARD+E syndrome.**

Ward-Romano syndrome   Abnormal prolongation of the Q-T interval on the ECG, leading to cardiac arrhythmia and reduction of cerebral perfusion sufficient to cause **occasional seizures,** as in **Stokes-Adams attacks.**[4443]

warfarin embryopathy   A congenital dysmorphic syndrome occurring in infants born to mothers treated with warfarin during pregnancy.

The clinical features include microcephaly, blindness with optic atrophy, seizures, hypotonia, epiphyseal lesions, and mental and developmental delay.[1467]

Warkany syndrome   (trisomy 8 syndrome) A congenital dysmorphic syndrome with great phenotypic variability, characterized by facial and skeletal anomalies and by any combination of mild physical and mental retardation, corneal opacities, nystagmus, callosal agenesis, aqueductal stenosis with hydrocephalus, seizures, and developing hypertonia.[1332]

warm-up effect   The reduction in myotonic stiffness and weakness with exercise; a peripheral rather than a central phenomenon due to altered excitation and contractile performance.[1123] **Paradoxical myotonia** represents the opposite condition, the myotonia worsening with activity.

warning headache   See **sentinel headache.**

Wartenberg cheiralgia paresthetica   (nocturnal arm dysesthesias, tired arm syndrome) Pain, paresthesias, and numbness following intercurrent stretching or compression of peripheral nerves and described as a syndrome of the superficial radial nerves.[5859]

Handcuff neuropathy is identical.[5303,5856]

Wartenberg migrant sensory neuritis   A self-limiting condition characterized by the occurrence of pain and numbness in the territory of sensory nerves that have suffered a stretching injury.[3708]

Wartenberg pendulum test   With the patient sitting with the legs hanging over the side of the bench, the examiner extends the knee and then drops it to swing freely under the action of gravity. The pattern of the swinging movements reflects the balance of suprasegmental motor influences (mainly affecting the quadriceps), and is decreased with spasticity.

The test was originally introduced by Wartenberg for assessing rigidity in patients with **Parkinson disease,**[5861] in whom a marked reduction in the maximum velocity of the first swing has been shown, while the reduction in spastic limbs is less so.[801, 802]

Wartenberg,   Robert   (1887–1956)   Lithuanian-American neurologist who graduated *cum laude* from Rostock, worked with **Foerster** and headed the neurology service at Freiburg before emigrating to the United States in 1935 (when his teaching permit had been withdrawn by the Nazi government). He was eventually made clinical professor at San Francisco University, where he built and led a strong teaching, research, and clinical service.

His publications were eclectic; initially, they were much influenced by the epidemic encephalitis raging in Europe, while later he became interested in the employment of new technologies for the examination of neurological disease, and in the clinical examination. In this area, his book *The Examination of Reflexes* was acclaimed as a perfect simplification of a previously complex subject. He was a superb clinical neurologist, and some of his clinical insights are indicated in the following entries.[4967,4495] His facility with the English language was admirable, but his detailed editorial corrections of F.M.R. **Walshe**'s *Diseases of the Nervous System* were not appreciated by its author.

Wartenberg signs   1. Decreased arm swing on walking, in cases of pyramidal, cerebellar, or basal ganglion disease. 2. Active flexion of the terminal phalanges of the four fingers of a paretic hand about a firm object, or against resistance offered by the examiner's fingers similarly flexed, is followed by adduction, flexion, and opposition of the thumb (in a normal extremity the thumb remains in abduction and extension); a pathological associated movement in pyramidal tract disease.[5858] 3. Intense pruritus of the nostrils and the tip of the nose felt by patients with cerebral tumor.[5854] 4. Abduction of the little finger in cases of ulnar nerve palsy[5855] (Wartenberg's oriental prayer sign). 5. Reduced vibration felt in the upper eyelid when the patient with facial palsy closes his or her eyes.[5853] 6. The "useless arm" as a sign of a parietal plaque in **multiple sclerosis.** 7. The **finger flexor reflex** (a pyramidal sign with excessive flexion of the fingers). 8. Diminished abduction of the thumb in cases of median nerve palsy.

Wartenberg syndrome   1. See **Parry-Romberg syndrome.** 2. Brachialgia statica paresthetica. See **carpal tunnel syndrome**[5856]

Wartenberg wheel   A small wheel upon a handle, set with radially projecting spikes, which is run over the surface of the skin in testing superficial pain sensation. Use of the instrument is ill advised today because of its capacity for transmitting such diseases as AIDS and hepatitis.

Wartenberg winking-jaw phenomenon   (corneomandibular reflex, pterygocorneal reflex, reverse Marcus Gunn phenomenon, inverse Marcus Gunn phenomenon) Involuntary deviation of the jaw to the opposite side when the cornea is stimulated; seen with supranuclear lesions of the fifth cranial nerve.[5860]

Wassermann, August Paul von   (1866–1925) German bacteriologist, who worked mainly in Berlin. The Wassermann reaction for the diagnosis of syphilis, a modification of the Bordet-Gengou complement-fixation reaction, was described in 1906.

wasting   Atrophy of skin or muscle.

water babies   A term applied to children suffering from pitressin-resistant diabetes insipidus, fancifully emulating the title of the classic children's book by Charles Kingsley.

Waterhouse, Rupert   (1873–1958) English physician who in 1911 gave the definitive account of the syndrome bearing his name.[5868] Friedreichsen (see next entry) published 7 years later.

Waterhouse-Friedreichsen syndrome   Adrenal hemorrhage leading to adrenal failure, complicating meningococcemia. The condition was first described by Dr. Arthur Voelcker (1861–1946), an English physician, in a brief report in 1894.

The major clinical features are petechiae leading to extensive purpura, hypotensive hypovolemic shock, and reducing consciousness up to coma.[5868]

watershed areas   The boundary zones between the territories of the three major cerebral arteries (anterior/middle, middle/posterior) of the brain, representing the sites most likely to show evidence of infarction when cerebral perfusion is globally diminished, as occurs with impaired cardiac output and decreased perfusion pressure.

watershed infarcts   (border-zone, borderline, distal field, extraterritorial, low-flow, or terminal zone infarcts) Cerebral infarcts of two types, each occurring at the point furthest from the systemic arterial supply: The *macro*-type occurs between the territories of supply of the major arteries (anterior, middle, and posterior cerebral). The *micro*-watershed infarct is located between the columnar, penetrating arteries of the cortex. Both usually occur as a result of systemic hypotension with critical reduction in cerebral blood flow. In addition, "internal" watershed infarcts occur in the centrum semi-ovale between the arterial territories of the deep branches of the basal cerebral arteries and those of the superficial pia-arachnoid plexus and also between the territories of the major arteries supplying the cerebellum.[960]

See also **transcortical aphasia.**

Watson-Schwarz test   A chemical reaction of value in the diagnosis of acute intermittent porphyria.[5402]

wave   A transient change in voltage represented as a line of differing directions over time.

wave-and-spike phantom   See **phantom spike and wave.**

waveform   The shape of a wave.

We Move   A coalition of organizations with interests in movement disorders. Web site: http://www.wemove.org.

weakness   A decrease in the force of muscular activity exerted in the performance of a resisted task, as judged by the patient or the examiner.

weakness of one leg with ease of falling   A **lacunar syndrome** suspected to be due to a lesion of the brainstem, in which the hypertensive patient notes mild weakness of one leg, or of the arm and leg, with a marked tendency to fall toward that side.[1853,1867]

wear and tear pigment   See **lipofuscin.**

wearing-off effect   See **end-of-dose deterioration.**

weaver mutant   A murine mutation causing ataxia.

Weaver syndrome   A dysmorphic syndrome, manifesting also accelerated skeletal maturation, flat occiput, hypertelorism, hoarse voice, camptodactyly and clinodactyly, congenital cardiac anomalies, hypertonia, and mental and developmental delay.[5881]

Weaver-Williams syndrome   A congenital dysmorphic syndrome, characterized also by deafness, dental and skeletal malformations, microcephaly, and mental and developmental delay.[337]

Weber, Ernst Heinrich   (1795–1878) German anatomist and physiologist, born and educated in Wittenberg, whence he graduated with a thesis on the sympathetic nerves.

Weber, Frederick Parkes   (1863–1962) The son of Sir Hermann David Weber, he studied medicine at Cambridge and St. Bartholomew's Hospital, London, as well as in Paris, and Vienna and was a prolific writer with over 1200 papers published. Neurological publications included studies of amyotrophies and cerebral tumors but he is best known for his description of *multiple hereditary developmental angiomata (telangiectases) of the skin and mucous membranes associated with recurring haemorrhages* (**Rendu-Osler- Weber hemangiomatosis**) (Lancet, London, 1907;**2**:160–162), **Weber-**

Christian disease, *Weber disease* (localized epidermolysis bullosa), and the **Klippel-Trenaunay-Weber syndrome.**

Frederick Parkes Weber

Weber law   (Weber-Fechner law) The variation in the intensity of a stimulus that causes the least appreciable change in sensation maintains an approximately fixed ratio to the strength of the whole stimulus already acting. Thus, perception is proportional to stimulus strength. This designates the relationship between the magnitude of the stimulus and that of the response, the sensation being a logarithmic function of the stimulus as the sensation increases only arithmetically when the stimuli increase geometrically.[5817] The law was elaborated by E.H. Weber.

Weber, Sir Herman David   (1823–1918) German-English physician who was born in Germany and graduated in medicine from Bonn. He became enamored of England and emigrated there, entering as a student at Guy's Hospital to qualify again. Thereafter, he created a successful practice in London; his patients included five prime ministers.

His own clinical research output was also notable (e.g., the **cerebral peduncle syndrome**), but it was his son, Frederick Parkes **Weber** (1863–1962) whose name is applied to more syndromes.

Weber syndrome   (Weber-Gubler syndrome, Leyden paralysis, hemiplegia alternans superior peduncularis, syndrome of the cerebral peduncle) Unilateral third nerve palsy with contralateral hemiparesis, due to a lesion of the mesencephalon.[5885] The syndrome is named for H.D. Weber who described it in 1863, though Gubler had already described it 4 years previously.

Weber test   A test of auditory function. A vibrating tuning fork placed in the scalp in the midline should be heard equally by each ear but will be heard more loudly in the ear affected by conduction (middle ear) deafness. In the presence of nerve deafness, the sound will be localized to the normal ear. Thus, if the sound is heard more loudly in the right ear, then either there is conductive deafness on the right or nerve deafness on the left, and tests of acuity will be needed to determine which is the case. The test was described by E.H. Weber in 1834.

Weber-Christian disease   (relapsing panniculitis) A syndrome of later adult life characterized by repetitive episodes of pain felt in fatty subcutaneous tissue nodules, mainly over the thighs and hips.[5884] Myopathy is an uncommon complication. The syndrome was named after H.D. Weber.

Weber-Gubler syndrome   See **cerebral peduncle syndrome.**

WEBINO syndrome   See **wall-eyed bilateral internuclear ophthalmoplegia syndrome.**

Webster rating scale   A rating scale designed to provide a semiquantitative assessment of the disabilities of patients with **Parkinson disease.** The items scored are *bradykinesia, rigidity, posture, arm-swing, gait, tremor, facial movement, seborrhea, speech,* and *self-care.* As with other scales, this one provides a template for the physical examination and arbitrarily selects common clinical features for scrutiny. See also **Hoehn and Yahr scale, Columbia Rating scale, Unified Rating scale.**

Wechsler Adult Intelligence Scale   (WAIS) A classic psychometric instrument in use for over 30 years, but requiring both training and experience to administer reliably. It is composed of six verbal and five (nonverbal) performance subtests, yielding verbal, performance, and composite (intelligence quotient) scores.

A relative retention of abilities on the verbal as opposed to the performance items is commonly used as an indicator of a decline in cognitive functioning. Scores on the information and vocabulary subtests are the best measures of original ability, or "that ubiquitous test factor which appears to be the statistical counterpart of learning capacity plus mental alertness, speed and efficiency." The scale has been revised (WAIS-R), mainly with respect to scoring.[5889]

The *Wechsler Intelligence Scale for Children* is a variant form of this test battery.

Wechsler Memory Scale   A standardized measurement tool for the assessment of aspects of memory including information and orientation, mental control, visual pattern reproduction, and digit recall forwards and reversed.[5887] A revised version is now available.

weckblitz   Noise-induced phosphenes, occurring in the hypnagogic state and commonly associated with disease of the eye or optic nerve.

wedge hemianopia   A sectoral field loss caused by a lesion of the lateral geniculate body.

weekend migraine   The occurrence of caffeine-withdrawal headaches in people who do not go to the office on weekends.

Wegener granulomatosis   A granulomatous vasculitis of the upper respiratory tract accompanied by systemic necrotizing vasculitis of arteries and veins, with eventual necrotizing pulmonary vasculitis and glomerulonephritis.[1751] Neurological complications include cranial and peripheral neuropathies, meningism, diabetes insipidus, and focal lesions of the brain or cord (stroke, seizures, cerebritis), and occur in a quarter of all cases.[1508,4143]

Dr. Friedreich Wegener (b. 1907) was a German pathologist.

Weichselbaum, Anton   (1845–1920) German physician.

Weichselbaum syndrome   Cerebrospinal (meningococcal) meningitis.

Weigel test   A modified color-sorting test, in which blocks are sorted according to any one of five principles which can be derived.[4663]

Weigert, Karl   (1843–1905) German professor of pathology at Frankfort. Weigert's myelin stain (1882) was modified by Jakob Pal 6 years later and is known now as the *Weigert-Pal stain,* but his own modification of the van Gieson/hematoxylin stain is still in use.

weightlifters migraine   An acute exertional headache.[4371] See **benign exertional headache.**

Weil disease   Infection by *Leptospira icterohaemorrhagica,* usually from rodents or other small mammals. The clinical manifestations include fever, severe headache with meningism, widespread petechiae later running into purpura, conjunctival hemorrhages, jaundice due to hepatic necrosis, myalgia, myoglobinuria, and encephalopathy with cranial nerve palsies and drowsiness, progressing (if untreated) to coma.

Weil, M.P.   (b. 1884) French physician.

Weil stain   An iron-alum-hematoxylin method for staining myelin sheaths, now superseded by more effective methods.

Weill-Marchesani syndrome   (brachydactylyspheroplakia) A recessively inherited congenital dysmorphic syndrome, manifesting also short stature, broad skull, dental anomalies, brachydactyly, myopia, ectopia lentis, and sometimes glaucoma leading to blindness.[5893]

The syndrome was further defined by Oswald Marchesani (1900–1952), an Austrian ophthalmologist working in Münster, in 1939

Weill-Reys syndrome   See **Adie pupil, Holmes-Adie syndrome.**

Weir Mitchell, Silas   (1829–1914) American physiologist, neurologist, and novelist. He was regarded by his father as "wanting in nearly all the qualities that go to make a success in Medicine," but he was stimulated to investigate the nervous system by Claude **Bernard,** under whom he had studied in Paris for a year after graduation from Jefferson Medical College and before returning to Philadelphia.

He published extensively in pharmacology, toxicology, and physiology both before and after his experience as a contract surgeon to the Union forces in the American Civil War, but it was his experiences in what became a 400-bed neurological hospital under his direction that led to his greatest work, *Gunshot Wounds and Other Injuries of Nerves* (1864), later enlarged as *Injuries of Nerves and Their Consequences* (1872),[3910] which became a standard text internationally. In this book, Weir Mitchell described ascending neuritis, pressure effects upon peripheral nerves, neural anatomy and physiology, trophic changes, the overlap of cutaneous sensation, referred sensation, and current forms of treatment with accounts of 66 patients. A final chapter described **causalgia** in complete detail. The 1864 edition also contains an excellent description of what we call **Horner syndrome.** Nearly 30 of the patients originally described there were subsequently reexamined by his son Dr. John Mitchell (1857–1917) and his findings were published in the book *Remote Consequences of Injuries to Nerves* (1895).

After the war, Weir Mitchell practiced successfully as a neurologist and continued to publish extensively on the topics of muscle stretch reflexes (he described what amounts to the **Jendrassik maneuver**), ankle clonus, erythromelalgia, epilepsy, hysteria and malingering, the circle of Willis, the cerebellum, and numerous other subjects.

In the latter half of his life, he published nearly a score of historical novels as well as books of poetry, a biography of George Washington, and other medical and historical tracts, the total amounting to over 250 publications between 1852 and 1917. He was elected a Fellow of the Royal Society (London) on the recommendation of Sir William **Osler,** whose appointment as professor of clinical medicine in Philadelphia he had assisted. The two were close friends and Osler, in his obituary of Mitchell, quoted Dr. Samuel **Johnson**'s remark about Richard Mead: "No man ever lived more in the sunshine of life",[3759] while perhaps less charitably, **Cushing** remarked that he was vain, but had much to be vain about.

Weir Mitchell syndrome   (erythromelalgia) The sudden onset of a vasomotor disorder causing pain, redness, and thickening of the terminal phalanges and nail beds in the hands and feet, and engorgement of the peripheral veins. The pain is worsened by heat and relieved by cold. The temperature sense may be diminished.

Weir Mitchell treatment   Rest in isolation, exercise, good food, and massage as a treatment for hysteria.

Weisenberg syndrome   See **glossopharyngeal neuralgia.**

Weisenberg-Sicard-Robineau syndrome   See **Collet-Sicard syndrome.**

Weiss sign   Contraction of the facial muscles when they are tapped lightly, as occurs in tetany, neurasthenia, hyperthyroidism, and hysteria.[5904]

Weiss, Soma   (1898–1942) Hungarian-American physician and physiologist who emigrated to the United States in 1920 and trained in medicine at Cornell. After further work in Boston, he was appointed professor of the theory and practice of physick and physician-in-chief at the Peter Bent Brigham Hospital.

Most of his publications were concerned with cardiovascular disease, including the elucidation of the mechanism of **carotid sinus syncope.**[5905]

Weiss syndrome   1. A rare congenital syndrome characterized by congenital deafness, dwarfism, obesity and hypogenitalism, sometimes with mental retardation, described by Dr. E. Weiss in 1932.[5902] 2. A dominantly inherited syndrome characterized by craniosynostosis, medially deviated great toes, and syndactyly.[5903]

Weiss-Charcot-Baker syndrome   See **carotid sinus hypersensitivity.**[5905]

Welander distal myopathy   A dominantly inherited distal myopathy with adult onset, mapped to 2p13.[55] It is complicated by mild disturbances of temperature sensation.[5908] See also **distal muscular dystrophy.**

Welander-Kugelberg-Wohlfart syndrome   See **hereditary motor neuropathy, type 3.**

well-leg compartment syndrome   A syndrome resulting from incorrect positioning of the leg, almost exclusively associated with maintenance of the lithotomy or hemilithotomy position for 2 hours or more during surgery and due to direct external compression and vascular insuffiency or hypoperfusion of the calf muscles, or a combination of the two. The common pathway may be hypo-oxygenation, leading to local ischemia, tissue edema, and a fulminant compartment syndrome.[2547]

Wepfer, Johann Jakob   (1620–1695). German physician. He wrote the first major treatise on stroke in 1658, in which he showed that the *rete mirabile* does not exist in the human; described intra- and extracranial occlusion of the carotid artery, transient ischemic attacks, and reversible ischemic neurological deficits; and established that most cases of apoplexy were due to intracerebral hemorrhage or vascular occlusion.

He seems to have been unaware of the decussation of the motor pathways as in cases of stroke; he usually looked for the pathology on the same side as the paralysis, a mistake corrected during his lifetime by Antonio Maria **Valsalva** (1666–1738).

Werdnig, Guido   (1844–1919) Austrian neurologist who spent most of his professional life in Graz or

Vienna, and who, independently of **Hoffmann,** published a series of papers between 1891 and 1900 on the clinical and pathological findings in infants suffering from the disease named for him.

Werdnig-Hoffmann disease   See **hereditary motor neuropathy, type 1.**

Werner, Otto   German physician who, while still a medical student at Kiel, described the syndrome named for him in four siblings.

Werner syndrome   See **progeria.**[5922]

Wernicke aphasia   (Bastian aphasia, dissociated aphasia, auditory receptive dysphasia, cortical receptive aphasia)[5923] A form of fluent aphasia containing verbal and phonemic **paraphasias,** in which comprehension, repetition, and naming are severely impaired and writing is poor, while grammar, articulation, prosody, and phrase length are often normal.

It was described by Wernicke in 1874 (but also by Bastian in 1869), and occurs with large lesions of the posterior temporal, inferior parietal, and lateral posterior temporal lobes. It has also been described with a right hemisphere lesion (*dissociated aphasia*). The composer Ravel was so afflicted.

Wernicke cramp   A rare form of local muscle cramp precipitated by movement, described by Wernicke in a lecture-demonstration in 1904.[5926]

Wernicke hemianopic pupil   Loss of the pupillary reflex when a thin pencil of light is shone exclusively upon the "blind" side of the retina, indicating that the lesion is anterior to the point at which the pupillary fibers leave the optic tract for the superior colliculus, because when the lesion is more posterior, these fibers are spared, and so pupillary constriction still occurs even when the "blind" retina is stimulated.[5925]

Wernicke, Karl   (1848–1905) German neuropsychiatrist, born in Silesia and dying (after a bicycle accident) in Thuringia. He studied medicine at Breslau and, on graduating in 1870, worked there and in Vienna under Meynert. He was later assistant to **Westphal** in Berlin and, in 1885, was elected to the faculty in neurology and psychiatry in Berlin, then Breslau, and, shortly before his death, Halle.

He left neurology such major legacies as his description of the encephalopathy named for him, and the anatomy and phenomenology of dysphasia (1874); he conceived that sensory aphasia was due to damage to the left temporal lobe where auditory images were stored, motor dysphasia to lesions of Broca's area, conduction aphasia to the pathways between them, and total dysphasia to lesions of both areas. The encephalopathy (which he first described in his major textbook in 1881) was named for him and for **Korsakoff,** although it had been recognized previously by **Gayet** in 1875. He also described the major cerebral

convolutions, predicted the occurrence of pseudobulbar palsy, demonstrated the existence of a brainstem center for lateral gaze, and helped to establish the concept of unilateral cerebral dominance.

Wernicke-Korsakoff encephalopathy   (Wernicke syndrome, polioencephalitis hemorrhagica superior, Meynert amentia, Gayet disease, Gayet-Wernicke syndrome) The association of nystagmus, ophthalmoplegia, cerebellar signs, neuropathy, and inability to record new information ("loss of recent memory") as a result of thiamine deficiency, with bilateral pinhead-sized hemorrhages in the mamillary bodies and in the periventricular and periaqueductal gray matter.

This classical syndrome was first described by a Swedish physician, Magnus Huss (1807–1890), who had spent the greater part of his career in the study of alcoholic diseases. **Strümpell** in 1883 and **Charcot** in the following year also called attention to the association of mental manifestations and polyneuropathy in alcoholism, while Charles Gayet described the pathology in 1875.

Wernicke[5924] described three cases: the first a seamstress who had developed pyloric stenosis after swallowing sulfuric acid; the other two were alcoholics. He named the disease *acute superior hemorrhagic polioencephalitis*, considering it to be an infectious process. **Meynert's** account of the amnesic syndrome was as accurate as **Korsakoff's** but published a year later, in 1890. Korsakoff considered the pathology to be cortical and probably vascular.[3135, 5758] The role of vitamin deficiency in the causation was only established following the studies of thiamine deficiency in pigeons conducted by Peters in 1936.

Diagnostic criteria have been suggested[868] as follows:
Two of the following features are present:
  Dietary deficiencies
  Oculomotor abnormalities
  Cerebellar dysfunctiomn
  Altered mental state or mild memory impairment
In a *variant* form, the condition is associated with paraneoplastic nutritional deficiency states.

Wernicke-Mann paralysis   A form of hemiparesis with remarkable variability in the severity of involvement of different muscle groups, or the inequality of weakness in different muscle groups in a paretic limb during recovery.

The sign was described by these authors in 1889 and 1896, respectively.[4979] The peronei; knee flexors; extensors of the elbow, wrists, and fingers; and supinators are muscle groups in which functional recovery is least, compared with their antagonists,[574] and leads to the typical posture of the patient with unilateral spastic hemiparesis.

Wernicke's area   The posterior part of the auditory association cortex together with the heteromodal cortex on the banks of the superior temporal sulcus, and part of the inferior parietal lobule. Damage to this region leads to **Wernicke aphasia.**

West Haven–Yale Multidimensional Pain inventory

A series of 12 scales examining the impact of pain on people's lives, the responses of others to their communications about pain, and the extent to which they are able to participate in usual daily activities.[3013]

West Indian (Jamaican) amblyopia   Optic atrophy occurring in subjects with **Jamaican neuropathy.**

West Indian spastic-ataxic syndrome   The insidious onset of deafness, visual scotomas, optic atrophy, ataxia, and spasticity associated with HTLV-1 infection. Some patients have more spasticity, some have more ataxia.[3952] See **tropical spastic paraparesis.**

West Nile encephalitis   Direct infection of brain due to a flavivirus member of the togavirus group of arboviruses, endemic in Israel and Egypt, but also farther east and west, mainly affecting elderly adults.

West syndrome   (infantile spasms, massive infantile spasms, blitz-nick-salaam krämpfe) A degenerative epileptic syndrome of infancy or childhood with onset before the age of 1 year (max. 4–7 months), characterized by brief muscle contractions resembling massive myoclonic attacks, sometimes with tonic or atonic components, and accompanied by a characteristic chaotic EEG appearance of high-voltage bursts of slow waves and spikes pattern known as **hypsarrhythmia.**[5929] Microphthalmia, colobomas of the optic nerve and retina with optic atrophy, pigmentary retinopathy, strabismus, nystagmus, dementia, microcephaly, and callosal abnormalities have also been recorded in affected children. The cause of the condition is not known.

Usually the syndrome consists of a characteristic triad: infantile spasms, arrest of psychomotor development, and hypsarrhythmia, although any one element may be missing. The spasms may be flexor, extensor, lightning, or simple nodding, but most commonly they are mixed. The age of onset peaks between 4 and 7 months and is always before the end of the first year. Boys are more commonly affected. The prognosis is generally poor.

The syndrome may be divided between two groups. The *symptomatic* group, characterized by the previous existence of brain damage signs (psychomotor retardation, neurological signs, radiological signs, or other types of seizures) or by a known etiology (metabolic, dysgenetic, or infectious, or due to perinatally acquired disease or tumors.[2182] A smaller, *cryptogenic* group is characterized by a lack of previous signs of brain damage and of known etiology. The prognosis appears to be partly based on early therapy with adrenocorticotrophic hormone or oral steroids. (Adapted from Commission for Classification and Terminology, ILAE. Proposal for revised classifications of epilepsies and epileptic syndromes. *Epilepsia* 1989;**30**:389–399.[1114])

Variants include the following:

Infantile spasms, hemimegalencephaly, and hemihypsarrhythmia A congenital epileptic syndrome manifesting infantile spasms with hypsarrhythmia, polymicrogyria, megalencephaly, and heterotopias.

Infantile spasms, X-linked (OMIM 308350) An inherited form in which the onset of infantile spasms, myoclonic seizures, and mental and developmental deterioration is in the first few months of life.[1041]

Forms characterized by spasms and mental retardation without hypsarrhythmia but with paroxysmal EEG abnormalities; with spasms and hypsarrhythmia but without mental retardation; with hypsarrhythmia and mental retardation but without spasms; with mental retardation, hypsarrhythmia, and staring seizures (see **Lennox-Gastaut syndrome**) with onset before 3 months of age; and **Aicardi syndrome.** See also **salaam attacks.**

West, W.J.   (1794–) English general practitioner working in Tunbridge Wells, whose son James was affected by repetitive flexion seizures (*salaam attacks* in the words of Sir Charles Clarke, whom he had consulted), pareses, and mental deterioration. He reported the syndrome in a letter to the *Lancet* in 1841.

Western Aphasia battery   A formal, validated scale for assessing language, in particular spontaneous speech, naming, repetition, comprehension of oral language, reading, and writing, but also apraxia and constructional and visuospatial tasks.[3018]

Western equine encephalitis   Direct infection of brain by an α-virus member of the togavirus group, a virus with a reservoir in birds and small rodents. The condition is seen mainly in the central and western United States and in Southern Canada. The major vector is a mosquito; despite the name, horses play no role in transmission.

Clinically, the encephalitis is relatively mild and subclinical infection is common. The usual course in adults is for the mild encephalitis to lead to recovery within 10 days. The illness may be more serious in small children, among whom many exhibit seizures, pyramidal signs, or behavioral problems.[1828]

Westphal, Alexander Karl Otto   (1863–1941) German physician, the son of Karl Westphal. He trained at Berlin and studied with **Erb** and others in psychiatry and neurology, eventually becoming professor of neurology at Bonn. He described pathologic sleep attacks as well as the phenomena now given his name.

Westphal, Karl Friedreich Otto   (1833–1890) German psychiatrist, neurologist, and anatomist who held the chair of psychiatry in Berlin, where his son became professor of neurology. He gave the first account of what is now known as **Wilson disease** (which he called pseudosclerosis) in 1883, and at the same time as **Erb** described muscle stretch reflexes in any detail.

Westphal maneuver   The use of kinesthetic clues to identify large print, by dint of sweeping movements of the eyes or of the head and neck, named for A.K.O. Westphal.

Westphal nucleus   See **Edinger-Westphal nucleus.** Edinger's paper (1885) was 2 years earlier than that of K.F.O. Westphal.

Westphal reflex   See **knee jerk.**

Westphal sign   Abolition of the knee jerks in **tabes dorsalis,** named after K.F.O. Westphal. **Erb** described the same thing independently, but at the same time.

Westphal syndrome   1. Agoraphobia; the dread of open spaces nicely described by Westphal in 1872, but also previously noted by the Dutch physician Pieter Forest (1522–1597) in 1592 and by many others subsequently (Wepfer in 1727, de Sauvages in 1768, Stoll in 1788, Herz in 1791, Bruck in 1832, Reynolds in 1855, Delasiauve in 1854, Perroud in 1863, and Kohler in 1867). This is thus a prime example of an eponymous attribution which is wholly unjustified, although one must credit Westphal with the generation of the term and with an accurate description.

The author defends the inclusion of this condition in a book that claims a neurological leaning on the grounds that patients complaining of dizziness or vertigo commonly present to neurologists and are ultimately found to have agoraphobia.

2. See **familial periodic paralysis.**

Westphal-Leyden syndrome   See **acute cerebellar ataxia,** described by Leyden in 1890,[3391] 13 years after the shorter account of A.K.O. Westphal.

Westphal-Piltz phenomenon   (paradoxical pupil phenomenon) Contraction followed by dilatation of the pupil after forceful eye closure, when the tension of the orbicularis muscle is increased,[5932] named after A.K.O. Westphal.

Westphal-Strümpell pseudosclerosis   See **Wilson disease.** Westphal described most of the neurological features in 1883,[5934] and **Strümpell** the same 15 years later (but still without remarking on the hepatic cirrhosis, which was the particular contribution of S.A.K. **Wilson** in 1912).

wet beriberi   Cardiac failure with edema as a result of thiamine deficiency.

wheelchair palsy   A form of compression neuropathy of the radial nerve at the level of the elbow. See also **posterior interosseous syndrome.**

whiplash amnesia   Transient loss of memory following extension-flexion injury of the cervical spine. The mechanism is unknown.[1854]

whiplash injury   (cervical acceleration injury syndrome) An acceleration/deceleration mechanism of energy transfer to the neck, described by Crowe in 1928 and more fully by Gay and Abbott in 1953. It may result from rear-end or side-impact motor vehicle colli-sions but can also occur during diving or other mishaps. In humans, the injury is usually of the hyperextension-flexion type.[4380] The impact may result in bony or soft tissue injuries (*whiplash injuries*) which in turn may lead to a variety of clinical manifestations (*whiplash-associated disorders*).[5298] The definition should exclude damage to the cervical disks, the nerve roots, or the spinal cord.[865,3531]

The pathology is not known but cervical facet (zygo-apophyseal) joint strain has been incriminated as the source of the pain. The more common symptoms include neck, head, and thoracic pain; dizziness; tinnitus; blurred vision; psychological distress; impaired concentration; and memory disturbances. For unknown reasons, up to 20% of subjects fail to return to normal capacity within a year; this is most likely if there is reduced range of motion of the neck.[622,2946] There is no good evidence that the persistence of symptoms is associated with a search for compensation, nor with psychogenic factors. Patients with whiplash-associated headache are not significantly different from those with other forms of post-traumatic headache or with whiplash-associated neck pain without headache but have higher scores on somatization, obsessive-compulsive, depression, and hostility subscales, and the global severity, implying that patients with whiplash-associated headache suffer psychological distress mainly as a result of chronic pain.

One may speculate that the lack of such symptoms in people who participate in, e.g., demolition derbies or professional sports with extreme body contact may be explained by a state of anticipatory readiness in such situations, such that a protective degree of muscle contraction is in place prior to each "hit," unlike the surprise impacts of motor vehicle collisions in the general public. A biopsychosocial explanation synthesizing physical and societal perceptive causes has been proposed.[1798]

A *variant* of the syndrome is the *whiplash–shaken infant syndrome*, a form of nonaccidental injury to infants presenting with a suspiciously uncertain history from the parents or guardians that is at odds with the physical findings; evidence of epileptic seizures; retinal hemorrhages; CT or MRI scan findings of intradural surface hemorrhages; and new or healing rib or limb bone fractures.[151, 865]

Whipple, Allen Oldfather   (b. 1881) American surgeon who practiced in New York.

Whipple disease   An infective enteropathy caused by a small, rod-shaped organism cross-reacting with streptococci and characterized by the presence of macrophages laden with foamy periodic acid-Schiff (PAS)-positive material in cells of all organs. It was described by George Whipple in 1907.

Typical clinical features include malabsorption, fever, arthralgias, and lymphadenopathy occurring as an indolent disorder of older men. Features reflecting CNS involvement comprise progressive lethargy and hypersomnia, dementia, memory loss, ocular and facial myoclonus, increased intracranial pressure, and supranuclear gaze palsies. Oculomasticatory and oculofacioskeletal myorhythmias are considered to be diagnostic signs.[171] Those with possible CNS Whipple's disease should undergo small bowel biopsy.

Evidence of hypogonadotrophic hypogonadism may be detected. In the CNS, the unculturable PAS-positive, rod-shaped inclusions within macrophages (*tropheryma whippelii*) are found in the temporal lobes; scattered cortical and subcortical lymphocytic infiltrates[2395,5240] and MRI lesions are also described. The condition usually responds to protracted antibiotic treatment.[3479]

Whipple, George Hoyt   (b. 1878) American physician who worked at Johns Hopkins University.

Whipple triad   Confusion, faintness, seizures, or coma in the fasting state; hypoglycemia; and recovery with administration of glucose,[5936] named after A.O. Whipple. But most postprandial symptoms are not due to hypoglycemia.

whispering   The utterance of language without vibration of the vocal cords.

whispering dysphonia   (whispering dystonia) 1. A dominantly inherited syndrome characterized by the onset in childhood or adult life of facial spasms, bulbar palsies, torticollis, and an inability to converse normally in anything above a whisper, although affected subjects can yell under emotional stress. Other dystonic symptoms often eventually supervene.[4336] See **hereditary whispering dysphonia.** 2. That form of dystonia in which the muscles of the larynx are involved, producing adduction of the vocal cords and whispered speech.

whispering dystonia   See **whispering dysphonia.**

whistle-smile sign   (Hanes sign) Failure of the patient to smile when asked by the examiner to whistle; suggested as a sign of **Parkinson disease.**[2412]

whistling-face syndrome   (craniocarpotarsal dysplasia, Freeman-Sheldon syndrome) A dominantly inherited or sporadic congenital dysmorphism, characterized by microstomia, flat mid-face, high palate, talipes equinovarus, and ulnar deviation of the fingers. Strabismus, ptosis, and hypertelorism may also be present.

It was described in 1938 by Freeman and Sheldon,[1942] while the name used here was applied independently by Burian in 1963.

white centered retinal hemorrhages   (Roth spots) Small retinal hemorrhages seen in sepsis such as bacterial endocarditis, and in subarachnoid hemorrhage, leukemia, myeloma, diabetes, and anemia. They were first described by Litten in 1880; the retinal lesions described by Roth are now thought to have been cytoid bodies.[5739]

white cerebellum sign   A CT appearance in children with acute cerebral edema in which there is loss of the normal gray–white matter differentiation, obliteration of cortical sulci, and diffuse low density but sparing of the cerebellum and basal ganglia, which appear relatively hyperdense.

white-matter medullary infarcts   Infarcts in the centrum semi-ovale or the external/extreme capsule due to embolism or small vessel disease. Clinically, hemiparesis of variable severity is the main feature.

white muscles   The light-colored striated muscles, best seen in animals or birds; such muscles are composed mainly of type 2 myofibrils with fast-twitch capacity, and are seen particularly in the phasically contracting limb muscles of humans. Compare with **red muscles.**

white rami   B fibers of the sympathetic efferent system, bearing nicotinic cholinergic synapses at the ganglia.

white-liver disease   See **Reye syndrome.**

Whole Brain Atlas   A Web site providing anatomical images of the central nervous system, at http://www.med.harvard.edu/AANLIB/home.html

Whytt disease   Acute hydrocephalus resulting from tuberculous meningitis.

Whytt reflex   Loss of the pupillary reaction to light due to damage to the superior corpora quadrigemina.[5047]

Robert Whytt

Whytt, Robert   (1714–1766) Scottish physician, who became professor of the Institutes of Medicine at Edinburgh at the age of 33. He was elected a Fellow of the Royal Society and later president of the Royal College of Physicians of Edinburgh.[186]

Whytt demonstrated reflex activity in frogs and in 1751 was the first to describe the pupillary light reflex and its anatomy.[5955] He also wrote a full description of the clinical features of increased intracranial pressure, probably in patients with communicating hydrocephalus resulting from tuberculous meningitis, and described "dropsy of the brain" (cerebral edema), transient monocular blindness and diphtheria.[5956] In 1764 he published the first textbook of neurology since that of Thomas **Willis.**[793,5204]

wicket rhythm   An EEG finding, consisting of a fragment of mu-like rhythm, occurring singly or in trains during wakefulness or sleep and recorded in temporal lobe regions. The phenomenon has no clinical significance.[3075]

wicket spikes   Benign EEG phenomena comprising a brief run of mu-like rhythm, occurring asymmetrically in the temporal regions of adults in alert or drowsy states.[4638] They have no known clinical significance. See **mu rhythm.**

Wide Range Achievement test   A brief test of reading, spelling, and arithmetic, used as an objective assessment of academic progress.[2818]

Widowitz sign   See **Cantelli sign.**

Wieacker syndrome   (contractures, muscle atrophy, and ocular lesions syndrome) A congenital, X-linked recessive dysmorphic syndrome characterized also by abnormal pupils, strabismus, ptosis, dysarthria, clubfoot, muscle contractures, neural or myopathic weakness, scoliosis, and mental and developmental delay.[5959] See **Cogan syndrome** (definition 1).

Wildervanck syndrome   (Franceschetti-Klein-Wildervanck syndrome, cervico-osteofacial syndrome, cervico-oculo-acoustic syndrome) An X-linked dominant disorder seen almost exclusively in females and characterized by deaf-mutism, **Klippel-Feil syndrome, Duane retraction syndrome,** facial dysmorphism, and abnormal tethering of the hair.

Dysraphism, skeletal deformities, deafness, torticollis, spina bifida occulta, and psychomotor delay may also be associated.[5969]

Wilhelmsen-Lynch disease   A dominantly inherited neurologic multisystem disease characterized by dementia, parkinsonism, amyotrophy, and behavioral disinhibition.[3531]

Wilks, Sir Samuel   (1824–1911) English physician to Guy's Hospital. He was a general physician who, like his colleague Richard **Bright,** was unusually interested in neurological problems. He published accounts of alcoholic paraplegia[5974] and of bulbar palsy,[5975] as well as a major summation of neurological knowledge in his collected *Lectures on Diseases of the Nervous System* (London, 1878).

Williams syndrome   (elfin face syndrome, infantile hypercalcemia) A genetic dysmorphic syndrome manifesting short stature, idiopathic hypercalcemia, congenital heart disease such as supravalvular aortic stenosis or coarctation, pulmonary stenosis and peripheral arterial stenoses, craniosynostosis with microcephaly, blue irides with a stellate pattern, strabismus, and a constellation of facial dysmorphisms such as medial eyebrow flare, malar flattening, elongated philtrum, full lips, upturned nasal tip, and low nasal bridge resulting in the "pixie face." Dental anomalies, skeletal contractures and synostoses, and retardation of mental and somatic growth with relative preservation of affective skills are other characteristics.[4051,5981] Neurological features include disproportionate skills in music and language, squint, muscle hypertonia, and hyperreflexia.

The syndrome results from a deletion in band 7q11.23, the gene locus for elastin. It has been suggested that the folklore surrounding pixies, elves, and leprechauns and their musical talents may be based on the features of this syndrome.[3344]

Williams Syndrome Association   A charitable organization in this field. Address: P.O. Box 297, Clawson, MI 48017-0297. Tel: 248-541-3630. E-mail: Tmonkaba@aol.com. Web site: http://www.williams-syndrome.org/.

Willis headache   A vascular headache following a stroke, possibly as a result of increased blood flow through the branches of the external carotid artery when the internal is occluded, or in the vessels at the base of the brain (which do have pain fiber innervation) in the presence of occlusion of one of the arteries contributing to the circle of Willis. It may also occur on the side opposite that of the internal carotid artery occlusion, suggesting increased flow, presumably as a result of increased demand.

Willis, Thomas   (1621–1675) English physician who took up arms in defense of King Charles I before entering upon the study of medicine. He later practiced in Oxford, obtaining the Sedlian Chair of Natural Philosophy at the university in 1660 as a result of family connections and patronage, then even more than now a common method. On moving to London in 1666, he obtained an appointment as physician to the family of the Duke of York (later King James II), in which eminent position he did not long remain on account of the forthrightness of his clinical diagnoses.

He was a founder of the Royal Society. Like **Sylvius,** he ascribed behavioral functions to the cortex rather than to the ventricles of the brain. His name is given to the arterial anastomotic circle at the base of the brain (**circle of Willis**), which he described in precise detail, along with a reclassification of the cranial nerves into nine pairs and a description of the sympathetic chain, in his "*Cerebri Anatome*" (1664), for which Sir Christopher Wren drew many of the plates, and which, with great political acumen, he dedicated to the Archbishop of Canterbury.

Willis described the eleventh cranial nerve, which was known by his name for some years thereafter, and the ciliary ganglion, thalamus, lentiform body, corpus striatum, and intercostal nerves. He also described meningococcal meningitis, **hysteria, general paresis, narcolepsy,** and a body of physiological observations in his *De Anima Brutorum* (*Two Discourses of the Soul of Brutes which is the Vital and Sensitive (soul) of Man*; London, 1672).[5987] Other observations concerned the intercostal and spinal nerves (1684) and the differentiation of diabetes insipidus and diabetes mellitus in 1674. He distinguished between cerebral and meningeal inflammation and gave a good clinical description of **myasthenia gravis** in his book *The London Practice of Physick* (London, 1685)

He described the epidemiology of (probably) meningococcal meningitis; carotid occlusion with headache (**Willis headache**); transient ischemic attacks ("the irradiation of the spirits is wont . . . to be interrupted with little clouds, as it were, scattered here and there"); migraine; vertebral occlusion; epilepsy (due to "an explosion of the animal spirits in the brain"); focal seizures; parkinsonism; palilalia; torsion **dystonia;** referred pain; **internuclear ophthalmoplegia;** post-traumatic dementia; and traumatic quadriplegia.[2565,2755,5989]

Again like Sylvius, he denied that either the *rete mirabile* or the ventricles were the site of production of "animal spirits," although he did consider that these were secreted by the cortex. The word *neurology* was his invention; he derived this from the Greek name for a tendon, sinew, or bowstring and defined it as "the doctrine of the nerves."[2693]

Willis discounted the existence of Galen's channels from intracranial to extracranial and introduced the concept of CSF absorption into the veins as well as through the infundibulum; he suggested active CSF secretion by the choroid, but still accepted drainage through the nose until this was refuted by Richard Lower.[2693,5457]

Thomas Willis

Willvonseder syndrome   (dementia, vertical gaze palsy, copper dysmetabolism syndrome) A dysmorphic syndrome of abnormal copper metabolism presenting in childhood with speech defect, vertical gaze palsy, splenomegaly, platelet abnormalities, dementia, sleep disorders, and cerebellar ataxia.[5992]

Wilson disease   (Westphal-Strümpell syndrome, Hall disease, cerebral pseudosclerosis, hepatolenticular degeneration, progressive lenticular degeneration, Gowers tetanoid chorea) A recessively inherited syndrome linked to markers on chromosome 13 (13q14.21), originally described in 1861 by Friedrich **Frerichs** (1819–1885), by **Westphal** (also in Germany) in 1883, and by von **Strümpell** in 1898, but only widely recognized after the independent report by Wilson in 1912, in which, however, the characteristic corneal changes were not described.[5999]

The essential features are due to the deposition of copper in the basal ganglia, corneas, liver, and kidneys, and comprise **Kayser-Fleischer rings,** evidence of hepatic cirrhosis and its complications, and progressive incoordination of fine movements, such as those required for handwriting and speech. Sunflower cataracts may also be seen. Dystonias, chorea or athetosis, pyramidal and cerebellar signs, parkinsonian features, dysarthria, mental deterioration, psychiatric syndromes, seizures, and flapping tremor of the arms and hands are the other major features. Low serum ceruloplasmin and bound serum copper levels, and high tissue and urine copper levels are diagnostic.[1149,2507] On T2-weighted MRI scans, a bilateral hyperintense stripe is classically seen in each putamen.

The disease has been subdivided into two types. In *pseudosclerosis*, dysarthria and the flapping wing-beating tremor are accompanied by cirrhosis, which is asymptomatic and progresses slowly. In the *juvenile* type, onset is also during childhood or adolescence, but hepatic involvement is obvious and the first neurological sign is usually dystonia, while the flapping tremor is rare.[1395]

Since the disease is eminently treatable if detected early (using agents to chelate and excrete copper), the index of suspicion should be high in young people manifesting any involuntary movement disorder whatsoever.

In an X-linked variety, the clinical findings (dementia, dysarthria, gait disturbance, tremor, vertical gaze paresis, hypersomnia, splenomegaly) are similar, but Kayser-Fleischer rings are absent, ceruloplasmin levels are normal, and the metabolic disorder is copper depletion due to abnormal membrane transport.[2146,5992]

Involuntary movements such as dystonia, myoclonus, athetosis, dysarthria, and rapid orobuccal movements occur in the presence of slightly low urinary and serum copper levels.[5466]

See also **acquired (non-Wilsonian) hepatocerebral degeneration, Menkes syndrome, hepatic encephalopathy.**

Wilson, Samuel Alexander Kinnier (1874–1937) Irish-American neurologist, born in the United States, who trained at Edinburgh and in Europe with Pierre **Marie** and others before going to the **National Hospital** in 1904. He practiced there for the rest of his life, the first "pure" neurologist in the United Kingdom, holding successively more senior appointments despite unfriendly relationships with most of his contemporaries. He was also variously on the staff of the Westminster and King's College Hospitals and was editor of the *British Journal of Neurology* before founding the *Journal of Neurology* (*Neurosurgery*) *and Psychiatry,* the first issue of which appeared just after his death.

His fame was early achieved by his description in 1912 of the disease bearing his name, but rests also upon his superbly lucid textbook *Neurology* (edited by A.N. Bruce), published in 1940, which is filled with historical fact and a distillate of his clinical wisdom, and upon his other studies on the basal ganglia, the extrapyramidal system (so named by him), apraxia,[5998] and aphasia.

Wilson sign   See **pronator sign.**

Wilson's Disease Association   A charitable organization providing support and information on this condition. Address: P.O. Box 75324, Washington, DC 20013. Tel: 203-775-9666. Web site: http://www.wilsonsdisease.org/.

Wilson-Vogt syndrome   See **Vogt syndrome.**

windmill nystagmus   (alternating windmill nystagmus) A form of **periodic alternating nystagmus** seen in some patients with severe or total visual loss, and characterized by vertical and horizontal oscillations that are out of phase in the two eyes.[4902]

wing-beating tremor   A proximal, wide-amplitude, regular tremor of the upper limbs due to lesions of the dentatorubral pathway; it is best elicited with the shoulders abducted and the elbows flexed, at which the elbows move up and down.

Winiwater-Buerger disease   (Buerger disease) Thromboangiitis obliterans of the cerebral as well as of the peripheral vessels. An entity of doubtful validity. Most cases are actually due to either atherosclerosis or other forms of angiitis.

wink reflex   See **orbicularis oculi reflex.**

winking jaw   See **Wartenberg winking-jaw phenomenon.**

Winkleman disease   (Winkleman-Dercum disease) See **progressive pallidal atrophy, Hallervorden-Spatz disease.**

Winkleman sign   Described as a mild, permanent hyperextension of the great toe on the side affected by pyramidal tract disease, but more commonly evidence of disease of the basal ganglia.

Winkleman-Dercum disease   See **Winkleman disease.**

wire electrodes   Thin wires that are insulated except for the tips, which are bare, and which are inserted into a muscle through a needle for kinesiologic EMG studies, in which they are superior to surface electrodes because they are less affected by **cross talk** from adjacent muscles.

WISC-R   Acronym for the Wechsler Intelligence Scale for Children–Revised, a compound instrument for the assessment of intelligence with 12 verbal or performance subtests adapted from the **WAIS** for use in children over the age of 7 years. Verbal subtests examine information, similarities, arithmetic, vocabulary, comprehension, and digit span; performance tests are of picture arrangement and completion, block design, object assembly, coding, and maze drawing.[5888]

Below this age, the Revised Wechsler Preschool and Primary Scale of Intelligence (**WPPSI-R**), which has a parallel structure, can be employed.[5890]

Wisconsin Card Sorting test   A test of ability to respond selectively to different aspects of a situation. In this case, the color, form, and number of designs printed on cards shown to the subject have to be matched by the subject, using response cards, on which are printed the same symbols in various colors and numbers. The subject is told when he or she makes a correct match and when he or she is wrong, and is expected to learn from these clues which cards to use to make the match in future; only the rules are changed after 10 successful matches, so that, successively, form, then color and then number are the criteria for matching successfully.[2259]

The test is sensitive in detecting lesions of the dorsolateral regions of the frontal lobes.[2258]

Wishart, John (1782–1834) Scottish surgeon who graduated in medicine at Edinburgh where he returned to practice after study in Europe, working with **Argyll Robertson.** He was at some time president of the Royal College of Surgeons at Edinburgh. His contributions were mainly in the areas of ophthalmia neonatorum, ophthalmic surgery, and methods of pupillary dilation.

Wishart syndrome   Multiple meningiomas or neurilemmomas of the eighth cranial nerves or of the spinal roots, or a glioma associated with neurofibromatosis. See **neurofibromatosis.**

withdrawal emergent dyskinesias   A transient syndrome seen usually in children, characterized by the occurrence of chorea and ataxia with autonomic hyperreactivity when neuroleptic agents are suddenly withdrawn.[2027]

withdrawal reflex   A painful stimulus to the sole of the foot will cause withdrawal of the stimulated limb and sometimes also of the unstimulated limb.[6064]

Wittmarck-Ekbom syndrome   See **restless legs syndrome.**

witzelsucht   A German term for a state of unwonted and unwarranted cheerfulness, characterized by mild euphoria, jocularity, and an abnormal tendency to make rhyming or punning word associations. Frontal lobe disease (cortical atrophy, tumor) is usually responsible.

wobbler mouse   A murine mutation, with some features resembling those of **amyotrophic lateral sclerosis.**

Wohlfarht-Kugelberg-Welander disease   See **hereditary motor neuropathy, type 3.**

Wohwill-Andrade syndrome   See **Andrade neuropathy.**

Wolff, Harold G.   (1898–1963) American neurologist, born in New York and educated at Harvard, who worked mainly at Bellvue and became Anne Parrish Titzel Professor of Neurology at Cornell and director of the neurological service at the New York Hospital.

His best-remembered studies were those dealing with aspects of headache, psychosomatic diseases, and pain, and for his studies with Stewart Wolf on Alexis St. Martin, whose stomach wall had been eventrated since a childhood accident; the secretions of the stomach and its vascularity were observed during the daily activities of St. Martin and the influences upon them were reported in a series of classic studies. Wolff was editor of the *Archives of Neurology* from its inception to his death and an important figure in American neurological research and administration.

Wolfflin nodules   Small regular and uniform spots found in the periphery of the iris in 10%–25% of normal subjects, and, apart from their similarity with **Brushfield spots,** of no clinical significance.[5984]

Wolf-Hirschorn syndrome   (deletion at 4p.16.3, midline fusion defect syndrome) A chromosomal dysmorphic syndrome characterized by low birth weight, failure to thrive, asymmetrical microcephaly, micrognathia, abnormal ear structure, hypertelorism, and midline fusion defects such as cleft palate and defects in the scalp.[5968]

Myoclonic and other seizures, strabismus, hypotonia, and insensitivity to pain are also reported.

Wolfing reflex   (atz, mastication reflex: OMIM 194190) Sucking, chewing, and swallowing movements, representing an exaggerated **sucking reflex;** seen in subjects with severe diffuse cortical disease or with bilateral corticobulbar lesions.

Wolfram syndrome   (DIDMOAD) A rare, recessively inherited syndrome presenting in youth with widespread cerebral atrophy, characterized by the presence of four cardinal signs: **D**iabetes **I**nsipidus, **D**iabetes **M**ellitus, **O**ptic **A**trophy and nerve **D**eafness. Numerous other neurological, endocrine, and urinary tract abnormalities are also found, but variably.[4586,6024]

Wolman disease   A lysosomal storage disease (an inborn error of metabolism) due to absence of acid lipase, presenting in infancy and characterized by hepatosplenomegaly, steatorrhea, anemia, and adrenal calcifications. There is a heavy deposition of cholesterol esters and triglycerides in many tissues.[6025]

Woltman sign   Slowness of both the contraction and the relaxation of muscles in hypothyroid patients, best seen as the "hung-up" ankle jerk and occurring because of mechanical factors and slowness of contraction time, as in myotonia and pseudomyotonia.

Dr. H.W. Woltman (1889–1964) was an American physician.

Woodcock-Johnson Scales of Independent Behavior   A set of scales used in assessing children's abilities, based on data acquired by interviewing the parents and by assessing motor and communication skills, social interaction, and personal and community independence.[3]

Woodhouse syndrome   (hypogonadism, alopecia, diabetes, and deafness) A congenital dysmorphic syndrome characterized by alopecia, endocrinopathy, sensorineural deafness, hypogonadotropic hypogonadism, and mental and developmental delay.[337]

Woods-Pendleton syndrome   A familial condition manifesting dystonia, dysequilibrium, and speech disturbance observed during a famine in China but not reported in the Western hemisphere since (Osler, quoted by Durham[1563]).

woodtrimmer's disease   A syndrome of transient tremor resulting from overexposure to the mycotoxins contained in sawdust. See **tremorgenic encephalopathy.**

Woon syndrome   A congenital dysmorphic syndrome characterized also by spinal, skeletal, and gastrointestinal malformations, brachycephaly, and craniosynostosis. See **craniosynostosis.**

word blindness   1. (developmental dyslexia) The term suggested by Rudolph Berlin (1833–1897), a German ophthalmologist, for the difficulties experienced by children in mastering the comprehension and production of written words. The degree of dyslexia is variable; it has been estimated that 10% of all children have some degree of congenital language difficulty. Errors in reading, spelling, and writing occur in the presence of normal recognition of letters and understanding of the meaning of pictures, objects, and diagrams. The condition is somewhat susceptible to steady and prolonged educational effort. See **alexia.**

2. **Aphasia** (here, an inability to understand the language value of written symbols), as suggested by Adolf Kussmaul (1822–1902), a German physician, in 1877.

word deafness (developmental receptive aphasia, verbal auditory agnosia, auditory imperception, central deafness) The inability to understand the accepted content and symbolic meaning of words heard; difficulty in the comprehension and discrimination of spoken language, while spontaneous speech, reading, writing, and comprehension of nonlanguage sounds are relatively intact.

Repetition is also affected, but reading, writing, and spontaneous speech are not. *Pure word deafness* is described, but appears to be a vanishing rarity. The condition was first described by **Bastian** in 1869 and attributed to disturbance of the auditory perceptive center in the first temporal convolution; Lichtheim applied the name in 1885. The condition is somewhat susceptible to steady and prolonged educational effort.[828]

Word List Generation test A test of word fluency, perseveration, and concentration (and indirectly of intelligence), in which subjects generate as many words within a category as they can think of (e.g., words beginning with *D*, items to be found in a supermarket, or names of animals or of plants) within a defined period of time, usually 1 minute.[5300]

word list recall A standard, sensitive method of testing recent memory (new learning), as in the assessment of mild-to-moderate age-related cognitive dysfunction. Usually up to 10 three-letter words (which may be nonsense words) are presented, and the number recalled after a delay, with or without distraction during this time, represents the subject's score.

word production anomia Difficulty in word-finding, which, however, is assisted by phonetic or semantic cues, and seen in aphasics with dominant frontal lobe lesions.[464] See also **anomia.**

word rests See **stereotypy.**

word-form dyslexia An acquired form of dyslexia characterized by letter-by-letter reading, whole-word reading being impossible. Reading is this exceptionally slow. It is considered to be due to a lesion of the system whereby a visual word-form is obtained.[5090]

word-selection anomia See **anomia.**

work shift change The occurrence of excessive sleepiness and impaired work performance during a subject's conventional sleep–wake schedule, when daytime activities are rescheduled to that period, as occasioned by shift work, and of insomnia with shortened and fragmented sleep during the new sleep period. (See also ASDA Diagnostic Classification,[234] **sleep disorders.**)

working memory The process whereby information is temporarily stored, and manipulated. This requires a number of interrelated systems including a central executive system controlling an articulatory loop (which is concerned with the storage of speech) and a third system that maintains and manipulates visuospatial material.[1475]

The *structural capacity* of working memory refers to the number of distinct informational unts that can be remembered at one time; while the *operational capacity* is the number of processing operations that can be performed while still preserving the products of earlier operations.[4890]

See also **short-term memory.**

World Federation of Neurology An international organization for the advancement of research and education in neurology. Address: 12 Chandos Street, London W1G 9DR, UK. Tel: +44 20 7323 4011. Web site: http://www.elsevier.com/homepage/sah/wfnnew/default.htm.

World Federation of Neurology Research Committee on Parkinsonism and Related Disorders An international research committee of 37 members established by the **World Federation of Neurology** to promote and monitor research developments, and to foster communication among neuroscientists in this field. It sponsors occasional symposia on Parkinson disease. Web site: http://www.elsevier.com/inca/publications/store/3/0/5/4/1/.

World Federation of Neurosurgical Societies An organization including all national neurosurgical societies, based at: Academic Hospital, Radboud, PO Box 9101, NL-6500 HB Nijmegen, The Netherlands. Web site: http://www.wfns.org/.

World Health Organization Handicap Scale Six scales, based on six "survival roles," each intended to classify the circumstances in which individuals find themselves as a result of disease. Each scale has nine levels, 0 reflecting the best and 8 the worst functional state. Detailed descriptions are given in an accompanying manual. The concept of Handicap refers to discordance between the individual's performance or status and the expectations of the individual or of the particular group of which he or she is a member.

The scales deal with *orientation, physical independence, mobility, occupation, social integration,* and *economic self-sufficiency,* using semantic gradations.[6040]

The Organization's web site is at http://www.who.int/.

World of Multiple Sclerosis A Web site maintained by the Multiple Sclerosis International Federation, providing information and advice particularly to people with multiple sclerosis, at http://www.ifmss.org.uk/.

World Muscle Society An international, multidisciplinary, scientific society, dedicated to the advancement and dissemination of knowledge in the field of neuromuscular disorders. Web site: http://www.ior.it/wms/.

Worldwide Education & Awareness for Movement Disorders (WE MOVE) A charitable organization in this field. Address: 204 West 84th St., New York,

NY 10024. Tel: 800-437-6682. Web site: http://www.wemove.org/.

Worm disease Bulbar **tetanus.** See also **cephalic tetanus.**

Worm, Ole (1588–1654) Danish anatomist.

Wormian bones Small areas of bone lying in the cranial sutures like islands in a river, described by Ole **Worm** and named for him by Thomas Bartholin, his nephew, in 1656.[4979]

Worster-Drought syndrome 1. (congenital suprabulbar palsy) A dominantly inherited congenital syndrome of weakness of the face, soft palate, and tongue, sometimes complicated by seizures and mental retardation.[335] See **congenital suprabulbar paresis.** 2. (familial spastic paraparesis and dementia) A dominantly inherited spastic syndrome with onset in mature adult life, characterized by slowly progressive dysarthria, spastic paraparesis, and dementia with widespread ischemic damage to the deep white matter and corpus callosum.[6043] See also **familial multi-infarct dementia, multi-infarct dementia.**

Worster-Drought-Allen syndrome (congenital auditory imperception, idiotic aphasia, atavistic speech, congenital pure word deafness) A congenital syndrome in which the child who has normal hearing is unable to comprehend spoken language but can lip read and can repeat sounds and words that he or she hears, but not a long series of them. Speech is absent or very defective and the comprehension of written language at least slightly impaired. Inability to appreciate musical sounds may also be found.[6042]

WPPSI-R Acronym for the **W**echsler **P**reschool and **P**rimary **S**cale of **I**ntelligence (**R**evised), an instrument adapted from the **WISC-R** for use in children between 3 and 7 years of age. Subtests include information, arithmetic, vocabulary, similarities, geometric design, design recognition, animal pegs, and sentences.[5890]

Wren, Sir Christopher (1632–1723) English scientist, anatomist, artist, and architect. He was the illustrator for **Willis'** book *Cerebri Anatome.*

Wright maneuver Hyperabduction and elevation of the arms as a test for the vascular form of the **thoracic outlet syndrome.** Obliteration of the radial pulse is the end point sought but as this may also occur in normal subjects, the two sides have to be compared. See also **Adson test.**

wrinkly skin syndrome A recessively inherited congenital disorder of connective tissue, characterized by short stature, skeletal malformations, premature aging, wrinkled skin, optic atrophy, pigmentary retinopathy, myopia, microcephaly, and mental and developmental delay.[2065]

Wrisberg, Heinrich (1739–1808) Professor of anatomy at Göttingen, where he was **Soemerring's** assistant. The nerve of Wrisberg is the nervus intermedius, the sensory component of the seventh nerve. Wrisberg was also the first to identify the medial cutaneous nerve of the arm and he gave a good account of the phrenic, vagus, and trigeminal nerves.

wrist drop A persistent posture of flexion of the wrist due to loss of power in the radial-innervated long extensor muscles of the forearm. The lesion is high in the upper arm or in the brachial plexus, as the branch of the nerve to the extensor carpi radialis longus comes off above the elbow.

wrist extension reflex Contraction of the extensor muscles of the arm when they are tapped, with the arm supported and the arm hanging flexed; this represents a normal phenomenon when just visible and a sign of pyramidal tract disease when increased in amplitude.

wrist flexion reflex Contraction of the long flexor muscles of the arm when they are tapped at the volar aspect of the wrist, with the arm supported in supination; this represents a normal phenomenon when just visible and a sign of pyramidal tract disease when increased in amplitude.

wrist sign See **Chaddock reflex.**

writers' cramp (scrivener's palsy, *la crampe des écrivains*, graphospasm, mogographia) A focal (occupational) dystonia usually manifest in adults who earn their living by writing, typing, or otherwise communicating language mechanically, preventing the further performance of writing tasks because of clumsiness, cramp, aching, tremor, "freezing," or involuntary movement of the hand.[2904,4576]

It was first described in detail by **Bell** in 1830, and although in fact a focal dystonia, it was long considered to be psychogenic in origin. It differs only in form and site from other occupational cramps, which have been listed as affecting people in at least 55 different activities.

In the *simple* form of writer's cramp, only writing is affected. In the *dystonic* form, the disorder spills over into other activities. Psychiatric morbidity is not increased among such patients.[5110] A (complex) rating scale to assess the benefit of local botulinus toxin injection into the forearm muscle has been published.[6013]

A *variant* is a familial form with onset in adult life.[337] See also **myoclonic writers' cramp.**

writing tremor A variant of **essential tremor** characterized by the adult onset of tremor at 5–6 Hz while writing, and occasionally complicated by other dystonias or by myoclonic seizures. See **primary writing tremor.**

wrong-way deviation 1. Deviation of the eyes *away from* the side of the lesion and *toward* the paretic side in patients with medial thalamic hemorrhage who have blood in the third ventricle.[1847] The usual, though not invariable, finding with supratentorial lesions is that the eyes deviate toward the side of the cerebral lesion and away from the paretic limbs. 2. Acute hemiparesis should be accompanied by deviation of the protruded tongue to the paretic side; a minority of patients with hysterical hemiparesis protrude their tongue toward the normal side. Such wrong-way deviation, however, also occurs in **Jackson syndrome,** in which a low medullary lesion damages the twelfth cranial nerve nucleus and the pyramidal tract which has not yet crossed.[2980]

wry head   See **plagiocephaly.**

wry neck   See **torticollis.**

Wyatt syndrome   See **Sturge-Weber syndrome.**

Wyatt-Brushfield disease   See **Sturge-Weber syndrome.**

Wyburn-Mason syndrome   (Bonnet-Déchaum-Blanc syndrome, retinocephalic angiomatosis, cerebroretinal arteriovenous aneurysms, multiple cerebroretinal arteriovenous malformations) Tortuosity of the retinal vessels unilaterally, with cirsoid aneurysms or huge overgrowths of the vessels; arteriovenous angiomas of the optic nerve, thalamus, and mesencephalon; and often trigeminal vascular nevi.

Clinically, the main presenting features are headache, facial palsy and hydrocephalus with oculomotor paresis, visual field deficits, and hemangiomas of the optic disk, due to brainstem and subarachnoid hemorrhages.[656,6054] See **Bonnet syndrome.**

Wynter, Walter Essex   (1860–1945) A physician at the Middlesex Hospital, London, and sometime editor of the *British Medical Journal.* While on the junior staff of the Middlesex Hospital he made the first attempt at lumbar puncture (reported by him in the *Lancet* on May 2, 1891). Each of his four patients had meningitis, and each died.

xanthinuric myopathy A syndrome due to xanthine oxidase deficiency, characterized by proximal weakness, wasting, and muscle discomfort, with electrical and biopsy evidence of myopathy. Electron microscopy study reveals intracellular aggregates of crystalline material within muscle fibers.[958]

xanthochromia (from Gr, yellow + color) (of CSF) A yellow discoloration of the CSF, usually due to the presence of protein which has had time to absorb bilirubin from blood spilled into this foreign compartment. The protein level is commonly more than 300 mg/dl. When the protein level is very high but the cell count is low **albumino-cytological dissociation,** spinal block, **acute inflammatory demyelinating polyneuropathy,** and eighth nerve schwannomas are the most common causes.

xanthoma 1. (fibroxanthoma, fibrohistiocytoma) A benign tumor of histiocytes containing uni- or multinucleated cells and giant cells and usually attached to the dura mater. 2. (xanthosarcoma, malignant fibrous histiocytoma) A rare malignant form of fibroxanthoma.

xanthomatosis 1. See **cerebrotendinous xanthomatosis.** 2. See **Hand-Schüller-Christian disease** (generalized xanthomatosis).

xanthomatous neuropathy A rare complication of biliary cirrhosis in which cholesterol esters are deposited within the peripheral nerves.[3508]

xanthopsia A condition in which all visual perceptions have a yellow tinge, as occurs in chronic digitalis, sulfonamide, and other drug poisoning, as well as in jaundice and in eclampsia.

xanthurenic aciduria A hereditary disorder due to deficiency of the enzyme kyureninase, manifesting mental retardation, which is responsive to treatment with pyridoxine.

X-disease See **Murray valley encephalitis.**

xenografts Grafts taken from one species and placed in another. Human-to-mouse is the most common example.

xeroderma pigmentosum (Gr, dry + skin pigment) (xerodermic idiocy) A rare, recessively inherited heterogeneous **neurocutaneous syndrome** due to failure of DNA repair and manifested by extreme cutaneous sensitivity to ultraviolet light, with telangiectasias, pigment changes, keratoses, and skin malignancies of all types.

The condition was first described by Hebra and Kaposi in 1872. De Sanctis and Cacchione noted its association with mental retardation, microcephaly, hypogonadism, and dwarfism 60 years later.[1417] See **de Sanctis-Cacchione syndrome.**

Since then, seizures, cerebellar ataxia, choreoathetosis, dysarthria, deafness, spasticity, peripheral neuropathy, glycogen storage myopathy, dementia, areflexia, abnormal EEG, and neuropathic EMG and muscle biopsy findings have been added as components of the syndrome.[3898, 5572]

xeroderma with talipes equinovarus and enamel defects A congenital dysmorphic syndrome, a *variant* of xeroderma pigmentosum, manifesting also skeletal malformations, abnormalities of the hair, teeth, nails, and skin, and psychomotor retardation.[337]

xerodermic idiocy See **xeroderma pigmentosum.**

xerophthalmia An ocular disorder due to deficiency of vitamin A, and characterized by keratomalacia, night blindness, and Bitot spots.

xerostomia Dryness of the mouth.

XK-aproscencephaly A congenital dysmorphic syndrome characterized by cyclopia, cardiac and genital maldevelopment, microcephaly, and aproscencephaly or arhinencephaly.[337]

X-linked adrenoleukodystrophy See **adrenoleukodystrophy.**

X-linked bulbospinal neuronopathy (Kennedy syndrome, familial progressive bulbospinal muscular atrophy) A slowly progressive hereditary motor neuropathy with onset in young adult life, characterized by androgen insensitivity (gynecomastia, oligozoospermia, raised serum gonadotrophins), pelvic girdle and proximal limb weakness with postural tremor, prominent lingual and perioral fasciculations, hyporeflexia, and muscle cramps. Masseteric and facial weakness, dysphagia, and dysarthria appear later. EMG, sensory conduction, and biopsy studies show typical changes resulting from degeneration of the anterior horn cells and dorsal root ganglia.[1796,2448,3006]

Variants include the following:
A form in which hexosaminidase A and B deficiencies have been demonstrated, as in **Sandhoff disease.**[4233,5554]
A form resembling **hereditary spastic paraparesis**[3627]
X-linked spinal muscular atrophy with bulbar involvement A syndrome of proximal limb, facial, and bulbar weakness and wasting with adult onset, associated with gynecomastia and raised CSF protein levels, differing from *Kennedy syndrome* mainly in its later age of onset.[4705]

X-linked cerebellar ataxia An X-linked ataxic syndrome with onset in infancy. Pyramidal signs appear later and myoclonic seizures, ophthalmoplegia, sensorimotor peripheral neuropathy, lordosis, scoliosis, and pes cavus have been reported in association.[5290] See also **X-linked periodic ataxia, cerebellar ataxias.**

X-linked congenital muscle fiber hypotrophy with central nuclei.[245] See **centronuclear myopathies.**

X-linked congenital neural deafness An X-linked disease manifesting congenital severe neural hearing loss but normal vestibular function.[1405]

X-linked dominant myopathy A proximal myopathic syndrome seen only in females, since it is lethal in hemizygous boys.[2546]

X-linked early-onset neural deafness A sex-linked recessive syndrome of severe neural hearing loss with early onset.[3933]

X-linked external ophthalmoplegia and myopia A rare syndrome in males characterized by bilateral ptosis, weakness of the external ocular muscles, high myopia, ectopic pupils, hyporeflexia, and scoliosis.[4887] See also **familial static ophthalmoplegia.**

X-linked humeroperoneal muscular disease An inclusive term describing mild and slowly progressive muscular disorders so inherited, with onset in the first decade.

The clinical features include mainly distal neurogenic and proximal myopathic EMG findings and cardiomyopathy.[5871] See **Emery-Driefuss syndrome.**

X-linked hydrocephalus Familial **aqueductal stenosis** causing obstructive hydrocephalus, so inherited.[551]

X-linked leukodystrophies A large and ill-defined group of **peroxisomal diseases** in which cholesterol esters are deposited. These stain red with fat stains engendering the alternative term *sudanophilic leukodystrophy.* See **adrenoleukodystrophy, Pelizaeus-Merzbacher disease.**

X-linked lissencephaly and subcortical band heterotopias A genetically determined or sporadic condition presenting with mental retardation and epilepsy, mainly in females, and mapped to Xq22.3. See **also heterotopias, bilateral periventricular nodular heterotopia.**[1481]

X-linked mental retardation A nonspecific, non-syndromic condition of intellectual impairment associated with congenital micropcephaly and due to a mutation in the protein kinase gene.[565]

X-linked mental retardation with fragile site See **fragile-X syndrome.**

X-linked microcephaly A congenital dysmorphic syndrome manifesting also microcephaly, sensorineural deafness, psychomotor retardation, seizures, and spasticity.[337]

Obesity is present in a *variant* form.

X-linked moderate hearing loss A sex-linked disease manifesting the childhood onset of a slowly progressive, moderate neural hearing loss, but normal vestibular responses.[3441]

X-linked muscular dystrophy (Mabry muscular dystrophy) A pseudohypertrophic muscular dystrophy manifesting features similar to those of **Becker muscular dystrophy,** but with a later onset and slower course.[3537]

X-linked muscular dystrophy with humeropelvic distribution, contractures, and cardiomyopathy See **Emery-Dreifuss syndrome.**

X-linked myoclonic epilepsy with generalized spasticity and intellectual disability (XMESID) A rare X-linked recessive form of myoclonic epilepsy, presenting with spasticity and intellectual disability, while carrier women are hyperreflexic. It is associated with a missense mutation in *ARX* and is allelic with X-linked infantile spasms (ISSX; MIM 308350) in which polyalanine tract expansions represent the molecular defect. Mutations of *ARX* are associated with a wide range of phenotypes.

X-linked myopathies A group of muscle diseases sharing this pattern of inheritance. Such conditions include **Duchenne muscular dystrophy, Becker muscle dystrophy**[418] and related forms[3537]; **Emery-Driefuss syndrome,**[1650] **X-linked humeroperoneal muscular disease, X-linked dominant myopathy, dystrophin partial deficiency, Barth syndrome, X-linked myopathy with excessive autophagy,** and **McLeod syndrome,**[5444] as well as other X-linked disorders separately listed under this letter.

X-linked myopathy with excessive autophagy A congenital benign, slowly progressive, X-linked recessive proximal myopathy with onset in childhood or youth mapped to Xq28 with mild and slowly progressive limb-girdle weakness, slight increase in serum CK levels, and myopathic EMG. There is neither cardiac nor intellectual involvement. EMG and biopsy evidence suggestrs a vacuolar myopathy.[2908] For further data, access   http://www.neuro.wustl.edu/neuromuscular/maltbrain.html.

X-linked periodic ataxia A form of pyruvate dehydrogenase deficiency characterized by symptoms and pathology resembling those of **Leigh disease,** with intermittent episodes of ataxia and dysarthria lasting days, with onset in childhood and abating during adolescence.[3444]

X-linked pigmentary abnormalities and congenital deafness A congenital, X-linked recessive disease characterized by severe neural deafness, large irregular spots of hypo- and hyperpigmentation, and impaired vestibular function.[3124]

X-linked recessive congenital muscle fiber hypotrophy with central nuclei A fatal congenital myopathy with the features suggested by the title.[245] In a *variant* form, there is an added axonal neuropathy without segmental demyelination.[1336]

X-linked recessive myotubular myopathy (XLMTM; OMIM 310400) A rare congenital muscle disorder resulting from mutations in the *MTMl* gene located at Xq28, and characterized by severe hypotonia and generalized muscle weakness at birth in affected males, most of whom die within the first year of life from respiratory failure.[5741]

The characteristic muscle histopathology consists of small, rounded muscle cells with centrally located nuclei resembling fetal myotubes, suggesting that the disorder results from a defect in the structural organization or in the normal development of the muscle fibers. Autosomal centronuclear myopathies (CNM) are disorders with similar histopathological findings, but the age of onset is later with a progressive clinical course. For further data, access http://www.neuro.wustl.edu/neuromuscular/maltbrain.html.

X-linked recessive ophthalmoplegia and myopia
Complete or partial ophthalmoplegia with ptosis, abnormal pupillary shape, myopia, choroidoretinal degeneration, and sometime hyporeflexia.[4887]

X-linked scapuloperoneal muscular dystrophy
One of a heterogeneous group of diseases manifesting weakness and wasting of the proximal arm and distal leg muscles which may have a myopathic or a neurogenic etiology; in this case, an X-linked, childhood-onset muscular dystrophy manifesting joint contractures and pes cavus as well as the muscular involvement but without pseudohypertrophy.

Type 2 fiber group atrophy is detectable on muscle biopsy specimens.[5206] Progression is slow, but a lethal cardiomyopathy may develop in adult life.[497] The con-

dition is linked to deutan color blindness.[5544] See also **Emery-Driefuss syndrome;** the differences between these disorders are minimal.

X-linked sideroblastic anemia with ataxia   A very rare syndrome characterized by motor delay, ataxia with onset in early childhood, and dysarthria; these are almost nonprogressive until later adult life. The hematological features are ineffective erythropoiesis with marked iron loading of the red cell precursors.[2524]

X-linked spastic paraplegia   A congenital syndrome manifesting optic atrophy, strabismus, dysarthria, joint contractures, pyramidal signs, and psychomotor retardation. The responsible gene maps to Xq12–q22. See also **hereditary spastic paraparesis, hereditary motor neuropathy.**

X-linked spinal and bulbar muscular atrophy   See **X-linked bulbospinal neuronopathy.**

X-linked spinal muscular atrophy   See **X-linked bulbospinal neuronopathy.**

X-linked spinal muscular atrophy with bulbar involvement   See **X-Linked bulbospinal neuronopathy.**

X-linked spinobulbar muscular atrophy   See **X-linked bulbospinal neuronopathy.**

X-linked torsion dystonia   An X-linked dystonic syndrome of childhood or early adult onset, manifesting also sensorineural deafness and psychomotor retardation. See **dystonia.**

Xp21 myopathy   See **McLeod syndrome.**

Y

Yakolev, Paul Ivan (1894–1983) Russian-born neurologist and neuropathologist who trained at St. Petersburg, where at first he considered psychiatry as a career, but was dissuaded after listening to Pavlov's lectures. After graduating with high honors, he escaped from revolutionary Russia to Finland in 1919. After some time in England, he was later able to study in Paris with **Marie** and **Babinski**. After obtaining his MD degree in Paris, he went to America and was appointed to positions in neurology and neuropathology at the Boston City Hospital under Stanley **Cobb** and later at the Harvard Medical School.

He improved upon the methods then available for sectioning brains and published widely on cerebral malformations, mainly in the context of epilepsy. He eventually became clinical professor of neuropathology; his large collection of neuropathological specimens is now located at the Armed Forces Institute of Pathology, as it is regarded as a national resource.

Yakolev's most important publications were on the functional anatomy of the limbic system and of thalamocortical relationships, and on neuroanatomy.[3002]

Yale Children's inventory A child-rating instrument responsive to *DSM-III* terminology used to assess pediatric neurobehavioral disorders. The inventory rates attention, habituation, activity, impulsivity, tractability, academic performance, and fine motor skills.[5107]

yawning (chasma, oscedo) (Gr, open mouth, Lat, yawning) "A slow inspiration and depression of the lower jaw, followed by brief tonic spasm of the muscles of inspiration, of the depressors and elevators of the lower jaw, of some of the facial muscles and of the muscles of the neck so that the head is drawn backward" (Sir William **Gowers**). It can often be inhibited and frequently is associated with stretching.

Its occurrence is thought to be associated with an integrated discharge in a bulbospinal motor complex, which appears at a certain (depressed) level of excitability of the reticular activating system,[344] but the teleological benefit of this primitive movement pattern, a commonplace phenomenon halfway between a reflex and an expressive movement, is obscure.

Year Book Of Neurology and Neurosurgery An annual review book published by Elsevier. Web site: http://www.us.elsevierhealth.com/fcgi-bin/display page.pl?isbn= 05135117/.

yellow-blue color blindness (tritanopia) A dominantly inherited syndrome of confusion between blue-green and yellow-pink shades, considered due to a deficiency in the blue pigment in the retinal cones.[6049]

Yim syndrome A congenital dysmorphic syndrome, manifesting also severe skeletal and ocular maldevelopments, macrocephaly, cerebral atrophy, and hydrocephalus.[337]

yips Involuntary movements occurring during the execution of skilled, focused, finely controlled motor behavior, as in the game of golf. The movements emerge particularly during putting; golfers have used such descriptive terms for them as *yips, twitch, staggers, waggles, jitters, jerks* or "*them,*" suggesting that muscle spasms, myoclonus, cramps, or tremor may variously be responsible.[3740]

Such eminent golfers as Sam Snead and Ben Hogan are reported to have been afflicted. The movements probably represent a form of focal dystonia resembling those of other sporting activities such as **bowlers' cramp.**

yoga footdrop A common peroneal palsy resulting from remaining in the customary cross-legged position for a prolonged period. See also **lotus footdrop.**

Yolken syndrome A congenital dysmorphic syndrome, manifesting also genital and skeletal maldevelopments, deafness, blindness, and microcephaly.[337]

Yom Kippur headache A generalized non-throbbing headache experienced in the middle of the day and associated with fasting. It is thought to reflect the effects of dehydration and is relieved by lying down.[4008]

Yoshimura reflex Yet another way of eliciting the plantar response, this time by stimulating the middle of the sole. Bekhterev, Guillain, Sicard, and others have also found that a noxious stimulus here is an effective way of eliciting the response.

For neurologists who aspire to immortality, the bad news is that there is scarcely a square inch of the foot left for *de novo* stimulation, interpretation, and publication.

Young syndrome A dominantly inherited distal form of **hereditary motor neuropathy** with onset in adolescence, affecting the arms before the legs and associated with laryngeal paresis.[6092] 2. (macrocephaly and callosal agenesis) A congenital dysmorphic syndrome manifesting also intestinal and cerebellar abnormalities, hydrocephalus, and mental and developmental delay.[337]

young-onset Parkinson disease Arbitrarily defined as that form of otherwise typical **Parkinson disease** which produces symptoms between the ages of 21 and 39 inclusively and which is either sporadic or dominantly inherited. *Dominantly inherited early-onset parkinsonism* is one *variant.*

Although similar to Parkinson disease in older patients, slower progression of symptoms, an onset with dystonia, a greater incidence of L-dopa-related fluctuations, and the earlier appearance of dyskinesias, as with

juvenile parkinsonian syndromes, are distinguishing characteristics.[2157]

yo-yo-ing Rapid fluctuations in the clinical status of parkinsonian patients on long-term L-dopa therapy.[3645] See **on-off phenomenon, fluctuations.**

Yunis-Varon craniocleidal dysostosis plus A recessively inherited congenital dysmorphic syndrome, characterized also by severe skeletal maldevelopments, including brachydactyly and absence of the thumbs, dolichocephaly, scaphocephaly, and microcephaly with delayed closure of the fontanelles.[6100]

Zackai syndrome A congenital dysmorphic syndrome, manifesting also microcephaly, fusion of cervical vertebrae, and psychomotor retardation.[337] See also **Klippel-Feil syndrome.**

Zadik syndrome A congenital dysmorphic syndrome, manifesting also hypothyroidism; abnormalities of the teeth, skin, and skeleton; dermoid cysts; strabismus; and extra fontanelles in the skull.[337]

Zange-Kindler syndrome (cerebrospinal block syndrome, cisternal block syndrome) Arrest of CSF flow through the cisterna magna due to chronic meningitis or to mass lesions such as tumor and abscess, producing early signs of compromise of brainstem function and obstructive hydrocephalus.[6104]

Zappert syndrome (Zappert-Heller syndrome) See **acute cerebellar ataxia, cerebellar ataxias** (*variants*).

Zazzo test A test of attention and visuomotor abilities in which the subject is required within a 2-minute period to mark every box with each of two particular designs on them, such boxes being randomly placed among a thousand boxes with 25 different designs printed on a chart placed before the subject.[6108]

zebra body myopathy An inherited myopathy characterized by congenital onset, weak fetal movements, mild and nonprogressive proximal myopathic weakness, atrophy, hypotonia, areflexia, raised serum creatine kinase levels, and the presence of targets and nemaline rods in type 2 fibers in extraocular muscle biopsy specimens.[3229]

The zebra bodies are thin actin filaments, arranged parallel to the plasma membranes. See also **congenital myopathies with intracytoplasmic inclusions.**

Zeh syndrome The association of acalculia, dysgraphia, and non-comprehension of facial expression in pictures.[1177, 6114]

zeitgebers Indicators of the passage of time, required to synchronize the circadian rhythms. They include mealtimes, shifts, broadcasts, clocks, etc.

Zellweger, H.V. (1909–1990) Swiss geneticist, pediatrician, and neurologist who trained in Hamburg, Rome, and Berlin before graduating from Zurich in 1934. After residency training in Switzerland and a period spent with Dr. Albert Schweitzer in Africa, he moved to the United States as a Rockefeller Fellow, and, after further experience in Lebanon, returned to Iowa where he later became professor of pediatrics. He founded one of the earliest neuromuscular clinics and was instrumental in founding regional genetic counselling services in his state. He was the author of *Chromosomes of Man* and of *Genetics in Neurology*, each in collaboration.

Zellweger syndrome 1. (cerebrohepatorenal syndrome) A rare, recessively inherited disorder due to the deficiency of multiple peroxisomes and, therefore, of the enzymes contained there. It is characterized by dysgenesis of the cerebral cortex (micropolygyria, macrogyria, heterotopias), lissencephaly, callosal agenesis, cerebellar and olivary dysplasias, and white matter degeneration (sudanophilic leukodystrophy), as well as renal cortical cysts, hepatic periportal fibrosis, and bone pathology. Other clinical features include low birth weight, hypertelorism, abnormal ears, an open metopic suture, and generalized hypotonia.[379, 1359, 4353]

Three genotypes are recognized on the basis of peroxisomal disorder complementation groups.[4009] The chromosomal abnormality is at 7q11.23. Clinical manifestations in each include congenital facial dysmorphism, megalencephaly, multifocal seizures, cataract, optic atrophy, hepatomegaly, hypotonia, areflexia, and diminution of motor activity in infancy; death ensues within a few months.

The clinical and morphological features strongly resemble those of other **peroxisomal disorders.**[690]

2. The combination of **narcolepsy** and petit mal epilepsy.[6117]

Zeman-King syndrome (anterior midline structure syndrome) The association of slowly progressive intellectual deterioration and affective lability, associated with a paroxysmal confusional state, gait ataxia, vertigo, weakness, nystagmus, pyramidal signs and disturbances of sensation due to tumors of the septal region.

The syndrome was first described by the American neurologists Wolfgang Zeman and Frederick King in 1958,[6122] who noted that an English physician, W.B. Ransom, had already described the same findings in a heterogeneous group of patients in 1895.

Zenker fluid A fixative for pathological specimens, compounded by Friedrich Albert Zenker (1825–1898), a German pathologist. The active ingredients are mercuric chloride and potassium dichromate.[4979]

Zenker paralysis Peroneal nerve palsy.

zickzakbewegungen See **square-wave jerks/oscillations.**

Ziehen, Georg Theodor (1862–1924) German psychiatrist, professor at Jena, who described **dystonia** in the same year as **Oppenheim.**

Ziehen syndrome (Ziehen-Oppenheim disease) See **dystonia.**

Zimmer syndrome (tetra-amelia with multiple malformations) A congenital dysmorphic syndrome, manifesting also severe ocular and skeletal maldevelopments, hydrocephalus, and agenesis of the corpus callosum.[337]

Zimmerlin dystrophy Hereditary muscular dystrophy with onset in the shoulder girdle.[6129] See **scapulohumeral muscular dystrophy.**

Zimmerlin, F. (1858–1932) Swiss physician in Basel who gave an early account of **scapulohumeral muscular dystrophy.**

Zonana syndrome A congenital dysmorphic syndrome, manifesting also hypotonia, nystagmus, and psychomotor retardation.[337]

zoster arteritis (Gr, a girdle). Contralateral hemiparesis occurring weeks after the onset of herpes zoster ophthalmicus. It is considered that the virus infects the appropriate artery directly, spreading by way of the first division of the fifth nerve, and causing a necrotizing arteritis with occlusion, producing characteristic radiological findings.[3766]

Zung self-rating depression scale A popular self-rating inventory which lists 20 attitudes (for example,

"I feel downhearted, blue, and sad") which the patient scores (alone or with an interviewer) according to the frequency with which the patient experiences them. Eight items relate to physiological disturbances, the remainder to affect and to psychological and psychomotor changes.[6138]

The test yields unusually high scores in subjects older than 65 years, and so is best not employed for individual screening or for the evaluation of change in depressive symptoms in the elderly. See also **depression rating scales, Hamilton rating scale.**

Zunich syndrome A congenital dysmorphic syndrome, manifesting also retinal colobomas, ichthyosis, seizures, and psychomotor delay.[337]

zygomatic reflex Deviation of the mandible to the side on which the zygoma is tapped; a sign of bilateral corticobulbar tract lesions.

Envoi

While you and i have lips and voices which
are for kissing and to sing with,
who cares if some oneeyed sonofabitch
invents an instrument to measure Spring with?

e.e. cummings

References

1. *The Lennox-Gastaut Syndrome*. Niedermeyer, E. (ed.) New York: Alan R. Liss, 1988.

2. *Disablement in the Community*. Patrick DL (ed.) Appendices 1, 2. Oxford: Oxford University Press, 1989.

3. *Pediatric Neurology*. Slaiman KF, Ashwal, S. (eds.) St. Louis: C.V. Mosby, 1989.

4. *Craniofacial Malformations*. Edinburgh: Churchill, 1990.

5. *Neuro-Ophthalmology*. Philadelphia: Lippincott, 1990.

6. Weller RO, *Systemic Pathology of the Nervous System, Muscle and Eyes*. Edinburgh: Churchill Livingstone, 1990.

7. *The Founders of Child Neurology*. San Francisco: Norman Publishing, 1990.

8. Proceedings of a Consensus Development Conference on Standardized Measures in Diabetic Neuropathy. *Neurology* 1992;**42**:1823–39.

9. *Dictionary of Biological Psychology*. London: Routledge, 2001.

10. AAEM subcommittee. Glossary of terms in electrodiagnostic medicine. *Muscle Nerv* 2001;**Suppl. 10**:S5–S28.

11. AAN AIDS Task Force. Research criteria for diagnosis of chronic inflammatory demyelinating polyneuropathy (CIDP). *Neurology* 1991;**41**:617–8.

12. AAN Quality Standards Subcommittee. Practice parameters: carpal tunnel syndrome [unpublished]. 1993.

13. AAN Therapeutic and Technology Assessment Committee. The clinical usefulness of botulinus toxin A in treating neurologic disorders. *Neurology* 1990;**40**:1332–6.

14. AAN Therapeutic and Technology Assessment Committee. Assessment: posturography [unpublished]. 1993.

15. AAN Therapeutic and Technology Assessment Committee. Melodic intonation therapy. *Neurology* 1994;**44**:566–8.

16. Aase JM, Smith DW. Congenital anemia and triplalangeal thumbs: a new syndrome. *J. Pediatr* 1969;**74**:417.

17. Abadie CA. *Traité des Maladies des Yeux*. O.D. in: Paris, 1877.

18. Abarbanel JM, Bashan N, Potashnik R, et al. Adult muscle phosphorylase "b" kinase deficiency. *Neurology* 1986;**36**:560–2.

19. Abbie AA. The clinical significance of the anterior choroidal artery. *Brain* 1933;**56**:233–46.

20. Abboud FM. Neurocardiogenic syncope. *N Engl J Med* 1993;**328**:1117–20.

21. Abe K, Fujimura H, Tatsumi C, et al. Eyelid "apraxia" in patients with motor neuron disease. *J Neurol Neurosurg Psychiatry* 1995;**59**:629–32.

22. Abel LA, Parker L, Daroff RB, et al. End point nystagmus. *Invest Ophthalmol* 1978;**17**:539–44.

23. Abel LA, Traccis S, Dell'Osso LF. Square wave oscillation. The relation of saccadic intrusions and oscillations. *Neuroophthalmology* 1984;**4**:21.

24. Aberfeld DC. The hypertrophic degeneration of the olives. *Acta Neurol Scand* 1966;**42**:296–306.

25. Aberfeld DC, Hinterbuchner LP, Schneider M. Myotonia, dwarfism, diffuse bone disease and unusual ocular and facial abnormalities (a new syndrome). *Brain* 1965;**88**:313–22.

26. Aberfeld DC, Namba T. Progressive ophthalmoplegia in Kugelberg-Welander disease. *Arch Neurol* 1969;**20**:253–6.

27. Abid F, Hall R, Hudgson P, et al. Möbius syndrome, peripheral neuropathy and hypogonadotrophic hypogonadism. *J Neurol Sci* 1978;**35**:309–15.

28. Abrahamson J, Bell L. Carotid-cavernous-fistula syndrome. *Am J Ophthalmol* 1955;**39**:521.

29. Absher JR, Benson DF. Disconnection syndromes. *Neurology* 1993;**43**:862–7.

30. Achard J. *Rev Neurol* (Paris) 1924;**41**:270–6.

31. Achenbach T, Edelbrock C. The child behavior profile II. Boys aged 12–16 and girls aged 6–11 and 12–16. *J Consult Clin Psychol* 1979;**47**:223.

32. Ackerknecht EH. The history of the discovery of the vegetative (autonomic) nervous system. *Med Hist* 1974;**18**:1–8.

33. Adamolekun B. Epidemiological studies of the etiology of a seasonal ataxia in Nigerians. *Neurology* 1993;**43**:1419.

34. Adams CBT. Hemispherectomy—a modification. *J Neurol Neurosurg Psychiatry* 1983;**46**:61–9.

35. Adams D. Hereditary and acquired amyloid neuropathies. *J Neurol* 2001;**248**:647–57.

36. Adams RD. Cases of diseases of the heart, accompanied with pathological observations. *Dublin Hosp Rep* 1827;**4**:353–453.

37. Adams RD. Striatonigral degeneration. *J Neuropathol Exp Neurol* 1964;**24**:584–608.

38. Adams RD, Fisher CM, Hakim S, et al. Symptomatic occult hydrocephalus with "normal" cerebrospinal fluid pressure: a treatable syndrome. *N Engl J Med* 1965;**273**:117–26.

39. Adams RJ, Meador KJ, Sethi KD, et al. Graded neurological scale for use in acute hemispheric stroke protocols. *Stroke* 1987;**18**:665–9.

40. Addonizio G, Susman VL, Roth SD. Neuroleptic malignant syndrome: review and analysis of 115 cases. *Biol Psychiatry* 1987;**22**:1004–20.

41. Adie WJ. Pseudo-Argyll Robertson pupils with absent tendon reflexes: a benign disorder simulating tabes dorsalis. *BMJ* 1931;**1**:928–30.

42. Adie WJ, Critchley M. Forced grasping and groping. *Brain* 1927;**50**:142–70.

43. Adler FH, Schie HC. The site of the disturbance in tonic pupils. *Trans Am Ophthalmol Soc* 1940;**38**:183–9.

44. Adolfsson R, Forsell A, Johansson G. Hereditary polycystic osteodysplasia with progressive dementia in Sweden. *Lancet* 1978;**i**:120.

45. Adornato BT, Carlini WG. Pushing palsy: a case of self-induced bilateral peroneal palsy induced during natural childbirth. *Neurology* 1992;**42**:936–7.

46. Adour KK. Mona Lisa syndrome: solving the enigma of the Gioconda smile. *Ann Otol Rhinol Laryngol* 1989;**98**:196–9.

47. Adrian ED. General principles of nervous activity. *Brain* 1947;**70**:1–17.

48. Adrian ED, Forbes A. The all-or-nothing response of sensory nerve fibres. *J Physiol* 1922;**56**:301–30.

49. Adrilq A, Lopez MV. Paroxysmal aphasias. *Epilepsia* 1988;**29**: 630–4.

50. Adson AW, Coffey JR. Cervical rib: a new method of anterior approach for relief of symptoms by division of the scalenus anticus. *Ann Surg* 1927;**85**:839–57.

51. Affi AK, Rebeiz JJ, Mire J, et al. The myopathology of the prune belly syndrome. *J Neurol Sci* 1972;**15**:153–65.

52. Afifi AK. Idiopathic hyperCKemia revisited. *J Child Neurol* 1998;**13**:251–2.

53. Aguayo A, Nair CPV, Bray GM. Peripheral nerve abnormalities in Riley-Day syndrome. *Arch Neurol* 1971; **24**:105–16.

54. Aguilar L, et al. A new syndrome characterized by mental retardation, epilepsy, palpebral conjunctival telangiectasias and IgA deficiency. *Clin Genet* 1978;**13**:154–8.

55. Ahlberg G, Borg K, Edstrom L, et al. Welander hereditary distal myopathy: a molecular genetic comparison to hereditary myopathies with inclusion bodies. *Neuromuscul Disord* 1998;**8**:111–4.

56. Aicardi J. *Epilepsy in Children.* New York: Raven Press, 1986.

57. Aicardi J. Alternating hemiplegia of childhood. *Int Pediatr* 1987;**2**:115–9.

58. Aicardi J. *Diseases of the Nervous System in Infancy and Childhood.* London: MacKeith Press, 1992.

59. Aicardi J. The place of neuronal migration abnormalities in child neurology. *Can J Neurol Sci* 1994;**21**:185–93.

60. Aicardi J, Barbosa C, Andermann E, et al. Ataxia-ocular motor apraxia: a syndrome mimicking ataxia-telangiectasia. *Ann Neurol* 1988;**24**:497–502.

61. Aicardi J, Goutieres F. A progressive familial encephalopathy in infancy with calcifications of the basal ganglia and chronic cerebrospinal fluid lymphocytosis. *Ann Neurol* 1984;**15**:49–54.

62. Ainiala H, Loukkala J, Peltola J, et al. The prevalence of neuropsychiatric syndromes in systemic lupus erythematosus. *Neurology* 2001;**57**:496–500.

63. Aird C, McIntosh RAC. Shakespeare's Richard III and the Ellis-van Creveld syndrome. *Practitioner (Lond)* 1978;**220**:656–62.

64. Ajax ET. Trapshooters cramp. *Arch Neurol* 1982;**39**:131.

65. Akesson HO. Cutis verticis gyrata and mental deficiency in Sweden. *Acta Med Scand* 1964;**175**:115–27.

66. Alafuzoff I. The pathology of dementias: an overview. *Acta Neurol Scand Suppl* 1992;**139**:8–15.

67. Alajouanine T. Quatre cas d'une affection congénitale caracterisée par un double pied bot, une double paralysie faciale et une double paralysie de la sixième paire. *Rev Neurol (Paris)* 1930;**2**:501–11.

68. Alajouanine T. Baillarger and Jackson: the principle of Baillarger and Jackson in aphasia. *J Neurol Neurosurg Psychiatry* 1960;**23**:191–3.

69. Alajouanine T. Trouble with expressive language activities in aphasia, and their relationship with apraxias [in French]. *Rev Neurol (Paris)* 1960;**102**:604–33.

70. Alajouanine T. Dostoiewski's epilepsy. *Brain* 1963;**86**:209–18.

71. Alam CN, Merskey H. Neuralgia: the history of a meaning. *Pain Res Manage* 1996;**1**:165–72.

72. Alayza Escardo F. Arnold's neuralgia. *JAMA* 1966;**161**:391.

73. Alba A, Trainor FS, Ritter W, et al. A clinical rating scale for Parkinson patients. *J Chron Dis* 1968;**21**:507–22.

74. Alberca R, Montero C, Ibanez A, et al. Progressive bulbar paralysis associated with neural deafness. *Arch Neurol* 1980;**37**:214–6.

75. Alberca R, Romero M, Chaparro J. Jerking stiff man syndrome. *J Neurol Neurosurg Psychiatry* 1982;**45**:1159–60.

76. Albers JW, Allan AA, Bastron JA, et al. Limb myokymia. *Muscle Nerve* 1981;**4**:494–504.

77. Albers JW, Kelly JJ. Acquired inflammatory demyelinating polyneuropathy: clinical and electrodiagnostic features. *Muscle Nerve* 1989;**12**:435–51.

78. Albers-Schonberg HE. Projections-rontgenbilder einer seltenen knochenerkrankung. *Fortschr Geb Rontgenstr* 1903;**7**:158–9.

79. Albert M, Cohen C. The Test for Severe Impairment: an instrument for the assessment of patients with severe cognitive dysfunction. *J Am Geriatr Soc* 1992;**40**:449–53.

80. Albert ML. A simple test of visual neglect. *Neurology* 1973;**23**: 658–64.

81. Albert ML. Henry Hécaen, MD: neurologist–neuropsychologist 1912–1983. *Arch Neurol* 1984;**41**:458–9.

82. Albert ML, Feldman RG, Willis AL. The "subcortical dementia" of progressive supranuclear palsy. *J Neurol Neurosurg Psychiatry* 1974;**37**:121–30.

83. Albert ML, Reches A, Silverberg R. Associative visual agnosia without alexia. *Neurology* 1975;**25**:322–6.

84. Albert ML, Sparks RW, Helm NA. Melodic intonation therapy for aphasia. *Arch Neurol* 1973;**29**:130–1.

85. Albert MS, Butters N, Levin J. Temporal gradients in the retrograde amnesia of patients with alcoholic Korsakoff's disease. *Arch Neurol* 1979;**36**:211.

86. Albright F, Butler AM, Hampton AO, et al. Syndrome characterized by osteitis fibrosa disseminata, areas of pigmentation and endocrine dysfunction, with precocious puberty in females. *N Engl J Med* 1937;**216**:727.

87. Albright F, et al. Pseudo-hypoparathyroidism—example of "Seabright bantam" syndrome. *Endocrinology* 1942;**30**:922–32.

88. Alcock NS. A note on the pathology of senile chorea (non-hereditary). *Brain* 1936;**59**:376–87.

89. Al-Deeb SM, Yaqub BA, Sharif HS, et al. Neurobrucellosis. *Neurology* 1989;**39**:498–501.

90. Al-Din ASN, Anderson M, Bickerstaff ER, et al. Brainstem encephalitis and the syndrome of Miller Fisher: a clinical study. *Brain* 1982;**105**:481–95.

91. Aldrich MS. Diagnostic aspects of narcolepsy. *Neurology* 1998; **50**:S2–S7.

92. Aldrich MS, Alessi AG, Beck RW, Gilman S. Cortical blindness: etiology, diagnosis and prognosis. *Ann Neurol* 1987;**21**:149–58.

93. Aldrich MS, Beck RW, Albers JW. Familial recurrent Bell's palsy with ocular motor palsies. *Neurology* 1987;**37**:1369–71.

94. Aleck KA, Shapiro LJ. Genetic–metabolic considerations in the sick neonate. *Pediatr Clin North Am* 1978;**25**:431–51.

95. Aleksic S, Budzilovich GN, Chou A, et al. Congenital ophthalmoplegia in oculo-auriculo-vertebral dysplasia–hemifacial microsomia (Goldenhar-Gorlin syndrome). *Neurology* 1976;**26**:638–44.

96. Alexander MP. Mild traumatic brain injury. *Neurology* 1995;**45**: 1253–60.

97. Alexander WS. Progressive fibrinoid degeneration of fibrillary astrocytes associated with mental retardation in a hydrocephalic infant. *Brain* 1949;**72**:373–81.

98. Alexopoulos GS, Abrams RC, Young RC, et al. Cornell scale for depression in dementia. *Biol Psychiatry* 1988;**23**:271–84.

99. Alfonso I, et al. Spinal cord involvement in encephalocutaneous lipomatosis. *Pediatr Neurol* 1986;**2**:380–4.

100. Alford CA, Stagno S, Reynolds DW. Congenital toxoplasmosis: clinical, laboratory, and therapeutic considerations, with special reference to subclinical case. *Bull NY Acad Med* 1974;**50**:160–81.

101. Al-Hakim M, Katirji MB, Osorio I, et al. Cerebral venous thrombosis in paroxysmal nocturnal hemaglobinuria. *Neurology* 1993;**43**: 742–6.

102. Alhalabi M, Moore PM. Serial angiography in isolated angiitis of the nervous system. *Neurology* 1994;**44**:1221–6.

103. Ali-Khan Z, Irving RT, Wignall N, et al. Imported sparganosis in Canada. *CMAJ* 1973;**108**:590–3.

104. Alison MR, Sarraf CE. Apoptosis: a gene-directed programme of cell death. *J R.Coll Phys Lond* 1992;**26**:25.

105. Allan JD, et al. A disease, probably hereditary, characterized by severe mental deficiency and a constant gross abnormality of aminoacid metabolism. *Lancet* 1958;**1**:182–7.

106. Allbutt TG. On the ophthalmoscopic signs of spinal disease. *Lancet* 1870;**1**:76.

107. Allen CMC. Clinical diagnosis of the acute stroke syndrome. *Q J Med* 1983;**52**:515–23.

108. Allen CMC. Predicting the outcome of acute stroke. *J Neurol Neurosurg Psychiatry* 1984;**47**:457–80.

109. Allen IM. Speech defects apparently congenital in origin. *Br J Child Dis* 1932;**29**:98.

110. Allen IV, Dermott E, Connally J, et al. A study of a patient with the amyotrophic form of Creutzfeldt-Jakob disease. *Brain* 1971;**94**: 715–24.

111. Allen RJ, Young W, Read S, et al. "Galactosemic encephalopathy": the effect of early versus late neonatal detection and treatment on neurological outcome. *Ann Neurol* 1991;**30**:465.

112. Allen T, Carman H. Homonymous hemianoptic paracentral scotoma. *Arch Ophthalmol Berlin* 1938;**20**:846–9.

113. Allgrove J, Clayden.GS, Grant DB, et al. Familial glucocorticoid deficiency with achalasia of the cardia and deficient tear production. *Lancet* 1978;**1**:1284–6.

114. Allison RS. Perseveration as a sign of diffuse and focal brain damage. *BMJ* 1966;**2**:1027–32.

115. Allison RS, Millar J. Prevalence and familial incidence of disseminated sclerosis. *Ulster Med.J* 1954;**Suppl 23**:1–92.

116. Allman P. Crying and laughing after brain damage [letter]. *J Neurol Neurosurg Psychiatry* 1990;**53**:1439–40.

117. Al-Lozi MT, Pestronk A, Yee WC, et al. Rapidly evolving myopathy with myosin deficient muscle fibers. *Ann Neurol* 1994;**35**:273–9.

118. Al-Shahwan SA, Singh B, Riela A, et al. Hemisomatic spasms in children. *Neurology* 1994;**44**:1332–3.

119. Allsop JL, Martins L, Lebris H. Neurological manifesations of ciguatera [in French]. *Rev Neurol (Paris)* 1986;**142**:590–7.

120. Alpers BJ. Diffuse progressive degeneration of the gray matter of the cerebrum. *Arch Neurol* 1931;**25**:469–505.

121. Alpers BJ, Grant FC. The clinical syndrome of corpus callosum. *J Nerv Ment Dis* 1931;**121**:205–14.

122. Alpers BJ, Yaskin BJ. The Bruns syndrome. *J Nerv Ment Dis* 1944;**100**:115–34.

123. Alpert JN. Failure of fixation suppression: a pathologic effect of vision on caloric nystagmus. *Neurology* 1974;**24**:891–6.

124. Alpert JN, Coats AC, Perusquia E. Saccadic nystagmus in cerebellar cortical atrophy. *Neurology* 1975;**25**:676–80.

125. Alport AC. Hereditary familial congenital hemorrhagic nephritis. *BMJ* 1927;**1**:504–6.

126. Alston W, Angel RW, Fink FS, et al. Motor activity following the silent period in human muscle. *J Physiol* 1967;**190**:189.

127. Alstrom CH, Hallgren B, Nilsson LB, et al. Retinal degeneration combined with obesity, diabetes mellitus and neurogenous deafness. *Acta Psychiatr Scand Neurol Suppl* 1959;**129**.

128. Alter M. The digiti quinti sign of mild hemiparesis. *Neurology* 1973;**23**:503–5.

129. Alter M, Schaumann B. Hereditary amyotropic lateral sclerosis. A report of two families. *Euro Neurol* 1976;**14**:250–65.

130. Altrocchi PH. Spontaneous oral-facial dyskinesia. *Arch Neurol* 1972;**36**:506.

131. Alvarez SL, Jacobs NA, Murray IJ. Visual changes mediated by beer in retrobulbar neuritis—an investigative report. *Br. J. Ophthalmol* 1986;**70**:141–6.

132. Alvord EC, Lofton S. Gliomas of optic nerve or chiasm. *J Neurosurg* 1988;**68**:85–98.

133. Alzheimer A. Uber eine eigenartige Erkrangkung der Hirnrinde. *Allg Z Psychiatr* 1907;**64**:146–8.

134. Amalric P. A new type of tapetoretinal degeneration in the course of deaf-mutism. *Bull Fr Soc Ophthalmol* 1960;**73**:196–212.

135. Amato AA, Barohn RJ. Hereditary neuropathy with liability to pressure palsies: assocation with central nervous system demyelination. *Muscle Nerve* 1996;**19**:770–3.

136. Amato AA, Jackson CE, Ridings LW, et al. Childhood-onset oculopharygodistal myopathy with chronic instestinal pseudo-obstruction. *Muscle Nerve* 1995;**18**:842–7.

137. Amato AA, Kagan-Hallet K, Jackson CE, et al. The wide spectrum of myofibrillar myopathy suggests a multifactorial etiology and pathogenesis. *Neurology* 1998;**51**:1646–55.

138. Ambler MW, Trice J, Grauerholz J, et al. Infantile osteopetrosis and neuronal storage disease. *Neurology* 1983;**33**:437–41.

139. Ameli NO. Avicenna and trigeminal neuralgia. *J Neurol Sci* 1965;**2**:105–7.

140. American Academy of Neurology. The Dolman-Delcato treatment of neurologically handicapped children. *Neurology* 1968;**18**:1214–6.

141. American Academy of Neurology. Assessment: thermography in neurologic practice. *Neurology* 1990;**40**:523–5.

142. American Academy of Neurology. Assessment and management of patients in the persistent vegetative state. *Neurology* 1995;**45**:1015–8.

143. American Academy of Neurology AIDS Task Force. Nomenclature and case definitions for neurological manifestations of HIV type 1 infection. *Neurology* 1991;**41**:778–85.

143a. American Academy of Neurology Quality Standards Committee. *Practice Parameters*; Carpal Tunnel Syndrome, 1993.

144. American Academy of Neurology Quality Standards Committee. *Practice parameters*: lumbar puncture. *Neurology* 1993;**43**:625–7.

145. American Academy of Neurology Therapeutics subcommittee. Assessment: positron emission tomography. *Neurology* 1991;**41**:163–7.

146. American Academy of Electrodiagnostic Medicine. AAEE glossary of terms in clinical electromyography. *Muscle Nerve* 1987;**10S**: G5–G23.

147. American Diabetes Association. Report and recommendations of the San Antonio Conference on Diabetic Neuropathy. *Muscle Nerve* 1988;**11**:661–7.

148. American Neurological Association Committee on Ethical Affairs. Persistent vegetative state. *Ann Neurol* 1993;**33**:386–90.

150. American Psychiatric Association. *Diagnostic and Statistical Manual of Mental Disorders*, 4th ed. (DSM-IV Text Revision). Washington, DC: American Psychiatric Association, 2000.

151. American Society of Pediatric Surgeons. Identifying the infant with nonaccidental central nervous system injury (the whiplash-shake syndrome). *Pediatr Neurosurg* 1993;**19**:170.

152. Ames FR, Saffer D. The sunflower syndrome. *J Neurol Sci* 1983;**59**: 1–11.

153. Amico L, Caplan LR, Thomas C. Cerebrovascular complications of mucinous cancers. *Neurology* 1989;**39**:522–6.

154. Amiel-Tison C, Grenier A. *Neurological Assessment During the First Year of Life*. New York: Oxford University Press, 1986.

155. Aminoff MJ. Acanthocytosis and neurological disease. *Brain* 1972; **95**:749–60.

156. Aminoff MJ. Vascular anomalies in intracranial dura mater. *Brain* 1973;**96**:601–2.

157. Aminoff MJ, Dedo HH, Izdebski K. Clinical aspects of spasmodic dysphonia. *J Neurol Neurosurg Psychiatry* 1978;**41**:361–5.

158. Amir RE, van den Veyver IB, Wan M, et al. Rett syndrome is caused by mutations in X-linked MECP2, encoding methyl-CpG-binding protein 2. *Nat Genet* 1999;**23**:185–8.

159. Amit R, Bashan N, Abarbanel JM, et al. Fatal familial infantile glycogen storage disease: multisystem phosphofructokinase deficiency. *Muscle Nerve* 1992;**15**:455–8.

160. Amit R, Glick B, Itzchak Y, et al. Acute severe combined demyelination. *Childs Nerv Syst* 1992;**8**:354–6.

161. Amoiridis G. Median–ulnar nerve communications and anomalous innervation of the intrinsic hand muscles: an electrophysiological study. *Muscle Nerve* 1993;**15**:576–9.

162. Andermann E, Andermann F, Silver K, et al. Benign familial nocturnal alternating hemiplegia of childhood. *Neurology* 1994;**44**:1812–4.

163. Andermann E, et al. Agenesis of the corpus callosum with sensorimotor neuropathy. In Littlefield JW, ed. *Vth International Conference on Birth Defects*, Amsterdam: Excerpta Medica, 1977.

164. Andermann F. Nicolaus Friedreich and degenerative atrophy of the posterior columns of the spinal cord. *Can J Neurol Sci* 1976;**3**:275–7.

165. Andermann F, Andermann E. Excessive startle syndromes: startle disease, jumping, and statle epilepsy. In Fahn S, Marsden CD, van Woert M, eds. *Myoclonus*, pp. 321–328. New York: Raven Press, 1984.

166a. Andermann F, Andermann E, Carpenter S, et al. Action myoclonus-renal failure: a new autosomal recessive syndrome in three families. *Adv Neurol* 1986;**43**:87–103.

167. Andermann F, Keene DL, Andermann A, Quesney LF. Startle disease or hyperekplexia. *Brain* 1980;**103**:985–97.

168. Andermann F, Olivier A, Melanson D, et al. Epilepsy due to focal cortical dysplasia with macrogyria and the forme fruste of tuberous sclerosis: a study of 15 patients. In Wolf P, Dam M, Janz D, et al., eds. *Advances in Epileptology*, pp 35–8. New York: Raven Press, 1987.

169. Andersen DH. Familial cirrhosis of the liver with storage of abnormal glycogen. *Lab Invest* 1956;**5**:11–20.

170. Anderson B, McCann SM. The effects of hypothalamic lesions on the water intake of the dog. *Acta Physiol Scand* 1956;**35**:312–20.

171. Anderson M. Neurology of Whipple's disease. *J Neurol Neurosurg Psychiatry* 2000;**68**:2–5.

172. Anderson W. A case of "angiokeratoma". *Br J Dermatol* 1898; **10**:113.

173. Andersson M, Alvarez-Cermeno J, Bernadi G, et al. Cerebrospinal fluid in the diagnosis of multiple sclerosis: a consensus report. *J Neurol Neurosurg Psychiatry* 1994;**57**:897–902.

174. Andrade C. A peculiar form of peripheral neuropathy. *Brain* 1952;**75**:408–27.

175. Andrade C, Araki S, Block WD, et al. Hereditary amyloidosis. *Arthritis Rheum* 1970;**13**:902–15.

176. Andrasik F, Blanchard EB, Arena JG, et al. Psychological functioning in headache sufferers. *Psychosom Med* 1982;**44**:171–82.

177. Andres PL, Hedlund W, Finison L, et al. Quantitative motor assessment in amyotrophic lateral sclerosis. *Neurology* 1986;**36**:937–41.

178. Andres PL, Skerry LM, Munsat TL. Measurement of strength in neuromuscular disease. In Munsat TL, ed. *Quantification of Neurologic Deficit*, pp 87–100. Boston: Butterworths, 1989.

179. André-Thomas. Atrophie lamellaire des cellules de Purkinje. *Rev Neurol (Paris)* 1905;**13**:917–24.

180. Andrews PI, Massey J, Howard JF, et al. Race, sex and puberty influence onset, severity and outcome in juvenile myasthenia gravis. *Neurology* 1994;**44**:1208–14.

181. Angel RW. Shortening reaction in patients with cerebellar ataxia. *Ann Neurol* 1982;**11**:2722–278.

182. Angelman H. Puppet children. *Dev Med Child Neurol.* 1965; **7**:681–8.

183. Angelucci A. Di una sindrome sconosciuta negli infermi di cattaro primaverile. *Arch Ottal* 1897;**4**:270.

184. Anon. Eosinophilia-myalgia syndrome and L-tryptophan containing products. *MMWR Morb Mortal Wkly Rep* 1989;**38**:785.

185. Anon. Obituary. *J Neurophysiol* 1942;**5**:1–17.

186. Anon. Richard Whytt [editorial]. *JAMA* 1964;**189**:150–1.

187. Anthony JH, Procopis PG, Ouvrier RA. Benign acute childhood myositis. *Neurology* 1979;**29**:1068–71.

188. Anton G. Ueber den Ausdruck der Gemuthsbewegungen beim gesunden und kranken Menschen. *Psychiatr Wochenschr* 1900;**17**: 165–9.

189. Antonaci F, Ghimmai S, Bono G, et al. Cervicogenic headache: evaluation of the original criteria. *Cephalalgia* 2001;**21**:583.

190. Antozzi C, Garavaglia B, Mora M, et al. Late-onset riboflavine-responsive myopathy with combined multiple acyl coenzyme A dehydrogenase and respiratory chain deficiency. *Neurology* 1994;**44**:2153–8.

191. Anzil AP, Gessaga E. Late-life cavitating dystrophy of cortical and cerebellar white matter. *Eur Neurol* 1972;**7**:79–94.

192. Apert E. De l'acrocephalosyndactylie. *Bull Soc Med Hop Paris.* 1906;**23**:1310–30.

193. Apgar V. A proposal for a new method of evaluation of the newborn infant. *Anesthesiol Analg* 1953;**32**:260–7.

194. Appel V, et al. A rating scale for amyotrophic lateral sclerosis. *Arch Neurol* 1987;**22**:328–33.

195. Appelt J, et al. Tetraphokomelie mit Lippen-Kiefer-Gaumenspalte und Clitorishhypertrophie—ein Syndrom. *Padiat Padol* 1966;**2**:119–24.

196. Appen RE, Wray SH, Cogan DG. Central retinal artery occlusions. *Am J Ophthalmol* 1975;**79**:374–81.

197. Appenzeller O, Amick L. Paralysis with paradoxic myotonia. *Trans Am Neurol Assoc* 1972;**97**:245–7.

198. Appenzeller O, Biehl JP. Mouthing in the elderly: a cerebellar sign. *J Neurol Sci* 1968;**6**:249–60.

199. Appenzeller O, Hanson JC. Parietal ataxia. *Arch Neurol* 1966;**15**: 264–9.

200. Appenzeller O, Kornfeld M. Macrodactyly and localized hypertrophic neuropathy. *Neurology* 1974;**24**:767–71.

201. Appenzeller O, Parks RD, MacGee J. Peripheral neuropathy in chronic disease of the respiratory tract. *Am J Med* 1968;**44**:873–80.

202. Appleton RE, Panayiotopoulos CP, Acomb BA, et al. Eyelid myoclonia with typical absences: an epilepsy syndrome. *J Neurol Neurosurg Psychiatry* 1993;**56**:1312–6.

203. Apuzzo MLJ, Davey LM, Manuelidise EE. Pineal apoplexy associated with anticoagulant therapy. *J Neurosurg* 1976;**45**:223–6.

204. Aran FA. Récherches sur un maladie non encore décrite du système musculaire (atrophie musculaire progressive). *Arch Gen Med Paris* 1850;**24**:172–214.

205. Arbisser A, et al. A syndrome manifested by brittle hair, with morphologic and biochemical abnormalities, developmental delay and normal stature. *Birth Defects* 1976;**12**:219–28.

206. Arden JB, Barrada A, Kelsey JH. New clinical test of retinal function based on the standing potential of the eye. *Br J Ophthalmol* 1962;**46**:449–67.

207. Ardinger HH, Bell WE. Hypomelanosis of Ito. *Arch Neurol* 1986;**43**:848–50.

208. Arend R, Handzel L, Weiss B. Dysphatic stuttering. *Folia Phoniatr Logop* 1962;**14**:55–66.

209. Aretaeus. On epilepsy. In Adams F, trans., ed. *Extant Works*, London: 1856.

210. Arezzo JC, Schaumberg HH. The use of the Optacon as a screening device for detecting sensory loss in individuals exposed to neurotoxins. *J Occup Med* 1980;**22**:461–4.

211. Argov Z, Navon R. Clinical and genetic variations in the syndrome of adult GM2 gangliosidosis resulting from hexosaminidase A deficiency. *Ann Neurol* 1984;**16**:14–20.

212. Argyll Robertson J. Four cases of spinal myosis. With remarks on the action of light on the pupil. *Edinb Med J* 1869;**15**:487–93.

213. Arias D, Passarge E, Engle MA, et al. Human chromosomal deletion; two patients with the 4p syndrome. *J Pediatr* 1970;**76**:82–8.

214. Arieff AJ, Tigay EL, Kurtz JF. The Hoover Sign. *Arch Neurol* 1961;**5**:673–8.

215. Arjundas G. Experiences with neuromuscular disorders in South India. *Neurology (Bombay)* 1977;**25**:1–18.

216. Armendares S, Antillar F, del Castillo V, et al. A newly recognized inherited syndrome of dwarfism, craniosynostosis, retinitis pigmentosa, and multiple congenital malformations. *J Pediatr* 1974;**85**:872–3.

217. Armon C. The alternating eye deviation sign. *Neurology* 1991;**41**: 1845.

218. Armon C, Radtke RA, Friedman AH. Inhibitory simple partial (non-convulsive) status epilepticus after intracranial surgery. *J Neurol Neurosurg Psychiatry* 2000;**69**:18–24.

219. Armstrong D, Sachis P, Bryan C, et al. Pathological features of persistent infantile sleep apnea with reference to the pathology of sudden infant death syndrome. *Ann Neurol* 1982;**12**:169–74.

220. Arnason BGW. Inflammatory polyradiculoneuritis. In Dyck PJ, Thomas PK, Lambert EH, eds. *Peripheral Neuropathy*, pp 1110–48. Philadelphia: W.B. Saunders, 1975.

221. Arnold J. Myelocyste, Transposition von Gewebskeinem und Sympodie. *Beitr Pathol Anat* 1894;**16**:1–28.

222. Arnoldi CC, Brodsky AE, Cauchoix J, et al. Lumbar spinal stenosis and nerve root entrapment syndromes: definition and classification. *Clin Orthop* 1976;**115**:4–5.

223. Arts WFM, Busch HFM, van de Brand HJ, et al. Hereditary neuralgic amyotrophy. *J Neurol Sci* 1983;**62**:261–79.

224. Arts WFM, Loonen MCB, Sengers RCA, et al. X-linked ataxia, weakness, deafness and loss of vision in early childhood with a fatal course. *Ann Neurol* 1993;**33**:535–9.

225. Arvanitakis Z, Wszolek ZK. Recent advances in the understanding of tau protein and movement disorders. *Curr Opin Neurol* 2001;**14**:491–7.

226. Asberg MA, Montgomery SA, Perris C, et al. A comprehensive psychopathological rating scale. *Acta Psychiatr Neurol Scand Suppl* 1978;**271**:S5–S27.

227. Asbury AK. Renaut bodies—a forgotten endoneurial structue? *J Neuropathol Exp Neurol* 1973;**324**:334–43.

228. Asbury AK, Arnason BGW, Karp H, et al. Criteria for the diagnosis of Guillain-Barre syndrome. *Ann Neurol* 1978;**3**:565–6.

229. Asbury AK, Cornblath DR. Assessment of current diagnostic criteria for Guillain-Barré syndrome. *Ann Neurol* 1990;**27**:S21–S24.

230. Asbury AK, Picard EH, Baringer JR. Sensory perineuritis. *Arch Neurol* 1972;**26**:302–12.

231. Asbury AK, Prensky AL. Graphogenic epilepsy. *Trans Amer Neurol Assoc* 1963;**88**:193–4.

232. Asbury AK, Victor M, Adams RD. Uremic polyneuropathy. *Arch Neurol* 1963;**8**:413–28.

233. Aschoff JC, Becker W, Rettelbach R. Voluntary nystagmus in five generations. *J Neurol Neurosurg Psychiatry* 1976;**39**:300–4.

234. ASDA Diagnostic Classification Steering Committee. *The International Classification of Sleep Disorders Diagnostic and Coding Manual.* Rochester, MN: American Sleep Disorders Association, 1990.

235. Aserinsky E, Kleitman N. Regularly occurring periods of eye motility and concomitant phenomena during sleep. *Science* 1953;**118**:273–4.

236. Ashe J, Hain TC, Zee DS, et al. Microsaccadic flutter. *Brain* 1991;**114**:461–72.

237. Asher R. Myxoedematous madness. *BMJ* 1949;**ii**:555–62.

238. Asher R. Munchausen's syndrome. *Lancet* 1951;**1**:339–41.

239. Asher SW, Berg BO. Progressive hemifacial atrophy: report of three cases, including one observed over 43 years, and computed tomographic findings. *Arch Neurol* 1982;**39**:44–6.

240. Asherson N. Trotter's syndrome and associated lesions. *J Laryngol Otol* 1951;**65**:349–66.

241. Ashizawa T, Butler IJ, Harati Y, et al. A dominantly inherited syndrome with continuous motor neuron discharges. *Ann Neurol* 1983;**13**:285–90.

242. Ashizawa T, Rolak LA, Hines M. Spastic pure motor monoparesis. *Ann Neurol* 1986;**20**:638–41.

243. Ashwal S, Thrasher TV, Rice DR, et al. A new form of sea-blue histiocytosis associated with progressive anterior horn cell and axonal degeneration. *Ann Neurol* 1984;**16**:184–92.

244. Askanas V, Engel WK, Kwan HH, et al. Autosomal dominant syndrome of lipid neuromyopathy with normal carnitine: successful treatment with long-chain fatty acid–free diet. *Neurology* 1985;**35**:66–72.

245. Askanas V, Engel WK, Reddy NB, et al. X-linked recessive congenital muscle fiber hypotrophy with central nuclei. *Arch Neurol* 1979;**36**:604–9.

246. Askenasy H, Wijsenbeek H, Hertzberger E. Retraction nystagmus and retraction of the eyelids due to arteriovenous aneurysm of the midbrain. *Arch Neurol Psychiatry* 1953;**69**:236.

247. Askenasy JJM. Sleep hiccup. *Sleep* 1988;**11**:187–94.

248. Assmann H, Bielenstein H, Hobs H, et al. Beobachtungen und Untersuchungen bei der Haffkrankheit. *Dtsch Med Wochenschr* 1933;**59**:122–6.

249. Association of Sleep Disorder Centers. Diagnostic classification of sleep and arousal disorders. *Sleep* 1979;**2**:1–137.

250. Astrom K-E, Mancall EL, Richardson EP jr. Progressive multifocal leuko-encephalopathy: a hitherto unrecognized complication of chronic lymphatic leukaemia and Hodgkin's disease. *Brain* 1958;**81**:93–111.

251. Astrup J, Siesjo BK, Symon L. Thresholds in cerebral ischemia: the ischemic penumbra. *Stroke* 1981;**12**:723–5.

252. Atchison PR, Thompson PD, Frackowiak RS, et al. The syndrome of gait ignition failure: a report of six cases. *Mov Disord* 1993;**8**:285–92.

253. Atkin A, Bender MB. Lightning eye movements (ocular myoclonus). *J Neurol Sci* 1964;**1**:2–12.

254. Atkin BM, Buist NRM, Utter MF, et al. Pyruvate carboxylate deficiency and lactic acidosis in a child without Leigh's disease. *Pediatr Res* 1979;**13**:109.

255. Atkin JF, Flaitz K, Patil S, et al. An X-linked mental retardation syndrome. *Am J Med Genet* 1985;**21**:697–705.

256. Auberger G, Ratzlaff T, Lunkes A, et al. A gene for autosomal dominant paroxysmal choreoathetosis/spasticity (CSE) maps to the vixcinity of a potassium channel gene cluster on chromosome 1p. *Genomics* 1996;**31**:90–4.

257. Aubert H. *Physiologie der Netzhaut.* Breslau: Morgenstern, 1865.

258. Auerbach SH. Central razzle: a central auditory pain syndrome? *Arch Neurol* 1981;**38**:671.

259. Auer-Grumbach M, Strasser-Fuchs S, Wagner K, et al. Roussy Levy syndrome is a phenotypic variant of Charcot-Marie-Tooth syndrome associated with a duplication on chromosome 17p11.2. *J Neurol Sci* 1998;**154**:72–5.

260. Auger RA, Daube JR, Gomez MR, et al. Hereditary form of sustained muscle activity of peripheral nerve origin causing generalized myokymia and muscle stiffness. *Ann Neurol* 1984;**15**:13–21.

261. Auger RG. Diseases associated with excess motor unit activity. *Muscle Nerve* 1994;**17**:1250–63.

262. Aujesky, A. Ueber eine neue Infektionskrankheit bei Haustieren. *Zentralbl Bakteriol* 1902;**32**:535–557.

263. Aula P, Autio S, Raivio KO, et al. "Salla disease": a new lysosomal storage disorder. *Arch Neurol* 1979;**36**:88–94.

264. Auranen M, Villanova M, Muntoni F, et al. X-linked vacuolar myopathies: two separate loci and refined genetic mapping. *Ann Neurol* 2000;**47**:666–9.

265. Ausman JI, Shrontz CE, Pearce JE, et al. Vertebrobasilar insufficiency: a review. *Arch Neurol* 1985;**42**:803–8.

266. Austin EJ, Wilkus RJ, Longstreth WT. Etiology and prognosis of alpha coma. *Neurology* 1988;**38**:773–7.

267. Austin J. Studies in metachromatic leukodystrophy. XII. Multiple sulfatase deficiency. *Arch Neurol* 1973;**28**:258–64.

268. Austin J, Armstrong D, Fouch S, et al. Metachromatic leukodystrophy (MLD). *Arch Neurol* 1968;**18**:225–40.

269. Avellis G. Klinische Beitrage zur halbseitigen Kehlkopflamung. *Berl Klin Wochenschr* 1891;**40**:1–26.

270. Averback P. Primary cerebral venous thrombosis in young adults: the diverse manifestations of an underrecognized disease. *Ann Neurol* 1978;**3**:81–6.

271. Averbuch-Heller L, Zivotovsky AZ, Das VE, et al. Investigations of the pathogenesis of acquired pendular nystagmus. *Brain* 1995;**118**:369–78.

272. Aver'ianov I, Il'ina NA, Nechkina NP, et al. Ophthalmoplegia plus (multisystem mitochondrial cytopathy) in childhood. *Zh Nevropatol Psikiatr* 1983;**83**:1624–8.

273. Avoni P, Monari L, Carelli V, et al. Congenital encephalomyopathy with epilepsy, chorioretinitis, basal ganglia involvement and muscle minicores. *Ann Neurol* 2000;**47**:399.

274. Awang DVC. Feverfew. *Pharm J* 1987;**239**:487.

275. Axenfeld T. Cyclic oculomotor paralysis. *Klin Monatsbl Augenheilkd* 1901;**39**:64–73.

276. Ay H, Buonanno FS, Price BH, et al. Sensory alien hand syndrome: case report and review of the literature. *J Neurol Neurosurg Psychiatry* 1998;**65**:366–9.

277. Azouvi P, Bergigo C, Robel L, et al. Slowly progressive apraxia: two case studies. *J Neurol* 1993;**240**:347–50.

278. Azzarelli B, Roessmann U. Diffuse anoxic myelopathy. *Neurology* 1977;**27**:1049–52.

279. Baar HS, Gabriel AM. Sex linked spastic paraplegia. *Am J Ment Defic* 1966;**71**:13–8.

280. Baastrup CI. On the spinous processes of the lumbar vertebra and the soft tissues between them, and on pathological changes in that region. *Acta Radiol* 1933;**14**:52–4.

281. Babel J. Association d'un diabete juvenile insulino-dependant et d'atrophie optique. *Rev Med Suisse Rom* 1980;**100**:337–41.

282. Babikian V, Ropper AH. Binswanger's disease: a review. *Stroke* 1987;**18**:2–12.

283. Babinski J. Sur le réflexe cutane plantaire dans certains affections organique de système nerveux central. *C R Soc Biol* 1896;**48**:207–8.

284. Babinski J. Des troubles pupillaires dans les anevrismes de l'aorte. *Bull Soc Hop Paris* 1901;**18**:1121–4.

285. Babinski J. De l'équilibre volitionnel statique et de l'équilibre volitionnel cinétique. *Rev Neurol (Paris)* 1902;**10**:470–4.

286. Babinski J. Hemispasme faciale peripherique. *Nouv Icon Salpet* 1905;**18**:418–23.

287. Babinski J. Contribution a l'étude des troubles mentaux dans l'hemiplégie organique cérébrale (anosognosie). *Rev Neurol (Paris)* 1914;**22**:845–8.

288. Babinski J, Froment JC. *Bull Acad Med Paris* 1916;**75**:40–7.

289. Babinski J, Nageotte J. Hemiasynergie, lateropulsion et miosis bulbaire. *Nouv Icon Salpet* 1902;**5**:492.

290. Bahill AT, Hsu FK, Stark L. Glissadic overshoots are due to pulse width errors. *Arch Neurol* 1978;**35**:138–42.

291. Bahill AT, Troost BT. Types of saccadic eye movements. *Neurology* 1979;**29**:1150–2.

292. Bailey P. Reflections aroused by an unusual tumor of the cerebellum. *J Mt Sinai Hosp* 1942;**9**:299–310.

293. Bailey P, Cushing HW. Medulloblastoma cerebelli: a common type of midcerebellar glioma in childhood. *Arch Neurol Psychiatry* 1925; **14**:192–225.

294. Bailey P, Cushing HW. *A Classification of the Tumors of the Glioma Group on a Histogenetic Basis with a Correlated Study of Prognosis.* Philadelphia: J.B. Lippincott, 1926.

295. Bailey RO, Dentinger MP, Tome ME, et al. Benign muscular dystrophy with contractures. *Acta Neurol Scand* 1986;**73**:439–43.

296. Bailey RO, Markules DL, Hans MTS. Infantile facioscapulohumeral muscular dystrophy. *Acta Neurol Scand* 1986;**74**:51–8.

297. Baillarger J-G-F. General paralysis—a new symptom [in French]. *Gaz Hop Civ Milit* 1850;**2**:225.

298. Baillarger J-G-F. *Récherches sur L'anatomie, la Physiologie et la Pathologie du Système Nerveux.* Paris: Victor Masson, 1872.

299. Bain P. A combined clinical and neurophysiological approach to the study of patients with tremor. *J Neurol Neurosurg Psychiatry* 1993;**69**:839–44.

300. Bain P, Brin M, Deuschl G, et al. Criteria for the diagnosis of essential tremor. *Neurology* 2000;**54(Suppl 4)**:S7.

301. Baker AB, Adams JM. Lipomatosis of the central nervous system. *Am J Cancer* 1938;**34**:214.

302. Baker GA, Smith DF, Dewey M, et al. The development of a seizure severity scale as an outcome measure in epilepsy. *Epilepsy Res* 1991;**8**:245–51.

303. Baker RS, Ross PA, Baumann RJ. Neurologic complications of the epidermal nevus syndrome. *Arch Neurol* 1987;**44**:227–32.

304. Balasubramanian M, Ramamurthi B. An unusual location of Guinea worm infestation. *J Neurosurg* 1965;**23**:537.

305. Balduzzi O. A new reflex of the contralateral adductor muscles. *Rev Neurol (Paris)* 1926;**2**:243–6.

306. Bale JF. Human cytomegalovirus infection and disorders of the nervous system. *Arch Neurol* 1984;**41**:310–20.

307. Balestrini MR, Cavaletti G, D'Angelo A, Tredici G. Infantile hereditary neuropathy with hypomyelination: report of two siblings with different expressivity. *Neuropediatrics* 1991;**22**:65–70.

308. Balint R. Seelenlahmung des "Schauens", optische Ataxia, raumliche Storung der Aufmerskameit. *Monatschr Psychiatr Neurol* 1909; **25**:51–81.

309. Baller F. Radiusaplasie und Inzucht. *Z Menschl Vererb Konstit Lehre* 1950;**29**:782–90.

310. Ballet G. External ophthalmoplegia and bulbar palsy. *Rev Med Paris* 1888;**8**:337, 513–355, 546.

311. Balo J. Encephalitis periaxalis concentrica. *Arch Neurol* 1928; **19**:242–64.

312. Baloh RB. Charles Skinner Hallpike and the beginnings of neurotology. *Neurology* 2000;**54**:2138–46.

313. Baloh RB, Foster CA, Yue Q, et al. Familial migraine with vertigo and essential tremor. *Neurology* 1996;**46**:458–60.

314. Baloh RB, Jacobson K, Honrubia V. Horizontal semicircular canal variant of benign positional vertigo. *Neurology* 1993;**43**:2542–9.

315. Baloh RB, Yue Q, Jacobson KM, et.al. Persistent direction-changing positional nystagmus. *Neurology* 1995;**45**:1297–301.

316. Baloh RW, DeRossett SE, Cloughesy TF, et al. Novel brainstem syndrome associated with prostate carcinoma. *Neurology* 1993;**43**: 2591–6.

317. Baloh RW, Furman JMR, Yee RD. Dorsal midbrain syndrome: clinical and oculographic findings. *Neurology* 1985;**35**:54–60.

318. Baloh RW, Honrubia V, Jacobson K. Benign positional vertigo. *Neurology* 1987;**37**:371–8.

319. Baloh RW, Jacobson K, Fife T. Familial vestibulopathy. *Neurology* 1994;**44**:20–5.

320. Baloh RW, Konrad HR, Dirks D, et al. Cerebellar-pontine angle tumors. *Arch Neurol* 1976;**33**:507–12.

321. Baloh RW, Sills AW, Kumley WE, et al. Quantitative measurement of saccade amplitude, duration and velocity. *Neurology* 1975;**25**: 1065–70.

322. Bamberger H von. Saltatorischer Refelexkrampf, eine merkwurdige Form vom Spinal-Irritation. *Wien Med Wochenschr* 1859;**9**:49–67.

323. Bamford JM. Interobserver agreement for the assessment of handicap in stroke. *Stroke* 1989;**20**:828.

324. Bamford JM, Sandercock P, Dennis M, et al. Classification and natural history of clinically identifiable subtypes of cerebral infarction. *Lancet* 1991;**337**:1521–6.

325. Bancaud J. Kojewnikow's syndrome (epilepsia partialis continua) in children. In Roger J, Dravet C, Bureau M, et al., eds. *Epileptic Syndromes*, pp 286–98. London: John Libbey, 1985.

326. Banfield GK, Crate ID, Griffiths CL. Long-term sequelae of Palmar-Plantar erythrodysaesthesia syndrome secondary to 5–fluouracil therapy. *J R Soc Med* 1995;**88**:365P-57P.

327. Banker BQ, Chester CS. Ischemic infarction of thigh muscle in the diabetic patient. *Neurology* 1973;**23**:667–77.

328. Banker BQ, Victor M, Adams RD. Arthrogryposis multiplex due to congenital muscular dystrophy. *Brain* 1957;**80**:319–34.

329. Banks G, Short P, Martinez AJ, et al. The alien hand syndrome. *Arch Neurol* 1989;**46**:456–9.

330. Bannister R, Davis B, Holly E, et al. Defective cardiovascular reflexes and supersensitivity to sympathomimetic drugs in autonomic failure. *Brain* 1979;**102**:144–9.

331. Bannwarth A. Chronische lymphocytare Meningitis, entzundliche Polyneuritis und "Rheumatismus." *Arch Psychiatr (Berlin)* 1941;**113**: 284–376.

332. Baquis GD, Pessin MS, Scott RM. Limb shaking—a carotid TIA. *Stroke* 1985;**16**:444–8.

333. Barac B. Vertiginous epileptic attacks and so-called vestibulogenic seizures. *Epilepsia* 1968;**9**:137–44.

334. Baraitser M. The orofaciodigital (OFD) syndromes. *J Med Genet* 1986;**23**:116–9.

335. Baraitser M. *The Genetics of Neurological Disorders.* Oxford: Oxford University Press, 1990.

336. Baraitser M, Burn J, Fixsen J. A female infant with features of Mohr and Majewsky syndromes: variable expression, a genetic compound or a distinct entity. *J Med Genet* 1983;**20**:65–7.

337. Baraitser M, Tomiwa K, Wilson J, et al. A database of genetically determined neurological conditions for clinicians. *J Neurol Neurosurg Psychiatry* 1989;**52**:106–7.

338. Baraitser M, Winter RM, Brett EM. Greig cephalopolysyndactyly: report of 13 affected individuals in three families. *Clin Genet* 1983;**24**: 257–65.

339. Barany R. Vestibularapparat und Centralnervensystem. *Med Klin Berlin* 1911;**7**:1818–21.

340. Barbeau A. Distribution of ataxia in Quebec. In Sobue I, ed. *Spinocerebellar Degeneration*, pp 120–2. Tokyo: Tokyo University Press, 1980.

341. Barber HS. Myalgic syndrome with constitutional effects: polymyalgia rheumatica. *Ann Rheum Dis* 1957;**16**:230–7.

342. Barbieri F, Pellechia MT, Esposito E, et al. l. Adult onset familial laryngeal abductor paralysis, cerebellar ataxia and pure motor neuropathy. *Neurology* 2001;**56**:1412–4.

343. Barbieri F, Santangelo R, Capperelli G, et al. Autosomal recessive motor and sensory neuropathy with excessive myelin outfolding in two siblings. *Can J Neurol Sci* 1994;**21**:29–33.

344. Barbizet J. Yawning. *J Neurol Neurosurg Psychiatry* 1958;**21**:203–9.

345. Barcia-Goyanes JJ, Calvo W, Barcia-Salorio JL. A new method for exploration of the cerebral circulation. *Rev Esp Otoneurooftal* 1953;**12**: 241–6.

346. Bardet G. Sur un syndrome d'obesity congenitale avec polydactylie et retinite pigmentaire. Paris: Thesis, Université de Paris, 1920.

347. Bardosi A, DiMauro S, Servidei S, et al. Myo-neuro-gastro-intestine-encephalopathy. *Muscle Nerve* 1986;**9**:177–81.

348. Bardwick PA, Zvaifler NJ, Gill GN, et al. Plasma cell dyscrasia with polyneuropathy, organomegaly, M protein and skin changes; the POEMS syndrome. *Medicine* 1980;**59**:311–22.

349. Barer N, Nouri F. Measurement of activities of daily living. *Clin Rehabil* 1990;**3**:179–87.

350. Barjon P, Labauger R, Cazaban R, et al. Primary optic atrophy, hearing loss and juvenile diabetes mellitus. *Diabetes* 1964;**11**:231–7.

351. Barker RA, Revesz T, Thom M, et al. Review of 23 patients affected by the stiff man syndrome: clinical division into stiff trunk (man) syndrome, stiff limb syndrome and progressive encephalomyelitis with rigidity. *J Neurol Neurosurg Psychiatry* 1998;**65**:633–40.

352. Barkhaus PE, Morgan O. Jamaican neuropathy: an electrophysiological study. *Muscle Nerve* 1988;**11**:380–5.

352a. Barkhof F, Filippi M, Miller DH. et al. Comparison of MR imaging criteria at first presentation to predict conversion to clinically definite multiple sclerosis. *Brain* 1997;**120**:2059–69.

353. Barkovich AH, Jackson DE, Boyer RS. Band heterotopias: a newly recognized neuronal migration anomaly. *Radiology* 1989;**171**:455–8.

354. Barkovich AJ, Chuang SH. Unilateral megalencephaly. *Am J Neuroradiol* 1990;**11**:523–31.

355. Barkovich AJ, Kock TK, Carrol CL. The spectrum of lissencephaly: report of 10 patients analyzed by magnetic resonance imaging. *Ann Neurol* 1991;**30**:139–46.

356. Barkovich AJ, Kuzniecky R. Gray matter heterotopia. *Neurology* 2000;**55**:1603–8.

357. Barkovich AJ, Kuzniecky R, Bollen AW, et al. Focal transmantle dysplasia: a specific malformation of cortical development. *Neurology* 1997;**49**:1148–52.

358. Barkovich AJ, Kuzniecky R, Jackson GG, et al. Classification system for malformations of cortical development. *Neurology* 2001;**57**: 2168–78.

359. Barlow CF. *Headaches and Migraine in Childhood.* Philadelphia: J.B. Lippincott, 1984.

360. Barmada MA, Moosy J, Painter M. Pontosubicular necrosis and hyperoxemia. *Pediatrics* 1980;**66**:840.

361. Barnard RI, Scholz RO. Ophthalmoplegia and retinal degeneration. *Am J Ophthalmol* 1944;**27**:621–4.

362. Barnes D, Misra VP, Young EP, et al. An adult onset hexosaminidase A deficiency syndrome with sensory neuropathy and internuclear ophthalmoplegia. *J Neurol Neurosurg Psychiatry* 1991;**54**:1112–3.

363. Barnes HD. Further South African cases of porphyrinuria. *S Afr J Clin Sci* 1951;**2**:117–69.

364. Barnes MP, Saunders M, Walls TJ. The syndrome of Karl Ludwig Kahlbaum. *J Neurol Neurosurg Psychiatry* 1986;**49**:991.

365. Barnett HJM, Wortzman G, Gladstone RM, et al. Diversion and reversal of cerebral blood flow. *Neurology* 1970;**20**:1–14.

366. Barohn RJ, Kissel JT, Warmolts JR, et al. Chronic inflammatory demyelinating polyradiculopathy: clinical characteristics, course, and recommendations for diagnostic criteria. *Arch Neurol* 1989;**46**:878–84.

367. Barohn RJ, Miller RG, Griggs RC. Autosomal recessive distal dystrophy. *Neurology* 1991;**41**:1365–70.

368. Baron DN, Dent CE, Harris H, Hart EW, Jepson JB. Hereditary pellagra-like skin rash with temporary cerebellar ataxia, constant renal amino-aciduria and other bizarre biochemical features. *Lancet* 1956; **2**:421–8.

369. Baron JC, Bousser M-G, Comar D, et al. "Crossed cerebellar diaschisis" in human supratentorial brain infarction. *Trans Am Neurol Assoc* 1980;**105**:459–61.

370. Baron JC, Busser M-G, Comar D, et al. Crossed cerebellar diaschisis in human supratentorial infarction. *Ann Neurol* 1980;**8**:128.

371. Baron R, Levine JD, Fields HL. Causalgia and reflex sympathetic dystrophy: does the sympathetic nervous system contribute to the generation of pain? *Muscle Nerve* 1999;**22**:678–95.

372. Barre JA. Chronic vertebral arthritis and medullar disturbances; chronic vertebral arthritis and tumor of the spinal cord. *Paris Med* 1925;**2**:226.

373. Barre MJ. Sur un syndrome sympathique cervical posterieur et sa cause frequent, l'artrite cervicale. *Rev Neurol (Paris)* 1926;**1**:1246–8.

374. Barrows HS. Neurological eponyms. *Arch Neurol* 1960;**3**:91–7.

375. Barry DT, Gooch J. Evoked acoustic signals as a measure of contractile properties of muscles. *Muscle Nerve* 1986;**9**:651a.

376. Barsky RJ, Borus JF. Functional somatic syndromes. *Ann Intern Med* 1999;**130**:910–21.

377. Bart RS, Pumphrey RE. Knuckle pads, leukonychia and deafness: a dominantly inherited syndrome. *N Engl J Med* 1967;**276**:202–7.

378. Barth PG, Blennow G, Lenard HG, et al. The syndrome of autosomal recessive pontocerebellar hypoplasia, microcephaly and extrapyramidal dyskinesia (pontocerebellar hypoplasia type 2). *Neurology* 1995;**45**:311–7.

379. Barth PG, Gootjes J, Bode H, et al. Late onset white matter disease in peroxisome biogenesis disorder. *Neurology* 2001;**57**:1949–55.

380. Barth PG, Hoffmann GF, Jaeken J, et al. L-2-hydroxyglutaric acidemia: a novel inherited neurometabolic disease. *Ann Neurol* 1992;**32**:66–71.

381. Bassen FA, Kornzweig AL. Malformation of the erythrocytes in a case of atypical retinitis pigmentosa. *Blood* 1950;**5**:381–7.

382. Bassetti C, Bogousslavsky J, Mattle H, et al. Medial medullary stroke: report of seven patients and review of the literature. *Neurology* 1997;**48**:882–90.

383. Bassetti C, Bogousslavsky J, Regli F. Sensory syndromes on parietal stroke. *Neurology* 1993;**43**:1942–9.

384. Bassoe CF. The skinache syndrome. *J R Soc Med* 1995;**88**:565–9.

385. Bassoe HH. Familial congenital muscular dystrophy with gonadal dysgenesis. *J Clin Endocrinol* 1956;**16**:1614–21.

386. Bastian AJ, Mink JW, Kaufman JA, et al. Posterior vermal split syndrome. *Ann Neurol* 1998;**44**:601–10.

387. Bastian HC. On the various forms of loss of speech in cerebral disease. *Br Med Chir Rev* 1869;**43**:209–36.

388. Bastian HC. On the symptomatology of total transverse lesions of the spinal cord, with special reference to the condition of the various reflexes. *Med Chir Trans* 1890;**73**:151–217.

389. Bateman DE, Saunders M. Cyclic oculomotor palsy: description of a case and hypothesis of the mechanism. *J Neurol Neurosurg Psychiatry* 1983;**46**:451–3.

390. Batshaw ML. Inborn errors of urea synthesis. *Ann Neurol* 1994; **35**:133–41.

391. Battaglia A, Gurrieri F, Bertini E, et al. The inv dup(15) syndrome. *Neurology* 1997;**48**:1081–6.

392. Batten FE. Cerebral degeneration with symmetrical changes in the maculae in two members of a family. *Trans Ophthalmol Soc UK 1903;* **23**:386–390.

393. Batten FE. Acute poliomyelitis. *Brain* 1916;**39**:115–211.

394. Battistella PA, et al. Carnitine deficiency induced during haemodialysis. *Lancet* 1978;**i**:939.

395. Baumann N, Turpin J-C. Adult-onset leukodystrophies. *J Neurol* 2000;**247**:751–9.

396. Baumgarten M, Becker R, Gauthier S. Validity and reliability of the dementia behavior disturbance scale. *J Am Geriatr Soc* 1990;**38**:221.

397. Baumgartner MR, Poll-The BT, Verhoeven NM, et al. Clinical approach to genetic peroxisomal disorders: a series of 27 patients. *Ann Neurol* 1998;**44**:720–30.

398. Bautista J, Rafel E, Castilla JM, et al. Hereditary distal myopathy with onset in early infancy. *J Neurol Sci* 1978;**37**:149–58.

399. Baxter DM, Warrington EK. Ideational agraphia: a single case study. *J Neurol Neurosurg Psychiatry* 1986;**369**:374.

400. Baxter DW, Olszewski J. Congenital universal insensitivity to pain. *Brain* 1983;**83**:381–93.

401. Bay E. Disturbances of visual perception and their examination. *Brain* 1953;**76**:515–50.

402. Bayle ALJ. Récherches sur la maladie mentale. Thesis, Université de Paris, 1822.

403. Beal MF, Fisher CM. Neoplastic angioendotheliosis. *J Neurol Sci* 1982;**53**:359–75.

404. Beal MF, Richardson EP Jr. Primary lateral sclerosis: a case report. *Arch Neurol* 1981;**38**:630–3.

405. Beall SS, Patten BM, Janovik J. Familial calcification of the brain, iron storage and porphyria: a new syndrome. *Ann Neurol* 1984;**16**:137.

406. Beard GM. Neurasthenia, or nervous exhaustion. *Boston Med Surg J* 1869;**80**:217–21.

407. Beard GM. Remarks on "jumpers" or "jumping frenchmen". *J Nerv Ment Dis* 1878;**5**:526.

408. Beard GM. *A Practical Treatise on Nervous Exhaustion (Neurasthenia).* New York: W. Wood & Co., 1880.

409. Beatty RA. The piriformis muscle syndrome: a simple diagnostic maneuver. *Neurosurgery* 1994;**34**:512–4.

410. Beauchesne P, Pialat J, Duthel R, et al. Aggressive treatment with complete remission in primary diffuse leptomeningeal gliomatosis—a case report. *J Neurooncol* 1998;**37**:161–7.

411. Beauvieux J. Quelques aspects de syncinésies oculaires. *Concours Med* 1952;**74**:369–72.

412. Beauvois M-F, Derouesne J. Lexical or orthographic agraphia. *Brain* 1981;**104**:21–49.

413. Beck AT, Ward CH, Mendelson M, et al. An inventory for measuring depression. *Arch Gen Psychiatry* 1961;**4**:561–71.

414. Beck K. The syndrome of anterior spinal artery thrombosis. *Dtsch Z Nervenklinik* 1952;164–86.

415. Becker DP, Grossman RG, McLaurin RL, et al. Head injuries—panel 3. *Arch Neurol* 1979;**36**:750–8.

416. Becker GD, Davis JL, Parell J. Pseudocaloric nystagmus. *Arch Neurol* 1978;**35**:93–4.

417. Becker LE. Synaptic dysgenesis. *Can J Neurol Sci* 1991;**18**:170–180.

418. Becker PE. Neue Ergebnisse der Genetik der Muskeldystrophien. *Acta Genet* 1957;**7**:303–10.

419. Beckham JC, Krug LM, Penzien DB, et al. The relationship of ovarian steroids, headache activity and menstrual distress: a pilot study with female migraineurs. *Headache* 1992;**32**:292–7.

420. Beckman E. A celebrated case of cerebral injury. *Bull Med Hist* 1945;**17**:521–6.

421. Beede HE, Newcomb RW. Lower motor neurone paralysis in association with asthma. *Johns Hopkins Med J* 1980;**147**:186–7.

422. Beeson D, Newland C, Croxen R, et al. Congenital myasthenic syndromes. Studies of the AChR and other candidate genes. *Ann NY Acad Sci.* 1998;**841**:181–3.

423. Beeson D, Palace J, Vincent A. Congenital myasthenic syndromes. *Curr Opin Neurol* 1997;**10**:402–7.

424. Beevor CE. The cerebral arterial supply. *Brain* 1907;**30**:403.

425. Begbie J. Remarks on rheumatism and chorea: their relation and treatment. *Month J Med Sci* 1847;**7**:740–54.

426. Beghi E, Kurland LT, Mulder DW, et al. Brachial plexus neuropathy in the population of Rochester, Minnesota, 1970–1981. *Ann Neurol* 1985;**18**:320–3.

427. Behcet H. Uber rezidivierende, aphthose durch ein Virus verurasachte Geschwure am Mund, am Auge und an dem Genitalien. *Dermatol Wochenschr* 1937;**105**:1152–7.

428. Behr C. Die komplizierte, hereditar-familiare Optikusatrophie des Kindesalters. Ein bisher nicht beschriebener Symptomkomplex. *Klin Monatsbl Augenheilkd* 1909;**47**:138–60.

429. Behr C. Die Heredodegeneration der Makula. *Klin Monatsbl Augenheilkd* 1920;**65**:465–505.

430. Behrman S. Vestibular epilepsy. *Brain* 1955;**78**:471–86.

431. Behrman S. Pathology of papilledema. *Brain* 1966;**89**:1–14.

432. Beighton P, et al. Osteoglophonic dwarfism. *Pediatr Radiol* 1980;**10**:46–50.

433. Beighton PH, Hamersma H, Raad M. Oculodento-osseous dysplesia—variability of expression within a large family. *Clin Genet* 1979;**16**:169–77.

434. Bejsovec M, Kulenda Z, Ponca E. Familial intrauterine convulsions in pyridoxine dependency. *Arch Dis Child* 1967;**42**:201–7.

435. Bekhterev VM. Die Bedeutung der Sehhugel auf Grund von experimentalen und pathologischen Daten. *Virchows Arch Pathol Anat Physiol* 1887;**110**:102–54.

436. Belafsky MA, Rosman NP, Miller P, et al. Prolonged epileptic twilight state. *Neurology* 1978;**28**:239–45.

437. Belal S, Cancel G, Stevanin G, et al. Clinical and genetic analysis of a Tunisian family with autosomal dominant cerebellar ataxia type 1 linked to the SCA2 locus. *Neurology* 1994;**44**:1423–6.

437a. Bell, C. Idea for a new anatomy of the brain. London: Strahan and Preston, 1811.

438. Bell C. On the nerves: giving an account of some experiments on their structure and functions which lead to a new arrangement of the system. *Phil Trans R Soc Lond* 1821;**111**:398–424.

439. Bell C. On the motions of the eye, an illustration of the uses of the muscles and nerves of the orbit. *Phil Trans R Soc Lond* 1823;**113**:166–86.

440. Bell HS. Cruciate paralysis. *J Neurosurg* 1970;**33**:376–90.

441. Bell JA, Fielder AR, Viney S. Congenital double elevator palsy in identical twins. *J Clin Neuroophthalmol* 1990;**10**:38–40.

442. Bell R, Font RL. Granulomatous anterior uveitis caused by coccidioides immitis. *Am J Ophthalmol* 1972;**74**:93–8.

443. Bell SP, Frankel A, Brown EA. Cholesterol emboli syndrome—uncommon or unrecognized? *J R Soc Med* 1997;**90**:543–6.

444. Bell WE, Van Allen MW. Agenesis of the corpus callosum with associated facial abnormalities. *Neurology* 1959;**9**:694–8.

445. Belman AL, Lantos G, Houroupian D, et al. AIDS; Calcification of the Basal Ganglia in Infants and Children. *Neurology* 1986;**36**:1192.

446. Benbadis SR, Lancman ME, King LM, et al. Preictal pseudosleep: a new finding in psychogenic seizures. *Neurology* 1996;**47**:63–7.

447. Bender L. *A Visual Motor Gestalt Test and Its Clinical Use.* New York: American Orthopsychiatric Association, 1938.

448. Bender MB. Syndrome of isolated episode of confusion with amnesia. *J Hillside Hosp* 1956;**5**:212–5.

449. Bender MB. Oscillopsia. *Arch Neurol* 1965;**13**:204–13.

450. Bender MB, Fink M, Green M. Patterns in perception on simultaneous test of face and hand. *Arch Neurol Psychiatry* 1951;**66**:355–62.

451. Bender MB, Stacy C, Cohen J. Agraphesthesia. *J Neurol Sci* 1982;**53**:531–55.

452. Bender MD. Polyopia and monocular diplopia of cerebral origin. *Arch Neurol Psychiatry* 1945;**54**:323.

453. Benedek L. Zwangsmassig Schreien in Anfallen als postencephalitische Hyperkinese. *Z Ges Neurol Psychiatr* 1925;**98**:17–26.

454. Benedikt M. Tremblement avec paralysie croissée du moteur oculaire commun. *Bull Soc Med Hop Paris* 1889;**3**:547–8.

455. Benhaiem-Sigaux N, Gray F, Gherardi R, et al. Expanding cerebellar lacunes due to dilatation of the perivascular space associated with Binswanger's subcortical arteriosclerotic encephalopathy. *Stroke* 1987;**18**:1087–92.

456. Ben Hamida M, Belal S, Sirugo G, et al. Friedreich's ataxia phenotype not linked to chromosome 9 and associated with selective autosomal recessive vitamin E deficiency in two inbred Tunisian families. *Neurology* 1993;**43**:2179–83.

457. Ben Hamida M, Fardeau M, Attia N. Severe childhood muscular dystrophy affecting both sexes and frequent in Tunisia. *Muscle Nerve* 1983;**6**:469.

458. Bennett BM, Bong DM, Spargo BH. Neuropsychiatric problems in mixed connective tissue disease. *Am J Med* 1978;**65**:955–62.

459. Bennett DA, Wilson RS, Gilley DW, et al. Clinical diagnosis of Binswanger's disease. *J Neurol Neurosurg Psychiatry* 1990;**53**:961–5.

460. Bennett NM. Murray Valley encephalitis,1974. Clinical features. *Med J Aust* 1976;**ii**:446–50.

461. Benomar A, Le Guern E, Durr A, et al. Autosomal dominant cerebellar ataxia with retinal degeneration (ADCA type II) is genetically different from ADCA type I. *Ann Neurol* 1994;**35**:439–44.

462. Benson DF. The aphasias and related disturbances. In Baker AB, Baker LH, eds. *Clinical Neurology*, pp 1–26. New York: Harper and Row, 1971.

463. Benson DF. The third alexia. *Arch Neurol* 1977;**34**:327–31.

464. Benson DF. Neurologic correlates of anomia. In Whitaker H, ed. *Studies in Neurolinguistics*, pp 293–328. New York: Academic Press, 1979.

465. Benson DF, Davis JR, Synder BD. Posterior cortical atrophy. *Arch Neurol* 1988;**45**:789–93.

466. Benson DF, Djenderedjian A, Miller BL, et al. Neural basis of confabulation. *Neurology* 1996;**46**:1239–43.

467. Benson DF, Geschwind N. The alexias. In Vinken PJ, Bruyn GW, eds. *Handbook of Neurology*, pp 112–40. Amsterdam: North Holland Publishing, 1969.

468. Benson DF, Geschwind N. Aphasia and related disorders: a clinical approach. In Mesulam M-M, ed. *Principles of Behavioral Neurology*, pp 193–238. Philadelphia: F.A. Davis, 1985.

469. Benstead TJ, Grant IA. Charcot-Marie-Tooth disease and related inherited peripheral neuropathies. *Can J Neurol Sci* 2001;**28**:199–214.

470. Bentley JF, Smith JR. Developmental posterior enteric remnants and spinal malformations: the split notochord syndrome. *Arch Dis Child* 1960;**35**:76–86.

471. Benton AL. Differential behavioral effects in frontal lobe disease. *Neuropsychologia* 1968;**6**:53–60.

472. Benton AL. *Revised Visual Retention Test: Clinical and Experimental Applications.* New York: Psychological Corporation, 1974.

473. Benton AL. Historical notes on hemispheric dominance. *Arch Neurol* 1977;**34**:127–9.

474. Benton AL, Hamsher KDS, Varney N, et al. *Contributions to Neuropsychological Assessment.* New York: Oxford University Press, 1983.

475. Benton AL, Joynt RJ. Early descriptions of aphasia. *Arch Neurol* 1960;**3**:205–22.

476. Benton AL, Levin HS. An experimental study of 'obscuration'. *Neurology* 1972;**22:**1176–81.

477. Benton JW, Nellhaus G, Huttenlocher PR, et al. The bobble-head doll syndrome: report of a unique truncal tremor associated with third ventricular cyst and hydrocephalus in children. *Neurology* 1966;**16:** 725–9.

478. Benzer A, Mitterschliffthaler G, Marosi M, et al. Prediction of non-survival after trauma: Innsbruck coma scale. *Lancet* 1991;**338:** 977–8.

479. Beradinelli W. An undiagnosed endocrine metabolic syndrome. *J Clin Endocrinol* 1954;**14:**193.

480. Berant W, Berant N. Radioulnar synostosis and craniosynostosis syndromes. *Birth Defects* 1992;**11:**137–89.

481. Berchtold MW, Brinkmeier H, Muntener M, et al. Calcium ions in skeletal muscle: its crucial role for muscle function, plasticity and disease. *Physiol Rev* 2000;**80:**1215–65.

482. Berciano J. Olivopontocerebellar atrophy. *J Neurol Sci* 1982;**53:** 253–72.

483. Berenberg RA, Pellock JM, DiMauro S, et al. Lumping or splitting? "Ophthalmoplegia plus" or Kearns-Sayre syndrome? *Ann Neurol* 1977;**1:**37–54.

484. Beresford OD, Graham AM. Chorea gravidarum. *J Obstet Gynecol Br Empire* 1950;**57:**616–25.

485. Berg AT, Panayiotopoulos CP. Diversity in epilepsy and a newly recognized benign childhood syndrome. *Neurlogy* 2000;**55:**1073–4.

486. Berg BO, Rosenberg S, Asbury AK. Giant axonal neuropathy. *Pediatrics* 1972;**49:**894–9.

487. Berg L. Clinical dementia rating (CDR). *Psychopharmacol Bull* 1988;**24:**637.

488. Berg L. Mild senile dementia of the Alzheimer type: diagnostic criteria and natural history. *Mt Sinai J Med* 1988;**55:**87–96.

489. Berg MJ, Williams LS. The transient syndrome of headache with neurologic deficits and CSF lymphomatosis. *Neurology* 1995;**45:** 1648–54.

490. Bergara C. Un nuevo signo de paralisis facial. *Rev Espec Asoc Med Argent* 1929;**4:**556–60.

491. Berger E. Pupillary and other disturbances in tabes. *Arch Augenheilkd* 1889;**19:**305–53.

492. Berger J. Uber das Elektrenkephalogramm des Menschen. *Arch Psychiatr Nervenkr* 1929;**87:**527–70.

493. Berger J, Moser HW, Forss-Petter S. Leukodystrophies: recent developments in genetics, molecular biology, pathogenesis and treatment. *Curr Opin Neurol* 2001;**14:**305–12.

494. Berger L, Luc, Richard. L'ésthesioneuroepitheliome olfactif. *Bull Assoc Fr Etude Cancer* 1924;**13:**410–21.

495. Berger MS, Wilson CB. Epidermoid cysts of the posterior fossa. *J Neurosurg* 1985;**62:**214–9.

496. Bergia B, Sybers HD, Butler IJ. Familial lethal cardiomyopathy with mental retardation and scapulo-peroneal muscular dystrophy. *J Neurol Neurosurg Psychiatry* 1986;**49:**1423–6.

497. Bergia B, Sybers HD, Butler IJ, et al. Lethal cardiomyopathy with motor retardation and scapuloperoneal muscular dystrophy. *J Neurol Neurosurg Psychiatry* 1986;**49:**1423–6.

498. Berginer VM, Salen G, Shefer S. Cerebrotendinous xanthomatosis. *Neurol Clin* 1989;**7:**55–74.

499. Bergner M, Bobbit RA, Carter J, et al. The Sickness Impact Profile. Development and final revision of a health status measure. *Med Care* 1981;**19:**787–805.

500. Bergstedt M, Johansson S, Muller R. Hereditary spastic ataxia with central retinal degeneration and vestibular impairment. *Neurology* 1962;**12:**124–32.

501. Beri M, Klugman MR, Kohler JA, et al. Anterior ischemic optic neuropathy: VII. Incidence of bilaterality and various influencing factors. *Ophthalmology* 1987;**94:**1020–8.

502. Beric A. Central pain: "new" syndromes and their evaluation. *Muscle Nerve* 1994;**16:**1017–24.

503. Beric A, Light JK. Anorgasmia in anterior spinal cord syndrome. *J Neurol Neurosurg Psychiatry* 1993;**56:**548–51.

504. Berkovic S, Carpenter S, Andermann F, et al. Kufs' disease: a critical reappraisal. *Brain* 1988;**111:**27–62.

505. Berkovic S, et al. Progressive myoclonus epilepsies: specific causes and diagnosis. *N Engl J Med* 1986;**315:**296–305.

506. Berkovic S, McIntosh AM, Howell RA, et al. Familial temporal lobe epilepsy: a common disorder identified in twins. *Ann Neurol* 1996;**40:**227–235.

507. Berkovic SF, Scheffer IE. Genetics of the epilepsies. *Curr Opin Neurol* 1999;**12:**177–82.

508. Berkowitz BW. Matutinal vertigo: clinical characteristics and possible management. *Arch Neurol* 1985;**42:**874–7.

509. Berlin C. Congenital generalized melanoleucoderma associated with hypodontia, hypotrichosis, stunted growth, and mental retardation occurring in two brothers and two sisters. *Dermatologica* 1961; **123:**227–43.

510. Berlin L. A peroneal muscle stretch reflex. *Neurology* 1971;**21:** 1177–8.

511. Berlin R. *Eine besondere Art der Wortblindheit.* Wiesbaden: J.F. Bergmann, 1887.

512. Berlit P. Car toll neuropathy. *J Neurol Neurosurg Psychiatry* 1993;**56:**1329.

513. Berman B. Voluntary propulsion of the eyeballs. *Arch Intern Med* 1966;**117:**648.

514. Berman ER, Livni N, Shapira E, et al. Congenital corneal clouding with abnormal systemic storage bodies: a new variant of mucolipidosis. *J Pediatr* 1974;**84:**519–26.

515. Berman W, Haslam RHA, Konigsmark BW, et al. A new familial syndrome with ataxia, hearing loss, and mental retardation. *Arch Neurol* 1973;**29:**258–61.

516. Bermils C, Tassin S, Brvela J-M, et al. Idiopathic recurrent myoglobinuria and persistent weakness. *Neurology* 1983;**33:**1613–5.

517. Bernard C. Experience sur les fonctions de la portion cephalique du grand sympathique. *C R Soc Biol* 1854;**5:**77.

518. Bernard C. Des phenomenes oculo-pupillaires produits par la section du nerf sympathique cervical; ils sont independents des phenomenes vasculaires caloriques de la tete. *C R Acad Sci (Paris)* 1862; **55:**381–8.

519. Bernhardt M. Ueber isoliert im Gebiete des N. cutaneous femoris externus vorkommende Parasthesien. *Neurol Centralbl* 1895;**14:**242–4.

520. Bernstein EF, Browse NL. The CHAT classification of stroke. *Ann Surg* 1989;**209:**242–8.

521. Berrios GE. Depressive pseudodementia or melancholic dementia: a 19th century view. *J Neurol Neurosurg Psychiatry* 1985;**48:**393–400.

522. Berry H. Examination of the central portion of the visual fields at the bedside. *Br J Ophthalmol* 1963;**47:**435–40.

523. Berry H, MacDonald EA, Mrazek AC. Accessory nerve palsy: a review of 23 cases. *Can J Neurol Sci* 1991;**18:**337–41.

524. Bertola L, Pedrocca A. Oste opatie nevralgiformi lombosciatalgiche a localizzazioni vertebrali e paravertebrali (Sindrome del Camera). *Minerva Orthop* 1953;**4:**215–8.

525. Bertolotti M. Les syndromes lombo-ischialgiques d'origine vertébrale. *Rev Neurol (Paris)* 1922;**38:**1112–25.

526. Bertoni JM, Schwartzman RJ, Van Horn G, et al. Asterixis and encephalopathy following metrizamide myelography: investigations into possible mechanisms and review of the literature. *Ann Neurol* 1981;**9:**366–70.

527. Bertoni JM, von Loh S, Allen RJ. The Aicardi syndrome: report of 4 cases and review of the literature. *Ann Neurol* 1979;**5:**475–82.

528. Bertorini T, Woodhouse C, Horner L. Muscle hypertrophy secondary to the tethered cord syndrome. *Muscle Nerve* 1994;**17:**331–5.

529. Bertorini T, Yeh Y-Y, Trevisan C, et al. Carnitine palmitoyl transferase deficiency: myoglobinuria and respiratory failure. *Neurology* 1980;**30:**263–71.

530. Bertrand J. Anatomico-clinical study of Ollivier's disease. Lyon, France: Université de Lyon, 1932.

531. Besana G, Comi G, del Maschio A, et al. Electrophysiological and MRI evaluation of neurological involvement in Behçet's disease. *J Neurol Neurosurg Psychiatry* 1989;**52:**749–54.

532. Bessman SP, Baldwin R. Imidazole aminoaciduria in cerebromacular degeneration. *Science* 1962;**135:**789–91.

533. Bethlem J, Van Gool J, Hulsmann WC, Meijer AEFH. Familial non-progressive myopathy with muscle cramps after exertion. *Brain* 1966;**89:**569–88.

534. Bethlem J, Van Wijngaarden GK. The incidence of ringed fibres and sarcoplasmic masses in normal and diseased muscle. *J Neurol Neurosurg Psychiatry* 1963;**26**:326–32.

535. Bethlem J, Van Wijngaarden GK. Centronuclear myopathy with type 1 fiber atrophy and myotubes. *Arch Neurol* 1970;**23**:70–3.

536. Betz VA. Anatomischer Nachweis zweiter Gehirncentra. *Zentralbl Med Wiss* 1874;**12**:578–95.

537. Beversdorf BQ, Heilman K. Facilitatory paratonia and fromtal lobe functioning. *Neurology* 1998;**51**:968–71.

538. Bhagat K, Vallance P. Nitric oxide 9 years on. *J R Soc Med* 1996;**89**:667–73.

539. Bhandari B, Gupta BM, Garg AR. Touch epilepsy. *Indian J Pediatr* 1973;**40**:111–3.

540. Bharucha NE, Morgan-Hughes JA. Chronic focal polymyositis in the adult. *J Neurol Neurosurg Psychiatry* 1981;**44**:419–25.

541. Bhatia KP. The paroxysmal dyskinesias. *J Neurol* 1999;**246**:149–55.

542. Bhatia KP, Quinn N, Marsden CD. Clinical features and natural history of axial predominant adult onset primary dystonia. *J Neurol Neurosurg Psychiatry* 1997;**63**:788–91.

543. Bhatia KP, Soland VL, Bhatt MH, et al. Paroxysmal exercise-induced dystonia: eight new sporadic cases and a review of the literature. *Mov Disord* 1997;**12**:1007–12.

544. Bianchi E, et al. A family with Saethre-Chotzen syndrome. *Am J Med Genet* 1985;**22**:649–58.

545. Bianchi L. La sindrome parietale. *Med Ital* 1911;**9**:187,243–333.

546. Bianchine JW, Lewis RC. The MASA syndrome: a new heritable mental retardation syndrome. *Clin Genet* 1974;**21**:123–9.

547. Biary N, Cleeves L, Findley LJ, et al. Post-traumatic tremor. *Neurology* 1989;**39**:103–6.

548. Bichat MFX. Nerfs de la vie organique. In *Traité d'Anatomie Descriptive*, p 319. Paris: Masson, 1802.

549. Bicjnese AR, May W, Hickey WF, et al. Early childhood hepatocerebral degeneration misdiagnosed as valproate toxicity. *Ann Neurol* 1992;**32**:767–75.

550. Bick RL, Baker WF. Anticardiolipin antibodies and thrombosis. *Hematol Oncol Clin North Am* 1992;**6**:1287–99.

551. Bickers DS, Adams RD. Hereditary stenosis of the aqueduct of Sylvius as a cause of congenital hydrocephalus. *Brain* 1949;**72**:246–62.

552. Bickerstaff ER. Basilar artery migraine. *Lancet* 1961;**1**:15–7.

553. Bickerstaff ER, Cloake PCP. Mesencephalitis and rhombencephalitis. *BMJ* 1951;**2**:77–81.

554. Bickford RG. Sensory precipitation of seizures. *J Mich State Med Soc* 1954;**53**:1018–20.

555. Bickford RG, Billinger TW, Fleming NI, et al. The compressed spectral array (CSA): a pictorial EEG. *Proc San Diego Biomed Symp* 1972;**11**:365–70.

556. Bickford RG, Klass DW, Whelan JL, et al. Reading epilepsy: clinical and electrographic studies of a new syndrome. *Trans Am Neurol Assoc* 1956;**81**:100–2.

557. Bickford RG, Sem-Jacobsen CW, Whithe PT, et al. Some observations on the mechanism of photic and photo-metrazol activation. *Electroencephalogr Clin Neurophysiol* 1952;**4**:275–82.

558. Bickford RG, Whelan JL, Klass DW, et al. Reading epilepsy: clinical and EEG studies of a new syndrome. *Trans Am Neurol Assoc* 1956;**8**:100–2.

559. Bicknell JM, Holland JV. Neurologic manifestations of Cogan syndrome. *Neurology* 1978;**28**:278–81.

560. Bielschowsky A. Die Innervation der Musculi recti interni als Seitenwender. *Ber Dtsch Ophthalmol Ges* 1902;**30**:164–71.

561. Bielschowsky M. Uber spatinfantilefamiliare amautotische Idiotie mit Kleinhirnsymptomen. *Dtsch Z Nervenklinik* 1914;**50**:7–29.

562. Biemond A. Brachydactyly, nystagmus and cerebellar ataxia: a familial syndrome. *Ned Tschr Geneesk* 1934;**78**:1423.

563. Biemond A. Het syndroom van Laurence-Biedl en een aanverwant, nieuw syndroom. *Ned Tschr Geneesk* 1934;**78**:1801–9.

564. Biemond A. La forme radiculo-cordonalle posterieure des dégénerescences spino-cerebelleuses. *Rev Neurol (Paris)* 1954;**91**:3–21.

565. Bienvenu T, des Portes V, McDonell N, et al. Missense mutation in PAK3, R67C, causes X-linked non-specific mental retardation. *Am J Med Genet* 2000;**93**:294–8.

566. Bignami A, MacCagnami F, Zappella M, et al. Familial infantile spasms and hypsarrhythmia associated with leukodystrophy. *J Neurol Neurosurg Psychiatry* 1966;**29**:129–34.

567. Bill PLA, Cole G, Proctor NSF. Centronuclear myopathy. *J Neurol Neurosurg Psychiatry* 1979;**42**:548–56.

568. Biller J, Sand JJ, Corbett JJ, et al. Syndrome of the paramedian thalamic arteries: clinical and neuroimaging correlation. *Clin Neuroophthalmol* 1985;**5**:217 23.

569. Billiard M, Guilleminault C, Dement WC. A menstruation-linked periodic hypersomnia. *Neurology* 1975;**25**:436–43.

570. Bilous RW, Murty G, Parkinson DB, et al. Brief report: autosomal dominant familial hypoparathyroidism, sensorineural deafness and renal dyspslasia. *N Engl J Med* 1992;**327**:1069–74.

571. Binder JR, Lazar RM, Tatemichi TK, et al. Left hemiparalexia. *Neurology* 1992;**42**:562–9.

572. Bindl L, Emons D, Haverkamp F, et al. Das Megazystis-Mikrokolon-intestinale Hypoperistaltik-Syndrom: eine Neuropathie? *Z Kinderchir* 1989;**44**:249–52.

573. Bing J, Neel AV. Two cases of hyperglobulinemia with affection of the central nervous system on a toxi-infectious basis. (myelitis, polyradiculitis, spinal-fluid change). *Acta Med Scand* 1936;**88**:492–506.

574. Bing R. *Textbook of Nervous Diseases.* London: Kimpton, 1939.

575. Binnie CD, Macgillivray BB. Brain mapping—useful tool or dangerous toy? *J Neurol Neurosurg Psychiatry* 1992;**55**:527–9.

576. Binnie CD, Prior PF. Electroencephalography. *J Neurol Neurosurg Psychiatry* 1994;**57**:1308–19.

577. Binswanger OL. Die Abgrenzung der allgemeinen progressiven Paralyse. *Berl Klin Wochenschr* 1894;**31**:1103–5.

578. Biot C. Contribution to the study of Cheyne-Stokes breathing. *Lyon Med* 1876;**23**:517–28, 561–7.

579. Biousse V, Bousser M-G. The myth of carotidynia. *Neurology* 1994;**44**:993–5.

580. Biran I, Cohen O, Diment J, et al. Focal, steroid responsive myositis causing droppped head syndrome. *Muscle Nerve* 1999;**22**:769–71.

581. Birch-Machin MA, Taylor RW, Cochran B, et al. Late-onset optic atrophy, ataxia and a myopathy associated with a mutation of a complex II gene. *Ann Neurol* 2000;**48**:330–5.

582. Bird AV. Schistosomiasis of the central nervous system. In Vinken PJ, Bruyn GW, eds. *Handbook of Clinical Neurology, Vol. 35*, pp 231–41. Amsterdam: Elsevier/North Holland Biomedical Press, 1978.

583. Bird TA. Nicolaus A. Friedreich's description of peripheral facial nerve paralysis in 1798. *J Neurol Neurosurg Psychiatry* 1979;**42**:56–8.

584. Bird TD, Carlson CB, Hall JG. Familial essential (benign) chorea. *J Med Genet* 1976;**13**:357–62.

585. Bird TD, Koerker RM, Leaird BJ, et al. Lipomembranous polycystic osteodysplasia (brain, bone and fat disease): a genetic cause of presenile dementia. *Neurology* 1983;**33**:81–6.

586. Birke RN. Congenital ptosis; a classification of 200 cases. *Arch Ophthalmol* 1949;**41**:188.

587. Birnbaum G. Chronisch-progressive Chorea mit Kleinhirnatrophie. *Arch Psychiatrie (Berlin)* 1941;**114**:160–82.

588. Bischoff A, Flerz U, Regli F, et al. Fabry disease [in German]. *Fall Klin Wochenschr* 1968;**46**:666–71.

589. Bishop D. Test for reception of grammar. Manchester, UK: University of Manchester, 1990.

590. Bisno AL, Stevens DL. Streptococcal infections of skin and soft tissues. *N Engl J Med* 1996;**334**:240–5.

591. Bjerrum JP. *Vejledning i anveldesen of ojespejlet.* Copenhagen: Priors, 1890.

592. Bjornstadt R. *Pili Torti and Sensory-Neural Loss of Hearing.* Copenhagen: Scandinavian Dermatology Association, 1965.

593. Black DN, Booth F, Watters GV, et al. Leukoencephalopathy among native Indian infants in northern Quebec and Manitoba. *Ann Neurol* 1988;**24**:490–6.

594. Black DN, Watters GV, Andermann E, et al. Encephalitis among Cree children in Northern Quebec. *Ann Neurol* 1988;**24**:483–9.

595. Black DW. Pathological laughter. *J Nerv Ment Dis* 1982;**170**:67–71.

596. Black PM. Brain tumors. *N Engl J Med* 1991;**324**:1471–6.

597. Blackburn CRB, McLeod JG. CNS lesions in cystinuria. *Arch Neurol* 1977;**34**:638–9.

598. Bladin CF, Alexandrov AV, Murphy J, et al. The Toronto Stenosis Index. *Can J Neurol Sci* 1994;**21**(**Suppl 2**):S7.

599. Blanchet P. Unilateral lumbar polyradiculopathy with sympathetic features [in French]. *Presse Med* 1945;**53**:383–4.

600. Blass JP. Inborn errors of pyruvate metabolism. In Stanbury JB, Wyngaarden JB, Fredrickson DS, et al., eds. *The Metabolic Basis of Inherited Disease*, pp. 193–203. New York: McGraw-Hill, 1983.

601. Blau EB. Ectodermal dysplasia, osteosclerosis, atrial septal defect, malabsorption, neutropenia, growth and mental retardation: the Cote-Katsantoni syndrome? *Am J Med Genet* 1987;**26**:729–32.

602. Bleicher RJ, Sherman HF, Latenser BA. Bilateral gluteal compartment syndrome. *J Trauma* 1997;**42**:118–22.

603. Blessed G, Tomlinson BE, Roth M. The association between quantitative measures of dementia and of senile change in the cerebral grey matter of elderly subjects. *Br J Psychiatry* 1968;**114**:797.

604. Blethen SL, Weldon VV. Hypopituitarism and septo-optic dysplasia in first cousins. *Am J Med Genet* 1985;**21**:123–9.

604a. Bliss M. William Osler: *A Life in Medicine*. Toronto: University of Toronto Press, 1999.

605. Bloch B. Eigentumliche bisher nicht beschriebene Pigmentaffekton (Incontinentia pigmenti). *Schweiz Med Wochenschr* 1926;**56**:404–5.

606. Blocq P. Sur une affection caracterisée par de l'astasie et de l'abasie. *Arch Neurol (Paris)* 1888;**15**:24–51.

607. Bloor K. Gustatory sweating and other responses after cervicothoracic sympathectomy. *Brain* 1969;**92**:137–46.

608. Blume G, Pestronk A, Goodnough LT. Anti-MAG antibody-associated polyneuropathies. *Neurology* 1995;**45**:1577–80.

609. Blume RS, Wolff SM. The Chediak-Higashi syndrome: studies in four patients and a review of the literature. *Medicine* 1972;**51**:247–80.

610. Blume WT. Clinical and electroencephalographic correlates of the multiple independent spike foci pattern in children. *Ann Neurol* 1978;**4**:541–7.

611. Blume WT. Hemispheroic epilepsy. *Brain* 1996;**121**:1937–49.

612. Blume WT. Clinical and basic neurophysiology of generalized epilepsies. *Can J Neurol Sci* 2002;**29**:6–18.

613. Blume WT, Kaibara M. The "start-stop-start" phenomenon in subdural recordings of epileptic patients. *Neurology* 1991;**41 Suppl**:261.

614. Blumenthal HJ. Great auricular neurlgia. *Headache* 1992;**32**:413–5.

615. Blumstein SE, Alexander MP, Ryalls JH, et al. On the nature of the foreign accent syndrome: a case study. *Brain Lang* 1987;**31**:215–44.

616. Bobker DH, Deloughery TG. Natural killer cell leukemia presenting with a peripheral neuropathy. *Neurology* 1993;**43**:1853–4.

616a. Boder H, Sidgwick R. Ataxia-telangiectasia; dermatological aspects. Trans Los Angeles Derm. *Soc Arch Derm* 1958;**78**:402–5.

617. Bodian D. A new method for staining nerve fibers and nerve endings in mounted paraffin sections. *Anat Rec* 1936;**65**:89–97.

618. Bodner RA, Lynch TLL, et al. Serotonin syndrome. *Neurology* 1995;**45**:219–23.

619. Boehme DH, Cottrel JC, Leonberg SC, et al. A dominant form of neuronal ceroid lipofuscinosis. *Brain* 1971;**94**:745–60.

620. Boeri R, Passerini A. The megadolichobasilar anomaly. *J Neurol Sci* 1964;**1**:475–84.

621. Bogduk N, Marsland A. On the concept of third occipital headache. *J Neurol Neurosurg Psychiatry* 1986;**49**:775–80.

622. Bogduk N, Teasell R. Whiplash. *Arch Neurol* 2000;**57**:590–1.

623. Boghen DR, Chartrand J-P, Laflamme P, et al. Primary aberrant third nerve regeneration. *Ann Neurol* 1979;**6**:415–8.

624. Boghen DR, Glaser JS. Ischaemic optic neuropathy: the clinical profile and natural history. *Brain* 1975;**98**:689–708.

625. Bogorad FA. [A syndrome of crocodile tears]. *Vrach Delo* 1928;**11**:1328–30.

626. Bogousslavsky J, Gaio J-M, Caplan LR, et al. Encephalopathy, deafness and blindness in young women; a distinct retinocochleocerebral arteriolopathy? *J Neurol Neurosurg Psychiatry* 1989;**52**:43–6.

627. Bogousslavsky J, Kumral E, Regli F, et al. Acute hemiconcern: a right anterior parietal syndrome. *J Neurol Neurosurg Psychiatry* 1995;**58**:428–32.

628. Bogousslavsky J, Maeder P, Regli F, et al. Pure midbrain infarction. *Neurology* 1994;**44**:2032–40.

629. Bogousslavsky J, Martin R, Moulin T. Homolateral ataxia and crural paresis: a syndrome of anterior cerebral artery territory infarction. *J Neurol Neurosurg Psychiatry* 1992;**55**:1146–9.

630. Bogousslavsky J, Regli F. Response-to-next-patient-stimulation: a right hemisphere syndrome. *Neurology* 1988;**38**:1225–7.

631. Bogousslavsky J, Regli F. Capsular genu syndrome. *Neurology* 1990;**40**:1499–502.

632. Bogousslavsky J, Regli F. Centrum ovale infarcts: subcortical infarction in the superficial territory of the middle cerebral artery. *Neurology* 1992;**42**:1992–8.

633. Bogousslavsky J, Regli F, Uske A. Thalamic infarcts—clinical syndromes, etiology, and prognosis. *Neurology* 1988;**38**:837–47.

634. Bogousslavsky J, Regli F, Van Melle G, et al. Migraine stroke. *Neurology* 1988;**38**:223–7.

635. Bogousslavsky J, Regli F, Zografos L, et al. Optico-cerebral syndrome: simultaneous hemodynamic infarction of optic nerve and brain. *Neurology* 1987;**37**:263–8.

636. Bogousslavsky J, Regli F, Zogratos L, et al. Optico-cerebral syndrome. *Neurology* 1987;**37**:263–8.

637. Bohan A, Peter JB. Polymyositis and dermatomyositis. *N Engl J Med* 1975;**292**:344–7.

638. Bohan A, Peter JB, Bowman RL, et al. A computer assisted analysis of 153 patients with polymyositis and dermatomyositis. *Medicine* 1977;**56**:255–86.

639. Bohannon RW, Andrews AW. Interrater reliability of hand-held dynamometry. *Phys Ther* 1987;**67**:931–3.

640. Bohm E, Strang RR. Glossopharyngeal neuralgia. *Brain* 1962;**85**:371–88.

641. Boland RP. The neurocristopathies. *Hum Neurobiol* 1974;**5**:409–28.

642. Bolger G, Bojanic S, Sheahan N, et al. Ocular microtremor (OMT): a new neurophysiological approach to multiple sclerosis. *J Neurol Neurosurg Psychiatry* 2000;**68**:639–42.

643. Boller F. Johann Baptist Schmidt: a pioneer in the history of aphasia. *Arch Neurol* 1977;**34**:306–7.

644. Boller F, Bignolo LA. Latent sensory aphasia in hemisphere-damaged patients; an experimental study with the Token test. *Brain* 1966;**89**:815–31.

645. Boller F, Cole M, Kim Y, et al. Optic ataxia: clinical-radiological correlations with the EMI scan. *J Neurol Neurosurg Psychiatry* 1975;**38**:954–8.

646. Boller F, Keefe NC, Zoccolotti P. Luigi Galvani, body electricity and the "galvanic skin response". *Neurology* 1989;**39**:868–70.

647. Boller F, Segarra JM. Spino-pontine degeneration. *Eur Neurol* 1969;**2**:356–73.

648. Bolton CF, McFarlane RM. Human pneumatic tourniquet paralysis. *Neurology* 1978;**28**:787–93.

649. Bolton CF, Young GB, Zochodne DW. The neurological complications of sepsis. *Ann Neurol* 1993;**33**:94–100.

650. Bond MR, Pilowsky I. The subjective assessment of pain and its relationship to the administration of analgesics in patients with advanced cancer. *J Psychosom Res* 1966;**10**:203–7.

651. Bondin G, Barbizet J. D'association epilepsie-endocrinopathie. *Rev Neurol (Paris)* 1954;**91**:330–47.

652. Bonhoeffer KL. Ein Beitrag zur Localisation der Choreatischen Bewegungen. *Monatschr Psychiatr Neurol* 1897;**1**:6–41.

653. Bonkalo A. Hypersomnia, a discussion of psychiatric implication based on three cases. *Br J Psychiatry* 1968;**114**:69–75.

653a. Bonneau D, Toutain A, Laquerriere A, et al. X-linked lissencephaly with absent corpus callosum and ambiguous genitalia (XLAG): clinical, magnetic resonance imaging, and neuropathological findings. *Ann Neurol* 2002;**51**:340–9.

654. Bonnet C. *Essai analytique sur les facultés de l'ame.* Copenhagen: TA Philibert, 1760.

655. Bonnet P. Les syndromes trigeminosympathiques. *Arch Ophthalmol (Paris)* 1956;**16**:361–79.

656. Bonnet P, Dechaume J, Blanc E. L'aneurysme cirsoide de la retine (aneurysme racemeux). Ses relations avec l'aneurysme cirsoide de la face et avec l'aneurysme cirsoide du cerveau. *J Med Lyon* 1937;**18**:163–78.

657. Bonnet P, Dechaume J, Blanc E. L'aneurisme cirsoide de la retine (aneurisme racemeux) ses relations avec l'aneurisme cirsoide du cerveau. *Bull Fr Soc Ophthalmol* 1938;**51**:521–4.

658. Bonnette H, Roelofs R, Olson WH. Multicore disease: report of a case with onset in middle age. *Neurology* 1974;**24**:1039–44.

659. Bonney G. The value of axon responses in determining the site of the lesion in traction injuries of the brachial plexus. *Brain* 1954;**77**:588–609.

660. Bonnier P. Un nouveau syndrome bulbaire. *Presse Med* 1903;**11**: 174–7.

661. Booker HE, Forster FM, Klove H. Extinction factors in startle (acousticomotor) seizures. *Neurology* 1965;**15**:1095–103.

662. Boothroyd A. Developments in speech audiometry. *Sound* 1968;**2**:3.

663. Bordarier C, Aicardi J, Goutieres F. Congenital hydrocephalus and eye abnormalities with severe developmental brain defects: Warburg's syndrome. *Ann Neurol* 1984;**16**:60–5.

664. Bordini C, Antonaci F, Stovner LJ, et al. "Hemicrania continua": a clinical review. *Headache* 1991;**31**:20–6.

665. Borenstein S, Desmedt J. Local cooling in myasthenia. *Arch Neurol* 1975;**32**:1152–157.

666. Borjeson M, Forssman H, Lehmann O. An X-linked recessively inherited syndrome characterized by grave mental deficiency, epilepsy and endocrine disorder. *Acta Med Scand* 1962;**171**:13–21.

667. Born JD. The Glasgow-Liege Scale. Prognostic value and evolution of motor response and brain stem reflexes after severe head injury. *Acta Neurochir* 1988;**91**:1–11.

668. Borrett D, Becker LE. Alexander's disease. A disease of astrocytes. *Brain* 1985;**108**:367–85.

669. Borries T. Otogene encephalitis. *Z Ges Neurol Psychiatrie* 1921;**70**: 93–101.

670. Bors E. Urological aspects of rehabilitation in spinal cord Injuries. *JAMA* 1951;**146**:225–9.

671. Botez MI. [The tonic palmar reflex]. *Acta Neurol Psychiatr Belg* 1957;**57**:551–61.

672. Botez MI. Two visual systems in clinical neurology: readaptive role of the primitive system in visual agnostic patients. *Eur Neurol* 1975;**13**:101.

673. Botez MI, Serbanescu T, Vernea I. Visual static agnosia with special reference to literal agnosic alexia. *Neurology* 1964;**14**:1101–11.

674. Bots GTAM, Staal A. Amyotrophic lateral sclerosis-dementia complex, neuroaxonal dystrophy and Hallervorden Spatz disease. *Neurology* 1973;**23**:35–9.

675. Bottini G, Sterzi R, Vallar G. Directional hypokinesia in spatial neglect: a case study. *J Neurol Neurosurg Psychiatry* 1992;**55**:562–5.

676. Bouchard J-P, Barbeau A, Bouchard R, Bouchard RW. Autosomal recessive spastic ataxia of Charlevoix-Saguenay. *Can J Neurol Sci* 1978;**5**:61–9.

677. Bougneres PF, Saudubray JM, Marsac C, et al. Fasting hypoglycemia resulting from hepatic carnitine palmitoyltransferase deficiency. *J Pediatr* 1981;**98**:742–6.

678. Bouillaud JB. Récherches cliniques propres a démontrer que la perte de la parôle correspond a la lésion des lobules anteriores de cerveau. *Arch Gen Med Paris* 1825;**8**:25.

679. Bouma PAD, Westendorp RGJ, van Dijk JG, et al. The outcome of absence epilepsy: a meta-analysis. *Neurology* 1996;**47**:802–8.

680. Bour H, Tutin M, Pasquier P. The central nervous system and carbon monoxide poisoning. 1. Clinical data with reference to 20 fatal cases. *Prog Brain Res* 1967;**24**:1.

681. Bourne RB, Rorabeck CH. Compartment syndromes of the lower leg. *Clin Orthop Rel Res* 1988;**40**:97–104.

682. Bourneville DM. Contribution a l'étude de l'idiotie. *Arch Neurol (Paris)* 1880;**1**:69–91.

683. Bourneville DM, Brissaud E. Encephalite ou sclerose tubereuse des circonvolutions cérébrales. *Arch Neurol (Paris)* 1880;**1**:397–412.

684. Bourque CN, Anderson BA, del Campo CM, et al. Sensorimotor perineuritis—an autoimmune disease? *Can J Neurol Sci* 1985;**12**: 129–33.

685. Bousser M-G. Cerebral venous thrombosis: diagnosis and management. *J Neurol* 2000;**247**:252–8.

686. Bousser M-G, Chiras J, Bories J, et al. Cerebral venous thrombosis—a review of 38 cases. *Stroke* 1985;**16**:199–213.

687. Boustany RMN, et al. Autosomal dominant familial spastic paraplegia. *Neurology* 1987;**37**:910.

688. Bouwsma G, Van Wijngaarden GIC. Spinal muscular atrophy with hypertrophy of the calves. *J Neurol Sci* 1980;**44**:275–9.

689. Bowen P, Conradi GJ. Syndrome of skeletal and genitourinary anomalies with unusual facies and failure to thrive in Hutterite sibs. *Birth Defects* 1976;**12**:101–8.

690. Bowen P, et al. A familial syndrome of multiple congenital defects. *Bull Johns Hopkins Hosp* 1964;**114**:402–14.

691. Bower BD, Jeavons PM. The "happy puppet" syndrome. *Arch Dis Child* 1967;**42**:298–302.

692. Bower JH, Hammack JE, McDonnell SK, et al. The neurological complications of B-cell chronic lymphocytic leukemia. *Neurology* 1997;**48**:407–12.

693. Bower S, Dennis M, Warlow C, et al. Long-term prognosis of transient lone bilateral blindness in adolescents and young adults. *J Neurol Neurosurg Psychiatry* 1994;**57**:734–6.

694. Boyd Y, Buckle VJ. Cytogenetic heterogeneity of translocations associated with Duchenne muscular dystrophy. *Clin Genet* 1986;**29**: 108–15.

695. Boylan KB, Ferriero DM, Greco CM, et al. Congenital hypomyelination neuropathy with arthrogryposis multiplex. *Ann Neurol* 1992;**31**:337–40.

696. Boyle RS, Shakir RA, Weir AI, McInnes A. Inverted knee jerk: a neglected localising sign in spinal cord disease. *J Neurol Neurosurg Psychiatry* 1979;**42**:1005–7.

697. Braakhekke JP, Bruin MId, Stegeman DF, et al. The second wind phenomenon in McArdle's disease. *Brain* 1986;**109**:1087–101.

698. Brackstone M, Patterson SD, Kertesz A. Triple E syndrome: bilateral locked posterior fracture dislocation of the shoulders. *Neurology* 2001;**56**:1403–4.

699. Bradley WG, Chad DA, Verghese JP, et al. Painful lumbosacral plexopathy with elevated erythrocyte sedimentation rate: a treatable inflammatory syndrome. *Ann Neurol* 1984;**15**:457–64.

700. Bradley WG, Fewings JD, Cumming WJK, et al. Delayed myeloradiculopathy produced by spinal irradiation in the rat. *J Neurol Sci* 1977;**31**:51.

701. Bradley WG, Hudgson P, Gardner-Medwin D, et al. The syndrome of myosclerosis. *J Neurol Neurosurg Psychiatry* 1973;**36**:651–60.

702. Bradley WG, Madrid R, Thrush DC. Recurrent brachial plexus neuropathy. *Brain* 1975;**98**:381–98.

703. Braham J, Sadeh M, Sarova-Pinhas I. Skin wrinkling on immersion of hands: a test of sympathetic function. *Arch Neurol* 1979;**36**: 113–4.

704. Braheny, S. Hangman's vs non-hangman's fracture. Personal communication, 1993.

705. Braille L. Procéde pour écrire au moyen des points. Paris: 1837.

706. Brain WR. On the rotated or "cerebellar" posture of the head. *Brain* 1926;**49**:61–76.

707. Brain WR. Visual disorientation with special reference to lesions of the right cerebral hemisphere. *Brain* 1941;**64**:244–72.

708. Brain WR. The physiological basis of consciousness. *Brain* 1958;**81**:426–55.

709. Brain WR, Curran RD. The grasp-reflex of the foot. *Brain* 1932;**55**:347–56.

710. Brain WR, Northfield D, Wilkinson M. The neurological manifestations of cervical spondylosis. *Brain* 1952;**75**:187–225.

711. Brain WR, Wilkinson M. Subacute cerebellar degeneration associated with neoplasms. *Brain* 1965;**88**:465–78.

712. Brais B. The third left frontal convolution plays no role in language: Pierre Marie and the Paris debate on aphasia (1906–1908). *Neurology* 1992;**42**:690.

713. Brait K, Fahn S, Schwarz GA. Sporadic and familial parkinsonism and motor neurone disease. *Neurology* 1973;**23**:990–1002.

714. Bramwell B. *The Diseases of the Spinal Cord.* Edinburgh: Maclachlan and Stewart, 1882.

715. Brancatelli G, Lagalla R. Reversal sign after cardiopulmonary arrest. *J Neurol Neurosurg Psychiatry* 2000;**68**:525.

716. Branch LG, Meyers AR. Assessing physical function in the elderly. *Clin Geriatr Med* 1987;**3**:29–51.

717. Branconnier RJ. A computerized battery for behavioural assessment in Alzheimer's disease. In Poon LW, Crook T, Davis KL, et al., eds. *Handbook for Clinical Memory Assessment in Older Adults*, pp 189–96. Washington, DC: American Psychological Association, 1986.

718. Brandel J-P, Delasnerie-Lauprêtre N, Laplanche J-P, et al. Diagnosis of Creutzfeldt-Jakob disease. *Neurology* 2000;**54**:1095–9.

719. Brandt IK, Hsia YE, Clement DH, et al. Proprionic acidemia (ketotic hyperglycinemia). *Pediatrics* 1974;**53**:391–5.

720. Brandt J. The Hopkins Verbal Learning Test. Development of a new memory test with six equivalent forms. *Clin Psychol* 1991;**5**:125–42.

721. Brandt NJ. Symptoms and signs in organic acidurias. *J Inherit Metab Dis* 1984;**Suppl 1**:23–7.

722. Brandt NJ, Brandt S, Christensen E, et al. Glutamic aciduria in progressive choreo-athetosis. *Clin Genet* 1978;**13**:77–80.

723. Brandt NJ, Terenius L, Jacobsen BB, et al. Hyper-endorphin syndrome in a child with necrotizing encephalomyelopathy. *N Engl J Med* 1980;**303**:914–6.

724. Brandt S, Carlsen N, Glenting P, et al. Encephalopathia myoclonica infantilis (Kinsbourne) and neuroblastoma in children. A report of three cases. *Dev Med Child Neurol* 1974;**16**:286–94.

725. Brandt T. Phobic postural vertigo. *Neurology* 1996;**46**:1515–9.

726. Brandt T, Bronstein AM. Cervical vertigo. *J Neurol Neurosurg Psychiatry* 2001;**71**:8–12.

727. Brandt T, Daroff RB. The multisensory physiological and pathological vertigo syndromes. *Ann Neurol* 1980;**7**:195–203.

728. Brashear A, DeLeon D, Bressman SB, et al. Rapid-onset dystonia-parkinsonism in a second family. *Neurology* 1997;**48**:1066–9.

729. Bray PF, Bale JF, Anderson RE. Progressive neurological disease associated with chronic cytomegalovirus infection. *Ann Neurol* 1981;**9**:499–502.

730. Brazis PW, Masdeu JC, Biller J. *Localization in Clinical Neurology.* Boston: Little, Brown, 1990.

731. Brazis PW, Volger JB, Shaw KE. The "numb cheek–limp lower lid" syndrome. *Neurology* 1991;**41**:327–8.

732. Breathnach CS. Sir Gordon Holmes. *Med Hist* 1975;**19**:194–200.

733. Bregeat P, Juge P, Pouliquen Y, et al. A propos d'une angiomatose orbito-thalamencéphalique. *Bull Fr Soc Ophthalmol* 1958;581–94.

734. Bremer FW. On the etiology of syringomyelia and the dysraphic state. *Dtsch Klin Nervenheilk* 1926;**95**:1–103.

735. Bremer FW. Cerveau isolé et physiologie du sommeil. *C R Soc Biol* 1935;**118**:1235–41.

736. Brenner RP, Atkinson R. Generalised paroxysmal fast activity: electroencephalographic and clinical features. *Ann Neurol* 1982;**11**:386–90.

737. Bresolin N, Miranda A, Chang HW, et al. Phosphoglycerate kinase deficiency myopathy. *Muscle Nerve* 1984;**5**:542–55.

738. Bressman S. Dystonia. *Curr Opin Neurol Neurosurg* 1998;**11**:363–72.

739. Bressman S, Fahn S. Essential myoclonus. *Adv Neurol* 1986;**43**:287–94.

739a. Bret P, Guyotat J, Chazal J. Is normal pressure hydrocephalus a valid concept in 2002? A reappraisal in five questions and proposal for a new designation of the syndrome as "chronic hydrocephalus". *J Neurol Neurosurg Psychiatry* 2002;**73**:9–12.

740. Brett EM. On a particular mode of onset of epilepsy in childhood. *J Neurol Sci* 1967;**4**:315–38.

741. Brewerton DA, Sandifer PH, Sweetnam DR. Idiopathic pes cavus. *BMJ* 1963;**1**:659–61.

742. Brey RL. Antiphospholipid antibodies and ischemic stroke. *Heart Dis Stroke* 1992;**1**:379–82.

743. Brice JEH. Congenital varicella resulting from infection during second trimester of pregnancy. *Arch Dis Child* 1976;**51**:474–6.

744. Brickner RM. Oscillopsia: a new symptom commonly occurring in multiple sclerosis. *Arch Neurol Psychiatry* 1936;**36**:586–9.

745. Bright R. Fatal epilepsy, from suppuration between the dura mater and arachnoid in consequence of blood having been effused in that situation. *Guys Hosp Rep* 1836;**1**:36–40.

746. Brill AA. Piblokto or hysteria among Peary's Eskimos. *J Nerv Ment Dis* 1913;**40**:514–20.

747. Brinker KR, Paulson G, Monath TP, et al. St. Louis encephalitis in Ohio, September 1975. Clinical and EEG studies in 16 cases. *Arch Intern Med* 1979;**139**:561–6.

748. Brinkman C. Lesions in supplementary motor area interfere with a monkey's performance of a bimanual co-ordination task. *Neurosci Lett* 1981;**27**:267.

749. Brinkmann R, Von Cramon D, Schultz H. The Munich Coma Scale (MCS). *J Neurol Neurosurg Psychiatry* 1976;**39**:788–93.

750. Briquet P. Traité clinique et thérapeutique de l'hysteria. B. Baillhèveertils: Paris, 1859.

751. Brissaud E. La chorée variable des dégénérés. *Rev Neurol (Paris)* 1896;**4**:417–31.

752. Brissaud E. L'infantilisme vrai. *Nouv Icon Salpet* 1907;**20**:1–17.

753. Brissaud E. La sinistrose. *Bull Med Chir Accid Trav* 1908;**2**:97–109.

754. Brissaud E, Lereboullet P. Deux cas d'hemicraniose. *Rev Neurol (Paris)* 1903;**11**:37–40.

755. Brissaud E, Marie P. De la déviation faciale dans l'hémiplegie hysterique. *Prog Med (Paris)* 1887;**15**:84,128–85, 131.

756. Brissaud E, Sicard JA. L'hemispasme facial alterne. *Presse Med* 1908;**16**:234–6.

757. Brissaud EA, Sicard J. Type special de syndrome alterne. *Rev Neurol (Paris)* 1908;**16**:86.

758. Brissaud EW. Spasmodic laughing and crying. *Rev Sci Paris* 1894;**1**:38–46.

759. Britton JW, Uitti RJ, Ahlskog JE, et al. Hereditary late-onset chorea without significant dementia. *Neurology* 1995;**45**:443–7.

760. Broadbent DE, Cooper PF, FitzGerald P, et al. The cognitive failures questionnaire and its correlates. *Br J Clin Psychol* 1982;**21**:1–16.

761. Broadbent W. Hughlings Jackson as pioneer in nervous physiology and pathology. *Brain* 1903;**26**:305–66.

762. Broadbent WH. On ingravescent apoplexy. *Proc R Med Chir Soc* 1876;**8**:103–8.

763. Broca P-P. Remarques sur le siège de la faculté du language articulé, suivie d'une observation d'aphemie (perte de la parôle). *Bull Soc Anat Paris* 1861;**36**:330–57.

764. Broca P-P. Sur le siége de la faculté de language articule. *Bull Soc Anthrop Paris* 1865;**6**:398–407.

765. Brockmann K, Wang D, Korenke CG, et al. Autosomal dominant Glut-1 deficiency syndrome and familial epilepsy. *Ann Neurol* 2001;**50**:476–85.

766. Brody IA. Muscle contracture induced by exercise: a syndrome attributed to decreased relaxation factor. *N Engl J Med* 1969;**2821**:187–92.

767. Brogna CG, Lee SI, Dreifuss FE. Pilomotor seizures: magnetic resonance imaging and electroencephalographic localization of originating focus. *Arch Neurol* 1986;**43**:1085–6.

768. Bromberg MB. Comparison of electrodiagnostic criteria for primary demyelination in chronic polyneuropathy. *Muscle Nerve* 1991;**14**:968–76.

769. Bronstein AM. Visual vertigo syndrome: clinical and posturography findings. *J Neurol Neurosurg Psychiatry* 1995;**59**:472–6.

770. Bronstein AM, Gresty MA, Mossman SS. Pendular pseudonystagmus arising as a combination of head tremor and vestibular failure. *Neurology* 1992;**42**:1527–31.

771. Bronstein AM, Hood JD. The cervico-ocular reflex in normal subjects and patients with absent vestibular function. *Brain Res* 1986;**373**:399–408.

772. Brooke MH. Congenital fiber type disproportion. In Kakulas BA, ed. *Proceedings of the 2nd International Congress on Muscle Diseases, Perth, Australia, Part 2*, pp 147–59. Amsterdam: Excerpta Medica, 1973.

773. Brooke MH. *A Clinician's View of Neuromuscular Diseases.* Baltimore: Williams & Wilkins, 1986.

774. Brooke MH, Carroll JE, Davis JE, et al. The prolonged exercise test. *Neurology* 1979;**29**:636–43.

775. Brooke MH, et al. Clinical investigation in Duchenne dystrophy: 2. Determination of the "power" of therapeutic trials based on the natural history. *Muscle Nerve* 1983;**6**:91–103.

776. Brooke MH, King-Engel W. Histological biopsy with regard to fiber types. *Neurology* 1969;**19**:591–605.

777. Brooke MH, Miller R. Fatigue testing. *Muscle Nerve* 1990;**S13**:S35–S37.

778. Brooke MH, Neville HE. Reducing body myopathy. *Neurology* 1972;**22**:829–40.

779. Brookeman JR. MRI: physical principles and glossary. *Va Med* 1986;**113**:343–6.

780. Brooks DJ. PET: its clinical role in neurology. *J Neurol Neurosurg Psychiatry* 1991;**54**:1–5.

781. Brooks JSJ, Freeman M, Enterline HT. Malignant triton tumours. *Cancer* 1985;**55**:2543–9.

782. Brossard J. Clinical study of a Hereditary type of progressive muscular atrophy beginning in the legs [in French]. Paris: Université de Paris, 1886.

783. Broughton R, Tolentino M, Krelina M. Fragmentary pathological myoclonus in NREM sleep: a report of 38 cases. *Electroencephalogr Clin Neurophysiol* 1985;**61**:123–33.

784. Broughton RJ. Pathological fragmentary myoclonus, intensified "hypnic jerks' and hypnagogic foot tremor: three unusual sleep-related disorders. In Koella WP, Obal F, Schulz H, et al., eds. *Sleep 1986*, pp 240–3. Stuttgart: Fischer Verlag, 1988.

785. Broughton RJ. Sleep attacks, naps, and sleepiness in medical disorders. In Dinges DF, Broughton RJ, eds. *Sleep and Alertness: Chronological, Behavioral, and Medical Aspects of Napping*, pp 267–98. New York: Raven Press, 1989.

786. Broughton RJ, Hasan J, Dunham W. Anterior slow alpha of drowsiness EEG patterns do not represent the alpha rhythm. *Can J Neurol Sci* 1994;**21**(**Suppl 2**):S30.

787. Brousolle E, Tommasi M, Mauguiere F, et al. Progressive anarthria with secondary parkinsonism: a clinicopathological case report. *J Neurol Neurosurg Psychiatry* 1992;**55**:577–80.

788. Brouwer OF, Padberg GW, Ruys CJM, et al. Hearing loss in facioscapulohumeral muscular dystrophy. *Neurology* 1991;**41**:1878–81.

789. Brown CL, Symmers D. Acute serous encephalitis. A newly recognized disease of children. *Am J Dis Child* 1925;**29**:174–81.

790. Brown GC, Shields JA, Patty BE, et al. Congenital pits of the optic nerve head. *Arch Ophthalmol* 1979;**97**:1341–4.

791. Brown GK, Scholem RD, Croll HB, et al. Sulfite oxidase deficiency: clinical, neuroradiologic and biochemical features in two new patients. *Neurology* 1989;**39**:252–7.

792. Brown J, Lantos P, Stratton M, et al. Familial progressive supranuclear palsy. *J Neurol Neurosurg Psychiatry* 1993;**56**:473–6.

793. Brown JA, Braun MA, Namey TC. Pyriformis syndrome in a 10–year old boy. *Neurosurgery* 1988;**23**:117–9.

794. Brown JR. The early years of the American Academy of Neurology. *Neurology* 1974;**24**:1–9.

795. Brown JW, Podosin R. A syndrome of the neural crest. *Arch Neurol* 1966;**15**:294–301.

796. Brown M, Asbury AK. Diabetic neuropathy. *Ann Neurol* 1984;**15**:2–12.

797. Brown P, Marsden CD. The stiff man and stiff man plus syndromes. *J Neurol* 1999;**246**:648–52.

798. Brown P, Rothwell JC. New observations on the normal auditory startle reflex in man. *Brain* 1991;**114**:1891–902.

799. Brown P, Rothwell JC, Marsden CD. The stiff leg syndrome. *J Neurol Neurosurg Psychiatry* 1997;**62**:31–7.

800. Brown RA, Lawson DA, Leslie GC, et al. Does the Wartenberg Pendulum Test differentiate quantitatively between spasticity and rigidity? A study in elderly stroke and parkinsonian patients. *J Neurosurg Psychiatry* 1988;**51**:1178–86.

801. Brown RA, Lawson DA, Leslie GC, et al. Observations on the applicability of the Wartenberg Pendulum test to healthy elderly subjects. *J Neurol Neurosurg Psychiatry* 1988;**51**:1171–7.

802. Brown RG, Jahanshahi M, Marsden CD. The execution of bimanual movements in patients with Parkinson's, Huntington's and cerebellar disease. *J Neurol Neurosurg Psychiatry* 1993;**56**:295–7.

803. Brown RJ, Trimble MR. Dissociative psychopathology, nonepileptic seizures and neurology. *J Neurol Neurosurg Psychiatry* 2000;**69**:285–91.

804. Brown WF, Yates SK. Percutaneous localization of conduction abnormalities in human entrapment neuropathies. *Can J Neurol Sci* 1982;**9**:391–400.

805. Browne CD, Nolan BM, Faithfull DK. Occupational repetition strain injuries: guidelines for diagnosis and management. *Med J Aust* 1984;**140**:329–332.

806. Browne F, Bayer JF. Familial nephrosis associated with deafness and urinary tract anomalies in siblings. *J Pediatr* 1962;**60**:33.

807. Browne TR, Mirsky AF. Absence (petit mal) seizures. In Browne TR, Feldman RG, eds. *Epilepsy, Diagnosis and Management*, pp 61–74. Boston: Little, Brown, 1983.

808. Brownell AKW, Severson DL, Thompson CD. Cold-induced rhabdomyolysis in carnitine palmitoyl transferase deficiency. *Can J Neurol Sci* 1979;**6**:367–70.

809. Brown-Sequard CE. De la transmission croisée des impressions sensitives par la moelle épinière. *C R Soc Biol* 1850;**2**:33–4.

810. Brudzinski J. Un signe nouveau sur les membres inferieurs dans les meningites chez les enfants. *Arch Med Enf Paris* 1909;**12**:745.

811. Brudzinski J. A new symptom of tuberculous meningitis and irritation in children. *Berl Klin Wochenschr* 1916;**53**:686–90.

812. Brugger P, Agosti R, Regard MN, et al. Heautoscopy, epilepsy and suicide. *J Neurophysiol* 1994;**57**:838–9.

813. Brumback RA, Staton RD, Susaq ME. Exercise-induced pain, stiffness and tubular aggregation in skeletal muscle. *J Neurol Neurosurg Psychiatry* 1981;**44**:250–4.

814. Brun A, Englund B, Mann DMA, Neary D, et al. Consensus on clinical and neuropathological criteria for fronto-temporal dementia. *J Neurol Neurosurg Psychiatry* 1994;**57**.

815. Bruni J, Bilbao JM, Pritzker KP, et al. Myopathy associated with amyloid. *Can J Neurol Sci* 1977;**4**:77–9.

816. Bruns L. Gait disorders in frontal lobe tumors. *Dtsch Med Wochenschr* 1892;**18**:138–40.

817. Bruns L. Neuropathologische Demonstrationen. *Neurol Zentralbl* 1902;**21**:561–7.

818. Bruns L, Cramer A, Ziehen T. *Handbuch der Nervenkrankheiten im Kindesalter*. Berlin: S. Karger, 1912.

819. Brushfield T. Mongolism. *Br J Dis Child* 1924;**21**:241–58.

820. Brushfield T, Wyatt W. Hemiplegia associated with extensive naevus and mental defect. *Br J Dis Child* 1927;**24**:98–106.

821. Brust JCM. Music and language. *Brain* 1980;**103**:367–92.

822. Brust JCM, Behrens MM. Release hallucinations as the major symptom of posterior cerebral artery occlusion. *Ann Neurol* 1977;**2**:432–6.

823. Brust JCM, List TA, Catalaro LW, et al. Ocular myasthenia gravis mimicking progressive external ophthalmoplegia. *Neurology* 1974;**24**:755–60.

824. Bruyn GW, Staathof LJA, Raymakers GMJ. Mollaret's meningitis: differential diagnosis and diagnostic pitfalls. *Neurology* 1962;**12**:745–53.

825. Bruyn GW, Vielvoye GJ, Went LJ. Hereditary spastic dystonia: a new mitochondrial encephalopathy? *J Neurol Sci* 1991;**103**:195–202.

826. Bryceson ADM, Parry EHO, Perine PL, et al. Louse-borne relapsing fever. A clinical and laboratory study of 62 cases and a reconsideration of the literature. *Q J Med* 1970;**39**:129–70.

828. Buchman AS, Garron DC, Trost-Cardamone JE, et al. Word deafness: one hundred years later. *J Neurol Neurosurg Psychiatry* 1986;**49**:489–99.

829. Buckley DJ, Hall MS, Penney S. Shuddering attacks mimicking infantile spasms. *Can J Neurol Sci* 1994;**21**(**Suppl 2**):S33–S34.

830. Budd MA, Tanaka K, Holmes LB, et al. Isovaleric acidemia. *N Engl J Med* 1967;**277**:321–7.

831. Budka H. Cerebral pathology in AIDS. *Curr Opin Neurol Neurosurg* 1992;**5**:917–23.

832. Bull JWD, Nixon WLB, Pratt RTC. The radiological criteria and familial occurrence of primary basilar impression. *Brain* 1955;**78**:229–47.

833. Bullard DE. Diencephalic seizures: responsiveness to bromocriptine and morphine. *Ann Neurol* 1987;**21**:609–11.

834. Bundey S. A genetic study of infantile and juvenile myasthenia gravis. *J Neurol Neurosurg Psychiatry* 1972;**35**:41–51.

835. Bundey S, Griffiths MI. Recurrent risks of families of children with symmetrical spasticity. *Dev Med Child Neurol* 1977;**19**:179–81.

836. Bundey S, Harrison MJG, Marsden CD. A genetic study of torsion dystonia. *J Med Genet* 1975;**12**:12–19.

837. Burde RM. Amaurosis fugax. *J Clin Neuroophthalmol* 1989;**9**:185–9.

838. Burger PC, Vogel FS, Green SB, et al. Glioblastoma multiforme and anaplastic astrocytoma: pathologic criteria and prognostic implications. *Cancer* 1985;**56**:1106–011.

839. Burke D, Andrews CJ, Lance JW. Tonic vibration reflex in spasticity, Parkinson's disease, and normal subjects. *J Neurol Neurosurg Psychiatry* 1972;**35**:477–86.

840. Burke RE, Brin MF, Fahn S, et al. Analysis of the clinical course of non-Jewish, autosomal dominant torsion dystonia. *Mov Disord* 1986;**1**:163–78.

841. Burke RE, Fahn S, Jankovic J, et al. Tardive dystonia: late-onset and persistent dystonia caused by antipsychotic drugs. *Neurology* 1982;**32**:1335–46.

842. Burke RE, Fahn S, Marsden CD, et al. Validity and reliability of a rating scale for the primary torsion dystonias. *Neurology* 1985;**35**:73–7.

843. Burke RE, Kang UJ, Fahn S. Tardive akathisia: motor phenomena and treatment. *Neurology* 1987;**37**(Suppl):124–5.

844. Burneo JG, Shatz R, Nikolaoa IH, et al. Amusement park stroke. *Neurology* 2000;**55**:564–5.

845. Burnett C, Commons RR, Albright F, et al. Hypercalcemia without hypercalciuria or hypophosphatemia, calcinosis and renal insufficiency: a syndrome following prolonged intake of milk and alkali. *N Engl J Med* 1949;**240**:787–94.

846. Burnham HH. Anterior ethmoidal nerve syndrome; referred pain and headache from lateral nasal wall. *Arch Otolaryngol* 1949;**50**:640–6.

847. Burnier LR. A new hypophysial syndrome. *Ann Ophthalmol* 1912;**21**:263–73.

848. Burns FS. A case of generalised congenital erythroderma. *J Cutan Dis* 1915;**32**:255.

849. Burns RJ, Bretag AH, Blumbergs PC, et al. Benign familial disease with muscle mounding and rippling. *J Neurol Neurosurg Psychiatry* 1994;**57**:344–7.

850. Burton MJ, Brochwitz-Lewinski M. L. Frey and the auriculotemporal syndrome. *J R Soc Med* 1991;**84**:619–20.

851. Burwell CS, Robin ED, Whaley RD, Bickemann AG. Extreme obesity associated with alveolar hypoventilation—a Pickwickian syndrome. *Am J Med* 1956;**21**:811.

852. Buschke F. Selective reminding for analysis of memory and learning. *J Verb Learn Verb Behav* 1973;**12**:543–50.

853. Buschke H. Cued recall in amnesia. *J Clin Neuropsychol* 1984;**6**:433–40.

854. Buschke H, Kuslansky G, Katz M, et al. Screening for dementia witrh the Memory Impairment Screen. *Neurology* 1999;**52**:231–8.

855. Butinar D, Zidar J, Leonardis L, et al. Hereditary auditory, vestibular, motor and sensory neuropathy in a Slovenian Roma (Gypsy) kindred. *Ann Neurol* 1999;**46**:36–44.

856. Butterworth B, Warrington EK. Two routes to repetition: evidence from a case of 'deep dysphasia'. *Neurocase* 1995;**1**:55–66.

857. Butterworth T, Strean LP. The ichthyosiform genodermatosis. *Postgrad Med J* 1965;**37**:175.

858. Buzzard T. On the simulation of hysteria by organic disease of the nervous system. *Brain* 1890;**13**:1–44.

859. Bynke O, Hillman J. Role of transsphenoidal operation in the management of pituitary adenomas with surasellar extension. *Arch Neurochir* 1989;**100**:50–5.

860. Byrne E, Thomas PK, Zilkha KJ. Familial extrapyramidal disease with polyneuropathy. *J Neurol Neurosurg Psychiatry* 1982;**45**:372–4.

861. Byrne E, White O, Cook M. Familial dystonic choreoathetosis with myokymia: a sleep responsive disorder. *J Neurol Neurosurg Psychiatry* 1991;**54**:1090–2.

862. Byrne EJ. Diffuse Lewy body disease: clinical features in 15 cases. *J Neurol Neurosurg Psychiatry* 1989;**52**:709–17.

863. Bywaters EGL. The Cheshire cat syndrome. *Postgrad Med J* 1968;**44**:19–22.

864. Bywaters EGL, Beall D. Crush injuries with impairment of renal function. *BMJ* 1941;**1**:427–32.

865. Caffey J. The whiplash–shaken infant syndrome. *Pediatrics* 1974;**54**:396–403.

867. Caffey J, Silverman WA. Infantile cortical hyperostosis. *AJR Am J Roentgenol* 1945;**54**:1–16.

868. Caine D, Halliday GM, Kril JJ, et al. Operational criteria for the classification of chronic alcoholics: identification of Wernicke's encephalopathy. *J Neurol Neurosurg Psychiatry* 1997;**62**:51–60.

869. Cairns H. Surgical aspects of meningitis. *BMJ* 1949;**1**:969–76.

870. Cairns H, Oldfield RC, Pennybacker JB, Whitteridge D. Akinetic mutism with an epidermoid cyst of the 3rd ventricle. *Brain* 1941;**64**:273–90.

871. Calabrese LO, Mallek JA. Primary angiitis of the central nervous system. Report of 8 new cases, review of the literature, and proposal for diagnostic criteria. *Medicine* 1988;**67**:20–39.

872. Calabresi PA, Silvestri G, DiMauro S, et al. Ekbom's syndrome: lipomas, ataxia, and neuropathy with MERRF. *Muscle Nerve* 1994;**17**:943–5.

872a. Call GK, Fleming MC, Sealfon S, et al. Reversible cerebral segmental vasoconstriction. *Stroke*. 1988;**19**:1159–70.

873. Calleja J, Carpizo R, Berciano J. Orgasmic epilepsy. *Epilepsia* 1988;**29**:635–9.

874. Calne DB, Pallis CA. Vibratory sense: a critical review. *Brain* 1966;**89**:723–46.

875. Calne DB, Snow BJ, Lee C. Criteria for diagnosing Parkinson's disease. *Ann Neurol* 1992;**32**:S125–S127.

876. Calvert RJ, Caplin G. The Houssay syndrome. *BMJ* 1957;**2**:71–4.

877. Cambier J, Dehen H. Imitation synkinesia and sensory control of movement. *Neurology* 1977;**27**:646–9.

878. Camfield PR, Metrakos K, Andermann F. Basilar migraine, seizures, and severe epileptiform EEG abnormalities. *Neurology* 1978;**28**:584–8.

879. Camins MB, Mount LA. Primary suprasellar atypical teratoma. *Brain* 1974;**97**:447.

880. Campbell AMG, Rosenberg LE, Snodgrass PJ, et al. Orthinine transcarbamylase deficiency: a cause of lethal neonatal hyperammonemia in males. *N Engl J Med* 1973;**288**:1–6.

881. Campbell AMG, Williams CR, Barltrop D. Motor neurone disease and exposure to lead. *J Neurol Neurosurg Psychiatry* 1970;**33**:877–85.

882. Campbell WW. The numb cheek syndrome: a sign of infraorbital neuropathy. *Neurology* 1986;**36**:421–3.

883. Campbell WW. Ulnar neuropathy at the elbow. *Muscle Nerve* 2000;**23**:450–2.

884. Campbell WW, Buschbacher R, Pridgeon RM, et al. Selective finger drop in cervical radiculopathy: the pseudopseudoulnar claw hand. *Muscle Nerve* 1995;**18**:108–10.

885. Camponovo F, Meier C. Neuropathy of vasculitic origin in a case of Garin-Boujadoux-Bannwarth syndrome with positive borrelia antibody response. *J Neurol* 1986;**233**:69–72.

886. Canadian Medical Association. Eating disorders: anorexia nervosa and bulimia. Ottawa, Canada: Dept. of Communications and Government Relations, 1989.

887. Canavan M. Schilder's encephalitis periaxalis diffusa. Report of a case in a child aged sixteen and one-half months. *Arch Neurol* 1931;**25**:299–308.

888. Cancilla PA, Kalyanaraman K, Verity MA, et al. Familial myopathy with probably lysis of myofibrils in type 1 fibre. *Neurol Minneap* 1971;**21**:579–85.

889. Canter GJ, De la Torre R, Mier M. A method for evaluating disability in Parkinson disease. *J Nerv Ment Dis* 1961;**133**:143–7.

890. Cantu JM, et al. Autosomal recessive microcephaly associated with chorioretinopathy. *Hum Genet* 1977;**36**:243–7.

891. Cantwell RJ. Congenital sensorineural deafness associated with onycho-osteodystrophy and mental retardation. *Humangenetik* 1975;**26**:261–5.

892. Capetto JR, et al. A syndrome of arterial occlusive retinopathy and encephalopathy. *Am J Ophthalmol* 1984;**98**:189–202.

893. Capgras J. L'illusion des "sosies" dans une délire systematisée chronique. *Ann Med Psychol* 1923;**81**:186.

894. Capistrant TD, Gumnit RJ. Thermography and extracranial vascular disease. *Arch Neurol* 1970;**22**:499–503.

895. Caplan LR. Ptosis. *J Neurol Neurosurg Psychiatry* 1974;**37**:1–7.

896. Caplan LR. "Top of the basilar" syndrome. *Neurology* 1980;**30**:72–9.

897. Caplan LR. Bilateral distal vertebral artery occlusion. *Neurology* 1983;**33**:552–8.

898. Caplan LR. TGA criteria: what's in a name? *Neurology* 1986;**36**:1625.

899. Caplan LR. Intracranial branch atheromatous disease. *Neurology* 1989;**39:**1246–50.

900. Caplan LR. Charles Foix—the first modern stroke neurolgist. *Stroke* 1990;**21:**348–56.

901. Caplan LR. Binswanger's disease revisited. *Neurology* 1995;**45:** 626–33.

902. Caplan LR, Gorelick PB. "Salt and pepper on the face" pain in acute brainstem ischemia. *Ann Neurol* 1983;**13:**344–7.

903. Carfi J, Ma DM. Posterior interosseous syndrome revisited. *Muscle Nerve* 1985;**8:**499–502.

904. Carleton A, Biggs R. Diffuse mesodermal pigmentation with cranial abnormality. *Br J Dermatol* 1948;**60:**102.

905. Carmel PW. Tumors of the third ventricle. *Acta Neurochir* 1985;**75:**136–46.

906. Carney JA, Bianco AJ jr, Sizemore GW, et al. Multiple endocrine neoplasia with skeletal manifestations. *J Bone Jt Surg* 1981;**63:**405–10.

907. Carney JA, Gordon H, Carpenter PC, et al. The complex of myxomas, spotty pigmentation, and endocrine overactivity. *Medicine* 1985;**64:**270–83.

908. Carney LR. The dimple sign in peroneal palsy. *Neurology* 1967;**17:** 922.

909. Carney RG jr. Incontinentia pigmenti. *Arch Dermatol* 1976;**112:** 535–42.

910. Carol WL, Godfried EG, Prakken JR, et al. v. Recklinghausensche Neurofibromatosis, Atrophodermia vermiculata und kongenitale Herzanomalie als Hauptkennizeichen eines familiar-hereditaren Syndroms. *Dermatologica* 1940;**81:**345–65.

911. Carota A, Rossetti AO, Karapanayiotides T, et al. Catastrophic reaction in acute stroke: a reflex behaviour in aphasic patients. *Neurology* 2001;**57:**1902–5.

912. Carota A, Staub F, Bogousslavsky J. Emotions, behaviours and mood changes in stroke. *Curr Opin Neurol* 2002;**15:**57–69.

913. Carpay JA, Vermeulen J, Stropink J, et al. Seizure severity in children with epilepsy: a parent-completed sacale compared with clinical attacks. *Epilepsia* 1997;**38:**346–52.

914. Carpenter G. Two sisters showing malformation of the skull and other congenital abnormalities. *Rep Soc Study Dis Child (Lond)* 1901;**1:**110–8.

915. Carpenter S, Karpati G, Rothman S, et al. The childhood type of dermatomyositis. *Neurology* 1976;**26:**952–62.

916. Carpio A, Placencia M, Santillan F, et al. A proposal for classification of neurocysticercosis. *Can J Neurol Sci* 1994;**21:**43–7.

917. Carr RE, Ripps H, Sequal IM, et al. Visual function in congenital night-blindness. *Invest Ophthalmol* 1976;**5:**508.

918. Carraro A. [Congenital absence of the tibia and deafness in 4 siblings]. *Ch di Org di Movimento* 1931;**16:**429–38.

920. Carr-Locke DL, Nair HJ. Neurological presentation of psittacosis during a small outbreak in Leicestershire. *BMJ* 1976;**ii:**853–4.

921. Carroll FD. Optic nerve complications of cataract extraction. *Trans Am Acad Ophthal Otolaryngol* 1973; **77:**623.

922. Carroll GJ, Willis K, Peter JB. Penicillamine-induced polymyositis or dermatomyositis. *J Rheumatol* 1987;**14:**995–9.

923. Carroll JE, Brooke MH, DeVivo DC, et al. Biochemical and physiologic consequences of carnitine palmityl transfersase deficiency. *Muscle Nerve* 1978;**1:**103–10.

924. Carroll JE, Shumate JB, Brooke MH, et al. Riboflavine-responsive lipid myopathy and carnitine deficiency. *Neurology* 1981;**31:**1557–9.

925. Carroll RA, Bornstein SS, Hoffman SG. Rehabilitation networking: a solution for the future. In Granger CV, Gresham GE, eds. *Functional Assessment in Rehabilitation Medicine*, pp 364–77. Baltimore: Williams and Wilkins, 1984.

926. Carruthers A, Carruthers J, Wright P. Necrotizing fasciitis with polymyositis. *BMJ* 1975;**3:**355–6.

927. Carskadon MA, Dement WC, Mitler MM, et al. Guidelines for the Multiple Sleep Latency Test. *Sleep* 1986;**9:**519–24.

928. Carson NA, Scally BG, Neill DW, et al. Saccharopinuria: a new inborn error of lysine metabolism. *Nature* 1968;**218:**679.

929. Carter RF, et al. Primary amebic meningoencephalitis. *Rep R Soc Trop Med Hygiene* 1972;**66:**193.

930. Carton H, Kayembe K, Kabeya, et al. Epidemic spastic paraparesis in Bandundu (Zaire). *J Neurol Neurosurg Psychiatry* 1986;**49:**620–7.

931. Casaer P. *Migraine and Other Headaches.* Pearl River, NJ: Parthenon, 1989.

932. Caselli RJ, Boeve BF, Scheithauer BW, et al. Nonvasculitic autoimmune inflammatory meningoencephalitis (NAIM): a reversible form of encephalopathy. *Neurology* 1999;**53:**1579–81.

933. Caselli RJ, Hunder GG, Whisnant JP. Neurologic disease in biopsy-proven giant cell (temporal) arteritis. *Neurology* 1988;**38:**352–8.

934. Caselli RJ, Jack CR. Asymmetric cortical degenerative syndromes: a proposed clinical classification. *Arch Neurol* 1992;**49:**770–80.

935. Caselli RJ, Jack CR, Peterson RC, et al. Assymetric cortical degenerative syndromes: clinical and radiologic correlations. *Neurology* 1992;**42:**1462–8.

936. Caselli RJ, Windebank AJ, Peterson RC, et al. Rapidly progressive aphasic dementia and motor neuron disease (MND): six new cases of a distinctive clinical syndrome. *Neurology* 1991;**41(Suppl):**176.

937. Cassidy SB. Prader-Willi syndrome: characteristics, management, and etiology. *Ala J Med Sci* 1987;**24:**169–75.

938. Castillo M, Davis PC, Takei Y, et al. Intracranial ganglioglioma: MR, CT, and clinical findings in 18 patients. *AJR Am J Roentgenol* 1990;**154:**607–12.

939. Cavanagh JB. Peripheral nerve changes in orthocresyl phosphate poisoning in the rat. *J Pathol Bacteriol* 1964;**87:**365–83.

940. Cavanagh JB. The 'dying-back' process: a common denominator in many naturally occurring and toxic neuropathies. *Arch Pathol Lab Med* 1979;**103:**659–64.

941. Cavanagh JB, et al. The effects of thallium salts, with particular reference to the nervous system changes. *Q J Med* 1974;**43:**293.

942. Cavanagh NPC, Eames RA, Galvin RJ, et al. Hereditary sensory neuropathy with spastic paraplegia. *Brain* 1979;**102:**79–94.

943. Cavanagh NPC, Yates DAH, Sutcliffe J. Thenar hypoplasia with associated radiologic abnormalities. *Muscle Nerve* 1979;**2:**431–6.

944. Cederbaum SD, et al. Argininosuccinic aciduria. *Am J Ment Defic* 1973;**77:**395–404.

945. Celani MG, Righetti E, Migliacci R, et al. Comparability and validity of two clinical scores in the early differential diagnosis of acute stroke. *BMJ* 1994;**308:**1674–6.

946. Celesia GC. Disorders of membrane channels or channelopathies. *Clin Neurophysiol* 2001;**112:**2–18.

947. Celesia GC, Andermann F, Wiglesworth FW, Robb JP. Monomelic myopathy. *Arch Neurol* 1967;**17:**69–77.

948. Cerebral Embolism Task Force. Cardiogenic brain embolism. *Arch Neurol* 1986;**43:**71–84.

949. Cervero F, Iggo A. The substantia gelatinosa of the spinal cord. *Brain* 1980;**103:**717–72.

950. Cestan EJM, Chenais J. Du miosis dans certains lesions bulbaires en foyer (hemiplégie du type Avellis associés au syndrome oculaire sympathique). *Gaz Hop Paris* 1903;**76:**1229–33.

951. Chabriat H, Levy C, Taillia H, et.al. Patterns of MRI lesions in CADASIL. *Neurology* 1998;**51:**452–7.

952. Chad DA, Lacomis D. Critically ill patients with newly acquired weakness: the clinico-pathological spectrum. *Ann Neurol* 1994;**35:**257–9.

953. Chaddock CG. A preliminary communication concerning a new diagnostic nervous sign. *Interstate Med* 1911;**18:**742–6.

954. Chadwick D, Clear DB, Eldridge P, et al. Golf ball epilepsy. *J Neurol Neurosurg Psychiatry* 2000;**68:**251–2.

955. Chalela JA, Kasner SE. The fogging effect. *Neurology* 2000;**55:**315.

956. Chalk CH, Mills KR, Jacobs JM, et al. Familial multiple symmetric lipomatosis with peripheral neuropathy. *Neurology* 1990;**40:** 1246–50.

957. Chalk CH, Windebank AJ, Kimmel DW, et al. The distinctive clinical features of paraneoplastic sensory neuropathy. *Can J Neurol Sci* 1992;**19:**346–51.

958. Chalmers RA, Johnson M, Pallis CA, et al. Xanthenuria with myopathy. *Q J Med* 1969;**38:**493–512.

959. Chalmers RM, Bird AC, Harding AE. Autosomal ldominant optic atrophy with asymptomatic peripheral neuropathy. *J Neurol Neurosurg Psychiatry* 1996;**60:**195–6.

960. Chambers BR, Bladin CF. Internal watershed infarction. In Donnan GA, Norrving B, Bamford JM, eds. *Lacunar and Other Subcortical Infarctions*, pp 139–48. Oxford: Oxford University Press, 1995.

961. Chan CC, Egbert PR, Herrick MK, et al. Oculocerebral malformations: a reappraisal of Walker's "lissencephaly". *Arch Neurol* 1980;**37**:104–8.

962. Chan DKY, Hung WT, Wong A, et al. Validating a screening questionnaire for parkinsonism in Australia. *J Neurol Neurosurg Psychiatry* 2000;**69**:117–20.

963. Chanarin I, et al. Chanarin-Miranda syndrome: lipid storage myopathy and congenital ichthyosis. *BMJ* 1975;**1**:203.

964. Chancellor MB, Lavelle J, Ozawa H, et al. Ice water test in the urodynamic evaluation of spinal cord injured patients. *Tech Urol* 1998;**4**:87–91.

965. Chandler D, Angelicheva D, Heather L, et al. Hereditary motor and sensory neuropathy-Lom (HMSNL); refined genetic mapping in Romani (Gypsy) families from several European countries. *Neuromusc Disord* 2000;**10**:584–91.

966. Chang CM, Yu CW, Fong KY, et al. N-hexane neuropathy in off-set printers. *J Neurol Neurosurg Psychiatry* 1993;**56**:538–42.

967. Chapman SB, Rosenberg RN, Weiner MF, et al. Autosomal dominant progressive syndrome of motor-speech loss without dementia. *Neurology* 1997;**49**:1298–306.

968. Chapple CC. A duosyndrome of the laryngeal nerve. *J Dis Child* 1956;**91**:14–8.

969. Charcot J-M. Histologie de la sclèrose en plaques. *Gaz Hop Paris* 1868;**41**:554–558.

970. Charcot J-M. Sur quelques arthropathies qui paraissent dépendre d'une lésion du cerveau ou de la moelle épinière. *Arch Physiol* (*Paris*) 1868;**1**:161–78.

971. Charcot J-M. Leçons sur les maladies du système nerveux faites a la Salpêtrière. A. Delahnye: Paris, 1872.

972. Charcot J-M. Séance du 13 mai. *C R Soc Biol* 1873;**serie 5e iii,1871**:32–8.

973. Charcot J-M. Des amyotrophies spinales chroniques. *Prog Med* (*Paris*) 1874;**2**:573–4.

974. Charcot J-M. On chorea in old people [in French]. *Med Times Gaz* 1878;**1**:245–6.

975. Charcot J-M. Diagnostic des formes frustes de la sclèrose en plaques. *Prog Med* (*Paris*) 1879;**7**:97–9.

976. Charcot J-M. Du vertige larynge. *Prog Med* (*Paris*) 1879;**7**:317–9.

977. Charcot J-M. Un cas de suppression brusque et isolée de la vision mentale des objects (formes et couleurs). *Prog Med* (*Paris*) 1883;**11**:568.

978. Charcot J-M. *Clinical Lectures on Diseases of the Nervous System.* London: The New Syndenham Society, 1889.

979. Charcot J-M, Bouchard A. Douleurs fulgurantes de l'ataxie sans incoordination des mouvements; sclérose commençante des cordons posterièures de la moèle épinière. *Gaz Med* (*Paris*) 1866;**21**:122–4.

980. Charcot J-M, Joffroy A. Deux cas d'atrophie musculaire progressive avec lesions de la substance grise et des faisceaux anterolateraux de la moelle épinière. *Arch Physiol Norm Pathol* (*Paris*) 1869;**2**:354–67.

981. Charcot J-M, Marie P. Sur une forme particulière d'atrophie musculaire progressive, souvent familiale, débutant par les pieds et les jambes et attéignant plus tard les mains. *Rev Med Paris* 1886;**6**:97–138.

982. Charleston AJ, Andserson NE, Willoughby EW. Idiopathic steroid responsive chronic lymphocytic meningitis—clinical features and long-term outcome in 17 patients. *Aust NZ J Med* 1998;**28**:784–9.

983. Charlin C. Le syndrome du nerf nasal. *Ann Ocul* 1931;**168**:86.

984. Charnas LR, Luciano CA, Dalakas M, et al. Distal vacuolar myopathy in nephropathic cystinosis. *Ann Neurol* 1994;**35**:181–8.

985. Charnas LR, Marini JC. Communicating hydrocephalus, basilar invagination and other features in osteogenesis imperfecta. *Neurology* 1993;**43**:2603–8.

986. Charous DI, Saxe BI. The Landry Guillain Barré syndrome: report of an unusual case. *N Engl J Med* 1962;**267**:1334–8.

987. Chaslin P. Note sur l'anatomie pathologique de l'epilepsie dite essentielle. La sclerose nevroglique. *C R Soc Biol* 1889;**1**:169–71.

988. Chassaignac P. De la paralysie douloureuse des jeunes enfants. *Arch Gen Med Paris* 1856;**1**:653–69.

989. Chatrian GE, Bergamini L, Dondey M, et al. A glossary of terms most commonly used by clinical electroencephalographers. *Electroencephalogr Clin Neurophysiol* 1974;**37**:538–48.

990. Chatrian GE, Shaw C-M, Leffman H. The significance of periodic, lateralized epileptiform discharges in EEG: an electrographic, clinical, and pathologic study. *Electroencephalogr Clin Neurophysiol* 1964;**17**:177–93.

991. Chavanay J-A, Brunhes J. Syndromes cephalgiques et psychoneurotiques avec calcification de la faux du cerveau. *Rev Neurol* (*Paris*) 1938;**69**:113–31.

992. Chavanay J-A, Taptas JN, Haggenmuiller D. Les faux syndromes alternes d'origine hemispherique; l'hemiplegia cruciata par lesions corticales bilaterales. *Presse Med* 1952;**60**:1126–8.

993. Chee K-Y, Sachdev P. A controlled study of sensory tics in Gilles de la Tourette syndrome and obsessive-compulsive using a structured interview. *J Neurol Neurosurg Psychiatry* 1997;**62**:188–92.

994. Chelluri L, Jastremski MS. Bilateral optic atrophy after cardiac arrest in a patient with acute respiratory failure on positive pressure ventilation. *Rescucitation* 1998;**16**:45–8.

995. Chen HC, Marcharani U. Hashimoto's encephalopathy. *South Med J* 2000;**93**:504–6.

996. Chen R, Collins S, Remtulla H, et al. Phrenic nerve conduction study in normal subjects. *Muscle Nerve* 1995;**18**:330–5.

997. Chen R, Sahjpaul R, Del Maestro RF, et al. Initial enlargement of the opposite pupil as a false localizing sign in intraparenchymal frontal hemorrhages. *J Neurol Neurosurg Psychiatry* 1994;**57**:1126–8.

998. Cherington M. Botulism: clinical and therapeutic observations. *Rocky Mt Med J* 1972;**69**:55–8.

999. Cherington M. Botulism: ten year experience. *Arch Neurol* 1974;**30**:432–7.

1000. Cherington M. Anterior interosseous nerve syndrome straight thumb sign. *Neurology* 1977;**27**:800–1.

1001. Cherington M, Yarnell P, Hallmark D. MRI in lightning encephalopathy. *Neurology* 1993;**43**:1437–8.

1002. Chesney PJ, Davis JP, Purdy WK, et al. Clinical manifestations of toxic shock syndrome. *JAMA* 1981;**246**:741–8.

1003. Chester EM, Agamanolis DP, Banker BQ, et al. Hypertensive encephalopathy: a clinicopathologic study of 20 cases. *Neurology* 1978;**28**:928–39.

1004. Cheyne J. *The English Malady, or a Treatise of Nervous Diseases of All Kinds, as Spleen and Vapours, Lowness of Hypochondriacal Distempers* etc. London: Powell, 1773.

1005. Cheyne J. A case of apoplexy in whch the fleshy part of the heart was converted into fat. *Dublin Hosp Rep* 1818;**2**:216–23.

1006. Chia L-G, Chu F-L. A clinical and genetic study of patients with PCB poisoning. *J Neurol Neurosurg Psychiatry* 1985;**48**:894–901.

1007. Chiappa KH, Gladstone KJ, Young RR. Brain stem auditory evoked responses: studies of waveform variations in 50 normal human subjects. *Arch Neurol* 1979;**36**:81–7.

1008. Chiappa KH, Ropper AH. Evoked potentials in clinical medicine. *N Engl J Med* 1982;**306**:1140–50, 1205–1211.

1009. Chiari H. Concerning changes in the cerebellum due to hydrocephalus of the cerebrum. *Dtsch Med Wochenschr* 1891;**17**:1172–5.

1010. Chiba S, Saitoh M, Hatanaka Y, et al. Autosomal dominant muscle cramp syndrome in a Japanese family. *J Neurol Neurosurg Psychiatry* 1999;**67**:116–9.

1011. Childs B, Nyhan WR, Borden M, et al. Idiopathic hyperglycinemia and hyperglycinuria. *Pediatrics* 1961;**27**:522–38.

1012. Chinnery PF, Johnson MA, Walls TJ, et al. A novel autosomal dominant distal myopathy with early respiratory failure: clinico-pathologic characteristics and exclusion of linkage to candidate genetic loci. *Ann Neurol* 2001;**49**:443–52.

1013. Chiray P, Foix C, Nicolesco I. Hemi-tremblement du type de la sclérose en plaques par lesion rubro-thalamo-sous-thalamique. *Ann Med* 1923;**14**:173–91.

1014. Chitanondh H, Rosen L. Fatal eosinophilic encephalomyelitis caused by the nematode Gnathostoma sphingerum. *Am J Trop Med* 1967;**16**:638.

1015. Chodzko W. On a new symptom of organic CNS lesions [in French]. *Rev Neurol* (*Paris*) 1936;**65**:131–4.

1016. Chokroverty S, Bruetman ME, Berger V, et al. Progressive dialytic encephalopathy. *J Neurol Neurosurg Psychiatry* 1976;**39**:411–9.

1017. Chokroverty S, Khedekar R, Derby B, et al. Pathology of olivopontocerebellar atrophy with glutamate dehydrogenase deficiency. *Neurology* 1984;**34**:1451–5.

1018. Chokroverty S, Reyes MG, Rubino FA, et al. Hemiplegic amyotrophy: muscle and motor point biopsy study. *Arch Neurol* 1976;**33**:104–10.

1019. Chokroverty S, Walters A, Zimmerman T, et al. Propriospinal myoclonus. *Neurology* 1992;**42**:1591–5.

1020. Chollet P, Rigal J-P, Pignide L. Une complication méconnue de l'hyperthyroidie; la neuropathie péripherique. *Presse Med* 1971;**79**:145.

1021. Cholod EJ, Haust MD, Hudson AJ, et al. Myopathy in primary familial hyperparathyroidism. *Am J Med* 1970;**48**:700–7.

1022. Chou SM. Myxovirus-like structures in a case of human chronic polymyositis. *Science* 1967;**158**:1453.

1023. Chouinard G, Ross-Chouinard A, Annable L, et al. The Extrapyramidal Symptom Rating Scale. *Can J Neurol Sci* 1980;**7**:233.

1024. Chow CW, Frerman FE, Goodman SI, et al. Striatal degeneration in glutaric acidemia type 2. *Acta Neuropathol* 1989;**77**:554–6.

1025. Chretien JH, Fermaglich J, Garagusi VF. Ciguatera poisoning: presentation as a neurologic disorder. *Arch Neurol* 1981;**38**:783.

1026. Christian JC, Bixsler D, Blythe SC, et al. Familial telecanthus with associated abnormalities. *Birth Defects* 1969;**5**:82.

1027. Christian JC, et al. X-linked skeletal dyspslasia with mental retardation. *Clin Genet* 1977;**11**:128–36.

1028. Christian JC, et al. The adducted thumbs syndrome: an autosomal recessive disease with arthrogryposis, dysmyelination, craniostenosis, and cleft palate. *Clin Genet* 1971;**2**:95–103.

1029. Christodoulou K, Zamba E, Tsingis M, et al. A novel form of distal hereditary motor neuropathy maps to chromosome 9p21.1–p12. *Ann Neurol* 2000;**48**:877–84.

1030. Chroni E, Panayiotopoulos CP. F tacheodispersion. *J Neurol Neurosurg Psychiatry* 1993;**56**:1103–8.

1031. Chui HC, Victoroff JI, Margolin D, et al. Criteria for the diagnosis of ischemic vascular dementia. *World Neurol* 1992;**7**:12–13.

1032. Chung MH, Sum J, Morrell MJ, et al. Intracerebral involvement in scleroderma en coup de sabre: report of a case with neuropathologic findings. *Ann Neurol* 1995;**37**:679–81.

1033. Chung SJ, Kim JS, Lee MC. Syndrome of cerebral spinal fluid hypovolemia. *Neurology* 2000;**55**:1321–7.

1034. Chusid J, DeGutierrez-Mahoney CG. Syndrome of bilateral vestibular paralysis. *J Nerv Ment Dis* 1946;**103**:172–80.

1035. Chutkow JG. Posterior femoral cutaneous neuralgia. *Muscle Nerve* 1988;**11**:1146–8.

1036. Chutkow JG, Heffner RR jr, Kramer AA, Edwards JA. Adult-onset autosomal dominant limb-girdle muscular dystrophy. *Ann Neurol* 1986;**20**:240–8.

1037. Chvostek F. Beitrag zur Tetanie. *Wien Med Presse* 1876;**17**:1201–3.

1038. Cilicchia CF, Gol A, Ericksen EE. Diffuse central nervous system involvement in papulosis atrophica maligna. *Neurology* 1962;**12**:503–9.

1039. Cincotta M, Borgheresi A, Liotta P, et al. Reorganization of the motor cortex in a patient with congenital hemiparesis and mirror movements. *Neurlogy* 2000;**55**:129–31.

1040. Citak KA, Dickoff DJ, Simpson DM. Progressive sensory radiculopathy responsive to corticosteroid therapy. *Muscle Nerve* 1993;**16**:679–80.

1041. Claes S, Devrient.K., Lagae L, et al. The X-linked infantile spasms syndrome. *Ann Neurol* 1997;**42**:360–4.

1042. Clancy RR, Kurtz MB, Baker D, et al. Neurologic manifestations of the organoid nevus syndrome. *Arch Neurol* 1985;**42**:236–40.

1043. Clara R, Lowenthal A. Familial and congenital lysine-cystinuria with benign myopathy and dwarfism. *J Neurol Sci* 1966;**3**:433–4.

1044. Clark JR, d'Agostino AN, Wilson J, et al. Autosomal dominant myofibrillar inclusion body myopathy. *Neurol Minneap* 1978;**28**:399.

1045. Clarke CRA, Harrison MJG. Neurological manifestations of Paget's disease. *J Neurol Sci* 1978;**38**:171–8.

1046. Clarke E. Apoplexy in the Hippocratic writings. *Bull Hist Med* 1963;**37**:301–14.

1047. Clarke E, Bearn JG. The spiral nerve bands of Fontana. *Brain* 1972;**95**:1–20.

1048. Clarke E, Dewhurst K. *An Illustrated History of Brain Function.* Oxford: Sandford Publications, 1972.

1049. Clarke TH, Saunders BS, Feldman B. Pyridoxine-dependent seizures requiring high doses of pyridoxine for control. *Am J Dis Child* 1979;**133**:963.

1050. Clarren SK, Alvord EC, Sumi SM, et al. Brain malformations related to prenatal exposure to alcohol. *J Pediatr* 1978;**92**:64.

1051. Classification Committee I. Classification of Headache Disorders, Cranial Neuralgias and Facial Pain; and Diagnostic Criteria for Primary Headache Disorders. *Cephalalgia* 1988;**8(Suppl)**:1–96.

1052. Claude H. Syndrome pedonculaire de la région du noyau rouge. *Rev Neurol (Paris)* 1912;**23**:311–3.

1053. Claude H, Lhermitte JJ. Le syndrome infundibulaire dans les tumeurs de l'encéphale. *Presse Med* 1918.

1054. Clay SA, Ramseyer JC, Fishman LS, et al. Acute infantile motor unit disorder. *Arch Neurol* 1977;**34**:226–43.

1055. Cleckley H. *The Mask of Sanity.* St. Louis: C.V. Mosby, 1964.

1056. Cleland JB, Campbell AW. The Australian epidemics of an acute polio-encephalomyelitis (X disease). In *Report of the Director General of Public Health, New South Wales*, pp 150–280. 1917.

1057. Clemens PR, Yamamoto M, Engel AG. Adult phosphorylase b kinase deficiency. *Ann Neurol* 1990;**28**:529–38.

1058. Clements SD, Peters JE. Minimal brain dysfunctions in school-age child. *Arch Gen Psychiatry* 1962;**6**:185–97.

1059. Clouston HC. A hereditary ectodermal dystrophy. *CMAJ* 1929;**21**:18–31.

1060. Co S. Intractable sneezing: case report and literature review. *Arch Neurol* 1979;**36**:111–2.

1061. Cobb S. Haemangioma of the spinal cord associated with skin naevi of the same metamere. *Ann Surg* 1915;**62**:641–9.

1062. Cobb S, Bereday M. Familial system diseases of the neuraxis. *Trans Am Neurol Assoc* 1953;**78**:12–4.

1063. Cobben JM, de Visser M, Scheffer H, et al. Confirmation of clinical diagnosis in requests for prenatal prediction of SMA type 1. *J Neurol Neurosurg Psychiatry* 1993;**56**:319–21.

1063a. Cochrane DD, Poskitt KJ, Normal MG. Surgical implications of cerebral dysgenesis. *Can J Neurol Sci* 1991;**18**:181–95.

1064. Cockayne EA. Dwarfism with retinal atrophy and deafness. *Arch Dis Child* 1936;**11**:1–8.

1065. Cockel R, Hill EE, Rushton DI, et al. Familial steatorrhea with calcfification of the basal ganglia and mental retardation. *Q J Med* 1973;**42**:771–83.

1066. Coers C, Telerman-Toppet N, Durdu J. Neurogenic benign fasciculations, pseudomyotonia, and pseudotetany: a disease in search of a name. *Arch Neurol* 1981;**38**:282–7.

1067. Coers C, Telerman-Toppet N, Gerard J-M. Terminal innervation ratio in neuromuscular disease: methods and controls. *Arch Neurol* 1973;**29**:210–4.

1068. Coffin GS. A syndrome of retarded development with characteristic appearance. *Am J Dis Child* 1968;**115**:698–702.

1069. Cogan DG. Syndrome of nonsyphilitic interstitial keratitis and vestibuloauditory symptoms. *Arch Ophthalmol* 1945;**33**:144–9.

1070. Cogan DG. A type of congenital motor apraxia presenting jerky head movements. *Am J Ophthalmol* 1953;**36**:433–41.

1071. Cogan DG. Ocular dysmetria, flutter-like oscillations of the eyes and opsoclonus. *Arch Ophthalmol* 1954;**51**:318–35.

1072. Cogan DG. *Neurology of the Ocular Muscles.* Springfield, IL: Charles C. Thomas, 1956.

1073. Cogan DG. Hemianopia and associated symptoms due to parieto-temporal lesions. *Am J Ophthalmol* 1960;**50**:1056–66.

1074. Cogan DG. Myasthenia gravis. A review of the disease and a description of lid twitch as a characteristic sign. *Arch Ophthalmol* 1965;**74**:217–21.

1075. Cogan DG. Opsoclonus, body tremulousness and benign encephalitis. *Arch Ophthalmol* 1968;**79**:545–51.

1076. Cogan DG, Adams RD. Type of paralysis of conjugate gaze (ocular motor apraxia). *Arch Ophthalmol* 1953;**50**:434–42.

1077. Cogan DG, Chu FC, Reingold DB. Ocular signs of cerebellar disease. *Arch Ophthalmol* 1982;**100**:755.

1078. Cogan DG, Freese CG. Spasm of the near reflex. *Arch Ophthalmol* 1955;**54**:752–9.

1079. Coggins CH, Lillington GA, Gray CP. Micturition syncope. *Arch Intern Med* 1964;**113**:14–8.

1080. Cohen D. Magnetoencephalography: evidence of magnetic fields produced by alpha rhythm currents. *Science* 1968;**161**:784–6.

1081. Cohen HA, Nussinovitch M, Ashkenazi A, et al. Benign abducens nerve palsy of childhood. *Pediatr Neurol* 1993;**9**:394–5.

1082. Cohen HA, Nussinovitch M, Ashkenazi A, et al. Benign paroxysmal torticollis in infancy. *Pediatr Neurol* 1993;**9**:488–90.

1083. Cohen L, Benoit N, Van Eeeckhout P, et al. Pure progressive aphemia. *J Neurol Neurosurg Psychiatry* 1993;**56**:923–4.

1084. Cohen LG, Hallett M. Hand cramps. *Neurology* 1988;**38**:1005–12.

1085. Cohen M, Campbell R, Yaghmai F. Neuropathological abnnormalities in developmental dysphasia. *Ann Neurol* 1989;**25**:567–70.

1086. Cohen M, Lanska D, Roessmann U, et al. Amyloidoma of the CNS. *Neurology* 1992;**42**:2019–23.

1087. Cohen MM, et al. Syndrome with cephalocele. *Teratology* 1982;**25**:161–72.

1088. Cohen MM Jr Craniosynostosis and syndromes with craniosynostosis: incidence, genetics, penetrance, variability, and new syndrome updating. *Birth Defects* 1979;**15**:13–63.

1089. Cohen MM Jr. *The Child with Multiple Birth Defects.* New York: Raven Press, 1982.

1090. Cohen MM Jr, Gorlin RJ. Prader-Willi syndrome. *Am J Dis Child* 1969;**117**:213–8.

1091. Cohen MM Jr, et al. A new syndrome with hypotonia, obesity, mental deficiency and facial, oral, ocular and limb anomalies. *J Pediatr* 1973;**83**:280–4.

1092. Cohn R. Phantom vision. *Arch Neurol* 1971;**25**:468–71.

1093. Cohn R. Eyeball movements in homonymous hemianopia following simultaneous bitemporal object presentation. *Neurology* 1972;**22**:12–4.

1094. Cohn R, Neumann MA, Wood DH. Prosopagnosia: a clinical study. *Ann Neurol* 1977;**1**:177–82.

1095. Colby MY, Kearns TP. Radiation therapy of pituitary adenomas with associated visual impairment. *Proc. Staff Meet Mayo Clin* 1962;**37**:15.

1096. Colebatch JG, Halmagyi GM, Skuse NF. Myogenic potentials generated by a click-evoked vestibulocollic reflex. *J Neurol Neurosurg Psychiatry* 1994;**57**:190–7.

1097. Coleman AE, Norman DJ. OKT3 encephalopathy. *Ann Neurol* 1990;**28**:837–8.

1098. Coleman DI, Gambetti P, DiMauro S. Muscle in Lafora disease. *Arch Neurol* 1974;**31**:396–406.

1099. Coleman RJ, Russon L, Blanshard K, et al. Useless hand of Oppenheim—magnetic resonance imaging findings. *Postgrad Med J* 1993;**69**:149–50.

1100. Coleman RM. Periodic Nocturnal Myoclonus in Disorders of Sleep and Wakefulness. Ann Arbor, MI: Yeshiva University Microfilms, 1979.

1101. Coleman RM, Pollak CP, Weitzman ED. Periodic movements in sleep (nocturnal myoclonus): relation to sleep disorders. *Ann Neurol* 1980;**8**:416–21.

1102. Collen FM. Rivermead Mobility Index. *Int Disabil Stud* 1991;**13**:50–4.

1103. Collet FJ. Sur un nouveau syndrome paralytique pharyngo-larynge par blessure de guerre (hemiplegie glosso-laryngo-scapulopharyngée). *Lyon Med* 1915;**124**:121–9.

1104. Collier J. Epilepsy. In Bett WR, ed. *A Short History of Some Common Diseases*, pp 119–36. Oxford: Oxford University Press, 1934.

1105. Collier M. Ophthalmological findings in Kartagener syndrome. *Bull Fr Soc Ophthalmol* 1961;**74**:429–47.

1106. Collins ET. Case with symmetrical congenital notches in the outer parts of each lower lid and defective development of the malar bones. *Trans Ophthalmol Soc UK* 1900;**20**:190.

1107. Collins MP, Mendell JR, Periquet MI, et al. Superficial peroneal nerve/peroneus brevis muscle biopsy in vasculitic neuropathy. *Neurology* 2000;**55**:636–43.

1108. Collins SJ, Ahlskog JE, Parisi J, et al. Progressive supranuclear palsy: neuropathologically based diagnostic clinical criteria. *J Neurol Neurosurg Psychiatry* 1995;**58**:167–73.

1109. Coltheart M, Patterson K, Marshall JC. *Deep Dyslexia.* London: Routledge and Kegan Paul, 1980.

1110. Combs JT, Grunt JA, Brandt IK. New syndrome of neonatal hypoglycemia, association with visceromegaly, macroglossia, microcephaly and abnormal umbilicus. *N Engl J Med* 1966;**275**:236–43.

1111. Comi G, Fortunato F, Lucchiari S, et al. Beta-enolase deficiency, a new metabolic myopathy of distal glycolysis. *Ann Neurol* 2001;**50**:202–7.

1112. Comi G, Testa D, Cornelio F, et al. Potassium depletion myopathy. *Muscle Nerve* 1985;**8**:17–21.

1113. Comings DE, Amromin GD. Autosomal dominant insensitivity to pain with hyperplastic myelinopathy. *Neurology* 1974;**24**:838–48.

1114. Commission for Classification and Terminology I. Proposal for revised classification of epilepsies and epileptic syndromes. *Epilepsia* 1989;**30**:389–99.

1115. Commission of Epidemiology and Prognosis I. Guidelines for epidemiological studies in epilepsy. *Epilepsia* 1993;**34**:592–6.

1116. Confavreux C, Compston DAS, Hommes OR, et al. EDMUS, a European database for multiple sclerosis. *J Neurol Neurosurg Psychiatry* 1992;**55**:671–6.

1117. Conics BW, Hollander MB, Berlin CI. Familial neural hearing loss and atopic dermatitis. *JAMA* 1968;**204**:953.

1118. Connett MC, Lansche JM. Fibromuscular hyperplasia of the internal carotid artery. *Ann Surg* 1969;**162**:59–62.

1119. Connolly AM, Dodson WE, Prensky AL, et al. Course and outcome of acute cerebellar ataxia. *Ann Neurol* 1994;**35**:673–9.

1120. Conradi E. Hypoplastic fetal chondrodystrophia [in German]. *Jahrb Kinderheilkol* 1914;**80**:86–7.

1121. Consensus Panel. Report and Recommendations of the San Antonio Conference on Diabetic Neuropathy. *Diabetes* 1988;**37**:1000–4.

1122. Cook AW, Nathan PW, Smith MC. Sensory consequences of commissural myelotomy. *Brain* 1984;**107**:547–68.

1123. Cooper RG, Stokes MJ, Edwards RHT. Physiological characteristics of the "warm-up" effect of activity in patients with myotonic dystrophy. *J Neurol Neurosurg Psychiatry* 1988;**51**:1134–41.

1124. Coplan J. *The Early Language Milestone Scale.* Austin, TX: PRO-ED, Inc., 1987.

1125. Coppack SW, Watkins PJ. The natural history of diabetic femoral neuropathy. *Q J Med* 1991;**79**:307–13.

1126. Coppeto JR, Lessell S. A familial syndrome of dystonia, blepharospasm, and pigmentary retinopathy. *Neurology* 1990;**40**:1359–63.

1127. Corbett JJ, Butler AB, Kaufman B. "Sneeze syncope," basilar invagination and Arnold-Chiari type I malformation. *J Neurol Neurosurg Psychiatry* 1976;**39**:381–4.

1128. Corbett JJ, Schatz NJ, Shults WT, et al. Slowly alternating skew deviation. *Ann Neurol* 1981;**10**:540–6.

1129. Corbin D, Martyr T, Graham AC. Migraine coma. *J Neurol Neurosurg Psychiatry* 1991;**54**:744.

1130. Corbin D, Williams A, Johnson AP. Dystonia complicated by respiratory obstruction. *J Neurol Neurosurg Psychiatry* 1987;**50**:1707.

1131. Cori GT. Biochemical aspects of glycogen deposition disease. *Bibl Pediatr Basel* 1958;**66**:344–58.

1132. Corkin S. Aquisition of motor skill after bilateral medial temporal lobe excision. *Neuropsychologia* 1968;**6**:255–65.

1133. Cormand B, Pihko H, Bayés M, et al. Clinical and genetic distinction between Walker-Warburg syndrome and muscle-eye-brain disease. *Neurology* 2001;**56**:1059–69.

1134. Cornblath DR, Chaudhry V, Carter K, et al. Total neuropathy score. *Neurology* 1999;**53**:1660–4.

1135. Cornblath DR, et al. Radiculopathy in AIDS. *Ann Neurol* 1987;**21**:32.

1136. Corsellis JAN, Goldberg GJ, Norton AR. "Limbic encephalitis" and its association with carcinoma. *Brain* 1968;**91**:481–96.

1137. Cortez MA, McKerlie C, Snead OC. A model of atypical absence seizures. *Neurology* 2001;**56**:341–9.

1138. Cossa PM, Berard-Badier M, Camuzard S, et al. Familial polyradiculopathy syndrome [in French]. *Rev Neurol (Paris)* 1957;**97**:450–65.

1139. Costeff H, Elpeleg O, Apter N, et al. 3-Methylglutaconic aciduria in "optic atrophy plus". *Ann Neurol* 1993;**33**:103–4.

1140. Costen JB. A syndrome of ear and sinus symptoms dependent upon disturbed function of the temporo-mandibular joint. *Ann Otol Rhinol* 1934;**43**:1–15.

1141. Coté R, Battista RN, Wolfson C, et al. The Canadian Neurological Scale: validation and reliability assessment. *Neurology* 1989;**39**:638–43.

1142. Cotugno D. *A Treatise of the Nervous Sciatia or Nervous Hip Gout.* London: Wilkie, 1775.

1143. Coulter DL, Allen RJ. Benign neonatal sleep myoclonus. *Arch Neurol* 1982;**39**:191–2.

1144. Coulter DL, Beals TF, Allan IJ. Neurotrichosis: hair abnormalities associated with neurological disease. *Dev Med Child Neurol* 1982;**24**:634.

1145. Courtois A. Unilateral reflex flexion of the leg with flexion of the neck in cases of coma due to focal cerebral lesions [in French]. *Ann Med Psychol* 1931;**89**:506–11.

1146. Courville CB. *Birth and Brain Damage.* Pasadena,TX: M.F. Courville, 1971.

1147. Coutinho A, Andrade C. Autosomal dominant system degeneration in Portuguese families of the Azores Islands. *Neurology* 1978;**28**: 703–9.

1148. Coutinho P, Barros J, Zemmouri R, et al. Clinical heterogeneity of autosomal recessive spastic paraplegias: analysis of 106 patients in 46 families. *Arch Neurol* 1999;**56**:943–9.

1149. Cox DW. Factors influencing ceruloplasmin levels in normal individuals. *J Lab Clin Med* 1966;**68**:893–904.

1150. Cox JM. *Low Back Pain: Mechanism, Diagnosis and Treatment.* Baltimore: Williams and Wilkins, 1985.

1151. Cox TA. Pupillary escape. *Neurology* 1992;**42**:1271–3.

1152. Cox TM. Hereditary fructose intolerance. *Q J Med* 1988;**68**: 585–94.

1153. Coyle PK, Wolinsky JS. Characterization of immune complexes in progressive rubella panencephalitis. *Ann Neurol* 1981;**9**:557–62.

1154. Cram RH. A sign of sciatic nerve pressure. *J Bone Jt Surg* 1905; **35B**:192.

1155. Cramer JA, French J. Quantitative assessment of seizure severity for clinical trials: a review of approaches to seizure components. *Epilepsia* 2001;**42**:119–29.

1156. Crandall BF. A familial syndrome of deafness, alopecia and hypogonadism. *J Pediatr* 1973;**82**:461–5.

1157. Cravens G, Kline DG. Posterior interosseous nerve palsies. *Neurosurgery* 1990;**27**:397–402.

1158. Cravioto H, Feigin I. Noninfectious granulomatous angiitis with a predilection for the nervous system. *Neurology* 1959;**9**:599–609.

1159. Cremer PD, Halmagyi GM, Goadsby PJ. Secondary cluster headache responsive to sumatriptan. *J Neurol Neurosurg Psychiatry* 1995;**59**:633–634. 1995.

1160. Cremers FPM, Molloy CM, van der Pol DJR, et al. An autosomal homologue of the choroideremia gene colocalizes with the Usher syndrome type II locus on the distal part pf chromosome 1q. *Hum Mol Genet* 1992;**1**:71–5.

1161. Creston RN, Godwin-Austen RB. Transient global amnesia in four brothers. *J Neurol Neurosurg Psychiatry* 1982;**45**:375–7.

1162. Creutzfeldt HG. On a peculiar type of disease of the central nervous system: a preliminary communication [in German]. *Z Ges Neurol Psychiatr* 1920;**57**:1–18.

1163. Crevits L, Vander Ecken H. Ocular lateropulsion in Wallenburg's syndrome. *Acta Neurol Scand* 1982;**65**:219.

1164. Crimlisk H. The little imitator-porphyria: a neuropsychiatric disorder. *J Neurol Neurosurg Psychiatry* 1997;**62**:319–28.

1165. Crino PB, Henske EP. New developments in the neurobiology of the tuberous sclerosis complex. *Neurology* 1999;**53**:1384–90.

1166. Critchley M. The anterior cerebral artery and its syndromes. *Brain* 1930;**53**:120–65.

1167. Critchley M. Musicogenic epilepsy. *Brain* 1937;**60**:13–27.

1168. Critchley M. Spastic dysphonia("inspiratory speech"). *Brain* 1939;**62**:96–103.

1169. Critchley M. *The Language of Gesture.* London: Edward Arnold, 1939.

1170. Critchley M. Types of visual perseveration: paliopsia and illusory visual spread. *Brain* 1951;**74**:267–99.

1171. Critchley M. *The Parietal Lobes.* London: Edward Arnold, 1953.

1172. Critchley M. *Aphasiology and Other Disorders of Speech.* London: Edward Arnold, 1957.

1173. Critchley M. Head's contribution to aphasia. *Brain* 1961;**84**: 551–60.

1174. Critchley M. Periodic hypersomnia and megaphagia in adolescent males. *Brain* 1962;**85**:627–56.

1175. Critchley M. Acquired anomalies of colour perception of central origin. *Brain* 1965;**88**:711–24.

1176. Critchley M. Neurology's debt to F.J. Gall. *BMJ* 1965;**2**:775–81.

1177. Critchley M. The enigma of Gerstmann's syndrome. *Brain* 1966; **89**:183–98.

1178. Critchley M. *Aphasiology and Other aspects of Language.* London: Edward Arnold, 1970.

1179. Critchley M. *Aphasiology and Other Disorders of Speech.* London: Edward Arnold, 1980.

1180. Critchley M. And all the daughters of musick shall be brought low: language function in the elderly. *Arch Neurol* 1984;**41**:1135–9.

1181. Critchley M, Earl CJC. Tuberose sclerosis and allied conditions. *Brain* 1932;**55**:311–46.

1182. Critchley M, Henson RA. *Music and the Brain—Studies in the Neurology of Music.* London: Heinemann, 1977.

1183. Crock HV. Isolated lumbar disk resorption as a cause of nerve root canal stenosis. *Clin Orthop* 1976;**115**:109–15.

1184. Crock HV. Internal disk disruption; a challenge to disc prolapse fifty years on. *Spine* 1986;**11**:650–3.

1185. Crocker AC, Farber S. Niemann Pick disease: a review of 18 patients. *Medicine* 1958;**37**:1–95.

1186. Croft PB, Urich H, Wilkinson M. Peripheral neuropathy of sensorimotor type associated with malignant disease. *Brain* 1967;**90**:31.

1187. Croft PB, Wilkinson M. The course and prognosis in some types of carcinomatous neuromyopathy. *Brain* 1969;**92**:1.

1188. Crome L, et al. Congenital cataracts, renal tubular necrosis and encephalopathy in two sisters. *Arch Dis Child* 1963;**38**:505–15.

1189. Crome L, Hanefeld F, Patrick D, et al. Late onset globoid cell leukodystrophy. *Brain* 1973;**96**:841–8.

1190. Crome L, Williams C. The problem of familial multilocular encephalomalacia. *Acta Pediatr Scand* 1960;**49**:175.

1191. Crook TH, Bartus RT, Ferris SH, et al. Age-associated memory impairment: proposed diagnostic criteria and measures of clinical change: report of a National Institute of Mental Health work group. *Dev Neuropsychol* 1986;**2**:261–76.

1192. Crook TH, Ferris SH, McCarthy M. The Misplaced Objects Task: a brief test for memory dysfunction in the aged. *J Am Geriatr Soc* 1979;**7**:284–7.

1193. Crook TH, Larrabee GJ. Age-associated memory impairment: diagnostic criteria and treatment strategies. *Psychopharmacol Bull* 1988;**2**:509–14.

1194. Crosby L, Parsons LC. Clinical neurological assessment tool. *Heart Lung* 1989;**18**:121–9.

1195. Cross HE, McKusick VA. The Mast syndrome. *Arch Neurol* 1967;**16**:1–13.

1196. Cross HE, McKusick VA. The Troyer syndrome: a recessive form of spastic paraplegia with distal muscle wasting. *Arch Neurol* 1967;**16**: 473–85.

1197. Cross HE, McKusick VA, Breen W. A new oculocerebral syndrome with hypopigmentation. *J Pediatr* 1967;**70**:398–406.

1198. Crouzon E. De l'acrocephalosyndactylie. *Bull Soc Med Hop Paris* 1906;**23**:1310–30.

1199. Crouzon O. Dysostose cranio-faciale hereditaire. *Bull Soc Med Hop Paris* 1912;**33**:545–55.

1200. Crouzon O, Justin-Besancon L-E. Post-traumatic parkinsonism [in French]. *Presse Med* 1929;**37**:1325–7.

1201. Crow RS. Peripheral neuritis in myelomatosis. *BMJ* 1956;**2**: 802–4.

1202. Croxen R, Newland C, Betty M, et al. Novel functional e-subunit polypeptide generated by a single nucleotide deletion in acetylcholine receptor deficiency congenital myasthenic syndrome. *Ann Neurol* 1999;**46**:639–47.

1203. Cruchet JR. *Traité des Torticollis Spasmodiques.* Paris: Masson, 1907.

1204. Cruchet JR, Moutier J, Calmettes R. Quarante cas d'encephalomyelite subaîgue. *Bull Soc Med Hop Paris* 1917;**41**:814–6.

1205. Crue BL. *Medulloblastoma.* Springfield IL: Charles C. Thomas, 1958.

1206. Cruickshank JK, Rudge P, Dalgleish AG, et al. Tropical spastic paraparesis and human T-cell lymphotropic virus type 1 in the United Kingdom. *Brain* 1989;**112**:1057.

1207. Cruveilhier J. *Anatomie Pathologique du Corps Humain*. Paris: Bailliere, 1829.

1208. Cruz Martinez A, Conde MCP, Ferrer MT, et al. Neuromuscular disorders in a new toxic syndrome. *Muscle Nerve* 1984;**7**:12–22.

1209. Cuba Neuropathy Field Investigation Team. Epidemic optic neuropathy in Cuba—clinical characterization and risk factors. *N Engl J Med* 1995;**333**:1176–82.

1210. Cuetter AC, Bartoszek DM. The thoracic outlet syndrome: controversies, overdiagnosis, overtreatment and recommendations for management. *Muscle Nerve* 1989;**12**:410–9.

1211. Cumming WJK. Lipid myopathy. *J Neurol Sci* 1984;**64**:73–7.

1212. Cumming WJK, Weiser R, Teoh R, et al. Localized nodular myositis: a clinical and pathological variant of polymyositis. *Q J Med* 1977;**46**:531–46.

1212a. Cummings CJ, Zoghbi HY. Fourteen and counting: unraveling trinucleotide repeat diseases. *Hum Molec Genet* 2000;**9**:906–16.

1213. Cummings J, Benson DF, LoVerne S. Reversible dementias. *JAMA* 1980;**243**:2434–9.

1214. Cummings JL, Gittinger JW Jr. Central dazzle: a thalamic syndrome? *Arch Neurol* 1981;**38**:372–4.

1215. Cummings JL, Mega M, Gray K, et al. The neuropsychiatric inventory. *Neurology* 1994;**44**:2308–14.

1216. Cummings JL, Syndulko K, Goldberg Z, et al. Palinopsia reconsidered. *Neurology* 1982;**32**:444–7.

1218. Cummings JN, Kremer M. Clinical effects of hypoglycemia. In *Biochemical Aspects of Neurological Disorders*, pp 159–68. Philadelphia: Lippincott, 1965.

1219. Cuneo RA, Caronna JJ, Pitts L, et al. Upward transtentorial herniation: seven cases and a literature review. *Arch Neurol* 1979;**36**:618–23.

1220. Cunliffe WJ, Hudgson P, Fulthorpe JJ, et al. A calcitonin-secreting medullary thyroid carcinoma associated with mucosal neuromas, marfanoid features, myopathy and pigmentation. *Am J Med* 1970;**48**:120–6.

1221. Curless RG, Flynn JT, Olsen KR, et al. Leber congenital amaurosis in siblings with diffuse demyelination. *Pediatr Neurol* 1991;**7**:223–5.

1222. Curran T, Grewal K, Frecker M. Dystonia, acanthocytosis, basal ganglia 'calcification' and eye abnormalities (DACE syndrome). Personal communication, 1993.

1223. Currie S, Noronha M, Harriman DGF. In *Abstracts of the 3rd World Congress on Muscle Diseases*. Amsterdam: Excerpta Medica, p 12, 1974.

1224. Currie S, Roberts AH, Urich H. The nosological position of concentric lacunar leucoencephalopathy. *J Neurol Neurosurg Psychiatry* 1970;**33**:131–7.

1225. Currier RD, Giles CL, DeJong RN. Some comments on Wallenberg's lateral medullary syndrome. *Neurology* 1961;**11**:778–91.

1226. Curschmann H. Ueber die diagnostische Bedeutung des Babinskischen Phaenomens im praeuraemischen Zustand. *Munch Med Wochenschr* 1911;**39**:2054–7.

1227. Curtius F. Kongenitaler partieller Riesenwuchsmit endocrinen Storungen. *Arch Klin Med* 1925;**147**:310–9.

1228. Cushing HW. Concerning a definite regulatory system mechanism of the vasomotor center which controls blood pressure during cerebral compression. *John Hopkins Hosp Bull* 1901;**12**:290–2.

1229. Cushing HW. *Tumors of the Nervus Acousticus and the Syndrome of the Cerebellopontine Angle*. Philadelphia: W.B. Saunders, 1917.

1230. Cushing HW. The meningiomas (*dural endotheliomas*): their source and favoured seats of origin. *Brain* 1922;**5**:282–316.

1231. Cushing HW. The chiasmal syndrome of primary optic atrophy with bitemporal field defects in adults with a normal sella turcica. *Arch Ophthalmol* 1930;**3**:505–51.

1232. Cushing HW. The basophil adenomas of the pituitary body and their clinical manifestations (pituitary basophilism). *Bull Johns Hopkins Hosp* 1932;**50**:137–95.

1233. Cushing HW, Walker CB. Distortions of the visual fields in cases of brain tumour. *Brain* 1915;**37**:341–400.

1234. Cusimano MD, Bilbao JM, Cohen SM. Hypertrophic brachial plexus neuritis: a pathological study of two cases. *Ann Neurol* 1988;**24**:615–22.

1235. Cutler EA, et al. A familial thyrocerebral-renal syndrome. *Birth Defects* 1978;**14**:265–74.

1236. Cutler RWP, Spertell RB. Cerebrospinal fluid: a selective review. *Ann Neurol* 1982;**11**:1–10.

1237. Cytowic RE. *Synesthesia: A Union of the Senses*. New York: Springer-Verlag, 1988.

1238. Cytowic RE. Synesthesia: phenomenology and neuropsychology: a review of current knowledge. *Psyche* 1995;**2**:723–93.

1239. D'Addario R, Greenberg J, O'Neill JE, et al. Pneumocephalus: an unusual cause. *J Neurol Neurosurg Psychiatry* 1974;**37**:271–4.

1240. Daentl DL, Berg BO, Layzer RB, et al. A new familial arthrogryposis without weakness. *Neurology* 1974;**24**:55–60.

1241. Dalakas M. Progress in inflammatory myopathies: good but not good enough. *J Neurol Neurosurg Psychiatry* 2001;**70**:569–73.

1242. Dalakas MC. Chronic idiopathic ataxic neuropathy. *Ann Neurol* 1986;**19**:545–54.

1243. Dalakas MC, Elder G, Hallett M, et al. A long-term follow-up study of patients with post-poliomyelitis neuromuscular symptoms. *N Engl J Med* 1986;**314**:959–63.

1244. Dalakas MC, et al. Late post-polio muscular atrophy. *Rev Infect Dis* 1984;**6 Suppl 2**:s562.

1245. Dalakas MC, Hallett M. Post-polio muscular atrophy. In Plum F, ed. *Advances in Contemporary Neurology*, pp 61–83. Philadelphia: F.A. Davis, 1988.

1246. Dalal PM. The aortic arch syndrome. In Spillane JD, ed. *Tropical Neurology*, pp 92–8. London: Oxford University Press, 1973.

1247. Dalby MA. Epilepsy and 3 per second spike wave rhythms. A clinical, EEG and prognostic analysis of 346 patients. *Acta Neurol Scand, Suppl* 1969;**40 Suppl**:1–183.

1248. Dal Canto MC, Rapin I, Suzuki K. Neuronal storage disease with chorea and curvilinear bodies. *Neurology* 1974;**24**:1026.

1249. D'Alessio JG, Rosenblum M. The Bezold-Jarisch reflex. *Anesthiol Analg* 1996;**83**:201–2.

1250. Daley ML, Swank RL, Ellison CM. Flicker fusion thresholds in multiple sclerosis: a functional measure of neurological damage. *Arch Neurol* 1979;**36**:292–5.

1251. Dalla Bernardina B, Bureau M, Dravet C, et al. Epilepsie benigne de l'enfant avec crises a semeiologie affective. *Rev Electroencephalogr Neurophysiol Clin* 1980;**10**:8–18.

1252. Dalmau J, Posner JB. Neurologic paraneoplastic antibodies (anti-Yo; anti-Hu; anti-Ri). *Neurology* 1994;**44**:2241–6.

1253. Dalmau JO, Posner JB. Paraneoplastic syndromes. *Arch Neurol* 1999;**56**:405–8.

1254. Dalton J. Extraordinary facts relating to the vision of colours with observations. *Mem Lit Phil Soc (Manchester)* 1798;**5**:28–45.

1255. Dalton K, Dalton MJT. Characteristics of pyridoxine overdose neuropathy syndrome. *Acta Neurol Scand* 1987;**76**:8–11.

1256. Daly DD. Uncinate fits. *Neurology* 1958;**8**:250–60.

1257. Daly RF, Forster FM. Inheritance of reading epilepsy. *Neurol Minneap* 1975;**25**:1051–4.

1258. Damas-Mora J, Skelton-Robinson, Jenner FA. The Charles Bonnet syndrome in perspective. *Psychol Med* 1982;**12**:251–61.

1259. Damasio AR. Autism. *Arch Neurol* 1984;**41**:481.

1260. Damasio AR. Disorders of complex visual processing: agnosias, achromatopsia, Balint's syndrome, and related difficulties of orientation and construction. In Mesulam M-M, ed. *Principles of Behavioral Neurology*, pp 259–89. Philadelphia: F.A. Davis, 1985.

1261. Damasio AR. Aphasia. *N Engl J Med* 1992;**326**:531–9.

1262. Damasio AR, Damasio H, Rizzo M, et al. Aphasia with non-hemorrhagic lesions in the basal ganglia and internal capsule. *Arch Neurol* 1982;**39**:15–20.

1263. Damasio AR, Damasio H, Van Hoesen GW. Prosopagnosia: anatomic basis and behavioral mechanisms. *Neurology* 1982;**32**:331–41.

1264. Damasio AR, Galaburda AM. Norman Geschwind. *Arch Neurol* 1985;**42**:500–4.

1265. Damasio H, Damasio AR. The anatomical basis of conduction aphasia. *Brain* 1980;**103**:337–50.

1266. Dan D, Grubb BP, Mouhaffel AH, et al. Use of serotonin re-uptake inhibitors as primary therapy for carotid sinus hypersensitivity. *Clin Electrophysiol* 1997;**20**:1633–5.

1267. Dana CL. Hereditary tremor, a hitherto undescribed form of motor neurosis. *Am J Med Sci* 1887;**94**:386–93.

1268. Dana CL. The degenerative diseases of the spinal cord with the description of a new type. *J Nerv Ment Dis* 1891;**18**:205–16.

1269. Dana Consortium. Clinical confirmation of the American Academy of Neurology algorithm for HIV-1–associated cognitive/motor disorder. *Neurology* 1996;**47**:1247–53.

1270. Dandy WE. Ventriculography following the injection of air into the cerebral ventricles. *Ann Surg* 1918;**68**:5–11.

1271. Dandy WE. Rontgenography of the brain after the injection of air into the spinal canal. *Ann Surg* 1919;**70**:397–403.

1272. Dandy WE. The diagnosis and treatment of hydrocephalus due to occlusion of the foramina of Luschka and Magendie. *Surg Gynecol Obstet* 1921;**32**:112–24.

1273. Danek A, Rubio JP, Rampoldi L, et al. McLeod neuroacanthocytosis: genotype and phenotype. *Ann Neurol* 2001;**50**:755–64.

1274. Danielssen DC, Boeck CW. *Om Spedalskheden.* Christiana: Grondahl, 1847.

1275. Danon MJ, Carpenter S, Manaligod R, et al. Fatal infantile glycogen storage disease. *Neurology* 1981;**31**:1302–7.

1276. Danon MJ, Oh SJ, DiMauro S, et al. Lysosomal glycogen storage diseases with normal acid maltase. *Neurology* 1981;**31**:51–7.

1277. Danpure J, Angelini C, Vergani L. Enzymic diagnosis of primary hyperoxaluria, type 1 by measurement of hepatic alanine:glyoxalate aminotransferase activity. *Lancet* 1987;**1**:289–91.

1278. Danta G. Familial carpal tunnel syndrome with onset in childhood. *J Neurol Neurosurg Psychiatry* 1975;**38**:350–5.

1279. Danta G, Hilton RC, Lynch PG. Chronic progressive external ophthalmoplegia. *Brain* 1975;**98**:473–92.

1280. Danzl DF, Pozos RS. Accidental hypothermia. *N Engl J Med* 1994;**331**:1756–60.

1281. Daras M, Koppel BS, Atos-Radzien E. Cocaine-induced choreoathetoid movements (crack dancing). *Neurology* 1994;**44**:751–2.

1282. Darby DY, Domman GA, Saling MA. Primary interventricular hemorrhage. *Neurology* 1988;**38**:68–75.

1283. Darin N, Kyllerman M, Wahlstrom J, et al. Autosomal dominant myopathy with congenital joint contractures, ophthalmoplegia and rimmed vacuoles. *Ann Neurol* 1998;**44**:242–8.

1284. Darley FL, Aronson AE, Brown JR. Differential diagnostic pattern of dysarthria. *J Speech Hear Res* 1969;**12**:246–9.

1285. Darley FL, Aronson AE, Brown JR. *Audioseminars in Speech Pathology—Motor Speech Disorders.* Philadelphia: W.B. Saunders, 1975.

1286. Darnell RB, Arbit E. Reversible diencephalic dysfunction. *Neurology* 1993;**43**:579–82.

1287. Daroff R. Ocular oscillations. *Ann Otol Rhinol* 1977;**86**:1–6.

1288. Daroff RB. The office tensilon test for ocular myasthenia gravis. *Arch Neurol* 1986;**43**:843–4.

1289. Daroff RB, Deller JJ, Kastl AJ, et al. Cerebral malaria. *JAMA* 1967;**202**:679–82.

1290. Daroff RB, Hoyt WF. Supranuclear disorders of ocular motor control systems in man. In Bach-y-Rita P, Collins CC, Hyde JE, eds. *The Control of Eye Movements,* pp 191–5. New York: Academic Press, 1971.

1291. Daroff RB, Hoyt WF, Sanders MD, et al. Gaze-evoked eyelid and ocular nystagmus inhibited by the near reflex. *J Neurol Neurosurg Psychiatry* 1968;**31**:362–7.

1292. Darsee JR. Mitral valve prolapse and ophthalmoplegia; a progressive cardio-neurologic syndrome. *Ann Intern Med* 1980;**92**:735.

1293. Darsee JR, Miklozek L, Heynsfield S, et al. Mitral valve prolapse and ophthalmolegia. *Ann Intern Med* 1980;**92**:735–41.

1294. Darwish H, Sarnat HB, Archer C, et al. Congenital cervical spinal muscular atrophy. *Muscle Nerve* 1981;**4**:106–10.

1295. Dastur DK, Manghani DK, Osuntokun BO, et al. Neuromuscular and related changes in malnutrition. *J Neurol Sci* 1982;**55**:207–30.

1296. Dastur DK, Udani PM. The pathology and pathogenesis of tuberculous encephalopathy. *Acta Neuropathol* 1992;**6**:311–26.

1297. Dau PC. Plasmapheresis: therapeutic or experimental procedure? *Arch Neurol* 1984;**41**:647–53.

1298. Daube JR. Rucksack paralysis. *JAMA* 1969;**208**:2447–52.

1299. Daube JR, Peters HA. Hereditary essential myoclonus. *Arch Neurol* 1966;**15**:587–94.

1300. Dauer WT, Burke RE, Greene P, et al. Current concepts on the clinical features, aetiology and management of idiopathic cervical dystonia. *Brain* 1996;**121**:547–60.

1301. Daum RS, Lamm PH, Mamer OA, et al. A 'new' disorder of isoleucine catabolism. *Lancet* 1971;**2**:1289–90.

1302. Daum RS, Scriver CR, Mamer OA, et al. An inherited disorder of isoleucine catabolism causing accumulation of alpha methylacetoacetate and alpha-methyl-beta-hydroxybutyrate, and intermittent acidosis. *Pediatr Res* 1973;**7**:149.

1303. Daumas-Duport C. Histological grading of gliomas. *Curr Opin Neurol Neurosurg* 1992;**5**:924–31.

1304. Daumas-Duport C, Scheithauer B, O'Fallon J, et al. Grading of astrocytomas: a simple and reproducible method. *Cancer* 1988;**62**: 2152–65.

1305. D'Avanzo R, Scuotto A, Natale M, et al. Transient 'cerebellar' mutism in lesions of the mesencephalic-cerebellar region. *Acta Neurol* 1993;**15**:289–94.

1306. David AS, Jeste DV, Folstein MF, et al. Voluntary movement dysfunction in Huntington's disease and tardive dyskinesia. *Acta Neurol Scand* 1987;**75**:130–9.

1307. David DJ, Proudman TW. Cephaloceles: classification, pathology and management. *World J Surg* 1989;**13**:349–57.

1308. David NJ. Optokinetic nystagmus. *J Clin Neuroophthalmol.* 1989; **9**:258–66.

1309. David TJ. Nature and etiology of the Poland anomaly. *N Engl J Med* 1972;**287**:487–9.

1310. Davidenkow S. Scapuloperoneal amyotrophy. *Arch Neurol Psychiatry* 1939;**41**:694–701.

1311. Davidson G. Time agnosia. *J Nerv Ment Dis* 1941;**94**:336–43.

1312. Davidson S. Cryptococcal spinal arachnoiditis. *J Neurol Neurosurg Psychiatry* 1968;**31**:76.

1313. Davis FA, Bergen D, Schauf C, et al. Movement phosphenes in optic neuritis: a new clinical sign. *Neurology* 1967;**26**:1100–4.

1314. Davis MJ, Cilo M, Plaitakis A, et al. Trichinosis: severe myopathic involvement with recovery. *Neurology* 1976;**26**:37–40.

1315. Dawson G. Glycosphingolipid levels in an unusual neurovisceral storage disease: lactosylceramidosis. *J Lipid Res* 1972;**13**:207–19.

1316. Dax M. Lesions de la moitie gauche de l'encéphale coincident avec l'oublie des signes de la pensée. *Gaz Hebd Med Chir* 1865;**2**:259.

1317. Day JW, Raskin NH. Thunderclap headache: symptom of unruptured cerebral aneurysm. *Lancet* 1986;**ii**:1247–8.

1318. Dayan AD, Williams R. Demyelinating peripheral neuropathy in liver disease. *Lancet* 1967;**2**:133–4.

1319. D'Costa DF, Abbott RJ, Pye IF, et al. The apomorphine test in parkinsonian syndromes. *J Neurol Neurosurg Psychiatry* 1991;**54**:870–2.

1320. Deady JP, Morrell AJ, Sutton GA. Recognising aponeurotic ptosis. *J Neurol Neurosurg Psychiatry* 1989;**52**:996–8.

1321. Dearborn G. A case of congenital general pure analgesia. *J Nerv Ment Dis* 1932;**75**:612–5.

1322. de Barsy AM, Moens E, Dierckx L. Dwarfism, oligophrenia and degeneration of the elastic tissue in skin and cornea: a new syndrome? *Helv Pediatr Acta* 1968;**23**:305–13.

1323. DeBassio WA, Kemper TL, Knoefel JE. Coffin-Siris syndrome: neuropathological findings. *Arch Neurol* 1985;**42**:350–3.

1324. Debré R, Semelaigne G. Hypertrophie musculaire generalisée du petit enfant. *Bull Soc Pediatr Paris* 1934;**32**:699–706.

1325. Dechambre A. Memoire sur la curabilité du ramollissement cérébral. *Gaz Med (Paris)* 1838;**6**:305–14.

1326. DeCroix JP, Graveleau Ph, Masson M, et al. Infarction in the territory of the anterior choroidal artery: a clinical and computerized tomographic study of 16 cases. *Brain* 1986;**109**:1071–85.

1327. De Gasperi R, Gama Sosa MA, Battinisti S, et al. Late onset GM2 gangliosidosis. *Neurology* 1996;**47**:547–52.

1328. deGirolami U, Haas ML, Richardson EP jr. Subacute diencephalic angioencephalopathy—a clinico-pathologic case study. *J Neurol Sci* 1974;**22**:197–210.

1329. Degos R, Delort J, Tricot R. Dermatite papulo-squameuse atrophiante. *Bull Soc France Dermatol Syph* 1942;**49**:148–281.

1330. Degoul F, Pou-Serradell A, Lloreta J, et al. Myo-leukoencephalopathy in twins: study of 3243 myopathy, encephalopathy, lactic acidosis and strokelike episodes of mitochondrial mutation. *Ann Neurol* 1994;**35**:365–70.

1331. DeGrouchy J, Royer P, Salmon Ch, et al. Deletion partielle des bras longs du chromosome 18. *Pathol Biol* 1964;**12**:5–79.

1332. de Grouchy J, Turleau C, Leonard C. Etude en fluorescence d'une trisomy C mosaïque, probablement 8:46, XY-47, XY:8+. *Ann Genet* 1971;**14**:69.

1333. de Haan R, Aaronson N, Limburg M, et al. Measuring quality of life in stroke. *Stroke* 1993;**24**:320–7.

1334. de Haan RJ. Clinimetrics in stroke. Thesis, University of Amsterdam, 1994.

1335. Dehan M, Quilleron D, Navelet Y, et al. Les convulsions du cinquième jour de vie: un nouveau syndrome? *Arch Fr Pediatr* 1977;**34**:730–42.

1336. Dehkharghani F, Sarnat H, Brewster M, et al. Congenital muscle fiber type disproportion in Krabbe's leukodystrophy. *Arch Neurol* 1981;**38**:585–7.

1337. Dejean MC. Le syndrome du plancher de l'orbite. *Bull Fr Soc Ophthalmol* 1935;**48**:473–85.

1338. Déjerine JJ. Sur un cas de paraplégie par névrites périphèriques, chez un ataxique morphiomane. *C R Soc Biol* 1887;**4**:137–43.

1339. Déjerine JJ. Sur un cas de cécité verbal avec agraphie, suivie d'autopsie. *C R Soc Biol* 1891;**3**:197–201.

1340. Déjerine JJ. *Diseases of the Spinal Cord* [in French]. Paris: Baillière, 1909.

1341. Déjerine JJ. *Sèmiologie des Affections du Système Nerveux.* Paris: Masson, 1914.

1342. Déjerine JJ, Déjerine-Klumpke H. *Anatomie des Centres Nerveux.* Paris: J. Rueff, 1901.

1343. Déjerine JJ, Mouzon J. Two cases of a sensory cortical syndrome [in French]. *Rev Neurol (Paris)* 1914;**28**:388–92.

1344. Déjerine JJ, Roussy G. Le syndrome thalamique. *Rev Neurol (Paris)* 1906;**14**:521–32.

1345. Déjerine JJ, Sottas J. Sur la névrite interstitielle hypertrophique et progressive de l'enfant. *C R Soc Biol* 1890;**2**:43–53.

1346. Déjerine JJ, Thomas A. L'atrophie olivo-ponto-cerebelleuse. *Nouv Icon Salpet* 1900;**13**:330–70.

1347. De Jong JGY. Over families met hereditaires disposities tpt het optreden van neuritiden gecorreleerd met migraine. *Psychiatr Neurol (Belg)* 1947;**50**:60–76.

1348. De Jong JGY, Sloof JL, van der Erden AAJJ. A family with paramyotonia congenita with the report of an autopsy. *Acta Neurol Scand* 1973;**49**:480–94.

1349. De Jong R. *The Neurological Examination.* New York: Harper & Row, 1967.

1349a. De Jong R. *The Neurological Examination.* Hagerstown, MD: Harper & Row, 1979.

1350. Dejoun HH. *Experimental Catatonia.* Baltimore: Williams and Wilkins, 1945.

1351. Dekaban AS. Anencephaly in human embryos. *J Neuropathol Exp Neurol* 1963;**22**:533.

1352. Delacourte A, Buée L. Tau pathology: a marker of neurodegenerative disorders. *Curr Opin Neurol* 2000;**13**:371–6.

1353. de la Monte SM, Horowitz SA, Larocque AA, et al. Keyhole aqueduct syndrome. *Arch Neurol* 1986;**43**:926–9.

1354. Delaney P. Neurologic Manifestations of Sarcoidosis. *Ann Intern Med* 1977;**87**:336–45.

1355. de Lange C. Sur un type nouveau de dégénération (typus amstelodamnus). *Arch Med Enf Paris* 1933;**36**:713–9.

1356. de Lange C. Congenital hypertrophy of the muscles, extrapyramidal motor disturbances and mental deficiency. A clinical entity. *Am J Dis Child* 1934;**48**:243–68.

1357. Del Brutto OH, Rajshekhar V, White AC, et al. Proposed diagnostic criteria for neurocysticercosis. *Neurology* 2001;**57**:177–83.

1358. Del Brutto OH, Wadia NH, Dumas M, et al. Proposal of diagnostic criteria for human cysticercosis and neurocysticercosis. *J Neurol Sci* 1996;**142**:1–6.

1359. De Leon GA, Grover WD, Huff DS, et al. Globoid cells, glial nodules and peculiar fibrillary changes in the cerebro-hepato-renal syndrome of Zellweger. *Ann Neurol* 1977;**2**:473–84.

1360. Deleu D, Buisseret T, Ebinger G. Vertical one and a half syndrome. *Arch Neurol* 1989;**46**:1361–3.

1361. Delgado-Escueta AV. Epileptogenic paroxysms: modern approaches and clinical correlations. *Neurology* 1979;**29**:1014–22.

1362. Delgado-Escueta AV, Greenberg D. Classification of the epilepsies for genetic studies. *Ann Neurol* 1984;**16 Suppl**:1–11.

1363. Delis DC, Kramer JH, Kaplan E, et al. *The California Verbal Learning Test.* New York: Psychological Corporation, 1987.

1364. DeLisa JA, Saeed MA. The tarsal tunnel syndrome. *Muscle Nerve* 1983;**6**:664–70.

1365. De Lisi L. Su di un fenomeno motorio costante del sonno normale: le mioclonie ipniche fisiologiche. *Riv Pat Nerv Ment* 1932;**39**:481–96.

1366. Delitto A. Isokinetic dynamometry. *Muscle Nerve* 1990;**S53–S57**.

1367. Delleman JW, Oorthuys JWE. Orbital cysts in addition to congenital cerebral and focal dermal malformations: a new entity? *Clin Genet* 1984;**25**:470–2.

1368. Dell'Osso LF. Nystagmus, saccadic intrusions/oscillations and oscillopsia. In Lessell S, van Dalen JTW, eds. *Current Neuro-ophthalmology,* pp 153–91. St. Louis: Mosby-Year Book, 1991.

1369. Dell'Osso LF, Schmidt D, Daroff RB. Latent, manifest latent and congenital nystagmus. *Arch Ophthalmol* 1979;**97**:1877–85.

1370. Dell'Osso LF, Troost BT, Daroff RB. Macro square wave jerks. *Neurology* 1975;**25**:975–9.

1371. Dell'Osso LF, Weissman BM, Leigh RJ, et al. Hereditary congenital nystagmus and gaze-holding failure. *Neurology* 1993;**43**:1741–9.

1372. DeLong GR, Bean SC, Brown FR. Acquired reversible autistic syndrome in acute encephalopathic illness in children. *Arch Neurol* 1981;**38**:191–4.

1373. Delwaide PJ, Pepin JL, Maertens de Noordhout A. The audiospinal reaction in parkinsonian patients reflects functional changes in reticular nuclei. *Ann Neurol* 1993;**33**:63–9.

1374. DeMarco P, Tassinari CA. Extreme somatosensory evoked potential (ESEP): an EEG sign forecasting the possible occurrence of seizures in children. *Epilepsia* 1981;**22**:569–75.

1375. de Melo A, Krauss GL, Niedermeyer E. Spindle coma: observations and thoughts. *Clin Electroencephalogr* 1990;**21**:151–61.

1376. Demeurisse G, Demol O, Robaye E. Motor evaluation in vascular hemiplegia. *Eur Neurol* 1980;**19**:382–9.

1377. DeMeyer W, Zeman W, Palmer CG. The face predicts the brain: diagnostic significance of median facial anomalies for holoprosencephaly. *Pediatrics* 1964;**34**:256–63.

1378. Demirkiran M, Jankovic J. Paroxysmal dyskinesias: clinical features and classification. *Ann Neurol* 1995;**38**:571–9.

1379. de Morsier G. Pathologie du diencephale. Le syndrome psychologique et le syndrome sensori-moteur. *Schweiz Arch Neur* 1944;**54**:161–226.

1380. de Morsier G. Median cranioencephalic dysraphias and olfactogenital dysplasia. *World Neurol* 1962;**3**:485–506.

1381. de Morsier G. Contribution a l'étude clinique des alterations de la formation reticulée: le syndrome sensori-moteur et psychologique. *J Neurol Sci* 1966;**4**:15–49.

1382. de Morsier G. Amyotrophic lateral sclerosis with Pick disease. *Rev Neurol (Paris)* 1967;**116**:373.

1383. Dempsey JA, Skatrud JB. A sleep induced apneic threshold and its consequences. *Am Rev Respir Dis* 1986;**133**:1163–70.

1384. De Myer W. Megalencephaly: types, clinical syndromes, and management. *Pediatr Neurol* 1986;**2**:321.

1385. Dengler R, Wohlfarth K, Zierz S, et al. Muscle fatigue, lactate and pyruvate in mitochondrial myopathy with progressive external ophthalmoplegia. *Muscle Nerve* 1996;**19**:456–62.

1386. Denier C, Ducros A, Vahedi K, et al. High prevalence of CACNA1A truncations and broader clinical spectrum in episodic ataxia type 2. *Neurology* 1999;**52**:1816–21.

1387. Denmark A. An example of symptoms resembling tic Douleureux produced by a wound in the radial nerve. *Med Chir Trans* 1813;**3**:48–52.

1388. Dennie C. Partial paralysis of the lower extremities in children accompanied by backward mental development. *Am J Syph* 1929;**13**:157–63.

1389. Dennis M, Bamford JM, Sandercock P, Warlow CP. A comparison of risk factors and prognosis for transient ischemic attacks and minor ischemic strokes. *Stroke* 1989;**20**:1494–9.

1390. Dennis M, Warlow C. Migraine aura without headache; transient ischemic attack or not? *J Neurol Neurosurg Psychiatry* 1992;**55**: 437–40.

1391. Denny-Brown D. Primary sensory neuropathy with muscular changes by carcinoma. *J Neurol* 1948;**11**:73–87.

1392. Denny-Brown D. Hereditary sensory radicular neuropathy. *J Neurol Neurosurg Psychiatry* 1951;**14**:237–52.

1393. Denny-Brown D. Recurrent cerebrovascular episodes. *Arch Neurol* 1960;**2**:194–210.

1394. Denny-Brown D. *The Basal Ganglia*. Oxford: Oxford University Press, 1962.

1395. Denny-Brown D. Hepato-lenticular degeneration (Wilson's disease). Two different components. *N Engl J Med* 1964;**270**:1149.

1396. Denny-Brown D. The release of deep pain by nerve injury. *Brain* 1965;**88**:725–38.

1397. Denny-Brown D. Clinical symptomatology of diseases of the basal ganglia. In Vinken PJ, Bruyn GW, eds. *Handbook of Clinical Neurology*, pp 133–72. Amsterdam: North Holland, 1975.

1398. Denny-Brown D. Spasm of visual fixation. In Rose FC, ed. *Physiological Aspects of Clinical Neurology*, p 68. Oxford: Blackwell, 1977.

1399. Denny-Brown D, Banker BQ. Amorphosynthesis from left parietal lesions. *Arch Neurol Psychiatry* 1954;**71**:302–13.

1400. Denny-Brown D, Chambers RA. Pseudo-thalamic syndrome. *Res Publ Assoc Nerv Ment Dis*. 1958;**36**:35.

1401. Denny-Brown D, Foley JM. Myokymia and benign fasciculations of muscular cramps. *Trans Am Acad Physicians* 1948;**61**:88–96.

1402. Denny-Brown D, Rose AS, Sahs AL. *Centennial Anniversary Volume, American Neurological Association*. New York: Springer-Verlag, 1975.

1403. Deonna TW. *Neuropediatrics* 1986;**17**:81–5.

1404. Deonna TW. Paroxysmal disorders which may be migraine or may be confused with it. In Hockaday JM, ed. *Migraine in Childhood*, pp 75–87. London: Butterworths, 1988.

1405. Deraemaeker R. Sex-linked congenital deafness. *Acta Genet* 1958;**8**:228–31.

1406. Dercum FX. A subcutaneous connective tissue dystrophy of the arms and neck, associated with symptoms ressembling myxedema. *University Med Mag* 1888;**1**:140–50.

1407. Dercum FX. Three cases of an hitherto unclassified affection resembling in its grosser aspects obesity, but associated with special nervous symptoms, adiposis dolorosa. *Am J Med Sci* 1892;**104**:521–35.

1408. De Renzi E. Slowly progressive visual agnosia or apraxia without dementia. *Cortex* 1986;**22**:171–80.

1409. De Renzi E, Faglione P. Normative data and screening power of a shortened version of the Token Test. *Cortex* 1978;**14**:41–9.

1410. De Renzi E, Ferrari C. The reporter's test: a sensitive test to detect expressive disturbances in aphasics. *Cortex* 1978;**14**:279–93.

1411. De Renzi E, Gentilini M, Bazolli C. Eyelid movement disorders and motor impersistence on acute hemisphere disease. *Neurology* 1986;**36**:414.

1412. De Renzi E, Vignolo LA. The Token Test: a sensitive test to detect disturbances in aphasics. *Brain* 1962;**85**:665.

1413. Derkay CS, Bramhall TC. Epstein-Barr viral infectious mononucleosis. *Otolaryngol Head Neck Surg* 1995;**113**:334–7.

1415. Derogatis LR, Spencer PM. *The Brief Symptom Inventory (BSI)[md]Administration, Scoring and Procedures Manual*. Baltimore: Clinical Psychometric Research, 1982.

1416. Desai BT, Porter RJ, Penry JK. Psychogenic seizures: a study of 42 attacks in six patients, with intensive monitoring. *Arch Neurol* 1982;**39**:202–9.

1417. DeSanctis C, Cacchione A. L'idiozia xerodermica. *Riv Sperimentale Freniatria Med Leg Alienazione* 1932;**56**:269–92.

1418. Desforges JF. Medical problems associated with underwater diving. *N Engl J Med* 1992;**326**:30–5.

1419. de Silva RN. A diagnostic sign in migraine? *J R Soc Med* 2001; **94**:286–7.

1420. Desmond NM, Wilson GS, Melnick JL, et al. Congenital rubella encephalitis. *J Pediatr* 1967;**71**:311.

1421. Destee A, Cassim F, Defebvre L, et al. Hereditary chin trembling or hereditary chin myoclonus. *J Neurol Neurosurg Psychiatry* 1997;**63**: 804–7.

1422. Deuschl G, Bain P, Brin M. Consensus Statement of the Movement Disorder Society on Tremor. *Mov Disord* 1998;**13**:2–23.

1423. Devereaux MW, Kleane JR, Davis RL. Automatic respiratory failure associated with infarction of the medulla. *Arch Neurol* 1973;**29**: 46–52.

1424. Devic ME. Myélite aîgue dorso-lombaire avec névrite optique. Autopsie. *Cong Fr Med Lyon* 1894;**1**:434–9.

1425. de Visser M, Scholte HR, Schutgens RS, et al. Riboflavine responsive hereditary storage myopathy and glutaric aciduria type II of early adult onset. *Neurology* 1986;**36**:367–72.

1426. Dewey RB, Maraganore DM. Isolated eyelid-opening apraxia. *Neurology* 1994;**44**:1752–4.

1427. DeWitt LD, Wechsler L. Transcranial Doppler. *Stroke* 1988;**19**: 915–21.

1428. De Wytt CN, Dickson PL, Holt GW. Cryptococcal meningitis. *J Neurol Sci* 1982;**53**:283–92.

1429. de Yebenes JG, Vacquez A, Rabarro J, et al. Hereditary branchial myoclonus with spastic paraparesis and cerebellar ataxia. *Neurology* 1988;**38**:569–72.

1430. Diamond S, Markham CH. Evaluating the evaluations: or how to weigh the scales of parkinsonian disability. *Neurology* 1983;**33**: 1098–9.

1431. Diaz-Arrastia R, Younger DS, Hair L, et al. Neurolymphomatosis. *Neurology* 1992;**42**:1136–41.

1432. Di Chiro G, Reames PM, Matthews WB. RISA-ventriculography and RISA-cisternography. *Neurology* 1964;**14**:185–91.

1433. Dick AP, Massey EW. Neurological presentations of decompression sickness and air embolism in sport divers. *Neurology* 1985;**35**: 667–71.

1434. Dick AP, Stevenson CJ. Hereditary spastic paraplegia. Report of a family with associated extrapyramidal signs. *Lancet* 1953;**i**:921–3.

1435. Dick JPR, Cantello R, Buruma O, et al. The Bereitschaftspotential, L-dopa and Parkinson's disease. *Electroencephalogr Clin Neurophysiol* 1987;**66**:263–74.

1436. Di Costanzo A, Tedeschi G, Di Salle F, et al. Pineal cysts: an incidental MRI finding? *J Neurol Neurosurg Psychiatry* 1993;**56**:207–8.

1437. Dide M. [Persisting amnesia, pure speech loss and atopagnosia with bilateral lingual lobe lesions [in French]. *Rev Neurol (Paris)* 1902;**10**:676–80.

1438. Dide M. Les désorientations temporo-spatiale et la préponderance de l'hemisphere droit dans les agnoso-akinesies proprioceptives. *Encephale* 1938;**33**:276–94.

1439. Di Donato D, Garavaglieri B, Striociuglio P, et al. Multisystem triglyceride storage disease is due to a specific defect in the degradation of endocellularly synthesized triglycerides. *Neurology* 1988;**38**:1107–10.

1440. Di Donato S, Gellera C, Peluchetti D, et al. Normalization of short-chain acylcoenzyme A dehydrogenase. *Arch Neurol* 1989;**25**: 479–84.

1441. Dieterich M, Brandt T. Wallenberg's syndrome. *Ann Neurol* 1992;**31**:399–408.

1442. Dieterich M, Brandt T. Ocular torsion and tilt of subjective visual vertical are sensitive brainstem signs. *Ann Neurol* 1993;**33**:292–9.

1443. Dieterich M, Brandt T. Episodic vertigo related to migraine (90 cases): vestibular migraine? *J Neurol* 1999;**246**:883–92.

1444. DiGeorge AM. A new concept of the cellular basis of immunity. *J Pediatr* 1965;**67**:907–8.

1445. Di Lazzaro V, Restuccia D, Nardone R, et al. Preliminnary observations on a new trigeminal reflex. *Neurology* 1996;**46**:479–85.

1446. Diliberti JH, et al. The fetal valproate syndrome. *Am J Med Genet* 1984;**19**:473–81.

1447. Dillmann U, Heide G, Dietz B, et al. Hereditary motor and sensory neuropathy with spastic paraplegia and optic atrophy; report on a family. *J Neurol* 1997;**244**:562–5.

1448. DiMauro S, Bonilla E, Zeviani M, et al. Mitochondrial myopathies. *Ann Neurol* 1985;**17**:521–38.

1449. DiMauro S, Bresolin N. Newly recognized defects in distal glycolysis. In Engel WK, Banker BQ, eds. *Myology*, pp 1619–51. New York: McGraw-Hill, 1986.

1450. DiMauro S, Dalakas MC, Miranda AF. Phosphoglycerate kinase deficiency, another cause of recurrent myoglobinuria. *Ann Neurol* 1983;**13**:11–19.

1451. DiMauro S, DiMauro PMM. Muscle carnitine palmityltransferase deficiency and myoglobinuria. *Science* 1973;**182**:929–31.

1452. DiMauro S, et al. Metabolic myopathies. *Am J Med Genet* 1986;**25**:635–51.

1453. DiMauro S, Hartlege PL. Fatal infantile form of muscle phosphorylase deficiency. *Neurology* 1978;**28**:1124–9.

1454. DiMauro S, Hartwig GB, Hays A, et al. Debrancher deficiency: neuromuscular disorder in 5 adults. *Ann Neurol* 1979;**5**:422–36.

1455. DiMauro S, Mendell JR, Sahenk Z, et al. Fatal infantile mitochondrial myopathy and renal dysfunction due to cytochrome c oxidase deficiency. *Neurology* 1980;**30**:795–804.

1456. DiMauro S, Miranda AF, Hays AF, et al. Myoadenylate deaminase deficiency. *J Neurol Sci* 1980;**47**:191–202.

1457. DiMauro S, Miranda AF, Olarte M, et al. Muscle phosphoglycerate mutase deficiency. *Neurology* 1982;**32**:584–91.

1458. DiMauro S, Schotland DL, Bonilla E, et al. Progressive ophthalmoplegia, glycogen storage and abnormal mitochondria. *Arch Neurol* 1973;**29**:170–9.

1459. DiMauro S, Trevisan C, Hays A. Disorders of lipid metabolism in muscle. *Muscle Nerve* 1980;**3**:369–88.

1460. Dimsdale H. Hereditary optic atrophy in family with keratodermia palmaris et plantaris (tylosis). *Proc Roy Soc Med* 1949;**42**:796.

1461. Dinarello CA, et al. New concepts on the pathogenesis of fever. *Rev Infect Dis* 1988;**10**:1.

1462. Dincer P, Leturcq F, Richard I, et al. A biochemical, clinical and genetic study of autosomal recessive limb girdle muscular dystrophies in Turkey. *Ann Neurol* 1997;**42**:222–9.

1463. Diniz MA, Cunha L, Goncalves F, et al. Two cases of stiff man syndrome with tremor. *J Neurol* 1986;**142**:918–20.

1464. Dinsdale HB. Hypertensive encephalopathy. *Stroke* 1982;**13**:717–9.

1465. DiNubile MJ. Septic thrombosis of the cavernous sinuses—neurological review. *Arch Neurol* 1988;**45**:567–74.

1466. Direkze M, Fernando BL. Transient anterior horn cell dysfunction in diphenylhydantoin therapy. *Eur Neurol* 1977;**15**:131.

1467. Di Saia PJ. Pregnancy and delivery of a patient with Starr-Edwards mitral valve prosthesis. *Obstet Gynecol* 1966;**28**:469–71.

1473. Disertori B, Ducati A, Piazza M, et al. Brainstem auditory evoked potentials in a case of "Manto syndrome" or spasmodic torticollis with thoracic outlet syndrome. *Ital J Neurol Sci* 1982;**3**:359–63.

1474. Dix MR. Modern tests of vestibular function, with special reference to their value in clinical practice. *BMJ* 1969;**270**:317.

1475. Dobbs AR, Rule BG. Adult age differences in working memory. *Psychol Aging* 1989;**4**:500–503.

1476. Dobkin BH, Verity MA. Spinal muscular atrophy with bulbar palsy. *Neurology* 1976;**26**:754.

1477. Dobkin BH, Verity MA. Familial neuromuscular disease with type I fiber hypoplasia, tubular aggregates, cardiomyopathy and myasthenic features. *Neurology* 1978;**28**:1135–40.

1478. Dobson J. *Anatomical Eponyms*. London: Bailliere, Tindall & Cox, 1946.

1479. Dobyn WB, Pagon RA, Armstrong D, et al. Diagnostic criteria for Walker-Warburg syndrome. *Am J Med Genet* 1989;**32**:195–210.

1480. Dobyns WB. The neurogenetics of lissencephaly. *Neurol Clin* 1989;**7**:89–105.

1481. Dobyns WB, Andermann E, Andermann F, et al. X-linked malformations of neuroonal migration. *Neurology* 1996;**47**:331–9.

1482. Dobyns WB, et al. Familial cavernous malformations of the central nervous system and retina. *Ann Neurol* 1987;**21**:578–83.

1483. Dobyns WB, Ozelius LJ, Kramer PL, et al. Rapid-onset dystonia-parkinsonism. *Neurology* 1993;**43**:2596–602.

1484. Dobyns WB, Stratton RF, Greenberg F. Syndromes with lissencephaly. I: Miller-Dieker and Norman-Roberts syndromes with isolated lissencephaly. *Am J Med Genet* 1984;**18**:509–26.

1485. Dodick DW. Thunderclap headache. *J Neurol Neurosurg Psychiatry* 2002;**72**:6–11.

1486. Dodwell DG, Jampol LM, et al. Optic nerve involvement associated with multiple evanescent white-dot syndrome. *Ophthalmology* 1990;**97**:862–8.

1487. Donaghy M. Classification and clincial features of motor neurone diseases and motor neuropathies in adults. *J Neurol* 1999;**246**:331–3.

1488. Donaghy M, Hakin RN, Bamford JM, et al. Hereditary sensory neuropathy with neurotrophic keratitis. *Brain* 1987;**110**:563–83.

1489. Donaldson IM. Volvular epilepsy: a distinctive and underreported seizure type. *Arch Neurol* 1986;**43**:260–2.

1490. Donat JR, Auger R. Familial periodic ataxia. *Arch Neurol* 1979;**36**:568–9.

1491. Donnan GA, Bladin PF, Berkovic S, et al. The stroke syndrome of striatocapsular infarction. *Brain* 1991;**114**:51–70.

1492. Donnan GA, O'Malley HM, Quang L, et al. The capsular warning syndrome. *Neurology* 1993;**43**:957–62.

1493. Donofrio PD. Monomelic amyotrophy. *Muscle Nerve* 1994;**17**:1129–34.

1494. Donohue WL. Dysendocrinism. *J Pediatr* 1948;**32**:739–48.

1495. Dooley JM, Gordon K, Camfield P. The rushes. *Clin Pediatr* 1990;**29**:536–8.

1496. Doose H, Baier WK. Epilepsy with primarily generalized myoclonic-astatic seizures. *Eur J Pediatr* 1987;**146**:550–4.

1497. Doose H, Gerken H, Leonhardt R, et al. Centrencephalic myoclonic-astatic petit mal. *Neuropediatrics* 1970;**2**:59–78.

1498. Dorfman LJ, Forno LS. Paraneoplastic encephalomyelitis. *Acta Neurol Scand* 1972;**48**:556–74.

1499. Dorfman LJ, Pedley TA, Tharp BR, et al. Juvenile neuroaxonal dystrophy: clinical, electrophysiological and neuropathological features. *Ann Neurol* 1978;**3**:419–28.

1500. Doshi R, Fowler T. Proximal myopathy due to carcinomatous metastasis in muscle. *J Neurol Neurosurg Psychiatry* 1983;**46**:358–60.

1501. Doty RL, Sharman P, Dann M. Development of the Univeraity of Pennsylvania Smell Identification Test. *Physiol Behav* 1984;**32**:489–502.

1502. Douglas AC, MacLeod JG, Matthews JD. Symptomatic sarcoidosis of skeletal muscle. *J Neurol Neurosurg Psychiatry* 1973;**36**:1034–40.

1503. Douglas EF, White PT. Abdominal epilepsy: a reappraisal. *J Pediatr* 1951;**78**:59–67.

1504. Douglas VI. Attentional and cognitive problems. In Rutter M, ed. *Developmental Neuropsychiatry*, pp. 280–329. New York: The Guilford Press, 1983.

1505. Down JL. Marriages of consanguinity in relation to degeneration of race. *Lond Hosp Clin Lect Rep* 1866;**3**:224–36.

1506. Doyle JB. Neurologic complications of serum sickness. *Am J Med Sci* 1933;**185**:484–92.

1507. Drachman D, Banker BQ. Arthrogryposis multiplex congenita. *Arch Neurol* 1961;**5**:89–105.

1508. Drachman DA. Neurological complications of Wegener's granulomatosis. *Arch Neurol* 1963;**8**:145–55.

1509. Drachman DA. Ophthalmoplegia plus: the neurodegenerative disorders associated with progressive external ophthalmoplegia. *Arch Neurol* 1968;**18**:654–74.

1510. Drachman DA. New criteria for the diagnosis of vascular dementia; do we know enough yet? *Neurology* 1993;**43**:243–5.

1511. Drachman DA, Hart CW. Approach to the dizzy patient. *Neurology* 1972;**22**:323–34.

1512. Drachman DA, Richardson EP jr. Aqueductal narrowing, congenital and acquired. *Arch Neurol* 1961;**5**:552–9.

1513. Drake CG. Report of a World Federation of Neurosurgeons Committee on a Universal Subarachnoid Hemorrhage Scale. *J Neurosurg* 1988;**68**:1985–6.

1514. Drake ME, Jackson RL, Miller CA. Paroxysmal choreoathetosis after head injury. *J Neurol Neurosurg Psychiatry* 1986;**49**:837–8.

1515. Dreifuss FE. Discussion of absence and photosensitive epilepsy. In Roger J, Dravet C, Bureau M, et al., eds. *Epileptic Syndromes in Infancy, Childhood and Adolescence*, pp 237–41. London: John Libbey, 1985.

1516. Dreifuss FE. The epilepsies: clinical implications of the international classification. *Epilepsia* 1990;**31**:S3–S10.

1517. Drislane FW. Evidence against permanent neurological damage from nonconvulsive status epilepticus. *J Clin Neurophysiol* 1999;**16**:323–31.

1518. Druckman R, Chao D, Alvord EC. A case of atonic cerebral diplegia with lissencephaly. *Neurology* 1959;**9**:806–14.

1519. Drummond KN, et al. The Blue Diaper syndrome: familial hypocalcemia with nephrocalcinosis and indicanuria. *Am J Med* 1964;**37**:928–48.

1520. Drummond PD, Lance JW. Site of autonomic deficit in harlequin syndrome: local autonomic failure affecting the arm and the face. *Ann Neurol* 1993;**34**:814–6.

1521. Druschky K-F. Hereditary putaminal necrosis. In Vinken PJ, Bruyn GW, Klawans HL, eds. *Extrapyramidal Disorders. Handbook of Clinical Neurology, Vol. 5*, pp 493–8. Amsterdam: Elsevier Science Publishers, 1986.

1522. Duane A. Congenital deficiency of abduction, associated with impairment of adduction, retraction movements, contraction of the palpebral fissure and oblique movements of the eye. *Arch Ophthalmol* 1905;**34**:133–59.

1523. Dubini A. Primi cenni sulla corea elettrica. *Ann Univ Med (Milano)* 1846;**117**:5–50.

1524. Dubois B, Slachevsky A, Litvan I, et al. The FAB. *Neurology* 2000;**55**:1621–6.

1525. Dubois G, Mussini J-M, Auclair M, et al. Adult sphingomyelinase deficiency. *Neurology* 1990;**40**:132–6.

1526. Dubourg O, Barhoumi C, Azzedine H, et al. Clinical, electrophysiological and genetic study of a family with autosomal dominant hereditary sensory neuropathy and predominant weakness. *Muscle Nerve* 2000;**23**:1508–14.

1527. Dubowitz L, Dubowitz V. The neurological assessment of the preterm and full-term newborn infant. In Dubowitz L, Dubowitz V, eds. *Clinics in Developmental Medicine*, London: Heinemann, 1981.

1528. Dubowitz LMS, Dubowitz V, Goldberg C. Scoring system for neurologic criteria. *J Pediatr* 1970;**77**:1.

1529. Dubowitz V. Familial low birthweight dwarfism with an unusual facies and a skin eruption. *J Med Genet* 1965;**2**:12–7.

1530. Dubowitz V. Pseudo-muscular dystrophy. In Research Committee of the Muscular Dystrophy Group of Great Britain, ed. *Research in Muscular Dystrophy. Proceedings of the Third Symposium. Research Committee of the Muscular Dystrophy Group of Great Britain*, pp 57–73. London: Pitman Medical, 1965.

1531. Dubowitz V. Rigid spine syndrome: a muscle syndrome in search of a mname. *Proc R Soc Med* 1973;**66**:219.

1532. Dubowitz V. What is muscular dystrophy? *J R Coll Physicians* 2000;**34**:464–8.

1533. Dubowitz V, Brooke MH. *Muscle Biopsy: A Modern Approach.* London: W.B. Saunders, 1973.

1534. Dubrovsky T, Curless R, Scott G, et al. Cerebral aneurysmal arteriopathy in childhood AIDS. *Neurology* 1998;**51**:560–45.

1535. Duchenne de Boulogne GBA. De l'ataxie locomotrice progressive; récherches sur une maladie caracterisée spécialement par les troubles généraux de la coordination des mouvements. *Arch Gen Med Paris* 1858;**12**:641–52.

1536. Duchenne de Boulogne GBA. Paralysie musculaire progressive de la langue, du voile, du palais et des lèvres, affection non encore décrite comme espéce morbide distincte. *Arch Gen Med Paris* 1860;**16**:283–96.

1537. Duchenne de Boulogne GBA. Récherches sur la paralysie musculaire pseudohypertrophique ou paralysie myo-sclerosique. *Arch Gen Med Paris* 1868;**11**:5–25.

1538. Duchenne de Boulogne GBA. *De L'electrisation Localisee et de Son Application a la Pathologie et a la Therapeutique.* Paris: J.B. Baillière, 1872.

1539. Duchowny M, Jayakar P, Resnick T, et al. Posterior temporal epilepsy: electroclinical features. *Ann Neurol* 1994;**35**:427–31.

1540. Duddung BA, Gorlin RJ. The oto-palato-digital syndrome. *Am J Dis Child* 1967;**113**:214–21.

1541. Duffy CJ. The legacy of association cortex. *Neurology* 1984;**34**:192–7.

1542. Duffy CJ. Implicit memory. *Neurology* 1997;**49**:1200–2.

1543. Duffy FH, Burchfiel JL, Lombroso CT. Brain electrical activity mapping (BEAM): a method for extending the clinical utility of EEG and evoked potential data. *Ann Neurol* 1979;**5**:309–21.

1544. Duffy PE, Sassin JF, Summers DS, et al. Rhombencephalitis due to *Listeria monocytogenes*. *Neurology* 1964;**14**:1067–72.

1545. Duhamel B. From the mermaid to anal imperforation: the syndrome of caudal regression. *Arch Dis Child* 1961;**36**:152–5.

1546. Dulcan MK. Attention deficit disorder: evaluation and treatment. *Pediatr Ann* 1985;**14**:383–400.

1547. Dumitru D, DeLisa JA. AAEM Minimonograph #10: Volume Conduction. *Muscle Nerve* 1991;**14**:605–24.

1548. Duncan JS. Idiopathic generalized epilepsies with typical absences. *J Neurol* 1997;**244**:403–11.

1549. Duncan JS, Sander JWA. The Chalfont Seizure Severity Scale. *J Neurol Neurosurg Psychiatry* 1991;**54**:873–6.

1550. Dunn HG. Ataxia-telangiectasia. *Dev Med Child Neurol* 1973;**15**:324.

1551. Dunn LM. *Expanded Manual for the Peabody Picture Vocabulary Test.* Minneapolis: American Guidance Service, 1970.

1552. Dunne JW, Summers QA, Stewart Wynne EG. Non-convulsive status epilepticus: a prospective study in an adult population. *Q J Med* 1987;**62**:117–26.

1553. Du Pasquier R, Vingerhoets F, Safran AB, et al. Periodic downbeat nystagmus. *Neurology* 1998;**51**:1478–80.

1554. du Petit P. A memoir showing that the intercostal nerves supply branches to the eyes. *Mem Acad Sci Paris* 1727;**1**:1–19.

1555. Duplay ES. De la peri-arthrite scapulo-humerale et des raideurs de l'épaule qui en sont la consequence. *Arch Gen Med Paris* 1872;**20**:513–42.

1556. Dupre E. Le meningisme. *Cong Fr Med Lyon* 1894;**1**:411–23.

1557. Duran M, Wadman SK. Thiamine responsive inborn errors of metabolism. *J Inherit Metab Dis* 1985;**8(Suppl 1)**:70.

1558. Durand N, Favre J. Lymphogranulomatose inguinale subaïgue d'origine génitale probable peut-être vénérienne. *Bull Soc Med Hop Paris* 1913;**35**:274–88.

1559. Durand P, Borrone C, Della Cella G. A new mucopolysaccharide lipid storage disease? *Lancet* 1966;**ii**:1313–4.

1560. Durand P, Zunin C. Associazione de agenesia del setto pelluciodo, cranio lacunare, spina bifida ed altri segni malformativi. *Minerva Pediatr* 1955;**7**:1249–56.

1561. Duret H. Récherches anatomiques sur la circulation de l'encèphale. *Arch Physiol Norm Pathol (Paris)* 1874;**1**:60, 316–664, 919.

1562. Duret H. *Etudes Experimentales et Cliniques sur les Traumatismes Cerebraux.* Paris: V. Adrien Delahaye, 1878.

1563. Durham RH. *Encyclopedia of Medical Syndromes.* New York: Paul Hoeber, 1960.

1564. Durr A, Brice A, Serdaru M, et al. The phenotype of "pure" autosomal dominant spastic paraplegia. *Neurology* 1994;**44**:1274–7.

1565. Duvoisin RC, Golbe LI, Lepore FE. Progressive supranuclear palsy. *Can J Neurol Sci* 1987;**14**:547–54.

1566. Dwork AJ, Balmaceda C, Fazzini OD, et al. Dominantly inherited, early-onset parkinsonism: neuropathology of a new form. *Neurology* 1993;**43**:69–74.

1567. Dyck PJ. Inherited neuronal degeneration and atrophy affecting peripheral motor, sensory, and autonomic neurons. In Dyck PJ, Thomas PK, Lambert EH, eds. *Peripheral Neuropathy*, pp 825–67. Philadelphia: W.B. Saunders, 1975.

1568. Dyck PJ. Detection, characterization and staging of polyneuropathy: assessed in diabetics. *Muscle Nerve* 1988;**11**:21–32.

1569. Dyck PJ. Hypoxic neuropathy: does hypoxia play a role in diabetic neuropathy? *Neurology* 1989;**39**:111–8.

1570. Dyck PJ, Benstead TJ, Conn DL, et al. Nonsystemic vasculitic neuropathy. *Brain* 1987;**110**:843–54.

1571. Dyck PJ, Carney JA, Sizemore GW, et al. Multiple endocrine neoplasia, type 2b: phenotype recognition; neurological features and their pathological basis. *Ann Neurol* 1979;**6**:302–14.

1572. Dyck PJ, Conn DL, Okazaki H. Necrotizing angiopathic neuropathy. *Mayo Clin Proc* 1972;**47**:461–75.

1573. Dyck PJ, Curtis DJ, Buskek W, et al. Description of Minnesota thermal disks and normal values of cutaneous thermal discrimination in man. *Neurology* 1974;**24**:325–30.

1574. Dyck PJ, Karnes J, O'Brien PC, et al. Neuropathy symptom profile in health, motor neurone disease, diabetic neuropathy and amyloidosis. *Neurology* 1986;**36**:1300–8.

1575. Dyck PJ, Kratz KM, Lehman KA, et al. The Rochester Diabetic Neuropathy Study. *Neurology* 1991;**41**:799–807.

1576. Dyck PJ, Lambert EH. Lower motor and primary sensory neuron diseases with peroneal muscular atrophy. I. Neurologic, genetic and electrophysiological findings in hereditary polyneuropathies. *Arch Neurol* 1968;**80**:603–18.

1577. Dyck PJ, Lambert EH. Polyneuropathy associated with hypothyroidism. *J Neuropathol Exp Neurol* 1970;**29**:631–58.

1578. Dyck PJ, Litchy WJ, Minnerath S, et al. Hereditary motor and sensory neuropathy with diaphragm and vocal cord paresis. *Ann Neurol* 1994;**35**:608–15.

1579. Dyck PJ, Norell JE, Dyck PJ jr. Non-diabetic lumbosacral radiculoplexus neuropathy: natural history, outcome and comparison with the diabetic variety. *Brain* 2001;**124**:1197–207.

1580. Dyck PJ, Sherman WR, Hallcher LM, et al. Human diabetic endoneurial sorbitol, fructose and myo-inositol related to sural nerve morphometry. *Ann Neurol* 1980;**8**:590–6.

1581. Dyck PJ, Yao JK, Knickerbocker DE, et al. Multisystem neuronal degeneration, hepatosplenomegaly and adrenocortical deficiency associated with reduced tissue arachidonic acid. *Neurology* 1981;**31**:925–34.

1582. Dyel J. [Differentiation between optic neuritis in Bright's disease from that due to cerebral tumor]. *Semin Med* 1901;**21**:247.

1583. Dyggve HV, Melchior JC, Clausen J, et al. Morquio-Ulrich's disease. An inborn error of metabolism. *Arch Dis Child* 1962;**37**:525–34.

1584. Dyke CG, Davidoff LM, Masson CB. Cerebral hemiatrophy with homolateral hypertrophy of the skull and sinuses. *Surg Gynecol Obstet* 1933;**57**:588–600.

1585. Dyken P, Kolar O. Dancing eyes, dancing feet: infantile polymyoclonia. *Brain* 1968;**91**:305–20.

1586. Dyken P, Krawiecki N. Neurodegenerative diseases of infancy and childhood. *Ann Neurol* 1983;**13**:351–64.

1587. Dyken PR, Miller M. *Facial Features of Neurologic Disease*. St. Louis: C.V. Mosby, 1980.

1588. Dyken PR, Morales V, John-Sanchez F, et al. Chronic toxoplasmosis of the central nervous system: another neurological "degenerative" disease. *Proc Child Neurol Soc* 1976;**5**:27.

1589. Dzierzynsky W. Dystrophia periostalic hyperplastica familiaris. *Zentrabl Ges Neurol Psychiatr* 1913;**20**:547.

1590. Eadie MJ. Olivopontocerebellar degeneration (Menzel type). In Vincken PJ, Bruyn GW, eds. *Handbook of Clinical Neurology*, pp 433–49. Amsterdam: North Holland, 1975.

1591. Eagle WW. Facial pain from an elongated styloid process. *Arch Otolaryngol* 1948;**47**:630–40.

1592. Eagleton WP. *Cavernous Sinus Thrombosis*. New York: Macmillan, 1926.

1593. Eales H. Cases of retinal hemorrhage, associated with epistaxis and constipation. *Birmingh Med Rev* 1880;**9**:262–73.

1594. Eames P. Hysteria following brain injury. *J Neurol Neurosurg Psychiatry* 1992;**55**:1046–53.

1595. Earl CJC, Fullerton PM, Wakefield GS, et al. Hereditary neuropathy with liability to pressure palsies. *Q J Med* 1964;**33**:481–98.

1596. Eastman JR, Bixler D. Facio-cardio-renal syndrome. *Clin Genet* 1977;**11**:424–30.

1596a. Eaton LM, Lambert EH. Electromyography and electrical stimulation of nerves in diseases of the motor unit. *JAMA* 1957;**162**:1117–24.

1597. Ebers GC. Optic neuritis and multiple sclerosis. *Arch Neurol* 1985;**42**:702–4.

1598. Ebke M, Dichgans M, Bergmann M, et al. CADASIL: skin biopsy allows diagnosis in early stages. *Acta Neurol Scand* 1997;**95**:351–7.

1599. Ebrahim S, Nouri F, Barer D. Measuring disability after stroke. *J Epidemiol Commun Health* 1985;**39**:86–9.

1600. Eccles JC, Gibson WC. *Sherrington: His Life and Thought*. Berlin: Springer, 1979.

1601. Edelman RR, Warach S. Magnetic resonance imaging. *N Engl J Med* 1993;**328**:708, 785–16, 791.

1602. Edelson RN, Levy DE. Transient benign pupillary dilatation in young adults. *Arch Neurol* 1974;**31**:12–4.

1603. Edmeads J. The cervical spine and headache. *Neurology* 1988; **38**:1874–8.

1604. Edmeads J. Headache of cervical origin. *Rev Prat* 1990;**40**:399–402.

1605. Edstrom L, Thornell LE, Eriksson A. A new type of hereditary distal myopathy with characteristic sarcoplasmic bodies and intermediate (skeletin) filaments. *J Neurol Sci* 1980;**47**:171–90.

1606. Edwards JA, Sethi PK, Scoma AJ, et al. A new familial syndrome characterized by pigmentary retinopathy, hypogonadism, mental retardation, nerve deafness, and glucose intolerance. *Am J Med* 1976;**60**:23–32.

1607. Edwards JH. Sign of the Cheshire cat. *Lancet* 1987;**2**:581.

1608. Edwards JH, Harnden DG, Cameron AH, et al. A new trisomic syndrome. *Lancet* 1960;**1**:787–90.

1609. Edwards WG, Lincoln CR, Bassett FH, et al. The tarsal tunnel syndrome, diagnosis and treatment. *JAMA* 1969;**207**:716–20.

1610. Efron R. An extension of the Pulfrich effect. *Brain* 1963;**86**:295–300.

1611. Egas Moniz AC. L'encéphalographie arterielle, son importance dans la localisation des tumeurs cérébrales. *Rev Neurol (Paris)* 1927;**2**:72–90.

1612. Egas Moniz AC. Essai d'un traitement chirurgical de certaines psychoses. *Bull Acad Med Paris* 1936;**115**:385–92.

1613. Ehle A, Co S, Jones MG. Clinical correlates of midline spikes: an analysis of 21 patients. *Arch Neurol* 1981;**38**:355–7.

1614. Ehlers E. Cutis laxa. *Dermatol Z* 1901;**8**:173.

1615. Ehrenkranz NJ, Ventura AK. Venezuelan equine encephalitis virus infection in man. *Annu Rev Med* 1974;**25**:9–14.

1616. Ehrenpeis P. *Hirschsprung's Disease*. Chicago: Year Book Medical, 1970.

1617. Ehret H. Ueber eine functionelle Lahrmungsform der Peronealmuskeln traumatischen Ursprunges. *Arch Unfallheilkd (Stuttgart)* 1898; **2**:32–56.

1618. Eidelberg D, Sotrel A, Vogel H, et al. Progressive polyradiculopathy in aquired immune deficiency syndrome. *Neurology* 1986;**36**:912–6.

1619. Eisen A, Shtybel W. Clinical experience with transcranial magnetic stimulation. *Muscle Nerve* 1990;**13**:995–1011.

1620. Eisendrath SJ, Rand DC, Feldman MC. Factitious disorders in the legal setting. In Feldman MC, Eisendrath SJ, eds. *The Spectrum of Factitious Disorders*, pp 65–82. American Psychiatric Press, 1996.

1621. Eisenson J. *Examination for Aphasia*. New York: Psychological Corporation, 1954.

1622. Eisler T, Wilson JH. Muscle fibre-type disproportion: report of a family with symptomatic and asymptomatic members. *Arch Neurol* 1978;**35**:823–6.

1623. Ekbom KA. Asthenia crurum paresthetica ("irritable legs"). A new syndrome consisting of weakness, sensation of cold and nocturnal paresthesia in the legs, responding to a certain extent to treatment in general. *Acta Med Scand* 1944;**118**:197–209.

1624. Ekbom KA. Restless legs. A clinical study of a hitherto overlooked disease in the legs characterized by peculiar paresthesia (anxietas tibiarum), pain and weakness and occurring in two main forms, asthenia crurum paraesthetica and asthenia crurum dolorosa. A short review of paraesthesias in general. *Acta Med Scand* 1945;**158**(Suppl):1–123.

1625. Ekbom KA. Hereditary ataxia, photomyoclonus, skeletal deformities and lipoma. *Acta Neurol Scand* 1975;**51**:393–404.

1626. Hed R, Lundmark C, Fahlgrer H, et al. Muscular affections in chronic alcoholism. *Acta Med Scand* 1962;**171**:585–99.

1627. Ekbom KA, Hed R, Kirstein L, et al. Muscular affections in chronic alcoholism. *Arch Neurol* 1964;**10**:449–58.

1628. Ekbom KA, Jernelius B, Kugelberg E. Perioral reflexes. *Neurology* 1952;**2**:103–11.

1629. El Masry WS, Biyani A. Incidence, management and outcome of post-traumatic syringomyelia. *J Neurol Neurosurg Psychiatry* 1996;**60**:141–6.

1630. Elble RJ. Diagnostic criteria for esstential tremor and differential diagnosis. *Neurology* 2000;**54**(Suppl 4):S2–S6.

1631. Eldjarn L, Jellum E, Stokke O. Betahydroxyvaleric aciduria and betamethyl crotanyl glycinuria: a new inborn error of metabolism. *Lancet* 1970;**2**:54–5.

1632. Eldridge R, Anayiotos CP, Schlesinger S, et al. Hereditary adult-onset leukodystrophy simulating chronic progressive multiple sclerosis. *N Engl J Med* 1984;**311**:948–53.

1633. Elia M, Musumeci SA, Ferri R, et al. Familial cortical tremor, epilepsy and mental retardation; a distinct clinical entity? *Arch Neurol* 1998;**55**:1569–73.

1634. Elkon D, Hightower SI, Lim ML, et al. Esthesioneuroblastoma. *Cancer* 1979;**44:**1087–94.

1635. Ellenberg M. Diabetic neuropathic cachexia. *Diabetes* 1974;**23:** 418–23.

1636. Ellenberger C. Modern perimetry in neuro-ophthalmic diagnosis. *Arch Neurol* 1974;**30:**193–201.

1637. Ellenberger C, Messner KH. Papillophlebitis: benign retinopathy resembling papilledema or papillitis. *Ann Neurol* 1978;**3:**438–44.

1638. Eller KM, Kuller JA. Fetal porencephaly: a review of etiology, diagnosis and prognosis. *Obstet Gynecol Surv* 1995;**50:**684–7.

1639. Ellie E, Julien J, Ferrer X. Familial idiopathic striopallidodentate calcifications. *Neurology* 1989;**39:**381–5.

1640. Ellis K, Speed J, Balbierz JM. Post-craniectomy intracranial hypotension: potential impact on rehabilitation. *Brain Inj* 1998;**12:**895–9.

1641. Ellis RWB, van Crefeld S. A syndrome characterized by ectodermal dysplasia, polydactyly, chondrodro-dysplasia and congenital morbus cordis. *Arch Dis Child* 1940;**15:**65.

1642. Ellis SJ, Small M. Denial of illness in stroke. *Stroke* 1993;**24:** 757–9.

1643. Ellison PH, Farina MA. Progressive central nervous system deterioration: a complication of advanced chronic lung disease and prematurity. *Ann Neurol* 1980;**8:**43–6.

1644. Ellner JJ. Chronic meningitis. In Mandell GL, Douglas RG, Bennett JE, eds. *Principles and Practice of Infectious Diseases,* pp 573–9. New York: John Wiley & Sons, 1985.

1645. Elsahy NI, Waters WR. The brachio-skeleto-genital syndrome. *Plast Reconstr Surg* 1971;**48:**542–50.

1646. Elsberg CA. Experiences in spinal surgery. Observations upon 60 laminectomies in spinal disease. *Surg Gynecol Obstet* 1931;**16:**117.

1647. Elschnig A. Nystagmus retractorius, ein cerebrales Herdsymptom. *Med Klin Berlin* 1913;**1:**8–11.

1648. Elston JS. A new variant of blepharospasm. *J Neurol Neurosurg Psychiatry* 1992;**55:**369–71.

1649. Elston JS, Casgranje F, Lees AJ. The relationship between eye-winking tics, frequent eye-blinking and blepharospasm. *J Neurol Neurosurg Psychiatry* 1989;**52:**477–80.

1650. Emery AEH, Dreifuss FE. Unusual type of benign X-linked muscular dystrophy. *J Neurol Neurosurg Psychiatry* 1966;**29:**338–42.

1651. Emslie-Smith AM, Engel AG. Necrotizing myopathy with pipestem capillaries, microvascular deposition of the complement membrane attack complex (MAC), and minimal cellular infiltration. *Neurology* 1991;**41:**936–9.

1652. Enderby PM, Wood VA, Wade DT, Langton-Hewer RL. The Frenchay Aphasia Screening Test: a short, simple test for aphasia appropriate for non-specialists. *Int Rehabil Med* 1987;**8:**166–70.

1653. Endicott J, Spitzer RL. A diagnostic interview for affective disorders and schizophrenia. *Arch Gen Psychiatry* 1978;**35:**837–44.

1654. Enevoldson TP, Sanders MD, Harding AE. Autosomal dominant cerebellar ataxia with pigmentary macular dystrophy: a clinical and genetic study of eight families. *Brain* 1994;**117:**445–460.

1655. Eng L, Vanderhaegen J, Bignami A, et al. An acidic protein isolated from fibrous astrocytes. *Brain Res* 1971;**28:**351–4.

1656. Engel AG. Late onset rod myopathy (a new syndrome?). Light and electron microscopic observations in two cases. *Mayo Clin Proc* 1966;**41:**713–41.

1657. Engel AG. Acid maltase deficiency in adults: studies in four cases of a syndrome which may mimic muscular dystrophy or other myopathies. *Brain* 1970;**93:**599–616.

1658. Engel AG. Myasthenia gravis and myasthenic syndromes. *Ann Neurol* 1984;**16:**519–34.

1659. Engel AG. Congenital myasthenic syndromes. *Neurol Clin* 1994;**12:**401–37.

1660. Engel AG, Angelini C. Carnitine deficiency of human skeletal muscle with associated lipid storage myopathy: a new syndrome. *Science* 1973;**173:**899–902.

1661. Engel AG, Angelini C, Gomez MR. Fingerprint body myopathy: a newly recognized congenital muscle disease. *Mayo Clin Proc* 1972; **47:**377–88.

1662. Engel AG, Banker BQ, eds. *Myology.* New York: McGraw-Hill, 1986.

1663. Engel AG, Gomez MR. Congenital myopathy associated with multifocal degeneration of muscle fibers. *Trans Am Neurol Assoc* 1966;**91:**222–3.

1666. Engel AG, Gomez MR, Groover RV. Multicore disease: a recently recognized congenital myopathy associated with multifocal degeneration of muscle fibres. *Mayo Clin Proc* 1971;**46:**666–81.

1667. Engel AG, Gomez MR, Seybold ME, et al. The spectrum and diagnosis of acid maltase deficiency. *Neurology* 1973;**23:**95–106.

1668. Engel AG, Lambert EH, Gomez MR. A new myasthenic syndrome with end-plate acetylcholinesterase deficiency, small nerve terminals, and reduced acetylcholine release. *Ann Neurol* 1977;**1:**315–30.

1669. Engel AG, Lambert EH, Mulder DM, et al. Recently recognized congenital myasthenic syndromes: (a) end-plate acetylcholine (ACh) esterase deficiency (b) putative abnormality of the ACh induced ion channel (c) putative defect of ACh resynthesis or mobilization—clinical features, ultrastructure and cytochemistry. *Ann NY Acad Sci* 1981;**377:**614–639.

1670. Engel AG, Lambert EH, Mulder DM, et al. A newly recognised congenital myasthenic syndrome attributed to a prolonged open time of the actylcholine-induced ion channel. *Ann Neurol* 1982;**11:**553–69.

1671. Engel AG, Uchitel OD, Walls TJ. Newly recognized congenital myasthenic syndrome associated with high conductance and fast closure of the acetylcholine channel. *Ann Neurol* 1993;**34:**38–47.

1672. Engel J Jr, Rapin I, Giblin DR. Electrophysiological studies in two patients with cherry-red spot-myoclonus syndrome. *Epilepsia* 1977;**18:**73–87.

1672a. Engel J Jr. Update on surgical treatment of the epilepsies. Summary of the Second International Palm Desert Conference on the Surgical Treatment of the Epilepsies (1992). *Neurology* 1993;**43:**1612–7.

1673. Engel M, Carmel PW, Chutorian AM. Increased intraventricular pressure without ventriculomegaly in children with shunts: "normal volume" hydrocephalus. *Neurosurgery* 1979;**5:**549–52.

1674. Engel WK. Muscle target fibers: a newly recognized sign of denervation. *Nature* 1961;**191:**389–90.

1675. Engel WK. Brief, small, abundant motor-unit action potentials. *Neurology* 1975;**25:**173–6.

1676. Engel WK, Dorman JD, Levy RI, et al. Neuropathy in Tangier disease: a-lipoprotein deficiency manifesting as familial recurrent neuropathy and intestinal lipid storage. *Arch Neurol* 1967;**17:**1–9.

1677. Engel WK, et al. A recently recognized congenital myopathy associated with multifocal degeneration of muscle fibers. *Mayo Clin Proc* 1971;**46:**666–81.

1678. Engel WK, Eyerman EL, Williams HE. Late onset type of skeletal muscle phosphorylase deficiency. A new familial variety with completely and partially affected subjects. *N Engl J Med* 1963;**268:**135–7.

1679. Engel WK, Gold GN, Karpati G. Type I fiber hypotrophy and central nuclei. *Arch Neurol* 1968;**18:**435–44.

1680. Engel WK, Hawley RJ. Focal lesions of muscle in peripheral vascular disease. *J Neurol* 1977;**215:**161–8.

1681. Engel WK, Kurland LT, Klatzo I. An inherited disease similar to amyotrophic lateral sclerosis with a pattern of posterior column involvement. *Brain* 1959;**82:**203–20.

1682. England AC, Denny-Brown D. Severe sensory changes and trophic disorder, in peroneal muscular atrophy (Charcot-Marie-Tooth type). *Arch Neurol Psychiatry* 1952;**67:**1–22.

1683. Enzinger FM, Dulcey F. Proliferative myositis. Report of 33 cases. *Cancer* 1967;**20:**2213–23.

1684. Epley JM. Particle repositioning for benign paroxysmal positional vertigo. *Otolaryngol Clin North Am* 1996;**29:**323–31.

1685. Epstein CJ. Werners syndrome. *Medicine* 1966;**45:**177–221.

1686. Epstein SH. History of the Boston Society of Psychiatry and Neurology. *Arch Neurol* 1985;**42:**391–2.

1687. Erb WH. Uber eine eigentumliche Lokalisation von Lahmung im Plexus brachialis. *Verh Naturh Med Ver Heidelberg* 1874;**2:**130–7.

1688. Erb WH. Ueber einen wenig bekannten spinalen Symptomencomplex. *Berl Klin Wochenschr* 1875;**12:**357–9.

1689. Erb WH. Ueber die spastische Spinalparalyse (tabès dorsal spasmodique Charot). *Virchows Arch Pathol Anat Physiol Klin Med Berl* 1877;**70:**241–67.

1690. Erb WH. Casuistik der bulbaren Lahmungen. *Arch Psychiatrie (Berlin)* 1879;**9:**325–50.

1691. Erb WH. Ueber einen eigenthumlichen bulbaren Symptomenkomplex. *Arch Psychiatr Nervenkr* 1879;**9:**172–3.

1692. Erb WH. Ueber die "juvenile Form" der progressiven Muskelatrophie, ihre Beziehungen zur sogenannten Pseudohypertrophie der Muskeln. *Arch Klin Med* 1884;**34:**467–519.

1693. Erb WH. Ueber syphilitische Spinalparalyse. *Neurol Zentrabl* 1892;**11**:161–8.

1694. Erba G, Browne TR. Atypical absence, myoclonic, atonic, and tonic seizures and the "Lennox-Gastaut syndrome". In Browne TR, Feldman RG, eds. *Epilepsy, Diagnosis and Management*, pp 75–94. Boston: Little, Brown, 1983.

1695. Erdheim J. On complications of acromegaly [in German]. *Virchows Arch Pathol Anat Physiol* 1931;**281**:197–296.

1696. Erickson TC. Neurogenic hyperthermia. *Brain* 1998;**172**:1039.

1697. Erikson A. Hereditary syndrome consisting of recurrent attacks resembling brachial plexus neuritis, special features and cleft palate. *Acta Pediatr Scand* 1974;**63**:885–8.

1698. Erkinjuntti T, Haltia M, Palo J, et al. Accuracy of the clinical diagnosis of vascular dementia. *J Neurol Neurosurg Psychiatry* 1988;**51**:1037–44.

1699. Eronen M, et al. A digito-reno-cerebral syndrome. *Am J Med Genet* 1985;**22**:281–5.

1700. Ertekin C, Reel F. Bulbocavernosus reflex in normal men and in patients with neurogenic bladder and/or impotence. *J Neurol Sci* 1976;**28**:1–15.

1701. Erzigkeit H. The SKT—a short cognitive performance test as an instrument for the assessment of clinical efficacy of cognition enhancers. In Berenger M, Reisberg B, eds. *Diagnosis and Treatment of Senile Dementia*, p 164. Berlin: Springer-Verlag, 1989.

1702. Escobar V, et al. Multiple pterygium syndrome. *Am J Dis Child* 1978;**132**:609–11.

1703. Escueta AV, Boxley J, Stubbs N, et al. Prolonged twilight state and automatisms: a case report. *Neurology* 1974;**24**:331–9.

1704. Espildora-Luque C. Sindrome oftalmico-silviano (ceguera monocular y hemiplejia alternas). *Arch Oft Hisp Am* 1934;**34**:616–21.

1705. Esquirol JE-D. *Des Maladies Mentales Considerées Sous les Rapports Medical, Hygenique et Medico-legal*. Paris: Bailliere, 1838.

1706. Estanol BV, Marin OSM. Mechanism of the inverted supinator reflex: a clinical and neurophysiological study. *J Neurol Neurosurg Psychiatry* 1976;**39**:905–8.

1707. Esterly NB, McKusick VA. Stiff skin syndrome. *Pediatrics* 1971;**47**:360–9.

1708. Ethelberg S. Symptomatic "cataplexy" or chalastic fits in cortical lesion of the frontal lobe. *Brain* 1950;**73**:499–512.

1709. Etiemble J, Picort Ceal, Simeon J. Inherited erythrocyte PFK deficiency. *Hum Genet* 1980;**55**:383–90.

1710. Eulenberg A. Uber eine familiare durch 6 Generationen verfolgbare Form kongenitaler Paramyotonie. *Zentralbl Neurol* 1886;**5**:265.

1711. Eunson LH, Rea R, Zuberi SM, et al. Clinical, expression and genetic studies of mutations in the potassium channel gene *KCNA1* reveal new phenotypic variability. *Ann Neurol* 2000;**48**:647–56.

1712. European Malignant Hyperpyrexia Group. A protocol for the investigation of malignant hyperpyrexia (MH) susceptibility. *Br J Anaesth* 1984;**56**:1267–9.

1713. Evans BK, Donley DK. Pseudohypoparathyroidism, parkinsonism syndrome, with no basal ganglia calcification. *J Neurol Neurosurg Psychiatry* 1988;**51**:709–13.

1714. Evans BM, Milen M. Potassium losing nephritis presenting as a case of periodic paralysis. *BMJ* 1954;**2**:1067.

1715. Evans DGR, Mason S, Huson SM, et al. Spinal and cutaneous schwannomatosis is a variant form of type 2 neurofibromatosis: a clinical and molecular study. *J Neurol Neurosurg Psychiatry* 1997;**62**:361–6.

1716. Evans J. Rocking at night. *J Child Psychol Psychiatry* 1961;**2**:71–85.

1717. Evans PR. Referred itch (Mitempfidungen). *BMJ* 1976;**2**:839–41.

1718. Evans RW. The postconcussion syndrome and the sequelae of mild head injury. *Neurol Clin* 1992;**10**:815–47.

1719. Eve FR. Pterygoid-levator synkinesis. *J Clin Neuroophthalmol* 1987;**7**:61–2.

1720. Everett HC. Sneezing in response to light. *Neurology* 1964;**14**:483–90.

1721. Ewer RW, Bissonnette RP, Brakel FJ, et al. Tetanic neuromyopathy and renal failure. *JAMA* 1965;**192**:1117–20.

1722. Ewing DJ, Campbell IW, Murray A, et al. Immediate heart rate response to standing: simple test for autonomic neuropathy in diabetes. *BMJ* 1978;**1**:145–7.

1723. Ewing DJ, Irving IB, Kerr F, et al. Cardiovascular responses to sustained handgrip in normal subjects and in subjects with diabetes mellitus: a test of autonomic function. *Clin Sci Mol Med* 1974;**46**:295–306.

1724. Eymard B, Hauw J-J. Mitochondrial encephalomyelopathies. *Curr Opin Neurol Neurosurg*. 1992;**5**:909–16.

1725. Eymard B, Romero N, Leturcq F, et al. Primary adhalinopathy: (alpha-sarcoglycanopathy). *Neurology* 1997;**48**:1227–34.

1725a. Eysenck HJ, Eysenck SGB. *Handbook of the Eysenck Personality Inventory*. London: University of London Press, 1964.

1726. Fabbrini G, Juncos J, Mourdian MM, et al. Levadopa pharmacokinetic mechanisms and motor fluctuations in Parkinson disease. *Ann Neurol* 1987;**21**:370–6.

1727. Fabian TC, Hoots AV, Stanford DS, et al. Fat embolism syndrome. *Crit Care Med* 1990;**18**:42–6.

1728. Fabry J. Ein Beitrag zur Kenntnis der Purpura haemorrhagica nodularis (Purpura papulosa haemorrhagica Hebrae). *Arch Dermatol Syph* 1898;**43**:187–200.

1729. Fahn S. Rating scales for blepharospasm. *Adv Ophthalm Reconstr Surg* 1985;**4**:97–101.

1730. Fahn S. Generalized dystonia: concept and treatment. *Clin Neuropharmacol* 1986;**9** (**Suppl 2**):S37–S48.

1731. Fahn, S. AAN Course Manual, 1989 [unpublished].

1732. Fahn S. Clinical variants of idiopathic torsion dystonia. *J Neurol Neurosurg Psychiatry* 1989;**Suppl:**96–100.

1733. Fahn S, Marsden CD, Calne DB. Classification and investigation of dystonias. In Marsden CD, Fahn S, eds. *Movement Disorders 2*, pp 332–58. Butterworth, 1987.

1734. Fahr T. Idiopathische Verkalkung der Hirngefasse. *Zentralbl Allg Pathol* 1930;**50**:129–33.

1735. Falconer MA. Mesial temporal (Ammon's horn) sclerosis as a common cause of epilepsy. *Lancet* 1974;**2**:767–70.

1736. Falconer MA, Taylor DC. Surgical Treatment of drug-resistant epilepsy due to mesial temporal lobe sclerosis. *Arch Neurol* 1968;**19**:353–61.

1737. Falconer MA, Weddell G. Costoclavicular compression of the subclavian artery and vein. Relation to the scalenus anticus syndrome. *Lancet* 1943;**2**:539–43.

1738. Fallon MD, Teitelbaum SL. Hypophosphatasia: clinicopathologic comparison of the infantile, childhood and adult forms. *Medicine* 1984;**63**:12–24.

1739. Falls HF. Sex-linked ocular albinism displaying typical fundus changes in female heterozygotes. *Am J Ophthalmol* 1951;**34**:41.

1740. Fanconi G. Familial infantile pernicious anemia [in German]. *Jahrb Kinderheilkd* 1927;**117**:257–80.

1741. Fanconi G, Turler U. Kongenitale Kleinhirnatrophie mit supranuclearen Störungen der Motilität der Augenmuskeln. *Helv Pediatr Acta* 1951;**6**:475–83.

1742. Fara M, et al. Dysmorphic oto-facio-cervical abnormalities. *Acta Chir Orthop Traum Cech* 1967;**34**:511–20.

1743. Farber S. A lipid metabolic disorder—disseminated lipogranulomatosis—a syndrome with similarity to, and important differences from, Nieman-Pick and Hand-Schuller-Christian disease. *Am J Dis Child* 1952;**84**:499–500.

1744. Fardeau M. Some orthodox and non-orthodox considerations on congenital myopathies. In Ellinson RJ, Murray NMF, Halliday AM, eds. *The London Symposia (EEG Suppl 39)*, pp 85–90. Amsterdam: Elsevier Science Publishers, 1987.

1745. Fardin P, Negrin P, Sparta S, et al. Posterior interosseous nerve neuropathy: clinical and electromyographic aspects. *Electromyogr Clin Neurophysiol* 1992;**32**:229–34.

1746. Farlow MR, DeMyer W, Dlouhy S, et al. X-linked recessive inheritance of ataxia and adult onset dementia. *Neurology* 1987;**37**:602–7.

1747. Farrar JJ, Yen LM, Cook T, et al. Tetanus. *J Neurol Neurosurg Psychiatry* 2000;**69**:292–301.

1748. Farrell DF, Starr A. Delayed neurologic sequelae of electrical injuries. *Neurology* 1968;**18**:601–6.

1749. Fasler JJ, Rose FC. West Indian amblyopia. *Postgrad Med J* 1980;**56**:494.

1750. Fauci AS, Haynes BF, Katz P. The spectrum of vasculitis: clinical, pathologic, immunologic, and therapeutic considerations. *Ann Intern Med* 1978;**89**:660–76.

1751. Fauci AS, Wolff SM. Wegener's granulomatosis: studies in eighteen patients and a review of the literature. *Medicine* 1973;**52**:535–61.

1752. Faull K, Bolton P, Halpern B, et al. Patient with defect in leucine metabolism. *N Engl J Med* 1976;**294**:1013.

1753. Fazio M. Eredetarieta della paralisi bulbare progressiva. *Rif Med* 1892;**8**:327.

1754. Fearnley JM, Lees AJ. Striatonigral degeneration. *Brain* 1990;**113**:1823–42.

1755. Feasby TE, Burton SR, Hahn AF. Obstetrical lumbosacral plexus injury. *Muscle Nerve* 1992;**15**:937–40.

1756. Feasby TE, Gilbert JJ, Brown WF, et al. An acute axonal form of Guillain-Barré polyneuropathy. *Brain* 1986;**109**:1115–26.

1757. Feder HM, Gerber MA. Saxophone headaches. *N Engl J Med* 1991;**325**:1888.

1758. Federico A, Cecio A, Apponi Battini G, et al. Macular cherry-red spot and myoclonus syndrome: juvenile form of sialidosis. *J Neurol Sci* 1980;**48**:157–69.

1759. Federico A, Guazzi G, Gruschelli C, et al. Glycopeptidosis: a new inherited disorder of glycoconjugate metabolism affecting the central nervous system. *J Inher Metab Dis* 1981;**4**:141–2.

1760. Feeney DM, Baron JC. Diaschisis. *Stroke* 1986;**17**:817–30.

1761. Feeney DM, Walker AE. The prediction of posttraumatic epilepsy: a mathematical approach. *Arch Neurol* 1979;**36**:8–12.

1762. Feibel JH, Campa JF. Thyrotoxic neuropathy (Basedow's paraplegia). *J Neurol Neurosurg Psychiatry* 1976;**39**:491–7.

1763. Feigin I, Pena CE, Budzilovich GN. The infantile spongy degenerations. *Neurology* 1968;**18**:153–66.

1764. Feinberg TE, Haber LD, Leeds NE. Verbal asomatognosia. *Neurology* 1990;**40**:1391–4.

1765. Feinberg TE, Shapiro AK, Shapiro E. Paroxysmal myoclonic dystonia with vocalisations: new entity or variant of preexisting syndromes? *J Neurol Neurosurg Psychiatry* 1986;**49**:52–7.

1766. Feindel W. Herbert Henri Jasper (1906–1999): an appreciation. *Can J Neurol Sci* 1999;**26**:224–9.

1767. Feit H, Glasberg M, Ireton C, et al. Peripheral neuropathy and starvation after gastric partitioning for morbid obesity. *Ann Intern Med* 1982;**96**:453–5.

1768. Feit H, Silbergleit A, Schneider LB, et al. Vocal cord and pharyngeal weakness with autosomal dominant distal myopathy: clinical description and gene localization to 5q31. *Am J Hum Genet* 1998;**63**:1732–42.

1769. Feldman EL, Russell JW, Sullivan KA, et al. New insights into the pathogenesis of diabetic neuropathy. *Curr Opin Neurol* 1999;**12**:553–63.

1770. Feldman EL, Stevens MJ. Clinical testing in diabetic peripheral neuropathy. *Can J Neurol Sci* 1994;**21**:S3–S7.

1771. Feldman GL, Weaver DD, Lovrein EW. The fetal trimethadione syndrome. *Am J Dis Child* 1977;**131**:1389–92.

1772. Feldman H, Kertesz A. Diagnosis, classification and natural history of degenerative dementias. *Can J Neurol Sci* 2001;**28**:S17–S27.

1773. Feldman H, Schulzer M, Wang S, et al. The Functional Rating Scale in Alzheimer's disease assessment: a longitudinal study. In Iqbal K, Mortimer JA, Winblad B, et al., eds. *Research Advances in Alzheimer's Disease and Related Disorders*, pp 235–41. Chichester: John Wiley and Sons, 1995.

1774. Feldman M, Todman L, Bender MB. `Flight of colours' in lesions of the visual system. *J Neurol Neurosurg Psychiatry* 1974;**37**:1265–72.

1775. Feldman MD. The syndrome of anticholinergic intoxication. *Am Fam Physician* 1986;**34**:113–6.

1776. Feldman MJ, Drasgow J. *The Visual–Verbal Test*. Los Angeles: Western Psychological Services, 1959.

1777. Felice K, Meredith C, Bonz N, et al. Autosomal dominant distal myopathy not linked to the known distal myopathy loci. *Neuromusc Disord* 1999;**9**:59–65.

1778. Felice KJ, North WA, Moore SA, et al. FSH dystrophy 4q35 deletion in patients presenting with facial-sparing scapular myopathy. *Neurology* 2000;**54**:1927–31.

1779. Felice KJ, Schwarta RC, Brown CA, et al. Autosomal dominant Emery-Dreifuss dystrophy due to mutations in rod domain of the lamin A/C gene. *Neurology* 2000;**55**:275–80.

1780. Fenichel GM. Clinical syndromes of myasthenia in infancy and childhood: a review. *Arch Neurol* 1978;**35**:97–103.

1781. Fenichel GM. Congenital muscular dystrophies. *Neurol Clin* 1988;**6**:519–28.

1782. Fenichel GM, Emery ES, Hunt P. Neurogenic atrophy simulating facioscapulohumeral dystrophy. *Arch Neurol* 1967;**17**:257–60.

1783. Fenichel GM, Olson WH, Kilroy AW. Hereditary dystonia associated with unique features in skeletal muscle. *Adv Neurol* 1971;**25**:552–9.

1784. Fenichel GM, Sul YC, Kilroy AW, et al. An autosomal dominant dystrophy with humero-pelvic distribution and cardiomyopathy. *Neurology* 1982;**32**:1399–401.

1785. Féré C. Note sur les modifications de la résistance éléctrique sous l'influence des excitations sensorielles et des emotions. *C R Soc Biol* 1888;**6**:217–19.

1786. Féré MC. Le fou rire prodromique. *Rev Neurol (Paris)* 1903;**11**:353.

1787. Ferell MR, Smallberg G, Lesis LD, et al. A benign motor neuron disorder: delayed cramps and fasciculations after poliomyelitis or myelitis. *Ann Neurol* 1982;**11**:423–7.

1788. Ferguson F, Critchley M. A clinical study of an heredo-familial disease ressembling disseminated sclerosis. *Brain* 1929;**52**:203–25.

1789. Ferguson IT, Mahon M, Cinnings WJK. An adult case of Andersen's disease—type IV glycogenosis. *J Neurol Sci* 1983;**60**:337–51.

1790. Feringa ER, Weatherbee L. Hypertrophic granulomatous cranial pachymenigitis causing progressive blindness in a chronic dialysis patient. *J Neurol Neurosurg Psychiatry* 1975;**38**:1170–6.

1791. Fernandes CM, Daya MR. A roller coaster headache: case report. *J Trauma* 1994;**37**:1007–10.

1792. Fernandez HH, Friedman JH. Punding on L-dopa. *Mov Disord* 1999;**14**:836–8.

1793. Fernandez M, Raskind W, Matsushita M, et al. Hereditary benign chorea. *Neurology* 2001;**57**:106–10.

1794. Fernandez M, Raskind W, Wolff J, et al. Familial dyskinesia and facial myokymia (FDFM): a novel movement disorder. *Ann Neurol* 2001;**49**:486–92.

1795. Fernandez-Alvarez E. Transient movement disorders in children. *J Neurol* 1998;**245**:1–5.

1796. Ferrante MA, Wilbourn AJ. The characteristic electrodiagnostic features of Kennedy's disease. *Muscle Nerve* 1997;**20**:323–9.

1797. Ferrari G, Taddei L, Vivenza C, et al. Paraparesis in hereditary multiple exostoses. *Neurology* 1979;**29**:973–7.

1798. Ferrari R, Schrader H. The late whiplash syndrome: a biopsychological approach. *J Neurol Neurosurg Psychiatry* 2001;**70**:722–6.

1799. Ferreiro A, Estournet B, Chateau D, et al. Multi-minicore disease—searching for boundaries: phenotype analysis of 38 cases. *Ann Neurol* 2000;**48**:745–57.

1800. Ferrier D. Experimental researches in cerebral physiology and pathology. *The West Riding Lunatic Asylum Medical Reports* 1873;**3**:30.

1801. Ferriman D. *Acrocephaly and Acrocephalosyndactyly*. London: Oxford University Press, 1941.

1802. Ferris SH, Crook TH, Clarke E, et al. Facial recognition of memory deficits in normal aging and senile dementia. *J Gerontol* 1988;**35**:707–14.

1803. Ferris SH, Flicker C, Reisberg B. NYU computerized test battery for assessing cognition in aging and dementia. *Psychopharmacol Bull* 1988;**24**:699.

1804. Ferro JM, Kertesz A, Black SE. Subcortical neglect: quantitation, anatomy, and recovery. *Neurology* 1987;**37**:1487.

1805. Fetell MR, Smallberg G, Lewis L, et al. A benign motor neurone disorder: delayed cramps and fasciculations after poliomyelitis or myelitis. *Ann Neurol* 1982;**11**:423–7.

1806. Feuerstein RC, Mims LC. Linear nevus sebaceous with convulsions and mental retardation. *Am J Dis Child* 1962;**104**:675–9.

1807. Feyrter F. Uber eine eigenartige Geschwulstform des Nervengewebes im menschlichen Verdauungsschlauch. *Virchows Arch* 1935;**295**:480–501.

1808. Fidueira F. Cephaloplegic syndrome in children [in French]. *Arch Med Enf Paris* 1919;**22**:113–25.

1809. Fidzianska A, Badurska B, Ryniewicz B, et al. "Cap disease": new congenital myopathy. *Neurology* 1981;**31**:1113–20.

1810. Field CE. Albers-Schonberg disease. A typical case. *Proc R Soc Med* 1939;**32**:3220–4.

1811. Fields WS, Lemak NA. Joint study of extracranial arterial occlusion: VII. subclavian steal: a review of 168 cases. *JAMA* 1972;**222**:1139–43.

1812. Fiero RA, Groth M, Hurewitz A, et al. Chronic hemoptysis: an unusual manifestation of fungal sinusitis. *South Med J* 1995;**88**:782–5.

1813. Fife TD, Baloh RB. Disequilibrium of unknown cause in older people. *Ann Neurol* 1993;**34**:694–702.

1814. Filipek PA, Accardo PJ, Ashwal S, et al. Practice parameter: screening and diagnosis of autism. *Neurology* 2000;**55**:468–79.

1815. Filippi M, Campi A, Martinelli V, et al. Transitional progressive multiple sclerosis: MRI and MTI findings. *Acta Neurol Scand* 1995;**92**:178–82.

1816. Filla A, De Michele G, Cocozza S, et al. Early onset autosomal dominant dementia with ataxia, extrapyramidal features and epilepsy. *Neurology* 2002;**58**:922–8.

1817. Filley CM, Kleinschmidt-DeMasters BK. Toxic leukoencephalopathy. *N Engl J Med* 2001;**345**:425–32.

1818. Findlay JM, Hao C, Emery D. Non-atherosclerotic fusiform cerebral aneurysms. *Can J Neurol Sci* 2002;**29**:41–8.

1819. Findley LJ, Gresty MA. Tremor. In Harrison MJG, ed. *Contemporary Neurology*, London: Butterworths, 1983.

1820. Findley LJ, Koller WC. Essential tremor: a review. *Neurology* 1987;**37**:1194–7.

1821. Fine EJ, Wongjirad C. The ulnar flexion maneuver [unpublished]. 1985.

1822. Fine JD, Arndt KA. The TORCH syndrome: a clinical review. *J Am Acad Dermatol* 1985;**12**:697–706.

1823. Finisterer J, Milvay E. Lactate stress testing in 155 patients with mitochondriopathy. *Can J Neurol Sci* 2002;**29**:49–53.

1824. Fink JK, Filling-Katz MR, Sokol J, et al. Clinical spectrum of Niemann-Pick disease. *Neurology* 1989;**39**:1040–9.

1825. Fink JK, Heiman-Paterson T. Hereditary spastic paraplegias: advances in genetic research. *Neurology* 1996;**46**:1507–14.

1826. Fink JN. Localization of the "sneeze center". *Neurology* 2001;**56**:138.

1827. Fink M, Green MA, Bender MB. The face-hand test as a diagnostic sign of organic mental syndrome. *Neurology* 1952;**2**:46–58.

1828. Finley KH. Post-encephalitic manifestations in viral encephalitis. In Field WS, Blattner RL, eds. *Viral Encephalitis*, pp. 69–94. Springfield, Il.: C.C. Thomas, 1958.

1829. Firkin BG, Whitworth JA. *Dictionary of Medical Eponyms*. Lancashire UK: The Parthenon Publishing Group, 1987.

1830. Fischer-Perroudon C, Mouret J, Jouvet M. Four months without sleep (agrypnia) in a case of "chorée fibrillaire de Morvan"—improvement after 5HTP. In Chase MH, Stern WC, Walter PL, eds. *Sleep Research*, p 148. Los Angeles: Brain Information Systems, UCLA, 1973.

1831. Fischer-Perroudon C, Mouret J, Jouvet M. Sur un cas d'agrypnie (4 mois sans sommeil) au cours d'une maladie de Morvan. Effet favorable du 5–hydroxytryptophane. *Electroencephalogr Clin Neurophysiol* 1974;**36**:1–18.

1832.. Fischer H. A familial syndrome [in German]. *Dermatol Z (Berlin)* 1921;**32–33**:114–42.

1833. Fischer MH, Gerritsen T, Opitz JM. Aminoadipic aciduria; a non-deleterious inborn metabolic defect. *Humangenetik* 1974;**24**:265–70.

1834. Fischer P-A, Enzensberger W. Neurological complications in AIDS. *J Neurol* 1987;**234**:269–79.

1835. Fischer-Williams M, Bosanquet FD, Daniel PM. Carcinomatosis of the meninges. *Brain* 1955;**78**:42–58.

1836. Fisher A, Gresty MA, Chambers B, Rudge P. Primary position upbeating nystagmus. *Brain* 1983;**106**:949–64.

1837. Fisher CM. Lacunes: small deep cerebral infarctions. *Neurology* 1954;**15**:774–84.

1838. Fisher CM. An unusual variant of acute idiopathic polyneuritis (syndrome of ophthalmoplegia, ataxia and areflexia). *N Engl J Med* 1956;**255**:57–65.

1839. Fisher CM. Left hemiplegia and motor impersistence. *J Nerv Ment Dis* 1956;**123**:201–18.

1840. Fisher CM. A simple test of cordination in the fingers. *Neurology* 1960;**10**:745–6.

1841. Fisher CM. An improved test of motor coordination in the lower limbs. *Neurology* 1961;**11**:335–6.

1842. Fisher CM. Concerning recurrent transient cerebral ischemic attacks. *CMAJ* 1962;**86**:1091–9.

1843. Fisher CM. Ocular bobbing. *Arch Neurol* 1964;**11**:543–6.

1844. Fisher CM. Pure sensory stroke involving face, arm and leg. *Neurology* 1965;**15**:76–80.

1845. Fisher CM. Concussion amnesia. *Neurology* 1966;**16**:826–30.

1846. Fisher CM. A lacunar stroke. *Neurology* 1967;**17**:614–7.

1847. Fisher CM. Some neuro-ophthalmological observations. *J Neurol Neurosurg Psychiatry* 1967;**30**:383–92.

1848. Fisher CM. Nonsense speech—amphigory. *Trans Am Neurol Assoc* 1970;**95**:238–40.

1849. Fisher CM. Pure spastic paralysis of corticospinal origin. *Can J Neurol Sci* 1977;**4**:251–8.

1850. Fisher CM. Transient paralytic attacks of obscure nature: the question of non-convulsive seizure paralysis. *Can J Neurol Sci* 1978;**5**:267–73.

1851. Fisher CM. Oval pupils. *Arch Neurol* 1980;**37**:502–3.

1852. Fisher CM. Disorientation for place. *Arch Neurol* 1982;**39**:33–6.

1853. Fisher CM. Lacunar strokes and infarcts: a review. *Neurology* 1982;**32**:871–6.

1854. Fisher CM. Whiplash amnesia. *Neurology* 1982;**32**:667–8.

1855. Fisher CM. Cataclysmic migraine. *Can J Neurol Sci* 1986;**13**:1–5.

1856. Fisher CM. Late-life migraine accompaniments—further experience. *Stroke* 1986;**17**:1033–42.

1857. Fisher CM. The posterior cerebral artery syndrome. *Can J Neurol Sci* 1986;**13**:232–9.

1858. Fisher CM. Neurologic fragments. 1. Clinical observations in demented patients. *Neurology* 1988;**38**:1868–73.

1859. Fisher CM. The 'herald hemiparesis' of basilar artery occlusion. *Arch Neurol* 1988;**45**:1301–3.

1860. Fisher CM. Neurologic fragments. II. Remarks on anosognosia, confabulation, memory, and other topics; and an appendix on self-observation. *Neurology* 1989;**39**:127–32.

1861. Fisher CM. Transient monocular blindness versus amaurosis fugax. *Neurology* 1989;**39**:1622–4.

1862. Fisher CM. Visual hallucinations on eye closure associated with atropine toxicity. A neurological analysis and comparison with other visual hallucinations. *Can J Neurol Sci* 1991;**18**:18–27.

1863. Fisher CM. Brain herniation: a revision of clasical concepts. *Can J Neurol Sci* 1995;**22**:83–91.

1864. Fisher CM. Alien hand phenomena: a review with the addition of six personal cases. *Can J Neurol Sci* 2000;**27**:192–203.

1865. Fisher CM, Adams RD. Transient global amnesia. *Acta Neurol Scand* 1964;**40**:1–83.

1866. Fisher CM, Cole M. Homolateral ataxia and crural paresis: a vascular syndrome. *J Neurol Neurosurg Psychiatry* 1965;**28**:48–55.

1867. Fisher CM, Curry HB. Pure motor hemiplegia of vascular origin. *Arch Neurol* 1965;**13**:30–44.

1868. Fisher CM. Binswanger's encephalopathy: a review. *J Neurol* 1989;**236**:65–79.

1869. Fisher M, Mateer JE, Ullrich I, et al. Pyramidal tract deficits and polyneuropathy in hyperparathyroidism. *Amer J Med* 1985;**78**:1041–4.

1870. Fisher M, Sargent J, Drachman D. Familial inverted choreoathetosis. *Neurology* 1979;**29**:1627–31.

1871. Fisher O. Zur Frage der anatomischen Grundlage der Athetose double und der posthemiplegischen Bewegungsstorung uberhaupt. *Z Ges Neurol Psychiatr* 1911;**7**:463.

1872. Fishman LM, Zybert PA. Electrophysiological evidence of pyriformis syndrome. *Arch Phys Med Rehab* 1992;**73**:359–64.

1873. Fishman LS, Samson JH, Sperling D. Primary alveolar hypoventilation syndrome (Ondine's curse). *Am J Dis Child* 1965;**110**:155–61.

1874. Fishman MA, et al. Lacunar skull deformity and intelligence. *J Pediatr* 1977;**59**:296.

1875. Fishman RA. *Cerebrospinal Fluid in Diseases of the Nervous System*. Philadelphia: W.B. Saunders, 1980.

1876. Fisk JD, Pontefract A, Ritvo PG, et al. The impact of fatigue on patients with multiple sclerosis. *Can J Neurol Sci* 1994;**21**:9–14.

1877. Fitch N, Karpati G, Pinsky L. Congenital blepharophimosis, joint contractures and muscular hypotonia. *Neurology* 1971;**21**:1215–20.

1878. Fitzsimmons JS, et al. Four brothers with mental retardation, spastic paraplegia and palmoplantar hyperkeratosis. *Clin Genet* 1983;**23**:329–35.

1879. Flamm ES. The dilated pupil and head trauma. *Med Hist* 1972; **16**:194–8.

1880. Flamm ES. The neurology of Jean Cruveilhier. *Med Hist* 1973; **17**:343–55.

1881. Flanagan DE, Ibrahim AE, Ellison DW, et al. Inflammatory hypophysitis: the spectrum of disease. *Acta Neurochir (Wien)* 2002;**144**: 47–56.

1881a. Flanigan K, Gardner K, Alderson K, et al. Autosomal dominant spinocerebellar ataxia with sensory axonal neuropathy (SCA4): clinical description and genetic localization to chromosome 16q22.1. *Am J Hum Genet* 1996;**59**:392–9.

1882. Flanigan KM, Kerr L, Bromberg MB, et al. Congenital muscular dystrophy with rigid spine syndrome: a clinical, pathological, radiological, and genetic study. *Ann Neurol* 2000;**47**:152–61.

1883. Flatau E. *Atlas des Menschlichen Gehirns und des Faserverlaufes.* Berlin: S. Karger, 1894.

1884. Flatau E. On an epidemic of disseminated inflammation of the nervous system. *Encephale* 1929;**25**:619–60.

1885. Fletcher WA, Imes RK, Goodman D, et al. Acute idiopathic blind spot enlargement. A big blind spot syndrome without disc edema. *Arch Ophthalmol* 1988;**106**:44–9.

1886. Fletcher WA, Sharpe JA. Saccadic eye movement dysfunction in Alzheimer's disease. *Ann Neurol* 1986;**20**:464.

1887. Fleury P, Hageman G. A dominantly inherited lower motor neurone disorder presenting at birth with associated arthrogryposis. *J Neurol Neurosurg Psychiatry* 1985;**48**:1037–48.

1888. Flink EB, McCollister R, Prasad AS, et al. Evidences for clinical magnesium deficiency. *Ann Intern Med* 1957;**47**:956–68.

1889. Flourens MJP. *Récherches Experimentales sur les Propriétés et les Fonctions du Système Nerveux dans les Animaux Vertèbres.* Paris: J.B. Bailliere, 1842.

1890. Floyd P, Ayyar DR, Barwick DD. Myopathy in chronic renal failure. *Q J Med* 1974;**43**:509–23.

1891. Flynn P, Aird RB. A neuroectodermal syndrome of dominant inheritance. *J Neurol Sci* 1965;**2**:161–82.

1892. Foerster O. Der atonisch-astatische Typus der infantilen Cerebrallahmung. *Arch Klin Med* 1909;**48**:216–44.

1893. Foerster O. The dermatomes in man. *Brain* 1933;**56**:1–39.

1894. Foix C. Syndrome de la paroi externe du sinus caverneux. *Rev Neurol (Paris)* 1922;**38**:827–32.

1895. Foix C. Le syndromes de la région thalamique. *Presse Med* 1925;**33**:113–7.

1896. Foix C, Alajouanine T. Myélite necrotique subaigue (myélite contrale angiohypertrophique a evolution progressive). *Rev Neurol (Paris)* 1926;**2**:1–42.

1897. Foix C, Chavanay J-A, Marie J. Diplegie facio-linguo-masticatrice d'origine cortico-sous-corticale sans paralysie des membres. *Rev Neurol (Paris)* 1926;**33**:214–9.

1898. Foix C, Chavany H, Hillemand P, et al. Obliteration de l'artere choroidienne anterieure. Ramollissment de son territoire cerebral. Hemiplegie, hemianesthesie, hemianopsie. *Bull Fr Soc Ophthal* 1925; 221–3.

1899. Foldes FF, Klonymus DH, Maisel W, et al. A new curare test for diangosis of myasthenia gravis. *JAMA* 1968;**203**:183–8.

1900. Foley J. The athetoid syndrome: A review of a personal series. *J Neurol Neurosurg Psychiatry* 1983;**46**:289–98.

1901. Foley JM. Calcification of the corpus striatum and dentate nuclei occurring in a family. *J Neurol Neurosurg Psychiatry* 1951;**14**: 253–61.

1902. Foley JM. Benign forms of intracranial hypertension—"toxic" and "otitic" hydrocephalus. *Brain* 1955;**78**:1–41.

1903. Foley JM. Derek Ernest Denny-Brown, 1901–1981. *Ann Neurol* 1982;**11**:413–9.

1904. Foley JM, Watson CW, Adams RD. Significance of the electroencephalographic changes in hepatic coma. *Trans Am Neurol Assoc* 1950;**75**:161–4.

1905. Folstein MF, Folstein SE, McHugh PR. Mini-Mental State. A practical method for grading the cognitive state of patients for the clinician. *J Psychiatr Res* 1975;**12**:189–98.

1906. Folstein MF, Luria R. Reliability, validity, and clinical application of the visual analogue mood scale. *Psychol Med* 1973;**3**:479.

1907. Folstein SE, Leigh RJ, Parhad IM, Folstein MF. The diagnosis of Huntington's disease. *Neurology* 1986;**36**:1279–83.

1908. Fontaine A, Azouvi P, Remy P, et al. Functional anatomy of neuropsychological deficit after severe traumatic brain injury. *Neurology* 1999;**53**:1963–8.

1909. Ford CV. A type of disability neurosis: the Humpty-Dumpty syndrome. *Int J Psychiatr Med* 1978;**8**:285–93.

1910. Ford FR, Wilkins L. Congenital universal insensitiveness to pain: a clinical report of three cases in children, with discussion of the literature. *Bull Johns Hopkins Hosp* 1938;**62**:448–66.

1911. Forsius H, Eriksson AW. A new X-linked syndrome [in German]. *Klin Monatsbl Augenheilkd* 1964;**144**:447.

1912. Forster FM, Hansotia P, Cleeland CS, et al. A case of voice induced epilepsy treated by conditioning. *Neurology* 1969;**19**:325–31.

1913. Forsythe WI. Congenital hereditary vertical nystagmus. *J Neurol Neurosurg Psychiatry* 1955;**18**:196–8.

1914. Fothergill J. Of a painful affection of the face. *Med Obs Ing* 1773; **5**:129.

1915. Fothergill J. *A concise and Systematic Account of a Painful Affection of the Nerves of the Face, Commonly Called Tic Douloureux.* London: C. Dilly, 1794.

1916. Fotopoulos A. Spinal muscular atrophy with Huntington disease. *Psychiatr Neurol Med Psychol (Leipzig)* 1966;**18**:129.

1917. Fountain RB. Familial bone abnormalities, deaf mutism, mental retardation and skin granuloma. *Proc R Soc Med* 1974;**67**:878–9.

1918. Fourman P. Hereditary deafness in a family with ear pits. *BMJ* 1955;**2**:13542–1356.

1919. Fourney DR, Tong KA, Macoulay RJB, et al. Spinal angiolipoma. *Can J Neurol Sci* 2001;**28**:82–8.

1920. Foville A. Note sur un paralysie peu connu dans certains muscles de l'oeil et sa liason avec quelques points de l'anatomie et la physiologie de la protuberance annulaire. *Bull Soc Anat Paris* 1858;**30**: 393–414.

1921. Fowler EPA. A method for the early detection of otosclerosis: a study of sounds well above threshold. *Arch Otolaryngol* 1936;**24**:731.

1922. Fowler HL. Machado-Joseph-Azorean disease: a ten year study. *Arch Neurol* 1984;**41**:921–5.

1923. Fowler M, Dow R, White TA, et al. Congenital hydrocephalus–hydrancephaly in five siblings with autopsy studies: a new disease. *Dev Med Child Neurol* 1972;**14**:173–88.

1924. Fowler WM, Layzer RB, Taylor RG, et al. The Schwartz-Jampel syndrome. *J Neurol Sci* 1974;**22**:127–46.

1925. Fox AJ, Vinuela F. Neurological deficit from an inoperable arteriovenous malformation: an indication for therapeutic embolization? *Arch Neurol* 1986;**43**:510–1.

1926. Fox RH, Wilkins DC, Bell JA, et al. Spontaneous periodic hypothermia: diencephalic epilepsy. *BMJ* 1973;**2**:693–5.

1927. Francalcini P, Eymard-Pierre E, Dionisi-Vici C, et al. Fatal infantile leukodystrophy: a severe variant of CACH/VWM syndrome, allelic to chromosome 3q27. *Neurology* 2001;**57**:265–70.

1928. Francis DA, Bronstein AM, Rudge P, et al. The site of brainstem lesions causing semicircular canal paresis: an MRI study. *J Neurol Neurosurg Psychiatry* 1992;**55**:446–9.

1929. Francis DA, Heron JR. Ocular flutter in suspected multiple sclerosis: a presenting paroxysmal manifestation. *Postgrad Med J* 1985; **61**:333–4.

1930. Francois J. Oculo-cutaneous angiomatosis of Lawford. *Acta Neurol Psychiatr Belg* 1951;**8**:503–20.

1931. Francois J. The phakomatoses: introduction. In Vincken PJ, Bruyn GW, eds. *Handbook of Clinical Neurology, Vol. 14*, pp. 1–18. Amsterdam: North Holland Publishing, 1972.

1932. Frank JW, Kuschner BJ, France TD. Paradoxical pupillary phenomena: a review of patients with pupillary constriction to darkness. *Arch Ophthalmol* 1988;**106**:1564.

1933. Frankel HL, Hancock DO, Hyslop G, et al. The value of postural reduction in the initial management of closed injuries of the spine with paraplegia and tetraplegia. *Paraplegia* 1969;**7**:179–92.

1934. Frankenburg WK, Dodds J, Archer P, et al. Denver II. *Denver Developmental Materials* 1990.

1935. Frankl-Hochwart J. Uber Diagnose der Zirbeldrusentumoren. *Dtsch Z Nervenklinik* 1909;**37**:455–65.

1936. Fraser CL. Hepatic encephalopathy. *N Engl J Med* 1985;**313**: 865–73.

1937. Fraser FC, Lytwyn A. Spectrum of abnormalities in the Meckel syndrome. *Am J Med Genet* 1981;**9**:67–73.

1938. Fraser JL, Olney RK. The relative diagnostic sensitivity of different F-wave parameters in various polyneuropathies. *Muscle Nerve* 1992;**15**:912–8.

1939. Fredrickson DS, Altrocchi PH, Avioli LV, et al. Tangier disease. *Ann Intern Med* 1961;**55**:1016–31.

1940. Freedman BJ. *Just a Word, Doctor.* Oxford: Oxford University Press, 1987.

1941. Freedman M, Alexander MP, Naeser MA. Anatomic basis of transcortical motor aphasia. *Neurology* 1984;**34**:409–17.

1942. Freeman EA, Sheldon JH. Cranio-carpo-tarsal dystrophy. An undescribed congenital formation. *Arch Dis Child* 1938;**13**:277–83.

1943. Freeman JE, et al. Somnolence after prophylactic cranial irradiation in children with acute lymphoblastic leukaemia. *BMJ* 1973;**4**: 523–5.

1944. Freeman JM, Finkelstein JD, Mudd SH, et al. Homocystinuria presenting as reversible "schizophrenia": a new defect in methionine metabolism with reduced methylene-tetrahydrofolate reductase activity. *Pediatr Res* 1972;**6**:423.

1945. Freeman RW, Bleecker ML, Comstock GW, et al. Validation of self-administered questionnaire for study of peripheral neuropathy. *Am J Epidemiol* 1985;**121**:291–300.

1946. Freeman T, Gathercole CE. Perseveration: the clinical symptoms in chronic schizophrenia and organic dementia. *Br J Psychiatry* 1966; **112**:27–32.

1947. Freeman W, Watts JW. Prefrontal lobotomy in agitated depression. Report of a case. *Med Ann Distr Columbia* 1936;**5**:326–8.

1948. Frei KP, Patronas N, Crutchfield KE, et al. Mucolipidosis type IV. *Neurology* 1998;**51**:565–9.

1949. Freiberg AH. Sciatic pain and its relief by operations on muscle and fascia. *Arch Surg* 1937;**34**:337–49.

1950. Freire-Maia N, et al. The neurofaciodigitorenal (NFDR) syndrome. *Am J Med Genet* 1982;**11**:329–36.

1951. Freke J. A case of extraordinary exostoses on the back of a boy. *Phil Trans R Soc Lond* 1740;**41**:369–70.

1952. Frey E. Hereditary quivering of the chin [in German]. *Dtsch Z Nervenheilkd* 1930;**115**:9–26.

1953. Frey L. Le syndrome du nerf auriculo-temporal. *Rev Neurol (Paris)* 1923;**2**:97–104.

1954. Friedburg D. Pseudoneuritis und Drusenpapille beim Alport-Syndrom. *Klin Monatsbl Augenheilk* 1968;**152**:379.

1955. Friede RL. *Developmental Neuropathology.* Vienna: Springer-Verlag, 1975.

1956. Friedmann M. On the pathology and anatomy of widespread chronic encephalitis [in German]. C. Fromme: Vienna, 1883.

1957. Friedmann M. Ueber die nicht epileptischen absenscen oder kurzen narkoleptischen Anfalle. *Dtsch Z Nervenklinik* 1906;**30**:462–92.

1958. Friedreich N. Uber degenerative Atrophie der spinalen Hiterstrange. *Virchows Arch Pathol Anat Physiol Klin Med Berlin* 1863;**26**: 391–419.

1959. Friedreich N. Ueber congenitale halbseitige Kopfhypertrophie. *Virchows Arch Pathol Anat Physiol Klin Med Berlin.* 1863;**28**:474–81.

1960. Friedreich N. Paramyoclonus multiplex. *Virchows Arch Pathol Anat Physiol Berlin* 1881;**86**:421–30.

1961. Friis ML, Lund M. Stress convulsions. *Arch Neurol* 1974;**31**: 155–9.

1962. Frijns CJM, Van Deutekom J, Frants RR, et al. Dominant congenital benign spinal muscular atrophy. *Muscle Nerve* 1994;**17**:192–7.

1963. Frisen L. Quadruple sectoranopia and sectorial optic atrophy: a syndrome of the distal anterior choroidal artery. *J Neurol Neurosurg Psychiatry* 1979;**42**:590–4.

1964. Frisoni GB. Structural imaging in the clinical diagnosis of Alzheimer's disease: problems and tools. *J Neurol Neurosurg Psychiatry* 2001;**70**:711–8.

1965. Frith JA, McLeod JG, Nicholson GA, et al. Peroneal muscular atrophy with pyramidal tract features (hereditary motor and sensory neuropathy type V). *J Neurol Neurosurg Psychiatry* 1994;**57**:1343–6.

1966. Fritsch GT, Hitzig E. Ueber die elektrische Erregbarkeit des Grosshirns. *Arch Anat Physiol Wiss Med* 1870;**37**:300–32.

1967. Frohlich A. Ein Fall von Tumor der Hypophysis cerebri ohne Akromegalie. *Wien Klin Rdsch* 1901;**15**:883–906.

1968. Froin G. Inflammations meningees avec reactions chromique, fibrineuse et cytologique du liquide cephalo-rachidien. *Gaz Hop Paris* 1903;**76**:1005–6.

1969. Froment JC. La préhension dans les paralysies du nerf cubital et le signe du pouce. *Presse Med* 1915;**23**:409.

1970. Froment JC, Gardene H. La rigidité et la rue dentée Parkinsoniene s'effacent au repos. *Rev Neurol (Paris)* 1926;**1**:52–3.

1971. Fromm GH, Graff-Radford SB, Terrence CF, et al. Pre-trigeminal neuralgia. *Neurology* 1990;**40**:1493–5.

1971a. Frontali M. Spinocerebellar ataxia type 6: channelopathy or glutamine repeat disorder? *Brain Res Bull* 2001;**56**:227–31.

1972. Fry JH. Overuse syndrome in musicians—100 years ago: an historical review. *Med J Aust* 1986;**145**:620–5.

1973. Frydman M, et al. Oculo-palato-cerebral dwarfism: a new syndrome. *Clin Genet* 1985;**27**:414–9.

1974. Frymoyer JW. Back pain and sciatica. *N Engl J Med* 1988;**318**: 291–300.

1975. Frymoyer JW, Selby DK. Segmental instability: rationale for treatment. *Spine* 1985;**10**:280–6.

1976. Fryns JP, et al. A new lethal syndrome with cloudy corneae, diaphragmatic defects and distal limb deformities. *Hum Genet* 1979;**50**: 65–70.

1977. Fugl-Meyer AR, Jaasko L, Leyman I, et al. The post-stroke hemiplegic patient: 1. A method for evaluation of physical performance. *Scand J Rehabil Med* 1975;**7**:13–31.

1978. Fujii T, Okuno T, Ito M, et al. Non-Menkes–type copper deficiency with regression, lactic acidosis, and granulocytopenia. *Neurology* 1991;**41**:1263–6.

1979. Fujita T, Kanno T, Kobayashi S. *The Paraneuron.* Tokyo and London: Springer, 1988.

1980. Fukatsu R, Yamadori A, Fujii T. Impaired recall and preserved encoding in prominent amnesic syndrome: a case of basal forebrain amnesia. *Neurology* 1998;**50**:541.

1981. Fukazawa T, Sasaki H, Kikuchi S, et al. Dominantly inherited leukodystrophy showing cerebellar deficits and spastic paraparesis: a new entity? *J Neurol* 1997;**244**:446–9.

1982. Fukuda K, Tanaka T, Hyodo S, et al. Hyperphenylalaninaemia due to impaired dihydropterin biosynthesis: leukocyte function and effect of tetrahydrobiopterin therapy. *J Inherit Metab Dis* 1985;**8**:49–52.

1983. Fukuhara N. Myoclonus epilepsy and mitochondrial myopathy. In Scarlato G, Cerri C, eds. *Mitochondrial Pathology in Muscle Diseases,* pp 89–110. Padova: Piccin, 1983.

1984. Fukuhara N, Kumamoto T, Hirahara H, Tsubaki T. A new myopathy with tubulomembranous inclusions. *J Neurol Sci* 1981;**50**: 95–107.

1985. Fukunaga H, Osame M, Igata A. A case of nemaline myopathy with ophthalmoplegia and mitochondrial abnormalities. *J Neurol Sci* 1980;**46**:169–77.

1986. Fukutate T, Kita K, Sakakibara R, et al. Late onset hereditary ataxia with global thermoanalgesia and absence of fungiform papillae on the tongue in a Japanese family. *Brain* 1996;**119**:1011–21.

1987. Fukuyama Y, Audo T, Yokota J. Acute fulminant myoglobinuria polymyositis with picornavirus-like crystala. *J Neurol Neurosurg Psychiatry* 1977;**40**:775–81.

1988. Fukuyama Y, Osaw M, Suzuki H. Congenital muscular dystrophy of the Fukuyama type—clinical, genetic, and pathological considerations. *Brain Dev* 1981;**3**:1–29.

1989. Fuld PA, Katzman R, Davies P, et al. Intrusions as a sign of Alzheimer dementia: chemical and pathological verification. *Ann Neurol* 1982;**11**:155–9.

1990. Fuller GN, Marshall A, Flint J, et al. Migraine madness: recurrent psychosis after migraine. *J Neurol Neurosurg Psychiatry* 1993;**56**: 416–8.

1991. Fullerton PM, Gilliatt RW. Axon reflexes in human motor nerve fibres. *J Neurol Neurosurg Psychiatry* 1965;**28**:1–11.

1992. Funakoshi M, Goto K, Arahata K. Epilepsy and mental retardation ina subset of early onset 4q35-facioscapulohumeral muscular dystrophy. *Neurology* 1998;**50**:1791–4.

1993. Furman JMR, Crumrine PK, Reinmuth O. Epileptic nystagmus. *Ann Neurol* 1990;**27**:686–8.

1994. Furman JMR, et al. Infantile cerebellar atrophy. *Ann Neurol* 1985;**17**:399–402.

1995. Furman JMR, Jacob RG. Psychiatric dizziness. *Neurology* 1997; **48**:1161–6.

1996. Furst W, Ostrum HW. Platybasia, Klippel-Feil syndrome and Sprengel's deformity. *AJR Am J Roentgenol* 1942;**47**:588–90.

1997. Furukawa T. Numb chin syndrome in the elderly. *J Neurol Neurosurg Psychiatry* 1990;**53**:173.

1998. Furukawa T, Akagami N, Maruyama S. Chronic neurogenic quadriceps amyotrophy. *Ann Neurol* 1977;**2**:528–30.

1999. Furukawa T, Takogi A, Nakao K, et al. Hereditary muscular atrophy with ataxia, retinitis pigmentosa and diabetes mellitus. *Neurology* 1968;**18**:942–7.

2000. Furukawa T, Toyokura V. Congenital hypotonic-sclerotic muscular dystrophy. *J Med Genet* 1977;**14**:426–9.

2001. Furukawa T, Toyokura Y. Alternating Horner's syndrome. *Arch Neurol* 1974;**30**:311–4.

2002. Fuzukawa T, Sasaki H, Kikuchi S, et al. Dominantly inherited leukodystrophy showing cerebellar deficits and spastic paraparesis: a new entity? *J Neurol* 1997;**244**:446–9.

2003. Gafni J, Fischel B, Reit R, et al. Amyloidotic polyneuropathy in a Jewish family. *Q J Med* 1985;**55**:33–43.

2004. Gagliardi ART, et al. GAPO syndrome: report of three affected brothers. *Am J Med Genet* 1984;**19**:217–23.

2005. Gaillard JM. Electrophysiological semeiology of sleep. *Experientia* 1980;**36**:3–7.

2006. Gainer JV Jr, Chou SM, Chadduck WM. Familial cerebral sarcomas. *Arch Neurol* 1975;**32**:665–8.

2007. Gajusdek DC, Zigas V. Degenerative disease of the central nervous system in New Guinea. The endemic occurrence of "Kuru" in the native population. *N Engl J Med* 1957;**257**:974–8.

2008. Galer BS. Neuropathic pain of peripheral origin. *Neurology* 1995; **45**:S17–S25.

2009. Galer BS, Jensen MP. Development and preliminary validation of a pain measure specific to neuropathic pain. *Neurology* 1997;**48**: 332–8.

2009a. Gall FJ, Spurzheim JC. Anatomie et physiologie du système nerveux en général et du cerveau en particulier. Paris: F. Schoell, 1810–1819.

2010. Gallai V, Hockaday JM, Hughes JT, et al. Ponto-bulbar syndrome with deafness (Brown-Vialetto-Van Laere syndrome). *J Neurol Sci* 1981;**50**:259–75.

2010a. Gallo J-M. Kennedy's disease: a triplet repeat disorder or a motor neuron disease? *Brain Res Bull* 2001;**56**:209–214.

2011. Gallop TR. Fronto-facio-nasal-dysostosis: a new autosomal recessive syndrome. *Am J Med Genet* 1981;**10**:409–12.

2012. Galton CJ, Gomez-Anson B, Antoun N, et al. Temporal Lobe Rating Scale: Application to Alzheimer's disease and frontal lobe dementia. *J Neurol Neurosurg Psychiatry* 2001;**70**:165–73.

2012a. Galvao R, Mendes-Soares L, Camara J, et al. Triplet repeats, RNA secondary structure and toxic gain-of-function models for pathogenesis. *Brain Res Bull* 2001;**56**:191–201.

2013. Galvin JE, Lee VM-Y, Trojanowski JQ. Synucleinopathies. *Arch Neurol* 2001;**58**:186–90.

2014. Gamstorp I. Adynamia episodica hereditaria. *Acta Pediatr Scand Suppl* 1956;**108**:1–126.

2015. Gamstorp I, Wohlfart G. Myokymia, hyperhydrosis, impaired muscle relaxation. *Acta Psychiatr Scand* 1959;**34**:181.

2016. Gancher ST, Nutt JG. Autosomal dominant episodic ataxia: a heterogenous syndrome. *Mov Disord* 1986;**1**:239–53.

2017. Gandevia SC, McCloskey DI. Sensations of heaviness. *Brain* 1977;**100**:345–54.

2018. Ganser SJA. Ueber einen eigenartigen hysterischen Dammerzustund. *Arch Psychiatr (Berlin)* 1898;**30**:633–40.

2019. Garcia HA, Milner-Brown HS, Fisher MA. "Turns" analysis in the physiologicall evaluation of neuromuscular disorders. *J Neurol Neurosurg Psychiatry* 1980;**43**:1091–7.

2020. Garcin R, Raverdy Ph, Delthil S, et al. Sur une affection heredo-familiale associant cataracte, atrophie optique, signes extra pyramidaux et certains stigmates de la maladie de Friedreich. *Rev Neurol (Paris)* 1961;**101**:373–9.

2021. Gardner RC. Confirmed case and diagnosis of pseudocarpal tunnel (sublimis) syndrome. *N Engl J Med* 1970;**282**:858.

2022. Gardner WJ. Cross talk—the paradoxical transmission of a nerve impulse. *Arch Neurol* 1966;**14**:149–56.

2023. Gardner WJ, Frazier CH. Bilateral acoustic neurofibromas. *Arch Neurol Psychiatry* 1930;**23**:266–302.

2024. Gardner-Medwin D, Johnston HM. Severe muscular dystrophy in girls. *J Neurol Sci* 1984;**64**:79–87.

2025. Gardner-Thorpe C. Muscle weakness due to sarcoid myopathy. *Neurology* 1972;**22**:917–28.

2026. Gardos G, Cole JO, Salomon M, et al. Clinical forms of severe tardive dyskinesia. *Am J Psychiatry* 1987;**144**:895–902.

2027. Gardos G, Simmelgaard H. Tardive dyskinesia during and following treatment. *Psychopharmacol Berlin* 1978;**59**:105–12.

2028. Gareis FJ, Mason JD. X-linked mental retardation associated with bilateral clasp-thumb anomaly. *Am J Med Genet* 1984;**17**:333–8.

2029. Garfield J. Brain abscesses and focal suppurative infections. In Vinken PJ, Bruyn GW, eds. *Handbook of Clinical Neurology*, Vol. 33 Pt. 1. Amsterdam: North Holland Publishing, 1978.

2030. Garfinkel PE. Anorexia nervosa and bulimia. *Med Clin North Am* 1987;**Nov 15**:2952–63.

2030a. Garfinkel PE. The validity of the distinction between bulimia with and without anorexia nervosa. *Am J Psychiatry* 1985;**143**:581–7.

2031. Garg BP. Colpocephaly: an error of morphogenesis? *Arch Neurol* 1982;**39**:243–6.

2032. Garies FJ, Johnson J. Inanition in infants associated with diencephalic neoplasms. *J Dis Child* 1965;**109**:349.

2033. Garland HG. Central nervous deficiency syndrome. *Proc R Soc Med* 1946;**39**:178–80.

2034. Garland HG, Astley CE. Hereditary spastic paraplegia with amyotrophy and pes cavus. *J Neurol Neurosurg Psychiatry* 1950;**13**:130–3.

2035. Garland HG, Taverner D. Diabetic myelopathy. *BMJ* 1953;**1**: 1405–8.

2036. Garlepp MJ, Dawkins RL, Christiansen FT. Penicillamine-induced myasthenia. *BMJ* 1983;**286**:338–40.

2037. Garlepp MJ, Mastaglia FL. Inclusion body myositis. *J Neurol Neurosurg Psychiatry* 1996;**60**:251–5.

2038. Garvey MA, Giedd J, Swedo SE. PANDAS: the search for environmental triggers of pediatric neuropsychiatric disorders. Lessons from rheumatic fever. *J Child Neurol* 1998;**13**:413–23.

2039. Gascon GG, Barlow CF. Juvenile migraine presenting as an acute confusional state. *Pediatrics* 1970;**45**:628–35.

2040. Gascon GG, Gilles FH. Limbic dementia. *J Neurol Neurosurg Psychiatry* 1973;**36**:421–30.

2041. Gascon GG, Lombroso CT. Epileptic (gelastic) laughter. *Epilepsia* 1971;**12**:63–76.

2042. Gass A, Barker GJ, Kidd D, et al. Correlation of magnetisation transfer ratio with clinical disability in multiple sclerosis. *Ann Neurol* 1994;**36**:62–7.

2043. Gass JD. The syndrome of keratoconjunctivitis, superficial monoliasis, idiopathic hypoparathyroidism and Addison's disease. *Am J Ophthalmol* 1962;**54**:660–74.

2044. Gass JD. Cavernous hemangioma of the retina: a neuro-oculocutaneous syndrome. *Am J Ophthalmol* 1971;**71**:799.

2045. Gass JMD. Acute posterior multifocal placoid pigment epithiliopathy. *Arch Ophthalmol* 1968;**80**:177–85.

2046. Gassell MM. False localising signs. *Arch Neurol* 1961;**4**:526–54.

2047. Gassell MM, Williams D. Visual function in patients with homonymous hemianopia. Part III. *Brain* 1963;**86**:229–60.

2048. Gastaut H. Le syndrome "hemiconvulsion-hemiplegie-epilepsie". *Rev Neurol (Paris)* 1957;**97**:37–52.

2049. Gastaut H. *Dictionary of Epilepsies. Part I: Definitions.* Geneva: World Health Organization, 1973.

2050. Gastaut H. Fyodor Dostoevsky's involuntary contribution to the symptomatology and prognosis of epilepsy. *Epilepsia* 1978;**19**:186–19.

2051. Gastaut H. A new type of epilepsy: benign partial epilepsy of childhood with occipital spike-waves. *Clin Electroencephalogr* 1982; **13**:13–22.

2052. Gastaut H. Classification of status epilepticus. In Delgado-Escueta AV, Wasterlain DG, Traimen DM, et al., eds. *Advances in Neurology, Vol. 34: Status Epilepticus*, p 75. New York: Raven Press, 1983.

2053. Gastaut H. Benign epilepsy of childhood with occipital paroxysms. In Roger J, Dravet C, Bureau M, et al., eds. *Epileptic Syndromes in Infancy, Childhood and Adolescence*, pp 159–70. London: John Libbey, 1985.

2054. Gastaut H, Broughton RJ. Paroxysmal psychological events and certain phases of sleep. *Percept Mot Skills* 1963;**17**:362.

2055. Gastaut H, Broughton RJ. *Epileptic Seizures*. Springfield, IL: C.C. Thomas, 1972.

2056. Gastaut H, Gastaut Y. Syncopes et convulsions. A propos de la nature syncopal de certains spasmes du sanglot et de certains convulsions essentielles, hyperthermiques et a froid. *Rev Neurol (Paris)* 1957;**96**:158–63.

2057. Gastaut H, Naquet, R. Etude electroencephalographique de l'insuffisance circulatoire cerebrale (ICC). In *Symposium International sur la Circulation Cerebrale*, pp. 163–191, 1966.

2058. Gastaut H, Roger J, Ouahchi S, et al. An electro-clinical study of generalized epileptic seizures of tonic expression. *Epilepsia* 1963;**4**: 15–44.

2059. Gates AI, McGintie WH. *Gates-McGintie Reading Exercises*. New York: Teachers College Press, 1965.

2060. Gatfield PD, Taller E, Hinton GG, et al. Hyperpipecolatemia. A new metabolic disorder associated with neuropathy and hepatomegaly: a case study. *CMAJ* 1968;**99**:1215–33.

2061. Gaucher PCE. De l'epithelioma primitif de la rate: hypertrophie idiopathique de la rate sans leucémie. Paris: University of Paris, 1882.

2062. Gaull GE, Bender AN, Vulovic D, et al. Methioninemia and myopathy: a new disorder. *Ann Neurol* 1980;**9**:423–32.

2063. Gautier-Smith PC. Neurological complications of glandular fever (infectious mononucleosis). *Brain* 1965;**88**:323–34.

2064. Gaymard B, Lafitte C, Gelot A, et al. Plus–minus lid syndrome. *J Neurol Neurosurg Psychiatry* 1992;**55**:846–8.

2065. Gazit E, et al. The wrinkly skin syndrome: a new heritable disorder of connective tissue. *Clin Genet* 1973;**4**:186–92.

2066. Geiger LR, Mancall EL, Penn AS, et al. Familial neuralgic amyotrophy: report of three families with review of the literature. *Brain* 1974;**97**:87–102.

2067. Gélineau JBE. De la narcolepsie. *Gaz Hop Paris* 1880;**53**:626–8.

2068. Gellis SS, Feingold M. Spondylothoracic dysplasia (costo-vertebral dysplasia, Jarcho Levin syndrome). *Am J Dis Child* 1976;**130**: 513–4.

2069. Gelwan MJ, Seidman M, Kupersmith MJ. Pseudo-pseudo Foster Kennedy syndrome. *J Clin Neuroophthalmol* 1985;**5**:209–12.

2070. Geminginani F. Spinocerebellar ataxia with localized amyotrophy of the hands, sensorineural deafness and spastic paraparesis in 2 brothers. *J Neurogenet* 1986;**3**:125–33.

2071. Gent M, Blakeley J, Easton JD, et al. Canadian-American Ticlopidine Study: Thrombo-embolic stroke. *Stroke* 1988;**19**:1203–10.

2072. Gerhardt C. Encephalitis; Stimmbandlahmung ohne Stimmveranderung. *Virchows Arch Pathol Anat Physiol Klin Med Berlin* 1863;**27**:309.

2073. Gerle B. Dynamite encephalosis. *Acta Psychiatr Neurol* 1946; **21**:319.

2074. Gerlier EF. Une epidémie de vértige paralysant. *Rev Med Suisse Rom* 1887;**7**:5–29.

2075. Gershanik OS, Nygaard TG. Parkinson's disease beginning before age 40. *Adv Neurol* 1990;**53**:251–8.

2076. Gerstmann J. Fingeragnosie und isolierte Agraphie—ein neues Syndrom. *Z Ges Neurol Psychiatrie* 1927;**108**:152–77.

2077. Gerstmann J, Straussler E, Scheinker IM. Uber eine eigenartige hereditar-familiare Erkrankung des Zentralnervensystems zugleich ein Beitrag zur Frage des vorzeitigen lokalen Alterns. *Z Neurol* 1936;**154**: 736–62.

2078. Gertz MA, Kyle RA. Myopathy in primary systemic amyloidosis. *J Neurol Neurosurg Psychiatry* 1999;**60**:655–60.

2079. Geschwind DH, Perlman S, Figueroa K, et al. Spinocerebellar ataxia type 6. *Neurology* 1997;**49**:1247–51.

2080. Geschwind N. Disconnexion syndromes in animals and man. *Brain* 1965;**88**:237–94.

2082. Geschwind N. Derek Ernest Denny-Brown. *J Neurol Sci* 1982; **53**:137–9.

2083. Geschwind N, Galaburda AM. Cerebral lateralization: biological mechanisms, associations, and pathology: I–III. A hypothesis and a program for research. *Arch Neurol* 1985;**42**:428–59, 521–52, 634–54.

2084. Geschwind N, Sherwin I. Language-induced epilepsy. *Arch Neurol* 1967;**16**:25–31.

2085. Geyelin HR, Penfield W. Cerebral calcification and epilepsy. *Arch Neurol Psychiatry* 1929;**21**:1020–43.

2086. Geyer JD, Payne TA, Drury I. The value of pelvic thrusting in the diagnosis of seizures and pseudoseizures. *Neurology* 2000;**54**:227–9.

2087. Gfeller JD, Chibnall JT, Duckro JN. Postconcussion symptoms and cognitive functioning in posttraumatic headache patients. *Headache* 1994;**34**:503–7.

2088. Ghadimi H, Bimington VI, Pecora F. Hyperlysinemia associated with retardation. *N Engl J Med* 1965;**273**:723–9.

2089. Gherardi R, Chretien F, Delfau-Larue M-H, et al. Neuropathy in diffuse infiltrative lymphocytosis syndrome. *Neurology* 1998;**50**: 1041–4.

2090. Ghika-Schmid F, Bogousslavsky J. The acute behavioral syndrome of anterior thalamic infarction: a prospective study of 12 cases. *Ann Neurol* 2000;**48**:220–7.

2091. Ghosh D, Mohanty GPS. Ictal deafness—a report of three cases. *Seizure* 2001;**10**:130–3.

2092. Giacino JT, Ashwal S, Chinnery PF, et al. The minimally conscious state. *Neurology* 2002;**58**:349–53.

2093. Giacino JT, Kezmarsky MA, DeLuca J, et al. Monitoring rate of recovery to predict outcome in minimally responsive patients. *Arch Phys Med Rehabil* 1991;**72**:897–901.

2094. Gibb WRG. Neuropathology in movement disorders. *J Neurol Neurosurg Psychiatry* 1989;**Suppl**:55–67.

2095. Gibb WRG, Esiri MM, Lees AJ. Clinical and pathological features of diffuse cortical Lewy body disease (Lewy body dementia). *Brain* 1987;**110**:1131–53.

2096. Gibb WRG, Lees AJ. The clinical phenomenon of akathisia. *J Neurol Neurosurg Psychiatry* 1986;**49**:861–6.

2097. Gibb WRG, Luthert PJ, Janota I, Lantos PL. Cortical Lewy body dementia: clinical features and classification. *J Neurol Neurosurg Psychiatry* 1989;**52**:185–92.

2098. Gibb WRG, Mountjoy CQ, Mann DMA, Lees AJ. A pathological study of the association between Lewy body disease and Alzheimer's disease. *J Neurol Neurosurg Psychiatry* 1989;**52**:701–8.

2099. Gibb WRG, Narabayashi H, Yokochi M, et al. New pathologic observations in juvenile onset parkinsonism with dystonia. *Neurology* 1991;**41**:820–2.

2100. Gibberd FB, Gavrilescu K. A familial neuropathy associated with a paraprotein in serum, CSF and urine. *Neurology* 1966;**16**:130–44.

2101. Gibbon NO. Nomenclature of neurogenic bladder. *Urology* 1976; **8**:423–31.

2102. Gibbons A. The Chinese paralytic syndrome. *Science* 1991; **253**:26.

2103. Gibbs FA, Davis H, Lennox WG. The electroencephalagram in epilepsy and in conditions of impaired consciousness. *Arch Neurol Psychiatry* 1935;**34**:1133.

2104. Gibbs RC, Frank SB. Keratoma hereditaria mutilans (Vohwinkel syndrome). *Arch Dermatol* 1966;**94**:619.

2105. Gibson T, Noris W. Skin fragments removed by injection needles. *Lancet* 1958;**2**:983.

2106. Gieron MA, Korthais JK, Koussett BG. Facio-scapulo-humeral dystrophy with cochlear hearing loss and tortuosity of the retinal veins. *Am J Med Genet* 1985;**22**:143–7.

2107. Giladi N, Turezkite T, Harel D. Myelopathy as a complication of diabetes mellitus. *Isr J Med Sci* 1991;**27**:316–9.

2108. Gilbert GJ. Ménière's syndrome and cluster headache. Recurrent paroxysmal focal vasodilatation. *JAMA* 1965;**191**:691–4.

2109. Gilbert GJ. Lightning-induced robotic speech. *Neurology* 1994; **44**:991.

2110. Gilbert GJ, McEntee WJ, Glaser GH. Familial myoclonus and ataxia; pathophysiologic implications. *Neurology* 1963;**13**:365.

2111. Gilbert JG, Levee RF. Patterns of declining memory. *J Gerontol* 1971;**26**:70.

2112. Gilchrist JM, Ambler MW, Agatiello P. Steroid-responsive tubular aggregate myopathy. *Muscle Nerve* 1991;**14**:233–6.

2113. Gilchrist JM, Leschner RT. Humeroperoneal myopathy. *Arch Neurol* 1986;**43**:734–5.

2114. Gilden DH, Beinlich BR, Rubinstein EM, et al. Varicella-zoster virus myelitis. *Neurology* 1994;**44**:1818–23.

2115. Gilden DH, Dueland AN, Cohrs R, et al. Preherpetic neuralgia. *Neurology* 1991;**41**:1215–8.

2116. Gillepsy T III, Gillespy T Jr, Revak C. Progressive senile scoliosis: seven cases of increasing spinal curves in elderly patients. *Skeletal Radiol* 1985;**13**:280–6.

2117. Gilles FH, Averil DR, Kerr CS. Neonatal endotoxin encephalopathy. *Ann Neurol* 1977;**2**:49–56.

2118. Gillespie FD. Aniridia, cerebellar ataxia and oligophrenia in siblings. *Arch Ophthalmol* 1965;**73**:338–41.

2119. Gilliam F, Steinhoff BJ, Bitterman HJ, et al. Adult myoclonic epilepsy: a distinct syndrome of idiopathic generalized epilepsy. *Neurology* 2000;**55**:1030–3.

2120. Gilliam F, Wyllie E. Ictal amaurosis: MRI, EEG and clinical features. *Neurology* 1995;**45**:1619–21.

2121. Gilman S, Horenstein S. Familial amyotrophic dystonic paraplegia. *Brain* 1964;**87**:51–66.

2122. Gilman S, Little R, Johanns J, et al. Evolution of sporadic olivopontocerebellar atrophy into multiple system atrophy. *Neurology* 2000;**55**:527–32.

2123. Gilman S, Low PA, Quinn N, et al. Consensus statement on the diagnosis of multiple system atrophy. *J Auton Nerv Syst* 1998;**74**:189–92.

2124. Ginsberg L, DiFerrante DT, Caskey CT, et al. Glucosamine-6–SO₄ sulfatase deficiency: a new mucopolysaccharidosis. *Clin Res* 1977;**25**:471a.

2125. Giraud P, Thobois S, Hermier M, et al. Intravenous hypertrophic Paccioni granulations: differentiation from venous dural thrombosis. *J Neurol Neurosurg Psychiatry* 2001;**70**:700–1.

2126. Giroud M, Creisson E, Fayolle H, et al. Homolateral ataxia and crural paresis: a crossed cerebral–cerebellar diaschisis. *J Neurol Neurosurg Psychiatry* 1994;**57**:221–222.

2127. Giroux JM, Barbeau A. Erythrokeratodemia with ataxia. *Arch Dermatol* 1972;**106**:183–8.

2128. Gisselin S, Kyle RA, Dyck PJ. Neuropathy associated with monoclonal gammopathy of undetermined significance. *Ann Neurol* 1991; **30**:54–61.

2129. Gittinger JWJr. Functional hemianopsia: a historical perspective. *Surv Ophthalmol* 1988;**32**:427–32.

2130. Gitzelmann R. Deficiency of erythrocyte galactokinase in a patient with galactose diabetes. *Lancet* 1965;**2**:670.

2131. Giurgea CE. The nootropic concept—twenty years on. In *Proceedings of the Third Congress, International Psychogeriatric Association*, #369, 1987.

2132. Gladstone RM. Development and significance of heterochromia iridis. *Arch Neurol* 1969;**21**:184–92.

2133. Glaser JS. *Clinical Neuroophthalmology*. Philadelphia, J.B. Lippincott, 1990.

2134. Glaser JS, Savino PJ, Sumers KD, et al. The photostress recovery test in the clinical assessment of visual function. *Am J Ophthalmol* 1977;**83**:255–60.

2135. Glasgow BJ, Brown HH, Hannah JB, et al. Ocular pathologic findings in neonatal adrenoleukodystrophy. *Ophthalmology* 1987;**94**: 1054–60.

2136. Glass J, Hochberb FH, Miller DC. Intravascular lymphomatosis: a systemic disease with neurologic manifestations. *Cancer* 1993;**71**: 3156–64.

2137. Glass JD, Levey AI, Rothstein JD. The dysarthria–clumsy hand syndrome: a distinct entity related to pontine infarction. *Arch Neurol* 1990;**27**:487–94.

2138. Glew RH, Basu A, Prence EM, Remaley AT. Lysosomal storage diseases. *Lab Invest* 1985;**53**:250–69.

2139. Glick B, Shapira Y, Stein A, et al. Congenital fiber type disproportion. *Ann Neurol* 1984;**16**:405–6.

2140. Gloor P. Consciousness. *Epilepsia* 1986;**27** Suppl 2:S14–S26.

2141. Goadsby PJ, Lance JW. Clinicopathological correlation in a case of painful ophthalmoplegia: Tolosa-Hunt syndrome. *J Neurol Neurosurg Psychiatry* 1989;**52**:1290–3.

2142. Goadsby PJ, Lipton RB. A review of paroxysmal hemicranias, SUNCT syndrome and other short-lasting headaches with autonomic features, including new cases. *Brain* 1997;**120**:193–209.

2144. Godtfredsen E. Ophthalmological and neurological symptoms in malignant naso-pharyngeal tumors. *Acta Pathol Microbiol Scand* 1944;**Suppl 55**:120–85.

2145. Godtfredsen E. Ophthalmoneurological symptoms in malignant naso-pharyngeal tumors. *Br J Ophthalmol* 1947;**31**:78–100.

2146. Godwin-Austen RB, Robinson A, Evans K, Lascelles PT. An unusual neurological disorder of copper metabolism clinically resembling Wilson's disease but biochemically a distinct entity. *J Neurol Sci* 1978;**39**:85–98.

2147. Goebel HH. Desmin-related neuromuscular disorders. *Muscle Nerve* 1995;**18**:1306–20.

2148. Goebel HH, d'Agostino AN, Wilson J, et al. Spheroid body myopathy revisited. *Muscle Nerve* 1997;**20**:1127–36.

2149. Goebel HH, et al. Subacute necrotizing encephalomyelopathy (Leigh's disease). *Muscle Nerve* 1986;**9**:1657.

2150. Goebel HH, Heipertz R, Scholz W, et al. Juvenile Huntington's chorea: clinical ultrastructural and biochemical studies. *Neurol Minneap* 1978;**28**:23–31.

2151. Goebel HH, Lenard HG, Langenbeck U, et al. A form of congenital muscular dystrophy. *Brain Dev* 1980;**2**:387–400.

2152. Goebel HH, Muller J, DeMyer W. Myopathy associated with Marfan syndrome. *Neurology* 1973;**23**:1257–68.

2153. Goeminne F. A new, probably X-linked syndrome: congenital muscular torticollis, multiple keloids, cryptorchidism and renal dysplasia. *Acta Genet (Roma)* 1968;**17**:439.

2154. Goetz CG. *Charcot the Clinician*. New York: Raven Press, 1987.

2155. Goetz CG, Tanner CM, Wilson RS, et al. Tourette Rating Scale. *Neurology* 1987;**37**:1542–4.

2156. Golabi M, Rosen L. A new X-linked mental retardation–overgrowth syndrome. *Am J Med Genet* 1984;**17**:345–58.

2157. Golbe LI. Young-onset Parkinson's disease: a clinical review. *Neurology* 1991;**41**:168–73.

2158. Golbe LI, Lazzarini AM, Schwarz KO, et al. Autosomal dominant parkinsonism with benign course and typical Lewy-body pathology. *Neurology* 1993;**43**:2222–7.

2159. Gold M, Shuren J, Heilman KM. Proximal intentional neglect: a case study. *J Neurol Neurosurg Psychiatry* 1994;**57**:1395–400.

2160. Goldberg G. Supplementary motor area structure and function: review and hypotheses. *Behav Brain Sci* 1985;**8**:567–615.

2161. Goldberg MF, Cotlier E, Fichenscher LG, et al. Macular cherry-red spot, corneal clouding and β-galactosidase deficiency. *Arch Intern Med* 1971;**128**:387–98.

2162. Golden CJ. A standardized version of Luria's neuropsychological tests. In Filskov S, Boll TJ, eds. *Handbook of Clinical Neuropsychology*, New York: Wiley-Interscience, 1981.

2163. Golden GM. Tics and Tourettes: a continuum of symptoms. *Ann Neurol* 1978;**4**:145–8.

2164. Golden GS. Stroke syndromes in childhood. *Neurol Clin* 1985; **3**:59–75.

2165. Goldenhar M. Associations malformatives de l'oeil et de l'oreille, en particulier le syndrome dermoide epibulbaire-appendices auriculaires-fistula auris congenita et ses relations avec la dysostose mandibulo-faciale. *J Genet Hum* 1952;**1**:243–83.

2166. Goldfield M, Sussman O. The 1959 outbreak of eastern encephalitis in New Jersey. 1. Introduction and description of outbreak. *Am J Epidemiol* 1968;**87**:1–10.

2167. Goldfischer SL, Collins J, Rapin I, et al. Pseudo-Zellweger syndrome: deficiencies in several peroxisomal oxidative activities. *J Pediatr* 1986;**108**:25–32.

2168. Goldhammer Y, Lawton Smith J. Acquired intermittent Brown's syndrome. *Neurology* 1974;**24**:666–8.

2169. Goldhammer Y, Smith JL. Optic nerve anomalies in basal encephalocele. *Arch Ophthalmol* 1975;**93**:115–8.

2170. Goldie WD, Holtzman D, Suzuki K. Chronic hexosaminidase A and B deficiency. *Ann Neurol* 1977;**2**:156–8.

2171. Goldman RL. Gliomyosarcoma of the cerebrum. *Am J Clin Pathol* 1969;**52**:741–4.

2172. Goldstein K. Acute cerebellitis [in German]. *Munch Med Wochenschr* 1915;**92**:1439–42.

2173. Goldstein K. Account of the symptoms and lesions of the cerebellum. *Arch Psychiatr Nervenkr* 1916;**56**:466–521.

2174. Goldstein K. *Language and Language Disturbances*. New York: Grune and Stratton, 1948.

2175. Goldstein LB, Bertels C, Davis JN. Interrater reliability of the NIH stroke scale. *Arch Neurol* 1989;**46**:660–2.

2176. Gollin ES. Developmental studies of visual recognition of incomplete objects. *Percept Mot Skills* 1960;**11**:289.

2177. Goltz RW. Focal dermal hypoplasia. *Arch Dermatol* 1962; **86**:708–17.

2178. Gomez CR, Gomez SM, Selhorst JB. Acute thalamic esotropia. *Neurology* 1988;**38**:1759.

2179. Gomez MR. *Tuberous Sclerosis*. New York: Raven Press, 1979.

2180. Gomez MR, Clermont V, Bernstein J. Progressive bulbar paralysis in childhood. *Arch Neurol* 1962;**6**:317–23.

2181. Gomez MR, Engel AG, Dyck PJ. Progressive ataxia, retinal degeneration, neuromyopathy, and mental subnormality in a patient with true hypoparathyroidism, dwarfism, malabsorption and cholelithiasis. *Neurology* 1972;**22**:849–55.

2182. Gomez MR, Klass DW. Epilepsies of infancy and childhood. *Ann Neurol* 1983;**13**:113–24.

2183. Gomez-Aranda F, Canadillas F, Marti-Masso JF, et al. Pseudomigraine with temporary neurological symptoms and lymphocytic pleocytosis. A report of 50 cases. *Brain* 1997;**120**:1105–13.

2184. Gomori AJ, Partnow AJ, Houroupian DS, et al. Ataxic form of Creutzfeldt-Jakob disease. *Arch Neurol* 1973;**29**:318–23.

2185. Gonce M, Delwaide PJ. Exteroceptive reflex myoclonus: clinical and electrophysiological study. *J Neurol Neurosurg Psychiatry* 1986;**49**: 1195–8.

2186. Gonzalez J, Lacomis D, Kramer DJ. Mushroom myopathy. *Muscle Nerve* 1996;**19**:790–2.

2187. Gooddy W. On the nature of pain. *Brain* 1957;**80**:118–31.

2188. Gooddy W, Reinhold M. The function of the cerebral cortex. *Brain* 1954;**77**:416–26.

2189. Goodenough DJ, Fariello RG, Annis BL, et al. Familial and acquired paroxysmal dyskinesias. A proposed classification with delineation of clinical features. *Arch Neurol* 1978;**35**:827–31.

2190. Goodglass H, Berko J. Agrammatism and inflectional morphology in English. *J Speech Hear Res* 1960;**3**:257–67.

2191. Goodglass H, Kaplan E. *The Assessment of Aphasia and Related Disorders*. Philadelphia: Lea & Febiger, 1972.

2192. Goodglass H, Kaplan E. *The Assessment of Aphasia and Related Disorders*. Philadelphia: Lea & Febiger, 1983.

2193. Goodin DS, Squires KC, Henderson BH, et al. Age-related variations in evoked potentials to auditory stimuli in normal human subjects. *Electroencephalogr Clin Neurophysiol* 1978;**44**:447–58.

2194. Goodkin DE, Hertsgaard D, Seminary J. Upper extremity function im multiple sclerosis: improving assessment sensitivity with box and block and nine-hole peg tests. *Arch Phys Med Rehabil* 1988;**69**: 850–4.

2195. Goodman BW. Temporal arteritis. *Am J Med* 1979;**77**:839–52.

2196. Goodman G, Ripps H, Siegal IM. Cone dysfunction syndromes. *Arch Ophthalmol* 1963;**70**:214.

2197. Goodman RM, et al. Camptodactyly: occurrence in two new genetic syndromes and its relationship to other syndromes. *J Med Genet* 1972;**9**:203–12.

2198. Goodman RM, Lockareff S, Gwinup G. Hereditary congenital deafness with onychodystrophy. *Arch Otolaryngol* 1969;**90**:474.

2199. Goodman SI, Mace JW, Pollak S. Serum gamma-glutamyl transpeptidase deficiency. *Lancet* 1971;**1**:234.

2200. Goodwin JA, Kansu T. Vulpian's sign: conjugate eye deviation in acute cerebral hemisphere lesions. *Neurology* 1986;**36**:711–2.

2201. Gopalan C. The "burning feet" syndrome. *Indian Med Gaz* 1946; **81**:22–6.

2202. Gordon A. A new reflex: paradoxic flexor reflex. Its diagnostic value. *Am Med* 1904;**8**:971.

2203. Gordon A. Paradoxical flexor reflexes and their relationship with the knee jerk and the Babinski response. *Rev Neurol (Paris)* 1904; **21**:1083.

2204. Gordon AM, Capute AJ, Konigsmark BW. Progressive quadriparesis, mental retardation, retinitis pigmentosa and hearing loss—report of 2 sibs. *Johns Hopkins Med J* 1976;**138**:142–5.

2206. Gordon KE, Masotti RE, Waddell WR. Tremorgenic encephalopathy: a role of mycotoxins in the production of CNS disease in humans? *Can J Neurol Sci* 1993;**20**:237–9.

2207. Gordon NS, Marsden HB, Noronha MJ. Neuronal ceroid lipofuscinosis (Batten's disease). *Arch Dis Child* 1972;**47**:285–91.

2208. Gorelick PB, Rosenberg M, Pagano RJ. Enhanced ptosis in myasthenia gravis. *Arch Neurol* 1981;**38**:531.

2209. Gorelick PB, Sullivan M, Lansky L. Cerebral auscultation. *Neurology* 1987;**37**:1523–4.

2210. Gorelick PB, Zych D. Corning, James Leonard and the early history of spinal puncture. *Neurology* 1987;**37**:672–4.

2211. Goren H, Steinberg MC, Farbourg GH. Familial oculoleptomeningeal amyloidosis. *Brain* 1980;**103**:473–8.

2212. Gorham DR. A proverbs test for clinical and experimental use. *Psychol Rep* 1956;**1**:1.

2213. Gorlin RJ. Some facial syndromes. *Birth Defects* 1969;**5**:65–76.

2214. Gorlin RJ, Chaudhry AP, Moss ML. Craniofacial dysostosis, patent ductus arteriosus, hypertrichosis hypoplasia of labia majora, dental and eye anomalies, a new syndrome? *J Pediatr* 1960;**56**:778–85.

2215. Gorlin RJ, Cohen MM Jr. Frontometaphyseal dysplasia: a new syndrome. *Am J Dis Child* 1969;**118**:487–94.

2216. Gorlin RJ, et al. Genetic craniotubular bone dysplasias and hyperostoses: a critical analysis. *Birth Defects* 1969;**5**:79–95.

2217. Gorlin RJ, et al. Multiple lentigines syndrome, complex comprising multiple lentigines, electrocardiographic conduction abnormalities, ocular hypertelorism, pulmonary stenosis, abnormalities of genitalia, retardation of growth, sensorineural deafness, and autosomal dominant hereditary pattern. *Am J Dis Child* 1969;**117**:652–62.

2218. Gorlin RJ, Jue R, Jacobsen K, et al. Oculoauriculovertebral dysplasia. *J Pediatr* 1963;**63**:991–9.

2219. Gorlin RJ, Pindborg JJ, Cohen MM Jr. *Syndromes of the Head and Neck*. New York: McGraw-Hill, 1976.

2220. Gorlin RJ, Psaume J. Orodigitofacial dysostosis—a new syndrome. *J Pediatr* 1962;**61**:250.

2221. Gorlin RJ, Sedano H, Anderson VE. The syndrome of palmaroplantar hyperkeratosis and premature periodontal destruction of the teeth, a clinical and genetic analysis of the Papillon-Lefevre syndrome. *J Pediatr* 1964;**65**:895–908.

2222. Gorlin RJ, Sedano HO. Multiple nevoid basal cell carcinoma syndrome. In Vincken PJ, Bruyn GW, eds. *Handbook of Clinical Neurology*, Vol. 14, pp. 455–73. Amsterdam: North Holland Publishing, 1972.

2223. Gorlin RJ, Vickers RA, Kelln E, et al. The multiple basal cell nevi syndrome. *Cancer* 1965;**18**:89.

2224. Gormley JB. Treatment of postspinal headache. *Anesthesiology* 1960;**21**:565–6.

2225. Gormley RK. Low back pain with special reference to the articular facets with presentation of an operative procedure. *Coll Papers Mayo Clin* 1933;**25**:813–23.

2226. Gorson KC, Ropper AH, Adelmann LS, et al. Chronic motor axonal neuropathy: pathological evidence of inflammatory polyradiculoneuropathy. *Muscle Nerve* 1999;**22**:266–270.

2227. Gospe SM, Lazaro RP, Lava NS, et al. Familial X-linked myalgia and cramps. *Neurology* 1989;**39**:1277–80.

2228. Gotham JE, Wein H, Meyer JS. Clinical studies of neuropathy due to macroglobulinemia (Waldenstrom's syndrome). *CMAJ* 1963;**89**: 806.

2229. Goto I, Kanazawa Y, Kobagashi T, et al. Oculopharyngeal myopathy with distal and cardiomyopathy. *J Neurol Neurosurg Psychiatry* 1977;**40**:600–7.

2230. Goto I, Nakai H, Tabira T, et al. Juvenile neurogenic muscular atrophy with lysosomal deficiencies: a new variant or a variant of mucopolysaccharidosis? *J Neurol* 1983;**229**:45–54.

2231. Gottschaldt K. Uber den Einfluss, der Erfahrung auf die Wahrnehmung von Figuren. *Psychol Forsch* 1928;**8**:18–317.

2232. Gouider R, LeGuern E, Emile J, et al. Hereditary neuralgic amyotrophy and hereditary neuropathy with liability to pressure palsies. *Neurology* 1994;**44**:2250–2.

2233. Gourie-Devi M, Suresh TG, Shankar SK. Monomelic amyotrophy. *Arch Neurol* 1984;**41**:388–94.

2234. Goutieres F, Aicardi J, Farakas E. Anterior horn cell disease associated with pontocerebellar hypoplasia in infants. *J Neurol Neurosurg Psychiatry* 1977;**40**:370–8.

2235. Goutieres F, Bogicevic D, Aicardi J. A predominantly cervical form of spinal muscular atrophy. *J Neurol Neurosurg Psychiatry* 1991; **54**:223–5.

2236. Gouw LG, Digre KB, Harris CP, et al. Autosomal dominant cerebellar ataxia with retinal degeneration. *Neurology* 1994;**44**:1441–7.

2237. Gowers WG. *The Border-Land of Epilepsy.* London: Churchill, 1907.

2238. Gowers WR. On saltatoric spasm. *Lancet* 1877;**2**:42,152–45,155.

2239. Gowers WR. *Epilepsy and Other Chronic Convulsive Diseases.* London: J & A. Churchill, 1881.

2240. Gowers WR. *A Manual of Diseases of the Nervous System.* Philadelphia: Blakiston, 1888.

2241. Gowers WR. Myopathy of a distal form. *BMJ* 1902;**2**:89–92.

2242. Gowers WR. Vasovagal attacks. *Lancet* 1907;**1**:1551.

2243. Gowland C, Stratford P, Ward M, et al. Measuring physical impairment and disability with the Chedoke-McMaster Stroke Assessment. *Stroke* 1993;**24**:58–63.

2244. Goyal RK, Hirano I. The enteric nervous system. *N Engl J Med* 1996;**334**:1106–15.

2245. Goyer RA, Reynolds J, Burke J, et al. Hereditary renal disease with neurosensory hearing loss, prolinuria and ichthyosis. *Am J Med Sci* 1968;**256**:166–79.

2245a. Grabczyk E, Kumari D, Usdin K. Fragile X syndrome and Friedreich's ataxia: Two different paradigms for repeated induced transcript insufficiency. *Brain Res Bull* 2001;**56**:367–73.

2246. Grabow JD, Chou SM. Thyrotropic hormone deficiency with polyneuropathy. *Arch Neurol* 1968;**19**:284–91.

2247. Gradenigo G. Sulla leptomeningite circonscritta e sulla paralisi dell'abducente di origine attica. *Gior Acad Med Torino* 1904;**4**:59–84.

2249. Graf CJ. Spontaneous carotid-cavernous fistula. *Arch Neurol* 1965;**13**:662–72.

2250. Graff-Radford NR. A recessively inherited ataxia with episodes of dystonia. *J Neurol Neurosurg Psychiatry* 1986;**49**:591–4.

2251. Graff-Radford NR, Tranel D, Van Hoesen GW, et al. Diencephalic amnesia. *Brain* 1990;**113**:1–25.

2252. Graham FK, Kendall BS. Memory for Designs Test: revised general manual. *Percept Mot Skills* 1960;**11**:147–88.

2253. Graham J, Greenwood R, Lecky B. Cortical deafness: a case report and review of the literature. *J Neurol Sci* 1980;**48**:35–49.

2254. Graham K, Paterson K, Hodges JR. Progressive pure anomia: insufficient activation of phonology by meaning. *Neurocase* 1995;**1**: 25–38.

2255. Grand MG, Kaine J, Fulling K, et al. Cerebroretinal vasculapathy: a new hereditary syndrome. *Ophthalmology* 1988;**95**:649–59.

2256. Grandas F, Elston J, Quinn N. Blepharospasm; a review of 264 patients. *J Neurol Neurosurg Psychiatry* 1988;**51**:767–72.

2257. Grant AC, Hunter S, Partin WC. A case of acutre monocytic ehrlicosis with prominent neurologic signs. *Neurology* 1997;**48**: 1619–23.

2258. Grant DA, Berg EA. A behavioural analysis of degree of reinforcement and ease of shifting to new responses in a Weigl-type card sorting problem. *J Exp Psychol* 1948;**38**:404–11.

2259. Grant DA, Berg EA. *The Wisconsin Card Sort Test Random Layout: Directions for Administration and Scoring.* Madison, WI: Wells Printing Co, 1980.

2260. Graus F, et al. Neuronal antinuclear antibody in sensory neuropathy from lung cancer. *Neurology* 1985;**35**:538–43.

2261. Gray F, Eisenbaum JF, Gherardi R, et al. Luyso-pallido-nigral atrophy and amyotrophic lateral sclerosis. *Acta Neuropathol* 1985;**66**: 78–82.

2262. Gray F, Louarn F, Gherardi R, et al. Adult form of Leigh's disease: a clinicopathological study with CT scan examination. *J Neurol Neurosurg Psychiatry* 1984;**47**:1211–5.

2263. Green AJE, Thompson EJ, Stewart GE, et al. Use of 14–3–3 and other brain-specific proteins in CSF in the diagnosis of variant Creutzfeldt-Jakob disease. *J Neurol Neurosurg Psychiatry* 2001;**70**: 744–8.

2264. Green JB. Pilomotor seizures. *Neurology* 1984;**34**:837–9.

2265. Green JS, Parfrey PS, Harnett JD, et al. The cardinal manifestations of Bardet-Biedl syndrome, a form of Laurence-Moon-Biedl syndrome. *N Engl J Med* 1989;**321**:1002–10.

2266. Greenberg R. Dream interruption insomnia. *J Nerv Ment Dis* 1967;**144**:18–21.

2267. Greenfield ADM, Sheperd JT, Whelen RF. The part played by the nervous system in the response to cold of the circulation through the finger tip. *Clin Sci* 1951;**10**:347–60.

2268. Greenfield JG. A form of progressive cerebral sclerosis in infants associated with primary degeneration of the interfascicular glia. *J Neurol Psychopathol* 1933;**13**:289–302.

2269. Greenfield JG. Encephalitis and encephalomyelitis in England and Wales during the last decade. *Brain* 1950;**73**:141–66.

2270. Greenfield JG. *The Spinocerebellar Degenerations.* Oxford: Oxford University Press, 1954.

2271. Greenfield JG, Matthews WB. Post-encephalitic parkinsonism with amyotrophy. *J Neurol Neurosurg Psychiatry* 1954;**17**:50–6.

2272. Greenfield JG, Turner JWA. Acute and subacute necrotic myelitis. *Brain* 1939;**62**:227–52.

2273. Greenhouse AH, Bicknell JM, Pesch RN, et al. Myotonia, myokymia, hyperhidrosis and wasting of muscle. *Neurology* 1967; **17**:263–8.

2274. Greenwood RS, Nelson JS. Atypical neuronal ceroid lipofuscinosis. *Neurology* 1978;**28**:710–7.

2275. Greer HD, Massey EW. Neurologic injury from undersea diving. *Neurol Clin* 1992;**10**:1031–45.

2276. Gregg N. Congenital cataract following German measles in the mother. *Trans Ophthalmol Soc Aust* 1941;**3**:35.

2277. Greig DM. Hypertelorism, a hitherto undifferentiated congenital cranio-facial deformity. *Edinb Med J* 1924;**31**:560–93.

2278. Gresty MA, Ell JJ, Findley LJ. Acquired pendular nystagmus: its characteristics, localizing value and pathophysiology. *J Neurol Neurosurg Psychiatry* 1982;**45**:431.

2279. Gribbin B, Pickering TG, Sleight P, et al. Effect of age and high blood pressure on baroreflex sensitivity in man. *Circ Respir* 1971; **29**:424–31.

2280. Griesinger W. Ueber Muskelhypertrophie. *Arch Heilkd* 1865; **6**:1–13.

2281. Griffin JW, Goren E, Schaumberg HH, et al. Adrenomyeloneuropathy; a probable variant of adrenoleukodystrophy. *Neurology* 1977;**27**:1107–13.

2282. Griffiths RA, Mortimer TF, Oppenheimer DR, Spalding JMK. Congophilic angiopathy of the brain; a clinical and pathological report on two siblings. *J Neurol Neurosurg Psychiatry* 1982;**45**:396–408.

2283. Griggs RC, Askanas V, DiMauro S, et al. Inclusion body myositis and myopathies. *Ann Neurol* 1995;**38**:705–13.

2284. Griggs RC, Moxley RT, Lafrance RA, et al. Hereditary paroxysmal ataxia: response to acetazolamide. *Neurology* 1978;**28**:1259–64.

2285. Grisold W, Drlicek M. Paraneoplastic neuropathy. *Curr Opin Neurol* 1999;**12**:617–25.

2286. Groenblad E. Angioid streaks—pseudoxanthoma elasticum. *Acta Ophthalmol Kopenhagen* 1929;**7**:329.

2287. Grompe M, St. Louis M, Demers SI, et al. A single mutation of the fumarylacetoacetate hydrolase gene in French Canadians with hereditary tyrosinemia type 1. *N Engl J Med* 1994;**331**:353–7.

2288. Gronwall DMA. Paced Auditory Serial–Addition Task: a measure of recovery from concussion. *Percept Mot Skills* 1977;**44**: 367–73.

2289. Gross DW, Rajput AH, Yeung M. Distal hereditary upper limb muscular atrophy. *J Neurol Neurosurg Psychiatry* 1998;**64**:217–20.

2290. Gross KB, Skrivanek JA, Carlson KC, et al. Familial amyotrophic chorea with acanthocytosis: new clinical and laboratory invstigations. *Arch Neurol* 1985;**42**:753–6.

2291. Gross MLP, et al. Rejection encephalopathy. An acute neurological syndrome complicating renal transplantations. *J Neurol Sci* 1982;**56**:23–34.

2292. Grove AS. Evaluation of exophthalmos. *N Engl J Med* 1975; **292**:1005.

2293. Grubb BP, Kosinski DJ, Boehm K, et al. The postural orthostatic tachycardia syndrome: a neurocardiogenic variant identified during head-up tilt table testing. *Pacing Clin Electrophysiol* 1997;**20**:2205–12.

2294. Gruber GB. Gruber syndrome [in German]. *Beitr Pathol Anat* 1934;**93**:459.

2295. Gruber R, et al. Experiments with anti-siphon device in shunt therapy of pediatric hydrocephalus. *J Neurosurg* 1984;**61**:156–62.

2296. Grunnett ML. Gomori's trichrome stain: its use with myelin sheaths. *Arch Neurol* 1978;**35**:692.

2297. Grunnett ML, Bale JF. Brain abnormalities in infants with Potter syndrome (oligohydramnios tetrad). *Neurology* 1981;**31**:1571–4.

2298. Guarino JR. Auscultatory percussion of the head. *BMJ* 1982;**284**:1075–7.

2299. Guarnaschelli J. "Fallen fontanelle" (caida de mollera): a variant of the battered child syndrome. *JAMA* 1972;**222**:1545–6.

2300. Guazzi GC, D'Amore I, van Hoef F, et al. Type III chronic GM1 gangliosidosis presenting as infantile choreo-athetosis and dementia without epilepsy in three sisters. *Neurology* 1988;**38**:1124–7.

2301. Guberman A. Clinical significance of the corneomandibular reflex. *Arch Neurol* 1982;**39**:578–80.

2302. Guberman A, Catching J. Swallow syncope. *Can J Neurol Sci* 1986;**13**:267–9.

2303. Gubermann A, Stuss D. The syndrome of bilateral paramedian infarction. *Neurology* 1983;**33**:540–6.

2304. Gubler AM. De l'hemiplegie alterne envisagée comme signe de lesion de la protuberance annulaire et comme preuve de la decussation des nerfs faciaux. *Gaz Hebd Med Chir* 1856;**3**:749.

2305. Gudden BAL. Experimentaluntersuchungen uber das peripherische und centrale Nernensystem. *Arch Psychiatrie (Berlin)* 1870;**2**:693–723.

2306. Guérin JR. Récherches sur les déformités congenitales chex les monstres. Paris: 46 v de Vaugivard, 1880.

2307. Guerreiro MM, Andermann E, Guerrini R, et al. Familial perisylvian polymicrogyria: a new familial syndrome of cortical maldevelopment. *Ann Neurol* 2000;**48**:39–48.

2308. Guerrini R, Barkovich AJ, Sztriha L, et al. Bilateral frontal polymicrogyria. *Neurology* 2000;**54**:909–13.

2309. Guerrini R, Bureau M, Mattei M-G, et al. Trisomy 12p syndrome: a chromosomal disorder associated with generalized 3 Hz spike and wave discharges. *Epilepsia* 1990;**31**:557–66.

2310. Guerrini R, Dobyns WB. Bilateral periventricular nodular heterotopia with mental retardation and frontonasal malformation. *Neurology* 1998;**51**:499–503.

2311. Guerrini R, Dravet C, Genton P, et al. Epileptic negative myoclonus. *Neurology* 1993;**43**:1078–83.

2312. Guggenheim MA, McCabe ERB, Rogi M, et al. Glycerol kinase deficiency with neuromusculoskeletal and adrenal abnormalities. *Ann Neurol* 1980;**7**:441–9.

2313. Guignon G. L'oedème bleu des hysteriques. *Progr Med (Paris)* 1890;**12**:259–64.

2314. Guillain G. On a clinical form of syphilis affecting the neuraxis and lying between tabes, GPI and myelitis [in French]. *C R Soc Biol* 1905;**63**:49–51.

2315. Guillain G, Alajouanine R, Garcin R. Le syndrome paralytique unilateral global des nerfs craniens. *Bull Soc Hop Paris* 1926;**50**:456–60.

2316. Guillain G, Barre J, Strohl A. Sur un syndrome de radiculonévrite avec hyperalbuminose du liquide cerebro-rachidien sans réaction cellulaire. Remarques sur les caractères cliniques et graphiques des réflexes tendineux. *Bull Soc Med Hop Paris* 1916;**40**:1462–70.

2317. Guillain G, Bertrand I, Lerebouillet J. Myoclonies arythmiques unilaterale des membres par lesion de noyau dentele du cervelet. *Rev Neurol (Paris)* 1934;**2**:73–8.

2318. Guillain G, Mollaret P. Deux cas de myoclonies synchrones et rhythmees velo-pharyngo-laryngo-oculo-diaphragmatiques. *Rev Neurol (Paris)* 1931;**2**:545–66.

2319. Guillamo J-S, Doz F, Delattre J-Y. Brain stem gliomas. *Curr Opin Neurol* 2001;**14**:711–5.

2320. Guilleminault C. Narcolepsy 1985. *Sleep* 1986;**9**:99–291.

2321. Guilleminault C, Billiard M, Montplaisir J, Dement WC. Altered states of consciousness in disorders of daytime sleepiness. *J Neurol Sci* 1975;**26**:377–93.

2322. Guilleminault C, Dement WC. 235 cases of excessive daytime sleepiness. *J Neurol Sci* 1977;**31**:13–27.

2323. Guilleminault C, Eldridge FL, Phillips JR, et al. Two occult cases of insomnia and their therapeutic problems. *Arch Gen Psychiatry* 1976;**33**:1241–5.

2324. Guilleminault C, Phillips R, Dement WC. A syndrome of hypersomnia with automatic behaviour. *Electroencephalogr Clin Neurophysiol* 1975;**38**:403.

2325. Guilleminault C, Stoohs R, Quera-Salva M-A. Sleep-related obstructive and nonobstructive apneas and neurologic disorders. *Neurology* 1992;**42 (Suppl 6)**:53–60.

2326. Guiloff RJ. Evidence for linkage of type I hereditary motor and sensory neuropathy to the Duffy locus on chromosome 1. *Ann Hum Genet* 1982;**46**:25–7.

2327. Guinter RH, Hernreid LS, Kaplan AM. Infantile neurogenic muscular atrophy with prolonged survival. *J Pediatr* 1977;**90**:95–7.

2328. Gulick EE. Model confirmation of the MS-related symptom checklist. *Nurs Res* 1989;**38**:147–53.

2329. Gull WW. Case of progressive atrophy of the muscles of the hands: enlargement of the ventricle of the cord in the cervical region, with atrophy of the gray matter. *Guys Hosp Rep* 1862;**8**:244–50.

2330. Gull WW. On a cretinoid state supervening in adult life in women. *Trans Clin Soc Lond* 1874;**7**:180–5.

2331. Gullstrand A. Om Braunlinier vid Astigmatism. *Nord Ophthalmol Tidsskr Kjobenh* 1890;**3**:1–18.

2332. Gultekin SH, Rosenfeld MR, Voltz R, et al. Paraneoplastic limbic encephalitis: neurological symptoms, immunological findings and tumour association in 50 patients. *Brain* 2000;**123**:1481–94.

2333. Gumpert J, Hansotia P, Upton ARM. Gelastic epilepsy. *J Neurol Neurosurg Psychiatry* 1970;**33**:479–83.

2334. Gunderson CH, Lehmann CR, Sidell FR, et al. Nerve agents: a review. *Neurology* 1992;**42**:946–50.

2335. Gunn RM. Congenital ptosis with peculiar associated movements of the affected lid. *Trans Ophthalmol Soc UK* 1883;**3**:283–7.

2336. Gurdjian ES. History of occlusive cerebrovascular disease. 1. From Wepfer to Moniz. *Arch Neurol* 1979;**36**:340–3.

2337. Gurel L, Linn MW, Linn BB. Physical and mental impairment-of-function in the aged: The PAMIE Scale. *J Gerontol* 1972;**27**:83–90.

2338. Gurland B, Golden RR, Teresi JA, et al. The SHORT-CARE: an efficient instrument for the assessment of depression, dementia and disability. *J Gerontol* 1984;**39**:166–9.

2339. Gurland B, Kuriansky J, Sharpe L, et al. The comprehensive assessment and referral evaluation (CARE). Rationale, development and reliability. *Int J Aging Hum Dev* 1977;**81**:9–42.

2340. Gurney GE. Chronic bilateral benign hypertrophy of masseter muscles. *Am J Surg* 1947;**73**:137–9.

2341. Gustafson L. Clinical classification of dementia conditions. *Acta Neurol Scand Suppl* 1992;**139**:16–20.

2342. Gutmann L. Management of the quinizarine sweat test. *Postgrad Med J* 1947;**23**:332–6.

2343. Gutmann L. Facial and limb myokymia. *Muscle Nerve* 1991;**14**:1043–9.

2344. Gutmann L, Libell D, Gutmann L. When is myokymia neuromyotonia? *Muscle Nerve* 2001;**24**:151–3.

2345. Guze BH, Baxter LR. Neuroleptic malignant syndrome. *N Engl J Med* 1985;**313**:163–6.

2346. Guzzetta F, Ferriere G, Lyon G. Congenital hypomyelination polyneuropathy. *Brain* 1982;**105**:395–416.

2347. Gwinn-Hardy K, Chen JY, Liu H-C, et al. Spinocerebellar ataxia type 2 with parkinsonism in ethnic Chinese. *Neurology* 2000;**55**:800–5.

2348. Haan J, Roos RAC, Algra PR, et al. Hereditary cerebral hemorrhage with amyloidosis–Dutch type. *Brain* 1990;**113**:1251–67.

2349. Haar F, Dyken P. Hereditary nonprogressive athetotic hemiplegia: a new syndrome. *Neurology* 1977;**27**:849–54.

2350. Haas DC. Chronic post-traumatic headaches classified and compared with natural headaches. *Cephalalgia* 1996;**16**:486–93.

2351. Haas DC, Lourie H. Delayed deterioration of consciousness after trivial head injury in childhood. *BMJ* 1984;**289**:1625.

2352. Haas RH, Robinson A, Evans K, et al. An X-linked disease of the nervous system with disordered copper metabolism and features differing from Menkes disease. *Neurology* 1981;**31**:852–9.

2353. Habel A. Typus Edinburgensis? *Pediatrics* 1974;**53**:425–30.

2354. Haberland C, Perou J. Encephalocraniocutaneous lipomatosis. *Arch Neurol* 1970;**22**:144.

2355. Hachinski VC. Classification of stroke for clinical trials. *Stroke* 1990;**21 Suppl**:II-27–II-29.

2356. Hachinski VC, Iloff L, Zilkha K, et al. Multi-infarct dementia. *Arch Neurol* 1975;**32**:632–7.

2357. Hachinski VC, Lassen N, et al. Multi-infarct dementia. *Lancet* 1974;**2**:207–9.

2358. Hachinski VC, Potter P, Merskey H. Leuko-araiosis. *Arch Neurol* 1987;**44**:21–3.

2359. Hackett PH, Rennie D. Acute mountain sickness. *Semin Respir Med* 1983;**5**:132–9.

2360. Hackett PH, Yarnell PR, Hill R. High altitude cerebral edema evaluated with magnetic resonance imaging: clinical correlation and pathophysiology. *JAMA* 1998;**280**:1920–5.

2361. Hadden RDM, Cornblath DR, Hughes RAC, et al. Electrophysiological classification of Guillain-Barré syndrome: clinical associations and outcome. *Ann Neurol* 1998;**44**:780–8.

2362. Haddock DRW, Ebrahim GJ, Kappur BB. Ataxic neurological syndrome found in Tanganyika. *BMJ* 1962;**2**:1442–3.

2363. Hademenos GJ, Alberts MJ, Awad I, et al. Advances in the genetics of cerebrovascular disease and stroke. *Neurology* 2001;**56**:997–1008.

2363a. Hadjivassiliou M, Grunewald RA, Davies-Jones GA. Gluten sensitivity as a neurological illness. *J Neurol Neurosurg Psychiatry* 2002;**72**:560–3.

2364. Haenel H. Ein neues Tabessymptom. *Neurol Zentrabl.* 1909;**28**:1199.

2365. Haerer AF, Currier RD. Mirror movements. *Neurology* 1966;**16**:737–60.

2366. Haerer AF, Currier RD, Jackson JF. Hereditary nonprogressive chorea of early onset. *N Engl J Med* 1967;**276**:1220–4.

2367. Hagberg B, Aicardi J, Dias K, Ramos O. A progressive syndrome of autism, dementia ataxia and loss of purposeful hand use in girls: Rett's syndrome: report of 35 cases. *Ann Neurol* 1983;**14**:471–9.

2368. Hagberg B, Sanner G, Steen G. The dyseqilibrium syndrome in cerebral palsy. *Acta Pediatr Scand* 1972;**61 Suppl 226**:1–63.

2369. Hageman G, Ippel PF, te Nijenhuis FCAM. Autosomal dominant congenital Horner's syndrome in a Dutch family. *J Neurol Neurosurg Psychiatry* 1992;**55**:28–30.

2370. Hageman G, Ramaekers V, Hilhorst BGJ, et al. Congenital cervical spinal muscular atrophy: a non-familial, non-progressive condition of the upper limbs. *J Neurol Neurosurg Psychiatry* 1993;**56**:365–8.

2371. Haig AJ, Talley C, Grobler LJ, et al. Paraspinal mapping: quantified needle electromyography in lumbar radiculopathy. *Muscle Nerve* 1993;**16**:477–84.

2372. Hainfellner JA, Schmidbauer M, Schmutzhard E, et al. Devic's neuromyelitis optica and Schilder's myelinoclastic diffuse sclerosis. *J Neurol Neurosurg Psychiatry* 1992;**55**:1194–6.

2373. Hajdu N, Kauntze R. Cranio-skeletal dysplasia. *Br J Radiol* 1948;**21**:42–8.

2374. Haley EC Jr, Brashear HR, Barth JT, et al. Deep cerebral venous thrombosis. *Arch Neurol* 1989;**46**:337–40.

2375. Hall AJ. Encephalitis lethargica. *Lancet* 1923;**1**:731.

2376. Hall BD. Choanal atresia and associated multiple anomalies. *J Pediatr* 1979;**95**:395–8.

2377. Hall BM, Walsh JC, Horvath JS, et al. Peripheral neuropathy complicating primary hyperoxaluria. *J Neurol Sci* 1976;**29**:343–9.

2378. Hall JAS. Diphtheritic pseuodotabes. *West Indian Med J* 1963;**12**:47.

2379. Hall JG, Pellester PD, et al. Congenital hypothalamic hamartoblastoma, hypopituitarism, imperforate anus and post-axial polydactyly—a new syndrome? *Am J Med Genet* 1980;**7**:47–74.

2380. Hall JG, Reed SD, Scott CI, et al. Three distinct types of X-linked arthrogryposis seen in 6 families. *Clin Genet* 1982;**21**:81–97.

2381. Hall M. On the reflex function of the medulla oblongata and medulla spinalis. *Phil Trans R Soc Lond* 1833;**123**:635–59.

2382. Hallermann W. Bird-like face and congenital cataract. *Klin Monatsbl Augenheilkd* 1948;**113**:315–8.

2383. Hallervorden J, Spatz H. Einartige Erkrankung im extrapyramidalen System mit besonderer Beteiligung des Globus pallidus und der Substantia nigra: ein Beitrag zu den Beziehungen zwischen diesen beiden Zentren. *Z Ges Neurol Psychiatr* 1922;**79**:254–302.

2384. Hallett M. Myoclonus: relation to epilepsy. *Epilepsia* 1985;**26(Suppl 1)**:s67–s77.

2385. Hallett M. The pathophysiology of myoclonus. *Trends Neurosci* 1987;**10**:69–73.

2386. Hallett M. NINDS Myotatic Reflex Scale. *Neurology* 1993;**43**:2923.

2387. Hallett M, Chadwick D, Marsden CD. Ballistic movement overflow myoclonus: a form of essential myoclonus. *Brain* 1977;**100**:299–312.

2388. Hallett M, Cogan DG. Episodic unilateral mydriasis in otherwise normal patients. *Arch Ophthalmol* 1970;**84**:130–6.

2389. Hallpike JF. Superior orbital fissure syndrome. *J Neurol Neurosurg Psychiatry* 1973;**36**:486–90.

2390. Halmagyi GM, Curthoys IS, Gresty MA, et al. Hemi see-saw nystagmus due to unilateral diencephalic lesion. *Ann Neurol* 1987;**Suppl 22**:147.

2391. Halmagyi GM, Gresty MA, Gibson WPR. Ocular tilt reaction with peripheral vestibular lesion. *Ann Neurol* 1979;**6**:80–3.

2392. Halmagyi GM, Gresty MA, Leech J. Reversed optokinetic nystagmus (OKN): mechanism and clinical significance. *Ann Neurol* 1980;**7**:429–35.

2393. Halmagyi GM, Rudge P, Gresty MA, et al. Downbeating nystagmus: a review of 62 cases. *Arch Neurol* 1983;**40**:777–84.

2394. Halmagyi MB, Evans WA, Hallinan JM. Failure of downward gaze: the site and nature of the lesion. *Arch Neurol* 1978;**35**:22–6.

2395. Halperin JJ, Landis DMD, Kleinman GM. Whipple disease of the nervous system. *Neurology* 1982;**32**:612–7.

2396. Halperin JJ, Logigian EL, Finkel MF, et al. Practice parameters for the diagnosis of patients with nervous system Lyme borreliosis (Lyme disease). *Neurology* 1996;**46**:619–27.

2397. Halpern L, Bental E. Epileptic cephalea. *Neurology* 1958;**8**:615–20.

2398. Halstead WC. *Brain and Intelligence.* Chicago: University of Chicago Press, 1947.

2399. Halstead WC, Wepman JM. The Halstead-Wepman Aphasia Screening Test. *J Speech Hear Dis* 1959;**14**:9–15.

2400. Haltia M, Somer H, Palo J, et al. Neuronal intranuclear inclusion disease in identical twins. *Ann Neurol* 1984;**15**:316–21.

2401. Haltia T, Palo J, Haltia M, et al. Juvenile metachromatic leukodystrophy. *Arch Neurol* 1980;**37**:42–6.

2402. Hamida MB, Fardeau M, Attia N. Severe childhood muscular dystrophy affecting both sexes and frequent in Tunisia. *Muscle Nerve* 1983;**6**:469–72.

2403. Hamida MB, Hentati F, Hamida CB. Hereditary motor system diseases (chronic juvenile amyotrophic lateral sclerosis). *Brain* 1990;**113**:347–63.

2404. Hamilton M. A rating scale for depression. *J Neurol Neurosurg Psychiatry* 1960;**23**:56–62.

2405. Hamilton M. Development of a rating scale for primary depressive illness. *Br J Soc Clin Psychol* 1967;**6**:278–96.

2406. Hamilton SR, Liu B, Parsons RE, et al. The molecular basis of Turcot's syndrome. *N Engl J Med* 1995;**332**:839–47.

2407. Hammans SR. The inherites ataxias and the new genetics. *J Neurol Neurosurg Psychiatry* 1996;**61**:327–332.

2408. Hammond WA. Athetosis. *Med Times Gaz* 1871;**2**:747–8.

2409. Hanaway J, Lee SI, Netsky MG. Pachygyria: relation of findings to modern embryologic concepts. *Neurology* 1968;**18**:791–9.

2410. Hand A. Polyuria and tuberculosis. *Arch Pediatiatr* 1893;**10**:673–5.

2411. Handforth A, Nag S, Sharp D, et al. Paraneoplastic subacute necrotic myelopathy. *Can J Neurol Sci* 1983;**10**:204–7.

2412. Hane FM. The whistle-smile reflex in the parkinsonian syndrome. *JAMA* 1989;**121**:1152.

2413. Hanigan WC, Winer SJ. Saxophone headache. *N Engl J Med* 1991;**325**:1888–9.

2414. Hankey GJ. Isolated angiitis/angiopathy of the central nervous system. *Cerebrovasc Dis* 1991;**1**:2–15.

2415. Hankey GJ, Edis RH. The utility of testing tactile perception of direction of scratch as a sensitive clinical sign of posterior column dysfunction in spinal cord disorders. *J Neurol Neurosurg Psychiatry* 1989;**52**:395–8.

2416. Hankey GJ, Warlow CP. Symptomatic carotid ischaemic events: safest and most cost effective way of selecting patients for angiography, before carotid endarterectomy. *BMJ* 1990;**300**:1485–90.

2417. Hansen GH. Indberetning til det Norske medicinske Selskab i Christiania om en med understottelseof selskabet foretagen rise for at anstille undersogelser angaende spedalskhedens arsager, tildels udforte sammen med forstander Hartwig. *Norsk* 1874;**4**(**Suppl**):1–88.

2418. Hansen L, Salmon D, Galasko D, et al. The Lewy body variant of Alzheimer's disease. *Neurology* 1990;**40**:1–8.

2419. Hansen LA, Galasko D. Lewy body disease. *Curr Opin Neurol Neurosurg* 1992;**5**:889–94.

2420. Hansen SL, Borelli-Moller L, Strange P, et al. Ophthalmoplegic migraine: diagnostic criteria, incidence of hospitalization and possible etiology. *Acta Neurol Scand* 1990;**81**:54–60.

2421. Hanson PA, Chodos R. Hemiparetic seizures. *Neurology* 1978;**28**:920–3.

2422. Hanson PA, Farber RE, Armstrong RA. Distal muscle wasting, nephritis and deafness. *Neurology* 1970;**20**:427–34.

2423. Hanson PA, Mastrianni AF, Post L. Neonatal ophthalmoplegia with microfibers: a reversible myopathy? *Neurology* 1977;**27**:974–80.

2424. Hanson PA, Mincy JE. Adolescent familial cramps. *Neurology* 1975;**25**:454–8.

2425. Hanson PA, Rowland LP. Möbius' syndrome with facioscapulo-humeral muscular dystrophy. *Arch Neurol* 1971;**24**:31–9.

2426. Hanson PA, Urizar RE. Ultrastructural lesions of muscle and immunofluorescent deposits in vessels in Reye's syndrome: a preliminary report of serial muscle biopsies. *Arch Neurol* 1977;**1**:431–7.

2428. Hansotia P. Spindle coma. *Neurology* 1981;**31**:83–7.

2429. Harada E. A clinical study of non-suppurative choroiditis. Acute diffuse choroiditis [in Japanese]. *Acta Soc Ophthalmol Japan* 1926;**30**:356.

2430. Haravuori H, Makela-Bengs P, Udd B, et al. Assignment of the tibial muscular dystrophy locus to chromosome 2q31. *Am J Hum Genet* 1998;**62**:620–6.

2431. Harbison JW, Lessell S, Selhorst JB. Neuro-ophthalmology of sphenoid sinus carcinoma. *Brain* 1984;**107**:855–70.

2432. Harcherik DF, Leckman JF, Detleor J, et al. A new instrument for clinical studies of Tourette's syndrome. *J Amer Acad Child Psychiatry* 1984;**23**:153–60.

2433. Hardesty WH, Roberts B, Toole JF, et al. Studies of carotid blood flow in man. *N Engl J Med* 1960;**263**:944–6.

2434. Hardie RJ, Lees AJ, Stern GM. On–off fluctuations in Parkinson's disease: a clinical and neuropharmacological study. *Brain* 1984;**107**:487–506.

2435. Hardie RJ, Pullon HWH, Harding AE, et al. Neuroacanthocytosis. *Brain* 1991;**114**:13–49.

2436. Harding AE. "Idiopathic" late-onset cerebellar ataxia: a clinical and genetic study of 36 families. *J Neurol Sci* 1981;**50**:259–71.

2437. Harding AE. Friedreich's ataxia: a clinical and genetic study of 90 families with an analysis of early diagnostic criteria and intrafamilial clustering of clinical features. *Brain* 1981;**104**:589–620.

2438. Harding AE. The clinical features and classification of the late onset autosomal dominant cerebellar ataxias. *Brain* 1982;**105**:1–28.

2439. Harding AE. *The Spinocerebellar Degenerations and Related Disorders.* Edinburgh: Livingstone, 1983.

2440. Harding AE. Clinical features and classification of inherited ataxias. In Harding AE, Deufel T, eds. *Advances in Neurology,* pp 1–14. New York: Raven Press, 1993.

2441. Harding AE. From the syndrome of Charcot, Marie and Tooth to disorders of peripheral myelin proteins. *Brain* 1995;**118**:809–18.

2442. Harding AE, Bradbury PG, Murray NMF. Chronic asymmetrical spinal muscular atrophy. *J Neurol Sci* 1983;**59**:69–83.

2443. Harding AE, Diengdoh JV, Lees AJ. Autosomal recessive late onset multisystem disorder with cerebellar cortical atrophy at necropsy. *J Neurol Neurosurg Psychiatry* 1984;**47**:853–6.

2444. Harding AE, Muller DPR, Thomas PK, et al. Spinocerebellar degeneration secondary to chronic intestinal malabsorption: a vitamin E deficiency syndrome. *Ann Neurol* 1982;**12**:419–24.

2445. Harding AE, Thomas PK. Hereditary distal spinal muscular atrophy. *J Neurol Sci* 1980;**45**:337–48.

2446. Harding AE, Thomas PK. The clinical features of hereditary motor and sensory neuropathy types I and II. *Brain* 1980;**103**:259–80.

2447. Harding AE, Thomas PK. Progressive muscular atrophy with pyramidal features. *J Neurol Neurosurg Psychiatry* 1984;**47**:168–72.

2448. Harding AE, Thomas PK, Baraitser M, et al. X-linked recessive bulbospinal neuronopathy: a report of 10 cases. *J Neurol Neurosurg Psychiatry* 1982;**45**:1012–9.

2449. Harding BN. Familial olivopontocerebellar atrophy with neonatal onset: a recesssively inherited syndrome with systemic and biochemical abnormalities. *J Neurol Neurosurg Psychiatry* 1988;**51**:385–90.

2450. Hardison J. Are the jumping Frenchmen of Maine goosey? *JAMA* 1980;**70**:244.

2451. Hare ES. Tumour involving certain Nerves. *Lond Med Gaz* 1838;**1**:16–8.

2452. Harik SI, Ghandour MH, Farah FS, Affi AK. Postganglionic cholinergic dysautonomia. *Ann Neurol* 1977;**1**:393–6.

2453. Harley RD, Rodriguez MM, Crawford JS. Congenital fibrosis of the extraocular muscles. *Trans Am Ophthalmol Soc* 1978;**76**:197.

2454. Harlow JW. Passage of an iron rod through the head. *Boston Med Surg J* 1848;**20**:381.

2455. Harmon DC. Case discussion. *N Engl J Med* 1994;**331**:1079–84.

2456. Harnett JD, Green JS, Cramer BC, et al. The spectrum of renal disease in Laurence-Moon-Biedel syndrome. *N Engl J Med* 1988;**319**:615–8.

2457. Harper A. *Myotonic Dystrophy.* London: W.B. Saunders, 1988.

2458. Harper CM. Hemifacial spasm: preoperative diagnosis and intraoperative management. *Muscle Nerve* 1991;**14**:213–8.

2459. Harriman DGF. The histochemistry of reactive masticatory muscle hypertrophy. *Muscle Nerve* 1996;**19**:1447–56.

2460. Harriman DGF, et al. Ekbom syndrome "restless legs". *Brain* 1970;**93**:393.

2461. Harriman DGF, Sumner DW, Ellis FR. Malignant hyperpyrexia myopathy. *Q J Med* 1973;**42**:639–64.

2462. Harris H, Penrose LS, Thomas DHH. Cystathioninuria. *Am J Hum Genet* 1959;**23**:442.

2463. Harris W. *Neuritis and Neuralgia.* London: Oxford University Press, 1926.

2464. Harrison MJG. Muscle wasting after prolonged hypoglycemic coma; case report with electrophysiological data. *J Neurol Neurosurg Psychiatry* 1976;**39**:465–70.

2465. Hart MN, Earle KM. Primitive neuroectodermal tumors of the brain in children. *Cancer* 1973;**32**:890–7.

2466. Hart MN, Malamud N, Ellis WG. The Dandy-Walker syndrome. *Neurology* 1972;**22**:771–80.

2467. Hart RG, Gardner DP, Howieson J. Acoustic tumors: atypical features and recent diagnostic tests. *Neurology* 1983;**33**:211–21.

2468. Hart RG, Kanter MC. Acute autonomic neuropathy: two cases and a clinical review. *Arch Intern Med* 1990;**150**:2373–6.

2469. Hart ZH, Sahashi K, Lambert EH, et al. A congenital familial myasthenic syndrome caused by a presynaptic defect of transmitter resynthesis or mobilization. *Neurology* 1979;**29**:556–7.

2470. Hartmann E, Baekeland F, Zwilling GR. Psychological differences between long and short sleepers. *Arch Gen Psychiatry* 1972;**26**:463–8.

2471. Hartmann F. Beitrage zur Apraxielehre. *Monatschr Psychiatr Neurol* 1907;**21**:97–118.

2472. Harvey CC, Haworth JC, Lorber J. A new heredofamilial neurological syndrome. *Arch Dis Child* 1955;**30**:338–44.

2473. Harvey DG, Torack RM, Rosenbaum HE. Amyotrophic lateral sclerosis with ophthalmoplegia. *Arch Neurol* 1979;**36**:615–7.

2474. Harwood RH, Gompertz P, Ebrahim S. Handicap one year after stroke: validity of a new scale. *J Neurol Neurosurg Psychiatry* 1994;**57**:825–9.

2475. Hathaway SR, McKinley JC. *The Minnesota Multiphasic Personality Inventory Manual.* New York: Psychological Corporation, 1951.

2476. Hauptmann A. Luminal bei Epilepsie. *Munch Med Wochenschr* 1912;**59**:1907–9.

2477. Hauri P. *The Sleep Disorders.* Kalamazoo: Upjohn (Scope), 1982.

2478. Hauri P, Fischer J. Persistent psychophysiological (learned) insomnia. *Sleep* 1986;**9**:38–53.

2479. Hauser SL, Dawson DM, Lehrich JR, et al. Intensive immunosuppression in progressive multiple sclerosis. *N Engl J Med* 1983;**308**:173–80.

2480. Hauw J-J, Daniel SE, Dickson D, et al. Preliminary NINDS neuropathologic criteria for Steele-Richardson-Olszewski syndrome (progressive supranuclear palsy). *Neurology* 1994;**44**:2015–9.

2481. Hauw J-J, De Baecque C, Hausser-Hauw C, et al. Chromatolysis in alchoholic encephalopathies. Pellagra-like changes in 22 cases. *Brain* 1988;**111**:843–57.

2482. Haven H. Neurocirculatory scalenus anticus syndrome in presence of developmental anomaly of first rib. *Yale J Biol Med* 1939;**11**:443–8.

2483. Hawkes CH, Thorpe JW. Acute polyneuropathy due to lightning injury. *J Neurol Neurosurg Psychiatry* 1992;**55**:388–90.

2484. Haworth C, Evans DIK, Mitra J, et al. Thiamine responsive anemia: study of two further cases. *Br J Haematol* 1982;**50**:549.

2485. Haxton HA. Gustatory sweating. *Brain* 1948;**71**:16–25.

2486. Hayashi Y, Nagashima K, Urano Y, et al. Spinocerebellar degeneration with prominent involvement of the motor neurone system. *Acta Neuropathol* 1986;**70**:82–5.

2487. Hayden R, Grossman M. Rectal, ocular, and submaxillary pain: a familial autonomic disorder related to proctalgia fugax. Report of a family. *Am J Dis Child* 1959;**97**:479–82.

2488. Hayes DJ, Lecky BRF, Landon DN, et al. A new mitochondrial myopathy. *Brain* 1984;**107**:1165–77.

2489. Hayes DJ, Taylor DJ, Bore PJ, et al. An unusual metabolic myopathy—a malate-aspartate shuttle defect. *J Neurol Sci* 1987;**82**:27–39.

2490. Haymaker W. Oskar and Cecile Vogt. *Arch Neurol* 1961;**4**:675–84.

2491. Hayman M, Harvey AS, Hopkins IJ. Paroxysmal tonic upgaze: a reappraisal of outcome. *Ann Neurol* 1998;**43**:514–20.

2492. Head H. On disturbances of sensation with especial reference to the pain of visceral disease. *Brain* 1893;**16**:1–133.

2493. Head H. Hughlings Jackson on aphasia and kindred disorders of speech. *Brain* 1915;**38**:1–42.

2494. Head H. Sensation and the cerebral cortex. *Brain* 1918;**41**:57–253.

2495. Head H. Some principles of neurology. *Brain* 1918;**41**:344–54.

2496. Head H. *Aphasia and Kindred Disorders of Speech.* Cambridge, UK: Cambridge, 1926.

2497. Head H, Campbell AW. The pathology of herpes zoster and its bearing on sensory localisation. *Brain* 1900;**23**:353–523.

2498. Head H, Holmes G. Sensory disturbances from cerebral lesions. *Brain* 1911;**34**:102–254.

2499. Head H, Riddoch G. The automatic bladder, excessive sweating and some other reflex conditions in gross injuries of the spinal cord. *Brain* 1917;**40**:188–263.

2500. Head H, Sherren J. The consequences of injury to the peripheral nerves in man. *Brain* 1905;**28**:118–338.

2501. Healton EB, Brust JCM, Kerr DL, et al. Presumably autosomal dominant motor system degeneration in a presumably non-Portuguese family. *Neurology* 1980;**30**:1084–9.

2502. Heathfield KWG, Turner JWA. Syphilitic wrist-drop. *Lancet* 1951;**2**:566–9.

2503. Hebb DO. Intelligence, brain function and the theory of mind. *Brain* 1959;**82**:260–75.

2504. Heberden W. Of the night-blindness or nyctalopia. *Med Trans Coll Phys Lond* 1768;**1**:60–3.

2505. Hecaen H, Angelergues R, Houillier S. Les varietes cliniques des acalculies au cours des lesions retrorolandiques: approche statistique du probleme. *Rev Neurol (Paris)* 1961;**105**:85–103.

2506. Hécaen H, Penfield W, Bertrand C, et al. The syndrome of apractognosia due to lesions of the minor cerebral hemisphere. *AMA Arch Neurol Psychiatry* 1956;**75**:400–34.

2507. Heckman J, Saffer D. Abnormal copper metabolism: another "non-Wilson's" case. *Neurology* 1988;**38**:1493–5.

2509. Hedley-Whyte T. Case records of the MGH: case 30:1992. *N Engl J Med* 1992;**327**:265–7.

2510. Heerfordt CF. Uber eine "Febris uveo-parotidea subchronica", and der Glandula parotis und der Uvea des Auges lokalisiert und haufig mit Paresen cerebrospinaler Nerven komplizert. *Graefes Arch Ophthalmol* 1909;**70**:254–73.

2511. Heffner HE. Ferrier and the study of auditory cortex. *Arch Neurol* 1987;**44**:218–21.

2512. Heffner RR Jr. Myopathy of embolic type in patients with carcinoma. *Neurology* 1971;**21**:841–6.

2513. Heffner RR Jr, Barron SA. Polymyositis beginning as a focal process. *Arch Neurol* 1981;**38**:439–42.

2514. Heggie P, et al. Cerebro-ocular dysplasia–muscular dystrophy syndrome. *Arch Ophthalmol* 1987;**105**:520–4.

2515. Heidenhain A. Klinische und anatomische Untersuchungen uber eine eigenartige organische Erkrankung des Zentralnervensystems im Praesenium. *Z Ges Neurol Psychiatrie* 1929;**118**:49–114.

2516. Heilman KM. Orthostatic tremor. *Arch Neurol* 1984;**41**:880–1.

2517. Heilman KM, Rothi L, McFarling DA, et al. Transcortical sensory apahasia with relatively spared spontaneous speech and naming. *Arch Neurol* 1981;**38**:236–9.

2518. Heilman KM, Scholes R, Watson RT. Auditory affective agnosia: disturbed comprehension of affective speech. *J Neurol Neurosurg Psychiatry* 1975;**38**:69–72.

2519. Heilman KM, Valenstein E. Mechanisms underlying hemispatial neglect. *Ann Neurol* 1979;**5**:166–70.

2520. Heilman KM, Watson R, Valenstein E. Neglect and related disorders. In Heilman K, Valenstein E, eds. *Clinical Neuropsychology*, pp 243–93. New York: Oxford University Press, 1985.

2521. Heimburger RF, Reitan RM. Easily administered written test for lateralizing brain lesions. *J Neurosurg* 1961;**18**:301–12.

2522. Heine J. *Beobachtungenuber Lahrmungstande der untern Extremitaten und deren Behandlung.* Stuttgart: Kohler, 1840.

2523. Heller T. Ueber Dementia infantilis. *Z Kinderforsch* 1930;**37**:661–7.

2524. Hellier KD, Hatchwell E, Duncombe AS, et al. X-linked sideroblastic anaemia with ataxia: another mitochondrial disease? *J Neurol Neurosurg Psychiatry* 2001;**70**:65–9.

2525. Helm NA, Butler RB, Benson DF. Acquired stuttering. *Neurology* 1978;**28**:1159–65.

2526. Helmchen C, Glasauer S, Buttner U. Pathological torsional eye deviation during voluntary saccades: a violation of Listing's law. *J Neurol Neurosurg Psychiatry* 1997;**62**:253–60.

2527. Helmes E, Csapo KG, Short JA. Standardization and validation of the Multidimensional Observation Scale for Elderly Subjects (MOSES). *J Gerontol* 1987;**42**:395–405.

2528. Helm-Estabrooks N, Fitzpatrick PM, Barresi B. Visual action therapy for global aphasia. *J Speech Hear Dis* 1982;**47**:385–9.

2529. Helmholtz HLF von. Beschreibung eines Augen-Spiegels zur Untersuchung der Netzhaut im lebenden Auge. Berlin: A. Forstner, 1851.

2530. Helweg-Larsen HF, Ludvigsen K. Congenital familial anhidrosis and neurolabyrinthitis. *Acta Dermatol Vener Stockh* 1946;**26**:489–505.

2531. Henderson VW. Speech fluency in crossed aphasia. *Brain* 1983;**106**:837–57.

2532. Henderson VW. Jules Déjèrine and the third alexia. *Arch Neurol* 1984;**41**:430–2.

2533. Henderson VW. Paul Broca's less heralded contributions to aphasia research: historical perspective and contemporary relevance. *Arch Neurol* 1986;**43**:609–12.

2534. Henderson WR, Smyth GE. Phantom limbs. *J Neurol Neurosurg Psychiatry* 1948;**11**:88.

2535. Henkind P, Siegel IM, Carr RE. Mesodermal dysgenesis of the anterior segment: Rieger's anolamy. *Arch Ophthalmol* 1965;**73**:810.

2536. Henley FA. Pelvic colectomy for obstinate constipation. *Proc R Soc Med* 1967;**60**:806–7.

2537. Hennebert C. Reactions vestibularies dans les labyrinthes hérédo-syphilitiques. *Arch Int Laryngol (Paris)* 1909;**28**:93–6.

2538. Hennebert C. Vestibularreaction auf die Pneumonitische. *Ohr Rhinolaryngol* 1909;**8**:532.

2539. Henson JW. Spinal cord gliomas. *Curr Opin Neurol* 2001;**14**:679–82.

2540. Henson RA. Henry Head's work on sensation. *Brain* 1961;**84**:535–50.

2541. Henson RA. Henry Head: his influence on the development of ideas on sensation. *Br Med Bull* 1977;**33**:91–6.

2542. Henson RA. The editors of *Brain*. *Practitioner (Lond)* 1978;**221**:639–44.

2543. Henson RA, Hoffman HL, Urich H. Encephalomyelitis with carcinoma. *Brain* 1965;**88**:449–64.

2544. Henson RA, Russell DS, Wilkinson M. Carcinomatous neuropathy and myopathy: a clinical and pathological study. *Brain* 1954;**77**:82–121.

2545. Henson RA, Urich H. *Cancer and the Nervous System: The Neurological Manifestations of Systemic Malignant Disease.* Oxford: Blackwell Scientific, 1982.

2546. Henson TE, Muller J, DeMyer WE. Hereditary myopathy limited to females. *Arch Neurol* 1967;**17**:238–47.

2547. Heppenstall B, Tan V. Well-leg compartment syndrome. *Lancet* 1999;**354**:970–1.

2548. Herman E. Neurological syndromes in typhus fever. *J Nerv Ment Dis* 1949;**109**:25–36.

2549. Hernandez A, et al. Cortical blindness, growth and psychomotor retardation and postaxial polydactyly. *Clin Genet* 1985;**28**:251–4.

2550. Herrick JB. Peculiar elongated and sickle-shaped red corpuscles in a case of severe anemia. *Arch Intern Med* 1910;**6**:517.

2551. Herrmann C, Anguilar M, Sacks O. Hereditary photomyoclonus associated with diabetes mellitus, deafness, nephropathy and cerebral dysfunction. *Neurology* 1964;**14**:213–21.

2552. Herrmann J, et al. A familial dysmorphogenetic syndrome of limb deformities, characteristic facial appearance and associated anomalies: the "pseudothalidomide" or SC-syndrome. *Birth Defects* 1969;**5**:81–9.

2553. Herrmann J, Opitz JM. An unusual form of acrocephalosyndactyly. *Birth Defects* 1969;**5**:39–42.

2554. Hers HG. Etudes enzymatiques sur fragments hepatiques: application a la classification des glycogenoses. *Rev Int Hepatol* 1959;**9**:35–55.

2555. Hersch EL. Development and application of the extended scale for dementia. *J Am Geriatr Soc* 1979;**26**:348.

2556. Hershey AD, Powers SW, Vockell A-LB, et al. PedMIDAS. *Neurology* 2001;**57**:2034–9.

2557. Herskovitz S, Lipton RB, Lantos G. Neuro-Behçet's disease. *Neurology* 1988;**38**:1714–20.

2558. Herskovitz S, Loh F, Berger AR, et al. Erythromelalgia: association with hereditary sensory neuropathy and response to amitryptline. *Neurology* 1993;**43**:621–2.

2559. Hertzman PA, Blevins WL, Mayer J, et al. Association of the eosinophilia–myalgia syndrome with the ingestion of tryptophan. *N Engl J Med* 1990;**322**:869–73.

2560. Herva R, Leisti J, Kerkinen P, et al. A lethal autosomal recessive syndrome of multiple congenital contractures. *Am J Med Genet* 1985;**20**:431–439.

2561. Herxheimer A. Gustatory sweating and piloerection. *BMJ* 1958;**1**:688–9.

2562. Hess DC. Stroke associated with antiphospholipid antibodies. *Stroke* 1992;**23** (**Suppl 1**):23–8.

2563. Heymans A, Nelck G, Oorthuys JWE, et al. Rhizomelic chondrodysplasia punctata. *N Engl J Med* 1985;**313**:187–8.

2564. Hicks EP. Hereditary perforating ulcer of the foot. *Lancet* 1922;**1**:319–21.

2565. Hierons R. Willis' contribution to clinical medicine and neurology. *J Neurol Sci* 1967;**4**:1–13.

2566. Hietaharju A, Jaaskelainen S, Kalimo H. Peripheral neuromuscular manifestations in systemic sclerosis (scleroderma). *Muscle Nerve* 1993;**16**:1204–12.

2567. Higashi K, et al. Cerebral paragonimiasis. *J Neurosurg* 1971;**34**:515.

2568. Higgins JJ, Kaneski CR, Bernadini I. Pyridoxine-responsive hyper-β-alaninemia associated with Cohen's syndrome. *Neurology* 1994;**44**:1728–32.

2569. Higgins JJ, Morton DH, Patronas N, et al. An autosomal recessive disorder with posterior column ataxia and retinitis pigmentosa. *Neurology* 1997;**49**:1717–20.

2570. Higgins JJ, Patterson M, Papadopoulos NM, et al. Hypoprebetalipoproteinemia, acanthocytosis, retinitis pigmentosa and pallidal degeneration (HARP syndrome). *Neurology* 1991;**41**(**Suppl 1**):243.

2571. Higgins JJ, Rosen DR, Loveless JM, et al. A gene for nonsyndromic mental retardation maps to chromosome 3p25–pter. *Neurology* 2000;**55**:335–40.

2572. Hilden T, Svendsen TL. Electrolyte disturbance in beer drinkers. *Lancet* 1975;**2**:245–7.

2573. Hilger JA. Carotid pain. *Laryngol Rhinol Otol* 1949;**59**:829–38.

2574. Hillbom M, Muuronen A, Holm L, et al. The clinical versus radiological diagnosis of alcoholic cerebellar degeneration. *J Neurol Sci* 1986;**73**:45–53.

2575. Hillemand P. Charles Foix and his Life Work [in French]. *Clio Med* 1976;**11**:269–87.

2576. Hilliquin P, Menkes CJ, Laoussadi S, et al. Camptocormia in the elderly. A new entity with paravertebral muscle involvement? [in French]. *Rev Rheum Mal Osteoarthritis* 1992;**59**:169–75.

2577. Hinchey J, Chaves C, Appignani B, et al. A reversible posterior leukoencephalopathy syndrome. *N Engl J Med* 1996;**334**:494–500.

2578. Hippel E von. Vorstellung eines Patienten mit einem sehr ungewohnlichen Aderhautleiden. In *Bericht* über die 24. Versammlung der *Ophthlalmogischen Gesedlschaft in Heidelberg,* p 269. 1895.

2579. Hippocrates. The sacred disease. In Jones WHS, Withington ET, eds. *Works,* pp 127–83. London: 1990.

2580. Hirano A, Kurland LT, Krooth RS, et al. Parkinsonism–dementia complex, endemic disease on island of Guam. I. Clinical features. *Brain* 1961;**84**:642–61.

2581. Hirano A, Kurland LT, Sayre GP. Familial amyotrophic lateral sclerosis. *Arch Neurol* 1967;**16**:232–43.

2582. Hirano M, Ott BR, Raps EC, et al. Acute quadriplegic myopathy: a complication of treatment with steroids, non-depolarizing blocking agents, or both. *Neurology* 1992;**42**:2082–7.

2583. Hirano M, Ricci E, Koenigsburger MR. MELAS: an original case and clinical criteria for diagnosis. *Neuromusc Disord* 1992;**2**:125–35.

2584. Hirayama K, Tomonaga M, Kitano K, et al. Focal cervical poliopathy causing juvenile muscular atrophy of the distal upper extremity. *J Neurol Neurosurg Psychiatry* 1987;**50**:285–90.

2585. Hirayama K, Toyakura Y, Tsubaki T. Juvenile muscular atrophy of unilateral upper extremity; a new clinical entity. *Psychiatry Neurol* (*Japan*) 1959;**6140**:2190–7.

2586. Hirayama T, Takemitsu Y. Isolated paralysis of the descending branch of the posterior interosseous nerve. *J Bone Jt Surg* 1988;**70–A**:1402–3.

2587. Hirsch AE, Ommaya AK, Mahone RH. Tolerance of subhuman primate brain to cerebral concussion. In Gurdijan ES, Lange WA, Patrick LM, et al., eds. *Impact Injury and Crash Protection,* pp 352–71. Springfield, IL: C.C. Thomas, 1970.

2588. Hirschowitz BI, Groll A, Ceballos R. Hereditary nerve deafness in three sisters with absent gastric motility, small bowel diverticulitis and ulceration and progressive sensory neuropathy. *Birth Defects* 1972;**8**(**2**):27–41.

2589. Hisanaga K, Hosokawa M, Sato N, et al. "Neuro-sweet disease". *Arch Neurol* 1999;**56**:1010–3.

2590. Hitchings RA, Corbett AA, Winklemam J, et al. Hemorrhages with optic nerve drusen. *Arch Neurol* 1976;**33**:675–7.

2591. Hjorth RJ, Willison RG. The electromyogram in facial myokymia and hemifacial spasm. *J Neurol Sci* 1973;**20**:117–26.

2592. Ho K-L, Meyer KR. The medial medullary syndrome. *Arch Neurol* 1981;**38**:385–7.

2592a. Ho TW et al. Guillain-Barré syndrome in northern China. Relationship to *Campylobacter jejuni* infection and anti-glyolipid antibodies. *Brain* 1995;**118**:597–605.

2593. Ho SS, Berkovic SF, Newton MR, et al. Parietal lobe epilepsy. *Neurology* 1994;**44**:2277–84.

2594. Hobart JC, Thompson AJ. The five item Barthel Index. *J Neurol Neurosurg Psychiatry* 2001;**71**:225–30.

2594a. Hochberg MC, for the Diagnostic and Therapeutic Criteria Committee of the American College of Rheumatology. Updating the American College of Rheumatology revised criteria for the classification of systemic lupus erythematosus [letter]. *Arthritis Rheum* 1997;**40**:1725.

2595. Hochsinger C. Concerning tetany in children. *Verh Ges Kinderheilkd* 1900;**16**:107–15.

2596. Hockaday JM, Whitty CWM. Patterns of referred pain in the normal subject. *Brain* 1967;**90**:481–96.

2597. Hoddes E, Zarcone V, Smythe H, et al. Quantification of sleepiness: a new approach. *Psychophysiology* 1973;**10**:431–6.

2598. Hoehn MH, Yahr MD. Parkinsonism: onset, progression and mortality. *Neurology* 1967;**17**:427–42.

2599. Hoffman EP, Festoff BW, Gijon LT Jr, et al. Amyotrophic lateral sclerosis due to HIV. *N Engl J Med* 1985;**313**:324.

2600. Hoffman EP, Fischbeck KH, Brown RH, et al. Characterization of dystrophin in muscle biopsy specimens from patients with Duchenne's or Becker's muscular dystrophy. *N Engl J Med* 1988;**318:** 1363–8.

2601. Hoffmann J. Ueber chronische spinale Muskelatrophie im Kindesalter, auf familiarer Basis. *Dtsch Z Nervenklinik* 1891;**1:**95–120.

2602. Hoffmann J. Weiterer Beitrag zur Lehre von der Tetanie. *Dtsch Z Nervenklinik* 1897;**9:**278–80.

2603. Hoffmann J, et al. Hoffmann syndrome (adults). *Dtsch Z Nervenheilk* 1897;**9:**278.

2605. Hoffmann PM, Stuart WH, Earle KM, et al. Hereditary late-onset cerebellar degeneration. *Neurology* 1971;**21:**771–7.

2606. Hogan EL, Krigman MR. Herpes myelitis. *Arch Neurol* 1973; **29:**309–13.

2607. Hogan PJ, Greenberg MK, McCarty GE. Neurological complications of lymphomatoid granulomatosis. *Neurology* 1981;**31:**619–20.

2608. Hognestad S. Hereditary nerve deafness associated with diabetes. *Acta Otolaryngol* 1967;**64:**219.

2609. Hogrel J-Y, Laforêt P, Yaou RB, et al. A non-ischemic forearm exercise test for the screening of patients with exercise intolerance. *Neurology* 2001;**56:**1733–8.

2610. Hohol MJ, Orav EJ, Weiner HL. Disease steps in multiple sclerosis: a longitudinal study comparing disease steps and EDSS to evaluate disease progression. *Multi Scler* 1999;**5:**349–54.

2611. Hoke A, Rewcastle NB, Zochodne DW. Acute quadriplegic myopathy unrelated to steroids or paralyzing agents: quantitative EMG studies. *Can J Neurol Sci* 1999;**26:**325–9.

2612. Holbrook M, Skilbeck CE. An activities index for use with stroke patients. *Age Ageing* 1983;**12:**166–70.

2613. Holden JD. The Russell-Silver's dwarf. *Dev Med Child Neurol* 1967;**9:**457–9.

2614. Holden KR, Dekaban AS. Neurological involvement in nevus unis lateralis and nevus linearis sebaceus. *Neurology* 1972;**22:**879–87.

2615. Hollander H, Levy JA. Neurologic abnormalities and recovery of human immunodeficiency virus from cerebrospinal fluid. *Ann Intern Med* 1987;**106:**692–5.

2616. Hollenhorst RW. The Neuro-ophthalmology of strokes. In Smith JL, ed. *Neuro-Ophthalmology*, p 109. St. Louis: C.V. Mosby, 1965.

2617. Hollenhorst RW, Svien HJ, Benoit CF. Unilateral blindness occurring during anesthesia for neurosurgical operations. *Arch Ophthalmol* 1954;**52:**819.

2618. Holman CB. Radiologic manifestations of glioma of the optic nerve and chiasm. *Am J Radiol* 1959;**82:**462.

2619. Holmes G. A form of familial degeneration of the cerebellum. *Brain* 1907;**30:**466–89.

2620. Holmes G. The symptoms of acute cerebellar injuries due to gunshot injuries. *Brain* 1917;**40:**461–535.

2621. Holmes G. Disturbances of visual orientation. *Br J Ophthalmol* 1918;**2:**449–68.

2622. Holmes G. Spasm of fixation. *Trans Ophthalmol Soc UK* 1930; **50:**253–62.

2623. Holmes G. Partial iridoplegia associated with symptoms of other disease of the nervous system. *Trans Ophthalmol Soc UK* 1931;**51:** 209–24.

2624. Holmes G. The cerebral integration of the ocular movements. *BMJ* 1938;**2:**107–12.

2625. Holmes G. The cerebellum of man. *Brain* 1939;**62:**1–30.

2626. Holmes G. *The National Hospital, Queen Square 1860–1948.* London: Livingstone, 1954.

2627. Holmes G. *Selected Papers of Gordon Holmes.* Oxford: Oxford University Press, 1979.

2628. Holmes G, Lister WT. Disturbances of vision from cerebral lesions. *Brain* 1916;**39:**35–73.

2629. Holmes G, Russman J. Shuddering attacks. *Am J Dis Child* 1986;**140:**72–3.

2630. Holmes GL, Logan WJ. A syndrome of infantile CNS degeneration. *Am J Dis Child* 1980;**134:**262–6.

2631. Holmes GL, McKeever M, Adamson M. Absence seizures in children: clinical and electroencephalographic features. *Ann Neurol* 1987;**21:**268–73.

2632. Holmes GP, Kaplan JE, Gantz NM, et al. Chronic fatigue syndrome: a working case definition. *Ann Intern Med* 1988;**108:**387–9.

2632a. Holmes SE, O'Heam E, Ross CA, et al. SCA12: An unusual mutation leads to an unusual spinocerebellar ataxia. *Brain Res Bull* 2001; **56:**397–403.

2633. Holtermuller K, Wiedemann HR. Kleeblattschadel-Syndrom. *Med Wochenschr* 1960;**14:**439–46.

2634. Homeida J, et al. Dapsone motor neuropathy. *BMJ* 1980; **281:**1180.

2635. Homen EA. Eine eigenthumliche Familienkrankheit, unter der Form einer progressiven Dementia, mit besonderem anatomischen Befund. *Neurol Zentrabl* 1890;**9:**514–8.

2636. Hood JD, Kayan A, Leech J. Rebound nystagmus. *Brain* 1973;**96:**507–26.

2637. Hood JD, Korres S. Vestibular suppression in peripheral and central vestibular disorders. *Brain* 1979;**102:**785–804.

2638. Hooft C, DeLacey P, Herpol J, et al. Familial hypolipidemia and retarded development without steatorrhea. *Helv Pediatr Acta* 1962;**17:**1.

2639. Hooper HE. *The Hooper Visual Organization Test Manual.* Los Angeles: Western Psychological Services, 1958.

2640. Hooshmand H, Martinez AJ, Rosenblum WI. Arthrogryposis multiplex congenita. *Arch Neurol* 1971;**24:**561–70.

2641. Hootnick D, Holmes LB. Familial polysyndactyly and craniofacial anomalies. *Clin Genet* 1972;**3:**128–34.

2642. Hoover CF. A new sign for the detection of malingering and functional paresis of the lower extremities. *JAMA* 1908;**51:**746.

2643. Hopf H. Topodiagnostic value of brainstem reflexes. *Muscle Nerve* 1994;**17:**475–84.

2644. Hopf HC. Peripheral neuropathy in acrodermatitis chronica atrophicans. *J Neurol Neurosurg Psychiatry* 1975;**38:**452–8.

2645. Hopf HC, Ehrrich J, Hundemer H. The pterygoid reflex in man and its clinical application. *Muscle Nerve* 1992;**15:**1278–83.

2646. Hopkins A, Rudge P. Hyperpathia in the cervical cord syndrome. *J Neurol Neurosurg Psychiatry* 1973;**36:**637–42.

2647. Hopkins AP, Harvey PKP. Chronic benign lymphocytic meningitis. *J Neurol Sci* 1973;**18:**443–53.

2648. Hopkins AP, Michael WF. Spinal myoclonus. *J Neurol Neurosurg Psychiatry* 1974;**37:**1112–5.

2649. Hopkins IJ. A new syndrome: poliomyelitis-like illness associated with acute asthma. *Aust Paediatr J* 1974;**10:**273–6.

2650. Hopkins IJ, Turner B. Spongy glio-neural dystrophy: a degenerative disease of the nervous system. *J Neurol Neurosurg Psychiatry* 1973;**36:**50–6.

2651. Hopper KD, et al. Poland-Möbius syndrome. *South Med J* 1985;**78:**523–7.

2652. Hormes JT, Filley CM, Rosenberg NL. Neurological sequelae of chronic solvent vapor abuse. *Neurology* 1986;**36:**698–702.

2653. Horn JL. Psychometric studies of aging and intelligence. In Gershon S, Raskin A, eds. *Aging*, pp 19–43. New York: Raven Press, 1975.

2654. Horner F. Uber ein Form von Ptosis. *Klin Monatsbl Augenheilkd* 1869;**7:**193–8.

2655. Horner J, Massey EW. Dynamic spelling alexia. *J Neurol Neurosurg Psychiatry* 1986;**49:**455–7.

2656. Horoupian DS. Hereditary sensory neuropathy with deafness. *Neurology* 1989;**39:**244–8.

2657. Horowitz SH, Schmalbruch H. Autosomal dominant distal myopathy with desmin storage: a clinicopathologic and electrophysiologic study of a large kinship. *Muscle Nerve* 1994;**17:**151–60.

2658. Horsley VAH. *The Structure and Functions of the Brain and Spinal Cord.* London: Charles Griffin and Co., 1892.

2659. Horsley VAH. The Linacre lecture on the function of the so-called motor area of the brain. *BMJ* 1909;**2:**125–32.

2660. Horsley VAH, Clarke RH. The structure and functions of the cerebellum examined by a new method. *Brain* 1908;**31:**45–124.

2661. Horten BC, Rubinstein LJ. Primary cerebral neuroblastoma; a clinicopathological study of 35 cases. *Brain* 1976;**99:**735–56.

2662. Horton BT, Magath TB, Brown GE. Arteritis of the temporal vessels. A previously undescribed form. *Arch Intern Med* 1934;**53:**400–9.

2663. Horton JC, Hoyt WF. Occipital visual field defects respecting the horizontal meridian: a hallmark of extrastriate cortical lesions [unpublished]. 1990.

2664. Horwich MS, Cho L, Poro RS, Posner JB. Subacute sensory neuropathy: a remote effect of carcinoma. *Ann Neurol* 1977;**2**:7–19.

2665. Hosking G. Special forms: variants of migraine in childhood. In Hockaday JM, ed. *Migraine in Childhood*, pp 35–53. London: Butterworths, 1988.

2666. Hoskins TA, Squires JE. Developmental assessment: a test for gross motor and reflex development. *Phys Ther* 1973;**2**:117–26.

2667. How A, Dent PB, Liao SK, et al. Antineuronal antibodies in neuropsychiatric systemic lupus erythematosus. *Arthritis Rheum* 1985; **28**:789–95.

2668. Howard RS, Greenwood R, Gawler J, et al. A familial disorder associated with palatal myoclonus, other brainstem signs, tetraparesis, ataxia and Rosenthal fiber formation. *J Neurol Neurosurg Psychiatry* 1993;**56**:977–81.

2669. Howe JR, Miller CA. Midbrain deafness following head injury. *Neurology* 1975;**25**:286–9.

2670. Howell JT, Monto RW. Syndrome of anemia, dysphagia, and glossitis (Plummer-Vinson syndrome). *N Engl J Med* 1953;**249**: 1009–12.

2671. Howell SJL, Owen L, Chadwick DW. Pseudostatus epilepticus. *Q J Med* 1989;**71**:507–19.

2672. Howlett WP, Brubaker GR, Mlingi N, et al. Konzo, an epidemic upper motor neurone disease studied in Tanzania. *Brain* 1990;**113**: 223–35.

2673. Howship J. *Practical Remarks on the Discrimination and Appearance of Surgical Disease*. London: Churchill, 1840.

2674. Hsia YE, et al. Genetics of the Meckel syndrome (dysencephalia splanchnocystica). *Pediatrics* 1971;**48**:237–47.

2675. Huang C-C, Chu N-S, Chen T-J, et al. Acute hemorrhagic leucoencephalitis with a prolonged clinical course. *J Neurol Neurosurg Psychiatry* 1988;**51**:870–4.

2676. Huang C-C, Chu N-S, Lu C-S, et al. Long-term progression in chronic manganism. *Neurology* 1998;**50**:698–700.

2677. Huang C, Broe G. Isolated facial palsy; a new lacunar syndrome. *J Neurol Neurosurg Psychiatry* 1984;**47**:84–6.

2678. Hubble JP, Busenbark KL, Koller WC. Essential tremor. *Clin Neuropharmacol* 1989;**12**:453–82.

2679. Huber A. Electrophysiology of the retraction syndromes. *Br J Ophthalmol* 1974;**58**:293.

2680. Huber SJ, Paulson GW. The concept of subcortical dementia. *Am J Psychiatry* 1985;**142**:1312–7.

2681. Huchard H. Character and mental state of hysterics. *Arch Neurol* 1882;**3**:187–211.

2682. Hudgins RJ, Edwards MSB, Ousterhouk DK, et al. Pediatric neurosurgical implications of the amniotic band syndrome. *Pediatr Neurosci* 1986;**12**:232–9.

2683. Hudgson P. Subacute or chronic proximal metabolic myopathies. *BMJ* 1984;**1**:585.

2684. Hudgson P, Peter JB. Classification (of polymyositis). *Clin Rheum Dis* 1984;**10**:3–8.

2685. Hudson AJ. Amyotrophic lateral sclerosis and its association with dementia, parkinsonism and other neurological disorders. *Brain* 1981;**104**:217–47.

2686. Hudson AJ, Brown WF, Gilbert JJ. The muscular pain–fasciculation syndrome. *Neurology* 1978;**28**:1105–9.

2687. Hudson AJ, Grace GM. Misidentification syndromes related to face-specific area in the fusiform gyrus. *J Neurol Neurosurg Psychiatry* 2000;**69**:645–8.

2688. Hug G, Bove KE, Soukup S. Lethal neonatal multiorgan deficiency of carnitine palmitoyltransferase II. *N Engl J Med* 1991;**325**: 1862–4.

2689. Hugh AE. Trickle arteriography. *BMJ* 1970;**2**:574–6.

2690. Hughes CA, Byrne PC, Webb S, et al. SPG15, a new locus for autosomal recessive complicated HSP on chromosome 14q. *Neurology* 2001;**56**:1230–3.

2691. Hughes CP, Berg L, Danziger WL, et al. A new clinical scale for the staging of dementia. *Br J Psychiatry* 1982;**140**:566–72.

2693. Hughes JT. *Thomas Willis 1621–1675. His Life and Work*. London: Royal Society of Medicine Services, 1991.

2694. Hughes JT, Oppenheimer DR. Superficial siderosis of the central nervous system. A report on nine cases with autopsy. *Acta Neuropathol* 1969;**13**:556–74.

2695. Hughes RAC, Bensa S, Willison H, et al. Randomized controlled trial of intravenous immunoglobulin versus oral prednisolone in chronic inflammatory demyelinating polyneuropathy. *Ann Neurol* 2001;**50**:195–201.

2696. Hughes RAC, Newsom-Davis J, Perkin GD, et al. Controlled trial of prednisolone in acute polyneuropathy. *Lancet* 1978;**2**:750–3.

2697. Hughes RAC, Sanders E, Hall S, et al. Subacute idiopathic demyelinating polyradiculoneuropathy. *Arch Neurol* 1992;**49**:612–6.

2698. Humphreys P, Whiting S, Pham B. Hemiparetic cerebral palsy: Clinical pattern and imaging in prediction of outcome. *Can J Neurol Sci* 2000;**27**:210–9.

2699. Hund E. Neurological complications of sepsis: critical illness polyneuropathy and myopathy. *J Neurol* 2001;**248**:929–34.

2700. Hunt AD. Pyridoxine dependency: report of a case of intractable convulsions in an infant, controlled by pyridoxine. *Pediatrics* 1954; **13**:140–5.

2701. Hunt JR. On herpetic inflammation of the geniculate ganglion. A new syndrome and its complications. *J Nerv Ment Dis* 1907;**34**:73–96.

2702. Hunt JR. Dyssynergia cerebellaris progressiva—a chronic progressive form of cerebellar tremor. *Brain* 1914;**37**:247–68.

2703. Hunt JR. Progressive atrophy of the globus pallidus (primary atrophy of the pallidal system). *Brain* 1917;**40**:58–148.

2704. Hunt JR. Dyssynergia cerebellaris myoclonica—primary atrophy of the dentate system: a contribution to the pathology and symptomatology of the cerebellum. *Brain* 1921;**44**:490–538.

2705. Hunt JR. On the occurence of static seizures in epilepsy. *J Nerv Ment Dis* 1922;**56**:351–6.

2706. Hunt WE, Hess RM. Surgical risks as related to time of intervention in the repair of intracranial aneurysms. *J Neurosurg* 1968;**28**: 14–20.

2707. Hunter AG, et al. Absence of cerebellar granular layer, mental retardation, tapetoretinal degeneration, and progressive glomerulopathy: an autosomal recessive ocular-renal-cerebellar syndrome. *Am J Med Genet* 1982;**11**:383–95.

2708. Hunter AGW, McAlpine PJ, Rudd NL, et al. A "new" syndrome of mental retardation with characteristic facies and brachyphalangy. *J Med Genet* 1977;**14**:430–7.

2709. Hunter C. A rare disease in two brothers. *Proc R Soc Med* 1917;**10**:104–16.

2710. Huntington G. On chorea. *Med Surg Rep* 1872;**26**:317–21.

2711. Huott AD, Madison DS, Niedermeyer E. Occipital lobe epilepsy. *Eur Neurol* 1974;**11**:325–39.

2712. Hurler G. Uber einen Typ multipler Abartungen vorwiegend am Skelettsystem. *Z Kinderheilkd* 1919;**24**:220–34.

2713. Hurst EW. Acute haemorrhagic leucoencephalitis; previously undefined entity. *Med J Aust* 1941;**2**:1–6.

2714. Huson SM, Harper PS, Hourihan MD, et al. Cerebellar haemangioblastoma and von Hippel–Lindau disease. *Brain* 1986;**109**: 1297–310.

2715. Hutchinson J. On the different forms of inflammation of the eye consequent on inherited syphilis. *Ophthalmol Hosp Rep* 1858;**1**:191, 226–30, 244.

2716. Hutchinson J. Report on the effect of infantile syphilis in marring the development of teeth. *Trans Pathol Soc Lond* 1858;**9**:449–55.

2717. Hutchinson J. Case of congenital absence of hair with atrophic condition of the skin and its appendages. *Lancet* 1886;**1**:923.

2718. Hutchinson R. Suprarenal sarcoma in children with metastasis in the skull. *Q J Med* 1907;**1**:33.

2719. Huttenlocher PR, Gilles FH. Infantile neuroaxonal dystrophy. *Neurology* 1967;**17**:1174–84.

2720. Hwang YM, Lee MC, Suh DC, et al. Coxiella (Q-fever)-associated myelopathy. *Neurology* 1993;**43**:338–42.

2721. Hyland K, Surtees RAH, Rodeck C, et al. Aromatic L-amino acid decarboxylase deficiency: clinical features, diagnosis, and treatment of a new inborn error of neurotransmitter amine synthesis. *Neurology* 1992;**42**:1980–8.

2722. Hymas N, Lees A, Bolton D, et al. The neurology of obsessional slowness. *Brain* 1991;**114**:2203–33.

2723. IASP Taxonomy Committee. Classification of chronic pain. *Pain* 1986;**27**:S1–S226.

2724. Iglesias S, Chapon F, Baron J-C. Familial Occipital Calcifications, hemorrhagic strokes, leukoencephalopathy, dementia and external carotoid dysplasia. *Neurology* 2000;**55**:1661–7.

2725. Iizuka R, et al. Dentato-rubro-pallido-luysian atrophy. *J Neurol Neurosurg Psychiatry* 1984;**47**:1288–98.

2726. Ikeda A, Kakigi R, Funai N, et al. Cortical tremor: a variant of cortical reflex myoclonus. *Neurology* 1990;**40**:1561–5.

2727. Ikeda K, Iwasaki Y, Kinoshita M. Amyotrophic lateral sclerosis associated with isolated adrenocorticotrophic hormone deficiency. *Muscle Nerve* 1995;**18**:111–3.

2728. Ikeda S, Yakazi M, Takei Y, et al. Type II (adult onset) cit-rullinemia: clinical pictures and the therapeutic effect of liver trans-plantation. *J Neurol Neurosurg Psychiatry* 2001;**71**:663–70.

2729. Ikida S, Kondo K, Oguchi K, et al. Adult fucosidosis. *Neurology* 1984;**334**:451–4.

2730. Iliceto G, Thompson PD, Day BL, et al. Diaphragmatic flutter, the moving umbilicus syndrome and "belly-dancers' dyskinesia". *Mov Disord* 1990;**5**:15–22.

2731. Illa I, Serrano-Munuera C, Gallardo E, et al. Distal anterior com-partment myopathy: a dysferlin mutation causing a new muscular dys-trophy phenotype. *Ann Neurol* 2001;**49**:130–4.

2732. Illingworth RS. *The Development of the Infant and the Young Child: Normal and Abnormal.* Edinburgh: Churchill Livingstone, 1987.

2733. Illis LS. Central pain. *BMJ* 1990;**300**:1284–6.

2734. Ince B, Petty GW, Brown JR Jr, et al. Dolichoectasia of the in-tracranial arteries in patients with first ischemic stroke. *Neurology* 1998;**50**:1694–8.

2734a. Ince PG, Duffey P, Cochrane HR et al. Relapsing ischemic en-cephaloenteropathy and cryoglobulinemia. *Neurology* 2000;28;**55**:1579–81.

2735. Indo T, Takahashi A. Swimmer's migraine. *Headache* 1990;**30**:485–7.

2736. Ingall TJ, McLeod JG, Tamura N. Autonomic function and un-myelinated fibres in chronic inflammatory demyelinating polyradicu-loneuropathy. *Muscle Nerve* 1990;**13**:70–6.

2737. Inghilleri M, Bernadelli A, Cioni B, et al. The conduction veloc-ity of the corticospinal tract in man. In Rossini PM, Marsden CD, eds. *Non-Invasive Stimulation of Brain and Spinal Cord,* pp 123–30. New York: Alan R. Liss, 1988.

2738. Ingle VN, Talwalker YB, Neil JV. Bilateral congenital anoph-thalmos. *J Pediatr* 1966;**33**:149.

2739. Ingram TTS. *Paediatric Aspects of Cerebral Palsy.* Edinburgh: Liv-ingstone, 1964.

2740. Ingram TTS, Naughton JA. Paediatric and psychological aspects of cerebral palsy associated with hydrocephalus. *Dev Med Child Neu-rol* 1962;**4**:287–92.

2741. Ingvar DH, Nyman GE. Epilepsia arithmetices. *Neurology* 1962;**12**:282–7.

2742. Inomata H, Kato M. Vogt-Koyanagi-Harada disease. In Bruyn GW, Vinken PJ, eds. *Handbook of Clinical Neurology,* pp 611–26. Am-sterdam: Elsevier, 1989.

2744. Inouye SK, van Dyck CH, Alessi CA, et al. Clarifying confusion: the confusion assessment method. *Ann Intern Med* 1990;**113**:941–8.

2745. International Continence Society Standardisation Committee. Fourth Report on the Standardisation of Terminology of Lower Uri-nary Tract Dysfunction. *Br J Urol* 1981;**53**:333.

2746. International Federation of Multiple Sclerosis Societies. Minimal record of disability for multiple sclerosis. *Acta Neurol Scand Suppl* 1984;**101**:15–217.

2747. Ionasescu V. Oculogastrointestinal muscular dystrophy. *Am J Med Genet* 1983;**15**:103–12.

2748. Ionasescu VV, Burns TL, Searby C, et al. X-linked dominant Charcot-Marie-Tooth neuropathy with 15 cases in a family genetic link-age study. *Muscle Nerve* 1988;**11**:1154–6.

2749. Iqbal A, Alter M, Lee SH. Pseudoxanthoma elasticum: a review of neurological complications. *Ann Neurol* 1978;**4**:18–20.

2750. Iragui VJ. The Charcot-Bouchard controversy. *Arch Neurol* 1986;**43**:290–5.

2751. Isaacs B, Kennie AT. The Set Test as an aid to the detection of dementia in old people. *Br J Psychiatry* 1973;**123**:467–70.

2752. Isaacs H. A syndrome of continuous muscle fibre activity. *J Neu-rol Neurosurg Psychiatry* 1961;**24**:319–25.

2753. Isgren WP. Normocalcemic tetany. A problem of erethism. *Neu-rology* 1976;**26**:825–34.

2754. Ishihara S. Tests for colour-blindness. Tokio: Kanehawa Shup-pan Co. Ltd., 1917.

2755. Isler H. Thomas Willis' two chapters on headache of 1672: a first attempt to apply the "new science" to this topic. *Headache* 1986;**26**:95–8.

2756. Ismael SS, Ameranco G, Bayle B, et al. Postpartum lumbosacral plexopathy limited to autonomic and perineal manifestations: clinical and electrophyiological study of 19 patients. *J Neurol Neurosurg Psy-chiatry* 2000;**68**:771–3.

2757. Isozaki E, Naito A, Horiguchi S, et al. Early diagnosis and stage classification of vocal cord abductor paralysis in patients with multiple system atrophy. *J Neurol Neurosurg Psychiatry* 1996;**60**:399–402.

2758. Israels S, Haworth JC, Dunn HG, et al. Lactic acidosis in child-hood. *Adv Pediatr* 1976;**22**:267–303.

2759. Itigaki S, McGeer PL, Akiyama H, et al. A case of adult onset de-mentia with argyrophilic grains. *Ann Neurol* 1989;**26**:685–9.

2760. Ito M. Nevus fusco-ceruleus acromio-deltoideus. *Tohoku J Exp Med* 1954;**60**:10.

2761. Ives EJ, Houston CS. Autosomal recessive microcephaly and mi-cromelia in Cree Indians. *Am J Med Genet* 1980;**7**:351–60.

2762. Iwashita H, Ohnishi A, Asada M, et al. Polyneuropathy, skin hy-perpigmentation, edema and hypertrichosis in localised osteosclerotic myeloma. *Neurology* 1977;**27**:675–81.

2763. Jablecki CK. Lateral antebrachial cutaneous neuropathy in a windsurfer. *Muscle Nerve* 1999;**22**:944–5.

2764. Jablonski S. *Illustrated Dictionary of Eponymic Syndromes and Diseases and Their Synonyms.* Philadelphia: W.B. Saunders, 1969.

2765. Jablonski S. *Jablonski's Dictionary of Syndromes and Eponymic Diseases.* Malabar, FL: Krieger, 1991.

2766. Jabre JF. Surface recording of the H-reflex of the flexor carpi ra-dialis. *Muscle Nerve* 1981;**4**:435–8.

2767. Jabre JF. Concentric macro electromyography. *Muscle Nerve* 1991;**14**:820–5.

2768. Jabre JF, Bryan RW. Bent-knee pulling in the diagnosis of up-per lumbar root lesions. *Arch Neurol* 1982;**39**:669–70.

2769. Jackson AC. Acute viral infections. *Curr Opin Neurol* 1995;**8**:170–4.

2770. Jackson AC, Gilbert JJ, Young GB, Bolton CF. The en-cephalopathy of sepsis. *Can J Neurol Sci* 1985;**12**:303–7.

2771. Jackson CE, Amato AA, Barohn RJ. Isolated vitamin E deficiency. *Muscle Nerve* 1996;**19**:1161–5.

2772. Jackson CE, Barohn RJ. Improvement of the Exercise Test in thy-rotoxic periodic paralysis. *Muscle Nerve* 1992;**15**:1069–71.

2773. Jackson CE, et al. "Brittle" hair with short stature, intellectual impairment with decreased fertility; an autosomal recessive syndrome in an Amish kindred. *Pediatrics* 1974;**54**:201–7.

2774. Jackson JH. Unilateral epileptiform seizures, attended by tem-porary defect of sight. *Med Times Gaz* 1863;**1**:588.

2775. Jackson JH. Case of paralysis of the tongue from haemorrhage in the medulla oblongata. *Lancet* 1872; **2**:770–3.

2776. Jackson JH. Contribution to the comparative study of convul-sions. *Brain* 1886;**9**:1–23.

2777. Jackson JH. On a particular variety of epilepsy. *Brain* 1889;**11**:179–207.

2778. Jackson JH. Case of tumor of the middle lobe of the cerebellum: cerebellar paralysis with rigidity (cerebellar attitude), occasional tetanus-like seizures. *Brain* 1906;**29**:425–40.

2779. Jackson MJ, Schaefer JA, Johnson MA, et al. Presentation and clinical investigation of mitochondrial respiratory chain disease. *Brain* 1995;**118**:339–57.

2780. Jacobs EB, Landing BH, Thomas W. Vernicomyelia. Its bearing on theories of genesis of the Arnold-Chiari complex. *Am J Pathol* 1961;**39**:345–53.

2781. Jacobs JW, Bernhard MR, Delgado A, et al. Screening for organic mental syndromes in the medically ill. *Ann Intern Med* 1977;**86**:40–6.

2782. Jacobs L. Visual allesthesia. *Neurology* 1980;**30**:1059–63.

2783. Jacobs L, Grossman MD. Three primitive reflexes in normal adults. *Neurology* 1980;**30**:184–8.

2784. Jacobsen P. Ptosis, oligomimia and motor dysphasia in mental retardation. *Lancet* 1966;**1**:1379.

2785. Jacobson GP, Ramadan NR, Aggarwal SK, et al. The Henry Ford Hospital Headache Disability Inventory. *Neurology* 1994;**44**:837–42.

2786. Jacobson PL, Farmer TW. The hypernormal CT scan in dementia. *Neurology* 1979;**29**:1522–7.

2787. Jacobson RI. Classification of craniosynostosis. *Neurol Clin* 1985;**3**:117.

2788. Jacod M. Sur la propagation intracranienne des sarcomes de la trompe d'Eustache, syndrome du carrefour petro-sphenoidal, paralysie des 2, 3, 4, 5, et 6 paires craniennes. *Rev Neurol (Paris)* 1921;**37**:33–8.

2789. Jacome DE. Synkinetic blepharoclonus. *J Neuroophthalmol* 2000; **20**:276–84.

2790. Jacome DE. Dracula's teeth syndrome. *Headache* 2001;**41**:892–4.

2791. Jacome DE, FitzGerald R. Monocular ictal nystagmus. *Arch Neurol* 1982;**39**:653–6.

2792. Jacome DE, Risko M. Pseudocataplexy: gelastic-atonic seizures. *Neurology* 1984;**34**:1381–3.

2793. Jadassohn J, Lewandowski K. Pachyonychia congenita. In Neisser A, Jacobi E, eds. *Ikonographia Dermatologica*, p 29. Berlin: Urban & Schwarzenberg, 1906.

2794. Jaeken J, Carchon H. Congenital disorders of glycosylation; the rapidly growing tip of the iceberg. *Curr Opin Neurol* 2001;**14**:811–5.

2795. Jafari H, Couratier P, Camu W. Motor neuron disease after electrical injury. *J Neurol Neurosurg Psychiatry* 2001;**71**:265–7.

2796. Jaffe HL. Osteoid osteoma. Benign osteoblastic tumor composed of osteoid (atypical bone). *Arch Surg* 1935;**31**:709–28.

2797. Jahanshahi M, Hunter M, Philips C. The Headache Scale: an examination of its reliability and validity. *Headache* 1986;**26**:76–82.

2798. Jakob AM. Ueber eigenartige Erkrankungen des Zentralnervensystems mit bemerkenswertem anatomischem Befunde. *Z Ges Neurol Psychiatr* 1921;**64**:147–228.

2799. Jamal JA, Hansen S, Apertopoulos Feal. The "Gulf War syndrome". Is there evidence of dysfunction of the nervous system? *J Neurol Neurosurg Psychiatry* 1996;**60**:449–51.

2800. James DG, Sharma OP. Neurologic complications of sarcoidosis. *Proc R Soc Med* 1967;**60**:1169–70.

2801. James PB. Dysbarism; the medical problems from high and low atmospheric pressures. *J R Coll Physicians* 1993;**27**:367–74.

2802. James W. *Textbook of Psychology*. London: Macmillan, 1892.

2803. Jamieson PW, Katorji MB. Idiopathic generalized myokimia. *Muscle Nerve* 1994;**17**:42–51.

2804. Jampel RS, et al. Ophthalmoplegia and retinal degeneration associated with spinocerebellar ataxia. *Arch Ophthalmol* 1961;**6**:247–59.

2805. Jankovic J. Neuroacanthocytosis syndrome. *Neurology* 1985; **35**:1679.

2806. Jankovic J. Post-traumatic movement disorders. *Neurology* 1994; **44**:2006–14.

2807. Jankovic J, Fahn S. The phenomenology of tics. *Mov Disord* 1986; **1**:17–26.

2808. Jankovic J, Ford J. Blepharospasm and oro-facial-cervical dystonia: clinical and pharmacological findings in 100 patients. *Ann Neurol* 1983;**13**:407–11.

2809. Jankovic J, Kirkpatric JB, Blomquist KA. Late-onset Hallervorden-Spatz disease presenting as familial parkinsonism. *Neurology* 1985;**35**:227–34.

2810. Jankovic J, Leder S, Warner D, et al. Cervical dystonia: clinical findings and associated movement disorders. *Neurology* 1991;**41**: 1088–91.

2811. Jankovic J, Rivera VM. Hereditary myoclonus and progressive distal muscular atrophy. *Ann Neurol* 1979;**6**:227–31.

2811a. Jankovic J, Schwartz KS, Ondo W. Re-emergent tremor of Parkinson's disease. *J Neurol Neurosurg Psychiatry* 1999;**67**:646–650.

2812. Jannetta PJ. Hemifacial spasm. In Samii M, Jannetta PJ, eds. *The Cranial Nerves*, pp 484–93. Berlin: Springer-Verlag, 1981.

2813. Jannetta PJ, Moller MB, Moller AR. Disabling positional vertigo. *N Engl J Med* 1984;**310**:1700–5.

2814. Janz D. Epilepsy with impulsive petit mal (juvenile myoclonic epilepsy). *Acta Neurol Scand* 1985;**72**:339–59.

2815. Jaretzki AI, Barohn RJ, Ernstoff RM, et al. Myasthenia gravis: recommendations for clinical research standards. *Ann Thorac Surg* 2000;**70**:327–34.

2816. Jarrell HR. Vegas neuropathy. *N Engl J Med* 1981;**319**:1487.

2817. Jasper HH, Van Buren J. Interrelationships between cortex and subcortical structures: clinical electroencephalographic studies. *Electroencephalogr Clin Neurophysiol* 1953;**4**:168–202.

2818. Jastakj S. *The Wide Range Achievement Test*. Wilmington, DE: Guidance Associates, 1965.

2819. Jayam AV, Hass WK, Carr RE, Kumar AJ. Saturday night retinopathy. *J Neurol Sci* 1974;**22**:413–8.

2820. Jeavons PM. Nosological problems of myoclonic epilepsies in childhood and adolescence. *Dev Med Child Neurol* 1977;**19**:3–8.

2821. Jeavons PM, Harding GFA. Television epilepsy. *Lancet* 1970;**2**: 926–7.

2822. Jefferson G. Compression of the chiasma, optic nerves and optic tracts by intracranial aneurysms. *Brain* 1937;**60**:444–97.

2823. Jefferson G. On the saccular aneurysms of the internal carotid artery in the cavernous sinus. *Br J Surg* 1938;**26**:267–302.

2824. Jefferson G. Memories of Hugh Cairns. *J Neurol Neurosurg Psychiatry* 1959;**22**:155–66.

2825. Jeffreys R. Clinical and surgical aspects of posterior fossa haemangioblastomata. *J Neurol Neurosurg Psychiatry* 1975;**38**:105–11.

2826. Jelliffe SE. Sigmund Freud as a neurologist. *J Nerv Ment Dis* 1937; **85**:696–711.

2827. Jellinek EH. The orbital pseudotumour syndrome and its differentiation from endocrine exophthalmos. *Brain* 1969;**92**:35–58.

2828. Jellinek EH, Kelly RE. Cerebellar syndrome in myxoedema. *Lancet* 1960;**2**:225–7.

2829. Jellinger K. [Progressive pallidal atrophy]. *J Neurol Sci* 1968;**6**: 19–44.

2830. Jellinger K, Neumayer E. Progressive vascular myelopathy. *Acta Neurol Psychiatr Belg* 1962;**62**:944.

2831. Jellinger K, Seitelberger F. Protracted post-traumatic encephalopathy. Pathology, pathogenesis and clinical implications. *J Neurol Sci* 1970;**10**:51–94.

2832. Jellinger K, Seitelberger F. Spongy glioneural dystrophy in infancy and childhood. *Acta Neuropathol* 1970;**16**:125–40.

2833. Jen J, Cohen AH, Yue Q, et al. Hereditary endotheliopathy with retinopathy, nephropathy and stroke (HERNS). *Neurology* 1997;**49**: 1322–30.

2834. Jendrassik E. Beitrage zur Lehre von den Sehnenreflexen. *Arch Klin Med* 1883;**33**:177–99.

2835. Jenis EH, Lindquist RR, Lister RC. New congenital myopathy with crystalline intranuclear inclusions. *Arch Neurol* 1969;**20**:281–7.

2836. Jenkins JE. The Mozart effect. *J R Soc Med* 2001;**94**:170–2.

2837. Jenkyn LR, Walsh DB, Culver RG, Reeves AG. Clinical signs in diffuse cerebral dysfunction. *J Neurol Neurosurg Psychiatry* 1977;**40**: 956–66.

2838. Jenkyn LR, Walsh DB, Walsh BT, et al. The nuchocephalic reflex. *J Neurol Neurosurg Psychiatry* 1975; **38**:561–6.

2839. Jennekens FGI, Busch HFM, van Hemel NM. Inflammatory myopathy in scapulo-ilio-peroneal atrophy with cardiomyopathy. *Brain* 1975;**98**:709–22.

2840. Jennekens FGI, Veldman H, Vroegindeweij-Claessens LJHM, et al. Congenital oculo-bulbar palsy. *J Neurol Neurosurg Psychiatry* 1992; **55**:404–6.

2841. Jennekens FGI, Wokke JHJ. Proximal weakness of the extremities as main feature of amyloid myopathy. *J Neurol Neurosurg Psychiatry* 1987;**50**:1353–8.

2842. Jennett B. Post-traumatic epilepsy. *Arch Neurol* 1974;**30**:396–8.

2843. Jennett B. *Epilepsy After Non-Missile Head Injuries*. London: Heinemann, 1975.

2844. Jennett B, Bond M. Assessment of outcome after severe brain damage. *Lancet* 1975;**1**:480.

2845. Jennett B, Teasedale G, Braakman R, et al. Prognosis in series of patients with severe head injury. *Neurosurgery* 1979;**4**:283–300.

2846. Jennum P, Friberg L, Fuglsang-Frederiksen A, et al. Speech localization using repetitive transcranial magnetic stimulation. *Neurology* 1994;**44**:269–273.

2847. Jensen PK. Nerve deafness, optic nerve atrophy, and dementia: a new X-linked recessive syndrome? *Am J Med Genet* 1981;**9**:55–60.

2848. Jequier M, Deonna TW. A propos des dégénérescences neurosensorielles. *Schweiz Arch Neurol Psychiatrie* 1973;**112**:219–27.

2849. Jerritsen T, Waisman HA. Hypersarcosinemia. *N Engl J Med* 1966;**275**:66.

2850. Jerusalem F, Angelini C, Engel AG, et al. Mitochondria-lipid-glycogen (MLG) disease of muscle. *Arch Neurol* 1973;**29**:162–9.

2851. Jerusalem F, Engel AG, Gomez MR. Sarcotubular myopathy. *Neurology* 1973;**23**:897–906.

2852. Jerusalem F, Ludin H, Bischoff A, Hartmann G. Cytoplasmic body neuromyopathy presenting as respiratory failure and weight loss. *J Neurol Sci* 1979;**441**:1–9.

2853. Jerusalem F, Spiess H, Baumgartner G. Lipid storage myopathy with normal carnitine levels. *J Neurol Sci* 1975;**24**:273–82.

2854. Jervell A, Lange-Nielson F. Congenital deaf-mutism, functional heart disease with prolongation of the Q-T interval, and sudden death. *Am Heart J* 1957;**54**:59–68.

2855. Jervis GA. Early familial cerebellar degeneration (report of three cases in one family). *J Nerv Ment Dis* 1950;**111**:398–407.

2856. Jestico JV, Urry PA, Efphimiou J. An hereditary sensory and autonomic neuropathy transmitted as an X-linked recessive trait. *J Neurol Neurosurg Psychiatry* 1985;**48**:1259–64.

2857. Jeune M, et al. Syndrome familial associant ataxie, surdité et oligophrenic sclerose myocardique d'evolution fatale chez l'un des enfants. *Pediatrie* 1963;**18**:984–7.

2858. Jewsbury ECO. Insensitivity to pain. *Brain* 1951;**74**:336–53.

2859. Jia J, Pollock M. Cold nerve injury is enhanced by intermittent cooling. *Muscle Nerve* 1999;**22**:1644–52.

2860. Jobsis GJ, Boers JM, Barth PG, et al. Bethlehem myopathy: a slowly progrressive congenital muscular dystrophy with contractures. *Brain* 1999;**122**:649–55.

2861. Joffroy A. Nature et traitement du goitre exophthalmique. *Prog Med (Paris)* 1893;**18**:477–80.

2862. Jog MS, Lang AE. Chronic acquired hepatocerebral degeneration: case reports and new insights. *Mov Disord* 1995;**10**:714–22.

2863. Johnson J. Thomsen and myotonia congenita. *Med Hist* 1968;**12**:190–4.

2864. Johnson KP, Lepow ML, Johnson RT. California encephalitis. 1. Clinical and epidemiological studies. *Neurology* 1968;**18**:250–4.

2865. Johnson LC, Karpan W. Autonomic correlates of the spontaneous K-complex. *Psychophysiology* 1968;**4**:444–52.

2866. Johnson LV. Adherence syndrome: pseudoparalysis of lateral or superior rectus muscles. *Arch Ophthalmol Berlin* 1950;**44**:870–8.

2867. Johnson PC, Rolak LA, Hamilton RH, et al. Paraneoplastic vasculitis of nerve: a remote effect of cancer. *Ann Neurol* 1979;**5**:437–44.

2868. Johnson RJ, Bonfiglio M. Lipofibromatous hamartoma of the median nerve. *J Bone Jt Surg* 1969;**51A**:984.

2869. Johnson RT. The pathogenesis of acute viral encephalitis and postinfectious encephalomyelitis. *J Infect Dis* 1987;**155**:359–64.

2870. Johnson RV, Kaplan SR, Blailock ZR. Cerebral venous thrombosis in paroxysmal nocturnal hemoglobinuria. *Neurology* 1970;**20**:681–6.

2870a. Johnson TM, Moore HJ. A Cranial nerve X and XII paralysis (Tapia's syndrome) after an interscalene brachial plexus block for a left shoulder Mumford procedure. *Anesthesiology* 1999;**90**:311–2.

2871. Johnson WG. The clinical spectrum of hexoaminidase deficiency diseases. *Neurology* 1981;**31**:1453–6.

2872. Johnson WG, Chutorian AM, Miranda A. A new juvenile hexosaminidase deficiency disease presenting as cerebellar ataxia. *Neurology* 1977;**27**:1012–6.

2873. Johnson WG, Wigger HJ, Karp HR, et al. Juvenile spinal muscular atrophy: a new hexosaminidase deficiency phenotype. *Ann Neurol* 1982;**11**:11–6.

2874. Johnston AW, Mckay E. X-linked muscular dystrophy with contractures. *J Med Genet* 1986;**23**:591–5.

2875. Johnston JC, Rosenbaum DM, Picone CM, et al. Apraxia of eyelid opening secondary to right hemishere infarction. *Ann Neurol* 1989;**25**:622.

2876. Johnston W, Karpati G, Carpenter S. Late-onset mitochondriall myopathy. *Ann Neurol* 1995;**37**:16–23.

2877. Joliffe N, et al. Nicotinic acid deficiency encephalopathy. *JAMA* 1940;**114**:307–12.

2878. Jolly F. Pseudoparalysis myasthenica. *Neurol Zentralbl* 1895;**14**:34–6.

2879. Jones HR. EMG evaluation of the floppy infant: differential diagnosis and technical aspects. *Muscle Nerve* 1990;**13**:338–47.

2880. Joplin RJ. The proper digital nerve, vitallium stem arthroplasty and some thoughts about foot surgery in general. *Clin Orthop* 1971;**76**:199–212.

2881. Jordan A, Kelsall AR. Observations on a case of idiopathic hypoparathyroidism. *Arch Intern Med* 1951;**87**:242–58.

2882. Jordan BD. Neurologic aspects of boxing. *Arch Neurol* 1987;**44**:453–9.

2883. Jorgenson RJ. Ectodermal dysplasia with hypotrichosis, hypohydrosis, defective teeth, and unusual dermatoglyphics (Basan syndrome?). *Birth Defects* 1974;**10**:323–5.

2884. Joseph R, et al. Maladie familiale associant des convulsions a debut tres précoce, une hyperalbuminorachie et une hyperaminoaciduruie. *Arch Fr Pediatr* 1958;**15**:374–87.

2885. Joubert M, Eisenring JJ, Robb JP, Andermann F. Familial agenesis of the cerebellar vermis. *Neurology* 1969;**19**:813–25.

2886. Joutel A, Tournier-Lasserve E, Bousser MG, et al. Hemiplegic migraine [in French]. *Presse Med* 1995;**24**:411–4.

2887. Juba A. Contribution to the pathology of ballism. *Psychiatr Neurol (Belg)* 1957;**134**:81–96.

2888. Juberg RC, Hayward JR. A new familial syndrome of oral, cranial, and digital anomalies. *J Pediatr* 1969;**74**:755–62.

2889. Juberg RC, Hellman CD. A new familial form of convulsive didorder and mental retardation, limited to females. *J Pediatr* 1971;**79**:726–32.

2890. Juguilon A, Chad DA, Bradley WG, et al. Familial granulovacuolar lobular myopathy with electrical myotonia. *J Neurol Sci* 1983;**62**:261–79.

2891. Julien J, Vital C, Deleplanque B, et al. Subacute familial thalamic atrophy with memory disorders and complete insomnia. *Rev Neurol (Paris)* 1990;**146**:173–8.

2892. Julien J, Vital C, Vallant J, et al. Inclusion body myositis. *J Neurol Sci* 1982;**55**:15–24.

2893. Juncos JL, Beal MF. Idiopathic cranial polyneuropathy. *Brain* 1987;**110**:197–211.

2894. Juneja I, Yovic A. Hepatic decerebration. *Neurology* 1972;**22**:537–9.

2895. Jung HH, Hergersberg M, Kneifel S, et al. McLeod syndrome: a novel mutation, predominant psychiatric manifestations and distinct striatal imaging findings. *Ann Neurol* 2001;**49**:384–92.

2896. Jusic A, Dogan S, Stojanovic V. Hereditary persistent distal cramps. *J Neurol Neurosurg Psychiatry* 1972;**35**:379–84.

2897. Juvonen V, Hietala M, Paivarinta M, et al. Clinical and genetic findings in Finnish ataxia patients with the spinocerebellar ataxia 8 repeat expansion. *Ann Neurol* 2000;**48**:354–61.

2898. Kachi T, Rothwell JC, Cowan JM, et al. Writing tremor: its relation to benign essential tremor. *J Neurol Neurosurg Psychiatry* 1985;**48**:545–50.

2899. Kachi T, Sobue G, Yamamoto M, et al. Sensory conduction study in chronic sensory ataxic neuropathy. *J Neurol Neurosurg Psychiatry* 1994;**57**:941–944.

2900. Kaeser HE. Scapuloperoneal muscular atrophy. *Brain* 1965;**88**:407–18.

2901. Kahn A, Mozin MJ, Rebuffat E, et al. Difficulty in initiating and maintaining sleep associated with cows milk allergy in infants. *Sleep* 1987;**10**:116–21.

2902. Kahn E. A neurologic syndrome in infants recovering from malnutrition. *Arch Dis Child* 1954;**29**:256–61.

2903. Kahn RL, Goldfarb AI, Pollack M, Peck A. Brief objective measures for the determination of mental status in the aged. *Am J Psychiatry* 1960;**117**:326–8.

2904. Kaji R. Facts and fancies on writer's cramp. *Muscle Nerve* 2000;**23**:1313–5.

2905. Kakigi R, Shibasaki H. Generator mechanism of giant somatosensory potentials in cortical reflex myoclonus. *Brain* 1987;**110**:1359–73.

2906. Zakzanis KF. Ideomotor prosodic apraxia. *J Neurol Neurosurg Psychiatry* 1999;**67**:694–5.

2907. Kales A, Jacobson A, Paulson MJ, et al. Somnambulism. *Arch Gen Psychiatry* 1966;**14**:586–94.

2908. Kalimo H, Savontaus M-L, Lang H, et al. X-linked myopathy with excessive autophagy: a new hereditary muscle disease. *Ann Neurol* 1988;**23**:258–65.

2909. Kalkers NF, de Groot V, Lazeron RHC, et al. MS functional composite. *Neurology* 2000;**54**:1233–9.

2910. Kallmann FJ, et al. The genetic aspects of primary eunuchoidism. *Am J Ment Defic* 1943;**48**:203–36.

2911. Kalpakian B, Choy AE, Sparkes RS, et al. Duane syndrome associated with features of the cat-eye syndrome and mosaicism for a supernumerary chromosome probably derived from number 22. *J Pediatr Ophthalmol Strabismus* 1988;**25**:293–7.

2912. Kamaki M, Kawamura M, Moriya H, et al. Crossed homonymous hemianopia and crossed left hemispatial neglect in a case of Marchiafava-Bignami disease. *J Neurol Neurosurg Psychiatry* 1993;**56**:1027–32.

2913. Kane RE. Neurologic deficits following eepidural and spinal anesthesia. *Anesthesiol Analg* 1981;**60**:150–61.

2914. Kanemoto K, Watanabe Y, Tsuji T, et al. Rub epilepsy: a somatosensory evoked reflex epilepsy induced by prolonged cuteneous stimulation. *J Neurol Neurosurg Psychiatry* 2001;**70**:541–3.

2915. Kanjilal GC. Spontaneous cerebral ventriculostium: two cases. *J Neurol Neurosurg Psychiatry* 1972;**35**:676–81.

2916. Kanner L. Autistic disturbances of affective contact. *Nerv Child* 1943;**2**:217.

2917. Kanno T, Sudo K, Takeuchi I, et al. Hereditary deficiency of lactate dehydrogenase M subunit. *Clin Chem Acta* 1980;**108**:267–76.

2918. Kanouchi T, Yokota T, Kamata T, et al. Central pathway of photic reflex myoclonus. *J Neurol Neurosurg Psychiatry* 1997;**62**:414–7.

2919. Kantarjian AD. A syndrome clinically resembling amyotrophic lateral sclerosis following mercurialism. *Neurology* 1961;**11**:639–44.

2920. Kantola IM, Tarssanen LT. Diagnosis of familial hypokalemic periodic paralysis: role of the potassium exercise test. *Neurology* 1992;**42**:2158–61.

2921. Kaplan E, Goodglass H, Weintraub S. *The Boston Naming Test*. Philadelphia: Lea & Febiger, 1983.

2922. Kaplan H. Collateral circulation of the brain. *Neurology* 1961;**11**:S9–S15.

2923. Kaplan KG, Barasch E, Hirschfeld A, et al. Spinal epidural lipomatosis. *Neurology* 1989;**39**:1031–4.

2924. Kaplan P. X linked recessive inheritance of agenesis of the corpus callosum. *J Med Genet* 1983;**20**:122–4.

2925. Kaplan P, Genoud D, Ho TW, et al. Etiology, neurologic correlations and prognosis in alpha coma. *Aust NZ J Med* 1979;**9**:448–50.

2926. Kaplan RE, Lacey DJ. Bengn familial neonatal and infantile seizures. *Am J Med Genet* 1983;**16**:595–9.

2927. Kapur N. The coin-in-the-hand test. *J Neurol Neurosurg Psychiatry* 1993;**56**:385–6.

2928. Kapur N. Transient epileptic amnesia—a clinical update and a reformulation. *J Neurol Neurosurg Psychiatry* 1993;**56**:1184–90.

2929. Kar NC, Pearson CM, Verity MA. Muscle fructose 1.6 diphosphate deficiency associated with an atypical central core disease. *J Neurol Sci* 1980;**48**:243–56.

2930. Karacan I. Painful nocturnal penile erections. *JAMA* 1971;**215**:1831.

2931. Karadimas CL, Greenstein P, Sue CM, et al. Recurrent myoglobinuria due to a missense mutation in the *COX1* gene of mitochondrial DNA. *Neurology* 2000;**55**:644–9.

2932. Karch SB, Urich H. Medulloepithelioma: definition of an entity. *J Neuropathol Exp Neurol* 1972;**31**:27–53.

2933. Karnath H-O, Ferber S, Dichgans J. The origin of contraversive pushing. *Neurology* 2000;**55**:1298–304.

2934. Karnofsky DA, Burchenal JH, Armistead GC, et al. Triethylene melamine in the treatment of malignant disease. *Arch Intern Med* 1951;**87**:477–516.

2935. Karp BI, Hallett M. Extracorporeal 'phantom' tics in Tourettes syndrome. *Neurology* 1996;**46**:38–40.

2936. Karpati G, Carpenter S. Idiopathic inflammatory myopathies. *Curr Opin Neurol Neurosurg* 1988;**1**:806–14.

2937. Karpati G, Carpenter S, Eisen A, et al. Multiple peripheral nerve entrapments. *Arch Neurol* 1974;**31**:418–22.

2938. Karpati G, Carpenter S, Engel AG, et al. The syndrome of systemic carnitine deficiency. *Neurology* 1975;**25**:16–24.

2939. Karpati G, Carpenter S, Larbrisseau A, Lafontaine R. The Kearns-Shy syndrome. *J Neurol Sci* 1973;**19**:133–51.

2940. Karpati G, Carpenter S, Wolfe LS, et al. Juvenile dystonic lipidosis: an unusual form of neurovisceral storage disease. *Neurology* 1977;**27**:32–42.

2941. Karpati G, Engel WK. "Type grouping" in skeletal muscles after experimental reinnervation. *Neurology* 1968;**18**:447–55.

2942. Karpati G, et al. Myopathy caused by a deficiency of calcium-ATP in sarcoplasmic reticulum. *Ann Neurol* 1986;**20**:33–49.

2943. Karsch J. Erbliche Augenmissbildung in Verbindung mit Spalyhand und -Fuss. *Z Augenheilkd* 1936;**89**:274–9.

2944. Karson CN. Spontaneous eye-blink rates and dopaminergic systems. *Brain* 1983;**106**:643–53.

2945. Kasarskis EJ, Winslow M. When did Lou Gehrig's personal illness begin? *Neurology* 1989;**39**:1243–5.

2946. Kasch H, Bach FW, Jensen TS. Handicap after acute whiplash injury. *Neurology* 2001;**56**:1637–43.

2947. Kase CS. Case records of the M.G.H. (cerebral amyloid angiopathy). *N Engl J Med* 1988;**318**:623–31.

2948. Kasim S, Moo LR, Zschocke J, et al. Phenylketonuria presenting in adulthood as progressive spastic paraparesis with dementia. *J Neurol Neurosurg Psychiatry* 2001;**71**:795–7.

2949. Kasman M, Bernstein L, Schulman S. Chronic polyradiculoneuropathy of infancy. *Neurology* 1976;**26**:565–73.

2950. Katz DA, Naseem A, Horoupian DS, et al. Familial multisystem atrophy with possible thalamic dementia. *Neurology* 1984;**34**:1213–7.

2951. Katz DI, Alexander MP, Mandell AM. Dementia following strokes in the mesencephalon and diencephalon. *Arch Neurol* 1987;**44**:1127–33.

2952. Katz JD, Ropper AH. Progressive necrotic myelopathy. *Arch Neurol* 2000;**57**:355–361.

2953. Katz JS, Saperstein DS, Gronseth G, et al. Distal acquired demyelinating symmetric neuropathy. *Neurology* 2000;**54**:615–20.

2954. Katz JS, Wolfe GI, Anderss PB, et al. Brachial amyotrophic diplegia—a slowly progressive motor neurone disorder. *Neurology* 1999;**53**:1071–6.

2955. Katz MM, Lyerly SB. Methods of measuring adjustment and social behaviour in the community 1. *Psychol Rep* 1963;**13**:503–35.

2956. Katz S. Assessing self-maintenance: activities of daily living, mobility and instrumental activities of daily living. *J Am Geriatr Soc* 1983;**31**:721.

2957. Katz S, Ford AB, Moskowitz RW, et al. Studies of illness in the aged: the index of ADL—a standardized measure of biological and psychosocial function. *JAMA* 1963;**185**:914–9.

2958. Katzin RC. Arm rolling test. *Neurology* 1995;**45**:203.

2959. Katzman R. Alzheimer's disease. *N Engl J Med* 1986;**314**:964–73.

2960. Kaufman B. The "empty sella turcica": a manifestation of the intrasellar subarachnoid space. *Radiology* 1968;**90**:931–41.

2961. Kaufman DK, Kimmel DW, Parisi J, et al. A familial syndrome with cutaneous malignant melanoma and cerebral astrocytoma. *Neurology* 1993;**43**:1728–31.

2962. Kaufman MD. Masticatory spasm in facial hemiatrophy. *Ann Neurol* 1980;**7**:585–7.

2963. Kaufman MD, Hopkins LC, Hurwitz BJ. Progressive sensory neuropathy in patients without carcinoma. *Ann Neurol* 1981;**9**:237–42.

2964. Kaufman RL, et al. An oculocerebral facial syndrome. *Birth Defects* 1971;**7**:135–8.

2965. Kaufman S, et al. Phenylketonuria due to a deficiency of dihydropteridine reductase. *N Engl J Med* 1975;**293**:785.

2966. Kaufman S, et al. Hyperphenylalaninemia due to a deficiency of biopterin. *N Engl J Med* 1978;**299**:673.

2967. Kaufmann WE, Galaburda AM. Cerebrocortical microdysgenesis in neurologically normal subjects: a histopathologic study. *Neurology* 1989;**39**:238–44.

2968. Kavanaugh GJ, Svien HJ, Holman CB, et al. "Pseudoclaudication" syndrome produced by compression of the cauda equina. *JAMA* 1968;**206**:2477–81.

2969. Kawamura M, Hirayama K, Shinohara Y, et al. Alloesthesia. *Brain* 1987;**110**:225–36.

2970. Kawanami T, Kato T, Daimon M, et al. Hereditary ceruloplasmin deficiency: clinicopathological study of a patient. *J Neurol Neurosurg Psychiatry* 1996;**61**:506–9.

2971. Kayden NJ, Reagan TJ, Mize CE, et al. Diffuse cerebral sclerosis erroneously reported as Refsum's disease. *Arch Neurol* 1973;**28**:304–7.

2972. Kaye JA. Diagnostic challenges in dementia. *Neurology* 1998;**51** (**Suppl 1**):S45–S52.

2973. Kaye K, Grigsby J, Robbins LJ, et al. Prediction of independent functioning and behavior problems in geriatric patients. *J Am Geriatr Soc* 1990;**38**:1304–10.

2974. Kayser B. Ueber einen Fall von angeborener grunlicher Verfarbung der Cornea. *Klin Monatsbl Augenheilkd* 1902;**40**:22–5.

2975. Keane JR. Spastic eyelids: failure of levator inhibition in unconscious states. *Arch Neurol* 1975;**32**:695–8.

2976. Keane JR. Gaze-evoked blepharoclonus. *Ann Neurol* 1978;**3**:243–5.

2977. Keane JR. Neuro-ophthalmologic signs and symptoms of hysteria. *Neurology* 1982;**32**:757–62.

2978. Keane JR. Galloping tongue: post-traumatic, episodic, rhythmic movements. *Neurology* 1984;**34**:251–2.

2979. Keane JR. Pretectal pseudobobbing: five patients with "V"-pattern convergence nystagmus. *Arch Neurol* 1985;**42**:592–4.

2980. Keane JR. Wrong-way deviation of the tongue with hysterical hemiparesis. *Neurology* 1986;**36**:1406–7.

2981. Keane JR. Lid opening apraxia in Wilson's disease. *J Clin Neuroophthalmol* 1988;**8**:31.

2982. Keane JR. Neurectasy. *Neurology* 1990;**40**:829–31.

2983. Keane JR. The pretectal syndrome: 206 patients. *Neurology* 1990;**40**:684–90.

2984. Keane JR, Itabashi HH. Upbeat nystagmus: clinicopathologic study of two patients. *Neurology* 1987;**37**:491.

2985. Kearns TP. Differential diagnosis of central retinal vein obstruction. *Ophthalmology* 1983;**90**:475–80.

2986. Kearns TP, Sayre GP. Retinitis pigmentosa, external ophthalmoplegia and complete heart block. *Arch Ophthalmol Berlin* 1958;**60**:280–9.

2987. Keay AJ, Lewis IC. The Bonnevie-Ullrich syndrome. *Arch Dis Child* 1954;**29**:424.

2988. Keesey JC. Contemporary opinions about Mary Walker. *Neurology* 1998;**51**:1433–9.

2989. Keime-Guibert F, Napolitano M, Delattre J-Y. Neurological complications of radiotherapy and chemotherapy. *J Neurol* 1998;**245**:695–708.

2990. Keipert JA, et al. A new syndrome of broad terminal phalanges and facial abnormalities. *Aust Paediatr J* 1973;**9**:10–3.

2990a. Keith NM, Wagener HP, Barker NW. Some different types of essential hypertension: Their course and prognosis. *Am J Med Sci* 1939;**197**:332–43.

2991. Keith RA, Granger CV, Hamilton BB, Sherwin FS. The functional independence measure: a new tool for rehabilitation. In Eisenberg MG, Grzesiak RC, eds. *Advances in Clinical Rehabilitation*. New York: Springer-Verlag, 1987;**1**:6–18.

2992. Keller M, Hiltbrunner B, Dill C, et al. Reversible neuropsychological deficits after mild traumatic brain injury. *J Neurol Neurosurg Psychiatry* 2000;**68**:761–4.

2993. Kelley RI, et al. Neonatal adrenoleukodystrophy: new cases, biochemical studies and differentiation from Zellweger and related perioxysomal polydystrophy syndromes. *Am J Med Genet* 1986;**23**:869–901.

2994. Kelley RI, Moser HW. Hyperpipecolic acidemia in neonatal adrenoleukodystrophy. *Am J Med Genet* 1984;**19**:791–5.

2995. Kelley EC. *Encyclopedia of Medical Sources.* Baltimore: Williams and Wilkins, 1948.

2996. Kelly JJ. Peripheral neuropathies associated with monoclonal proteins: a clinical review. *Muscle Nerve* 1985;**8**:138–50.

2997. Kelly JP, Rosenberg JH. Diagnosis and management of concussion in sports. *Neurology* 1997;**48**:575–80.

2998. Kelly R. Colloid cysts of the third ventricle. *Brain* 1951;**74**:23–65.

2999. Kelly RI, Data NS, Dobyns WB, et al. Neonatal adrenoleukodystrophy. *Am J Med Genet* 1986;**23**:869.

3000. Kelly RI, et al. The association of the DiGeorge anomaly with partial monosomy of chromosome 22. *J Pediatr* 1982;**101**:197.

3001. Kelly TE. Teratogenicity of anticonvulsant drugs. *Am J Med Genet* 1984;**19**:413–34.

3002. Kemper T. Paul Ivan Yakovlev: 1894–1983. *Arch Neurol* 1984;**41**:536–40.

3003. Kennard C, Swash M. Acute viral encephalitis. *Brain* 1981;**104**:129–48.

3004. Kennaway NG, Buist NRM. Metabolic studies in a patient with hepatic cytosol tyrosine aminotransferase deficiency. *Pediatr Res* 1971;**5**:287.

3005. Kennedy F. Retrobulbar neuritis as an exact diagnostic sign of certain tumors and abscesses in the frontal lobes. *Am J Med* 1911;**142**:355–68.

3006. Kennedy WR, Alter M, Sung JH. Progressive proximal spinal and bulbar muscular atrophy of late onset. A sex-linked recessive trait. *Neurology* 1968;**18**:671–80.

3007. Kennedy WR, Sakuta M, Sutherland D, et al. Quantitation of the sweating defect in diabetes mellitus. *Ann Neurol* 1984;**15**:482–8.

3008. Kerkhoff G. Neurovisual rehabilitation: recent developments and future directions. *J Neurol Neurosurg Psychiatry* 2000;**68**:691–706.

3009. Kern WH. Proliferative myositis: a pseudosarcomatous reaction to injury. *Arch Pathol* 1960;**69**:209–16.

3010. Kernig VM. Ein Krankheitssymptom der acuten Meningitis. *St Petersb Med Wochenschr* 1882;**7**:398.

3011. Kernohan JW, Sayre GP. *Atlas of Tumor Pathology: Tumors of the CNS.* Washington, DC: Armed Forces Institute of Pathology, 1993.

3012. Kernohan JW, Woltman HW. Incisura of the crus due to contralateral brain tumour. *Arch Neurol Psychiatry* 1929;**21**:274–87.

3013. Kerns RD, Turk DC, Rudy TE. The West Haven-Yale Multidimensional Pain Inventory. *Pain* 1985;**23**:345–56.

3014. Kerr A, Derbes VJ. The syndrome of cough syncope. *Ann Intern Med* 1953;**39**:1240–53.

3015. Kerr GW, Parke TR. Scombroid poisoning—a pseudoallergic syndrome. *J R Soc Med* 1998;**91**:83–4.

3016. Kerrigan JF, Aleck KA, Tarby TJ, et al. Fumaric aciduria: clinical and imaging features. *Ann Neurol* 2000;**47**:583–8.

3017. Kertesz A. Paroxysmal kinesigenic choreoathetosis. *Neurology* 1967;**17**:680–90.

3018. Kertesz A. *The Western Aphasia Battery.* New York: Grune and Stratton, 1982.

3019. Kertesz A, Benson F. Neologistic jargon—a clinicopathological study. *Cortex* 1970;**6**:362–86.

3020. Kertesz A, Davidson W, Fox H. Frontal Behavioral Inventory: diagnostic criteria for frontal lobe dementia. *Can J Neurol Sci* 1997;**24**:29–36.

3021. Kertesz A, Hudson L, MacKenzie IRA, et al. The pathology and nosology of primary progressive aphasia. *Neurology* 1994;**44**:2065–72.

3022. Kertesz A, Martinez-Lage P, Davidson W, et al. The corticobasal degeneration syndrome overlaps progressive aphasia and frontotemporal dementia. *Neurology* 2000;**55**:1368–75.

3023. Kertesz A, Nicholson I, Cancelliere A, et al. Motor impersistence: a right-hemisphere syndrome. *Neurology* 1985;**35**:662–6.

3024. Kertesz A, Poole E. The Aphasia Quotient: the taxonomic approach to measurement of aphasic disability. *Can J Neurol Sci* 1974;**1**:7–16.

3025. Kertesz A, Sheppard A, MacKenzie R. Localization in transcortical sensory aphasia. *Arch Neurol* 1982;**39**:475–8.

3026. Keshavan MS. The ear wigglers: tics of the ear in ten patients. *Am J Psychiatry* 1988;**145**:1462–3.

3027. Keutel J, et al. Eine wahrscheinlich autosomal recessive vererbte Skeletmissbildung mit Humeroradialsynostose. *Humangenetik* 1970;**9**:43–53.

3028. Keynes G. The history of myasthenia gravis. *Med Hist* 1961;**5**:313–25.

3029. Khaleeli AA, Levy RD, Edwards RH, et al. The neuromuscular features of acromegaly: a clinical and pathological study. *J Neurol Neurosurg Psychiatry* 1984;**47**:1009–115.

3030. Khalifeh RR, Zellweger H. Hereditary sensory neuropathy with spinal cord disease. *Neurol Minneap* 1963;**13**:405–11.

3031. Khurana RK, Watabiki S, Hebel JR, et al. Cold face test in the assessment of trigeminal-brainstem-vagal function in humans. *Ann Neurol* 1980;**7**:144–9.

3031a. Khurana VG, Perez-Terzic CM, Petersen R, et al. Singing paraplegia: A distinctive manifestation of a spinal dural arteriovenous fistula. *Neurology* 2002;**58**:279–81.

3032. Kibler RF, Rose FC. Peripheral neuropathy in the collagen diseases. *BMJ* 1960;**1**:1781–1784.

3033. Kidd D, Steuer A, Denman AM, et al. Neurological complications in Behçet's syndrome. *Brain* 1999;**122**:2183–94.

3034. Kidd M. An electron microscopical study of a case of atypical cerebral lipidosis. *Acta Neuropathol* 1967;**9**:70.

3035. Kienbock R. Kritik der sogenannten "traumatischen Syringomyelie". *Jahrb Psychiatr* 1902;**21**:50–210.

3036. Kilgare S, Laker GW. Hallervorden-Spatz syndrome and brain iron metabolism. *Arch Neurol Psychiatry* 1946;**56**:401.

3037. Kiloh LG, Nevin S. Progressive dystrophy of external ocular muscles (ocular myopathy). *Brain* 1951;**74**:115–43.

3038. Kiloh LG, Nevin S. Isolated neuritis of the anterior interosseous nerve. *BMJ* 1952;**1**:850–1.

3039. Kim JH, Shucart WA, Haimovici H. Symptomatic arachnoid diverticula. *Arch Neurol* 1974;**31**:35–7.

3040. Kim JS. Smile-wink phenomenon. *J Neurol* 2001;**248**:389–93.

3041. Kim JY, Lee KW, Roh JK, et al. A clinical study of benign focal amyotrophy. *J Korean Med Sci* 1994; **9**:145–54.

3042. Kim YJ, Pakiam AS-I, Lang AE. Historical and clinical features of psychogenic tremor: a review of 70 cases. *Can J Neurol Sci* 1999;**2**: 190–5.

3043. Kim JS, Lopez I, DiPatre DL, et al. Internal auditory artery infarction. *Neurology* 1999;**52**:40–4.

3044. Kimoff RJ, Cosio MG, McGregor M. Clinical features and treatment of obstructive sleep apnea. *CMAJ* 1991;**144**:689–95.

3045. Kimura J. *Electrodiagnosis in Diseases of Nerve and Muscle.* Philadelphia: F.A. Davis, 1983.

3046. Kindler P. Morning glory syndrome: unusual congenital disk abnormality. *Am J Ophthalmol* 1970;**69**:376.

3047. Kindstrand E, Nilsson BY, Hovmark A, et al. Peripheral neuropathy in acrodermatitis chronica atrophicans—a late borrelia manifestation. *Acta Neurol Scand* 1997;**95**:338–45.

3048. King JO, Denborough MA. Anesthetic induced malignant hyperexia in children. *J Pediatr* 1973;**83**:37–40.

3049. Kingston W, Moxley RT, Griggs RC, et al. Flier syndrome: muscle cramps, acanthocytosis nigricans, acral hypertrophy and insulin resistance. *Ann Neurol* 1982;**12**:79.

3050. Kinney H, Burger PC, Vogel FSY. Subacute diencephalic angioencephalopathy: report of an additional case. *J Neurol Sci* 1980; **45**:73–81.

3051. Kinney HC, Filiano JJ, Brazy JE, et al. Congenital apnea with medullary and olivary hypoplasia. *Clin Neuropathol* 1989;**8**:163–73.

3052. Kinsbourne M. Myoclonic encephalopathy of infants. *J Neurol Neurosurg Psychiatry* 1962;**25**:271–6.

3053. Kinsbourne M. Hiatus hernia with contortions of the neck. *Lancet* 1964;**1**:1058–61.

3054. Kinsbourne M. The cerebral basis of lateral asymmetries in attention. *Acta Psychol* 1970;**33**:193–201.

3055. Kinsbourne M, Warrington EK. A study of finger agnosia. *Brain* 1962;**85**:47–66.

3056. Kinsella SM, Tuckey JP. Perioperative bradycardia and asystole: relationship to vasovagal syncope and the Bezold-Jarisch reflex. *Br J Anaesth* 2001;**86**:859–68.

3056a. Kinton L, Johnson MR, Smith SJ, et al. Partial epilepsy with pericentral spikes: A new familial epilepsy syndrome with evidence for linkage to chromosome 4p15. *Ann Neurol* 2002;**51**:740–9.

3057. Kirby DM, Crawford M, Cleary MA, et al. Respiratory chain complex 1 deficiency: an underdiagnosed energy generation disorder. *Neurology* 1999;**52**:1255–64.

3058. Kirk A, Boyle CAJ. Radial neglect is caused by vertical neglect of an internal representation. *Can J Neurol Sci* 1994;**21**(**Suppl 2**):S51.

3059. Kirk A, Heilman KM. Auricular myoclonus. *Can J Neurol Sci* 1991;**18**:503–4.

3060. Kirkham TH. The ocular symptomatology of pituitary tumours. *Proc R Soc Med* 1972;**65**:517–8.

3061. Kirshner HS, Tanridag O, Thurman L, et al. Progressive aphasia without dementia: two cases with focal spongiform degeneration. *Ann Neurol* 1987;**22**:527–32.

3062. Kisch B. Horners syndrome: an American discovery. *Bull Med Hist* 1951;**25**:284–8.

3063. Kish SJ, Dixon LM, Burnham WM, et al. Brain neurotransmitters in glycine encephalopathy. *Ann Neurol* 1988;**24**:458–61.

3064. Kissel P, Arnould G, André JM. Incidence des accidents vasculaires cerebraux au cours des conjonctivo dysplasies hereditaires. *J Genet Hum* 1972;**29**:151–67.

3065. Kistler JP, Lott IT, Kolodny EH, et al. Mannosidosis: new clinical presentation, enzyme studies, and carbohydrate analysis. *Arch Neurol* 1977;**34**:45–51.

3066. Kitagawa M, Fukushima J, Tashiro K. Relationship between antisaccades and the clinical symptoms in Parkinson's disease. *Neurology* 1994;**44**:2285–9.

3067. Kitamoto T, Amano N, Terao Y, et al. A new inherited prion disease (PrP-P105L mutation) showing spastic paraparesis. *Ann Neurol* 1993;**34**:808–13.

3068. Kite WC. Seizures associated with the Catlin mark. *Neurology* 1961;**11**:345–8.

3069. Kitka DG, Breuer A, Wilbourn AJ. Thoracic root pain in diabetes. *Ann Neurol* 1982;**11**:80–3.

3070. Kiuru S, Seppalainen A-M. Neuropathy in familial amyloidosis, Finnish type (FAF): electrophysiological studies. *Muscle Nerve* 1994;**17**: 299–304.

3071. Kivlin JD, Sanborn GE, Myers GG. The cherry-red spot in Tay-Sachs and other storage diseases. *Ann Neurol* 1985;**17**:356–60.

3072. Kiwaki T, Umehara F, Takashima H, et al. Hereditary motor and sensory neuropathy with myelin folding and juvenile onset glaucoma. *Neurology* 2000;**55**:392–7.

3073. Kjellin K. Familial spastic paraplegia with amyotrophy, oligophrenia and central retinal degeneration. *Arch Neurol* 1959;**1**: 133–40.

3074. Kjer P. Infantile optic atrophy with dominant mode of inheritance. *Acta Ophthalmol* 1959;**Suppl 54**:1.

3075. Klass DW, Westmoreland BF. Nonepileptogenic epileptiform electroencephalographic activity. *Ann Neurol* 1985;**18**:627–35.

3076. Klatzky RL. *Human Memory.* San Francisco: W.H. Freeman, 1980.

3077. Klawans HL. Hemiparkinsonism as a late complication of hemiatrophy: a new syndrome. *Neurology* 1981;**31**:625–8.

3078. Klein D. *Arch Julius Klaus-Stift* 1947;**22**:336.

3079. Klein R, Hadow JE, DeLuca C. Familial congenital disorder resembling stiff-man syndrome. *Am J Dis Child* 1972;**124**:730–1.

3080. Kleine W. Periodische Schlafsucht. *Monatschr Psychiatr* 1925; **57**:285–320.

3081. Kleist K. Gegenhalten (motorischer Negativsmus) Zwangsgreifen und Thalamus Opticus. *Monatschr Psychiatrie Neurol* 1927; **65**:317.

3082. Kline LB, Hoyt WF. The Tolosa-Hunt syndrome. *J Neurol Neurosurg Psychiatry* 2001;**71**:577–82.3083. Klingele TC, Burde RM, Rappazzo JA, et al. Paraneoplastic retinopathy. *J Clin Neuroophthalmol* 1984;**4**:239–45.

3084. Klingman WO, Hodges RG. Acute ataxia of unknown origin in children. *J Pediatr* 1944;**24**:536–43.

3085. Klintworth GK. The neurological manifestations of osteopetrosis. *Neurology* 1963;**13**:512–9.

3086. Klippel M. Concerning spontaneous thumb flexion in hemiplegic contractures. *Rev Neurol (Paris)* 1909;**17**:506–7.

3087. Klippel M, Feil A. Un cas d'absence des vertèbres cervicales avec cage thoracic remontant jusqu'a la base du crâne (cage thoracique cervicale). *Nouv Icon Salpet* 1912;**25**:223–50.

3088. Klippel M, Felstein E. L'hypertrophie cranienne simple familiale. *Nouv Icon Salpet* 1913;**26**:445–51.

3089. Klippel M, Trenaunay P. Du noevus variqueux osteohypertrophique. *Arch Gen Med Paris* 1900;**3**:641–72.

3090. Klockgether T, Ludkte R, Kramer B, et al. The natural history of degenerative ataxia: a retrospective study in 466 patients. *Brain* 1998; **121**:589–600.

3091. Kloepfer HW. Kloepfer syndrome, *Proceedings of the 10th International Conference on Genetics*, Toronto: University of Toronto Press, 1958–9;**1**:146.

3092. Kluin KJ, Foster NL, Berent S, et al. Perceptual analysis of speech disorders in progressive supranuclear palsy. *Neurology* 1993;**43**:563–6.

3093. Kluver H, Bucy PC. "Psychic blindness" and other symptoms following bilateral temporal lobectomy in rhesus monkeys. *Am J Physiol* 1937;**119**:352–3.

3094. Knapp HJ. On the formation of dark angioid streaks as an unusual metamorphosis of retinal hemorrhage. *Arch Ophthalmol* 1892;**21**:289–92.

3095. Knapp PC. Astasia-abasia, with the report of a case of paroxysmal trepidant abasia, associated with paralysis agitans. *J Nerv Ment Dis* 1891;**17**:673–703.

3096. Knaus WA, Draper EA, Wagner DP, et al. APACHE II: a severity of disease classification system. *Crit Care Med* 1985;**13**:818–29.

3097. Knaus WA, et al. Trauma severity classification. *Crit Care Med* 1985;**13**:818–29.

3098. Knight RSG, Anslow P, Theaker JM. Neoplastic angioendotheliosis: a case of subacute dementia with unusual cerebral CT appearances and a review of the literature. *J Neurol Neurosurg Psychiatry* 1987;**50**:1022–8.

3099. Knopman DS, Knapp MJ, Gracon SI, et al. The Clinician Interview-Based Impression (CIBI). *Neurology* 1994;**44**:2315–21.

3100. Knopman DS, Mastri AR, Frey WH, et al. Dementia lacking distinctive histological features. *Neurology* 1990;**40**:251–6.

3101. Knopman DS, Sung JH, Davis D. Progressive familial leukodystrophy of late onset. *Neurology* 1996;**46**:429–34.

3102. Knox DL. Ischemic ocular inflammation. *Am J Ophthalmol* 1965;**60**:995–1001.

3103. Knox DL, Clark DB, Schuster FF. Benign VI nerve palsies in children. *Pediatrics* 1967;**40**:560–4.

3104. Kny E. Concerning paramyoclonus multiplex (Friedreich). *Arch Psychiatr Nervenkr* 1888;**19** :577–90.

3105. Kobari M, Nogawa S, Sugimoto Y, et al. Familial idiopathic brain calcification with autosomal dominant inheritance. *Neurology* 1997;**48**:645–9.

3106. Kobayashi JS, Clarke M, Sullivan T. Familial congenital corneal anesthesia. *Can J Neurol Sci* 1993;**Suppl 2**:S37.

3107. Kobayashi O, Hayashi Y, Arahata K, et al. Congenital muscular dystrophy. *Neurology* 1996;**46**:815–8.

3108. Kobori JA, Herrick MK, Urich H. Arhinencephaly. *Brain* 1987;**110**:237–60.

3109. Kocher T. Zur Verhuntung des Cretinismus und cretinoider Zustande nach neuen Forschungen. *Dtsch Z Nervenklinik* 1892;**34**:556–626.

3110. Koebbe CJ, Sherman JD, Warnick RE. Distant wounded glioma syndrome: report of two cases. *Neurosurgery* 2001;**48**:940–3.

3111. Koehler PJ, Endtz LJ. Between Magendie and Brown-Séquard: Isaac van Deen's spinal hemisections. *Neurology* 1989;**39**:446–8.

3112. Koeppen AH, Dickson AC, Chu RC, et al. The pathogenesis of superficial siderosis of the central nervous system. *Ann Neurol* 1993;**34**:646–53.

3113. Koerber HL. Ueber drei Falle von Retraktionsbewegung des Bulbus. *Ophthalmol Klin* 1903;**7**:65–7.

3114. Kohlschutter A, Chappuis D, Meier C, et al. Familial epilepsy and yellow teeth—a disease of the CNS associated with enamel hypoplasia. *Helv Pediatr Acta* 1974;**29**:283–94.

3115. Koizumi J, Ofuku K, Sakuma K, et al. CNS changes in Usher's syndrome with mental disorder: CT, MRS, and PET findings. *J Neurol Neurosurg Psychiatry* 1988;**51**:987–90.

3116. Koizumi K, Levine DG, Brooks CM. Effect of tetrodotoxin (puffer fish toxin) on the central nervous system. *Neurology* 1967;**17**:395–404.

3117. Koller WC. Adult onset foot dystonia. *Neurology* 1984;**34**:703.

3118. Koller WC. How accurately can Parkinson's disease be diagnosed? *Neurology* 1992;**42(Suppl)**:6–16.

3119. Kolmel HW. Complex visual hallucinations in the hemianopic field. *J Neurol Neurosurg Psychiatry* 1985;**48**:29–38.

3120. Kolodny EH. Agenesis of the corpus callosum: a marker for inherited metabolic disease? *Neurology* 1989;**39**:847–8.

3121. Kolodny EH, Cable WJL. Inborn errors of metabolism. *Ann Neurol* 1982;**11**:221–32.

3122. Komar J, Varga B. Syndrome of the rectus abdominis muscle. *J Neurol* 1975;**210**:121–5.

3123. Kondo K, Tsubaki T, Sakamoto F. The Ryukyan muscular atrophy. *J Neurol Sci* 1970;**11**:359–82.

3124. Konigsmark BW. Hereditary deafness in man. *N Engl J Med* 1969;**281**:713–20.

3125. Konigsmark BW, Weiner LP. The olivopontocerebellar atrophies: a review. *Medicine* 1970;**49**:227–41.

3126. Kono N, et al. Amyotrophy with acute haemorrhagic conjunctivitis. *J Infect Dis* 1974;**129**:590.

3127. Konrad PN, et al. Gamma glutamyl cysteine deficiency. *N Engl J Med* 1972;**286**:557.

3128. Kopell HP, Thompson WAL. *Peripheral Entrapment Neuropathies.* Malabar: Robert Krieger, 1976.

3129. Kopell HP, Thompson WAL, Postel AH. Entrapment neuropathy of the ilioinguinal nerve. *N Engl J Med* 1962;**266**:16.

3130. Korein J, Codder DR, Mowrey FH. The clinical syndrome of paroxysmal paralytic myoglobinuria. *Neurology* 1959;**9**:767–85.

3131. Korenblat P, Wedner H, Whyte M, et al. "Systemic mastocytosis". *Arch Intern Med* 1984;**144**:2249–53.

3132. Korf B, Waldman JK, Levy HL, et al. Bilateral lucency of the globus pallidus complicating methylmalonic acidemia. *Ann Neurol* 1986;**20**:364–6.

3133. Kori SH. Interventional neurology. *Neurology* 1993;**43**:2395–9.

3134. Kors EE, Terwindt GM, Vermeulen FLMG, et al. Delayed cerebral edema and fatal coma after minor head trauma: role of the *CACNA1A* calcium channel subunit gene and relationship with familial hemiplegic migraine. *Ann Neurol* 2001;**49**:753–60.

3135. Korsakov SS. Ob. alkogol'nom paraliche. *Vest Psikhiat* 1887;**4**.

3136. Korten JJ, Notermans SLH, Frenken CWGM, et al. Familial essential myoclonus. *Brain* 1974;**97**:131–8.

3137. Kosaka K. Diffuse neurofibrillary tangles with calcification: a new presenile dementia. *J Neurol Neurosurg Psychiatry* 1994;**57**:594–6.

3138. Koski L, Lacoboni MN, Mazziotta JC. Deconstructing stroke: understanding disorders of intentional movement after stroke. *Curr Opin Neurol* 2002;**15**:71–77.

3139. Koskinen T, Sainio K, Rapola J, et al. Sensory neuropathy in infantile onset spinocerebellar ataxia (IOSCA). *Muscle Nerve* 1994;**17**:509–15.

3140. Kost GJ, Verity MA. A new variant of late-onset myophopsphorylase deficiency. *Muscle Nerve* 1980;**3**:195–201.

3141. Kost RG, Strauss SE. Postherpetic neuralgia: pathogenesis, treatment and prevention. *N Engl J Med* 1996;**335**:32–42.

3142. Kothari MJ, Macintosh K, Heistand M, et al. Medial antebrachial cutaneous sensory studies in the evaluation of neurogenic thoracic outlet syndrome. *Muscle Nerve* 1998;**21**:647–9.

3143. Kousseff BG. Sacral meningocele with conotruncal heart defects: a possible autosomal recessive trait. *Pediatrics* 1984;**74**:395–8.

3144. Koutras A. Myositis with Kawasaki's disease. *Am J Dis Child* 1982;**136**:78–9.

3145. Kovanen J, Somer Heal, Schroeder P. Acute myopathy associated with gasoline sniffing. *Neurology* 1983;**33**:629.

3146. Kozhevnikov AY. Osobyi: vid kortikalnoi epilepsii. *Med Obozr* 1894;**42**:97–118.

3147. Kozlowski K, Maroteaux P, Spranger J. La dysostose spondylometaphysaire. *Presse Med* 1967;**75**:2769–74.

3148. Krabbe KH. A new familial infantile form of diffuse brain sclerosis. *Brain* 1916;**39**:74–114.

3148a. Krabbe KH. Focal and meningeal angiomatosis associated with calcifications of brain cortex. *Arch Neurol Psychiatr* 1934;**32**:737–55.

3149. Krabbe KH. Congenital generalised muscular atrophies. *Acta Psychiatr Scand* 1958;**33**:94.

3150. Kral VA. Senescent forgetfulness: benign and malignant. *CMAJ* 1962;**86**:257–60.

3151. Kramer JH, Reed BR, Mungas D, et al. Executive dysfunction in subcortical ischaemic vascular disease. *J Neurol Neurosurg Psychiatry* 2002;**72**:217–20.

3152. Kramer RE, Luders H, Goldstick LP, et al. Ictus emeticus: an electroclinical analysis. *Neurology* 1988;**38**:1048–52.

3153. Krams M, Quinton R, Mayston MJ, et al. Mirror movements in X-Linked Kallmann's syndrome. II. A PET study. *Brain* 1997;**120**:1217–29.

3154. Krane RJ, Siroky MB. *Clinical Neuro-Urology.* Boston: Little, Brown, 1979.

3155. Krarup C, Stewart JD, Sumner AJ, et al. A syndrome of asymmetric limb weakness with motor conduction block. *Neurology* 1990;**40:** 118–27.

3156. Kratz R, Brooke MH. *Distal Myopathy.* Amsterdam: North-Holland, 1979.

3157. Krause AC. Congenital encephalo-ophthalmic dysplasia. *Arch Ophthalmol Berlin* 1946;**36:**387–444.

3158. Krayenbuhl H, Siebermann R. Small vascular malformations as a cause of primary intracerebral hemorrhage. *J Neurosurg* 1965;**22:**7–20.

3159. Kretschmer E. Das apallische Syndrom. *Z Ges Neurol* 1940;**169:** 576–9.

3160. Kriegstein AR. The pathogenesis of epilepsy: relevance to therapy. *Curr Opin Neurol Neurosurg* 1988;**1:**200–5.

3161. Krill AE, Kline BA. Retinal syndrome. *Arch Ophthalmol* 1965; **74:**496.

3162. Krill AE, Smith VC, Pokorny J. Further studies supporting the identity of congenital tritanopia and hereditary dominant optic atrophy. *Invest Ophthalmol* 1971;**10:**457–65.

3163. Krishaber M. *Gaz Hebd Med Chir* 1872.

3164. Kritschevsky M, Squire LR. Permanent global amnesia with unknown etiology. *Neurology* 1993;**43:**326–32.

3165. Krugliak L, Gadofi N, Behan AJ. Neuropathic form of arthrygryposis multiplex congenita. *J Neurol Sci* 1978;**37:**179–85.

3166. Kruiansky J, Gurland B. The performance test of activities of daily living. *Int J Aging Hum Dev* 1976;**7:**343–52.

3167. Krumholz A. Nonepileptic seizures: diagnosis and management. *Neurology* 1999;**53:**S76–S83.

3168. Krumholz A, Bergey GK, Nathanson N. John Hughlings Jackson's observations on 'lower level' or 'pontobulbar' fits and their relevance to current concepts of seizures and myoclonus. *Neurology* 1994; **44:**1527–30.

3169. Krupp LB, Elkins LE. Fatigue and declines in cognitive functioning in multiple sclerosis. *Neurology* 2000;**55:**934–939.

3170. Krupp LB LaRocca NG, Muir-Nash J, et al. The fatigue severity scale. Application to patients with multiple sclerosis and systemic lupus erythematosus. *Arch Neurol* 1989;**46:**1121–3.

3171. Krupp LB, Pollina DA. Mechanisms and management of fatigue in progressive neurological disorders. *Curr Opin Neurol* 1996;**9:**456–60.

3172. Ksiasek SM, Repka MX, Maguire A, et al. Divisional oculomotor nerve paresis caused by intrinsic brainstem disease. *Ann Neurol* 1989;**26:**714–8.

3173. Ku A, Kern H, Lachman E, et al. Sciatic nerve impingement from piriformis hematoma due to prolonged labor. *Muscle Nerve* 1995; **18:**789–90.

3174. Kuban KCK, Leviton A. Cerebral palsy. *N Engl J Med* 1994; **330:**188–95.

3175. Kubik CS, Adams RD. Subdural empyema. *Brain* 1943;**66:**18–42.

3176. Kudo T. Spontaneous occlusion of the circle of Willis. *Neurology* 1968;**18:**485–96.

3177. Kudrow L. *Cluster Headache: Diagnosis and Management.* New York: Oxford University Press, 1980.

3178. Kudrow L, Esperanca P, Vijayan N. Episodic paroxysmal hemicrania? *Cephalalgia* 1987;**7:**197–201.

3179. Kufs A. Uber heredopofamiliare Angiomatose des Gehirns und der Retina, ihre Beziehungen zueinader und Angiomatose der Haut. *Zentralbl Ges Neurol Psychiatr* 1928;**112:**651–86.

3180. Kufs H. Uber eine Spatform der amaurotischen Idiotie und ihre heredofamiliaren Grundlagen. *Z Ges Neurol Psychiatr* 1925;**95:**169–88.

3181. Kugelberg E. Facial reflexes. *Brain* 1952;**75:**385–96.

3182. Kugelberg E, Hagbarth KE. Spinal mechanism of the abdominal and erector spinae skin reflexes. *Brain* 1958;**81:**290–304.

3183. Kugelberg E, Welander L. Heredofamilial juvenile muscular atrophy simulating muscular dystrophy. *Arch Neurol Psychiatry* 1956;**75:** 500–9.

3184. Kuijpers HC, Bleijenberg G. The spastic pelvic floor syndrome: a cause of constipation. *Dis Colon Rectum* 1985;**28:**669–72.

3185. Kulenkampff C. Ein eigentumliches Syndrom im oralen Bereich bei Megaphenapplikation. *Nervenarzt* 1956;**27:**178–80.

3186. Kulisevsky J, Marti-Fabregas J, Grau JM. Spasms of amputation stumps. *J Neurol Neurosurg Psychiatry* 1992;**55:**626–7.

3187. Kun LE. Postirradiation myelopathy in children. *Ann Neurol* 1979;**5:**106.

3188. Kuncl RW, Wiggins WW. Toxic myopathies. *Neurol Clin* 1988;**6:** 593–619.

3189. Kunishio K, Yamamoto Y, Sunami N. Histologic investigation of a case of meningoangiomatosis not associated with von Recklinghausen's disease. *Surg Neurol* 1987;**27:**575–9.

3190. Kunitz SC, Gross CR, Heyman A, et al. The pilot stroke data bank: definition, design, and data. *Stroke* 1984;**15:**740–6.

3191. Kuntzer T, Van Melle G, Regli F. Clinical and prognostic features in unilateral femoral neuropathies. *Muscle Nerve* 1997;**20:**205–11.

3192. Kuriansky JB, Gurland BJ, Fleiss JL, et al. The assessment of self-care capacity in geriatric psychiatric patients by objective and subjective methods. *J Clin Psychol* 1990;**32:**95–102.

3193. Kurihara T, Landau WM, Torack RM. Progressive supranuclear palsy with action myoclonus, seizures. *Neurology* 1974;**24:**219–23.

3194. Kurlan R. Tourette's syndrome: current concepts. *Neurology* 1989;**39:**1625–30.

3195. Kurlan R. Tourette's syndrome and PANDAs. *Neurology* 1998; **50:**1530–4.

3196. Kurlan R, Behr J, Medved L, et al. Transient tic disorder and the spectrum of Tourette's syndrome. *Arch Neurol* 1989;**45:**1200–1.

3197. Kurlan R, Behr J, Shoulson I. Hereditary myoclonus and chorea: the spectrum of hereditary nonprogressive hyperkinetic movement disorders. *Mov Disord* 1987;**2:**301–6.

3198. Kurtzke JF. Rating neurological impairment in multiple sclerosis: an expanded disability status scale (EDSS). *Neurology* 1983;**33:** 1444–52.

3199. Kurtzke JF. Neuroepidemiology. *Ann Neurol* 1984;**16:**265–77.

3200. Kurtzke JF. Optic neuritis or multiple sclerosis. *Arch Neurol* 1985;**42:**704–10.

3201. Kushner MJ, Parrish M, Burke A, et al. Nystagmus in motor neurone disease. *Ann Neurol* 1984;**16:**71–7.

3202. Kussmaul A. Die Storungen der Sprache. Versuch einer Pathologie der Sprache. In von Ziemssen HW, ed. *Handbuch der Speciellen Pathologie und Therapie,* pp 211–2. Lepzig: FCW Vogel, 1881.

3203. Kuter I. Systemic mastocytosis. *N Engl J Med* 1992;**326:**472–81.

3204. Kuzniecky R, Andermann F, Guerrini R, et al. The epileptic spectrum in the congenital bilateral perisylvian syndrome. *Neurology* 1994; **44:**379–85.

3205. Kuzniecky R, Andermann F, Tampieri D, et al. Bilateral cerebral macrogyria: epilepsy, pseudobulbar palsy, and mental retardation—a recognisable neuronal migration disorder. *Ann Neurol* 1989;**25:**547–54.

3206. Kuzniecky R, Berkovic S, Andermann F, et al. Focal cortical myoclonus and rolandic cortical dysplasia: clarification by magnetic resonance imaging. *Ann Neurol* 1988;**23:**317–25.

3207. Kuzuhara S, Kanakawa I, Sasaki H, et al. Gerstmann-Straussler-Scheinker's disease. *Ann Neurol* 1983;**14:**216–25.

3208. Kwok RHM. Chinese restaurant syndrome. *N Engl J Med* 1968; **278:**1122.

3209. Kwon SE, Heilman K. Ipsilateral neglect in a patient following a unilateral frontal lesion. *Neurology* 1991;**41:**2001–4.

3210. Kyle RA, Bayrd ED. Benign monoclonal gammopathy (monoclonal gammopathy of undetermined significance). In *The Monoclonal Gammopathies,* pp 284–368. Springfield, Ill: C.C. Thomas, 1976.

3211. Kyriakides T, Silberstein JM, Jongpiputvanich S, et al. The clinical significance of type 1 fiber predominance. *Muscle Nerve* 1993;**16:** 418–23.

3212. La Spada AR, Paulson HL, Fishbeck KH. Trinucleotide repeat expansion in neurological disease. *Ann Neurol* 1994;**36:**814–22.

3213. LaBan MM, Viola SL, Femminineo AF, et al. Restless legs syndrome associated with diminished cardiopulmonary compliance and lumbar spinal stenosis—a motor concomitant of Vespers curse. *Arch Phys Med Rehabil* 1990;**71:**384–8.

3214. Labrune P, Lacroix C, Goutieres F, et al. Extensive brain calcifications, leukodystrophy and formation of parenchymal cysts. *Neurology* 1996;**46:**1297–301.

3215. Lacerte D, Gagné F, Copty M. Intracranial chondroma. Report of cases and review of the literature. *Can J Neurol Sci* 1996;**23:**132–137.

3216. Lach B, Russell NA, Benoit B, Atack D. Cellular blue nevus (melanocytoma) of the spinal meninges. *Neurosurgery* 1988;**22:**773–80.

3217. Lacheretz M, Walbum CH, Tourgis R. L'acrocephalosynankie. A propos d'une observation avec synostoses multiples. *Pediatrie* 1974; **29:**169–77.

3218. Lacomis D, Smith TW, Chad DA. Acute myopathy and neuropathy in status asthmaticus: case report and literature review. *Muscle Nerve* 1993;**16:**84–90.

3219. Lacomis D, Zochodne DW, Bird SJ. Critical illness myopathy. *Muscle Nerve* 2000;**23:**1785–8.

3220. Lacruz F, Artieda J, Pastor MA, et al. The anatomical basis of somaesthetic temporal discrimination in humans. *J Neurol Neurosurg Psychiatry* 1991;**54:**1077–81.

3221. Lacson AG, Seshia SS, Sarnat HB, et al. Autosomal recessive, fatal infantile hypertrophic musular dystrophy among Canadian natives. *Can J Neurol Sci* 1994;**21:**203–212.

3222. Ladame P. Friedreich's disease. *Brain* 1890;**13:**467–537.

3223. Lader MH, Montagu JD. The psycho-galvanic reflex: a pharmacological study of the peripheral mechanism. *J Neurol Neurosurg Psychiatry* 1962;**25:**126–33.

3224. Lafora GR. Beitrag zur Histopathologie der myoklonischen Epilepsie. *Z Ges Neurol Psychiatr* 1911;**6:**1–14.

3225. Lagier R, Cox JN. Pseudomalignant myositis ossificans. *Hum Pathol* 1975;**6:**653–65.

3226. Lagueny P, et al. Amyotrophy after radiotherapy. *Rev Neurol (Paris)* 1985;**141:**222.

3227. Laing NG, Laing BA, Meredith C, et al. Autosomal dominant distal myopathy: linkage to chromosome 14. *Am J Hum Genet* 1995;**56:** 422–7.

3228. Lairy GC, Harrison A, Leger EM. Foyers EEG biocciptaux asynchrones de pointes chez l'enfant mal voyant et aveugle d'age scolaire. *Rev Neurol (Paris)* 1964;**111:**351–3.

3229. Lake BD, Wilson J. Zebra body myopathy. *J Neurol Sci* 1975;**24:** 437–46.

3230. Lambert CD, Young JRB. Hypertrophy of the branchial muscles. *J Neurol Neurosurg Psychiatry* 1976;**39:**810–6.

3231. Lambert EH, Eaton LM, Rooke ED. Myasthenia associated with small-cell carcinoma of the bronchus. *Am J Physiol* 1956;**187:**612–3.

3232. Lambert EH, Eaton lM, Roche ED. Defects of neuromuscular conduction associated with malignant neoplasms. *Am J Physiol* 1956; **189:**612–3.

3233. Lamey P-J, Lamb AB. Prospective study of aetiological factors in burning mouth syndrome. *BMJ* 1988;**296:**1243–6.

3234. Lance JW. Familial paroxysmal dystonic choreoathetosis and its differentiation from related syndromes. *Ann Neurol* 1977;**2:**285–93.

3235. Lance JW. Spasticity. In Feldman RG, Young RR, Koella WP, eds. *Spasticity: Disordered Motor Control*, p. 485. Chicago: Year Book Medical Publishers, 1980.

3236. Lance JW. Symposium synopsis. In Feldman RG, Young RR, Koella WP, eds. *Spasticity: Disordered Motor Control*, pp 485–94. Chicago: Year Book Medical Publishers, 1980.

3237. Lance JW. Solved and unsolved headache problems. *Headache* 1991;**31:**439–445.

3238. Lance JW. The red ear syndrome. *Neurology* 1996;**47:**617–20.

3239. Lance JW. Transient sensations of impending loss of consciousness: the "blip" syndrome. *J Neurol Neurosurg Psychiatry* 1996;**60:** 437–8.

3240. Lance JW, Adams RD. The syndrome of intention or action myoclonus as a sequel to hypoxic encephalopathy. *Brain* 1963;**86:**111–36.

3241. Lance JW, Anthony M. Neck-tongue syndrome on sudden turning of the head. *J Neurol Neurosurg Psychiatry* 1980;**43:**97–101.

3242. Lance JW, Burke D, Pollard J. Hyperexcitability of motor and sensory neurons in neuromyotonia. *Ann Neurol* 1979;**5:**523–32.

3243. Lance JW, Drummond PD, Gandevia SC, Morris JGL. Harlequin syndrome: the sudden onset of unilateral flushing and sweating. *J Neurol Neurosurg Psychiatry* 1988;**51:**635–42.

3244. Landau WM. Spasticity: the fable of a neurological demon and the emperor's new therapy. *Arch Neurol* 1974;**31:**217–9.

3245. Landau WM. Au clair de lacune. *Neurology* 1989;**39:**725–30.

3246. Landau WM. Reflex dementia: disinhibited primitive thinking. *Neurology* 1989;**39:**133–7.

3247. Landau WM, Kleffner FR. Syndrome of acquired aphasia with convulsive disorder in children. *Neurology* 1957;**7:**523–30.

3248. Landau WM, Torack RM, Guggenheim MA. Congenital retardation and later evolution to a seizure disorder, orofacial dysplasia and amyotrophy. *Neurology* 1976;**26:**869–73.

3249. Lander CM, Eadie MJ, Tyrer JH. Hereditary motor peripheral neuropathy predominantly affecting the arms. *J Neurol Sci* 1976;**28:** 389–94.

3250. Landi G, Motto C, Cella E, et al. Pathogenetic and prognostic features of lacunar transient ischemic attack syndromes. *J Neurol Neurosurg Psychiatry* 1993;**56:**1265–70.

3251. Landing BH, Shirkley HS. A syndrome of recurrent infection and infiltration of viscera by pigmented lipid histiocytes. *Pediatrics* 1957;**20:** 431–8.

3252. Landis DMD, Rosenberg RN, Landis C. Olivopontocerebellar degeneration. *Arch Neurol* 1974;**31:**295–307.

3253. Landouzy L. De la sciatique et de l'atrophie musculaire qui peut la compliquer. *Arch Gen Med Paris* 1875;**1:**303–25.

3254. Landouzy L. De la déviation conjugée des yeux et de la rotation de la tête par excitation ou paralysie des 6e et 11e paires. *Bull Soc Anat Paris* 1879;**54:**293–352.

3255. Landouzy L. De la myopathie atrophique progressive; myopathie sans neuropathie, débutant d'ordinaire dans l'enfance par la face. *Rev Med Paris* 1885;**5:**81–117.

3256. Landouzy L. Camptodactylie. *Presse Med* 1906;**14:**251–3.

3257. Landrieu P, Said G. Niemann-Pick disease. *Acta Neuropathol* 1984;**63:**66–71.

3258. Landry de Thézillat JPO. Note sur la paralysie ascendante aigue. *Gaz Med Hebd Chir* 1859;**6:**472–4.

3259. Landsborough D. St. Paul and temporal lobe epilepsy. *J Neurol Neurosurg Psychiatry* 1987;**50:**659–64.

3260. Lane RJM. Cardiogenic dementia. *Lancet* 1977;**i:**27–8.

3261. Lane RJM, Mastaglia FL. Malignant hyperpyrexia. *Lancet* 1978;**2:**562.

3262. Lang AE. Psychogenic dystonia: a review of 18 cases. *Can J Neurol Sci* 1995;**22:**136–43.

3263. Lang AE, Consky E, Sandor P. Signing tics. *Ann Neurol* 1993; **33:**212–5.

3264. Lang AH, Hirvasniemi A, Siivola J, et al. Neurophysiological findings in the northern epilepsy syndrome. *Acta Neurol Scand* 1997; **95:**1–8.

3265. Lang H, Wurzburg U. Creatine kinase, an enzyme of many forms. *Clin Chem* 1982;**28:**1439–47.

3266. Lange C. Die Ausflockung kolloidalen Goldes durch Zebrospinalflussgeit bei luetischen Affektionen des Zentralnervensystems. *Z Chemotherap* 1912;**1:**44–78.

3267. Langley JN. The autonomic nervous system. *Brain* 1903;**26:**1–26.

3268. Langley JN, Sherrington CS. *J Physiol* 1891;**12:**278.

3269. Langston JW, Dorfman LJ, Forno LS. Encephalomyeloneuritis in the absence of cancer. *Neurology* 1975;**25:**633–7.

3270. Lanska D, Remler BF. Benign paroxysmal positioning vertigo. *Neurology* 1997;**48:**1167–77.

3271. Lanska DJ. The history of reflex hammers. *Neurology* 1989; **39:**1542–9.

3272. Lanska DJ, Currier RD, Cohen M, et al. Familial progressive subcortical gliosis. *Neurology* 1994;**44:**1633–43.

3273. Lanska DJ, Goetz C. Romberg's sign. *Neurology* 2000;**55:**1201–6.

3274. Lanthier S, Lortie A, Michaud J, et al. Isolated angiitis of the CNS in children. *Neurology* 2001;**56:**837–42.

3275. Lantos PL, Papp MI. Cellular pathology of multiple system atrophy: a review. *J Neurol Neurosurg Psychiatry* 1994;**47:**129–33.

3276. Lapresle J, Annabi A. OPCA with velopharyngolaryngeal paralysis. *J Neuropathol Exp Neurol* 1979;**38:**401–6.

3277. Larbrisseau A, Vanasse M, Brochu P, et al. The Andermann syndrome: agenesis of the corpus callosum associated with mental retardation and progressive sensorimotor neuropathy. *Can J Neurol Sci* 1984;**11:**257–61.

3277a. Larkin K, Fardaei M. Myotonic dystrophy—A multigene disorder. *Brain Res Bull* 2001;**56:**389–95.

3278. Larrabee GJ, Crook TH. A computerized everyday memory Battery for assessing treatment effects. *Psychopharmacol Bull* 1988;**24:** 695–7.

3279. Larrabee GJ, Pathy MSJ, Bayer A, et al. Memory clinics: state of the art and future prospects. In Bergener M, Finkel SI, eds. *Clinical and Scientific Psychogeriatrics*, pp. 83–97. Berlin: Springer-Verlag, 1988.

3280. Larsen R, Ashwal S, Peckham N. Incontinentia pigmenti and anterior horn cell degeneration. *Neurology* 1987;**37**:446–50.

3281. Larsen R, Ashwall S, Peckham N. Infantile spinal muscular atrophy in incontinentia pigmenti. *Neurology* 1987;**37**:446–50.

3283. Lascelles RG, Baker IA, Thomas PK. Hereditary polyneuropathy of Roussy-Levy type with associated cardiomyopathy. *Guys Hosp Rep* 1970;**119**:253–62.

3284. Lasègue E-C. Considerations sur la sciatique. *Arch Gen Med Paris* 1852;**28**:129–50.

3285. Lasègue E-C. De l'anesthesie et de l'ataxie hysteriques. *Arch Gen Med Paris* 1864;**3**:385–402.

3286. Lasègue E-C. Des hysteriques peripheriques. *Arch Gen Med Paris* 1878;**1**:641–56.

3287. Lashley KS. Brain mechanisms and intelligence: a quantitative study of injuries to the brain. Chicago: University of Chicago, 1929.

3288. Lassen NA. The luxury-perfusion syndrome and its possible relation to acute metabolic acidosis localised with the brain. *Lancet* 1966;**2**:1113–5.

3289. Latham AD, Munro TA. Familial myoclonus epilepsy associated with deaf mutism in a family showing other psychobiological abnormalities. *Ann Eugen* 1937;**8**:166–75.

3290. Latov S, et al. Peripheral neuropathy and anti-MAG antibodies. *C R C Crit Rev Clin Neurobiol* 1988;**3**:301–31.

3291. Laurence JZ, Moon RC. Four cases of "retinitis pigmentosa", occurring in the same family, and accompanied by general imperfections of development. *Ophthalmol Rev Lond* 1866;**2**:32–41.

3292. Lauritzen M. Cortical spreading depression as a putative migraine mechanism. *Trends Neurosci* 1987;**8**–13.

3293. Laursen J, Fode K, Dahlerup B. Spinal epidural hematomas. *Clin Neurol Neurosurg* 1987;**89**:247–53.

3294. Laux W. In memoriam—Hans-Gerhard Creutzfeldt. *Med Klin Berlin* 1965;**60**:553–5554.

3295. Lavade T, Graber D, Flurin V, et al. Human beta-mannosidase deficiency associated with peripheral neuropathy. *Ann Neurol* 1994;**35**:116–9.

3296. Law EM, Masterson JG. Partial deletion of chromosome 18. *Lancet* 1966;**2**:1137.

3297. Lawford JB. Naevus of left side of face, nevus of choroid, subretinal hemorrhage and detached retina in left eye. *Trans Ophthalmol Soc UK* 1885;**5**:136–9.

3298. Lawton MP, Brody EM. Assessment of elder people: self-maintaining and instrumental activities of daily living. *Gerontologist* 1969;**9**:179–86.

3299. Lawton MP, Moss M, Fulcomer M, et al. A research and service oriented multilevel assessment instrument. *J Gerontol* 1982;**37**:91–9.

3300. Laxova R, et al. A further example of lethal autosomal recessive condition in sibs. *J Ment Defic Res* 1972;**16**:139–43.

3301. Layzer RB. *Neuromuscular Manifestations of Systemic Disease*. Philadelphia: F.A. Davis, 1985.

3302. Layzer RB. The origin of muscle fasciculations and cramps. *Muscle Nerve* 1994;**17**:1243–9.

3303. Layzer RB, Rowland LP, Ranney HM. Muscle phosphofructokinase deficiency. *Arch Neurol* 1967;**17**:512–23.

3304. Layzer RB, Shearn MA, Satya-Murti S. Eosinophilic polymyositis. *Ann Neurol* 1977;**1**:65–71.

3305. Lazare A. Conversion symptoms. *N Engl J Med* 1981;**305**:745–8.

3306. Lazarevic LK. Ischias postica Cotunnii. *Allg Wien Med Z* 1884;**29**:425.

3307. Lazawow PB, Moser HW. Disorders of peroxisomal biogenesis. In Scriver CR, ed. *The Metabolic Basis of Inherited Disease*, New York: McGraw-Hill, 1989.

3308. Leao AAP. Spreading depression of activity in the cerebral cortex. *J Physiol* 1944;**7**:358–90.

3309. Leber T. Beitrage zur Kenntniss der atrophischen Veranderungen des Sehnerven nebst Bemerkungen uber die normale Structur des Nerven. *Arch Ophthalmol Berlin* 1868;**14**:164–76.

3310. Leber T. Uber hereditare und kongenital-angelegte Sehnervenleiden. *Arch Ophthalmol Berlin* 1871;**17**:249–91.

3311. Lechtenberg R, Shulman A. The neurologic implications of tinnitus. *Arch Neurol* 1984;**41**:718–21.

3312. Lederman RJ, Calabrese LH. Overuse syndromes in instrumentalists. *Med Probl Perform Art* 1986;**1**:7–11.

3313. Le Douarin NM. Embryonic chimeyas: a tool for studying the development of the nervous and immune systems. *Proc R Soc Med* 1988;**235**:1–17.

3314. Lee BI, Lesser RP, Pippinger CE, et al. Familial paroxysmal hypnogenic dystonia. *Neurology* 1985;**35**:1357–60.

3315. Lee EK, Maselli RA, Ellis WG, et al. Morvan's fibrillary chorea: a paraneoplastic manifestation of thymoma. *J Neurol Neurosurg Psychiatry* 1998;**65**:857–62.

3316. Lee J, Gresty M. A case of "voluntary nystagmus" and head tremor. *J Neurol Neurosurg Psychiatry* 1993;**56**:1321–2.

3317. Lee YS, Yip WCL. A fatal congenital myopathy with severe type 1 fibre atrophy, central nuclei and multicores. *J Neurol Sci* 1981;**50**:227–90.

3318. Leech J, Gresty MA, Hess K, et al. Gaze failure, drifting eye movements, and centripetal nystagmus in cerebellar diseases. *Br J Ophthalmol* 1977;**61**:774–81.

3319. Lees AJ. Familial static ophthalmoplegia. *J Neurol Neurosurg Psychiatry* 1960;**23**:46.

3320. Lees AJ. *Tics and Related Disorders*. Edinburgh: Churchill Livingstone, 1985.

3321. Le Forestier N, Moulonguet A, Maisonobe T, et al. True neurogenic thoracic outlet syndrome: electrophysiological diagnosis in six cases. *Muscle Nerve* 1998;**21**:1129–34.

3323. Lehmann-Horn F, Rüdel R. Hereditary nondystrophic myotonias and periodic paralyses. *Curr Opin Neurol* 1995;**8**:402–10.

3324. Lehoczky T, Fodors T. Clinical significance of dissociation of the abdominal reflexes. *Neurology* 1953;**3**:453–9.

3325. Leichtenstern OML. Concerning epidemic meningitis [in German]. *Dtsch Med Wochenschr* 1885;**11**:537–40.

3326. Leigh D. Subacute necrotizing encephalomyelopathy in an infant. *J Neurol Neurosurg Psychiatry* 1951;**14**:216–21.

3327. Leigh RJ, Foley JM, Remler BF, et al. Oculogyric crises: a syndrome of thought disorder and ocular deviation. *Ann Neurol* 1987;**22**:13–17.

3328. Leigh RJ, Robinson DA, Zee DS. A hypothetical explanation for periodic alternating nystagmus: instability in the optokinetic-vestibular system. *Ann NY Acad Sci* 1981;**374**:619.

3329. Leigh RJ, Tusa RJ. Disturbance of smooth pursuit caused by infarction of occipito-parietal cortex. *Ann Neurol* 1985;**17**:185.

3330. Leigh RJ, Zee DS. *The Neurology of Eye Movements*. Philadelphia: F.A. Davis, 1991.

3331. Leiguarda R, Starkstein S, Nogues M, et al. Paroxysmal alien hand syndrome. *J Neurol Neurosurg Psychiatry* 1993;**56**:788–92.

3332. Leiguarda RC, Marsden CD. Limb apraxias. *Brain* 2000;**123**:860–79.

3333. Leis AA, Ross MA, Summers AK. Psychogenic seizures: ictal characteristics and diagnostic pitfalls. *Neurology* 1992;**42**:95–9.

3334. Leisti J, et al. The floating harbor syndrome. *Birth Defects* 1975;**11**:305.

3335. Lejeune J, LaFourcade J, Berger R, et al. Three cases of deletion of the short arm of chromosome 5 [in French]. *C R Acad Sci (Paris)* 1963;**257**:3098.

3336. Lejonne P, Lhermitte JJ. Olivo-rubro-cerebellar atrophy [in French]. *Nouv Icon Salpet* 1909;**2**:605–19.

3337. Leli DA, Furlow TW, Falgout JE. Benign familial chorea. *J Neurol Neurosurg Psychiatry* 1984;**47**:471–4.

3338. LeMarquand HS, Hausmann W, Hemsted EH. Myxoedema as a cause of death: report of two cases. *BMJ* 1953;**1**:704–6.

3339. Lemierre A-A, Boltanski E, Justin-Besancon L-E. Les polynevrites alcoolo-tuberculeuses. *Bull Acad Med Paris* 1931;**105**:676–8.

3340. Lemieux G, Neemeh JA. Charcot-Maric-Tooth disease and nephritis. *CMAJ* 1967;**97**:1193–8.

3341. Lempert T. Syncope. Phenomenology and differentiation from epileptic seizures. *Nervenarzt* 1997;**68**:620.

3342. Lempert T, Bauer MS, Schmidt D. Syncope: a videometric analysis of 56 episodes of transient cerebral hypoxia. *Ann Neurol* 1994;**36**:233–7.

3343. Lendon CL, Lynch T, Norton J, et al. Hereditary dysphasic disinhibition dementia. *Neurology* 1998;**50**:1546–55.

3344. Lenhoff HM, Wang PP, Greenberg F, et al. Williams syndrome and the brain. *Sci Am* 1997;**277**:63–73.

3345. Lennox WG. *Epilepsy and Related Disorders.* Boston: Little, Brown, 1960.

3346. Lenoble E, Aubineau E. Une variété nouvelle de myoclonie congénitale pouvant être héréditaire et familiale a nystagmus constant. *Rev Med Paris* 1906;**26**:471–515.

3347. Lenz W. Recessiv-geschlechtsgebundene Mikrophthalmie mit multiplen Missbildungen. *Z Kinderheilkd* 1955;**77**:384–90.

3348. Leonard JV, Schapira AHV. Mitochondrial respiratoiry chain disorders I: mitochondrial DNA defects. *Lancet* 2000;**355**:299–304.

3348a. Leonard JV, Schapira AHV. Mitochondrial respiratory chain disorders II: neurodegenerative disorders and nuclear gene defects. *Lancet* 2000;**355**:389–94.

3349. Leone M, D'Amico D, Grazzi L, et al. Cervicogenic headache: a critical review of the current diagnostic criteria. *Pain* 1998;**78**:1–5.

3350. Leonhard K. Agraphia and constructional apraxia [in German]. *Arch Psychiatr Z Neurol* 1952;**188**:504–10.

3351. Lepore F. Bilateral cerebral ptosis. *Neurology* 1987;**37**:1043–6.

3352. Lerche H, Weber YG, Baier H, et al. Generalized epilepsy with febrile seizures plus. *Neurology* 2001;**57**:1191–8.

3353. Leri A. A reflex phenomenon in the arm [in French]. *Rev Neurol (Paris)* 1913;**25**:277.

3354. Leriche R. Resection of the aorto-iliac bifurcation and bilateral sympathectomy for distal aortic arteritis [in French]. *Presse Med* 1940;**48**:601–4.

3355. Lerman P, Kivity S. Benign focal epilepsy of childhood: a follow-up study of 100 recovered patients. *Arch Neurol* 1975;**32**:261–4.

3356. Lerman P, Kivity S. The benign focal epilepsies of childhood. In Pedley TA, Meldrum BS, eds. *Recent Advances in Epilepsy–3*, pp 137–56. Edinburgh: Churchill Livingstone, 1986.

3357. Lermoyez M. La vertige qui fait entendre (angiospasme labyrinthique). *Presse Med* 1919;**27**:1–3.

3358. Leroy MR. Syndrome of lilliputian hallucinations. *J Nerv Ment Dis* 1922;**56**:325–33.

3359. Lesch M, Nyhan WL. A familial disorder of uric acid metabolism and central nervous system function. *Am J Med* 1964;**36**:561–70.

3360. Lescher FG. The nervous complications of infective hepatitis. *BMJ* 1944;**1**:554.

3361. Lessell S. Supranuclear paralysis of monocular elevation. *Neurology* 1975;**25**:1134–43.

3362. Lessell S, Lessell IM, Rizzo IJF. Ocular neuromyotonia after radiation therapy. *Am J Ophthalmol* 1986;**102**:766–70.

3363. Lessell S, Wolf PA, Benson MD, et al. Scalloped pupils in familial amyloidosis. *N Engl J Med* 1975;**293**:914–5.

3364. Leuzzi V, De Negri AM, Gallucci M, et al. Bilateral striatal necrosis, dystonia and optic atrophy in two siblings. *J Neurol Neurosurg Psychiatry* 1992;**55**:16–9.

3365. Leuzzi V, Rinna A, Gallucci M., et al. Ataxia, deafness, leukodystrophy: inherited disorder of the white matter in three related patients. *Neurology* 2000;**54**:2325–8.

3366. Levenson JL. Neuroleptic malignant syndrome. *Am J Psychiatry* 1985;**142**:1137–45.

3367. Levic ZM, Stefanovic BS, Nikolic MZ, et al. Progressive nuclear ophthalmoplegia associated with mental deficiency, lingua scrotalis, and other neurologic and ophthalmologic signs in a family. *Neurology* 1975;**25**:68–71.

3368. Levin AB. A simple test of cardiac function based upon the heart rate changes during the Vansalva maneuver. *Am J Cardiol* 1966;**18**:90–9.

3369. Levin BE. The clinical significance of spontaneous pulsations of the retinal vein. *Arch Neurol* 1978;**35**:37–40.

3370. Levin HS, High WM, Goethe AE, et al. The Neurobehavioral Rating Scale. *J Neurol Neurosurg Psychiatry* 1987;**50**:183–93.

3371. Levin HS, O'Donnell VM, Grossman RG. The Galveston Orientation and Aphasia Test. *J Nerv Ment Dis* 1979;**167**:675–84.

3372. Levin KH, Wilbourn AJ, Maggiano HJ. Cervical rib and median sternotomy-related brachial plexopathies: a reassessment. *Neurology* 1998;**50**:1407–13.

3373. Levin LS, et al. A heritable syndrome of craniosynostosis, short, thin hair, dental abnormalities, and short limbs: cranioectodermal dysplasia. *J Pediatr* 1977;**90**:55–61.

3373a. Levin M. Periodic hypersomnolence and morbid hunger. *Brain* 10036;**62**:494–503.

3374. Levin SL. The syndrome of isolated disturbance of the tympanic nerve. *Arch Neurol* 1983;**40**:106–8.

3375. Levine DN, Lee JM, Fisher CM. The visual variant of Alzheimer's disease. *Neurology* 1993;**43**:305–13.

3376. Levine IM, Estes JW, Looney JM. Hereditary neurological disease with acanthocytosis. *Arch Neurol* 1968;**19**:403–9.

3377. Levine SR, Welch KMA. Cerebrovascular ischemia associated with lupus anticoagulant. *Stroke* 1987;**18**:257–63.

3378. Levine SR, Welch KMA. Antiphospholipid antibodies. *Ann Neurol* 1989;**26**:386–9.

3379. Levine T, Pestronk A. Inflammatory myopathy with cytochrome oxidase negative muscle fibers: methotrexate treatment. *Muscle Nerve* 1998;**21**:1724–8.

3380. Leviton A, Gilles FH. An epidemiologic study of perinatal telencephalic leucoencephalopathy in an autopsy population. *J Neurol Sci* 1973;**18**:53–66.

3381. Levy DE. Transient CNS deficits. *Neurology* 1988;**38**:831–6.

3382. Levy IS, Wright JE, Lloyd GAS. Orbital and retro-orbital pseudotumors. *Mod Prob Ophthalmol* 1975;**14**:364–7.

3383. Levy ML, Cummings JL, Fairbanks LA, et al. Apathy is not depression. *J Neuropsychiatry Clin Neurosci* 1998;**10**:314–9.

3384. Lewis AJ, Besant DF. Muscular dystrophy in infancy. *J Pediatr* 1962;**60**:376–84.

3385. Lewis DW, Tucker SH. Central nervous system involvement in cat scratch disease. *Pediatrics* 1986;**77**:714–21.

3386. Lewis JM, Kline LB. Periodic alternating nystagmus with periodic alternating skew deviation. *J Clin Neuroophthalmol* 1983;**3**:115.

3387. Lewis P. Familial orthostatic hypotension. *Brain* 1964;**87**:719–28.

3388. Lewis RA, Sumner AJ, Brown MJ. Multifocal demyelinating neuropathy with conduction block. *Neurology* 1982;**32**:958–64.

3389. Lewy FH. Zur pathologischen Anatomie der Paralysis agitans. *Dtsch Z Nervenklinik* 1913;**50**:50.

3390. Leyden E. *Klinik der Ruckenmarks-Krankheiten* 1876;**2**.

3390a. Leyden E v. [On poliomyelitis and neuritis] *Z klin Med* 1879–1880;**1**:387–434.

3391. Leyden E. Ueber acute Ataxie. *Z Klin Med* 1890;**18**:576–87.

3392. Lezak MD. *Neuropsychological Assessment.* New York: Oxford University Press, 1983.

3393. Lhermitte F. "Utilization behaviour" and its relation to lesions of the frontal lobes. *Brain* 1983;**106**:237–55.

3393a. Lhermitte F. Human anatomy and the frontal lobes. Part II: Patient behavior in complex and social situations: the "environmental dependency syndrome." *Ann Neurol* 1986;**19**:335–43.

3394. Lhermitte F, Pillon B, Serdaru M. Human autonomy and the frontal lobes. Part I: Imitation and utilization behavior: a neuropsychological study of 75 patients. *Ann Neurol* 1986;**19**:326–34.

3395. Lhermitte JJ. Les maladies du sommeil et des narcolepsies. *J Neurol* 1910;**15**:1–17.

3396. Lhermitte JJ. L'encéphalite léthargique: anatomie et physiologie pathologiques. *Arch Ophthalmol Berlin* 1921;**38**.

3397. Lhermitte JJ, Cornil L, Quesnel. Le syndrome de la degeneration pyramido-pallidale progressive. *Rev Neurol (Paris)* 1920;**27**:262–9.

3398. Lhermitte JJ, Delthil, Garnier. Syndrome contralateral du noyau rouge avec hallucinations visuelles et auditives. *Rev Neurol (Paris)* 1938;**70**:623–8.

3399. Lhermitte JJ, Levy G. L'hallucinose pedonculaire. *Rev Neurol (Paris)* 1931;**55**:312–8.

3400. Lhermitte JJ, McAlpine D. A clinical and pathological resume of combined disease of the pyramidal and extrapyramidal systems with especial reference to a new syndrome. *Brain* 1926;**49**:157–81.

3401. Lhermitte JJ, Nicholas M. Les douleurs a type de decharge electrique consecutives a la flexion cephalique dans la sclerose en plaques. Un cas de forme sensitive de la sclerose multiple. *Rev Neurol (Paris)* 1924;**2**:56–62.

3402. Libman LJ, Matthews JH. "Oblongata" crises in tabes dorsalis. *J Neurol Neurosurg Psychiatry* 1976;**39:**1240–1.

3403. Lichtenstein H, Knorr A. Uber einige Falle von fortschreitender Schwerhorigkeit bei hereditarer Ataxie. *Dtsch Z Nervenklinik* 1930;**114:** 1–28.

3404. Lichtheim L. Ueber Aphasie. *Arch Klin Med* 1885;**36:**204–68.

3405. Liddell EGT, Sherrington CS. Reflexes in response to stretch (myotatic reflexes). *Proc R Soc Med* 1924;**B96:**212–42.

3406. Lidge RT, Bechtol RC, Lambert CM. Congenital muscular torticollis; etiology and pathology. *J Bone Jt Surg* 1957;**39A:**1165–82.

3406a. Lieberman AP, Fischbeck KH. Triplet repeat expansion in neuromuscular disease. *Muscle Nerve* 2000;**23:**843–50.

3407. Liebow AS, Carrington CRB, Friedman RJ. Lymphomatoid granulomatosis. *Hum Pathol* 1972;**3:**457–538.

3408. Liepert J, Kotterba S, Tegenthoff M, et al. Central fatigue assessed by transcranial stimulation. *Muscle Nerve* 1996;**19:**1429–34.

3409. Liepmann HK. Das Krankheitsbild der Apraxie (motorischen Asymbolie) auf Grund eines Falles von einseitiger Apraxie. *Monatschr Psychiatr Neurol* 1900;**8:**15,102,182.

3410. Lilly R, Cummings JL, Benson DF, et al. The human Kluver-Bucy syndrome. *Neurology* 1983;**33:**1141–5.

3411. Lim J, Yagnik P, Schraeder P, et al. Ictal catatonia as a manifestation of nonconvulsive status epilepticus. *J Neurol Neurosurg Psychiatry* 1986;**49:**833–6.

3412. Lin JT-Y, Ziegler DK, Lai C-W, Bayer W. Convulsive syncope in blood donors. *Ann Neurol* 1982;**11:**525–8.

3413. Lincoln N, Leadbitter D. Assessment of motor function in stroke patients. *Physiotherapy* 1979;**65:**48–51.

3414. Lincoln NB. The Speech Questionnaire: an assessment of functional language ability. *Int Rehabil Med* 1982;**4:**114–7.

3415. Lincoln NB, Edmans JA. A re-validation of the Rivermead ADL scale for elderly patients with stroke. *Age Ageing* 1990;**19:**9–24.

3416. Lindenov H. *The Aetiology of Deaf-Mutism with Special Reference to Heredity.* Copenhagen: Munksgard, 1945.

3417. Lindenstrom E, Boysen G, Waage Christiansen L, et al. Reliability of Scandinavian Neurological Stroke Scale. *Cerebrovasc Dis* 1991; **1:**103–7.

3418. Lindgren K-A, Manninen H, Rytkonen H. Thoracic outlet syndrome—a functional disturbance of the thoracic upper aperture? *Muscle Nerve* 1995;**18:**526–30.

3419. Lindsberg J, Hallenbeck JM, Feuerstein G. Platelet-activating factor in brain injury. *Ann Neurol* 1991;**30:**117–29.

3420. Lingam S, Read S, Hart EW. Hereditary stiff-baby syndrome. *Am J Dis Child* 1981;**135:**909–11.

3421. Lingjaerde O, Bratlid T, Hansen T. Insomnia during the dark period in northern Norway: an explorative controlled trial with light treatment. *Acta Psychiatr Neurol* 1985;**71:**506–12.

3422. Linn MW, Linn BS. The Rapid Disability Rating Scale 2. *J Am Geriatr Soc* 1982;**30:**378–82.

3423. Lippa CF, Zhukareva V, Kararai T, et al. Frontotemporal dementia with novel tau pathology and a Glu342Val *tau* mutation. *Ann Neurol* 2000;**48:**850–8.

3424. Lisak RP, Lebeau J, Tucker SH. Hyperkalemic periodic paralysis and cardiac arrhythmia. *Neurology* 1972;**22:**810–5.

3425. Lishman WA. Cerebral disorder in alcoholism. *Brain* 1981; **104:**1–20.

3426. Lishman WA. What is neuropsychiatry? *J Neurol Neurosurg Psychiatry* 1992;**55:**983–5.

3427. Lishman WA, Russell WR. The brachial neuropathies. *Lancet* 1961;**2:**941–7.

3428. Lison M, Kombrut B, Feinstein A, et al. Progressive spastic paraparesis, vitiligo, premature graying and distict facial appearance: a new genetic syndrome in three sibs. *Am J Med Genet* 1981;**9:**361–7.

3429. Lissauer H. Ein Fall von Seelenblindheit nebst einem Beitrag zur Theorie derselban. *Arch Psychiatrie Nervenkr* 1890;**21:**222–70.

3429a. Lissauer H. Beitrag zur Pathologischen Anatomia der Tabes dorsalis und zem Fazerdauf in menschlichen Rüchermark. *Neurol Zbl* 1885;**4:**245–6.

3430. List CF. Neurologic syndromes accompanying developmental anomalies of occipital bone, atlas, and axis. *Arch Neurol Psychiatry* 1941;**45:**577–616.

3431. List CF. Interhemispheric subdural suppuration. *J Neurosurg* 1950;**7:**313–24.

3432. Lister GD, Belso LB, Clivert HE. The radial tunnel syndrome. *J Hand Surg* 1979;**4:**52.

3433. Little BW, Brown PW, Rodgers-Johnson P, et al. Familial myoclonic dementia masquerading as Creutzfeldt-Jakob disease. *Ann Neurol* 1986;**20:**231–6.

3434. Little BW, Park DP. Oculopharyngeal muscular dystrophy. *J Neurol Sci* 1982;**53:**145–58.

3435. Little JR, Opitz JM. The G syndrome. *Am J Dis Child* 1971; **121:**505–7.

3436. Little WJ. Course of lectures on the deformities of the human frame. Lecture IX. *Lancet* 1843;**1:**350–4.

3437. Little WJ. On the influence of abnormal parturition, difficult labours, premature birth, and asphyxia neonatorum on the mental and physical condition of the child especially in relation to deformities. *Trans Obstet Soc Lond* 1861;**3:**293–344.

3438. Litvan I, Agid Y, Calne DB, et al. Clinical research criteria for the diagnosis of progressive supranuclear palsy (Steele-Richardson-Olszewski syndrome). *Neurology* 1996;**47:**1–9.

3439. Litvan I, Agid Y, Goetz C, et al. Accuracy of the clinical diagnosis of corticobasal degeneration. *Neurology* 1997;**48:**119–25.

3440. Litvan I, Mangone CA, Werden W, et al. Reliability of the NINDS Myotatic Reflex Scale. *Neurology* 1996;**47:**969–72.

3441. Livan M. Contributo alla conoscenza della sordita ereditarie. *Arch Ital Otol* 1961;**72:**331–9.

3442. Livingston S, Torres I. Photic epilepsy: report of an unusual case and review of the literature. *Clin Pediatr* 1964;**3:**304–7.

3443. Livingston WK. Back disabilities due to strain of multifidus muscle; cases treated by novocain injection. *West J Surg* 1941;**49:**259–65.

3444. Livingstone IR, Gardner-Medwin D, Watkins PJ. Familial intermittent ataxia with possible X-linked recessive Inheritance. *J Neurol Sci* 1984;**64:**89–97.

3445. Livingstone MG, Livingstone HM. The Glasgow Assessment Schedule: clinical and research asssessment of head injury outcome. *Int Rehabil Med* 1985;**7:**145–9.

3446. Lloyd AR, Hales JP, Gandevia SC. Muscle strength, endurance and recovery in the post-infection fatigue syndrome. *J Neurol Neurosurg Psychiatry* 1988;**51:**1316–22.

3447. Lloyd KG, Hornykiewicz O, Davidson L, et al. Biochemical evidence of dysfunction of brain transmitters in the Lesch-Nyhan syndrome. *N Engl J Med* 1981;**305:**1106–11.

3448. Lloyd ME, Spector TD, Howard R. Osteoporosis in neurological disorders. *J Neurol Neurosurg Psychiatry* 2000;**68:**543–9.

3449. Lobstein J. *De l'appairaissment des os.* Paris: Traite de l'anatomie pathologique, 1833.

3450. Lockwood AH. Medical problems of musicians. *N Engl J Med* 1989;**320:**221–7.

3451. Locock C. In discussion, Sieveking EH. Analysis of 52 cases of epilepsy observed by the author. *Lancet* 1857;**1:**527–8.

3452. Lodder J, Baard WC. Paraballism caused by bilateral hemorrhagic infarction in basal ganglia. *Neurology* 1981;**31:**484–6.

3453. Loeb C, Gandolfo C, Mancardi GL, et al. The lacunar syndromes: a review with personal contribution. In Meyer JS, Lechner H, Eichorn O, eds. *Cerebrovascular Disease: Research and Clinical Management,* pp 107–56. Amsterdam: Elsevier, 1986.

3454. Loeffen J, Elpeleg O, Smeitink J, et al. Mutations in the complex 1 *NDUFS2* gene of patients with cardiomyopathy and encephalomyopathy. *Ann Neurol* 2001;**49:**195–201.

3455. Loewen SC, Anderson BA. Reliability of the modified motor assessment scale and the Barthel Index. *Phys Ther* 1988;**68:**1077–81.

3456. Loewenfeld IE, Thompson HS. Oculomotor paresis with cyclic spasms. *Surv Ophthalmol* 1975;**20:**81.

3457. Logan JL, Harveyson KB, Wisdom GB, et al. Hereditary caeruloplasmin deficiency, dementia and diabetes mellitus. *Q J Med* 1994;**87:**663–70.

3458. Logigian EL, Kolodny EH, Griffith JF, et al. Myoclonus epilepsy in two brothers. *Brain* 1986;**109:**411–29.

3459. Logothetis J, Constantoulakis M, Economidou J, et al. Thalassemia major (homozygous bete-thalassemia). *Neurology* 1972;**22:** 294–304.

3460. Logsdail SJ, Toone BK. Post-ictal psychosis: a clinical and phenomenological description. Br J Psychiatry 1988;152:246–52.

3461. Loiseau H, Marchal C, Vital A, et al. Occurrence of polyglucosan bodies in temporal lobe epilepsy. J Neurol Neurosurg Psychiatry 1992; 55:1092–3.

3462. Loiseau J, Loiseau P, Duclo B, et al. A survey of epileptic disorders in South West France: seizures in elderly patients. Ann Neurol 1990;27:231–8.

3463. Loiseau P, Guyot M, Loiseau H, et al. Eating seizures. Epilepsia 1986;27:161–3.

3464. Lombroso CT. Sylvian seizures and midtemporal spike foci in children. Arch Neurol 1967;17:52–9.

3465. Lombroso CT, Fejerman N. Benign polymyoclonus of early infancy. Ann Neurol 1977;1:138–43.

3466. Lombroso CT, Lerman P. Breathholding spells (cyanotic and pallid infantile syncope). Pediatrics 1967;39:563–81.

3467. Long RR, Sargent JC, Pappas AM, et al. Pitcher's arm: an electrodiagnostic enigma. Muscle Nerve 1996;19:1276–81.

3468. Loonen MCB, Busch HFM, Koster JF, et al. A family with different forms of acid maltase deficiency glycogenosis type II. Neurology 1981;31:1209–16.

3469. Lopez JR, Adornato BT, Hoyt WF. Entomopia: a remarkable case of cerebral polyopia. Neurology 1993;43:2145–6.

3470. Lopez PF, Lawton Smith J. Leber's optic atrophy. J Clin Neuroophthalmol 1986;6:144–52.

3471. Lopez-Hernandez A. Craniosynostosis, ataxia, trigeminal anaesthesia and parietal alopecia with pons-vermis fusion anomaly (atresia of the fourth ventricle). Report of two cases. Neuropediatrics 1982; 13:99–102.

3472. Lord SM, Barnsley L, Walis BJ, et al. Third occipital nerve headache: a prevalence study. J Neurol Neurosurg Psychiatry 1994;57: 1187–90.

3473. Lorentzen SE. Drusen of the optic disk, an irregularly dominant hereditary affection. Acta Ophthalmol 1961;39:626–43.

3474. Loseth S, Torbergsen T, Brautaset N, et al. A new non-dystrophic painful myotonia with dominant inheritance. J Neurol Neurosurg Psychiatry 2001;71:419.

3475. Lossos A, Barash V, Soffer D, et al. Hereditary branching enzyme dysfunction in adult polyglucosan body disease: a possible metabolic cause in two patients. Ann Neurol 1991;30:655–62.

3476. Lossos A, Cooperman H, Soffer D, et al. Hereditary leukoencephalopathy and palmoplantar keratoderma. Neurology 1995;45: 331–7.

3477. Lotz BP, Stubgen J-P. The rigid spine syndrome: a vacuolar variant. Muscle Nerve 1993;16:530–6.

3478. Louis ED, Lynch T, Ford B, et al. Delayed onset cerebellar syndrome. Arch Neurol 1996;53:450–4.

3479. Louis ED, Lynch T, Kaufmann P, et al. Diagnostic guidelines in central nervous system Whipple's disease. Ann Neurol 1996;40:561–8.

3480. Louis-Bar D. Sur un syndrome progressif comprenant des telangiectasies capillaires cutanees et conjontivales symmetriques, a disposition naevoide et des troubles cerebelleux. Confin Neurol 1941;4: 32–42.

3481. Louis-Bar D, Legros J. Les hypertrophies partielles avec angiome (syndrome de Klippel-Trenaunay) et leurs rapports avec les phacomatoses. Confin Neurol 1946;7–8:245.

3482. Love S, Duchen LW. Familial cerebellar ataxia with cerebrovascular amyloid. J Neurol Neurosurg Psychiatry 1982;45:271–3.

3483. Lovell HW. Familial progressive bulbar paralysis. Arch Neurol Psychiatry 1932;28:394–8.

3484. Low PA, Burke WJ, McLeod JG. Congenital sensory neuropathy with selective loss of small myelinated nerve fibers. Ann Neurol 1978;3:179–82.

3485. Low PA, Dyck PJ, Lambert EH, et al. Acute panautonomic neuropathy. Ann Neurol 1983;13:412.

3486. Low PA, et al. The sympathetic nervous system in diabetic neuropathy. Brain 1975;98:341–56.

3487. Low PA, Fealey RD, Sheps SG, et al. Chronic idiopathic anhidrosis. Ann Neurol 1985;18:344–8.

3488. Lowden JA, O'Brien JS. Sialidosis: a review of human neuraminidase deficiency. Am J Hum Genet 1979;31:1–18.

3489. Lowe CU, Terrey M, MacLachlan EA. Organic aciduria, decreased renal ammonia production, hydrophthalmos, and mental retardation. A clinical entity. Am J Dis Child 1952;83:164–84.

3490. Lowe J, Spillantini MG. Non-Alzheimer degenerative dementias. Brain Pathol 1998;8:295–7.

3491. Lowenberg K, Hill TS. Diffuse sclerosis with preserved myelin islands. Arch Neurol Psychiatry 1933;29:1232–45.

3492. Lowenstein O, Levine AS. Pupillographic studies. Arch Ophthalmol Berlin 1944;31:74–94.

3493. Lowenthal A. [On a congenital and familial form of generalized muscle sclerosis with blepharoptosis]. Acta Neurol Psychiatr Belg 1952; 52:141–55.

3494. Lowenthal A. Striopallidodentate calcifications. In Vinken PJ, Bruyn GW, Klawans HL, eds. Extrapyramidal Disorders. Handbook of Clinical Neurology, Vol. 5, pp 417–36. Amsterdam: Elsevier Science Publishers, 1986.

3495. Lowry RB. Congenital absence of the fibula and craniosynostosis in sibs. J Med Genet 1972;9:227–9.

3496. Lowry RB, Wood BJ. Syndrome of epiphyseal dysplasia, short stature, microcephaly and nystagmus. Clin Genet 1975;8:269–74.

3497. Lubbers WJ, Brunt ERP, Scheffer H, et al. Hereditary myokymia and paroxysmal ataxia linked to chromosome 12 is responsive to acetazolamide. J Neurol Neurosurg Psychiatry 1995;59:400–5.

3498. Lubin B. Depression Adjectives Checklist (Manual). San Diego: Educational and Industrial Testing Service, 1967.

3499. Lubkin V. The inverse Marcus Gunn phenomenon: an electromyographic contribution. Arch Neurol 1978;35:249.

3500. Lublin FD, Tsairis P, Streletz LJ, et al. Myokymia and impaired muscular relaxation with continuous motor unit activity. J Neurol Neurosurg Psychiatry 1979;42:557–62.

3501. Lubs M-LE, Bauer MS, Formas ME, et al. Lisch nodules in neurofibromatosis type 1. N Engl J Med 1991;324:1264–5.

3502. Luccelli F, De Renzi E. Primary dyscalculia after a medial frontal lesion of the left hemisphere. J Neurol Neurosurg Psychiatry 1993; 56:304–7.

3503. Lucchelli F, De Renzi E, Perani D, et al. Primary amnesia of insidious onset with subseqent stabilisation. J Neurol Neurosurg Psychiatry 1994;57:1366–70.

3504. Luders H, Lesser RP, Dinner DS, et al. The second sensory area in humans: evoked potential and electrical stimulation studies. Ann Neurol 1985;17:177–84.

3505. Ludlow CL. Children's language disorders: recent research advances. Ann Neurol 1980;7:497–507.

3506. Ludolph AC, Hugon J, Dwivedi MP, et al. Studies on the aetiology and pathogenesis of motor neuron diseases. I. Lathyrism: clinical findings in established cases. Brain 1987;110:149–66.

3507. Ludwig CL, Smith MT, Godfrey AD, et al. A clinicopathological study of 323 patients with oligodendrogliomas. Ann Neurol 1986;19: 15–21.

3508. Ludwig J, Dyck PJ, LaRusso NF. Xanthomatous neuropathy of liver. Hum Pathol 1982;137:1049–51.

3509. Luft R, et al. A case of severe hypermetabolism of nonthyroid origin with a defect in the maintenance of mitochondrial respiratory control: a correlated clinical, biochemical, and morphological study. J Clin Invest 1962;41:1776–804.

3510. Lugaresi E. Abnormal movements occurring during sleep (AAN course handout) [unpublished]. 1989.

3511. Lugaresi E, Cirignotta F. Hypnogenic paroxysmal dystonia: epileptic seizure or a new syndrome? Sleep 1981;4:129–38.

3512. Lugaresi E, Cirignotta F, Montagna P. Occipital lobe epilepsy with scotosensitive seizures: the role of central vision. Epilepsia 1984;25: 115–20.

3513. Lugaresi E, Cirignotta F, Montagna P. Nocturnal paroxysmal dystonia. J Neurol Neurosurg Psychiatry 1986;49:375–80.

3514. Lugaresi E, Coccagna G, Gambi D, et al. Symond's nocturnal myoclonus. Electroencephalogr Clin Neurophysiol 1967;23:289.

3515. Lugaresi E, Pazzaglia P, Roger J. Evolution and prognosis of petit mal. In Harris P, Mawdsley C, eds. Epilepsy: Proceedings of the Hans Berger Centenary, pp 151–3. Edinburgh: Churchill Livingstone, 1974.

3516. Lundberg A. Myalgia cruris epidemica. Acta Pediatr Scand 1957; 46:18.

3517. Lundberg N. Continuous recording and control of ventricular fluid pressure in neurosurgical practice. *Acta Psychiatr Neurol* 1960;**36:** 1–193.

3518. Lundberg PO. Hererditary polyneuropathy, oligophrenia, premature menopause and acromicria. *Eur Neurol* 1971;**5:**84–98.

3519. Lundberg PO, Westerberg CE. A hereditary neurological disease with facial spasm. *J Neurol Sci* 1968;**8:**85–100.

3520. Lundberg PO, Wranne I, Brun A. A family with optic atrophy and neurological symptoms. *Acta Neurol Scand* 1967;**43:**87–105.

3521. Luria AR. *Human Brain and Psychological Processes.* New York: Harper & Row, 1966.

3522. Luria AR. *The Mind of a Mnemonist.* New York: Basic Books, 1968.

3523. Luscher E. Function of the stapedius muscle [in German]. *Z Hals Nasen Ohrenheilkd* 1929;**105:**23.

3524. Luscher TF, Lie JT, Stanson AW, et al. Arterial fibromuscular dysplasia. *Mayo Clin Proc* 1987;**62:**931–52.

3525. Luxon LM. Disorders of hearing. In Asbury AK, McKhann GM, McDonald WI, eds. *Diseases of the Nervous System,* pp 544–60. Philadelphia: W.B. Saunders, 1987.

3526. Lyell A. Delusions of parasitosis. *Br J Dermatol* 1983;**108:**489.

3527. Lying-Tunell U. Quantitative methods of estimating CSF flow. *Radiol Clin North Am* 1974;**12:**503–11.

3528. Lyle DJ. The ocular syndrome of cataract and papilledema in the manifest form of parathyroid deficiency. *Am J Ophthalmol* 1948;**31:**580.

3529. Lynch DR, Chance PF. Inherited peripheral neuropathies. *Neurologist* 1997;**3:**277–92.

3530. Lynch PG, Bansal DV. Granulomatous polymyositis. *J Neurol Sci* 1973;**18:**1–9.

3531. Lynch T, Sano M, Marder KS, et al. Clinical characteristics of a family with chromosome 17–linked disinhibition-dementia-parkinsonism-amyotrophy complex. *Neurology* 1994;**44:**1878–84.

3532. Lyon G, Arita F, Le Galloudec E, et al. A Disorder of axonal development, necrotizing myopathy, cardiomyopathy and cataracts: a new familial disease. *Ann Neurol* 1990;**27:**193–9.

3533. Lyon G, Ponsot G, Lebon P. Acute measles encephalitis of the delayed type. *Ann Neurol* 1977;**2:**322–7.

3534. Lyon LW. Neurological manifestations of cat-scratch disease. Report of a case and review of the literature. *Arch Neurol* 1971;**25:**23–7.

3535. Lyons JB. *The Citizen Surgeon: A Biography of Sir Victor Horsley.* London: Dawnay, 1966.

3536. Lyons JB. Sir Victor Horsley. *Med Hist* 1967;**11:**361–73.

3537. Mabry CC, Roeckel IE, Munich RL, et al. X-linked pseudohypertrophic muscular dystrophy with a late onset and slow progression. *N Engl J Med* 1965;**273:**1062–70.

3538. Macalpine I, Hunter R. A clinical reassessment of the insanity of King George III and some of its historical implications. *Bull Inst Hist Res* 1967;**40:**166–85.

3539. Maccario M, et al. A sibship with neuroaxonal dystrophy and renal tubular acidosis. *Ann Neurol* 1983;**13:**608–15.

3540. Maccario M, Lustman LI. Paroxysmal nocturnal dystonia presenting as excessive daytime somnolence. *Arch Neurol* 1990;**47:**291–4.

3541. MacCollin M, De Vivo DC, Moser AB, et al. Ataxia and peripheral neuropathy: a benign variant of peroxisome dysgenesis. *Ann Neurol* 1990;**28:**833–6.

3542. MacCollin M, Woodfin W, Kronn D, et al. Schwannomatosis: a clinical and pathologic study. *Neurology* 1996;**46:**1072–9.

3543. MacDermot KD, Walker RWH. Autosomal recesative hereditary motor and sensory neuropathy with mental retardation, optic atrophy and pyramidal signs. *J Neurol Neurosurg Psychiatry* 1987;**50:**1342–7.

3544. MacDonald RL, Deck JHN. Immunohistochemistry of ecchordosis physaliphora and chordoma. *Can J Neurol Sci* 1990;**17:**420–423.

3545. Mace CJ, Trimble MR. "Hysteria", "functional", or "psychogenic"? A survey of British neurologists' preferences. *J R Soc Med* 1991;**84:**471–5.

3546. Mace JW, Sponaugle HD, Mitsunaga RY, et al. Congenital hereditary non-progressive external ophthalmoplegia. *Am J Dis Child* 1971; **122:**261–3.

3547. MacEwen W. A consideration of the means we possess for distinguishing between coma arising from alcoholic intoxication and that produced by apoplexy, fracture of the base of the skull, and other causes. *Glasgow Med J* 1879;**2:**1.

3548. MacEwen W. *Pyogenic Infective Diseases of the Brain and Spinal Cord.* Glasgow: J Maclehose & Sons, 1893.

3549. MacFarlin DE, Strober W, Waldmann TA. Ataxia telangiectasia. *Medicine* 1972;**51:**281–314.

3550. Mack WJ, Freed DM, Williams BW. Boston Naming Test: shortened version for use in Alzheimer's disease. *J Gerontol* 1992;**47:**154–8.

3551. Mackay RP. Congenital demyelinating encephalopathy. *Arch Neurol Psychiatry* 1940;**43:**111–8.

3552. MacKeith RC. The placing response and primary walking. *Guys Hosp Gaz* 1965;**79:**394.

3553. Mackenzie I. The clinical presentation of the cerebral angioma. *Brain* 1953;**76:**184–214.

3554. Mackenzie S. Two cases of associated paralysis of the tongue, soft palate and vocal chord on the same side. *Trans Clin Soc Lond* 1886;**19:** 317–9.

3555. Mackin GA, Bird SJ, Adams CA, et al. EMG indicators of critical illness myopathy following prolonged neuromuscular blockade and high dose corticosteroids. *Muscle Nerve* 1994;**17:**168 (abstract).

3556. Maclaren NK, Max SR, Cornblath M, et al. GM3 gangliosidosis: a novel human sphingolipodystrophy. *Pediatrics* 1976;**57:**106–11.

3557. MacLean JB, Sassin JF. Paroxysmal vertical ocular dyskinesia. *Arch Neurol* 1973;**29:**117–9.

3558. MacLeod PM, Wood S, Jan JE, et al. Progressive cerebellar ataxia, spasticity, psychomotor retardation and hexosaminidase deficiency in a 10–year old child: juvenile Sandhoff disease. *Neurology* 1977;**27:** 571–3.

3559. MacPherson RI. Craniodiaphyseal dysplasia a disease or group of diseases? *J Can Assoc Radiol* 1974;**25:**22.

3560. Madonick MJ, Gilbert S, Stern WZ. Partial agenesis of septum pellucidum with cave of septum pellucidum. *Arch Neurol* 1964;**11:** 324–9.

3561. Madrid R, Bradley WG. The pathology of neuropathies with focal thickenings of the myelin sheath (Tomaculous neuropathy). *J Neurol Sci* 1975;**25:**415–48.

3562. Maeda K, Horiguchi S, Hosokawa M. History of the studies on occupational cervicobrachial disorder in Japan and remaining problems. *J Hum Ergol* 1982;**11:**17–29.

3563. Magee KR, DeJong RN. Hereditary distal myopathy with onset in infancy. *Arch Neurol* 1965;**13:**387–90.

3564. Magee R. Genitofemoral causalgia. *CMAJ* 1942;**46:**326–9.

3565. Magendie F. Memoire sur un liquide qui se trouve dans le crane et le canal vertebral de l'homme et des animaux mammiferes. *J Physiol Exp* 1825;**5:**27.

3566. Maguadda A, Bernardino BD, de Marco P, et al. Bilateral occipital calcification, epilepsy and celiac disease: clinical and neuroimaging features of a new syndrome. *J Neurol Neurosurg Psychiatry* 1993;**56:**885–9.

3567. Magy L, Birouk N, Vallat JM, et al. Hereditary thermosensitive neuropathy. *Neurology* 1997;**48:**1684–90.

3568. Mahjneh I, Udd B, Haravuori H, et al. A distinct phenotype of distal myopathy in a large Finnish family. *J Neurol* 2000;**3:**247.

3569. Mahloudji M, Livingston KE. Familial and congenital simple anhidrosis. *Am J Dis Child* 1967;**134:**77.

3570. Mahloudji M, Pikielny RT. Paramyoclonus multiplex. *Trans Am Neurol Assoc* 1966;**91:**289–90.

3571. Mahloudji M, Pikielny RT. Hereditary essential myoclonus. *Brain* 1967;**90:**669–74.

3572. Mahloudji M, Teasdall RD, Adamkiewicz JJ, et al. The genetic amyloidoses: with particular reference to hereditary neuropathic amyloidosis, type II (Indiana Rukavina type). *Medicine* 1969;**48:**1–37.

3573. Mahoney FI, Barthel DW. Functional evaluation: the Barthel Index. *Md State Med J* 1965;**14:**61–5.

3574. Mahowald MW, Ettinger MG. Things that go bump in the night: the parasomnias revisited. *J Clin Neurophysiol* 1990;**7:**119–43.

3575. Mahowald MW, Schenck CH. REM sleep behavior disorder. In Kryger MH, Roth T, Dement WC, eds. *Principles and Practice of Sleep Medicine,* Philadelphia: W.B. Saunders, 1989.

3576. Mahowald MW, Schenck CH. Dissociated states of wakefulness and sleep. *Neurology* 1992;**42:**44–52.

3577. Mai FM, Merskey H. Briquet's concept of hysteria: an historical perspective. *Can J Psychiatry* 1981;**26:**57–63.

3578. Maigne R. *Douleur d'origine vertébrale et traitment par manipulation.* Paris: Expansion Scientifique, 1977.

3579. Mailander JC. Hereditary gustatory sweating. *JAMA* 1967;**202:**203–4.

3580. Mainzer F, Saldino RM, Ozonoff MB, et al. Familial nephropathy associated with retinitis pigmentosa, cerebellar ataxia and skeletal abnormalities. *Am J Med* 1970;**49:**556–62.

3581. Maitland CG, Abiko S, Hoyt WF, et al. Chiasmal apoplexy: report of four cases. *J Neurosurg* 1982;**56:**118–22.

3582. Majewski F, et al. Polysyndactyly . . . an original syndrome? [in German]. *Z Kinderheilkd* 1971;**111:**118–38.

3583. Makin GJV, Brown WF, Ebers GC. C7 radiculopathy: importance of scapular winging in clinical diagnosis. *J Neurol Neurosurg Psychiatry* 1986;**49:**640–4.

3584. Malm J, Kristensen B, Karlsson T, et al. The predictive value of cerebrospinal fluid dynamic tests in patients with the idiopathic hydrocephalus syndrome. *Arch Neurol* 1995;**52:**783–9.

3585. Mancall EL, Patel AN, Hirschorn AM. Hypertrophic branchial myopathy. *Neurology* 1974;**24:**1166–70.

3586. Manchanda R, Miller H, McLachlan RS. Post-ictal psychosis after right temporal lobectomy. *J Neurol Neurosurg Psychiatry* 1993;**56:**277–9.

3587. Mandler RN, Davis LE, Jeffery DR, et al. Devic's neuromyelitis optica: a clinicopathological study of 8 patients. *Ann Neurol* 1993;**34:**168.

3588. Manford M, Andermann F. Complex visual hallucinations. Clinical and neurobiological insights. *Brain* 1992;**121:**1819–40.

3589. Manford MRA, Fish DR, Shorvon SD. Startle provoked epileptic seizures: features in 19 patients. *J Neurol Neurosurg Psychiatry* 1996;**61:**151–6.

3590. Mann L. Concerning some physical signs after brain contusion [in German]. *Dtsch Med Wochenschr* 1931;**57:**2072–5.

3591. Mann MD, MacFarlane CM, Verburg CJ, et al. The bromide partition test and CSF adenosine deaminase activity in the diagnosis of tuberculosis meningitis in children. *S Afr Med J* 1982;**62:**431–3.

3592. Mann SC, Caroff SN, Blein HR, et al. Lethal catatonia. *Am J Psychiatry* 1986;**143:**1374–81.

3593. Manni JJ, Scaf JJ, Huygen PLM, et al. Hyperostosis cranialis interna: a new hereditary syndrome with cranial nerve entrapment. *N Engl J Med* 1990;**322:**450.

3594. Manor-Esperrilat M, Gothe B, Adams N, et al. Familial sleep apnea plus syndrome. *Neurology* 1988;**38:**190–3.

3595. Manschot S, van Passel L, Buskens E, et al. Mayo and NINDS scales for assessment of tendon reflexes: between observer agreement and implications for communication. *J Neurol Neurosurg Psychiatry* 1998;**64:**253–5.

3596. Mansour AH, Shoch D, Logani S. Optic disk size in ischemic optic neuropathy. *Am J Ophthalmol* 1988;**106:**587–9.

3597. Manta P, Kalfakis N, Bassilopoulos D, et al. An unusual case of lower motor neurone disease. *J Neurol* 1983;**230:**141–2.

3598. Manta P, Kalfakis N, Vassipoulos D, et al. Neuropathy of vasculitic origin in a case of Garin-Boujadoux-Bannwarth syndrome with a positive Borrelia antibody response. *J Neurol* 1986;**233:**69–72.

3599. Manto M, Goldman S, Bodur H. Cerebellar syndrome associated with Hashimoto's encephalopathy. *Rev Neurol (Paris)* 1996;**152:**202–4.

3600. Manzur AY, Keyes RD, Bennett M, et al. Progressive axial muscle rigidity during infancy: a new entity. *Can J Neurol Sci* 1994;**21(Suppl 2):**S34.

3601. Mao C-C, Coull BM, Golper AC, et al. Anterior operculum syndrome. *Neurology* 1989;**39:**1169–72.

3602. Maraist TA, Soloman DH, Barohn RJ, et al. Thalamic ataxia. *Neurology* 1991;**41 Suppl 1:**125.

3603. Marburg O. Die sogenannte "akute multiple Sklerose". *Jahrb Psychiatr Neurol* 1906;**27:**211–312.

3604. Marchall C. Some clinical correlates of the wave and spike phantom. *Electroencephalogr Clin Neurophysiol* 1955;**77:**633–43.

3605. Marchiafava E, Bignami A. Sopra un alterazione del corpo calloso osservata da sogetti alcolisti. *Riv Pat Nerv Alienazione* 1903;**8:**544–9.

3606. Marden PM, Walker WA. A new generalized connective tissue syndrome. *Am J Dis Child* 1966;**112:**225–8.

3607. Marelli FL. Lichtheim syndrome: neurologic study. *Rev Argent Neurol Psquiat Rosario* 1942;**7:**143.

3608. Marfan ABJ. A case of congenital deformation of all four limbs [in French]. *Bull Soc Med Hop Paris* 1896;**13:**220.

3609. Margo CE, Levy MH, Beck RW. Bilateral idiopathic inflamation of the optic nerve sheaths. *Ophthalmology* 1989;**96:**200–6.

3610. Margolis E. A new hereditary syndrome—sex-linked deaf mutism associated with total albinism. *Acta Genet* 1962;**12:**12.

3611. Margolis RL, O'Hearn E, Rosenblatt A, et al. A disorder similar to Huntington's disease is associated with a novel CAG repeat expansion. *Ann Neurol* 2001;**50:**373–80.

3612. Maridort P. Un nouveau sign d'alcoolisme. *Med Mod* 1900; **11:**397.

3613. Marie J, See G. Hydrocephalie aigue benigne du nourrisson apres ingestion d'une dose massive et unique de vitamine A et D. *Arch Fr Pediatr* 1951;**8:**563–5.

3614. Marie P. Sur l'heredo-ataxie cerebelleuse. *Semin Med* 1893; **13:**444–7.

3615. Marie P. Existe-t-il une atrophie musculaire progressive Aran-Duchenne? *Rev Neurol (Paris)* 1897;**5:**686.

3616. Marie P. Revision de la question de l'aphasie; la troisieme circonvolution frontale gauche ne joue aucun role special dans la fonction du language. *Semin Med* 1906;**26:**241.

3617. Marie P, Foix C. Symmetrical and centrilobar intracerebral sclerosis [in French]. *Rev Neurol (Paris)* 1914;**27:**1–16.

3618. Marie P, Meige ET, Patrikios H. Paralysie radiale disociée simulant une griffe cubitale. *Rev Neurol (Paris)* 1917;**24:**123–4.

3619. Marin Amat M. Contribucion al esudio de la curabilidad de las paralisis oculares de origen traumatico—substitucion funcional del VII par el V par craneal. *Arch Oft Hisp Am* 1918;**18:**70–99.

3620. Marin R, Dillingham TR, Chang CM, et al. Extensor digitorum brevis reflex in normals and patients with radiculopathies. *Muscle Nerve* 1995;**18:**52–9.

3621. Marinacci AA, von Hagen KO. Misleading all median hand. *Arch Neurol* 1965;**12:**80–3.

3622. Marinesco G. Succulent hand and muscle atrophy in syringomyelia [in French]. Paris: Université de Paris, 1897.

3623. Marinesco G, Draganesco S, Vasili U. Nouvelle maladie familiale caracterise par une cataracte congenitale et un arret du developpement somato-neuro-psychique. *Encephale* 1931;**26:**97–109.

3624. Marin-Padilla M. Cephalic axial skeletal-neural dysraphic disorders: embryology and pathology. *Can J Neurol Sci* 1991;**18:**153–69.

3625. Marin-Padilla M, Parisi J, Armstrong D, et al. Shaken infant syndrome: developmental neuropathology, progtressive cortical dysplasia and epilepsy. *Acta Neuropathol (Berl)* 2002;**103:**321–32.

3626. Marion MH, Gledhill RF. Spasms of amputation stumps: a report of two cases. *Mov Disord* 1989;**4:**354–8.

3627. Maris T, Androulidakis EJ, Tzagournissakis M, et al. X-linked adrenoleukodystrophy presenting a neurologically pure familial spastic paraparesis. *Neurology* 1994;**45:**1101–4.

3628. Markand ON, Daly DD. Juvenile type of slowly progressive bulbar palsy: report of a case. *Neurology* 1971;**21:**753–8.

3629. Markesbery WR, Griggs RC, Herr B. Distal myopathy: electron microscopic and histochemical studies. *Neurology* 1977;**27:**727–35.

3630. Markesbery WR, Griggs RC, Leach RP, et al. Late onset hereditary distal myopathy. *Neurology* 1974;**23:**127–34.

3631. Markson EW, Levitz G. A Guttman scale to assess memory loss among the elderly. *Gerontologist* 1973;**13:**337–40.

3632. Markson L, Jarman P, Bril V. Response to therapy in demyelinating motor neuropathy. *Muscle Nerve* 1998;**21:**1769–71.

3633. Maroon JC. Burning hands in football spinal cord injuries. *JAMA* 1977;**238:**2049–51.

3634. Maroteaux P. Le syndrome camptomyelique. *Presse Med* 1971; **79:**1157–62.

3635. Maroteaux P, Lamy M. Pyknodysostosis [in French]. *Presse Med* 1962;**70:**999.

3636. Maroteaux P, Lamy M. Hurler's disease, Morquio's disease, and related mucopolysaccharidoses. *J Pediatr* 1965;**67:**312–23.

3637. Marquez S, Turley JJ, Peters WJ. Neuropathy in burn patients. *Brain* 1993;**116**:471–83.

3638. Mars H, Lewis LA, Robertson AL, et al. Familial hypo-β-lipoproteinemia. *Am J Med* 1969;**46**:886–900.

3639. Marsden CD. Blepharospasm-oromandibular dystonia syndrome (Brueghel's syndrome): a variant of adult-onset torsion dystonia? *J Neurol Neurosurg Psychiatry* 1976;**39**:1204–9.

3640. Marsden CD. The problem of adult-onset idiopathic torsion dystonia and other isolated dyskinesias in adult life. In Eldridge R, Fahn S, eds. *Advances in Neurology; Dystonia,* pp 259–76. New York: Raven Press, 1976.

3641. Marsden CD. The focal dystonias. *Clin Neuropharmacol* 1986;**9** (**Suppl 2**):S49–S60.

3642. Marsden CD, Harrison MJG. Idiopathic torsion dystonia (dystonia musculorum deformans). *Brain* 1974;**97**:793–810.

3643. Marsden CD, Obeso JA, Rothwell JC. Benign essential tremor is not a single entity. In Yahr MD, ed. *Current Concepts in Parkinson's Disease,* pp 31–6. Amsterdam: Excerpta Medica, 1983.

3644. Marsden CD, Obeso JA, Zarranz JJ, et al. The anatomical basis of symptomatic hemidystonia. *Brain* 1985;**108**:463–83.

3645. Marsden CD, Parkes JD. "On-off" effects in patients with Parkinson's disease on chronic levodopa therapy. *Lancet* 1976;**1**:292–6.

3646. Marsden CD, Reynolds EH, Parsons V. Myopathy associated with anticonvulsant osteomalacia. *BMJ* 1973;**4**:526–7.

3647. Marseille Consensus Group. Classification of progressive myoclonus epilepsies and related disorders. *Ann Neurol* 1990;**28**:113–6.

3648. Marshall J. Observations of reflex changes in the lower limbs in spastic paraplegia in man. *Brain* 1954;**77**:290–304.

3649. Marshall J. Dominant saddle nose, cataract and hearing loss. *Am J Ophthalmol* 1958;**45**:143–56.

3650. Marshall JC, Newcombe F. Patterns of paralexia—a psycholinguistic approach. *J Psychol Res* 1973;**2**:175–99.

3651. Marshall LF, Marshall LB, Klauber MR, et al. The diagnosis of head injury requires a classification based on computed axial tomography. *J Neurotrauma* 1992;**9**(**Suppl 1**):S287–S292.

3652. Martensson B. Dominant hereditary nerve deafness. *Acta Otorhinolaryngol (Belg)* 1960;**52**:270–4.

3653. Martin J-J, Brucher J-M, Evrard Ph, et al. On an autosomal dominant form of retino-cerebellar degeneration: an autopsy study of four patients in a Belgian family. *Neurology* 1991;**41**(**Suppl**):424.

3654. Martin J, Swash M. Myopathy with absence of muscle glycogen and neutral lipid in the neuroleptic malignant syndrome. *J Neurol* 1987;**235**:120–1.

3655. Martin JP. Fits of laughter (sham mirth) in organic cerebral disease. *Brain* 1950;**73**:453–64.

3656. Martin JP. Tilting reactions and disorders of the basal ganglia. *Brain* 1965;**88**:855–74.

3657. Martinelli P, Fabbri R, Gabellini AS. Familial hypertrophy of the masseter muscles. *J Neurol* 1987;**234**:251–3.

3658. Martinez AC. Slimmer's paralysis: electrophysiological evidence of compressive lesion. *Eur Neurol* 1987;**26**:189.

3659. Martinez BA, Lake BD. Childhood nemaline myopathy—a review of clinical presentation in relation to prognosis. *Dev Med Child Neurol* 1987;**29**:815–20.

3660. Martinsson T, Darin N, Kyllerman M, et al. Dominant hereditary inclusion-body myopathy gene (*IBM3*) maps to chromosome region 17p13.1. *Am J Hum Genet* 1999;**64**:1420–6.

3661. Martsolf JT, Cracco JB, Carpenter GG, et al. Pfeiffer syndrome: an unusual type of acrocephalosyndactyly with broad thumbs and great toes. *Am J Dis Child* 1971;**121**:257–62.

3662. Martsolf JT, et al. Severe mental retardation, cataracts, short stature and primary hypogonadism in two brothers. *Am J Med Genet* 1978;**1**:291–9.

3663. Martuza RL, Eldridge R. Neurofibromatosis 2. *N Engl J Med* 1988;**318**:684–8.

3664. Martyn CN, Ewing DJ. Pupil cycle time: a simple way of measuring an autonomic reflex. *J Neurol Neurosurg Psychiatry* 1986;**49**: 771–4.

3665. Marxmiller J, Trenkle I, Ashwal S. Rud syndrome revisited. *Dev Med Child Neurol* 1985;**27**:335–43.

3666. Mas JL, Dilouya A, de Recondo J. A familial disorder with subcortical ischemic strokes, dementia and leukoencephalopathy. *Neurology* 1992;**42**:1015–9.

3667. Masdeu JC, et al. Pseudo-abducens palsy with midbrain lesions. *Trans Am Neurol Assoc* 1981;**105**:184.

3668. Masdeu JC, Gorelick PB. Thalamic astasia: inability to stand after unilateral thalamic lesions. *Ann Neurol* 1988;**23**:596–603.

3669. Masdeu JC, Quinto C, Olivera C, et al. Open-ring imaging sign. *Neurology* 2000;**54**:1427–33.

3670. Masdeu JC, Ross ER. Medullary satiety. *Neurology* 1988;**38**: 1643–5.

3671. Maselli RA, Kong DZ, Bowe CM, et al. Presynaptic congenital myasthenic syndrome due to quantal release deficiency. *Neurology* 2001;**57**:279–89.

3672. Maselli RA, Rosenberg RS, Spire J-P. Episodic nocturnal wanderings in non-epileptic young patients. *Sleep* 1988;**11**:156–61.

3673. Maset AL, Marmarou A, Ward JD, et al. Pressure-volume index in head injury. *J Neurosurg* 1987;**67**:832–40.

3674. Mass A. Retinopathy, encephalopathy and deafness. *Neurology* 1988;**38**(**Suppl 1**):215.

3675. Massey EW. Familial occurrence of meralgia paresthetica. *Arch Neurol* 1978;**35**:182.

3676. Massey EW. Effort headache in runners. *Headache* 1982;**22**: 99–100.

3677. Massey EW, Brannon WL, Friedman AJ, Pleet AB. Cylindroma (adenoid cyctic carcinoma) causing unilateral cranial neuropathy. *South Med J* 1979;**72**:1003–5.

3678. Massey EW, Brannon WL, Moreland M. Nevus of ota and intracranial arteriovenous malformation. *Neurology* 1979;**29**:1625–7.

3679. Massey EW, Massey J. Elongated styloid process (Eagle's syndrome) causing hemicrania. *Headache* 1979;**19**:339.

3680. Massey EW, McHenry LC Jr. Hysteroepilepsy in the nineteenth century: Charcot and Gowers. *Neurology* 1986;**36**:65–7.

3681. Massey EW, Moore J, Schold SC. Mental neuropathy from systemic cancer. *Neurology* 1981;**31**:1277–81.

3682. Massey EW, Schoenberg B. Foster Kennedy syndrome. *Arch Neurol* 1984;**41**:658–9.

3683. Massion-Verniory L, Dumont E, Potvin AM. Retinite pigmentaire familiale compliquée d'une amyotrophie neurale. *Rev Neurol (Paris)* 1946;**78**:561–71.

3684. Masson C, Henin D, Hauw JJ, et al. Cranial pachmeningitis of unknown origin. *Neurology* 1993;**43**:1329–34.

3685. Mastaglia FL, Barwick DD, Hall R. Myopathy in acromegaly. *Lancet* 1970;**2**:907–9.

3686. Mastaglia FL, Laing NG. Distal myopathies: clinical and molecular diagnosis and classification. *J Neurol Neurosurg Psychiatry* 1999;**67**:703–9.

3687. Mastaglia FL, Ojeda V. Inflammatory myopathies: parts 1 and 2. *Ann Neurol* 1985;**17**:215–27, 317–323.

3688. Mastaglia FL, Walton JN. Inflammatory myopathies. In Mastaglia FL, Walton JN, eds. *Skeletal Muscle Pathology,* pp 360–92. Edinburgh: Churchill Livingstone, 1991.

3689. Masters CL, Harris JO, Gajusdek DC, et al. Creutzfeldt-Jakob disease: patterns of worldwide occurrence and the significance of familial and sporadic clustering. *Ann Neurol* 1979;**5**:177–88.

3690. Masucci EF, Kurtzke JF, Saini N. Myorhythmia: a widespread movement disorder. *Brain* 1984;**107**:53–79.

3691. Masuzugawa S, Kuzuhara S, Natita Y, et al. Autosomal dominant hyaline body myopathy presenting as scapuloperoneal syndrome. *Neurology* 1997;**48**:253–7.

3692. Mata M, Dorovini-Zis K, Wilson M, et al. New form of familial Parkinson-dementia syndrome. *Neurology* 1983;**33**:1439–43.

3693. Mathers SE, Kempster PA, Swash M, Lees AJ. Constipation and paradoxical puborectalis contraction in anismus and Parkinson's disease: a dystonic phenomenon? *J Neurol Neurosurg Psychiatry* 1988;**51**: 1503–7.

3694. Mathew NT, Meyer JS, Rivera VM, et al. Double blind evaluation of glycerol treatment in acute cerebral infarction. *Lancet* 1972;**2**: 1327–9.

3695. Mathew NT, Tietgen NE, Lucker C, et al. Serotonin syndrome complicating migraine pharmacotherapy. *Cephalalgia* 1996;**16**:323–7.

3696. Mathiesen B, Reumert T. Blue jeans syndrome. *Ugersk Laeger* 1981;**143**:1333.

3697. Mathuranath PS, Nestor PJ, Berrios GE, et al. A brief cognitive test battery to differentiate Alzheimer's disease and frontotemporal dementia. *Neurology* 2000;**55**:1613–20.

3698. Matison R, Mayeux R, Rosen J, et al. "Tip-of-the-tongue" phenomenon in Parkinson's disese. *Neurology* 1982;**32**:567–70.

3699. Matson DD. *Neurosurgery of Infancy and Childhood.* Springfield, IL: C.C. Thomas, 1969.

3700. Matsumoto J, Fuhr P, Nigro M, et al. Physiological abnormalities in hereditary hyperekplexia. *Ann Neurol* 1992;**32**:41–50.

3701. Matsumoto S. Cheiro-oral syndrome with bilateral involvement: a study of pontine lesions by high-resolution MRI. *J Neurol Neurosurg Psychiatry* 1989;**52**:792–4.

3702. Matsunaga M, Inokudi T, Ohnishi A, et al. Oculopharyngeal involvement in familial neurogenic muscular atrophy. *J Neurol Neurosurg Psychiatry* 1973;**36**:104–11.

3703. Matsuo F, Ajax ET. Palatal myoclonus and denervation supersensitivity in the central nervous system. *Ann Neurol* 1979;**5**:72–8.

3704. Matsuura T, Achari M, Khajavi M, et al. Mapping of the gene for a novel spinocerebellar ataxia with pure cerebellar signs and epilepsy. *Ann Neurol* 1999;**45**:407–11.

3705. Matthews BJ, Crutchfield MB. Painful nocturnal penile erections associated with rapid eye movement sleep. *Sleep* 1987;**10**:184–7.

3706. Matthews WB. Sarcoidosis of the nervous system. *J Neurol Neurosurg Psychiatry* 1965;**28**:23.

3707. Matthews WB. Footballer's migraine. *BMJ* 1972;**2**:326–7.

3708. Matthews WB, Esiri MM. The migrant sensory neuritis of Wartenberg. *J Neurol Neurosurg Psychiatry* 1983;**46**:1–4.

3709. Matthews WB, Howell DA, Stevens DL. Progressive myoclonus epilepsy without Lafora bodies. *J Neurol Neurosurg Psychiatry* 1969;**32**:116–22.

3710. Matthews WB, Rundle AT. Familial cerebellar ataxia and hypogonadism. *Brain* 1964;**87**:463–8.

3711. Mattis S. Mental status examination for organic mental syndrome in the elderly patient. In Bellak L, Karasu TB, eds. *Geriatric Psychiatry: A Handbook for Psychiatrists and Primary Care Physicians.*, pp 77–121. New York: Grune & Stratton, 1976.

3712. Mauguiere F, Courjon J. Somatosensory epilepsy: a review of 127 cases. *Brain* 1978;**101**:307–32.

3713. Maumenee AE. Congenital hereditary corneal dystrophy. *Am J Ophthalmol* 1960;**50**:1114–24.

3714. Maxwell RE. Surgical control of chronic migrainous neuralgia by ganglio-rhizolysis. *J Neurosurg* 1982;**57**:459–66.

3715. May DL, White DL. Familial myoclonus, cerebellar ataxia and deafness; specific genetically determined disease. *Arch Neurol* 1968;**19**:331–8.

3716. Mayer C, Ostheimer S. *Arch Psychiatr Nervenkr* 1918;**59**:462–83.

3717. Mayer EA, Schuffler MD, Rotter JI, et al. Familial visceral neuropathy with autosomal dominant transmission. *Gastroenterology* 1986;**91**:1528–35.

3718. Mayer-Gross W. Some observations on apraxia. *Proc R Soc Med* 1935;**28**:1203–12.

3719. Mayeux R, Alexander MP, Benson DF, et al. Poriomania. *Neurology* 1979;**29**:1616–9.

3720. Maynard R, Garrel S. Les crises de nouveau-ne; intêret de la polygraphie. *Rev Electroencephalogr Neurophysiol Clin* 1983;**13**:219–23.

3721. Maytum CK. Tetany caused by functional dyspnea with hyperventilation: report of a case. *Proc Staff Meet Mayo Clin* 1933;**8**:282–4.

3722. Mazars G. Criteria for identifying cingulate epilepsies. *Epilepsia* 1970;**11**:41–7.

3723. Mbakop A, et al. Lethal multiple pterygium syndrome: report of a new case with hydraencephaly. *Am J Med Genet* 1986;**25**:575–9.

3724. McAllister VL, Kendle BL, Bull JW. Symptomatic vertebral hemangiomas. *Brain* 1975;**98**:71.

3725. McAlpine D, Araki S. Minamata disease: an unusual neurological disorder caused by contaminated fish. *Lancet* 1958;**2**:629–31.

3726. McArdle B. Myopathy due to a defect in muscle glycogen breakdown. *Clin Sci (Lond)* 1951;**10**:13–35.

3727. McArthur J, Harrison MJG, HIV-associated dementia. In Appel SH, ed. *Current Neurology*, pp 231–74. St. Louis: C.V. Mosby, 1994.

3728. McArthur JB. Neurologic manifestations of AIDS. *Medicine* 1987;**66**:407–37.

3729. McCarthy RA, Evans JJ, Hodges JR. Topographic amnesia: spatial memory disorder, perceptual dysfunction, or category specific semantic memory impairment? *J Neurol Neurosurg Psychiatry* 1996;**60**:318–25.

3730. McCarthy RA, Warrington EK. The double dissociation of short-term memory for lists and sentences. Evidence from aphasia. *Brain* 1987;**110**:1545–63.

3731. McCauley SR, Levin HS, Vanier M, et al. The Neurobehavioural Rating Scale revised: sensitivity and validity in closed head injury assessment. *J Neurol Neurosurg Psychiatry* 2001;**71**:643–51.

3732. McComas AJ. Motor unit estimation: anxieties and achievements. *Muscle Nerve* 1995;**18**:369–79.

3733. McCombe PA, Pollard JD, McLeod JG. Chronic inflammatory demyelinating polyradiculoneuropathy: a clinical and electrophysiological study of 92 cases. *Brain* 1987;**110**:1617–30.

3734. McCormick GF, Zee C-S, Heiden J. Cysticercosis cerebri: review of 127 cases. *Arch Neurol* 1982;**39**:534–9.

3735. McCormick K, et al. Partial pyruvate decarboxylase deficiency with profound lactic acidosis and hyperammonemia: response to dichloroacetate acid benzoate. *Am Med Genet* 1985;**22**:291–9.

3736. McCormick WF, Lemmi H. Familial degeneration of the pallidonigral system. *Neurology* 1965;**15**:141–53.

3737. McCrory PR, Berkovic S. Concussion. *Neurology* 2001;**57**:2283–9.

3738. McCrory PR, Berkovic SF. Second impact syndrome. *Neurology* 1998;**50**:677–83.

3739. McCune DJ, Bruch H. Osteodystrophia fibrosa. *Am J Dis Child* 1937;**54**:806–12.

3740. McDaniel KD, Cummings JL, Shain S. The "yips": a focal dystonia of golfers. *Neurology* 1989;**39**:192–5.

3741. McDermott CJ, White K, Bushby K, et al. Hereditary spastic paraparesis: a review of new developments. *J Neurol Neurosurg Psychiatry* 2000;**69**:150–69.

3742. McDonald JW, Bautista RE, Gutmann DH. Pseudocervical cord syndromes. *Arch Neurol* 1996;**53**.

3743. McDonald WI, Compston DAS, Edan G, et al. Recommended diagnostic criteria for multiple sclerosis: guidelines from the International Panel on the Diagnosis of Multiple Sclerosis. *Ann Neurol* 2001;**50**:121–7.

3744. McDonald WI, Halliday AM. Diagnosis and classification of multiple sclerosis. *Br Med Bull* 1977;**33**:4–9.

3745. McDowell F, Lee JE, Swift T, et al. Treatment of Parkinson's syndrome with levodopa. *Ann Intern Med* 1970;**72**:29–35.

3746. McEntee WJ, Biber MP, Perl DP, et al. Diencephalic amnesia: a reappraisal. *J Neurol Neurosurg Psychiatry* 1976;**39**:436–41.

3747. McEntee WJ, Crook TH. Age-associated memory impairment. *Neurology* 1990;**40**:526–30.

3748. McEntee WJ, Mancall EL. Neuromyositis: a reappraisal. *Neurology* 1965;**15**:69–75.

3749. McFarland HR, Wood WG, Drowns BV, et al. Papulosis atrophicans maligna (Kohlmeier-Degos disease): a disseminated occlusive vasculopathy. *Ann Neurol* 1978;**3**:388–92.

3750. McFarland RA. Air travel across time zones. *Am Sci* 1975;**63**:23–30.

3751. McFarlin DE, Strober W, Barlow M, et al. The immunological deficiency state in ataxia-telangiectasia. *Res Publ Assoc Nerv Ment Dis* 1972;**49**:275–92.

3752. McFarling DA, Susac JO. Hoquet diabolique: intractable hiccups as a manifestation of multiple sclerosis. *Neurology* 1979;**29**:797–801.

3753. McGee DA, Van Patter HJ, Marotta J, et al. Subpial cerebral siderosis. *Neurology* 1962;**12**:108–13.

3754. McGeer EG, McGeer PL. The dystonias. *Can J Neurol Sci* 1988;**15**:447–85.

3755. McGeoch KL, Gilmour WH, Taylor W. Sensorineural objective tests in the assessment of hand–arm vibration syndrome. *Occup Environ Med* 1994;**51**:57–61.

3756. McGovern FH. Association of nerve deafness and retinitis pigmentosa. *Acta Otolaryngol* 1942;**36**:827–36.

3757. McGuire SA, Fischbeck KH. Autosomal recessive Duchenne-like muscular dystrophy: molecular and histochemical results. *Muscle Nerve* 1991;**14**:1209–12.

3758. McHenry LC. Rheoencephalography. *Neurology* 1965;**15**:507–17.

3759. McHenry LC Jr. Introduction. In Weir Mitchell S, ed. *Injuries to Nerves*, New York: Dover (Reprint), 1965.

3760. McHenry LC Jr. *Garrison's History of Neurology.* Springfield, IL: Charles C. Thomas, 1969.

3761. McHugh HE, Souden KA, Levitt MN. Facial paralysis and muscle agenesis in the newborn. *Arch Otolaryngol* 1969;**89**:131.

3762. McJunkin JE, de los Reyes EC, Irazuzta JE, et al. La Crosse encephalitis in children. *N Engl J Med* 2001;**344**:801–7.

3763. McKeith IG, Fairbairn AF, Rothwell RA, et al. An evaluation of the predictive validity and inter-rater reliability of clinical diagnostic criteria for senile dementia of the Lewy body type. *Neurology* 1994;**44**:872–7.

3764. McKeith IG, Galasko D, Kosaka K, et al. Consensus guidelines for the clinical and pathological diagnosis of dementia with Lewy bodies. *Neurology* 1996;**47**:1113–24.

3765. McKenna P, Warrington EK. Testing for nominal dysphasia. *J Neurol Neurosurg Psychiatry* 1980;**43**:781–8.

3766. McKenzie RA, Forbes GS, Karnes WE. Angiographic findings in herpes zoster arteritis. *Ann Neurol* 1981;**10**:458–64.

3767. McKhann A, et al. Clinical and electrophysiological aspects of acute paralytic diseases of children and young adults in northern China. *Lancet* 1991;**338**:593–7.

3768. McKhann GM, Cornblath DR, Griffin JW, et al. Acute motor axonal neuropathy: a frequent cause of acute flaccid paralysis in China. *Ann Neurol* 1993;**33**:333–42.

3769. McKusick VA. Dwarfism in the Amish: 1. The Ellis-van Creveld syndrome. *Bull Johns Hopkins Hosp* 1964;**115**:306–36.

3770. McKusick VA. *Mendelian Inheritance in Man.* Baltimore: Johns Hopkins University Press, 1983.

3771. McKusick VA, et al. Chorioretinopathy with hereditary microcephaly. *Arch Ophthalmol* 1966;**75**:597–600.

3772. McLachan RS, Girvin JP, Blume WT, et al. Rasmussen's chronic encephalitis in adults. *Arch Neurol* 1993;**50**:269–74.

3773. McLaurin RL. Parietal cephaloceles. *Neurology* 1964;**14**:764–72.

3774. McLeod JG, Baker WdC, et al. Centronuclear myopathy with autosomal dominant inheritance. *J Neurol Sci* 1972;**15**:375–87.

3775. McLeod JG, Low PA, Morgan JA. Charcot-Marie-Tooth disease with Leber optic atrophy. *Neurology* 1978;**28**:179–84.

3776. McLeod JG, Tuck RR. Disorders of the autonomic nervous system, part 1. Pathophysiology and clinical features. *Ann Neurol* 1987;**21**:419–30.

3777. McLeod JG, Tuck RR. Disorders of the autonomic nervous system, part 2. Investigation and treatment. *Ann Neurol* 1987;**21**:519–29.

3778. McLeod JG, Tuck RR, Pollard JD, et al. Chronic polyneuropathy of unknown cause. *J Neurol Neurosurg Psychiatry* 1984;**47**:530–5.

3779. McLeod JG, Walsh JC. Peripheral neuropathy associated with lymphomas and other reticuloses. In Dyck PJ, Thomas PK, Lambert EH, Bunge R, eds. *Peripheral Neuropathy*, pp 2192–203. Philadelphia: W.B. Saunders, 1984.

3780. McManis PG, Lambert EH, Daube JR. The exercise test in periodic paralysis. *Muscle Nerve* 1986;**9**:704–10.

3781. McManis PG, Sharborough FW. Orthostatic tremor: clinical and electrophysiological characteristica. *Muscle Nerve* 1993;**16**:1254–60.

3782. McMaster KR, Powers JM, Hennigar GR, et al. Nervous system involvement in type IV glycogenosis. *Arch Pathol Lab Med* 1979;**103**:105.

3783. McMenemey WH, et al. Two examples of presenile dementia (Pick's disease and Stern-Garcin syndrome) with a history of trauma. *Arch Psychiatr Nervenkr* 1965;**207**:128–40.

3784. McMurray WC, Rathbun JC, Mohyuddin F, et al. Citrullinuria. *Pediatrics* 1963;**32**:347–57.

3785. McNair D, Lorr M, Droppleman LF. *Profile of Mood States, Bipolar Form.* San Diego: Educational and Industrial Testing Service, 1971.

3786. McNamara JO. Kindling: An animal model of complex partial epilepsy. *Ann Neurol* 1984;**16**(Suppl):S72–S76.

3787. McNamara JO, Curran JR, Hideo H, et al. Congenital ichthyosis with spastic paraplegia of adult onset. *Arch Neurol* 1975;**32**:699–701.

3788. McNaughton S. *Communicating with Blissymbolics.* Don Mills, Ontario Canada: Blissymbolics Cummunication International, 1985.

3789. McQuarrie I. Idiopathic spontaneously occurring hypoglycemia in infants. *Am J Dis Child* 1954;**87**:399–428.

3790. McQuillen MP. Familial limb-girdle myasthenia. *Brain* 1966;**89**:121–32.

3791. McQuillen MP, Cantor H, O'Rourke JR. Myasthenic syndrome associated with antibiotics. *Arch Neurol* 1968;**18**:402–15.

3792. Mead S, James-Galton M, Revesz T, et al. Familial British dementia with amyloid angiopathy. Early clinical, neuro-psychological and imaging findings. *Brain* 2000;**123**:975–99.

3793. Mead S, Proukakis C, Wood N, et al. A large family with hereditary spastic paraparesis due to a frame shift mutation of the spastin (*SPG4*) gene. *J Neurol Neurosurg Psychiatry* 2001;**71**:788–91.

3794. Meador KJ, Loring DW. The Wada Test. *Neurology* 1999;**52**:1535–6.

3795. Meador KJ, Watson RT, Bowers D, et al. Hypometria with hemispatial and limb motor neglect. *Brain* 1986;**109**:293–305.

3796. Meadow R. Fictitious epilepsy. *Lancet* 1984;**2**:25–8.

3797. Meadow SR. Who's to blame—mothers, Munchausen or medicine? *J R Coll Physicians* 1994;**28**:332–7.

3798. Meadows JC. Dysphagia in unilateral cerebral lesions. *J Neurol Neurosurg Psychiatry* 1973;**36**:853–60.

3799. Meadows JC. Observations of a case of monocular diplopia of cerebral origin. *J Neurol Sci* 1973;**18**:249.

3800. Meadows JC, Marsden CD, Harriman DGF. Chronic spinal muscular atrophy in adults, Part I. (The Kugelberg-Welander syndrome). *J Neurol Sci* 1969;**9**:527–50.

3801. Medina JL, Diamond S. Cluster headache variant: spectrum of a new headache syndrome. *Arch Neurol* 1981;**38**:705–9.

3802. Medlock MD, Cruse RS, Winek SJ, et al. A 10–year experience with postpump chorea. *Ann Neurol* 1993; **34**:820–6.

3803. Medori R, Fritscher HJ, le Blanc A, et al. Fatal familial insomnia: a prion disease with a mutation at codon 178 of the prion protein gene. *Neurology* 1992;**32**:444–9.

3804. Meenakashisundaram E, Jagganathan K, Ramamurthi B. Clinical pattern of motor neurone disease in younger age groups. *Neurology (Bombay)* 1970;**8**(Suppl 1):109.

3805. Mega MS, Masterman DL, Benson DF, et al. Dementia with Lewy bodies. *Neurology* 1996;**47**:1403–9.

3806. Mehegan CC, Driefuss MB. Hyperlexia. *Neurology* 1092;**22**:1105–11.

3807. Mehler M. The rostral basilar artery syndrome. *Neurology* 1989;**39**:9–16.

3808. Mehler MF. Complete visual inversion in vertebrobasilar ischemic disease. *J Neurol Neurosurg Psychiatry* 1988;**51**:1235–41.

3809. Mehler MF. The clinical spectrum of ocular bobbing and ocular dipping. *J Neurol Neurosurg Psychiatry* 1988;**51**:725–7.

3810. Mei Liu H, Loew JM, Hunt CE. Congenital central hypoventilation syndrome: a pathologic study of the neuromuscular system. *Neurology* 1978;**28**:1013–9.

3811. Meier C, et al. Spinal muscular atrophy with phenylketonuria. *Dev Med Child Neurol* 1975;**17**:625.

3812. Meier C, Vodlony W, Gatsch M, et al. Nemaline myopathy appearing in adults as cardiomyopathy. *Arch Neurol* 1984;**41**:443–5.

3813. Meierkord H, Shorvon S. Variations on a theme—singing as an epileptic automatism. *J Neurol Neurosurg Psychiatry* 1991;**54**:1114–6.

3814. Meige H. Les convulsions de la face, une forme clinique de convulsion faciale, bilaterale et mediane. *Rev Neurol (Paris)* 1910;**20**:437–43.

3815. Meissner I, Sapir S, Kokmen E, et al. The paramedian diencephalic syndrome: a dynamic phenomenon. *Stroke* 1987;**18**:380–5.

3816. Melberg A, Oldfors A, Bloomstrom-Lundqvist C, et al. Autosomal dominant myofibrillar myopathy with arrhythmogenic right ventricular cardiomyopathy linked to chromosome 10q. *Ann Neurol* 1999; **46**:684–92.

3817. Meleney F. Hemolytic streptococcal gangrene. *Arch Surg* 1924; **9**:317–64.

3818. Melins RB, Balfour HH, Turino GM, Winters RW. Failure of automatic control of ventilation (Ondine's curse). *Medicine* 1973;**49**:487.

3819. Melkersson E. Ett fall av recidiverande facialispares i samband med angioneurotiskt odem. *Hygiea* 1928;**90:**737–41.

3820. Mellarup E, Fog T, Raun N, et al. The socio-economic scale. *Acta Neurol Scand Suppl* 1981;**S87:**130–8.

3821. Mellon CD, Carter JE, Owen DB. Ollier's disease and Maffuci's syndrome: distinct entities or a continuum? *J Neurol* 1988;**235:**376–8.

3822. Melo TP, Bogousslavsky J. Hemiataxia-hypesthesia: a thalamic stroke. *J Neurol Neurosurg Psychiatry* 1992;**55:**581–4.

3823. Melotte G. Idiopathic paralysis of the facial nerve. *Arch Neurol* 1981;**38:**349–53.

3824. Melzack R. The McGill Pain Questionnaire: major properties and scoring methods. *Pain* 1975;**1:**277–99.

3825. Melzack R, Wall PD. On the nature of cutaneous sensory mechanisms. *Brain* 1962;**85:**331–56.

3826. Melzack R, Wall PD. Pain mechanisms; a new theory. *Science* 1965;**150:**971–9.

3827. Mendaz MF, Selwood A, Mastri AR, et al. Pick's disease versus Alzheimer's disease. *Neurology* 1993;**43:**289–92.

3828. Mendel K. Ein Reflex ein Fussrucken. *Neurol Zentrlabl* 1904; **23:**197–8.

3829. Mendell JR, Florence J. Manual muscle testing. *Muscle Nerve* 1990;**13(Suppl):**S16–S20.

3830. Mendell JR, Kilkin S, Kissel JT, et al. Evidence for central nervous system demyelination in chronic inflammatory demyelinating polyneuropathy. *Neurology* 1987;**37:**1291–4.

3831. Mendez MF, Cherrier MM, Perryman KM. Epileptic forced thinking from left frontal lesions. *Neurology* 1996;**47:**79–83.

3832. Mendez MF, Zander BA. Dementia presenting with aphasia: clinical characteristics. *J Neurol Neurosurg Psychiatry* 1991;**54:**542–5.

3833. Mengel MC, Konigsmark BW, Berlin CI. Recessive early onset neural deafness. *Acta Otolaryngol* 1967;**64:**313–26.

3834. Ménière P. Sur une forme particulière de surdité grave dependant d'une lesion de l'oreille interne. *Gaz Med (Paris)* 1861;**16:**21.

3835. Menkes JH. *Textbook of Child Neurology.* Philadelphia: Lea and Febiger, 1985.

3836. Menkes JH, Alter M, Stiegleder GK, et al. A sex-linked recessive disorder with retardation of growth, peculiar hair, and focal cerebral and cerebellar degeneration. *Pediatrics* 1962;**29:**764–79.

3837. Menkes JH, Hurst PL, Craig JM. A new syndrome: progressive familial infantile cerebral dysfunction associated with an unusual urinary substance. *Pediatrics* 1954;**14:**462–7.

3838. Menkes JH, Philippart M, Clark DB. Hereditary partial agenesis of corpus callosum. *Arch Neurol* 1964;**11:**198–208.

3839. Menzel P. Beitrag zur Kenntniss der hereditaren Ataxie und Kleinhirnatrophie. *Arch Psychiatr (Berlin)* 1891;**22:**160–90.

3840. Meola G, Sansone V, Radice S, et al. A family with an unusual myotonic and myopathic phenotype and no CTG expansion (proximal myotonic myopathy syndrome): a challenge for future molecular studies. *Neuromusc Dis* 1996;**6:**143–50.

3841. Meredith J, Grantham E. Cervical spine trauma associated with injury to the head and shoulder girdle. *Am J Surg* 1940;**49:**203.

3842. Meretoja J. Familial systemic paramyloidosis. *Ann Clin Res* 1969; **1:**314–24.

3843. Meretoja J, Teppo L. Histopathological findings of familial amyloidosis with cranial neuropathy as principal manifestation. *Acta Pathol Microbiol Scand* 1971;**79:**432–40.

3844. Merlevede K, Theys P, van Hees J. Diagnosis of ulnar neuropathy: a new approach. *Muscle Nerve* 2000;**23:**478–81.

3845. Merritt HH, Putnam TJ. Sodium diphenylhydantoinate in the treatment of convulsive disorders. *JAMA* 1938;**111:**1068.

3846. Mertens H-G, Zschocke S. Neuromyotonie. *Klin Wochenschr* 1965;**43:**917–25.

3847. Merwarth HR. Hemiplegia of cortical or venous origin (occlusion of Rolandic veins). *Brooklyn Hosp J* 1940;**2:**193–212.

3848. Mestre D, Blin O, Serratrice GT. Contrast sensitivity is increased in a case of nonparkinsonian freezing gait. *Neurology* 1992;**42:**189–94.

3849. Mesulam M-M. Slowly progressive aphasia without generalised dementia. *Ann Neurol* 1982;**11:**592–8.

3850. Mesulam M-M. Norman Geschwind, 1926–1984. *Ann Neurol* 1985;**18:**98–100.

3851. Mesulam M-M. *Principles of Behavioral Neurology.* Philadelphia: F.A. Davis, 1985.

3852. Mesulam M-M. Frontal cortex and behavior. *Ann Neurol* 1986; **19:**320–5.

3853. Mesulam M-M. Primary progressive aphasia. *Ann Neurol* 2001; **49:**425–32.

3854. Metcalfe RA, Macdermott N, Chalmers RJG. Restless red legs. *J Neurol Neurosurg Psychiatry* 1986;**49:**820–3.

3855. Mettinger KL, Ericson K. Fibromuscular dyspasia and the brain: observations on angiographic, clinical, and genetic characteristics. *Stroke* 1982;**13:**46–58.

3856. Meyer A. Karl Friedrich Burbach and his place in the history of neuroanatomy. *J Neurol Neurosurg Psychiatry* 1970;**33:**553–61.

3857. Meyer A. The frontal lobe syndrome, the aphasias and related conditions (a contribution to the history of cortical localization). *Brain* 1974;**97:**565–600.

3858. Meyer A, Leigh D, Bagg CF. Heidenhain's disease. *J Neurol Neurosurg Psychiatry* 1954;**17:**129–31.

3859. Meyer B-U, Irlbacker K, Meierkord H. Analysis of stimuli triggering attacks of paroxysmal dystonia induced by exertion. *J Neurol Neurosurg Psychiatry* 2001;**70:**247–51.

3860. Meyer JS, Portnoy HD. Post-epileptic paralysis: a clinical and experimental study. *Brain* 1959;**82:**162–85.

3861. Meyer-Betz F. Beobachtungen an einem eigenartigen mit Muskellahmungen verbundenem Fall von Hamoglobinurie. *Arch Klin Med* 1910;**101:**85–127.

3862. Meyers R. The extrapyramidal system. *Neurology* 1953;**3:**627–55.

3862a. Meynert TH. Der Bau der Gross-Himrinde und Seine örtlichen verschiederheiten. *Vjschr Psychiatr* 1867;1:77–93;198–217; and 2: 88–113.

3863. Meyrier A, Fardeau M, Richet G. Acute asymmertical neuritis asociated with rapid ultrafiltration dialysis. *BMJ* 1972;**2:**252–4.

3864. Michel D, Laurent B, Convers P, et al. Cortical pain: clinical, electrophysiological and mapping study in 12 cases. *Rev Neurol (Paris)* 1990;**146:**405–14.

3865. Michel P-J. Linea fusca. A study of 13 cases. *Ann Dermatol Syph* 1958;**85:**509–21.

3866. Michiels JJ, Koudstaal PJ, Mulder AH, et al. Transient neurologic and ocular manifestations in primary thrombocythemia. *Neurology* 1993;**43:**1107–10.

3867. Mickey MR, Ellison GW, Myers LW, et al. An illness severity score for multiple sclerosis. *Neurology* 1984;**34:**1343–7.

3868. Middleton PJ, Alexander RM, Szymanski MT. Severe myositis during recovery from influenza. *Lancet* 1970;**2:**533–5.

3869. Midroni G, Dyck PJ. Chronic inflammatory demyelinating polyradiculoneuropathy. *Neurology* 1996;**46:**1206–1212.

3870. Mietens C, Weber H. A syndrome characterized by corneal opacity, nystagmus, flexion contracture of the elbows, growth failure and mental retardation. *J Pediatr* 1966;**69:**624.

3871. Mikati MA, Maguire H, Barlow CF, et al. A syndrome of autosomal dominant alternating hemiplegia: clinical presentation mimicking intractable epilepsy; chromosomal studies; and physiologic investigations. *Neurology* 1992;**42:**2251–7.

3872. Miles JH, et al. Macrocephaly with hamatomas: Bannayan-Zonana syndrome. *Am J Med Genet* 1984;**19:**225–34.

3873. Milhorat AT. Studies in disease of muscle. XIV Progressive muscular atrophy of peroneal type associated with atrophy of the optic nerves; report on a family. *Arch Neurol Psychiatry* 1943;**50:**279–87.

3874. Milhorat TH. *Pediatric Neurosurgery.* Philadelphia: F.A. Davis, 1978.

3875. Millard A. Extrait du Rapport. *Bull Soc Anat Paris* 1855;**30:**206.

3876. Miller A, Nathanson N. Rabies: recent advances in pathogenesis and control. *Ann Neurol* 1977;**2:**511–9.

3877. Miller A, Texidor T. Precordial catch. *JAMA* 1955;**159:**1364–5.

3878. Miller BL, Ikonte C, Ponton M, et al. A study of the Lund-Manchester research criteria for fronto-tempoal dementias. *Neurology* 1997;**48:**937–42.

3879. Miller GM, Sears JC, Guggenheim MA, et al. Schizencephaly: a clinical and CT study. *Neurology* 1984;**34:**997–1001.

3880. Miller JD. Intracranial pressure monitoring. *Arch Neurol* 1985; **42:**1191–3.

3881. Miller JQ. Lissencephaly in two siblings. *Neurology* 1963;**13**: 841–50.

3882. Miller JQ, Price TR. The nervous system in Rocky Mountain spotted fever. *Neurology* 1972;**22**:561–6.

3883. Miller LA, McLachan RS, Bouwer S, et al. Amygdalar sclerosis: preoperative indicators and outcome after temporal lobectomy. *J Neurol Neurosurg Psychiatry* 1994;**57**:1099–105.

3884. Miller ME, Kido D, Horner F. Cavum vergae. *Arch Neurol* 1986; **43**:821.

3885. Miller MT, Ray V, Owens P, et al. Möbius and Möbius-like syndromes (TTV-OFM, OMLH). *J Pediatr Ophthalmol Strabismus* 1989; **26**:176–88.

3886. Miller RG, Layzer RB, Mellenthen MA, et al. Emery-Dreifuss muscular dystrophy with autosomal dominant transmission. *Neurology* 1985;**35**:1230–3.

3887. Miller RG, Nielsen SL, Sumner AJ. Hereditary sensory neuropathy and tonic pupils. *Neurology* 1976;**26**:931–5.

3888. Miller RM, Sparkes RS. Segmental neurofibromatosis. *Arch Dermatol* 1977;**113**:837–8.

3889. Miller SD, Thompson HS. Edge-light pupil cycle time. *Br J Ophthalmol* 1978;**72**:495–500.

3890. Miller TA, Mogyoros I, Burke D. Homonymous and heteronymous monosynaptic reflexes in biceps brachii. *Muscle Nerve* 1995; **18**:585–92.

3891. Miller VT, Rothrock JF, Pearce LA, et al. Ishemic stroke in patients with atrial fibrillation. *Neurology* 1993;**43**:332–36.

3892. Millikan CH, Siekert RG. Studies in cerebrovascular disease. 1. The syndrome of intermittent insufficiency of the basilar arterial system. *Proc Mayo Clin* 1955;**30**:61–8.

3893. Millns JL, Dicken CH. Hereditary acrolabial telangiectasia. A report of familial blue lips, nails and nipples. *Arch Dermatol Chicago* 1979;**115**:474–8.

3894. Mills CK. Unilateral ascending paralysis and unilateral descending paralysis. Their clinical varieties and their pathological causes. *JAMA* 1906;**47**:1638–45.

3895. Mills JA. Systemic lupus erythematosus. *N Engl J Med* 1994; **330**:1871–9.

3896. Mills KR, Murray NMF. Corticospinal tract conduction time in multiple sclerosis. *Ann Neurol* 1985;**18**:601–5.

3897. Milner B. Interhemispheric differences in the localization of psychological processes in man. *Br Med Bull* 1971;**27**:272.

3898. Mimaki T, Itoh N, Abe J, et al. Neurological manifestations in xeroderma pigmentosum. *Ann Neurol* 1986;**20**:70–5.

3899. Minauf E, Jellinger K. Amyotrophy in sporadic Pick disease. *Arch Psychiatrie Nervenkr* 1969;**212**:279.

3900. Minchin R. Primary lateral sclerosis of South India; lathyrism without lathyrus. *BMJ* 1940;**1**:253–5.

3901. Minor L. Central hematomyelia [in German]. *Arch Psychiatrie Nervenkr* 1892;**24**:693–729.

3902. Minor LB, Solomon D, Zinreich JS, et al. Sound and/or pressure induced vertigo due to bone dehiscence of the superior semicircular canal. *Arch Otolaryngol* 1998;**124**:249–58.

3903. Mirra SS, Heyman A, McKeel D, et al. The Consortium to Establish a Registry of Alzheimer's Disease II. *Neurology* 1991;**41**:479–86.

3904. Misiewick JJ, Waller SL, Anthony PP, et al. Achalasia of the cardia. *Q J Med* 1969;**38**:17.

3905. Mitchell J, Weller RO, Evans H, et al. Buckthorn neuropathy: Effects of intraneural injection of Karwinskia humboldtiana toxins. *Neuropathol Appl Neurobiol* 1978;**4**:85–97.

3906. Mitchell DM, Olcszak SA. Remission from a syndrome indistinguishable from motor neurone disease after resection of a bronchial carcinoma. *BMJ* 1979;**2**:176–7.

3907. Mitchell G, Larochelle J, Lambert M, et al. Neurologic crises in hereditary tyrosinemia. *N Engl J Med* 1990;**322**:432.

3908. Mitchell RG. The Landau reaction. *Dev Med Child Neurol* 1962;**4**:65.

3909. Mitchell SW. Phantom limbs. *Lippincotts Mag* 1871;**8**:563–9.

3910. Mitchell SW. *Injuries of Nerves and Their Consequences.* Philadelphia: J.B. Lippincott, 1872.

3911. Mitchell SW. On some of the disorders of sleep. *Va Med Monthly* 1876;**2**:769–81.

3912. Mitler MM, Gujavarty KS, Browman CP. Maintenance of wakefulness test: a polysomnographic test for evaluating treatement in patients with excessive somnolence. *Electroencephalogr Clin Neurophysiol* 1982;**53**:658–61.

3913. Mitros FA, Schuffler MD, Teja K, et al. Pathologic features of familial visceral myopathy. *Hum Pathol* 1982;**13**:825–33.

3914. Mitsumoto H, Adelmann LS, Liu HC. A case of congenital Werdnig Hoffman disease with glial bundles in spinal roots. *Ann Neurol* 1982;**11**:214–6.

3915. Mitsumoto H, Estes ML, Wilbourn AJ, et al. Perineurial cell hypertrophic mononeuropathy manifesting as carpal tunnel syndrome. *Muscle Nerve* 1992;**15**:1364–8.

3916. Mitsumoto H, Sliman RH, Schafer IA, et al. Motor neurone disease and adult hexosaminidase—a deficiency in two families; evidence for multisystem degeneration. *Arch Neurol* 1985;**17**:378–85.

3917. Mitsumoto H, Wilbourn AJ, Subramony SH. Generalized myokymia and gold therapy. *Arch Neurol* 1982;**39**:449–50.

3918. Miwa H, Hatori K, Kondo T, et al. Thalamic tremor. *Neurology* 1996;**46**:75–9.

3919. Miwa H, Yamaji Y, Abe H, et al. Evaluation of the somatosensory evoked blink response in patients with neurological disorders. *J Neurol Neurosurg Psychiatry* 1996;**60**:539–43.

3920. Miyajima H, Nishimura Y, Mizoguchi K, et al. Familial apoceruloplasmin deficiency associated with blepharospasm and retinal degeneration. *Neurology* 1987;**37**:761–7.

3921. Miyoshi K, Kawai H, Masaru I, et al. Autosomal recessive distal muscular dystrophy as a new type of progressive muscular dystrophy. *Brain* 1986;**109**:31–54.

3922. Miyoshi K, Matsuoka T, Mizushima S. Familial holotopistic striatal necrosis. *Acta Neuropathol* 1969;**13**:240–9.

3923. Mizuguchi M, Mikkaichi K, Noma S, et al. Acute necrotizing encephalopathy of childhood: a new syndrome presenting with multifocal symmetric brain lesions. *J Neurol Neurosurg Psychiatry* 1995;**58**: 555–61.

3924. Mizuno Y, Hattori N, Mori H, et al. Parkin and Parkinson's disease. *Curr Opin Neurol* 2001;**14**:477–82.

3925. Mizusawa H, Tagaki A, Sugita H, et al. Mounding phenomenon: an experimental study in vitro. *Neurology* 1983;**33**:90–3.

3926. Möbius PJ. Ueber periodisch wiederkehrende Oculomotoriuslahmung. *Berl Klin Wochenschr* 1884;**21**:604–8.

3927. Möbius PJ. Ueber angeborene doppelseitige Abducens-facialis Lahmung. *Munch Med Wochenschr* 1888;**35**:108–11.

3928. Modarres H, Samuel M, Schon F. Isolated finger flexion: a novel form of focal neuromyotonia. *J Neurol Neurosurg Psychiatry* 2000; **69**:110–3.

3929. Moerman P, Fryns JP, Godderis P, et al. Multiple ankyloses, facial anomalies, and pulmonary hypoplasia associated with severe antenatal spinal muscular atrophy. *J Pediatr* 1983;**103**:238–41.

3930. Moersch FP, Woltman HW. Progressive fluctuating muscular rigidity and spasm ("stiff man syndrome"): report of a case and some observations in 13 other cases. *Mayo Clin Proc* 1956;**31**:421–7.

3931. Moessinger AC. Fetal akinesia deformation sequence: an animal model. *Pediatrics* 1983;**72**:857–63.

3932. Mohnot D, Snead OC, Benton JW. Burn encephalopathy in children. *Ann Neurol* 1982;**12**:42–7.

3933. Mohr J, Magerpy K. Sex-linked deafness of a possibly new type. *Acta Genet* 1960;**10**:54–62.

3934. Mohr JP. Distal field infarction. *Neurology* 1969;**12**:279.

3935. Mohr JP, Barnett HJM. Classification of ischemic strokes. In Barnett HJM, Stein BM, Mohr JP, Yatsu FM, eds. *Stroke: Pathophysiology, Diagnosis, and Management, Vol. 1*, pp 281–91. New York: Churchill Livingstone, 1986.

3936. Mohr JP, et al. Right hemianopia with memory and color deficits in circumscribed left posterior cerebral artery territory infarction. *Neurology* 1971;**21**:1104–6.

3937. Mohr JP, Pessin MS, Finkelstein S, et al. Broca's aphasia: pathological and clinical. *Neurology* 1978;**28**:311–24.

3938. Mohr OL. An hereditary sublethal syndrome in man. *Avhandinger ugitt av det Norske Videnskaps*, Oslo: Norsk Videnskaps, 1941.

3939. Mokri B. Raeder's paratrigeminal syndrome: original concept and subsequent deviations. *Arch Neurol* 1982;**39**:395–9.

3940. Moldaver J. Tourniquet paralysis syndrome. *Arch Surg* 1954;**68:** 136–44.

3941. Molinari GF. Lobar hemorrhages. *Stroke* 1993;**24:**523 526.

3942. Moll JWB, Antoine JC, Brashear HR, et al. Guidelines on the detection of paraneoplastic anti-neuronal–specific antibodies. *Neurology* 1995;**45:**1937–41.

3943. Moll JWB, Henzen-Logmans SC, Splinter TAW, et al. Diagnostic value of anti-neuronal antibodies for paraneoplastic disorders of the nervous system. *J Neurol Neurosurg Psychiatry* 1990;**53:**940–3.

3944. Mollaret P. La méningite endothélio-leucocytaire multirécurrente bénigne. *Bull Soc Med Paris* 1944;**60:**121–2.

3945. Mollica F, Pavone L. Hyperprolinemia: a disease which does not need treatment. *Acta Pediatr Scand* 1976;**65:**206.

3946. Mom AM, Polak M, Fabitero JL, et al. Psoriatic myopathy. *Dermatologia* 1970;**140:**214–8.

3947. Monakow K von. *Gehirnpathologie.* Vienna: Holder, 1905.

3948. Monakow K von. Biologisches und Morphogenetisches uber die Mikrocephalia vera. *Schweiz Arch Neurol Psychiatr* 1926;**18:**3–39.

3949. Monbrun A, Benisty A. Symptoms in war-injured eyes. *Rev Neurol (Paris)* 1916;**23:**906–11.

3950. Monday K, Jankovic J. Psychogenic myoclonus. *Neurology* 1993; **43:**349–52.

3951. Monnens L, Heymans H. Peroxisomal disorders: clinical characterization. *J Inherit Metab Dis* 1987;**10(Suppl):**23–32.

3952. Monrad-Krohn GH. Dysprosody or altered melody of language. *Brain* 1947;**70:**405–15.

3953. Monrad-Krohn GH. *The Clinical Examination of the Nervous System.* New York: Paul B. Hoeber, 1955.

3954. Montagna P. Nocturnal paroxysmal dystonia and nocturnal wandering. *Neurology* 1992;**42:**61–7.

3955. Montagna P. Motor Tinel sign: a new localizing sign in entrapment neuropathy. *Muscle Nerve* 1994;**17:**1493–4.

3956. Montgomery RD, Cruickshank EK, Robertson WB, et al. Clinical and pathological observations on Jamaican neuropathy; a report on 206 cases. *Brain* 1964;**87:**425–62.

3957. Montgomery SA, Asberg MA. A new depression scale designed to be sensitive to change. *Br J Psychiatry* 1979;**134:**382–9.

3958. Montoya G, Dohn DF, Mercer RD. Arteriovenous malformation of the vein of Galen as a cause of heart failure and hydrocephalus in infants. *Neurology* 1971;**21:**1054–8.

3959. Montplaisir J, Godbout R. Restless legs syndrome and periodic movements during sleep. In Kryger MH, Roth T, Dement WC, eds. *Principles and Practice of Sleep Medicine,* pp 402–9. Philadelphia: W.B.Saunders, 1989.

3960. Monytigiani A, Cencetti S, Bandinelli G, et al. The "harlequin sign". Case description and review of the literature. *Ann Ital Med Int* 1998;**13:**173–5.

3961. Moore MT. Paroxysmal abdominal pain. *JAMA* 1944;**124:**561–3.

3962. Moore PM, Cupps TR. Neurological complications of vasculitis. *Ann Neurol* 1983;**14:**155.

3963. Moore RF. Physiology and pathology of the pupil reactions. *Trans Ophthalmol Soc UK* 1924;**44:**38–43.

3964. Moore RF. Subjective "lightning streaks". *Br J Ophthalmol* 1947; **31:**46.

3965. Moosa A, Dubowitz V. Peripheral neuropathy in Cockayne's syndrome. *Arch Dis Child* 1970;**45:**674–7.

3966. Mora M, Lambert EH, Engel AG. Synaptic vesicle abnormality in familial infantile myasthenia. *Neurology* 1987;**37:**206–14.

3967. Moran LJ, Mefferd RB. Repetitive psychometric measures. *Psychol Rep* 1959;**5:**269–75.

3968. Moran NF, Fish DR, Kitchen N, et al. Supratentorial cavernous hemangiomas and epilepsy; a review of the literature and case series. *J Neurol Neurosurg Psychiatry* 1999;**66:**561–8.

3969. Morariu MA, Taranu. Clinico-genetic consideration of basilar impression. *Stud Cerc Neurol* 1968;**13:**441.

3970. Morel F. Hyperostosis frontalis interna, its clinical signs and associated symptoms. *Schweiz Med Wochenschr* 1937;**67:**1235–7.

3971. Morel F. A special anatomo-clinical form of chronic alcoholism: alcoholic laminated cortical sclerosis. *Rev Neurol (Paris)* 1939;**71:**280–8.

3972. Morel F, Wildi E. Disseminated nodular dysgenesis of the frontal cortex. *Rev Neurol (Paris)* 1952;**87:**251–70.

3973. Moretti G, Manzoni GC, Carrarra MD, et al. "Benign recurrent vertigo" and its connection with migraine. *Headache* 1980;**20:**344–6.

3974. Moretti G, Manzoni GC, Mainini P, et al. Empty sella headache. *Headache* 1981;**21:**211–7.

3975. Morgagni GB. *De sedibus et causis morborum peranatomen indagatis libri quinque.* Venetiis: Remondiniana, 1769.

3976. Morgan D, Williams B. Syringobulbia: a surgical appraisal. *J Neurol Neurosurg Psychiatry* 1992;**55:**1132–41.

3977. Morgan JP, Penovich P. Jamaica ginger paralysis: forty-seven year follow-up. *Arch Neurol* 1978;**35:**530–2.

3978. Morgan WC. The probably systemic nature of Mikulicz's syndrome and its relation to Sjogren's syndrome. *N Engl J Med* 1954;**251:**5.

3979. Morgan-Hughes JA. Mitochondrial and lipid storage myopathies. In Engel AG, Banker BQ, eds. *Myology,* pp 1709–43. New York: McGraw Hill, 1993.

3980. Morgan-Hughes JA, Darvenica P, Kahn SM, et al. A mitochondrial myopathy characterized by a deficiency in reducible cytochrome b. *Brain* 1977;**11:**617–40.

3981. Morgan-Hughes JA, Darveniza P, Landon DN, et al. A mitochondrial myopathy with a deficiency of respiratory chain NADH-Co-Q reductase activity. *J Neurol Sci* 1979;**43:**27–46.

3982. Morgan-Hughes JA, Hayes DJ, Clark JB, et al. Mitochondrial encephalomyelopathies. *Brain* 1982;**105:**553–82.

3983. Morgan-Hughes JA, Hayes DJ, Cooper M, et al. Mitochondrial myopathies: deficiencies localised to complex I and complex III of the mitochondrial respiratory chain. *Biochem Soc Trans* 1985;**13:**648–50.

3984. Morgan-Hughes JA, Lecky BRF, Murray NMF, et al. Alterations in the number and affinity of junctional acetylcholine receptors in a myopathy with tubular aggregates. *Brain* 1981;**104:**279–95.

3985. Morgan-Hughes JA, Mair WGP, Lascelles PT. A disorder of skeletal muscle associated with tubular aggregates. *Brain* 1970;**93:** 873–80.

3986. Morgenlander JC, Goldstein RB. Recurrent transient ischemic attacks and stroke associated with an internal carotid argery web. *Stroke* 1991;**22:**94–8.

3987. Mori E, Yamadori A. Rejection behaviour; a human homologue of the abnormal behaviour of Denny-Brown and Chambers' monkey with bilateral parietal ablation. *J Neurol Neurosurg Psychiatry* 1989;**52:** 1260–6.

3988. Morin C, Dubé J, Robinson BH, et al. Stroke-like episodes in autosomal recessive cytochrome oxidase deficiency. *Ann Neurol* 1999; **45:**389–92.

3989. Morin P, Lechevalier B, Bianco C. Atophie cerebelleuse et lesions pallido-luyso-nigriques avec corps de Lewy. *Rev Neurol (Paris)* 1980; **136:**381–90.

3990. Morita H, Ikeda S, Yamamoto K, et al. Hereditary ceruloplasmin deficiency with hemosiderosis: a clinicopathological study of a Japanese family. *Ann Neurol* 1995;**37:**646–56.

3991. Morley JS, Miles JB, Wells JC, et al. Paradoxical pain. *Lancet* 1992;**340:**1045.

3992. Morquio L. Sur une forme de dystrophie osseuse familiale. *Bull Soc Pediatr Paris* 1929;**27:**145–152.

3993. Morquio L. Sur une forme de dystrophie osseuse familiale. *Arch Med Enf Paris* 1929;**32:**129–40.

3994. Morris HH, Dinner DS, Luders H, et al. Supplementary motor seizures: clinical and electroencephalographic findings. *Neurology* 1988; **38:**1075–82.

3995. Morris HH, Peters BH. Pronator syndrome: clinical and electrophysiological features of seven cases. *J Neurol Neurosurg Psychiatry* 1976;**39:**461–4.

3996. Morris JC, Cole M, Banker BQ, et al. Hereditary dysphasic dementia and the Pick-Alzheimer spectrum. *Ann Neurol* 1984;**16:**455–66.

3997. Morris JC, Heyman A, Mohs RC, et al. The consortium to establish a registry for Alzheimer's disease (CERAD). Part 1. Clinical and neuropsychological assessment of Alzheimer's disease. *Neurology* 1989;**39:**1159–65.

3998. Morris JC, Mohs RC, Rogers H, et al. CERAD clinical and psychological assessment of Alzheimer's disease. *Psychopharmacol Bull* 1988;**24:**641–51.

3999. Morrow MJ, Sharpe JA. Torsional nystagmus in the lateral medullary syndrome. *Ann Neurol* 1988;**24:**390–8.

4000. Morse WI, Cochrane WA, Landrigan PL. Familial hypoparathyroidism with pernicious anemia, steatorrhea and adrenocortical insufficiency. *N Engl J Med* 1961;**264**:1021–6.

4001. Morton LT. *A Medical Bibliography*. London: Andre Deutsch, 1970.

4002. Morton TG. A peculiar and painful affection of the fourth metatarsalphalangeal articulation. *Am J Med Sci* 1876;**71**:37–45.

4003. Moruzzi G, Magoun HW. Brain stem reticular formation and activation of EEG. *Electroencephalogr Clin Neurophysiol* 1949;**1**:455–73.

4004. Morvan AM. De la parésie analgésique à panaris des extrémites supérieures ou paréso-analgésie des extrémites supérieures. *Gaz Med Hebd Chir* 1883;**20**:580–583, 590–594.

4005. Morvan AM. De la chorée fibrillaire. *Gaz Med Hebd Chir* 1890;**27**:173–176, 186–189.

4006. Mosberg WH. The Klippel-Feil syndrome: etiology and treatment of neurologic signs. *J Nerv Ment Dis* 1953;**117**:479–91.

4007. Moschcowitz E. An acute febrile pleiochromic anemia with hyaline thrombosis of the terminal arterioles and capillaries. An undescribed disease. *Arch Intern Med* 1925;**36**:89–93.

4008. Mosek A, Korcyzn AD. Yom Kippur headache. *Neurology* 1995;**45**:1953–5.

4009. Moseley I. *Magnetic Resonance Imaging in Diseases of the Nervous System*. Oxford: Blackwell, 1988.

4010. Moseley JL, Molinari JF, Walker AE. Respirator brain. Report of a survey and review of current concepts. *Arch Pathol Lab Med* 1976;**100**:61–4.

4011. Moser IIW. The peroxisome: nervous system role of a previously underrated organelle. *Neurology* 1988;**38**:1617–27.

4012. Moser HW, Moser AB, Kawamura N, et al. Adrenoleukodystrophy: elevated C26 fatty acid in cultured skin fibroblasts. *Ann Neurol* 1980;**7**:542–9.

4013. Moser HW, Naidu S, Kumar AJ, et al. The adrenoleukodystrophies. *Crit Rev Clin Neurobiol* 1987;**3**:29–88.

4014. Moskowitz MA, Henrikson BM, Beyerl BD. Headache. In Rose C, ed. *Handbook of Clinical Neurology*, pp 107–16. Amsterdam: Elsevier, 1986.

4015. Moskowitz MA, Winickoff RN, Heinz ER. Familial calcification of the basal ganglions. *N Engl J Med* 1971;**285**:72–7.

4016. Moss M, Albert M, Butters N, et al. Differential patterns of memory loss in patients with Alzheimer's disease, Huntington's disease and alcoholic Korsakoff's syndrome. *Arch Neurol* 1986;**43**:239–46.

4017. Moss-Morris R, Petrie KJ, Large RG, et al. Neuropsychological deficits in chronic fatigue syndrome: artifact or reality? *J Neurol Neurosurg Psychiatry* 1996;**60**:474–7.

4018. Motta J, Guilleminault C. Cardiac dysfunction during sleep. *Ann Clin Res* 1985;**17**:190–8.

4019. Mount LA, Reback S. Familial paroxysmal choreoathetosis. Preliminary report on a hitherto undescribed clinical syndrome. *Arch Neurol* 1940;**44**:841–7.

4020. Mouradian MM. Recent advances in the genetics and pathogenesis of Parkinson disease. *Neurology* 2002;**58**:179–85.

4021. Mouret JB, Renaud P, Quenin D, et al. Monoamines et regulation de la vigilance. In Girard P, Couteaux R, eds. *Les Mediateurs Chimiques*, p 139. Paris: Masson, 1972.

4022. Moxley RT. Functional testing. *Muscle Nerve* 1990;**13**(Suppl): S26–S29.

4023. Moy S, Opfer-Gehrking TL, Proper CJ. The venoarteriolar reflex in diabetic and other neuropathies. *Neurology* 1989;**39**:1490–2.

4024. Moynahan EJ. Familial congenital alopecia, epilepsy, mental retardation with unusual electroencephalograms. *Proc R Soc Med* 1962;**551**:411–2.

4025. Mozaffar T, Pestronk A. Myopathy with anti-Jo-1 antibodies: pathology in perimysium and neighbouring muscle fibres. *J Neurol Neurosurg Psychiatry* 2000;**68**:472–8.

4026. Mozes M, Ramon Y, Jahr J. The anterior tibial syndrome. *J Bone Jt Surg* 1962;**44-A**:730–5.

4027. Mrak RE, Griebel M, Brodsky MC. Broad A band disease: a new benign congenital myopathy. *Muscle Nerve* 1996;**19**:587–94.

4028. Mrak RE, Lange B, Brodsky MC. Broad A bands of striated muscle in Leber's congenital amaurosis: a new congenital myopathy? *Neurology* 1993;**43**:838–41.

4030. Mrissa N, Belal S, Ben Hamida M, et al. Linkage to chromosome 13q11–12 of an autosomal recessive cerebellar ataxia in a Tunisian family. *Neurology* 2000;**54**:1408–14.

4031. Mubarak SJ, Hargens SR. *Compartment Syndromes and Volkmann's Contracture*. Philadelphia: W.B. Saunders, 1981.

4032. Muckle TJ, Wells M. Urticaria, deafness, and amyloidosis; a new heredo-familial syndrome. *Q J Med* 1962;**31**:235–48.

4033. Mulder DW, Baskan JA, Lambert EH. Hyperinsulin neuronopathy. *Neurology* 1956;**6**:627–35.

4034. Mulder DW, Daly DD, Bailey AA. Visceral epilepsy. *Arch Intern Med* 1954;**91**:481–93.

4035. Mulder DW, Kurland LT, Offord KP, et al. Familial adult motor neurone disease. *Neurology* 1986;**36**:511–7.

4036. Mulleners WM, Verhagen WI, Bartels RH. Cerebral salt wasting syndrome. *J Neurol Neurosurg Psychiatry* 1996;**60**:234–5.

4037. Muller E. Ueber einige weniger bekannte Verlaufdformen der Multiplen Sklerose. *Neurol Zentralbl* 1905;**24**:593–601.

4038. Muller J, Zeman W. Dégenérescence systematisée opticocochleo-dentelée. *Acta Neuropathol* 1965;**5**:26–39.

4039. Muller M, Hubbard SL, Provias J, et al. Malignant rhabdoid tumour of the pineal region. *Can J Neurol Sci* 1994;**21**:277.

4040. Mulvey BE, Reilly LA. Familial syringomyelia and status dysraphicus. *Ann Intern Med* 1942;**16**:966.

4041. Munchau A, Valente EM, Shahidi GA, et al. A new family with paroxysmal exercise induced dystonia and migraine: a clinical and genetic study. *J Neurol Neurosurg Psychiatry* 2000;**68**:609–14.

4042. Munchmeyer E. Ueber Myositis ossificans progressiva. *Z Rat Med* 1869;**34**:9–41.

4043. Munoz-Garcia D, Ludwin SK. Adult-onset neuronal intranuclear hyaline inclusion disease. *Neurology* 1986;**36**:785–90.

4044. Munoz-Malaga A, Bautista J, Salazar JA, et al. Lipomatosis, proximal myopathy and the mitochondrial 8344 mutation. A lipid storage myopathy? *Muscle Nerve* 2000;**23**:538–42.

4045. Munsat TL. A standardized forearm ischemic exercise test. *Neurology* 1970;**20**:1171–8.

4046. Murachi S, Nogami H, Oki T, et al. The trichorhinophalangeal syndrome with exostoses; four additional patients without mental retardation and a review of the literature. *Am J Med Genet* 1984;**19**:111.

4047. Muratov W. Pathogenesis of post-apoplectic chorea. *Monatschr Psychiatr Neurol*. 1899;**5**:180–92.

4048. Murphy SF, Drachman DB. The oculopharyngeal syndrome. *JAMA* 1968;**203**:1003–8.

4049. Murray TJ. Congenital sensory neuropathy. *Brain* 1973;**96**:387–94.

4050. Murri A. Degeneratione cerebellare da intossicazione endogena. *Riv Crit Clin Med* 1900;**1**:593–609.

4051. Myers AR, Willis PW. Clinical spectrum of supravalvular aortic stenosis. *Arch Intern Med* 1966;**118**:553–61.

4052. Myerson A. Contralateral periosteal reflexes of the arm. *J Nerv Ment Dis* 1914;**41**:162–4.

4053. Myhrman G. The secondary wave; a forgotten muscular phenomenon. *Acta Med Scand* 1939;**98**:542–60.

4054. Nachemson A. Lumbar spine instability; a critical update and symposium summary. *Spine* 1985;**10**:290–1.

4055. Nadeau SE, Trobe JD. Pupil sparing in oculomotor palsy: a brief review. *Ann Neurol* 1983;**13**:143–8.

4056. Nadkarni N, Lisak RP. Guillain-Barré syndrome with bilateral optic neuritis and central white matter disease. *Neurology* 1993;**43**:842–3.

4057. Nadler HL, Egan TJ. Deficiency of lysosomal acid phosphatase. *N Engl J Med* 1970;**282**:303–7.

4058. Nadol JB Jr, Burgess B. Cochleosaccular degeneration of the inner ear and progressive cataracts inherited as an autosomal dominant trait. *Laryngoscope* 1982;**92**:1028–37.

4059. Naffziger HC. Subdural fluid accumulation following head injury. *JAMA* 1924;**82**:1751–2.

4060. Naffziger HC. The scalenus syndrome. *Surg Gynecol Obstet* 1937;**64**:119–20.

4061. Nagamitsu S, Matsuura T, Khajavi M, et al. A "dystrophic" variant of autosomal recessive myotonia congenita caused by novel mutations in the *CLCN1* gene. *Neurology* 2000;**55**:1697–703.

4062. Naidu S, Hoefler G, Watkins PA, et al. Neonatal seizures and retardation in a girl with biochemical features of X-linked adrenoleukodystrophy; a possible new disease entity. *Neurology* 1988;**38**: 1100–7.

4063. Nakada T, Knight RT, Mani RL. Intermittent venous claudication of the upper extremity; the pectoralis minor syndrome. *Ann Neurol* 1982;**11**:433–4.

4064. Nakada T, Kwee IL. Oculopalatal myoclonus. *Brain* 1986;**109**: 431–41.

4065. Nakada T, Kwee IL. See-saw nystagmus—role of visuovestibular interaction in its pathogenesis. *J Clin Neuroophthalmol* 1988;**8**:171.

4066. Nakajima M, Hirayama K. Midcervical central cord syndrome: numb and clumsy hands due to midline cervical disc protrusion at the C3–4 intervertebral level. *J Neurol Neurosurg Psychiatry* 1995;**58**: 607–13.

4066a. Nakamura K, Jeong S-Y, Uchihara T, et al. SCA 17; a novel autosomal dominant cerebellar ataxia caused by an expanded polyglutamine in TATA-binding protein. *Hum Molec Genet* 2001;**10**:1441–48.

4067. Nakano KK, Dawson DM, Spence A. Machado disease. *Neurology* 1972;**22**:49–55.

4068. Nakano T, Ikeda S, Condo K, et al. Adult GM 1–gangliosidosis. *Arch Neurol* 1985;**35**:875–80.

4069. Namba T, Brown SB, Grob D. Neonatal myasthenia gravis. *Pediatrics* 1970;**45**:488–504.

4070. Namba T, Brunner NG, Brown SB. Familial myasthenia gravis: report of 27 patients in 12 families and review of 164 patients in 73 families. *Arch Neurol* 1971;**25**:49–60.

4071. Namba T, Brunner NG, Grob N. Idiopathic giant cell polymyositis: report of a case and review of the syndrome. *Arch Neurol* 1974;**31**:27–30.

4072. Nance WE, et al. X-linked mixed deafness with congenital fixation of the stapedial footplate and perilymphatic gusher. *Birth Defects* 1971;**7(4)**:64–9.

4073. Narabayashi H, Imai H, Yokochi M, et al. Cases of pure akinesia without rigidity and tremor and with no effect by L-dopa therapy. In Birkmayer W, Horniekiewicz O, eds. *Advances in Parkinsonism*, pp 335–42. Basel: Roche, 1976.

4074. Nardocci N, Zorzi G, Farina L, et al. Infantile neuroaxonal dystrophy. *Neurology* 1999;**52**:1472–8.

4075. Nashold BS, Ostdahl RH, Bullitt E, et al. Dorsal root entry zone lesions: a new neurosurgical therapy for deafferentation pain. In Bonica JJ, ed. *Advances in Pain Research and Therapy*, pp 739–50. New York: Raven Press, 1983.

4076. Nathan PW, Smith MC. The rubrospinal and central tegmental tracts in man. *Brain* 1982;**105**:223–69.

4077. Nathan PW, Smith MC, Cook AW. Sensory effects in man of lesions of the posterior columns and of some other afferent pathways. *Brain* 1986;**109**:1003–41.

4078. Nathanson M. Lou Gehrig. *Neurology* 1986;**36**:1349.

4079. National Institute of Neurological and Communicative Diseases and Stroke. Diagnostic criteria for Alzheimer disease. *Neurology* 1988;**38**:360–5.

4080. National Institute of Neurological Disorders and Stroke. Classification of cerebrovascular diseases III. *Stroke* 1990;**21**:637–76.

4081. Nausieda PA, Weiner WJ, Klawans HL. Dystonic foot response of Parkinsonism. *Arch Neurol* 1980;**37**:132–6.

4082. Navon R, Khosravi R, Korczyn T, et al. A new mutation in the *HEXA* gene associated with a spinal muscular atrophy phenotype. *Neurology* 1995;**45**:539–43.

4083. Neary D, Snowden JS, Gustafson L, et al. Frontotemporal lobar degeneration. *Neurology* 1998;**5157**:1546–54.

4083a. Nechiporuk A, Lopes-Cendes I, Nechiporuk T, et al. Genetic mapping of the spinocerebellar ataxia type 2 gene on human chromosome 12. *Neurology* 1996;**46**:1731–5.

4084. Needles W. Pseudotabes pituitaria. *J Nerv Ment Dis* 1934;**80**: 651–7.

4085. Neelon FA, Goree JA, Lebovitz HE. The primary empty sella: clinical and radiographic characteristics and endocrine function. *Medicine* 1973;**52**:73–92.

4086. Negro C. *Clinical and Pathological Study of the Nervous System*. Torino: Lattes, 1912.

4087. Neill CA, Dingwall MM. A syndrome resembling progeria. *Arch Dis Child* 1950;**25**:213–21.

4088. Nellhaus G. Composite international and inter-racial graphs. *Pediatrics* 1968;**41**:106.

4089. Nelson DA, Landau WM. Jaws: diversities of gnathological history and temporomandibular joint enterprise. *J Neurol Neurosurg Psychiatry* 1999;**67**:141–7.

4090. Nelson DH, Meakin JW, Dealy JB, et al. ACTH-producing tumour of the pituitary gland. *N Engl J Med* 1958;**259**:161–4.

4091. Nelson HE. Wisconsin Card Sorting Test. *Cortex* 1976;**12**: 313–24.

4092. Nelson I, Hanna MG, Alsamjari N, et al. A new mitochondrial DNA mutation associated with progressive dementia and chorea: a clinical, pathological and genetic study. *Ann Neurol* 1995;**37**:400–3.

4093. Nelson JR. The minimal ice water caloric test. *Neurology* 1970; **20**:577–85.

4094. Nelson JS, Prensky AL. Sporadic juvenile amyotrophic lateral sclerosis. *Arch Neurol* 1972;**27**:300–6.

4095. Nelson KB, Ellenberg JH. The asymptomatic newborn and risk of cerebral palsy. *Am J Dis Child* 1987;**141**:1333.

4096. Nelson M, Lessell S, Sadun AA. Optic nerve hypoplasia and maternal diabetes mellitus. *Arch Neurol* 1986;**43**:20–5.

4097. Nelson MM, Thompson AJ. The acrocallosal syndrome. *Am J Med Genet* 1982;**12**:195–9.

4098. Nemni R, Bottacci E, Fazio R, et al. Polyneuropathy in hypothyroidism. *J Neurol Neurosurg Psychiatry* 1987;**50**:1454–60.

4099. Nemni R, Galassi G, Cohen M, et al. Symmetrical sarcoid polyneuropathy. *Neurology* 1981;**31**:1217–23.

4100. Neng T, Yi C, Xiu-Bao Z, et al. Acute infectious torticollis. *Neurology* 1983;**33**:1344–6.

4101. Neri V. On a new sign of organic hemiplegia [in French]. *Nouv Icon Salpet* 1910;**23**:88–9.

4102. Neu RL, Kajii T, Gardner LI, et al. A lethal syndrome of microcephaly with multiple genetic anomalies in three siblings. *Pediatrics* 1971;**47**:610–2.

4103. Neufeld MY, Blumen SC, Nisipeanu P, et al. Lingual seizures. *Epilepsia* 1988;**29**:20–33.

4104. Neumann MA, Cohn R. Progressive subcortical gliosis—a rare form of presenile dementia. *Brain* 1967;**90**:405–17.

4105. Neuzelius C. Spontaneous cerebrospinal fluid otorrhea due to congenital malformation. *Acta Otolaryngol* 1951;**39**:314.

4106. Neville BGR, Boyd SG. Selective epileptic gait disorder. *J Neurol Neurosurg Psychiatry* 1995;**58**:371–3.

4107. Neville HE, Baumbach LL, Ringel SP, et al. Familial inclusion body myositis. *Neurology* 1992;**42**:897–902.

4108. Neville HE, Ringel SP, Guggenheim MA, et al. Ultrastructure and histochemical abnormalities of skeletal muscle in patients with chronic vitamin E deficiency. *Neurology* 1983;**33**:483–8.

4109. Nevin S. Gliomatosis cerebri. *Brain* 1938;**61**:170–91.

4110. Nevin S, Jones DP. Rapidly progressive cerebral degeneration (subacute vascular encephalopathy) with mental disorder, focal disturbances, and myoclonic epilepsy. *J Neurol Neurosurg Psychiatry* 1954; **17**:148–59.

4111. Nevin S, McMenemey WH, Behrman S, Jones DP. Subacute spongiform encephalopathy. *Brain* 1960;**83**:519–63.

4112. New GB, Eric JB. Dermoid cysts of head and neck. *Surg Gynecol Obstet* 1937;**65**:48.

4113. Newman LC, Lipton RB, Russell M, et al. Hemicrania continua: attacks may alternate sides. *Headache* 1992;**32**:237–8.

4114. Newman LC, Lipton RB, Solomon S. Hemicrania continua. *Neurology* 1994;**44**:2111–4.

4115. Newman NJ, Lessell S, Winterkorn MS. Optic chiasmal neuritis. *Neurology* 1991;**41**:1203–10.

4116. Newman NM, Tornambe PE, Corbett JJ. Ophthalmoscopy of the retinal nerve fiber layer: use in detection of neurologic disease. *Arch Neurol* 1982;**39**:226–33.

4117. Newman PH. Sprung back. *J Bone Jt Surg* 1952;**34B**:30–7.

4118. Newmark J, Hochberg FH. Isolated painless manual incoordination in 57 musicians. *J Neurol Neurosurg Psychiatry* 1987;**50**:291–5.

4119. Newsom-Davis J. Diseases of the nervous system. In Campbell EJJM, Agostoni E, Newsom Davis J, eds. *The Respiratory Muscles*, pp 314–27. London: Lloyd-Luke, 1970.

4120. Newton CRJC, Hien TT, White N. Cerebral malaria. *J Neurol Neurosurg Psychiatry* 2000;**69**:433–41.

4121. Newton CRJC, Warrell DJ. Neurological manifestations of falciparum malaria. *Ann Neurol* 1998;**43**:695–702.

4122. Newton FH, Rosenberg RN, Lampert PW, et al. Neurologic involvement in Urbach-Wiethe's disease (lipoid proteinosis). *Neurology* 1971;**21**:1205–13.

4123. Newton RW. Intracranial pressure and its monitoring in childhood; a review. *J R Soc Med* 1987;**80**:566–70.

4124. Neyman J. Statistics—servant of all sciences. *Science* 1955;**122**:401.

4125. Nezelof C, Dupont F, Jankers F, et al. A lethal familial syndrome associating arthrogryposis multiplex congenita, renal dysfunction and a cholestatic and pigmentary liver disease. *J Pediatr* 1979;**94**:258–90.

4126. Nguyen DK, Botez MI. Diaschisis and neurobehavior. *Can J Neurol Sci* 1998;**25**:5–12.

4127. Nichols FL, Holdsworth DE, Reinfrank RF. Familial hypocalcemia latent tetany and calcification of the basal ganglia: report of a kindred. *Am J Med* 1961;**30**:518–28.

4128. Nickel SN, Frame B, Bebin J, et al. Myxedema neuropathy and myopathy. *Neurology* 1961;**11**:125–37.

4129. Nicolao P, Xiang F, Gunnarsson LG, et al. Autosomal dominant myopathy with proximal weakness and early respiratory muscle involvement maps to chromosome 2q. *Am J Hum Genet* 1999;**64**:788–92.

4130. Nielsen JM. *Agnosia, Apraxia, and Aphasia*. New York: Hoeber, 1946.

4131. Nielsen JM. Tornado epilepsy simulating Ménière's syndrome. *Neurology* 1959;**9**:794–6.

4132. Nielsen VK, Friis ML, Johnsen T. Electromyographic distinction between paramyotonia congenita and myotonia congenita: effect of cold. *Neurology* 1982;**32**:827–32.

4133. Nielson JM. A subacute generalized neuromuscular exhaustion syndrome. *JAMA* 1940;**126**:801–6.

4134. Niemann A. Ein unbekanntes Krankheitsbild. *Jahrb Kinderheilkd* 1914;**79**:1–10.

4135. Nighoghossian N, Derex L, Loire R, et al. Giant Lambl excrescences. *Arch Neurol* 1997;**54**:41–4.

4136. Nihira K, Foster R, Shellhaas M, et al. *American Association of Mental Deficiency Adaptive Behavior Scale, 1974 Revision*. Washington, DC: AAMD, 1975.

4137. Niikawa N, Fukushima Y, Taniguchin M, et al. Chromosome abnormalities involving 11p13 and low erythrocyte catalase activity. *Hum Genet* 1982;**60**:373–5.

4138. Niikawa N, Matsuura N, Fukushima Y, et al. Kabuki make-up syndrome. *J Pediatr* 1981;**99**:565–9.

4139. Nikoskelainen EK, Marttila RJ, Huoponen K, et al. Leber's "plus"; neurological abnormalities in patients with Leber's hereditary optic neuropathy. *J Neurol Neurosurg Psychiatry* 1995;**59**:160–4.

4140. NINCDS Ad Hoc Committee. Classification of headaches. *Ann Neurol* 1978;**3**:565.

4141. NINCDS Ad Hoc Committee. Classification of cerebrovascular disease. *Stroke* 1990;**21**:637–76.

4142. Nishimura RN, Barranger JA. Neurological complications of Gaucher's disease, type 3. *Arch Neurol* 1980;**37**:92–3.

4143. Nishino H, Rubino FA, DeRemee RA, et al. Neurological involvement in Wegener's granulomatosis: an analysis of 324 consecutive patients at the Mayo Clinic. *Ann Neurol* 1993;**33**:4–9.

4144. Nissen JJ, Jones PA, Signorini DF, et al. Glasgow Head Injury Prediction Program: an independent assessment. *J Neurol Neurosurg Psychiatry* 1999;**67**:796–9.

4145. Nix WA, Butler IJ, Roontga S, et al. Persistent unilateral tibialis anterior muscle hypertrophy with complex repetitive discharges and myalgia. *Neurology* 1992;**42**:602–6.

4146. Noachtar S, Holthausen H, Luders HO. Epileptic negative myoclonus. *Neurology* 1997;**49**:1534–7.

4147. Noad KB, Haymaker W. The neurological features of Tsutsugamushi fever, with special reference to deafness. *Brain* 1953;**76**:113–31.

4148. Nobile-Orakio E, Baldini L, Barbieri S. Treatment of patients with neuropathy and anti-MAG IgM M-proteins. *Ann Neurol* 1988;**24**:93–7.

4149. Nobunga M, Yoskioka K, Yasuda M, et al. Clinical studies of polymyalgia rheumatica. A proposal of diagnostic crieteria. *Jpn J Med* 1989;**28**:452–6.

4150. Nogen AG. Congenital muscular disease and abnormal findings on computerized tomography. *Dev Med Child Neurol* 1980;**22**:658–63.

4151. Nomizu S, Person DA, Saito C, et al. A unique case of reducing body myopathy. *Muscle Nerve* 1992;**15**:463–6.

4152. Nonaka I. Distal myopathies. *Curr Opin Neurol* 1999;**12**:493–9.

4153. Nonaka I, Sunohara N, Satoyoshi E, et al. Autosomal recessive distal muscular dystrophy: a comparative study with distal myopathy with rimmed vacuole formation. *Ann Neurol* 1985;**17**:51–9.

4154. Noonan JA. Hypertelorism with Turner phenotype. *Am J Dis Child* 1968;**116**:373–80.

4155. Nordborg C, Conradi N, Sourander P, et al. A new type of nonprogressive sensory neuropathy in children with atypical dysautonomia. *Acta Neuropathol* 1981;**55**:135–41.

4156. Norenberg MD, Leslie KO, Robertson AS. Association between rise in serum sodium and central pontine myelinolysis. *Ann Neurol* 1982;**11**:128–35.

4157. Norman MG, Roberts M, et al. Lissencephaly. *Can J Neurol Sci* 1976;**3**:39–46.

4158. Norman RM, Tingey AH. Syndrome of microencephaly, striocerebellar calcification and leukodystrophy. *J Neurol Neurosurg Psychiatry* 1966;**29**:157–63.

4159. Norman RM, Urich H. Cerebellar hypoplasia associated with systemic degeneration early in life. *J Neurol Neurosurg Psychiatry* 1958;**159**:166.

4160. Norman RM, Wood N. A congenital form of amaurotic familial idiocy. *J Neurol Neurosurg Psychiatry* 1941;**4**:175–90.

4161. Norre ME, Stevens A. Cervical vertigo. *Acta Otorhinolaryngol (Belg)* 1987;**41**:436.

4162. Norregaard J, Bulow PM, Danneskiold-Samsoe B. Muscle strength, voluntary activation, twitch properties and endurance in patients with fibromyalgia. *J Neurol Neurosurg Psychiatry* 1994;**57**:1106–11.

4163. Norrie G. Causes of blindness in children. *Acta Ophthalmol Kopenhagen* 1927;**5**:363–4.

4164. Norris FH. Amyotrophic lateral sclerosis score. *Neurology* 1974;**24**:721–8.

4165. Norris FH, Panner BJ. Hypothyroid myopathy. *Arch Neurol* 1966;**14**:574–89.

4166. Norris FH, Panner BJ, Stormont JM. Thyrotoxic periodic paralysis; metabolic and ultrastructural studies. *Arch Neurol* 1968;**19**:88–98.

4167. Norton JV, Zager E, Grady JF. Erythromelalgia: diagnosis and classification. *J Foot Ankle Surg* 1999;**38**:238–41.

4168. Noseworthy JH, Ebers GC, Leigh RJ, et al. Torsional nystagmus: quantitative features and possible pathogenesis. *Neurology* 1988;**38**:992–4.

4169. Noseworthy JH, Heffernan LP, Ross JB. Acne fulminans with inflammatory myopathy. *Ann Neurol* 1980;**8**:67–9.

4170. Notermans NC, Fransses H, Eurelings M, et al. Diagnostic criteria for demyelinating polyneuropathy associated with monoclonal gammopathy. *Muscle Nerve* 2000;**23**:73–9.

4171. Noth J, Dietz V, Mauritz K-H. Cyclist's palsy. *J Neurol Sci* 1980;**47**:111–6.

4172. Nothnagel CWH. On vasomotor neuroses. *Arch Klin Med* 1867;**2**:173–91.

4173. Nothnagel H. *Topische Diagnostik der Gehirnkrankheiten*. Berlin: Hischwalden, 1879.

4174. Nouri FM, Lincoln NB. An extended activities of daily living scale for stroke patients. *Clin Rehabil* 1987;**1**:301–5.

4175. Noviaka I, Sunohara N, Isiki S, et al. Familial distal myopathy with rimmed vacuoles and lamellar (myeloid) body formation. *J Neurol Neurosurg Psychiatry* 1981;**51**:141–55.

4176. Novotny HR, Alvis DL. A method of photographing fluorescence in circulating blood of the human eye. *Am J Ophthalmol* 1960;**50**:176.

4177. Nowak DA, Widenka DC. Neurosarcoidosis: a review of its intracranial manifestations. *J Neurol* 2001;**248**:363–72.

4178. Nudleman K, Andermann E, Andermann F, et al. The Hemi 3 syndrome. *Brain* 1984;**107**:533–46.

4179. Nukada H, McMorran PD, Shimizu J. Acute inflammatory demyelination in reperfusion nerve injury. *Ann Neurol* 2000;**47**:71–9.

4180. Nutt JG, Marsden CD, Thompson PD. Human walking and higher-level gait disorders, particularly in the elderly. *Neurology* 1993;**43**:268–79.

4181. Nygaard TG, Marsden CD, Duvoisin RC. Dopa-responsive dystonia. *Adv Neurol* 1988;**50**:377–84.

4182. Nygaard TG, Raymond D, Chen C, et al. Localization of a gene for myoclonus-dystonia to chromosome 7q21–q31. *Ann Neurol* 1999; **46**:794–8.

4183. Obal A. Nutritional amblyopia. *Am J Ophthalmol* 1951;**34**: 857–65.

4184. Oberklaid F, Danks DM, Mayne V, et al. Asphyxiating thoracic dysplasia. *Arch Dis Child* 1977;**52**:758–65.

4185. Oberman HA. Chemodectomas (nonchromaffin paraganglioma) of head and neck. *Cancer* 1968;**21**:838–51.

4186. Obersteiner H. On allochiria, a peculiar sensory disorder. *Brain* 1881;**4**:153–63.

4187. Obeso JA, Rothwell JC, Lang AE, et al. Myoclonic dystonia. *Neurology* 1983;**33**:825–30.

4188. O'Brien JG, et al. Juvenile GM1 gangliosidosis. Clinical, pathological, chemical and enzymatic studies. *Clin Genet* 1972;**3**:411–34.

4189. O'Brien JS. The gangliosidoses. In Stanbury JS, Wyngaarden JB, Frederickson DS, et al., eds. *The Metabolic Basis of Inherited Disease*, p 952. New York: McGraw-Hill, 1983.

4190. O'Brien MD, Upton ARM. Anterior interosseous nerve syndrome. *J Neurol Neurosurg Psychiatry* 1972;**35**:531–6.

4191. O'Brien TJ, Cascino GD, So EL, et al. Incidence and clinical consequences of the purple glove syndrome in patients receiving intravenous phenytoin. *Neurology* 1998;**51**:1034–9.

4192. Ochipa C, Rothi LJG, Heilman KM. Conduction apraxia. *J Neurol Neurosurg Psychiatry* 1994;**57**:1241–4.

4193. Ochoa JL. Positive sensory symptoms in neuropathy; mechanisms and aspects of treatment. In Asbury AK, Thomas PK, eds. *Peripheral Nerve Disorders 2*, pp 44–58. Oxford: Butterworth-Heinemann, 1995.

4194. Ochoa JL, Yarnitsky D. Mechanical hyperalgesias in neuropathic pain patients: dynamic and static subtypes. *Ann Neurol* 1993;**33**:465–72.

4195. Ochs S. The early history of nerve regeneration, beginning with Cruickshank's observations in 1776. *Med Hist* 1977;**21**:261–74.

4196. Ochsner A, Gage M, DeBakey M. Scalenus anticus (Naffziger) syndrome. *Am J Surg* 1935;**28**:669.

4197. O'Connell JEA, Du Boulay EPGH. Binasal hemianopia. *J Neurol Neurosurg Psychiatry* 1973;**36**:697–709.

4198. O'Connell JEA, Turner JWA. Basilar impression of the skull. *Brain* 1950;**73**:405–25.

4199. Odaka M, Yuki N, Hirata K. Anti-GQ1b antibody syndrome: clinical and immunological range. *J Neurol Neurosurg Psychiatry* 2001;**70**:50–5.

4200. O'Donnell PP, Leschner RT, Campbell WW. Hypertrophia musculorum vera in familial ataxia. *Arch Neurol* 1986;**43**:146–7.

4201. O'Duffy J. Propos pour le diagnostic de la maladie de Behçet. *Rev Med (Bruxelles)* 1974;**36**:2371–8.

4202. O'Duffy JD, Goldstein NP. Neurologic involvement in seven patients with Behçet's disease. *Am J Med* 1976;**61**:170–8.

4203. Oerlemans WG, de Visser M. Dropped head syndrome and bent spine syndrome: two separate clinical entities or different manifestations of axial myopathy? *J Neurol Neurosurg Psychiatry* 1998;**65**:258–9.

4204. Offen ML, Davidoff RA, Troost BT, et al. Dacrystic epilepsy. *J Neurol Neurosurg Psychiatry* 1976;**39**:829–34.

4205. Offenbacher H, Fazekas F, Schmidt R, et al. Assessment of MRI criteria for a diagnosis of MS. *Neurology* 1993;**43**:905–9.

4206. Oguni H, Olivier A, Andermann F, et al. Anterior callosotomy in the treatment of medically intractable epilepsies: a study of 43 patients with a mean follow-up of 39 months. *Ann Neurol* 1991;**30**: 357–364.

4207. Ogunyemi AO, Dreifuss FE. Syndromes of epilepsy in childhood and adolescence. *J Child Neurol* 1988; **35**:214–24.

4208. Ogunyemi AO, Murphy D. The pinky finger in neurological diagnosis. *Can J Neurol Sci* 1999;(**Suppl 2**):S44.

4209. Oh SJ, Birmingham AL, Danon MJ, et al. Mitochondrial myelomyopathy (3–M syndrome). *Neurology* 1991;**41**(**Suppl 1**):178.

4210. Oh SJ, Claussen GC, Kim DS. Motor and sensory demyelinating mononeuropathy multiplex (multifocal motor and sensory demyelinating neuropathy): a separate entity or a variant of chronic inflammatory demyelinating polyneuropathy? *J Periph Nerv Syst* 1997;**2**: 362–9.

4211. Oh SJ, Claussen GC, Ryan H, et al. Multifocal sensory demyelinating neuropathy: a heretofore unrecognized entity. *Ann Neurol* 2000; **48**:468.

4212. Oh SJ, Darron MJ. Nonprogressive congenital neuromuscular disease with uniform type 1 fiber. *Arch Neurol* 1983;**40**:147–50.

4213. Oh SJ, Dwyer DS, Bradley RJ. Overlap myasthenia gravis and Eaton-Lambert syndrome. *Neurology* 1987;**37**:1411–4.

4214. Oh SJ, Joy JL, Kuruoglu R. "Chronic sensory demyelinating neuropathy": chronic inflammatory demyelinating polyneuropathy presenting as a pure sensory neuropathy. *J Neurol Neurosurg Psychiatry* 1992;**55**:677–80.

4215. Oh SJ, Kuruoglu R. Chronic limb-girdle myasthenia gravis. *Neurology* 1992;**42**:1153–6.

4216. Oh SJ, Kwon KH, Hah JS, et al. Lateral plantar neuropathy. *Muscle Nerve* 1999;**22**:1234–8.

4217. Oh SJ, LaGanke C, Claussen GC. Sensory Guillain-Barré syndrome. *Neurology* 2001;**56**:82–6.

4218. Oh SJ, Lee KW. Medial plantar neuropathy. *Neurology* 1987;**37**: 1408–10.

4219. Oh SJ, Myers GJ, Wilson ER, et al. A benign form of reducing body myopathy. *Muscle Nerve* 1983;**6**:278–82.

4220. Ohara S, Kondo K, Morita H, et al. Progressive supranuclear palsy-like syndrome in two siblings of a consanguineous marriage. *Neurology* 1992;**42**:1009–14.

4221. O'Hearn E, Holmes SE, Cavert PC, et al. SCA-12: tremor with associated cerebellar and cortical atrophy is associated with a CAG repeat expansion. *Neurology* 2001;**56**:299–303.

4222. Ohkawa S, Yamasaki H, Tabuchi M, et.al. Eyebrow lifting test. *J Neurol Neurosurg Psychiatry* 1997;**63**:256–7.

4223. Ohlsson L. Congenital renal disease, deafness, and myopia in one family. *Acta Med Scand* 1963;**174**:77–84.

4224. Ohno K, Engel AG, Brengman JM, et al. The spectrum of mutations causing end-plate acetylcholinesterase deficiency. *Ann Neurol* 2000;**47**:162–70.

4225. Ohta M, Ellefson RD, Lambert EH, et al. Hereditary sensory neuropathy type II. *Arch Neurol* 1973;**29**:23–37.

4226. Ohtahara S, Ishida T, Oka E, et al. On the age-dependent epileptic syndromes: the early infantile encephalopathy with suppression burst. *Brain Dev* 1976;**8**:270–88.

4227. Ohtahara S, Yamatogi Y, Ohtsuka Y, et al. Prognosis of West syndrome with special reference to Lennox syndrome: a developmental study. In Wada J, Penry JK, eds. *Advances in Epileptology: The Xth Epilepsy International Symposium*, pp 149–54. New York: Raven Press, 1980.

4228. Oka Y, Fukui K, Shoda D, et al. Cerebral cysticercosis manifesting as hydrocephalus—case report. *Neurol Med Chir (Tokyo)* 1996;**36**: 654–8.

4229. Okajima T, Yamamura S, Hamada K, et al. Chronic autonomic and sensory neuropathy. *Neurology* 1983;**33**:1061–4.

4230. Okihiro MM, et al. Duane syndrome and congenital upper limb anomalies. *Arch Neurol* 1977;**34**:174–9.

4231. O'Leary CP, Willison H. Autoimmune ataxic neuropathies (sensory ganglionopathies). *Curr Opin Neurol* 1997;**10**:366–70.

4232. Olney RK. Neuropathies in connective tissue disease. *Muscle Nerve* 1992;**15**:531–42.

4233. Olney RK, Aminoff MJ, So YT. Clinical and electrodiagnostic features of X-linked recessive bulbospinal neuronopathy. *Neurology* 1991;**41**:823–7.

4234. Olson LC, Bourgeois CH, Cotton RB, et al. Encephalopathy and fatty degeneration of the viscera in northeastern Thailand: clinical syndrome and epidemiology. *Pediatrics* 1971;**47**:707.

4235. Olson WH, Bardin CW, Walsh GC, et al. Moebius syndrome. *Neurology* 1970;**20**:1002–8.

4236. Omae T, Tsuchiya T, Yamaguchi T. Cheiro-oral syndrome due to lesions in the corona radiata. *Stroke* 1992;**23**:599–601.

4237. Omenn GS. Familial reticuloendotheliosis with eosinophilia. *N Engl J Med* 1965;**273**:427–32.

4238. Ommaya AK, et al. Nontraumatic cerebrospinal fluid rhinorrhea. *J Neurol Neurosurg Psychiatry* 1968;**31**:214–25.

4239. Onanoff M. Du réflexe "bulbo-caverneux". *Paris Soc Biol* 1890; **2**:215–7.

4240. O'Neill B, Butler AB, Young E, et al. Adult onset GM2 gangliosidosis. *Neurol Minneap* 1978;**28**:117–1123.

4241. O'Neill BP, Aronson AE, Pearson BW, et al. Superior laryngeal neuralgia: carotidynia or just another pain in the neck? *Headache* 1982;**22**:6–9.

4242. O'Neill BP, Illig JJ. Primary central nervous system lymphoma. *Mayo Clin Proc* 1989;**64**:1005–20.

4243. O'Neill JH, Murray NMF, Newsom-Davis J. The Lambert-Eaton myasthenic syndrome. *Brain* 1988;**111**:577–96.

4244. Oonk JGW, Van der Helm HJ, Martin JJ. Spinocerebellar degeneration: hexosaminidase A and B deficiency in two adult sisters. *Neurology* 1979;**29**:380–3.

4245. Opalski A. Nowy zespol podopuszkowy. Zespol czesciowy tetnicy kregowo-rezeniowej tylnej. *Pol Tyg Lek* 1946;**1**:397–402.

4246. Opitz JM, Frias JL, Gutenberger JE, et al. The G syndrome of multiple congenital anomalies. The clinical delineation of birth defects ll malformation syndromes. *Birth Defects* 1969;**V**:95–101.

4247. Opitz JM, Johnson RC, McCreadie SR, et al. The C syndrome of multiple congenital anomalies. *Birth Defects* 1969;**5**:161–6.

4248. Opitz JM, Kaveggia EG. The FG syndrome. An X-linked recessive syndrome of multiple congenital anomalies and mental retardation. *S Kinderheilkd* 1974;**117**:1–18.

4249. Oppenheim G. Multiple system atrophy. *J Neurol Neurosurg Psychiatry* 1989;**28**:34.

4250. Oppenheim H. Ueber allgemeine und localisierte Atonie der Muskulatur(Myatonie) im fruhen Kindersalter. Vorlaufige Mitteilung. *Monatschr Psychiatr* 1900;**8**:232–3.

4251. Oppenheim H. Zur Pathologie der Hautreflexe an den unteren Extremitaten. *Monatschr Psychiatr Neurol* 1902;**12**:421–3.

4252. Oppenheim H. Ueber eine eigenartige Krampfkrankheit des kindlichen und jugendlichen Alters (Dysbasia lordotica progressiva, Dystonia musculorum deformans). *Zentralbl Nervenheilkd* 1911;**30**:1090–109.

4253. Oppenheim H, Vogt C. Wesen und Localisation der kongennitalen und infantilen Pseudobulbarparalyse. *Jahrb Psychol Neurol* 1911;**18**:293–308.

4254. Oppenheimer DR. A benign "tumour" of the cerebellum. *J Neurol Neurosurg Psychiatry* 1955;**18**:199–213.

4255. Oppenheimer DR. Diseases of the basal ganglia, cerebellum and motor neurons. In Blackwood W, Corsellis JAN, eds. *Greenfield's Neuropathology*, p 615. London: Arnold, 1976.

4256. Optiz JM, Johnsons RC, McCreadie SR, et al. The syndrome of multiple congenital anomalies. *Birth Defects* 1969;**5**:161–6.

4257. Orgogozo JM. Evaluation of treatments in ischemic-stroke patients. In Amery WK, Bousser MG, Rose FC, eds. *Clinical Trial Methodology in Stroke*, pp 35–53. London: Balliere Tindall, 1989.

4258. Orgogozo JM. A unified form for neurological scoring of hemispheric stroke with motor impairment. *Stroke* 1992;**23**:1678–9.

4259. Orgogozo JM, Bougousslavsky J. Lacunar syndromes. In Toole JF, ed. *Handbook of Clinical Neurology*, Amsterdam: North Holland, 1989;**10**:235–69.

4260. Ormandy L. Scapulocostal syndrome. *Va Med Q* 1994;**121**:105–8.

4260a. Orr HT, Chung MY, Banfi S, et al. Expansion of an unstable trinucleotide CAG repeat in spinocerebellar ataxia type 1. *Nat Genet* 1993;**4**:221–6.

4261. Orrell RW, Marsden CD. The neck-tongue syndrome. *J Neurol Neurosurg Psychiatry* 1994;**57**:348–52.

4262. Orschansky J. Tabes dorsalis und das Kniewinkelphänomen. *Neurol Centralbl* 1906;**25**:401–5.

4263. Ortiz-Arduan A, Martin-Lionch N. Supermarket neuropathy. *Muscle Nerve* 1991;**14**:785.

4264. Ortner N. Recurrenslahmung bei Mitralstenose. *Wien Klin Wochenschr* 1897;**10**:753–5.

4265. Orzechowski K, Walichiewicz T. [Operated cyst of the cerebellum]. *Lwowski Tygodnik Lekarski* 1913;**8**:219–27.

4266. Osher RH, Griggs RC. Orbicularis fatigue: the "peek" sign of myasthenia gravis. *Arch Ophthalmol* 1979;**97**:677.

4267. Osher RH, Shields JA, Schatz MJ. Axial myopia: a neglected case of proptosis. *Arch Neurol* 1978;**35**:237–41.

4268. Ostberg O. Study of interindividual differences in circadian fatigue patterns of shift workers. *Br J Industr Med* 1973;**30**:341–51.

4269. Oster G. Phosphenes. *Sci Am* 1970;**222**:82.

4270. Oster J. Growing pain: a symptom and its significance. *Dan Med Bull* 1972;**19**:72–9.

4271. O'Sullivan DJ, McLeod JG. Spinal muscular atrophy, sporadic, confined to hands. *J Neurol Neurosurg Psychiatry* 1978;**41**:653–8.

4272. Osuntokun BO. An ataxic neuropathy in Nigeria: a clinical, biochemical and electrophysiological study. *Brain* 1968;**91**:215–48.

4273. Osuntokun BO, Odeku EL, Luzzato L. Congenital pain asymbolia and auditory imperception. *J Neurol Neurosurg Psychiatry* 1968; **31**:291–6.

4274. Oswald I. Sudden bodily jerks on falling asleep. *Brain* 1959; **82**:92–102.

4275. Otsubo H, Chitoku S, Ochi A, et al. Malignant rolandic-sylvian epilepsy in children. *Neurology* 2001;**57**:590–6.

4276. Ott BR, Saver JL. Unilateral amnesic stroke. *Stroke* 1993;**24**:1033–42.

4277. Ouachi K, Arita M, Kayden H, et al. Ataxia with isolated vitamin E deficiency is caused by mutations in alpha-tocopherol transfer protein. *Nat Genet* 1995;**9**:141–5.

4278. Ouvrier RA. Progressive dystonia with marked diurnal fluctuation. *Ann Neurol* 1978;**4**:412–7.

4279. Ouvrier RA, et al. HMSN III, autosomal recessive inheritance. *Brain* 1987;**110**:121.

4280. Ouzonellis T. Some Notes on quail myopathy. *J Amer Med Ass* 1970;**211**:1186–7.

4281. Overall JE, Gorham DR. Introduction—the Brief Psychiatric Rating Scale. *Psychopharmacol Bull* 1988;**24**:97–9.

4282. Owen CA, Woody PR, Mubarak SJ, et al. Gluteal compartment syndromes. A report of three cases and management utilising the wick catheter. *Clin Orthop* 1978;**132**:57–60.

4283. Oxbury JM, Oxbury SM, Humphrey NK. Varieties of colour anomia. *Brain* 1969;**92**:847–60.

4284. Oxbury JM, Whitty CWM. The syndrome of isolated epileptic status. *J Neurol Neurosurg Psychiatry* 1971;**34**:182–4.

4285. Ozawa E, Noguchi S, Mizuno Y, et al. From dystrophinopathy to sarcoglycanopathy: evolution of a concept of muscular dystrophy. *Muscle Nerve* 1998;**21**:421–38.

4286. Ozawa K, Saida K, Saida T, et al. Familial neuropathy with dementia, retinitis pigmentosa and dysautonomia. *Neurology* 1985;**35**:1184–7.

4287. Pace JB, Nagle D. Piriform syndrome. *West J Med* 1976;**124**:435–9.

4288. Pachner AR, Delaney E. The polymerase chain reaction in the diagnosis of Lyme neuroborreliosis. *Ann Neurol* 1993;**34**:544–50.

4289. Pacia SV, Devinsky O, Lucioano DJ, et al. The prolonged QT syndrome presenting as epilepsy. *Neurology* 1994;**44**:1408–10.

4290. Packman S, Sweetman L, Baker H, et al. The neonatal form of biotin-responsive multiple carboxylase deficiency. *J Pediatr* 1981;**99**:418–20.

4291. Padberg GW, Schot JDL, Vielvoye GJ, et al. Lhermitte—Duclos disease and Cowden disease: a single phakomatosis. *Ann Neurol* 1991; **29**:517–23.

4292. Page IH. A syndrome simulating diencephalic stimulation occurring in patients with essential hypertension. *Am J Med Sci* 1935;**190**:9–14.

4293. Page NGR, Bolger JP, Sanders MD. Auditory evoked phosphenes in optic nerve disease. *J Neurol Neurosurg Psychiatry* 1982;**45**:7–12.

4294. Pageot N, Vial C, Chazot G, et al. Progressive chorea and amyotrophy without acanthocytes: a new case of Fotopoulos syndrome? *J Neurol* 2000;**247**:392–4.

4295. Pagon RA. Retinitis pigmentosa. *Surv Ophthalmol* 1988;**33**:137–77.

4296. Paige DG, Clayton P, Bowron A, et al. Richner-Hanhart syndrome. *J R Soc Med* 1992;**85**:759–60.

4297. Paine RS. Evaluation of familial biochemically determined mental retardation in children, with special reference to amino-aciduria. *N Engl J Med* 1960;**262**:658–65.

4298. Paine RS, Efron ML. Atypical variants of "ataxia-telangiectasia syndrome". *Dev Med Child Neurol.* 1963;**5**:14–23.

4299. Pakalnis A, Drake ME, John K, et al. Forced normalization: acute psychosis after seizure control in seven patients. *Arch Neurol* 1987;**44**: 289–92.

4300. Pakarinen S. Incidence, etiology, and prognosis of primary subarachnoid hemorrhage. *Acta Neurol Scand* 1967;**43**(**Suppl 29**):1–28.

4301. Pakiam AS-I, Parry GJ. Multifocal motor neuropathy without overt conduction block. *Muscle Nerve* 1998;**21**:243–5.

4302. Palace J, Wiles CM, Newsom-Davis J. 3,4–diaminopyridine in the treatment of congenital (hereditary) myasthenia. *J Neurol Neurosurg Psychiatry* 1991;**54**:1069–72.

4303. Paladini D, Dellantonio R, Cinti A, et al. Axillary neuropathy in volleyball players: report of two cases and literature review. *J Neurol Neurosurg Psychiatry* 1996;**60**:345–7.

4304. Palau F, De Michele G, Vilchez JJ, et al. Early onset ataxia with cardiomyopathy and retained tendon reflexes maps to the Friedreich's ataxia locus on chromosome 9q. *Ann Neurol* 1995;**37**:359–362.

4305. Palix C, Coignet J. A case of congenital neuropathy with absence of myelin in the peripheral nervous system [in French]. *Pediatrie* 1978; **33**:201–7.

4306. Pallis CA, Scott JT. Peripheral neuropathy in rheumatoid arthritis. *BMJ* 1965;**1**:1141–7.

4307. Pallister PD, et al. The W syndrome. Studies of malformation syndromes of man XXVIII. *Birth Defects* 1974;**10**(**7**):51–60.

4308. Pallister PD et al. The Pallister mosaic syndrome. *Birth Defects* 1977;**13**(**13B**):103–10.

4309. Palmer EP. Transient global amnesia and the amnestic syndromes. *Med Clin North Am* 1986;**70**:1361–74.

4310. Palmer JJ. Radiation myelopathy. *Brain* 1972;**95**:109–22.

4311. Palmini A, Andermann F, Aicardi J, et al. Diffuse cortical dysplasia, or the "double cortex" syndrome. *Neurology* 1991;**41**:1656–62.

4312. Palmucci L, Mongini T, Doriguzzi C, et al. Familial autosomal recessive rigid spine syndrome with neurogenic facio-scapulo-peroneal muscle atrophy. *J Neurol Neurosurg Psychiatry* 1991;**54**:42–5.

4313. Paloneva J, Autti T, Raininko R, et al. CNS manifestations of Nasu-Hakola disease. *Neurology* 2001;**56**:1552–8.

4314. Palthe PM van Wulfften. A peculiar reflex phenomenon. *Brain* 1925;**48**:476–91.

4314a. Palthe PM van Wulfften. Leiodystonia, an endocrine-autonomic neurosis of the tropros. *Brain* 1933;**56**:479–90.

4315. Pampiglione G, Maia M. Syndrome of rapid irregular movements of eyes and limbs in childhood. *BMJ* 1972;**1**:469–73.

4316. Panayiotopoulos CP. Benign childhood epilepsy with occipital paroxysms: a 15–year prospective study. *Ann Neurol* 1989;**26**:51–6.

4317. Panayiotopoulos CP. Benign childhood partial epilepsies: benign childhood seizure susceptibility syndromes. *J Neurol Neurosurg Psychiatry* 1993;**56**:2–5.

4318. Panayiotopoulos CP. Early-onset benign childhood occipital seizure susceptibility syndrome: a syndrome to recognize. *Epilepsia* 1999;**40**:621–30.

4319. Panayiotopoulos CP, Chroni E. F waves in clinical neurophysiology: a review, methodological issues and overall value in peripheral neuropathies. *Electroencephalogr Clin Neurophysiol* 1996;**101**:365–74.

4320. Pancoast HK. Superior pulmonary sulcus tumor. Tumor characterized by pain, Horner's syndrome, destruction of bone and atrophy of hand muscles. *JAMA* 1932;**99**:1391–6.

4320a. Pandolfo M. Molecular pathogenesis of Friedreich ataxia. *Arch Neurol* 1999;**56**:1201–08.

4321. Pansini S. On a cerebellar syndrome with dysarthria in acute malaria. *Rif Med* 1901;**4**:458–62.

4322. Pant SS, Benton JW, Dodge PR. Unilateral pupillary dilatation during and immediately following seizures. *Neurology* 1966;**16**:837–40.

4323. Paparella MM. The cause (multifactorial inheritance) and pathogenesis (endolymphatic malabsorption) of Meniere's disease and its symptoms. *Acta Otolaryngol* 1985;**99**:445–51.

4324. Paparella MM, Elfiky FM. Mondini's deafness. *Arch Otolaryngol* 1972;**95**:134–40.

4325. Papez JW. A proposed mechanism of emotion. *Arch Neurol Psychiatry* 1937;**38**:725–43.

4326. Paping RHL, Annyas AA, Mouji JJA. Nasopharyngeal torticollis (Grisel's syndrome). *Ned Tschr Geneesk* 1985;**129**:1787–90.

4327. Paradiso G, Micheli F, Taratuto AL, et al. Familial bulbospinal neuronopathy with optic atrophy: a distinct entity. *J Neurol Neurosurg Psychiatry* 1996;**61**:196–9.

4328. Pareja JA, Antonaci F, Vincent M. The hemicrania continua diagnosis. *Cephalalgia* 2001;**21**:940–6.

4328a. Pareja JA, Caminero AB, Serra J, et al. Numular headache: A coin-shaped cephalgia. *Neurology* 2002;**58**:1678–9.

4329. Pareja JA, Vincent M, Antonaci F, et al. Hemicrania continua: diagnostic criteria and nosologic status. *Cephalalgia* 2001;**21**:874–7.

4330. Pareyson D. Charcot-Marie-Tooth disease and related neuropathies: molecular basis for distinction and diagnosis. *Muscle Nerve* 1999;**22**:1498–509.

4331. Parinaud H. Paralysie des mouvements associés des yeux. *Arch Neurol (Paris)* 1883;**5**:145–72.

4332. Parinaud H. Paralysie de la convergence. *Ann Ocul Paris* 1886;**95**: 205–6.

4333. Parisi JE, Collins GH, Kim C, et al. Prenatal symmetric thalamic degeneration with flexion spasticity at birth. *Ann Neurol* 1983;**13**:94.

4334. Parjiale JR, Hudgins TH, Fishman LM. The piriformis syndrome. *Am J Orthop* 1996;**25**:819–23.

4335. Park TA, Del·Toro DR. Isolated inferior calcaneal neuropathy. *Muscle Nerve* 1996;**19**:106–8.

4336. Parker N. Hereditary whispering dysphonia. *J Neurol Neurosurg Psychiatry* 1985;**48**:218–24.

4337. Parkes JD. *Sleep and Its Disorders.* London: W.B. Saunders, 1985.

4338. Parkinson D. Concussion. *Mayo Clin Proc* 1977;**52**:492–6.

4339. Parkinson J. *An Essay on the Shaking Palsy.* London: Whittingham and Rowland, 1817.

4340. Parks AG. Anorectal incontinence. *Proc R Soc Med* 1975;**68**: 681–90.

4341. Parmelee AH. Critical evaluation of the Moro reflex. *Pediatrics* 1964;**33**:773.

4342. Parr J, Terry TM, Larner J. Symptomatic hypoglycemia, visceral fatty acid metamorphosis and aglycogenosis in an infant lacking glycogen synthetase and phosphorylase. *Pediatrics* 1965;**35**:770.

4343. Parrott JMJ. Sur une pseudo-paralysie causée par une alteration du système osseux chez les nouveau-nés atteints de syphilis hereditaire. *Arch Physiol (Paris)* 1871;**4**:319–33.

4344. Parrott JMJ. Lesions of the skull as a result of congenital syphilis. *Prog Med (Paris)* 1879;**7**:268–9.

4345. Parrott JMJ. On a pupillary phenomenon observed in certain pathological states in infancy. *Rev Med Paris* 1882;**2**:809–24.

4346. Parry CH. *Collections from the Unpublished Medical Writings.* London: Underwood, 1825.

4347. Parry GJ. Are multifocal motor neuropathy and Lewis-Sumner syndrome distinct nosologic entities? *Muscle Nerve* 1999;**22**:557–9.

4348. Parsonage MJ, Turner JWA. Neuralgic amotrophy, the shoulder girdle syndrome. *Lancet* 1948;**1**:973–8.

4349. Parziale JR, Hudgins TH, Fishman LM. The piriformis syndrome. *Am J Orthop* 1996;**25**:819–23.

4350. Pascucci RC. Head trauma in the child. *Intensive Care Med* 1988; **14**:185–95.

4351. Pascuzzi RM, Gratianne R, Azzarelli B, et al. Schwartz-Jampel syndrome with dominant inheritance. *Muscle Nerve* 1990;**13**:1152–63.

4352. Pashayan HA. A family with blepharo-naso-facial malformations. *Am J Dis Child* 1973;**125**:389–93.

4353. Passarge E, McAdams AJ. Cerebro-hepato-renal syndrome: a newly recognized hereditary disorder of multiple congenital defects, including sudanophilic leukodystrophy, cirrhosis of the liver, and polycystic kidneys. *J Pediatr* 1967;**71**:691–702.

4354. Passouant P. Historical Note. Doctor Gélineau (1828–1906): narcolepsy centennial. *Sleep* 1981;**4**:241–6.

4355. Passwell JL, Ziplowski D, Nelson A, et al. A syndrome characterized by congenital ichthyosis, erythroderma, mental retardation, dwarfism and generalized aminoaciduria. *J Pediatr* 1973;**82**:466–71.

4356. Patau K, Smith DW, Therman E, et al. Multiple congenital anomaly caused by an extra autosome. *Lancet* 1960;**1**:790–3.

4357. Patel AN, Razzak ZA, Dastur DK. Disuse atrophy of human skeletal muscles. *Arch Neurol* 1969;**20**:413–21.

4358. Patel H, Berry K, McLeod P, et al. Cytoplasmic body myopathy. *J Neurol Sci* 1983;**60**:281–92.

4359. Paterson D, Carmichael EA. Form of familial cerebral degeneration chiefly affecting the lenticular nucleus. *Brain* 1924;**47**:207–31.

4360. Paterson D, Greenfield JG. Erythroedema polyneuritis (the so-called Pink disease). *Q J Med* 1923;**65**:6–18.

4361. Paton JY, Swaminathan S, Sargent CW, et al. Hypoxic and hypercapneic ventilatory responses in awake children with congenital central hypoventilation syndrome. *Am Rev Respir Dis* 1989;**140**:368–72.

4362. Patry G, Lyagoubi S, Tassinari CA. Subclinical "electrical status epilepticus" induced by sleep in children. *Arch Neurol* 1971;**24**:242–52.

4363. Patten BM, Pages M. Severe neurological disease associated with hyperparathyroidism. *Ann Neurol* 1984;**15**:453–6.

4364. Patterson JH. Presentation of a patient with leprechaunism. *Birth Defects* 1969;**5(4)**:117–21.

4365. Patterson JR, Grabois M. Locked-in syndrome: a review of 139 cases. *Stroke* 1986;**17**:758–64.

4366. Pattie AH, Gileard CJ. A brief psychogeriatric assessment schedule. *Br J Psychiatry* 1975;**127**:289–93.

4367. Pattison EM. Uveomeningoencephalitic syndrome (Vogt-Koyanagi-Harada). *Arch Neurol* 1965;**12**:197–205.

4368. Paty DW, Blume WT, Brown WF, et al. Chronic progressive myelopathy: investigation with CSF electrophoresis, evoked potentials, and CT scan. *Ann Neurol* 1979;**6**:419–24.

4369. Paul JR. *A History of Poliomyelitis.* New Haven: Yale University Press, 1971.

4370. Paulson G, Gottlieb G. Developmental reflexes: the reappearance of foetal and neonatal reflexes in aged patients. *Brain* 1968;**91**:37–52.

4371. Paulson GW. Weightlifter's headache. *Headache* 1983;**23**:193–4.

4372. Pavlakis SG, Phillips PC, DiMauro S, et al. Mitochondrial myopathy, encephalopathy, lactic acidosis, and strokelike episodes: a distinctive clinical syndrome. *Ann Neurol* 1984;**16**:481–8.

4373. Pavone L, Curatolo P, Rizzo R, et al. Epidermal nevus syndrome: a neurologic variant with hemimegalencephaly, gyral malformation, mental retardation, seizures, and facial hemihypertrophy. *Neurology* 1991;**41**:266–271.

4374. Pavone P, Parano E, Polizzi A, et al. Colobomatous microphthalmia, microcephaly with cerebellar hypoplasia: a new clincal syndrome. *Ann Neurol* 2000;**48**:530.

4375. Payne EE, Spillane JD. The cervical spine: an anatomico-pathological study of 70 specimens (using a special technique) with particular reference to the problem of cervical spondylosis. *Brain* 1957;**80**:571–96.

4376. Pearce JMS. Needle-in-the-eye syndrome. *World Med* 1979;**14**:77–8.

4377. Pearce JMS. Historical aspects of migraine. *J Neurol Neurosurg Psychiatry* 1986;**49**:1097–103.

4378. Pearce JMS. Aspects of the history of Parkinson's disease. *J Neurol Neurosurg Psychiatry* 1989;**Suppl**:6–10.

4379. Pearce JMS. Clinical features of the exploding head syndrome. *J Neurol Neurosurg Psychiatry* 1989;**52**:907–10.

4380. Pearce JMS. Whiplash injury: a reappraisal. *J Neurol Neurosurg Psychiatry* 1989;**52**:1329–31.

4381. Pearlman AL, Birch J, Meadows JC. Cerebral color blindness: an acquired defect in hue discrimination. *Ann Neurol* 1979;**5**:253–61.

4382. Pearn JH. Neurology of ciguatera. *J Neurol Neurosurg Psychiatry* 2001;**70**:4–8.

4383. Pearn JH, Gardner-Medwin D, Wilson J. A clinical study of chronic childhood spinal muscular atrophy. *J Neurol Sci* 1978;**38**:23–37.

4384. Pearn JH, Hudgson P, Walton JN. A clinical and genetic study of spinal muscular atrophy of adult onset. *Brain* 1978;**101**:591–606.

4385. Pearson CM. The periodic paralyses; differential features and pathological observations in permanent myopathic weakness. *Brain* 1963;**87**:341.

4386. Pebenito R, Feretti C, Chaudary RR, et al. Idiopathic torsion dystonia associated with lesions of the basal ganglia. *Clin Pediatr* 1984;**23**:232.

4387. Pederson E. Epidemic vertigo: clinical picture, epidemiology and relation to encephalitis. *Brain* 1959;**82**:566–80.

4388. Pedley TA, Guilleminault C. Episodic nocturnal wanderings responsive to anticonvulsant drug therapy. *Ann Neurol* 1977;**2**:30–5.

4389. Pedraza S, Gamez J, Rovira A, et al. MRI findings in Mobius syndrome: correlation with clinical features. *Neurology* 2000;**55**:1058–60.

4390. Peiris JB, Senviratne KN, Wickremasinghe HR, et al. Nonfamilial juvenile distal spinal muscular atrophy of upper extremity. *J Neurol Neurosurg Psychiatry* 1989;**52**:314–9.

4391. Pelayo R, Barasch E, Kang H, et al. Progressively intractable seizures, focal alopecia and hemimegalencephaly. *Neurology* 1994;**44**:969–71.

4392. Peled R, Lavie P. Paroxysmal awakenings from sleep associated with excessive daytime somnolence: a form of nocturnal epilepsy. *Neurology* 1986;**36**:95–8.

4393. Pelizaeus F. Ueber eine eigentumliche Form spastischer Lahmung mit Cerebralerscheinungen auf hereditarer Grundlage (multiple Sklerose). *Arch Psychiatr (Berlin)* 1885;**16**:698–710.

4394. Pellechia MT, Scala R, Filla A, et al. Idiopathic cerebellar ataxia associated with celiac disease: lack of distinctive neurological features. *J Neurol Neurosurg Psychiatry* 1999;**66**:32–5.

4395. Pellissier JF, Pouget J, de Victor B, et al. Tomaculous neuropathy. Histopathologic study and electro-clinical correlations in 10 cases. *Rev Neurol (Paris)* 1987;**143**:263–78.

4396. Pelmear PL, Taylor W. Hand-arm vibration syndrome. *J Fam Pract* 1994;**38**:180–5.

4397. Pelz DM, Fox AJ, Vinuela F. Digital subtraction angiography: current clinical applications. *Stroke* 1985;**16**:528–36.

4398. Pena CE, Miller F, Budzilovich GN. Arthrogryposis multiplex congenita. *Neurology* 1968;**18**:926–30.

4399. Pena SDJ, Shokeir MHK. Syndrome of campodactyly, multiple ankyloses, facial anomalies, and pulmonary hypoplasia: a lethal condition. *J Pediatr* 1974;**85**:373–5.

4400. Pendred V. Deaf-mutism and goitre. *Lancet* 1896;**2**:532.

4401. Penfield W. Diencephalic autonomic epilepsy. *Arch Neurol Psychiatry* 1929;**22**:358–74.

4402. Penfield W. Engrams in the human brain. *Proc R Soc Med* 1968;**61**:831–40.

4403. Penfield W, Perot P. The brain's record of auditory and visual experience. *Brain* 1963;**86**:595–696.

4404. Penfield W, Ward A. Calcifying epileptogenic lesions. *Arch Neurol Psychiatry* 1948;**60**:20–36.

4405. Penfield W, Welch K. The supplementary motor area in the cerebral cortex of man. *Trans Am Neurol Assoc* 1949;**74**:179–269.

4406. Penfield W, Welch K. The supplementary motor area of the cerebral cortex: a clinical and experimental study. *Arch Neurol Psychiatry* 1951;**66**:289–317.

4407. Penisson-Besnier I, Dumez C, Chateau D, et al. Autosomal dominant late adult onset distal leg myopathy. *Neuromusc Disord* 1998;**8**:459–66.

4408. Percy ME, Thompson MW. Creatine kinase—no phospho—please. *Muscle Nerve* 1981;**4**:271–3.

4409. Peress NS, DiMauro S, Roxburgh VA. Adult polysaccharidosis: clinicopathological, ultrastructural, and biochemical features. *Arch Neurol* 1979;**36**:840–5.

4410. Perheentupa J, et al. Mulibrey nanism, an autosomal recessive syndrome with pericardial constriction. *Lancet* 1973;**2**:351–5.

4411. Perheentupa J, Visakorpi JK. Protein intolerance with deficient transport of basic amino acids. *Lancet* 1965;**2**:813.

4412. Peripheral Neuropathy Association. Quantitative sensory testing. *Neurology* 1993;**43**:1050–2.

4413. Perot P, Feindel W, Lloyd-Smith D. Hematomyelia as a complication of syringomyelia: Gowers' syringal haemorrhage. Case report. *J Neurosurg* 1966;**25**:447–51.

4414. Perret G. The epidemiology and clinical course of arteriovenous malformations. In Pia HW, Gleave JRW, Grote E, et al., eds. *Cerebral Angiomas: Advances in Diagnosis and Therapy*, pp 21–6. New York: Springer-Verlag, 1975.

4415. Perry TL, Bratty PJA, Hansen S, et al. Hereditary mental depression and parkinsonism with taurine deficiency. *Arch Neurol* 1975;**32**:108–13.

4416. Perry TL, Hansen S, Tischler B, et al. Carnosinemia: a new metabolic disorder associated with neurologic disease and mental defect. *N Engl J Med* 1967;**277**:1219–27.

4417. Pestronk A, et al. Polyneuropathy syndromes associated with serum antibodies to sulfatide and myelin associated glycoprotein. *Neurology* 1991;**41**:357–62.

4418. Pestronk A, Lopate G, Kornberg AJ, et al. Distal lower motor neuron syndrome with high-titer serum IgM anti GM1 antibodies. *Neurology* 1994;**44**:2027–31.

4419. Petajan JH. Antigravity posture for analysis of motor unit recruitment: the 45 degree test. *Muscle Nerve* 1990;**13**:355–9.

4420. Petajan JH, Danforth RC, D'Allesio D, et al. Progressive sudomotor denervation and Adie's syndrome. *Neurology* 1965;**15**:172.

4421. Petajan JH, Momberger GL, Aase J, et al. Arthrogryposis syndrome (Kuskokwim disease) in the Eskimo. *JAMA* 1969;**209**:1481.

4422. Petersen RB, Tabaton M, Berg L, et al. Analysis of the prion protein gene in thalamic dementia. *Neurology* 1992;**42**:1859–63.

4423. Petersen RB, Tabaton M, Chen SG, et al. Familial progressive subcortical gliosis. *Neurology* 1995;**45**:1062–7.

4424. Peterson LR, Peterson MJ. Short-term retention of individual verbal items. *J Exp Psychol* 1959;**58**:193–8.

4425. Petito CK, Navia BA, Cho BD, et al. Vacuolar myelopathy pathologically resembling subacute combined degeneration in patients with the acquired immunodeficiency syndrome. *N Engl J Med* 1985;**312**:874–9.

4426. Pettigrew LC, Jankovic J. Hemidystonia: a report of 22 patients and a review of the literature. *J Neurol Neurosurg Psychiatry* 1985;**48**:650–7.

4427. Petty RKH, Harding AE, Morgan-Hughes JA. The clinical features of mitochondrial myopathy. *Brain* 1986;**109**:915–38.

4428. Petzold A, Thom M, Powell M, et al. Relapsing intracranial Rosai-Dorfman disease. *J Neurol Neurosurg Psychiatry* 2001;**71**:538–41.

4429. Pfeiffer E. A short portable mental status questionnaire for the assessment of organic brain deficit in elderly patients. *J Am Geriatr Soc* 1975;**23**:433–41.

4430. Phalen GS, Kendrick JI. Compression of the median nerve in the carpal tunnel. *JAMA* 1957;**614**:524–30.

4431. Phelps CD, et al. The diagnosis and prognosis of atypical carotid-cavernous fistula (red-eyed shunt syndrome). *Am J Ophthalmol* 1982;**93**:423–36.

4432. Phillips CI, Griffiths DL. Macular coloboma and skeletal abnormality. *Br J Ophthalmol* 1969;**53**:346–9.

4433. Phillips CJ, Smith B. The draw-a-man test: A study in scoring methods, validity and norms with English children at five and eleven years. *J Child Psychol Psychiatry* 1973;**14**:123–35.

4434. Phillips DG. The shoulder girdle disc. *J Neurol Neurosurg Psychiatry* 1976;**39**:817–20.

4435. Phillips JA, McLean WT, Huntley CC. Co-existing Guillain-Barre and visceral larva migrans syndromes. *Pediatrics* 1969;**44**:142–3.

4436. Phillips LHI. Familial long thoracic nerve palsy: a manifestation of brachial plexus neuropathy. *Neurology* 1986;**36**:1251–3.

4437. Piccolo F, Roberds SL, Jeanpierre M, et al. Primary adhalinopathy: a common cause of autosomal recessive muscular dystrophy of variable severity. *Nat Genet* 1995;**10**:243–5.

4438. Pick A. Clinical studies III. On reduplicative paramnesia. *Brain* 1903;**26**:260–7.

4439. Pick L. *Gaucher's disease* [in German]. Berlin: Springer, 1926.

4440. Pickett JB, Schmidley JW. Sputtering positive potentials in the EMG. *Neurology* 1980;**30**:215–8.

4441. Pietrantoni L. Neuralgic and anesthetic zones in the face and mouth as early signs of malignancies of the paranasal cavities. *Arch Ital Otol* 1948;**59**:105–28.

4442. Pietz J. Neurological aspects of adult phenylketonuria. *Curr Opin Neurol* 1998;**11**:679–88.

4443. Pignata C, Farina V, Andria G, et al. Prolonged Q-T interval syndrome presenting as idiopathic epilepsy. *Neuropediatrics* 1983;**14**:235–6.

4444. Pihko H, Lehtinen I, Tikkanen H, et al. Progressive unilateral hypertrophic myopathy: a case study. *Muscle Nerve* 1993;**16**:63–8.

4445. Pilley SF, Thompson HS. Pupillary dilatation lag in Horner's syndrome. *Br J Ophthalmol* 1975;**59**:731–5.

4446. Pillon B, Signoret JL, Lhermitte F. Associative visual agnosia: role of the left hemisphere in visual perception. *Rev Neurol (Paris)* 1981;**137**:831.

4447. Piltz J. Concerning a pupillary reflex. *Neurol Zentrlabl* 1899;**18**:14–7.

4448. Pinard J-M, Motte J, Chiron C, et al. Subcortical laminar heterotopia and lissencephaly in two families: a single X-linked doninant gene. *J Neurol Neurosurg Psychiatry* 1994;**57**:914–20.

4449. Pinckers A. Patterned dystrophies of the retinal pigment epithelium. *Ophthalmol Paediatr Genet* 1988;**9**:77–114.

4450. Pinckers AJL. Leber's congenital amaurosis as conceived by Leber. *Ophthalmologia* 1979;**179**:48–51.

4451. Pincus JH, Chutorian AM. Familial benign chorea with intention tremor: a clinical entity. *J Pediatr* 1967;**70**:724.

4452. Pineda M, et al. Family agenesis of the corpus callosum with hypothermia and apnoeic spells. *Neuropediatrics* 1984;**15**:63–7.

4453. Pinel P. *Traite Medico-philosophique sur L'alienation Mentale ou la Manie.* Paris: Richard, Caille, & Ravier, 1801.

4454. Pinsky L, Finlayson MH, Libman I, et al. Familial amyotrophic lateral sclerosis with dementia. *Clin Genet* 1975;**7**:186–91.

4455. Pitt DB, Rogers JG, Danks DM. Mental retardation, unusual face and intrauterine growth retardation. A new recessive syndrome? *Am J Med Genet* 1984;**19**:307–13.

4456. Pitt P, Hamilton EBD. Myositis ossificans progressiva. *J R Soc Med* 1984;**77**:68–70.

4457. Pittock SJ, Joyce C, O'Keane V, et al. Rapid-onset dystonia-parkinsonism. *Neurology* 2000;**55**:991–5.

4458. Plant GT. The fortification spectra of migraine. *BMJ* 1986;**293**:1613–6.

4459. Plaster NM, Uyama E, Uchino M, et al. Genetic localization of the familial adult myoclonic epilepsy (FAME) gene to chromosome 8q24. *Neurology* 1999;**53**:1180–3.

4460. Platt BS, Burgess RC. Beriberi. *Fed Proc* 1958;**17**:3–56.

4461. Pleet AB, Massey EW. Notalgia paresthetica. *Neurology* 1978;**28**:1310–1.

4462. Pleet AB, Massey EW. Palmaris brevis sign in neuropathy of the deep palmar branch of the ulnar nerve. *Ann Neurol* 1978;**3**:469.

4463. Plum F. Mechanisms of "central" hyperventilation. *Ann Neurol* 1982;**11**:636–7.

4464. Plum F. Other disorders of consciousness. *Curr Opin Neurol Neurosurg.* 1989;**2**:236–9.

4465. Plum F, Brown HW, Snoep E. Neurologic significance of posthyperventilation apnea. *JAMA* 1962;**181**:1050–5.

4466. Plum F, Posner JB. *The Diagnosis of Stupor and Coma.* Philadelphia: F.A. Davis, 1987.

4467. Plum F, Van Uitert R. Nonendocrine diseases and disorders of the hypothalamus. In Reichlin S, Baldessarini RJ, Martin JB, eds. *The Hypothalamus,* pp 415–73. New York: Raven Press, 1978.

4468. Plutchik R, Conte H, Lieberman M, et al. Reliability and validity of a scale for assessing the functioning of geriatric patients. *J Am Geriatr Soc* 1971;**19**:614–23.

4469. Poch GF, Sica EP, Taratuto A, et al. Hypertrophia musculorum vera. Study of a family. *J Neurol Sci* 1971;**12**:53–61.

4470. Podoll K, Robinson D. Illusory splitting as visual aura symptom in migraine. *Cephalalgia* 2000;**20**:228–32.

4471. Podreka I, Suess E, Goldenberg G, et al. Initial experience with technetium-99m HM-PAO and SPECT. *J Nucl Med* 1987;**28**:1657–66.

4472. Poeck K, Orgass B. The concept of the body schema. A critical review with some experimental results. *Cortex* 1971;**7**:254–77.

4473. Poels PJE, Wevers RA, et al. Exertional rhabdomyolysis in a patient with calcium adenosine triphosphatase deficiency. *J Neurol Neurosurg Psychiatry* 1993;**56**:823–6.

4474. Poewe W, Willeit H, Surgon E. The rigid spine syndrome. *J Neurol Neurosurg Psychiatry* 1985;**48**:887–9.

4475. Pohowalla JN, Kaul KK, Bhandari NR, Singh SD. Infantile "meningoencephalitic syndrome". *Indian J Pediatr* 1960;**27**:49.

4476. Poland A. Deficiency of the pectoral muscles. *Guys Hosp Rep* 1841;**6**:191–3.

4477. Polinsky J. Sympathotonic orthostatic hypotension. *Neurology* 1981;**31**:1–7.

4478. Poll-The B, Aicardi J, Girot R, et al. Neurological findings in triosephophate isomerase deficiency. *Ann Neurol* 1985;**17**:439–43.

4479. Pollack L, Klein C, Rabey J-M. The distance shortening phenomenon or the lazy arm sign as a subtle pyramidal sign. *Arch Neurol* 1997;**54:**935.

4480. Pollard WE, Bobbitt RA, Bergner M. The Sickness Impact Profile: reliability of a health status measure. *Med Care* 1976;**14:**146–55.

4481. Pollen RH. Cat-scratch encephalitis. *Neurology* 1968;**18:**1031–3.

4482. Pollitt RJ, Jenna FA, Mersky H. Aspartal glycosaminuria: an inborn error of metabolism associated with mental defect. *Lancet* 1968;**2:**253.

4483. Pollock M, Kies B. Benign hereditary cerebellar ataxia and extensive thermoanalgesia. *Brain* 1990;**113:**857–65.

4485. Pollock M, Nukada H, Frith RW, et al. Peripheral neuropathy in Tangier disease. *Brain* 1983;**106:**911–28.

4486. Polo A, Manganotti P, Zanette G, et al. Polyneuritis cranialis: clinical and electrophysiological findings. *J Neurol Neurosurg Psychiatry* 1992;**55:**398–400.

4487. Pomeranz HD, Lessell S. Palinopsia and palinopia in the absence of drugs or cerebral disease. *Neurology* 2000;**54:**855–9.

4488. Pompe JC. Over idiopatische hypertophie van het hart. *Ned Tschr Geneesk* 1932;**76:**304–5.

4489. Poppelreuter W. *Die psychischen Schadigungen durch Kopfschuss im Kriege 1914–16.* Leipzig: Verlag von Leopold Voss, 1917.

4490. Poppi M, Giuliani G, Gambari PI, et al. A hazard of craniotomy in the sitting position: the posterior compartment syndrome of the thigh. *J Neurosurg* 1989;**71:**618–9.

4491. Porch BE. *Porch Index of Communicative Ability.* Palo Alto: Consulting Psychologists Press, 1967.

4492. Porot A. Hemorragie limitée du pedoncle cerebelleux superieur droit; hemisyndrome cerebelleux direct. *Lyon Med* 1906;**106:**1137–41.

4493. Portenoy RK. Mechanisms of clinical pain. In Portenoy RK, ed. *Neurologic Clinics, Vol. 7. Pain: Mechanisms and Syndromes,* p 205. Philadelphia: W.B. Saunders, 1989.

4494. Portenoy RK, Duma C, Foley KM. Acute herpetic and postherpetic neuralgia: clinical review and current management. *Ann Neurol* 1986;**20:**651–64.

4495. Porter L, Wartenberg R. The man. *J Nerv Ment Dis* 1952;**116:** 469–74.

4496. Porteus SD. *Porteus Maze Test.* Palo Alto: Pacific Books, 1933.

4497. Portmann M, Aran JM. Electro-cochleography. *Laryngoscope* 1971;**81:**899.

4498. Posas HN Jr, Rivner MH. Deep peroneal sensory neuropathy. *Muscle Nerve* 1992;**15:**745–6.

4499. Poser CM. Myelinoclastic and diffuse sclerosis. In Vincken PJ, Bruyn GW, eds. *Handbook of Clinical Neurology,* p 469. Amsterdam: North Holland, 1970.

4500. Poser CM. Diseases of the myelin sheath. In Baker AB, Baker LH, eds. *Clinical Neurology,* pp 80–104. Hagerstown, MD: Harper & Row, 1978.

4501. Poser CM. Dysmyelination revisited. *Arch Neurol* 1978;**35:**401–8.

4502. Poser CM. Criteria for the diagnosis of the Guillain-Barre syndrome: a critique. *J Neurol Sci* 1981;**52:**191–9.

4503. Poser CM. Notes on the pathogenesis of subacute sclerosing panencephalitis. *J Neurol Sci* 1990;**95:**219–24.

4504. Poser CM, Paty DW, Scheinberg L, et al. New diagnostic criteria for multiple sclerosis: guidelines for research protocols. *Ann Neurol* 1983;**13:**227–31.

4505. Poser CM, Paty DW, Scheinberg L, et al. The Diagnosis of Multiple Sclerosis. New York: Thieme-Stratton, 1984.

4506. Poser CM, van Bogaert L. Natural history and evolution of the concept of shilders diffuse sclerosis. *Acta Psychiatr Neurol* 1956;**31:** 285–331.

4507. Poskanzer DC, Kerr DNS. A third type of periodic paralysis with normokalemia and a favourable response to sodium chloride. *Am J Med* 1961;**31:**328–42.

4508. Posner JB. Paraneoplastic cerebellar degeneration. *Can J Neurol Sci* 1993;**20:**S117–S122.

4509. Pott P. *Remarks on that kind of palsy of the lower limbs which is frequently found to accompany a curvature of the spine and is supposed to be caused by it, together with its method of cure.* London: Johnson, 1779.

4510. Potzl O. Word- and color-blindness. *Zentralbl Neurol* 1919; **52:**241.

4511. Potzl O, Sittig O. Klinische Befunde mit Hertwig-Magendiescher Augeneinstellung. *Z Ges Neurol Psychiatr* 1925;**95:**701.

4512. Power H, Sedgwick LW. *Lexicon of Medicine and the Allied Sciences.* London: The New Sydenham Society, 1882.

4513. Poza JJ, Saenz A, Martinez-Gil A, et al. Autosomal dominant lateral temporal lobe epilepsy: clinical and genetic study of a large Basque pedigree linked to chromosome 10q. *Ann Neurol* 1999;**45:**182–8.

4514. Pranzatelli MR, Huang Y, Tate E, et al. Cerebrospinal fluid 5-hydroxyindoeacetic acid and homovanillic acid in the pediatric opsoclonus-myoclonus syndrome. *Ann Neurol* 1995;**37:**189–97.

4515. Prasad A, Kaye EM, Alroy J. Electron microscopic examination of skin biopsy as a cost-effective tool in the diagnosis of lysosomal storage diseases. *J Child Neurol* 1996;**11:**301–8.

4516. Prasad AN, Prasad C, Stafstrom C. Recent advances in the genetics of epilepsy: insights from human and animal studies. *Epilepsia* 1999;**40:**1329–52.

4517. Prechtl HF, Stemmer CJ. The choreiform syndrome in children. *Dev Med Child Neurol* 1962;**4:**119.

4518. Prendes JL, Rosenberg SJ. Rip van Winkle syndrome: confusion and irresistible somnolence after stroke. *South Med J* 1986;**179:**1162–4.

4518a. Prengler M, Pavlakis SG, Prohovnik I, et al. Sickle cell disease: The neurological complications. *Ann Neurol* 2002;**51:**543–52.

4519. Preobrashenski PA. Syphilitic paraplegia with dissociated disturbance of sensation. *Zh Nevropatol Psikiatr* 1904;**4:**388.

4520. Preston DC, Kelly JJ. "Pseudospasticity" in Guillain-Barre syndrome. *Neurology* 1991;**41:**131–4.

4521. Preston NW. Toxicity of pertussis vaccine. *BMJ* 1982;**284:** 1817–8.

4522. Prevost J-L. On conjugate deviation of the eyes and rotation of the head in some cases of hemiplegia. Paris: Thése de Paris, 1868.

4523. Price BH, Mesulam M-M. Behavioral manifestations of central pontine myelinolysis. *Arch Neurol* 1987;**44:**671–3.

4524. Price RW, Brew BJ. The AIDS-dementia complex. *J Infect Dis* 1988;**158:**1079–83.

4525. Price TR, Netsky MG. Myxedema and ataxia. *Neurology* 1966; **16:**957–62.

4526. Prichard JW, Brass LM. New anatomical and functional imaging methods. *Ann Neurol* 1992;**32:**395–400.

4527. Prineas JW, Hall R, Barwick DD, et al. Myopathy associated with pigmentation following adrenalectomy for Cushing disease. *Q J Med* 1968;**37:**63–77.

4528. Pringle CE, Belden J, Veitch JE, et al. Multifocal motor neuropathy presenting as ophthalmoplegia. *Muscle Nerve* 1997;**20:**347–51.

4529. Pringle CE, Hudson AJ, Munoz KC, et al. Primary lateral sclerosis. *Brain* 1992;**115:**495–520.

4530. Pritchard C, Flynn JT, Smith JL. Waveform characteristics of vertical oscillations in long standing visual loss. *J Pediatr Ophthalmol Strabismus* 1988;**25:**233–6.

4531. Probst A, et al. Sensory ganglioneuropathy in infantile muscular atrophy. *Neuropediatrics* 1981;**12:**215–31.

4532. Prusiner S. Prions and neurodegenerative diseases. *N Engl J Med* 1987;**317:**1571–80.

4533. Prusiner S. Prion diseases of humans and animals. *J R Coll Physicians* 1993;**28:**1–30.

4534. Prusiner SB. Neurodegenerative disease and prions. *N Engl J Med* 2001;**344:**1516–25.

4535. Prynn WL, Kates DE, Pollack CV. Gluteal compartment syndrome. *Ann Emerg Med* 1994;**24:**1180–3.

4536. Pryse-Phillips WEM. Bowlers cramp. *Med J Aust* 1967;**1:**61–2.

4537. Pryse-Phillips WEM. An olfactory reference syndrome. *Acta Psychiatr Scand* 1971;**47:**484–509.

4538. Pryse-Phillips WEM. Validation of a diagnostic sign in carpal tunnel syndrome. *J Neurol Neurosurg Psychiatry* 1984;**47:**870–2.

4539. Pryse-Phillips WEM, Johnson GJ, Larsen B. Incomplete manifestations of myotonic dystrophy in a large kinship in Labrador. *Ann Neurol* 1982;**8:**582–91.

4540. Przelomski MM, O'Rourke E, Grady GF, et al. Eastern equine encephalitis in Massachusetts. *Neurology* 1988;**38:**736–9.

4541. Psychopharmacology Research Branch N. *ECDEU Assessment Manual for Psychopharmacology.* Revised DEW Publication No. ADM

76–338. Rockville, MD: Department of Health, Education and Welfare, 1976.

4542. Ptacek LJ, Johnson KJ, Griggs RC. Genetics and physiology of the myotonia muscle disorders. *N Engl J Med* 1993;**328:**482–9.

4543. Puce A, Kalnins RM, Berkovic S, et al. Limbic P3 potentials, seizure localization and surgical pathology in temporal lobe epilepsy. *Ann Neurol* 1989;**26:**377–85.

4544. Pullicino PM, Jacobs L. Palpebromandibular synkinesia. *Ann Neurol* 1991;**30:**318.

4545. Pullicino PM, Jacobs L, McCall WD, et al. Spontaneous palpebromandibular synkinesia: a localizing clinical sign. *Ann Neurol* 1994;**35:**222–8.

4546. Purdy A, Hahn AF, Barnett HJM, et al. Familial fatal parkinsonism with alveolar hypoventilation and mental depression. *Ann Neurol* 1979;**6:**523–31.

4547. Purves-Stewart JPM. Paralysis agitans, with an account of a new symptom. *Lancet* 1898;**2:**1258–60.

4548. Putnam JJ. A series of cases of paraesthesia, mainly of the hands, of periodical recurrence, and possibly of vaso-motor origin. *Arch Med (New York)* 1880;**4:**147–62.

4549. Putnam JJ. A group of cases of system sclerosis of the spinal cord, associated with diffuse collateral degeneration; occurring in enfeebled persons past middle life, and especially in women; studied with particular reference to etiology. *J Nerv Ment Dis* 1891;**16:**69.

4550. Putnam T. The progressive confusional syndrome following injuries to cervical portion of the spinal cord. *Science* 1937;**86:**542–3.

4551. Pyeritz RE, Conant, J. *The Marfan Syndrome. I.* New York: National Marfan Foundation, 1984.

4552. Pyeritz RE, McKusick VA. The Marfan syndrome: diagnosis and management. *N Engl J Med* 1979;**300:**772–7.

4553. Pyle E. Case of unusual bone development. *J Bone Jt Surg* 1931;**13:**874–80.

4554. Quality Standards Committee of the American Academy of Neurology. The management of concussions in sports. *Neurology* 1997;**48:**581–5.

4555. Quarles RH, Weiss MD. Autoantibodies associated with peripheral neuropathy. *Muscle Nerve* 1999;**22:**800–22.

4556. Quay HC, Peterson DR. *Interim Manual for the Revised Behavior Problem Checklist.* Coral Gables, FL: University of Miami, 1983.

4557. Queckenstedt H. Diagnosis of compression of the spinal cord [in German]. *Dtsch Z Nervenklinik* 1916;**55:**325–33.

4558. Queckenstedt H. Changes in spinal fluid in peripheral neuritis [in German]. *Dtsch Z Nervenklinik* 1917;**57:**316–29.

4559. Quincke H. Die Lumbarpunction des Hydrocephalus. *Klin Wochenschr* 1891;**28:**929–33.

4560. Quinn N. Multiple system atrophy—the nature of the beast. *J Neurol Neurosurg Psychiatry* 1989;**Suppl:**78–89.

4561. Quinn N, Wenning G, Marsden CD. The Shy-Drager syndrome. *Arch Neurol* 1995;**52.:**656–7.

4562. Quinn NP. Classification of fluctuations in patients with Parkinson's disease. *Neurology* 1998;**51**(**Suppl 2**):S25–S29.

4563. Quinn NP, Rothwell JC, Thompson PD, Marsden CD. Hereditary myoclonic dystonia. In Fahn S, et al., eds. *Advances in Neurology*, pp 391–6. New York: Raven Press, 1988.

4564. Qureshi AI, Choudhry MA, Akbar MS, et al. Plasma exchange versus intravenous immunoglobulin treatment in myasthenic crisis. *Neurology* 1999;**52:**629–32.

4565. Qureshi HI, Tuhrim S, Broderick JP, et al. Spontaneous intracerebral hemorrhage. *N Engl J Med* 2001;**344:**1450–60.

4566. Rabin BA, Griffin JW, Crain BJ, et al. Autosomal dominant juvenile amyotrophic lateral sclerosis. *Brain* 1999;**122**(Pt 8):1550.

4567. Rademaker GGJ. On the lengthening and shortening reactions and their occurrence in man. *Brain* 1947;**70:**109–26.

4568. Radloff LS. The CES-D Scale. *Appl Psychol Meas* 1977;**1:**385–401.

4569. Raeder JG. Paratrigeminal paralysis of oculo-pupillary sympathetic. *Brain* 1924;**47:**149–58.

4570. Ragge NK, Hoyt WF. Midbrain myasthenia: fatigable ptosis, 'lid twitch' sign, and ophthalmoparesis from a dorsal midbrain glioma. *Neurology* 1992;**42:**917–9.

4571. Rail D, Scholtz C, Swash M. Post-encephalitic parkinsonism: current experience. *J Neurol Neurosurg Psychiatry* 1981;**44:**670–6.

4572. Raimondi AJ, Hirschauer J. Head injury in the infant and toddler: Coma Scoring and Outcome Scale. *Childs Brain* 1984;**11:**12–35.

4573. Raitta C, Perheentupa J. Congenital ophthalmoplegia plus. *Neuroophthalmology* 1985;**5:**27–31.

4574. Ramachandran VS, Altschuler EL, Hillyer S. Mirror agnosia. *Proc R Soc Lond* 1997;**264:**645–7.

4575. Ramat S, Zee DS, Minor L, et al. Translational vestibulo-ocular reflex evoked by a "head heave" stimulus. *Ann NY Acad Sci* 2001;**942:**95–113.

4576. Ramazzini M. *Diseases of Scribes and Notaries.* Privately printed, 1713.

4577. Ramirez F, Arana IR. [The hypothalamic crossroads syndrome]. *Ann Faculty Med Univ Montevideo* 1952;**37:**109.

4578. Ramon Y Cajal S. *Manual de Anatomia Patologica General.* Madrid: N. Moya, 1909.

4579. Ramon Y Cajal S. *Recollections of My Life.* London: MIT Press, 1989.

4580. Ramos Arroyo MA, Weaver DD, Beals RK. Congenital contractural arachnodactyly. *Clin Genet* 1985;**27:**570–81.

4581. Rana PVS, Wadia RS. The Marin-Amat syndrome: an unusual facial synkinesia. *J Neurol Neurosurg Psychiatry* 1985;**48:**939–41.

4582. Ranalli PJ, Sharpe JA. Contrapulsion of saccades and ipsilateral ataxia: a unilateral disorder of the rostral cerebellum. *Ann Neurol* 1986;**20:**311.

4583. Ranalli PJ, Sharpe JA. Upbeat nystagmus and the ventral tegmental pathway of the upward vestibulo-ocular reflex. *Neurology* 1988;**38:**1329–30.

4584. Rand RW, Crowdall PH. Central spinal cord syndrome in hyperextension injuries of the cervical spine. *J Bone Jt Surg* 1962;**44:**1415.

4585. Rando TA, Fishman RA. Spontaneous intracranial hypotension: report of two cases and review of the literature. *Neurology* 1992;**42:**481–7.

4586. Rando TA, Horton JC, Layzer RB. Wolfram syndrome. *Neurology* 1992;**42:**1220–4.

4587. Rangel-Guerra R, Martinez HR, Saenz C. Mucormycosis: report of 11 cases. *Arch Neurol* 1985;**42:**578–81.

4588. Rankin J. Cerebrovascular accidents in patients over the age of 60: II. prognosis. *Scot Med J* 1957;**2:**200–15.

4589. Rantamaki M, Krahe R, Paetau A, et al. Adult-onset autosmal recessive ataxia with thalamic lesions in a Finnish family. *Neurology* 2001;**57:**1043–9.

4589a. Ranum LP, Schut LF, Lundgren JK, et al. Spinocerebellar ataxia type 5 in a family descended from the grandparents of President Lincoln maps to chromosome 11. *Nat Genet* 1994;**8:**280–4.

4590. Rao KC, Kanipp HC, Waggoner EJ. CT findings in cerebral sinus and venous thrombosis. *Radiology* 1981;**140:**391–75.

4591. Rao SM, Devinsky O, Grafman J, et al. Viscosity and social cohesion in temporal lobe epilepsy. *J Neurol Neurosurg Psychiatry* 1992;**55:**149–52.

4592. Rapcsak SZ, Polster MR, Glisky ML, et al. False recognition of unfamiliar faces following right hemisphere damage: neuropsychological and anatomical observations. *Cortex* 1996;**32:**593–611.

4593. Rapin I, Goldfischer S, Katzman R, et al. The cherry-red spot–myoclonus syndrome. *Ann Neurol* 1978;**3:**234–42.

4594. Rapin I, Susuki K, Valsamis MP. Adult (chronic) Gm2–angliosidosis—atypical spinocerebellar degeneration in a Jewish sibship. *Arch Neurol* 1976;**33:**120–30.

4595. Rapoport AM. Analgesic rebound headache. *Headache* 1988;**28:**662–5.

4596. Rappaport M, Hall KM, Hopkins K, et al. Disability rating scale for severe head trauma: Coma to community. *Arch Phys Med Rehabil* 1982;**63:**118–23.

4597. Rapcsak S, Cimino CR, Heilman KM. Altitudinal neglect. *Neurology* 1988;**38:**277–81.

4598. Rasdolsky I. Dorsal-Pontins Tumorsyndrom. *Z Ges Neurol Psychiatr* 1935;**152:**530–7.

4599. Rask MR. Superior gluteal nerve entrapment syndrome. *Muscle Nerve* 1980;**3:**304–7.

4600. Raskin A. *Validation of a Battery of Tests to Assess Psychopathology in the Elderly.* London: John Levi, 1985.

4601. Raskin A, Crook TH. Mood Scales–Elderly. *Psychopharmacol Bull* 1988;**24**:727–32.

4602. Raskin NH. Hypnic headache. *Headache* 1988;**28**:534–6.

4603. Raskin NH. The cough headache syndrome: treatment. *Neurology* 1995;**45**:1784.

4604. Raskin NH, Schwartz RK. Icepick-like pain. *Neurology* 1980; **30**:203–5.

4605. Raskind RH. Problems at the reading distance. *Am Orthop J* 1976;**26**:53.

4606. Rasmussen A, Matsuura T, Ruano L, et al. Clinical and genetic analysis of four mexican families with spinocerebellar ataxia type 10. *Ann Neurol* 2001;**50**:234–9.

4607. Rasmussen T, Olszewski J, Lloyd-Smith D. Focal seizures due to chronic localised encephalitides. *Neurology* 1958;**8**:435–45.

4608. Raven JC. *Guide to the Standard Progressive Matrices*. New York: The Psychological Corporation, 1956.

4609. Raven JC. *Guide to Using the Coloured Progressive Matrices*. New York: The Psychological Corporation, 1956.

4610. Ravits J. Autonomic system testing. *Muscle Nerve* 1997;**20**: 919–37.

4611. Ravits J, Hallett M, Baker M, et al. Primary writing tremor and myoclonic writer's cramp. *Neurology* 1985;**35**:1387–91.

4612. Raymond AA, Fish DR, Stevens JM, et al. Subependymal heterotopia: a distinct neuronal migration disorder associated with epilepsy. *J Neurol Neurosurg Psychiatry* 1994;**57**:1195–202.

4613. Raymond F, Cestan R. Trois observations de paralysie des mouvements associés des globes oculaires. *Rev Neurol (Paris)* 1901;**9**:70–7.

4614. Raymond GV. Peroxisomal disorders. *Curr Opin Neurol* 2001; **14**:783–7.

4615. Raynaud M. *De l'asphyxie locale et de la gangrène symmetrique des extremities*. Paris: Rignoux, 1862.

4616. Reagan TJ, Thomas JE, Colby MY Jr. Chronic progressive radiation myelopathy. *JAMA* 1968;**203**:106–10.

4617. Rebeiz JJ, Kolodny EH, Richardson EP Jr. Corticodentatonigral degeneration with neuronal achromasia. *Arch Neurol* 1968;**18**:20–33.

4618. Rebollo M, Val JF, Garijo F, et al. Livedo reticularis and cerebrovascular lesions (Sneddon's syndrome). *Brain* 1983;**106**:965–79.

4619. Rebouche J, Engel AG. Systemic carnitine deficiency. *Neurology* 1981;**31**:813–8.

4620. Rechtschaffen A, Kales A. *A Manual of Standardized Terminology, Techniques and Scoring for Sleep Stages of Human Subjects*. Washington, DC: Department of Health, Education and Welfare, 1968.

4621. Recklinghausen FD. *Uber die multiplen Fibrome der Haut und ihre Beziehungen zu den Neuromen*. Berlin: Festschr. R. Virchow, 1882.

4622. Reddy AN. The stethoscope neuropathy. *Ann Intern Med* 1987; **106**:913.

4623. Redekop GJ, Del Maestro RF. Diagnosis and management of spinal epidural abscess. *Can J Neurol Sci* 1992;**19**:180–7.

4624. Reding MJ, Orto L, Willensky P, et al. The dexamethasone suppression test: an indicator of depression in stroke but not a predictor of rehabilitation outcome. *Arch Neurol* 1985;**42**:209–12.

4625. Redlich FC, Dorsey JF. Denial of blindness by patients with cerebral disease. *Arch Neurol Psychiatry* 1945;**53**:407.

4626. Reed DM, Kurland LT. Muscle fasciculations in a healthy population. *Arch Neurol* 1963;**9**:363–7.

4627. Reed LA, Grabowski TJ, Schmidt ML, et al. Autosomal dominant dementia with widespread neurofibrillary tangles. *Ann Neurol* 1997;**42**:564–72.

4628. Reed WB, Stone VM, Boder E, et al. Hereditary syndrome with auditory and dermatological manifestations. *Arch Dermatol* 1967;**95**: 456–61.

4629. Rees JR, et al. Lentiginosis and left atrial myxoma. *Br Heart J* 1973;**35**:874–6.

4630. Refetoff S, DeWind LT, DeGroot LJ. Familial syndrome combining deaf-mutism, stipple deficiencies, goitre and abnormally high PBI: possible target organ refractory to thyroid hormone. *J Clin Endocrinol* 1967;**27**:279.

4631. Refsum S. Heredoataxia hemeralopica polyneuritiformis—et tidligere ikke beskrevet familiaert syndrome? En forelobig moddelelse. *Nord Med* 1945;**28**:2682–5.

4632. Regard M, Landis T. Gourmand syndrome. *Neurology* 1997; **48**:1185–90.

4633. Regueiro AM, Segurado OG, Mata P, et al. Acquired selective signature dysgraphia. *Ann Neurol* 1992;**31**:115.

4634. Reichert FL. Tympanic plexus neuralgia. True tic douloureux of the ear or so-called geniculate ganglion neuralgia: cure effected by intracranial section of the glossopharyngeal nerve. *JAMA* 1933;**100**: 1744–6.

4635. Reichmann H, Goebel HH, Schneider C, et al. Familial mixed congenital myopathy with rigid spine phenotype. *Muscle Nerve* 1997;**20**:411–6.

4636. Reid E. The hereditary spastic paraplegias. *J Neurol* 1999; **246**:995–1003.

4637. Reid RL, Quigley ME, Yen SSC. Pituitary apoplexy: a review. *Arch Neurol* 1985;**42**:712–9.

4638. Reiher J, Lebel M. Wicket spikes: clinical correlates of a previously undescribed EEG pattern. *Can J Neurol Sci* 1977;**4**:39–47.

4639. Reik L, Steere AC, Bartenhagen NH, Shope RE, Malawista SE. Neurologic abnormalities of Lyme disease. *Medicine* 1979;**58**:281–94.

4640. Reinfeld H, Louis S. Unilateral asterixis. *NY State J Med* 1983; **83**:206–8.

4641. Reinhold M. A case of auditory agnosia. *Brain* 1950;**73**:203–23.

4642. Reis DJ. The palmo-mental reflex. A fragment of a general nociceptive skin reflex: a physiological study in normal man. *Arch Neurol* 1961;**4**:486–98.

4643. Reis J, Eber A-M, Warter J-M, et al. Alternating nystagmus and infectious mononucleosis. *Neuroophthalmology* 1989;**9**:289–92.

4644. Reisberg B. Functional assessment staging (FAST). *Psychopharmacol Bull* 1988;**24**:653.

4645. Reisberg B, Borenstein J, Franssen E, et al. BEHAVE-AD: A clinical rating scale for assessment of pharmacologically remediable behavioral symptomatology in Alzheimer's disease. In Altman HJ, ed. *Alzheimer's Disease: Problems, Prospects, and Perspectives*, p 1. New York: Plenum Press, 1987.

4646. Reisberg B, Ferris SH. The Brief Cognitive Rating Scale (BCRS). *Psychopharmacol Bull* 1988;**24**:629.

4647. Reisberg B, Ferris SH, De Leon MJ, et al. The Global Deterioration Scale in assessment of primary degenerative dementia. *Am J Psychiatry* 1982;**139**:1136–9.

4648. Reisberg B, Ferris SH, De Leon MJ, et al. The Global Deterioration Scale (GDS). *Psychopharmacol Bull* 1988;**24**:661–663.

4649. Reisberg B, London E, Ferris SH, et al. The Brief Cognitive Rating Scale: language, motoric and mood concomitants in primary degenerative dementia. *Psychopharmacol Bull* 1983;**19**:702–8.

4650. Reisecker F, Lebelhuber F, Lexner R, et al. A sporadic form of hereditary neuropathy with liability to pressure palsies. *Neurology* 1994; **44**:753–5.

4651. Reisman LE, Kashara S, Chung C-Y, et al. Antimongolism. *Lancet* 1966;**1**:394.

4652. Reisner SH, et al. Cutis laxa associated with severe intrauterine growth retardation and congenital dislocation of the hip. *Acta Pediatr Scand* 1971;**60**:357.

4653. Reitan RM. Validity of the trail-making test as an indication of organic brain damage. *Percept Mot Skills* 1958;**8**:271.

4654. Reitan RM, Davison LA. *Clinical Neuropsychology: Current Status and Applications*. Tucson: Neuropsychology Press, 1985.

4655. Reitan RM, Wolfson D. *The Halstead-Reitan Neuropsychological Test Battery: Theory and Clinical Interpretation*. Tucson: Neuropsychology Press, 1985.

4656. Reivich M, Holling HE, Roberts B, et al. Reversal of blood flow through the vertebral artery and its affect on cerebral circulation. *N Engl J Med* 1961;**265**:878–85.

4657. Remak E. Zur Pathogenese der Bleilahmungen. *Arch Psychiatr (Berlin)* 1878;**6**:1–56.

4658. Remillard GM, Andermann F, Rhi-Sausi A, et al. Facial asymmetry in patients with temporal lobe epilepsy. *Neurology* 1977;**27**: 109–14.

4659. Remillard GM, Ethier R, Andermann F. Temporal lobe epilepsy and perinatal occlusion of the posterior cerebral artery. A syndrome analogous to infantile hemiplegia and a demonstrable etiology in some patients with temporal lobe epilepsy. *Neurology* 1974;**24**:1001–9.

4660. Renehan AG, Booth C, Potten CS. What is apoptosis and why is it important? *BMJ* 2001;**322**:1536–8.

4661. Renfrew S, Melville ID. The somatic sense of space (choraesthesia) and its threshold. *Brain* 1960;**83**:93–112.

4662. Rennert OM, Greer M. Hereditary fructosemia. *Neurology* 1970;**20**:421–5.

4663. Rensi E, Faglione P, Savoiardo M. The influence of aphasia and of the hemisphere side of the cerebral lesion on abstract thinking. *Cortex* 1966;**2**:399–420.

4664. Requena I, Arias M, Lopez-Ibor L, et al. Cavernomas of the central nervous system: clinical and neuroimaging manifestations in 47 patients. *J Neurol Neurosurg Psychiatry* 1991;**54**:590–4.

4665. Requena I, Indakoextea B, Lema C, et al. Coma associated with migraine. *Rev Neurol (Paris)* 1999;**29**:1048–51.

4666. Reszel PA, Janes JM, Spittell JA. Ischemic necrosis of the peroneal musculature: a lateral compartment syndrome; report of a case. *Proc Staff Meet Mayo Clin* 1963;**38**:130–6.

4667. Rett Syndrome Diagnostic Criteria Working Group. Diagnostic criteria for Rett syndrome. *Ann Neurol* 1988;**23**:425–8.

4668. Retzlaff JA, Kearns TP, Howard FM, et al. Lancaster red-green testing in evaluation of edrophonium effect in myasthenia gravis. *Am J Ophthalmol* 1969;**67**:13–21.

4669. Revilliod JLA. Left hemiplegia in a left-hander from embolism of the brachiocephalic trunk; orbicularis sign. *Rev Med Suisse Rom* 1889;**9**:595–606.

4670. Rey A. L'examen psychological en cas d'encephalopathie traumatique. *Arch Psychiol Norm Pathol (Paris)* 1941;**28**:286–340.

4671. Rey A. *L'examen Clinique en Psychologie*. Paris: Presses Universitaires de France, 1964.

4672. Reye RD, Morgan G, Baral J. Encephalopathy and fatty degeneration of the viscera. *Lancet* 1963;**2**:749–52.

4673. Reyes MG, Noronha P, Thomas V, et al. Myositis of chronic graft-versus-host disease. *Neurology* 1983;**33**:1222–4.

4674. Reynolds DW, Stagno S, Stubbs G, et al. Inapparent congenital cytomegalovirus infection with elevated cord IgM levels: causal relation with auditory and mental deficiency. *N Engl J Med* 1974;**290**:291–6.

4675. Richards BW, Rundle AT. A familial hormonal disorder associated with mental deficiency, deaf mutism and ataxia. *J Ment Defic* 1959;**3**:33–55.

4676. Richardson JK, Forman GM, Riley B. An electrophysiological exploration of the double crush hypothesis. *Muscle Nerve* 1999;**22**:71–7.

4677. Richieri-Costa A, et al. Adult proximal spinal muscular atrophy. *Am J Med Genet* 1981;**9**:119–23.

4678. Richman DP, Agius MA. Acquired myasthenia gravis: immunopathology. *Neurol Clin* 1994;**12**:273–4.

4679. Ricker K, Kock MC, Lehmann-Horn F, et al. Proximal myotonic myopathy. *Arch Neurol* 1995;**52**:25–31.

4680. Ricker K, Lehmann-Horn F, Moxley RT. Myotonia fluctuans. *Arch Neurol* 1990;**47**:268–72.

4681. Ricker K, Mertens H-G. Okulare neuromyotonie. *Klin Monatsbl Augenheilk* 1970;**156**:837.

4682. Ricker K, Moxley RT, Rohkamm R. Rippling muscle disease. *Arch Neurol* 1989;**46**:405–8.

4683. Riddoch G. The reflex functions of the completely divided spinal cord in man, compared with those associated with less severe lesions. *Brain* 1917;**40**:264–402.

4684. Riddoch G. Visual disorientation in homonymous half-fields. *Brain* 1935;**58**:376–82.

4685. Riddoch G. Phantom limbs and body shape. *Brain* 1941;**64**:197–222.

4686. Ridley A, Kennard C, Scholtz CL, et al. Omnipause neurons in two cases of opsoclonus associated with oat cell carcinoma of the lung. *Brain* 1987;**110**:1699.

4687. Rieder H. Die "Steintrager-Lahmung." Eine Form der combinirten Armnerven- oder Brachialplexus-Lahmung. *Munch Med Wochenschr* 1893;**40**:121–3.

4688. Riegel W. On alternating mydriasis. *Dtsch Z Nervenklinik* 1900;**17**:169–70.

4689. Rieger H. Beitrage zur Kenntnis seltener Missbildungen der Iris. *Arch Ophthalmol Berlin* 1935;**133**:602.

4690. Riese W. The early history of aphasia. *Bull Med Hist* 1947;**21**:322–34.

4691. Riese W. The sources of Hughlings Jackson's view on aphasia. *Brain* 1965;**88**:811–22.

4692. Riggs JE, Klingberg WG, Flink EB, et al. Cardioskeletal mitochondrial myopathy associated with chronic magnesium deficiency. *Neurology* 1992;**42**:128–30.

4693. Riggs JE, Schochet SS, Fakadi AV, et al. Mitochondrial encephalomyopathy with decreased succinate cytochrome reductase activity. *Neurology* 1984;**34**:48–53.

4694. Riggs JE, Schochet SS, Gutmann L, et al. Lysosomal glycogen storage disease with acid maltase deficiency. *Neurology* 1983;**33**:873–7.

4695. Riley CM, Day RL, Greeley DM, et al. Central autonomic dysfunction with defective lacrymation: report of 5 cases. *Pediatrics* 1949;**3**:468–78.

4696. Riley CM, Shwachman H. Unusual osseous disease with neurologic changes. *Am J Dis Child* 1960;**150**–4.

4697. Riley DE, Lang AE. Non-Parkinson akinetic-rigid syndromes. *Curr Opin Neurol* 1996;**9**:321–6.

4698. Riley HD, Smith WR. Macrocephaly, pseudopapilledema, and multiple hemangiomata. *Pediatrics* 1960;**26**:293–300.

4699. Rimel RW, Giodani B, Barth JT, et al. Disability caused by minor head injury. *Neurosurgery* 1981;**9**:221–8.

4700. Riminton DS, Chambers ST, Parkin PJ, et al. Inclusion body myositis presenting solely as dysphagia. *Neurology* 1993;**43**:1241–3.

4701. Ringel SP, Bailey OT. Rathke's cleft cyst. *J Neurol Neurosurg Psychiatry* 1972;**35**:693–7.

4702. Ringel SP, Claman HN. Amyloid-associated muscle pseudohypertrophy. *Arch Neurol* 1982;**39**:413–7.

4703. Ringel SP, Forstot JZ, Tau EM, et al. Sjogren's syndrome with polymyositis or dermatomyositis. *Arch Neurol* 1982;**39**:157–68.

4704. Ringel SP, Kenny CE, Neville HE, et al. Spectrum of inclusion body myositis. *Arch Neurol* 1987;**44**:1154–7.

4705. Ringel SP, Lava NS, Treihaft MM, et al. Late onset X-linked recessive spinal and bulbar muscular atrophy. *Muscle Nerve* 1978;**1**:297–307.

4706. Ringel SP, Neville HE, Duster MC, et al. A new congenital neuromuscular disease with trilaminar muscle fibers. *Neurology* 1978;**28**:282–9.

4707. Ringertz N. Grading of gliomas. *Acta Pathol Microbiol Scand* 1950;**27**:51–64.

4708. Ringrose RE, et al. Hemihypertrophy. *Pediatrics* 1965;**36**:434–48.

4708a. Rinne FHA. *Beitr. zur Physiologie des menschlichen Ohres.* Vierteljahrsschrift fur die praktische Heilkunde (Prague) 1855;**45**:71–123 and **46**:45–72.

4709. Riordan-Eva P, Sanders MD, Govan GG, et al. The clinical features of Leber's hereditary optic neuropathy defined by the presence of a pathogenic mitochondrial mutation. *Brain* 1995;**118**:319–37.

4710. Ripps H, Noble KG, Greenstein VC, et al. Progressive cone dystrophy. *Ophthalmology* 1987;**94**:1401.

4711. Riser M, Geraud J, Ducoudray J, et al. Dolicho-carotide interne avec syndrome vertigineux. *Rev Neurol (Paris)* 1951;**85**:145–7.

4712. Risk WS, Bosch EP, Kimura J, et al. Chronic tetanus: clinical report and histochemistry of muscle. *Muscle Nerve* 1981;**4**:363–6.

4713. Rivers WH, Head H. A human experiment in nerve division. *Brain* 1908;**31**:323–450.

4714. Rizzo M, Hurtig R, Damasio AR. The role of scanpaths in facial recognition and learning. *Ann Neurol* 1987;**22**:41–5.

4715. Roach ES, Gomez MR, Northrup MH. Tuberous Sclerosis Complex Consensus Conference: revised clinical diagnostic criteria. *J Child Neurol* 1998;**13**:624–8.

4716. Roaf R. Lateral flexion injuries of the cervical spine. *J Bone Jt Surg* 1963;**45**:36–8.

4717. Robb JP. A footnote to medical history: David Alexander Shirres on spinal cord regeneration. *Can J Neurol Sci* 1991;**18**:361–2.

4718. Roberts TA, Jenkyn LR, Reeves AG. On the notion of doll's eyes. *Arch Neurol* 1984;**41**:1242–3.

4719. Robertson A. On an interesting series of eye-symptoms in a case of spinal disease, with remarks on the action of Belladonna on the iris, etc. *Edinb Med J* 1868;**14**:696–708.

4720. Robertson D, Hollister AS, Biaggioni I, et al. The diagnosis and treatment of baroreflex failure. *N Engl J Med* 1993;**329**:1449–55.

4721. Robertson MM, Banerjee S, Kurlan R, et al. The Tourette Syndrome Diagnostic Confidence Index. *Neurology* 1999;**53**:2108–12.

4722. Robertson WC, Fariello RG. Eating epilepsy associated with a deep forebrain glioma. *Ann Neurol* 1979;**6**:271–3.

4723. Robertson WE, Robertson HF. *Diagnostic Signs, Reflexes and Syndromes.* Philadelphia: F.A. Davis, 1947.

4724. Robin P. La glossoptose: son diagnostic, ses conséquences, son traitement. *J Med (Paris)* 1923;**43**:235–7.

4725. Robins LN, Helzer JE, Croughan J, et al. NIMH Diagnostic Interview Schedule. *Arch Gen Psychiatry* 1981;**38**:381–9.

4726. Robinson B, Johnson R, Abernethy D, et al. Familial distal dysautonomia. *J Neurol Neurosurg Psychiatry* 1989;**52**:1281–5.

4727. Robinson D. Pyriformis syndrome in relation to sciatic pain. *Am J Surg* 1947;**73**:355–8.

4728. Robinson DA, Zee DS, Hain TC, et al. Alexander's law: its behavior and origin in the human vestibulo-ocular reflex. *Ann Neurol* 1984;**16**:714–22.

4729. Robinson G, Blair J, Cipolotti L. Dynamic aphasia: an inability to select between competing verbal responses? *Brain* 1998;**121**:77–89.

4730. Robinson GC, Miller JR, Bensimon JR. Familial ectodermal dysplasia with sensorineural deafness and other anomalies. *Pediatrics* 1962;**30**:797.

4731. Robinson LK, et al. Carpenter syndrome; natural history and clinical spectrum. *Am J Med Genet* 1985;**20**:461–9.

4732. Robinson RO, Thornett CEE. Benign hereditary chorea response to steroids. *Dev Med Child Neurol* 1985;**27**:814–6.

4733. Robitaille Y, Carpenter S, Karpati G, et al. A distinct form of adult polyglucosan body disease with massive involvement of central and peripheral neuronal processes and astrocytes. A report of four cases and a review of the occurrence of polyglucosan bodies in other conditions such as Laflora's disease and normal ageing. *Brain* 1980;**103**:315–36.

4734. Rochon-Duvigneau A. Some cases of paralysis of all the orbital nerves. *Arch Ophthalmol Berlin* 1896;**16**:746–60.

4735. Rockwood K, Parhad I, Hachinski V, et al. Diagnosis of vascular dementia. *Can J Neurol Sci* 1994;**21**:358–64.

4736. Rodiet A, Cans F. Differentiation of toxic and general paralytic cerebral diseases. *Ann Med Psychol* 1906;**4**:408–20.

4737. Rodriquez B, Rodriquez BR, Oreggia A. A new type of peduncular syndrome. *Am J Ophthalmol* 1946;**29**:511.

4738. Roelcke U, Hornstein C, Hund E, et al. "Sunbath polyneuritis": subacute axonal polyneuropathy in perazine-treated patients after intense sun exposure. *Muscle Nerve* 1996;**19**:438–41.

4739. Roessmann U, Schwartz JF. Familial striatal degeneration. *Arch Neurol* 1973;**29**:314–7.

4740. Roger J, Dravet C, Bureau M, et al. *Epileptic Syndromes in Infancy, Childhood and Adolescence.* London & Paris: John Libby Eurotext, 1985.

4741. Roger J, Genton P, Bureau M, et al. Dyssynergia cerebellaris myoclonica (Ramsay Hunt's syndrome) associated with epilepsy: a study of 32 cases. *Neuropediatrics* 1987;**18**:117.

4742. Rogers L. The posterior fossa compression syndrome. *BMJ* 1933;**2**:100–1.

4743. Rohkamm R, Boxler K, Ricker K, et al. A dominantly inherited myopathy with excessive tubular aggregates. *Neurology* 1983;**33**:331–6.

4744. Rolak LA. The flight of colors test in multiple sclerosis. *Arch Neurol* 1985;**42**:759–60.

4745. Roland PE. Lack of appreciation of compressibility. *J Neurol Sci* 1973;**20**:51–61.

4746. Roles NC, Maudsley RH. Radial tunnel syndrome: resistant tennis elbow as nerve entrapment. *J Bone Jt Surg* 1972;**54**:499–508.

4747. Rollet J, Colrat. Syndrome de l'apex orbitaire (ophthalmoplegie sensorio-sensitivo-motrice d'origine traumatique). *Bull Soc Ophthalmol Lyon* 1926;**16**:13–4.

4748. Roman G. Epidemic neuropathy in Cuba: a public health problem related to the Cuban Democracy Act of the United States. *Neuroepidemiology* 1998;**17**:111–5.

4749. Roman G, Fisher M, Perl DP, et al. Neurological manifestations of hereditary hemorrhagic telangiectasia (Rendu-Osler-Weber disease): report of 2 cases and review of the literature. *Ann Neurol* 1978;**4**:130–44.

4750. Roman GC, Roman LN, Spencer PS, et al. Tropical spastic paraparesis—a neuroepidemiological study in Colombia. *Ann Neurol* 1985;**17**:361–5.

4751. Roman GC, Spencer PS, Schoenberg BS. Tropical myeloneuropathies. *Neurology* 1985;**35**:1158–70.

4752. Roman GC, Tatemichi TK, Erkinjuntti T, et al. Vascular dementia: diagnostic criteria for research studies. *Neurology* 1993;**43**:250–60.

4753. Romberg MH. *Klinische Ergebnisse.* Berlin: A. Förstner, 1846.

4754. Romberg MH. *Lehrbuch der Nervenkrankheiten des Menschen.* Berlin: Duncker, 1846.

4755. Romberg MH. Hyperesthesia of the nerves of muscular sense. In Sieveking EH, ed. *Manual of the Nervous Diseases of Man,* pp. 226–227. London: Sydenham Society, 1853.

4756. Romeo G. Enzymatic defects of hereditary porphyrias: an explanation of dominance at a molecular level. *Hum Genet* 1977;**39**:261–76.

4757. Ron MA. Somatisation in neurological practice. *J Neurol Neurosurg Psychiatry* 1994;**57**:1161–4.

4758. Rondot P, Marchand MP, Dellatolas G. Spasmodic torticollis—review of 220 patients. *Can J Neurol Sci* 1991;**18**:143–51.

4759. Rondot P, Recondo JD, Dumas JLR. Visuomotor ataxia. *Brain* 1977;**100**:355–76.

4760. Ronen GM, Rosales TO, Connolly M, et al. Seizure characteristics in chromosome 20 benign familial neonatal convulsions. *Neurology* 1993;**43**:1355–60.

4761. Roos DB. Thoracic outlet syndrome. *Muscle Nerve* 1999;**22**:126–9.

4762. Roos RA, van Dijk JC. Reflex-epilepsy induced by immersion in hot water. Case report and review of the literature. *Eur Neurol* 1988;**28**:6–10.

4763. Ropper AH. Case records of the Massachusetts General Hospital #35–1981. *N Engl J Med* 1981;**305**:507–14.

4764. Ropper AH. Ocular dipping in anoxic coma. *Arch Neurol* 1981;**38**:297–9.

4765. Ropper AH. Self-grasping: a focal neurological sign. *Ann Neurol* 1982;**12**:575–7.

4766. Ropper AH. Unusual spontaneous movements in brain-dead patients. *Neurology* 1984;**34**:1089–92.

4767. Ropper AH. In favor of intracranial pressure monitoring and aggressive therapy in neurologic practice. *Arch Neurol* 1985;**42**:1194–5.

4768. Ropper AH. Seronegative, non-neoplastic acute cerebellar degeneration. *Neurology* 1993;**43**:1602–5.

4769. Ropper AH. Syndrome of transtentorial herniation: is vertical displacement necessary? *J Neurol Neurosurg Psychiatry* 1993;**56**:932–5.

4770. Ropper AH, Davis KR. Lobar cerebral hemorrhages: acute clinical syndromes in 26 cases. *Ann Neurol* 1980;**8**:141–7.

4771. Ropper AH, Poskanzer DC. The prognosis of acute and subacute transverse myelopathy based on early signs and symptoms. *Ann Neurol* 1978;**4**:51–9.

4772. Ropper AH, Wijdicks EFM, Truax BT. *Guillain-Barré Syndrome.* Philadelphia: F.A. Davis, 1991.

4773. Roscher A, Hofler S, Hofler G, et al. Neonatal adrenoleukodystrophy (ALD) and cerebral-hepato-renal syndrome (CHRS): genetic complementation analysis of impaired peroxisomal plasmalogen biosynthesis. In *24th International Symposium, Society for the Study of Inborn Errors in Metabolism,* Boston: MTP Press, 1986.

4774. Rose BD. Hypoosmolal states—hyponatremia. In *Clinical Physiology of Acid-Base and Electrolyte Disorders,* pp. 651–94. New York: McGraw-Hill, 1989.

4775. Rose E. Ueber den Starrkrampf. *Pitha-Billroths Handbuch,* 1870;1–118.

4776. Rosemberg S. Neuropathology of S. Paulo south coast epidemic encephalitis. *J Neurol Sci* 1980;**45**:1–12.

4777. Rosen S. Tic douloureux of the chorda tympani. *Arch Neurol Psychiatry* 1953;**69**:275–8.

4778. Rosen SM, et al. Hemodialysis disequilibrium. *BMJ* 1964;**2**:672–5.

4779. Rosen WG, Mohs RC, Davis KL. A new rating scale for Alzheimer's disease. *Am J Psychiatry* 1984;**14**:1356–64.

4780. Rosen WG, Terry RD, Fuld PA, et al. Pathological verification of ischemic score in differentiation of dementias. *Ann Neurol* 1980;**7**:486–8.

4781. Rosenbach O. Ein Beitrag zur sympt. cerebraler Hemiplegien. *Arch Psychiatr (Berlin)* 1876;**6**:845.

4782. Rosenbaum DH, Siegel M, Barr WB, et al. Epileptic aphasia. *Neurology* 1986;**36**:822–5.

4783. Rosenberg AL, Bergstrom L, Troost BT, et al. Hyperuricemia and neurological deficits. *N Engl J Med* 1970;**282**:992–7.

4784. Rosenberg LE, Durant JL, Elsas LJ. Familial iminoglycinuria: an inborn error of renal tubular transport. *N Engl J Med* 1968;**278**:1407–13.

4785. Rosenberg ML. Congenital trigeminal anesthesia. *Brain* 1984;**107**:1073–82.

4786. Rosenberg ML, Clark JB. Familial trembling of the chin. *Neurology* 1987;**37**(**Suppl 1**):190.

4787. Rosenberg ML, Glaser JS. Superior oblique myokymia. *Ann Neurol* 1983;**13**:667–9.

4788. Rosenberg NL, Neville HE, Ringel SP. Tubular aggregates: their association with neuromuscular diseases, including the syndrome of myalgias/cramps. *Arch Neurol* 1985;**42**:973–6.

4789. Rosenberg R, Fowler HL. Spinal muscular atrophy with Joseph disease. *Neurology* 1981;**31**:1124.

4790. Rosenberg R, Greenberg J. Linear scleroderma as a cause for hemiatrophy. *Ann Neurol* 1979;**5**:307.

4791. Rosenberg RN, Chutorian AM. Familial opticoacoustic nerve degeneration and polyneuropathy. *Neurology* 1967;**17**:827–32.

4792. Rosenberg RN, Green JB, White CL, et al. Dominantly inherited dementia and parkinsonism, with Non-Alzheimer amyloid plaques. *Ann Neurol* 1989;**25**:152–8.

4793. Rosenberg RN, Grossman A. Hereditary ataxia. In Johnson WG, ed. *Neurologic Clinics*, pp 25–36. Philadelphia: W.B. Saunders, 1989.

4794. Rosenberg RN, Nyhan WL, Bay C, et al. Autosomal dominant striatonigral degeneration. *Neurology* 1976;**26**:703–14.

4795. Rosenberg RN, Nyhan WL, Borg C, et al. Autosomal dominant striato-nigral degeneration: a clinicopathological and biochemical study of a new genetic disease. *Neurology* 1976;**26**:703–14.

4796. Rosenberg S, Lancellotti CLP, Anta F, et al. Progressive bulbar paralysis of childhood (Fazio-Londe disease) with deafness. *Eur Neurol* 1982;**21**:84–9.

4797. Rosenblatt B, Kaplan P. A distinctive facies in neurofibromatosis. *Am J Human Genet* 1983;**35**(**6**):115A.

4798. Rosenthal R, Hall JA, Archer D, et al. *The PONS Test Manual*. New York: Irvington Publishers, 1979.

4799. Rosow I, Breslau N. A Guttman scale for the aged. *J Gerontol* 1966;**21**:556–9.

4800. Ross AT. Progressive selective sudomotor denervation; a case with coexisting Adie's syndrome. *Neurology* 1959;**8**:809–17.

4801. Ross ED. The aprosodias: functional–anatomic organization of the affective components of language in the right hemisphere. *Arch Neurol* 1981;**38**:561–9.

4802. Ross MA, Miller RG, Berchert L, et al. Toward earlier diagnosis of amyotrophic lateral sclerosis. *Neurology* 1998;**50**:768–72.

4803. Ross RT. Transient tumor attacks. *Arch Neurol* 1983;**40**:633–6.

4804. Rossi F, Triggs WJ, Gooch J, et al. Bilateral medial pectoral neuropathy in a weight lifter. *Muscle Nerve* 1999;**22**:1597–9.

4805. Rossi G, Macchi G, Porro M, et al. Fatal familial insomnia. *Neurology* 1998;**50**:688–92.

4806. Rossi PW, Kleiferts S, Reding MJ. Fresnel prisms improve visual perception in stroke patients with homonymous hemianopia or unilateral visual neglect. *Neurology* 1990;**40**:1597–9.

4807. Rossolimo GI. De la myotonie atrophique: contribution a la theorie des myopathies. *Nouv Icon Salpet* 1902;**15**:63–77.

4808. Rosvold HE, Mirsky AF, Sarason I, et al. A continuous performance test of brain damage. *J Clin Consult Psychol* 1956;**20**:343.

4809. Rot WK. *Meralgia Paresthetica*. Berlin: S. Karger, 1895.

4810. Roth B. Functional hypersomnia. In Guilleminault C, Dement WC, Passouant P, eds. *Advances in Sleep Research*, pp 333–50. New York: Spectrum, 1976.

4811. Roth B, Bruhova S, Berkova L. Familial sleep paralysis. *Arch Suisse Neurol Neurochir Psychiatr* 1968;**102**:321–30.

4812. Roth B, Nevsimalova S, Rechtschaffen A. Hypersomnia with "sleep drunkenness". *Arch Gen Psychiatr* 1972;**26**:456–62.

4813. Roth CJ, Williams HE. The muscular variant of Pompe's disease. *J Pediatr* 1967;**71**:567–73.

4814. Roth M, Tym E, Mountjoy MQ. CAMDEX: a standardised instrument for the diagnosis of mental disorder in the elderly with special reference to the early detection of dementia. *Br J Psychiatry* 1986;**149**:698–709.

4815. Rothi LJ, McFarling DA, Heilman KM. Conduction aphasia, syntactic alexia, and the anatomy of syntactic comprehension. *Arch Neurol* 1982;**39**:272–5.

4816. Rothi LJG, Mack L, Heilman KM. Pantomime agnosia. *J Neurol Neurosurg Psychiatry* 1986;**49**:451–4.

4817. Rothman S. Physiology of itching. *Physiol Rev* 1941;**21**:357–81.

4818. Rothstein TL, Alvord EC. Posterior internuclear ophthalmoplegia. *Arch Neurol* 1971;**24**:191–202.

4819. Rothwell JC, Traub MM, Marsden CD. Primary writing tremor. *J Neurol Neurosurg Psychiatry* 1979;**42**:1106–14.

4820. Rothwell P. Investigation of sensory or motor symptoms: frequency of neurological pathology depends on side of symptoms. *J Neurol Neurosurg Psychiatry* 1994;**57**:1401–2.

4821. Rotthauwe HW, Kowalewski S, Mumenthaler M. Congenital muscle dystrophy [in German]. *Z Kinderheilkd* 1969;**106**:131–62.

4822. Roussy G, Cornil L. Névrite hypertrophique progressive nonfamilial de l'adulte. *Ann Med* 1919;**6**:296–305.

4823. Roussy G, Levy G. Sept cas d'une maladie particulaire: troubles de la marche, pieds bots et areflexie tendineuse generalisée, avec accessoirement, legère maladresse des mains. *Rev Neurol (Paris)* 1926;**1**:427–50.

4824. Roussy G, Lhermitte JJ. *Les Blessures de la Moelle et de la Queue de Cheval.* Paris: Masson, 1918.

4825. Rowland LP. Myoglobinuria. *Can J Neurol Sci* 1984;**11**:1–6.

4826. Rowland LP. Cramps, spasms and muscle stiffness. *Rev Neurol (Paris)* 1985;**141**:261–73.

4827. Rowland LP, Fetel M, Olarte A, et al. Emery-Dreifuss muscular dystrophy. *Ann Neurol* 1979;**5**:111–7.

4828. Rowland LP, Greer M. Toxoplasmosis. *Neurology* 1961;**11**:367.

4829. Rowland LP, Penn AS. Myoglobinuria. *Med Clin North Am* 1972;**56**:1233–4.

4830. Rowland LP, Shneider NA. Amyotrophic lateral sclerosis. *N Engl J Med* 2001;**344**:1688–99.

4831. Roy FH. *Ocular Syndromes and Systemic Diseases.* Philadelphia: W.B. Saunders, 1989.

4832. Roy PR, Emanual R, Ismail SA, et al. Hereditary prolongation of the Q-T interval: genetic observations. *Am J Cardiol* 1976;**37**:237–43.

4833. Royall DR, Cabello M, Polk M. Executive dyscontrol: an important factor affecting the level of care received by elderly retirees. *J Am Geriatr Soc* 1988;**46**:1519–24.

4834. Royall DR, Chiodo LK, Polk M. Correlates of disability among elderly retirees with "sub-clinical" cognitive impairment. *J Gerontol* 2000;**55A**:M541–M546.

4835. Royall DR, Cordes JA, Polk M. CLOX: an executive drawing task. *J Neurol Neurosurg Psychiatry* 1999;**64**:588–94.

4836. Royall DR, Mahurin RK, Gray KF. Bedside assessment of executive cognitive impairment: the executive interview. *J Am Geriatr Soc* 1992;**40**:1221–6.

4837. Rozear MP, Pericak-Vance S, Pericaz-Vance MA, et al. Hereditary motor and sensory neuropathy, X-linked. *Neurology* 1987;**37**:1460–5.

4838. Rubens O, Logina I, Kravale I, et al. Peripheral neuropathy in chronic occupational inorganic lead exposure: a clinical and electrophysiological study. *J Neurol Neurosurg Psychiatry* 2001;**71**:200–4.

4839. Rubenstein JH, Taybi H. Broad thumbs and toes and facial abnormalities. *Am J Dis Child* 1963;**105**:588.

4840. Rubin SA, Sylves P, Vogel M, et al. Borna disease virus-induced hippocampal dentate gyrus damage is associated with spatial learning and memory deficits. *Brain Res Bull* 1998;**48**:23–30.

4841. Rubin SE, Wagner RS. Ocular torticollis. *Surv Ophthalmol* 1986;**30**:366.

4842. Rubinstein AE, Weinapel SF. Acute hypokalemic myopathy of alcoholism. *Arch Neurol* 1977;**34**:553–5.

4843. Rubio-Golalbo ME, Smeitink JA, Ruitenbeek W, et al. Spinal muscular atrophy-like picture, cardiomyopathy, and cytochrome c oxidase deficiency. *Neurology* 1999;**52**:383–6.

4844. Ruchoux MM, Maurage CA. CADASIL. Cerebral autosomal dominant arteriopathy with subcortical infarcts and leukoencephalopathy. *J Neuropathol Exp Neurol* 1997;**56**:947–64.

4845. Rud E. Et tilfaelde af infantilisme med tetani, epilepsi, polyneuritis, ichthyosis og anaemi of pernicios type. *Hospitalstidende* 1927;**70**:525–38.

4846. Rudick RA, Cutter G, Baier M, et al. Use of the Multiple Sclerosis Functional Composite to predict disability in relapsing MS. *Neurology* 2001;**56**:1324–30.

4847. Ruggieri M, Tigano G, Mazzone D, et al. Involvement of the white matter in hypomelanosis of Ito. *Neurology* 1996;**46**:485–92.

4848. Rukavina JG, Block WD, Jackson CF, et al. Amyloidosis type II. *Medicine (Baltimore)* 1956;**35**:239–334.

4849. Rush PJ, Inman R, Bernstein M, et al. Isolated vasculitis of the central nervous system in a patient with celiac disease. *Am J Med* 1986;**81**:1092–4.

4850. Rushton AR, Genel G. Hereditary ectodermal dysplasia, olivopontocerebellar degeneration, short stature and hypogonadism. *J Med Genet* 1981;**18**:335–9.

4851. Rushworth G. Observations on blink reflexes. *J Neurol Neurosurg Psychiatry* 1962;**25**:93–108.

4852. Russell AA. A diencephalic syndrome of emaciation in infancy and childhood. *Arch Dis Child* 1951;**26**:274.

4852a. Bigner DD, Mclendon RE, Bruner JM (eds). *Russell and Rubinstein's Pathology of Tumors of the Nervous System, Sixth Edition.* New York: Oxford University Press, 1998.

4853. Russell DS, Marshall AHE, Smith FB. Microgliomatosis. *Brain* 1948;**71**:1–15.

4854. Russell EW. A multiple scoring method for the assessment of complex memory functions. *J Consult Clin Psychol* 1975;**43**:800–9.

4855. Russell GFM. Bulimia nervosa: an ominous variant of anorexia nervosa. *Psychol Med* 1979;**9**:429–48.

4856. Russell JSR, Batten FE, Collier J. Subacute combined degeneration of the spinal cord. *Brain* 1900;**23**:39–110.

4857. Russo LS, Aron A, Anderson PJ. Alexander's disease: a report and reappraisal. *Neurology* 1976;**26**:607–14.

4858. Russomano S, Herbison GJ, Baliga A, et al. Riche-Cannieu anastomosis with partial transection of the median nerve. *Muscle Nerve* 1995;**18**:120–2.

4859. Ruvalcaba RHA, Reichert A, Smith DW. A new familial syndrome with osseous dysplasia and mental deficiency. *J Pediatr* 1971;**79**:450–5.

4860. Ryan AJ, Stephens RE. *Dance Medicine. A Comprehensive Guide.* Chicago: Pluribus Press, 1987.

4861. Ryan MM, Schnell C, Strickland CD, et al. Nemaline myopathy; a clinical study of 143 cases. *Ann Neurol* 2001;**50**:312–20.

4862. Rylander G. Psychoses and the punding and choreiform syndromes in addiction to central stimulant drugs. *Psychiatr Neurol Neurochir (Amst)* 1972;**75**:203–12.

4863. Sabin TD, Swift TR. Leprosy. In Dyck PJ, Thomas PK, Lambert EH, eds. *Peripheral Neuropathy*, p 1198. Philadelphia: W.B. Saunders, 1975.

4864. Sabra AF, Hallett M. Action tremor with alternating activity in antagonist muscles. *Neurology* 1984;**34**:151–6.

4865. Sachdev P, Loneragan C. Low dose apomorphine challenge in tardive akathisia. *Neurology* 1993;**43**:544–7.

4866. Sachdev PS, Smith JS, Angus-Lepan H, et al. Pseudodementia twelve years on. *J Neurol Neurosurg Psychiatry* 1990;**53**:254–9.

4867. Sachs B. On arrested cerebral development, with special reference to its cortical pathology. *J Nerv Ment Dis* 1887;**14**:541–53.

4868. Sachs GM, Raynor EM, Schefner JM. The all ulnar motor hand without forearm anastomosis. *Muscle Nerve* 1995;**19**:309–13.

4869. Sadeghian H. Mount Fuji sign in tension pneumocephalus. *Arch Neurol* 2000;**57**:1366.

4870. Sadeh M, Blatt I, Goldhammer Y. Single fiber EMG in a congenital myasthenic syndrome associated with facial malformations. *Muscle Nerve* 1993;**16**:177–80.

4871. Sadun AA, Currie JN, Lessell S. Transient visual obscurations with elevated optic discs. *Ann Neurol* 1984;**16**:489–94.

4872. Saenger A. On a form of myotonic pupil. *Neurol Centralbl* 1902;**21**:1137–8.

4873. Saenz-Lope E, Herranz FJ, Masdeu JC. Startle epilepsy: a clinical study. *Ann Neurol* 1984;**16**:78–81.

4874. Saethre H. Ein Beitrag zum Turmschadelproblem (Pathogenese, Erblichkeit und Symptomatolgie). *Dtsch Z Nervenheilkd* 1931;**117**:533–55.

4875. Safdari H, Richardson EPj. Subacute necrotizing polioencephalopathy. *Arch Neurol* 1979;**36**:638–42.

4876. Sagin K. Le réfléxe de la malleole éxterne et le phénomène de Piostrowski. *Rev Neurol (Paris)* 1927;**1**:319–25.

4877. Sahgal V, Sahgal S. A new congenital myopathy: a morphological, cytochemical and histochemical study. *Acta Neuropathol* 1977;**37**:255.

4878. Said G. A clinicopathological study of acrodystrophic neuropathies. *Muscle Nerve* 1980;**3**:491–501.

4879. Said G, Goulon-Goeau C, Lacroix C, et al. Nerve biopsy findings in different patterns of proximal diabetic neuropathy. *Ann Neurol* 1994;**35**:559–69.

4880. Saiz A, Arpa J, Sagasta A, et al. Autoantibodies to glutamic acid decarboxylase in three patients with cerebellar ataxia, late onset insulin dependent diabetes mellitus and polyendocrine abnormality. *Neurology* 1997;**49**:1026–30.

4881. Saka E, Saygi S, Ciger A, et al. Circling seizures. *Seizure* 1996;**5**:299–302.

4882. Sakati N, et al. A new syndrome with acrocephalopolysyndactyly, cardiac disease, and distinctive defects of the ear, skin, and lower limbs. *J Pediatr* 1971;**79**:104–9.

4883. Sakuraba H, Suzuki Y, Akagi M, et al. Beta galactosidase–neuraminidase deficiency (galactosialidosis): clinical, pathological, and enzymatic studies in a postmortem case. *Ann Neurol* 1983;**13**:497–503.

4884. Salanova V, Andermann F, Rasmussen T, et al. Parietal lobe epilepsy. *Brain* 1995;**118**:607–27.

4885. Salbert BA, Pellock JM, Wolf B. Characterization of seizures associated with biotinidase deficiency. *Neurology* 1993;**43**:1351–5.

4886. Saldino RM, Mainzer F. Cone-shaped epiphyses in siblings with hereditary renal disease and retinitis pigmentosa. *Radiology* 1971;**98**:39–45.

4887. Salleras A, Ortiz J, Zarate JC. Recessive sex-linked inheritance of external ophthalmoplegia and myopia coincident with other dysplasias. *Br J Ophthalmol* 1950;**34**:662.

4888. Salman MS, Ackerley C, Senger C, et al. New insights into the pathogenesis of molybdenum cofactor deficiency. *Can J Neurol Sci* 2002;**29**:91–6.

4889. Salonen R, Herva R, Norio R. The hydrolethalus syndrome: delineation of a "new", lethal malformation syndrome based on 28 patients. *Clin Genet* 1981;**19**:321–30.

4890. Salthouse TA, Mitchell DRD. Structural and operational capacities in integrative spatial ability. *Psychol Aging* 1989;**4**:18–25.

4891. Salus R. Acquired retraction movements of the globe. *Arch Augenheilkd* 1910;**68**:61–76.

4892. Samii A, Pal PK, Schulzer M, et al. Post-traumatic cervical dystonia: a distinct entity? *Can J Neurol Sci* 2000;**27**:55–9.

4893. Samples JR, Howard FM, Okazaki H. Syringomesencephalia: report of a case. *Arch Neurol* 1983;**40**:757–9.

4894. Samuels OB, Duffy CJ, Griggs RC. Cacacusis: frightening echoes in neurologic disease. *Neurology* 1996;**46(Suppl)**:A293–A294.

4895. Sanborn GE, Magargal L. *Neuro-Ophthalmology enters the Nineties.* Hialeah: Dutton, 1988.

4896. Sander HW, Tavoulareas GP, Quinto CM, et al. The exercise test distinguishes myotonic myopathy from myotonic dystrophy. *Muscle Nerve* 1997;**20**:2325–237.

4897. Sander JE, Layzer RB, Goldsobel AB. Congenital stiff man syndrome. *Ann Neurol* 1980;**8**:195–7.

4898. Sander JE, Sharp FR. Lumbosacral plexus neuritis. *Neurology* 1981;**31**:470–3.

4899. Sander S, Ouvrier RA, McLeod JG, et al. Clinical syndromes associated with tomacula or myelin swellings in sural nerve biopsies. *J Neurol Neurosurg Psychiatry* 2000;**68**:483–8.

4900. Sanders DB. Myotonia congenita with painful muscle contractions. *Arch Neurol* 1976;**33**:580–2.

4901. Sanders DB, Stalberg E. Single-fiber electromyography. *Muscle Nerve* 1996;**19**:1069–83.

4902. Sanders MD. Alternating windmill nystagmus. In Smith JL, Glaser JS, eds. *Neuro-Ophthalmology*, pp 133–6. St. Louis: C.V. Mosby, 1973.

4903. Sanders MD. Retinal arteritis, retinal vasculitis and autoimmune retinal vasculitis. *Eye* 1987;**1**:441.

4904. Sanders MD, Hoyt WF, Daroff RB. Lid nystagmus evoked by ocular convergence: an ocular electromyographic study. *J Neurol Neurosurg Psychiatry* 1968;**31**:368–71.

4905. Sandhoff K, Andreae U, Jatkewitz H. Deficient hexosaminidase activity in an exceptional case of Tay-Sachs disease with additional storage of kidney globoside in visceral organs. *Life Sci* 1968;**7**:283–8.

4906. Sandhoff K, Harzer K, Wassle W, et al. Enzyme alteration and lipid storage in three variants of Tay-Sachs disease. *J Neurochem* 1971;**18**:2469.

4907. Sandok BA, Houser OW, Baker HL, et al. Fibromuscular dysplasia: neurologic disorders associated with disease involving the great muscles in the neck. *Arch Neurol* 1971;**24**:462–6.

4908. Sandson J, Albert ML. Varieties of perseveration. *Neuropsychologia* 1984;**22**:715–32.

4909. Sandvig K. Pseudoglaucoma of autosomal dominant inheritance. *Acta Ophthalmol Kopenhagen* 1961;**39**:33.

4910. Sanfilippo SJ, et al. Mental retardation associated with mucopolysacchariduria (heparitin sulfate type). *J Pediatr* 1963;**63**:832–8.

4911. San Pedro EC, Mountz JM, Ojha B, et al. Anterior cingulate gyrus epilepsy: the role of SPECT in seizure localization. *Epilepsia* 2000;**41**:594–600.

4912. Santavuori P, Haltia M, Rapola J, Raitta C. Infantile type of socalled neuronal ceroid-lipofuscinosis. *J Neurol Sci* 1973;**18**:257–67.

4913. Santavuori P, Leisti J, Kruus J, et al. Muscle, eye and brain disease: a new syndrome. *Doc Ophthalmol* 1978;**17**:393–6.

4914. Saper JR. The mixed headache syndrome: a new perspective. *Headache* 1982;**22**:284–6.

4915. Saper JR. Daily chronic headache. *Neurol Clin* 1990;**8**:891–901.

4916. Saper JR, Holt JF. Cranial metaphyseal dysplasia: a cause of recurrent bilateral facial palsy. *Arch Neurol* 1974;**31**:204–7.

4917. Saperstein DS, Amato AA, Wolfe GI, et al. Multifocal acquired demyelinating sensory and motor neuropathy: the Lewis-Sumner syndrome. *Muscle Nerve* 1999;**22**:560–6.

4918. Saperstein DS, Katz JS, Barohn RJ. Clinical spectrum of chronic acquired demyelinating polyneuropathies. *Muscle Nerve* 2001;**24**:311–24.

4919. Sarnat H, Morrissey RT. Idiopathic torticollis, sternocleidomastoid myopathy and accessory neuropathy. *Muscle Nerve* 1981;**4**:374.

4920. Sarnat HB, Case ME, Graviss R. Sacral agenesis. *Neurology* 1976;**26**:1124–9.

4921. Sasanuma S, Monoi H. The syndrome of Gogi (word-meaning) aphasia. *Neurology* 1975;**25**:627–32.

4922. Satoh A, Tsuijihata M, Yokimura T. Myasthenia gravis associated with the Satayoshi syndrome. *Neurology* 1983;**33**:1209–11.

4923. Satoh T, Harada Y. Electrophysiological study on tooth-grinding during sleep. *Electroencephalogr Clin Neurophysiol* 1973;**35**:267–75.

4924. Satoyoshi E. A syndrome of progressive muscle spasm, alopecia and diarrhea. *Neurology* 1978;**28**:458–71.

4925. Satoyoshi E, Kinoshita M. Oculopharyngodistal myopathy: report of four families. *Arch Neurol* 1977;**34**:89–92.

4926. Satoyoshi E, Kowa H. A myopathy due to glycolytic abnormality. *Arch Neurol* 1967;**17**:248–55.

4927. Satoyoshi E, Yamada K. Recurrent muscle pains of central origin. *Arch Neurol* 1967;**16**:254–64.

4928. Satran R. Déjèrine-Sottas disease revisited. *Arch Neurol* 1980;**37**:67–8.

4929. Satya-Murti S, Navada S, Eames F. Central nervous system involvement in blue-rubber-bleb-nevus syndrome. *Arch Neurol* 1986;**43**:1184–6.

4930. Saunders-Pullman R, Shriberg J, Heiman G, et al. Myoclonus dystonia. *Neurology* 2002;**58**:242–5.

4931. Sauvineau J. Un nouveau type de paralysie associé des mouvements horizontal des yeux. *Ann Ocul Paris* 1895;**113**:363–4.

4932. Savage DCL, Forbes M, Pearce GW. Idiopathic rhabdomyolysis. *Arch Dis Child* 1971;**46**:594–607.

4933. Sawayama T, Kurihara T, Araki S. Non-invasive cardiovascular findings in familial amyloid polyneuropathy. *Br Heart J* 1978;**40**:1288–92.

4934. Sawyer RN, Hanna JP, Ruff RL, et al. Asymmetry of forearm rolling as a sign of unilateral cerebral dysfunction. *Neurology* 1993;**43**:1596–8.

4935. Saxton J, Swihart AA. Neuropsychological assessment of the severely impaired elderly patient. *Clin Geriatr Med* 1989;**5**:531–43.

4936. Say B, Meyer J. Familial trigonocephaly associated with short stature and development delay. *Am J Dis Child* 1981;**135**:711–2.

4937. Scaglione C, Salvi F, Riguzzi P, et al. Symptomatic unruptured capillary telangiectasia of the brain stem: report of three cases and a review of the literature. *J Neurol Neurosurg Psychiatry* 2001;**71**:390–3.

4938. Scarfone H, McComas AJ, Pape K, et al. Denervation and reinnervation in congenital brachial palsy. *Muscle Nerve* 1999;**22**:600–7.

4939. Scarrfe R. *J Nerv Ment Dis* 1947;**106**:605–7.

4940. Schady W, Meara RJ. Hereditary progressive chorea without dementia. *J Neurol Neurosurg Psychiatry* 1988;**51**:295–7.

4941. Schady W, Smith CML. Sensory neuropathy in hereditary spastic paraplegia. *J Neurol Neurosurg Psychiatry* 1994;**57**:693–8.

4942. Schaefer M. On an antagonistic reflex. *Neurol Zentralbl* 1899;**18**:1016–8.

4943. Schapira AHV. Inborn and induced defects of mitochondria. *Arch Neurol* 1998;**55**:1293–6.

4944. Scharli AF, Meier-Ruge W. Localized and disseminated forms of neuronal intestinal dysplasia mimicking Hirschsprung's disease. *J Pediatr Surg* 1981;**16**:164–70.

4945. Schaul N, Luders H, Sachdev KK. Generalized bilaterally synchronous bursts of slow waves in the EEG. *Arch Neurol* 1981;**38**:690–2.

4946. Scheffer IE, Lones L, Pozzebon M, et al. Autosomal dominant rolandic epilepsy and speech dyspraxia: a new syndrome with anticipation. *Ann Neurol* 1995;**38**:633–42.

4947. Scheffer IE, Phillips HA, Mulley J, et al. Autosomal dominant partial epilepsy with variable foci is not allelic with autosomal dominant frontal lobe epilepsy. *Epilepsia* 1995;**36**(**Suppl 3**):S28.

4948. Scheffer IE, Phillips HA, O'Brien CE, et al. Familial partial epilepsy with variable foci. *Ann Neurol* 1998;**44**:890–9.

4949. Scheie HG, et al. A new recognized forme fruste of Hurler's disease (gargoylism). *Am J Ophthalmol* 1962;**53**:753–69.

4950. Scheinberg P. Dementia due to vascular disease—a multifactorial disorder. *Stroke* 1988;**19**:1291–9.

4951. Scheinker IM. Subependymoma: a newly-recognized tumor of subependymal origin. *J Neurosurg* 1945;**2**:232–40.

4952. Schelhaas HJ, Ippel PF, Beemer FA, et al. Similarities and differences in the phenotype, genotype and pathogenesis of different spinocerebellar ataxias. *Eur J Neurol* 2000;**7**:309–314.

4953. Schellack J, Fulenwider JT, Olson RA, et al. The carotid sinus syndrome: a frequently overlooked cause of syncope in the elderly. *J Vasc Surg* 1986;**4**:376–83.

4954. Schenck CH, Bundle SR, Mahowald MW. Human REM sleep chronic behaviour disorders; a new category of parasomnia. *Sleep Res* 1985;**14**:208.

4955. Schenck CH, Mahowald MW. REM sleep parasomnias. *Neurol Clin* 1996;**14**:697–718.

4956. Schenck CH, Milner DM, Hurwitz TD, et al. Dissociative disorders presenting as somnambulism: polysomnographic, video and clinical documentation (8 cases). *Dissociation* 1989;**2**:194–204.

4957. Schenkenberg T, Bradford DC, Ajax ET. Line bisection and unilateral visual neglect in patients with neurological impairment. *Neurology* 1980;**30**:509–17.

4958. Schenone A, Mancardi GL. Molecular basis of inherited neuropathies. *Curr Opin Neurol* 1999;**12**:603–16.

4959. Schiff HB, Alexander MP, Naeser MA, et al. Aphemia; clininal–anatomical correlations. *Arch Neurol* 1983;**40**:720–7.

4960. Schiffmann R, Moller JR, Trapp BD, et al. Childhood ataxia with diffuse central nervous system hypomyelination. *Ann Neurol* 1994;**35**:331–40.

4962. Schilder P. Zur Kenntnis der sogenannten diffusen Sklerose (uber Encephalitis periaxialis diffusa). *Z Neurol* 1912;**10**:1–60.

4963. Schilder P. Notes on psychopathology of pain in neuroses and psychoses. *Psych Anal Rev* 1931;**18**:1–22.

4964. Schiller F. The reflex hammer. *Med Hist* 1967;**11**:75–85.

4965. Schiller F. Coenesthesis. *Bull Hist Med* 1984;**58**:496–515.

4966. Schiller F. The inveterate paradox of dreaming. *Arch Neurol* 1985;**42**:903–6.

4967. Schiller F, Wartenberg R. The neurologist. *J Nerv Ment Dis* 1952;**116**:480–7.

4968. Schimke RN, et al. A new X-linked syndrome comprising progressive basal ganglion dysfunction, mental and growth retardation, external ophthalmoplegia, postnatal microcephaly and deafness. *Am J Med Genet* 1984;**17**:323–32.

4969. Schindler RJ, Feinberg TE, Flanagan NG, et al. Two syndromes of the alien hand. *Neurology* 1991;**41(Suppl 1)**:187.

4970. Schinzel A. Post-axial polydactyly, hallux duplication, absence of the corpus callosum, macrocephaly and severe mental retardation: a new syndrome. *Helv Pediatr Acta* 1979;**34**:141–6.

4971. Schinzel A, Hayashi K, Schmid W. Further delineation of the clinical picture of trisomy for the distal segment of chromosome 13. *Hum Genet* 1976;**32**:1–12.

4972. Schlitt M, Dempsey PJ, Robinson RK. Cervical butterfly-block vertebra. A case report. *Clin Imaging* 1989;**13**:167–70.

4973. Schmahmann JD, Sherman JC. The cerebellar cognitive affective syndrome. *Brain* 1996;**121**:561–79.

4974. Schmand B, Lindeboom J, Schagen S, et al. Cognitive complaints after whiplash injury: the impact of malingering. *J Neurol Neurosurg Psychiatry* 1998;**64**:339–43.

4975. Schmidley JW, Levinsohn MW, Maratto V. Infantile X-linked ataxia and deafness. *Neurology* 1987;**37**:1344–9.

4976. Schmidt A. Doppelseitige Accessormslahmung bei Syringomyelie. *Dtsch Med Wochenschr* 1892;**18**:606–8.

4977. Schmidt D. Ocular myasthenia. In Daroff RB, Neetens A, eds. *Neurological Organization of Ocular Movement*, pp. 353–380. Berkeley: Kugler and Ghedini, 1990.

4978. Schmidt D, Dell'Osso LF, Abel LA, et al. Myasthenia gravis: dynamic changes in saccadic wavefor, gain and velocity. *Exp Neurol* 1980; **68**:365.

4979. Schmidt JE. *Medical Discoveries*. Springfield: Charles C. Thomas, 1959.

4980. Schmidt S, Hertfelder H-J, von Speigel T, et al. Lethal capillary leak syndrome after a single administration of interferon beta-1b. *Neurology* 1999;**53**:220–3.

4981. Schmitt HP, Bersch W, Feustel HP. Acute abdominal rhabdomyolysis after body building exercise. *Muscle Nerve* 1983;**6**:228–32.

4982. Schmitt HP, Emser W, Heimes C. Familial occurrence of amyotrophic lateral sclerosis, parkinsonism, and dementia. *Ann Neurol* 1984;**16**:642–8.

4983. Schneider H. On an epidemic of serous meningitis [in German]. *Wien Klin Wochenschr* 1831;**44**:350–2.

4984. Schneider RC, Cherry G, Pantek H. The syndrome of acute central cervical spinal cord injury. *J Neurosurg* 1954;**11**:546–77.

4985. Schnider A, Benson DF, Rosner LJ. Callosal disconnection in multiple sclerosis. *Neurology* 1993;**43**:1243–5.

4986. Schoenberg B, Massey EW. Tapia's syndrome. *Arch Neurol* 1979; **36**:257–60.

4987. Schold SC, Cho E-S, Somasundaram M, et al. Subacute motor neuropathy: a remote effect of lymphoma. *Ann Neurol* 1979;**5**:271–87.

4988. Scholte HR, Jennekens FGI, Bonvy JJBJ. Carnitine palmitoyl transferase II deficiency with normal carnitine palmitoyl transferase I in skeletal muscle and leucocytes. *J Neurol Sci* 1979;**40**:39–51.

4989. Scholtz CL, Swash M. Cerebellar degeneration in dominantly inherited spastic paraplegia. *J Neurol Neurosurg Psychiatry* 1985;**48**:145–9.

4990. Schon F, Blau JN. Post-epileptic headache and migraine. *J Neurol Neurosurg Psychiatry* 1987;**50**:1148–52.

4991. Schondorf R, Low PA. Idiopathic postural orthostatic tachycardia syndrome: an attenuated form of acute pandyautonomia? *Neurology* 1993;**43**:132–7.

4992. Schooler NR, Kane JM. Research diagnoses for tardive dyskinesia. *Arch Gen Psychiatry* 1982;**39**:486–7.

4993. Schott GD. Distant referral of cutaneous sensation. *Exp Neurol* 1973;**1**:451–6.

4994. Schott GD. Some neurological observations on Leonardo da Vinci's handwriting. *J Neurol Sci* 1979;**42**:321–9.

4995. Schott GD. A chronic and painless form of idiopathic brachial plexus neuropathy. *J Neurol Neurosurg Psychiatry* 1983;**46**:555–7.

4996. Schott GD. Mechanisms of causalgia and related clinical conditions: the role of the central and of the sympathetic nervous systems. *Brain* 1986;**109**:717–38.

4997. Schott GD. Reflex sympathetic dystrophy. *J Neurol Neurosurg Psychiatry* 2001;**71**:291–5.

4998. Schott GD, Wills MR. Myopathy in hypophosphatemic osteomalacia presenting in adult life. *J Neurol Neurosurg Psychiatry* 1975;**38**: 297–304.

4999. Schott GD, Wyke MA. Obligatory bimanual associated movements. *J Neurol Sci* 1977;**33**:301–12.

5000. Schrag A, Selai C, Jahanshahi M, et al. The EG-5D—a generic quality of life measure—is a useful instrument to measure quality of life in patients with Parkinson's disease. *J Neurol Neurosurg Psychiatry* 2000;**68**:67–73.

5001. Schreiber MM, McGregor JG. Pseudolymphoma syndrome. A sensitivity to anticonvulsant drugs. *Arch Dermatol* 1968;**97**:297–300.

5002. Schroder JM, Kramer KG, Hopf HC. Granular nuclear inclusion body disease. *Muscle Nerve* 1985;**8**:52–9.

5003. Schroeder AH. Diagnostico del quiste hidatico cerbral y su tratamiento. *An Inst Neurol (Montevideo)* 1941;**3**:11–38.

5004. Schroeder AH, Medoc J. Vertebral hydatidosis. *J Nerv Ment Dis* 1952;**116**:1025–45.

5005. Schubert R, Cracco JB. Familial rectal pain: a type of reflex epilepsy? *Ann Neurol* 1992;**32**:824–6.

5006. Schuell H. *Differential Diagnosis of Aphasia with the Minnesota Test*. Minneapolis: University of Minnesota Press, 1965.

5007. Schuffler M, Pagon RA, Schwartz R, et al. Visceral myopathy of the gastrointestinal and genitourinary tracts in infants. *Gastroenterology* 1988;**94**:892–8.

5008. Schulman LM, David NJ, Weiner WJ. Psychosis as the initial manifestation of adult-onset Niemann-Pick disease. *Neurology* 1995;**45**: 1739–43.

5009. Schulz U, O'Leary CP. Spinal AVM, epidermal nevus and rhabdomyosarcoma: a rare neurocutaneous syndrome? *Neurology* 2001;**56**: 395–7.

5010. Schulz V, Ward D, Moulin DE. Segmental hyperhidrosis as a manifestation of spinal and paraspinal disease. *Can J Neurol Sci* 1998;**25**: 325–7.

5011. Schumacher GA, Beebe G, Kibler RF, et al. Problems of experimental trials of therapy in multiple sclerosis: Report by the Panel on the Evaluation of Experimental Trials of Therapy in Multiple Sclerosis. *Ann NY Acad Sci.* 1965;**122**:552–68.

5012. Schuman JS, Lieberman KV, Friedman AH, et al. Senior-Loken syndrome (familial renal-retinal dystrophy) and Coats' disease. *Am J Ophthalmol* 1985;**100**:822–5.

5013. Schurch B, Wichmann W, Rossier AB. Post-traumatic syringomyelia (cystic myelopathy): a prospective study of 449 patients with spinal cord injury. *J Neurol Neurosurg Psychiatry* 1996;**60**:61–7.

5014. Schurr PH. The Cairns tradition. *J Neurol Neurosurg Psychiatry* 1990;**53**:188–93.

5015. Schut JW, Haymaker W. Hereditary ataxia: a pathologic study of five cases of common ancestry. *J Neuropathol Clin Neurol* 1951;**1**: 183–213.

5016. Schwalbe MW. Eine eigentumliche tonische Krampfform mit hysterischen Symptomen. Berlin: Inaugural dissertation, 1907.

5017. Schwankhaus JD, Parisi J, Gulledge WR, et al. Hereditary adult-onset Alexander's disease with palatal myoclonus, spastic paraparesis and cerebellar ataxia. *Neurology* 1995;**45**:2266–71.

5018. Schwartz AS, Marchok PL, Flynn RE. A sensitive test for tactile extinction: results in patients with parietal and frontal lobe disease. *J Neurol Neurosurg Psychiatry* 1977;**402**:228–33.

5019. Schwartz CE, Vollmer T, Lee H, et al. Reliability and validity of two self-report measures of impairment and disability for MS. *Neurology* 1999;**52**:63–70.

5020. Schwartz E. Craniometaphyseal dysplasia. *AJR Am J Roentgenol* 1960;**84**:461–6.

5021. Schwartz GE. Geriatric evaluation by Relatives Rating Instrument. *Psychol Rep* 1983;**53**:479–88.

5022. Schwartz HG, O'Leary J. Section of the spinothalamic tract in the medulla with observations on the pathway for pain. *Surgery* 1941;**9**:183–93.

5023. Schwartz JT, Brumback RJ, Lakatos M. Acute compartment syndrome of the thigh. *Am J Med Genet* 1999;**85**:147–56.

5024. Schwartz M, et al. Postviral fatigue syndrome or benign postinfection myositis. *BMJ* 1978;**2**:1256.

5025. Schwartz MA, Selhorst JB, Ochs AL, et al. Oculomasticatory myorhythmia: a unique movement disorder occurring in Whipple's disease. *Ann Neurol* 1986;**20**:677–83.

5026. Schwartz MS, Swash M. Scapulo-peroneal atrophy with sensory involvement; Davidenkow's syndrome. *J Neurol Neurosurg Psychiatry* 1975;**38**:1063–7.

5027. Schwartz O, Jampel R. Congenital blepharophimosis associated with a unique generalized myopathy. *Arch Ophthalmol* 1962;**68**:52–7.

5028. Schwartz RA, Tedesco AS, Stern LZ, et al. Myopathy associated with sclerodermal facial hemiatrophy. *Arch Neurol* 1981;**38**:592–4.

5029. Schwartz S, Mohr A, Knauth M, et al. Acute disseminated encephalomyelitis. *Neurology* 2001;**56**:1313–8.

5030. Schwartzman RJ, McLellan TL. Reflex sympathetic dystrophy: a review. *Arch Neurol* 1987;**44**:555–61.

5031. Scoppetta C, Vaccario ML, Casali C, et al. Distal muscle dystrophy with autosomal recessive inheritance. *Muscle Nerve* 1984;**7**:478–81.

5032. Scott CR, Bryant JI: Graham CB. A new craniodigital syndrome with mental retardation. *J Pediatr* 1971;**78**:658–63.

5033. Scott DGI. Classification and treatment of systemic vasculitis. *Br J Rheumatol* 1988;**27**:251.

5034. Scott O, Macartney FJ, Deverall PB. Sick sinus syndrome in children. *Arch Dis Child* 1976;**51**:100–5.

5035. Scott OM, Goddard C, Dubowitz V. Quantitation of muscle function in children: a prospective study in Duchenne muscular dystrophy. *Muscle Nerve* 1982;**5**:291–301.

5036. Scott RM, Brody JA. Benign early-onset Parkinsons disease: a syndrome distinct from classic post-encephalitis Parkinson disease. *Neurology* 1970;**20**:400.

5037. Scott TF. Neurosarcoidosis. *Neurology* 1993;**43**:8–12.

5038. Scott TF, Yager JG, Gross JA. Handcuff neuropathy revisited. *Muscle Nerve* 1989;**12**:219–20.

5039. Scottish Motor Neurone Disease Research Group. The Scottish Motor Neurone Disease Register. *J Neurol Neurosurg Psychiatry* 1992;**55**:536–41.

5040. Scribanu N, Kennedy C. Familial syndrome with dystonia, nerve deafness and possible intellectual impairment. *Adv Neurol* 1976;**14**:235–43.

5041. Scrimgeour EM, Mastaglia FL. Oculopharyngeal and distal myopathy. A case study from Papua New Guinea. *Am J Med Genet* 1984;**17**:763–71.

5042. Scriver CR, Levy HL. Histidinemia 1. *J Inherit Metab Dis* 1983;**6**:51.

5043. Scriver CR, Pueschel S, Davis E. Hyperbetaalaninemia associated with beta aminoaciduria and gamma aminoaciduria. *N Engl J Med* 1966;**174**:636.

5044. Seashore CE, Lewis D, Saetveit DL. *Seashore Measures of Musical Talents.* New York: The Psychological Corporation, 1960.

5045. Sebire G, DeVistor D, Hualt G, et al. Coma associated with intense bursts of abnormal movements and long-lasting cognitive disturbances: an acute encephalopathy of obscure origin. *J Pediatr* 1992;**121**:845–51.

5046. Seckel HPG. *Bird-headed Dwarfs: Studies in Developmental Anthropology Including Human Proportions.* Springfield, IL: C.C. Thomas, 1960.

5047. Seckersen ALG. Neuroscience biographies [unpublished]. 1989.

5048. Seddon HJ. Three types of nerve injury. *Brain* 1943;**66**:237–88.

5049. Seeligmuller O. Ueber spastiche spinale Paralysen bei Kindern. *Amtl Ber Dtsch Naturforsch Aertze* 1877;**50**:299.

5050. Seeligmuller O. On syphilitic neuralgia. *Dtsch Med Wochenschr* 1883;**9**:624–5.

5051. Seemenova E, et al. Familial microcephaly with normal intelligence, immunodeficiency and risk for lymphoreticular malignancies: a new autosomal recessive syndrome. *Am J Med Genet* 1985;**20**:639–48.

5052. Segawa M, Hosaka A, Miyagawa F, et al. Hereditary progressive dystonia with marked diurnal fluctuation. *Adv Neurol* 1976;**14**:215–33.

5053. Seitelberger E. Pelizaeus-Merzbacher disease. In Vincken PJ, Bruyn GW, eds. *Handbook of Clinical Neurology*, pp 150–202. Amsterdam: North Holland Publishing Co., 1990.

5054. Seitelberger F. Eine unbekannte Form von infantiler lipoidspeicher Krankheit des Gehirns. In *Proceedings of the 1st International Congress of Neuropathology (Turin)* 1952;**3**:323–33.

5055. Seitelberger F, Simma A. On the pigment variant of amaurotic idiocy. In Aronson SM, Volk BM, eds. *Cerebral Sphingolipidoses*, pp 29–47. New York: Academic Press, 1962.

5056. Seitz RJ, et al. Congenital Leigh's disease: panencephalomyelopathy and peripheral neuropathy. *Acta Neuropathol* 1984;**64**:167–71.

5057. Selcen D, Stilling G, Engel AG. The earliest pathological alterations in dysferlinopathy. *Neurology* 2001;**56**:1472–81.

5058. Selhorst JB, Hoyt WF, Feinsod M, et al. Midbrain corectopia. *Arch Neurol* 1976;**33**:193–5.

5059. Selhorst JB, Stark L, Ochs A, et al. Disorders of cerebellar oculomotor control: II. Macrosaccadic oscillation. An oculographic control system and clinico-anatomical analysis. *Brain* 1976;**99**:509–22.

5060. Selye H. The general adaptation syndrome and the diseases of adaptation. *J Clin Endocrinol* 1946;**6**:117–230.

5061. Selye H. *The Physiology and Pathology of Exposure to Stress; A Treatise Based on the Concepts of the General-Adaptation Syndrome and the Diseases of Adaptation.* Montreal: Acta, 1950.

5062. Selye H, Gabbiani G, Tuchweber B. Neurotropic calcergy. *Neurology* 1964;**14**:1084–90.

5063. Semon F. On the proclivity of the abductor fibers of the recurrent laryngeal nerve to become affected sooner than the adductor fibers, or even exclusively, in cases of undoubted central or peripheral injury or disease of the roots or trunks of the pneumogastric, spinal accessory, or recurrent nerves. *Arch Laryngol* 1881;**2**:197–222.

5064. Semont A, Freyss G, Vitte E. Curing the BPPV with a liberatory maneuver. *Adv Otorhinolaryngol* 1988;**42**:290–3.

5065. Sencer W. Neurological manifestations of the malabsorption syndrome. *J Mt Sinai Hosp* 1957;**24**:331.

5066. Senelick RC. Ping-pong alternating gaze deviation. *Neurology* 1976;**26**:532–5.

5067. Sen Gupta PC, Sanyal NN, Battacharya B, et al. Avitaminosis in Kala-Azar: preliminary observations. *Indian Med Gaz* 1952;**87**:444.

5068. Serdaru M, Chiras J, Cujas M, et al. Isolated benign vasculitis or migrainous vasospasm? *J Neurol Neurosurg Psychiatry* 1984;**47**:73–6.

5069. Sergent J. A new look at the human split brain. *Brain* 1987;**110**:1375–92.

5070. Sergott RC. Neuro-ophthalmic evaluation of the red orbit syndrome. *Neurol Clin* 1983;**1**:897–908.

5071. Serra S, Millgren SI, Bergsholm R, et al. Amyotrophic choreoacanthocytosis. *Acta Neurol Scand* 1986;**66**:78–82.

5072. Serratrice GT, Azulay J-P, serratrice J, et al. Palmaris brevis spasm syndrome. *J Neurol Neurosurg Psychiatry* 1999;**59**:182–4.

5073. Serratrice GT, Pellissier JF, Cros D, et al. Relapsing eosinophilic perimyositis. *J Rheumatol* 1980;**7**:199–205.

5074. Serratrice GT, Pouget J, Pellissier JF. Bent spine syndrome. *J Neurol Neurosurg Psychiatry* 1996;**60**:51–4.

5075. Serratrice GT, Toga M, Pellissier JF. Chronic spinal muscular atrophy and pallidonigral degeneration: report of a case. *Neurology* 1983;**33**:306–10.

5076. Serratrice J, Gastaut JL, Dubois D. Peripheral neurogenic atrophy in Marinesco-Garland syndrome [in French]. *Rev Neurol (Paris)* 1973;**128**:432–41.

5077. Servidei S, Capon F, Spinazzola M, et al. A distinctive autosomal dominant vacuolar neuromyopathy linked to 19p13. *Neurology* 1999;**53**:830–7.

5078. Servidei S, Zeviani M, Manfredi G, et al. Dominantly inherited mitochondrial myopathy with multiple deletions of mitochondrial DNA: clinical, morphologic, and biochemical studies. *Neurology* 1991;**41**:1053–9.

5079. Sethi KD, Rivner MH, Swift TR. Ice pack test for myasthenia gravis. *Neurology* 1987;**37**:1383–5.

5080. Sethi PK, Rao TS. Gelastic, quiritanian and cursive epilepsy. *J Neurol Neurosurg Psychiatry* 1976;**39**:823–8.

5081. Severinghaus JW, Mitchell RA. Ondine's curse—failure of respiratory center automaticity while awake. *Clin Res* 1962;**10**:122.

5082. Seybold ME. The office Tensilon Test for ocular myasthenia gravis. *Arch Neurol* 1986;**43**:842–3.

5083. Seyffarth H. The reaction to passive straining of joints (bending reflex) in patients with frontal lobe lesions. *Brain* 1953;**76**:457–72.

5084. Seyffarth H, Denny-Brown D. The grasp reflex and the instinctive grasp reaction. *Brain* 1948;**71**:109–83.

5085. Shabtai F, Halbrecht I. Bloom's syndrome, missing Y, hypogonadism and cancer. *Clin Genet* 1980;**18**:93.

5086. Shader RI, Harmantz JS, Salzman C. A new scale for assessment in geriatric populations: Sandoz Clinical Assessment-Geriatric. *J Am Geriatr Soc* 1974;**22**:107–13.

5087. Shakir RA, Al-Din ASN, Araj GF, et al. Clinical categories of neurobrucellosis. *Brain* 1987;**110**:213–23.

5088. Shallice T. Phonological agraphia and the lexical route in writing. *Brain* 1981;**104**:413–29.

5089. Shallice T, Burgess PW. Deficits in strategy application following frontal lobe damage in man. *Brain* 1991;**114**:727–41.

5090. Shallice T, Warrington EK. Word form dyslexia. *Brain* 1980;**103**:99–112.

5091. Shane E, McClane KA, Olarte MR, et al. Hypoparathyroidism and elevated muscle enzymes. *Neurology* 1980;**30**:192–195.

5092. Shapiro AK, Shapiro ES, Young JG. *Gilles de la Tourette Syndrome.* New York: Raven Press, 1988.

5093. Shapiro K, Shulman K. Facial nevi associated with anomalous venous return and hydrocephalus. *J Neurosurg* 1976;**45**:20–5.

5094. Shapiro LJ, et al. Metachromatic leukodystrophy without arylsulfatase A deficiency. *Pediatr Res* 1979;**13**:1179–81.

5095. Shapiro WR, Williams GH, Plum F. Spontaneous recurrent hypothermia accompanying agenesis of the corpus callosum. *Brain* 1969;**92**:423–36.

5096. Sharief MK, Hentges R, Ciardi M. Intrathecal immune response in patients with post-polio syndrome. *N Engl J Med* 1991;**325**:749–55.

5097. Sharp FR, Rando TA, Greenberg SA, et al. Pseudochoreoathetosis. Movements associated with loss of proprioception. *Arch Neurol* 1994;**51**:1103–1109.

5098. Sharpe JA, Hoyt WF, Rosenberg ML. Convergence-evoked nystagmus. *Neurology* 1990;**40**:161–2.

5099. Sharpe JA, Lo AW. Voluntary and visual control of the vestibulo-ocular reflex after cerebral hemidecortication. *Ann Neurol* 1981;**10**:164–72.

5100. Sharpe JA, Rosenberg MA, Hoyt WF, et al. Paralytic pontine exotropia. *Neurology* 1974;**24**:1076–81.

5101. Sharpe JA, Silversides JL, Blair RDG. Familial paralysis of horizontal gaze. *Neurology* 1975;**25**:1035–40.

5102. Shaw C-M, Alvord EC. Cava septi pellucidi et vergae: their normal and pathological states. *Brain* 1969;**92**:213–24.

5103. Shaw EB, et al. Aminopterin-induced fetal malformation. *Am J Dis Child* 1968;**115**:477.

5104. Shaw MDM, Russell JA, Grossart KW. The changing pattern od spinal arachnoiditis. *J Neurol Neurosurg Psychiatry* 1978;**41**:97–107.

5105. Shaw MW, Falls HF, Neil JV. Congenital aniridia. *Am J Hum Genet* 1960;**12**:389.

5106. Shaw PJ, Walls TJ, Newman PK, et al. Hashimoto's encephalopathy: a steroid responsive disorder associated with high antithyroid antibody titers—report of 5 cases. *Neurology* 1991;**41**:228–33.

5107. Shaywitz SE, Shaywitz BA, Schell C, et al. Concurrent and predictive validity of the Yale Children's Inventory: an instrument to assess children with attentional deficits and learning disabilities. *Pediatrics* 1988;**81**:562.

5108. Sheaff HM. Hereditary myokymia. *Arch Neurol Psychiatry* 1952;**68**:236–47.

5109. Sheehan HL. Atypical hypopituitarism. *Proc R Soc Med* 1961;**54**:43–8.

5110. Sheehy MP, Marsden CD. Writer's cramp—a focal dystonia. *Brain* 1982;**105**:461–80.

5111. Sheldon JH. On the natural history of falls in old age. *BMJ* 1960;**2**:1685–90.

5112. Shelley ED, Shelley WB. The fish odor syndrome. *JAMA* 1984;**251**:253–6.

5113. Shelley WB, Livingood CS. Familial multiple nevi flammei. *Arch Dermatol Syph* 1949;**59**:343–5.

5114. Shelton P, Knopman DS. Isolated gait apraxia with bilateral posterior subcortical lesions. *Neurology* 1986;**36(Suppl)**:164.

5115. Sher JH, Rimalovski AB, Athanassiades TJ, et al. Familial centronuclear myopathy: a clinical and pathological study. *Neurol Minneap* 1967;**17**:727–42.

5116. Sheridan MD. *The Developmental Progress of Infants and Young Children. 2*, 1968. London, UK: Ministry of Health.

5117. Sherman L, Goldberg M, Larson FC. The Achilles reflex: a diagnostic test of thyroid function. *Lancet* 1963;**1**:243–5.

5118. Sherrington CS. Decerebrate rigidity, and reflex coordination of movements. *J Physiol* 1898;**22**:319–32.

5119. Sherrington CS. *The Integrative Action of the Nervous System.* New Haven: Yale University Press, 1906.

5120. Sherrington CS. On plastic tonus and proprioceptive reflexes. *Q J Exp Physiol* 1909;**2**:109–56.

5121. Sherrington CS. *The Brain and its Mechanisms.* Cambridge, UK: Cambridge University Press, 1933.

5122. Sherrington CS. *Selected Writings of Sir Charles Sherrington.* Oxford: Oxford University Press, 1979.

5123. Shetan AH, Lawton Smith J, O'Connor P, et al. The phantom optic nerve. *J Clin Neuroophthalmol* 1985;**5**:209–12.

5124. Shevell M. Racial hygiene, active euthanasia, and Julius Hallervorden. *Neurology* 1992;**42**:2214–9.

5125. Shevell M. Familial acephalgic migraines. *Neurology* 1997;**48**:776–7.

5126. Shevell M, Rosenblatt B, Silver K, et al. Congenital inflammatory myopathy. *Neurology* 1990;**40**:1111–4.

5127. Shibasaki H. Electrophysiologic studies of myoclonus. *Muscle Nerve* 1988;**11**:899–907.

5128. Shibasaki H. Electrophysiological studies of myoclonus. *Muscle Nerve* 2000;**23**:321–35.

5129. Shibasaki H, et al. Pigmentary degeneration of the retina in heredodegenerative neurological disease. *Acta Neurol Scand* 1979;**59**:331–42.

5130. Shibasaki H, Yamashita Y, Neshige R, et al. Pathogenesis of somatosensory evoked potentials in progressive myoclonic epilepsy. *Brain* 1985;**108**:225–40.

5131. Shibasaki Y, et al. Linkage of autosomal recessive familial spastic paraplegia with mental impairment and thin corpus callosum to chromosome 15q13–15. *Ann Neurol* 2000;**48**:108–12.

5132. Shields CL, Eagle RC Jr. Pseudo-Schnabel's cavernous degeneration of the optic nerve secondary to intraocular silicone oil. *Arch Ophthalmol* 1989;**107**:714–7.

5133. Shih VE, Efron ML, Moser HW. Hyperornithinemia, hyperammonemia and homocitrullinuria: a new disorder of amino acid metabolism associated with myoclonic seizures and mental retardation. *Am J Dis Child* 1969;**117**:83.

5134. Shilkin KB, Chen BTM, Khoo OT. Rhabdomyolysis caused by hornet venom. *BMJ* 1972;**1**:156.

5135. Shin RK, Galetta SL, Ting TY, et al. Ross syndrome plus. *Neurology* 2000;**55**:1841–6.

5136. Shinar D, Cross CR, Price TR, et al. Screening for depression in stroke patients: the Reliability and Validity of the Center for Epidemiologic Studies Depression Scale. *Stroke* 1986;**17**:241–5.

5137. Shipley WC. *Institute of Living Scale.* Los Angeles: Western Psychological Services, 1946.

5138. Shore JW, McCord CD. Anatomical changes in involutional blepharoptosis. *Am J Ophthalmol* 1984;**98**:21.

5139. Short DW. Tardy median nerve palsy following injury. *Glasgow Med J* 1951;**32**:315.

5140. Shorvon HJ. The depersonalisation syndrome. *Proc R Soc Med* 1946;**39**:779–92.

5141. Shuaib A, Becker WJ. Variants of Guillain-Barré syndrome: Miller Fisher syndrome, facial diplegia and multiple cranial nerve palsies. *Can J Neurol Sci* 1987;**14**:611–6.

5142. Shuaib A, Paasuke RT, Brownell AKW. Central core disease. *Medicine* 1987;**66**:389–96.

5143. Shulman DI, Martinez CR, Bercu BB, et al. Hypothalamic–pituitary dysfunction in primary empty sella syndrome in childhood. *J Pediatr* 1986;**108**:540.

5144. Shulman LE. Diffuse fasciitis with eosinophilia: a new syndrome. *Arthritis Rheum* 1977;**20S:**S205–S215.

5145. Shuman RM, Leech RW, Scott CR. The neuropathology of the nonketotic and ketotic hyperglycinemias: three cases. *Neurology* 1978; **28:**139–46.

5146. Shuman RM, Selednik LJ. Periventricular leukomalacia: a one-year autopsy study. *Arch Neurol* 1980;**37:**231–5.

5147. Shuren J, Geldmacher D, Heilman KM. Nonoptic aphasia. *Neurology* 1993;**43:**1900–7.

5148. Shy GM, Drager GA. A neurological syndrome associated with orthostatic hyotension. *Arch Neurol* 1960;**2:**511–27.

5149. Shy GM, Engel WK, Somers JE, et al. Nemaline myopathy, a new congenital myopathy. *Brain* 1963;**86:**793–810.

5150. Shy GM, et al. A generalized disorder of nervous system, skeletal muscle and heart resembling Refsum's syndrome and Hurler's syndrome. *Am J Med* 1967;**42:**163.

5151. Shy GM, Gonatas NK, Perez M. Two childhood myopathies with abnormal mitochondria: I. megaconial myopathy. II. Pleoconial myopathy. *Brain* 1966;**89:**133–58.

5152. Shy GM, Magee KR. A new congenital non-progressive myopathy. *Brain* 1956;**79:**610–21.

5153. Shy ME, Rowland LP, Smith T, et al. Motor neurone disease and plasma cell dyscrasia. *Neurology* 1986;**36:**1429–32.

5154. Siddall PJ, McClelland J. Non-painful sensory phenomena after spinal cord injury. *J Neurol Neurosurg Psychiatry* 1999;**66:**617–22.

5155. Siemen HW. Siemen syndrome [in German]. *Arch Dermatol Syph* 1926;**152:**372–80.

5156. Silberstein SD. Tension-type headaches. *Headache* 1994;**34:** S2–S7.

5157. Silberstein SD, Lipton RB, Sliwinski M, et al. Classification of daily and near-daily headaches. *Neurology* 1996;**47:**871–5.

5158. Silburn PA, Nicholson GA, Teh BT, et al. Charcot-Marie-Tooth disease and Noonan syndrome with giant proximal nerve hypertrophy. *Neurology* 1998;**50:**1067–73.

5159. Silver JR. Familial spastic paraplegia with amyotrophy of the hands. *Ann Hum Genet* 1966;**30:**69–73.

5160. Silver MM, Gilbert JJ, Stewart S, et al. Morphologic and morphometric analysis of muscle in X-linked myotubular myopathy. *Hum Pathol* 1986;**17:**1167–78.

5161. Silverman FN, et al. Cerebro-costo-mandibular syndrome. *J Pediatr* 1980;**97:**406–16.

5162. Silverman IE, Liu GT, Volpe NJ, et al. The crossed paralyses. *Arch Neurol* 1994;**52:**635–8.

5163. Silverstein A, Siltzbach LE. Muscle involvement in sarcoidosis. *Arch Neurol* 1969;**21:**235–41.

5164. Silvis SE, Paragas PD. Paresthesias, weakness, seizures and hypophosphatemia in patients receiving hyperalimentation. *Gastroenterology* 1972;**62:**513–20.

5165. Sima AAF, Caplan M, D'Amato CJ, et al. Fulminant multiple system atrophy in a young adult presenting as motor neurone disease. *Neurology* 1993;**43:**2031–5.

5166. Simell O, et al. Lysinuria protein intolerance. *Am J Med* 1975; **59:**229.

5167. Simmonds NJ, Hoffbrand BI. Contracturing granulomatous myositis: a separate entity. *J Neurol Neurosurg Psychiatry* 1990;**53:** 998–1000.

5168. Simon DB, Ringel SP, Sufit RL. Clinical spectrum of fascial inflammation. *Muscle Nerve* 1982;**5:**525–37.

5169. Simon F, Slatt BK. Light-induced nystagmus. *Can J Ophthalmol* 1971;**6:**128–32.

5170. Simon LT, Horoupian DS, Dorfman LJ, et al. Polyneuropathy, ophthalmoplegia, leukoencephalopathy, and intestinal pseudo-obstruction: POLIP syndrome. *Ann Neurol* 1990;**28:**349–60.

5171. Simon LT, Ricuarte GA, Forno LS. Chronic idiopathic ataxic neuropathy. *Acta Neuropathol* 1989;**79:**104–7.

5172. Simon RP. Neurosyphilis. *Arch Neurol* 1985;**42:**606–13.

5173. Simone DA, Alreja M, LaMotte RH. Psychophysical studies of the itch sensation and itchy skin ("allokinesis") produced by intracutaneous injection of histamine. *Somatosens Mot Res* 1991;**8:**271–9.

5174. Simons RC. Resolution of the latah paradox. *J Nerv Ment Dis* 1980;**168:**195–206.

5175. Simpson CA. Practical use of the ring finger in sensory conduction for the early carpal tunnel syndrome. *Can J Neurol Sci* 1978;**5:**353.

5176. Simpson DM. Pseudoneurogenic thoracic outlet syndrome. *Muscle Nerve* 1994;**17:**242–4.

5177. Simpson DM, Bender AN, Farraye J, et al. Human immunodeficiency virus wasting syndrome may represent a treatable myopathy. *Neurology* 1990;**40:**535–8.

5178. Simpson DM, Olney RK. Peripheral neuropathies asociated with human immunodeficiency virus infection. In Dyck PJ, ed. *Neurological Clinics; Peripheral Neuropathy*, pp 685–711. Philadelphia: W.B. Saunders, 1992.

5179. Simpson GM, Lee JH, Zoubokb L. A rating scale of tardive dyskinesia. *Psychopharmacol Berlin* 1979;**64:**171–9.

5180. Sinclair DC. Cutaneous sensation and the doctrine of specific energy. *Brain* 1955;**78:**584–614.

5181. Singer HS, Naidu S. Rett syndrome. *Neurology* 2001;**56:**582–5.

5182. Singh A, Jolly SS, Bansal BC. Skeletal fluorosis and its neurological complications. *Lancet* 1961;**1:**197.

5183. Singh B, Jamil A, Al-Shahwah SA, et al. Choroido-cerebral calcification syndrome with retardation. *Neurology* 1993;**43:**2387–9.

5184. Singh H, Sham R. Heredofamilial ataxia with muscle fasciculations. *Br J Cln Pract* 1964;**18:**91–2.

5185. Singh N, Grewal MS, Austin JH. Familial anosmia. *Arch Neurol* 1970;**22:**40–4.

5186. Singh N, Sachdev KK, Susheela AK. Juvenile muscular atrophy localized to arms. *Arch Neurol* 1980;**37:**297–9.

5187. Singh R, Scheffer IE, Crossland K, et al. Generalized epilepsy with febrile seizures plus: a common childhood-onset genetic epilepsy syndrome. *Ann Neurol* 1999;**45:**75–81.

5188. Singleton EB, et al. Peripheral dysostosis. *AJR Am J Roentgenol* 1960;**84:**499–505.

5189. Sinha D, Zemlan FP, Nelson S, et al. A new scale for assessing behavioral agitation in dementia. *Psychiatry Res* 1992;**41:**73–88.

5190. Sinniah D, Lin HP, Loh TG. Inhibitory epilepsy. *Aust NZ J Med* 1979;**9:**448–50.

5191. Sipe JC, Knobler RL, Braheny SL, et al. A neurological rating scale for use in multiple sclerosis. *Neurology* 1984;**34:**1368–72.

5192. Sipila I, Simell O, Rapola J, et al. Gyrate atrophy of the choroid and retina with hyperornithinemia: tubular aggregates and type 2 fiber atrophy in muscle. *Neurology* 1979;**29:**996–1005.

5193. Siqueira EB, Murray KJ. Calcified aneurysm of the vein of Galen. *Neurochirurgia* 1972;**15:**106–12.

5194. Siva A. Vasculitis of the nervous system. *J Neurol* 2001;**248:** 451–68.

5195. Sjaastad O, Apfelbaum R, Caskey W, et al. Chronic paroxysmal hemicrania: the clinical manifestations. *Uppsala J Med Psychiatr* 1980; **31:**27–35.

5196. Sjaastad O, Berstad J, Gjesdahl P, et al. Homocarnosinosis. *Acta Neurol Scand* 1976;**53:**275–90.

5197. Sjaastad O, deSouza CD, Fragoso YD, et al. Cluster headache: on the significance of so-called minibouts. *Cephalalgia* 1988;**8:**285–91.

5198. Sjaastad O, Fredriksen TA, Pfaffenrath V. Cervicogenic headache: diagnostic criteria. *Headache* 1990;**30:**725–6.

5199. Sjaastad O, Saunte C, Salveson R, et al. Shortlasting, unilateral neuralgiform headache attacks with conjunctival injection, tearing, sweating, and rhinorrhea. *Cephalalgia* 1989;**9:**147–56.

5200. Sjaastad O, Spierings ELH. Hemicrania continua: another headache absolutely responsive to indomethacin. *Cephalalgia* 1984;**4:** 65–70.

5201. Sjögren HSC. Zur Kenntnis der Keratoconjunctivitis sicca (Keratitis filiformis bei Hypofunktion der Tranendrusen). *Acta Ophthalmol Kopenhagen* 1933;**2:**151.

5202. Sjögren T, Larsson T. Oligophrenia in combination with congenital ichthyosis and spastic disorders. A clinical and genetic study. *Acta Psychiatr Neurol Suppl* 1957;**113:**1–112.

5203. Skelton AK, Fried RA. Headphone neuralgia. *N Engl J Med* 1995; **333:**1786–7.

5204. Skinner HA. *The Origin of Medical Terms*. Baltimore: Williams and Wilkins, 1949.

5205. Skipper JJ, Barnes GR. Eye movements induced by linear acceleration are modified by visualisation of imaginary targets. *Acta Otolaryngol Suppl* 1989;**468:**289–93.

5206. Skre H. Unusual type of neural muscular atrophy with a possible X-linked inheritance pattern. *Acta Neurol Scand* 1978;**58**:249–60.

5207. Slater E. Diagnosis of hysteria. *BMJ* 1965;**1**:1395–9.

5208. Slater E, Beard AW, Glitheroe E. The schizophrenia-like psychosis of epilepsy. *Br J Psychiatry* 1963;**109**:95–150.

5209. Sluder G. The role of the sphenopalatine (or Meckel's) ganglion in nasal headaches. *NY Med J* 1908;**87**:989–90.

5210. Sly WS, Lang R, Avioli J, et al. Recessive osteopetrosis: new clinical phenotype. *Am J Hum Genet* 1972;**24**:34A.

5211. Sly WS, Quinton BA, McAlister WH, et al. Beta glucuronidase deficiency. *J Pediatr* 1973;**82**:249–57.

5212. Smaje JC, McLellan DL. Depth sense aesthesiometry: an advance in the clinical assessment of sensation of the hands. *J Neurol Neurosurg Psychiatry* 1981;**44**:950–6.

5213. Small RG. Coats' disease and muscular dystrophy. *Trans Am Acad Ophthalmol Otolaryngol* 1968;**72**:225–31.

5214. Smith A. *Symbol Digit Modalities Test Manual*. Los Angeles: Western Psychological Services, 1973.

5215. Smith AB. Unilateral hereditary deafness. *Lancet* 1939;**2**:1172–3.

5216. Smith AJ, Strang LB. An inborn error of metabolism with the urinary excretion of alpha-hydroxy-butyric acid and phenylpyruvic acid. *Arch Dis Child* 1958;**33**:109–13.

5217. Smith BE. Inflammatory sensory polyganglionopathies. In Dyck PJ, ed. *Neurological Clinics: Peripheral Neuropathy*, pp 735–59. Philadelphia: W.B. Saunders, 1992.

5218. Smith CG, Linell EA. Microgyria: a case report. *Neurology* 1959;**9**:689–93.

5219. Smith DB, Sidman R, Hencke J. A reliable method for localizing both depth and superficially generated EEG potentials. *Neurology* 1983;**33**(**Suppl 2**):70.

5220. Smith DP. Diagnostic criteria in dominantly inherited juvenile optic atrophy. *Am J Optom* 1972;**49**:183.

5221. Smith DW. The 18 trisomy and 13 trisomy syndromes. *Birth Defects* 1969;**5**:67–71.

5222. Smith DW. *Recognizable Patterns of Human Malformations*. Philadelphia: W.B. Saunders, 1976.

5223. Smith DW, Lemli L, Opitz JM. Newly recognized syndrome of multiple congenital anomalies. *J Pediatr* 1964;**64**:210–7.

5224. Smith GM, Egbert LD, Markowitz RA, et al. An experimental pain method sensitive to morphine in man: the submaximal effort tourniquet technique. *J Pharmacol Exp Ther* 1966;**154**:324–32.

5225. Smith I, Clayton BE, Wolff OH. New variant of phenylketonuria with progressive neurological illness unresponsive to phenylalanine restriction. *Lancet* 1975;**i**:1108.

5226. Smith IS, Kahn SN, Lacey BW, et al. Chronic demyelinating polyneuropathy associated with benign IgM paraproteinemia. *Brain* 1983;**106**:169.

5227. Smith J. Accessory enteric formations: a classification and nomenclature. *Arch Dis Child* 1960;**35**:87.

5228. Smith J, Zellweger H, Affi AK. Muscular form of glycogenosis type II (Pompe). *Neurology* 1967;**17**:537–49.

5229. Smith JK, Gonda VE, Malamud N. Unusual form of cerebellar ataxia. Combined dentato-rubral and pallido-Luysian degeneration. *Neurology* 1958;**8**:205–9.

5230. Smith JL. Whence pseudotumor cerebri? *J Clin Neuroophthalmol* 1985;**5**:55–6.

5231. Smith JL, Cogan DG. Internuclear ophthalmoplegia—a review of 58 cases. *Arch Ophthalmol* 1959;**61**:687.

5232. Smith JL, David NJ. Internuclear ophthalmoplegia: two new clinical signs. *Neurology* 1964;**14**:307.

5233. Smith JL, David NJ, Klintworth GK. Skew deviation. *Neurology* 1964;**14**:96–105.

5234. Smith JL, Flynn JT, Spiro JT. Monocular vertical oscillations of amblyopia. *J Clin Neuroophthalmol* 1982;**2**:85–91.

5235. Smith LA, Moersch HJ, Love JG. Superior laryngeal neuralgia. *Proc Staff Meet Mayo Clin* 1941;**16**:164–7.

5236. Smith ME, Katz DA, Harris JO, et al. Systemic histiocytosis presenting as multiple sclerosis. *Ann Neurol* 1993;**33**:549–54.

5237. Smith MT, Huntington HW. Inverse cerebellum and occipital encephalocele: a dorsal fusion defect. *Neurology* 1977;**27**:246–51.

5238. Smith NJ, Espir ML, Matthews WB. Familial myoclonus epilepsy with ataxia and added features of Friedreich's ataxia and peroneal muscular atrophy. *Brain* 1978;**101**:461–72.

5239. Smith R, Stern G. Myopathy, osteomalacia and hyperparathyroidism. *Brain* 1967;**90**:593–602.

5240. Smith WT, French JM, Gottsman M, et al. Cerebral complications of Whipple's disease. *Brain* 1965;**88**:137–50.

5241. Smithy DC, Mitchell DA, Peterson GW, et al. Medial brachial fascial compartment syndrome: anatomic basis of neuropathy after transaxillary arteriopathy. *Radiology* 1989;**173**:149–54.

5242. Sneddon IB. Cerebrovascular lesions and livedo reticularis. *Br J Dermatol* 1965;**77**:180–5.

5243. Sneddon W, Mellor CS, Martin JR. Hypertryptophanemia in two mentally subnormal siblings. *N Engl J Med* 1982;**307**:1405.

5244. Snider WD, Simpson DM, Nielsen S, et al. Neurological complications of acquired immunodeficiency syndrome. *Ann Neurol* 1983;**14**:403–18.

5245. Snorrason E. Cranial deformation in the reign of Akhnaton. *Bull Med Hist* 1946;**20**:601–10.

5246. Snyder TM, Little BW, Roman-Campos G, et al. Successful treatment of familial idiopathic lipid storage myopathy with L-carnitine and a modified lipid diet. *Neurology* 1982;**32**:1106–15.

5247. Snyderman SE. Clinical aspects of disorders of the urea cycle. *Pediatrics* 1981;**68**:284–9.

5248. Snyderman SE, et al. Argininemia. *J Pediatr* 1975;**90**:563.

5249. So YT, Olney RK. Acute lumbosacral polyradiculopathy in acquired immunodeficiency syndrome: experience in 23 patients. *Ann Neurol* 1994;**35**:53–8.

5249a. Sobrido M-J, Cholfin JA, Perlman S, et al. SCA8 repeat expansions in ataxia: A controversial association. *Neurology* 2001;**57**:1310–12.

5250. Sobue I, Saito N, Lida M, et al. Juvenile type of distal and segmental muscular atrophy of upper extremities. *Ann Neurol* 1978;**3**:429–32.

5251. Soffer D, Grotsky HW, Rapin I, et al. Cockayne syndrome: unusual neuropathological findings and review of the literature. *Ann Neurol* 1979;**6**:340–8.

5252. Sogg RL, Hoyt WF, Boldrey E. Spastic paretic facial contracture. *Neurology* 1963;**13**:607–12.

5253. Solders G, Andersson T, Borin Y, et al. Electroneurography index: a standardized neurophysiological method to assess peripheral nerve function in patients with polyneuropathy. *Muscle Nerve* 1993;**16**:941–6.

5254. Solomon DH, Barohn RJ, Bazan C, et al. The thalamic ataxia syndrome. *Neurology* 1994;**44**:810–4.

5255. Solomon GE, Hilal SK, Gold AP, Carter S. Natural history of acute hemiplegia in childhood. *Brain* 1970;**93**:107–20.

5256. Solomon S, Karfunkel P, Gugliemo KM. Migraine-cluster headache syndrome. *Headache* 1985;**25**:236–9.

5257. Solomon T, Dung NM, Kneen R, et al. Japanese encephalitis. *J Neurol Neurosurg Psychiatry* 2000;**68**:405–15.

5258. Sommer C, Ringelstein EB, Biniek R, et al. Adult *Toxocara canis* encephalitis. *J Neurol Neurosurg Psychiatry* 1994;**57**:229–31.

5259. Sonninen V, Savontaus M-L. Hereditary multi-infarct dementia. *Eur Neurol* 1987;**27**:209–15.

5260. Sorenson EJ, Sima AAF, Blaivas M, et al. Clinical features of perineuritis. *Muscle Nerve* 1997;**20**:1153–7.

5261. Sotaniemi KA. Slimmer's paralysis—peroneal neuropathy during weight reduction. *J Neurol Neurosurg Psychiatry* 1984;**47**:564–6.

5262. Sotos JF, Dodge PR, Muirhead D, et al. Cerebral giantism in childhood, a report of two cases and a review of the literature. *N Engl J Med* 1964;**271**:109–16.

5263. Souques AA. Congenital absence of the pectoralis major and minor muscles. *Nouv Icon Salpet* 1902;**15**:131–7.

5264. Souques AA. On the interosseous or digital phenomenon in organic hemiplegia. *Bull Soc Med Hop Paris* 1907;**24**:677–8.

5265. Souques AA. Palilalie. *Rev Neurol (Paris)* 1908;**16**:340–2.

5266. Souques AA. Rapport sur les syndromes parkinsoniens. *Rev Neurol (Paris)* 1921;**28**:534–73.

5267. Souques M, Rosanoff-Saloff M. Camptocormia: incurvation of the trunk following trauma of the back and lumbar region; morphological considerations. *Rev Neurol (Paris)* 1914;**28**:937–9.

5268. Spaide RF, Klara PM, Restuccia RD. Spasmus nutans as a presenting sign of arachnoid cyst. *Pediatr Neurosci* 1986;**12:**311–4.

5269. Sparrow SS, Cicchetti DV. Diagnostic uses of the Vineland Adaptive Behavior Scales. *J Pediatr Psychol* 1985;**10:**215–25.

5270. Spector GJ, Druck NS, Gado M. Neurologic manifestations of glomus tumours in the head and neck. *Arch Neurol* 1976;**33:**270–4.

5271. Spencer PS. Guam ALS/parkinsonism-dementia: a long latency neurotoxic disorder caused by "slow toxin(s)" in food? *Can J Neurol Sci* 1987;**14:**347–57.

5272. Spencer PS, Nunen PB, Hugar J, et al. Guam amyotrophic lateral sclerosis–parkinsonism–dementia linked to a plant excitant neurotoxin. *Science* 1987;**237:**517–22.

5273. Spencer SE, Walker FO, Moore SA. Chorea-amyotrophy with chronic hemolytic anemia. *Neurology* 1987;**37:**645–9.

5274. Spens T. History of a case in which there took place a remarkable slowness of the pulse. *Med Commentaries Edinb* 1793;**7:**458–65.

5275. Spetzler RF, Martin NH. A proposed grading system of arteriovenous malformations. *J Neurosurg* 1986;**65:**476–83.

5276. Spiegel EA, Wycic HT, Orchinik C, et al. Thalamic chronotaraxis. *Am J Psychiatry* 1956;**113:**97–105.

5277. Spielman FJ. Post-lumbar puncture headache. *Headache* 1982;**22:**280–3.

5278. Spilker B, Molinek FR Jr, Johnston KA, et al. Quality of life bibliography and indexes. *Med.Care* 1990;**28:**DS1–DS77.

5279. Spillane JD. Familial pes cavus and absent ankle jerks. *Brain* 1940;**63:**275–90.

5280. Spillane JD. *The Doctrine of the Nerves.* Oxford: Oxford Medical Publications, 1981.

5281. Spillane JD, Nathan PW, Kelly RE, Marsden CD. Painful legs and moving toes. *Brain* 1971;**94:**541–56.

5282. Spillane JD, Pallis CA, Jones AM. Developmental abnormalities in the region of the foramen magnum. *Brain* 1957;**80:**11–48.

5283. Spillane JD, Urich H. Trigeminal neuropathy with nasal ulceration; report of two cases and one necropsy. *J Neurol Neurosurg Psychiatry* 1976;**39:**105–13.

5284. Spillane JD, Wells CEC. Isolated trigeminal neuropathy: a report of 16 cases. *Brain* 1959;**82:**391–416.

5285. Spiller WG. Epidural ascending spinal paralysis. *Rev Neurol Psychiatr* 1911;**9:**494–8.

5286. Spiller WG. Akinesia algera. *Arch Neurol Psychiatry* 1933;**30:**842–84.

5287. Spiller WG, Martin E. The treatment of persistent pain of organic origin in the lower part of the body by division of the anterolateral column of the spinal cord. *JAMA* 1912;**58:**1489–90.

5288. Spina-Franca A, Mattosinho-Franca LC. Chagas disease and the nervous system. In Spillane JD, ed. *Tropical Neurology,* pp 397–407. London: Oxford University Press, 1973.

5289. Spinella GM, Sheridan PH. Research initiatives on Machado-Joseph disease: National Institute of Neurological Disorders and Stroke Workshop summary. *Neurology* 1992;**42:**2048–51.

5290. Spira PJ, McLeod JG, Evans WE. A spinocerebellar degeneration with X-linked inheritance. *Brain* 1979;**102:**27–41.

5291. Spire J-P, Maselli RA. Episodic nocturnal wandering: further evidence of an epileptic disorder. *Neurology* 1983;**33**(Suppl 2):215.

5292. Spiro A. Minipolymyoclonus: a neglected sign in childhood spinal muscular atrophy. *Neurology* 1970;**20:**1124–6.

5293. Spiro AJ, Fogelson MH, Goldberg AC. Microcephaly and mental subnormality in chronic progressive spinal muscular atrophy of childhood. *Dev Med Child Neurol* 1967;**9:**594–601.

5294. Spiro AJ, Shy GM, Gonatas NK. Myotubular myopathy. *Arch Neurol* 1966;**14:**1–14.

5296. Spitz MC, Jankovic J, Killian JM, et al. Familial tic disorder, Parkinson disease, motor neurone disease and acanthocytosis. *Neurology* 1985;**35:**366–70.

5297. Spitzer K, Thie A, Caplan LR, Kunze K. The TOPOSCOUT Expert System for Stroke Diagnosis. *Stroke* 1989;**20:**1195–201.

5298. Spitzer WO, Skovron MI, Salmi LR, et al. Scientific monograph of the Quebec Task Force on Whiplash-Associated Disorders. *Spine* 1995;**20**(Suppl):1S–73S.

5299. Spoor TC, Hartel WC. Orbital myositis. *J Clin Neuroophthalmol* 1983;**3:**67–74.

5300. Spreen O, Benton AL. Neurosensory Center Comprehensive Examination for Aphasia. Victoria, B.C., Canada: Neuropsychological Laboratory, Department of Psychology, University of Victoria, 1969.

5301. Spreen O, Benton AL. Neurosensory Center Comprehensive Examination for Aphasia. Victoria, B.C., Canada: Neuropsychological Laboratory, Department of Psychology, University of Victoria, 1977.

5302. Sprenger JW, et al. Cerebrodigital syndrome: a newly recognized formal genesis syndrome in three patients. *Am J Med Genet* 1985;**13:**24.

5303. Sprofkin BE. Cheiralgia paresthetica—Wartenberg's disease. *Neurology* 1954;**4:**857–62.

5304. Spruance SL, Bailey A. Colorado tick fever. A review of 115 laboratory confirmed cases. *Arch Intern Med* 1973;**131:**288–93.

5305. Squire LR. Remote memory as affected by aging. *Neuropsychologia* 1974;**12:**429–35.

5306. Srinivasan R, Rhodes J. The median-ulnar anastomosis (Martin-Gruber) in normal and congenitally abnormal fetuses. *Arch Neurol* 1981;**38:**418–9.

5307. Staal A, Went LW. Juvenile amyotrophic lateral sclerosis–dementia complex in a Dutch family. *Neurol Minneap* 1968;**18:**800–6.

5308. Stacy M, Cardodo F, Jankovic J. Tardive stereotypy and other movement disorders in tardive dyskinesias. *Neurology* 1993;**43:**937–41.

5309. Stacy M, Jankovic J. Tardive tremor. *Mov Disord* 1992;**7:**53–7.

5310. Stahl SM, Layzer RB, Aminoff MJ, et al. Continuous cataplexy in a patient with a midbrain tumor: the limp man syndrome. *Neurology* 1980;**30:**1115–8.

5311. Stalberg E. Macro EMG. *Muscle Nerve* 1983;**6:**619–30.

5312. Stalberg E, Bischoff C, Falck B. Outliers, a way to detect abnormality in quantitative EMG. *Muscle Nerve* 1994;**17:**392–9.

5313. Stalberg E, Chu J, Bril V, et al. Automatic analysis of the EMG interference pattern. *Electroencephalogr Clin Neurophysiol* 1983;**56:**672–81.

5314. Stam J. The tibialis anterior reflex in healthy subjects and in L5 radicular compression. *J Neurol Neurosurg Psychiatry* 1988;**51:**397–402.

5315. Stanley CH. New genetic defects in mitochondrial fatty acid oxidation and carnitine deficiency. *Adv Pediatr* 1987;**34:**59.

5316. Stanton-Hicks M, Janig W, Hassenbrusch S, et al. Reflex sympathetic dystrophy: changing concepts and taxonomy. *Pain* 1995;**63:**127–33.

5317. Stanzac DE, White DE, White JG, et al. Comprehensive Level of Consciousness Scale. *J Neurosurg* 1984;**60:**955–60.

5318. Stapleton SR, Harkness W, Wilking PR, et al. Gliomyosarcoma: an immunohostochemical analysis. *J Neurol Neurosurg Psychiatry* 1992;**55:**728–30.

5319. Stargardt KB. On progressive familial macular degeneration [in German]. *Graefe's Arch Ophthalmol* 1909;**71:**534–51.

5320. Stark P. Etude clinique et genétique d'une famille atteinte d'atrophie musculaire progressive neuronale (amyotrophie de Charcot-Marie). *J Genet Hum* 1958;**7:**1–32.

5321. Starkstein S, Federoff JP, Price TR, et al. Catastrophic reaction after cerebrovascular lesions: frequency, correlates and validation of a scale. *J Psychiatr Clin Neurosci* 1993;**5:**189–94.

5322. Starmark J-E, Stalhammar D, Holmgren E. The Reaction Level Scale (RLS85). Manual and guidelines. *Acta Neurochir* 1988;**91:**12–20.

5323. Starr A, Picton TW, Sininger Y, et al. Auditory neuropathy. *Brain* 1996;**119:**741–53.

5324. Staunton T, Andermann F, Melanson D, et al. Focal macrogyria: a recognizable developmental disorder presenting with intractable focal seizures. *Ann Neurol* 1983;**14:**152A.

5325. Staunton TG. A left-sided hemisensory phenomenon more common in women. *Can J Neurol Sci* 1994;**21**(Suppl 2):S.38.

5326. Staunton TG. Traumatic pudendal neuropathy and the dimple sign. *Can J Neurol Sci* 1994;**21**(Suppl 2):S.63.

5327. Steegman AT, Roberts DJ. The syndrome of the anterior choroidal artery. *JAMA* 1935;**104:**1695–7.

5328. Steele JC, Richardson JC, Olszewski J. Progressive supranuclear palsy. A heterogeneous degeneration involving the brain stem, basal ganglia and cerebellum with vertical gaze and pseudobulbar palsy, nuchal dystonia and dementia. *Arch Neurol* 1964;**10:**333–59.

5329. Steere AC. Lyme disease. *N Engl J Med* 1989;**321:**586–96.

5330. Stein BM, Wolpert SM. Arteriovenous malformations of the brain. 1. Current concepts and treatment. *Arch Neurol* 1980;**37:**1–5.

5331. Steinman GS, Rorke LB, Brown MJ. Infantile neuronal degeneration masquerading as Werdnig-Hoffmann disease. *Ann Neurol* 1980; **8**:317–24.

5332. Stengel E. Loss of spatial orientation, constructional apraxia and Gerstmann's syndrome. *J Ment Sci* 1944;**90**:753.

5333. Stephens FE. Hereditary nerve deafness. *Am J Hum Genet* 1949; **1**:37–51.

5334. Stephens J, Hoover ML, Denst J. On familial ataxia, neural amyotrophy and their association with progressive external ophthalmoplegia. *Brain* 1958;**81**:556–66.

5335. Stephens RE. The biomechanical aspects of injuries in elite ballet dancers. In *La Récherche en Danse*, pp 226–8. Paris: University of Paris, Sorbonne, 1986.

5336. Sterling W. A finger phenomenon like that of Rossolimo or Babinski [in German]. *Rev Neurol (Paris)* 1926;**2**:82–8.

5337. Sterman AB, Schaumberg HH, Asbury AK. The acute sensory neuronopathy syndrome: a distinct clinical entity. *Ann Neurol* 1980;**7**:354–8.

5338. Sterman MB, McGinty DJ, Harper PM, et al. Developmental comparison of sleep EEG power spectral patterns in infants at high and at low risk for sudden death. *Electroencephalogr Clin Neurophysiol* 1982;**53**:166–81.

5339. Stern BJ, Krumholz A, Johns C, et al. Sarcoidosis and its neurological manifestations. *Arch Neurol* 1985;**42**:909–17.

5340. Stern JM. The epilepsy of trisomy 9p. *Neurology* 1996;**47**:821–4.

5341. Stern K. Severe dementia associated with bilateral, symmetrical degeneration of the thalamus. *Brain* 1939;**62**:157–70.

5342. Stern LZ, Hall SW. Tornwaldt's disease. *Neurology* 1972;**22**:1182–5.

5343. Stern MB. The clinical characteristics of Parkinson's disease and parkinsonian syndromes: diagnosis and assessment. In Stern MB, Hurtig HM, eds. *The Comprehensive Management of Parkinson's Disease*, pp 33–41. New York: PMA Publishing Corp., 1988.

5344. Sternbach H. The serotonin syndrome. *Am J Psychiatry* 1991; **148**:705–13.

5345. Sternbach H. The serotonin syndrome. *Neurology* 1998;**51**:276–9.

5346. Sternberg D. High-speed scanning in human memory. *Science* 1966;**153**:652.

5347. Stevanin G, Durr A, David G, et al. Clinical and molecular features of spinocerebellar ataxia type 6. *Neurology* 1997;**49**:1243–6.

5348. Stevens DL, Matthews WB. Cryptogenic drop attacks: an affliction of women. *BMJ* 1973;**1**:439–42.

5349. Stevens H. Jumping Frenchmen of Maine. *Arch Neurol* 1965; **12**:311–4.

5350. Stevenson VL, Hardie RJ. Acanthocytosis and neurological disorders. *J Neurol* 2001;**248**:87–94.

5351. Stewart BM. The hypertrophic neuropathy of acromegaly. *Arch Neurol* 1966;**14**:107–10.

5352. Stewart JD. Diabetic truncal neuropathy: topography of the sensory deficit. *Ann Neurol* 1989;**25**:233–8.

5353. Stewart JD, Low PA, Fealey RD. Distal small fiber neuropathy: results of tests of sweating and autonomic cardiovascular reflexes. *Muscle Nerve* 1992;**15**:661–2.

5354. Stewart JM, Bergstrom L. Familial hand abnormality and sensorineural deafness. *J Pediatr* 1971;**78**:102–10.

5355. Stewart PM, Hensley WJ. Acute polymyopathy. *BMJ* 1981;**283**:1578.

5356. Stewart RM, Turnell G, Ehle A. Familial spastic paraplegia, peroneal neuropathy and crural hypopigmentation: a new neurocutaneous syndrome. *Neurology* 1981;**31**:754–7.

5357. Stewart TG, Holmes G. Symptomatology of cerebellar tumours; a study of forty cases. *Brain* 1904;**27**:522–91.

5358. Stibler H, Blennow G, Kristiannsson B, et al. Carbohydrate-deficient glycoprotein syndrome: clinical expression in adults with a new metabolic disease. *J Neurol Neurosurg Psychiatry* 1994;**57**:552–6.

5359. Stickler GB, et al. Hereditary progressive arthro-ophthalmopathy. *Mayo Clin Proc* 1965;**40**:433–55.

5360. Stickroot FL, Schaeffer RL, Bergo HL. Myasthenia gravis occurring in an infant of a myasthenic mother. *JAMA* 1942;**120**:1207–9.

5361. Stocks P. Facial spasm inherited through four generations. *Biometrika* 1923;**14**:311–5.

5362. Stogbauer F, Young P, Kuhlenbaumer G, et al. Autosomal dominannt burning feet syndrome. *J Neurol Neurosurg Psychiatry* 1999; **67**:78–81.

5363. Stokes W. Observations on some cases of permanently slow pulse. *Q J Med Sci (Dublin)* 1846;**2**:73–85.

5364. Stokke O, et al. Beta-methyl-crotonol-CoA-carboxylase deficiency: new metabolic error in lysine degradation. *Pediatrics* 1972; **49**:726.

5365. Stoll BA, Andrews JT. Radiation-induced peripheral neuropathy. *BMJ* 1966;**1**:834–6.

5366. Stone BW, Wilson B, Wroot A, et al. The assessment of visuospatial neglect after acute stroke. *J Neurol Neurosurg Psychiatry* 1991; **54**:345–50.

5367. Stone SP, Halligan PW, Wilson B, et al. Performance of age-matched controls on a battery of visuo-spatial neglect tests. *J Neurol Neurosurg Psychiatry* 1991;**54**:341–4.

5368. Stopford J. Neuritis produced by a wristlet watch. *Lancet* 1922;**1**:993.

5369. Storch E. On an atypical form of progressive paralysis. *Monatschr Psychiatr Neurol* 1901;**9**:401–34.

5370. Stores G. Dramatic parasomnias. *J R Soc Med* 2001;**94**:173–6.

5371. Storey E, Gardner RJM, Knigyht MA, et al. A new autososmal dominant pure cerebellar ataxia. *Neurology* 2001;**57**:1913–5.

5372. Stormorken H, Sjaastad O, Langslet A, et al. A new syndrome: thrombocytopathia, muscle fatigue, asplenia, miosis, migraine, dyslexia and ichthyosis. *Clin Genet* 1985;**28**:367–74.

5373. Stothers HH. Prosper Ménière. *Ann Otol Rhinol* 1961;**70**:319–37.

5374. Stowens D. Neuroblastoma and related tumors. *Arch Pathol* 1957;**63**:451–9.

5375. Stracciari A, Lorusso S, Pazzaglia P. Transient topographical amnesia. *J Neurol Neurosurg Psychiatry* 1994;**57**:1423–5.

5376. Strachan H. On a form of multiple neuritis prevalent in the West Indies. *Practitioner (Lond)* 1897;**59**:477–84.

5377. Strauss L, Churg J, Zak FG. Cutaneous lesions of allergic granulomatosis: a histiopathologic study. *J Invest Dermatol* 1951;**17**:349–59.

5378. Streib EW. AAEE minimonograph #27: differential diagnosis of myotonic syndromes. *Muscle Nerve* 1987; **10**:603–15.

5379. Streib EW, Sun SF, Yarkowski T. Transient paresis in myotonic syndromes: a simplified electrophysiological approach. *Muscle Nerve* 1982;**5**:719–23.

5380. Strobos RRJ, Torre Edl, Martin JF. Symmetrical calcification of the basal ganglia with familial ataxia and pigmentary macular degeneration. *Brain* 1957;**80**:313–8.

5381. Strominger MB, Mincy EJ, Strominger NL. Bilateral internuclear movements ophthalmoplegia with absence of convergent eye movements—clinicopathologic correlation. *J Clin Neuroophthalmol* 1986; **6**:57.

5382. Strong E, Davila J. The cluneal nerve syndrome. *Indust Med* 1957;**26**:417–29.

5383. Strong MJ. The evidence for ALS as a multisystems disorder of limited phenotypic expression. *Can J Neurol Sci* 2001;**28**:283–98.

5384. Stroop JR. Studies of interference in serial verbal reactions. *J Exp Psychol* 1935;**18**:643.

5385. Strother CM, Sackett JF, Crummy AB, et al. Clinical applications of computerized fluoroscopy; the extracranial carotid arteries. *Radiology* 1980;**136**:781–3.

5386. Strumpell EAGG von. Beitrage zur Pathologie des Ruckenmarks. *Arch Psychiat (Berlin)* 1880;**10**:676–717.

5387. Strumpell EAGG von. On acute encephalitis in children. *Jahrb Kinderheilkd* 1885;**22**:173–8.

5388. Strumpell EAGG von. Uber eine bestimmte Form der primaren kombinierten Systemerkrankungen des Ruckenmarks. *Arch Psychiatr (Berlin)* 1886;**17**:217–38.

5389. Strumpell EAGG von. Ueber primare acute Encephalitis. *Arch Klin Med* 1890;**47**:53–74.

5390. Strumpell EAGG von. On the tibialis phenomenon and muscle synergies in spastic pareses. *Dtsch Z Nervenklinik* 1901;**20**:436–44.

5391. Strupp M, Arbusow V. Acute vestibulopathy. *Curr Opin Neurol* 2001;**14**:11–20.

5392. Stuart JM, Bergstrom L. Familial hand abnormality and sensorineural deafness. *J Pediatr* 1971;**78:**102.

5393. Stübgen J-P. Limb girdle muscular dystrophy; description of a phenotype. *Muscle Nerve* 1994;**17:**1449–55.

5394. Stübgen J-P. Neuromuscular disorders in systemic malignancy and its treatment. *Muscle Nerve* 1995;**18:**636–48.

5395. Stunkard AJ, Grace WJ, Wolfe HG. The night eating syndrome. *Am J Med* 1955;**7:**78–86.

5396. Sturge WA. A case of partial epilepsy apparently due to a lesion of one of the vasomotor centers of the brain. *Clin Soc Trans* 1879; **12:**162.

5397. Sturtevant FM. Zinc deficiency, acrodermatitis enteropathica, optic atrophy, subacute myelo-optic neuropathy and 5, 7–dihalo-8–quinolinols. *Pediatrics* 1980;**65:**610–3.

5398. Sturznegger M, Newell DW, Douville CM, et al. Transcranial and Doppler findings in adolescent stretch syncope. *J Neurol Neurosurg Psychiatry* 1995;**58:**367–70.

5400. Suarez GA, Kelly JJ. The Dropped head syndrome. *Neurology* 1992;**42:**1625–7.

5401. Suarez GA, Opfer-Gehrking TL, Offord KP, et al. The autonomic symptom profile. *Neurology* 1999;**53:**523–8.

5402. Suarez JI, Cohen ML, Larkin J, et al. Acute intermittent porphyria: clinicopathologic correlation. *Neurology* 1997;**48:**1678–83.

5403. Subramony SH, Filla A. Autosomal dominant spinocerebellar ataxias ad infinitum? *Neurology* 2001;**56:**287–9.

5404. Sudeck P. Ueber die acute entzundliche Knochenatrophie. *Arch Klin Chir Berlin* 1900;**62:**147–56.

5405. Sugar HS. The cryptophthalmos–syndactyly syndrome. *Am J Ophthalmol* 1968;**66:**897–9.

5406. Sugarman GI, Katakia M, Menkes JH. See-saw winking in a familial oro-facio-digital syndrome. *Clin Genet* 1971;**2:**248–54.

5407. Sugiura K, Muraoka K, Chishiki T, et al. The Edinburgh-2 Coma Scale; a new scale for assessing impaired consciousness. *Neurosurgery* 1983;**12:**411–5.

5408. Sugiura Y, Aoki T, Sugiyama Y, et al. Temperature-sensitive sodium channelopathy with heat-induced myotonia and cold-induced paralysis. *Neurology* 2000;**54:**2179–81.

5409. Sullivan HC, Kaminski HJ, Maas EF, et al. Lateral deviation of the eyes on forced lid closure in patients with cerebral lesions. *Arch Neurol* 1991;**48:**310–1.

5410. Sullivan JJL, Edgley K, Dehoux E. A survey of multiple sclerosis, Part 1: Perceived cognitive problems and compensatory strategy use. *Can J Rehabil* 1990;**4:**99–105.

5411. Sumi SM, Bird TD, Nochlin D, et al. Familial presenile dementia with psychosis associated with cortical neurofibrillary tangles and degeneration of the amygdala. *Neurology* 1992;**42:**120–7.

5412. Summerskill WHJ. Aguecheek's disease. *Lancet* 1955;**2:**288.

5413. Summerskill WHJ, Molnar GD. Eye signs in hepatic cirrhosis. *N Engl J Med* 1962;**266:**1244.

5414. Summitt RL. Recessive acrocephalosyndactyly with normal intelligence. *Birth Defects* 1969;**5:**35–8.

5415. Sunderland A, Tinson D, Bradley L, et al. Arm function after stroke. *J Neurol Neurosurg Psychiatry* 1989;**52:**1267–72.

5416. Sunderland S. A classification of peripheral nerve injuries producing loss of function. *Brain* 1951;**74:**491–516.

5417. Sunderland T, Hill JL, Lawlor BA, et al. NIMH Dementia Mood Assessment Scale (DMAS). *Psychopharmacol Bull* 1988;**24:**747.

5418. Sung JH, Ramirez-Lassepas M, Mastro AR, et al. An unusual degenerative disorder of neurons associated with a novel intranuclear hyaline inclusion (neuronal intranuclear hyaline inclusion disease). *J Neuropathol Exp Neurol* 1980;**39:**107–30.

5419. Sunohara N, Mano Y, Ando K, et al. Idiopathic dystonia-parkinsonism with marked diurnal fluctuation of symptoms. *Ann Neurol* 1985;**17:**39–45.

5420. Suomalainen A, Majander A, Wallin M, et al. Autosomal dominant progressive external ophthalmoplegia with multiple deletions of mtDNA. *Neurology* 1997;**48:**1244–1253.

5421. Surtees R. Inherited ion channel disorders. *Eur J Pediatr* 2000; **159:**S199–S203.

5422. Susac JO. Susac's syndrome. *Neurology* 1994;**44:**591–3.

5423. Susuki J, Kodama N. Moyamoya disease—a review. *Stroke* 1983;**14:**104–8.

5424. Sutherland JM. Familial spastic paraplegia: its relationship to mental and cardiac abnormalities. *Lancet* 1957;**ii:**169–70.

5425. Sutherland JM, Tyrer JH, Eadie MJ. Atrophie spino-cerebelleuse familiale avec mydriase fixé. *Rev Neurol (Paris)* 1963;**108:**439–42.

5426. Sutherling WW, Hershman LM, Miller JQ, et al. Seizures induced by playing music. *Neurology* 1980;**30:**1001–4.

5427. Sutton GG, Mayer RF. Focal reflex myoclonus. *J Neurol Neurosurg Psychiatry* 1974;**37:**207–17.

5428. Sutton JR. Mountain sickness. *Neurol Clin* 1992;**10:**1015–30.

5429. Sutton T. *Tracts on delirium tremens, on peritonitis, and on some other internal inflammatory infections, and on the gout.* London: Underwood, 1813.

5430. Suzuki J, Takaku A. Cerebrovascular moyamoya disease. *Arch Neurol* 1969;**20:**277–99.

5431. Svien HJ. Jugular foramen syndrome and allied syndromes. *Neurology* 1963;**13:**796–809.

5432. Swaiman K. Hallervorden-Spatz syndrome and brain iron metabolism. *Arch Neurol* 1991;**48:**1285–93.

5433. Swaiman KF, Garg BP, Lockman LA. Sea-blue histiocyte and posterior column dysfunction: a familial disorder. *Neurol Minneap* 1975;**25:**1084–7.

5434. Swan KC. A squint syndrome. *Arch Ophthalmol Berlin* 1947; **37:**149–54.

5435. Swan KC. Syndrome of congenital epiblepharon and inferior oblique insufficiency. *Am J Ophthalmol* 1955;**39:**130–6.

5436. Swanson AG. Congenital insensitivity to pain with anhidrosis. *Arch Neurol* 1963;**8:**299–306.

5437. Swartz MN. The chronic fatigue syndrome—one entity or many? *N Engl J Med* 1988;**319:**1726–7.

5438. Swash M. Acute fatal carcinomatous neuromyopathy. *Arch Neurol* 1974;**30:**324–6.

5439. Swash M. John Hughlings-Jackson: a sesquicentennial tribute. *J Neurol Neurosurg Psychiatry* 1986;**49:**981–5.

5440. Swash M, Fox KP, Davidson AR. Carcinoid myopathy. *Arch Neurol* 1975;**32:**572–4.

5441. Swash M, Heathfield W. Quadriceps myopathy. A variant of the limb girdle dystrophy syndrome. *J Neurol Neurosurg Psychiatry* 1983; **46:**355–7.

5442. Swash M, Schwartz MS. Familial multicore disease with focal loss of cross striations and ophthalmoplegia. *J Neurol Sci* 1981;**52:**1–10.

5443. Swash M, Schwartz MS. *Neuromuscular Diseases.* London: Springer-Verlag, 1988.

5444. Swash M, Schwartz MS, Carter ND, et al. Benign X-linked myopathy with acanthocytes (McLeod syndrome). *Brain* 1983;**106:**717–33.

5445. Swash M, van der Noorts S, Craig JW. Late onset proximal myopathy with diabetes mellitus in 4 sisters. *Neurology* 1970;**20:**694–9.

5446. Swedo SE, Leonard HL, Rapoport JL, et al. A double-blind comparison of clomipramine and desipramine in the treatment of trichotillomania (hair-pulling). *N Engl J Med* 1989;**321:**497–501.

5447. Sweeney CJ, Gilden DH. Ramsay Hunt syndrome. *J Neurol Neurosurg Psychiatry* 2001;**71:**149–54.

5448. Sweet RA, Nimgaonkar VL, Devlin B, et al. Increased familial risk of the psychotic phenotype of Alzheimer disease. *Neurology* 2002; **58:**907–11.

5449. Swift TR, Leschner RT, Gross JA. Arm-diaphragm synkinesis: electrodiagnostic studies of aberrant regeneration of phrenic motor neurons. *Neurology* 1980;**30:**339–44.

5450. Swift TR, Nichols FT. The droopy shoulder syndrome. *Neurology* 1984;**34:**212–5.

5451. Swisher H. Semantic pragmatic syndrome. *Neuropsychologica* 1972;**10:**137.

5452. Sydenham T. *Schedula monitoria de novae febris ingressu.* London: Kettleby, 1636.

5453. Sylvester PE. Some unusual findings in a patient with Friedreich's ataxia. *Arch Dis Child* 1958;**33:**217–21.

5454. Symmans WA, Beresford CH, Bruton D, et al. Cyclic eosinophilic myositis and hyperimmunoglobuinemia E. *Ann Intern Med* 1986;**104:**26–32.

5455. Symonds CP. Otitic hydrocephalus. *Brain* 1931;**54**:55.

5456. Symonds CP. Nocturnal myoclonus. *J Neurol Neurosurg Psychiatry* 1953;**16**:166–71.

5457. Symonds CP. Thomas Willis. *BMJ* 1955;**1**:119–23.

5458. Symonds CP. A particular variety of headache. *Brain* 1956;**79**: 217–32.

5459. Symonds CP. Cough headache. *Brain* 1956;**79**:557–68.

5460. Symonds CP. Excitation and inhibition in epilepsy. *Brain* 1959; **82**:133–46.

5461. Symonds CP. *Studies in Neurology.* London: Oxford University Press, 1970.

5462. Synek VM. Prognostically important EEG coma patterns in diffuse anoxic and traumatic encephalopathies in adults. *J Clin Neurophysiol* 1988;**5**:161–74.

5463. Taaka K, Kean EA, Johnson B. Jamaican vomiting sickness: biochemical investigation of two cases. *N Engl J Med* 1976;**295**:461–7.

5464. Tabuenca JM. Toxic–allergic syndrome caused by ingestion of rapeseed oil denatured with aniline. *Lancet* 1981;**2**:567.

5465. Tada K, Wada Y, Arakawa T. Hypervalinemia. *Am J Dis Child* 1967;**113**:64.

5466. Tagawa A, Ono S, Shibata M, et al. A new neurological entity manifesting as involuntary movements and dysarthria with possible abnormal copper metabolism. *J Neurol Neurosurg Psychiatry* 2001;**71**: 780–3.

5467. Tahmoush AJ, Alopnso RJ, Tarmoush GP. Cramp-fasciculation syndrome: a treatable hyperexcitable peripheral nerve disorder. *Neurology* 1991;**41**:1021–4.

5468. Tahmoush AJ, Alpers DH, Feigin RD, et al. Hartnup disease. *Arch Neurol* 1976;**33**:797–807.

5469. Takahashi H, Nakamura H, Okada E. Hereditary amyotrophic lateral sclerosis, histochemical and electron microscopic study of hyaline inclusions in motor neurones. *Arch Neurol* 1972;**27**:292–9.

5470. Takahashi H, Ohama E, Naito H, et al. Hereditary dentatorubral-pallidoluysian atrophy. *Neurology* 1988;**38**:1065–70.

5471. Takahata N, Ito K, Yoshimura Y, et al. Familial chorea and myoclonus epilepsy. *Neurol Minneap* 1978;**28**:913–9.

5472. Takamori M, Gutmann L, Crosby TW, et al. Myasthenic syndrome with hypothyroidism. *Arch Neurol* 1972;**26**:326–35.

5473. Takayasu MA. A Case with peculiar changes in the central retinal vessels. *Am J Med* 1962;**32**:379.

5473a. Takeuchi M. Occlusive disease of the carotid artery. *Rec Adv Res Nervous System* 1961;**60**:121–22.

5474. Talks SJ, Elston JS. Oculopalatal myoclonus; eye movement studies. *Eye* 1997;**11**:19–24.

5475. Tallaksen CME, Dürr A, Brice A. Recent advances in hereditary spastic paraplegia. *Curr Opin Neurol* 2001;**14**:457–63.

5476. Talma S. On acquired myotonia [in German]. *Dtsch Z Nervenklinik* 1892;**2**:210–6.

5477. Talwar D, Smith SA. CAMFAK syndrome: a demyelinating disease similar to Cockayne's syndrome. *Am J Med Genet* 1989;**34**:194–8.

5478. Tan E-K, Jankovic J. Tardive and idiopathic oromandiblar dystonia: a clinical comparison. *J Neurol Neurosurg Psychiatry* 2000;**68**: 186–90.

5479. Tan EM, Cohen AS, Fines JF, et al. The 1982 revised criteria for the diagnosis of systemic lupus erythematosus. *Arthritis Rheum* 1982; **25**:1271–7.

5480. Tan N, Urich H. Postictal cerebral hemiatrophy: with a contribution to the problem of crossed cerebellar atrophy. *Acta Neuropathol* 1984;**62**:332–9.

5481. Tanaka K, Shimazu S, Oya N, et al. Muscular form of glycogenosis type II (Pompe's disease). *Pediatrics* 1979;**63**:124.

5482. Tanaka Y, Albert ML, Hara H, et al. Forced hyperphasia and environmental dependency syndrome. *J Neurol Neurosurg Psychiatry* 2000;**68**:224–6.

5483. Tandan R, Bradley WG. Amyotrophic lateral sclerosis: Part 1. Clinical features, pathology, and ethical issues in management. *Ann Neurol* 1985;**18**:271–80.

5484. Tandan R, Taylor R, Adesina A, et al. Benign autosomal dominant syndrome of neuronal Charcot-Marie-Tooth disease, ptosis, parkinsonism and dementia. *Neurology* 1990;**40**:773–9.

5485. Tandon PN, Bajpai BC. The Infantile tremor syndrome. In Spillane JD, ed. *Tropical Neurology*, pp 114–9. London: Oxford University Press, 1973.

5486. Tandon PN, Pathak SN. Tuberculosis of the CNS. In Spillane JD, ed. *Tropical Neurology*, pp 37–62. London: Oxford University Press, 1973.

5487. Tani T, Yamamoto H, Kimura J. Cervical spondylotic myelopathy in elderly people: a high incidence of conduction block at C3–4 or C4–5. *J Neurol Neurosurg Psychiatry* 1999;**66**:456–64.

5488. Taori GM, Iyer GV. Neurological complications in tropical sprue. In Spillane JD, ed. *Tropical Neurology*, pp 73–7. London: Oxford University Press, 1973.

5489. Taphoorn MJB, Tulleken CAF, Jansen GH, et al. A "soap-bubble" tumour in the brain: isolated cerebral immunocytoma. *J Neurol Neurosurg Psychiatry* 1998;**65**:217.

5490. Tapia Garcia A. Un caso de paralisis del lado derecho de la laringe y de la lengua, con paralisis del esterno-cleido-mastoidea y trapecio del mismo lado; accompanado de hemiplejia total temporal del lado izquierdo del cuerpo. *Siglo Med Madrid* 1905;**52**:211–3.

5491. Tarlov IM. Cysts (perineurial) of the sacral roots. Another cause (removable) of sciatic pain. *JAMA* 1948;**138**:740–4.

5492. Tarui S, et al. Typical form of glycogenosis type 7 (Tarui's disease) due to phosphofructokinase deficiency, lack of M subunit. *Biochem Biophys Res Commun* 1965;**19**:571.

5493. Tarui S, Kono N, Kuwajima M, et al. Type VII glycogenoses. *Monogr Hum Genet* 1978;**9**:42–7.

5494. Tashiro K. Reversed Chaddock method: a new method to elicit the upgoing great toe. *J Neurol Neurosurg Psychiatry* 1986;**49**:1321.

5495. Tassinari CA, Bureau M. Epilepsy with myoclonic absences. In Roger J, Bureau M, eds. *Epileptic Syndromes in Infancy, Childhood and Adolescence*, London: Eurotext, 1985.

5496. Tassinari CA, Michelucci R, Genton P, et al. Dyssynergia cerebellaris myoclonica (Ramsay Hunt syndrome): a condition unrelated to mitochondrial encephalomyopathies. *J Neurol Neurosurg Psychiatry* 1989;**52**:262–5.

5497. Tatemichi TK, Desmond DW, Prohovnik I, et al. Confusion and memory loss from capsular genu infarction. *Neurology* 1992;**42**: 1966–79.

5498. Tatum WO, Coker SB, Ghobrial M, Adb-Allah S. The open opercular sign: diagnosis and significance. *Ann Neurol* 1989;**25**:196–9.

5499. Tawil R, Figlwwicz DA, Griggs RC, et al. Facioscapulohumeral dystrophy: a distinct regional myopathy with a novel molecular pathogenesis. *Ann Neurol* 1998;**43**:279–82.

5500. Tawil R, Ptacek LJ, Pavlakis SG, et al. Andersen's syndrome: potassium sensitive periodic paralysis, ventricular ectopy, and dysmorphic features. *Ann Neurol* 1994;**35**:326–30.

5501. Tay CH. Ichthyosiform erythroderma, hair shaft abnormalities and mental and growth retardation. *Arch Dermatol* 1971;**104**:4–13.

5502. Tay CH, Tan YT, Cheah JS, et al. Ocular palsies of obscure origin in South East Asia. *J Neurol Neurosurg Psychiatry* 1974;**37**:739–44.

5503. Tay W. Symmetrical changes in the region of the yellow spot in each eye of an infant. *Trans Ophthalmol Soc UK* 1880;**1**:55–7.

5504. Taybi H. Generalized skeletal dysplasia with multiple anomalies. *AJR Am J Roentgenol* 1962;**88**:450.

5505. Taylor D, Falconer M, Bruton C, et al. Focal dysplasia of the cerebral cortex in epilepsy. *J Neurol Neurosurg Psychiatry* 1971;**34**: 369–87.

5506. Taylor D, Lewis S. Delirium. *J Neurol Neurosurg Psychiatry* 1993; **56**:742–51.

5507. Taylor DA, Carroll JE, Smith ME, et al. Facioscapulohumeral dystrophy associated with hearing loss and Coats' syndrome. *Ann Neurol* 1982;**12**:395–8.

5508. Taylor DC. One hundred years of epilepsy surgery: Sir Victor Horsley's contribution. *J Neurol Neurosurg Psychiatry* 1986;**49**:485–8.

5509. Taylor DC, Marsh SM. Hughlings Jackson's Dr. Z. The paradigm of temporal lobe epilepsy. *J Neurol Neurosurg Psychiatry* 1980;**43**: 758–67.

5510. Taylor HA, Thomas GH, Miller CS, et al. Mucolipidosis III (pseudo-Hurler polydystrophy). Cytological and ultrastructural observations in cultural fibroblast cells. *Clin Genet* 1973;**4**:388–97.

5511. Taylor J. The ophthalmological observations of Hughlings Jackson and their bearing on nervous and other diseases. *Brain* 1915;**38**: 391–417.

5512. Taylor KL, Sandberg E, Baum KF. Medial medullary syndrome and meningovascular syphilis. *Neurology* 1994;**44**:2231–5.

5513. Taylor RA. Heredofamilial mononeuritis multiplex with brachial predilection. *Brain* 1960;**83**:113–37.

5514. Taylor W. The hand-arm vibration syndrome. *J R Soc Med* 1993; **86**:101–4.

5515. Teasedale G, Jennett B. Assessment of coma and impaired consciousness. A practical scale. *Lancet* 1974;**2**:81–4.

5516. Tein I, De Vivo DC, Hale DE, et al. Short-chain L-3–hydroxy-acyl-CoA dehydrogenase deficiency in muscle: a new cause for recurrent myoglobinuria and encephalopathy. *Ann Neurol* 1991;**30**:415–9.

5517. Teitelbaum JS, Zatorre RJ, Carpenter S, et al. Neurologic sequelae of domoic acid intoxication due to the ingestion of contaminated mussels. *N Engl J Med* 1990;**322**:1781–7.

5518. Telerman-Toppet N, Khoubesserian P, Bacq M, et al. Unclassified familial myopathy resembling Steinert disease, without myotonia. *Muscle Nerve* 1984;**7**:439–41.

5519. Telfer MA, et al. Dominant piebald trait (white forelock and leucoderma) with neurological impairment. *Am J Hum Genet* 1971;**23**: 383–9.

5520. Temkin O. Gall and the phrenological movement. *Bull Med Hist* 1947;**21**:275–321.

5521. Temtamy SA. Hand malformations. *J Pediatr* 1974;**85**:345–9.

5522. Temtamy SA, McKusick VA. Synopsis of hand malformations with particular emphasis on genetic factors. *Birth Defects* 1969;**V**: 125–84.

5523. Tenconi R, et al. Chorio-retinal dysplasia, microcephaly, and mental retardation. An autosomal dominant syndrome. *Clin Genet* 1981;**20**:347–51.

5524. Teng EL, Chui HC. The modified Mini-Mental State (3MS) Examination. *J Clin Psychiatry* 1987;**48**:314–8.

5525. Terrence CF, Rao GR, Pepper JA. Neurogenic pulmonary edema in unexpected, unexplained death of epileptic patients. *Ann Neurol* 1980;**9**:458–64.

5526. Terson A. An unusual ophthalmoscopic sign [in French]. *Ann Ocul* 1912;**147**:410–7.

5527. Terwindt GM, Hann J, Ophoff RA, et al. Clinical and genetic analysis of a large Dutch family with autosomal dominant vascular retinopathy, migraine and Raynaud's phenomenon. *Brain* 1998;**121**: 303–16.

5528. Tessitore E, Tessitore A. Tolosa-Hunt syndrome preceded by facial palsy. *Headache* 2000;**40**:393–6.

5529. The Multi-Society Task Force on PVS. Medical aspects of the persistent vegetative state (2). *N Engl J Med* 1994;**330**:1572–9.

5530. The Quality Standards Subcommittee of the American Academy of Neurology. Practice parameters for determining brain death in adults (summary statement). *Neurology* 1995;**45**:1012–4.

5531. Theodorakis GN, Markianos M, Livanis EG, et al. Central serotonergic responsiveness in neurocardiogenic syncope: a clomipramine test challenge. *Circulation* 1998;**98**:2724–30.

5532. Theodore WH, Porter RJ, Penryk JK. Complex partial seizures: clinical characteristics and differential diagnosis. *Neurology* 1983;**33**: 1115–21.

5533. Theunissen EJJM, Huygen PLM, Verhagen WIM. Familial vestibulocerebellar dysfunction: a new syndrome? *J Neurol Sci* 1989;**89**: 149–55.

5534. Thévenard A. L'acropathie ulcéro-mutilante familiale. *Rev Neurol* 1942;**74**:193–212.

5535. Thiebaut F. Spastic paraplegia and tendinous xanthomata with CSF cholesterinosis [in French]. *Rev Neurol (Paris)* 1942;**74**:313–5.

5536. Thomas A. Atrophie lamellaire des cellules de Purkinje. *Rev Neurol (Paris)* 1905;**13**:917–24.

5537. Thomas HL. *Hunterian Oration*. London: Royal College of Surgeons, 1827.

5538. Thomas JE, Howard FM. Herpes zoster. *Neurology* 1972;**22**: 459–66.

5539. Thomas JE, Klass DW. 6 Hz spike and wave pattern. *Electroencephalogr Clin Neurophysiol* 1968;**23**:591.

5540. Thomas JE, Schirger A. Idiopathic orthostatic hypotension. *Arch Neurol* 1970;**22**:289–93.

5541. Thomas JE, Schirger A, Fealey RD, et al. Orthostatic hypotension. *Mayo Clin Proc* 1981;**56**:117–25.

5542. Thomas P, Beaumanoir A, Genton P, et al. "De novo" absence status of late onset: report of 11 cases. *Neurology* 1992;**42**:104–10.

5543. Thomas PK. Tropical neuropathies. *J Neurol* 1997;**244**:475–82.

5544. Thomas PK, Calne DB, Elliott CF. X-linked scapulo-peroneal syndrome. *J Neurol Neurosurg Psychiatry* 1972;**35**:208–15.

5545. Thomas PK, Claus D, Jaspert A, et al. Focal upper limb demyelinating neuropathy. *Brain* 1996;**119**:765–74.

5546. Thomas PK, Claus D, King RHM. Autosomal recessive type II hereditary motor and sensory neuropathy with acrodystrophy. *J Neurol* 1999;**246**:107–12.

5547. Thomas PK, Kalaydjieva L, Youl B, et al. Hereditary motor and sensory neuropathy-Russe. *Ann Neurol* 2001;**50**:452–7.

5548. Thomas PK, Ormerod IEC. Hereditary neuralgic amyotrophy associated with a relapsing multifocal sensory neuropathy. *J Neurol Neurosurg Psychiatry* 1993;**56**:107–9.

5549. Thomas PK, Schaumberg HH, Spencer PS, et al. Central-distal axonopathy syndromes: newly recognized models of naturally occurring human degenerative disease. *Ann Neurol* 1984;**15**:313–5.

5550. Thomas PK, Schott GD, Morgan-Hughes JA. Adult-onset scapulo-peroneal myopathy. *J Neurol Neurosurg Psychiatry* 1975;**38**: 1008–15.

5551. Thomas PK, Walker JG. Xanthomatous neuropathy in primary biliary cirrhosis. *Brain* 1965;**88**:1079.

5552. Thomas PK, Walker RWH, Rudge P, et al. Chronic demyelinating peripheral neuropathy associated with multifocal central nervous system demyelination. *Brain* 1987;**110**:53–76.

5553. Thomas PK, Workman JM, Thage O. Behr's syndrome. A family exhibiting pseudodominant inheritance. *J Neurol Sci* 1984;**64**: 137–48.

5554. Thomas PK, Young E, King RHM. Sandhoff disease mimicking adult-onset bulbospinal neuronopathy. *J Neurol Neurosurg Psychiatry* 1989;**52**:1103–6.

5555. Thomas PS, Carson NAJ. Homocystinuria; the evolution of skeletal changes in relation to treatment. *Ann Radiol* 1978;**21**:95–104.

5556. Thomas SV. Neurological aspects of eclampsia. *J Neurol Sci* 1998;**155**:37–43.

5557. Thomasen E. Myotonia, Thomsen's disease (Myotonia Congenita?), Paramyotonia and Dystrophia Myotonica. Danmark: Universitetforlaget i Aarhus, 1992.

5558. Thomashevsky AJ, Horwitz SJ, Feingold MH. Acute autonomic neuropathy. *Neurology* 1972;**22**:251–5.

5559. Thomke F, Hopf HC. Pontine lesions mimicking acute peripheral vestibulopathy. *J Neurol Neurosurg Psychiatry* 1999;**66**:340–9.

5560. Thompson AJ, Kermode AG, Wicks D, et al. Major differences in the dynamics of primary and secondary multiple sclerosis. *Ann Neurol* 1991;**29**:53–62.

5561. Thompson AJ, Montalban X, Barkhof F, et al. Diagnostic criteria for primary progressive multiple sclerosis: a position paper. *Ann Neurol* 2000;**47**:831–5.

5562. Thompson BM, Corbett JJ, Kline LB, et al. Pseudo-Horner's syndrome. *Arch Neurol* 1982;**39**:108–11.

5563. Thompson CE. Infantile myositis. *Dev Med Child Neurol* 1982; **24**:307–13.

5564. Thompson HC. Associated movements in hemiplegia: their origin and physiological significance. *Brain* 1903;**26**:514–23.

5565. Thompson HS. Binasal field loss. In Thompson HS, ed. *Neuro-Ophthalmology*, pp 82–5. Baltimore: Williams and Wilkins, 1979.

5566. Thompson HS, Zackon DH, Czarnecki JSC. Tadpole-shaped pupils caused by segmental spasm of the iris dilator muscle. *Am J Ophthalmol* 1983;**96**:467.

5567. Thompson P, Obeso JA, Delgado G, et al. Focal dystonia of the jaw and the differential diagnosis of unilateral jaw and masticatory spasm. *J Neurol Neurosurg Psychiatry* 1986;**49**:651–6.

5568. Thompson PN, Carroll WM. Hemimasticatory spasm—a peripheral paroxysmal cranial neuropathy? *J Neurol Neurosurg Psychiatry* 1983;**46**:274–6.

5569. Thomsen J. Tonische Krampfe in willkurlich beweglichen Muskeln in Folge von ererbter psychischer Disposition (Ataxia muscularis?). *Arch Psychiatr (Berlin)* 1875;**6**:706–18.

5570. Thomson MS. Poikiloderma congenitale. *Br J Dermatol* 1936;**48**: 221–34.

5571. Thrush DC. Congenital insensitivity to pain. *Brain* 1973;**96:** 369–86.

5572. Thrush DC, Holt H, Bradley WG, et al. Neurological manifestations of xeroderma pigmentosum in two siblings. *J Neurol Sci* 1974;**22:** 91–104.

5573. Thrush DC, Morris CJ, Salmon MV. Paramyotonia congenita: a clinical, histochemical and pathological study. *Brain* 1972;**95:**537–52.

5574. Thudichum JLW. *A Treatise on the Chemical Constitution of the Brain.* London: Bailliere, Tindall and Cox, 1884.

5575. Thurston SE, Leigh RJ, Crawford T, et al. Two distinct deficits of visual tracking caused by unilateral lesions of cerebral cortex in humans. *Ann Neurol* 1988;**23:**266–73.

5576. Thuy LF, et al. Multiple carboxylase deficiency due to deficiency of biotinidase. *J Neurogenet* 1986;**3:**357–63.

5577. Thyagarajan D, Bressman S, Bruno C, et al. A novel mitochondrial 12SrRNA point mutation in parkinsonism, deafness and neuropathy. *Ann Neurol* 2000;**48:**730–6.

5578. Thyagarajan D, Shanske S, Vazquez-Memiji M, et al. A novel mitochondrial ATPase 6 point mutation in familial bilateral striatal necrosis. *Ann Neurol* 1995;**38:**468–72.

5579. Tibbetts RW. Spasmodic torticollis. *J Psychosom Res* 1971;**15:** 461–9.

5580. Tibbles JAR, Cohen MM Jr. The proteus syndrome; the Elephant Man diagnosed. *BMJ* 1986;**293:**683.

5581. Tiberin P, Beller AJ. Observations on so-called brain stones or cerebral calculi. *Neurology* 1963;**13:**464–76.

5582. Tien R, Arieff AI, Kucharczyk W, et al. Hyponatremic encephalopathy: is central pontine myelinolysis a component? *Am J Med* 1992;**92:**513–22.

5583. Tietz W. A syndrome of dominant deaf-mutism associated with albinism showing dominant autosomal inheritance. *Am J Hum Genet* 1963;**15:**259–64.

5584. Tijssen CC, van Gisbergen JAM, Schulte BPM. Conjugate eye deviation: side, site, and size of hemispheric lesion. *Neurology* 1991;**41:** 846–50.

5585. Tijssen MAJ, Brown P, Morris HR, et al. Late-onset startle induced tics. *J Neurol Neurosurg Psychiatry* 1999;**67:**782–4.

5586. Tiliket C, Ventre-Dominey J, Vighetto A, et al. Room tilt illusion. *Arch Neurol* 1996;**53:**1259–64.

5587. Tilikete C, Vial C, Niederlaender M, et al. Idiopathic ocular neuromyotonia: a neurovascular compression syndrome? *J Neurol Neurosurg Psychiatry* 2000;**69:**642–4.

5588. Tim RW, Sanders DB. Repetitive nerve stimulation studies in the Lambert-Eaton myasthenic syndrome. *Muscle Nerve* 1994;**17:** 995–1001.

5589. Tindall RSA, et al. Preliminary results of a trial of cyclosporine in myasthenia gravis. *N Engl J Med* 1987;**316:**719–24.

5590. Tinel J. *Les Blessures des Nerfs.* Paris: Masson, 1916.

5591. Tinetti ME, Williams TF, Mayewski R. Fall risk index for elderly patients based on number of chronic disabilities. *Am J Med* 1986;**80:** 429–34.

5591a. Tintoré M, Rovira A, Martinez M. et al. Isolated demyelinating syndromes; comparison of different MR imaging criteria to predict conversion to clinically definite multiple sclerosis. *Am J Neuroradiol* 2000;**21:**702–6.

5592. Tinuper P, Montagna P, Cortelli P, et al. Idiopathic recurring stupor: a case with possible involvement of the gamma-aminobutyric acid. *Ann Neurol* 1992;**31:**503–6.

5593. Tinuper P, Montagna P, Plazzi G, et al. Idiopathic recurring stupor. *Neurology* 1994;**44:**621–5.

5594. Tipton RE, Gorlin RJ. Growth retardation, alopecia, pseudoanodontia, and optic atrophy—The GAPO syndrome: report of a patient and review of the literature. *Am J Med Genet* 1984;**19:**209–16.

5595. Toda T, Yoshioka M, Nakahori Y, et al. Genetic identity of Fukayama-type congenital muscular dystrophy and Walker-Warburg syndrome. *Ann Neurol* 1995;**37:**99–101.

5596. Todd J. The syndrome of Alice in Wonderland. *CMAJ* 1955;**73:** 701–4.

5597. Todd RB. *Clinical Lectures on Paralysis, Certain Diseases of the Brain.* London: Churchill, 1856.

5598. Tollner U, et al. Hepta-octatarso-dactyly combined with multiple malformations. *Eur J Pediatr* 1981;**136:**207–10.

5599. Tolone S. La sindroma alterna parabulbar laterale. *J Nerv Ment Dis* 1952;**116:**1017–22.

5600. Tolosa ES. Periarteritic lesions of the cavernous syphon with clinical features of a carotid infraclinoid syndrome. *J Neurol Neurosurg Psychiatry* 1954;**17:**300–2.

5601. Tolosa ES. Clinical features of Meige's disease (idiopathic orofacial dystonia). *Arch Neurol* 1981;**38:**147–51.

5602. Toma S, Shiozawa Z. Amyotrophic cervical myelopathy in adolescence. *J Neurol Neurosurg Psychiatry* 1995;**58:**56–64.

5603. Tomasulo RA. Aberrant conduction in human nerve: ephaptic transmission? *Neurology* 1982;**32:**712–9.

5603a. Tome FM, Fardeau M. Hereditary inclusion body myopathies. *Curr Opin Neurol* 1998;**11:**453–9.

5604. Tomsak RL, et al. Bilateral central scotomas. In Smith JL, ed. *Neuro-Ophthalmology Focus,* New York: Manor, 1982.

5605. Tondeur M, Ubert J, Vamos E, et al. Infantile form of sialic acid storage disorder. *Eur J Pediatr* 1982;**139:**142–7.

5606. Toole JF, Weeks FD. Stimulation of the carotid sinus in man. *Am J Med* 1959;**27:**952.

5607. Topcu M, Gartioux C, Ribierre P, et al. Vacuoliting megalencephalic leukoencephalopathy with subcortical cysts, mapped to chromosome 22qtel. *Am J Hum Genet* 2000;**66:**733–9.

5608. Torack RM. Historical aspects of normal and abnormal brain fluids. 1. Cerebrospinal fluid. *Arch Neurol* 1982;**39:**197–201.

5609. Torack RM. Historical aspects of normal and abnormal brain fluids. 2. Hydrocehalus. *Arch Neurol* 1982;**39:**276–9.

5610. Torack RM. Historical aspects of normal and abnormal brain fluids. 3. Cerebral edema. *Arch Neurol* 1982;**39:**355–7.

5611. Torack RM, Morris JC. Mesolimbocortical dementia: a clinicopathologic case study of a putative disorder. *Arch Neurol* 1986;**43:** 1074–8.

5612. Torkildsen A. A new palliative operation in cases of inoperable occlusion of the Sylvian aqueduct. *Acta Chiurg Scand* 1939;**82:**117–24.

5613. Tosi L, Rigoli G, Beltramello A. Fibrocartilaginous embolism of the spinal cord: a clinical and pathological reconsideration. *J Neurol Neurosurg Psychiatry* 1996;**60:**55–60.

5614. Tosun F, Gerek M, Ozkaptan Y. Nasal surgery for contact point headaches. *Headache* 2000;**40:**237–40.

5615. Tourette G de la. Étude sur une affection nerveuse caracterisée par l'incordination motrice accompagné d'echolalie et de coprolalie. *Arch Neurol (Paris)* 1885;**9:**19,-153.

5616. Tournev I, Kalydjieva L, Youl B, et al. Congenital cataracts facial dysmorphism neuropathy syndrome, a novel complex genetic disease in Balkan gypsies: clinical and electrophysiological observations. *Ann Neurol* 1999;**45:**742–50.

5617. Tournier-Lasserve E, Iba-Zizen M-T, Romero N, et al. Autosomal dominant syndrome with strokelike episodes and leukoencephalopathy. *Stroke* 1991;**22:**1297–302.

5618. Towfighi J, Gonatas NK, Pleasure D, et al. Glue sniffer's neuropathy. *Neurology* 1976;**26:**238–43.

5619. Townsend JJ, Wolinsky JS, Baringer JR, et al. Acquired toxoplasmosis: a neglected cause of treatable nervous system disease. *Arch Neurol* 1975;**32:**335–43.

5620. Toyokura Y, Takasu T. Clinical features of SMON. *Jpn J Med Sci Biol* 1975;**28:**87–99.

5621. Tramer T. *Schweiz Arch Neurol Psychiatr* 1945;**55:**306–16.

5622. Tranchant C, Auclair M, Mohr M, et al. A new peroxisomal disease with impaired phytanic and pipecolic acid oxidation. *Neurology* 1993;**43:**2044–8.

5623. Tranebjaerg L, Schwartz C, Eriksen H, et al. A new X-linked recessive deafness syndrome with blindness, dydtonias, fractures and mental deficiency is linked to Xq 22. *J Med Genet* 1995;**32:**257–63.

5624. Tranier S, Durey A, Chevallier B, et al. Value of somatosensory evoked potentials in saphenous entrapement neuropathy. *J Neurol Neurosurg Psychiatry* 1992;**55:**461–5.

5625. Traquair HM. Bitemporal hemiopia: the later stages and the special features of the scotoma. With an examination of current theories of the mechanism of production of the field defects. *Br J Ophthalmol* 1917;**1:**216–39, 281–94.

5626. Traquair HM. *An Introduction to Clinical Perimetry.* London: Henry Kimptom, 1957.

5627. Travers RF. Limbic epilepsy. *J R Soc Med* 1991;**84**:454–6.

5628. Treft RL, et al. Dominant optic atrophy, deafness, ptosis, ophthalmoplegia, dystaxy and myopathy. *Ophthalmology* 1984;**91**:908–15.

5629. Trelles JO. Aspects neurologiques de la verruga peruvienne. *Rev Neurol (Paris)* 1955;**93**:357–68.

5630. Trendelenburg F. Ueber den Gang bei angeborener Huftgelenksluxation. *Dtsch Med Wochenschr* 1895;**21**:21–4.

5631. Trenel J. Quelques observations sur le délire aigu. *Presse Med* 1930;**2**:257–68.

5632. Trethowan WH, Enoch M. *Some Uncommon Psychiatric Syndromes.* Bristol: John Wright, 1970.

5633. Trevathan E, et al. Diagnostic criteria for Rett syndrome. *Ann Neurol* 1988;**23**:425–8.

5634. Triarhou LC, Cerro MD. Freud's contribution to neuroanatomy. *Arch Neurol* 1985;**42**:282–7.

5635. Triggs WJ, Beric A, Butler IJ, et al. A congenital myasthenic syndrome refractory to acetylcholinesterase inhibitors. *Muscle Nerve* 1992;**15**:267–72.

5636. Triggs WJ, Owens J, Gilmore RL, et al. Central conduction abnromalities after electrical injury. *Muscle Nerve* 1994;**17**:1068–70.

5637. Triggs WJ, Roe CR, Rhead WJ, et al. Neuropsychiatric manifestations of defect in mitochondrial beta oxidation response to riboflavin. *J Neurol Neurosurg Psychiatry* 1992;**55**:209–11.

5638. Tritschler HJ, Andreeta F, Moraes CT, et al.. Mitochondrial myopathy of childhood onset associated with depletion of mitochondrial DNA. *Neurology* 1992;**42**:209–17.

5639. Trobe JD, Acosta PC, Krischer JP, et al. Confrontation field techniques in the detection of anterior visual pathway lesions. *Ann Neurol* 1981;**10**:28–34.

5640. Trockel U, et al. Multiple exercise-related mononeuropathy with abdominal colic. *J Neurol Sci* 1983;**60**:431–42.

5641. Trommer BL, Homer D, Mikhael MA. Cerebral vasospasm and eclampsia. *Stroke* 1988;**19**:326–9.

5642. Troost BT, Newton TH. Occipital lobe arteriovenous malformations. *Arch Ophthalmol* 1975;**93**:250.

5643. Troost BT, Troost EG. Functional paralysis of horizontal gaze. *Neurology* 1979;**29**:82.

5644. Trosch RM, Hasbani M, Brass LM. "Bottoms up" dissection. *N Engl J Med* 1989;**320**:1564–5.

5645. Trotter W. On certain clinically obscure malignant tumours of the naso-pharyngeal wall. *BMJ* 1911;**2**:1057–9.

5646. Trotter W. Chronic subdural haematoma. *Am J Dis Child* 1930; **39**:980.

5647. Trouillas P, Brudon F, Froment JC, et al. Cerebellar imitation synkineses. *Rev Neurol (Paris)* 1990;**146**:107–15.

5648. Trousseau A. *Clinique Medicale de l'Hotel Dieu de Paris.* Paris: J.B. Bailliere, 1861.

5649. Trowell HC, Davies JNP, Dean RFA. *Kwashiorkor.* London: Edward Arnold, 1954.

5650. Tsrubaki T, Tiyokura Y, Tsukagoshi H. *Jpn J Med* 1965;**4**:181.

5651. Truswell AS. Osteopetrosis with syndactyly: a morphological variant of Albers-Schonberg's disease. *J Bone Jt Surg* 1958;**40**:208–18.

5652. Trzepacz PT, Baker RW, Greenhouse JA. A symptom rating scale for delirium. *J Psychiatr Res* 1987;**23**:89–97.

5653. Tsai SY. Eponym and identity. *Arch Gen Psychiatry* 1968;**19**: 104–9.

5654. Tsao CY, Mendell JR. The childhood muscular dystrophies: making order out of chaos. *Semin Neurol* 1999;**19**:9–23.

5655. Tsementzis SA, Hitchcock ER. The spoon test; a simple bedside test for assessing sudomotor autonomic failure. *J Neurol Neurosurg Psychiatry* 1985;**48**:378–80.

5656. Tsujino S, Kanazawa N, Ohashi T, et al. Three novel mutations in the *ORNT1* gene of Japanese patients with the HHH syndrome. *Ann Neurol* 2000;**47**:625–31.

5657. Tsujino T, Tonin P, Shanske S, et al. A splice junction mutation in a new myopathic variant of phosphoglycerate kinase deficiency (PGK North Carolina). *Ann Neurol* 1994;**35**:349–53.

5658. Tsukagoshi H. Spinal muscular atrophy, X-linked, juvenile, proximal. *Neurology* 1970;**20**:1188.

5659. Tsunoda I, Awano H, Kayama H, et al. Idiopathic AA amyloidosis manifested by autonomic neuropathy, vestibulocochleopathy and lattice corneal dystrophy. *J Neurol Neurosurg Psychiatry* 1994;**57**:635–7.

5660. Tuck RR, McLeod JG. Retinitis pigmentosa, ataxia, and peripheral neuropathy. *J Neurol Neurosurg Psychiatry* 1983;**46**:206–13.

5661. Tuck RR, McLeod JG, Basten A. Total lipodystrophy. A report of a case with peripheral neuropathy and glomerulonephritis. *Aust NZ J Med* 1983;**13**:65–9.

5662. Tucker T. Central nervous system AIDS. *J Neurol Sci* 1989;**89**: 119–33.

5663. Tucker T, Layzer RB, Miller RG, et al. Subacute reversible motor neuron disease. *Neurology* 1991;**41**:1541–4.

5663a. Tuckett RP. Neurophysiology and neuroanatomy of pruritis. In Bernhard, JD, ed. *Itch*, pp 1–22. New York: McGraw-Hill, 1994.

5664. Tukahashi K, Ohama E, Nerito H, et al. Hereditary dentatorubral-pallido-luysian atrophy. *Neurology* 1988;**38**:1065–70.

5665. Tumarkin A. The otolithic catastrophe. *BMJ* 1936;**2**:175.

5666. Tunbridge RE, Paley RG. Primary optic atrophy in diabetes mellitus. *Diabetes* 1956;**5**:295–6.

5667. Tunkel AR, Kaye D. Infective endocarditis. *Neurol Clin* 1993; **11**:419–40.

5668. Turnbull GK, Hoare C, Ritvo PG, et al. The assessment of bowel and bladder dysfunction in clinic-attending MS patients. Department of Medicine Research Symposium, Dalhousie University, Halifax, Canada, 1995.

5669. Turner JWA. The relationship between amyotonia congenita and congenital myopathy. *Brain* 1940;**63**:163–77.

5670. Turner JWA. On amytonia congenita. *Brain* 1949;**72**:25–34.

5671. Tyler HR. Abnormalities of perception with defective eye movements. *Cortex* 1968;**4**:154–70.

5672. Tyler HR, Tyler KL. Charles Edouard Brown-Séquard. *Neurology* 1984;**34**:1231–6.

5673. Tyrrell P, Rossor M. The association of gegenhalten in the upper limb with dyspraxia. *J Neurol Neurosurg Psychiatry* 1988;**51**:995–7.

5674. Tyrrell PJ. Hypertonia of opposition. *J Neurol Neurosurg Psychiatry* 1988;**51**:995–7.

5675. Tyrrell PJ, Feher MD, Rossor MN. Sciatic nerve damage due to toilet seat entrapment: another Saturday night palsy. *J Neurol Neurosurg Psychiatry* 1989;**52**:1113–4.

5676. Tyson J, Ellis D, Fairbrother U, et al. Hereditary demyelinating neuropathy of infancy: a genetically complex sysndrome. *Brain* 199; **120**:47–63.

5677. Uchihara T, Tsukagoshi H. Jolt accentuation of headache: the most sensitive sign of CSF pleocytosis. *Headache* 1991;**31**:167–71.

5678. Uchitel O, Engel AG, Walls TJ, et al. Congenital myasthenic syndromes:II. Syndrome attributed to abnormal interaction of acetylcholine with its receptor. *Muscle Nerve* 1993;**16**:1293–301.

5679. Udd B, Griggs RC. Distal myopathies. *Curr Opin Neurol* 2001; **14**:561–6.

5680. Udd B, Krahe R, Walgren-Petersson C, et al. Proximal myotonic dystrophy—a family with autosomal dominant muscular dystrophy, cataracts, hearing loss and hypogonadism: heterogeneity of proximal myotonic syndromes? *Neuromusc Disord* 1997;**7**:217–28.

5681. Udd B, Partanen J, Haloinen P, et al. Tibial muscular dystrophy: Late adult–onset distal myopathy in 66 Finnish patients. *Arch Neurol* 1993;**50**:604–8.

5682. Ugawa Y, Inoue K, Takamura T, et al. Accumulation of glycogen in Sural nerve axons in adult-onset type III glycogenosis. *Ann Neurol* 1986;**19**:294–7.

5683. Uhthoff W. Untersuchungen uber die bei der multiplen Herdsklerose vorkommenden Augenstorungen. *Arch Psychiatr Nervenkr* 1889;**21**:303–410.

5684. Ullrich O. Kongenitale, atonisch-sklerotische Muskel Dystrophie. *Z Ges Neurol Psychiatr* 1930;**126**:171–201.

5684a. Umapathi T, Chaudhry V, Cornblath D, et al. Head drop and camptocormia. *J Neurol Neurosurg Psychiatr* 2002;**72**:1–7.

5685. Uncini A, Sabatelli M, Mignogna T, et al. Chronic progressive steroid responsive axonal polyneuropathy: a CIDP variant or a primary axonal disorder? *Muscle Nerve* 1996;**19**:365–371.

5686. Uncini A, Servidei S, Silvestri G, et al. Ophthalmoplegia, demyelinating neuropathy, leukoencephalopathy, myopathy and gastrointestinal dysfunction with multiple deletions of mitochondrial DNA. *Muscle Nerve* 1994;**17**:667–74.

5687. Ungar-Sargon JY, Lovelace RE, Brust JCM. Spastic paraplegia-paraparesis. *J Neurol Sci* 1980;**46**:1–12.

5688. Unverricht H. Dermatomyositis acuta. *Dtsch Med Wochenschr* 1891;**17**:41–4.

5689. Unverricht H. *Die Myoclonie.* Leipzig: Franz Deuticke, 1891.

5690. Upshaw BY, Montgomery H. Hereditary anhidrotic ectodermal dysplasia. *Arch Dermatol* 1949;**60**:1170.

5691. Upton ARM, McComas AJ. The double crush in nerve entrapment syndromes. *Lancet* 1973;**2**:359–62.

5692. Urich H, Wilkinson M. Necrosis of muscle with carcinoma; myositis or myopathy? *J Neurol Neurosurg Psychiatry* 1970;**33**:398–407.

5693. Ursell MR, Marras CL, Farb R, et al. Recurrent intracranial hemorrhage due to postpartum cerebral angiopathy: implications for management. *Stroke* 1998;**29**:1995–8.

5694. Usher CH. On the inheritance of retinitis pigmentosa, with notes of cases. *R Lond Ophthalmol Hosp Rep* 1914;**19**:130–236.

5695. Vail HH. Vidian neuralgia. *Ann Otolaryngol* 1932;**41**:837.

5696. Vajsar J, Becker LE, Freedom RM, et al. Familial desminopathy: myopathy with accumulation of desmin-type intermediate filaments. *J Neurol Neurosurg Psychiatry* 1993;**56**:644–8.

5697. Valleix FLI. *Traite des Nevralgies ou Affections Douloureuses des Nerfs.* Paris: J.B. Bailliere, 1841.

5698. Van Acker R. Rett syndrome: a review of current knowledge. *Autism Dev Dis* 1991;**21**:381–406.

5699. Van Allen MW, Blodi FC. Neurologic aspects of the Möbius syndrome. *Neurology* 1960;**10**:249–59.

5700. Van Allen MW, et al. Amyloidosis type III. *Neurology* 1969;**19**:10.

5701. Van Allen MW, Frohlich JA, Davis JR. Inherited predisposition to generalized amyloidosis. Clinical and pathological study of a family with neuropathy, nephropathy and peptic ulcer. *Neurol Minneap* 1969;**19**:10–25.

5702. van Bogaert L. Tendinous areflexia without pupillary changes. *J Neurol Psychiatry* 1939;**29**:193–202.

5703. van Bogaert L. Une leuco-encephalite sclerosante subaigue. *J Neurol* 1945;**8**:101–20.

5704. van Bogaert L. La mélanose neurocutanée diffuse heredofamiliale. *Bull Acad R Med Belg 6th Series* 1948;**13**:397.

5705. van Bogaert L. Spinal cholesterolosis. *Brain* 1965;**88**:687–96.

5706. van Bogaert L, Divry P. Sur une maladie familiale caracterisée par une angiomatose diffuse cortico-meningée et une demyelinisation de la substance blanche du centre ovale. *Bruxelles Med* 1945;**25**:1090–1.

5707. van Bogaert L, Moreau M. Combination of Charcot-Marie-Tooth neuropathy and Friedreich ataxia [in French]. *Encéphale* 1939;**1**:312–20.

5708. van Bogaert L, Scherer HJ, Epstein E. *Une Forme Cérébrale de la Cholesterinose Generaliseé.* Paris: Masson, 1937.

5709. van Bogaert L, Theorides J. *Constantin von Economo—The Man and the Scientist.* Vienna: Springer Verlag, 1979.

5710. van Buchem FSP, Hadders HN, Ubbens R. An uncommon, familial systemic disease of the skeleton. *Acta Radiol* 1955;**44**:109–20.

5711. Vance JM. The many faces of Charcot-Marie-Tooth disease. *Arch Neurol* 2000;**57**:638–40.

5712. van den Bergh PYK, Thonnard J-L, Duprez T, et al. Chronic demyelinating hypertrophic brachial plexus neuropathy. *Muscle Nerve* 2000;**23**:283–8.

5713. Van den Berg-Vos RM, Franssen H, Wokke JHJ, et al. Multifocal motor neuropathy: diagnostic criteria that predict the response to immunoglobulin treatment. *Ann Neurol* 2000;**48**:919–26.

5714. Van den Berg-Vos RM, Van den Berg LH, Franssen H, et al. Multifocal inflammatory demyelinating neuropathy. *Neurology* 2000; **54**:26–32.

5715. Van den Burg W, Saan RJ, Deelman BG. 15–Woordetest. *Provisional Manual.* Groningen: University Hospital, 1985.

5716. Van der Eecken H, Adams RD, van Bogaert L. Striato-pallidal degeneration. An hitherto undescribed lesion in paralysis agitans. *J Neuropathol Exp Neurol* 1960;**19**:159–61.

5716a. van der Hoeve J. Signs in tuberose sclerosis. *Graefes Arch Clin Exp Ophthalmol* 1921;**105**:880–898.

5717. van der Hoeve J, Kleyn A. *Ned Tschr Geneesk* 1917;**1**:1003.

5718. van der Knapp MS, Barth PG, Gabreels FJ, et al. A new leukoencephalopathy with vanishing white matter. *Neurology* 1997;**48**:845–55.

5719. van der Knapp MS, Kamphorst W, Barth PG, et al. Phenotypic variation in leukoencephalopathy with vanishing white matter. *Neurology* 1998;**51**:540–7.

5719a. Van der Meche FG, van Gijn J. Hypotonia: an erroneous clinical concept? *Brain* 1986;**109**:1169–78.

5720. van der Ploeg RJO, Oosterhuis HJGH. The "make\break test" as a diagnostic tool in functional weakness. *J Neurol Neurosurg Psychiatry* 1991;**54**:248–51.

5721. Van der Viel HL, Van Gijn J. Horner's syndrome. *J Neurol Sci* 1982;**56**:293–8.

5722. Van der Zee SPM, et al. Citrullinaemia with a rapidly fatal neonatal outcome. *Arch Dis Child* 1971;**48**:847.

5723. van Dijk JG, Pondaag W, Malessy MJA. Obstetric lesions of the brachial plexus. *Muscle Nerve* 2001;**24**:1451–61.

5724. van Dongen HR, Catsman-Berrevoets CE, van Mourik M. The syndrome of 'cerebellar' mutism and subsequent dysarthria. *Neurology* 1994;**44**:2040–6.

5725. Van Dyke DH, Griggs RC, Murphy MJ, Goldstein MN. Hereditary myokymia and periodic ataxia. *J Neurol Sci* 1975;**25**:109–18.

5726. van Erven PMM, Cillessen JPM, Eekhoff EMW, et al. Leigh syndrome, a mitochondrial encephalo(myo)pathy. *Clin Neurol Neurosurg* 1987;**89**:217–30.

5727. van Geel BM, Assies J, Wanders RJA, Barth PG. X-linked adrenoleukodystrophy: clinical presentation, diagnosis and therpay. *J Neurol Neurosurg Psychiatry* 1997;**63**:4–14.

5728. Van Gijn J. Measurement of outcome in stroke prevention trials. *Cerebrovasc Dis* 1992;2(**Suppl 1**):23–34.

5729. Van Gijn J. The Babinski sign: the first hundred years. *J Neurol* 1996;**243**:675–83.

5730. Van Gijn J. Cerebral venous thrombosis: pathogenesis, presentation and prognosis. *J Roy Soc Med* 2000;**93**:230–3.

5731. Vanhatalo S, Riikonen R. Markedly elevated nitrate/nitrite levels in the cerebrospinal fluid of children with progressive encephalopathy with edema (PEHO syndrome). *Epilepsia* 2000;**41**:705–8.

5732. Van Hove JL, Kishnani PS, Demaerel P, et al. Acute hydrocephalus in nonketotic hyperglycemia. *Neurology* 2000;**54**:754–6.

5733. van Huffelen AC. A Tribute to Martinus Rulandus. *Arch Neurol* 1989;**46**:445–7.

5734. Van Laere JE. Paralysie bulbo-pontine chronique progressive familiâle avec surdité: un cas de syndrome de Klippel-Trenaunay dans la meme fratrie. *Rev Neurol (Paris)* 1966;**115**:289–95.

5735. VanLandingham KE, Heinz ER, Cavazos JE, et al. Magnetic resonance imaging evidence of hippocampal injury after prolonged focal febrile convulsions. *Ann Neurol* 1998;**43**:413–26.

5735a. Van Leewenhoek A. *Selected Works.* London: Nicol, 1798.

5736. Van Munster ETL, Joosten EMG, et al. The rigid spine syndrome. *J Neurol Neurosurg Psychiatry* 1986;**49**:1292–7.

5737. Vanneste JAL. Three decades of normal pressure hydrocephalus: are we wiser now? *J Neurol Neurosurg Psychiatry* 1994;**57**:1021–5.

5738. Van Praagh R. Diagnosis of kernicterus in the neonatal period. *Pediatrics* 1961;**28**:870–6.

5739. Van Uitert RL, Solomon GE. White-centered retinal hemorrhages: a sign of intracranial hemorrhage. *Neurology* 1979;**29**:236–9.

5740. van Vugt P, Paquier PF, Kees L, et al. Increased writing activity in neurological conditions: a review and clinical study. *J Neurol Neurosurg Psychiatry* 1996;**61**:510–4.

5741. Van Wijngaarden GK, Fleury P, Bethlem J, et al. Familial "myotubular" myopathy. *Neurology* 1969;**19**:901–8.

5742. van Zomeren AH, ten Duis H-J, Minderhoud JM, et al. Lightning stroke and neurophychological impairment: cases and questions. *J Neurol Neurosurg Psychiatry* 1998;**64**:763–9.

5743. Varma JS, Smith AN, McInnes A. Electrophysiological observations on the human pudendal–anal reflex. *J Neurol Neurosurg Psychiatry* 1986;**49**:1411–6.

5744. Vassilescu C, Alexianu M, Dan A. Neuronal type of Charcot-Marie-Tooth disease with a syndrome of continuous motor unit activity. *J Neurol Sci* 1984;**63**:11–25.

5745. Vazquez V, Sotelo J. The course of seizures after treatment for cerebral cysticercosis. *N Engl J Med* 1992;**327**:696–701.

5746. Veit C, Ware J. The structure of psychological distress and well-being in general populations. *J Consult Clin Psychol* 1983;**51**:730–732.

5747. Ventruto V, Di Garolamo R, Festa B, et al. Family study of inherited syndrome with multiple congenital deformities: symphalangism, carpal and tarsal fusion, brachydactyly, craniosynostosis, strabismus, hip osteochondritis. *J Med Genet* 1976;**13**:394–8.

5748. Verbiest H. Primaire stenose van het lumbale wervelkanal bij volwassenen, een nieur ziektebeeld. *Ned Tschr Geneesk* 1950;**94**:2415–33.

5749. Verdugo R, Ochoa JL. Quantitative somatosensory thermotest: a new method for functional evaluation of small calibre afferent channels. *Brain* 1992;**115**:893–913.

5750. Verhagen WIM, Horstink MWIM, Notermans SLH. Painful arm and moving fingers. *J Neurol Neurosurg Psychiatry* 1985;**481**:384–5.

5751. Verity MA, Roitberg B, Kepes JJ. Mesolimbocortical dementia: clinico-pathological studies on two cases. *J Neurol Neurosurg Psychiatry* 1990;**53**:492–5.

5752. Verma A, Bradley WG. High dose IVIg therapy in chronic progressive lumbosacral plexopathy. *Neurology* 1994;**44**:248–50.

5753. Verma P, Oger J. Treatment of acquired autoimmune myasthenia gravis. *Can J Neurol Sci* 1992;**19**:360–75.

5753a. Vermeer SE, van Dijk EJ, Koudstaal PJ, et al. Homocysteine, silent brain infarcts, and white matter lesions: The Rotterdam Scan Study. Ann Neurol 2002;**51**:285–9.

5754. Vernant JC, Cabre P, Smadja D, et al. Recurrent optic neuromyelitis with endocrinopathies. *Neurology* 1997;**48**:58–64.

5755. Vernet M. Les paralysies laryngées associés. Thesis, University of Lyon, 1916.

5756. Verrips A, et al. Spinal xanthomatosis: a variant of cerebrotendinous xanthomatosis. *Brain* 1999;**122**:1589–95.

5757. Vetrugno R, Provini F, Plazzi G, et al. Catathrenia (nocturnal groaning): a new type of parasomnia. *Neurology* 2001;**56**:681–3.

5758. Victor M. The Wernicke-Korsakoff syndrome. *Handb Clin Neurol* 1989;**28**:243–70.

5759. Victor M. Alcholic dementia. *Can J Neurol Sci* 1994;**21**:88–99.

5760. Vidailhet M. Paroxysmal dyskinesias as a paradigm of paroxysmal movement disorders. *Curr Opin Neurol* 2000;**13**:457–62.

5761. Viegas SF, Rimldi R, Scarborough M, et al. Acute compartment syndrome in the thigh. A case report and review of the literature. *Clin Orthop* 1988;**234**:232–4.

5762. Vignaendra V, Wilkus RJ, Copass MK, Chatrian GE. Electroencephalographic rhythms of alpha frequency in comatose patients after cardiac arrest. *Neurology* 1974;**24**:582–8.

5763. Vijayan N, Dreyfus PM. Posttraumatic dysautonomic cephalalgia: clinical observations and treatment. *Arch Neurol* 1975;**32**:649–52.

5764. Vijayan N, Watson C. Site of injury headache. *Headache* 1989;**29**:502–6.

5765. Villanova M, Louboutin JP, Chateau D, et al. X-linked vacuolated myopathy: complement membrane attack complex on surface membrane of injured muscle fibers. *Ann Neurol* 1995;**37**:637–45.

5766. Villaret M. Le syndrome nerveux de l'éspace retroparotidien posterieur. *Rev Neurol (Paris)* 1916;**23**:188–90.

5767. Vincent A, Cull-Candy SG, Newsom-Davis J, et al. Congenital myasthenia: end-plate acetylcholine receptors and electrophysiology in five cases. *Muscle Nerve* 1981;**4**:306–18.

5768. Vincent FM. Benign masturbatory cephalalgia. *Arch Neurol* 1982;**39**:673.

5769. Vinchon M, Blond S, Lejeune JP, et al. Association of Lhermitte-Duclos and Cowden Disease: report of a new case and review of the literature. *J Neurol Neurosurg Psychiatry* 1994;**57**:699–704.

5770. Virchow RLK. On the pathologic anatomy of children [in German]. *Virchows Arch Pathol Anat Physiol* 1867;**38**:129–38.

5771. Vitiello MV, Bliwise DL, Prinz PN. Sleep in Alzheimer's disease and the sundown syndrome. *Neurology* 1992;**42**(**Suppl 6**):83–94.

5772. Vodusek OB. Pudendal and bulbo-cavernosus reflexes in women. *Electroencephalogr Clin Neurophysiol* 1990;**77**:134–6.

5773. Vogel CM, Albin R, Albers JW. Lotus footdrop: sciatic neuropathy in the thigh. *Neurology* 1991;**41**:605–6.

5774. Vogel P, Gabriel M, Goebel HH, Dyck PJ. Hereditary motor sensory neuropathy type II with neurofilament accumulation. *Ann Neurol* 1985;**17**:455–61.

5775. Vogt A. Fruhzeitiges Ergrauen der Zilien ud Bemerkungen uber den sogenanten plotzlichen Eintritt dieser Veranderung. *Klin Monatsbl Augenheilk* 1906;**44**:228–42.

5776. Vogt C, Vogt O. Zur Lehre der Erkrankungen des striaten Systems. *J Psychol Neurol (Leipzig)* 1920;**25**:627–846.

5777. Vogt H. Uber familiare amaurotische Idiotie und verwandte Krankheitsbilder. *Monatschr Psychiatr* 1905;**18**:161–171, 310–357.

5778. Volkmann R von. Die ischamischen Muskellahmungen und Kontrakturen. *Zentralbl Chir* 1881;**8**:801–3.

5779. von Angyal L. Thumb-mouth agnosia: a special form of Gerstmann syndrome. *Confin Neurol.* 1940;**3**:245–52.

5780. Von Economo K. Encephalitis lethargica. *Wien Klin Wochenschr* 1917;**30**:581–5.

5781. Von Gierke E. Hepato-nephromegalia Glycogenica. *Beitr Pathol Anat* 1929;**82**:497–513.

5782. von Giesen H-J, Neuen-Jacob E, Dorries K, et al. Diagnostic criteria and clinical procedures in HIV-1 associated progressive multifocal leukoencephalopathy. *Arendt G Med Clin (Batrc)* 1999;**113**:210–4.

5783. von Giesen H-J, Stoll G, Koch MA, et al. Mixed axonal-demyelinating polyneuropathy as predominant manifestation of myotonic dystrophy. *Muscle Nerve* 1004;**17**:701–3.

5784. Von Graefe AF. Exceptionelles Verhalten des Gessichtsfeldes bei Pigmentatartung der Netzhaut. *Arch Ophthalmol Berlin* 1848;**4**:250.

5784a. Von Graefe AF. Ueber Based ou' sche Krankheit. *Dtsch Klinik* 1864;**16**:662–72.

5785. Von Graefe AF. Demonstration in der Berliner medizinischen Gesellschaft. *Berl Klin Wochenschr* 1868;**5**:127.

5786. Von Graefe AF. Verhandlungen artzlicher Gessellschaften. *Berl Klin Wochenschr* 1868;**5**:125–7.

5787. Vowles G, Scholtz CL. Diffuse axonal injury in early infancy. *J Clin Pathol* 1987;**40**:185–9.

5788. Vuardens P, Bogousslavsky J. Face-arm-trunk-leg sensory loss limited to the contralateral side in lateral medullary infarction; a new variant. *J Neurol Neurosurg Psychiatry* 1998;**65**:255–7.

5789. Waardenburg A. *Das menschliche Auge und seine Erblagen.* Haag: M. Nijhoff, 1932.

5790. Waardenburg PJ. A new syndrome combining developmental anomalies of the eyelids, eyebrows and nose root with pigmentary defects of the iris and head hair and with congenital deafness. *Am J Hum Genet* 1951;**3**:195–253.

5791. Waddell G, McCulloch JA, Kummell E, et al. Nonorganic physical signs in low back pain. *Spine* 1980;**5**:117–25.

5792. Wade DT. *Measurement in Neurological Rehabilitation.* Oxford: Oxford Medical, 1992.

5793. Wadia NH. Atlantoaxial dislocation. *Neurology (Bombay)* 1960;**8**:81.

5794. Wadia NH. An introduction to neurology in India. In Spillane JD, ed. *Tropical Neurology*, pp. 25–36. London: Oxford University Press, 1973.

5795. Wadia NH. Congenital atlanto-axial dislocation and its manifestations due to spinal cord compression. In Spillane JD, ed. *Tropical Neurology*, pp 99–107. London: Oxford University Press, 1973.

5796. Wadia NH, Ivari PF, Katrak SM. Amyotrophy with acute hemorrhagic conjunctivitis. *Lancet* 1972;**2**:970–1.

5797. Wadia NH, Swami RK. A new form of heredofamilial spinocerebellar degeneration with slow eye movements (nine families). *Brain* 1971;**94**:359–74.

5798. Wadia RS, Wadgaonkar SU, Amin RB, et al. An unusual family of benign "X" linked muscular dystrophy with cardiac involvement. *J Med Genet* 1976;**13**:352–6.

5799. Wadsworth TG. Tennis elbow. *BMJ* 1987;**294**:621–4.

5800. Waggoner RW, et al. Agenesis of white matter with idiocy. *Am J Ment Defic* 1942;**47**:20–4.

5801. Wagner EL. Fall einer seltenen Muskelkrankheit. *Arch.Heilk.* 1863;**4**:282–3.

5802. Wagner von Jauregg J. Ueber die Einwirkung der Malaria auf die progressive Paralyse. *Psychiatr Neurol (Belg)* 1918;**20**:132–134, 251–255.

5803. Wakai S, Ikehata M, Nihira H, et al. Obtundation status (Dravet) caused by complex partial status epilepticus in a patient with severe myoclonic epilepsy in infancy. *Epilepsia* 1996;**37**:1020–2.

5804. Walczak TS, Leppik IE, D'Amelio M, et al. Incidence and risk factors in sudden unexpected death in epilepsy. *Neurology* 2001;**56**:519–25.

5805. Waldenstrom J. Acute thyrotoxic encephalo- or myopathy, its cause and treatment. *Acta Med Scand* 1945;**121**:251–94.

5806. Waldenstrom J. Two interesting syndromes with hyperglobulinemia. Purpura, hyperglobinuria and macroglobulinemia [in German]. *Schweiz Med Wochenschr* 1948;**78**:927–8.

5807. Waldvogel D, Mattle HP, Sturzenegger M, et al. Pulsatile tinnitus: a review of 84 patients. *J Neurol* 1998;**245**:137–42.

5808. Walk D, Kang S-S, Horwitz A. Intermittent encephalopathy, reversible nerve conduction slowing, and MRI evidence of cerebral white matter disease in methylene tetrahydrofolate reductase deficiency. *Neurology* 1994;**44**:344–7.

5809. Walker FO. Voice fatigue in myasthenia gravis: the sinking pitch sign. *Neurology* 1997;**48**:1135–6.

5810. Walker MB. Treatment of myasthenia gravis with physostigmine. *Lancet* 1934;**1**:1200–1.

5811. Walker RW. Idiopathic intracranial hypertension: any light on the mechanism of the raised pressure? *J Neurol Neurosurg Psychiatry* 2001;**71**:1–5.

5812. Wall M, Rosenberg M, Richardson D. Gaze-evoked tinnitus. *Neurology* 1987;**37**:1034–6.

5813. Wall M, Wray SH. The one-and-a-half syndrome. A unilateral disorder of the pontine tegmentum: a study of 20 cases and review of the literature. *Neurology* 1983;**33**:971–80.

5814. Wall PD, Noordenbos W. Sensory functions which remain in nan after complete transection of dorsal columns. *Brain* 1977;**100**:641–53.

5815. Wallace MR, Dwulet FE, Conneally M, et al. Biochemical and molecular genetic characteristics of a new variant prealbumin associated with hereditary amyloidosis. *J Clin Invest* 1986;**78**:6–12.

5816. Wallenberg A. Acute Bulbaraffection (Embolie der Arteria cerebelli posterior inferior sinistra?). *Arch Psychiat (Berlin)* 1895;**27**:504–40.

5817. Waller AD. Points relating to the Weber-Fechner law. *Brain* 1895;**18**:200–16.

5818. Waller AV. Experiments on the section of the glossopharyngeal and hypoglossal nerves of the frog, and observations of the alterations produced thereby in the structure of their primitive fibers. *Phil Trans R Soc Lond* 1850;423–9.

5819. Wallgren-Pettersson C, Laing NG, Report of the 70th ENMC International Workshop: nemaline myopathy, 11–13 June, Naarden, The Netherlands. *Neuromusc Disord* 2000;**10**:299–306.

5820. Walser M. Urea cycle disorders and other hereditary hyperammonemic syndromes. In Stanbury JB, Wyngaarden JB, Fredrickson DS, et al., eds. *The Metabolic Basis of Inherited Disease*, pp 402–38. New York: McGraw-Hill, 1983.

5821. Walsh EG. Clonus: beats provoked by the application of a rhythmic force. *J Neurol Neurosurg Psychiatry* 1976;**39**:266–74.

5822. Walsh FB. Third nerve regeneration. *Br J Ophthalmol* 1957;**41**:577–98.

5823. Walsh FB, Gass JD. Concerning the optic nerve. *Am J Ophthalmol* 1960;**50**:1031–47.

5824. Walsh FB, Hoyt WF. *Clinical Neuro-Ophthalmology*. Baltimore: Williams & Wilkins, 1969.

5825. Walsh FB, King AB. Ocular signs of intracranial saccular aneurysms. *Arch Ophthalmol Berlin* 1942;**12**(Suppl):1–33.

5826. Walsh JC. Neuromyotonia; an unusual presentation of intrathoracic malignancy. *J Neurol Neurosurg Psychiatry* 1976;**39**:1086–91.

5827. Walshe F. Diagnosis of hysteria. *BMJ* 1965;**2**:1451–4.

5828. Walshe FMR. The physiological significance of the reflex phenomena in spastic paralysis of the lower limbs. *Brain* 1915;**37**:269–336.

5829. Walshe FMR. On certain tonic or postural reflexes in hemiplegia. *Brain* 1923;**46**:1–37.

5830. Walshe FMR. On the "syndrome of the premotor cortex" (Fulton) and the definition of the terms "premotor" and "motor": with a consideration of Jackson's views on the cortical representation of movements. *Brain* 1935;**58**:49–80.

5831. Walshe FMR. On the role of the pyramidal system in willed movements. *Brain* 1947;**70**:329–54.

5832. Walshe FMR. Contributions of John Hughlings Jackson to neurology: a brief introductions to his teachings. *Arch Neurol* 1961;**5**:119–31.

5833. Walshe FMR, Robertson EG. Observations upon the form and nature of the "grasping" movements and "tonic innervation" seen in certain cases of lesion of the frontal lobe. *Brain* 1933;**56**:40–70.

5834. Walter WG. Epilepsy. In Hill JDN, Parr G, eds. *Electroencephalography*, p 246. New York: Macmillan, 1950.

5835. Walter WG, Cooper R, Aldridge VJ. Contingent negative variation: an electrical sign of sensorimotor association and expectancy in the human brain. *Nature* 1964;**203**:380–4.

5835a. Walters AS, Hening WA, Shah SK, Chokroverty S. Painless legs and moving toes: A syndrome related to painful legs and moving toes? *Mov Disord* 1993;**8**:377–9.

5836. Walters AS. Toward a better definition of restless legs syndrome. *Mov Disord* 1995;**10**:634–42.

5837. Walton JN. Amyotonia congenita. A follow-up study. *Lancet* 1956;**1**:1023–8.

5838. Walton JN. The limp child. *J Neurol Neurosurg Psychiatry* 1957;**20**:144–54.

5839. Walton W. *Dictionary of Psychiatry*. Oxford: Blackwell, 1993.

5840. Waltz G, Harik SI, Kaufman B. Adult metachromatic leukodystrophy. *Arch Neurol* 1987;**44**:225–7.

5841. Wanamaker WM. Firearm recoil palsy. *Arch Neurol* 1974;**31**:208–9.

5842. War Department. *Army Individual Test Battery*. Washington, DC: Adjutant General's Office, 1944.

5843. Wardlaw JM, Dennis MS, Lindlay RI, et al. The validity of a simple clinical classification of acute ischaemic stroke. *J Neurol* 1996;**243**:274–9.

5844. Ware JC. Evaluation of impotence–monitoring periodic penile erections during sleep. *Psychiatr Clin North Am* 1987;**10**:675–86.

5845. Warier RP, et al. Opsomyoclonus and neuroblastoma. *Clin Pediatr* 1985;**24**:32.

5846. Warmolts JR, Mendell JR. Neurotonia: impulse-induced repetitive discharges in motor nerves in peripheral neuropathy. *Ann Neurol* 1980;**7**:245–50.

5847. Warner TT, Jarman P. The molecular genetics of the dystonias. *J Neurol Neurosurg Psychiatry* 1998;**64**:427–9.

5848. Warrell DA, Godfrey S, Olsen EJG. Giant cell arteritis with peripheral neuropathy. *Lancet* 1968;**1**:1010–3.

5849. Warren JD. Variations on the musical brain. *J R Soc Med* 1999;**92**:571–5.

5850. Warrington EK. *Warrington Recognition Memory Test*. Windsor, UK: NFER-Nelson, 1984.

5851. Warrington EK, Langdon D. Spelling dyslexia: a deficit of the visual word-form. *J Neurol Neurosurg Psychiatry* 1994;**57**:211–6.

5852. Warrington K, Shallice T. Category specific semantic impairments. *Brain* 1984;**107**:829–54.

5853. Wartenberg R. A sign of facial palsy [in German]. *Dtsch Z Nervenklinik* 1930;**116**:144–5.

5854. Wartenberg R. Nasal pruritis with cerebral tumours [in German]. *Klin Woschenschr* 1932;**11**:461.

5855. Wartenberg R. A sign of ulnar palsy. *JAMA* 1939;**112**:1688.

5856. Wartenberg R. Brachialgia statica paresthetica (nocturnal arm dysesthesias). *J Nerv Ment Dis* 1944; **99**:877–87.

5857. Wartenberg R. Progressive facial hemiatrophy. *Arch Neurol Psychiatry* 1945;**54**:75–96.

5858. Wartenberg R. *The Examination of Reflexes: A Simplification*. Chicago: The Year Book Publishers, 1945.

5859. Wartenberg R. Multiple sensory neuritis: a clinical entity. *Trans Am Neurol Assoc* 1946;**71**:101–4.

5860. Wartenberg R. Winking-jaw phenomenon. *Arch Neurol Psychiatry* 1948;**59**:734–53.

5861. Wartenberg R. Pendulousness of the legs as a diagnostic test. *Neurology* 1951;**1**:18–24.

5862. Wartenberg R. Digitalia paresthetica and gonyalgia paresthetica. *Neurology* 1954;**4**:106–15.

5863. Wartenberg R. On neurologic terminology, eponyms and the Lasègue sign. *Neurology* 1956;**6**:853–8.

5864. Warwick R. The so-called nucleus of convergence. *Brain* 1955;**78**:92–114.

5865. Wasserstrom WR, Glass JP, Posner JB. Diagnosis and treatment of leptomeningeal metastases from solid tumors: experience with 90 patients. *Cancer* 1982;**49**:759–72.

5866. Watanabe I, et al. Early lesion of Pelizaeus-Merzbacher's disease. Electron microscope and biochemical study. *J Neuropathol Exp Neurol* 1973;**32**:313–33.

5867. Watanabe T, Katamaya Y. Evaluation by magnetic resonance imaging of the entrapped temporal horn syndrome. *J Neurol Neurosurg Psychiatry* 1999;**66**:113.

5868. Waterhouse R. A case of suprarenal apoplexy. *Lancet* 1911;**1**:577–8.

5869. Waters CH, Miller CA. Autosomal dominant Lewy body parkinsonism in a four-generation family. *Ann Neurol* 1994;**35**:59–64.

5870. Waters CH, Takahashi H, Wilhelmsen KC, et al. Phenotypic expression of X-linked dystonia-parkinsonism (lubag) in two women. *Neurology* 1993;**43**:1555–8.

5871. Waters DD, Nutter DO, Hopkins LC, et al. Cardiac features of an unusual X-linked humeroperoneal neuromuscular disease. *N Engl J Med* 1975;**293**:1017–22.

5872. Watson CPN. Postherpetic neuralgia. In Portenoy RK, ed. *Neurologic Clinics, Vol. 7, Pain: Mechanisms and Syndromes*, p 231. Philadelphia: W.B. Saunders, 1989.

5873. Watson RT, Heilman KM. Callosal apraxia. *Brain* 1983;**106**:391–403.

5874. Watson RT, Valenstein E, Heilman KM. Thalamic neglect: possible role of the medial thalamus and nucleus reticularis in behavior. *Arch Neurol* 1981;**38**:501–6.

5875. Watson SR, Halmagyi GM, Colebatch JG. Vestibular hypersensitivity to sound (Tullio phenomenon): structural and functional assessment. *Neurology* 2000;**54**:722–8.

5876. Watters GV, Fitch N. Familial laryngeal abductor paralysis and psychomotor retardation. *Clin Genet* 1973;**4**:429–33.

5877. Waxman SG. The flexion-adduction sign in neuralgic amyotrophy. *Neurology* 1979;**29**:1301–4.

5878. Waxman SG, Geschwind N. Hypergraphia in temporal lobe epilepsy. *Neurology* 1974;**24**:629–36.

5879. Waziri M, et al. Abnormality of chromosome 11 in patients with features of Beckwith-Wiedermann syndrome. *J Pediatr* 1983;**102**:873.

5880. Weatherby E, Wiley NH. Left sided weakness, unequal blood presure in the two arms and left optic atrophy: a new syndrome? *J Nerv Ment Dis* 1940;**92**:151–6.

5881. Weaver DD, Graham B, Thomas IT, et al. A new overgrowth syndrome with accelerated skeletal maturation, unusual facies and camptodactly. *J Pediatr* 1974;**84**:547–52.

5882. Webb S, Coleman D, Byrne P, et al. Autosomal dominant hereditary spastic paraparesis with cognitive loss linked to chrosome 2p. *Brain* 1998;**121**:601–9.

5883. Webb WB, Agnew HW. Sleep and waking in a time-free environment. *Aerosp Med* 1974;**45**:617–22.

5884. Weber FP. A case of relapsing, non-suppurative nodular panniculitis, showing phagocytosis of subcutaneous fat-cells by macrophages. *Br J Dermatol* 1925;**37**:301–11.

5885. Weber H. A contribution to the pathology of the crura cerebri. *Med Chir Trans* 1863;**46**:121–39.

5886. Wechsler D. A standardised memory scale for clinical use. *J Psychol* 1954;**19**:87–95.

5888. Wechsler D. *The Wechsler Intelligence Scale for Children (Revised)*. New York: Psychological Corp., 1976.

5889. Wechsler D. *The Wechsler Adult Intelligence Scale (Revised)*. New York: Psychological Corp., 1986.

5890. Wechsler D. *The Wechsler Primary and Preschool Scale of Intelligence (Revised)*. New York: Psychological Corp., 1967.

5891. Wedemeyer L, Johnson CA, Keltner JL. Statokinetic dissociation in optic nerve disease. In Heijl A, ed. *Proceedings of the Eighth International Perimetric Society Meeting*, pp 9–14. Amsterdam: Kugler, 1989.

5892. Weglinski MR, Wedel DJ. Malignant hyperthermia testing in patients with persistently increased serum creatine kinase levels. *Anesthesiol Analg* 1997;**84**:1038–41.

5893. Weill G. Ectopia of the crystalline lens and general malformations [in French]. *Ann Ocul* 1932;**169**:21–44.

5894. Weiner LP, Konigsmark BW, Stoll J, et al. Hereditary olivopontocerebellar atrophy with retinal degeneration. *Arch Neurol* 1967;**16**:364–76.

5895. Weiner WJ, Koller WC, Perlik S, et al. Drug holiday and management of Parkinson disease. *Neurology* 1980;**30**:1257–61.

5896. Weiner WJ, Nora LM, Glantz RH. Elderly inpatients: postural reflex impairment. *Neurology* 1984;**34**:945–7.

5897. Weinstein EA, Kahn RL, Malitz S, Rozanski J. Delusional reduplication of parts of the body. *Brain* 1954;**77**:45–60.

5898. Weisberg LA. The syndrome of increased intracranial pressure without localizing signs: a reappraisal. *Neurology* 1975;**25**:85–8.

5899. Weisberg LA. Lacunar infarcts. Clinical and computed tomography correlations. *Arch Neurol* 1982;**39**:37–40.

5900. Weiser HG. The phenomenology of limbic seizures. In Weiser HG, Speckmann EJ, Engel J, eds. *The Epileptic Focus*, pp 113–36. London: John Libbey, 1987.

5901. Weiskrantz L. *Blindsight: A Case Study and Implications*. Oxford: Oxford University Press, 1986.

5902. Weiss E. Cerebral adiposity with nerve deafness, mental deficiency and genital dystrophy: a variant of the Lawrence-Biedl syndrome. *Am J Med Sci* 1932;**183**:268–72.

5903. Weiss L. Syndromes II. In Smith DW, ed. *Birth Defects*, pp 309–10. Amsterdam: Excerpta Medica, 1974.

5904. Weiss N. Zur Messung der Intensitat galvanischer Strome in der Elektrotherapie. *Zentralbl Ges Therap* 1883;**1**:9–14.

5905. Weiss S, Baker JB. The carotid sinus in health and disease: its role in the causation of fainting and convulsions. *Medicine* 1933;**12**:297–354.

5906. Weissleder R, et al. Limb girdle type muscular dystrophy associated with Wolff-Parkinson-White syndrome. *J Neurol Neurosurg Psychiatry* 1987;**50**:500–1.

5907. Weitzman ED, Czeisler CA, Coleman RM, et al. Delayed sleep phase syndrome: a chronobiological disorder with sleep-onset insomnia. *Arch Gen Psychiatry* 1985;**38**:737–46.

5908. Welander L. Myopathia distalis tarda heredetaria. *Acta Med Scand* 1951;**14 S265**:1–124.

5909. Welch JP, Alterman K. The syndrome of caudal dysplasia: a review. *Pediatr Pathol* 1984;**2**:313.

5910. Weleber RG, Beals RK. Hajdu-Cheney syndrome—report of two cases and review of the literature. *J Pediatr* 1976;**88**:243–9.

5911. Weleber RG, Tongue AC, Kennaway NG, et al. Ophthalmic manifestations of infantile phytanic acid storage disease. *Arch Ophthalmol* 1984;**102**:1317–21.

5912. Wellner VP, et al. Glutathione synthetase deficiency; an inborn error of metabolism. *Proc Natl Acad Sci USA* 1974;**71**:2505.

5913. Wells CR, Jankovic J. Familial spastic paraparesis and deafness: a new X-linked neurodegenerative disorder. *Arch Neurol* 1986;**43**:943–6.

5914. Wells GAH, Scott AC, Johnson CT, et al. A novel progressive spongiform encephalopathy in cattle. *Vet Rec* 1987;**121**:134–40.

5915. Wendel U, Rudiger HW, Pryzrembel H, et al. Alpha-ketoadipic aciduria: degradation studies with fibroblasts. *Clin Chem Acta* 1975;**58**:271.

5916. Wennberg R. Electroclinical analysis of postictal noserubbing. *Can J Neurol Sci* 2000;**27**:131–6.

5917. Wenning G, Ben-Schlomo Y, Hughes A, et al. What clinical features are most useful to distinguish definite multiple system atrophy from Parkinson's disease? *J Neurol Neurosurg Psychiatry* 2000;**68**:434–40.

5918. Werdnig G. Zwei fruhinfantile hereditare Falle von progressiver Muskelatrophie unter dem Bilde der Dystrophie, aber auf neurotischer Grundlage. *Arch Psychiatr (Berlin)* 1891;**22**:437–80.

5919. Werhahn KJ, Brown P, Thompson PD, et al. The clinical features and prognosis of chronic posthypoxic myoclonus. *Mov Disord* 1997;**12**:216–20.

5920. Wermer P. Genetic aspects of adenomatosis of endocrine glands. *Am J Med* 1954;**16**:363–71.

5921. Werner C-O. Lateral elbow pain and posterior interosseous nerve entrapment. *Acta Orthop Scand* 1979;**Suppl. 174:**1.

5922. Werner CWO. Ueber Katarackt in Verbindung mit Sclerodermie. *Diss Kiel* 1904.

5923. Wernicke K. Der aphasische Symptomenkomplex. Eine psychologische Studie auf anatomischer Basis. Breslau: M. Cohn, 1874.

5924. Wernicke K. Die acute Hamorrhagische der Polioencephalitis superior. In *Lehrbuch der Gehirnkrankheiten.* Kassel: Fischer, 1881.

5925. Wernicke K. Ueber hemiopische Pupillenreaction. *Fortschr Med* 1883;**1:**49–53.

5926. Wernicke K. A note on cramp-neurosis [in German]. *Berl Klin Wochenschr* 1904;**43:**1121–4.

5927. Wertham FL. A new sign of cerebellar diseases. *J Nerv Ment Dis* 1929;**69:**4986–93.

5928. Wertsch JJ, Sanger JR, Matloub HS. Pseudo anterior interosseous nerve syndrome. *Muscle Nerve* 1985;**8:**68–70.

5929. West WJ. On a peculiar form of infantile convulsions. *Lancet* 1840;**1:**724–5.

5930. Wester K, Hugdahl K. Arachnoid cysts of the left temporal fossa; impaired preoperative cognition and postoperative improvement. *J Neurol Neurosurg Psychiatry* 1995;**59:**293–8.

5931. Westheimer G, Blair SM. The ocular tilt reaction—a brainstem oculomotor routine. *Invest Ophthalmol* 1975;**14:**833–9.

5932. Westphal A. Ueber ein bischer nicht beschriebene Pupillenphanomen. *Neurol Centralbl* 1899;**18:**161–4.

5933. Westphal KFO. Die Agoraphobie, eine neuropathische Erscheinung. *Arch Psychiatr Nervenkr* 1871;**3:**138–61.

5934. Westphal KFO. Ueber eine dem Bilde der cerebrospinalen grauen Degeneration ahnliche Erkrankung des centralen Nervensystems ohne anatomischen Befund, nebst einigen Bemerkungen uber paradoxe Contraction. *Arch Psychiatr Nervenkr* 1883;**14:**87–134.

5935. Wexler N. Huntington's disease. *Curr Opin Neurol Neurosurg* 1988;**1:**319–23.

5936. Whipple AO. Criteria for diagnosis of islet cell adenoma. Surgery of the pancreas. *N Engl J Med* 1942;**226:**513–26.

5937. Whisnant JP, Cartlidge NEF, Elvebach LR. Carotid and vertebral-basilar transient ischemic attacks: effects of anticoagulants, hypertension, and cardiac disorders on survival and stroke occurrence—a population study. *Ann Neurol* 1978;**3:**107–15.

5938. White AA, McBride ME, Wiltse LL, et al. The management of patients with back pain and idiopathic vertebral sclerosis. *Spine* 1986;**11:**607–16.

5939. White BD, Firth JL. Anterior spinal hernia: an increasingly recognised cause of thoracic cord dysfunction. *J Neurol Neurosurg Psychiatry* 1994;**57:**1433–5.

5940. White BV. *Stanley Cobb: A Builder of the Modern Neurosciences.* Charlottesville, VA: University Press of Virginia, 1984.

5941. White HH, Rowland LP, Araki S, et al. Homocystinuria. *Arch Neurol* 1965;**13:**455–70.

5942. White JC. A case of keratosis (ichthyoses) follicularis. *J Cutan Dis* 1889;**7:**201–9.

5943. White JC, Langston JW, Pedley TA. Benign epileptiform transients of sleep. *Neurology* 1977;**27:**1061–8.

5944. White JC, Sweet WH. *Pain and the Neurosurgeon.* Springfield, IL: C.C. Thomas, 1989.

5945. Whitehouse PJ. The concept of subcortical dementia: another look. *Ann Neurol* 1986;**19:**1–6.

5946. Whiteley AM, Hauw J-J, Escourolle R. A pathological survey of 41 cases of acute intrinsic spinal cord disease. *J Neurol Sci* 1979;**42:** 229–42.

5947. Whiteley AM, Swash M, Urich H. Progressive encephalomyelitis with rigidity: its relation to "subacute myoclonic spinal neuronitis" and to the "stiff man syndrome". *Brain* 1976;**99:**27–42.

5948. Whiteside TCD, Graybiel A, Niven JI. Visual illusions of movement. *Brain* 1965;**88:**193–210.

5949. Whitley CB, et al. Warburg syndrome: lethal neurodysplasia with autosomal recessive inheritance. *J Pediatr* 1983;**102:**547–51.

5950. Whitley RJ, Nahmias AJ, Visintine AM, et al. The natural history of herpes simplex virus infection of mother and newborn. *Pediatrics* 1980;**66:**489–94.

5951. Whitman BW, Packer RJ. The photic sneeze reflex. *Neurology* 1993;**43:**868–71.

5952. Whitty CWM. On the so-called "laryngeal epilepsy". *Brain* 1943; **66:**43–54.

5953. WHO Study Group. Assessment of fracture risk and its application to screening for post-menopausal osteoporosis. *WHO Tech Rep Ser* 1994;**843:**1–129.

5954. Whyte KF, Alan MB, Jeffery AA, et al. Clinical features of the sleep apnoea, hypopnoea syndrome. *Q J Med* 1989;**72:**659–66.

5955. Whytt R. *An Essay on the Vital and Other Involuntary Motions of Animals.* Edinburgh: Hamilton, Balfour, and Neill, 1751.

5956. Whytt R. *Observations on the Dropsy in the Brain.* Edinburgh: J. Balfour, 1768.

5957. Wichman A, Frankl M, Kelly TE. Autosomal recessive congenital cerebellar hypoplasia. *Clin Genet* 1985;**27:**373–82.

5958. Wick B, Bedell HE. Magnitude and velocity of proximal vergence. *Invest Ophthamol Vis Sci* 1989;**30:**755–60.

5959. Wieacker P, Wolff G, et al. A new X-linked syndrome with muscle atrophy, congenital contractures and oculomotor apraxia. *Am J Med Genet* 1985;**20:**597–606.

5960. Wiebers DO, Swanson JW, Cascino TL, et al. Bilateral loss of vision in bright light. *Stroke* 1989;**20:**554–8.

5961. Wiese JA, Gentry LR, Menezes AH. Bobble head doll syndrome: review of the pathology and CSF dynamics. *Pediatr Neurol* 1985;**1:**361.

5962. Wigboldus JM, Bruyn GW. Hallervorden-Spatz disease. In Vinken PJ, Bruyn GW, eds. *System Disorders and Atrophies, Part I. Handbook of Clinical Neurology, Vol. 21,* pp 604–31. Oxford: North Holland Publishing Co., 1975.

5963. Wik B, Hillestad L. Deglutition syncope. *BMJ* 1975;**2:**747.

5964. Wilbourn AJ. Thoracic outlet syndrome is overdiagnosed. *Muscle Nerve* 1999;**22:**130–6.

5965. Wilbourn AJ, Aminoff MJ. The electrodiagnostic examination in patients with radiculopathies. *Muscle Nerve* 1998;**21:**1612–31.

5966. Wilbourn AJ, Furlan AJ, Hulley W, et al. Ischemic monomelic neuropathy. *Neurology* 1983;**33:**447–51.

5967. Wilbourn AJ, Sweeney PJ. Dissociated wasting of medial and lateral hand muscles with motor neurone disease. *Can J Neurol Sci* 1994;**21:**S9.

5968. Wilcox LM Jr, Bercovith K, Howard RO. Ophthalmic features of chromosome deletion 4p- (Wolf-Hirschorn syndrome). *Am J Ophthalmol* 1978;**86:**834.

5969. Wildervanck LS. Een cervico-oculo-acusticus syndroom. *Ned Tschr Geneesk* 1960;**104:**2600–5.

5970. Wiles CM, Karni Y. The measurement of strength in patients with peripheral neuromuscular disorders. *J Neurol Neurosurg Psychiatry* 1983;**46:**1006–13.

5971. Wilhelmsen KC, Weeks DE, Nygaard TG, et al. Genetic mapping of "Lubag" (X-linked dystonia-parkinsonism) in a Filipino kindred to the pericentromeric region of the X chromosome. *Ann Neurol* 1991;**29:**124–31.

5972. Wilkins DE, Hallett M, Erba G. Primary generalised epileptic myoclonus: a frequent manifestation of minipolymyoclonus of central origin. *J Neurol Neurosurg Psychiatry* 1985;**48:**506–16.

5973. Wilkinson IMS, Anderson JR, Holmes AE. Oligodendroglioma: an analysis of 42 cases. *J Neurol Neurosurg Psychiatry* 1987;**50:**304–12.

5974. Wilks S. Drunkard's or alcoholic paraplegia. *Med Times Gaz* 1868;**2:**470.

5975. Wilks S. On cerebritis, hysteria, and bulbar paralysis, as illustrative of arrest of function of the cerebro-spinal centres. *Guys Hosp Rep* 1877;**22:**7–55.

5976. Will AD, Sale EJ, Price S, et al. Quantitative measurement of the "milkmaid" sign in Huntington's disease. *Ann Neurol* 1991;**30:**320.

5977. Will RG. The spongiform encephalopathies. *J Neurol Neurosurg Psychiatry* 1991;**54:**761–3.

5978. Will RG. Prion-related disorders. *J R Coll Physicians* 1999;**33:** 311–5.

5979. Willemse J. Benign idiopathic dystonia with onset in the first year of life. *Dev Med Child Neurol* 1986;**28:**355–60.

5980. Williams AO, Osuntokun BO. Peripheral neuropathy in tropical (nutritional) ataxia in Nigeria. *Arch Neurol* 1969;**21:**475–92.

5981. Williams J, Barrett-Boyes B, Lowe J, et al. Supravalvular aortic stenosis. *Circulation* 1961;**24**:1311–8.

5982. Williams JC, et al. Progressive neurologic deterioration and renal failure due to storage of glutamyl ribose-5–phosphate. *N Engl J Med* 1984;**311**:152.

5983. Williams ME, Hadler NM, Earp JA. Manual ability as a marker of dependency in geriatric women. *J Chron Dis* 1982;**35**:115–22.

5984. Williams RDB. Brushfield spots and Wolfflin nodules in the iris: an appraisal in handicapped children. *Dev Med Child Neurol* 1981;**23**:646–50.

5985. Williamson PD, Boon PA, Thadani VM, et al. Parietal lobe epilepsy: diagnostic considerations and results of surgery. *Ann Neurol* 1992;**31**:193–201.

5986. Williamson PD, Spencer DD, Spencer SS, et al. Complex partial seizures of frontal lobe origin. *Ann Neurol* 1985;**18**:497–504.

5987. Willis T. *De anima brutorum.* London: R. Davis, 1672.

5988. Willis T. *The London Practice of Physick.* London: T. Basset, 1685.

5989. Willis T. *Willis' Oxford Lectures.* Oxford: Sandford Press, 1980.

5990. Willison HJ. Antiglycolipid antibodies in peripheral neuropathy: fact or fiction? *J Neurol Neurosurg Psychiatry* 1994;**57**:1303–6.

5991. Willoughby EW, Eason R. The crossed upgoing toe sign: a clinical study. *Ann Neurol* 1983;**14**:480–2.

5992. Willvonseder R, Goldstein NP, McCall JT, et al. A hereditary disorder with dementia, spastic dysarthria, vertical eye movement paresis, gait disturbance, splenomegaly and abnormal copper metabolism. *Neurology* 1973;**23**:1039–49.

5993. Wilson B, Cockburn J, Baddeley AD. *The Rivermead Behavioural Memory Test.* Reading, UK: Thames Valley Test Co., 1985.

5994. Wilson BA, Alderman N, Burgess P, et al. *Behavioural Assessment of the Dysexecutive Syndrome (BADS).* Bury St. Edmunds, UK: Thames Valley Test Co., 1996.

5995. Wilson BA, Cockburn J, Halligan P. *Behavioural Inattention Test.* Titchfield, Hants, UK: Thames Valley Test Company, 1987.

5996. Wilson MG, Towner JW, Forsman I, et al. Syndromes associated with deletion of the long arm of chromosome 18. *Am J Med Genet* 1979;**3**:155–74.

5997. Wilson MS, Wherrett BA, Mahdy MS. Powassan virus meningoencephalitis. *CMAJ* 1979;**121**:320–2.

5998. Wilson SAK. A contribution to the study of apraxia. *Brain* 1908;**31**:164.

5999. Wilson SAK. Progressive lenticular degeneration: a familial nervous disease associated with cirrhosis of the liver. *Brain* 1912;**34**:295–509.

6000. Wilson SAK. *Neurology.* London: Edward Arnold & Co., 1940.

6001. Wilson SAK, Walsh FMR. The phenomenon of tonic innervation and its relation to motor apraxia. *Brain* 1914;**37**:199–246.

6002. Winawer MR, Ottman R, Hauser WA, et al. Autosomal dominant partial epilepsy with auditory features: defiining the phenotype. *Neurology* 2000;**54**:2173–6.

6003. Winer JB. Bickerstaff's encephalitis and the Miller Fisher syndrome. *J Neurol Neurosurg Psychiatry* 2001;**71**:433–5.

6004. Wing JK, Cooper E, Sartorius N. *Measurements and Classification of Psychiatric Symptoms.* Cambridge, UK: Cambridge University Press, 1974.

6005. Winkelman NW. Progressive pallidal degeneration: a new clinicopathologic syndrome. *Arch Neurol Psychiatry* 1932;**27**:1–21.

6006. Winter HS. Case records of the Massachusetts General Hospital. *N Engl J Med* 1991;**325**:1865–73.

6007. Winter JH, Neville JB, Henderson AF, et al. Life-threatening respiratory failure due to a previously undescribed myopathy. *Q J Med* 1986;**61**:1171.

6008. Winterkorn JMS, Odel JG, Behrens MM. The sleep test for myasthenia gravis. *J Clin Neuroophthalmol* 1991;**11**:288–92.

6009. Wintzen AR, Plomb JJ, Molenaar PC, et al. Acquired slow-channel syndrome: a form of myasthenia gravis with prolonged open time of the acetylcholine receptor channel. *Ann Neurol* 1998;**44**:657–64.

6010. Wise BL, Smith M. Spinal arachnoiditis ossificans. *Arch Neurol* 1965;**13**:391–4.

6011. Wisniewski KE, French JH, Fernando S, et al. Fragile X syndrome: associated neurological abnormalities and developmental disabilities. *Ann Neurol* 1985;**18**:665–9.

6012. Wisniewski KE, Zhong N, Phillipart M. Pheno/genotypic correlations of neuronal ceroid lipofuscinosis. *Neurology* 2001;**57**:576–81.

6013. Wissel J, Kabus C, Klepsch S, et al. Botulinum toxin in writer's cramp: objective response evaluation in 31 patients. *J Neurol Neurosurg Psychiatry* 1996;**61**:172–5.

6014. Witt TN, Danek A, Hein MU, et al. McLeod syndrome: a distinct form of neuroacanthocytosis. *J Neurol* 1992;**239**:302–6.

6015. Wohlfart G. Zwei Falle von Dystrophia musculorum progressiva mit fibrillaren Zuckungen und atypischen Muskelbefund. *Dtsch Z Nervenklinik* 1942;**153**:189–204.

6016. Wohrle JC, Spengos K, Steinke W, et al. Alcohol-related acute axonal polyneuropathy: a differential diagnosis of Guillain-Barré syndrome. *Arch Neurol* 1998;**55**:1329–34.

6017. Wolf A, Morton BF. Ganglion cell tumours of the central nervous system. *NY Neurol Inst Bull* 1937;**6**:453–88.

6018. Wolf P. Juvenile absence epilepsy. In Roger J, Dravet C, Bureau M, et al., eds. *Epileptic Syndromes in Infancy, Childhood and Adolescence,* pp 242–6. London: John Libbey, 1985.

6019. Wolf P, Goosses R. Relation of photosensitivity to epileptic syndromes. *J Neurol Neurosurg Psychiatry* 1986;**49**:1386–91.

6020. Wolfe F, Smythe HA, Yunus MB, et al. The American College of Rheumatology 1990 Criteria for the Classification of Fibromyalgia. *Arthritis Rheum* 1990;**33**:160–72.

6021. Wolfe GI, Baker NS, Amato AA, et al. Chronic cryptogenic sensory polyneuropathy: clinical and laboratory characteristics. *Arch Neurol* 1999;**56**:540–7.

6022. Wolfe GI, Bank WJ. Pseudokyphosis in motor neuron disease corrected by the 'pocket sign'. *Muscle Nerve* 1994;**17**:1091.

6023. Wolff B, Grier RE, Lukvoy JRS, et al. Biotinidase deficiency; a novel vitamin recycling defect. *J Inherit Metab Dis* 1985;**8**(**Suppl 1**):53–8.

6024. Wolfram DJ. Diabetes mellitus and simple optic atrophy among siblings: report of four cases. *Proc Staff Meet Mayo Clin* 1938;**13**:715–8.

6025. Wolman M, et al. Primary familial xanthomatosis with involvement and calcification of the adrenals. *Pediatrics* 1961;**28**:742–57.

6026. Wolpe J. *Psychotherapy by Reciprocal Inhibition.* Stanford, CA: Stanford University Press, 1958.

6027. Wong KW, et al. Ocular involvement associated with chronic Epstein-Barr virus disease. *Arch Ophthalmol* 1987;**105**:788–92.

6028. Wong W, Tsuruda J, Kortman K, et al. *Practical MRI.* Rockville: Aspen Publishers, 1987.

6029. Wood DH. Cerebrovascular complications of sickle cell anemia. *Stroke* 1977;**9**:73–5.

6030. Wood M, Anderson M. *Neurological Infections.* London: W.B. Saunders, 1988.

6031. Wood N. Genes and parkinsonism. *J Neurol Neurosurg Psychiatry* 1997;**62**:305–9.

6032. Woodman R, Shin K, Pineo G. Primary non-Hodgkin's lymphoma of the brain: a review. *Medicine* 1985;**64**:425–30.

6033. Woods BT, Schaumberg HH. Nigro-spino-dentatal degeneration with nuclear ophthalmoplegia. *J Neurol Sci* 1972;**17**:149–66.

6034. Woody RC, et al. Ophthalmoplegic migraine in infancy. *Clin Pediatr* 1986;**25**:82–4.

6035. Woolf CM, Dolowitz DA, Aldous HE. Congenital deafness associated with piebaldness. *Arch Otolaryngol* 1965;**82**:244–50.

6036. Wooten GF, Lopes MBS, Harris WO, et al. Pallidoluysian atrophy. *Neurology* 1993;**43**:1764–8.

6037. World Federation of Neurology Ad Hoc Committee. Criteria for diagnosis of amyotrophic lateral sclerosis. *World Neurol* 1990;**5**:12.

6038. World Federation of Neurology Ad Hoc Committee. Classification of extrapyramidal disorders. *J Neurol Sci* 1981;**51**:311–27.

6039. World Federation of Neurology Classification Subcommittee. Classification of neuromuscular diseases. *J Neurol Sci* 1988;**86**:333–60.

6040. World Health Organization. *International Classification of Impairments, Disabilities and Handicaps.* Geneva: World Health Organization, 1980.

6041. World Health Organization. *The ICD-10 Classification of Mental and Behavioral Disorders.* Geneva: World Health Organization, 1992.

6042. Worster-Drought C, Allen IM. Congenital auditory imperception (congenital word deafness) and its relation to idioglossia and other speech defects. *J Neurol Psychopathol* 1930;**10**:193–235.

6043. Worster-Drought C, Greenfield JC, McMenemey WH. A form of familial presenile dementia with spastic paralysis. *Brain* 1940;**63**: 237–54.

6044. Worth HM, Wollin DG. Hyperostosis corticalis generalisata congenita. *J Can Assoc Radiol* 1966;**17**:67–74.

6045. Wray SH. Extracranial internal carotid disease. In Bernstein EF, ed. *Amaurosis Fugax*, New York: Springer-Verlag, 1987.

6046. Wray SH, Pavan-Langston D. A reevaluation of edrophomium chloride (Tensilon) tonography in the diagnosis of myasthenia gravis. *Neurology* 1971;**21**:586–93.

6047. Wright J, Morley DC. Encephalitis tremens. *Lancet* 1958;**1**: 871–3.

6048. Wright RA, Hermann RC, Parisi JE. Neurological manifestations of Erdheim-Chester disease. *J Neurol Neurosurg Psychiatry* 1999;**66**: 72–5.

6049. Wright WD. Characteristics of tritanopia. *J Optic Am* 1952; **42**:509.

6050. Wszolek ZK, Pfeiffer RF, Bhatt MH, et al. Rapidly progressive autosomal dominant parkinsonism and dementia with pallido-ponto-nigral degeneration. *Ann Neurol* 1992;**32**:312–20.

6051. Wulff EA, Simpson DM. Neuromuscular complications of the human immunodeficiency virus type 1 infection. *Semin Neurol* 1999;**19**:157–64.

6053. Wyatt HV. Injection paralysis. *Bull Hist Med* 1981;**55**:543–57.

6054. Wyburn-Mason R. Arterio-venous aneurysm of midbrain and retina, facial naevi and mental changes. *Brain* 1943;**66**:163–203.

6055. Wyllie E, Luders H, Morris HH, et al. The lateralizing significance of versive head and eye movements during epileptic seizures. *Neurology* 1986;**36**:606.

6056. Wynter E. Four cases of tubercular meningitis in which paracentesis of the theca vertebralis was performed for the relief of fluid pressure. *Lancet* 1:1891;981–2.

6057. Xiang F, Nicolao P, Chapon F, et al. A second locus for autosomal dominant myopathy with proximal muscle weakness and early respiratory muscle involvement: a likely chromosomal locus on 2q21. *Neuromusc Disord* 1999;**9**:308–12.

6058. Yaffe MG, Kaback M, Goldberg M, et al. An amyotrophic lateral sclerosis-like syndrome with hexosaminidase-A deficiency: a new type of GM2-gangliosidosis. *Neurology* 1979;**29**:611.

6059. Yagishita S, Itoh Y, Nakano T, et al. Pleomorphic intraneuronal polyglucosan bodies mainly restricted to the pallidum. *Acta Neuropathol* 1983;**62**:159–63.

6060. Yahr MD. A physician for all seasons. *Arch Neurol* 1978;**35**: 185–8.

6061. Yamada M, Ohno S, Okayasu I, et al. Chronic manganese poisoning. *Acta Neuropathol* 1986;**71**:273–8.

6062. Yamadori A, Mori E, Tabuchi M, et al. Hypergraphia: a right hemisphere syndrome. *J Neurol Neurosurg Psychiatry* 1986;**49**:1160–4.

6063. Yandell RW. Epidemic convulsions. *Brain* 1881;**4**:339–50.

6064. Yang DC. Neurologic status of newborn infants on first and third days of life. *Neurology* 1962;**12**:72–7.

6065. Yap CB, Mayo C, Barron K. "Ocular bobbing" in palatal myoclonus. *Arch Neurol* 1968;**18**:304–10.

6066. Yap PM. The latah reaction. Its pathodynamics and nosological position. *J Ment Sci* 1952;**98**:515–64.

6067. Yaqub BA, Al-Deeb SM, Daif AK, et al. Bickerstaff brainstem encephalitis. A grave non-demyelinating disease with benign prognosis. *J Neurol Sci* 1990;**96**:29–40.

6068. Yarnell PR, Lynch S. The 'ding': amnestic states in football trauma. *Neurology* 1973;**23**:196–7.

6069. Yasargil GM, Von Ammon K, Von Diem Ling A, et al. Central neurocytoma: histopathological variants and therapeutic approaches. *J Neurosurg* 1992;**76**:32–7.

6070. Yashon D, Beatty RA. Tethering of the conus medullaris within the sacrum. *J Neurol Neurosurg Psychiatry* 1966;**29**:244–50.

6071. Yassa R. The Pisa syndrome; a report of two cases. *Br J Psychiatry* 1984;**146**:93–5.

6072. Yasuda M, Takamatsu J, D'Souza I, et al. A novel mutation at position +12 in the intron following exon 10 of the *tau* gene in familial frontotemporal dementia (FTD-Kumamoto). *Ann Neurol* 2000;**47**: 422–9.

6073. Yates DW. Scoring systems for trauma. *BMJ* 1990;**301**:1090–4.

6074. Yatsu FM, Fields WS. Asymptomatic carotid bruits: stenosis or ulceration, a conservative approach. *Arch Neurol* 1985;**42**:383–5.

6075. Yee RD, Wong EK, Baloh RW, et al. A study of congenital nystagmus: waveforms. *Neurology* 1976;**26**:326–33.

6076. Yee WC, Hahn AF, Gilbert JJ. Adult onset scapuloperoneal myopathy: diagnostic value of nerve morphometry and multiple muscle biopsies. *J Neurol Neurosurg Psychiatry* 1988;**51**:808–13.

6077. Yeoman W. The relation of arthritis of the sacro-iliac joint to sciatica. *Lancet* 1928;**2**:1119–22.

6078. Yesavage JA, Brink TL. Development and validation of a geriatric depression screening scale: a preliminary report. *J Psychiatr Res* 1983;**17**:41.

6079. Yiannikas C, McLeod JG, Pollard JD, et al. Peripheral neuropathy associated with mitochondrial myopathies. *Ann Neurol* 1986;**20**: 249–57.

6080. Yip P-K. Bilateral ptosis, ataxia and areflexia—a variant of Fisher's syndrome. *J Neurol Neurosurg Psychiatry* 1991;**54**:1121.

6081. Yokochi M, et al. Juvenile parkinsonism—some clinical, pharmacological and neuropathological aspects. *Adv Neurol* 1984;**40**: 407–13.

6082. Yoshida J, Wakabayashi T, Okamoto S, et al. Tenascin in cerebrospinal fluid is a useful biomarker for the diagnosis of brain tumour. *J Neurol Neurosurg Psychiatry* 1994;**57**:1212–5.

6083. Yoshiyama A, Tokuymaru Y, Hattori T, et al. The pseudo-polyneuropathy type sensory disturbances in cervical spondylotic myelopathy. *Rinsho Shinkeigaku* 1995;**35**:141–6.

6084. Yoss RE, Corbin KB, MacCarty CS, et al. Significance of symptoms and signs in localization of involved roots in cervical disk protrusion. *Neurology* 1957;**7**:673–83.

6085. Yoss RE, Daly DD. Criteria for the diagnosis of the narcoleptic syndrome. *Mayo Clin Proc* 1957;**33**:320–8.

6086. Young AW, Robertson IH, Hellawell DJ, et al. Cotard delusion after brain injury. *Psychol Med* 1992; **22**:799–804.

6087. Young GB, Barr HWK, Blume WT. Painful Epileptic Seizures Involving the Second Sensory Area. *Ann Neurol* 1986;**19**:412.

6088. Young GB, Kark RM. Richard Bright, pioneer epileptologist. *Neurology* 1988;**38**:661–2.

6090. Young GB, McLachan RS, Kreeft JH, et al. An electroencephalographic classification for coma. *Can J Neurol Sci* 1997;**24**:320–5.

6091. Young GF, Leon-Barth CA, Green J. Familial hemiplegic migraine, retinal degeneration, deafness and nystagmus. *Arch Neurol* 1970;**23**:201–9.

6092. Young ID, Harper PS. Hereditary distal spinal muscular atrophy with vocal cord paralysis. *J Neurol Neurosurg Psychiatry* 1980;**43**:413–8.

6093. Young RR. Asterixis; one type of negative myoclonus. In Fahn S, ed. *Advances in Neurology: Myoclonus*, pp 123–53. New York: Raven Press, 1985.

6094. Young RR, Asbury AK, Corbett JL, et al. Pure pan-dysautonomia with recovery: description and discussion of diagnostic criteria. *Brain* 1975;**98**:613–36.

6095. Young SE, et al. The tilted disk syndrome. *Am J Ophthalmol* 1976;**82**:16–23.

6096. Yuen EC, Olney RK, So YT. Sciatic neuropathy. *Neurology* 1994; **44**:1669–74.

6097. Yuill GM, Lynch PG. Congenital non-progressive peripheral neuropathy with arthrogryposis multiplex. *J Neurol Neurosurg Psychiatry* 1974;**37**:316–23.

6098. Yukawa Y, Kate F. Isolated spinal cord sarcoidosis mimicking an intramedullary tumor. *Spinal Disord* 1999;**12**:530–3.

6099. Yung WA, Horten BC, Shapiro WR. Meningeal gliomatosis: a review of 12 cases. *Ann Neurol* 1980;**8**:605–8.

6100. Yunis E, Varon H. A new genetic syndrome. *Am J Dis Child* 1980;**134**:649–53.

6101. Yunus MB. Diagnosis, etiology and management of fibromyalgia syndrome: an update. *Compr Ther* 1988;**14**:8–20.

6102. Zaleski W, Hill A. Tyrosinosis: a new variant. *CMAJ* 1973;**108**: 477–84.

6103. Zalin A, Darby V, Vaughan S, et al. Primary neuropathic amyloidosis in three brothers. *BMJ* 1974;**1**:65–6.

6104. Zange J. On subarachnoid blockage in the region of the cerebromedullary cistern (cistern block) [in German]. *Munch Med Wochenschr* 1926;**173**:1150–2.

6105. Zappert J. Dementia infantilis (Heller). *Monatschr Kinderheilkd* 1921;**22**:389–97.

6106. Zaslavskii ES. [Scapulo-costal syndrome]. *Ortop Travmatol Protez* 1972;**33**:78–80.

6107. Zatz M, Vainzof M, Passos-Bueno MR. Limb-girdle muscular dystrophy: one gene with different phenotypes, one phenotype with different genes. *Curr Opin Neurol* 2000;**13**:511–7.

6108. Zazzo R. *Manuel pour l'examen Psychologique de l'enfant.* Neuchatel: Delachaux, Niestle, 1969.

6109. Zee DS. Adaptive control of eye movements: clinical implications. *Can J Neurol Sci* 1994;**21**:177–84.

6110. Zee DS, Chu FC, Leigh RJ, et al. Blink-saccade synkinesis. *Neurology* 1983;**33**:1233–6.

6111. Zee DS, Robinson DA. A hypothetical explanation of saccadic oscillations. *Ann Neurol* 1979;**5**:405.

6112. Zee DS, Yee RD, Cogan DG. Ocular motor abnormalities in hereditary cerebellar ataxia. *Brain* 1976;**99**:207–34.

6113. Zee DS, Yee RD, Singer HS. Congenital ocular motor apraxia. *Brain* 1977;**100**:581–99.

6114. Zeh W. Storung des ausdrucksenkennens beim Gerstmannschen Syndrom. *Arch Psychiatr Nervenkr* 1950;**185**:193–210.

6115. Zehender W, Ackermann E, Manz K. Eine Missbildung mit hautuberzogenen Augen oder Kryptophthalmus. *Klin Monatsbl Augenheilkd* 1872;**10**:225–34.

6116. Zeki S. Cerebral akinetopsia. *Brain* 1991;**114**:811–24.

6117. Zellweger H. Narcolepsy and epilepsy: case of narcolepsy with spike and waves in the EEG. *Helv Pediatr Acta* 1956;**11**:269–74.

6118. Zellweger H, Bell WE. Congenital muscular hypertrophy. *Neurology* 1959;**9**:160–6.

6119. Zellweger H, Simpson J, McCormick WF, et al. Spinal muscular atrophy with autosomal dominant inheritance. *Neurology* 1972;**22**:957–63.

6120. Zeman A, McLean B, Keir G, et al. The significance of serum oligoclonal bands in neurological diseases. *J Neurol Neurosurg Psychiatry* 1993;**56**:32–5.

6121. Zeman W. Historical development of the nosological concept of amaurotic familial idiocy. In Vincken PJ, Bruyn GW, eds. *Handbook of Clinical Neurology,* Vol. 10, pp. 212–32. Amsterdam: North Holland Publishing, 1970.

6122. Zeman W, King FA. Tumours of the septum pellucidum and adjacent structures with abnormal affective behavior: an anterior midline structure syndrome. *J Nerv Ment Dis* 1958;**127**:490–502.

6123. Zentner J, Wolf HK, Ostertun B, et al. Gangliogliomas: clinical, radiological and histopathological findings in 51 patients. *J Neurol Neurosurg Psychiatry* 1994;**57**:1497–1502.

6124. Zeviani M, Servidei S, Gellera C, et al. An autosomal dominant disorder with multiple deletions of mitochondrial DNA starting at the D-loop region. *Nature* 1989;**339**:309–11.

6125. Ziegler DK. Familial acephalgic migraine. *Neurology* 1995;**45**:2293–4.

6126. Ziegler DW, Schimke RN, Kepes JJ, et al. Late onset ataxia, rigidity and neuropathy. *Arch Neurol* 1972;**27**:52–66.

6127. Zifkin B, Andermann E, Andermann F, et al. An autosomal dominant syndrome of hemiplegic migraine, nystagmus, and tremor. *Ann Neurol* 1980;**8**:329–32.

6128. Zihl J, Von Cramon D. The contribution of the 'second visual system' to directed visual attention in man. *Brain* 1979;**102**:835–56.

6129. Zimmerlin F. On hereditary progressive muscular atrophy [in German]. *Z Klin Med* 1884;**7**:15–35.

6130. Zimprich F, Djamshidian A, Hainfellner J, et al. An autosomal dominant early adult onset distal muscular dystrophy. *Muscle Nerve* 2000;**23**:1876–9.

6131. Zinn AB, Kerr DS, Hoppel CL. Fumarase deficiency; a new cause of mitochondrial encephalopathy. *N Engl J Med* 1986;**315**:469–75.

6132. Zivin JA. Lateral cervical puncture: an alternative to lumbar puncture. *Neurology* 1978;**28**:616–8.

6133. Zochodne DW, Bolton CF, Wells GA, et al. Critical illness polyneuropathy. *Brain* 1987;**110**:819–42.

6134. Zochodne DW, Ramsay DA, Saly V, et al. Acute necrotizing myopathy of intensive care: electrophysiological features. *Muscle Nerve* 1994;**17**:285–92.

6135. Zorly T. Kofferath's syndrome. *Forum Med* (*Istanbul*) 1955;**1**:255–7.

6136. Zuckerman E, Peres MF, Kaup AO, et al. Chronic paroxysmal hemicrania-tic syndrome. *Neurology* 2000;**54**:1524–6.

6137. Zuckerman M, Lubin B. *Multiple Affect Adjective Checklist* (*Manual*). San Diego: Educational and Industrial Testing Service, 1965.

6138. Zung WAK. A self-rating depression scale. *Arch Gen Psychiatry* 1965;**12**:63–70.

6139. Zuniga G, Ropper AH, Frank J. Sarcoid peripheral neuropathy. *Neurology* 1991;**41**:1558–61.